7/2001

EDITED BY

ROBERT W. KIRK, D.V.M.

Professor of Medicine
Director, Veterinary Teaching Hospital
New York State College of Veterinary Medicine
Cornell University
Ithaca, New York

Special Therapy
Dermatologic Diseases

Consulting Editors

FREDERICK W. OEHME
Chemical and Physical Disorders

BRENDAN C. McKIERNAN
Respiratory Diseases

JOHN D. BONAGURA
Cardiovascular Diseases

ARTHUR I. HURVITZ
Hematology—Oncology—Immunology

CHARLES L. MARTIN
Ophthalmologic Diseases

MURRAY E. FOWLER
Diseases of Caged Birds and Exotic Pets

ALEXANDER DE LAHUNTA
Neurologic and Musculoskeletal Disorders

DONALD R. STROMBECK
Gastrointestinal Disorders

JOHN A. MULNIX
Endrocrine and Metabolic Disorders

CARL A. OSBORNE
Urinary Disorders

FREDRIC W. SCOTT
Infectious Diseases

DONALD H. LEIN
Reproductive Disorders

CURRENT VETERINARY THERAPY VIII

SMALL ANIMAL PRACTICE

1983

W. B. SAUNDERS COMPANY

PHILADELPHIA   LONDON   TORONTO   MEXICO CITY   RIO DE JANEIRO   SYDNEY   TOKYO

W. B. Saunders Company: West Washington Square
Philadelphia, PA   19105

1 St. Anne's Road
Eastbourne, East Sussex BN21 3UN, England

1 Goldthorne Avenue
Toronto, Ontario M8Z 5T9, Canada

Apartado 26370—Cedro 512
Mexico 4, D.F., Mexico

Rua Coronel Cabrita, 8
Sao Cristovao Caixa Postal 21176
Rio de Janeiro, Brazil

9 Waltham Street
Artarmon, N.S.W. 2064, Australia

Ichibancho, Central Bldg., 22-1 Ichibancho
Chiyoda-Ku, Tokyo 102, Japan

Listed here is the latest translated edition of this book together
with the language of the translation and the publisher.

Spanish (*3rd edition*)—Editorial Continental, Mexico

Japanese (*6th edition*)—Ishiyaku Publishers, Inc., Tokyo, Japan

Current Veterinary Therapy VIII   ISBN   0-7216-5465-7

Last digit is the print number: 9   8   7   6   5   4   3   2   1

CONTRIBUTORS

SHEHU U. ABDULLAHI, D.V.M., Ph.D.; Lecturer, Department of Veterinary Surgery and Medicine, Faculty of Veterinary Medicine, Ahmadu Bello University, Zaria, Nigeria; Director, Small Animal Medicine Section, Veterinary Teaching Hospital, Ahmadu Bello University, Zaria, Nigeria

GREGORY M. ACLAND, B.V.Sc.; Diplomate, American College of Veterinary Ophthalmologists; Assistant Research Professor, Scheie Eye Institute, Philadelphia, Pennsylvania; Assistant Research Professor, Department of Ophthalmology, School of Medicine, University of Pennsylvania, Philadelphia, Pennsylvania

W. M. ADAMS, D.V.M.; Diplomate, American College of Veterinary Radiology; Assistant Professor of Radiology, School of Veterinary Medicine, University of Wisconsin, Madison, Wisconsin

TIMOTHY A. ALLEN, D.V.M.; Diplomate, American College of Veterinary Internal Medicine; Assistant Professor, Department of Clinical Sciences, College of Veterinary Medicine and Biomedical Sciences, Colorado State University, Fort Collins, Colorado; Staff Member, Veterinary Teaching Hospital, Colorado State University, Fort Collins, Colorado

TERENCE C. AMIS, B.V.Sc., M.R.C.V.S., Ph.D.; Assistant Professor, Department of Medicine, School of Veterinary Medicine, University of California, Davis, California; Small Animal Internal Medicine Service, Veterinary Medical Teaching Hospital, School of Veterinary Medicine, University of California, Davis, California

ARTHUR L. ARONSON, D.V.M., Ph.D.; Professor and Head, Department of Anatomy, Physiological Sciences and Radiology, School of Veterinary Medicine, North Carolina State University, Raleigh, North Carolina

MARIE H. ATTLEBERGER, D.V.M., Ph.D.; Professor of Microbiology, School of Veterinary Medicine, Auburn University, Auburn, Alabama

E. MURL BAILEY, Jr., D.V.M., Ph.D.; Diplomate, American Board of Veterinary Toxicology; Professor of Veterinary Toxicology, Department of Veterinary Physiology and Pharmacology, College of Veterinary Medicine, Texas A&M University, College Station, Texas

THEODORE L. BAKER, Ph.D.; Director, Canine Narcolepsy Research Program, Department of Psychiatry and Behavioral Science, Stanford University School of Medicine, Stanford, California; Clinical Life Science Research Associate, Stanford University School of Medicine, Stanford, California

SANDY BALDWIN, D.V.M., M.S.; Graduate Research Assistant, New York State College of Veterinary Medicine, Cornell University, Ithaca, New York; Staff Member, Cornell Feline Health Center, Cornell University, Ithaca, New York

JEFFREY E. BARLOUGH, D.V.M.; Graduate Research Assistant, Department of Microbiology, New York State College of Veterinary Medicine, Cornell University, Ithaca, New York; Staff Member, Cornell Feline Health Center, Cornell University, Ithaca, New York

KATHLEEN P. BARRIE, D.V.M., M.S.; Diplomate, American College of Veterinary Ophthalmologists; Adjunct Assistant Professor, Department of Comparative Ophthalmology, College of Veterinary Medicine, University of Florida, Gainesville, Florida; Staff Ophthalmologist, Animal Eye Clinic, Sunshine Animal Hospital, Tampa, Florida

JEANNE A. BARSANTI, D.V.M., M.S.; Diplomate, American College of Veterinary Internal

Medicine; Associate Professor, Department of Small Animal Medicine, College of Veterinary Medicine, University of Georgia, Athens, Georgia; Internist, Small Animal Medicine, Veterinary Medical Teaching Hospital, College of Veterinary Medicine, University of Georgia, Athens, Georgia

CLAUDIA L. BARTON, D.V.M.; Diplomate, American College of Veterinary Internal Medicine; Associate Professor, Department of Small Animal Medicine and Surgery, College of Veterinary Medicine, Texas A&M University, College Station, Texas

TIMOTHY G. BAUER, D.V.M.; Lecturer, Department of Medicine, School of Veterinary Medicine, University of California, Davis, California; Private Practitioner, Seattle, Washington

VAL RICHARD BEASLEY, D.V.M..: Research Associate, Department of Veterinary Biosciences, College of Veterinary Medicine, University of Illinois, Urbana, Illinois

BONNIE V. BEAVER, B.S., D.V.M., M.S.; Professor, Department of Veterinary Anatomy, Texas A&M University College of Veterinary Medicine, College Station, Texas; Animal Behavior Specialist, Small Animal Clinic, Texas A&M University College of Veterinary Medicine, College Station, Texas

JOHN BENTINCK-SMITH, D.V.M.; Diplomate, American College of Veterinary Pathologists; Visiting Professor, Mississippi State University, Mississippi State, Mississippi

DANIEL M. BETTS, D.V.M., M.S.; Diplomate, American College of Veterinary Ophthalmologists; Associate Professor, Department of Veterinary Clinical Sciences, College of Veterinary Medicine, Iowa State University, Ames, Iowa; Associate Director, Veterinary Teaching Hospital, College of Veterinary Medicine, Iowa State University, Ames, Iowa

STEPHEN BISTNER, D.V.M.; Diplomate, American College of Veterinary Ophthalmologists; Associate Professor, Comparative Ophthalmology, School of Veterinary Medicine, University of Minnesota, St. Paul, Minnesota

JAMES L. BITTLE, D.V.M.; Professor, Department of Molecular Biology, Research Institute of Scripps Clinic, La Jolla, California

PAULE BLOUIN, D.M.V., Ph.D.; Diplomate, American College of Veterinary Ophthalmolo-

gists; Assistant Professor, Faculté de Médecine Vétérinaire, Université de Montréal, St. Hyacinthe, Quebec, Canada

WILLIAM J. BOEVER, D.V.M.; Adjunct Assistant Professor, College of Veterinary Medicine, University of Missouri, Columbia, Missouri; Senior Staff Veterinarian, St. Louis Zoological Park, St. Louis, Missouri

JOHN D. BONAGURA, D.V.M., M.S.; Diplomate, American College of Veterinary Internal Medicine (Cardiology, Internal Medicine); Assistant Professor, Department of Veterinary Clinical Sciences, The Ohio State University College of Veterinary Medicine, Columbus, Ohio; Staff Cardiologist, The Ohio State University Veterinary Teaching Hospital, Columbus, Ohio

JAMES J. BRACE, D.V.M.; Diplomate, American College of Veterinary Internal Medicine; Associate Professor of Medicine, University of Tennessee, College of Veterinary Medicine, Knoxville, Tennessee

DALE L. BROOKS, D.V.M., Ph.D.; Diplomate, American College of Laboratory Animal Medicine; Lecturer, Department of Medicine, School of Veterinary Medicine, University of California, Davis, California; Director, Animal Resources Service, School of Veterinary Medicine, University of California, Davis, California

NANCY O. BROWN, V.M.D.; Diplomate, American College of Veterinary Surgeons; Consultant, The Animal Medical Center, New York, New York; Private Practitioner, Hickory Veterinary Hospital, Plymouth Meeting, Pennsylvania

WILLIAM B. BUCK, D.V.M.; Diplomate, American Board of Veterinary Toxicology; Professor of Toxicology, College of Veterinary Medicine, University of Illinois, Urbana, Illinois; Director, Animal Poison Control Center, College of Veterinary Medicine, University of Illinois, Urbana, Illinois

SUSAN E. BUNCH, D.V.M., Ph.D.; Diplomate, American College of Veterinary Internal Medicine, Specialty of Internal Medicine; Assistant Professor of Medicine, School of Veterinary Medicine, North Carolina State University, Raleigh, North Carolina

MARK G. BURNS, D.V.M; Diplomate, American College of Veterinary Internal Medicine; Director, Tribeca-Soho Animal Hospital, New York, New York

COLIN F. BURROWS, B.Vet.Med., Ph.D., M.R.C.V.S.; Diplomate, American College of Veterinary Internal Medicine; Associate Professor of Medicine, Department of Medical Sciences, University of Florida, College of Veterinary Medicine, Gainesville, Florida

GEORGE E. BURROWS, D.V.M., Ph.D.; Professor, Clinical Pharmacology and Toxicology, Department of Physiological Sciences, College of Veterinary Medicine, Oklahoma State University, Stillwater, Oklahoma

MITCHELL BUSH, D.V.M.; Chief Veterinarian, National Zoological Park, Rock Creek Park, Washington, D.C.

CLAY A. CALVERT, D.V.M.; Diplomate, American College of Veterinary Internal Medicine; Associate Professor of Internal Medicine, College of Veterinary Medicine, University of Georgia, Athens, Georgia; Staff Member, Small Animal Hospital, College of Veterinary Medicine, University of Georgia, Athens, Georgia

THOMAS L. CARSON, D.V.M., M.S., Ph.D.; Diplomate, American Board of Veterinary Toxicology; Professor of Veterinary Pathology, Veterinary Diagnostic Laboratory, College of Veterinary Medicine, Iowa State University, Ames, Iowa

ARTHUR A. CASE, D.V.M.; Professor Emeritus of Veterinary Medicine and Surgery, Department of Veterinary Medicine and Surgery, College of Veterinary Medicine, The University of Missouri, Columbia, Missouri

DENNIS J. CHEW, D.V.M.; Diplomate, American College of Veterinary Internal Medicine; Assistant Professor of Medicine, Department of Clinical Sciences, College of Veterinary Medicine, The Ohio State University, Columbus, Ohio; Internist, Veterinary Teaching Hospital, Columbus, Ohio

CHERYL L. CHRISMAN, D.V.M., M.S.; Diplomate, American College of Veterinary Internal Medicine (Neurology); Associate Professor, Assistant Dean for Instruction, College of Veterinary Medicine, University of Florida, Gainesville, Florida; Chief of Neurology Service, Veterinary Medicine Teaching Hospital, University of Florida, Gainesville, Florida

DAVID B. CHURCH, B.V.Sc.; Lecturer, Department of Veterinary Clinical studies, University of Sydney, N.S.W., Australia

J. DERRELL CLARK, D.V.M., M.S., B.Sc.; Diplomate, American College of Laboratory Animal Medicine; Director, Animal Resources, Associate Professor of Medical Microbiology, College of Veterinary Medicine, University of Georgia, Athens, Georgia

R. M. CLEMMONS, D.V.M., Ph.D.; Assistant Professor of Clinical Medicine, College of Veterinary Medicine, University of Florida, Gainesville, Florida

CHRIS W. CLINTON, M.T.; Supervisor, Urolithiasis Laboratory, Baylor College of Medicine, Houston, Texas

SUSAN L. CLUBB, D.V.M.; Pet Farm Inc., Miami, Florida

P. W. CONCANNON, Ph.D.; Senior Research Associate, Department of Physiology, New York State College of Veterinary Medicine, Cornell University, Ithaca, New York

ROBERT W. COPPOCK, B.S., D.V.M., M.S.; Diplomate, American Board of Veterinary Toxicology; Veterinary Toxicologist, College of Veterinary Medicine, University of Illinois, Urbana, Illinois; R. W. Coppock and Assoc., Toxicology Consultants, Urbana, Illinois

LARRY M. CORNELIUS, D.V.M., Ph.D.; Diplomate, American College of Veterinary Internal Medicine (Internal Medicine); Professor of Small Animal Medicine, University of Georgia College of Veterinary Medicine, Athens, Georgia; Small Animal Internist, University of Georgia Veterinary Teaching Hospital, Athens, Georgia

SUSAN M. COTTER, D.V.M.; Diplomate, American College of Veterinary Internal Medicine; Associate Professor of Medicine, Tufts University, School of Veterinary Medicine, Boston, Massachusetts; Lecturer in Cancer Biology, Harvard University, School of Public Health, Boston, Massachusetts; Staff Member, Angell Memorial Animal Hospital, Boston, Massachusetts

LARRY D. COWGILL, D.V.M., Ph.D.; Diplomate, American College of Veterinary Internal Medicine; Associate Professor, Department of Medicine, School of Veterinary Medicine, University of California, Davis, California; Acting Chief, Section of Small Animal Medicine, Veterinary Medical Teaching Hospital, University of California, Davis, California

STEVEN E. CROW, D.V.M.; Diplomate, American College of Veterinary Internal Medicine; Associate Professor, Department of Small Animal Clinical Sciences, College of Veterinary Medicine, Michigan State University, East Lansing, Michigan; Staff Clinical Oncologist, Veterinary Clinical Center, Michigan State University, East Lansing, Michigan

ALEXANDER DE LAHUNTA, D.V.M., Ph.D.; Diplomate, American College of Veterinary Internal Medicine (Neurology); Professor of Anatomy, Chairman, Department of Clinical Sciences, New York State College of Veterinary Medicine, Cornell University, Ithaca, New York

WILLIAM C. DEMENT, M.D., Ph.D.; Professor of Psychiatry, Stanford University School of Medicine, Stanford, California; Director, Sleep Disorders Center, Department of Psychiatry and Behavioral Science, Stanford University School of Medicine, Stanford, California

ROBERT C. DeNOVO, Jr., D.V.M., M.S.; Diplomate, American College of Veterinary Internal Medicine; Assistant Professor of Veterinary Internal Medicine, Department of Urban Practice, College of Veterinary Medicine, University of Tennessee, Knoxville, Tennessee

STEPHEN P. DiBARTOLA, D.V.M.; Diplomate, American College of Veterinary Internal Medicine; Assistant Professor of Medicine, Department of Clinical Sciences, College of Veterinary Medicine, The Ohio State University, Columbus, Ohio; Small Animal Internist, Veterinary Teaching Hospital, Columbus, Ohio

ROBERT A. DIETERICH, D.V.M.; Professor of Veterinary Science, Institute of Arctic Biology, University of Alaska, Fairbanks, Alaska

FREDERICK H. DRAZNER, D.V.M.; Diplomate, American College of Veterinary Internal Medicine; Director of Services, Animal Specialty Services of Cook County, Chicago, Illinois; Chief of Staff, Wright Animal Hospital, Des Plaines, Illinois; Consultant, Immunologic Diagnostic Service, Chicago, Illinois; Consultant, Toxicology, Rush Medical School, Presbyterian St. Luke's Hospital, Chicago, Illinois

I. D. DUNCAN, B.V.M.S., Ph.D., M.R.C.V.S.; Associate Professor, Department of Medical Sciences, School of Veterinary Medicine, University of Wisconsin, Madison, Wisconsin

SANDRA EMANUELSON, D.V.M.; Small Animal, Exotic, and Avian Clinician, Cottage Veterinary Hospital, Walnut Creek, California

L. REED ENOS, Pharm.D.; Lecturer, Department of Medicine, School of Veterinary Medicine, University of California, Davis, California; Chief Pharmacist, Veterinary Medical Teaching Hospital, University of California, Davis, California

PHILIP K. ENSLEY, D.V.M.; Associate Veterinarian, Jennings Center for Zoological Medicine, Zoological Society of San Diego, San Diego, California

VALERIE A. FADOK, D.V.M.; Diplomate, American College of Veterinary Dermatology; Assistant Professor, University of Tennessee, College of Veterinary Medicine, Knoxville, Tennessee; Clinical Dermatologist, Small and Large Animal Clinic, University of Tennessee, Knoxville, Tennessee

GEORGE C. FARNBACK, V.M.D., Ph.D.; Assistant Professor of Neurology, School of Veterinary Medicine, University of Pennsylvania, Philadelphia, Pennsylvania

BRIAN R. H. FARROW, B.V.Sc., Ph.D., F.A.C.V.Sc., M.R.C.V.S.; Associate Professor of Veterinary Medicine, Department of Veterinary Clinical Studies, University of Sydney, N.S.W., Australia

CHARLES S. FARROW, D.V.M.; Diplomate, American College of Veterinary Radiology; Associate Professor of Radiology, Department of Anesthesiology, Radiology, and Surgery, Western College of Veterinary Medicine, University of Saskatchewan, Saskatoon, Saskatchewan, Canada; Chief, Special Clinical Services, Veterinary Teaching Hospital, Western College of Veterinary Medicine, University of Saskatchewan, Saskatoon, Saskatchewan, Canada

ROY T. FAULKNER, D.V.M., M.S.; Staff Surgeon, Skyway Animal Hospital, St. Petersburg, Florida

DANIEL A. FEENEY, D.V.M., M.S.; Diplomate, American College of Veterinary Radiology; Associate Professor of Veterinary Radiology, University of Minnesota College of Veterinary Medicine, St. Paul, Minnesota; Radiologist, Lewis Hospital for Companion Animals/University of Minnesota Veterinary Teaching Hospital, St. Paul, Minnesota

BERNARD F. FELDMAN, D.V.M., Ph.D.; Associate Professor of Clinical Pathology, School of Veterinary Medicine, University of California, Davis, California

WILLIAM R. FENNER, D.V.M.; Diplomate, American College of Veterinary Internal Medicine (Neurology); Assistant Professor, Department of Veterinary Clinical Sciences, College of Veterinary Medicine, The Ohio State University, Columbus, Ohio; Attending Staff Neurologist, Veterinary Teaching Hospital, The Ohio State University, Columbus, Ohio

DELMAR R. FINCO, D.V.M., Ph.D.; Diplomate, American College of Veterinary Internal Medicine; Professor, Department of Physiology and Pharmacology, University of Georgia, Athens, Georgia; Staff Member, University of Georgia Veterinary Teaching Hospital, Athens, Georgia

JAMES A. FLANDERS, D.V.M.; Instructor in Small Animal Surgery, New York State College of Veterinary Medicine, Cornell University, Ithaca, New York

RICHARD B. FORD, D.V.M., M.S.; Diplomate, American College of Veterinary Internal Medicine; Associate Professor, Internal Medicine, North Carolina State University, Raleigh, North Carolina

ARTHUR S. FOUTZ, Ph.D.; Research Scientist, C.N.R.S., Gif sur Yvette, France

MURRAY E. FOWLER, D.V.M.; Diplomate, American College of Veterinary Internal Medicine, American Board of Veterinary Toxicology; Professor and Chairman, Department of Medicine, School of Veterinary Medicine, University of California, Davis, California; Chief, Zoological Medicine Service, Veterinary Medical Teaching Hospital, School of Veterinary Medicine, University of California, Davis, California

PHILIP R. FOX, D.V.M., M.S.; Diplomate, American College of Veterinary Internal Medicine (Cardiology); Associate Staff, Department of Medicine, The Animal Medical Center, New York, New York

FREDRIC L. FRYE, D.V.M., M.S.; Clinical Professor of Medicine, Department of Medicine, School of Veterinary Medicine, University of California, Davis, California; Consultant, Steinhart Aquarium, California Academy of Sciences, San Francisco, California

CHUCK GALVIN, D.V.M.; Owner and Director of The Veterinary Hospital of Ignacio, Novato, California

WILLIAM GRANT, D.V.M.; Private Practitioner, Garden Grove, California

CRAIG E. GREENE, D.V.M., M.S..: Diplomate, American College of Veterinary Medicine; Associate Professor, Department of Small Animal Medicine, College of Veterinary Medicine, University of Georgia, Athens, Georgia; Staff Member, Veterinary Teaching Hospital, University of Georgia, Athens, Georgia

C. E. GRIFFIN, D.V.M.; Diplomate, American College of Veterinary Dermatology; Staff Member, Animal Dermatology Clinic, Garden Grove, California; Staff Member, Animal Dermatology Clinic, San Diego, California

I. R. GRIFFITHS, B.V.M.S., Ph.D., F.R.C.V.S.; Reader, Department of Surgery, Glasgow University Veterinary School, Glasgow, Scotland

STEPHEN L. GROSS, V.M.D.; Diplomate, American College of Veterinary Ophthalmologists; Staff Ophthalmologist, The Animal Medical Center, New York, New York; Senior Research Associate, Cornell University Medical College, New York, New York

RICHARD E. W. HALLIWELL, Ph.D., Vet.M.B., M.R.C.V.S.; Diplomate, American College of Veterinary Dermatology; Professor and Chairman, Department of Medical Sciences, University of Florida College of Veterinary Medicine, Gainesville, Florida

ROBERT M. HARDY, D.V.M., M.S.; Diplomate, American College of Veterinary Internal Medicine; Associate Professor, Department of Small Animal Clinical Sciences, College of Veterinary Medicine, University of Minnesota, St. Paul, Minnesota

NEIL K. HARPSTER, V.M.D.; Director of Cardiology, Angell Memorial Animal Hospital, Boston, Massachusetts

COLIN E. HARVEY, M.R.C.V.S.; Professor of Surgery, School of Veterinary Medicine, University of Pennsylvania, Philadelphia, Pennsylvania

H. JAY HARVEY, D.V.M.; Diplomate, American College of Veterinary Surgery; Assistant Professor of Surgery, New York State College of Veterinary Medicine, Cornell University, Ithaca, New York; Staff Member, Small Animal Clinic, New York State College of Veterinary Medicine, Cornell University, Ithaca, New York

STEVEN C. HASKINS, D.V.M., M.S.; Diplomate, American College of Veterinary Anesthesiologists; Associate Professor, Department of Veterinary Surgery, School of Veterinary Medicine, University of California, Davis, California; Anesthesiology and Critical Patient Care, Veterinary Medicine Teaching Hospital, University of California, Davis, California

AUDREY A. HAYES, V.M.D.; Diplomate, American College of Veterinary Internal Medicine; Staff Oncologist, Donaldson-Atwood Cancer Clinic, The Animal Medical Center, New York, New York

MELVIN L. HELPHREY, D.V.M.; (Formerly) Assistant Professor, Veterinary Clinical Sciences, College of Veterinary Medicine, The Ohio State University, Columbus, Ohio; Private Practitioner, Gulf Coast Veterinary Surgical Referral Service, Seminole, Florida

DWIGHT C. HIRSH, D.V.M., Ph.D.; Associate Professor, Department of Veterinary Microbiology and Immunology, School of Veterinary Medicine, University of California, Davis, California; Chief, Microbiology Services, Veterinary Medical Teaching Hospital, University of California, Davis, California

ARTHUR I. HURVITZ, D.V.M., Ph.D.; Adjunct Assistant Professor, College of Physicians and Surgeons, Columbia University, New York, New York; Consulting Veterinary Pathologist, The Rockefeller University, New York, New York; Chairman, Department of Pathology, and Director of Research, The Animal Medical Center, New York, New York

PETER J. IHRKE, V.M.D.; Diplomate, American College of Veterinary Dermatology; Assistant Professor of Dermatology and Allergy, Department of Medicine, University of California, Davis, California; Staff Member, Veterinary Medical Teaching Hospital, Small and Large Animal Clinic, Davis, California

JAN E. ILKIW, B.V.Sc; Senior Lecturer, Department of Veterinary Clinical Studies, University of Sydney, N.S.W., Australia

NITA L. IRBY, D.V.M.; (Formerly) Intern, New York State College of Veterinary Medicine, Cornell University, Ithaca, New York; Resident in Ophthalmology, School of Veterinary Medicine, University of Pennsylvania, Philadelphia, Pennsylvania

ELLIOTT R. JACOBSON, D.V.M., Ph.D.; Assistant Professor, Department of Special Clinical Sciences, University of Florida, Gainesville, Florida; Laboratory Animal and Wildlife Medicine Clinician, Veterinary Medical Teaching Hospital, University of Florida, Gainesville, Florida

K. ANN JEGLUM, V.M.D.; Assistant in Medical Oncology, School of Veterinary Medicine, University of Pennsylvania, Philadelphia, Pennsylvania; Head, Clinical Oncology Service, School of Veterinary Medicine, University of Pennsylvania, Philadelphia, Pennsylvania

JUDITH S. JOHNESSEE, M.S., D.V.M.; Diplomate, American College of Veterinary Internal Medicine; Staff Member, Westchester Veterinary Emergency Hospital, White Plains, New York

GARY R. JOHNSTON, D.V.M., M.S.; Diplomate, American College of Veterinary Radiology; Assistant Professor, Department of Small Animal Clinical Sciences, University of Minnesota, College of Veterinary Medicine, St. Paul, Minnesota

SHIRLEY D. JOHNSTON, D.V.M., Ph.D.; Diplomate, American College of Theriogenologists; Assistant Professor, Department of Small Animal Clinical Sciences, College of Veterinary Medicine, University of Minnesota, St. Paul, Minnesota; Staff Member, Lewis Hospital for Companion Animals, St. Paul, Minnesota

KENNETH KAGAN, V.M.D.; Diplomate, American College of Veterinary Surgeons; Assistant Professor of Small Animal Surgery, College of Veterinary Medicine, University of Florida, Gainesville, Florida; Staff Surgeon, Veterinary Medical Teaching Hospital, University of Florida, Gainesville, Florida

ANDREW J. KALLET, D.V.M.; Medical Resident, University of California, Davis, California; Staff Internist, Madera Pet Hospital, Corte Madera, California

RENEE L. KASWAN, D.V.M.; Clinical Resident in Ophthalmology, University of Georgia, College of Veterinary Medicine, Athens, Georgia; Clinical Resident in Ophthalmology, Small Animal Hospital, College of Veterinary Medicine, University of Georgia, Athens, Georgia

BRUCE W. KEENE, D.V.M., M.Sc.; Clinical Instructor of Medicine, The Ohio State University College of Veterinary Medicine, Columbus, Ohio

SUZANNE KENNEDY-STOSKOPF, D.V.M.; Post-Doctoral Fellow, Johns Hopkins University School of Medicine, Department of Neurology, Baltimore, Maryland

THOMAS J. KERN, D.V.M.; Diplomate, American College of Veterinary Ophthalmologists; (Formerly) Assistant Professor, Department of Clinical Sciences, New York State College of

Veterinary Medicine, Cornell University, Ithaca, New York; Assistant Professor of Comparative Ophthalmology; Department of Comparative Ophthalmology, College of Veterinary Medicine, University of Florida, Gainesville, Florida

KERRY L. KETRING, D.V.M.; Diplomate, American College of Veterinary Ophthalmologists; Staff Member, All Animal Eye Clinic, Cincinnati, Ohio; Staff Member, Animal Emergency Center, Lexington and Louisville, Kentucky; Dayton, Ohio; Indianapolis, Indiana

ROBERT W. KIRK, D.V.M.; Diplomate, American College of Veterinary Internal Medicine; Diplomate, American College of Veterinary Dermatology; Professor of Medicine, Director, Veterinary Teaching Hospital, New York State College of Veterinary Medicine, Cornell University, Ithaca, New York

MARK KITTLESON, D.V.M., Ph.D.; Diplomate, American College of Veterinary Internal Medicine (Cardiology); Assistant Professor, Department of Small Animal Clinical Sciences, Michigan State University, College of Veterinary Medicine, East Lansing, Michigan; Staff Cardiologist, Veterinary Clinical Center, Michigan State University, East Lansing, Michigan

JEFFREY S. KLAUSNER, D.V.M., M.S.; Diplomate, American College of Veterinary Internal Medicine; Associate Professor of Veterinary Internal Medicine, College of Veterinary Medicine, University of Minnesota, St. Paul, Minnesota; Veterinary Internist, Veterinary Teaching Hospital, College of Veterinary Medicine, University of Minnesota, St. Paul, Minnesota

CHARLES D. KNECHT, B.S., V.M.D., M.S.; Diplomate, American College of Veterinary Internal Medicine (Neurology); Diplomate, American College of Veterinary Surgeons; Professor and Head, Department of Small Animal Surgery and Medicine, School of Veterinary Medicine, Auburn University, Auburn, Alabama

GEORGE V. KOLLIAS, Jr., D.V.M., Ph.D.; Assistant Professor, Department of Special Clinical Sciences, College of Veterinary Medicine, University of Florida, Gainesville, Florida; Chief, Laboratory Animal and Wildlife Medicine Service, Veterinary Medical Teaching Service, University of Florida, Gainesville, Florida

JOE N. KORNEGAY, D.V.M., M.S., Ph.D.; Diplomate, American College of Veterinary Internal Medicine (Neurology); Associate Professor, North Carolina State University School of Veterinary Medicine, Raleigh, North Carolina

DAVID F. KOWALCZYK, V.M.D., Ph.D.; Assistant Professor of Pharmacology and Toxicology, University of Pennsylvania School of Veterinary Medicine, Philadelphia, Pennsylvania

DONALD R. KRAWIEC, D.V.M., M.S., Ph.D.; Assistant Professor of Veterinary Internal Medicine, Department of Veterinary Clinical Medicine, College of Veterinary Medicine, University of Illinois, Urbana, Illinois

G. A. KUNKLE, D.V.M.; Diplomate, American College of Veterinary Dermatology; Assistant Professor, College of Veterinary Medicine, University of Florida, Gainesville, Florida; Chief of Dermatology Service, Veterinary Medical Teaching Hospital, University of Florida, Gainesville, Florida

ROLF E. LARSEN, D.V.M., Ph.D.; Diplomate, American College of Theriogenologists; Assistant Professor, College of Veterinary Medicine, University of Florida, Gainesville, Florida

GEORGE E. LEES, D.V.M., M.S.; Diplomate, American College of Veterinary Internal Medicine; Associate Professor, Department of Small Animal Medicine and Surgery, College of Veterinary Medicine, Texas A&M University, College Station, Texas; Staff Member, Veterinary Teaching Hospital, College of Veterinary Medicine, Texas A&M University, College Station, Texas

DONALD H. LEIN, D.V.M., Ph.D.; Diplomate, American College of Veterinary Pathology; Associate Professor of Theriogenology and Pathology, New York State College of Veterinary Medicine, Cornell University, Ithaca, New York; Associate Director of Diagnostic Laboratory, New York State College of Veterinary Medicine, Cornell University, Ithaca, New York; Staff Member, Small Animal Clinic, New York State College of Veterinary Medicine, Cornell University, Ithaca, New York

FLORA E.F. LINDSAY, M.R.C.V.S.; Senior Lecturer, Department of Veterinary Anatomy, University of Glasgow Veterinary School, Glasgow, Scotland

GERALD V. LING, D.V.M.; Professor, Department of Medicine, School of Veterinary Medicine, University of California, Davis, California; Chief, Small Animal Internal Medicine, Veterinary Medical Teaching Hospital, University of California, Davis, California

ALAN J. LIPOWITZ, D.V.M., M.S.; Diplomate, American College of Veterinary Surgeons; Associate Professor of Surgery, College of Veterinary Medicine, University of Minnesota, St. Paul, Minnesota

BARRY LISSMAN, D.V.M.; Staff Member, Long Island Mobile Veterinary Clinic, Stony Brook, New York

W. EUGENE LLOYD, D.V.M., Ph.D.; Professor of Pathology/Toxicology, College of Veterinary Medicine, Iowa State University, Ames, Iowa; President, VET-A-MIX, Inc., Shenandoah, Iowa

DONALD G. LOW, D.V.M., Ph.D.; Diplomate, American College of Veterinary Internal Medicine; Professor of Medicine, School of Veterinary Medicine, University of California, Davis, California; Staff Member, Small Animal Medicine Service, Veterinary Medical Teaching Hospital, University of California, Davis, California

J.M. MacDONALD, D.V.M.; Diplomate, American College of Veterinary Dermatology; Assistant Professor, School of Veterinary Medicine, Auburn University, Auburn, Alabama; Staff Member, Small Animal Clinic, School of Veterinary Medicine, Auburn University, Auburn, Alabama

E. GREGORY MacEWAN, V.M.D.; Diplomate, American College of Veterinary Internal Medicine; Staff Oncologist, Department of Medicine, Head, Donaldson-Atwood Cancer Clinic, New York, New York; Adjunct Assistant Member, Memorial Sloan-Kettering Cancer Center, New York, New York; Medical Director, Humane Society of New York, New York, New York

BRUCE R. MADEWELL, V.M.D., M.S.; Diplomate, American College of Veterinary Internal Medicine; Associate Professor, Department of Veterinary Surgery, University of California, Davis, California; Staff Member, Veterinary Medical Teaching Hospital, University of California, Davis, California

MARY E. MAINSTER, D.V.M.; Staff Member, Broadway Animal Hospital, San Antonio, Texas

THOMAS O. MANNING, D.V.M. Diplomate, American College of Veterinary Internal Medicine (Dermatology); Assistant Professor of Comparative Dermatology, North Carolina State University, School of Veterinary Medicine, Raleigh, North Carolina; Staff Member, Large and Small Animal Hospital, North Carolina State University School of Veterinary Medicine, Raleigh, North Carolina

CHARLES L. MARTIN, D.V.M., M.S.; Diplomate, American College of Veterinary Ophthal-

mologists; Professor, Department of Small Animal Medicine, University of Georgia, Athens, Georgia; Chief, Medicine Service, Teaching Hospital, University of Georgia, Athens, Georgia

LAWRENCE E. MATHES, Ph.D.; Assistant Professor, Department of Veterinary Pathobiology, The Ohio State University College of Veterinary Medicine, Columbus, Ohio

ROBERT E. MATUS, D.V.M., M.S.; Diplomate, American College of Veterinary Internal Medicine; Clinical Service Head, Oncology Unit-DACC, The Animal Medical Center, New York, New York

PATRICK L. McDONOUGH, M.S.; Bacteriologist and Graduate Research Assistant, Diagnostic Laboratory, New York State College of Veterinary Medicine, Cornell University, Ithaca, New York

PATRICK J. McKEEVER, D.V.M., M.S.; Associate Professor of Veterinary Comparative Dermatology, College of Veterinary Medicine, University of Minnesota, St. Paul, Minnesota; Staff Member, University of Minnesota Veterinary Teaching Hospital, St. Paul, Minnesota

BRENDAN C. McKIERNAN, D.V.M.; Diplomate, American College of Veterinary Internal Medicine; Assistant Professor of Medicine, Department of Veterinary Clinical Medicine, College of Veterinary Medicine, University of Illinois, Urbana, Illinois

GAVIN L. MEERDINK, D.V.M.; Diplomate, American Board of Veterinary Toxicology; Associate Professor, College of Veterinary Medicine, Michigan State University, East Lansing, Michigan; Clinical Diagnostic Toxicologist, Veterinary Clinical Center, Animal Health Diagnostic Laboratory, East Lansing, Michigan

KAY G. MEHREN, B.V.Sc., D.V.M.; Associated Member of Faculty of Graduate Studies, Ontario Veterinary College, University of Guelph, Ontario, Canada; Head of Veterinary Services, Metro Toronto Zoo, Ontario, Canada

JANE E. MEIER, D.V.M.; Associate Veterinarian, Jennings Center for Zoological Medicine, Zoological Society of San Diego, San Diego, California

H. DWIGHT MERCER, D.V.M., Ph.D.; Professor, College of Veterinary Medicine, Mississippi State University, Starkville, Mississippi; Director and Coordinator of Programs, Animal Health Center, College of Veterinary Medicine, Mississippi State University, Mississippi State, Mississippi

DONALD J. MEUTEN, D.V.M., Ph.D.; Diplomate, American College of Veterinary Pathology; Assistant Professor, College of Veterinary Medicine, Texas A&M University, College Station, Texas

K.M. MEYERS, Ph.D.; Professor of Physiology, College of Veterinary Medicine, Washington State University, Pullman, Washington

WILLIAM H. MILLER, Jr., V.M.D.; Diplomate, American College of Veterinary Dermatology; Assistant Professor of Dermatology, University of Pennsylvania School of Veterinary Medicine, Philadelphia, Pennsylvania; Staff Member, Veterinary Hospital of the University of Pennsylvania, Philadelphia, Pennsylvania

MERRILL MITLER, Ph.D.; Director, Sleep Disorders Program, Health Sciences Center, State University of New York at Stony Brook, Stony Brook, New York

N. SYDNEY MOISE, D.V.M.; Diplomate, American College of Veterinary Internal Medicine; Instructor of Medicine, New York State College of Veterinary Medicine, Cornell University, Ithaca, New York

RONDA PROUTY MOORE, D.V.M.; Resident, Department of Pathology, Angell Memorial Animal Hospital, Boston, Massachusetts

MICHAEL E. MOUNT, D.V.M., Ph.D.; Assistant Professor of Veterinary Clinical Pathology, School of Veterinary Medicine, University of California, Davis, California.

WILLIAM W. MUIR, D.V.M., Ph.D.; Professor, The Ohio State University College of Veterinary Medicine, Columbus, Ohio; Head, Section of Anesthesiology, and Co-Director, Small Animal Intensive Care, The Ohio State University College of Veterinary Medicine, Columbus, Ohio

RONALD L. MULL, D.V.M., Ph.D.; Staff Research Toxicologist, Shell Development Co., Houston, Texas

GEORGE H. MULLER, D.V.M.; Diplomate, American College of Veterinary Dermatology; Diplomate, American College of Veterinary Internal Medicine; Professor of Clinical Dermatology, Stanford University, Stanford, California; Director, Muller Veterinary Hospital, Walnut Creek, California; Director, Veterinary Dermatology Clinic, Walnut Creek, California

JOHN A. MULNIX, D.V.M., M.S.; Owner, Carlson Animal Clinic, Fort Collins, Colorado; Referrals in Medicine, Anderson Animal Hospital, Lakewood, Colorado

ROBERT J. MUNGER, D.V.M.; Diplomate, American College of Veterinary Ophthalmologists; Assistant Professor, Veterinary Ophthalmology, Department of Urban Practice, College of Veterinary Medicine, University of Tennessee, Knoxville, Tennessee; Manager, Animal Husbandry, Alcon Laboratories, Fort Worth, Texas; Manager, Animal Ophthalmology Clinic, Dallas, Texas

T.M. NETT, Ph.D.; Associate Professor, Physiology, Colorado State University, Fort Collins, Colorado; Laboratory Director, Rothgerber Endocrinology Laboratory, Colorado State University, Fort Collins, Colorado

STEVEN S. NICHOLSON, D.V.M.; Associate Professor of Veterinary Toxicology, School of Veterinary Medicine, Louisiana State University, Baton Rouge, Louisiana

JOAN A. O'BRIEN, V.M.D.; Professor of Medicine, School of Veterinary Medicine, University of Pennsylvania, Philadelphia, Pennsylvania

TIMOTHY O'BRIEN, D.V.M.; Veterinary Medical Associate, Department of Veterinary Pathobiology, College of Veterinary Medicine, University of Minnesota, St. Paul, Minnesota

FREDERICK W. OEHME, D.V.M., Ph.D.; Professor of Toxicology, Medicine and Physiology, College of Veterinary Medicine, Kansas State University, Manhattan, Kansas; Director, Comparative Toxicology Laboratories, Kansas State University, Manhattan, Kansas

JOHN E. OLIVER, D.V.M., M.S., Ph.D.; Professor and Head, Department of Small Animal Medicine, College of Veterinary Medicine, University of Georgia, Athens, Georgia; Neurologist, Veterinary Medical Teaching Hospital, College of Veterinary Medicine, University of Georgia, Athens, Georgia

RICHARD G. OLSEN, Ph.D.; Professor, Department of Veterinary Pathobiology, The Ohio State University College of Veterinary Medicine, Columbus, Ohio

P.N. OLSON, D.V.M., M.S., Ph.D.; Diplomate, American College of Theriogenologists; Assistant Professor, Clinical Sciences, Colorado State University, Fort Collins, Colorado; Clinical Director, Rothgerber Endocrinology Laboratory, Colorado State University, Fort Collins, Colorado

LAURIE G. O'ROURKE, D.V.M.; Instructor in Residence, Department of Clinical Pathology, School of Veterinary Medicine, University of California, Davis, California

CARL A. OSBORNE, D.V.M., Ph.D.; Diplomate, American College of Veterinary Internal Medicine; Professor and Chairman, Department of Small Animal Clinical Sciences, College of Veterinary Medicine, University of Minnesota, St. Paul, Minnesota

GARY D. OSWEILER, D.V.M., M.S. Ph.D.; Professor of Veterinary Pathology, College of Veterinary Medicine, University of Missouri-Columbia, Columbia, Missouri; Staff Member, Veterinary Medical Diagnostic Laboratory, University of Missouri, Columbia, Missouri

NICHOLAS E. PALUMBO, B.S., D.V.M.; Professor and Chairman, Department of Comparative Medicine, School of Medicine, University of Hawaii, Honolulu, Hawaii

NIELS C. PEDERSEN, D.V.M., Ph.D.; Professor, School of Veterinary Medicine, University of California, Davis, California; Staff Clinician in Small Animal Medicine, Veterinary Medicine Teaching Hospital, University of California, Davis, California

PAUL L. PEMBERTON, B.V.Sc.; Department of Animal Husbandry, Faculty of Veterinary Science, University of Sydney, N.S.W., Australia; Private Practitioner, Avalon, N.S.W., Australia

S.F. PERRI, B.A.; Research Associate, Comparative Medicine, University of Hawaii at Manoa, Honolulu, Hawaii

MARK E. PETERSON, D.V.M.; Diplomate, American College of Veterinary Internal Medicine; Assistant Professor of Medicine, Department of Clinical Sciences, New York State College of Veterinary Medicine, Cornell University, Ithaca, New York; Staff Endocrinologist, Department of Medicine, The Animal Medical Center, New York, New York; Director of Clinical Medicine, Cornell University Center for Research Animal Resources, Cornell University Medical College, New York, New York; Associate Professor, Department of Radiology, Cornell University Medical College, New York, New York; Research Associate, Department of Medicine, Cornell University Medical College, New York, New York;

Assistant Director, Division of Laboratory Animal Medicine, Cornell University Medical College, New York, New York

LYNDSAY G. PHILLIPS, Jr., D.V.M.; Resident Veterinarian/Assistant Director, Henry Doorly Zoo, Omaha, Nebraska

CLYDE PITTS, D.V.M.; Private Practitioner, Studio City, California

ROGER P. PITTS, D.V.M.; Assistant Professor, School of Veterinary Medicine, University of Wisconsin, Madison, Wisconsin

ROY V. H. POLLOCK, D.V.M., Ph.D.; Assistant Professor of Microbiology, New York State College of Veterinary Medicine, Cornell University, Ithaca, New York

DAVID J. POLZIN, D.V.M., Ph.D.; Diplomate, American College of Veterinary Medicine (Internal Medicine); Assistant Professor, College of Veterinary Medicine, University of Minnesota, St. Paul, Minnesota; Staff Internist, Lewis Hospital for Companion Animals of the University of Minnesota, St. Paul, Minnesota

RAYMOND G. PRATA, D.V.M.; Diplomate, American College of Veterinary Surgeons; Director of Surgery, The Animal Medical Center, New York, New York

ANNIE K. PRESTWOOD, D.V.M., Ph.D.; Professor of Parasitology, College of Veterinary Medicine, University of Georgia, Athens, Georgia

JENNIFER E. PRICE, B.V.M., M.S. Ph.D.; Senior Lecturer, Department of Clinical Studies, Faculty of Veterinary Medicine, University of Nairobi, Nairobi, Kenya; Head of Small Animal Clinic, Department of Clinical Studies, Faculty of Veterinary Medicine, University of Nairobi, Nairobi, Kenya

JOHN F. RANDOLPH, D.V.M.; Diplomate, American College of Veterinary Internal Medicine; Assistant Professor of Medicine, Department of Clinical Sciences, New York State College of Veterinary Medicine, Cornell University, Ithaca, New York

CLARENCE A. RAWLINGS, D.V.M., M.S., Ph.D.; Diplomate, American College of Veterinary Surgeons; Professor, Departments of Small Animal Medicine and Physiology and Pharmacology, College of Veterinary Medicine, University of Georgia, Athens, Georgia; Chief of Staff, Small

Animal Surgery, Veterinary Teaching Hospital, College of Veterinary Medicine, University of Georgia, Athens, Georgia

PATRICK T. REDIG, D.V.M., Ph.D.; Assistant Professor, College of Veterinary Medicine, University of Minnesota, St. Paul, Minnesota; Medical Director, Raptor Research and Rehabilitation Program, College of Veterinary Medicine, University of Minnesota, St. Paul, Minnesota

LLOYD M. REEDY, D.V.M.; Diplomate, American College of Veterinary Dermatology; Clinical Associate Professor, Comparative Medicine, University of Texas Southwestern Medical School, Dallas, Texas; Owner, Animal Dermatology Clinic, Dallas, Texas

T. J. REIMERS, Ph.D.; Assistant Professor of Endocrinology and Director of the Endocrinology Laboratory, New York State College of Veterinary Medicine, Cornell University, Ithaca, New York

VICTOR T. RENDANO, Jr., V.M.D., M.Sc.; Diplomate, American College of Veterinary Radiology; Associate Professor, Department of Clinical Sciences, New York State College of Veterinary Medicine, Cornell University, Ithaca, New York

RALPH C. RICHARDSON, D.V.M.; Diplomate, American College of Veterinary Internal Medicine; Associate Professor, Internal Medicine, School of Veterinary Medicine, Purdue University, West Lafayette, Indiana; Chief, Clinical Oncology, Purdue Comparative Oncology Program, School of Veterinary Medicine, Purdue University, West Lafayette, Indiana

J. EDMOND RIVIERE, D.V.M., Ph.D.; Assistant Professor of Pharmacology and Toxicology, Department of Anatomy, Physiological Sciences and Radiology, School of Veterinary Medicine, North Carolina State University, Raleigh, North Carolina

JANE F. ROBENS, D.V.M.; Diplomate, American Board of Veterinary Toxicology

EDWARD L. ROBERSON, D.V.M., Ph.D.; Professor of Parasitology, College of Veterinary Medicine, University of Georgia, Athens, Georgia

Q. R. ROGERS, Ph.D.; Professor of Physiological Chemistry, School of Veterinary Medicine, University of California, Davis, California

ROBERT C. ROSENTHAL, D.V.M., M.S.; Diplomate, American College of Veterinary Internal Medicine; Research Associate, College of Veterinary Medicine, University of Illinois, Urbana, Illinois

ROD ROSYCHUK, D.V.M.; Diplomate, American College of Veterinary Internal Medicine; Assistant Professor, Department of Veterinary Clinical Medicine, College of Veterinary Medicine, University of Illinois, Urbana, Illinois; Staff Member, Small Animal Clinic, College of Veterinary Medicine, University of Illinois, Urbana, Illinois

PHILIP ROUDEBUSH, D.V.M.; Diplomate, American College of Veterinary Internal Medicine; Assistant Professor, College of Veterinary Medicine, Mississippi State University, Mississippi State, Mississippi

MARK E. RUSSO, V.M.D.; Diplomate, American College of Veterinary Internal Medicine (Neurology); Veterinary Neurology Referral Service, Kingston, Massachusetts

BARBARA ANN SAWYER, D.V.M.; Private Practitioner, Merced, California, Deceased

PAUL D. SAYER, B.V.M.S., F.R.C.V.S.; (Formerly) Senior Lecturer in Charge, Small Animal Clinic, Faculty of Veterinary Medicine, University of Nairobi, Nairobi, Kenya

M.C. SCHAEFFER, M.P.H.; Department of Physiological Chemistry, School of Veterinary Medicine, University of California, Davis California

WILLIAM D. SCHALL, D.V.M., M.S.; Diplomate, American College of Veterinary Internal Medicine (Internal Medicine); Professor of Internal Medicine, College of Veterinary Medicine, Michigan State University, East Lansing, Michigan; Internist, Veterinary Clinical Center, College of Veterinary Medicine, Michigan State University, East Lansing, Michigan

NORMAN R. SCHNEIDER, D.V.M., M.Sc.; Diplomate, American Board of Veterinary Toxicology; Associate Professor of Veterinary Science, University of Nebraska, Lincoln, Nebraska; Associate Professor of Pharmacodynamics and Toxicology, University of Nebraska Medical Center, Omaha, Nebraska

MICHAEL SCHOLLMEYER, D.V.M.; Director, Physiological Research Laboratories, Minneapolis, Minnesota

DANNY W. SCOTT, D.V.M.; Diplomate, American College of Veterinary Dermatology; Associate Professor of Medicine, New York State College of Veterinary Medicine, Cornell University, Ithaca, New York

FREDRIC W. SCOTT, D.V.M., Ph.D.; Diplomate, American College of Veterinary Internal Medicine; Professor of Virology, New York State College of Veterinary Medicine, Cornell University, Ithaca, New York

RICHARD C. SCOTT, D.V.M.; Diplomate, American College of Veterinary Internal Medicine; Staff, Department of Medicine, The Animal Medical Center, New York, New York

DAVID F. SENIOR, B.V.Sc.; Diplomate, American College of Veterinary Internal Medicine; Assistant Professor, College of Veterinary Medicine, University of Florida, Gainesville, Florida; Chief, Small Animal Intensive Care, and Clinician, Small Animal Medicine, Veterinary Medical Teaching Hospital, University of Florida, Gainesville, Florida

DONALD SHAW, D.V.M.; Private Practitioner, The Animal Eye Clinic, St. Paul, Minnesota

SANG J. SHIN, D.V.M.; Director of Microbiology Laboratory, Diagnostic Laboratory, New York State College of Veterinary Medicine, Cornell University, Ithaca, New York

STEPHEN T. SIMPSON, D.V.M., M.S.; Diplomate, American College of Veterinary Internal Medicine (Neurology); Assistant Professor of Veterinary Medicine, Auburn University School of Veterinary Medicine, Auburn, Alabama; Staff Member, Small Animal Clinic, Auburn University School of Veterinary Medicine, Auburn, Alabama

FRANCES O. SMITH, D.V.M.; Teaching Associate, College of Veterinary Medicine, University of Minnesota, St. Paul, Minnesota; Resident, Division of Theriogenology, College of Veterinary Medicine, University of Minnesota Lewis Hospital for Companion Animals, St. Paul, Minnesota

S. F. SODERBERG, D.V.M., Ph.D.; Staff Member, Northeast Veterinary Hospital, Detroit, Michigan

ANTHONY A. STANNARD, D.V.M., Ph.D.; Diplomate, American College of Veterinary Dermatology; Professor, School of Veterinary Medicine, University of California, Davis, California; Chief of Dermatology Service and Associate Director, Small Animal Clinic, Veterinary Medical Teaching Hospital, University of California, Davis, California

STEPHEN P. STEPHEN, B.S. Pharm. M.S.; Assistant Professor, College of Veterinary Medicine, Mississippi State University, Mississippi State, Mississippi; Chief Pharmacist, Animal Health Center, College of Veterinary Medicine, Mississippi State University, Mississippi State, Mississippi

MARILYN E. STIFF, M.S., D.V.M.; Diplomate, American College of Veterinary Internal Medicine; Clinician, Animal Medical Clinic, Inc., Lakeland, Florida

MICHAEL K. STOSKOPF, D.V.M.; Assistant Professor, Johns Hopkins University School of Medicine, Baltimore, Maryland; Chief Veterinarian, National Aquarium, Baltimore, Maryland

D. R. STROMBECK, D.V.M., Ph.D.; Professor of Medicine, School of Veterinary Medicine, University of California, Davis, California; Staff Member, Veterinary Medical Teaching Hospital, School of Veterinary Medicine, University of California, Davis, California

LARRY J. SWANGO, D.V.M., Ph.D.; Alumni Associate Professor of Virology, Department of Microbiology, School of Veterinary Medicine, Auburn University, Auburn, Alabama; Consultant to Auburn University Small Animal Clinic, Auburn, Alabama

GARY W. THAYER, D.V.M., M.S.; Diplomate, American College of Veterinary Internal Medicine; Assistant Professor, Department of Small Animal Medicine, College of Veterinary Medicine, University of Georgia, Athens, Georgia

RICHARD E. THOMAS, D.V.M.; Director, Town and Country Animal Clinic, Cheektowaga, New York; Veterinary Consultant, Roswell Park Memorial Institute, Buffalo, New York

WILLIAM P. THOMAS, D.V.M.; Diplomate, American College of Veterinary Internal Medicine (Cardiology); Assistant Professor, Department of Medicine, School of Veterinary Medicine, University of California, Davis, California; Chief, Cardiology Service, Veterinary Medical Teaching Hospital, University of California, Davis, California

JERRY A. THORNHILL, D.V.M.; Diplomate, American College of Veterinary Internal Medicine; Assistant Professor of Medicine, School of

Veterinary Medicine and Hemodialysis Laboratory, Institute of Interdisciplinary Engineering, Purdue University, West Lafayette, Indiana

THAD E. THORSON, D.V.M.; Staff Member, Long Beach Dog and Cat Hospital, Long Beach, California

DAVID C. TWEDT, D.V.M.; Diplomate, American College of Veterinary Internal Medicine; Associate Professor, Department of Clinical Sciences, College of Veterinary Medicine, Colorado State University, Fort Collins, Colorado

A. J. VENKER-van HAAGEN, D.V.M., Ph.D.; Lecturer, Small Animal Clinic, State University of Utrecht, Utrecht, The Netherlands

WILLIAM ARDENE VESTRE, D.V.M., M.S.; Diplomate, American College of Veterinary Ophthalmologists; Assistant Professor, Ophthalmology, School of Veterinary Medicine, Purdue University, West Lafayette, Indiana

BARBARA J. WATROUS, D.V.M.; Diplomate, American College of Veterinary Radiology; Assistant Professor, School of Veterinary Medicine, Oregon State University, Corvallis, Oregon; Head of Radiology, School of Veterinary Medicine, Oregon State University, Corvallis, Oregon

RICHARD C. WEISS, V.M.D., Ph.D.; Syntex Research, Mountain View, California

STEPHEN D. WHITE, D.V.M.; Assistant Professor, School of Veterinary Medicine, Tufts University, Boston, Massachusetts

JEFF R. WILCKE, D.V.M., M.S.; Assistant Professor, Division of Veterinary Biology and Clinical Studies, Virginia-Maryland Regional College of Veterinary Medicine, Virginia Polytechnic and

State University, Blacksburg, Virginia; Staff Member, Veterinary Medical Teaching Hospital, Virginia-Maryland Regional College of Veterinary Medicine, Virginia Polytechnic and State University, Blacksburg, Virginia

MICHAEL D. WILLARD, D.V.M., M.S.; Diplomate, American College of Veterinary Internal Medicine; Assistant Professor of Veterinary Medicine, Mississippi State University, College of Veterinary Medicine, Mississippi State, Mississippi; Internist, Animal Health Center, Mississippi State University, College of Veterinary Medicine, Mississippi State, Mississippi

THOMAS R. WOLSKI, D.V.M.; Doctoral Candidate and Research Assistant, New York State Veterinary College, Cornell University, Ithaca, New York; Animal Behavior Consultant, Ithaca, New York

GARY L. WOOD, D.V.M.; Diplomate, American College of Veterinary Internal Medicine (Cardiology); Cardiologist, Oregon Veterinary Specialty Clinic, Portland, Oregon; Cardiologist, Cardio-trace, Inc., Transtelephonic Electrocardiographic Monitoring, Portland, Oregon

ROBERT D. ZENOBLE, D.V.M., M.S.; Diplomate, American College of Veterinary Medicine; Associate Professor, Department of Small Animal Surgery and Medicine, Auburn University, Auburn, Alabama; Staff Member, Small Animal Clinic, School of Veterinary Medicine, Auburn, Alabama

JAMES F. ZIMMER, D.V.M., Ph.D.; Assistant Professor of Medicine, Department of Clinical Sciences, New York State College of Veterinary Medicine, Cornell University, Ithaca, New York

PREFACE

You, the readers, have continued to make *Current Veterinary Therapy* a popular textbook. We, the authors, hope we will continue to merit your trust in providing updated, authoritative ideas. We are reminded anew of the progress our profession continues to make as we compare each new edition with its predecessor. *CVT VIII* is no exception. This volume reaches a new high: 240 articles, 95 per cent completely new and the others appropriately updated.

In this volume, we continue our policy of referencing articles from the previous edition. This has received mixed reactions from our readers. Some feel this is a great idea—they have the previous edition—but others feel frustrated when the older edition is not available. Students with access to a library have no problem. We hope the reference to three-year-old data that are still current is helpful to the busy practitioner, and we join the overwhelming majority who like the idea of referencing articles from the previous edition.

This edition reflects new emphasis in the fields of immunology and oncology, contains articles on behavior and bonding, and places reproductive disorders in a new section for better identity.

The editor is grateful to many people: his wife, Helen, who toiled with him on sabbatic leave to revise two books at once; and the tremendously helpful staff of W. B. Saunders Company. Particularly, we are indebted to each contributor and consulting editor, without whom this book would not exist. We hope you continue to find our joint efforts useful.

ROBERT W. KIRK

CONTENTS

SECTION

3

RESPIRATORY DISEASES
Brendan C. McKiernan
Consulting Editor

SECTION
5
HEMATOLOGY—ONCOLOGY—IMMUNOLOGY
Arthur I. Hurvitz
Consulting Editor

SECTION
4
CARDIOVASCULAR DISEASES
John D. Bonagura
Consulting Editor

HEMATOLOGY

ONCOLOGY

SECTION
7
OPHTHALMOLOGIC DISEASES
Charles L. Martin
Consulting Editor

SECTION
6
DERMATOLOGIC DISEASES
Robert W. Kirk
Consulting Editor

SECTION
10
GASTROINTESTINAL DISORDERS
Donald R. Strombeck
Consulting Editor

SECTION

14

INFECTIOUS DISEASES

Fredric W. Scott
Consulting Editor

IMMUNIZATION

DIAGNOSTIC PROCEDURES

APPENDICES
Robert W. Kirk
Consulting Editor

NOTICE

Extraordinary efforts have been made by the authors, the editors, and the publisher of this book to insure that dosage recommendations are precise and in agreement with standards officially accepted at the time of publication.

It does happen, however, that dosage schedules are changed from time to time in the light of accumulating clinical experience and continuing laboratory studies. This is most likely to occur in the case of recently introduced products.

It is urged, therefore, that you check the manufacturer's recommendations for dosage, especially if the drug to be administered or prescribed is one that you use only infrequently or have not used for some time.

In addition, some drugs mentioned have been used by the authors as experimental drugs. Others have been used after official clearance for use in one species but not in others described here. This is particularly true for rare and exotic species. In these cases the authors have reported on their own considerable experience, but readers are urged to view the recommendations with discretion and precaution.

THE EDITORS

Section

1

SPECIAL THERAPY

ROBERT W. KIRK, D.V.M.

Consulting Editor

SHOCK

(The Pathophysiology and Management of the Circulatory Collapse States)

STEVE C. HASKINS, D.V.M.

Davis, California

CARDIOVASCULAR HOMEOSTASIS

The ability of the cardiovascular system to effectively transport blood and its constituent nutrients and metabolites to and from the various body organs in appropriate volumes and rates is dependent upon the coordinated interaction of several functions: blood pressure, arteriolar vasomotor tone and vascular volume capacity, blood volume, and cardiac output. The interdependency of each function is outlined in Table 1. Arterial blood pressure is important because it is normally the primary determinant of cerebral and coronary perfusion. Blood pressure is dependent on a proper balance between blood volume, cardiac output, and peripheral vasomotor tone. Impairment of one of these factors is usually compensated for by the other two so that an adequate blood pressure is maintained. If, however, the impairment is severe or if the compensatory processes are themselves debilitated by disease, excessive hypotension will develop and the patient may die from inadequate vital organ perfusion. The administration of general anesthetics (which are potent myocardial depressants and which tend to cause vasodilation) to a dehydrated patient (who is always hypovolemic) is an ideal way to demonstrate decompensation and precipitate severe hypotension. A mean systemic blood pressure of 60 mm Hg will usually provide an arteriovenous pressure differential sufficient for marginal cerebral and coronary perfusion. If the hypotension is produced by hemorrhagic hypovolemia, the compensatory peripheral vasoconstriction will cause impairment of visceral organ perfusion. If the hypotension is caused by peripheral vasodilation, visceral organ perfusion will be quite satisfactory.

Blood pressure predominantly regulates cerebral and coronary perfusion; peripheral vasomotor tone predominantly regulates visceral organ perfusion. When monitoring and treating cardiovascular disease, it is important to give appropriate attention to both factors. The measurement or calculation of any single parameter (blood pressure, peripheral vascular resistance, cardiac output, or blood vol-

ume) has a specific meaning, but it must be correlated with all of the other measurements of cardiovascular function before its overall importance to the patient can be determined. The measured cardiac output, for instance, can be higher than normal and still be relatively insufficient if it does not supply the perfusion needs of the hypermetabolic septic patient or if it does not maintain adequate blood pressure in patients with vasodilative hypotension.

HYPOTENSION VERSUS SHOCK

The difference between hypotension and shock has great conceptual importance with regard to the interpretation of cardiovascular measurements and the selection of a therapeutic focus. Hypotension is defined as low blood pressure; shock is defined as inadequate delivery of blood, oxygen, and energy substrates to the tissues. Since blood pressure predominantly influences cerebral and coronary perfusion, hypotension may be said to cause cerebral and myocardial shock. Arteriolar vasomotor tone predominantly influences perfusion of the other tissues, and vasoconstriction therefore causes thoracic and abdominal visceral organ shock. Hypotension and vasoconstriction commonly occur together, but they are not inextricably linked. Vasodilative hypotension is an example. When an animal loses vascular volume, compensatory changes will be instituted to support blood pressure. If these changes are not complete or rapid enough to restore blood pressure, the patient will die peracutely from inadequate perfusion of the brain and heart. If blood pressure can be maintained, then the patient will live at least temporarily. In this example, blood pressure may be maintained very much within the normal range, but at the expense of visceral organ perfusion (owing to peripheral vasoconstriction). If blood volume is not sufficiently restored by the intravascular redistribution of interstitial fluids or by the administration of exogenous fluids, the patient will die from inadequate visceral organ perfusion in about three to six hours. There are two distinctly different mechanisms regulating blood flow to various organs in the body; neither can be allowed to malfunction for long. Consideration must be given to both the adequacy of arterial blood pressure and the state of peripheral vasomotor tone when monitoring critically ill patients and selecting therapeutic preferences.

CAUSES OF SHOCK

Shock can be conveniently categorized into cardiogenic, hypovolemic, and septic causes. Cardiogenic shock may be caused by acute or chronic intrinsic congestive heart failure, endogenous or exogenous noxious agents, or, rarely, thromboembolic phenomena (see Table 1). Hypovolemic shock

Table 1. *Impairment of Cardiovascular Homeostasis*

Parameter	Cause of Impairment	Reason Impairment Is a Problem
Blood pressure	Peripheral vasodilation Hypovolemia Decreased cardiac output	Excessive hypotension reduces cerebral and coronary perfusion
Arteriolar vasomotor tone	Vasoconstriction (signs: pale color, prolonged capillary refill time, cool appendages, decreased urine output); sympathetic activation; sympathomimetic drugs or drugs that cause sympathetic activation; compensatory response to hypovolemia	Excessive vasoconstriction impairs visceral organ perfusion
	Vasodilation (signs: opposite of vasoconstriction) All anesthetic drugs but especially those with alpha-receptor blocking ability, e.g.. phenothiazines; hypermetabolic states such as hyperthermia and septic shock	Excessive vasodilation causes hypotension
Blood volume	Whole blood loss from the vascular fluid compartment (signs of vascular compartmental hypovolemia: tachycardia, weak pulse, vasoconstriction, and perhaps hypotension) Hypoproteinemia Extracellular fluid loss (signs of interstitial compartmental volume depletion: decreased skin turgor); diarrhea; vomition; diuresis; third-space accumulation (thoracic or abdominal cavities, at a fracture site, or via burns) Peripheral vasodilation and increased vascular volume capacity produces a relative hypovolemia	Hypovolemia predisposes to hypotension and causes compensatory peripheral vasoconstriction

Cardiac output	Decreased venous return
	    Surgical packing or positive pressure ventilation–induced collapse of large thoracic veins; hypovolemia or peripheral vasoconstriction; pericardial tamponade or inflow occlusion during surgery; gastric torsion
	Decreased contractility
	    Anesthetic drugs; hypoxia; exogenous or endogenous toxemia—myocardial depressant factors in shock; potassium, calcium, or pH disturbances; intrinsic heart failure
	Bradycardia
	    High vagal tone—endotracheal intubation, visceral or eyeball traction during surgery, drgus-narcotics, xylazine, too deep a level of anesthesia with any anesthetic, or anticholinesterases; atrioventricular conduction block or sick-sinus syndrome; electrolyte disturbances, severe hypoxia or hypothermia
	Severe arrhythmias
		Inadequate cardiac output causes hypotension

Table 2.   *Cardiovascular Patterns of Common Forms of Shock*

Parameter	Cause of Shock			
	Cardiogenic	*Hypovolemic*	*Septic**	*Endotoxic†*
Mean arterial pressure	Low	Low	Normal/low	Low
Cardiac output	Low	Low	Normal/high	Low
Peripheral vascular resistance	High	High	Low	High
Central venous pressure and pulmonary capillary wedge pressure	High	Low	Low	Low
Arterial oxygen tension	Low	Normal	Low	Normal
A/V oxygen content difference	Normal/decreased	Normal/decreased	Decreased	Normal/decreased
Pulmonary venous admixture	Normal	Normal	High	Normal
Lactic acidosis	High	High	High	High
Oxygen consumption	Low	Low	Low	Low

*The listed characteristics represent the early stages of septic shock, which may last for several days before decompensation intervenes; late stages resemble hypovolemic shock and homeostatic deterioration and will last only a few hours before death intervenes.

†Produced experimentally by the injection of a cell-wall lipopolysaccharide from gram negative bacteria.

may be caused by acute whole blood loss or chronic fluid loss from the vascular or extracellular fluid compartment (see Table 1). Septic shock may be caused by gram positive or negative bacteria, fungi, yeast, and viruses.

In contrast to the other forms of shock, septic shock begins as a hypermetabolic disorder associated with a dramatic increase in peripheral perfusion (Table 2). As the disorder progresses, tissue blood flow is unable to keep pace with high metabolic demands, and the character of the disorder comes to resemble hypovolemic vasoconstrictive shock. This represents preterminal cardiovascular decompensation. The progression of the disease state is often quite rapid, and the clinician should be constantly alert to the early signs of septic shock (Table 3). Early recognition and aggressive therapy are the keys to successful management of the patient with septic shock.

CONSEQUENCES OF SHOCK

The maintenance of cellular integrity is an energy-dependent process. Regardless of the specific energy substrate utilized by the various tissues (glucose, free fatty acids, or amino acids), oxidative metabolism is dependent on an adequate supply of blood and oxygen. When local blood flow and

Table 3.   *Early Signs of Septic Shock*

History of a recent surgical intervention or other invasive procedure (indwelling vascular or urinary catheter)
Hyperdynamic cardiopulmonary system (tachycardia, hyperventilation, respiratory alkalosis) (see also Table 2)
Hypermetabolic state (metabolic acidosis, hyperthermia)
CNS depression
Severe acute leukopenia (neutropenia)

either hypotension, vasoconstriction, or hypermetabolism, energy production is limited to anaerobic glycolysis. When energy stores become insufficient, cellular integrity and function begin to fail.

THE MICROCIRCULATION

Local tissue blood flow is normally modulated by autoregulatory mechanisms responsive to local demands for oxygen delivery and metabolite removal. In forms of shock-associated peripheral vasoconstriction, powerful sympathetic influences force the arteriolar sphincters to remain constricted in the face of increasing hypoxia and the appearance of noxious metabolic products (this is the vasoconstrictive phase of shock). Initially, vasoconstriction is beneficial to the patient as a whole with regard to blood pressure maintenance. The consequent visceral organ hypoperfusion eventually causes visceral organ failure. After a time, in the absence of energy, in the presence of a highly undesirable environment, and in spite of strong sympathetic stimulation, sphincters begin to dilate. Unfortunately, arteriolar sphincters dilate before venular sphincters and blood begins to pool in the capillary beds (this is the vasodilative or congestive phase of shock). This phenomenon is associated with a decrease in venous return and is a poor prognostic sign with regard to reversibility of the shock process. As the capillary endothelial membrane loses its integrity, increasing quantities of plasma and eventually whole red blood cells leak out of the vascular compartment, further decreasing venous return. Venous return and myocardial contractility progressively decline, as do cardiac output, blood pressure, and cerebral and coronary perfusion.

The red blood cells and platelets are normally repelled from each other and from the capillary endothelium by a surface electronegativity. In low flow states of shock when environmental hypoxia and acidosis are prominent, the red and white cells and the platelets begin to aggregate or sequester in the capillary beds of most organs. Aggregating platelets release (1) ADP, which causes further platelet aggregation as well as activation of the coagulation, fibrinolytic, and complement cascades; (2) serotonin, which causes vasoconstriction and increased capillary permeability; and (3) prostaglandins, which cause either vasoconstriction or vasodilation and increased capillary permeability. The white cells liberate (1) cationic proteins, which increase vascular permeability and degranulate mast cells (histamine causes vasodilation and increased capillary permeability); (2) lysosomal proteases, which digest collagen, elastic tissues, and the basement membrane; denature the phospholipid layer of cell walls; and decrease the surfactant properties of the alveolar surface fluid; (3) leukokinins, which increase capillary permeability; and (4) other mediators that further activate platelet aggregation and intravascular coagulation. The release of tissue thromboplastins from any degenerating cell further aggravates the intravascular coagulation.

Intracellular organelles are also susceptible to hypoxia. Lysosomes begin to leak proteolytic enzymes, which alter circulating plasma proteins to the extent that they deleteriously affect various organs of the body. One such altered protein is myocardial depressant factor (MDF), which has a negative inotropic effect on the heart; another is reticuloendothelial depressant substance (RDS). The pulmonary edema secondary to acute pancreatitis is also thought to be the result of such altered proteins. Lysosomal proteolytic enzymes also act on the surrounding cell structures.

THE BLOOD

Loss of red cell and plasma protein mass may be due to hemorrhage or may be a late event in all forms of shock as a result of capillary leakage of cells into the interstitium and gut lumen. Septic shock, in addition, causes a depletion of intraerythrocytic 2,3 DPG and a leftward shift of the oxygen-hemoglobin dissociation curve. Therapy with clear fluids may cause excessive hemodilution and may further reduce the oxygen-carrying and delivery capacity of the blood.

A neutropenic leukopenia is a common feature of early septic shock, but subsequently, and in all phases of hypovolemic shock, a neutrophilic leukocytosis should occur. Failure to manifest this leukocytosis in septic shock is a poor prognostic sign in humans.

THE RETICULOENDOTHELIAL SYSTEM

The reticuloendothelial (RE) system functions to scavenge circulating cellular debris, bacteria, fibrin split products, immune complexes, and other toxins. It is depressed in all forms of shock by hypoxia

and by depressant substances such as histamine, serotonin, bradykinin, and RDS. Infusion of cellular debris in poorly filtered stored blood transfusions may competitively interfere with RE function. General anesthesia may depress its ability to clear circulating debris. Fibrinectin, a plasma opsonic glycoprotein, appears to play an essential role in the ability of the RE system to phagocytize foreign debris. Depletion of circulating levels of fibrinectin is a common phenomenon in severe shock, and restoration of normal plasma levels has produced dramatic clinical improvement in human shock patients. The function of the RE system correlates closely with the clinical course and outcome of the shock state.

THE RESPIRATORY SYSTEM

A respiratory distress syndrome may develop somewhat in proportion to the severity and duration of the shock. Initial hypotension increases ventilation/perfusion mismatching and physiologic dead space. The compensatory arteriolar vasoconstriction decreases perfusion of some pulmonary capillary beds, and venular constriction may cause an elevated capillary hydrostatic pressure. Impaired capillary blood flow predisposes to red and white cell and platelet aggregation and sequestration, with all of the aforementioned consequences. The release of emboli, cellular debris, and vasoactive substances from extrapulmonary sources further aggravates the pulmonary compromise. Thromboembolic mechanical obstruction of the pulmonary microcirculation may further accentuate the maldistribution of pulmonary blood flow.

Fluids begin to leak into the interstitium and accumulate around the medium-sized arterioles and bronchioles, decreasing pulmonary compliance and increasing the work of breathing. When the interstitial fluid pressure increases to some critical point, fluid begins to leak into the small terminal airways and the alveoli. This increases the surface tension of the air spaces and, coupled with a decreased surfactant synthesis and activity, promotes alveolar and small airway collapse. Interstitial and airway infiltration with proteinaceous and cellular transudates contributes to hyaline membrane formation and pulmonary failure. The severity of the respiratory failure may be exaggerated by aggressive crystalloid fluid therapy, infusion of platelets and white cell aggregates in poorly filtered stored whole blood, or the prolonged administration of 100 per cent oxygen (oxygen toxicity). The progressive hypoxemia further impairs oxygenation of the rest of the body.

THE KIDNEYS

In all forms of shock associated with peripheral vasoconstriction, renal cortical blood flow is diminished (renal blood flow is increased in early septic shock). If the decrease is severe enough or prolonged enough, renal tubular epithelial cells will undergo hypoxic degeneration and will die. If sufficient numbers of nephrons are destroyed, acute anuric renal failure will result. Special attention should be given to the possibility of renal failure and to the presence of normal urine output during and immediately following resuscitation of a patient in the shock state. Clinical illness from the renal retention of waste metabolic products will not manifest itself for two to three days following the shock episode.

THE GASTROINTESTINAL TRACT

The gastrointestinal tract of the dog is particularly involved in the vasoconstrictive process of all forms of shock (including early septic shock). An increased portal venous resistance and centrilobular hepatocellular swelling cause portal hypertension and intestinal congestion. Hypoxia, as well as aggregation of white cells and platelets with the release of many vasoactive substances, causes degeneration and death of mucosal epithelial cells, which then separate and slough. Hydrochloric acid in the stomach and pancreatic proteases in the small intestine aid this degenerative process when the epithelial cells lose their protective layer of mucus in the early phases of shock. With progressive increases in capillary permeability, fluid, then plasma, and eventually whole blood are lost into the third space of the gut lumen. This can cause substantial reductions in the circulating blood volume. The mucosal epithelium becomes an ineffective barrier to the systemic absorption of noxious substances present in the gut lumen. The absorption of increasing quantities of these substances easily overwhelms the depressed RE system in the liver, and these noxious substances gain access to the systemic circulation.

THE LIVER

The extent of hepatic sinusoidal congestion, centrolobular necrosis, intrahepatic cholestasis, and post-shock liver enzyme elevation and dysfunction is approximately proportional to the severity and duration of the shock episode.

THE CENTRAL NERVOUS SYSTEM

The central nervous system is relatively spared during mild to moderate stages of early hypovolemic and cardiogenic shock. With progressive hypotension in the later stages of shock, there is a redistribution of cerebral blood flow away from the cerebral cortex in an attempt to preserve perfusion of the medulla and its essential functions. In endotoxic shock there is an early and persistent decrease in cerebral blood flow. Hypocapnia secondary to hyperventilation in the early phases of all types of shock further decreases cerebral blood flow. Hypoglycemia occurring in the intermediate and late stages of all types of shock deprives the brain of energy substrate and, in conjunction with the persistent hypoxia, promotes inadequate energy production. The clinical manifestation of inadequate cerebral energy production includes varying degrees of mental obtundation and ultimately coma and death.

THE HEART

The heart, in the absence of intrinsic failure, is relatively resistant to endogenous noxious materials such as acidosis, myocardial depressant factor, or leucine as long as blood pressure and coronary artery perfusion are maintained. Contractility and cardiac output are decreased in proportion to venous return in early hypovolemic or septic shock and are adversely affected by the hypoxia induced by hypotension and the poor coronary artery blood flow late in shock. Thus it is probably not heart failure *per se* that leads to the demise of the noncardiogenic shock patient. Visceral organ failure, extravasation of vascular volume, decreased venous return, and arteriolar vasodilation create a set of circumstances in which the heart can no longer perform adequately. The emphasis of therapy should therefore be directed at the noncardiac sources of systemic failure rather than the heart directly unless a component of intrinsic heart failure exists.

THE METABOLIC RESPONSE TO INJURY

The metabolic response to injury may be conceptually divided into three phases: (1) the shock phase just described, (2) the hypermetabolic catabolic phase, and (3) the tissue restorative anabolic phase. The characteristics of each phase are regulated by inevitable endogenous hormonal changes attempting to preserve vital organ perfusion in the shock phase and provide a continued source of energy substrates in the catabolic phase. If these compensatory homeostatic mechanisms are effective, tissue rebuilding will occur after the primary disease process is abated.

Energy expenditure is decreased during the shock phase (except in septic shock). Once the cardiovascular imbalance has been adequately managed, there will be an increased energy expenditure associated with the inflammatory process of any ongoing injury (fractures, soft tissue trauma, surgical procedures, sepsis, burn injury, or hypoxic injury from the shock state). Since endogenous glycogen stores are minimal, fat and protein must be catabolized to provide the necessary energy substrate to meet these increased energy requirements. These metabolic changes are vastly different from those seen in simple starvation, in which energy expenditure is low and protein catabolism is relatively spared. The magnitude of the increased energy expenditure during the hypermetabolic catabolic phase is directly proportional to the severity of the ongoing stress process; energy expenditure may be increased only 10 per cent during uncomplicated postoperative convalescence or it may be increased up to 100 per cent in severe sepsis or major third degree burns. Energy expenditure is directly proportional to the extent of the negative nitrogen balance and the rate of weight loss and muscle wasting during this phase. Adequate nutrition is therefore of some importance during this phase to minimize the extent of the tissue catabolism and the morbidities and mortalities associated with inadequate energy production and to reduce the convalescence requirements of the anabolic phase.

MONITORING THE CIRCULATORY COLLAPSE STATES

The initial examination of the shock or trauma patient should involve an assessment of the adequacy of function of the cardiovascular and respiratory systems by answering questions such as, Is the heart beating? Is it beating at an adequate rate (not too fast, not too slow)? Is it beating with or without arrhythmias? Is it putting out anything? What is the status of tissue perfusion? Is the patient breathing? Is it breathing at an adequate rate and volume? Is there any evidence of respiratory neuromuscular disease, loss of thoracic integrity, upper airway obstruction, pleural filling defect, or parenchymal disease? Is there any external or internal hemorrhage that requires immediate attention? Once these immediate life-threatening complications have been investigated and treated, if necessary, attention should be turned to evaluation of central and peripheral nervous system function, mouth and face trauma, fractures and lacerations, competence of the urinary system, abdominal pain, and other examinations attendant to a thorough physical exam.

Shock may be associated with a number of abnormalities (Table 4), which may be minimally to excessively involved in the disease process. It is the purpose of the thorough history and physical and laboratory examinations to determine the extent of the involvement. Interpretation and intercorrelation of each of the measurements help delineate which of the treatment options would be most efficacious for a particular patient.

THE CARDIOVASCULAR SYSTEM

There are a variety of ways in which normal cardiovascular function may be interfered with. Consequently, it is necessary to monitor a variety of parameters to properly assess the adequacy of cardiovascular function (Fig. 1, Table 5). Each parameter must be evaluated with regard to its individual meaning, but each value has greater importance when interpreted in the context of the recent past history of the patient, in comparison with previous measurements, and in conjunction with other measurements of cardiovascular function. It is important to understand the interrelationship between cardiac output, blood volume, and vasomotor tone and to appreciate the mechanisms by which drugs interact with disease processes so that appropriate and effective corrective therapy can be instituted.

HEART RATE AND RHYTHM

The importance of an abnormal heart rate lies in its effect on cardiac output. A simultaneously measured arterial blood pressure or cardiac output could differentiate those abnormal rates that are not jeopardizing the patient from those that are. In the absence of these measurements it is assumed that heart rates below 60 beats per minute (bpm) (dog and cat) and above 200 to 250 bpm (dog) or 250 to 300 bpm (cat) may have a deleterious effect on blood pressure and therefore may require definitive therapy. Trends of change in the heart rate have far greater importance than single measurements since they reflect a change in the disease-patient-therapy interaction.

The most common arrhythmia observed in critically ill or anesthetized patients (excluding bradycardia and tachycardia) is ventricular ectopic pacemaker activity. The importance of this arrhythmia is that it signals the existence of an underlying disorder that might lead to cardiac arrest if left to run its own course. Whenever irregularities in the rhythm of the heart are detected, they should be identified by electrocardiography and treated appropriately.

CONTRACTILITY AND CARDIAC OUTPUT

Mechanical performance of the heart can be roughly gauged by auscultation of the strength or loudness of each contraction. The routine use of heart sound amplifiers to audibly, continuously, and automatically monitor the rate, rhythm, and loudness of the heart in the anesthetized and critically ill recumbent patient can greatly contribute to effective management. More accurate measures of contractility, such as the maximum velocity of con-

Table 4. *Diagnostic and Therapeutic Considerations in Shock**

Abnormality	Treatment Options
1. Hypovolemia (relative or absolute)	1. Control blood or plasma loss Crystalloids Colloids (plasma, dextran) Whole blood
2. Anemia	2. Red cell transfusion (packed or whole blood)
3. Hypoproteinemia (low colloid oncotic pressure)	3. Colloids a. plasma b. dextrans
4. High peripheral resistance	4. Correction of hypovolemia Glucocorticoids Peripheral vasodilation a. phenothiazines b. minoxidil c. phentolamine d. phenoxybenzamine e. nitroprusside
5. Low output heart failure (acute or chronic)	5. Appropriate preload (fluid volume therapy) Decrease afterload (vasodilation) Cardiotonics: calcium, digitalis, beta-receptor stimulants Catecholamines: dobutamine, dopamine, isoproterenol, mephentermine
6. Oliguria/anuria	6. Correction of hypovolemia or vasoconstriction Diuretics a. furosemide b. mannitol or glucose c. dopamine
7. Hypoxemia	7. Oxygen supplementation (if ventilation is adequate) Ventilation therapy (if ventilation is inadequate)
8. Hypoglycemia	8. Glucose Insulin Potassium
9. Metabolic acidosis	9. Correct hypovolemia and vasoconstriction Sodium bicarbonate
10. Sepsis	10. Remove or drain and flush source of infection Antibiotics
11. Hypercoagulopathy	11. Treatment appropriate to underlying disease process Anticoagulants a. dextran or aspirin b. heparin
12. Consumption coagulopathy	12. Replacement therapy Treatment appropriate to underlying disease process Treatment appropriate to hypercoagulopathy

*For some therapeutic purposes there are several drugs that may be used. When the list is not preceded by a letter, it means that there is no way to predict which drug should be tried first owing to the large number of variables. Those lists that are lettered represent this author's probable choice order based on drug availability, least danger of deleterious consequences, and efficacy.

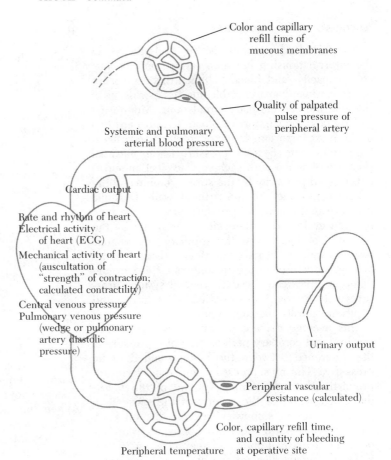

Color and capillary
refill time of
mucous membranes

Quality of palpated
pulse pressure of
peripheral artery

Systemic and pulmonary
arterial blood pressure

Cardiac output

Rate and rhythm of heart
Electrical activity
of heart (ECG)
Mechanical activity of heart
(auscultation of
"strength" of contraction;
calculated contractility)
Central venous pressure
Pulmonary venous pressure
(wedge or pulmonary
artery diastolic
pressure)

Urinary output

Peripheral vascular
resistance (calculated)

Color, capillary refill time,
and quantity of bleeding
Peripheral temperature   at operative site

Figure 1. Multiple parameters of cardiovascular function that could be monitored to assess performance.

traction (Vmax), the maximum rate of the ventricular pressure change during systole (dP/dt), ventricular or aortic pressure contour curves, systolic time intervals, ejection fraction, and ventricular end-diastolic pressure, have been utilized, although there is considerable debate with regard to which value most truly reflects myocardial contractile function. Cardiac output can be measured clinically with indicator-dilution techniques (indocyanin green dye, room temperature or iced saline, or radioactive isotopes) or by the Fick principle or Doppler ultrasonics.

Table 5. *Normal Canine Cardiovascular Values*

Heart rate	70–160 bpm
Cardiac output	150–180 ml/min/kg
Arterial blood pressure	
Systemic	
Systolic	100–160 mm Hg
Mean	70–120 mm Hg
Diastolic	50–100 mm Hg
Pulmonary	
Systolic	20–30 mm Hg
Mean	10–20 mm Hg
Diastolic	5–15 mm Hg
Central venous pressure	0–5 cm H_2O
Pulmonary artery wedge pressure	5–10 mm Hg
Oxygen consumption	5.0–8.0 ml/min/kg

Although the measurement of contractility and cardiac output may elude everyday practice, conceptualization of their importance in determining blood pressure and their impairment by some drugs and disease and enhancement by others must not. The normal heart is somewhat of an obligatory organ in that the cardiac output is directly dependent on venous return (end-diastolic filling volume or preload). Decreases or increases in venous return usually result in immediate decreases or increases in cardiac output, respectively. Inadequate circulating blood volume and insufficient venous return may be the most common causes of cardiovascular insufficiency. Excessive venous return or chronic congestive heart failure results in excessive preload and also diminishes cardiac output. Patients at risk for either condition should receive serial central venous pressure measurements and appropriate fluid therapy. Cardiac output is also diminished by decreases in contractility (hypoeffective heart, cardiogenic shock, acute and chronic heart failure) (see Table 1). Contractility and cardiac output are enhanced by endogenous and exogenous catecholamines, calcium, and optimal preload. Successful management of cardiovascular debilitation involves the application of an appropriate combination of "enhancers" in the face of the particular set of "depressors."

ARTERIAL BLOOD PRESSURE

Arterial blood pressure is the end-product of the interrelationship between cardiac output, vascular capacity, and blood volume. Blood pressure is predominantly responsible for the perfusion of the cerebral and coronary circulations. Monitoring and therapeutic support of blood pressure are two of the most important facets of an effective resuscitative endeavor. Systolic pressure is the maximal pressure obtained with each cardiac ejection and is determined primarily by the stroke volume and the elastic compliance of the arterial wall. Diastolic pressure is the minimal pressure prior to the next ejection cycle and is determined primarily by the "run-off" of blood into the capillary and venous systems and the heart rate. Mean pressure is the average pressure (approximately one-third of the difference between the diastolic and systolic pressures with normal pulse pressure wave forms) and is physiologically the most important force since it is this average driving pressure that determines cerebral and coronary perfusions. Pulse pressure is the difference between the systolic and diastolic pressures. The pulse pressure and wave form are proportional to the stroke volume of the heart; digital palpation of the quality of the pulse in a peripheral artery somewhat reflects this value. A weak, thready pulse is not proof of hypotension but of small stroke volumes and may occur with any tachycardia regardless of the absolute blood pressure.

Arterial blood pressure can be measured by indirect and direct techniques. Indirect sphygmomanometry involves the application of an occlusion cuff over an artery in a cylindrical appendage. Inflation of the cuff applies pressure to the underlying tissues and will totally occlude blood flow through the artery when the pressure exceeds the systolic blood pressure. As the cuff pressure is gradually decreased, blood will flow intermittently when the extraluminal pressure falls below the luminal systolic pressure. Systolic blood pressure is assumed to be represented by the cuff pressure at which blood flow or an arterial pulse can be detected distal to the occlusion cuff. Blood flow will be continuous when the extraluminal pressure decreases below diastolic pressure.

Indirect techniques require an artery that is large enough and superficial enough (e.g., dorsal metatarsal, ventral metatarsal and metacarpal, ulnar, and coccygeal arteries) so that pulsations can be determined by some external method. The dorsal metatarsal artery is the largest and most suitable artery for pulse pickup. The occlusion cuff should be placed snugly around the leg. If it is applied too tightly the pressure measurements will be erroneously low since the cuff itself will partially occlude the underlying artery and little additional cuff pressure will be required. If the cuff is too loose the pressure measurements will be erroneously high since excessive cuff pressure will be required to occlude the underlying artery.

There are several methods of determining blood flow distal to the occlusion cuff. The Korotkoff sounds can be auscultated during progressive deflation of the cuff if the artery is large enough or perhaps if a microphone is used. The first appearance of a clear tapping sound corresponds most closely to arterial systolic blood pressure. The tapping sound will then take on a swishing quality, which increases in intensity. The abrupt muffling or disappearance of this sound is the best index of diastolic blood pressure.

Digital palpation of the first pulse during cuff deflation corresponds approximately to the systolic blood pressure. The first appearance of definite needle oscillations on the manometer during cuff deflation is caused by the pulse wave hitting the cuff and corresponds approximately to systolic blood pressure.

Ultrasonic instrumentation has greatly facilitated accurate blood pressure measurements in small animals. A small piezoelectric crystal transmits ultrasound energy into the underlying tissues. Reflected energy is picked up by a receiving crystal. When the underlying tissues are moving, the reflected energy frequency is shifted slightly from that which was transmitted. This frequency difference is converted electronically to an audible signal. Some instruments measure blood flow* and are used for measuring systolic blood pressure. Other instruments measure movement of the arterial wall† and can be used for measuring both systolic and diastolic blood pressures. There is an excellent correlation between the measurements made by these instruments and direct arterial blood pressure measurements made over a wide range of blood pressures under ideal conditions.

All external techniques are, unfortunately, least accurate when the vessels are small, when the blood pressure is low, and when the vessels are constricted. Owing to the variabilities inherent in the technique, clinical measurements should be considered approximations of blood pressure rather than absolute accurate measurements.

Direct measurements of arterial blood pressure are more accurate and continuous compared with indirect methods but require the introduction of a catheter into an artery by percutaneous or cutdown procedure. The femoral, dorsal metatarsal, radial, and brachial arteries are available for percutaneous catheterization in the conscious dog. The lingual artery may be catheterized, and the carotid artery is available for surgical exposure in the anesthetized

---

*Parks Electronics, Beaverton, OR.
†Roche Medical Electronics, Cranbury, NJ; Sphygmetrics, Woodland Hills, CA.

dog. The femoral and carotid arteries are available for surgical exposure in the anesthetized cat.

Once the arterial catheter is in place, it may be attached to any of a variety of instruments for the measurement of blood pressure: (1) a long fluid administration set suspended from the ceiling; (2) an anaeroid manometer via a length of extension tubing or commercial or homemade diaphragm system; or (3) a pressure transducer and display device (write-out or oscilloscope) (Haskins, 1981). The first two methods measure mean blood pressure and are very economical. The last·method measures both systolic and diastolic pressures and facilitates continuous measurement with less ongoing maintenance. All methods are accurate assuming proper function of the measuring device, which should periodically be calibrated against a mercury column.

CENTRAL VENOUS PRESSURE

Central venous pressure (CVP) is the luminal pressure of the intrathoracic anterior vena cava. It is an indication of the ability of the heart to pump the quantity of fluids being returned to it and is an estimate of the relationship between blood volume and blood volume capacity. It should be measured whenever heart failure is suspected or rapid changes in blood volume are expected.

The CVP increases if the pump begins to fail, as seen with venoconstriction (a decrease in the volume capacity) and hypervolemia. The CVP decreases with vasodilation (an increase in the volume capacity) and hypovolemia. CVP measurements are affected by changes in pleural pressure during spontaneous (inspiration causes a synchronous decrease) or positive pressure (causes an increase) ventilation. A thoracotomy will increase the measured CVP by 2 to 6 cm H_2O. Obstructions to venous return peripheral to the site of measurement during upper abdominal or thoracic surgery decrease the measured CVP. Since the CVP is affected by many variables, all measurements must be related to the patient's recent past history, previous measurements, and other measurements of cardiovascular function before a proper interpretation can be made.

Catheters should be positioned in the anterior vena cava. Contact with the endocardium of the right atrium or the right ventricle should be avoided, since this may stimulate ectopic pacemaker activity. The proper placement of an unobstructed catheter can be verified by observing small fluctuations in the fluid meniscus within the manometer synchronous with the heart beat and larger excursions synchronous with ventilation.

Manometers for CVP measurements may be obtained commercially or may be constructed by taping extension tubing to a ruler with centimeter gradations. A rough estimation of the central venous pressure can be obtained by gradually lowering the fluid bottle until the fluid drip ceases (compare level of fluid in the drip reservoir with the "zero" point).

The "zero" point is estimated as a point on the manometer that is horizontally level with the end of the catheter. The difference between the level of the fluid meniscus in the column manometer after equilibration and the "zero" point is the CVP measurement (Haskins, 1981).

Normal central venous pressure is most commonly between 0 and 5 cm H_2O. Measurements in the range of 15 to 20 cm H_2O are too high, and serious efforts should be made to determine and treat the cause of the elevation. High normal CVP values may occur during hypovolemia owing to vasoconstriction; this does not contraindicate the administration of fluids when other parameters of cardiovascular function indicate hypovolemia. A test dose of fluids should be given. In some cases the CVP will actually decrease in response to fluid loading owing to the abatement of sympathetic venoconstriction. Further elevation of the CVP confirms that fluid loading was the wrong choice.

CVP is a measure of the filling pressure to the right side of the heart and may not accurately reflect events on the left side of the heart. Left heart failure may be associated with pulmonary edema with no change in the CVP measurement. The best clinical approach to obtaining knowledge with respect to the performance of the left heart is to pass a catheter (Silastic, polyethylene, or ballooned-tipped flow-directed) into the pulmonary artery via the jugular vein and force it to wedge into the periphery of the pulmonary arterial tree. The measured pressure is assumed to represent the·"back pressure" from the pulmonary veins. The balloon-tipped catheter is ideal for this purpose because it can be positioned so that when the balloon is deflated pulmonary artery pressure is measured and when it is inflated wedge pressure is measured. In the absence of tachycardia or wide pleural pressure swings, the pulmonary arterial diastolic pressure may be used to estimate the wedge pressure.

MEASURES OF PERIPHERAL PERFUSION

1. Capillary refill time (CRT) is the rate at which blood flows back into a capillary bed that has been digitally compressed and is determined specifically by arteriolar vasomotor tone. It is normally less than one second. It may be prolonged by any disorder that increases sympathetic tone and peripheral vasoconstriction (hypovolemia, hemorrhagic shock, pain, or the excitement stage of general anesthesia).

2. Pale color to the mucous membranes of the mouth and at the operative site; decrease or absence of bleeding at the operative site; both indicate vasoconstriction.

3. A decrease or absence of urinary output indicates decreased visceral organ perfusion.

4. A decrease in peripheral (skin, muscle, toe web) temperature and an increased difference between the core temperature and that of the periphery indicate peripheral vsoconstriction.

Measures of cardiovascular and respiratory function, the clinical level of mentation and reflex activity, body temperature, adequacy of urinary output, electrical activity of the heart, and appropriate radiographic investigations should be repeated as often as necessary to keep abreast of changing patient conditions.

LABORATORY EVALUATION

Since blood loss and hemodilutional anemia and hypoproteinemia are common problems in the shock patient, hematocrit and total protein measurements should be repeated frequently. White cell counts have some diagnostic and prognostic importance and should perhaps be repeated daily for the first several days. Screening tests that reflect the extent of visceral organ damage should be done: urea nitrogen or creatinine for urinary tract damage; ALT (alanine transaminase, formerly known as glutamic pyruvic transaminase) and ALP (alkaline phosphatase) for liver damage; AST (aspartate transaminase, formerly known as glutamic-oxaloacetic transaminase) or LDH (lactic dehydrogenase) for general tissue damage; and lipase or amylase for pancreatic damage. Electrolytes (sodium, potassium, and chloride) are not likely to be a problem in shock *per se* but should be evaluated if there is historical evidence that they are likely to be a problem (i.e., protracted vomiting, diarrhea, diuresis, or anorexia) or perhaps on a daily basis to monitor patient response to fluid therapy. Body weight and other parameters of hydration should be evaluated several times daily.

Laboratory evaluation of the acid-base status of the patient is of some importance, since all forms of shock are associated with metabolic acidosis and it would be therapeutically advantageous to be able to quantitate the amount of bicarbonate to administer. Metabolic acidosis is common. Acidemia, however, is less frequent, depending on the respiratory contribution to the acid-base balance. Hyperventilation-induced respiratory alkalosis secondary to hypotension and medullary hypoxia may generate an alkalemia in the face of a moderate to severe metabolic acidosis. In this example, bicarbonate therapy is not indicated as a first order of therapy and should await effective treatment of the underlying cause of the hyperventilation.

Laboratory instruments that measure bicarbonate (Oxford titrator) or total CO_2 (Harleco apparatus) provide information about the metabolic component but may be misleading if used to quantitate therapy without regard to the respiratory component. For this reason a complete arterial acid-base profile should be measured whenever possible. Commercial pH and blood gas analyzers also measure the arterial partial pressure of oxygen so that the oxygenating efficiency of the lungs can be simultaneously evaluated. An arterial blood sample can be stored in an ice water bath for several hours, to allow time for transport to a nearby facility for measurement, without important changes in the measured values owing to storage. Interpretation of pH and blood gas measurements is discussed in depth elsewhere.

Hyper- and hypocoagulation states occur in all forms of shock. *In vitro* whole blood clotting times, activated coagulation times, or partial thromboplastin times should be measured at periodic intervals to evaluate the performance of the coagulation cascade. Platelet numbers should be evaluated on a blood smear or by actual count and function estimated by measurement of bleeding time, observation of clot retraction, or platelet aggregometry. Measurement of fibrinogen concentration and fibrin split products is feasible and may provide important information with regard to the activity of the coagulation and fibrinolytic cascades. The causes and treatment of disturbances of blood coagulation are discussed in detail elsewhere.

Blood glucose is initially elevated in shock but becomes depressed in the middle and late stages of all forms of shock and should be monitored and supplemented when necessary.

TREATMENT OF SHOCK

The most important therapeutic component of shock and the circulatory collapse states is appropriate fluid therapy. In some cases, when effective fluid therapy is instituted early in the shock process, the patient responds well and there is no need to become involved in other in-depth monitoring procedures and therapeutic modalities. Patients that are not presented until much later in the shock process, that do not respond dramatically to initial fluid therapy, or that cannot sustain cardiovascular and respiratory homeostasis require more critical monitoring and more extensive therapeutic intervention.

Table 4 outlines the common categories of abnormalities associated with the various shock states and lists the treatment options available for each. The table could be used as a problem checklist. Repeated physical examinations and laboratory measurements during the progress of the treatment endeavor to define the extent of the patient's involvement with each abnormality.

FLUID THERAPY

The amount of fluids required for blood volume replacement is determined by the multiple measurements of cardiovascular function as previously discussed. The type of fluid to administer is determined by the balance of the measured constituents of the blood (Table 6). The choice of fluids for blood volume support should generally be those that are maintained within the extracellular fluid space or the vascular space. This excludes 5 per cent dextrose in water, tap water, and hypotonic sodium maintenance solutions. Although these may eventually be needed to correct intracellular volume deficits or hypernatremia, they are not efficient blood volume expanders and should not be used for this purpose. When administered in large volumes, these fluids cause intracellular edema. A multi-electrolyte sodium-containing crystalloid replacement solution is usually the fluid of choice to start replacement therapy. These fluids are relatively economical, can be administered fairly rapidly, and are good extracellular fluid volume expanders.

Crystalloid fluids cause dilution of blood particles such as red blood cells, protein, and coagulation factors (anemia and hypoproteinemia constitute the primary limiting factors to the administration of these fluids). When the packed cell volume falls below 20 per cent and further volume therapy is needed, the infusion of red blood cells is indicated. When the total plasma proteins fall below 3.0 to 3.5 gm/dl (assuming a normal albumin/globulin ratio)

and further volume therapy is needed, the infusion of plasma or a colloid substitute such as dextran 70 is indicated.

If, during an operative procedure or during maintenance fluid therapy, signs of moderate or severe hypovolemia or hypotension exist, a loading dose of fluids (start with lactated Ringer's or an equivalent solution unless contraindicated) should be administered. The dosage may range from 20 to 90 ml/kg of body weight in the dog and 10 to 60 ml/kg in the cat, depending on the needs of the patient. This loading dose of fluid should be administered rapidly (10 to 30 minutes, depending on the volume) so that optimal hemodynamics can be restored as soon as possible. Patients with normal heart and lungs are quite tolerant to fluid loading with regard to the development of airway and alveolar edema. Patients with pulmonary disease or heart failure may, however, be very sensitive to fluid loading. CVP measurements should be utilized to monitor the volume and rate of fluid administration if there is any doubt about the ability of the patient to tolerate the quantity of fluids in question. Rising values associated with rapid fluid administration indicate filling of the vascular volume capacity. Excessively high pressures (>15 cm H_2O) indicate overfilling of the vascular compartment. Fluids should also be administered with care in patients with renal failure and when colloid solutions are used.

A considerable depletion of blood volume (10 to 20 per cent) may occur before any overt signs of hypovolemia, hypotension, or shock are manifested

Table 6. *Important Considerations in Replacement Fluid Therapy**

Parameter	Applicable Measurement and Desired Level	Fluids of Choice if Measured Parameter is Outside Desired Level
Volume	Central venous pressure: 2 to 10 cm H_2O	1. Crystalloid sodium replacement solution (lactated Ringer's)†
	Arterial blood pressure: 70 to 120 mm Hg (mean)	2. Colloid expander (dextran, plasma)
	Pulse quality: strong Capillary refill time: <1 second Mucous membrane color: pink Normal skin turgor	3. Whole blood
Oxygen-carrying capacity	Packed cell volume: >20 per cent Hemoglobin: >7 gm/dl	1. Whole blood
Colloid oncotic pressure	Total plasma protein: >3.5 gm/dl	1. Colloid expander (plasma, dextran) 2. Whole blood
Osmolality	Sodium concentration: 130 to 160 mEq/L Serum osmolality: 270 to 330 mOsm/kg	1. Crystalloid sodium replacement solution to maintain (lactated Ringer's) or increase (saline) sodium concentration 2. Hypotonic solution to decrease osmolality (1/2 lactated Ringer's or saline and 1/2 5 per cent dextrose in water)
Viscosity	Packed cell volume: <60 per cent	1. Crystalloid sodium replacement solution (lactated Ringer's)

*Potassium and bicarbonate should be added as necessary.
†Lactated Ringer's solution or any equivalent isonatremic solution.

owing to the efficiency of compensatory mechanisms. Therefore, in repletion therapy, the rapid fluid administration should be continued somewhat beyond the point of restoration of the signs of acceptable cardiovascular performance. Recurrence of the signs of hypovolemia may be due to continued fluid loss at the original site, to a redistribution of the administered fluid out of the vascular compartment, or to renal excretion and indicates the need for further volume therapy.

There is no fluid that will fulfill all of the fluid requirements of all patients. Fluid therapy must be tailored to meet the needs of each patient. From the standpoint of volume requirements, there are a variety of fluids that have been shown to be efficacious. In many situations the logical choice of fluids represents an economical decision. The concentration of the constituent elements should be remeasured during acute replacement therapy as often as is necessary to assure that they remain within tolerable limits.

Sodium replacement solutions

Isotonic sodium replacement solutions, such as lactated Ringer's, Ringer's saline, and other equivalent solutions, are commonly used for blood volume support or, more accurately, extracellular volume support. Sodium freely diffuses across capillary membranes but is actively maintained outside of the cells.

During hemorrhagic shock, blood flow to the peripheral tissues is markedly slowed, blood viscosity is maximized, and adherence of red blood cells and platelets to each other and to the capillary endothelium is prominent. The administration of blood may enhance these effects. Crystalloid or colloid clear fluids cause hemodilution and help decrease the incidence of microcirculatory sludging. Excessive hemodilution should be avoided. In those patients with severe blood loss both crystalloid and whole blood administration may be necessary for successful resuscitation.

The obligate expansion of the interstitial fluid spaces associated with large volume crystalloid fluid infusion may be detrimental to the patient if it is excessive. The normal hormonal response during the shock and catabolic phases of injury promotes retention of these fluids and may facilitate accidental overloading. Interstitial lung edema decreases lung compliance and increases the work of breathing. Intracerebral edema causes varying degrees of depressed mentation. The potential for intraorgan interstitial edema to interfere with renal, hepatic, and gastrointestinal function is readily apparent. Subsequent to the initial restoration of intravascular and interstitial deficits and the balancing of plasma colloid oncotic pressure (as determined indirectly by total plasma protein measurements) and plasma osmolality (as determined by measured sodium concentration or osmolality), further crystalloid fluid-induced weight gain or subcutaneous edema production should be minimized. The more efficient colloidal solutions should be considered if further blood volume expansion is indicated.

Colloids

The efficiency of sodium replacement solutions for volume expansion is limited in that 75 to 80 per cent of the administered volume is distributed into the interstitial fluid compartment or excreted by the kidneys after about 30 minutes. This phenomenon may be clinically associated with the deterioration of cardiovascular parameters and may signal the need for further fluid administration. This may be in the form of more sodium replacement solution or colloid blood volume expanders such as dextran, plasma, or whole blood. Colloid blood volume expanders are fluids that contain particles of sufficient size that they do not rapidly leak through the vascular membranes; thus they are more efficient volume expanders than the crystalloid sodium solutions (Table 7).

Although glucose and mannitol may cause severe hypervolemia and appropriate precaution should be exercised when administering these agents rapidly, their duration of action is so transient that they are not recommended for use as blood volume expanders.

The dextrans are high molecular weight polysaccharides. Although they are produced in all molecular sizes, the two commonly marketed forms are low molecular weight dextran (average MW 40,000; 10 per cent solution) and high molecular weight dextran (average MW 70,000; 6 per cent solution). These are very hypertonic solutions (2.5 per cent dextran 40 and 3.5 per cent dextran 70 are approximately isotonic) and initially attract additional water into the vascular space, increasing the plasma volume more than the actual volume administered to the patient. The initial hypervolemic effects of dextran 40 are greater than those of dextran 70, but its plasma half-life is shorter owing to its smaller molecular size. Consequently the preferable agent for blood volume support and albumin-replacing plasma colloid oncotic pressure support is dextran 70. Both dextrans decrease red cell and platelet aggregation and therefore reduce the incidence of perioperative thrombosis. Dextran 40 decreases blood viscosity more than dextran 70 and should be used when improved microcirculatory blood flow and decreased peripheral vascular resistance are high priorities. Both agents may cause a hemorrhagic diathesis or excessive hypervolemia if given too fast or in too great a quantity. Gelatin and starch preparations are commercially available and have the same basic indications and precautions discussed for the dextrans (see Table 7).

Table 7. Colloid Plasma Expanders

Generic Product	Trade Name (Manufacturer)	Molecular Weight	Renal Excretion T1/2 (hrs)	Dosage*	Primary Uses and Indications	Precautions and Contraindications
Gelatin	Gelofusine 4% (Consolidated Chemicals)	30,000		20–30 ml/kg	Blood volume expansion Amino acid precursor	Hypervolemia Allergic reactions
	Haemacel 3.5% (Hoechst)	35,000				
Dextran	Gentran 40 (Travenol) Lomodex 40 (Fisons) Rheomacrodex (Pharmacia: Farillon)	40,000	3	20 ml/kg	Decrease blood viscosity and peripheral vascular resistance Decrease red cell and platelet aggregation Decrease thrombosis Marked, transient, blood volume expansion	Hemorrhagic diathesis if given too fast or too much Hypervolemia, congestive heart failure, and pulmonary edema Allergic reactions
	Gentran 70 (Travenol) Lomodex 70 (Fisons) Macrodex (Pharmacia: Farillon)	70,000	24	10–20 ml/kg/day	Same as dextran 40 except no change in viscosity More prolonged blood volume expansion	High doses may increase viscosity and vascular resistance (and afterload) Same as dextran 40 May interfere with crossmatching and blood typing procedures
Hydroxyethyl starch	Hetastarch 6%	400,000	24	10–20 ml/kg/day	Prolonged blood volume expansion	Same as dextran 40 and 70

*Must be administered over several hours to prevent vascular overload.

Plasma provides for more prolonged support of blood volume and colloid oncotic pressure. The natural half-life for canine albumin is 12 to 18 days, although this may be shortened by immune-mediated mechanisms. The other major advantage of plasma compared with dextran 70 is that the contained protein can serve as an energy substrate and can be utilized as an amino acid source for the construction of other protein molecules. To this end, the artificial colloid expanders should be considered as temporary replacements only and should not be used to the total exclusion of plasma or to the depletion of plasma proteins in diseases associated with transudative proteinaceous fluid losses.

Whole blood

Packed cell transfusions are primarily indicated in the anemic normovolemic patient. Whole blood transfusions are indicated in the anemic hypovolemic patient. Relatively large quantities of whole blood transfusions are necessary for meaningful elevation of hemoglobin concentration. For example, a 15-kg dog with a hemoglobin of 5 gm/dl has a blood volume of about 1350 ml and a hemoglobin mass of 67.5 gm. If it is desirable to increase the hemoglobin concentration to 10 gm/dl (a hemoglobin mass of 135 gm), 67.5 gm of hemoglobin must be infused. If the blood to be administered has, for example, a hemoglobin concentration of 15 gm/dl, 450 ml will need to be administered.

There are eight recognized canine erythrocytic antigens. All may cause a transfusion reaction on occasion, but only type A is antigenic enough to require routine consideration. Dogs have few problems with naturally occurring isoantibodies compared with humans. The A-positive antigen will stimulate the formation of antibodies in A-negative recipients. This will cause delayed destruction of red cells from the first transfusion and acute destruction of A-positive red cells from subsequent transfusions. These reactions will negate any beneficial effect of the transfusion and increase the metabolic requirements of the patient and may be toxic to the kidney. Dogs that are maintained for blood donor purposes should be typed to make sure they are A-negative. There has been little work done with feline blood groups. There are only three recognized red cell antigens, most of which are the same type. Blood typing in cats is less important than in dogs. Pretransfusion crossmatching and observation for hemolysis, vomiting, and icterus in the recipient are recommended when multiple transfusions are administered. The rapid infusion of homologous protein may cause a histamine-mediated reaction, which is manifested by urticaria, a rapid loss of the intravascular plasma protein, and possibly circulatory collapse.

The anticoagulants that are commonly used for *in vitro* transfer of blood are heparin, acid-citrate-dextrose (ACD), and citrate-phosphate-dextrose (CPD). CPD anticoagulant should be used if the blood is to be stored for any length of time. CPD anticoagulant is a better blood preservative than ACD. Red cell ATP and 2,3 DPG are maintained at higher levels for longer periods of time. CPD contains less citric acid, and therefore CPD-preserved blood produces less acidosis in the recipient.

When large transfusions are given, care should be exercised not to anticoagulate the recipient. If bleeding becomes a problem, protamine sulfate (Lilly) may be administered to counteract the effect of heparin (about 1 mg/mg of residual heparin, which has a half-life of two to four hours); or calcium to counteract the effect of the citrate (about 6 ml of 10 per cent CaCl per 67.5 ml of citrate solution). The cold temperature of stored blood may cause hypothermia in small patients receiving large quantities of blood. The blood can be warmed in a warm water bath ($< 42°$ C). Hyperkalemia in stored blood following the degeneration of stored red cells is not a problem in canine blood because of the low intraerythrocyte potassium concentration. When citrated fluids are administered at very rapid rates, they may have a marked negative inotropic effect (due to hypocalcemia). The magnitude of the cardiac depression is dependent upon the extent of free calcium binding and is accentuated by hypoxia and acidosis. It can be prevented by slowing the infusion rate and by the simultaneous administration of calcium chloride. The formation of microaggregates of platelets and fibrin in stored blood has been identified and may be responsible for pulmonary microvascular alterations when microfilters (20 to 50 μ) are not used. Platelets and a few other coagulation factors do not survive storage for more than a couple of days. If these factors are a required portion of the intended transfusion, fresh whole blood should be administered.

2,3 Diphosphoglycerate (2,3 DPG) is an important intraerythrocytic organic phosphate that affects the hemoglobin affinity for oxygen. A progressive depletion of 2,3 DPG occurs after one to two weeks of blood storage, resulting in an increased hemoglobin-oxygen affinity, which impairs the unloading of oxygen at the tissue level. When it can be foreseen that a blood transfusion will be necessary, it should be administered 6 to 12 hours before surgery so that there will be adequate time for the recipient to regenerate the 2,3 DPG in the transfused cells.

Glucocorticoids

Pharmacologic doses of glucocorticoids have been shown to improve survival in experimental animals, as well as clinically in humans, in all forms of shock (Shatney and Lillehei, 1981). They should be used early in the course of therapy in severely involved cases or in those in which initial fluid therapy alone is not expected to be totally curative. One of their most important effects relates to their ability to restore and stabilize vascular and lysosomal membrane integrity in all organs. Many of the deleterious effects of shock are related to capillary leakage of plasma and red cells into the interstitium and luminal spaces within the intestines, lungs, central nervous system, and other organs; and to the lysosomal leakage of proteolytic enzymes. Improved platelet and leukocyte membrane stability is probably responsible for decreased aggregation and sequestration of these cells in the microcirculation. The other important function of corticosteroids is their ability to reduce arteriolar and venular resistance and thus improve visceral and coronary blood flow and oxygenation, enhance venous return and cardiac output, and minimize lactic acid production.

Pharmacologic dosages (Table 8) should be administered over a ten-minute period and should be repeated at approximately 8- to 12-hour intervals for no more than one to two days and then stopped abruptly. With this dosage regimen there will be no residual depression of the pituitary-adrenal axis, the immune system, or wound healing. There is no evidence that any one glucocorticoid is more efficacious than any other.

VASODILATION

If low output heart failure persists subsequent to optimizing preload (mid range to high normal measurements of pulmonary capillary wedge pressure and central venous pressure) and there is evidence of high peripheral vascular resistance, pharmacologic vasodilation may be indicated. This will decrease mean and diastolic arterial pressure and decrease the pressure that the heart must pump against (afterload). It will also enhance venous return and diastolic ventricular filling (preload). The agents of choice, because of their established effectiveness and low morbidity, are pharmacologic doses of glucocorticoids. If their effectiveness is judged (by clinical signs or measurements) to be less than adequate, other, more potent, vasodilators could be used (Table 9). The vasodilation caused by these agents can be dramatic, and they should not be utilized without ongoing blood pressure measurements. An appropriate volume of fluids should be administered prior to their use to prevent undue hypotension. The phenothiazine tranquilizers, unfortunately, cause some depression of mental function, which may interfere with the evaluation of the patient's response to therapy.

Isoproterenol has peripheral vasodilating properties (beta-receptor stimulation), but its use should be limited to patients with coexisting bradycardia or poor myocardial contractility. It should not be used in patients exhibiting tachycardia or those without a fluid volume preload. Dopamine has peripheral vasodilating properties (dopaminergic-renal-receptor and beta-receptor stimulation) when used in small amounts (Table 10). Its primary use in this regard is to stimulate urine output when everything else has failed. In contrast to isoproterenol, when it is used in quantities sufficient to stimulate the cardiovascular system, its alpha-receptor stimulating properties will override the vasodilating effect discussed previously. Furosemide exhibits some mild vasodilating properties, which may be advantageous if the drug is being used as a diuretic.

CARDIOTONICS

If low output failure persists subsequent to optimizing preload and afterload, cardiotonic agents may be indicated. Glucagon increases cardiac output, lowers peripheral vascular resistance, and improves hepatic metabolic activity experimentally, but its clinical efficacy has not been established. Calcium and digitalis preparations improve cardiac contractility and output. The effects of calcium are transient but if found to be beneficial serve as indications for digitalization of the patient.

The use of catecholamines with potent alpha-receptor agonist activity (see Table 10) is not indicated for shock except as an initial treatment in the severely hypovolemic patient. When the patient is first presented it may be necessary to pharmacologically support blood pressure long enough to allow time for blood volume restitution.

Agents that cause vasodilation or minimal vasoconstriction should be used for more prolonged blood pressure support (dopamine, isoproterenol, dobutamine, or mephentermine; see Table 10). These agents may cause excessive hypertension and arrhythmias, and their use should be appropriately monitored to assure that they are effective in treating the hypotension without manifesting these adverse effects. It is not possible to predict or recommend which of these agents would be most appropriate for any particular situation because there are too many variables. The following discussion serves as a partial answer to this question. There is enough pharmacologic difference between the agents that there should be no hesitation in switching to another if the first does not bring about the desired changes or if it causes untoward effects.

Isoproterenol can be used if bradycardia or heart failure is the cause of the hypotension. It provides good vasodilation and tissue perfusion and, for this reason, may cause excessive hypotension if there is a large vasoconstrictive component to the disease process. Dosages of 0.01 to 0.06 µg/kg/min effectively increase contractility and cardiac output with

Text continued on page 22

Table 8.   *Characteristics of Common Glucocorticoid Agents*

Agent	Trade Name (Manufacturer)	Relative Glucocorticoid Activity	Relative Mineralo-corticoid Activity	Approximate Physiologic Replacement Dosage (mg/kg/day)	Pharmacologic Shock Dosage (mg/kg)	Approximate Duration of Action (hr)*
Dexamethasone sodium phosphate	Decadron Phosphate (Merck Sharp and Dohme) Hexadrol (Organon) Dexamethasone Sodium Phos (Med-Tech)	33.0	0	.01	4–6	10–12
Dexamethasone in polyethylene glycol†	Dexamethasone (Pfizer) Dexasone (Med-Tech; Beecham, Pitman-Moore)					
Methylprednisolone sodium succinate	Solu-Medrol (Upjohn)	5.0	0	.05–.06	30	10–12
Prednisolone sodium succinate	Solu-Delta-Cortef (Upjohn)	4.0	1	.05–.10	35	10–12
Prednisolone sodium phosphate	Codelsol (Merck Sharp and Dohme)					
Hydrocortisone sodium succinate	Solu-Cortef (Upjohn)	1.0	2	.25–.30	150	6–8

*Plasma half-life × 3.
†Cellular uptake may be slower than that of other steroidal preparations.

Table 9. *Vasodilating Agents*

Generic Name	Trade Name (Manufacturer)	Dosage and Mode of Administration	Maximum Effect (Plasma T1/2)	Mechanism of Vasodilation	Precautions and Contraindications
Phenothiazines	Acepromazine (Ayerst)	0.01–0.05 mg/kg IV	10–15 min (1–2 hr)	Alpha-receptor blockade	Hypotension
Minoxidil	(Upjohn)	2 mg/kg	60 min (4 hr)	Vascular smooth muscle relaxant	Hypotension
Phentolamine mesylate	Regitine (Ciba)	Dilute in saline; administer at 5–30 µg/kg/min	2 min (5 min)	Alpha-receptor blockade	Hypotension
Phenoxybenzamine	Dibenzyline (Smith, Kline and French)	0.5–1.0 mg/kg diluted in saline; administered over a 1-hour period	60 min (12 hr)	Alpha-receptor blockade	Hypotension
Nitroprusside	Nipride (Roche)	Dilute in D$_5$W; administer at 1 µg/kg/min	Immediate (1 min)	Vascular smooth muscle relaxant	Hypotension Denatured by light Avoid in hepatic or renal failure Increased plasma concentrations of cyanide and thiocyanate (keep dosage below 1.5 mg/kg/2 hr)

Table 10.   *Sympathomimetics Used for Cardiovascular Support*

Drug (Receptor Activity)	Trade Name (Manufacturer)	Myocardial Chronotropy and Inotropy	Peripheral Vasomotor Tone	Major Indication	Dosage (IV)
Catecholamines					
Epinephrine (α+++; β+++)	Adrenalin (Parke-Davis; Vitarine; Bristol)	Increased	Increased	Cardiac arrest resuscitation	0.05–0.5 mg (.5 to 5 ml 1:10,000 solution) for average-sized dog (15 kg)
Norepinephrine (α+++; β+)	Levophed bitartrate (Breon)	Variable	Increased	Vasoconstriction	0.10–1.0 mg for average-sized dog (15 kg)
Dopamine (dopa and β+++; α++)	Intropin (Arnar-Stone)	Increased	Variable	Blood pressure support ↑visceral perfusion	10–50 μg/kg/min 2.0–5 μg/kg/min 80–200 mg in 500 ml D$_5$W
Isoproterenol (α0; β+++)	Isuprel (Winthrop)	Increased	Decreased	Cardiac stimulation	0.4–1.0 mg in 500 ml D$_5$W (to effect; start 0.01 μg/kg/min)

Noncatecholamines					
Mephentermine (α+; β++)	Wyamine (Wyeth)	Increased	Variable	Blood pressure support	0.1–0.75 mg/kg
Metaraminol (α+++; β+)	Aramine (Merck Sharp and Dohme) Metaraminol bitartrate (Bristol; Invenex)	Variable	Increased	Vasoconstriction	0.1–0.2 mg/kg
Methoxamine (α+++; β0)	Vasoxyl (Burroughs Wellcome)	None	Increased	Vasoconstriction	0.1–0.2 mg/kg
Phenylephrine (α+++; β0)	Neo-Synephrine	None	Increased	Vasoconstriction	0.01–0.1 mg/kg
Dobutamine (α+; β+++)	Dobutrex (Lilly)	Increased	Variable	Blood pressure support	100–400 mg in 500 ml D₅W (to effect; start 5 µg/kg/min)
Ephedrine (α++; β+)	(Vitarine)	Increased	Variable	Blood pressure support	0.05–0.5 mg/kg IV, IM
Miscellaneous					
Calcium	(Bristol; Invenex; Vitarine)	Increased	Variable	Increase contractility	10% CaCl 1.5–2.0 ml 10% CaGluc 6–8 ml for average-sized dog
Digitalis Digoxin Digitoxin	(Wellcome) (Parke-Davis)	Increased	No direct effect	Increase contractility	Loading dose: 0.02–0.04 mg/kg divided into 4 doses over 48 hours Maintenance: 0.02–0.04 mg/kg divided b.i.d.
Glucagon	(Lilly)	Increased (variable effect on heart rate)	Decreased	Increase contractility	25–100 µg/kg/hr

minimal chronotropic effects in humans (Shoemaker, 1976). Higher dosages are associated with tachycardia and arrhythmias with little further improvement in cardiac output. When isoproterenol infusions are used without benefit of cardiac output measurements, the endpoint of the titration procedure (the highest infusion rate) should be (1) when the apparent peripheral tissue perfusion is maximized; (2) when the blood pressure has increased to an acceptable level; or (3) prior to the point at which it causes a marked tachycardia or arrhythmia. Prolonged administration of high dosages has been associated with myocardial necrosis in dogs and cats.

Dopamine causes less vasodilation than isoproterenol and in higher dosages may cause vasoconstriction. It can be used if isoproterenol causes excessive hypotension. It enhances myocardial contractility with less effect on heart rate compared with isoproterenol and should perhaps be used if the initial hypotension is not associated with bradycardia.

Dobutamine has minimal alpha-receptor and strong beta-receptor agonist activities and as such approximately splits the difference between isoproterenol and dopamine. It has less effect on heart rate than isoproterenol but about the same as dopamine. It promotes less peripheral vasoconstriction than dopamine but more than isoproterenol.

All of the previously mentioned agents have short durations of action (three to five minutes) and must therefore be given by constant infusion. They are very potent agents and are easy to overdose, but their effect is short-lived following cessation of the infusion.

Mephentermine has a much longer duration of action (30 minutes) and therefore can be given as an intermittent bolus. It has much less tendency to promote ventricular arrhythmias than any of the previously mentioned agents.

URINARY OUTPUT

Once all volume deficits have been restored, urinary output should be evaluated by frequent urinary bladder palpation or by an indwelling catheter. If urinary output is absent or below 1 ml/kg/ hr, diuretic therapy may be necessary. Furosemide (2.5 to 5.0 mg/kg) is a very effective inhibitor of sodium reabsorption in the ascending loop of Henle and also enhances renal blood flow by promoting vasodilation. If the initial dose does not cause a brisk diuresis, several repeat doses can be administered at 10- to 15-minute intervals. Mannitol or glucose osmotic diuretics (0.5 to 1 gm/kg) may occasionally be effective when furosemide is not. The next to the last resort is a low-dose dopamine infusion (2 to 5 μg/kg/min) to take advantage of its

dopaminergic renal vasodilating properties. A dose that is high enough to increase the heart rate or blood pressure or that causes arrhythmias is also high enough to cause renal vasoconstriction. These signs should be monitored, and the dopamine administration rate should be reduced if they occur. The last resort in the therapy of renal failure is peritoneal dialysis or hemodialysis. The complexity of these procedures underscores the importance of evaluation of renal function and institution of appropriate therapy to restore renal blood flow and urinary output early in the progress of treatment of the shock patient.

Urinary output is used to evaluate total renal blood flow. It does not necessarily prove adequate renal cortical blood flow, but short of extensive radiographic procedures it is the most efficacious clinical method of assessing renal blood flow.

GLUCOSE AND INSULIN

The hormonal response to trauma and shock is an elevation of corticosteroid, catecholamine, and glucagon levels and a decrease in insulin production. These hormonal changes promote hyperglycemia but inhibit peripheral glucose utilization. Hypoglycemia often develops as an intermediate or late event in all forms of shock. Supplemental administration of glucose or glucose and insulin promotes substrate uptake by the heart and brain and improves survival rates by supporting energy production. Insulin infusion must always be supplemented with glucose and potassium, and serial measurements of these components should be made to assure that they remain within acceptable limits.

Glucose should be infused as a 50 per cent solution via a central vein for as many hours as possible over the day at a rate of 0.3 to 2.0 gm/kg/ hr. Insulin should be added to the glucose infusion solution in quantities sufficient to prevent a glucose osmotic diuresis and hyperglycemia (up to about 0.3 unit/gm glucose). Since insulin adheres to the walls of glass bottles, plastic bags, and infusion sets, it is advisable to utilize the same setup for the full infusion period in question. If hyperglycemia develops, the infusion rate should be decreased and/ or the quantity of contained insulin should be increased (in small steps), depending on the severity of the hyperglycemia. The solution should contain potassium at an initial concentration of 20 mEq/L and increased as necessary (up to 60 mEq/L). The glucose solution bottle should be separate from the primary infusion bottle to facilitate control of its specific infusion rate. The glucose solution can mix with the main solution via a T-connector so that only one vein need be catheterized and so that the infused glucose concentration is diluted.

SODIUM BICARBONATE

Sodium bicarbonate is indicated to buffer the metabolic acidosis seen in shock. Its use should be restricted to those patients also manifesting acidemia. The respiratory alkalosis occurring in early shock may more than neutralize the metabolic acidosis and may result in an alkalemia. Alkalinizing therapy in such a patient would be an error. Substantiation of acidemia and definition of the extent of the metabolic acidosis by measurement of a complete acid-base profile (pH, pCO_2, base deficit, bicarbonate) would determine the alkalinizing needs of the patient. Bicarbonate infusion should be titrated to restore the blood pH to between 7.3 and 7.4.

In lieu of a completed acid-base profile, bicarbonate concentration can be estimated (Oxford titrator; Harleco apparatus) and bicarbonate deficit can be calculated. The degree of metabolic acidosis may be estimated (as mild, moderate, or severe) by clinical assessment of the degree and duration of the malperfusion of the peripheral tissues. If the patient is clinically hyperventilating, it may be wise not to administer any bicarbonate. Administer a small to medium-sized dose if the patient is not hyperventilating. If the patient is hypoventilating, intubate and begin positive pressure ventilation and administer a small to medium-sized dose of bicarbonate.

When the base deficit or bicarbonate deficit is known, the dose of sodium bicarbonate to administer is calculated by the following formula: base or bicarbonate deficit × 0.3 × kg body weight. If the extent of the acidosis must be based on a clinical estimation of the extent of tissue malperfusion, mild, moderate, and severe acidosis are equated with bicarbonate dosages of 1.0, 3.0, and 5.0 mEq/kg, respectively. These guidelines have a built-in margin of error to minimize iatrogenic alkalemia.

If the administration of sodium is contraindicated for reasons of hyperosmolality, tromethamine may be administered instead of sodium bicarbonate (Table 11).

ANTIBIOTICS

Sepsis is both a major cause and a consequence of shock. Invasive monitoring procedures expose the patient to an increased risk of infection. Antibiotics, like all other drugs, should not be used indiscriminately or in transient shock states that are rapidly corrected by appropriate fluid therapy. They are indicated for patients known to be septic or those who are highly suspected of becoming septic because of their extensive involvement in the shock state. Prolonged antibiotic therapy should be guided by culture and sensitivity testing in patients with known infections. Short-term therapy for the first one to two days until the sensitivity results return or for a total of one to two days in the difficult-to-treat shock patient with a high infection potential should include broad spectrum antibiotics. The causal organisms of the septicemias in our practice are approximately equally split between gram positive and gram negative organisms with a very few anaerobics. Gentamicin (3 mg/kg IM q6h) as a first choice or trimethoprimsulfadiazine (60 mg/kg IV q12h, initial dose 120 mg/kg) as a second choice (*Pseudomonas* and some *Klebsiella* are resistant) is most likely to be effective against the invading organism. It is common practice to add ampicillin (11 mg/kg IV or IM q6h) to cover anaerobic organisms.

ANTICOAGULANTS

Hypercoagulopathies are usually effectively treated by restoration of an effective circulating blood volume and therapy of the underlying disease process. Occasionally the release of systemic thromboplastin from hypoxic cellular damage and systemic aggregating factors from platelet aggregation causes the hypercoagulopathy to persist during and beyond the physiologic restoration of the patient. Under this circumstance specific anticoagulant therapy may be considered. Low molecular weight dextran and aspirin are the easiest and safest anticoagulants to administer (Table 12). However, their clinical effectiveness in this regard has not been proved. The administration of heparin is fraught with the dangers of overheparinization and bleeding and should probably not be attempted unless 24-hour-a-day observation and frequent monitoring (at least every four hours) of blood coagulation parameters can be arranged. Test tube or capillary tube clotting time, charcoal-activated coagulation time, or partial thromboplastin time may be used to evaluate coagulation. Bleeding time, clot retraction, or platelet aggregation may be used to evaluate platelet function. Sufficient anticoagulant should be administered to maintain the coagulation process in the range of 1.5 to 2.0 times normal. If heparinization is chosen as a modality of therapy, it should be administered in small doses frequently throughout the day or, preferably, continuously to avoid wide swings in coagulation times. If overheparinization occurs, stop the heparin infusion and allow time and metabolism to reduce the high blood heparin levels. If the bleeding is excessive and is not due to factor depletion, the heparin effect may be competitively inhibited with protamine sulfate. The proper dose of protamine is 1 mg/mg of active heparin. The normal plasma half-life of heparin is

Table 11.   Alkalinizing Agents*

Generic Name ("Trade Name")	Dosage	Mechanism of Alkalinization	Major Complications‡
Sodium bicarbonate (MW = 84.0) 1.26% sol is isotonic 1.4% sol = 167 mEq HCO$_3$/L 7.5% sol = 0.89 mEq/ml 8.4% sol = 1 mEq/ml	mEq bicarbonate to administer = a. base deficit† × 0.3 × kg bw b. 1–5 mEq/kg	Bicarbonate combines with hydrogen ion and shifts the carbonic acid equilibration to the left	Hypercapnia in the face of marginal ventilation CSF acidosis Hyperosmolality (intracellular dehydration and intracranial hemorrhage)
Sodium lactate (MW = 112.1) 1.68% sol is isotonic 1.85% sol = 165 mEq La/L	Same as for sodium bicarbonate	Metabolized in liver to pyruvate, consuming a hydrogen ion in the process (requires an oxygenated perfused liver and time)	Avoid in states of liver disease or dysfunction
Sodium acetate (MW = 82.0) 1.23% sol is isotonic	Same as for sodium bicarbonate	Metabolized in liver and muscle and consumes a hydrogen ion in the process	Vasodilation and hypotension Ketogenic
Trihydroxymethylaminomethane "THAM" "TRIS" "Tromethamine" "Trometamol" (MW = 121.1) 3.6% sol is isotonic 3.6% sol = 300 mEq THAM/L	mEq THAM to administer = a. base deficit × 0.4 × kg bw (due to larger volume of distribution) b. 2–6 mEq/kg	Combines with hydrogen ion to form cationic buffer and shifts the carbonic acid equilibration to the right	Hypocapnia and apnea Very irritating (avoid perivascular extravasation; administer in large veins in dilute solutions) Osmotic diuresis

*All agents are available from one or several of the following manufacturers: Abbott, Bristol, Cutter, Invenex, International Medication Systems, McGaw, Tera, Travenol.
†Use bicarbonate deficit if base deficit is not available.
‡Alkalosis is an implied but not stated major complication of any alkali therapy, as is an increased hemoglobin affinity for oxygen and its tendency to reduce plasma potassium concentration.

Table 12. *Anticoagulants*

Agent	Dosage and Mode of Administration	Mechanism of Anticoagulation
Aspirin	10 mg/kg PO q12h	Decreases platelet aggregation Decreases factor XII activity Inhibits prostaglandin production
Low molecular weight dextran (40)	2 ml/kg/hr up to 20 ml/kg	Decreases platelet aggregation Fibrinoplastic effect
Heparin	10 to 25 units/kg/hr	Inhibits factor X_a Inhibits thrombin formation

about two to four hours, and an approximation of the quantity of persistent heparin should be calculated. Excessive doses of protamine also cause bleeding. Utilizing the same infusion apparatus for the heparin for the full 24-hour period will help stabilize the quantity of drug received by the patient.

If the hypercoagulable state is not detected early in the process, coagulation factors may be consumed at a rate exceeding production and their plasma levels will become depleted. The absence of coagulation factors manifests as a hemorrhagic diathesis. Diagnosis is based on severely prolonged times of the coagulation tests, depleted platelet numbers and fibrinogen level, increased fibrin degradation products, and a history of a disease likely to induce coagulation (e.g., trauma, shock, hyperthermia, neoplasia, sepsis, heartworm infestation, extensive surgery). Treatment primarily involves replacement of the factors of coagulation with a fresh whole blood or plasma transfusion and correction of the underlying disease process. Secondary consideration may be given to treatment of the hypercoagulable state.

PROMISING NEW THERAPEUTIC CONCEPTS

There are several agents currently being investigated that demonstrate beneficial effects in the various shock states. Their clinical efficacy with regard to improved patient survival has not yet been established.

Carboxylic ionophores form cationic complexes that facilitate their transport across biologic membranes. Lasalocid (X-537A) forms a complex with calcium and transports it intracellularly. Monensin forms a complex primarily with sodium and increases intracellular sodium concentration, which in turn increases intracellular calcium concentration by a sodium-calcium exchange mechanism (Somani and Saini, 1981). Both agents cause an increased endogenous catecholamine release, myocardial contractility, cardiac output, arterial blood pressure, and coronary and visceral organ perfusion and a decrease in total peripheral resistance.

Verapamil, a slow-channel calcium blocker, has been reported to minimize the portal hypertension and duodenal mucosal necrosis and hemorrhage seen in canine hemorrhagic shock (Whalen et al., 1980). Its mechanism of action is not known. Whether the carboxylic ionophores enhance the intestinal lesions or the calcium blockers depress cardiovascular homeostasis remains to be determined.

Aspirin and indomethacin, inhibitors of prostaglandin synthesis, prevent the vascular constriction response associated with platelet aggregation but do not prevent and may even enhance pulmonary platelet aggregation. Their role in shock therapy is far from being elucidated.

Prostacyclin (PGI_2), synthesized by the vascular endothelial cells, has potent antiplatelet aggregating properties and is a vasodilator and a lysosomal enzyme stabilizer. Prostacyclin inhibits thromboxane-induced vasoconstriction. Thromboxane is released from degranulating platelets (Lefer, 1979). Prostacyclin improved the vascular response to endotoxin injection and improved survival but did not materially affect the incidence of the concurrent thrombocytopenia and granulocytopenia (Fletcher and Ramwell, 1980).

Aprotinin inhibits lysosomal proteolytic enzyme activity. It was associated with a more rapid regeneration of mitochondrial ATP compared with controls (Horpacsy and Schnells, 1980) and improved myocardial function (Davis et al., 1977) following repletion therapy in hemorrhagic shock.

Large dosages of naloxone have been reported to improve cardiovascular status and survival in canine hypovolemic shock (Vargish et al., 1980).

Fibrinectin supplementation has been reported to improve reticuloendothelial phagocytotic function and dramatically improve the patient's clinical condition in human septic shock (Scovill et al., 1978).

Fructose-1,6-diphosphate (FDP) has been reported to prevent ischemic EKG changes, to maintain myocardial ATP and creatine phosphate content, and to improve survival in canine hypotensive shock (Markov and Oglethorpe, 1981). FDP stimulates phosphofructokinase (PFK), which controls phosphorylation of fructose-6-phosphate during gly-

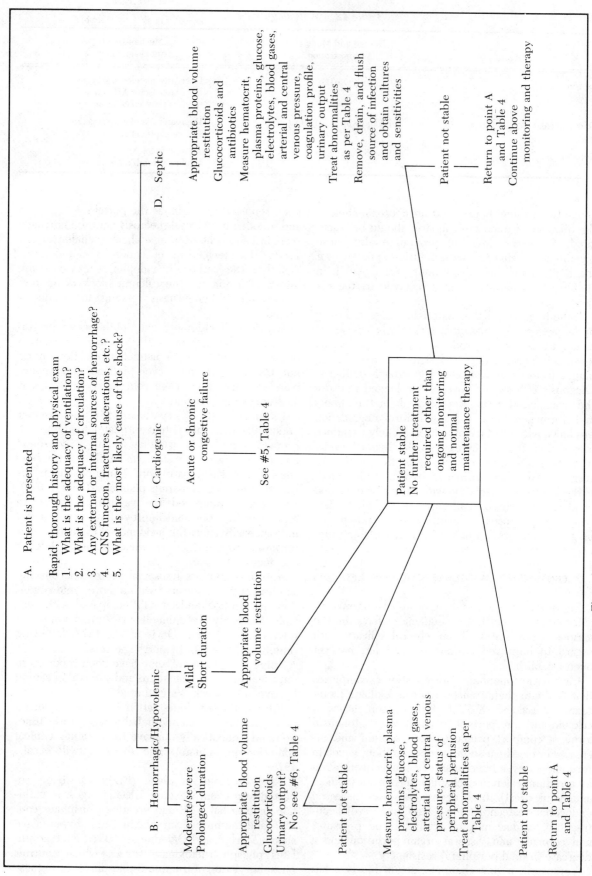

Figure 2. Overview of therapeutic considerations for the shock patient.

colysis. PFK is inhibited by the hypoxia and acidosis that occur during the shock state. FDP is then utilized as an energy substrate in the remainder of the glycolytic pathway. It also increases intraerythrocytic ATP and 2,3 DPG concentrations.

SUMMARY

I have, in the course of this article, presented many possible options with regard to therapy for the shock patient. Many patients do not require the extensive therapeutic intervention indicated in this article; others require at least that much. To help untangle the therapeutic web that has been woven, the following overview is offered (Fig. 2). This outline is a conceptual guide, not a recipe for the management of shock.

When the patient is first presented, obtain a complete history and perform a physical exam and appropriate laboratory tests. Define the status of the patient as completely as possible. Traumatic, hemorrhagic, and hypovolemic shock often respond quite well to simple fluid loading. Although it is common to start with crystalloid fluids, their indefinite administration without consideration of the hematocrit, plasma proteins, and interstitial fluid compartment overloading is an inappropriate approach to fluid therapy. Patients extensively involved with the shock process should at least receive pharmacologic doses of a glucocorticoid and an evaluation of urine output in addition to the fluids. Patients that do not respond to this therapy should receive more thorough monitoring and treatment appropriate to any detected disorders (see Table 4).

The emphasis of therapy in acute or chronic congestive heart failure involves effective control of contractility, preload, and afterload. The early management of this disorder is discussed in this article. The long-term management of congestive heart failure is discussed in more detail elsewhere. Myocardial infarction is a relatively rare event in animals, in contrast to humans. If it is suspected it should be treated in a manner similar to that for the human disease model (Shatney and Lillehei, 1981).

Septic shock is a rapidly progressive, highly lethal form of shock. If it is suspected (see Tables 2 and 3), therapy should be instituted immediately and should be aggressive in nature if the patient is to have any chance of surviving.

We have assumed that a patient may have hypovolemic, cardiogenic, or septic shock, but a single patient may have any or all of these in any combination. In addition, any or all of the complications listed in Table 4 may occur in each of the various forms of shock in any combination. It is necessary to first check those complications that are most likely to occur with each form of shock (see Fig. 2) and to investigate the possible existence of each of the complications (see Table 4) in patients refractory to the initial therapy. It is important to re-evaluate the physical signs and laboratory findings as often as is necessary to keep abreast of the changing status of the disease–patient response–therapy complex.

REFERENCES AND SUPPLEMENTAL READING

Davis, D., Hilewitz, H., and Rogel, S.: Humoral factors in shock causing bradycardia and myocardial depression. Circ. Shock 4:153, 1977.

Fletcher, J. R., and Ramwell, P. W.: The effects of prostacyclin (PGI_2) on endotoxin shock and endotoxin-induced platelet aggregation in dogs. Circ. Shock 7:299, 1980.

Haskins, S. C.: Standards and techniques of equipment utilization. *In* Sattler, F. P., Knowles, R. P., and Whittick, W. G. (eds.): *Veterinary Critical Care.* Philadelphia: Lea & Febiger, 1981, Chapter 3.

Horpacsy, G., and Schnells, G.: Energy metabolism and lysosomal events in hemorrhagic shock after aprotinin treatment. Circ. Shock 7:49, 1980.

Jennings, P. B., Whitten, N. J., and Sleeman, H. R.: The diagnosis and treatment of shock in the critical care patient. *In* Sattler, F. P., Knowles, R. P., and Whittick, W. G. (eds.): *Veterinary Critical Care.* Philadelphia: Lea & Febiger, 1981, Chapter 22.

Kolata, R. J., Burrows, C. F., and Soma, L. R.: Shock: pathophysiology and management. *In* Kirk, R. W. (ed.): *Current Veterinary Therapy VII.* Philadelphia: W. B. Saunders, 1980, pp. 32–48.

Lefer, A. M.: Role of the prostaglandin-thromboxane system in vascular homeostasis during shock. Circ. Shock 6:297, 1979.

Markov, A. K., and Oglethorpe, N.: Irreversible hemorrhagic shock: treatment and cardiac pathophysiology. Circ. Shock 8:9, 1981.

Scovill, W. A., Saba, T. M., et al.: Opsonic alpha2 surface binding glycoprotein therapy during sepsis. Ann. Surg. 188:521, 1978.

Shatney, C. H., and Lillehei, R. C.: Pathophysiology and treatment of circulatory shock. *In* Zschoche, D. A. (ed.): *Mosby's Comprehensive Review of Clinical Care,* 2nd ed. St. Louis: C. V. Mosby, 1981, Chapter 41.

Shoemaker, W. C.: Pathophysiology and therapy of shock states. *In* Berk, J. L., et al. (eds.): *Handbook of Critical Care.* Boston: Little, Brown and Co., 1976, Chapter 10.

Somani, P., and Saini, R. K.: A comparison of the cardiovascular, renal, and coronary effects of dopamine and monensin in endotoxic shock. Circ. Shock 8:451, 1981.

Vargish, T., Reynolds, P. G., et al.: Naloxone reversal of hypovolemic shock in dogs. Circ. Shock 7:31, 1980.

Whalen, G. F., Hackel, D. B., and Mikat, E.: Prevention of portal hypertension and small bowel hemorrhage in dogs treated with verapamil during hemorrhagic shock. Circ. Shock 7:399, 1980.

FLUID THERAPY

WILLIAM W. MUIR, D.V.M.,
and STEPHEN P. DIBARTOLA, D.V.M.

Columbus, Ohio

A variety of medical diseases and surgical complications can result in potentially lethal alterations in body fluid, electrolyte, and acid-base balance unless appropriate therapeutic measures are taken. The recognition and management of fluid and electrolyte disorders are dependent upon a knowledge of the physiologic processes governing fluid and electrolyte homeostasis. Fluid, electrolyte, and acid-base therapy is symptomatic and supportive and should be used in conjunction with and not as a substitute for more specific diagnostic and therapeutic procedures to identify and correct the primary problem. Owing to the lack of precise diagnostic techniques for the assessment of fluid requirements, several guidelines based on experimental studies and clinical experience have evolved to aid the veterinary clinician's approach to fluid therapy. The use of such guidelines or "rules of thumb" has become common practice in veterinary medicine today. These guidelines, in conjunction with proper patient evaluation (history, physical examination, and laboratory data) should be used to construct an objective therapeutic plan.

In the discussion that follows, we will describe the basis for and clinical significance of a variety of clinical and laboratory data used to evaluate fluid, electrolyte, acid-base, and caloric derangements in small animals. We have divided this material into categories of basic concepts and answers to commonly asked clinical questions. A discussion of fluid, electrolyte, and acid-base physiology will be followed by answers to the following questions: Is fluid therapy indicated? What type of fluid should be given? By what route (intravenous, subcutaneous, oral) should fluids be given? How fast should fluids be given? How much fluid should be given? The discussion will conclude with a description of techniques used to monitor fluid therapy and approaches to acid-base, electrolyte, and caloric therapy. Selected references are listed for those seeking a more comprehensive discussion of fluid, electrolyte, and acid-base disorders.

BASIC CONCEPTS

BODY FLUID COMPARTMENTS, VOLUMES, COMPOSITION, AND DISTRIBUTION

Terminology describing the compartmentalization of body water is anatomically based. Hence,

total body water (TBW), which represents approximately 60 per cent of total body weight in the adult animal, is divided into intracellular fluid (ICF: 50 per cent of TBW; 30 per cent of body weight) and extracellular fluid (ECF: 50 per cent of TBW; 30 per cent of body weight), which is further subdivided into the plasma volume (8 per cent of TBW; 5 per cent of body weight) and the interstitial fluid volume (37 per cent of TBW; 25 per cent of body weight) (Fig. 1). Interstitial fluid includes the fluid surrounding cells and that contained in dense connective tissue, cartilage, bone, and slowly equilibrating body compartments (e.g., cerebrospinal fluid, bile, gastrointestinal fluid). Cerebrospinal and gastrointestinal fluids and bile are referred to as transcellular fluid and are estimated to represent 5 per cent of TBW and 1 to 2 per cent of body weight. The transcellular fluid volume is not considered when calculating fluid deficits and has been omitted from Figure 1 for simplicity. Variations in the amount of total body water in normal animals are primarily due to differences in body fat, sex, and age. Obese animals have less TBW compared with lean animals of the same weight; male animals have slightly more TBW than females; and the TBW in neonates may be as great as 70 to 80 per cent of body weight.

Body fluid volumes are regulated by a variety of neuroendocrine reflex mechanisms. Maintenance of normal fluid volumes is dependent upon the appropriate regulation of fluid influx via the gastrointestinal system and fluid efflux via the gastrointestinal system, lungs, skin, and kidneys. Abnormalities in fluid volume and composition, therefore, result from diseases that affect the systems that regulate fluid influx and efflux. Dehydration occurs when water and electrolyte efflux exceeds influx. Dehydration is classified according to the type of fluid lost from the body and the tonicity of the fluid remaining in the body. Pure water loss and hypotonic fluid loss result in hypertonic dehydration with an increase in the tonicity of the remaining body fluids. Loss of hypertonic fluid or isotonic fluid with water replacement will result in hypotonic dehydration wherein the remaining body fluids are hypotonic. In isotonic dehydration, there is no osmotic stimulus for water movement between body compartments, and the remaining body fluids are unchanged in tonicity. The expected volume and tonicity changes in the extracellular and intracellular

28

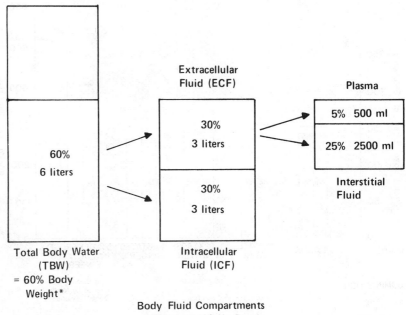

Figure 1. Distribution of body water.

Total Body Water
(TBW)
= 60% Body
Weight*

Body Fluid Compartments
Example, 10 Kg Beagle

* in very young dogs 70% body weight may be water

compartments with various types of dehydration are demonstrated in Figure 2. Note that in hypotonic dehydration, the intracellular compartment is actually overhydrated.

Knowledge of the electrolyte composition of body fluids and the rate at which intravenously administered fluids equilibrate with the ECF and TBW is essential in determining the electrolyte composition of the fluid to be administered and the maximum safe rate of fluid administration. The electrolyte composition of plasma and several commonly used fluid preparations is illustrated in Figure 3. The ECF volume represents approximately 30 per cent of the body weight, but for therapeutic reasons it may be divided into fast- and slow-equilibrating compartments. The fast-equilibrating compartment represents a volume slightly larger than the blood volume (plasma volume + red blood cells) and approximates 8 per cent of total body weight. The

clinical significance of this compartment becomes apparent when considering the rate of fluid administration. When balanced electrolyte solutions are administered intravenously, they equilibrate with the fast-equilibrating compartment in approximately 60 minutes, whereas the time for equilibration with the entire ECF volume or slow-equilibrating compartment is approximately 15 hours. The clinical implication of this concept is that the rate of intravenous fluid administration should not exceed 100 ml/kg/hr in the normal dog or cat. The response to higher rates of fluid administration will include tachycardia, increased urine production, restlessness, coughing, and dyspnea. Depending on the ambient temperature and the type of fluid administered, alterations in body temperature, packed cell volume, total plasma proteins, and serum electrolytes can be expected. Diseases and clinical procedures that markedly disturb the distribution of

Figure 2. Changes in volume and tonicity of body fluid compartments with different types of dehydration. ECF = extracellular fluid; ICF = intracellular fluid; N = normal.

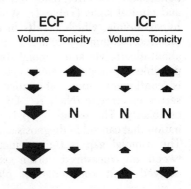

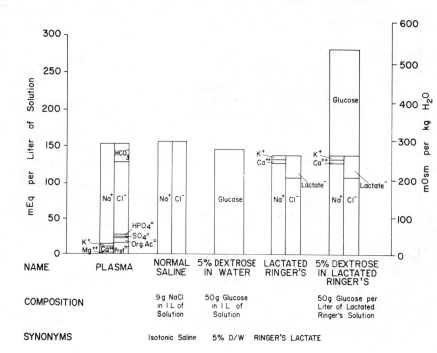

Figure 3. Electrolyte composition and osmolality of commonly used fluids. (Modified from Valtin: *Renal Dysfunction: Mechanisms Involved in Fluid and Solute Imbalance*. Boston: Little, Brown and Co., 1979.)

BODY FLUID ELECTROLYTE COMPOSITION

The distribution of fluids into body fluid compartments is dependent upon the ionic composition (types of electrolytes) and the number of particles (osmolality). Solutions containing approximately 300 mOsm/L are isosmotic with plasma (e.g., 0.9 per cent NaCl). Tonicity, which takes into consideration not only the number of particles (osmolality) but their permeability, is a third factor that determines fluid distribution. Solutions that are isotonic result in no net movement of water across the cell membrane (e.g., 0.9 per cent NaCl). Solutions containing urea, for example, may be isosmotic but, because they cross cell membranes and induce fluid shifts, are not considered isotonic.

A qualitative assessment of plasma electrolyte abnormalities is often made based on patient history and clinical signs (Table 1). With the exception of hyperkalemia, which results in classic clinical and electrocardiographic changes, quantitative guesses about electrolyte and osmolal abnormalities are impossible. Appropriate electrolyte therapy therefore is contingent upon laboratory determination of serum electrolyte (Na^+, K^+, Cl^-) composition and osmolality. The osmolal gap is a clinical determination that can aid in diagnosis and guide in therapy. The osmolal gap is the calculated difference between the measured serum osmolality and that derived from knowledge of plasma electrolytes,

glucose, and blood urea nitrogen (i.e., measured osmolality − calculated osmolality = osmolal gap). The osmolal gap increases (measured osmolality > calculated osmolality) when unmeasured, osmotically active solutes are present in plasma (e.g., ethylene glycol, lactic acid, infused hyperosmotic solutions). Clinically relevant decreases in the osmolal gap (measured osmolality < calculated osmolality) do not occur (Table 2).

ACID-BASE BALANCE

Normal acid-base balance (pH) is continuously being readjusted based on the production of volatile acids in the form of carbon dioxide (CO_2) and nonvolatile or fixed acids produced by metabolism. Blood buffers (bicarbonate, hemoglobin), the lungs, and the kidneys are responsible for maintaining normal blood pH. The blood buffer and pulmonary systems are quick to respond to derangements in blood pH, but they are only partially successful in restoring normal pH. Only the kidneys, whose response is comparatively slow, can completely correct alterations in blood pH to normal and regenerate titrated bicarbonate..

Severe abnormalities in acid-base balance are usually associated with abnormal serum electrolyte values and vice versa. The explanation for this relationship is based on the pH-dependent redistribution of charged particles (H^+, HCO_3^-, K^+, Cl^-) across cell membranes and the effects of acid-base and electrolyte derangements on renal function. Severe metabolic acidosis, for example, is often associated with hyperkalemia. In general, a change

Table 1. *Potential Fluid, Electrolyte, and Acid-Base Disorders Associated with Various Abnormalities**

Abnormality	Type of Dehydration	Electrolyte Balance	Acid-Base Status	Fluid Therapy
Simple dehydration, stress, exercise	Hypertonic	—	—	Half strength or balanced electrolyte solution; 5% glucose solution
Heat stroke	Hypertonic	K^+ variable Na^+ variable	Metabolic acidosis	Half strength electrolyte solution followed by balanced electrolyte solution
Anorexia	Isotonic	K^+ loss	Mild metabolic acidosis	Balanced electrolyte solution; KCl
Starvation	Isotonic	K^+ loss	Mild metabolic acidosis	Half strength or balanced electrolyte solution; KCl; calories
Vomiting	Isotonic or hypertonic	Na^+, K^+, and Cl^- loss	Metabolic alkalosis; metabolic acidosis chronically	Ringer's solution; 0.9% saline with KCl supplementation
Diarrhea	Isotonic or hypertonic	Na^+ loss K^+ loss chronically	Metabolic acidosis	Balanced electrolyte solution; HCO_3^-; KCl (if chronic)
Diabetes mellitus	Hypertonic	K^+ loss	Metabolic acidosis	Balanced electrolyte solutions; KCl
Cushing's disease	Isotonic	K^+ loss	Occasionally mild metabolic alkalosis	Balanced electrolyte solutions; KCl
Addison's disease	Isotonic or hypertonic	Na^+ loss K^+ retention	Metabolic acidosis	0.9% saline followed by balanced electrolyte solutions
Urethral obstruction	Isotonic or hypertonic	K^+ retention Na^+, Cl^- variable	Metabolic acidosis	0.9% saline followed by balanced electrolyte solution; KCl postobstruction
Acute renal failure	Isotonic or hypertonic (with vomiting)	K^+ retention Na^+, Cl^- variable	Metabolic acidosis	Balanced electrolyte solutions
Chronic renal failure	Isotonic or hypertonic (with vomiting)	Na^+, K^+, Cl^- variable	Metabolic acidosis	Balanced electrolyte solutions
Congestive heart failure	Plethoric (Na^+, H_2O retention early); hypotonic chronically	Na^+ retention (but dilutional hyponatremia)	Metabolic acidosis (chronically)	5% glucose solution
Hemorrhagic shock	Isotonic	—	Metabolic acidosis	Balanced electrolyte solutions; blood
Endotoxic shock	Isotonic	—	Metabolic acidosis	Balanced electrolyte solutions; 0.9% saline

*Adapted from Cornelius: J.A.V.M.A. 176:110. 1980.

Table 2. *Osmolal and Anion Gaps in Clinical Disorders of Fluid, Acid-Base, and Electrolyte Balance**

I. Osmolal gap = measured osmolality − calculated osmolality†
  A. Measured osmolality > calculated osmolality
    1. Measured osmolality normal; calculated osmolality decreased (decreased serum water content)
      a. Hyperlipidemia
      b. Hyperglobulinemia
    2. Measured osmolality elevated; calculated value normal or elevated (unmeasured osmoles)
      a. Infusion of hyperosmotic solutions (mannitol)
      b. Poisoning (ethylene glycol, salicylate, ethanol, methanol)
      c. Radiopaque dye
  B. Measured osmolality < calculated osmolality
    1. Laboratory or mathematical error
II. Metabolic acidosis and the anion gap: [$(Na^+ + K^+) - (Cl^- - HCO_3^-)$]
  A. Metabolic acidosis with increased anion gap (normochloremic metabolic acidosis)
    1. Lactic acidosis (lactate)
    2. Diabetic ketoacidosis (ketone production)
    3. Azotemic renal failure (phosphates, sulfates)
    4. Poisoning (ethylene glycol, salicylate, methanol)
  B. Metabolic acidosis with normal anion gap (hyperchloremic metabolic acidosis)
    1. Diarrhea
    2. Renal tubular acidosis
    3. Excessive use of carbonic anhydrase inhibitors (acetazolamide)
    4. Expansion acidosis (excessive 0.9% NaCl administration)
    5. Ammoniumn chloride administration

*Adapted from Feldman and Rosenberg: J.A.V.M.A. 178:396, 1981.
†Calculated osmolality =

$$1.86\,(Na^+ + K^+) + \frac{Glucose}{18} + \frac{BUN}{2.8} + 9$$

$$\text{Or (simplified)} = 2\,(Na^+) + \frac{Glucose}{20} + \frac{BUN}{3}$$

of 0.1 unit in the plasma pH produces an inverse change of 0.4 to 0.6 mEq/L in serum K^+.

Blood pH is dependent upon blood, pulmonary, and renal buffering systems. Abnormalities in one or all of these buffering systems can cause derangements in acid-base balance. Clinically, qualitative evidence suggesting acid-base abnormalities (e.g., vomiting, diarrhea) can occasionally be obtained from a good history. A physical examination provides minimal insight into acid-base problems and may be misleading. Hyperventilation, for example, may indicate excessive CO_2 elimination (respiratory alkalosis) and an increase in blood pH or may indicate a compensatory attempt to correct for the excessive production of or failure to eliminate fixed acids (metabolic acidosis).

Acid-base abnormalities are best evaluated by determination of pH and blood gases (CO_2 O_2) using sophisticated equipment. This equipment offers the veterinarian immediate knowledge of the patient's primary acid-base problem and guidelines for a quantitative approach to therapy. In addition to sophisticated equipment for determination of pH and blood gases, there are indirect methods for clinical evaluation of acid-base balance. For example, determination of urine pH is a crude method for assessing acid-base balance provided normal diets are fed and urinary tract infection does not exist. Generally, a urine pH below 5.0 indicates acidemia, whereas a urine pH above 8.0 suggests alkalemia. Disease-induced or iatrogenic derangements in serum potassium concentrations, however, can produce paradoxical relationships between plasma and urine pH (Table 3). The anion gap can also be used to indirectly assess acid-base status. The number of cations in the ECF equals the number of anions. Calculation of the difference between the commonly measured cations and anions [$(Na^+ + K^+) - (Cl^- + HCO_3^-)$] yields the number of unmeasured anions. The normal anion gap is 15 to 25 mEq/L in dogs and cats and represents the normal amount of unmeasured anions. The anion gap increases during normochloremic metabolic acidosis owing to increased acid production or decreased acid elimination (see Table 2). The Harleco CO_2 kit is a rapid, accurate, and inexpensive means for determining severe derangements in the plasma bicarbonate. Serum electrolytes can be determined by a flame photometer (Na^+, K^+) and a chloridometer (Cl^-).

Fluid, electrolyte, and acid-base therapy for the dog or cat with complicated cardiac, gastrointestinal, or renal disease poses special problems for the veterinary clinician. Accurate and quantitative information regarding therapy can only be obtained through appropriate laboratory evaluation. Although educated predictions regarding electrolyte and acid-base status are often used to guide initial therapy (see Table 1), they are no substitute for specific clinical laboratory tests. For example, it is generally true that dogs suffering from congestive

Table 3. *Renal Response to Plasma Acid-Base and Electrolyte Abnormalities**

Condition	Plasma pH	Renal Cell pH	Urine pH
Metabolic acidosis	↓	↓	Aciduria
Respiratory acidosis	↓	↓	Aciduria
Hyperkalemic metabolic acidosis	↓	↑	Alkaluria
Metabolic alkalosis	↑	↑	Alkaluria
Respiratory alkalosis	↑	↑	Alkaluria
Hypokalemic metabolic alkalosis	↑	↓	Aciduria

*Adapted from Koushanpour: *Renal Physiology: Principles and Functions.* Philadelphia: W. B. Saunders Co., 1976.

heart failure are overhydrated owing to salt and water retention. In addition, they may have prerenal azotemia and hyperkalemic metabolic acidosis due to diminished renal perfusion. If right heart failure is severe, liver congestion and hypoproteinemia may be present. Initial therapy should be designed to improve cardiac function (digitalis), reestablish renal blood flow, and optimize water elimination (diuretics). If therapy is successful, electrolyte and acid-base abnormalities generally will correct themselves. If, during the course of digitalis and diuretic therapy, the patient develops congestive symptoms, diarrhea, or vomiting, the clinician's ability to predict electrolyte or acid-base disturbances may become limited. If the patient's symptoms are due to inadequate therapy, hyperkalemic metabolic acidosis could be present. If, on the other hand, the signs are due to inappropriate therapy or drug intoxication, the patient could have hypochloremic, hypokalemic metabolic alkalosis. Similar examples can be envisioned for the patient with acute or chronic gastrointestinal or renal disease. Appreciation of this example should remind the reader that Table 1 is meant only as a guide and that there is no substitute for clinical laboratory tests.

IS FLUID THERAPY INDICATED?

For medical patients, the answer to this question depends on an assessment of the animal's hydration. The state of hydration is estimated by evaluating the history, physical examination, and simple laboratory tests. For the surgical patient, there may be additional indications for fluid therapy such as venous access for emergencies and establishment of a diuresis.

Historical information about the route of fluid loss will suggest the patient's electrolyte and acid-base derangements. The time period over which fluid losses occurred and an estimate of their magnitude should be ascertained. Information about food and water consumption, gastrointestinal losses (vomiting or diarrhea), urinary losses (polyuria), and traumatic losses (blood loss, extensive burns) should be obtained from the owner. Excessive insensible water losses (increased panting, fever) and third space losses (effusions, sequestration of fluid in an obstructed bowel segment) may be determined from the physical examination. In addition to the history, the clinician's knowledge of the suspected disease can aid in predicting the composition of the fluid lost (see Table 1).

The physical findings associated with fluid losses of from 5 to 15 per cent of body weight vary from subtle clinical changes (5 per cent) to signs of hypovolemic shock and impending death (15 per cent) (Table 4). The clinician may estimate the hydration deficit by evaluating skin turgor or plia-

bility, the moistness of the mucous membranes, the position of the eyes in their orbits, the heart rate, and the character of the peripheral pulses. This clinical assessment of hydration is potentially quite inaccurate. Detection of dehydration by skin turgor is dependent upon the animal's skin pliability prior to dehydration, the position of the animal when the skin is checked, the site used for evaluation, and the amount of subcutaneous fat. Skin pliability should be tested over the lumbar region with the dog in a standing position. When evaluated by skin turgor, obese animals may appear well-hydrated owing to excessive subcutaneous fat despite the presence of dehydration. On the other hand, emaciated animals may appear more dehydrated than they actually are due to a lack of subcutaneous and retrobulbar fat. A false impression of dehydration may also occur with persistent panting, which may dry the oral mucous membranes. When dehydration becomes severe (12 to 15 per cent body weight), signs of hypovolemic shock appear. These include lassitude, cool extremities, tachycardia, rapid and weak pulses, and prolonged capillary refill time. The urinary bladder should be small in a dehydrated animal with normal renal function. A large, urine-filled bladder in a severely dehydrated patient indicates failure of the normal renal concentrating mechanism.

Body weight recorded on a serial basis is an excellent indicator of hydration status, especially when fluid loss has been acute and the previous body weight has been recorded. Loss of 1 lb of body weight in such a setting indicates a fluid deficit of 500 ml. Loss of weight in chronic diseases includes loss of muscle mass as well as fluid loss. An anorexic animal may lose 0.1 to 0.3 kg body weight/day/1000 cal energy requirement. Losses in excess of this amount indicate fluid loss.

Table 4. *Clinical Signs of Dehydration**

Per Cent Dehydration	Clinical Signs
<5	Not detectable
5 to 6	Subtle loss of skin elasticity
6 to 8	Definite delay in return of skin to normal position Slight prolongation of capillary refill time Eyes possibly sunken in orbits Possibly dry mucous membranes
10 to 12	Tented skin stands in place Definite prolongation of capillary refill time Eyes sunken in orbits Dry mucous membranes Possibly signs of shock (tachycardia, cool extremities, rapid and weak pulses)
12 to 15	Definite signs of shock Death imminent

*Adapted from Cornelius: J.A.V.M.A. 176:110, 1980.

The hematocrit (PCV), total plasma proteins (TPP), and urine specific gravity are simple laboratory tools that can aid in the evaluation of hydration. It is important to obtain these parameters prior to initiation of fluid therapy. PCV and TPP should be evaluated together to minimize errors in interpretation. Table 5 shows possible interpretations for various combinations of PCV and TPP values. The hematocrit alone may be an unreliable indicator of hemoconcentration in water-deprived dogs, and although plasma proteins increase they may not be above the upper limit of the normal range. Urine specific gravity prior to fluid therapy is helpful as a preliminary evaluation of renal function. Urine specific gravity should be high (greater than 1.048) in a markedly dehydrated dog if renal function is normal. This may not be true if other disorders affecting renal concentrating ability, such as medullary washout of solute, are present. After fluid therapy has been initiated, urine specific gravity will fall into the isosthenuric range if rehydration has been achieved.

WHAT TYPE OF FLUID SHOULD BE GIVEN?

The veterinary practitioner can manage most animals requiring fluid therapy with one of three types of fluids: a balanced electrolyte solution such as lactated Ringer's solution, normal (0.9 per cent) saline, or 5 per cent dextrose in water. The solute composition of these fluids is compared with plasma in Figure 3. Supplementation of these fluids with KCl may be necessary when losses have included large amounts of potassium. The choice of fluid is dependent on the nature of the disease and the composition of the fluid lost. The clinician should attempt to replace fluid losses with a fluid that is similar in volume and electrolyte composition to that which has been lost from the body. For example, persistent vomition due to high gastrointestinal obstruction would be expected to result in losses of hydrochloric acid, potassium, sodium, and water, producing hypokalemic, hypochloremic metabolic alkalosis. The fluid of choice in this example would be 0.9 per cent NaCl with KCl supplementation. Other examples of fluid therapy in specific diseases are listed (see Table 1).

BY WHAT ROUTE SHOULD FLUIDS BE GIVEN?

The route of fluid therapy depends on the nature of the clinical disorder, its severity, and its duration. In general, when fluid loss is sudden or extensive, the intravenous route is preferred. The subcutaneous route is convenient for maintenance fluid therapy in small dogs and cats. This route is not recommended in extremely dehydrated animals because peripheral vasoconstriction may reduce absorption of the administered fluid. The volume that

Table 5. *Interpretation of Hematocrit and Plasma Protein Values*

PCV (%)	Total Plasma Proteins (gm/dl)	Interpretation
Increased	Increased	Dehydration
Increased	Normal or decreased	Splenic contraction Polycythemia Dehydration with pre-existing hypoproteinemia
Normal	Increased	Normal hydration with hyperproteinemia Anemia with dehydration
Decreased	Increased	Anemia with dehydration Anemia with pre-existing hyperproteinemia
Decreased	Normal	Nonblood loss anemia with normal hydration
Normal	Normal	Normal hydration Dehydration with pre-existing anemia and hypoproteinemia Acute hemorrhage Dehydration with secondary compartment shift
Decreased	Decreased	Blood loss Anemia and hypoproteinemia Overhydration

may be given is limited by skin elasticity, and only isotonic fluids are recommended. The subcutaneous administration of 5 per cent dextrose in water should be avoided because equilibration of extracellular fluid with a pool of electrolyte-free solution may lead to a temporary aggravation of electrolyte imbalance. Oral fluid therapy is useful for administering hypertonic fluids with high caloric density. This route should not be used, however, in the presence of vomition or diarrhea. The oral route is also inadequate in animals that have had sudden or extensive fluid losses.

HOW FAST MAY FLUIDS BE GIVEN?

The rate of fluid administration is dictated by the magnitude and rapidity of the fluid loss. Rapid or extensive losses demand rapid replacement. When necessary, fluids can be given safely at a rate slightly greater than one blood volume per hour (i.e., 100 ml/kg/hr). When fluids are given rapidly, it is necessary to monitor cardiovascular and renal function.

It is not usually necessary or desirable to replace the hydration deficit rapidly in chronic diseases. Instead, the hydration deficit may be calculated, the daily maintenance requirement of fluid added to this, and the total amount administered over 24 hours. An alternative approach is to replace the hydration deficit over the first few hours of treatment followed by maintenance therapy.

Whenever possible, fluid deficits should be replaced prior to anesthesia and surgery. During the induction and maintenance of anesthesia, prevention of hypovolemia and maintenance of renal blood flow are essential. Induction of a diuresis in this setting may be an important factor in the prevention of intraoperative acute renal failure. A basal fluid administration rate of 5 to 10 ml/kg/hr is recommended during anesthesia and surgery. During major surgery (e.g., exploratory laparotomy, thoracotomy), fluid administration at twice this basal rate is recommended.

HOW MUCH FLUID SHOULD BE GIVEN?

The initial assessment of hydration determines the volume of fluid needed to replace the hydration deficit (replacement requirement). Table 6 contains the calculation of the replacement requirement. This calculation underestimates the fluid requirement in hypovolemic shock in which the amount of fluid required for treatment may be two to four times the amount of blood lost due to vasodilatation and increased volume of distribution of fluid.

Coincident with or after replacement of the animal's hydration deficit, the maintenance fluid requirement must be administered. Maintenance fluid requirements are 40 to 60 ml/kg/day. Large dogs require the lower limit (40 ml/kg/day) and small dogs and cats the upper limit (60 ml/kg/day) of this range. Approximately two-thirds of the maintenance requirement represents sensible losses of fluid (urine output), and one-third represents insensible losses (fecal, cutaneous, and respiratory water loss). Daily maintenance for a 10-kg dog would be 600 ml, with 400 ml representing sensible loss and 200 ml insensible loss.

In addition to the hydration deficit (replacement requirement) and maintenance requirement, con-

temporary or ongoing losses must be considered. These are not always easily determined or quantitated in small animal medicine but can be very important in fluid therapy. An attempt should be made to estimate ongoing losses, which may include vomition, diarrhea, polyuria, large wounds or burns, drains, peritoneal or pleural losses, panting, fever, and blood loss. During surgical procedures, careful attention should be given to the amount of blood lost, drying of exposed tissues, and effusions removed by suction. Blood lost at surgery should be estimated and 3 ml of crystalloid solution administered for each milliliter of blood lost. Each 4 × 4 gauze sponge, when saturated with blood, represents a 15-ml blood loss. Contemporary losses must be estimated and carefully replaced along with the maintenance volume of fluid.

Repeated assessment of the patient by observation of clinical signs and determinations of weight, urine output, PCV, TPP, and urine specific gravity is mandatory in making appropriate readjustments of fluid therapy. Reasons for failure to achieve satisfactory rehydration include calculation errors, underestimation of the initial hydration deficit, contemporary losses larger than appreciated, infusion of fluid at an excessively rapid rate with consequent diuresis and obligatory urine loss, technical problems with the intravenous catheter, sensible losses larger than appreciated (e.g., polyuria), and insensible losses larger than appreciated (e.g., panting, fever). Failure to achieve successful hydration is an indication to increase the volume of fluid administered if renal and cardiovascular function are adequate. As a rule, the daily fluid volume may be increased by an amount equivalent to 5 per cent of body weight if the initial infusion fails to restore hydration.

MONITORING FLUID THERAPY

A complete physical examination including evaluation of skin turgor and careful thoracic auscultation should be performed once or twice daily on animals receiving fluid therapy. Hematocrit, plasma proteins, and body weight should be monitored. Animals receiving continuous fluid therapy should be weighed twice daily using the same scale. A gain or loss of 1 lb can be considered an excess or deficit of 500 ml fluid.

When fluids are administered intravenously at a rapid rate and renal function is in question, urine output should be monitored. Normal urine output is 1 to 2 ml/kg/hr. After the hydration deficit has been replaced, it may be prudent to divide daily fluid therapy into six four-hour intervals if the status of renal function is uncertain. The calculated insensible volume plus a volume equal to the urine output of the previous four hours is administered over each four-hour period. The risk of overhydra-

---

Table 6.   *Components of Fluid Therapy*

1. HYDRATION DEFICIT (REPLACEMENT REQUIREMENT)
   Body weight (lbs) × % dehydration as a decimal × 500* = deficit in milliliters
   Body weight (kg) × % dehydration as a decimal = deficit in liters

2. MAINTENANCE REQUIREMENT (40 to 60 ml/kg/day)
   a. Sensible losses (urine output): 27 to 40 ml/kg/day
   b. Insensible losses (fecal, cutaneous, respiratory): 13 to 20 ml/kg/day

3. CONTEMPORARY (ONGOING) LOSSES (e.g., vomition, diarrhea, polyuria)

---

*500 ml = 1 lb fluid.

tion is minimized, and fluid therapy will keep pace with urine output even if oliguria is present when this technique is used. If oliguria persists, an increase in the daily fluid volume by an amount equal to 5 per cent of body weight is justified on the assumption that the initial clinical estimation of dehydration was inaccurate. If oliguria does not respond to mild volume expansion, administration of increased volumes of fluid may result in pulmonary edema.

Measurement of central venous pressure (CVP) with a jugular catheter positioned at the level of the right atrium allows cardiovascular function to be monitored. Normal CVP is 0 to 5 cm H_2O. An increase in CVP of 2 cm H_2O during fluid therapy is an indication to decrease the rate of fluid administration or to stop fluid therapy temporarily. Sudden increases in CVP may indicate a failure of the cardiovascular system to effectively handle the fluid load and could result in pulmonary edema due to left heart failure. In addition to the volume of fluid administered, three other factors that may affect CVP are heart rate, vascular capacity, and cardiac contractility. A reduction in any of these three parameters can cause an increase in CVP.

Signs of overhydration occur when fluid is administered too rapidly. These include serous nasal discharge, chemosis, restlessness, cough, dyspnea, pulmonary edema, ascites, polyuria, exophthalmos, diarrhea, and vomition. Expected laboratory abnormalities include a reduction in hematocrit and plasma proteins and an increase in body weight.

When the intravenous route is chosen for fluid therapy, the clinician has made a commitment to careful, aseptic catheter placement and proper maintenance. The animal should be checked daily for cleanliness of the catheter site, fever, or cardiac murmurs. The catheter should be removed and an alternative site chosen every 48 to 72 hours. Complications related to catheter placement include bacterial endocarditis, thrombophlebitis, thromboembolism, and migration of a catheter fragment. When not in use, the catheter should be irrigated with a solution containing 5 units of heparin/ml 0.9 per cent NaCl ("heparinized saline").

SPECIFIC THERAPIES

POTASSIUM

Over 95 per cent of the body's potassium is located intracellularly, whereas only 2 to 5 per cent is present in the extracellular fluid. As a result, serum potassium values are not necessarily reliable indicators of total body stores of potassium. Clinical signs and causes of hypo- and hyperkalemia are presented in Tables 7 and 8.

Treatment of severe hyperkalemia must be prompt. Several techniques have been advocated to rapidly reverse the cardiotoxic effects of hyperkalemia. Intravenous administration of 1 to 2 mEq/kg of sodium bicarbonate potentiates the intracellular movement of potassium and the extracellular movement of hydrogen ions by its alkalinizing effect. The risks of hypervolemia and hyperosmolality due to the imposed sodium load must be considered when this technique is used, especially in cats and small dogs. A slow intravenous infusion of 0.5 ml/kg of a 10 per cent solution of calcium gluconate solution does not lower extracellular potassium levels but does antagonize the detrimental effects of hyperkalemia on the heart. Heart rhythm should be monitored when intravenously administering calcium gluconate. Glucose-containing solutions may be used in the initial treatment of hyperkalemia to promote the intracellular movement of potassium and glucose, thus decreasing the extracellular levels of potassium.

These techniques promptly lower serum potassium or reverse its cardiotoxic effects, but their duration of action is transient. A conscientious effort must be made to diagnose and treat the primary disease responsible for the hyperkalemia. If hyperkalemia is persistent, other steps must be taken to maintain sustained reduction in potassium levels. Sodium polystyrene sulfonate (Kayexalate) is an ion-exchange resin that may be given either orally or by retention enema to bind potassium in the gastrointestinal tract. If this is unsuccessful in controlling hyperkalemia, dialysis must be considered.

Parenteral potassium replacement may be given subcutaneously or intravenously. Solutions containing up to 30 mEq potassium per liter may be given subcutaneously without irritation. Return of alimentation after diagnosis and treatment of the primary disease responsible for hypokalemia will result in additional replacement of potassium deficits. When potassium loss has been severe and the patient is symptomatic for hypokalemia, potassium should be replaced intravenously. The approach presented in Table 9 is recommended for intravenous potassium supplementation, but to avoid cardiac rhythm disturbances, the infusion rate should not exceed 0.5 mEq/kg/hr.

SODIUM

Sodium is the major cation of the extracellular fluid, and preservation of the extracellular fluid volume depends on renal reabsorption of filtered sodium.' Serum sodium values indicate the amount of sodium relative to the amount of water in the extracellular fluid. Serum sodium values may be decreased, normal, or increased in dehydrated patients depending on the composition and tonicity of the fluid that has been lost (see Table 1 and Fig. 2). Therefore, serum sodium values do not neces-

Table 7. *Causes of Serum Electrolyte Abnormalities*

Hyperkalemia
Increased intake
High doses of potassium penicillin G intravenously
(1.7 mEq potassium/10^6 units penicillin)
Excessively rapid intravenous infusion of potassium
Inadequate mixing of potassium in flexible IV bags
KCl as a salt substitute during sodium restriction in
congestive heart failure
Decreased renal elimination
Oliguric acute renal failure
Terminal oliguric chronic renal failure
Hypoadrenocorticism (Addison's disease)
Use of potassium-sparing diuretics
Urinary tract obstruction
Ruptured urinary tract
Translocation from intracellular to extracellular
compartments
Metabolic acidosis
Rapid release of potassium from tissue during injury
or catabolic states

Hypokalemia
Decreased intake
Aberrant diet
Anorexia
Fluids deficient in potassium
Translocation from extracellular to intracellular
compartments
Glucose and insulin administration
Metabolic alkalosis
Excessive gastrointestinal losses
Chronic vomition
Overuse of laxatives, enemas, or exchange resins
Excessive urinary losses
Secondary hyperaldosteronism
Liver failure
Congestive heart failure
Nephrotic syndrome
Renal disease
Renal tubular acidosis
Post-obstructive diuresis
Chronic pyelonephritis
Drugs
Diuretics
Amphotericin B

Hypernatremia
Lack of water intake
Pure water loss
Salt poisoning
Administration of hypertonic sodium-containing fluids
Advanced chronic renal failure with very low glomerular
filtration rate (less than 5 per cent of normal)
Hypotonic fluid losses
Primary hyperaldosteronism (not reported in dog or cat)

Hyponatremia
In the OVERHYDRATED patient
Secondary hyperaldosteronism
Liver failure
Congestive heart failure
Nephrotic syndrome
Psychogenic polydipsia
Iatrogenic water load
Syndrome of inappropriate secretion of ADH (SIADH)
Central nervous system disease
Pulmonary disease
Drugs
Neoplasia
In the DEHYDRATED patient
Gastrointestinal losses
Isotonic losses with water replacement
Hypoadrenocorticism (Addison's disease)
Sodium-losing renal disease
Diuretic therapy
Hypertonic fluid loss
Burns
Large wounds
Body cavity lavage
Pseudohyponatremia
Multiple myeloma
Hyperlipidemia
Hyperglycemia

Table 8.   *Clinical Signs of Electrolyte Disturbances*

Hypokalemia	Hyponatremia
Weakness	Weakness
Paralytic ileus	Restlessness
Defective urinary	Muscular twitching
concentrating	Extreme thirst
ability	Signs of shock
Tachycardia	Seizures
Electrocardiographic	Anorexia
changes not	Vomition
consistent	Abdominal pain
	Paralytic ileus
	Electrocardiographic
	changes not
	consistent
Hyperkalemia	**Hypernatremia**
Weakness	Weakness
Cardiac arrhythmias	Extreme thirst
Characteristic	Muscular twitching
electrocardiographic	Depression
changes	Coma
	Seizures
	Electrocardiographic
	changes not
	consistent

sarily reflect the status of total body stores. Clinical signs and causes of hypo- and hypernatremia are listed in Tables 7 and 8.

Therapy for hyponatremia consists of infusion of sodium-containing fluids and termination of any infusion of sodium-poor fluid. In most cases, isotonic sodium solutions (0.9 per cent NaCl) will be adequate. Therapy for hypernatremia should consist of infusion of sodium-poor fluid (5 per cent dextrose or 2.5 per cent dextrose in 0.45 per cent saline) and termination of any sodium-rich infusion. Rapid lowering of extracellular fluid tonicity in animals with chronic hypertonicity may result in the development of an unfavorable osmotic gradient and overhydration of the brain. For this reason, therapy designed to lower serum sodium levels should be carried out slowly.

Table 9.   *Guidelines for Intravenous Potassium Supplementation* *

Serum Potassium (mEq/L)	mEq KCl to Add to 250 ml Fluid	Maximal Fluid Infusion Rate (ml/kg/hr)
<2.0	20	6
2.1 to 2.5	15	8
2.6 to 3.0	10	12
3.1 to 3.5	7	16

*From Dr. R. C. Scott, Animal Medical Center, New York, N.Y.

Note: DO NOT EXCEED 0.5 mEq/kg/hr.

ACID-BASE IMBALANCE

Attempts to correct severe acid-base abnormalities without proper laboratory support may result in a variety of iatrogenic acid-base, osmolal, and electrolyte disorders. Arterial or venous blood gas (pO_2, pCO_2) and pH determinations are the most accurate means of determining acid-base status. Measurements of plasma bicarbonate are useful in determining the presence and severity of metabolic acidosis. The anion gap and urine pH (see Tables 2 and 3) may aid indirectly in assessing a patient's acid-base status. The results of these clinical laboratory tests combined with pertinent historical and physical findings will guide fluid and electrolyte therapy.

A brief review of Table 1 indicates that the acid-base abnormality most frequently diagnosed in dogs and cats is metabolic acidosis. Metabolic acidosis occurs as a result of an increase in plasma nonvolatile (fixed) acids (renal failure, shock, diabetes mellitus) or loss of plasma bicarbonate ion (diarrhea). Balanced electrolyte solutions containing the salts of lactate or acetate can be used to treat mildly dehydrated or debilitated patients when metabolic acidosis is suspected. The presence of lactate in lactated Ringer's solution does not contribute to lactic acidosis but does require conversion by the liver to be effective as an alkalinizing agent. The alkalinizing properties of lactate are inhibited in the presence of severe metabolic acidosis (pH < 7.1) or severe liver disease.

Generally, treatment of the primary disease problem combined with adequate replacement and maintenance fluid therapy is adequate to restore plasma pH to normal in mild metabolic acidosis. When organ system disease or circulatory derangements are severe, appropriate fluid therapy and base replacement must be approached quantitatively. The patient's base deficit can be determined from a nomogram if blood pH and pCO_2 are known. Determination of total CO_2 (Harleco kit) is a simple, although less precise, method used to estimate the bicarbonate deficit (25 mEq/L − measured bicarbonate = bicarbonate deficit). Measurement of total CO_2, however, does not distinguish between respiratory and metabolic acid-base derangements. Either the base or bicarbonate deficit can be used to calculate the number of milliequivalents of bicarbonate therapy required. The patient's body weight in kilograms multiplied by 0.3 multiplied by the base or bicarbonate deficit equals the total bicarbonate therapy in milliequivalents (body weight in kg × 0.3 × bicarbonate deficit = mEq bicarbonate). The value 0.3 (30 per cent) represents the ECF and roughly estimates the fluid volume to which bicarbonate rapidly distributes. Formulas using a value of 0.6 (60 per cent) assume that bicarbonate distributes throughout the TBW. This latter value is used when bicarbonate is replaced over a period of 18 to 24 hours. Use of the factor 0.6 when calculating acute bicarbonate deficits for replacement therapy can result in metabolic alkalosis if intracellular acidosis is not severe. Excessive infusion of sodium bicarbonate may result in extracellular fluid hyperosmolality, intracranial hemorrhage, or coma. In addition, rapid bicarbonate infusions may cause paradoxical cerebrospinal fluid (CSF) acidosis, acute hypokalemia, and decreased blood oxygen availability.

The potential disadvantages of excessive infusion of bicarbonate argue against using "rules of thumb" when replacing bicarbonate. In situations in which the development of severe metabolic acidosis is obvious or imminent (cardiopulmonary arrest) and plasma bicarbonate determinations are not immediately available, a relatively safe approach is the intravenous administration of 1 mEq/kg sodium bicarbonate. Provided that breathing is adequate and appropriate fluids are administered to restore and maintain urine formation, this dose of bicarbonate can be repeated every 10 to 15 minutes until a total dose of 4 mEq/kg has been administered.

Therapeutic attempts to correct acid-base abnormalities other than metabolic acidosis should be directed toward the primary disease. For example, hypoventilation with resultant respiratory acidosis secondary to anesthesia should be managed by assisted breathing or respiratory stimulants; hyperventilation with resultant respiratory alkalosis secondary to pain should be managed wih analgesics; vomiting with resultant metabolic alkalosis should be managed by appropriate fluid therapy (see Table 1) and antiemetics.

NUTRITION

Many hospitalized animals exhibit variable degrees of protein-calorie malnutrition (PCM) in addition to fluid and electrolyte imbalances. The most common causes of PCM in dogs and cats are starvation and a prolonged metabolic response to injury. Causes of starvation include inadequate food supply, chronic anorexia, and gastrointestinal maldigestion or malabsorption. Metabolic rate and protein catabolism are usually decreased during starvation, whereas fatty acid metabolism increases, resulting in ketonuria (Fig. 4). The response to burns, trauma, and sepsis is a common cause for PCM in dogs and cats. The severity and rate of development of PCM is directly related to the type and severity of the infection or trauma.

Unlike starvation, metabolic rate and protein catabolism are increased following infection or trauma (see Fig. 4). The increase in metabolic rate is a collective neurohumoral response to injury that hastens tissue repair in the face of minimal nutritional support. This hypermetabolic state is followed

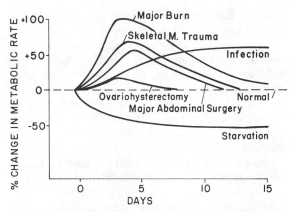

Figure 4. Changes in metabolic rate with various clinical disorders.

by an anabolic phase characterized by sudden improvement of the patient's appetite. PCM occurs when the hypermetabolic state becomes chronic (e.g., infection) or when adequate calories are not provided during the anabolic phase. The consequences of PCM are lethargy, muscle weakness, impaired wound healing, decubitus ulcers, poor immunocompetence, and nonregenerative anemia. In clinical practice, PCM should be assumed if the patient develops anorexia of several days (more than five days) duration, progressive weight loss (> 20 per cent), hypoalbuminemia, or nonregenerative anemia. Practical laboratory methods for monitoring nutritional status in the dog and cat are not developed at this time.

Nutritional therapy for the normal adult dog or cat is based on a knowledge of normal caloric and protein requirements. An average sized dog requires 50 Kcal/kg/day (Table 10). Adjustments in caloric requirements are based on size, exercise level, and age. Protein requirements are best supplied by providing protein as a percentage of the daily caloric intake. A normal adult dog requires 8 to 12 per cent of its daily calories as protein; an adult cat needs 15 to 20 per cent. During hypermetabolic states (see Fig. 4), protein requirements

Table 10.   *Caloric and Protein Requirements for Dogs*

Basal caloric requirement (Kcal/kg)	
Small	60
Medium	50
Large	40
Exercise	
Standing and walking	add 25 per cent
Normal activity	add 50 per cent
Vigorous exercise	add 100 per cent
Hypermetabolism (trauma, infection)	
Add 50 to 100 per cent; depending on estimated severity	
Hyperalimentation	
Enteral	add 50 per cent
Parenteral	add 75 per cent

increase. Parenteral and enteral hyperalimentation are techniques used to supply excess nutritional therapy to starving or severely traumatized dogs and cats. Hyperalimentation is indicated in animals that have been anorectic for longer than ten days, regardless of cause. Severe trauma victims or patients that have undergone prolonged and extensive surgical procedures may also benefit from hyperalimentation, particularly if malnutrition, anorexia, or infection is already present.

Enteral and parenteral routes are used for hyperalimentation. Enteral hyperalimentation is preferred when gastrointestinal integrity is normal. The most practical method for implementing enteral hyperalimentation is the pharyngostomy tube. The pharyngostomy tube enters the pharynx via a blunt incision made caudal to the mandible and rostral to the hyoid apparatus. The tube is passed to the level of the distal esophagus. The cardiac sphincter of the stomach is not entered to avoid reflux esophagitis. A needle-catheter jejunostomy can be used in surgical patients. A 16-gauge intravenous catheter is introduced into the lumen of the proximal jejunum via a 14-gauge needle at the time of abdominal surgery. The catheter is advanced into the lumen of the jejunum for 20 to 30 cm. The remaining catheter is then externalized through the abdominal wall, and the jejunostomy site is sutured to the abdominal wall. A liquid diet may then be administered by drip infusion similar to intravenous therapy. A predetermined quantity of liquid diet (Vivonex, Ensure) can be administered through the tube. Polymeric liquid diets (Ensure) require digestion but are preferred because of their osmolality and cost. Monomeric diets (Vivonex) are immediately absorbable but are hyperosmotic and costly. Liquid diets are generally formulated with a caloric density of 1 Kcal/ml. Liquid diet hyperalimentation will fulfill daily fluid requirements if supplementation is greater than 50 Kcal/kg.

Parenteral hyperalimentation is recommended when gastrointestinal disease is present or after extensive gastrointestinal surgery. Most parenteral hyperalimentation fluids incorporate glucose as a source of calories, hydrolyzed protein as a source of amino acids, a vitamin supplement, and variable amounts of potassium chloride depending on the patient's potassium status. Parenteral hyperalimentation fluids may be prepared by mixing 600 ml of 5 per cent hydrolyzed protein (Aminosol) with 400 ml of 50 per cent dextrose. To this solution is added 50 mEq of sodium chloride and 1 ml of a B-fortified injectable vitamin supplement. Between 20 and 40 mEq potassium chloride are added to the solution, depending on the patient's potassium status. The final 1-liter solution provides approximately 1 Kcal/ml. The total amount of solution required, therefore, is dependent upon the patient's daily caloric requirement (see Table 10) and is administered at a constant rate over 18 to 24 hours using a minidrip fluid administration unit. To allow ample time for adaptation to parenteral hyperalimentation, only 25 per cent of the patient's caloric requirement is administered on the first day. An additional 25 per cent is added each day so that the total calculated calories are administered by the fourth day.

Parenteral hyperalimentation solutions must be administered through large veins, preferably the jugular vein to minimize thrombophlebitis. A sterile Silastic catheter of at least 6 inches in length is surgically secured into the jugular vein. The catheter is then passed through a subcutaneous tunnel so as to emerge from the dorsal neck. The proximal end of the catheter is sutured in place, fitted with an appropriately sized needle and a three-way stopcock, and bandaged in place. Strict aseptic technique must be used to prevent bacterial contamination of the catheter and the parenteral fluid.

Hyperglycemia, glucosuria, and infection may be associated with parenteral hyperalimentation, and the patient should be monitored for these problems. In addition, the patient's hydration, temperature, and white blood cell count (WBC) should be closely followed. Additional noncaloric fluids can be administered through a different vein or subcutaneously. If infection occurs, the intravenous catheters should be removed and antibiotic therapy instituted.

SUGGESTED READING

Brasmer, T. H.: Fluid therapy in shock. J. A. V. M. A. 174:475, 1979.

Cornelius, L. M.: Fluid therapy in small animal practice. J. A. V. M. A. 176:110, 1980.

Cornelius, L. M., Finco, D. R., and Culver, D. H.: Physiologic effects of rapid infusion of Ringer's lactate solution into dogs. Am. J. Vet. Res. 39:1185, 1978.

Cornelius, L. M., and Rawlings, C. A.: Arterial blood gas and acid-base values in dogs with various diseases and signs of disease. J. A. V. M. A. 178:992, 1981.

Feldman, B. F., and Rosenberg, D. P.: Clinical use of anion and osmolal gaps in veterinary medicine. J. A. V. M. A. 178:396, 1981.

Finco, D. R.: Fluid therapy. *In* Kirk, R. W. (ed.): *Current Veterinary Therapy VI.* Philadelphia: W. B. Saunders Co., 1977, pp. 3–12.

Fleming, C. R., McGill, D. B., Hoffman, H. N., and Nelson, R. A.: Total parenteral nutrition. Mayo Clin. Proc. 51:187, 1976.

Hardy, R. M., and Osborne, C. A.: Water deprivation test in the dog: maximal normal values. J. A. V. M. A. 174:479, 1979.

Harrison, J. B., Sussman, H. H., and Pickering, D. E.: Fluid and electrolyte therapy in small animals. J. A. V. M. A. 137:637, 1960.

Hartsfield, S. M., Thurmon, J. C., and Benson, G. J.: Sodium bicarbonate and bicarbonate precursors for treatment of metabolic acidosis. J. A. V. M. A. 179:914, 1981.

Koushanpour, E.: *Renal Physiology: Principles and Functions.* Philadelphia: W. B. Saunders Co., 1976.

Valtin, H.: *Renal Dysfunction: Mechanisms Involved in Fluid and Solute Imbalance.* Boston: Little, Brown and Co., 1979.

PRINCIPLES OF ANTIMICROBIAL THERAPY

GERALD V. LING, D.V.M.,
and DWIGHT C. HIRSH, D.V.M.

Davis, California

If they could, colleagues of 40 years ago would look upon veterinarians of today engaged in the treatment of infectious disease and say that we are truly blessed. At our disposal today is a formidable array of extremely potent antimicrobial agents with which to successfully treat virtually any bacterial infection anywhere in the body of any animal. Concern on the part of veterinarians about infectious diseases caused by bacteria should be a thing of the past, as scarlet fever in children is to pediatricians. It is true that we are blessed with many powerful drugs. They are readily available at reasonable cost for use on any patient and for any reason. Why, then, do we not *feel* blessed?

With the increased utilization of antimicrobial agents have come several major problems that have complicated our everyday professional lives and the health of our patients. First, as the number and potency of the available antimicrobics have increased, our interest in, and our proficiency at, etiologic diagnosis of the infection being treated should also have increased. Unfortunately, this has not been the case. We have allowed the art and science of diagnosis of infectious disease to fall by the wayside while we prescribe course after course of ever more potent antimicrobics, often without a shred of evidence concerning what infection we are treating.

Second, many veterinarians express and/or practice the philosophy that all sick animals should be given therapeutic courses of one or more antimicrobics no matter how remote the possibility that their disease is caused by an infectious agent.

Third, the widespread use (or misuse) of antimicrobics has increased the incidence of undesirable drug interactions and toxic drug reactions. Many of these reactions can be avoided if antimicrobics are used only when they are specifically needed.

Through the injudicious use of antimicrobics, we have caused bacteria strains to form that are resistant to many available drugs. These resistant populations occur more often than is recognized both in our patients and in our veterinary hospitals.

Editor's Note: See *Current Veterinary Therapy VII*, pp. 2–16, for details of specific drug usage.

The rules governing when, what, how much, how often, and for how long as they pertain to antimicrobial therapy are really quite simple and are easily applied in clinical practice. It is precisely the need for veterinarians to understand and to utilize these rules, when contemplating the use of an antimicrobial agent, that was the stimulus for this article. We must recognize that the proper use of antimicrobial agents is extremely important, not only for the immediate success of therapy in our patients but also for human health and for the health of all pet and food-producing animals. If we as a profession do not become more conscious of the rules of antimicrobial therapy, our use of these drugs may someday be restricted by regulations imposed upon us by an outside agency.

COLLECTION AND HANDLING OF MICROBIOLOGIC SPECIMENS

The use of the microbiology laboratory as an aid in diagnosis and management of infectious disease has long been neglected by small animal veterinary clinicians. Microbiology has been classically taught as a basic science in veterinary schools, and its application to small animal practice problems has not been widely stressed. Consequently, demand by practitioners for microbiologic services from commercial laboratories has been minimal relative to the demand for blood chemistries and other clinical pathologic tests. This limited request for service has restricted the range of microbiologic services offered by commercial laboratories and the number of laboratories offering any service of this type because of the economics involved.

There is a growing tendency for veterinarians in private practice to conduct part of their microbiologic laboratory work in their own office rather than utilize a commercial lab. This practice is good or bad, depending on the viewpoint. The increasing commercial availability of attractively packaged culture kits or systems to veterinarians and physicians for office use has done much to awaken interest in using culture data to guide, support, and evaluate the results of antimicrobial therapy. A clear understanding of the limitations of these office culture systems and the criteria for validation of their results and an accurate interpretation of their results are essential, but unfortunately these are not universal among users of the systems. For example, it is usually beneficial to identify the infecting bacteria, but it is not possible to be accurate in the speciation of bacteria except in a very few of the systems currently available. If two or more bacterial species are present in the cultured material, there is little or no way to isolate and separate the individual species so that susceptibility test results can be accurately interpreted. Susceptibility test results will *always* be inaccurate unless certain test standards are met, e.g., the type of agar used, the age of the agar, and the depth of the agar in the plate. These standards are poorly controlled in the susceptibility test portion of most office culture systems. Additional test standards, such as the use of a standardized bacterial inoculum size, which is extremely important for test accuracy, may be difficult to incorporate into some culture systems because explicit directions and/or the necessary equipment and media are not included in the system package.

We recommend a combination of office and commercial microbiology testing for the overall best results. Inoculation of agar plates for primary isolation of aerobic bacteria or yeasts is often easiest if conducted in the office, whereas species identification and antimicrobial susceptibility testing should routinely be conducted by a commercial laboratory or a local human hospital laboratory employing trained microbiology personnel and quality control. Special requests or needs, such as viral or anaerobic bacterial isolations, must be conducted in commercial microbiology laboratories unless the veterinarian has advanced bacteriology or virology training.

Specimens for microbial culture must be collected and handled so that they are not altered by bacterial cell death, bacterial overgrowth, or contamination with extraneous bacteria. It is essential to obtain such specimens *before* beginning antimicrobial therapy. Material collected on sterile cotton swabs should be placed in a suitable transport medium (one that prevents overgrowth or death of bacteria during transport) if the microbiology tests are to be conducted by a commercial laboratory. Microbiologic laboratories usually supply their preferred transport medium for this purpose or recommend one that may be purchased from a supplier or a local human hospital. If transport medium is not to be used (e.g., urine for culture from which an estimation of numbers of bacteria per milliliter of urine is desired or if the specimen is to be cultured in the office), immediate refrigeration at 4° C in a closed, sterile container is necessary. Inoculation of media should take place within four hours of collection.

ANTIMICROBIAL SUSCEPTIBILITY TESTING

The terms "sensitive" and "resistant" are routinely used, albeit somewhat indiscriminately, when referring to bacterial susceptibility. They are terms relative to the infection site. Within an animal, a bacterial population may be sensitive (susceptible) to the concentration of an antimicrobic in one location but resistant in another. The most important factor here is the concentration of the antimicrobic that inhibits the infectious agent, either by killing it or by slowing its growth so that normal body defenses can take over. The concentration of any antimicrobic that must be attained at the infection site to achieve bacterial inhibition can be measured *in vitro* through the use of an antimicrobial susceptibility test. This concentration is called the minimum inhibitory concentration (MIC). If the MIC of an antimicrobic for the infecting bacteria *can* be achieved at the site of infection, the bacteria are said to be sensitive or susceptible. Conversely, if the MIC of an antimicrobic for a population of bacteria *cannot* be achieved at the site of infection, the bacteria are said to be resistant.

The results of antimicrobial susceptibility tests are used as a guide when choosing an antimicrobial agent for treatment of an infectious disease process. From the standpoint of clinical veterinary practice, a susceptibility test should only be used when an isolated bacterial species possesses traits that make prediction of its susceptibility difficult. Fortunately there are a limited number of bacterial species that possess such traits. In small animal practice, they include *Staphylococcus aureus* and members of the family Enterobacteriaceae. Other bacteria, with few exceptions, are predictably susceptible to certain antimicrobial agents at attainable tissue concentrations (Table 1).

Briefly, the mechanisms whereby *Staphylococcus aureus* and members of the family Enterobacteriaceae become resistant to antimicrobics are as follows. Certain *Staphylococcus aureus* isolates

Table 1. *Bacteria With Predictable Susceptibility to Certain Antimicrobial Agents*

Bacteria	Antimicrobial
Actinomyces spp.	Penicillin, ampicillin
Actinobacillus spp.	Penicillin, ampicillin
Pasteurella spp.	Penicillin, ampicillin
β-hemolytic streptococci*	Penicillin, ampicillin
Bordetella spp.	Ampicillin
Anaerobic bacteria†	Penicillin, ampicillin
Pseudomonas spp.	Gentamicin, amikacin

Streptococcus canis, Streptococcus zooepidemicus, and others.

†*Bacteroides* spp., *Peptostreptococcus* spp., *Fusobacterium* spp.

may possess an extrachromosomal piece of DNA containing genes that code for resistance to various antimicrobial agents. This DNA piece, called an R plasmid, can be gained or lost without damage to the bacterium possessing it. Transfer of an R plasmid from one *Staphylococcus aureus* to another is uncommon, but when it occurs the transfer is accomplished by a bacterial virus. It is difficult to predict whether a given isolate of *Staphylococcus aureus* will be susceptible to a given antimicrobic, since any number and combination of resistance genes can be carried by the R plasmids of this species. For example, the use of a specific antimicrobic will select for staphylococci that are resistant to tissue levels of that drug and also for various other resistance characteristics. The antimicrobial agents to which *Staphylococcus aureus* may be resistant through the presence of R plasmids include penicillin, tetracycline, chloramphenicol, erythromycin, and kanamycin. Resistance to methicillin and to other penicillinase-resistant penicillins may occur but is rare in *Staphylococcus aureus* isolates from animals, whereas R plasmids that encode for penicillinase production are common. Although penicillinase-resistant penicillins can be used to treat *Staphylococcus aureus* infections before susceptibility test results are known, their routine use against penicillin-sensitive strains (nonpenicillinase producers) is contraindicated. The unnecessary selective pressure placed on the bacterial population in this instance may lead to selection of one of the rare methicillin-resistant strains.

The so-called gram negative enterics, members of the family Enterobacteriaceae, include *Escherichia coli*, *Proteus* spp., *Enterobacter* spp., *Klebsiella* spp., and *Salmonella* spp. These organisms pose the greatest problem to veterinarians with regard to selection of an antimicrobial agent. They are almost always resistant to attainable tissue concentrations of penicillin. Owing to certain characteristics of the gram negative bacterial cell wall, sufficient penicillin cannot pass through the cell wall barrier unless the bacteria are exposed to concentrations far above those achieved in body tissues (concentrations that can only be attained in urine). Ampicillin, on the other hand, because of structural differences, is able to pass through the cell walls of these bacteria and exert its bacteriocidal action. The gram negative enterics also possess R plasmids that contain genes that code for resistance to nearly all of the commonly used antimicrobial agents. Since these genes may occur in any number and combination in a given population of bacteria, prediction of antimicrobial susceptibility is risky except in urinary tract infections. Bacterial resistance, mediated by R plasmids, has been shown to occur with ampicillin, tetracycline, chloramphenicol, sulfonamides, cephalosporins, trimethoprim sulfa, and the aminoglycosides (neomycin, kana-

mycin, gentamicin, streptomycin, and tobramycin). Penicillinase-resistant penicillins should not be used for treatment of this group of bacteria because they cannot pass through the gram negative cell wall. The R plasmids of the enteric group differ from those of *Staphylococcus aureus* in that they readily pass from one bacterium to another by a sexual process called conjugation. Conjugation between the same or different species within this group rapidly increases when a population of bacteria is exposed to residues of any antimicrobic. Thus, exposure to one antimicrobic may result in bacterial resistance to many other antimicrobics to which the bacteria may not have been exposed. This is of greatest importance in the fecal flora, since the feces provide the bacterial source of infections for many locations in the body, e.g., urinary tract, prostate, open wounds.

SELECTION OF AN ANTIMICROBIAL AGENT

The ideal antimicrobial agent is a drug that disrupts one or more of the essential life processes within bacterial cells at concentrations that do not damage membrane cells. This phenomenon is referred to as selective toxicity. The toxic effect of an antimicrobic on bacterial cells may be brought about by inhibition of cell wall synthesis, alteration of the permeability of bacterial cell membranes, or inhibition of the synthesis of genetic proteins and nucleic acids in bacterial cells (preventing bacterial replication). Penicillins and cephalosporins are two examples of antimicrobics that exert a bacteriocidal effect by selectively inhibiting cell wall synthesis, leading to cell lysis. Bacterial cell membrane permeability is altered by polymyxin, whereas fungal cell membranes are altered by amphotericin B and nystatin. Protein synthesis in bacteria is inhibited by many drugs including chloramphenicol, tetracycline, erythromycin, lincomycin, and the aminoglycosides such as gentamicin. Inhibition of nucleic acid (DNA) synthesis occurs in the presence of trimethoprim and the sulfonamides. Refer to the reading list at the end of this article for detailed references on drug/parasite interactions.

In addition to selective toxicity, other desirable criteria of the ideal antimicrobic include ease of client administration (which relates directly to dosage form), wide distribution in the body at therapeutic concentrations, and modest expense. It may not be possible to fulfill all of these criteria when selecting an antimicrobic for every situation. Whenever antimicrobial therapy is contemplated, however, these criteria should be routinely considered.

As discussed earlier, *Staphylococcus aureus* is the major gram positive bacterial species encountered in small animal practice to which susceptibility to penicillin cannot be predicted without *in vitro* testing. A three-year survey of *in vitro* bacterial susceptibility was recently completed at the University of California, Davis. Drugs surveyed included penicillin G, ampicillin, oxacillin, cephalothin, tetracycline, chloramphenicol, trimethoprim sulfa, erythromycin, carbenicillin, kanamycin, gentamicin, and amikacin. From the results of this survey, it can be predicted that, at attainable serum concentrations, oxacillin, cephalothin, chloramphenicol, trimethoprim sulfa, erythromycin, kanamycin, gentamicin, and amikacin would each be effective in the treatment of more than 90 per cent of *Staphylococcus aureus* isolates. Based on this survey, penicillin G and ampicillin were each less than 50 per cent effective.

In the portion of the survey that included members of the family Enterobacteriaceae (gram negative enterics), results indicated that only gentamicin and amikacin would be effective at attainable serum concentrations in the treatment of over 90 per cent of *Escherichia coli* isolates. Amikacin was the only drug tested to which more than 90 per cent of *Klebsiella* spp. isolates were susceptible, whereas amikacin, gentamicin, and trimethoprim sulfa were the only drugs tested to which 90 per cent or more of the *Proteus* spp. isolates were susceptible at attainable serum concentrations. Of the gram negative enterics less commonly encountered in small animal practice (*Salmonella* spp., *Enterobacter* spp., and so on), results indicated that only amikacin would be effective in more than 90 per cent of the isolates. The results of this survey clearly show that *in vitro* susceptibility testing *must* be conducted routinely on members of this family of bacteria for the veterinarian to be able to select an appropriate antimicrobic. Proper identification of the organism and knowledge of the distribution of each antimicrobic in the body are also essential for the proper selection of the most effective therapeutic agent (see Treatment of Urinary Tract Infections with Antimicrobial Agents for specific information regarding the urinary tract).

COMMON SENSE USE OF ANTIMICROBIAL THERAPY WHEN THE ETIOLOGIC AGENT IS UNDEFINED

If it were possible to routinely prescribe the correct antimicrobic on the basis of cultural and susceptibility test results, most therapeutic problems, other than toxic drug reactions, could be avoided. In small animal practice, however, antimicrobial therapy occasionally must be initiated before results of bacterial cultures and susceptibility tests are available. In these situations, the decision to initiate therapy with a specific antimicrobic must

be based on other factors. The site of bacterial infection established by history, a thorough physical examination, radiography, a gram stain of a smear of exudate, and so on, may be a guide for antimicrobic selection. If the infection site cannot be determined, establishment of lack of involvement of one or more body systems may be almost as helpful.

Certain bacterial species are frequently responsible for infections at specific locations in the body or infections involving specific body systems. The actual bacterial species involved may be influenced by geographic location, age, breed, sex, and environment. One example of this influence is otitis externa. The species of bacteria causing infection of the external ear canal can vary, depending on whether the infection is acute or chronic, whether it is induced by a foreign body, whether the pinnas of the ears are held erect or are allowed to dangle, whether there is hair growing in the external ear canals, and whether the ears have been recently treated or cleaned and how this was done. The most commonly isolated pathogens from the ears of dogs with otitis externa in our practice are staphylococci, *Pseudomonas aeruginosa*, *Proteus* spp., and *Pityrosporum* spp. A gram stained smear of exudate exhibiting many yeast forms or many gram positive cocci will greatly aid in the selection of the proper therapeutic agent. If gram negative rods predominate, a culture and organism identification test should be conducted.

Bacterial infections of the skin of both dogs and cats (other than cat bite abscesses) are most often caused by staphylococci (60 per cent) and *Escherichia coli* (20 per cent). Occasionally, one of the other gram negative enterics, *Pseudomonas* spp., or enterococci may contaminate a wound or superimpose itself on a chronic skin condition. Cat bite abscesses are most commonly caused by *Bacteroides* spp. (anaerobe), *Pasteurella* spp., or, less often, a member of the gram negative enteric group.

Bacteria most often isolated from tracheobronchial secretions in our practice include *Escherichia coli* (22 per cent), *Staphylococcus aureus* (18 per cent), *Bordetella bronchiseptica* (17 per cent), and *Klebsiella pneumoniae* (14 per cent). Other studies of bacterial pathogens isolated from small animals with respiratory disease in other regions of the US have yielded differing results, illustrating the important role that environment and locale play in influencing the species of bacterial pathogens associated with airway infections.

Septicemic patients that have had positive blood cultures have most frequently been infected with *Staphylococcus aureus* (37 per cent), *Escherichia coli* (20 per cent), and *Klebsiella pneumoniae* (11 per cent).

To reiterate, the two most frequently isolated

organisms in these commonly encountered diseases in small animal practice (i.e., otitis externa, bacterial infections of the skin, tracheobronchial infections) are *Staphylococcus aureus* and a member of the gram negative enteric group (except for bite wounds in cats). Prediction of antimicrobial susceptibility of these organisms without actual bacterial isolation and susceptibility testing is a risky business. The most frequently isolated organism in each disease previously mentioned makes up only a small percentage of the total number of isolates. The chance for error in blind prediction of the appropriate antimicrobic in any given situation is, therefore, compounded.

FEVER OF UNDETERMINED ORIGIN

Fever can occur in animals for a variety of reasons. In addition to bacterial infections, viral and fungal infections, certain immunologic diseases, neoplasia, exposure to excessive environmental temperature, excessive physical exertion, and persistent anxiety or fear are among the common causes of fever.

It seems to be an increasingly common veterinary practice to prescribe or administer an antimicrobial agent to patients with fever of any cause. Many, if not most, short-lived (one to five days) fevers in small animals are not caused by bacterial infections but rather by viral infections or other processes that lead to endogenous pyrogen release. These phenomena are nearly always short in duration, and the affected animal will routinely recover whether or not antimicrobics are administered.

A major problem resulting from the indiscriminate use of antimicrobial agents as previously mentioned is that antimicrobics, especially those given by mouth and those that are eliminated in active form via the gut, initiate a rapid increase in R plasmid–derived resistance of the gut microflora to many other antimicrobics. This high level of antimicrobial resistance persists for two months or more, and elements from this reservoir may subsequently infect a body system with resistant bacteria. An additional problem in some patients with persistent fever is that a diagnosis may be obscured by injudicious use of antimicrobics.

We believe that it is unnecessary to create a resistant fecal reservoir in most animals. We advocate restriction of the use of antimicrobics in animals with fever of undefined origin to those whose lives are thought to be in danger from sepsis and those whose fever is caused by bacterial infection of a specific site, organ, or body system (e.g., cat fight abscess, urinary tract infection) for which the causative organism can be deduced with a high degree of certainty with or without minimal office diagnostics (gram stained smear and so on).

THERAPEUTIC COMPLIANCE

It is important for veterinarians to know how to recognize situations that are likely to lead to poor therapeutic compliance. Careful specimen collection, accurate identification of an infectious agent, determination of its antimicrobial susceptibility, and selection of an appropriate antimicrobic may be all for naught if the client fails to comply with the dosing instructions. We have found no published data documenting the magnitude of noncompliance in small animal practice, but there is at least one unpublished study from which we can glean the problem. There also have been numerous compliance studies conducted in human medicine that may be applicable to veterinary practice.

Animals are given prescribed medications by their owners, who may demonstrate noncompliant behavior similar to that seen when medicating themselves or their children. We are convinced that therapeutic compliance is greatly increased if the veterinarian lucidly and completely explains to the client why a drug is prescribed. Time and again, in discussions with clients regarding past medications prescribed for their pet, it has come to light that drugs were not properly given at home either because the client did not understand the instructions for dosing or because the client could not follow the instructions on the label. Occasionally clients have admitted that they did not give the prescribed medication at all. The most frequent reasons for this surprising and frustrating behavior have been "I didn't know what it was for"; "I didn't know what it was"; "I didn't think it would help"; "a friend told me not to use it"; "I didn't know how to give it"; or "I couldn't give it." This last reason for noncompliance is commonly stated by clients, especially when ocular ointments were prescribed and tablets or capsules were prescribed for cats. A simple solution would be for the veterinarian, or a trained staff member, to demonstrate placement of ointment onto the conjunctivae or the pilling procedure when such medication is prescribed.

One additional reason given by clients for not giving medication has been "I didn't like (or trust) the doctor." This is most likely to occur when the client's regular veterinarian is not available and a relief veterinarian or another veterinarian in the practice with no previous association with the client sees the pet. It may also result from abrupt, strained, heated, or hurried contact with a new pet and client, which may give the client the impression that the veterinarian is callous and noncaring toward the pet and its medical problem.

Compliance is influenced by the physical characteristics of both the medication and the patient. Large tablets or capsules are difficult for even experienced animal handlers to give to cats and toy dogs. Pills of any size are difficult to give to small brachycephalic breeds. Prescribing oral solutions of antimicrobics may lead to increased compliance when pills are difficult to give but may decrease compliance in other situations because they are messy and sticky when spilled onto the fur around the mouth. Clients may have a personal aversion to capsules or tablets, to medication of a certain color or odor, or even to the name of a certain antimicrobial agent, and because of this they may not follow the veterinarian's directions. This problem may be avoided by asking the client if there is a type of medication (capsule, tablet, solution) that is easiest for him to give to the pet. It is rarely necessary to prescribe injectable antimicrobial agents for home use. This is fortunate for veterinarians, because many clients are frightened at the mere thought of injecting medication into an animal. Injectable antimicrobics should never be prescribed for home use without suitable instruction and demonstration of the proper injection technique by the veterinarian or a trained staff member. The client should then give the animal a trial injection of distilled water or saline, under the observation of the veterinarian or staff member, to demonstrate an understanding of the technique and proper proficiency in its application.

Compliance is influenced by the prescribed frequency of administration of a drug. It is often difficult for clients to remember when to give a dose of medication unless they are able to associate this activity with something that they do at about the same time each day. For example, if medication is to be given at eight-hour intervals, the veterinarian may suggest that doses be given before breakfast, before supper, and before bedtime, three reasonably constant interludes in the lives of nearly everyone. Similar association may be made with twice daily (before breakfast and after supper) and once daily administrations. Compliance may also be increased by dispensing a monthly calendar premarked with medication to be given at intervals greater than once a day, e.g., every other day or once a week.

Compliance is influenced by the duration of the course of therapy. Clients who must give medication to their pet for several weeks or months, as is necessary in diseases such as infectious discospondylitis, bacterial prostatitis, and nasal cryptococcosis, are likely to occasionally forget doses. Compliance may decrease or cease entirely as the signs of illness disappear and the pet appears normal to the owner unless the need for continued medication is frequently reinforced by the veterinarian. This reinforcement is perhaps best accomplished during follow-up examinations at not more than one-month intervals. Frequent telephone conversations with the client may also be effective. Lapses in compliance are also common with conditions requiring prophylactic or suppressive therapy, as may be needed in recurrent urinary tract infections, unless frequent positive reinforcement is given by the veterinarian.

Lastly, compliance may be influenced by the age, economic status, education, and emotional status of the client. Middle-aged, middle class, high school graduates have been singled out in studies of therapeutic compliance in human medicine as those most likely to comply with home treatment regimens. Young single people, the aged, the very poor or the very rich, and those with little education are most likely to ignore all or part of the therapeutic instructions given them regardless of whether the instructions are for themselves, their families, or their pets.

FAILURE OF ANTIMICROBIAL THERAPY

Failure to achieve the desired therapeutic outcome when using an antimicrobial agent to combat an infectious disease should be analyzed so that errors or omissions in diagnosis or management may be corrected and avoided in the future. Treatment failure may result from one or more of the following:

1. Failure to select an appropriate antimicrobic for the infecting bacterial species because of incorrect results of bacterial identification or susceptibility testing or because of sampling error, e.g., overgrowth of the culture plate with bacteria other than those causing the infection.

2. Failure to select an animicrobic that will attain needed concentrations of active drug at the site of infection. Example: bacterial prostatitis caused by streptococci that are susceptible to penicillin *in vitro*. Penicillin, however, is an unwise choice in this instance because it does not reach therapeutic concentrations in the prostate.

3. Failure to prescribe an antimicrobic frequently enough to maintain needed concentrations at the infection site.

4. Failure to prescribe an antimicrobic in high enough doses to maintain bacteriocidal or bacteriostatic concentrations at the infection site.

5. Failure to prescribe an antimicrobic for a sufficient period of time to allow the drug and the body defenses to interact to completely rid the infection site of the causative agent.

6. Failure of the patient to absorb the antimicrobic because of vomiting; because of interaction with residues of food, milk, or other medication in the gut; or because of a variety of intestinal diseases that affect absorption.

7. Development of acquired (R plasmid) resistance to the antimicrobic in the infecting bacterial population.

8. Failure of the patient to rid itself of the infection because of the presence of a foreign body acting as a nidus. Example: urinary tract infection persisting in the presence of cystic calculi.

9. Failure of the patient to rid itself of the infection because of impaired host defense mechanisms.

10. Failure of the patient to respond because of another underlying disease process at the infection site. Example: nasal cavity bacterial infection is invariably secondary to a neoplasm in the area.

SUPPLEMENTAL READING

Baggot, J. D.: *Principles of Drug Disposition in Domestic Animals: The Basis of Veterinary Clinical Pharmacology.* Philadelphia: W. B. Saunders Co., 1977.

Barry, A. L.: *The Antimicrobic Susceptibility Test: Principles and Practices.* Philadelphia: Lea & Febiger, 1976.

Blackwell, B.: Drug therapy: Patient compliance. N. Engl. J. Med. 289:249, 1973.

Gilman, A. G., Goodman, L. S., and Gilman, A.: *Goodman and Gilman's The Pharmacological Basis of Therapeutics,* 6th ed. New York: Macmillan Publishing Co., 1980, pp. 1080–1248.

Kagan, B. M.: *Antimicrobial Therapy,* 3rd ed. Philadelphia: W. B. Saunders Co., 1980.

MANAGING DISEASES OF THE EAR

A. J. VENKER-VAN HAAGEN, D.V.M.

Utrecht, The Netherlands

THE PINNA

Congenital Defects. The veterinarian is not often confronted with dogs or cats with misshapen pinnae, probably because these dogs or cats are already selected out directly after birth. More often the veterinarian is consulted concerning correction of hanging ears that are supposed to stand up and standing ears that are supposed to hang down. Since these are not strictly medical problems, they are not dealt with here.

Wounds. A tear in the pinna is usually presented as an emergency because the wound bleeds profusely and the animal will not stop shaking its head, causing the owner to panic. A small tear can be sutured under local anesthesia, but larger ones must be sutured under general anesthesia. Very fine interrupted sutures with atraumatic material are used to join skin to skin only, first on the inner side and then on the outer side. Good healing of the wound results without scar tissue contraction.

Othematoma. In most cases an othematoma occurs during the course of otitis externa and is caused by the animal scratching and shaking the ears. Surgical intervention should be delayed for about one week after the first manifestation of the othematoma so that bleeding can stop and the blood can clot. Under general anesthesia an S-shaped incision is made on the inner surface of the pinna, through both the skin and the cartilage. The S should be as large as the surface of the hematoma. Blood clots and fibrin are removed, and then interrupted mattress sutures of 2-0 chromic catgut are placed completely through the pinna to obliterate the hematoma cavity. The sutures should be ¾ cm wide and no more than ¾ cm apart and should be placed over the entire surface of the hematoma. The sutures should be tied on the outer surface. This method guarantees nice healing, and the pinna returns to its normal thinness several weeks after surgery. The sutures are removed after two weeks. An analgesic is prescribed for at least five days after surgery. The animal should be prevented from scratching the ear by use of a large bucket-shaped plastic collar rather than by bandaging the ear.

Abscesses. In cats, abscesses of the pinna are usually caused by a penetrating wound inflicted by the claw of another cat. The skin over the abscess should be opened, and the pus should be removed by gentle compression and flushing. An antibiotic should be administered for ten days, and, since *Pasteurella multocida* is usually cultured from the pus, penicillin G or ampicillin is usually appropriate.

Tumors. Pinna tumors are usually malignant. An exception is the histiocytoma or extragenital venereal tumor, which sometimes occurs on the ears of young dogs. Squamous cell carcinoma is particularly important in the white cat, because the tumor often appears as a nonhealing proliferative inflammation at the edge of the pinna. It is easily misdiagnosed as an inflammatory lesion, not only because of its slow progression but also because it is frequently bilateral. Amputation of the pinna is possible in the early stages but is not always accepted by the owner.

THE EXTERNAL EAR CANAL

A well-known congenital defect of the external ear canal is atresia of the canal. It is almost never well-advised to attempt surgical correction of such a defect. Even if a patent canal is achieved it almost always results in lifelong misery for the animal because of persistent otitis externa. In some cases one becomes aware of the atresia because hematogenous infection of the middle ear results in a fistula under the opening of the ear canal. In such cases the fistula is opened surgically, the middle ear is flushed with saline, and drainage is maintained for five days. An antibiotic selected on the basis of bacteriologic culture and sensitivity testing is administered for at least two weeks.

A disruption in the ear canal after *trauma* should certainly be repaired surgically. Interrupted atraumatic Vicryl sutures through the cartilage, but not penetrating the skin in the ear canal, will give very satisfactory results. The ear canal is exposed by a vertical incision through the skin over the vertical part of the canal.

Otitis externa

Inflammation of the external ear canal causes the dog or cat uneasiness and pain. Otitis externa in the dog or cat should be approached as a major disability, one that deserves the veterinarian's full attention and such time and effort as may be required.

Otitis externa is not so much a diagnosis as an indication of the location of a problem. There are so many ways in which the external ear can be affected, not only with regard to cause but also with regard to the way in which the dog or cat reacts. Some dogs will scratch and rub their ears and thereby inflict considerable trauma when a sign of inflammation can scarcely be found in the ear canal. The veterinarian is then confronted with a dog with painfully swollen ears and even a bleeding pinna, all brought about by discomfort from, for example, a ceruminous plug in the ear canal. Other dogs will not even scratch an ear that plays host to a huge mite invasion. Hence, even enlarging upon the notation "otitis externa" on the patient's record by noting the cause, such as bacterial or parasitic, falls short of an adequate description of the full extent of the problem.

We prefer to record the following information: general condition of the patient, condition of the pinna, condition of the orifice of the ear canal, the type of exudate, the width of the lumen of the canal, the condition of the lining of the canal, and the condition of the tympanic membrane. After the ear canal has been washed (see further), we again describe the width of the ear canal and the condition of the tympanic membrane. This recorded information is essential for objective evaluation of the results of treatment. The owner's comments on the results of treatment can be deceiving, since the treatment often consists of locally applied medications containing corticosteroids, which certainly diminish pruritus and pain but do not always change the pathologic condition of the ear canal.

Management of ear problems in the dog and cat begins with the case history, the first objective of which is to determine whether the problem is unilateral or bilateral and whether its onset was gradual or sudden. A unilateral disorder with a sudden onset marked by severe scratching is often associated with a foreign body such as a grass awn. A slowly developing unilateral disorder with pain and purulent discharge is often found to be due to a tumor within the ear. Equally important are the owner's impressions of the general condition of the animal and the past or present existence of skin diseases. A general examination of the patient should include the case history and the veterinarian's impression of the patient's general condition. The head and pinnae, the base of the pinna, the orifice of the ear canal, and the exudate should all be inspected. If the exudate is purulent, material is obtained for bacteriologic culturing.

An otoscopic examination always begins with an inspection of the unaffected or least affected ear. Similarly, if washing of the ear canal is needed, the least affected ear is handled first. After the ear is flushed the dog is allowed to shake its head, preferably in a corner of the room away from equipment and records. During this pause the first part of the report is recorded. The otoscopic examination is then repeated. If the tympanic membrane is not yet visible because of a ceruminous plug, the flushing and shaking are repeated. If there is an excess of hair growing in the opening of the ear canal, it is plucked out. Sometimes the tympanic membrane is not visible because of pathologic swelling or proliferation of the lining of the ear canal. In such cases treatment is begun following the scheme in Fig. 1. This general approach produces definitive results in a large proportion of disorders of the ear canal.

Examination and Cleaning. The dog or cat must be held by an experienced assistant. Most dogs and cats submit to the otoscopic examination easily when it is accompanied by petting and calming words, but they never like the flushing. The quality of the otoscope is most important. We prefer Welch Allyn*

---

*Welch Allyn, Inc., Skaneateles Falls, NY.

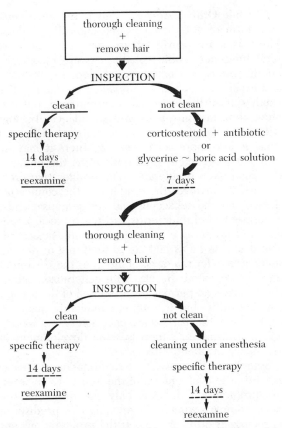

```
        ┌─────────────────────┐
        │  thorough cleaning  │
        │          +          │
        │    remove hair      │
        └─────────────────────┘
                   │
               INSPECTION
              ╱          ╲
           clean        not clean
             │              │
    specific therapy   corticosteroid + antibiotic
             │                   or
          14 days     glycerine ~ boric acid solution
             │                   │
        reexamine              7 days
                                 │
        ┌─────────────────────┐
        │  thorough cleaning  │
        │          +          │
        │    remove hair      │
        └─────────────────────┘
                   │
               INSPECTION
              ╱          ╲
           clean        not clean
             │              │
    specific therapy   cleaning under anesthesia
             │                │
          14 days       specific therapy
             │                │
        reexamine          14 days
                              │
                          reexamine
```

Figure 1. A general approach to managing diseases of the external ear.

otoscopes (Nos. 25.000 or 25.020), which have a fiber glass cone that transmits light and thus obviates the need for a light source in the path of vision. The illumination is good even in larger breeds of dogs. The range of the four sizes of the additional polypropylene specula (Nos. 24.302 to 24.305) is adequate for otoscopy in dogs and cats (disposable specula are quite inadequate). It is also possible to work through the cone of the otoscope under vision when the rectangular lens is slid aside halfway.

Cleaning of the ear canal is the most important part of the management of otitis externa and is essential in both diagnosis and treatment. Cleaning must be complete and yet must not be irritating to the ear canal. Cotton-tipped swabs are the *worst possible* aids for cleaning. Their cleaning function is doubtful, they push material inward, and the irritation they cause is severe, especially when used frequently.

Thorough flushing is best and is only possible with a fine and forceful stream of water. A very good instrument is the Elpa* otologic flusher designed for flushing the human ear (Fig. 2). This unit is connected permanently to a cold water supply

---

*Stümer, Haugerring 5, 8700 Würtzburg, W. Germany.

pipe, and its electrically heated, thermostatically controlled reservoir warms the water to 37 to 39° C. A flexible hose delivers water from the reservoir to a faucet handle with a second thermostat. Several types of cannulas can be attached to the handle. During flushing, the tip of the cannula is placed just within the horizontal part of the ear canal. The bayonet-type cannula is designed for flushing under observation through the otoscope, which we only do occasionally. Medication placed within the ear canal after flushing must be in a quantity sufficient to coat the entire surface of the ear canal. The only reliable way to achieve this is to completely fill the canal. Liquids or ointments packaged in disposable injectors are preferred. For successful treatment of otitis externa it is essential that the medication come into contact with the skin of a totally clean ear.

Parasitic Otitis Externa. This condition, seen in dogs and cats, is often caused by mite infestation (*Otodectes cynotis*). The mites appear to irritate the ceruminous glands in particular, because an excess of thick, dark brown cerumen always accompanies the mite infestation. The mites can easily be detected on this dark brown ceruminous background with an otoscope. When warmed by the light of the otoscope, the mites begin walking around. In treating mite infestation we first flush the ear canal until the tympanic membrane is in view. Then a 2 per cent lindane emulsion is applied both within the canal and on the pinna, particularly around the opening of the canal. The animal is then allowed to shake its head, after which all of the medication on the exterior surfaces is wiped away.

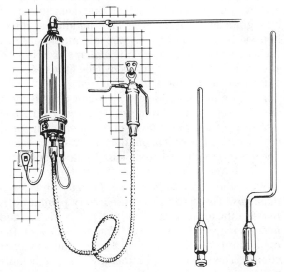

Figure 2. The otologic flusher. The unit is permanently connected to a cold water supply pipe, and its electrically heated, thermostatically controlled reservoir warms water to 37 to 39°C. A flexible hose delivers water from the reservoir to a faucet handle with a second thermostat. Several types of cannulas can be attached to the handle.

This is of particular importance in cats, because ingestion of lindane can cause epileptiform seizures. Following this antiparasitic treatment the external otitis is treated for five days by local application of wide spectrum antibiotics and a corticosteroid ointment. Weekly flea powder dusts or sprays are recommended to eliminate mites on the body. All animals in contact with the infested animal should be examined. One week after the initial treatment the ears are re-examined and, if necessary, are flushed again. In almost all cases no further treatment is needed.

Foreign Bodies. These are frequently seen in dogs but are rarely seen in cats. One of the most commonly seen foreign bodies is the grass awn, which works itself into the canal, stalk end first, so that only the tips of a few bristles, scarcely thicker than a hair, are seen with the otoscope. The case history is very helpful. Typically there is a sudden onset of severe scratching of the ear and vigorous shaking of the head while the dog is walking in a field and, upon returning home, rubbing of the ear on the floor. In the following days the itching diminishes and a purulent discharge appears. The ear becomes more and more painful, and the skin around the opening of the ear canal becomes red and swollen. If the veterinary examination is delayed for a long period it is quite possible that the veterinarian will not detect the grass awn immediately. If he also fails to consider the case history he may easily be misled into treating the problem as a primary bacterial otitis. If he follows the scheme in Fig. 1 he will certainly detect the grass awn at the second examination, but if he only follows the results of culture tests or tries one antibiotic after another, the cause of the condition may remain undetected for weeks. The resulting damage caused by a grass awn may even include middle ear infection via perforation of the tympanic membrane. In such cases systemic antibiotic therapy is required after removal of the foreign body (see Otitis Media).

Primary Purulent Otitis Externa. This condition is rare in dogs and cats. Purulent otitis is most often a sequela to chronic otitis externa but may also result from the growth of a tumor (or in cats, the growth of a polyp) in the external ear canal. The bacteria cultured from long-treated ear canals usually have a limited range of sensitivity to antibiotics; the most serious are *Proteus* and *Pseudomonas*. These bacteria cause a very painful otitis that is difficult to treat. The otitis is exudative and necrotizing, and there are large erosions of the epithelium of the ear canal and subcutaneous edema. The success of the therapy is unpredictable even when antibiotics indicated by culture and sensitivity testing are used. Ointments containing antibiotics and DMSO appear to be more effective in *Pseudomonas* infections but certainly not in all cases.

Chronic Otitis Externa. This is the most common form of otitis encountered clinically in dogs. There is more pruritus than pain. The effects of scratching and rubbing of the ears are recognized on the pinna as small areas of alopecia, redness, and excoriation, often accompanied by edema. The exudate from the ear canal is ceruminous, but it is often abnormal in quality and abundance. In dogs with generalized seborrhea the material in the ear canal is also more sebaceous; in others it may be rather dry cerumen. In chronic otitis the lining of the canal often proliferates. The proliferative process usually involves the epidermis, the connective tissue, and the sebaceous and ceruminous glands. Treatment of chronic otitis externa by local application of prednisone ointment is usually successful. The dose can be as high as 20 to 40 mg of prednisone/ear/day for ten days. Sometimes the treatment must be repeated. In dogs with generalized seborrhea there is no permanent resolution of the accompanying otitis, but it is often adequately managed by flushing the ear canals once every six weeks, which prevents or suppresses the development of secondary purulent otitis externa.

Sometimes there is severe deformation of the ear canal due to proliferation of the lining. Even when the proliferation involves only the orifice of the canal, the narrowing of the opening may predispose to recurrent otitis externa. If the proliferations are situated exclusively at the base of the pinna around the orifice, they can be removed surgically under general anesthesia. They should be excised carefully, taking care not to expose the cartilage. Electrocautery is contraindicated because it results in postoperative pain as well as subsequent scar tissue contraction. Surgical bleeding can be controlled by judicious cauterization of major vessels and a pressure bandage over the ear. When proliferations involve both the base of the pinna around the orifice and the vertical part of the ear canal, the lateral wall of the vertical part must be removed or transposed ventrally.

An aural resection (the Zepp operation) guarantees an optimal opening to the entrance of the horizontal part of the ear canal. Quite often the proliferation also involves the horizontal part of the canal. Conservative therapy with abundant corticosteroid ointment should be attempted first. This sometimes results in regression or disappearance of a large part of the proliferation. If the response is inadequate and particularly if there is no relief of pain, the entire ear canal must be removed. This surgical procedure is performed almost weekly in our clinic, and it is successful as long as there is no infection of the middle ear prior to surgery. Since other authors have had less satisfactory results, particularly because of postoperative fistulas, it may be useful to describe our method.

Two incisions are made in the skin over the

vertical part of the ear canal, one extending from the intertragic incisure to the ventral limit of the vertical canal (determined by palpation) and the second from the tragohelicine incisure to the same ventral point. The resulting triangular flap of skin is dissected free to its base at the opening of the canal and then removed. The vertical part of the ear cànal is then freed from the subcutaneous tissue and muscles. This dissection should proceed along the borderline between the cartilage and surrounding tissue, i.e., on the surface of the cartilage itself, to avoid unnecessary hemorrhage. The cartilage and the skin of the medial wall of the ear canal are separated from the cartilage and the skin at the inner side of the base of the pinna with strong scissors. All proliferations are included with the ear canal in this separation. The horizontal part of the ear canal is then separated from the surrounding tissues by dissecting close to the cartilage, as before. Appropriate care must be taken to avoid the facial nerve, which leaves the stylomastoid foramen and passes around the horizontal part of the ear canal in a rostral direction. In some cases the nerve is attached to the cartilage and must be separated from it very carefully. When the horizontal part of the ear canal has been freed from the surrounding tissues, its attachment to the osseus external acoustic meatus is easily palpated during slight movements of the canal. The cartilaginous part is separated from the osseus part with pointed scissors. The facial nerve must be protected during this procedure. Removal of the cartilaginous part of the ear canal is followed by a very important and time-consuming part of the operation, namely, the complete removal of all skin lining the osseus external ear canal. This is best accomplished with a small curette. When removal of the lining is complete, the tympanic membrane is also removed by curette.

The next step is the remodeling of the pinna. The caudal part of the pinna is folded forward, using the most natural folding point at the base of the pinna as the point of rotation. The most caudal part of the base of the pinna is folded against the rostral part of the base of the pinna, folding the pinna in the process. The caudal part of the base is then sutured to the rostral part of the base with interrupted Vicryl sutures, leaving the ends of the sutures long and lying inside the folded pinna. A Penrose drain is placed between the osseus external acoustic meatus and the ventral part of the skin incision, protruding 1 cm. The subcutaneous tissue and skin margins of the initial triangular incision are then sutured together. The Penrose drain remains in place for at least five days, and ampicillin is administered during this period.

The cosmetic effect of the naturally folded pinna is quite satisfactory. This operation is also indicated in cases of tumor of the ear canal, which may occur in dogs of all ages and in older cats. In young cats

apparent tumors in the ear canal are often found to be polyps arising from the middle ear. These can be removed through a ventral incision in the horizontal part of the canal. This is exposed via a vertical incision in the skin under the opening of the ear canal. The polyp is grasped with a small forceps, as close as possible to the osseus meatus, and removed by a short tug. The resulting hemorrhage is slight and stops spontaneously within a few minutes. The incision in the cartilage of the ear canal is closed with a continuous suture of atraumatic Vicryl, and then the subcutaneous tissue and skin are sutured. Ampicillin is administered for ten days, and if there is no infection of the middle ear there will be a regrowth of the tympanic membrane in three weeks.

THE TYMPANIC MEMBRANE

The pathology of the tympanic membrane is usually related to the pathology in the external ear canal or the middle ear. Chronic irritation results in thickening of the tympanic membrane. Spontaneous rupture does not occur often in dogs and cats as a consequence of otitis externa. However, it may occur in young dogs with purulent otitis media, and it often occurs in dogs with pyoderma and in young cats with a polyp arising in the middle ear. When accidental perforation of the tympanic membrane occurs and there is no middle ear infection, the membrane will heal in one to three weeks, depending on the size of the rupture.

THE MIDDLE EAR

Trauma to the middle ear can occur in an animal struck by an automobile. Blood is found in the ear canal, but the ear canal should not be flushed because there may be no natural barrier remaining between the external ear and the meninges and meningitis could result from flushing.

Otitis Media. This may arise hematogenously or by organisms entering via the auditory tube or a ruptured tympanic membrane. When the infection cannot be suppressed by systemic antibiotic therapy, flushing of the middle ear under general anesthesia is indicated. Under visual control through the otoscope, the middle ear is flushed with sterile 0.9 per cent NaCl solution by use of a 10-cc syringe and a cannula 10 cm long and 1 mm in diameter. Alternate flushing with 1 to 2 cc fluid under low pressure and careful drying of the middle ear by aspiration are continued until the aspirated fluid is completely clear. Systemic antibiotic therapy is then resumed for two weeks. The flushing must occasionally be repeated after two weeks, but in most cases there is visible regrowth or healing of the tympanic membrane by this time, indicating that the middle ear infection has been resolved.

In more erosive otitis media the facial nerve and the parasympathetic nerves that accompany it may be involved, resulting in facial paralysis, keratitis sicca, and dryness of the nasal membranes. These complications are reversible if the otitis media is resolved soon enough. Hence flushing is undertaken immediately, without the delay in a trial course of antibiotic therapy.

Tumors. Middle ear tumors are rare. They may cause chronic otitis media alone or in combination with facial paralysis, trigeminal paralysis, and vestibular dysfunction owing to their expansive or invasive growth. The most common, but still rare, tumors of the middle ear are glomus jugular tumors and sarcomas. Diagnosis is made by otoscopy, radiography, and scintigraphy. The prognosis is poor, either because of malignancy or because surgery is impracticable in animals.

THE LABYRINTH

Inherited deafness resulting from incomplete development of the cochlea is well known in the Dalmatian, the bull terrier, and the white cat. The deafness may be partial or total. Congenital deafness may also occur in other dogs or cats. The diagnosis of deafness can in principle be made in several ways, but the case history is often most important and is usually sufficient. The case history, combined with the finding that both ear canals are clean and both tympanic membranes are transparent, indicates that there is a developmental defect for which nothing therapeutic can be done.

Labyrinthitis. This sometimes occurs in the course of otitis media. In the acute stage there is a nystagmus and a severe loss of equilibrium. In most cases there is some degree of spontaneous compensation within the first three days, but there is almost always a definite partial or total loss of the perceptive function of the labyrinth, involving the vestibular organ as well as the cochlea. It is not yet known whether any immediate therapy would be beneficial. Degeneration of the perceptive cells is probably caused by toxic agents, which can pass through the membrane of the round window. The degeneration has been demonstrated after introduction of an antiseptic preparation containing chlorhexidine (Hibitane) in the middle ear. For this reason the ear canal should never be flushed with fluids other than water or 0.9 per cent NaCl solution. Furthermore, no medication (antibiotics, antiparasitics, or detergents) should be applied in the ear canal unless the tympanic membrane is known to be intact.

SUPPLEMENTAL READING

Aursnes, J.: Vestibular damage from chlorhexidine in guinea pigs. Acta Otolaryngol. 92:89, 1981.
Aursnes, J.: Cochlear damage from chlorhexidine in guinea pigs. Acta Otolaryngol. 92:259, 1981.
Zepp, C. P.: Surgical correction of diseases of the ear in the dog and cat. Vet. Rec. 61:643, 1949.

PREVENTING CANINE BEHAVIOR PROBLEMS

THOMAS R. WOLSKI, D.V.M.

Ithaca, New York

Treating behavior problems in pet dogs is a long and sometimes difficult process. The problem is often only a manifestation of deep-rooted defects in the pet-owner relationship or evidence of genetically based, nonmodifiable flaws in the dog's behavioral repertoire or temperament. Only in the last decade, however, has animal behavior become a formal part of most veterinarians' training. In the past, the resolution of many behavior problems has been left to the trainer or breeder, perhaps a derelict approach by the veterinary profession. In 1976, Wilbur reported that only 40 per cent of former dog owners lost their dogs to illness or old age. The rest had dogs that either ran away or were killed in accidents, given away, or taken to the local animal shelter. Accidental death and running away indicate lack of control over a pet, and the prevalence of all four of these categories may indicate widespread problems in the pet-owner bond. The majority of people giving up their dogs cited reasons indicating lack of both control of and commitment to their pet. Of the approximately 30,000,000 dog owners questioned, 19 per cent were described by Wilbur as "dissatisfied," and another 24 per cent as "worried." Those in the former category found more trouble than satisfaction in their pets, and those in the latter feared that their dog was potentially harmful because they were unable to control it.

Aggression is an uncomfortably common canine behavioral complaint. Fifty four per cent of canine behavior problems seen at the New York State Veterinary College from 1979 to 1981 presented with aggression as the primary complaint (Table 1); Borchelt (1982) reports a 66 per cent incidence of cases of aggressive behavior in the New York City area from 1978 to 1981.

Sorting out behavior problems, however, is a time-consuming process that usually starts with several hours of questioning, discussion, and demonstration. It sometimes requires professional re-training or conditioning of the pet. Most clinicians cannot afford this time, but, in view of the figures previously presented, they also cannot legitimately ignore the psychological needs of their patients. A reasonable approach might be for the clinician to be a source of information on preventive behavioral therapy. This information should be offered to puppy owners in conjunction with advice on preventive medicine and nutrition.

The recommendations that follow are drawn from four years' experience in behavior problem consulting. They are designed to help the new pet owner establish a healthy, rewarding relationship with his dog by: (1) preventing the purchase of the wrong dog for the wrong reason, (2) avoiding the formation of behaviorally dangerous pet-owner interaction patterns, and, (3) helping the owner start out with a sound environment in which to raise the new pet. The recommendations are presented as a series of questions the new dog owner should ask. Whenever possible, references are cited that are readily available to the client and are not necessarily scholarly discussions of the topic.

SHOULD I OWN A DOG?

Allowing for an 8 per cent annual inflation rate since 1976, figures compiled by Taylor (1976) indicate that a 15-kg dog presently costs $350 to care for in its first year and $240 each succeeding year. These figures do not include grooming, boarding, and the costs of illness or injury. A good pedigreed dog would probably cost a minimum of $100, and even a mediocre specimen of some breeds may cost two to four times that amount. Beyond the economic commitment, however, are the commitments in time and emotion. Dogs require walking (one-half to three hr/day), play (approximately one-half hr/day), training (one-quarter to one hr/day), and grooming (highly variable). The clinician might suggest that his client read *The Roger Caras Dog*

Table 1. A Summary of the Types of Behaviors Presented as the Primary Complaint to the New York State Veterinary College from 1979 to 1981

Behavior	Number	Per Cent
Aggression	98	54
Destructiveness	23	12
House soiling	29	16
Barking	10	6
Hyperactivity	7	4
Miscellaneous phobias, coprophagia, mounting	3	8
Total	170	100

Book, which compares the relative time needed daily to care for, exercise, and train each of the American Kennel Club (AKC) recognized breeds. Dogs are highly social animals and may respond to isolation and confinement with destructiveness and house soiling. These, in fact, are the second and third most common behavior problems seen in dogs (see Table 1).

A good pet-owner bond can only be established if there is a deep emotional commitment to the dog, and some clients need to be reminded that their pet will die before they will. The Monks of New Skete, in their excellent book *How To Be Your Dog's Best Friend*, discuss this topic well. In most cases, senior citizens moving into subsidized housing are forced to give the dog away or even have it euthanized.

A dog puts certain constraints on the owner's movements. Untrained, ill-behaved animals are not welcome anywhere, but all dogs are prohibited in many public facilities, hotels, and motels. A worrying owner may be reluctant to board the dog and may be forced to stay at home for the life of the dog or may repeatedly have to find and pay for a dog sitter.

Families should be realistic about who will care for the dog. It is unusual for the children to take more than minimal responsibility even though it may be "their dog." The parents, usually the mother, ends up with most or all of the dog care. As with all the points made previously, an unrealistic analysis of this consideration may lead to the dog being unaccepted or resented by one or more household members.

WHY DO I WANT A DOG?

There are good, acceptable, and poor reasons for obtaining a pet dog.

The first good reason to get a dog is companionship. A potential problem may arise if the dog is purchased as a child or spouse substitute; the owner may place unrealistic expectations on the dog. Dogs are neither moral nor rational in the human sense of these terms and may be incapable of human emotions such as love, hate, jealousy, or spitefulness. An owner will be repeatedly disappointed and confounded if he unreasonably insists on interpreting and predicting his dog's behavior in terms of human psychology. Fox's *Understanding Your Dog* and Sautter and Glover's *Behavior, Development, and Training of the Dog* might be good references for an owner confused on these points.

Another good reason to purchase a dog is for work and sport. These dogs are rarely presented with behavior problems.

An acceptable reason to buy a dog is for its object value. This dog provides little psychological benefit to its owner and usually will not be described by its owner as a problem, regardless of the dog's behavior.

Replacement for another dog is another acceptable reason for obtaining a dog. Owners are often unrealistic about the behavior of a new pup obtained soon after the loss of an old pet. The effort needed to train a new puppy has been forgotten. They had been immersed in the old dog's life and are so accustomed to all the idiosyncrasies of its behavior that they automatically assume the new dog will be the same. Most owners should probably wait several months before *considering* another pet, and sometimes several years are needed. The clinician should point out that a period of grief, sometimes prolonged, is normal (Monks of New Skete, 1978). Premature acquisition of a new dog might shorten this period of remembering and savoring the past relationship. It might be wise if the new dog was a different breed, a different color, or the opposite sex to visibly accentuate the difference between the memory of the old dog and the reality of the new one. If the clinician suspects the client might replace a pet too soon, he should discuss the situation with the client before the client decides to get a new dog.

Having a second (or third) dog is another acceptable reason for getting a dog. Owning two dogs is more difficult than most owners realize. The owner simply may not have the time to train two dogs simultaneously. Two dogs may be content with one another's company at the expense of the human-dog relationship. A hierarchy normally forms that is sometimes unstable. Repeated agonistic interactions may result, especially if the owner interferes by protecting or backing the "underdog." Competition for food or the owner's attention may be a constant source of stress. Vices acquired by one dog may be picked up by the other. Many abnormal behaviors are socially facilitated.

Protection is a poor reason to get a dog. Good protection dogs are highly stable, intelligent, and well-trained animals that are subjected to stringent selection standards before coming in contact with the public. Most police dogs, for example, are put through a minimum of 500 hours of training prior to street use. These dogs are taught to attack only on command and to unquestionably abort an attack on command. Clients seeking protection should be asked how reliable a protection source they need, whether they are willing to put in the hours of training necessary, and whether they are willing to destroy their pet if it proves dangerous or unstable. They should also be asked whether they consider trespassing to retrieve an errant baseball a major offense and whether their insurance policy will cover the expenses incurred if their dog maims or kills a child. In light of these questions, most people will rethink their needs. Most dogs will bark and alert owners to odd-hour disturbances and an alert, large, obviously controlled dog by one's side is all the protection most people really want or need. *An uncontrollable sentry-type dog is not protection; it is a liability.*

By all means, an owner should be discouraged from allowing his dog to protect an infant or young child. When infants grow up and start to walk, the nonthreatening baby, considered by the protective dog as part of its territory or as one of its possessions, is now transformed and may do unusual things such as throw objects or jump on the dog. The dog may respond violently. The dog is incapable of reliably discriminating whom it should protect the child from; a relative or neighborhood child may be defended against as readily as a potential kidnapper. Parents of young children should be instructed *never* to leave a dog alone in a room with a defenseless child (with a large dog this may mean a 5- to 7-year-old child).

WHAT TYPE OF DOG SHOULD I BUY?

The dichotomies are numerous: large or small, phlegmatic or frenetic, male or female, and purebred or mongrel are just a few. A large dog is usually not realistic in an urban setting or in some suburban locations unless the owner goes to great efforts to ensure that these athletic animals get adequate exercise. "Hyperactivity," destructiveness, self-mutilation, and aggression may all develop in a confined, bored dog. A very active dog may be too trying for an older person. A docile, quiet, retiring dog may aggravate another. Almost three-quarters of the cases of aggression seen at the New York State Veterinary College and reported by other behavior consultants (Borchelt, 1982; Beaver, 1982) involved male dogs (approximately 85 per cent of which were intact). Owners must be warned that males require especially conscientious training to ensure adequate control and dominance.

The question of purebred versus mongrel is complex and may be decided by the owner solely on the basis of what he or she wants the dog to look like. Not enough data are available to make definitive associations between certain breeds and problems nor to determine whether purebreds have more or fewer problems than mongrels. There may be an unfortunate bias built into the show ring competition that may result in the selection of dogs with more aggressive tendencies than is desirable. As Borchelt (1982) points out, a large proportion of the mating within a breed may be accomplished by the few males who are consistent show ring champions; and show standards sometimes specifically require dominant display postures such as upright body posture, erect ears, and forward tail and weight. In breeds without these standards, the selection for behavioral traits may be secondary to conformation. Lorenz noted this problem in his book *Man Meets Dog.* "Breeding to a strict standard of physical points," he suggests, "is incompatible with breeding for mental qualities." A very popular breed may be produced carelessly, and, as Lorenz again points out, "There is no single breed of dog the originally excellent mental qualities of which have not been completely destroyed as a result of becoming fashionable." Perhaps Lorenz overstated the point, but the veterinarian should probably recommend a specific breed, line, or breeder with extreme caution. He might restrict his recommendations to breeds raised locally and breeders whose breeding philosophy is known. Alternatively, the veterinarian can refer the client to an individual the clinician knows can be relied upon to give sound advice. This might be a local obedience school or kennel club representative.

Mixed-breed dogs are also heterogeneous in their behavioral tendencies. However, if the temperament of one or both parents of the pups is known, the veterinarian may be on safe ground in recommending or advising against a certain pup.

Caras clearly addresses the previously mentioned alternatives. He offers a very honest appraisal of each of the AKC breeds, including a description of what task the breed is designed to do. The book should probably be left in the clinician's waiting room for client use or even kept in stock for sale.

WHERE DO I BUY MY DOG?

There are several sources to avoid: Mail-order puppy mills and pet shops. The books by Caras and the Monks summarize the arguments against these sources. In most cases the buyer will get an unknown and unreliable product for his financial and emotional investment. The veterinarian should only recommend breeders known to him.

A client looking for an inexpensive dog should be steered toward the local animal shelter, but with several cautions. Dogs over 13 weeks old should be avoided; these have passed the peak socialization time (4 to 12 weeks) and may never be successfully incorporated into human society. This condition has been commonly referred to as "kennelitis." At best some of these become one-person dogs. An adult dog may be a good pet, but it may also have been given away because of some behavioral problem, which a mere change in environment will not correct. The 8- to 12-week-old puppy, however, may also have behaviors that are difficult to correct. Fear and avoidance develop at this stage of the socialization period, and pups in a shelter may become overly fearful and overreactive to other dogs and people. They may be considerably stressed by recent weaning and separation from littermates. In the shelter they may be surrounded by strange, sometimes threatening dogs and subjected to gruff kennel help and procedures or a teasing public. The pups learn to bark excessively, and they may habitually eliminate in their bedding. Although dogs raised in professional kennels where sound socialization practices are followed may be safely purchased at older ages, dogs from shelters should probably be adopted when six to eight weeks old (Hart, 1980; Monks of New Skete, 1978).

HOW SHOULD I CHOOSE A SPECIFIC PUPPY?

Clients should be advised that the first puppy to approach them and jump up on their legs or lap is probably the most dominant one of the litter. The runt and the pup pressed up against the back of the cage are poor choices, as they may be excessively timid or overreactive.

Campbell (1975) describes a simple five-step puppy test to evaluate the behavioral *potential* of a litter or selected pups. The test is conducted by the owner and consists of several following and restraint trials. Bartlett (1979) offers an expanded form of the test adding sound and touch sensitivity and retrieval steps. It is hoped that these tests will elicit responses useful in classifying the pup as passive or active, independent or socially attracted, and dominant or submissive. No data exist to justify using these simple, one-trial tests as predictors of adult behavior, but the simple appraisal may help the owner choose a puppy that better matches his own needs and personality.

HOW DO I GET READY FOR MY PUPPY AT HOME?

The puppy should be taken home only if someone will stay home with it all or most of the first week to facilitate housebreaking and socialization. This may mean taking a vacation from work. Family members should be in agreement as to where the puppy will sleep and where it will stay when no one is home. The best place for the pup at night is in the owner's bedroom in a box, cage, or crate, or tied to the bed; a hot water bottle and/or ticking clock may provide comfort, and the owner should reassure a crying puppy occasionally. The transition will be easier if the owner asks the breeder to separate the pup from its littermates and mother several days before picking it up. Never isolate the pup outdoors or in a basement; this is cruel to a young, social animal and represents an extreme stress. Owners planning on travelling with their dog should use a cage or crate from the beginning; in fact, most owners should consider crate training so as to have a safe place to leave a potentially destructive or house-soiling puppy in the owner's absence. Before the pup is brought home, all members of the household should work out what will be expected of the animal as a *dog*. Will it be permitted to bark at the sound of the doorbell, to jump on visitors, to sleep on the kids' beds, to beg from the table, to have puppies? Incredible tensions can develop or be brought to the surface if there is disagreement about what the dog is doing or where he is doing it.

A monotonous, palatable diet should be recommended to decrease the chances of feeding problems. A dog expecting the same food daily will be less likely to "hold out" for a special food or to beg or steal food from the table. Feeding should not be an emotionally charged event. There is some feeling that dogs that are not chronically hungry are less likely to be aggressive (Houpt, 1982).

Feeding and walking schedules should be discussed and agreed upon before these chores become the *de facto* burden of one family member.

HOW SHOULD I HANDLE THE FIRST FEW WEEKS AT HOME WITH THE PUP?

Do not overwhelm the puppy with attention. Over half its time should be spent sleeping. Introduction to the world should be as gradual and atraumatic as possible. This is especially important at the onset of the fear/avoidance reaction which is at eight to ten weeks of age. Acquaint the puppy to the house slowly. Freedom within the house should be earned and only allowed as the puppy learns to restrict his chewing and elimination habits. The pup should be tied or restricted to certain rooms, preferably those frequently used by the owners. Loeb and Loeb, *Supertraining Your Dog*, call this "preventive confinement." An owner facing feces on the floor and torn carpets daily will become frustrated and angry. He or she will not be in the mood to walk, play with, or train the dog.

Pet-owner bonding is critical. Perhaps the easiest bonding procedure is a simple "following" exercise. The pup is taken out and put on the ground. The owner turns and slowly walks away with or without gently calling the pup's name. Puppies will normally follow with little coaxing, just as they might follow their mother or a littermate. Without being domineering, the owner is establishing the foundation of the expected dominance order. Each family member should practice this exercise at least once daily for the first several weeks as part of normal play with the pup.

Pups should not be overly cuddled or protected, as some stress is normal for mental development (Fox, 1975). An overly fondled and protected puppy may end up as an overly dependent, hyperresponsive, or dominant dog, depending on its temperament and other rearing factors. Training by especially demonstrative owners becomes difficult. Physical rewards may be confusing to a dog accustomed to high levels of physical attention. Excessive physical attention by owners is part of the history of some dogs showing persistent masturbation as adults. Owners should not be discouraged from physical contact with their dogs, but some moderation is recommended. Some of the physical contact should be earned. For example, the pup may be petted only when it sits quietly, not while it is squirming or jumping.

The puppy should be introduced to all types of people and any conspecifics or heterospecifics that may be important to the dog as an adult before it completes its socialization development at 12 weeks. Single owners should make sure the dog is familiar with members of the opposite sex, and childless couples should invite children in to meet the pup. Puppies should interact with other dogs, cats, and even pet rodents. A gradual introduction to varied environments, such as crowded sidewalks, friends' homes, and the car, is desirable.

HOW DO I HOUSEBREAK MY PUPPY?

A conscientious owner can housebreak an eight-to ten-week-old puppy in one to three weeks. Pups should not be paper trained unless that will be the continued adult pattern. House training from the beginning not only eliminates the necessity of retraining the puppy later but also establishes the healthy habit of the owner walking his dog. Dog walking is a "quality" activity, a chance for dog-owner interaction that is often forgotten. We do not know how many owners of "normal" dogs walk them, but an almost constant part of the history of problem dogs is that they are not walked regularly. Housebreaking is greatly simplified by relying on the normal gastrocolic reflex; food intake is restricted to scheduled meals so that someone will be available to take the pup outside 15 to 30 minutes following the meal. Pups should also be taken out as they awaken and watched at other times as best as possible. Properly timed, elaborate praise is as essential as firm but not harsh correction of any "accidents." Owners can make a game out of the procedure by coupling a word or phrase (such as "Do it!") to the act of defecating or urinating. Not only will this speed things in inclement weather, but it will impress upon the owner how easily a dog can learn commands and how nonthreatening the process can be. A six- to ten-week-old pup confined to a cage or crate should not be expected not to foul its bedding unless feeding and watering are carefully regulated.

WHEN SHOULD I START TRAINING?

House training and training to follow should be started immediately, and there is no reason to delay more formal, but simple, training procedures. The pup can learn to discriminate between the *one* or *two* (never more) provided chew items and everything else in the house. He should be taught not to bite fingers or jump on people, as these can lead to annoying or dangerous behaviors later. A pup can retrieve small toys. Leash training can be started. If classes are available, the puppy and one owner should be enrolled in a puppy-training class when the pup is about three to four months old. This will introduce the pet and its owner to formal, novice exercises; provide a good socialization experience; and reinforce the dominant position of the owner/ handler. The owner will learn the capabilities of the pet and will be less likely to make excuses for its misbehavior.

Training should be a lifelong process. One of the best general training books is that written by the Monks of New Skete. It is clearly written, well-illustrated, logical, and behaviorally sound. *Supertraining Your Dog*, by Loeb and Loeb, and Strickland's *Expert Obedience Training for Dogs* are also excellent. Any dog will profit from proper obedience training.

Exercises that make the dog sit, lie down, shake, and roll over are particularly useful, as all express submissiveness to varying degrees. Quieting a fractious animal or stopping one from jumping up is much easier if "sit" or "down" commands are well ingrained. "Shake" and "roll over" are tricks that even children enjoy asking a dog to do, and repeated performance further cements the dog's hierarchical relation with the people giving the commands. Leash training is another form of dominance training, and owners should be encouraged to do all training on a lead for the first four to six months.

BY THE TIME MY DOG IS ONE YEAR OLD, WILL I PRETTY MUCH HAVE THE DOG I'LL ALWAYS HAVE?

Although the species matures sexually at 6 to 18 months and bitches seem to complete their social development within this time period, males do not usually complete this juvenile period of development and mature socially before 18 to 24 months. Whether male or female, however, the dog matures physically and eventually solidifies its social relationships and sense of position in the world during this extended juvenile period. Isolation is less damaging here than in the 4- to 12-week-old dog. But even at this time, isolation could result in a socially or sexually incompetent dog. Males in particular test social associations repeatedly. Although not static, the dominant or subordinate status (with regard to another dog or a person) becomes relatively stable once it is established at this time. Clients might be told they are dealing with the "teenager" mentality, to expect "rebellion," and to deal with it quickly and firmly if they expect to remain in control of their dog. Fox's *Understanding Your Dog* clearly explains canine body language. An informed owner need not wait for a full blown "attack" to interpret his dog's dominant and aggressive activity.

These questions are not the only ones a new dog owner might ask, but an honest evaluation of most or all of them should minimize the types of difficulties at least 40 per cent of the dog-owning public (the dissatisfied and worried types) are having now. Even if the veterinarian's help is limited to the recommendation of a good book, the advice will strengthen his working relationship with the client by helping make the pet-owner bond more sound and satisfying. Also, as the knowledge of animal behavior, including dog behavior, becomes increasingly scientific, the veterinarian is less justified in leaving behavioral recommendations to the dog breeder or trainer. Following a behavior problem prevention program with his clients should be professionally and personally rewarding.

REFERENCES AND SUPPLEMENTAL READING

Bartlett, M.: A novice looks at puppy attitude testing. Pure-Bred Dogs American Kennel Gazette March:31, 1979.

Beaver, B. V.: Canine aggression in retrospect. Appl. Anim. Ethol. in press, 1982.

Borchelt, P. L.: Aggressive behavior of dogs kept as companion animals: classification and influence of sex, reproductive status and breed. Appl. Anim. Ethol. in press, 1982.

Campbell, W.: *Behavior Problems in Dogs*. Santa Barbara: American Veterinary Publications, 1975.

Caras, R. A.: *The Roger Caras Dog Book*. New York: Holt, Rinehart and Winston, 1980.

Fox, M. W.: *Understanding Your Dog*. New York: Coward, McCann, and Geoghegan, 1972.

Fox, M. W.: The behaviour of dogs. *In* Hafez, E. S. E. (ed.): *The Behaviour of Domestic Animals*, 3rd ed. Baltimore: Williams & Wilkins Co., 1975.

Hart, B. L.: *Canine Behavior*. Santa Barbara: Veterinary Practice Publications, 1980.

Houpt, K. A.: Personal communication, 1982.

Loeb, J., and Loeb, P: *Supertraining Your Dog*. Englewood Cliffs, New Jersey: Prentice-Hall Inc., 1980.

Lorenz, K. Z.: *Man Meets Dog*. New York: Penguin Books, 1953.

Monks of New Skete: *How To Be Your Dog's Best Friend*. Boston: Little, Brown and Co., 1978.

Sautter, F. J., and Glover, J. A.: *Behavior, Development, and Training of the Dog*. New York: Arco Publishers, 1978.

Strickland, W. G.: *Expert Obedience Training for Dogs*. New York: Macmillan, 1976.

Taylor, D. H.: Pet owner education. Proceedings of the National Conference on Dog and Cat Control. Denver, 1976.

Wilbur, R. H.: Pets, pet ownership and animal control: social and psychological attitudes, 1975. Proceedings of the National Conference on Dog and Cat Control. Denver, 1976.

THERAPY OF BEHAVIOR PROBLEMS

BONNIE BEAVER, D.V.M.

College Station, Texas

There is no magic pill for pet behavior problems and, like other undesirable things, they tend not to go away if ignored. In reality, most of the behavior problems presented to practitioners can be satisfactorily modified if the veterinarian and pet owner are willing to spend a little time understanding how the problem originated and devising an appropriate therapeutic regimen.

Before any behavior problems can be solved, there are four behavior theories that must be understood. Although these theories are not universally accepted by veterinary ethologists, they offer an explanation of what is happening to the animal that the client can understand.

EXCESS ENERGY

Based on caloric intake and certain inherent factors, individual animals have a certain amount of energy to expend on a daily basis. In the wild, this energy would be used to hunt food, mate, groom, fight, and perform other survival activities. Since the expression of most of these natural activities is curtailed through domesticity, the energy is allowed to accumulate. Dogs that regularly play ball, jog, or live on large properties can expend their energy; however, those that are confined by themselves in small yards, houses, or apartments often do not have the opportunity to vent this energy in acceptable ways. The energy that normally would have been used for locomotion may instead be used for destructive chewing, excessive barking, "abnormal" mating behavior, prey chasing, or stereotyped pacing. Therefore, therapy for any problem behavior in which excessive energy might be a contributing factor should include some method to increase the amount of exercise the patient gets.

ROUTINE

Animals are creatures of habit, as the saying goes. Animals are very much attuned to daily events occurring at specific times. Most pets will readily remind an owner when it is time to wake up, go outside, be with the family, or be fed. They are also keenly aware of when the owner leaves for/and returns from work or school. When significant changes occur in the family's routine, and thus in

the pet's, problems result. Three of the most upsetting situations are the introduction of a new child into the family, the introduction of a new pet, and the death of an immediate family member. When routine changes are likely to occur (e.g., the family is expecting a child, children will soon be leaving the new summer puppy to go back to school, working people are about to retire), the owners should become aware of the pet's present routine and gradually change it to one that will fit in with the new lifestyle.

SOCIAL ATTENTION

Dogs are social animals and in the wild spend a great deal of each day in close proximity to pack members. In domestic environments, dogs have come to equate humans with pack members and, therefore, seek to spend a great deal of time near people. If the dog is in a good routine, certain times of each day will be devoted to contact between dog and owner. The dog learns that it will be with the family when they watch television at night or will play with the children when they come home from school.

When the dog is not on a schedule or when an interruption in the schedule occurs, the social contacts are erratic, resulting in problems. In some cases the dog seeks close contact whenever the person is home and is constantly underfoot. This leads to an unhappy owner who tries to shoo the dog away and an unhappy dog that tries harder for more social contact. A vicious negative cycle develops. For some dogs the negative cycle begins as an accident. A housebreaking accident can result from illness, not enough time outside, or a number of other factors. The owner comes home, finds the mess, and is angry with the dog. The dog that has chewed up something, dug a hole in the carpet, or vomited on the rug also has a perfectly logical excuse, but the owner is only concerned about the displeasure he experiences. The dog's nose is rubbed in the mess and it is scolded and isolated from the family outside. The dog may repeat the incident over the next few days generally for the same reasons. This results in the development of a negative attitude on the part of the owner and a dog that craves social acceptance. Regardless of how the negative cycle begins, the endpoint is the same. The dog learns that it must continue the specific behavior because negative attention is better than no attention.

At this point in the discussion of the problem, the owner will usually mention that when he returns home he "knows" the dog has done it again because it looks guilty. The animal carries on its normal, everyday routine until the owner's return. Only when two events are coupled, the problem behavior plus the owner, will the dog assume the submissive posture. The memory of committing a specific act only lasts 30 seconds past the action. Once the negative attitude has developed on the part of the owner, it must be stopped before the pet's behavior will change. The owner should reward simple, positive acts, such as sitting on command. Do not punish a negative behavior unless the animal is caught in the act. When the dog learns that there is no longer a reward for doing a particular act, it will shift its energies to actions that do get rewards. Of course, it is also important to get the dog on a routine with specific times for positive human interaction.

HORMONE THERAPY

For many years, the supposed "cure-all" for behavior problems has been castration. In more recent times a "magic pill" and injections have also been advocated as the answer for all behavior problems. Much to the frustration of veterinarians and owners, these have not solved most problems. Hormone therapy is useful in certain situations, and their results are generally good if used only in those cases (Beaver, 1982). Testosterone controls male sexually dimorphic behaviors. These male behaviors (mating, roaming, intermale aggression, and territorial marking) can also be exhibited by females and neutered animals to a lesser degree. The removal of testosterone decreases, but does not eliminate, the tendency to exhibit these male behaviors. Certain behaviors are learned, more so in dogs than in cats, so the chances of success decrease with increased patient age and experience. Castration is, of course, one way to remove the testosterone supply; however, this surgery is not possible in females and neutered males. In addition, certain owners are against the surgery.

The progestins have two primary actions that make them useful in certain behavior problems when castration is not the answer. They decrease serum testosterone levels, and they have an antianxiety calming action. If the antianxiety tranquilizer function is the primary reason for using a progestin, it would be better to try one of the drugs that is primarily an antianxiety tranquilizer. These generally work well in cats but are not as effective in dogs (Hart, 1974). The progestins also are antisper-

matogenic and are therefore contraindicated in breeding males. Long-term use has also resulted in uterine problems in females.

DESTRUCTIVE CHEWING

Destructive chewing by dogs is a common problem and one that can usually be corrected if caught early. Most frequently, this type of behavior appears in young dogs around six months of age or in breeds developed to use their mouth. There are a number of environmental events that can trigger this behavior, and each might be classified as something that "frustrates" the dog, if in fact "frustration" can be experienced by animals. Many of the offenders are large dogs or, at least, members of breeds developed to spend long days in the field. But now they are confined to a yard with a pesky neighboring cat or dog, or they are kept in the house during the day and watch television with the owner at night. These dogs experience great build-ups of energy, which are released through a normal channel as an undesirable behavior. Since these dogs are already mouth oriented, chewing is a natural outlet, and destructive chewing is the undesirable behavior. Owners may also inadvertently contribute to this mouth orientation by playing tug-of-war games and providing old socks and shoes as toys. Dogs cannot distinguish between the leather of old shoes or rawhide chewies and that of new shoes, jackets, and furniture.

The owner should begin therapy by removing all chewed objects and providing only one toy that is unique in composition (a nylon bone or rubber toy). Discourage mouth-oriented activities like tug-of-war games, bringing newspapers or slippers, and checking teeth numbers and bite. Put the dog on a strict routine that includes adequate exercise. If the damage is confined to one room, the owner should isolate the dog from that room while he is gone but allow the dog access to it when someone is there to immediately discipline a problem action.

Young puppies normally explore their environment with their mouth, just as young children do. To discourage the puppies from chewing on certain objects, divert their attention. They are behaving as expected, and normal behaviors should not be punished simply because they are unacceptable to the owner.

Another situation can result in destructive chewing by dogs while owners are away. Many people really make a fuss over their dogs immediately before leaving for work or immediately upon coming home. In these situations, the dog becomes worked up as the person gets ready to go, but then the animal suddenly finds itself excited and all alone. It must release this excitement in some way. Dogs anticipating the 5:30 return of the owner also build up excitement. This is first released by chewing, and only when the owner returns can it be released by jumping and licking. Both situations are treated by avoiding lively interactions with the pet immediately before leaving and after coming home. The owner should passively interact with the animal for at least 30 minutes before leaving and then simply say "Good-bye" and walk out. On returning, a "Hello" is sufficient, and only after changing clothes or starting supper (a new clue for the dog to anticipate) should interactions become lively. This also prevents destruction of the home when owners return late at night.

EXCESSIVE BARKING

Dogs of breeds that tend to bark often vocally relieve "frustrations" and release pent up energy. For some, this behavior is primarily nocturnal; for others, it occurs when the owner is away. The night barker is often suffering from a case of social isolation. The dog is alone most of the day and gets to be with the family only during the evening. Then at bedtime the dog is put out alone in the backyard. Frequently by accident the dog starts barking, perhaps at a passive cat, and the owners shout for quiet. The reward of social contact, even though negative, encourages more noise. Gradually the dog learns that continued barking might even result in being let into the house. Correcting this problem can take some time and effort. Following one technique, the animal can begin spending the night in the house and the owner can put it out for gradually increasing lengths of time each night, or the dog can receive a true negative reinforcement for barking, reserving words and contact for routine times when the owner wants to give social contact.

The day barker can be a special problem; often the owner only becomes concerned as a result of a neighbor and/or police complaints. In many cases the owner is not truly motivated to make the treatment work. "Frustration" is again the problem. The dog with excessive energy or one from a barking breed, such as a beagle, will often bark and howl when left by itself. For some of these dogs, the vocalizations occur shortly after the owner leaves or shortly before he returns. This pattern is similar to that seen in the dog that shows destructive chewing as a result of emotional owner departures or returns and can be dealt with in much the same way.

For the dog that barks all day while no one is home, a conscientiously applied retraining program is often successful. Initially, the owner walks out as if going to work, waits three to five minutes, and re-enters the house if the dog is not barking. Later in the day the same procedure is repeated using a five- to ten-minute interval. The owner should never enter or speak while the dog is barking or for several seconds immediately after it stops. The social reward comes from being quiet for increasingly long periods. After getting up to several hours of quiet, periods of absence should be varied so that the dog is never quite sure when the owner will return. Electric shock collars with remote control (not barking collars) have been used successfully on some dogs if the owner immediately gives a quick shock when the barking starts; however, these collars have several drawbacks and must be used very carefully. Some collars deliver excessive voltage, some dogs are extremely sensitive to shocks, and many owners do not use them properly. Increased exercise and training routines must also be stressed when correcting excessive barking.

PREY CHASING

Dogs that chase things can be very troublesome to pet owners, and if the object being chased is a small child, chasing can even be fatal. The canine urge to chase moving objects is strong; thus, dogs commonly chase cats, joggers, bikes, and cars. Often the dog will lie in ambush as an intended victim approaches and then initiate a chase as soon as the "prey" gets closest to the dog. Children that approach a dog and become afraid and those who are playing with the dog and then suddenly run away toward a new activity may initiate the prey chasing instinct. Dogs that chase poultry and livestock frequently use this same drive. The chasing may have begun as an outlet for the dog's extra energy, and because the behavior is self-rewarding, it is very likely to continue.

Treatment is difficult because outside rewards are not necessary and the behavior brings satisfaction. Only if the reward can be consistently made into a punishment is there a chance to stop the problem. If the joggers and bikers always stopped and suddenly rushed at the dog, it might find the behavior less rewarding. If the car always came to a screeching halt and the driver threw tin cans at the dog or jumped out, running toward and screaming at the animal, it might stop. Owners can tie long leads on the dog and haul it in with lots of "no" and "bad dog" and shaking each time a car passes. Eventually the owner will have to hide from the dog until it starts the chase so the dog will learn that it is still controlled even without human presence. Dogs that have killed chickens have had carcasses hung around their necks until the tissue rotted off, they have had meat laced with emetic stimulants, they have had livestock parts tied in their mouths, and they have been shot at. Needless to say, these methods are not highly successful in behavior modification.

The most conscientious owner can only expect a 40 per cent chance of success in treating prey-chasing dogs. The built-in natural reward is strong;

why else would dogs that have been hit by cars continue to chase them or dogs that have been shot with buckshot continue to chase sheep? Unique solutions may work in individual situations. A few geese in a flock of ducks may stop a duck-chasing dog. A front gate booby trapped with a tin can may work against a car chaser. In all cases, however, the longer the problem behavior has been practiced, the harder it will be to stop.

Cats also have a form of prey chasing that is unacceptable to most people. At times the cat will attack the ankles of owners or guests. This problem is almost exclusive of animals confined to the house that do not get an opportunity to hunt. As the energy normally used in hunting builds, the motion of passing feet is enough to initiate the attack. Treatment is usually accomplished by providing action toys for the cat and encouraging activity.

HOUSE SOILING

House soiling is the most common behavior complaint of cat owners and rates very high with dog owners as well. Assuming medical conditions have been eliminated as a causative factor, behavioral modification techniques can be employed to eliminate the problem.

Dogs, particularly males, that become "frustrated" by some event will often respond to that situation by urinating or defecating in or near an area associated with the event. This has been equated with marking of a territory or possession. A dog isolated from a guest because of its overly friendly nature may urinate on the chair occupied by the guest. A dog shut out of a room to prevent its black hairs from getting on the new carpet will frequently sneak in and defecate on the new carpet. A dog confined to the backyard because a houseguest does not like dogs may urinate on the guest's suitcase if it can sneak into the house. Frequently, house soiling leads to negative opinions of the dog, which, in turn, leads to more house soiling to get attention.

Most owners have tried burying the dog's nose in the spot and/or kicking the animal outside when they find the mess, but these remedies seldom work. The owner is mad and feels the pet "knew" it did wrong, so the negative cycle continues. To effectively treat the dog, the owner must not punish the animal unless it is caught in the act of soiling. Routine is also important. Efforts must be made to go out with the dog at normal times of elimination—after waking, after eating, after exercise, and before bed time—and to praise the accomplishment of normal, acceptable eliminations. Urine or feces

should be cleaned up in the house as soon as possible and the area deodorized to discourage recurrence. One note of caution: ammonia should not be used as the cleaning solution, because the ammonia in urine has the same smell. It is also important that the owner not mutter bad words or otherwise express a negative attitude toward the animal, because the dog is not making the same association that the owner is.

Cats will also house soil for reasons associated with "frustration." Tomcats use a standing posture to spray urine for a territorial mark. However, as with any sexually dimorphic behavior, neutered cats and females may also use the same behavior if they feel the situation warrants it. The invasion of an area by another cat, as happens when a new cat is introduced into a home or during the wanderings associated with mating, is the most common cause of soiling. Isolation of the new cat in a quiet room or of the offender from awareness of outside events may be useful. Castration and/or progestin therapy may help.

Some cats stop using the litter box for urination or defecation, but not both. In a number of cases the cat experienced pain, as with cystitis, and associated that pain with urinating in that location. A similar association could arise with the pain of temporary constipation. Litter boxes located elsewhere are used normally. Moving the litter box to a new location will cause the problem to disappear. Once the cat has consistently used the box for several weeks, it can be gradually inched back to the original location.

Occasionally cats stop using the litter box completely. The longer this is allowed to continue, the more difficult it becomes to correct. It is important to determine if the owner changed litter brands at about the time that the problem started. Some cats will not use chlorophyll litter. Litter boxes that are not cleaned often enough for a finicky cat can also initiate a house-soiling problem. Some owners solve the problem by merely moving the box or changing the type of litter to clay, shredded newspaper, or wood shavings. Cats with long-term problems may have to be retrained by confinement when the owner is not able to watch them. A combination of therapy and a conscientious owner can eliminate most feline house-soiling problems.

REFERENCES

Beaver, B. V.: *Veterinary Aspects of Feline Behavior.* St. Louis: C. V. Mosby, 1980.
Beaver, B. V.: Hormone therapy for behavior problems. V.M./S.A.C. 77:337, 1982.
Hart, B. L.: Behavioral effects of long-acting progestins. Fel. Pract. 4:8, 1974.

CANINE AND FELINE BEHAVIOR CONTROL: PROGESTIN THERAPY

PAUL L. PEMBERTON, B.V.Sc.

Avalon, N.S.W., Australia

INTRODUCTION

There is now no doubt that progestins are psychotropic hormones. Their exact role in the veterinary therapeutic saga is still being written, and, like players in any other drama, their performance varies. This article is concerned with trying to curb annoying habits in dogs and cats. Exact records have been kept and reports have been received from colleagues of over 2000 cases of social misbehavior in dogs and cats, and as far as possible these animals have been followed continuously since 1973. None of the patients has died of the behavior problem or the treatment, and although some of them have not responded to treatment, many have and are still alive today because their owners can now abide or even enjoy them.

The incidence of unacceptable behavior in dogs drops sharply after five years of age. This may have something to do with blood testosterone levels falling with age. There are many behavior problems that are not testosterone related, and studies done so far suggest that at the dose rate of 20 mg/kg, medroxyprogesterone acetate (MPA) does not act as an antiandrogen but increases blood testosterone levels while improving behavior. Although castration and training schools are recommended, many patients presented for psychotherapy have had failures with both. Much is yet to be learned about the causes of misbehavior in dogs; it is clear that lack of discipline in the first year of life is one cause and failure to let dogs be dogs, instead of substitute humans, is another.

We have treated, but not necessarily cured, the following conditions:

Extreme territorial aggression
Fighting
Raucous behavior tending toward viciousness
Biting children
Biting humans of any age or sex
Hyperkinesis hypermetria
Obsessive barking
Timidity with or without fear biting
Destructiveness
Inappropriate excretory activity
Unacceptable sexual activity
Roaming
Hole digging
Self-mutilation (acral lick)
Tail chasing
Phobias (storms, guns)
Frontal lobe epileptic-type behavior (rage syndrome)
Night howling in new pups
Anorexia nervosa
Severe false pregnancy following ovariohysterectomy
Extreme attention getting or jealousy
Killing poultry
The "nasty, dirty, little Chihuahua" syndrome
The "tense, jumpy, bad tempered, growling, snappy, Jekyll and Hyde" syndrome

The doses of progestins recommended in this article are higher than those recommended in the seventh edition of this book. Better, more consistent results are obtained at these higher doses, and some conditions, especially the personality problems, do not respond until the progestin has been given a second or third time. If the problem has a "learned" or "cerebral" component, good results will be more difficult to obtain than if the problem emanates from the interbrain as part of the animal's self- or species-preservation behavior. For example, it is easier to stop a dog from biting people intruding onto its territory than to stop its attention getting. The former was once a basic survival instinct, hypothalamic in origin, the latter a learned dependence on humans, probably controlled by the cerebral cortex and therefore not as susceptible to progestins.

Cats' behavior disorders are more truly neurotic, demonstrating failure to cope with their circumstances with useless and apparently unrelated activity. The best example is grooming too much because there is a new cat in the house.

There is no age predilection for cat neurosis. The results of progestin therapy are more predictable with cats than with dogs, probably because a cat's behavior is less influenced by humans than a dog's.

DEVELOPMENT OF AGGRESSION

NORMAL

Pups of age six weeks and older will wag their tails at every human they meet. They will lick anyone's face, given a chance. As they grow older they become more selective in their displays of affection, until by the end of puberty most dogs are only really affectionate with the members of their human family and other people they know well. Soon after this they begin protecting their human friends and what they consider to be their territory, which usually includes portions of the street. This protectiveness increases in intensity until the dog is about three years of age, when it often becomes a social nuisance. Three-year-old male dogs are the most likely to show excess territorial aggression toward tradespeople, other dogs, wildlife, and vehicles.

Aggression diminishes after five years of age. Lack of tolerance toward interference is sometimes seen in old age, as are urinary incontinence and poor vision and hearing. None of these senile changes responds to progestins.

Male dogs are more interested in what is happening outside the home than inside the home. They are more exploratory and like to travel far from home. Female dogs rarely wander far from home and are much more interested in events inside the house.

ABNORMAL

Some personality defects are observable from weaning. Puppies who do not wish to play or lie with their siblings are often also overly dependent on one human. Owners describe them as baby-like in their postures, clinging around the neck and continually following the owner. They never socialize properly with other dogs or people and are often the last of the litter to be sold. They are older when they are finally sold and so miss the critical age for forming strong bonds with their owner. They become fear biters and shrink away from the outstretched hand of friendship. They begin to bite at an age varying from a few weeks to two and one-half years. First they rush noisily at strangers, menacing them with their teeth. Next they begin to bite strange children, first on the hand and later on the face. If they are not controlled at this stage they begin to bite the children of the owner's family and, finally, everyone except the one human on whom they originally imprinted. There is a breed predilection for this behavior. Corgis, bassets, cattle dogs, and, lately, German shepherds seem to be finding it difficult to properly socialize with either dog or human. Such dogs are often surrendered to shelters, from whence they are recycled to well-meaning but unfortunate purchasers.

The second most common form of abnormal character development is extreme attention getting. This is manifested by the destruction of furnishings, sometimes to an astounding extent. Whole rooms full of carpets, tables, chairs, blinds, and curtains have frequently been destroyed by dogs who, from shortly after they were purchased, were quite unable to remain calm when alone. Owners report that such dogs cannot be left alone for more than ten minutes before they begin demolishing the house. The cause? Most owners of destructive dogs have no children. They punish the dog, often with quite spirited thrashings, but this is well after the behavior pattern has been established. The physical pain does not seem to bother these dogs. They seem to look for punishment to ensure their owner's full attention.

Since not all undisciplined dogs develop nasty personalities, there must be some hereditary basis for abnormal aggression. It is seen in inbred, outbred, and crossbred dogs of both sexes, neutered or whole. In cats, pedigreed animals develop unpleasant personalities more frequently than ordinary animals.

The prognosis for dogs and cats with inborn personality defects is guarded. Although most of them will improve with 20 mg/kg MPA, a second or third dose may need to be given a few weeks later. These animals are never really happy, likeable pets, yet strangely many clients love them and want them treated. They are, so to speak, "family."

The most difficult mental problems in dogs to treat are the syndromes that can be seen in child-substitute dogs belonging to ladies who will not discipline them. Among the small dogs there is the "nasty, dirty, little Chihuahua" who bites anyone who tries to touch him, is totally lacking in humor and playfulness, soils the house, and is endowed with disproportionately large reproductive organs. These dogs usually belong to older women. Among big dogs with mental problems, *young* female owners complain that the dog really has a nice personality except that, sometimes for no reason at all, it attacks and savagely bites children. The dog is perfectly behaved when with the owner but is very unreliable otherwise. These owners readily agree that the expression "Jekyll and Hyde" is an appropriate description of their dog.

These dogs sometimes respond to 20 mg/kg MPA, but it should be given to effect every two weeks and carries a guarded prognosis.

OTHER INDICATIONS FOR PROGESTIN THERAPY (Tables 1 and 2)

UNACCEPTABLE SEXUAL ACTIVITY

Although libido is basically a product of instinctive limbic-system function, sexual activity is also

Table 1. Psychotherapy in Dogs

Condition	Treatment	Supplementary Treatment
Personality defect, e.g., biting since weaning	MPA 20 mg/kg SC every three to six months	Gonadectomy; obedience training
Tail chasing	Alcohol injection between coccygeal vertebrae 1 and 2	
Hyperkinesis, destructive (barking, restlessness, uncontrollability, untrainability)	MPA 20 mg/kg SC	0.1 mg/kg flunitrazepam orally q12 to 24h until MPA takes effect
Anorexia nervosa, anorexia of chronic illness	Megestrol 4 mg/kg daily	Sensible dog or cat food
Timidity	MPA 20 mg/kg SC	Hysterectomy and gonadectomy
in greyhounds	Megestrol 4 mg/kg daily for eight days	Full training
Excessive instinctive aggression (biting people and dogs)	MPA 20 mg/kg SC every four to six months	Castration, short-term flunitrazepam therapy (0.1 mg/kg)
Sexual perversion	MPA 20 mg/kg SC	
Subepileptic episodes	MPA 20 mg/kg SC	Owner should not respond to howling in any way
Night howling in puppies	Megestrol 4 mg/kg daily	Gonadectomy
Roaming	MPA 20 mg/kg SC plus 12.5 to 25 mg Modicate (Prolixin, Squibb) IM	Repeat every two weeks until effect obtained
Attention getting, jealousy, possessiveness, and "Jekyll and Hyde" and 'nasty, dirty, little Chihuahua" syndromes	20 mg/kg MPA SC	

Table 2. Psychotherapy in Cats

Condition	Treatment	Supplementary Treatment
Persistent calling	MPA 50 mg SC every three to six months	
Overgrooming with/without eosinophilic ulcers	MPA 50 mg SC every three to six months	Flea control, change of home
Inappropriate urination	4 mg/kg megestrol daily to effect	
Claw marking of territory		
Viciousness		
Miliary dermatitis	Megestrol 2.5 to 5 mg once or twice a week	Perfect flea control
Fighting	MPA 50 mg SC every four to six months	Treat other cats
Psychosomatic skin disease	MPA 50 mg SC every five to 6 months	
Bizarre psychotic behavior	MPA 50 mg SC every five to 6 months	

greatly influenced by the gonadotropins, the sex hormones, and parts of the cerebral cortex. The sense of smell is important in canine sexual behavior, and it is interesting to note that the afferent olfactory tract has two branches, one to the cerebral cortex and one directly to the limbic system, the latter being unique among peripheral nerves.

Nearly all complaints about canine sexual behavior concern male dogs, but by no means only uncastrated male dogs, indicating that not all sexual behavior objectionable to humans is androgen-dependent. There seems to be no doubt that most of the so-called hypersexuality of male dogs is normal libido confused and frustrated by urban situations and the lack of unspayed females. Much of it, too, is due to a lack of owner control. A dog, for instance, that persists in mounting little boys has enough cortical control over its behavior to stop when told to do so, provided the command is firm enough.

Mounting behavior upsets humans more than any other sex-related behavior. In one study of male dogs in Sydney, Australia, 4 per cent of 416 dogs presented for euthanasia on the grounds of social misbehavior preferred to mount other male dogs, 8 per cent preferred to mount children or adults, and an additional 20 per cent numbered mounting as one of their faults but were not particular about what they mounted.

Excess territory marking by urination in the house is usually ascribed to sexual overactivity. Aggression is also frequently considered in the same category, but it is very hard to say whether urinating in the house or superaggressiveness in any one case is due to sexual frustration, territory marking, jealousy, learned behavior, or lack of discipline. The clinician should, therefore, avoid anticipating an improvement in house-training problems with the use of progestins on the assumption that these problems are based entirely on sex.

Masturbation is a rare complaint except in male dogs that are kept kenneled nearly all the time, e.g., racing greyhounds. It is usually performed by swinging the extruded penis from side to side, slapping the abdominal skin. Semen is found inside the dog's thighs and on the kennel walls. Dogs are secretive about masturbating, but their behavior may be discovered by the development of balanoposthitis and cystitis. Although masturbation responds well to progestin therapy, it is better to increase the workload of greyhounds in training, because progestins may cause loss of keenness to race.

Roaming and excessive barking may sometimes have a sexual basis, but they do not respond well to progestin therapy.

NIGHT HOWLING

Newly purchased pups are often presented to the clinician because they have howled all night for several successive nights. Dispensing phenothiazine-derivative tranquilizers to young pups distresses owners because of the degree of stupefaction produced. Frequently owners will call late at night, afraid that the pup is dying. Megestrol, 4 mg/kg orally daily, is quick acting enough to solve this problem, and only three or four days of treatment are necessary.

SPECIAL PROBLEMS OF GREYHOUNDS

Greyhounds occasionally try to bite other competitors during a race. Overuse of testosterone or anabolic steroids should be excluded as a cause before the dog is branded a "fighter." Trainers usually blame a real or imaginary painful physical condition, but this rarely is the case. Megestrol is the drug of choice because the dose rate is adjustable and because it can be withdrawn quickly in case of weight gain or a loss of interest in chasing.

Some greyhounds, usually female, are too timid or spoiled to be broken in. Megestrol therapy, 4 mg/kg once daily for a week, is effective, and such short-term therapy does not have any reproductive consequences.

URINE SPRAYING IN CATS

Inside and outside walls and trees may be sprayed with urine at the same height as the cat's urethra. This most often occurs for sexual reasons. It may be observed in castrated as well as uncastrated males. Spraying is most common in the mating season and responds better to progestin therapy than does inappropriate urination. MPA at 20 mg/kg once or megestrol at 4 mg/kg daily can be expected to cure spraying in up to 80 per cent of cats subjected to therapy. The remaining 20 per cent may need olfactory tractotomy.

SUCKING BLANKETS

This is a neurotic habit seen most often in inbred "fancy" cats. Animals with mild cases suck the tips of their tails. Those with severe cases suck their tails, dewclaws, toes, and footpads. Skin lesions typical of those of self-mutilation appear. Some badly affected animals will suckle inanimate objects such as a baby pacifier or "dummy." Although cats with these sucking habits respond well to six monthly injections of MPA, those that suck on or eat blankets do not. This condition is seen in the Siamese more often than in other breeds, and woolen blankets are usually preferred.

PSYCHOSES

Dogs and cats sometimes do not have a sense of what is real and what is not or what is reasonable and what is not. Some animals seem to see things that are not there or respond to stimuli that do not exist. This psychosis appears at a few weeks to a few years of age, sometimes, but not often, triggered by an actual event. The "fly catching" syndrome is a good example. Sufferers spend most of their lives staring intently into the middle distance and frequently reaching forward with their head to snap their jaws closed as if there were some flying organism there to be consumed. The experienced observer could not be blamed for believing that this is exactly what is happening. Alas, no such organism exists, and the cat continues snapping at thin air for most of its waking life. This condition is rare, and no concerted attempt has been made to correct it.

Tail chasing, on the other hand, is fairly common and is seen most often in bull terriers and German shepherds. A great deal of unrewarded effort has been expended to try to cure tail chasers. Progestins, tranquilizers, and anticonvulsants (particularly carbamazepine, phenytoin, and Primidone) do not have much effect. Injections of 70 per cent ethanol into the tail have been curative in all of the small number of bull terriers treated. Ethanol 0.5 ml is injected into the first caudal space. This leaves the motor nerve supply intact but anesthetizes the tail. To date, none of the treated tails have dropped off. Incidentally, tail amputation is not a successful treatment. Patients continue to chase the phantom tail.

Tail chasing is often first noticed after some physical trauma. One bull terrier in my experience began tail chasing after a caesarian section, and one German shepherd began after much local treatment for pemphigus vulgaris of the perianal skin. Even when the condition (sometimes known as "lacy anus") was correctly diagnosed and treated effectively with prednisolone at 6 mg/kg, the dog still chased its tail.

Siamese cats not uncommonly seem unable to stop "calling." The noise is more like a croak than a meow and is continued day and night at full volume, sometimes even when eating. They start calling in adolescence and continue all their lives. Phenobarbitone, 15 mg, and diazepam, 2 mg, together will reduce the noise volume and frequency temporarily. These very vocal cats usually have vacant personalities. They do not seem to care what is done to them. They do not seem to be making the noise for any particular reason. Neither punishment nor reward stops them. Most owners say that the cat always makes that noise and resignedly refer to the cat as being "mad," indicating that it has no redeeming features. MPA 50 mg subcutaneously once is curative in most cases but has to be repeated every three to six months and gives the cat an unattractive personality.

If these behaviors are similar to those seen in human psychoses, we should consider similar treatment. No work has yet been done on high-dose,

long-acting injectable phenothiazine derivatives in psychotic animals. For example, fluphenazine (Prolixin or Modicate) might be useful and should be tried.

NEUROSES

Maladaptions to stimuli commonly occur in dogs and cats. Cats behave normally until one or two other cats are introduced into the household. Then one of several things may happen. The normal adaptive behavior would be a fight, followed by mutual retreat and rearrangement of territory. Cats who fail to make this adjustment to conflict may begin overgrooming their hair with their tongues. This is interpreted by the owner as an indication that the cat has very "clean" habits. Soon the owner notices that every part of the cat that has been licked is stained a rusty red-brown by saliva and the cat's tongue, lips, and sometimes nose are worn into ulcers. In severe maladaptions the cat pulls at its hair with its incisor teeth, usually on the flanks, thighs, and tail. Large areas of skin are rendered almost hairless, and finally the skin succumbs to linear dermatitis on the limbs or eosinophilic plaques may develop anywhere on the body. This disease is most often called "psychogenic dermatitis." Humans who pull constantly at their hair because of unresolved inner conflict are said to have trichotillomania. The skin and hair problems are, however, only part of the feline territorially induced neurosis.

Other maladaptions include changes in excretory patterns. Neurotic cats will urinate on surfaces that they know will attract maximum attention from humans. They soil the bed cover, the dining table, the middle of the living room carpet, but never discrete locations like a corner. This kind of inappropriate urination is to be distinguished from the loss of bladder control that sometimes appears in senility or the tenesmus of the feline urologic syndrome.

Often, the cat's personality will change and it will become withdrawn, timid, and unaffectionate. It hides whenever strangers enter and hisses if any attempt is made to stroke it. Visual territory marking, i.e., scratching the furniture (often misinterpreted by owners as an attempt to sharpen the claws despite the obvious fact that it would, if anything, blunt them), increases.

Such cats respond very well to one subcutaneous injection of 50 mg MPA. Treatment usually has to be repeated every three to six months unless the cause of the neurosis is removed, that is, the other cats. It is interesting to note that "neurogenic dermatitis" was recognized in cats 30 years ago. Although the cause was not known and no chemotherapy was available, a move to a new household was often curative.

Vicious cats could probably be classified as maladjusted in that their senseless attacks on humans are unproductive and do not help them cope with life. There is also a strong hereditary component. Long-haired cats are usually more often vicious than short-haired cats; and purebred cats are vicious far more often than "ordinary" cats. The attacks begin when the cat is a kitten, occur without warning or provocation, and are designed not just as a gesture of malevolence but as a deliberate attempt to cause serious injury. These cats respond very well to a subcutaneous injection of 50 mg of MPA, which always has to be repeated every three to six months.

Miliary dermatitis is a well-recognized disease of cats that need not be described here. Assuming there are absolutely no fleas, it has been noticed that the appearance of the characteristic scabs on the head, neck, and back coincides with some social event in the cat's life. The arrival of a new dog, cat, or child in the house; the departure of a loved one; or even a change in the sleeping arrangements whereby the cat is encouraged to sleep outside instead of on the softest furniture are examples of precipitating causes of miliary dermatitis. Megestrol is the drug of choice because the owner can adjust the dose according to the condition of the cat's skin, stopping or starting therapy as circumstances change. This is impossible with a long-acting injection. Miliary dermatitis responds to MPA as well as megestrol, but it does not respond well to corticosteroids. This suggests a psychological basis, although there is no denying the antiallergic properties of progestins.

FIGHTING

"Normal" territorial fights are infrequent. Lorenz's classic work on aggression (1966) describes how territorial aggression diminishes as the distance from the center of the territory increases. This is provided the cat territories do not overlap. If they do, fighting becomes much more frequent, and the cats begin to show signs of excess trauma. Wounds, abscesses and dental and ocular injuries are common in situations of overcrowding and may even ruin the cat's life. Although MPA will decrease a cat's territorial requirements and aggression when given at a dose of 50 mg subcutaneously every four to six months, it does not solve the problem unless the other cats in the area are neutered and similarly treated.

HYPERKINESIS

Hyperkinesis is a neurosis of dogs that is increasing in incidence more rapidly than any other. This may be caused in part by the hyperkinetic behavior of the humans in the dog's family. Female dogs are more often affected than males. It is convenient to include the following under hyperkinesis: prolonged barking, repeated digging of holes, destruction of furniture, and an inability to keep still or be trained. It has not been described in cats (possibly because cats do not bark). Excessive barking of dogs is a major cause of ill will between neighbors.

Much of the overactivity could be curbed by physical punishment, but so many dogs are left alone for long periods of time that something else has to be done. Using tranquilizers alone is effective for only a week or so, as the dog rapidly becomes accustomed to such drugs as acetylpromazine, and owners do not like the depression it causes in their pets. MPA injected subcutaneously at 20 mg/kg is possibly more effective in this neurosis than in most others. During the week or two that it takes for a sufficient amount of MPA to reach and alter the functions of midbrain cells, some emergency control is necessary. Any tranquilizer will help, but for severe cases we use flunitrazepam (Rohypnol, Roche). This is a much more potent drug than nitrazepam and appears to have a much longer action. (Nitrazepam has a half-life of only three hours in dogs and even 10 mg IV will not quiet a hyperactive dog.) We discovered that dogs that barked in the hospital grew very quiet and ataxic after one or two flunitrazepam tablets and remained that way for 12 hours. An oral dose of 0.1 mg/kg seems to be adequate. Doubling this dose may produce a deep sleep from which it is difficult to rouse the dog for 12 hours.

ANOREXIA NERVOSA

Anorexia nervosa is responsive to progestin therapy. MPA, 20 mg/kg subcutaneously once, and 4 mg/kg daily, are both rapidly effective. The appetite is so stimulated by the progestin that it affords the owner an opportunity to teach the dog to eat commercial dry or soft moist food when it previously only ate small quantities of tasty human food. Megestrol daily also assists convalescent cats in regaining their appetite.

TIMIDITY

Extreme timidity is sometimes seen in dogs not properly socialized with humans at the critical age of 7 to 14 weeks. There is an hereditary factor in this behavior; it is more common in German shepherds and females. Histories of timid dogs will almost always reveal that they were not with their present owners as pups but came from some kind of dog shelter after six months of age. This is not to say that all recycled dogs are timid, just that most timid dogs may have been recycled. MPA, 20 mg/kg subcutaneously once, is very effective. Before treating with MPA, be sure that bitches and queens have had a total ovariohysterectomy, because prolonged use of progestins will cause a high percentage of pyometras. Megestrol is indicated in timid females whose uteri should remain intact, such as greyhounds. In this breed one week's therapy is usually sufficient, because the timidity is noticed at the commencement of training. The great increase in handling received under the influence of progestin during that week usually is enough to make the bitch confident.

Badly behaving dogs often do not have suitable owners. The owners lack the kind of personality that can dominate an aggressive dog or reassure a timid dog. They lack any understanding of the canine mind and are surprised to hear that they are the hard ones to teach in dog training schools. Dogs are often smarter than their owners, and cats are always more cunning. Progestins make dogs more obedient and cats less resistant to human influence. During the consultation at which the progestin is given, the clinician should explain to the owner that during the next few months his pet will be much more trainable. Repeat injections are sometimes not even necessary.

EXCESSIVE INSTINCTIVE BEHAVIOR

Through our study of the physiology of behavior, we have learned of an area in the midbrain whose purpose is self- and species-preservation. It is known that progestins affect the activity of brain cells in this area (Pemberton, 1980). Therefore, when irritating behavior originates in that area, progestins have a good chance of altering it.

Canine and feline male to male territorial aggression can be stopped by castration and/or progestin therapy. Dogs that bite humans entering their territory usually start with small children and work up to adults. They are instinctively guarding their territory and cannot be blamed if their territory includes the houses on either side and part of the street. They chase cars because the vehicle is a trespasser into their part of the street. The car always "runs away," and so the behavior is reinforced several times a day until it is such a source of satisfaction that it becomes virtually all the dog lives for. Neutered and progestin-filled car chasers improve greatly, especially if it can be arranged for a few cars to stop and reverse noisily toward the dog.

SUBEPILEPTIC EPISODES

MPA was first used as an anticonvulsant. It is quite effective against occasional jaw champing fits, running howling fits, and temporal lobe epilepsy. The running howling fit is characterized by a sudden unexplained onset of screaming or howling while running to hide somewhere, as if the dog had been stung or shot. Pre- and post-episodic behavior in-

cludes staying inside and remaining very close to the owner.

Temporal lobe epilepsy is brought on by excitement. The dog is involved in some activity or game, then suddenly viciously attacks one of the participants. This pattern may be followed by much mouth licking or dribbling. MPA, 20 mg/kg given once subcutaneously, gives good control and is easier for the client than daily administration of anticonvulsant tablets.

PSYCHOSOMATIC SKIN DISEASES

Dogs. Acral lick granulomata or dermatitis is caused by boredom. Progestins have no effect. The same applies to the habitual toe chewing seen in poodles and small terriers.

Cats. Moist dermatitis of the tip of the tail or the interdigital skin on one foot or the dewclaws can be mystifying until the history reveals that the cat spends each evening sitting watching television with its owner and contentedly sucking its tail, foot, or toe, much as its owner would a pipe. There is no use putting anything on the skin. MPA, 50 mg subcutaneously, will stop the habit after a week or so, but it will return in five months. Repeated injections work just as well, and one cat that has been on MPA since 1973 has come to no harm.

PHYSIOLOGY OF BEHAVIOR

There are many classic experiments that show that certain specific areas of the brain control behavior. The hypothalamus and related structures—older areas of the cerebrum that are located on the medial and ventral portions of the cerebral cortex—are grouped together and are called the limbic system. Different areas of the system have specific and separate functions. These include the control and regulation of (1) visceral and somatic reactions associated with defense and attack; (2) emotions, especially fear, anger, pleasure, and love; (3) fat, carbohydrate, and water metabolism; (4) body temperature; (5) gastric movements; (6) genital functions; (7) hunger, thirst, and satiety; (8) sleep rhythm; and (9) aggression.

The limbic system is also involved in the interpretation of sensations, whether pleasant or painful, and feelings of reward and punishment. Electric stimulation in certain areas soothes the animal and in other areas causes extreme pain, fear, and defense and escape reactions. The main reward centers are in the ventromedial nuclei of the hypothalamus. The principal centers for pain, punishment, and escape are in the midbrain and the periventricular area of the dorsomedial tegmentum, extending upward into the periventricular structures of the hypothalamus and thalamus.

Tranquilizers such as acetylpromazine inhibit both the reward and punishment centers, greatly decreasing the effective reactivity of the animal. The progestins MPA and megestrol appear to suppress only the pain and punishment centers, leaving the animal "happy" and still reactive to pleasant sensations.

Stimulation of the perifornical nuclei of the hypothalamus, which are the hypothalamic regions that give the most intense sensation of punishment, causes the animal (e.g., the cat) to assume a defensive posture, extend its claws, lift its tail, hiss, spit, growl, open its eyes wide, and dilate the pupils. Piloerection is also seen. The slightest provocation causes a savage attack. Stimulation of the more rostral area of the punishment center, that is, the midline preoptic and septal areas, causes fear and anxiety.

The opposite emotions and behavior, i.e., docility and tameness, appear when the reward centers are stimulated. Destructive lesions deliberately placed in the caudal hypothalamic nuclei cause hyperglycemia, glycosuria, drowsiness, and docility.

EFFECT OF PROGESTINS ON THE LIMBIC SYSTEM AND MIDBRAIN

CHEMICAL NATURE OF PROGESTINS

Natural progesterone is not active orally, but when injected it is fully metabolized in less than 24 hours. This property has hampered experimental work and therapeutic application.

In the 1950s, a new class of progesterone-like steroid chemicals with prolonged activity and enhanced oral effectiveness were synthesized. The increased availability of the progestins and our detailed knowledge of them result from their commercial value as human and animal contraceptives.

All progestins have the same basic steroid structure. Some have estrogenic effects and some have androgenic effects. Some have mixtures of the two effects, and some closely resemble progesterone.

MEGESTROL ACETATE

This is a very potent, quick-acting steroid with progestational and corticosteroid properties. It is metabolized mainly in the liver, with only 10 per cent excreted by the kidneys. For this reason it should not be given to cats that are suspected of having poor liver function. The half-life of megestrol acetate is eight days. It inhibits gonadotrophin release and release of leukotrophic factors and has a direct effect on the prostate and mammary glands. Gynecomastia is an uncommon complication of megestrol therapy. Lactation is stimulated by small doses and inhibited by large doses. Very large doses (10 mg/kg) used in behavior control cause male genital atrophy. Megestrol acetate is absorbed into receptor cells in the limbic system, altering their function to produce changes in sexual behavior, appetite, thirst, sleep, activity, and carbohydrate metabolism in both cats and dogs. The lethal dose in rats is 200 mg/kg. No fatalities have been recorded at the dose rates mentioned in this article, although one cat became temporarily symptomatically diabetic.*

MEDROXYPROGESTERONE ACETATE (MPA)

MPA is a hormonal inhibitor of gonadotrophin secretion with no androgenic or estrogenic activity. It reduces plasma testosterone by being metabolized by the same enzyme (5α-steroid reductase) that converts the prehormone testosterone into dehydrotestosterone and so acts by competitive inhibition. MPA also increases the rate of testosterone breakdown. MPA and megestrol have an action that castration does not. As progestins, they are absorbed onto binding macromolecules in the hypothalamic and preoptic areas of the limbic system, from where they directly influence behavior.

MPA is now used in human psychiatry in the treatment of such antisocial behaviors as assault, destructiveness, stealing, threats, and self-mutilation. Results are good. It is commonly used in jails. Sex offenders respond dramatically. Many different kinds of sexual aberrations, both homosexual and heterosexual, can be brought under control. Erotic and violent fantasies cease and the patients express great relief. Patients with the 47XYY karyotype suffering from aggressive antisocial behavior and very quick tempers say that the treatment has helped them. There is substantial evidence for the role of MPA in the treatment of human male aggression and deviant sexual behavior. It lowered blood testosterone level and controlled otherwise intractable behavior. Temporal lobe epileptics and men with severe angry-aggressive behavior disorders also responded well.

MPA has been used successfully to arrest obsessive homosexual pedophilic fantasies in humans, the psychological benefits outlasting the physiologic ones. This is also seen in dogs and cats. The physical side effects of increased sleep and appetite disappear in a few weeks, whereas the behavioral changes remain for months. Glucose intolerance has never been observed by us or recorded in the human or veterinary literature as a side effect of MPA. Some cats, who were probably slightly diabetic, became severely diabetic when given megestrol at 4 mg/kg. They recovered quickly on standard treatment for

---

*Editor's Note: I have seen iatrogenic Cushing's syndrome in cats given prolonged megestrol therapy.

ketoacidosis and did not require insulin thereafter. Mammary nodules have been reported in beagles treated with MPA over periods of up to four years.

MPA (4 mg/kg) injected into four "normal" male dogs reduced their circulating plasma testosterone level from an average of 4.08 mg/ml to 1.7 mg/ml after seven weeks. There was no adverse effect on their semen quality or a reduction in testicle size or libido. MPA, 20 mg/kg, reduces libido and produces a quieting effect in aggressive dogs. Once a dog reaches the stage at which it requires psychotherapy, most owners have long ago stopped worrying about the size of its testicles, and veterinarians should recommend that the dog not be used for breeding.

EXPECTATION OF SUCCESS

The clinician must guard against being talked into treating uncontrolled neurotic dogs presented by neurotic clients who are not suitable pet owners. Care, too, should be taken not to choose cats for progestin therapy in situations in which the owner or the other animals in the house are the sole cause of the abnormal behavior. Even in cases in which the limbic system is largely responsible, the effects of progestin therapy are surprisingly variable, and the prognosis is always guarded. In biting dogs, for instance, results vary from astounding success to complete failure. If progestins are effective in canine neurotics, they induce, among other things, increased obedience and trainability. Owners should take advantage of this and retrain their pets.

Because progestins may cause cystic endometrial hyperplasia, mucometra, or pyometra, depending on the dose rate and duration of administration, they should be used for behavior control in whole bitches for not longer than eight days. Thus, eight days of megestrol therapy is safe for a nervous young greyhound bitch. The prolonged effect of MPA (Depo-Provera, Upjohn; Perlutex, Leo; Promone E, Upjohn [UK, Australia]) or megestrol acetate (Ovaban, Schering; Ovarid, Glaxo [UK, Australia]) at the high dose necessary to cause a behavior change probably would not be safe for the uterus. It is wise to avoid progestin therapy in unspayed bitches, and it is surprising how rarely they require it.

Because of its very low solubility in tissue fluid, MPA is not fully absorbed, sometimes for a year or more. Clients should be informed that, quite often, especially in large dogs, the beneficial effects of MPA therapy may not be seen at all for two or three months after the injection. Megestrol, being faster acting than MPA, may be used during the interim. Diazepam (Valium, Roche) and nitrazepam (Mogadon, Roche) are sometimes useful in preventing forced euthanasia of the patient while the progestin is taking effect. Nitrazepam is particularly useful when sexual desire lies at the heart of the behavior problem.

THE OWNER

There is scarcely a mammal on earth whose behavior has not been interfered with by humans. It is impossible to isolate the behavior of a domestic dog or cat from that of the humans in its home. Attempts at chemical psychotherapy in companion animals are much more likely to be successful if the owners are reasonably sane.

BLOOD TESTOSTERONE LEVEL AND BEHAVIOR

The blood testosterone levels of dogs have been measured at various ages and during different stages of behavior therapy. The radioimmune assay technique was used. Thirty five dogs were studied, and each had his blood testosterone level measured once before and up to six times after treatment. All the dogs were less than three and one-half years old. The following conclusions can be drawn from the figures obtained:

1. The average blood testosterone level of aggressive young male dogs studied was 4.2 mg/ml.

2. The range was 1.2 to 10.0 mg/ml.

3. It is not possible to relate the severity of the aggression with the blood testosterone level except in those dogs that had been savage since weaning, in which case the blood testosterone level is always higher than average.

4. Castration reduces the blood testosterone level to 0.1 mg/ml within 12 hours.

5. MPA does not lower blood testosterone in uncastrated aggressive dogs at a dose of 20 mg/kg. It had no predictable effect on testosterone level at all; some stayed the same, some rose, and one fell (but only to 2 mg/ml). Despite this failure to reduce blood testosterone level, the behavior of all these dogs improved.

6. Castration alone does not stop fighting, biting, and territorial aggression consistently, and sometimes it takes up to one year to be effective.

7. The best treatment for aggressive male dogs is a combination of castration and MPA (20 mg/kg injected subcutaneously).

CONTRAINDICATIONS FOR PROGESTINS

1. Diabetes mellitus. Progestins also may occasionally precipitate incipient diabetes mellitus.

2. Pregnancy. It is claimed that megestrol is not teratogenic and does not prolong pregnancy. The same cannot be said for MPA. Depot injections of MPA can be given safely only to spayed bitches.

3. Estrus. The possibility of causing uterine disease must be considered.

4. Stud dogs. Progestins reduce libido but do not inhibit spermatogenesis completely. The time needed to return to normal is approximately the same as the duration of treatment.

SIDE EFFECTS OF PROGESTINS

The side effects of prolonged progestin therapy are similar to those seen with prolonged corticosteroid use. They are fairly obvious, and unless the client is warned of them he may cease therapy without first checking with the veterinarian. *Owners must be thoroughly appraised of side effects before the veterinarian prescribes progestins.* The side effects include the following:

1. Obesity. This may be due to (a) the drug's direct effect on the hunger and satiety areas of the hypothalamus; (b) decreased excretion of sodium by the kidney, leading to sodium and, thus, water retention; (c) altered carbohydrate metabolism, because, although the exact mechanism by which progestins alter carbohydrate metabolism is not known, they do have a glucocorticoid-like effect that, in the case of MPA, is prolonged and may be irreversible, and (d) decreased mental and physical activity. Obesity can be controlled by diet, exercise, and the quick establishment of the minimum effective dose. The subject of obesity is well covered in *Current Veterinary Therapy VII* and elsewhere in this volume.

2. Polydipsia. Patients will sometimes drink so much that they begin to urinate in the house. This problem usually only lasts a few days. If it persists, dose reduction is indicated.

3. Stump pyometra. Bitches and queens who have had ovariectomy or ovariectomy and partial hysterectomy are quite likely to develop pyometra in what is left of the uterus after prolonged high-dosage treatment.

4. Eosinopenia. In all 12 dogs in which hematologic studies were made before and after eight days of megestrol treatment at 4 mg/kg daily, eosinophils were reduced from an average of 7 per cent to nil. All these dogs were itchy at the commencement of therapy but much less so at the end.

5. Local alopecia. It is important to inject MPA into curly-haired breeds on a part of the body where it will not show, because the hair over the injection site sometimes falls out. It takes at least one year to grow back, and if it does it may be white and coarse.

6. Rebound effect. For about two weeks after the effects of progestin wear off, a small percentage of dogs and cats become much worse than they were before. This can be used as a guide to determine when the next injection is due.

REFERENCES AND SUPPLEMENTAL READING

Anderson, G., and Lewis, L.: Obesity. *In* Kirk, R. W. (ed.): *Current Veterinary Therapy VII*. Philadelphia: W. B. Saunders Co., 1980.

Evans, J. M.: Sexual behaviour patterns in dogs. Post-graduate Committee in Veterinary Science Proceedings, No. 37. Canine Medicine, Sydney, Australia, 1978.

Garben, H. A., Jockle, W., and Sulman, F. G.: Control of reproduction and undesirable social and sexual behaviour in dogs and cats. J. Small Anim. Pract. 14:151, 1973.

Hart, B. L.: Olfactory tractotomy for control of objectionable urine spraying and urine marking in cats. J.A.V.M.A. 179:231, 1981.

Iversen, I., et al. (eds.): *Handbook of Psychopharmacology*, Vol. 5. New York: Plenum Press, 1975.

Lorenz, C. T.: Aggression. New York: Methuen, 1966.

Pemberton, P. L.: The use of progestogens in certain behavioural abnormalities of dogs and cats. Post-graduate Committee in Veterinary Science Proceedings, No. 30. Neurology, Sydney, Australia, 1976.

COPING WITH THE DEATH OF A PET: CLIENT GRIEF

CLAUDIA L. BARTON, D.V.M.,
and BONNIE V. BEAVER, D.V.M.

College Station, Texas

Any veterinarian who practices companion animal medicine and surgery must learn to cope with client bereavement and grief over the loss of a beloved pet. This emotional response can range from completely acceptable, "normal" grief to a pathologic state requiring the assistance of a psychologist, psychiatrist, or other counselor. The degree of dependence of a client on a pet and the resultant outpouring of grief when the animal dies may sometimes amaze us as veterinarians, but we must attempt to understand this dependency.

CHANGING PSYCHOLOGICAL SUPPORT SYSTEMS

Certain conditions of modern life have contributed to the increased psychological closeness of our clients and their pets. First is the loss of the extended family unit. Today we are a mobile society, often with the closest of relatives scattered over the entire country. The traditional support network of parents, grandparents, sisters, brothers, and children has thus been rendered ineffective. Since man has a distinct psychological need for a "family" of some type, the veterinarian sees the pet assuming the role of a human substitute. Occasionally the pet is the person's closest social companion and entire support system. This is most often seen with elderly people. In the days when the extended family lived either under one roof or within a small town, the older person had many family members to depend on for social relationships; today, however, his or her children may live thousands of miles away and may visit once a year. The daily psychological needs of the elderly for companionship are fulfilled by the everpresent dog or cat.

Another factor contributing to a client's potential inability to deal with the death of a pet is the rarity of bereavement as a social situation in a person's life. Most people have little contact with death and few opportunities to be legitimately bereaved. Often, elderly relatives live far away and are visited infrequently; when they die, grief is transient, since their death does not make any difference in day-to-day, here-and-now life. So, for most people, bereavement is a stressful situation with which they have had little previous experience. The death of a pet is likely to be the first emotional loss of its type that many young and middle-aged adults have ex-

perienced. Certainly many children experience the death and loss of a pet as the first such experience.

Finally, modern society offers at least a modicum of social sanction and ritualized support to the person who has experienced the death of a close human family member. Outward expressions of grief are expected, even encouraged, and the funeral brings together family members to help the grieving individual cope. There is no such acceptance of grief over the death of a pet. The grieving person is looked upon as weak or silly if he grieves excessively. An overt display of grief over the loss of a pet is embarrassing to both the bereaved individual and others who witness it. After all, as people often say, it was "just a dog." Burial of a pet and pet funerals are regarded as childish or maudlin. For these reasons many pets are euthanatized and disposed of without the client ever seeing the body or receiving any expressions of sympathy from friends, coworkers, or family.

STAGES OF GRIEF

The veterinarian's response during the bereavement process can make a tremendous difference in the way the client copes with grief over the loss of a pet. If the veterinarian understands the process of human acceptance of death, he or she can deal more effectively with emotional outbursts when they occur. Elisabeth Kubler-Ross, in her classic treatise *On Death and Dying*, examined the stages of the grief process that the dying human experiences and found the same stages reflected in the family members of the dying individual. If the dog or cat is regarded as a human substitute, veterinarians may expect to see similar stages of grief in clients dealing with the announcement of their pet's terminal illness.

DEATH

Denial of the truth may be the first protective response of the client to the veterinarian's grave prognosis; he may insist that his pet's biopsy was misread or that the pathology laboratory sent the wrong report. The animal's eating, drinking, and otherwise normal behavior may be invoked as evidence that a terminal disease cannot be at hand. Such clients may "shop around" from veterinarian

72

to veterinarian in the vain hope that someone will tell them that the wrong diagnosis has been made. The veterinarian's best response to a client's denial of truth is to accept the possibility that a wrong diagnosis *may* have been made or that the possibility for cure might exist. This is necessary sometimes even when the doctor feels that the situation is hopeless. The veterinarian must re-biopsy the lesion, call the pathology laboratory to request the block of tissue for a second opinion, or refer the client to a specialist, even if the diagnosis is obviously correct. Often, the specialist will tell the client exactly—sometimes in the same words—what has been said by the client's veterinarian. If told of the incurability of a condition such as cancer, some owners will continue their denial by placing the animal on vitamins, special diets, or even laetrile, expressing great faith that the pet will improve on these ineffective regimens. Finally, however, the client will become assured of the truth of the situation, sometimes only by the pet's deterioration.

The likelihood of denial as a client reaction is usually greater if the dog's condition is acute. If the animal has been failing over a period of months, the client possibly expects to hear bad news and is emotionally braced for it. The most extreme denial reactions are seen when the client has no idea that the pet is ill at all. For example, a dog is presented for vaccination and the veterinarian discovers enlargement of all peripheral lymph nodes. Immediately, a cytologic aspirate of a lymph node is performed, and the shocked client is told ten minutes later that his dog has only a few months to live unless treated with expensive chemotherapy. In such an unexpected situation, the veterinarian is well advised to temper the shocking news by presenting the client with several possibilities for the diagnosis, including the most serious condition. A biopsy may then be taken, allowing the client a few days to accept the fact that a terminal disease is even being considered.

Unexpected death by trauma or during an elective surgical procedure may provoke shock and disbelief in the client, who experiences a stunned numbness. One client, when informed of the sudden death of her dog, began to sob hysterically over the telephone and hung up in the middle of the conversation. Repeated attempts to telephone her again were met only by a busy signal. Suddenly, she appeared at the clinic, cheerfully asking the receptionist if she might visit her pet. She had completely negated the previous telephone conversation. In this case the client's shock and disbelief lasted only a matter of hours, but for others the reaction may last for several days. The shock of acute bereavement is often described as a "cotton wool" time in which, as C.S. Lewis says, one "feels . . . mildly drunk or concussed." The range of reactions may run from verbal denial to complete incapacitation.

ANGER

Anger is a grief reaction that is commonly seen by the veterinarian. If handled inappropriately, this phase may be the most destructive to the client-veterinarian relationship. This anger may be displaced in three directions. First, it may be directed toward the veterinarian for being the deliverer of the bad news. The client, through an irrational reasoning process, may act as though it is the veterinarian's fault that the animal is dying. If the client has had a long relationship with his veterinarian, he may furiously demand to know why the diagnosis was not made sooner, in time to treat the disease. The veterinarian must be very careful at this stage not to take the expression of anger personally. Above all, the client's anger must not be met by a similar response from the veterinarian. Although it is sometimes difficult, the veterinarian must remain passive, merely stating the facts of the disease as they are. Rarely will a client later pursue accusations directed at the veterinarian during this phase of grief. More often, such an outburst will be followed by a profound apology a day or so later, the client saying that "I just lost my head for a moment."

Anger may also be directed against the pet itself, other family members, or even God. A pet may be blamed for imminent desertion of the family, causing a child to reject the animal completely, refusing to pet it or play with it ever again. Since it is difficult for a child to understand why parents cannot afford to treat an animal with an expensive medical or surgical regimen, the child will sometimes blame his parents for years for "killing my dog." For this reason, the veterinarian should be careful not to present treatment options to the client in the presence of small children. The parent must be allowed to choose euthanasia, if this is the only economical alternative, without the added stress and guilt imposed by young family members.

Finally, the client's anger may be directed against himself in the form of feelings of guilt. "If I had only come in sooner." "We never should have had this surgery done in the first place." These are expressions that veterinarians hear when a terminal condition has been diagnosed or an animal dies suddenly. Sometimes a client will search for ways in which he or his family may have contributed to the pet's condition. These may be totally unjustified. For example, a client called a year after her cat's death from metastatic mammary carcinoma, convinced that she had caused the cancer by smoking cigarettes while the cat sat in her lap. A client may feel guilty that financial resources are being diverted from the rest of the family for the care of the pet. It is apparent to most workers in the field of death and dying in humans that guilt is always present whether it is deserved or not. If possible, the veterinarian must help the client stop this self-recrimination. The owner must be assured, sometimes over and over, that the disease is not "anyone's fault." The client also must not be made to feel guilty if he selects euthanasia rather than treatment of the disease. Of course, in some instances, the client is obviously and incontrovertibly at fault, as in the case of the owner who runs over his cat with his car. These clients must be supported as well as possible with expressions of sympathy but will often take weeks or months to come to grips with their guilt.

GRIEF

At some point in the bereavement-acceptance process, the client will experience overt grief over his impending loss. The veterinarian will often hear a client say about his dog or cat, "I just don't think I can go on without him." This grief may take on extreme forms, sometimes to the point of threats of suicide. In general, however, the client ultimately accepts the inevitability of the animal's impending death and moves on to resolution. The veterinarian may help by enlisting the client's aid in caring for the animal and explaining the signs of pain and discomfort the animal will experience as the end approaches. Occasionally, a client will not accept euthanasia as an alternative to natural death. This can be a very difficult situation for the veterinarian, who is forced to watch an animal suffer when there is little that can be done to help it. In this instance, it may be gently pointed out to the client that the animal is in intractable pain and cannot recover. It may be suggested that the kindest last thing he can do for his pet as a friend is to relieve the pain and let the pet die with dignity. Occasionally, a veterinarian must send a hospitalized animal home for a few days to allow an owner to realize the real plight of the animal.

RESOLUTION

The final stage of the bereavement process is resolution. This stage is a kind of "positive submission," according to Kubler-Ross, "an acceptance of what you can't change with a sense of peace and serenity." The client is often emotionally drained and will be ready for euthanasia or death when the time comes. If the client reaches this phase before the pet dies, grieving has been completed and the ultimate death of the animal will usually be accepted with equanimity.

It is important to realize that the order, duration, and extent of the stages of grief vary greatly. Many clients will skip entire stages of this process, often suppressing their overt expressions of anger or grief. Some people seem outwardly to accept the situation, but a new outpouring of grief may be seen when the animal dies. For example, dogs under treatment for lymphosarcoma often feel and act so well that clients must be told over and over again that it is only a temporary remission. The client may express extreme disappointment when the animal's tumor exacerbates and the disease can no longer be brought into remission.

THE VETERINARIAN'S ROLE

During the process of bereavement over the loss of a pet, the veterinarian can give the owner tremendously important psychological support, which may make the difference in the client's ability to continue with his normal life. Often, the veterinarian's kindness and humane treatment of a pet will make a lasting impression on the client. This impression may extend beyond the client's personal veterinarian to veterinary medicine in general. Dr. Alton Hopkins, a small animal practitioner in Dallas, Texas, has expressed it this way:

In 25 years of practice, I have been involved in the birth of thousands of animals. I have made many difficult diagnoses and effected (at least in my mind) some near miraculous cures. I have performed surgeries, some very difficult and demanding. I have pioneered a few techniques that have saved a lot of animal suffering. To this date I have a dozen letters of gratitude and a few thank-you notes to show for all of these accomplishments.

On the other hand, I have received hundreds and hundreds of calls and letters and gifts expressing extreme gratitude and deep affection for my words, actions, attitude, concern, and understanding at the time of a pet's death. What this says about the human/companion animal bond I'm not sure, but it seems to me to say something like this:

The feelings of love, acceptance, dependence, empathy, sympathy, anger, fear, suspicion, concern in a relationship with a pet animal are readily accepted as normal by our culture.

But the sudden exacerbation of grief over loss of a pet comes as a total surprise to many of those experiencing it, and they don't really know how to handle it. I'm sure they are embarrassed by their actions, but at the same time they realize their reaction was spontaneous and real.

So these expressions of gratitude are really their way of saying: "Gee, doc, I felt like a fool acting that way over an animal, until your attitude told me what I felt and did was okay and not so weird after all."

And, by golly, that's *exactly* what I was trying to tell them.

What the veterinarian can do is *legitimize* the client's grief. In standing by the pet in both life and death, the practitioner renders the client an indispensable psychological service.

REFERENCES AND SUPPLEMENTAL READING

Hopkins, A.: Veterinarian offers sage advice on dealing with grieving clients. DVM 12:45, 1981.
Katcher, A. H., and Rosenberg, M. A.: Euthanasia and the management of the client's grief. Comp. Cont. Ed. 1:887, 1979.
Kubler-Ross, E.: *On Death and Dying.* New York: Macmillan Publishing Co., 1969.
Speak, P.: *Loss and Grief in Medicine.* London: Bailliere Tindall, 1978.

Section
2

CHEMICAL
AND
PHYSICAL
DISORDERS

FREDERICK W. OEHME, D.V.M.

Consulting Editor

COMMON POISONINGS IN SMALL ANIMAL PRACTICE

GARY D. OSWEILER, D.V.M.

Columbia, Missouri

Small animal poisoning is often associated with acute or peracute onset of severe clinical signs that progress rapidly to death or recovery. Many times, an animal's owner is not aware of access to foreign materials that could be toxic. In other instances, the client is firmly convinced that malicious poisoning had occurred. Dogs and cats previously in apparent good health may be found dead, and this situation frequently gives rise to suspicions of poisonings in the minds of client and veterinarian alike. There is also some tendency to consider as poisoning disease states that cannot be explained by other means. Perhaps the most common toxicologic diagnosis made is "poisoning" due to undetermined etiology.

Our view of what is a common poison is limited by the effort expended in gathering an accurate and detailed history, the thoroughness of the clinical and clinicopathologic exam, and the availability of confirmatory chemical analyses.

Circumstantial evidence has value if one can determine that animals have consumed or were definitely exposed to a particular toxic agent. Several types of evidence are usually important in determining which are the "common" confirmed poisonings. The veterinarian must decide, on the merits of each case, how much effort goes into reviewing the factors in a potential poisoning. When surveys or summaries are made concerning frequency of poisoning (or other diseases), one should always question the degree of certainty with which diagnoses were made.

In addition to lack of circumstantial or clinical evidence (on the clinician's part), lack of chemical or analytic data may be a problem. For some toxicants, such as plant toxins or animal venoms, diagnostic chemical analyses are not available or are not practical. In other cases, the cost of analyzing for many poisons is prohibitive.

CLASSIFICATION OF POISONS

Toxic materials may be classified in several ways. In many cases, it is useful to group them according to where they occur or why they are used. Thus, insecticides would be potential toxicants if the owner had just sprayed extensively for roaches, and plant poisoning is more likely if the season is spring and flowers, shrubs, and vines are abundant around the home.

Toxins may be grouped according to the following general headings:

A. Natural hazards
    1. Plants, seeds
    2. Fungi, algae
    3. Mycotoxins
    4. Zootoxins (snakes, toads, insects, etc.)
    5. Poisonous minerals in food or water
B. Man-made hazards
    1. Industrial contamination
    2. Pesticides and economic poisons
    3. Domestic materials
    4. Drugs
    5. Food and water

NATURAL TOXINS

Toxic plants and seeds are found in many homes and places of business. Although the dog and cat are not foragers, both species have been known to consume various plants or portions thereof (e.g., grass-eating dogs and catnip-loving cats). Poisoning by oleander, dumb cane, castor bean, chokecherry, jimsonweed, morning-glory, and mushrooms has been recorded to occur in small animals.

Fungi, mycotoxins, and blue-green algae have caused poisoning in pets. Most notable of the fungi are the *Amanita* spp. *A. phalloides* produces a fatal gastroenteric and hepatotoxic reaction, and *A. muscaria* causes signs that mimic cholinergic drugs and that are alleviated by atropine. Mycotoxins of *Aspergillus flavus* (aflatoxin) and *Penicillium* spp. are toxic to dogs, and outbreaks of aflatoxicosis from contaminated dog foods have been observed. Most effects of the aflatoxins are recorded in dogs and are exerted on the liver, kidney, and blood-vascular system. Diagnosis of mycotoxicosis is difficult, since effects may be delayed and a source of toxin may no longer be available. Algal blooms in late summer are associated with gastroenteritis, hepatotoxicity, and "fast death" in many species including dogs.

Certain toxic animals, insects, and snakes are a hazard to pets in some locations of North America. Most problems are reported from the southern and

76

southwestern United States. Snake bites (rattlesnake, copperhead, and coral snake) and toad poisoning from *Bufo* spp. are the most frequently reported problems. Animal venoms and toxins characteristically affect the nervous system, cause tissue necrosis, or induce hemorrhage, hemolysis, or an allergic response.

Mineral poisoning in food or water is rare in small animals. Arsenical contamination of grain or availability of rodent baits containing toxins such as phosphorus, arsenic, inorganic fluorides, or barium may occasionally occur. Cured meat or the water from cooked cured meats may be high in nitrites, and ingestion may result in methemoglobinemia. Since pets generally consume from the same water supply as man, acute water-borne poisoning is relatively rare.

MAN-MADE SOURCES OF POISONS FOR PET ANIMALS

Sources of potential poisons are legion and are exceeded in number only by the toxicants themselves. Some 2000 chemicals and drugs are considered dangerously toxic, and new chemicals with potential toxicity are being introduced at the rate of 1500 or more each year.

To consider even the broadest possibilities, one must be equipped with at least some ready reference works that give detailed information about the more common poisoning problems. In addition, it is helpful to know the areas in which the more toxic chemicals, plants, and venoms are found. Furthermore, the general clinical effects associated with toxic substances should be kept as a cross reference.

INDUSTRIAL CONTAMINATION

The gases, vapors, dusts, and water pollutants that plague man are available to the companion animals that share his environment. Carbon monoxide, oxides of nitrogen and sulfur, and various pneumoconioses should be considered when evaluating respiratory problems in small animals. Water pollutants such as nitrates have been associated experimentally with hydrocephalus in young dogs. However, little work has been done specifically relating pollutants to disease problems in the small animal population.

PESTICIDES AND ECONOMIC POISONS

These materials, especially the rodenticides and insecticides, appear most often as accidental and malicious poisons in small animals. This comes from the fact that they are designed to be toxic to similar biologic mechanisms and they are used largely by laymen in areas frequented by pets. Proper use and storage of such products would eliminate most of these problems.

The important economic poisons in small animal toxicology are discussed in individual chapters in this section.

DOMESTIC MATERIALS

A great number of products used in homes or businesses contain toxic materials. Many of these are listed in the article entitled "Potential Sources of Small Animal Poisoning." These materials are usually packaged and should not be available to pets if properly used and stored. Since most pets (perhaps primates excepted) do not remove caps or lids, and since they can be effectively locked away from these materials when in use, there is little excuse other than negligence for poisoning by these products. Many of these chemicals are volatile or corrosive, and often they are able to penetrate intact skin.

Clarke (1975) reports that overheated frying pans coated with nonstick materials emit a vapor toxic to birds. The fluorinated propellants (freons) may cause acute respiratory and cardiovascular abnormalities, with fatal consequences in pets.

Cats are peculiarly susceptible to many domestic products, and a good review of this subject has been written (Atkins and Johnson, 1975).

DRUGS

Pets occasionally gain access to drugs of abuse through living with an owner who is inclined to their use. Most common is the consumption of marijuana, generally with resultant nonfatal hallucination for one or two days.

Certain therapeutic agents intended for man may inadvertently or intentionally be given to pets. Excessive amounts of vitamin A, vitamin D, and aspirin may cause toxicosis, especially in cats, when given by well-meaning owners. Acetaminophen-containing pain killers may cause toxicosis in cats after consuming one or two of the 325-mg tablets. Barbiturates ("sleeping pills") or stimulants such as caffeine tablets have been carelessly left where pets could consume toxic amounts. A part of the anamnesis of any uncharacterized potential toxicosis in pets should include some determination of drug preparations used or kept in the household.

Generally, the side effects and therapeutic incompatibilities of veterinary drugs are known prior to their release. Individuals prescribing or using therapeutic agents should be familiar with the side effects, adverse reactions, and contraindications of all such drugs. A discussion of drug-induced and adverse reactions will be found in a separate chapter within this section.

FOOD AND WATER

Food poisoning or garbage intoxication is more frequently diagnosed than any other intoxication. Mold toxins, bacterial exotoxins, bacterial endotoxins, and toxic products from putrefaction may be involved separately or in concert with one another. Much more work is needed in studying the physiologic response of small animals to contaminated or tainted foods. This subject is treated more fully elsewhere in this section.

FREQUENCY OF SMALL ANIMAL POISONING

Humphreys (1978) reviewed veterinary literature over a 20-year period. Lead was cited as a commonly reported intoxicant of dogs. Other canine intoxicants of note were carbon monoxide, organophosphate and chlorinated hydrocarbon insecticides, paraquat, ethylene glycol, and theobromine. Caged pet birds were reported highly sensitive to polytetrafluoroethylene (PTFE) fumes from overheated Teflon frying pans.

In 1969, a survey of the American Animal Hospital Association membership and veterinary college teaching hospitals was conducted. Results are presented in Table 1. Surveys are only as good as the input data. In many cases, the diagnoses were not confirmed by chemical analyses nor was a source determined. However, the information does reflect the cases that clinically appeared to be caused by specific compounds.

The data presented in Table 1 are a composite of canine and feline poisoning. By far, the greater number of diagnosed toxicoses occurs in dogs. The peculiar sensitivity of cats to phenolics and chlorinated aryl-hydrocarbons, however, results in more frequent poisoning of cats by such compounds with ring structures, which they are unable to metabolize.

Except for the data reported in Table 1, comprehensive surveys of poisonings seen in veterinary

Table 1.   *Clinical Diagnoses of Small Animal Toxicoses in the United States**

	Northeast	Southeast	Southwest	West	Midwest	National Total
Rodenticides						
ANTU	0.4	1.0	0.3	1.1	0.5	0.7
Thallium	8.0	3.8	2.1	0.5	4.6	4.0
Warfarin	10.7	5.4	9.0	6.4	11.0	8.9
Strychnine	14.0	12.0	14.7	10.8	14.3	13.3
Compound 1080	0.0					
Zinc phosphide	0.5	0.2			0.2	0.2
Pesticides						
Arsenic	2.0	4.2	3.1	7.0	5.4	4.6
Chlorinated hydrocarbons	3.4	7.6	7.2	3.4	6.1	5.5
Organophosphates	8.6	13.9	8.5	3.3	9.2	8.6
Metaldehyde		0.4		19.2		3.8
Glycols						
Antifreeze	1.0	0.4	1.0		1.9	1.0
Heavy Metals						
Lead	3.0	0.6	0.3	0.5	4.0	2.1
Mercury					0.2	0.1
Miscellaneous						
Acid	0.0	0.6	0.8	0.5	1.1	0.7
Alkali	0.5	0.4	0.3	0.5	1.1	0.7
Phenols	0.0		0.5	0.16	1.2	0.5
Quarternary ammonia	0.4					0.1
Food intoxication	21.1	22.3	22.0	35.9	36.7	29.6
Phosphorus	0.0		0.3		0.2	0.1
Toxic plants	0.9		1.3	0.8	0.9	0.8
Fungi	21.9	3.0		1.8		4.7
Snakes	2.9	17.1	15.0	7.5	0.8	6.8
Toads	0.7	7.0	13.7	0.5	0.5	3.2
Percentage total	100.0	100.0	100.0	100.0	100.0	100.0
Total cases	559	498	387	610	1074	3128

*Percentage of total cases reported.

practices in North America have not been done. Available information about "common" poisonings is often the synthesis of impressions and experiences of individual toxicologists or clinicians. Summary reports of small animal poisonings are available chiefly through veterinary teaching clinics and diagnostic laboratories. Several of these will be reported. They are important as a reflection of relative clinical importance of various poisonings and because they represent different communities and environments.

Clinical data for acute poisonings in veterinary teaching clinics is probably similar to the routine clinical toxicoses seen in veterinary practices. Many of the poisonings are nonfatal, and a source is often apparent. Due to the acute nature of most small animal poisonings, it is assumed (not proved) that teaching clinic submissions represent the local community rather than long-distance referrals. By contrast, cases of poisoning reported from diagnostic laboratories are often based on pathologic or chemical evidence and reflect submission from a wide geographic area. Furthermore, they represent the fatal consequences of poisoning and often are not associated with an obvious source. Diagnostic laboratory findings should be considered not as the "most common poisonings" but as those that are serious enough to be submitted beyond the individual practice for assistance.

CLINICAL POISONING

The incidence of poisonings reported by three veterinary teaching hospitals is reported in Table 2. These data represent three different communities with populations ranging from 20,000 to 600,000. As much as possible, similar categories were grouped to aid in comparisons. It is apparent, however, that each clinic grouped and defined their diagnoses differently. Table 2 should be used only as a general comparative basis to demonstrate common and universally important toxicants. Certain generalizations and speculations are offered as follows.

1. Diagnosis of metal poisoning ranged from 2.2 to 25.7 per cent of toxicologic diagnoses, with lead and arsenic being the important individual toxicants. Minnesota reported an unusually high incidence of arsenic and lead poisoning in cats compared with traditional expectations. Perhaps this bears some relationship to the urban location and the demonstrated high rate of lead poisoning in urban dogs.

2. Insecticidal poisonings were mainly due to organophosphates rather than chlorinated hydrocarbons, reflecting the declining use of the latter category in recent years. Highest incidence was in

Kansas, where rural location and availability of crop insecticides could be factors.

3. Herbicide poisoning was rarely reported by any of the three clinics cited. This concurs with the known low acute toxicity of most common organic herbicides.

4. Rodenticides continue to be a major category of poisoning, especially for dogs. Of these the leader is still strychnine. Recently (1978), strychnine was declared a restricted use pesticide, but it is still available for some uses and as yet its incidence of poisoning remains high. The Kansas and Minnesota studies occurred during the time when Vacor was used. (Vacor was withdrawn from the market in 1979.)

5. Household and commercial products is a broad category of drugs, cosmetics, automotive products, home care products, and many other products generally available in homes. Collectively this accounts for a large group of poisonings. For many, the signs and lesions of intoxication are vague, and diagnosis depends on history of availability or consumption coupled with evidence of the chemical or its effects in the body. Of special note is the high prevalence of ethylene glycol (from antifreeze) poisoning reported from all three areas.

6. One clinic (Minnesota) reported a high incidence of abuse drug intoxication in dogs only (17.6 per cent). This may reflect the urban nature of the community or some differences in reporting such cases by various clinics.

7. Poisonous plants and fungi accounted for up to 16.6 per cent (in cats) of poisonings in Minnesota. Plants reported in that study included devil's ivy, goldenseal, Jerusalem cherry, black nightshade, European nightshade, mushroom, philodendron, mistletoe, green potatoes, poinsettia, and schefflera.

8. Both Kansas and Missouri reported high incidences of snake bite (13.5 and 15.8 per cent, respectively). In addition, Missouri data revealed insect stings involved in 16.9 per cent of all poisonings diagnosed.

Maddy and Winter (1980) reported in some detail on exposure to poisons for animals in the Los Angeles area. Table 3 summarizes their findings in dogs and cats. Findings are expressed as a percentage of total exposures reported. This work cannot be compared directly with the midwestern veterinary clinics reporting all classes of poisonings. However, it is a detailed analysis by category of pesticide and specific product involved. For example, five specific products were involved in both the arsenical incidents and the anticoagulant poisonings, whereas 14 different carbamates and 15 organophosphates were identified. Eleven of the 38 miscellaneous exposures were from herbicides. Since the area is a high pesticide use region, this detailed work is an excellent reference of the relative hazard to pets in such areas. They also report that in the last six years

Table 2. *Small Animal Poisoning at Three Veterinary Teaching Hospitals*

Location	Kansas State Univ.*		Univ. of Minnesota†		Univ. of Missouri‡
No. of Yrs. Reported	6		4		11
Period Covered	1975–1980		1974–1977		1965–1976
Species Reported	Dog	Cat	Dog	Cat	Dog
Total Reported	89	33	288	31	272
Toxicants Involved§					
Metals	2.2	0	11.0	25.7	13.6
Arsenic	0.0	0	4.1	12.9	5.9
Chromium	0.0	0	0.0	3.2	
Copper	0.0	0	0.0	0.0	
Iron	0.0	0	0.0	0.0	
Lead	2.2	0	5.2	6.4	5.9
Mercury	0.0	0	0.0	3.2	
Thallium	0.0	0	1.7	0.0	
Inorganics					2.2
Insecticides	27.4	49.8	5.2	9.6	7.4
Chlorinated hydrocarbons	1.1	12.0	0.7	0.0	
Organophosphates	11.2	30.3	3.8	6.4	
Carbamates	9.0	4.5	0.7	0.0	
Rotenone	0.0	0.0	0.0	3.2	
Other	3.4	3.0	0.0	0.0	
Herbicides	0.0	3.0	0.7	0.0	0.0
2,4D	0.0	0.0	0.7	0.0	
Rodenticides	23.5	3.0	52.8	19.4	22.0
Anticoagulants	6.7	0.0	1.4	9.7	
Fluoroacetate			0.7	0.0	
Strychnine	11.2	0.0	43.4	0.0	
Vacor	3.4	3.0	4.9	9.7	
Zinc phosphide			2.4	0.0	
Unspecified	2.2	0.0	0.0	0.0	
Household & Commercial Products	25.8	28.4	16.3	29.0	22.5
Aspirin	0.0	0.0	0.7	0.0	
Caffeine	0.0	0.0	1.0	0.0	
Carbon monoxide	0.0	0.0	1.0	0.0	
Ethylene glycol	19.1	18.2	7.3	19.4	10.7
Metaldehyde	0.0	0.0	0.7	0.0	
Nicotine	0.0	0.0	1.4	0.0	0.0
Phenolics	0.0	0.0	0.3	6.4	0.0
Solvents	0.0	6.1	0.0	0.0	0.0
Sulfonamides	0.0	0.0	1.0	0.0	0.0
Miscellaneous household	6.7	4.1	2.9	3.2	11.8
Abuse Drugs	1.0	0.0	7.6	0.0	0.0
Amphetamine	0.0	0.0	4.2	0.0	0.0
Caffeine	0.0	0.0	0.7	0.0	0.0
Cocaine	0.0	0.0	0.3	0.0	0.0
LSD	0.0	0.0	0.3	0.0	0.0
Marijuana	1.0	0.0	2.1	0.0	0.0
Poisonous Plants	0.0	3.0	5.6	16.1	1.4
Snake Bite	13.5	0.0	0.0	0.0	15.8
Insect Stings	4.5	0.0	0.0	0.0	16.9

*Barton and Oehme: Vet. Human Toxicol. 23:101, 1981.
†Stowe et al.: Paper presented to the 4th Biennial Toxicology Conference, 1978.
‡Webber and Acha: Unpublished data, 1978.
§Results reported are percentage of total poisonings for that location.

Table 3. *Poison Exposure of Small Animals by Pesticides in the Los Angeles Area**†

Pesticide	Dogs (244 incidents)	Cats (39 incidents)
Anticoagulants	20.9	12.8
Arsenicals	4.9	0.0
Carbamates	28.7	20.5
Chlorinated hydrocarbons	3.7	7.7
Metaldehyde	5.3	0.0
Organophosphates	11.1	35.0
Pentachlorophenol	0.4	0.0
Phosphorus	2.0	0.0
Strychnine	0.8	0.0
Thiocarbamates	1.6	0.0
Vacor	4.9	5.1
Miscellaneous	15.6	17.9

*Adapted from Maddy and Winter: Vet. Human Toxicol. 22, 409, 1980.

†Results are expressed as percentage of total pesticide exposures for each species.

there has been a tenfold reduction in snail bait poisoning of dogs. This is attributed to reformulation of the bait to make it less attractive to dogs. Such results should stimulate further interest in formulating baits and pesticides that are less attractive to pets while remaining attractive to pests.

EPIDEMIOLOGIC CHARACTERISTICS

Webber and Acha (1978), in reviewing case records of the University of Missouri, obtained epidemiologic and mortality data not generally covered in other studies. A summary of their findings includes the following.

1. *Attack Rate.* There were 458 poisonings out of 39,260 dogs examined, for an attack rate of 116.7/10,000 dog years at risk, or 1.17 per cent.

2. *Season.* There was no marked overall seasonal variation in poisonings reported. There were, however, seasonal variations for specific categories. Insect stings and snake bites were common in summer. Insecticide and rodenticide poisoning occurred more frequently in winter. Ethylene glycol incidence was highest in summer, contrasted with the higher incidence of ethylene glycol poisoning in winter for Minnesota.

3. *Sex.* There were no overall differences in poisoning when one sex was compared with the other.

4. *Age.* Dogs six months to two years of age had a significantly higher attack rate than the average, whereas the attack rate for dogs older than seven years was significantly lower.

5. *Mortality.* Mortality for 458 cases of poisoning was only 12 per cent. This was 0.14 per cent of all animals at risk for the 12-year period. Ethylene glycol mortality was 71 per cent, whereas the death rate for heavy metal intoxication was 18.5 per cent.

Insecticides caused death in 11 per cent of cases, and rodenticides, including strychnine, resulted in a 9 per cent death rate. Inadvertent exposure to human drugs was associated with a 7 per cent mortality rate. Snake bite accounted for 43 diagnoses in 11 years. Of these, four were identified as rattlesnake and 11 as copperhead. None of the bitten dogs died.

6. *Breed.* Pointers, dachshunds, and beagles specifically had a risk of poisoning twice that of mixed breed dogs.

7. *Source.* Of 106 poisonings determined to be due to carelessness or negligence, 69 per cent were related to baits or pesticides. "Poisons lying around the home" (e.g., ethylene glycol) accounted for 20 per cent, and therapeutic drugs (mostly for humans) accounted for 11 per cent of poisonings.

DIAGNOSTIC LABORATORIES

Diagnostic laboratory data focus on those poisonings that often result in fatalities, present difficult diagnostic problems for a clinician, or require corroboration because of legal or liability considerations.

Table 4. *Incidence of Common Poisonings in Dogs at Two Midwestern Veterinary Diagnostic Laboratories**

Toxicant	Laboratory Location	
	Iowa†	Missouri‡
Metals		
Antimony	—	1
Arsenic	6	4
Lead	10	8
Rodenticides		
Anticoagulants	7	5
Cyanide	—	1
Fluoroacetate	10	—
Strychnine	44	34
Thallium	<1	1
Vacor	—	—
Zinc phosphide	—	1
Insecticides		
Carbamates	2	—
Chlorinated hydrocarbons	3	3
Nicotine	—	1
Organophosphates	9	4
Herbicides		
Paraquat	—	1
Drugs		
Caffeine	—	1
Vitamin D	—	2
Miscellaneous		
Ethylene glycol	11	30

*Percentage of total cases reported.
†Meerdink: Unpublished data, 1978.
‡Osweiler: Unpublished data, 1981.

Table 4 compares data from two midwestern diagnostic laboratories based on poisonings confirmed by diagnostic procedures such as histopathology or analytic chemistry. Due to regional and population differences, diagnostic laboratory data from various states may differ markedly. Such data should be used in only a general sense to show broad trends. Again, from Table 4, the importance of metals, insecticides, rodenticides, and antifreeze as serious poisoning agents is evident.

Aside from the few generalizations made here, there is no definitive evidence of any one overwhelming toxicology problem. Certainly, clinical toxicoses of small animals pose a formidable diagnostic challenge. They must be dealt with clinically but can only be defined by a well-organized, coordinated gathering of evidence made in light of the potential hazards available and confirmed by chemical and clinical corroboration. The final task is to educate the client to avoid such hazards or to keep and use hazardous materials in their proper place.

REFERENCES AND SUPPLEMENTAL READING

Arena, J. M.: *Poisoning, Toxicology, Symptoms, Treatment*, 3rd ed. Springfield: Charles C Thomas, 1974.

Atkins, C. E., and Johnson, R. K.: Clinical toxicities of cats. Vet. Clin. North Am. 5:623, 1975.
Barton, J., and Oehme, F. W.: The incidence and characteristics of animal poisonings seen in Kansas State University from 1975 to 1980. Vet. Human Toxicol. 23:101, 1981.
Buck, W. B., Osweiler, G. D., and Van Gelder, G. A.: *Clinical and Diagnostic Veterinary Toxicology.* Dubuque, Iowa: Kendall-Hunt Publishing Co., 1973.
Clark, E. G. C.: Pets and poisons. J. Small Anim. Pract. 16:375, 1975.
Clarke, E. G. C., and Clarke, M. L.: *Garner's Veterinary Toxicology,* 3rd ed. Baltimore: The Williams & Wilkins Co., 1967.
Humphreys, D. J.: A review of recent trends in animal poisoning. Br. Vet. J. 134:128, 1978.
Kirk, R. W. (ed.): *Current Veterinary Therapy,* VII, Philadelphia: W. B. Saunders Co., 1977.
Kirk, R. W., and Bistner, S. I.: *Handbook of Veterinary Procedures and Emergency Treatment,* 2nd ed. Philadelphia: W. B. Saunders Co., 1975.
Maddy, K. T., Peoples, S. A., and Riddle, L. C.: Poisoning in dogs in California with pesticides. Calif. Vet. 31:9, 1977.
Maddy, K. T., and Winter, J.: Poisoning of animals in the Los Angeles area with pesticides during 1977. Vet. Human Toxicol. 22:409, 1980.
Malone, J. C.: Diagnosis and treatment of poisoning in dogs and cats. Vet. Rec. 84:161, 1969.
Meerdink, G.: Iowa Veterinary Medical Diagnostic Laboratory, Ames, Iowa, 1978. Unpublished data.
Osweiler, G.D.: Incidence and diagnostic considerations of major small animal toxicoses. J.A.M.A. 155:2011, 1969.
Osweiler, G. D.: Missouri Veterinary Medical Diagnostic Laboratory, Columbia, Missouri, 1981. Unpublished data.
Stowe, C. M., Fangmann, G., Arendt, T. D., et al.: The frequency of animal intoxications in Minnesota. Paper presented to the 4th Biennial Toxicology Conference, Logan, Utah. June 19–23, 1978.
Szabuniewicz, M.: Treatment of some common animal poisonings. Vet. Med. Small Anim. Clin. December 1971, pp. 1197–1205.
Webber, J. J., and Acha, S. M.: Poisonings, UMC Veterinary Clinic (1965–1976). Columbia, Missouri, 1978. Unpublished data.

EMERGENCY AND GENERAL TREATMENT OF POISONINGS*

E. MURL BAILEY, D.V.M.
College Station, Texas

Many acutely ill animals are diagnosed as poisoned when no other diagnosis can be readily ascertained. For this reason, the treatment and management of acutely ill animals should be directed toward preserving the life of the animal regardless of the etiology.

The veterinary clinician should direct his efforts toward treating the signs exhibited by the affected animal unless the correct diagnosis is obvious. Preexisting conditions and the diagnosis should be determined following stabilization of the patient.

Special goals of therapy in cases of intoxication include the following:

1. Emergency intervention and prevention of further exposure.

2. Delaying further absorption.
3. Application of specific antidotes.
4. Hastening elimination of the absorbed toxicant.
5. Supportive therapy.
6. Client education.

PRELIMINARY INSTRUCTIONS TO CLIENTS

Veterinarians are frequently contacted by telephone concerning an intoxicated animal. The preliminary instructions given at this time can be important to the success of subsequent therapeutic measures.

The client should be instructed to protect the

*Supported in part by Texas Agricultural Experiment Station, Project No. H-6255.

animal as well as the people in contact with the affected animal. This may include keeping the animal warm and avoiding any other stress phenomena. Onlookers should be warned about the condition of the animal, and it may be desirable to place a muzzle on the animal.

If the animal's exposure was topical, the client should be instructed to cleanse the animal's skin or eye with copious amounts of water. The client should also be instructed to be careful to avoid exposure to the toxicant and use some type of protective clothing if available, i.e., rubber gloves, apron, and so on.

In many instances, the client will be concerned about inducing emesis in the animal. The clinician should cite the contraindications to emesis, i.e., CNS depression and ingestion of petroleum distillates, acids, or alkalis. Emetic preparations and techniques readily available to the lay individual, such as hydrogen peroxide, table salt, and sticking the finger in the back of the animal's mouth, are generally ineffective and sometimes dangerous. One-half to two teaspoonfuls of syrup of ipecac may be administered if the animal is fully awake.

If the client is very insistent about administering medication, he should be advised to allow the animal to drink as much water as it wants. This will act as a diluent. In most cases, one may also advise the administration of milk or egg whites. Activated charcoal tablets may also be administered. The client should be cautioned not to administer anything by mouth if the animal is convulsing, depressed, or unconscious.

It is imperative that the client not waste time. The animal should be brought to the veterinarian as soon as possible (or the veterinarian should be summoned). The owner should be instructed to bring vomitus and/or suspected materials or their containers with the animal. The client should be advised to bring the specimens in clean plastic containers or glass jars and should be cautioned not to contaminate the material. In many instances valuable time can be saved by applying the proper therapeutic measure if the intoxicant is known. This material may also be valuable from a medicolegal aspect.

EMERGENCY INTERVENTION

The most important aspect of emergency treatment of intoxication is to ensure adequate physiologic functioning. All the antidotal procedures available to the clinician will be of no avail if the animal has lost one or all of its vital functions. This may include establishment of a patent airway, artificial respiration, cardiac massage (external or internal), and perhaps the application of defibrillation techniques. Following stabilization of the vital signs,

the clinician may proceed with subsequent therapeutic measures.

DELAYING ABSORPTION

Preventing the animal from absorbing additional intoxicant is a major factor in treating cases of poisoning. In many instances intoxication may be prevented if the animal was actually observed ingesting or coming in contact with suspected material. Removal of the animal from the affected environment is a necessary first step to prevent further absorption. It is hoped that bringing the animal to the veterinary clinic or hospital will serve this purpose. Preventing absorption may also entail washing the animal's skin to remove the noxious agent. If an external toxicant is involved, caution must be exercised to avoid contamination of persons handling the animal. In addition, the judicious use of emetics, gastric lavage techniques, adsorbents, and cathartics will aid in the prevention of further absorption of toxic materials that are ingested.

INDUCTION OF EMESIS

Emesis may be considered as a method of emptying the stomach of toxic materials. Some commonly available agents are not very reliable, and emesis may be of little value after one to two hours following exposure to a toxicant.

Syrup of ipecac is considered a general emetic. Its mechanism is gastric irritation and minor central nervous system stimulation. The dose for small animals is 1 to 2 ml/kg, but it is only about 50 per cent effective and not more than 15 ml (1 tablespoonful) should be used with even the largest dog. The dosage may be repeated in 20 minutes if vomiting does not occur. However, if the patient still does not vomit, lavage procedures should be instituted to recover the ipecac (syrup of ipecac can exert a cardiotoxic effect if it is not vomited but absorbed). This agent should never be used when activated charcoal is part of the therapeutic regimen, since it markedly reduces the effectiveness of the charcoal. The drug should not be confused with ipecac fluid extract, which is 14 times stronger than syrup of ipecac.

Other agents, such as copper sulfate, table salt, or hydrogen peroxide, have been advocated as locally acting emetics. However, the effectiveness of these agents is questionable.

Apomorphine is the most effective and most reliable emetic available. The effective dose in most small animals is 0.04 mg/kg IV or 0.08 mg/kg IM or SC. Apomorphine may cause respiratory depression, and protracted emesis may develop following its use. These signs can be effectively controlled with appropriate narcotic antagonists injected IV (naloxone, Narcan: 0.04 mg/kg; levallorphan, Lorfan: 0.02 mg/kg; or nalorphine, Nalline: 0.1 mg/kg). In addition to the general contraindications of emetics, apomorphine may be further contraindicated in cases in which additional CNS depression must be avoided.

The contraindications for induction of emesis are unconsciousness, severe depression, or intoxication by petroleum distillates, tranquilizers, or other antiemetics. If the time interval following exposure to the toxicant is greater than one to two hours, most of the toxicant will have passed into the duodenum.

Intoxication with acids or alkalis may be diagnosed when corrosive changes are present in and around the mouth, forepaws, and other areas on the cranial portion of the body. If emesis is induced, caustic agents could cause additional damage to the esophagus and oral cavity. In addition, these agents generally weaken the gastric wall, which could easily be ruptured during forceful emesis.

Activated charcoal may increase the efficacy of emesis. If charcoal is to be utilized, the clinician should first induce emesis with apomorphine, administer the charcoal, and then reinduce emesis with a subsequent IV dose of apomorphine (0.04 mg/kg).

Any vomitus should be saved for analysis, especially if there are any medicolegal considerations. The clinician should consider any intoxication as grounds for a possible court case and should conduct treatment accordingly.

GASTRIC LAVAGE

Gastric lavage is an emergency procedure that at times has been maligned as being relatively inefficient. Changes in technique (e.g., using a larger tube, more volume, and more frequent lavages) have made this a very reliable procedure when undertaken within two hours of exposure to an ingested toxicant.

The animal should be unconscious or under light anesthesia. A cuffed endotracheal tube should be placed within the trachea. The distal end of the tube should protrude 2 inches beyond the teeth. This will increase the animal's dead space but is required to prevent any inhalation of lavage fluid. The head and thorax should be lowered slightly but not enough to compromise respiration due to the weight of the abdominal viscera. The stomach tube should be premeasured from the tip of the animal's nose to the xiphoid cartilage. In all cases, as large a stomach tube as possible should be used. A good rule is to use the same size stomach tube as cuffed endotracheal tube (1 mm - 3 French). The volume of water or lavage solution to be used for each washing is 5 to 10 ml/kg of body weight. Following infusion of the solution, the fluid should be aspirated

from the stomach via the stomach tube with either a large aspirator bulb or a 50-ml syringe. The infusion and aspiration cycle of the lavage solution should be repeated 10 to 15 times. Activated charcoal in the solution will enhance the effectiveness of this procedure.

Some precautions to be taken with this technique include (1) using low pressure to prevent the forcing of the toxicant into the duodenum, (2) reducing the infused volume in obviously weakened stomachs, and (3) making sure not to force the stomach tube through either the esophagus or the stomach wall.

ADSORBENTS

Activated charcoal is probably the best adsorbing agent available to the practitioner. Although it does not detoxify toxicants, it will effectively prevent absorption of a toxicant if properly utilized. Activated charcoal can be effectively utilized with emetic and gastric lavage techniques.

The proper type of activated charcoal for treatment of intoxications is one of vegetable, not mineral or animal, origin. There are several types of activated charcoal available commercially: Norit (American Norit), Nuchar C (West Virginia Pulp and Paper), Darco G-60 (Atlas Chemical), and Activated Charcoal Powder, U.S.P. (J. T. Baker, City Chemical Corp., Humcolabs, Mallinckrodt, and Med-Corp., Inc.). Compressed activated charcoal tablets (5 gr) are also available (B. C. Crowley, Co. and Requa Mfg. Co.). These tablets are easier to handle than the powdered charcoal and are apparently almost as effective.

A bathtub or some other easily cleaned area is the best place to administer activated charcoal to small animals. The proper technique for utilizing activated charcoal is as follows. (1) Make a slurry of the charcoal using water. The proper dose is 2 to 8 gm/kg body weight in a concentration of 1 gm charcoal/5 to 10 ml water. (2) Administer the charcoal by a stomach tube using either a funnel or a large syringe. (3) Administer a cathartic of sodium sulfate 30 minutes following administration of the charcoal. This technique may be modified if the charcoal is used in conjunction with an emetic or lavage technique. However, with either technique some charcoal should remain in the stomach and should be followed by a cathartic to prevent desorption of the toxicant.

Activated charcoal is highly adsorptive for many toxicants including mercuric chloride, strychnine, other alkaloids including morphine and atropine, barbiturates, and ethylene glycol. It is ineffective against cyanide.

Syrup of ipecac will negate some of the adsorptive characteristics of the activated charcoal. The "universal antidote," consisting of 2 parts activated charcoal, 1 part MgO, and 1 part tannic acid, is very inefficient, since the MgO and tannic acid decrease the adsorptive capability of the charcoal. Burned or charred toast as described in some emergency texts is highly ineffective as an adsorbing agent.

CATHARTICS

Sodium sulfate is a more efficient agent for evacuation of the bowel than magnesium sulfate and is the preferred agent, especially with activated charcoal. There is also some danger of CNS depression owing to the magnesium ion, although the sodium ion may also precipitate a sodium ion intoxication or water deprivation syndrome. However, either agent may be used in an emergency. The oral dose of sodium sulfate is 1 gm/kg.

Mineral oil or vegetable oils are of value if lipid-soluble toxicants are involved. Mineral oil (liquid petrolatum) is inert and unlikely to be absorbed. Vegetable oil, however, is more likely to be absorbed and therefore may be contraindicated. Regardless of the type of oil utilized, its administration should be followed by a saline cathartic in 30 to 40 minutes.

A colonic lavage or high enema may be of value in hastening the elimination of toxicants from the gastrointestinal tract. Warm water with castile soap makes an excellent enema solution. Hexachlorophene soaps should be avoided. There are several commercially available enema preparations that act as osmotic agents. Care should be taken to avoid the induction of dehydration and electrolyte imbalances with overzealous treatment.

LOCALLY ACTING ANTIDOTES

There are numerous locally acting antidotes and therapeutic regimens reported to prevent the absorption of toxicants. The nonspecific antidotal procedures for some of the more common toxicants are described in Table 1.

SPECIFIC ANTIDOTES

There are a few specific antidotal agents available for some of the more common animal toxicants. A list of these specific antidotal procedures is presented in Table 2.

Caution should be exercised with the use of some of the more specific antidotes, since many of these agents are themselves toxic. In certain chronic metallic intoxications, such as lead poisoning, the use of chelating agents has precipitated the acute metallic intoxication. Consequently, the dosage of chelating agents should be reduced in some chronic metal intoxications.

ELIMINATION OF ABSORBED TOXICANTS

Absorbed toxicants are generally excreted via the kidneys. Some toxicants may be excreted by other routes (bile-feces, lung, other body secretions). Renal excretion can be manipulated in many instances. Urinary excretion of toxicants may be enhanced by the use of diuretics or by altering the pH of the urine.

The use of diuretics to enhance urinary excretion of toxicants requires adequate renal function and

Text continued on page 89

Table 1. *Locally Acting Antidotes Against Unabsorbed Poisons and Principles of Treatment*

Poison	Antidote and Dose or Concentration
Acids, corrosive	Internally; weak alkali — magnesium oxide solution (1:25 warm water); Milk of magnesia (1 to 15 ml). *Never give sodium bicarbonate!* Externally; flush with water. Apply paste of sodium bicarbonate.
Alkali, caustic	Weak acid — vinegar (diluted 1:4), 1% acetic acid or lemon juice given orally. Diluted albumin (4 to 6 egg whites to 1 qt tepid water) followed by an emetic and then a cathartic, because some compounds are soluble in excess albumin. Externally; flush with copious amounts of water and apply vinegar.
Alkaloids	Potassium permanganate (1:5000 to 1:10,000) for lavage and/or oral administration. Tannic acid or strong tea (200 to 500 mg in 30 to 60 ml of water) except in cases of poisoning by cocaine, nicotine, physostigmine, atropine, and morphine. Emetic or purgative should be used for prompt removal of tannates.

Table continued on following page

Table 1.   *Locally Acting Antidotes Against Unabsorbed Poisons
and Principles of Treatment (Continued)*

Poison	Antidote and Dose or Concentration
Arsenic	Sodium thiosulfate — 10% solution given orally (0.5 to 3.0 gm for small animals). Protein — evaporated milk, egg white, etc. Tannic acid or strong tea.
Barium salts	Sodium sulfate and magnesium sulfate (20% solution given orally). Dosage: 2 to 25 gm.
Bismuth salts	Acacia or gum arabic as mucilage.
Carbon tetrachloride	Empty stomach, give high protein and carbohydrate diet, maintain fluid and electrolyte balance. Hemodialysis is indicated in anuria. Epinephrine is contraindicated (ventricular fibrillation!).
Copper	Albumin (as for Alkali above). Sodium ferrocyanide in water (0.3 to 3.5 gm for small animals). Magnesium oxide (as for acids above).
Detergents, anionic (Na, K, NH_4^+-salts)	Milk or water followed by demulcent (oils, acacia, gelatin, starch, egg white, etc.)
Detergents, cationic (chlorides, iodides, etc.)	Soap (castile, etc.) dissolved in 4 times its bulk of hot water. Albumin (as for alkali above).
Fluoride	Calcium (milk, lime water, or powdered chalk mixed with water) given orally.
Formaldehyde	Ammonia water (0.2% orally) or ammonium acetate (1% for lavage). Starch — 1 part to 15 parts hot water added gradually. Gelatin soaked in water for one-half hour. Albumin (as for Alkali above). Sodium thiosulfate (as for Arsenic above).
Iron	Sodium bicarbonate — 1% for lavage.
Lead	Sodium or magnesium sulfate given orally. Sodium ferrocyanide (as for Copper above). Tannic acid (as for Alkaloids above). Albumin (as for Alkali above).
Mercury	Protein — milk, egg whites (as for Alkali above). Magnesium oxide (as for Acids above). Sodium formaldehyde sulfoxylate — 5% solution for lavage. Starch (as for Formaldehyde above). Activated charcoal — 5 to 50 gm.
Oxalic acid	Calcium — calcium hydroxide as 0.15% solution. Other alkalis are contraindicated because their salts are more soluble. Chalk or other calcium salts. Magnesium sulfate as cathartic. Maintain diuresis to prevent calcium oxalate deposition in kidney.
Petroleum distillates (aliphatic hydrocarbons)	Olive oil, other vegetable oils, or mineral oil given orally. After one-half hour, sodium sulfate as cathartic. Both emesis and lavage are contraindicated.
Phenol and cresols	Soap-and-water or alcohol lavage of skin. Sodium bicarbonate (0.5%) dressings. Activated charcoal and/or mineral oil given orally.
Phosphorus (white or yellow phosphides; red and black are nontoxic)	Copper sulfate (0.2 to 0.4% solution) or potassium permanganate (1:5000 solution) for lavage. Turpentine (preferably old oxidized) in gelatin capsules or floated on hot water. Give 2 ml 4 times at 15-minute intervals. Activated charcoal. Do not give vegetable oil cathartic. Remove all fat from diet.
Silver nitrate	Normal saline for lavage. Albumin (as for Alkali above).
Unknown (toxic plants, etc.)	Activated charcoal (replaces universal antidote). For small animals — 2 to 8 gm/kg in gelatin capsules or, via stomach pump, as a slurry in water. Follow by emetic or cathartic and repeat procedure.

Table 2. *Systemic Antidotes and Dosages*

Toxic Agent	Systemic Antidotes	Dosage and Method for Treatment
Acetaminophen	N-acetylcysteine (Mucomyst)	140 mg/kg orally (loading dose), then 7 mg/kg q4h for 17 additional doses.
Amphetamines	Chlorpromazine	1 mg/kg IM, IP, IV; administer only half dose if barbiturates have been given; blocks excitation.
Arsenic, mercury, and other heavy metals except silver, selenium, and thallium	Dimercaprol (BAL)	10% solution in oil; give small animals 2.5 to 5.0 mg/kg IM every 4 hours for 2 days, 3 times a day for the next 10 days or until recovery. NOTE: In severe acute poisoning, 5 mg/kg dosage should be given only first day.
	D-Penicillamine (Cuprimine)	Developed for chronic mercury poisoning, now seems most promising drug; no reports on dosage in animals. Dosage for man is 250 mg orally, every 6 hours for 10 days (3 to 4 mg/kg).
Atropine–belladonna alkaloids	Physostigmine salicylate	0.01 to 0.6 mg/kg. (Do not use neostigmine.)
Barbiturates	Pentylenetetrazol	10% solution; give small animals 10 to 20 mg/kg IV or IM, repeated at 15- to 30-minute intervals as needed.
	Doxapram	2% solution; give small animals 3 to 5 mg/kg IV only, repeated as necessary.
	Bemegride	3% solution; give small animals 5 to 10 mg/kg IV only, by slow infusion or in intermittent doses.
	NOTE: All the above are reliable only when depression is mild; in deeper levels of depression, artificial respiration (and oxygen) is preferable.	
Bromides	Chlorides (sodium or ammonium salts)	0.5 to 1.0 gm daily for several days; hasten excretion.
Carbon monoxide	Oxygen	Pure oxygen at normal or high pressure; artificial respiration; blood transfusion.
Cholinergic agents	Atropine sulfate	0.02 to 0.04 mg/kg, as needed.
Cholinesterase inhibitors	Atropine sulfate	Dosage is 0.2 mg/kg, repeated as needed for atropinization. Treat cyanosis (if present) first. Blocks only muscarinic effects. Atropine in oil may be injected for prolonged effect during the night. *Avoid atropine intoxication!*
Cholinergic agents and cholinesterase inhibitors (organophosphates, some carbamates; but not carbaryl, dimethan, or carbam piloxime, etc.)	Pralidoxime chloride (2-PAM)	2% solution; give 20 to 50 mg/kg IM or by slow IV injection (maximum dose is 500 mg/min), repeated as needed. 2-PAM alleviates nicotinic effect and regenerates cholinesterase. Morphine, succinylcholine, and phenothiazine tranquilizers are contraindicated.
Copper	D-Penicillamine (Cuprimine)	Dose for animals not established. Dose for man is 1 to 4 gm daily in divided doses (250-mg tablets).
Coumarin-derivative anticoagulants	Vitamin K₁ (Aquamephyton)	5% stable emulsion. 1 mg/kg IV in 5% dextrose. Give 5 mg/kg IM for 5 days.
	Whole blood or plasma	Blood transfusion, 25 ml/kg.
Curare (tubocurarine)	Neostigmine methylsulfate	Solution: 1:2000 or 1:5000 (1 ml = 0.5 mg or 2 mg). Dose is 0.005 mg/5 kg, SC. Follow with IV injection of a 1% solution of atropine (0.04 mg/kg). 1% solution; give 0.05 to 1.0 mg/kg IV.
	Edrophonium chloride (Tensilon)	1% solution; give 0.05 to 1.0 mg/kg IV.
	Artificial respiration	
Cyanide	Methemoglobin (sodium nitrite is used to form methemoglobin)	1% solution of sodium nitrite, dosage is 16 mg/kg IV. Follow with:
	Sodium thiosulfate	20% solution at dosage of 30 to 40 mg/kg IV. If treatment is repeated, use only sodium thiosulfate. NOTE: Both of the above may be given simultaneously as follows: 0.5 ml/kg of combination consisting of 10 gm sodium nitrite, 15 gm sodium thiosulfate, distilled water q.s. 250 ml. Dosage may be repeated once. If further treatment is required, give only 20% solution of sodium thiosulfate at level of 1 ml/kg.

Table continued on following page

In the formula for Vitamin K₁, this represents K_1.

Table 2.   *Systemic Antidotes and Dosages (Continued)*

Toxic Agent	Systemic Antidotes	Dosage and Method for Treatment
Digitalis glycosides, oleander, and Bufo toads	Potassium chloride	Dog: 0.5 to 2.0 gm, orally in divided doses, or in serious cases, as diluted solution given IV by slow drip (ECG control is essential).
	Phenytoin	25 mg/min IV until control is established.
	Propranolol (beta blocker)	0.5 to 1.0 mg/kg IV or IM as needed to control cardiac arrhythmias (ECG monitoring is essential).
	Atropine sulfate	0.02 to 0.04 mg/kg as needed for cholinergic control.
Fluoride	Calcium borogluconate	3 to 10 ml of 5 to 10% solution.
Fluoroacetate (compound 1080)	Glyceryl monoacetin	0.1 to 0.5 mg/kg IM hourly for several hours (total 2 to 4 mg/kg); or diluted (0.5 to 1.0%) IV (danger of hemolysis). Monoacetin is available only from chemical supply houses.
	Acetamide	Animal may be protected if acetamide is given prior to or simultaneously with 1080 (experimental).
	Phenobarbital or pentobarbital	May protect against lethal dose (experimental).
Hallucinogens (LSD, phencyclidine-PCP)	Diazepam (Valium)	As needed; avoid respiratory depression.
Heparin	Protamine sulfate	1% solution; give 1.0 to 1.5 mg to antagonize each 1 mg of heparin; slow IV injection. Reduce dose as time increases between heparin injection and start of treatment. (After 30 minutes give only 0.5 mg.)
Iron salts	Desferoxamine (Desferal)	Dose for animals not yet established. Dose for man is 5 gm of 5% solution given orally, then 20 mg/kg IM every 4 hours. In case of shock, dose is 40 mg/kg by IV drip over 4-hour period; may be repeated in 6 hours, then 15 mg/kg by drip every 8 hours.
Lead	Calcium disodium edate (EDTA) EDTA and BAL	Dosage: Maximum safe dose is 75 mg/kg/24 hours (only for severe case). EDTA is available in 20% solution; for IV drip, dilute in 5% glucose to 0.5%; for IM, add procaine to 20% solution to give 0.5% concentration of procaine. BAL is given as 10% solution in oil. Treatment: (1) In severe case (CNS involvement of > 100 mg Pb/100 gm whole blood), give 4 mg/kg. BAL only as initial dose; follow after 4 hours, and every 4 hours for 3 to 4 days, with BAL and EDTA (12.5 mg/kg) at separate IM sites; skip 2 or 3 days and then treat again for 3 to 4 days. (2) In subacute case or <100 mg Pb/100 gm whole blood, give only 50 mg EDTA/kg/24 hours for 3 to 5 days.
	Penicillamine (Cuprimine)	(3) May use following either (1) or (2) with 100 mg/kg/day orally for 1 to 4 weeks.
	Thiamine HCl	Experimental for nervous signs; 5 mg/kg IV, b.i.d., for 1 to 2 weeks; give slowly and watch for untoward reactions.
Metaldehyde	Diazepam (Valium) Triflupromazine Pentobarbital	2 to 5 mg/kg IV to control tremor. 0.2 to 2.0 mg/kg IV. To effect.
Methanol and ethylene glycol	Ethanol	Give IV, 1.1 gm/kg of 25% solution, then give 0.5 gm/kg every 4 hours for 4 days. To prevent or correct acidosis, use sodium bicarbonate IV. Sodium bicarbonate: 0.4 gm/kg. Activated charcoal: 5 gm/kg orally if soon after ingestion.
Methemoglobinemia-producing agents (nitrites, chlorates, etc.)	Methylene blue	1% solution (maximum concentration), given by *slow* IV injection, 8.8 mg/kg; repeat if necessary. To prevent fall in blood pressure in cases of nitrite poisoning, use a sympathomimetic drug (ephedrine, epinephrine, etc.).
Morphine and related drugs	Naloxone chloride (Narcan)	0.1 mg/kg IV. Do not repeat if respiration is not satisfactory.
	Levallorphan tartrate (Lorfan)	Give IV, 0.1 to 0.5 ml of solution containing 1 mg/ml. NOTE: Use either of the above antidotes only in acute poisoning. Artificial respiration may be indicated. Activated charcoal is also indicated.
Oxalates	Calcium	Treatment: 23% solution of calcium gluconate IV. Give 3 to 20 ml (to control hypocalcemia).

Table continued on opposite page

Table 2. *Systemic Antidotes and Dosages (Continued)*

Toxic Agent	Systemic Antidotes	Dosage and Method for Treatment
Phenothiazine derivatives	Methylamphetamine (Desoxyn)	0.1 to 0.2 mg/kg IV; also transfusion. Only available in tablet form.
	Diphenhydramine HCl	For CNS depression, 2 to 5 mg/kg IV for extrapyramidal signs.
Phytotoxins and botulin	Antitoxins (not available commercially)	As indicated for specific antitoxins. Examples of phytotoxins: ricin, abrin, robin, crotin.
Plants		Treat signs as necessary.
Red squill	Atropine sulfate, propranolol	As for digitalis glycosides poisoning above.
Snake bite (rattlesnake, copperhead, water moccasin)	Antivenin (Wyeth, Trivalent Crotalidae)	Caution: equine origin.
coral snake	Antivenin (Wyeth)	Caution: equine origin.
Spider bite (black widow)	Antivenin (Merck)	Caution: equine origin.
Strontium	Calcium salts	Usual dose of calcium borogluconate.
	Ammonium chloride	0.2 to 0.5 gm orally 3 to 4 times daily.
Strychnine and brucine	Pentobarbital	Give IP or IV to effect; higher dose is usually required than that required for anesthesia. Place animal in warm quiet room.
	Amobarbital	Give by slow IV injection to effect. Duration of sedation is usually 4 to 6 hrs.
	Methocarbamol (Robaxin) (guaifenesin)	10% solution; average first dose is 150 mg/kg IV (range: 40 to 300 mg), repeat half dose as needed.
	Glyceryl guaiacolate, guaifenesin	110 mg/kg IV, 5% solution. Repeat as necessary.
	Diazepam (Valium)	2 to 5 mg/kg to control convulsions, induce emesis; then use other agents.
Thallium	Diphenylthiocarbazone	Dog: 70 mg/kg orally, 3 times a day for 6 days. Hastens elimination, but is partially toxic.
	Prussian blue	0.2 mg/kg in 3 divided doses daily.
	Potassium chloride	Give simultaneously with thiocarbazone or Prussian blue, 2 to 6 gm orally daily in divided doses.

hydration of the affected animal. Once these requisites are established, diuretics are indicated. Monitoring of urinary output is essential in these animals, and a minimum urinary flow of 0.1 ml/kg/min is necessary. The diuretics of choice are mannitol and furosemide (Lasix). Both of these agents are very potent diuretics. The dosage for mannitol is 2 gm/kg/hr and for furosemide, 5 mg/kg q6–8 h. Again, hydration must be maintained for proper renal excretion.

Alteration of urinary pH to expedite the excretion of toxicants and foreign chemicals is a classic pharmacologic technique. The technique relies on the physiochemical phenomenon that ionized compounds do not readily traverse cell membranes and hence are not reabsorbed by the renal tubules. Consequently, acid compounds such as acetylsalicylic acid (aspirin) and some barbiturates remain ionized in alkaline urine, and alkaline compounds such as amphetamines remain ionized in acidic urine. As a result, urinary excretion of many toxic compounds may be enhanced by modifying the urine pH. Urinary acidifying agents include ammonium chloride (200 mg/kg/day in divided doses) and ethylenediamine dihydrochloride (Chloretham-ine, 1 to 2 tablets three times a day for the average-sized dog.) Sodium bicarbonate (5 mEq/kg/hr) may be used as an alkalinizing agent.

Peritoneal dialysis is indicated when an intoxicated animal exhibits oliguria or anuria. It is a rather time-consuming but effective technique for many conditions. The procedure requires the use of two separate solutions, and the solutions must be exchanged every 30 to 60 minutes. Two dialyzing solutions that may be used are 5 per cent dextrose in 0.45 per cent NaCl with 5 mEq/liter of potassium as potassium chloride, and 5 per cent dextrose in water with 44.6 mEq of bicarbonate and 5 mEq of potassium added. Other dialyzing solutions may be utilized.

The process of peritoneal dialysis involves (1) infusing 10 to 20 ml/kg of one dialyzing solution into the peritoneal cavity, (2) waiting the prescribed length of time, (3) withdrawing the first dialyzing solution, and (4) infusing the second solution. The infusion and withdrawal cycles with alternating solutions should be maintained for 12 to 24 hours or until normal renal function is restored. The pH of the dialyzing solutions may be altered to maintain the ionized state of the offending compound.

SUPPORTIVE MEASURES

Supportive measures are very important in intoxications. These measures include control of body temperature, maintenance of respiratory and cardiovascular function, control of acid-base imbalance, alleviation of pain, and control of central nervous system disorders.

BODY TEMPERATURE CONTROL

Hypothermia may be controlled by using blankets and by keeping the animal in a warm, draft-free cage. Infrared lamps or heating pads should be used with caution and under constant observation. A pad with circulating warm water may be of greater value and is less dangerous than lamps or conventional heating pads. This type of pad is convenient for both emergency and surgical use (Aquamatic K Pad, American Hospital Supply).

Hyperthermia is controlled through the use of ice bags, cold water baths, cold water enemas, or cold peritoneal dialysis solution. Regardless of the type of temperature control required, it is vitally important that the animal's body temperature be constantly monitored to ensure that overcorrection does not occur.

RESPIRATORY SUPPORT MEASURES

Adequate respiratory support requires the presence of an adequate patent airway, which may be obtained by using a cuffed endotracheal tube in an unconscious animal or by performing a tracheostomy under local anesthesia. An emergency tracheostomy tube may be made from a cuffed endotracheal tube that has been shortened to reduce the dead space.

A respirator, such as a Bird Respirator or an Ohio ventilator, is of great value in cases of respiratory depression; however, an anesthetic machine may be utilized with manual compression of the bag. A mixture of 50 per cent oxygen and 50 per cent room air is generally adequate unless there is a thickened respiratory membrane, in which case 100 per cent oxygen is necessary.

The use of analeptic drugs in cases of severe respiratory depression or apnea is questionable owing to the short duration of their effects and undesirable side effects. Positive pressure ventilatory support is of greater value.

CARDIOVASCULAR SUPPORT

Cardiovascular support requires the presence of an adequate circulating volume, adequate cardiac function, adequate tissue perfusion, and adequate acid-base balance. Blood volume and cardiac activity are of immediate concern. Perfusion and acid-base imbalance, although of no lesser importance, are not of immediate concern.

In the presence of hypovolemia due to loss of both cells and volume, whole blood is the necessary agent. A good rule is to give a sufficient quantity of whole blood to raise the packed cell volume to 75 per cent of the animal's estimated normal level (minimum—20 ml/kg).

Hypovolemia due to fluid loss alone can be treated with the administration of lactated Ringer's solution or plasma expanders. Central venous pressure should be monitored in these cases to prevent overloading the heart with too much volume too rapidly.

Tissue perfusion should also be monitored periodically to determine the adequacy of the replacement therapy. In some cases it may be necessary to administer massive doses of corticosteroids intravenously to restore adequate tissue perfusion (dexamethasone, Azium, 2 to 10 mg/kg).

Cardiac activity can be aided by the application of closed-chest cardiac massage for immediate cardiovascular support, but the administration of pharmaceutical agents that can stimulate ionotropic and chronotropic activity must also be undertaken in most instances. One of these agents is calcium gluconate infused very slowly intravenously. This agent is also reported to be a good nonspecific treatment in many toxicities. Other agents include glucagon, 25 to 50 μg/kg IV, and digoxin, 0.02 to 0.04 mg/kg IV. Care must be taken to avoid overdose with cardioactive agents, since they are highly toxic to the myocardium. The electrical activity of the heart should be closely monitored during administration of cardioactive agents.

ACID-BASE BALANCE

Control of acid-base balance problems is primarily a matter of physiologically maintaining an animal in a homeostatic condition. The most common acid-base disturbance seen in animals is acidosis, mainly of metabolic origin. However, acidosis or alkalosis may occur in cases of intoxication.

In correcting acidosis not of respiratory origin, sodium bicarbonate, administered IV at a dosage rate of 2 to 4 mEq/kg every 15 minutes, is the drug of choice. Other alkalinizing solutions include 1/6 molar sodium lactate, 16 to 32 ml/kg; lactated Ringer's solution, 120 ml/kg; or THAM buffer, 300 mg/kg. Bicarbonate is generally the easiest to administer with respect to volume and requires no metabolic conversion. Caution must be exercised with all alkalinizing agents to avoid the induction of alkalosis.

Alkalosis, unless drug induced, does not generally occur in animals. However, if alkalosis is present, the IV administration of 0.9 per cent NaCl (physiologic saline), 10 ml/kg, is usually sufficient for initial therapy. This should be followed by the oral administration of ammonium chloride, 200 mg/kg/day in divided doses. As in the case of acidosis, the clinician should be cautioned about the overtreatment of the alkalotic patient.

PAIN

Another important supportive measure in cases of intoxication is the control of pain. A minimal dose of morphine (dogs, 1 to 2 mg/kg; cats, 0.1 to 0.2 mg/kg) or meperidine (Demerol) (dogs, 5 to 10 mg/kg; cats, 1 to 2 mg/kg) is indicated in animals showing pain as a result of intoxication.

CENTRAL NERVOUS SYSTEM DISORDERS

Management of central nervous system (CNS) disorders, in cases of intoxication, is simple in appearance but complex in actuality. The type of therapy depends on the presence of hyperactivity. Either disorder can easily be turned into the opposite problem by overzealous therapeutic measures.

CNS Depression. CNS depression can also be considered respiratory depression, since the management of the two conditions is very similar. Although the IV administration of analeptic agents such as doxapram (Dopram), 3 to 5 mg/kg; bemegride (Mikedimide), 10 to 20 mg/kg; or pentylenetetrazol (Metrazol), 6 to 10 mg/kg is reported to be efficacious in these conditions, their actions are short lived, and CNS depression can return if the animal is not monitored continuously. Another disadvantage is that analeptics can induce convulsions. Artificial respiration or respiratory support is of greater value in animals exhibiting CNS depression and may be the treatment of choice for most CNS depression syndromes.

CNS Hyperactivity. Cases of CNS hyperactivity including convulsions can be managed by the administration of CNS depressants or tranquilizers. Pentobarbital sodium is generally the agent of choice for convulsions and hyperactivity. Care must

be taken, however, since in many cases a respiratory depressing dose may be required to alleviate the signs. In these cases, respiratory support is mandatory. Inhalant anesthetics have been reported as excellent for long-term management of CNS hyperactivity, but this removes the anesthetic machine from the surgery-room for extended periods. Central-acting skeletal muscle relaxants and minor tranquilizers have been reported for use with convulsant intoxicants. Some of these include methocarbamol (Robaxin), 110 mg/kg IV; glyceryl guaiacolate (Gecolate), 110 mg/kg IV; and diazepam (Valium), 0.5 to 1.5 mg/kg IV or IM. In other cases of CNS stimulation due to amphetamines and some hallucinogens such as LSD and phencyclidine, phenothiazine tranquilizers have produced adequate control. Regardless of the regimen of therapy for CNS hyperactivity, the animal should be placed in a quiet, dark room to prevent additional excitation due to auditory or visual stimuli.

POISON CONTROL CENTERS AND DIAGNOSTIC LABORATORIES

Poison control centers and/or animal diagnostic laboratories can be of great value to the clinician in cases of suspected intoxications, especially when labels or containers are presented with the acutely ill animal. *When the suspected compound and the signs exhibited by the animal do not concur, the signs should be treated and the label should be disregarded.*

The diagnosis should be confirmed by chemical analysis, even though this may occur after the fact. An accurate diagnosis, as well as detailed records, may help the veterinarian faced with subsequent cases poisoned by same intoxicant. Detailed records will also be invaluable in any medicolegal proceedings.

SUPPLEMENTAL READING

Buck, W. B., Osweiler, G. D., and VanGelden, G. A. (eds.): Clinical and Diagnostic Veterinary Toxicology, 2nd ed. Dubuque, Iowa: Kendal/Hunt, 1976.
Doull, J., Klaassen, C. D., and Amdur, M. O. (eds.): Casarett and Doull's Toxicology. The Basic Science of Poisons, 2nd ed. New York: Macmillan Co., 1980.
Oehme, F. W.: Symposium in clinical toxicology for the small animal practitioner. Clin. North Am. 5, 1, 1975.

EMERGENCY KIT FOR TREATMENT OF SMALL ANIMAL POISONING
(Antidotes, Drugs, Equipment)

FREDERICK W. OEHME, D.V.M.

Manhattan, Kansas

PARENTERAL SOLUTION
Amphetamine
Apomorphine
Atropine sulfate
Barbiturates (phenobarbital,
    pentobarbital)
3% Bemigride (Mikedimide)
Calcium borogluconate
Calcium disodium edetate
Calcium disodium edetate in
    5% dextrose
5% Dextrose
Diazepam (Valium)
Dimercaprol (BAL)
2% Doxapram (Dopram)
20% Ethanol
Glyceryl guaiacolate
Glyceryl monoacetate
Lactated Ringer's
10% Methocarbamol (Robaxin)
Neosynephrine
Nicotinamide (nicotinic acid, niacin)
Normal saline
10% Pentylenetetrazol
    (Metrazol)
Pralidoxine chloride (2-PAM,
    Protopam chloride)
Propranolol
Sedatives, tranquilizers
5% Sodium bicarbonate
Vitamin K_1
Whole blood, citrated
    (fresh within 2 weeks)

ORAL MEDICATIONS
Activated charcoal
0.2–0.4% Copper sulfate solution
Diphenylthiocarbazone
Egg whites, diluted
Hydrogen peroxide
Ipecac syrup
20% Magnesium sulfate solution
Milk of magnesia
Mineral oil
D-Penicillamine
Potassium chloride
1:10,000 Potassium
    permanganate solution
Prussian blue
Sodium chloride
Sodium ferrocyanide
20% Sodium sulfate solution
Tannic acid

MISCELLANEOUS ITEMS
Mild detergent
Oxygen
Sodium bicarbonate paste

EQUIPMENT
Aspirator bulb
Blankets
Endotracheal tubes, several sizes
Enema kit
Gauze rolls and tape
Intravenous catheters and stylets
Mechanical respirator or
    compression bag
Needles (hypodermic)
Stethoscope
Stomach tubes, several sizes
Syringes
Thermometers
Urinary catheters, various sizes
Venostomy kit

POTENTIAL SOURCES OF SMALL ANIMAL POISONINGS

GARY D. OSWEILER, D.V.M.

Columbia, Missouri

When a case of potential intoxication is presented, the first concerns are usually the accurate assessment of the clinical status of the animal and the prompt incorporation of procedures to support life and control clinical signs. Immediately thereafter, or concurrent with emergency management, a tentative diagnosis should be made.

Part of the input to determine that diagnosis is a review of potential toxicants to which an animal may have been exposed. Appropriate questioning of the owner may aid in establishing potential sources. From among the thousands of potentially toxic chemicals in the world, one usually attempts to consider those that are (1) in the animal's environment, (2) toxic enough to constitute a hazard if exposure occurs, (3) available to the animal, and (4) generally capable of causing the signs being manifested.

From the article "Common Poisonings in Small Animal Practice," it may be seen that the number of intoxications diagnosed is rather small and involves mainly natural toxins and economic poisons. Those toxins in the animal's environment generally include products in and around the home, those involved in pest control, and those that are available in the natural or altered environment. Key questions should be directed to the owner to establish what products, plants, or animals are kept or are available in or near the home. Recent use of such materials, where they are stored, and recollection of spillage should be reviewed with the client. The species, age, eating habits, and freedom of the affected animal should be known. For example, it is important to remember that the dog that roams the neighborhood nightly is exposed to "common sources" different from those of the constantly housed animal.

Each geographic area of North America has its own peculiar common sources, as detailed in the article on common poisonings. Indigenous plants, venomous reptiles, snail baits, rust inhibitors, and antifreeze solutions are but a few examples of toxicants that may be more prevalent in particular geographic areas.

Tables 1, 2, and 3 offer a broad review of the scope of commonly available substances that may occasionally be hazardous. These tables should be used to suggest specific potentially toxic agents found in many homes and businesses.

To consider which of the many toxicants available may be potentially dangerous, background data on reported exposures would be useful. Buck (1981) recently documented reports of animal exposures to various toxicants in the state of Illinois as well as from many other areas of North America. Table 4 is a summary of data from the Animal Poison Control Center, University of Illinois. Although the data do not reflect poisonings in each case, they can be used to gain some perspective on the commonly encountered toxicants for dogs and cats.

As with commonly diagnosed poisonings, Table 4 clearly shows the large portion of small animal toxicology that involves pesticides, plants, and metals as potential toxicants. Aside from the commonly considered categories just mentioned, notice that 24.3 per cent of all incidents reported involved

Text continued on page 97

Table 1. *Sources of Poisonous Plants*

LOCATION	EXAMPLES
House Plants	Daffodil, oleander, poinsettia, dumb cane, mistletoe, philodendron
Flower Garden	Delphinium, monkshood, foxglove, iris, lily-of-the-valley
Vegetable Garden	Rhubarb, spinach, tomato vine, sunburned potatoes
Ornamentals	Oleander, castor bean, daphne, golden chain, rhododendron, lantana
Trees and Shrubs	Cherry, peach, oak, elderberry, black locust
Woodland Plants	Jack-in-the-pulpit, moonseed, May apple, Dutchman's-breeches
Swamp Plants	Water hemlock, mushrooms
Field Plants	Buttercup, nightshade, poison hemlock, jimsonweed, pigweed
Range Plants	Locoweed, lupine, halogeton
Grain Contaminants	Crotalaria, corn cockle, ergot
Cultural Changes	Nitrate, cyanide, herbicides, insecticides

Table 2.   *Some Toxins of Zoologic Origin*

ORGANISMS	LOCATIONS	GENERAL PROBLEMS ENCOUNTERED
Snakes		
Pit vipers	Terrestrial; Eastern U.S.A.	Necrosis, inflammation,
Rattlesnake	through South Central,	anaphylaxis
Copperhead	Midwest, and Southwest	
Water moccasin		
Coral snake	Southeast U.S.A., mainly Florida	Neuroparalytic, loss of sensation
Lizards		
Gila monster	Terrestrial; primarily	Inflammation, vomition, shock
Mexican beaded lizard	Southwest U.S.A.	
Toads		
Bufo sp.	Terrestrial-aquatic; Southern and	Parotid glands exude a cardio-
	Southwestern U.S.A.	toxic and cholinergic toxin
Spiders		
Black widow	Terrestrial	Neuromuscular;
Brown recluse		wound heals with difficulty;
Tarantula		infection from the bite
Insects		
Fire ant	Terrestrial; Southern and	Painful, necrotizing bite;
Wasps	Southwestern U.S.A.	inflammation and anaphylaxis
Bees		
Invertebrates		
Jellyfish	Aquatic-marine	Pain, swelling, cramps, nausea,
Coral		CNS derangement
Sea anemone		
Sea urchin		Burning sensation, inflammation,
		paralysis
Vertebrates		
Fish	Aquatic-marine	Sharp pain, inflammation
Stingray		
Catfish		
Scorpion fish		

Table 3.   *Chemical Products Potentially Hazardous to Pets**

ARTS AND CRAFTS SUPPLIES
Antiquing Agents
  Methyl ethyl ketone
  Turpentine
Oil Paints and Tempera Paints
  Pigment salts of lead, arsenic, copper, and cadmium
Pencils, Indelible
  Crystal violet

PHOTOGRAPHIC SUPPLIES
Developers
  Borates
  Bromides
  Iodides
  Thiocyanates
Fixatives
  Sodium thiosulfate
Hardeners
  Aluminum chloride
  Formaldehyde

AUTOMOTIVE AND MACHINERY PRODUCTS
Antifreeze, Fuel System De-icer
  Ethylene glycol
  Isopropyl alcohol
  Methanol
  Rust inhibitors
    a. Borates
    b. Chromates
    c. Zinc chloride
Brake Fluids
  Butyl ethers of ethylene glycol and related glycols

Ethyl ethers of ethylene glycol and related glycols
Methyl ethers of ethylene glycol and related glycols
Carburetor Cleaners
  Cresol
  Ethylene dichloride
Corrosion Inhibitors
  Borates
  Sodium chromate
  Sodium nitrate
Engine and Motor Cleaners
  Cresol
  Ethylene dichloride
  Methylene chloride
Frost Removers
  Ethylene glycol
  Isopropyl alcohol
Lubricants
  Barium compounds
  Isopropyl alcohol
  Kerosene
  Lead compounds
  Stoddard solvent
Motor Fuel
  Gasoline
  Kerosene
  Tetraethyl lead
Radiator Cleaners
  Boric acid
  Oxalic acid
  Sodium chromate
Shock Absorber Fluids
  Petroleum ether

Table continued on opposite page

Table 3. *Chemical Products Potentially Hazardous to Pets (Continued)**

Tire Repair
Benzene
Windshield Washer
Ethylene glycol
Isopropyl alcohol
Methyl alcohol

CLEANERS, DISINFECTANTS, SANITIZERS

Cleaners, Bleaches, Polishes
Ammonium hydroxide
Benzene
Carbon tetrachloride
Hydrochloric acid
Methyl alcohol
Naphtha
Nitrobenzene
Oxalic acid
Phosphoric acid
Sodium fluoride
Sodium or potassium hydroxide
Sodium hypochlorite
Sodium perborate
Sulfuric acid
Trichloroethane
Turpentine
Disinfectants, Sanitizers
Acids
Alkalis
Hypochlorites
Iodophors
Paradichlorobenzene
Phenol, Cresols
Phenyl mercuric acetate
Pine oil
Quaternary ammonium

HEALTH AND BEAUTY AIDS

Athlete's Foot
Caprylic acid
Copper
Propionic acid
Sodium
Undecylenic acid
Zinc salts
Bath Preparations
Bath oils
Perfume
Sodium lauryl sulfate
Trisodium phosphate
Corn Removers
Phenoxyacetic acid
Salicylic acid
Deodorants and Antiperspirants
Alcohol
Aluminum chloride
Diet Pills
Amphetamines
Diuretics
Thyroid hormone
Eye Make-up
Boric acid
Peach kernel oil, q.s.
Hair Preparations
Cadmium chloride
Cupric chloride
Dyes, tints
Ferric chloride
Lead acetate
Permanent wave lotions

Pyrogallol
Silver nitrate
Thioglycolic acid
Headache
Aspirin
Phenacetin
Laxatives
IRRITANT OR STIMULANT LAXATIVES
Aloes
Aloin
Cascara sagrada
Liniments
Camphor
Chloroform
Oil of wintergreen (methyl salicylate)
Pine oil
Turpentine
Nailetics
Acetone
Alcohol
Benzene
Ethyl acetate
Nail enamel
Nail polish
Nail polish remover
Toluene
Tricresyl phosphate
Ointments
Benzoic acid
Borates
Caprylic acid
Menthol
Mercury compounds
Oil of wintergreen (methyl salicylate)
Phenols
Salicylic acid
Perfumes, Toilet Waters, and Colognes
Alcohol
Essential oils
Floral oils
Perfume essence
Shampoos
Sodium lauryl sulfate
Triethanolamine dodecyl sulfate
Shaving Lotions
Alcohol
Boric acid
Somnolents (Sleeping Pills)
Barbiturates
Bromides
Stimulants
Amphetamine
Caffeine
Suntan Lotions
Alcohol
Tannic acid and derivatives

PAINTS AND RELATED PRODUCTS

Caulking Compounds
Barium
Chlorinated biphenyl
Chromium
Lead
Mineral spirits
Petroleum distillate
Xylene
Driers
Cobalt compounds
Iron compounds

Table continued on following page

Table 3. *Chemical Products Potentially Hazardous to Pets (Continued)**

Manganese compounds
Vanadium compounds
Zinc compounds
Lacquer Thinners
Aliphatic hydrocarbons
Butyl acetate
Butyl alcohol
Toluene
Paint
Arsenic oxide
Coal tar
Cuprous oxide
Lead chromate
Petroleum ether
Pine oil
Red lead oxide
Zinc chromate
Paint Brush Cleaners
Benzene
Kerosene
Naphthas
Paint and Varnish Cleaners
Ethylene dichloride
Kerosene
Naphthalene
Trisodium phosphate
Paint and Varnish Removers
FLAMMABLE
Benzene
Cresols
Phenols
Toluene
NONFLAMMABLE
Methylene chloride
Toluene
Preservatives
BRUSH
Kerosene
Turpentine
CANVAS
2-Chlorophenylphenol
Pentachlorophenol
FLOOR
Magnesium fluorosilicate
WOOD
Copper naphthenate
Copper oleate
Mineral spirits
Pentachlorophenol
Zinc naphthenate

PEST CONTROL

Birds
Aminopyridine
Endrin
Toluidine
Fungicides
Captan
Copper compounds
Maneb
Mercurials
Pentachlorophenol
Thiram
Zineb
Insects and Spiders
Baygon
Carbaryl

Chlordane
Diazinon
Dichlorvos
Kelthane
Mirex
Paradichlorobenzene
Pyrethrins
Rotenone
Toxaphene
Lawn and Garden Weeds
Arsenic
Chlordane
Dacthal
Pentachlorophenol
2,4-D
Rats, Mice, Gophers, Moles
Arsenic
Barium carbonate
Dicoumarol
Phosphorus
Sodium fluoroacetate
Strychnine
Thallium (rare)
Warfarin
Zinc phosphide
Snails, Slugs
Metaldehyde

SAFETY PRODUCTS
Fire Extinguishers
LIQUID FIRE EXTINGUISHERS
Carbon tetrachloride
MISCELLANEOUS FIRE EXTINGUISHERS
Methylbromide
POWDER EXTINGUISHERS
Borax compounds
Nonskid Products
Stoddard solvent
Methyl ethyl ketone

SOLVENTS
Alcohols
Chlorinated Solvents
Carbon tetrachloride
Methylene chloride
Orthodichlorobenzene
Trichloroethylene
Esters
Amyl acetate
Ethyl acetate
Isopropyl acetate
Methyl acetate
Hydrocarbons
Aromatics, chiefly benzene, toluene and xylene
Naphthenes
Ketones
Acetone
Methyl ethyl ketone
Other Common Solvents
Aniline
Carbon disulphide
Cresylic acid
Kerosene
Mineral spirits
Phenols
Turpentine

*Adapted, in part, from Gleason et al.: *Clinical Toxicology of Commercial Products*, 4th ed., 1976.

Table 4. Categories and Incidence of Inquiries About Poisoning in Dogs and Cats*

Category	Dog†	Cat†
General	**58.3**	**70.0**
Insecticides	11.3	17.4
Rodenticides	15.0	8.3
Herbicides, fungicides	5.7	0.0
Plants	10.2	30.3
Solids, liquids, gases	7.7	6.4
Metals, minerals	4.9	0.0
Feed additives	1.4	0.0
Fertilizers, plant foods	2.0	4.6
Medications or Drug Ingestions	**9.7**	**14.6**
Athelmintics	3.1	2.7
Aspirin	1.2	7.3
Cardiovascular drugs	1.2	0.0
Miscellaneous internal medications	1.2	1.8
Psychopharmacologic Drugs	**4.1**	**0.7**
Tranquilizers	1.5	0.0
External Medications	**1.9**	**0.0**
Medicated creams and ointments	1.2	0.0
Household Product Ingestions	**13.8**	**14.7**
Soaps, detergents, cleaners	2.3	3.7
Corrosives, acid, alkali	2.3	2.7
Disinfectants, deodorizers	1.4	1.8
Shoe and leather treatments	1.2	0.0
Miscellaneous home and farm products	1.9	0.9
Petroleum products	2.2	3.7
Paints, stains, varnishes	1.4	0.9
Antifreeze	1.1	0.0
Metal or Mineral Ingestions	**4.9**	**0.0**
Arsenic	1.2	0.0
Lead	1.7	0.0
Other	1.5	0.0
Feed Additives	**3.6**	**0.0**
Monensin	1.2	0.0
Urea	2.2	0.0
Total Cases	**647**	**109**

*Data from W. B. Buck, 1981, for the period September, 1978 through June, 1981.

†All data expressed as percentage of total cases for each species. Toxicants comprising less than 1 per cent of inquiries are listed in text only.

medications or household products, categories generally considered important for children but less so for pets. Veterinarians should thus be prepared for some type of response to major problem chemicals in these categories. In the author's experience, these categories, although not always associated with toxicosis, do cause alarm for clients and generate many questions. Of note also is the 3.9 per cent incidence of inquires about psychopharmacologic drugs including illegal agents of abuse.

Some agents were consumed or contacted as a potential toxicant less than 1 per cent of the time. Among the general poison categories, cats had low exposure to herbicides, metals, and livestock feed additives. Both dogs and cats were involved with antibiotic, vitamin, and diet pill exposure. Marijuana was implicated for both dogs and cats, but only dogs had exposure to other abuse drugs including hashish, barbiturates, LSD, heroin, and antidepressants. For all other categories in Table 4, only solvents, thinners, and glues were reported for cats. Dog owners, however, generated questions about nail polish, nasal sprays, foot deodorizers, polishes, waxes, bleaches, solvents and thinners,

alcohols, glues, copper, mycotoxins, botulism, and snake bite (Buck, 1981).

When access or exposure to the materials listed is established, additional details may be found in this section or in the references listed at the end of this article.

Knowledge of sources and the pattern of exposure that occurred (e.g., accidental, malicious) can serve as a focus for education of the client in safe use of toxic materials to prevent further danger to either animals or man.

REFERENCES AND SUPPLEMENTAL READING

Arena, J. M.: *Poisoning. Toxicology, Symptoms, Treatments,* 3rd ed. Springfield: Charles C Thomas, 1974.

Atkins, C. E., and Johnson, R. K.: Clinical toxicities of cats. Vet. Clin. North Am. 5:623, 1975.

Buck, W. B., Osweiler, G. D., and Van Gelder, G. A.: *Clinical and Diagnostic Veterinary Toxicology,* Dubuque, Iowa: Kendall-Hunt Publishing Co., 2nd ed. 1976.

Buck, W. B.: Animal Poison Control Center, University of Illinois, Urbana, Illinois. Unpublished data. 1981.

Bureau of Veterinary Medicine: Memo. Summary of Adverse Reactions to Animal Drugs. BVMM-20, Rockville, Maryland, August, 1975.

Catcott, E. J. (ed.): *Canine Medicine.* Wheaton, Illinois: American Veterinary Publications, 1968.

Clarke, E. G. C.: Pets and poisons. J. Small Anim. Pract. 16:375, 1975.

Clarke, E. G. C., and Clarke, M. L.: *Garner's Veterinary Toxicology*, 3rd ed. Baltimore: The Williams & Wilkins Co., 1967.

Diechman, W. B., and Gerarde, H. W.: *Toxicology of Drugs and Chemicals*, 4th ed. New York: Academic Press, 1969.

Gleason, M. N., Gosselin, R. E., and Hodge, H. C.: *Clinical Toxicology of Commercial Products*, 4th ed. Baltimore: The Williams & Wilkins Co., 1976.

Kirk, R. W. (ed.): *Current Veterinary Therapy V*. Philadelphia: W. B. Saunders Co., 1974.

Kirk, R. W., and Bistner, S. T.: *Handbook of Veterinary Procedures and Emergency Treatment*, 2nd ed. Philadelphia: W. B. Saunders Co., 1975.

Malone, J. C.: Diagnosis and treatment of poisoning in dogs and cats. Vet. Rec. 84:161, 1969.

Osweiler, G. D.: Incidence and diagnostic considerations of major small animal toxicoses. J.A.V.M.A. 155:2011, 1969.

Radeleff, R. D.: *Veterinary Toxicology*, 2nd ed. Philadelphia: Lea & Febiger, 1970.

Robens, J. F.: Animal drug toxicities. Veterinary Toxicology Training and Review Workshop. Ames, Iowa, February 21–26, 1972.

Szabuniewiez, M.: *Treatment of some common animal poisonings*. Vet. Med. Small Anim. Clin. December, 1971. pp. 1197–1205.

STRYCHNINE POISONING

GARY D. OSWEILER, D.V.M.

Columbia, Missouri

SOURCE

Strychnine is an indole alkaloid. Commercial sources are derived from seeds of the plants *Strychnos nux-vomica* and *Strychnos ignatii*. It has been used as an animal poison since the 16th century (Franz, 1980).

Strychnine is currently used primarily as a ruminatoric (tartar emetic), stimulant, and pesticide. However, there is no modern rational basis for the use of strychnine in therapy. Principal pesticidal applications are for rat, gopher, mole, and coyote control. Many commercial forms are pelleted and dyed either bright green or red. Although strychnine is now a restricted use pesticide, it is still available and continues to be a major cause of canine poisoning.

TOXICITY

Strychnine is highly toxic to most domestic animals. The approximate oral lethal toxicity to various animals is as follows (Clarke and Clarke, 1967):

bovine	0.50 mg/kg
equine	1.00 mg/kg
porcine	0.5–1.00 mg/kg
canine	0.75 mg/kg
feline	2.00 mg/kg
fowl	5.00 mg/kg
rat	3.0 mg/kg

Parenteral strychnine is two to ten times more toxic than is oral strychnine, and strychnine alkaloid can be absorbed through mucous membranes.

The hazard of poisoning from strychnine is apparent when the commercial formulations containing 0.3 per cent strychnine are considered versus the toxicity values. At the 0.3 per cent level, each gram of bait contains 3 mg strychnine. Thus, 3 gm of bait could be lethal to a 12-kg dog. Strychnine has also been considered a secondary toxicant, killing pets that consume poisoned rodents or birds. Strychnine is stable in most environmental circumstances and would be expected to persist in soil, baits, and possibly poisoned rodents.

MECHANISM OF ACTION

The physiologic effect of strychnine is to allow uncontrolled and relatively diffuse spinal reflex activity to proceed basically unchecked. All striated muscle groups are affected, but the relatively more powerful extensors predominate to produce symmetric and generalized rigidity to tonic seizures. Gross and microscopic changes in the neurons, axons, and myelin sheaths have not been observed.

Strychnine appears to affect the central nervous system directly by selectively antagonizing certain types of spinal inhibition (Franz 1980). It interferes with post-synaptic inhibition in the spinal cord and medulla. Thus, the moderating and controlling effects in the reflex are eliminated. Examples of post-synaptic inhibition are the inhibitory influences between motor neurons of antagonistic muscle groups and the recurrent spinal inhibition mediated by Renshaw cells.

The amino acid glycine is an accepted inhibitory transmitter in the spinal cord and medulla. Strychnine reversibly and selectively antagonizes glycine in the spinal cord and medulla, possibly by a competitive type of antagonism (Franz 1980). Post-synaptic membrane permeability is changed, and the net effect is a reduction in the inhibitory post-synaptic potential normally controlled by glycine.

Sublethal but convulsant doses of strychnine have been shown to elevate blood pressure, heart rate, and right ventricular pulse pressure in barbiturate-anesthetized dogs. This cardiovascular effect can be abolished by combinations of alpha- and beta-adrenergic blocking agents and reduced significantly by diazepam (Sofola and Odusote, 1976).

CLINICAL SIGNS

Clinical signs of strychnine poisoning appear within ten minutes to two hours after ingestion of the poison. Speed of onset after ingestion may be altered by food taken with the alkaloid, because dilution of toxicant occurs. Furthermore, strychnine is a basic chemical, which is ionized (and thus nonabsorbable) in the stomach. Early signs of strychnine poisoning are apprehension, nervousness, tenseness, and stiffness. Palpation in early stages reveals a tense abdomen and rigid cervical musculature. Violent tetanic seizures may appear spontaneously or may be initiated by stimuli such as touch, sound, or sudden bright light. There is extreme and overpowering extensor rigidity causing the animal to assume a "sawhorse" stance. The strength of the tetanic spasm may throw the animal off its feet. The legs and body are stiff, the neck is arched, the ears are erect, and the lips are pulled back from the teeth. Breathing may cease momentarily. Duration of a tetanic convulsion may vary from a few seconds to a minute or more. Intermittent periods of relaxation are observed but become less frequent as the clinical course progresses. During convulsions, the pupils are dilated, and cyanotic mucous membranes indicate anoxia. Convulsive seizures become more frequent, and death eventually occurs from exhaustion or anoxia during a tetanic seizure. The entire course of the syndrome, if untreated, is often less than one to two hours (Osweiler, 1980).

PHYSIOPATHOLOGY

Rigor mortis occurs rapidly after death from strychnine poisoning. Relaxation of body musculature also follows in more rapid than normal succession. No gross or microscopic lesions characteristic of strychnine poisoning can be consistently detected. Cyanosis, petechial, or ecchymotic hemorrhages and traumatic lesions are evidence of a violent and hypoxic state. Characteristically, the stomach of strychnine-poisoned animals is filled with food or bait that has not been completely digested (Osweiler, 1980).

Absorbed strychnine is transported in the blood by both plasma and erythrocytes but is rapidly passed from blood to tissue. In some circumstances strychnine may be detected in blood as well as urine, although urine may contain higher concentrations (Gordon and Richards, 1979). It does not appear to concentrate in nervous tissue.

Excretion is accomplished in urine and via secretion into the stomach. The ionization of strychnine, a basic drug, is influenced by pH. Thus, ion trapping of strychnine occurs in the acid conditions of the stomach, and urinary excretion may be enhanced by acidification of the urine.

DIAGNOSIS

Tentative diagnosis is usually based on a history of ingestion, characteristic clinical signs, and lack of lesions. Similar clinical signs may be caused by chlorinated hydrocarbons, aminopyridine (an avicide), caffeine, amphetamine, metaldehyde, and hypocalcemia. All of these agents are characterized by some degree of hyperesthesia and muscular hypertonicity when ingested. Toxicants such as zinc phosphide, lead, fluoroacetate, and nicotine may cause seizures or tremors as part of a clinical pattern that includes effects in other systems.

Any dog found dead with no premonitory signs and no evidence of trauma should be considered a potential strychnine victim.

Samples for analysis should include stomach contents, liver, kidney, urine, and central nervous system. In addition, baits or vomitus should be kept for analysis. Most chemical confirmations of strychnine poisoning are from stomach contents or liver. In many cases, animals die so rapidly that urinary excretion has been insignificant. If urine or stomach contents cannot be obtained, blood may be an alternative, but less sensitive, specimen for testing (Gordon and Richards, 1979).

Presently, strychnine poisoning can be confirmed by laboratory procedures that are sensitive, specific, and reasonable in price. These include thin layer chromatography, ultraviolet spectrometry, gas-liquid chromatography, and, when necessary, mass spectroscopy (Oliver et al., 1979).

TREATMENT

Control of Seizures. Of prime concern in strychnine poisoning is the maintenance of relaxation and prevention of asphyxia. In emergency situations, pentobarbital in doses just sufficient to maintain relaxation is acceptable (Osweiler, 1980). However, prolonged maintenance of relaxation may be accomplished by a combination of agents to avoid complications from prolonged barbiturate administration.

Inhalation anesthesia has the advantages of being readily controllable, providing ready administration of oxygen, and maintaining a patent airway. However, inhalation techniques usually require barbiturate or other premedication and dedication of equipment to one animal for a considerable time (Bailey and Szabuniewiez, 1975). In addition, intubation and restraint of the animal for inhalant techniques are in themselves stimuli that may enhance seizure activity.

Muscle relaxants have been used in lieu of barbiturate anesthesia. Glyceryl guaiacolate ether (GGE), a centrally acting muscle relaxant, given in an IV dose of 110 mg/kg in either a 5 or 33⅓ per cent solution controls seizures for from 10 to 60 minutes. (Bailey and Szabuniewiez, 1975). Two to five or more subsequent doses may be necessary for maintenance at intervals ranging from 20 minutes to 6 hours. Interval and number of treatments vary depending on strychnine dose and other individual animal factors. The advantage of this procedure is that dogs become ambulatory shortly after treatment, thus reducing complications of prolonged recumbency.

Methocarbamol (Robaxin) has been employed to control strychnine seizures in dogs (Fountain, 1970). Intravenous injection of an average of 150 mg/kg successfully controlled strychnine seizures. A second dose averaging 90 mg/kg was given within 30 minutes to 2 hours. The need for subsequent treatments is again a matter of clinical judgement. As with GGE, methocarbamol therapy allows the patient to become ambulatory shortly after seizure control.

In man, diazepam has been used intravenously to successfully control seizures caused by strychnine (Maron et al., 1971). In some cases of estimated high doses of strychnine, diazepam did not effect control. Individual reports from veterinarians have indicated variable success with diazepam in controlling strychnine seizures. In addition, intravenous administration must be frequently repeated, necessitating close and nearly constant attendance to the patient.

Detoxification. Early induction of vomiting with apomorphine is recommended, provided the animal is not in a hyperesthetic or convulsive state. If anesthesia must be maintained, gastric lavage may be employed (see section on Emergency Therapy). Rapid recovery from strychnine toxicosis may be enhanced by prompt application of enterogastric lavage (Frye, 1974). This technique applies gastric lavage followed by enema and continued anal fluid administration with lavage tube in place until clear fluid flows from the esophageal tube. The result is complete gastrointestinal evacuation.

If anesthesia must be maintained, gastric lavage can be employed using 1 to 2 per cent tannic acid or 1:2000 potassium permanganate. Activated charcoal and sodium sulfate may be left in the stomach to aid adsorption and speed the elimination of the alkaloid. (Consult article on Emergency Therapy for dosages of charcoal and sodium sulfate.)

Forced diuresis with 5 per cent mannitol in 0.9 per cent sodium chloride administered at a rate of 7 mg/kg/hour and acidification of the urine with 150 mg/kg body weight of ammonium chloride orally will enhance urinary excretion of strychnine (Osweiler, 1980). These methods must follow establishment of adequate urine flow.

In addition to anticonvulsant and detoxification therapy, it may be advisable to closely monitor cardiac rate and blood pressure in the anesthetized animal. Evidence cited earlier shows marked pressor, inotropic, and chronotropic effects in barbiturate-anesthetized dogs. Agents that counteract this effect include alpha blockade with phentolamine (0.5 mg/kg); beta blockade with propranolol (0.5 to 1.0 mg/kg); and added sedation with diazepam (0.1 to 0.2 mg/kg) (Sofola and Odusote 1976). These agents are not advocated for general use in all strychnine poisonings but might be considered at the clinician's discretion if marked cardiovascular irregularities persist after seizure control.

Toxic doses of strychnine will be depleted from the body within 24 to 48 hours (Osweiler 1980). One must expect to continue maintenance relaxation and sedation for 12 to 48 hours. It should be emphasized that the sedation time can be considerably shortened if prompt and aggressive action is taken to clear the gastrointestinal tract, inactivate unabsorbed strychnine, and hasten elimination of alkaloid via diuresis and ion trapping.

When prompt and thorough action is taken, recovery of a high proportion of strychnine poisoning cases can be expected.

REFERENCES AND SUPPLEMENTAL READING

Bailey, E. M., and Szabuniewiez, M.: The use of glyceryl guaiacolate ether in the treatment of strychnine poisoning in the dog. Vet. Med. Small Anim. Clin 70:170, 1975.

Clarke, E. G. C., and Clarke, M. L.: *Garner's Veterinary Toxicology,* 3rd ed. Baltimore: The Williams & Wilkins Co., 1967.

Curtis, D. R., and Johnston, G. A. R.: Convulsant alkaloids. *In* Simpson, L. L., and Curtis, D. R. (eds.): *Neuropoisons,* Vol. 2, New York: Plenum Press, 1974.

Fountain, J. E.: A practitioner's experience with methocarbamol in the treatment of strychnine poisoning in dogs. Vet. Med. Small Anim. Clin. 65:718-719, 1970.

Franz, D.: Central nervous system stimulants. *In* Goodman, L. S., and Gilman, A. (eds.): *The Pharmacologic Basis of Therapeutics,* 6th ed. New York: Macmillan Co., 1980.

Frye, F. L.: Enterogastric lavage in small animal practice. Vet. Med. Small Anim. Clin 69:835, 1974.

Gordon, A. M., and Richards, D. W.: Strychnine intoxication. J.A.C.E.P. 8:520, 1979.

Maron, B. J., Krupp, J. R., and Tune, B.: Strychnine poisoning successfully treated with diazepam. J. Pediatr. 78:697, 1971.

Oliver, J. S., Smith H., and Watson, A. A.: Poisoning by strychnine. Med. Sci. Law. 19:134, 1979.

Osweiler, G. D.: Strychnine poisoning. *In* Kirk, R. W. (ed.): *Current Veterinary Therapy VII.* Philadelphia: W. B. Saunders Co., 1980.

Radeleff, R. D.: *Veterinary Toxicology.* Philadelphia: Lea & Febiger, 1964.

Sofola, O., and Odusote, K.: Sympathetic cardiovascular effects of experimental strychnine poisoning in dogs. J. Pharmacol. Exper. Ther. 196:29, 1976.

WARFARIN AND OTHER ANTICOAGULANT POISONINGS

VAL RICHARD BEASLEY, D.V.M.,
and WILLIAM B. BUCK, D.V.M.

Urbana, Illinois

MECHANISM OF ACTION

Warfarin, coumarin, indandione, and other anticoagulant rodenticide poisonings may occur in all mammals and birds. The toxicity of the compounds varies, and susceptibility differs from one species to another. Members of these anticoagulant classes are also used as human and equine pharmaceutical agents, to which animals may accidentally be exposed. Certain of these are excreted quite slowly. Warfarin has been used in the management of navicular disease in horses, and its anticoagulant properties may find future application in thromboembolic phenomena of small animals. These compounds may cross the placenta and may be excreted in milk, placing the offspring of exposed animals at risk.

Vitamin K functions as a cofactor in post-ribosomal modifications of some of the proteins involved in blood clotting (Fig. 1). These modifications are apparently a final touchup, probably a carboxylation, of factors II (prothrombin), VII, IX, and X. As vitamin K functions, it is changed back and forth from active vitamin K to "used" vitamin K epoxide. The primary mechanism of action of coumarin and indandione anticoagulants appears to be a competitive inhibition of the enzyme vitamin K epoxide reductase, which normally regenerates active vitamin K from the epoxide in this cycle.

CLINICAL SIGNS

Owing to the unavailability of natural, active vitamin K_2 in the body and resultant deficiencies of prothrombin and factors VII, IX, and X, hemorrhage results. The onset of hemorrhage does not take place until cofactors already in the blood are consumed. Depending on the species involved and the respective half-lives of clotting factors, defects in coagulation appear from two to five days after initial exposure. The mean half-lives for factors VII, IX, X, and II in the dog are 6.2, 13.9, 16.5, and 41 hours, respectively.

Many cases are subacute in nature, and animals are presented anemic and weak, with pale mucous membranes, dyspnea, hematemesis, epistaxis, or bloody feces. Scleral, conjunctival, and clinically evident diffuse subcutaneous hemorrhages are common. With severe blood loss profound weakness is observed. Blood loss and pulmonary or intrathoracic hemorrhage may cause dyspnea. Sometimes the onset may be acute, and occasionally animals are found dead without any premonitory signs noted. This may occur with hemorrhage in the pericardial

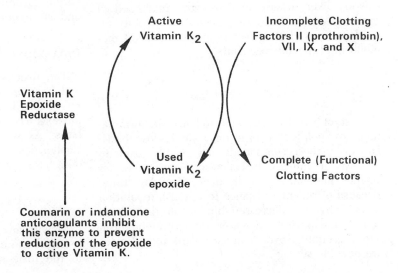

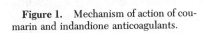

Figure 1. Mechanism of action of coumarin and indandione anticoagulants.

101

sac, mediastinum, thorax, abdomen, or cerebral vasculature. Warfarin has caused abortions in cattle and swollen, tender joints in swine.

PREDISPOSING FACTORS

These anticoagulants exist largely bound to serum albumin, and only the unbound fraction is pharmacologically active. Warfarin is 93 per cent protein bound in canine plasma. Therefore, substances that cause release from albumin result in increased clotting inhibition. A high lipid diet results in larger amounts of fatty acids in the blood, which progressively decreases the amount of bound warfarin. Drugs that are contraindicated include oxyphenbutazone and phenylbutazone, which in addition to displacing albumin-bound warfarin also decrease platelet aggregation. Diphenylhydantoin, sulfonamides, and corticosteroids also may displace anticoagulants from albumin. Uremia causes decreased serum protein binding, and renal failure may slow excretion of the unbound fraction.

Aspirin markedly diminishes platelet aggregation, although most other salicylates do not share this effect. Prolonged use of oral broad spectrum antibiotics possibly decreases vitamin K production by the gastrointestinal flora, and chloramphenicol may additionally reduce catabolism of the anticoagulant. Drugs contraindicated because of inhibition of hemostasis include promazine-type tranquilizers, sulfonamides, nitrofurans, local anesthetics, and antihistamines.

Drugs that increase fibrinolytic activity and are, therefore, contraindicated include testosterone, anderolone, anabolic steroids, corticosteroids, and epinephrine. Anoxia also increases fibrinolysis.

Viremia and live virus vaccines (2 to 14 days postvaccinal) cause a relative thrombocytopenia, which is undesirable, with decreased clotting from any agent. Newborn or debilitated animals are much more susceptible to these agents. Finally, pre-existing liver disease increases the likelihood of severe toxicosis owing to a decreased capacity for production of clotting factors and diminished metabolism of the anticoagulants.

SPECIFIC COMPOUNDS

Most of the anticoagulant rodenticide formulations are not highly toxic on a single-dose basis. However, these compounds may readily result in toxicosis if animals are allowed exposure to far smaller amounts repeatedly over a few days time. Because of rodent resistance to warfarin (evolution of bait shyness, decreased binding at the site of action, and possibly increased rates of metabolism and excretion), several anticoagulant rodenticides are now in use.

Table 1. *Some Values for Warfarin Toxicity in Various Species*

Species	Single Dose	Repeated Doses
Rats	50–100 mg/kg	1 mg/kg for 5 days
Dogs	5– 50 mg/kg	5 mg/kg for 5–15 days
Cats	5– 50 mg/kg	1 mg/kg for 5 days

COUMARIN-RELATED ANTICOAGULANTS

Warfarin. Synonyms and brand names: Warf 42, Compound 42, Coumafene, Rosex, Zoocoumarin, Kypfarin, RAX, Dethmor, D-con, Warficide, Prolin, Ratox, Tox-Hid, Warfarin-Plus, Raterex, Rat-Stop, Dethnel, Sulfarin, Rattanel, Marfrin, Banarat, Coumadin (pharmaceutical). Chemical name: 3(alpha-phenyl-beta-acetylethyl)-4 hydroxycoumarin. Prolin and Banarat contain sulfaquinoxaline.

Low level formulations include 0.025 per cent warfarin rat bait, and mouse poisons and rodent drinks contain 0.054 per cent warfarin. It should be borne in mind that stronger preparations such as 1 per cent throw packs, which are 40 times stronger than the usual rat bait, are sometimes used. Pharmaceutical preparations include 2-, 2.5-, 5-, 7.5-, and 10-mg tablets. Based on Table 1, a single dose LD_{50} of a 0.025 per cent bait in a 10-kg dog amounts to a high 2 kg of bait; however, only 0.05 kg (1.7 oz) of a 1 per cent bait contains the same amount of active ingredient. It follows that the commonly used 0.025 and 0.054 per cent baits are associated with toxicosis on a multiple-dose basis but not on a single-dose basis and that single-dose poisoning episodes are associated only with the highly concentrated formulations. Secondary poisoning from eating poisoned rodents is very uncommon and usually requires a diet of virtually only poisoned rodents. The half-life of warfarin in plasma is 14.5 hours in dogs.

Other coumarin-type anticoagulants (Table 2) vary in formulation, potency, and rate of excretion, and consequently the risk of exposure varies.

INDANDIONE ANTICOAGULANTS

The toxicity of the indandione products varies widely among compounds from 20 to 300 mg/kg in rats (Table 3). A general range of toxicity suggested for dogs has been 50 to 100 mg/kg on a single-dose basis. As with the coumarin anticoagulants, far smaller doses can cause hemorrhage on a multiple-dose basis.

CLINICAL DIAGNOSIS

As with any toxicosis, an attempt must be made to assess the exposure or opportunity for exposure to the toxic agent. If exposure is probable and

Table 2. *Preparations and Comparative Toxicity of Coumarin-Derived Anticoagulants Other Than Warfarin*

Generic Name	Synonyms, Brand Names: Chemical Name*	Formulations	Toxicity Data
Coumafuryl	Fumarin, Ratafin, Krumkil, Rat-a-way, Lurat, Tomarin, Fumasol: 3-[1-(2-Furanyl)-3-oxobutyl]-4-hydroxy-2H-1-benzopyran-2-one.	0.5% powder to be mixed with cornmeal, rolled oats, etc. at 1 part concentrate to 19 parts cereal to result in 0.025% coumafuryl.	Commonly used by exterminators. Oral LD_{50} (rat) is 25 mg/kg on a continuous feeding basis.
Brodifacoum	Talon, Talon G, Bolt, Havoc, Volid, Volak, PP 581, WBA 8119: 3-3(4'bromo(1-1'-biphenyl)-4-yl-1,2,3,4-tetrahydronaphthalyl)-4 hydroxy-2H-1-benzopyran-2-one.	Available in a ready-to-use grain base bait containing 50 ppm brodifacoum loose or in packs. Also may be pink like peppermint candy pellets. Volid contains 10 ppm brodifacoum.	Becoming more widely used. Acute oral LD_{50}s are 0.27, 0.25–1.0, and 25 mg/kg in rats, dogs, and cats, respectively. The compound is 40 to $200\times$ more potent than warfarin. May therefore have *single dose toxicity* and possibly secondary toxicity from eating poisoned rodents, especially in small dogs or cats.
Coumachlor	Coumachlor, Tomorin, Ratilan, G-23133: 3-[(1-chorophenyl)-3-oxbutyl]-4 hydroxy-2H-1-benzopyran-2-one.	0.03% bait. 1.0% tracking powder.	Not widely used. Acute oral LD_{50} (rat) 900–1200 mg/kg. LD_{50} over 2 to 3 weeks (rats) is 0.1–1 mg/kg/day. Highly toxic to dogs and pigs.
Difenacoum	Ratak, Neosorex, PP 580, WBA 8107: 3-(3-1, 1'-biphenyl-4-yl-1,2,3,4-tetrahydro-1-naphthylenyl)-4-hydroxy-2H-1-benzopyran-2-one.	0.005% bait.	Acute oral LD_{50} (rat) 1.8 mg/kg. Oral LD_{50}s in dog and cat reported as 50 and 100 mg/kg, respectively.
Coumatetralyl	Racumin, Bay 2564, Endox, Endrocid: 4-hydroxy-3-(1,2,3,4-tetra-hydro-1-naphthyl) coumarin.	Powder, liquid, ready-made bait.	Acute oral LD_{50} (rat) 16.5 mg/kg. Banana-like smell.
Bromadialone	Maki, Ratimus: (hydroxy-4-, coumarinyl-3)-3-phenyl(bromo-4-biphenyl-4)-1-propanol-1.	Ready-to-use baits or concentrate for mixing with cornmeal grains, etc. Finished bait = 0.005%.	LD_{50} multiple dose rat 1.125 mg/kg. *Single feeding mortality* of 90% in rats.
Dicumarol	Dicoumarol, Dicoumarin, Dicumol, Dufalone, Melitoxin, Bishydroxycoumarin: 3,3'-Methylenebis[4-hydroxy-2H-1-benzopyran-2-one].	Still available as a therapeutic agent; rodenticide use superseded by warfarin.	Acute oral LD_{50} (rat) 541.6 mg/kg. Originally isolated from spoiled sweet clover (*Melilotus*).
Acenocoumarol	Sintrom, Acenocoumarin, nicoumalone: 4-Hydroxy-3-[1-(4-nitrophenyl)-3-oxobutyl]-2H-i benzopyran-2-one.	Pharmaceutical agent.	Rapid GI absorption, maximum blood concentration in 3 hrs (human). I.P. LD_{50} (mice) 114.7 mg/kg. Half life in humans 8.2 to 8.7 hours.
Phenprocoumon	Phenprocouman N.F., Marcumar, Liquamar: 4-Hydroxy-3-(1-phenylpropyl)-2H-1-benzopyran-2-one.	Pharmaceutical agent.	Close relative of Dicoumarol. Half-life in humans 2.7 to 7 days.
Ethyl biscoumacetate	Tromexan, Dicumacyl, B.O.E.A., Tromexan Ethyl Acetate, Pelentan: 4-Hydroxy-alpha-(4-hydroxy-2-oxo-2H-1-benzopyran-3-yl)-2-oxo-2H-1-benzopyran-3-acetic acid ethyl ester.	Pharmaceutical agent.	LD_{50} (mice) 880 mg/kg.
Cyclocloumarol	4-hydroxycoumarin anticoagulant no. 63, Cumopyran, Cumopyrin: 3,4-Dihydro-2-methoxy-2-methyl-4-phenyl-2H, 5H-pyrano[3-2-c][1] benzopyran-5-one.	Pharmaceutical agent.	

*Chemical names vary, depending on the nomenclature system used.

Table 3.   *Preparations and Comparative Toxicity of Indandione Anticoagulants*

Generic Name	Synonyms, Brand Names: Chemical Name*	Formulations	Toxicity Data
Pindone	Chemrat, Pival, Pivaldione, Pivalyn, Pivacin, Tri-ban, Pivalyl Indandione, Pivalyl Valone: 2-(2,2-Dimethyl-1-oxopropyl)-1H-indene-1,3(2H)-dione.	0.2 or 5.0% powder to be mixed at 1 part concentrate to 19 parts bait. Also sold as baits of 0.025–0.075%. Pivalyn is water-soluble salt.	Still in common use. Usage has recently begun to decrease. Acute oral LD_{50} (rats) 280 mg/kg.
Chlorophacinone	Drat, Rozol, Rozol Tracking Powder, Caid, Microzul, Ramucide, Ratomet, Topitix, Raviac, LM 91, Liphadione: 2-[(4-Chlorophenyl)phenyl-acetyl]-1,3-indandione.	Oil concentrate for impregnating bait material, also dust concentrate, paraffin blocks, drinking water poison, tracking powder. Most common tracking powder = 2000 ppm.	Acute oral LD_{50} (rats) 20.5 mg/kg; lethal dosage rats 0.005%.
Diphenadione	Diphacinone, Diphacin 110, Diphacin 110A (2%), Diphacin 120, Promar, Pid, Ramik, Dipoxin, Oragulant, Solvan, Aidondin: 2-(Diphenylacetyl)-1H-indene-1,3(2H)-dione.	Apple, meat, and fish flavored baits. Most baits 0.005%. Others *0.1% bait, 0.1% water soluble,* 2% concentrate.	More potent than warfarin, especially in single-dose exposures. Duration of effect roughly $3\times$ as long as warfarin (human).
Valone	Isoval, Incco, PMP, Motomco Tracking Powder, Pivalyl Valone: 2-Isovaleryl-1,3-indandione.	Powder to be applied in paper-thin layer with squeeze bulb in protected areas or stationary bait boxes. Tracking powder concentration 2180 ppm.	Label caution not to breathe dust. Second most common tracking powder in use.
Anisindione	Miradon, Unidione, Unidone: 2-(4-Methoxyphenyl)-1H-indene-1,3(2H)-dione.	Pharmaceutical prep. 50-mg tablets.	
Naphthylindanedione	Radione	Rodenticide?	
Phenindione	Pindione, Bindan, Danilone, Anthrombon, Hedulin, Dindevan, Dineval, Diadilan, Hemolidione, Indon, Indema, Fenilin, Fenhydren, Rectadione, Diophindane, Cronodione, Thombasal, PID: 2-Phenyl-1H-indene-1,3(2H)-dione.	Pharmaceutical agent.	In addition to anticoagulant properties, fatal agranulocytosis, hepatitis, and hypersensitivity reactions may occur (human). Approximately 1/5 as potent as warfarin (human).

*Chemical names vary, depending on the nomenclature system used.

clinical signs are present, then tests of various clotting elements are used to help establish a clinical diagnosis.

Control samples should generally be submitted along with cases when dealing with human laboratories. Any test affected by factors II (prothrombin), VII, IX, or X may be affected by coumarin or indandione toxicosis. Typically in cases of coumarin or indandione poisoning, the activated coagulation time (ACT) and the activated partial thromboplastin time (APTT) are moderately prolonged and the prothrombin time (PT) is markedly prolonged. In some cases the PT may be prolonged before the APTT. The platelet count and fibrinogen estimate are normal or slightly to moderately reduced owing to associated hemorrhage. The fibrin/fibrinogen degradation products are usually within normal limits; however, subsequent to internal bleeding, activation of fibrinolysis may result in an increase in fibrin/fibrinogen degradation products. Confusion with disseminated intravascular coagulation (DIC) is possible when this occurs. However, hypofibrinogenemia and thrombocytopenia are usually not as severe in coumarin anticoagulant poisoning as in DIC. In equivocal cases, severe depletion of factor VII may be useful to confirm suspected anticoagulant toxicosis.

The packed cell volume (PCV) may be low if rehydration follows extensive or prolonged hemorrhage, and in such cases red blood cell morphology and indices often suggest a regenerative anemia. Hypoproteinemia may also occur owing to hemorrhage-associated losses.

SPECIFIC DIAGNOSIS

Anticoagulant analysis of blood and urine of live animals is worthwhile, and sometimes analysis of vomitus, bait, and feces is also helpful. When possible, confirmation of specific anticoagulants should be performed to pinpoint the source and avoid future exposure. False negative tests may occur, and failure to detect an anticoagulant is not uncommon owing to metabolism of the offending agent. Specimens for post-mortem analysis of coumarin or indandione toxicoses should include liver as the preferred tissue, but unclotted blood, stomach content, intestinal content, feces, spleen, and kidney should also be submitted. Tissues should be frozen during transport to the laboratory. Lesions most often include hemorrhages in the subcutaneous tissues, musculature, body cavities, and gastrointestinal tract.

Rarely, other vitamin K–responsive coagulapathies, such as chronic cholestasis, and malabsorption syndromes, which prevent absorption of the fat-soluble vitamin K, occur.

TREATMENT

When parenteral injections are necessary, the smallest possible needle should be used. The most effective therapeutic form of vitamin K is vitamin K_1, available as an injectable product (10 mg/cc) (AquaMEPHYTON Injection, Merck, Sharp & Dohme; also Veta K_1, Professional Veterinary Laboratories) and as tablets by the same manufacturers. This is a plant compound but is now synthesized. It may be given IM, SQ, or when serious hemorrhages are present, IV. IV administration should be slow, preferably diluted in a small amount of 5 per cent dextrose or dextrose and saline. The IV rate of administration should not exceed 0.1 mg/min/5 kg body weight. Vitamin K has low toxicity, but the pharmaceutical base of some preparations can induce shock when injected too rapidly or in an excessive dose. After IV injections, a temporary pressure wrap is desirable. A dosage of vitamin K_1 recommended for cats has been 15 to 25 mg. Dogs may be given as much as 5 mg/kg body weight. Another preparation, Konakion (Roche), is also available, but administration is limited to the IM route. Other synonyms for vitamin K_1 include phytonadione, phylloquinone, and phytomenadione. All forms of vitamin K_1 are oil soluble; therefore, oral forms require normal biliary function for absorption.

Vitamin K_1 is as effective as natural vitamin K_2 in the body. Vitamin K_1 begins to reverse the hypoprothrombinemia in about one hour, but several hours are needed for clotting factor production and full clinical response.

Other forms of vitamin K are not as prompt, not as potent, and not as prolonged in action as natural vitamin K_2 and the equally effective plant-originated K_1. One of these is vitamin K_3, which is synonymous with menadione N.F., menaphthone, Panosine, and Synkay. Vitamin K_3 dimethyl pyrimidinol bisulfite is a related compound and goes by the name Hetrazene. Vitamin K_3 sodium bisulfite U.S.P. is known as menadione sodium bisulfite, Hykinone, Klotogen, Clotin, and Vicasol. Menadione sodium diphosphate U.S.P. is synonymous with Synkayvite.

Vitamin K_4 is water soluble and, therefore, does not require bile or lipid for intestinal absorption. However, vitamin K_4 has approximately one-half the activity of K_3. Synonyms for vitamin K_4 include menadione acetate, acetomenaphthone, Prokayvit, and Kappaxin. Vitamin K_4 sodium diphosphate is also called menadiol diphosphate tetrasodium salt and Synkavit.

Vitamins K_3 and K_4 must be metabolically modified before they are of significant benefit. This often takes too long to be of benefit for the patient already demonstrating evidence of either hemorrhage or anemia. Therefore, vitamin K_1 is always preferred. Vitamin K_3 or K_4 is reserved for totally asymptomatic patients exposed within the last few hours. Even in this instance vitamins K_3 and K_4 are not as reliably effective as vitamin K_1.

When anemia and secondary tissue hypoxia are present the response to vitamin K is not as fast or as complete. Therefore, if significant hemorrhage or anemia is present whole blood administration is essential to provide the clotting factors and to correct anemia. Blood administered should be fresh (not over 24 hours old), preferably typed and crossmatched and given at a rate not faster than 4 to 6 ml/min for an average dog (Dodds, 1977). The total dose should be 10 to 20 ml/kg body weight depending on need. Half the dose is given fairly rapidly and the remainder by a slow drip. It may be helpful to keep a list of owners of larger dogs and cats who are willing to allow their animals to serve as blood donors in emergencies.

If hemorrhage has occurred into the thorax, as revealed by radiographs, drainage of the blood may be necessary. This decision must be made weighing the benefit of improved ventilation against the genuine risk of reinitiating hemorrhage by the thoracentesis. When adequate volumes of donor blood are not immediately available and blood must be removed from a body cavity, autotransfusion of this blood may be employed using a standard blood transfusion set to screen out small clots. This procedure provides the anemic animal cells but not the normal clotting factors that the patient also needs.

Oxygen may be needed prior to transfusion, but manual pumping of the chest is not advised. When intravenous fluid therapy is indicated (in addition to whole blood), balanced electrolyte solutions are preferred over saline. Of course, surgical procedures should be postponed until all clotting parameters have returned to normal except in cases of life-threatening intracranial hemorrhage, cardiac tamponade, or other similar circumstance in which decompression is essential.

For animals exposed within the last few hours, emesis should be induced followed by an injection of vitamin K_1 and oral vitamin K administration, preferably vitamin K_1, at a dose of 5 mg/kg body weight daily for two to three weeks. During the period of treatment a low fat diet (to minimize displacement from albumin) that is nonabrasive is indicated. A similar course of oral vitamin K and dietary therapy is indicated as a follow-up to in-hospital management of acute cases beginning after clotting parameters have returned to normal.

Treatment of these clinical syndromes is often unsuccessful, probably owing to failure to administer whole blood in the face of hemorrhage and the use of vitamins K_3 and K_4 in instances in which vitamin K_1 is indicated.

REFERENCES AND SUPPLEMENTAL READING

Atkins, C. E., and Johnson, R. K.: Clinical toxicities of cats, symposium on clinical toxicology for the small animal practitioner. Vet. Clin. North Am. 5:623, 1975.

Buck, W. B., Osweiler, G. D., and VanGelder, G. A.: *Warfarin and Other Anticoagulant Rodenticides in Clinical and Diagnostic Veterinary Toxicology*, 2nd ed. Dubuque, Iowa: Kendall Hunt, 1976, pp. 253–256.

Dodds, W. J.: The Diagnosis, Management and Treatment of Bleeding Disorders. Parts I and II. M.V.P. 58:680–684, 756–762, 1977.

Feldman, B. F.: Coagulopathies in small animals. J.A.V.M.A. 179:559, 1981.

Green, R. A., and Buck, W. B.: Warfarin and other anticoagulant poisonings. In Kirk, R. E. (eds.): *Current Veterinary Therapy VII.* Philadelphia: W. B. Saunders Co., 1980, pp. 131–134.

Kociba, G. J.: The diagnosis of hemostatic disorders, symposium on clinical laboratory medicine. Vet. Clin. North Am. 6:609, 1976.

Neff-Davis, C. A., Davis, L. E., and Gillette, E. L.: Warfarin in the dog: pharmacokinetics as related to clinical response. J. Vet. Pharmacol. Ther. 4:135, 1981.

METALDEHYDE POISONING

RONALD L. MULL, D.V.M.

Houston, Texas

Metaldehyde, a polymer of acetaldehyde, has been responsible for poisonings in children, livestock, horses, and dogs. Although cats are quite susceptible, metaldehyde poisoning has not been reported to be a problem in them. The toxic oral dose for most animals is in the range of 100 to 500 mg/kg. Although it has been used as a solid fuel in the past, the primary current use of metaldehyde is as a molluscicide in bait formulations. This is the usual form of exposure (snail and slug bait) encountered by the pet animal, and severe poisoning may follow ingestion of a few ounces of the bait. Metaldehyde is commonly used around vegetable crops, berries, and ornamentals. It seems likely that the increase in urban home gardens in recent years has resulted in increased pet exposure and subsequently more cases of metaldehyde poisoning.

Metaldehyde is apparently an attractant as well as a toxicant to snails and slugs. Bait formulators, however, have sought to make the baits more attractive to the mollusca by adding various food processing by-products (e.g., bran, molasses). Unfortunately, these additives also make the baits more attractive to dogs. A positive change is that the baits now usually contain only metaldehyde, generally in the range of 3.5 per cent concentration. In the recent past, the baits commonly contained metaldehyde in combination with calcium arsenate. Some baits now contain an organophosphorus or carbamate insecticide rather than the metaldehyde, which could result in somewhat similar signs of poisoning.

In the spring of 1973, there was an unusually large increase in cases of metaldehyde poisoning in dogs in California. California regulatory officials subsequently required that baits sold in the state be shown to be unattractive to dogs. Methods demonstrating the lack of attraction were promulgated based on research done at the University of California, Davis. The federal Environmental Protection Agency largely adopted the California regulations. Indications are, in California at least, that the incidence of metaldehyde bait poisoning has decreased markedly over the past several years, presumably because of the changes in the new bait formulations. One hopes that this is also the case nationwide as the older bait supplies become exhausted.

CLINICAL SIGNS

Depending on the amount of bait ingested and absorbed, the animal may be presented showing signs ranging from incoordination and anxiety with muscle fasciculations to continuous muscle spasms and prostration. Toxic effects are thought to be due primarily to absorption of acetaldehyde and other fragments of the polymer released by hydrolysis in the stomach, although some of the effects may be from the metaldehyde itself. Salivation, hyperesthesia, and muscle tremors are similar to those seen in strychnine poisoning and anticholinesterase insecticide poisoning. However, the muscle spasms cannot be initiated by external stimuli, as with strychnine poisoning, and cholinesterase blood levels will not be depressed. Marked hyperthermia also is common, with temperatures as high as 108°F reported. Severe acidosis may be an accompanying feature.

DIAGNOSIS AND TREATMENT

Goals of the clinician are to (1) stop absorption of the toxicant, (2) control the muscle tremors, and (3) provide supportive therapy to combat acidosis and dehydration. Emesis may be obtained by use of apomorphine, 0.04 mg/kg IV if the patient is ambulatory. This may be followed by (or supplanted by) light anesthesia that allows gastric lavage and controls muscle tremors. Care must be exercised to prevent aspiration of any vomitus.

The tremors can often be controlled by diazepam, 2 to 5 mg IV (repeat if necessary), or triflupromazine, 0.2 to 2.0 mg/kg IV. In severe cases, prolonged maintenance of light anesthesia with barbiturates in combination with muscle relaxants may be necessary. Lactated Ringer's Solution may be given to combat dehydration and acidosis. Intensive care may be required for up to 24 hours.

Necropsy of dogs that die acutely generally only shows slight to moderate inflammation of the gastric mucosa with hyperemia of the lungs, liver, and kidneys. If death is delayed for a few days, degenerative changes may be observed in the liver and brain.

As many as 50 per cent of cases presented may die if signs of poisoning are severe upon admission or if a large amount of bait has been consumed. Successful therapy is sometimes frustrated by the fact that some dogs appear to develop a liking for the baits; dogs have been poisoned again following discharge from the hospital.

Diagnosis usually depends on history of exposure to the baits or finding some of the pellets in the vomitus or stomach contents and is confirmed by analysis of the stomach contents. The odor of acetaldehyde may also be detected. Baits are available in both pelleted and meal formulations. The pellets seem to be far more hazardous than the meal to the dogs. Poisoning may be expected to occur most often during periods conducive to gardening activity, e.g., late afternoons, weekends, and holidays. Owners can minimize the hazard by confining their pets, using the meal formulations, and dispersing the bait well.

SUPPLEMENTAL READING

Harris, W. F.: Clinical toxicities of dogs. Vet. Clin. North Am. 5:605, 1975.
Jones, L. M., Booth, N. H., and McDonald, L. E. (eds.): *Veterinary Pharmacology and Therapeutics*, 4th ed. Ames, IA: Iowa State University Press, 1977.
Kitchell, R. L., et al.: Palatability studies of snail and slug bait poisons using dogs. J.A.V.M.A. 173:85, 1978.
Maddy, K. T.: Poisoning of dogs with metaldehyde in snail and slug poison bait. Calif. Vet. pp. 27–28, March 1955.
Udall, N. D.: The toxicity of the molluscicides metaldehyde and methiocarb to dogs. Vet. Rec. 93:420, 1978.

LEAD POISONING

DAVID F. KOWALCZYK, V.M.D.

Philadelphia, Pennsylvania

Lead poisoning in man has been recognized for thousands of years and has been implicated in such historic events as the decline of ancient Rome. The association of lead with clinical disease has been extremely difficult to make in the past owing to the ubiquitous nature of lead in the environment.

Lead poisoning in animals has probably occurred since its recognition in man, but only in the last 30 years have cases been well documented. Many of these cases were diagnosed post mortem. It was not until 1969 that the significance of lead poisoning in dogs was clearly recognized. Zook and associates reported that 1 of every 25 dogs under six months of age hospitalized at the Angell Memorial Animal Hospital (Boston) had been poisoned by lead (1977). In 1970, the hospital diagnosed 107 canine cases of lead toxicity.

At the School of Veterinary Medicine in Philadelphia, lead poisoning was rarely diagnosed until the availability of an in-house blood lead testing service in 1973. It is now the most common toxicity reported in dogs and cats.

The increased incidence of lead poisoning in dogs in the last few years has been the result of intensive screening programs and is not due to an actual increase in exposure to lead. The fault is not with the clinician's ability but with the nonspecific signs displayed during the early stages of lead poisoning (i.e., vomiting and anorexia). The most difficult aspect of lead poisoning is establishing the diagnosis.

ABSORPTION, DISTRIBUTION, AND EXCRETION OF LEAD

The most common route of entry of lead is through the gastrointestinal tract. Inhaled lead particles are cleared by ciliary action and are swallowed. In adult dogs and man, approximately 10 per cent of ingested lead is absorbed. However, in young animals, up to 90 per cent can be absorbed. The interaction of many nutritional factors with the bioavailability of lead has been well documented. An enhancement of lead absorption has been demonstrated with dietary deficiencies of calcium, zinc, iron, and protein. Lead dissolves at a much faster rate in an acid environment, such as the stomach, which thus enhances absorption. In bottom-feeding waterfowl, the ingestion of one to three shotgun pellets (which tend to remain in the gizzard) can be lethal.

Once the lead has been absorbed, it is carried by the red blood cells and distributed in the soft tissue. Over 90 per cent of the circulating lead is in the red blood cells. The presence of lead in the liver, kidney, central nervous system, and bone marrow causes the major signs of lead toxicity. Eventually, the lead redistributes to the bone, where it is biologically inert. However, this stored pool of lead may be mobilized if bone demineralization occurs (e.g., in acidosis or calcium deficiency) and can cause toxicity. The penetration of lead across the blood-brain barrier occurs more readily in the immature organism, accounting for the higher incidence of severe neurologic signs in the young animal. Lead can also cross the placenta and enter the mother's milk.

Lead is excreted very slowly from the whole body, predominantly via bile. The enterohepatic circulation of lead poisoning is not known. The elimination of lead through urine is minor unless chelating agents are being used (e.g., CaEDTA).

The measurement of blood lead can fluctuate greatly, depending on time of exposure, and it may not reflect tissue lead concentrations or the extent of lead toxicity. This is probably the reason for the poor correlation between blood-lead level and severity of clinical signs in dogs. Therefore, blood lead should not be the sole criterion in screening animals for lead exposure.

SOURCES OF LEAD

The sources of lead are varied and numerous, the most common being lead-containing paint. Interiors of dwellings painted before 1940 often contain layers of lead-based paint. Leaded paints are sometimes mistakenly used indoors and thus may be accessible to dogs in new as well as old dwellings. Exteriors of buildings (including dog houses) are frequently covered with lead paint, as are fences and painting materials. The lead salts in paint impart a sweet taste; thus their attractiveness to animals. Soil and vegetation may be contaminated with lead as a result of the weathering of lead pigments from painted structures.

Other sources of lead include linoleum, batteries, plumbing materials, putty, lead foil, solder, golf balls, certain roof coverings, lubricants, rug pads, acid (soft) drinking water from lead pipes or improperly glazed ceramic water bowls, and lead weights or objects such as fishing sinkers, drapery weights, and toys. Soil along streets and roadways may contain small amounts of lead from automobile exhaust fumes. Soil contaminated with lead from paint or auto exhausts is not a likely source of poisoning, but it may contribute somewhat to the total body burden of lead. Lead shot present subcutaneously or in muscle tissue usually becomes encapsulated and is biologically inert.

The history may or may not suggest exposure to lead. Recent remodeling of dwellings, especially old dilapidated houses, including removal of old paint, plaster, or linoleum, or application of new lead-based paints, is a common history. Remember that in cases displaying only mild gastrointestinal signs, the history may be the sole clue.

AGE

Lead poisoning may occur at any age, but most affected dogs are between two and eight months of age. Teething and the bizarre appetites of young dogs result in the gnawing on and ingestion of strange substances.

CLINICAL SIGNS

Clinical signs of lead poisoning in dogs are associated with the gastrointestinal and nervous systems. Usually both systems are clinically involved, but sometimes only one is. Very often, gastrointestinal signs are present for several days before the dog is examined, and they usually precede the neurologic signs. Such clinical signs in young dogs have led to erroneous diagnosis of canine distemper.

The most common gastrointestinal signs are vomiting, abdominal pain, and anorexia. Diarrhea and constipation are less frequently observed. The presence of abdominal pain or so-called "lead colic" is manifest by whining, restlessness, tensing of abdominal muscles, and crying when the abdomen is palpated. Many gastrointestinal upsets display the foregoing signs, but one should suspect lead toxicity if they persist for more than three days. Occasionally, megaesophagus has been associated with lead poisoning and is probably the result of esophageal paralysis.

The most common neurologic signs in order of frequency are convulsions, hysteria (characterized by barking and crying continuously, running in every direction, and indiscriminately biting at animate and inanimate objects), and other behavioral changes. Other neurologic signs are ataxia, blindness, and chomping of the jaws. Many dogs with hysteria or convulsions have increased rectal temperatures that decrease after the episode subsides.

The need for recognition of subtle neurologic deficits such as learning impairments, hyperactivity, and loss of visual discrimination during and after exposure to lead has only recently been appreciated. One investigation demonstrated residual neurologic deficits in sheep that were exposed to low levels of lead that never produced so-called "toxic blood-lead levels" (Van Gelder et al., 1973).

Differential diagnoses, based on history and clinical signs, include canine distemper, epilepsy, intestinal parasitism, nonspecific gastrointestinal disturbance, acute pancreatitis, encephalitis, vertebral problems, rabies, and other poisonings. Because of the high incidence of canine distemper in young dogs, the occurrence of convulsions with or without typical signs is usually attributed to canine distemper. However, recent investigations have found many of these cases to be the result of lead poisoning.

LABORATORY FINDINGS

One of the most helpful screening tests for the diagnosis of lead poisoning, without resorting to a quantitative test for lead, is examination of a stained blood smear. Of prime importance is the finding of large numbers of nucleated erythrocytes (5 to 40/100 white blood cells) without evidence of severe anemia—packed cell volume less than 30 per cent. This is considered to be nearly pathognomonic of lead poisoning. The nucleated erythrocytes are a relatively easy cell type to identify regardless of the staining procedure.

Other common abnormalities in red blood cell morphology are anisocytosis, polychromasia, poikilocytosis, target cells, and hypochromasia. The presence of basophilic stippling in red blood cells is another common feature, but detection depends on the staining procedure. One investigation at Angell Memorial Animal Hospital reported basophilic stippling in 94 per cent of lead-poisoned dogs (Zook et al., 1970); however, stippling was found in 42 per cent of dogs with other problems.

Red blood cell abnormalities usually precede clinical signs except in the very acute poisoning. Once chelation therapy has been started, these changes disappear quickly.

Moderate numbers of nucleated red blood cells and a few stippled red blood cells may be found in some dogs with marked and prolonged anemias—e.g., autoimmune hemolytic anemia. Older dogs that have visceral hemangiosarcomas are usually anemic and have numerous nucleated red blood cells but few or no stippled red blood cells.

The leukocyte counts are usually elevated because of a neutrophilic leukocytosis. It is important to correct the white blood cell count for the presence of nucleated erythrocytes; otherwise, exaggerated white blood cell counts will result.

Results of other laboratory tests, such as blood urea nitrogen, creatinine, transaminase, amylase, blood glucose, sedimentation rate, and Coomb's test, are normal. Bone marrow examination disclose an increase of erythroid elements. Elevated reticulocyte counts and the finding of many immature red blood cells in peripheral blood smears indicate early release or erythroid cells from the hyperplastic bone marrow. The urine usually contains granular casts. Often, mild proteinuria and sometimes glycosuria are found. The cerebrospinal fluid may have a normal pressure, protein, and cell content.

Other tests that have become very useful in human lead poisoning are related to detection of abnormalities in heme synthesis. The interference of lead at several enzymatic steps has proved to be a most sensitive indicator of biologic change. The accumulation of various substrates, such as aminolevulinic acid (urine) and zinc protoporphyrin (red blood cell), is commonly used as screening tests in high-risk children and lead-exposed workers. These tests reflect the presence and severity of lead poisoning. The substrate levels stay elevated despite fluctuations in blood-lead level. The concentration of zinc protoporphyrin has been shown to increase severalfold in cases of chronic lead poisoning in the horse, cow, and rabbit. However, in experimentally lead-poisoned dogs, the appearance of clinical signs was not well correlated with an increase in zinc protoporphyrin. This suggests that the sensitivity of dogs to lead is not reflected in porphyrin metabolism.

RADIOGRAPHIC FINDINGS

The most helpful radiographic finding is the presence of diffuse radiopaque material in the gastrointestinal tract. This material was found in over 60 per cent of the cases at the University of Pennsylvania. However, it should be emphasized that it is impossible to differentiate these radiodensities from bone chips or gravel. It is important to radiograph the animal, since chelation therapy has been shown to enhance intestinal absorption of lead.

The metaphyses of long bones may develop lead lines (metaphyseal sclerosis) in immature dogs. These radiopaque bands are best seen just proximal to the open epiphyses of the distal radius, ulna, and metacarpal bones. This is due to the incorporation of lead at the site of endochondral ossification, which stimulates active bone formation, causing a dense zone of mineralized cartilage. The lead lines are mainly the result of new bone formation and not the deposition of lead. Similar radiographic changes are reported in phosphorus and vitamin D intoxication.

The presence of lead lines is a difficult interpretation to make, even for radiologists and, as a diagnostic tool, has not been useful at our hospital.

DIAGNOSIS

Since the clinical signs of lead poisoning are not pathognomonic, a history detailing likelihood of exposure or the finding of many nucleated erythrocytes without anemia may be the first clue. Blood may be taken for lead analysis to confirm the diagnosis, but treatment for lead poisoning should be started.

The analysis of whole blood is the best single index for establishing a definitive diagnosis. Most laboratories require 10 ml of whole, oxalated, or heparinized blood in a clean, lead-free vial. Versenate (EDTA) anticoagulant interferes with some methods. The finding of 60 μg or more of lead/100 ml of blood (0.6 ppm) is virtually diagnostic of lead poisoning in dogs. Blood-lead values of 30 to 50 μg/100 ml (0.3 to 0.5 ppm) are abnormally high and indicate lead poisoning if associated with typical signs and hematologic findings. Baseline levels for lead range between 5 and 25 μg/100 ml (0.05 and 0.25 ppm). The small difference between background and toxic blood-lead levels make interpretation of this test difficult at the lower levels. The severity of clinical signs is usually not correlated with blood-lead content.

For post-mortem confirmation, analysis of liver for lead is the best diagnostic test. The upper limit of normal is 3.5 ppm (wet weight); 5 ppm or more is virtually diagnostic. Samples of hair or feces or single specimens of urine for lead analysis are not recommended. Urine specimens taken just before and 24 hours after starting chelation therapy (calcium disodium edetate, CaEDTA, at the dosage administered for regular treatment) disclose a ten- to sixtyfold increase in urine lead output in dogs with lead poisoning. Although this test is reliable, it is expensive and time consuming, and it is difficult to obtain the specimens.

TREATMENT

The purposes of therapy in lead poisoning are (1) to remove lead, if present, from the gastrointestinal tract so that further absorption is prevented, (2) to remove lead from the blood and body tissues rapidly, and (3) to alleviate marked neurologic signs.

Lead should be removed from the gastrointestinal tract prior to chelation therapy with enemas and emetics, as chelating agents can enhance the absorption of lead from the intestines. Lead-containing substances are often found in the large intestine. Large objects in the stomach may require surgery.

Chelating agents effectively remove heavy metals such as lead by forming nontoxic complexes with the metals that are rapidly excreted via the bile or urine. The chelating agent of choice is CaEDTA (calcium ethylenediaminetetraacetate), which has been shown to be effective in treating lead poisoning in a wide variety of animals. CaEDTA must be administered as the calcium chelate to prevent hypocalcemia. Renal damage has occurred in man owing to excessive CaEDTA; however, we have found no evidence of any side effects in dogs. Nonetheless, the daily dose should not exceed 2 gm, and therapy should not be continued for more than five consecutive days.

CaEDTA is given at the rate of 100 mg/kg of body weight daily for two to five days. The daily dose is divided into four equal portions and administered subcutaneously after dilution to a concentration of about 10 mg CaEDTA/ml of 5 per cent dextrose solution. Higher concentrations of CaEDTA can cause painful reactions at injection sites.

The use of CaEDTA has been extremely effective, with clinical improvement within 24 to 48 hours. Dogs that respond slowly or that have a pretreatment blood-lead level of more than 100 μg/100 ml (1.0 ppm) may need a second five-day treatment five days after completion of the first series. This second treatment prevents recurrence of clinical signs, provided the dog is not allowed to consume more lead after discharge from the hospital. Monitoring blood lead during treatment is not valuable, as the concentration of lead does not correlate with alleviation of clinical signs. This is probably due to CaEDTA's inability to cross cell membranes.

Penicillamine, an oral chelating agent of proven value in treating lead-poisoned children, offers promise for dogs. Penicillamine, given orally, has a distinct advantage over CaEDTA, which must be repeatedly injected subcutaneously, requiring hospitalization. Clinical trials to date indicate that penicillamine is effective in promoting urinary excretion of lead and alleviating clinical signs.

Penicillamine, given in a dose of 100 mg/kg body weight daily for one to two weeks, has some undesirable side effects such as vomiting, listlessness, and partial anorexia. To decrease the side effects, penicillamine should be given on an empty stomach in divided doses. Antiemetics have also proved useful (e.g., phenothiazines, antihistamines). The capsules may be dissolved in fruit juice (acidic) for ease of administration. At present, penicillamine can be recommended for dogs that are not seriously ill or that do not have marked neurologic disorders or persistent vomiting. If an owner refuses to hospitalize his dog, penicillamine can be prescribed; however, the owner should be warned that side effects may occur and that lead ingested while on treatment is apt to be absorbed more completely than it would be without treatment.

It seems that penicillamine might also be beneficial in combination with CaEDTA. It may be that CaEDTA needs to be given for only a few days, followed by penicillamine. This regimen should assure adequate hydration, promote renal function, and help reduce the care and cost of treatment. Penicillamine might also be useful in treating dogs that recovered slowly from a five-day course of CaEDTA or that had an initial blood-lead level of more than 100 μg/100 ml (1.0 ppm) and therefore should be treated again.

Dimercaprol (BAL) has been used successfully in combination with CaEDTA in children. It has seldom been used in lead-poisoned animals. However, it does offer the advantages of removing lead directly from red blood cells and excreting lead primarily via the bile (important if renal function is compromised).

SUPPORTIVE TREATMENT

The gastrointestinal signs (e.g., vomiting, diarrhea, anorexia) do not usually require specific drug therapy because they subside quickly after chelation therapy. However, the severe neurologic signs (e.g., convulsions) are due to cerebral edema and thus require immediate attention. Mannitol and dexamethasone are the agents of choice. Seizures and hysteria can be controlled with diazepam and/or pentobarbital intravenously. Permanent mental deficiencies and recurrent seizures are common sequelae of lead poisoning in children. Thus, it seems appropriate to treat lead encephalopathy in dogs as well, because these drugs not only appear to speed clinical recovery but may also prevent permanent brain damage.

PROGNOSIS

The prognosis in the majority of lead poisoning cases that undergo chelation therapy is favorable, with a dramatic improvement in 24 to 48 hours. Chelation therapy may thus be used as a diagnostic tool in cases of high suspicion when a blood-lead determination is impractical or delayed. Prognoses in cases treated promptly and adequately depend on the degree and duration of neurologic involvement and, to a lesser extent, the amount of lead found in the blood. Continuous or uncontrolled convulsions warrant an unfavorable prognosis. Dogs with 100 μg or more of lead/100 ml of blood tend to recover slowly, and signs may recur if a second course of therapy is not given. If there are no neurologic signs or if they are mild or readily controlled by ancillary treatment, the prognosis is favorable.

The prognosis in untreated cases that are only displaying gastrointestinal signs may be favorable if further exposure to lead is prevented. If the economic situation does not permit treatment with CaEDTA, a course of oral penicillamine may be advantageous.

PATHOLOGIC FINDINGS

Gross necropsy findings are generally not remarkable; however, careful examination may reveal chips of paint or other lead-containing substances in the gastrointestinal tract. White bands are sometimes found in transversely sectioned metaphyses of immature dogs. Microscopic study may disclose acid-fast intranuclear inclusion bodies in renal proximal tubular cells and less often in hepatocytes. These inclusions are essentially pathognomonic of lead poisoning but are not found in all cases. Lesions in the brain include degenerative changes in small vessels, hemorrhages, laminar necrosis, and proliferation of capillaries and gliosis in chronic encephalopathies.

VETERINARIAN'S OBLIGATION

Animals may manifest signs of toxicity before man when they are sharing the same environment. Birds have been used for years in mines as sensitive indicators of toxic gas accumulation. In the 1953 mercury poisoning outbreak in Japan, cats were dying a year before the disease was recognized in man. For lead poisoning, the young dog seems the most appropriate species because it shares the same environment and has eating habits (e.g., pica) similar to those of children. A recent study from Illinois indicated that an abnormally high blood-lead level in a family dog increased the probability sixfold of finding a child in the same family with an increased blood-lead level. At the University of Pennsylvania Veterinary School, owners with lead-poisoned dogs were advised to have children between one and five years of age checked for lead poisoning. A few children had blood-lead levels in the toxic range, even though they were not showing gross clinical signs.

When diagnosing canine lead poisoning to owners with small children, we strongly urge veterinarians to warn the family and/or family physician adequately. Most urban centers have free clinics for lead testing in children.

LEAD POISONING IN OTHER PETS

Cats are rarely poisoned by lead because, unlike dogs, they are very selective eaters and seldom gnaw on or ingest nonfood substances. Therefore, they are not subject to most sources of lead. Because of their fastidious fur-cleaning habits, however, they may ingest lead-containing dusts or other substances that contaminate their coat.

Parrots may pick at and ingest peeling paint or, if the bars of their cages are painted, they may ingest the paint while clambering about or trimming their beaks. At least two pet parrots and numerous zoo parrots are known to have died of lead poisoning. No hematologic changes were seen in the parrots studied. Any curious pet with indiscriminate eating habits and exposure to lead is a likely candidate for lead intoxication.

REFERENCES AND SUPPLEMENTAL READING

Buck, W. B., Osweiler, G. D., and Van Gelder, G. A.: *Clinical and Diagnostic Veterinary Toxicology*, 2nd ed. Dubuque, Iowa: Kendal-Hunt Publishing Co., 1976.

Carson, T. L. Van Gelder, G. A., Buck, W. B., and Hoffman, L. J.: Effects of low level lead ingestion in sheep. Clin. Toxicol. 6:389, 1973.

Clarke, E. G. C.: Lead poisoning in small animals. J. Small Anim. Pract. 14:183, 1973.

Finley, M. T., Dieter, M. P., and Locke, L. N.: Lead in tissues of mallard ducks dosed with two types of lead shot. Bull. Environ. Contamin. Toxicol. 16:261, 1976.

Grandjean, P., and Lintrup, J.: Erythrocyte-Zn-protoporphyrin as an indicator of lead exposure. Scand. J. Clin. Invest. 38:669, 1978.

Kowalczyk, D. F.: Lead poisoning in dogs at the University of Pennsylvania Veterinary Hospital. J.A.V.M.A. 168:428, 1976.

Mylroie, A. A., Moore, L., Olyai, B. S., and Anderson, M.: Increased susceptibility to lead toxicity in rats fed semipurified diets. Environ. Res. 15:57, 1978.

Pennumarthy, L., Oehme, F. W., and Galitzer, S. J.: Effects of chronic oral lead administration in young beagle dogs. J. Environ. Pathol. Toxicol. 3:465, 1980.

Schunk, K. L.: Lead poisoning in dogs. Small Anim. Vet. Med. Update 8:2, 1978.

Thomas, C. W., Rising, J. L., and Moore, J. K.: Blood lead concentrations of children and dogs from 83 Illinois families. J.A.V.M.A. 169:1237, 1976.

Van Gelder, G. A., Carson, T. L., Smith, R. M., Buck, W. B., and Karas, G. G.: Neurophysiologic and behavioral toxicologic testing to detect subclinical neurologic alterations induced by environmental toxicants. J.A.V.M.A. 163:1033, 1973.

Zook, B. C., Carpenter, J. L., and Kirk, R. W. (eds.): Current Veterinary Therapy VI. Philadelphia: W. B. Saunders Co., 1977.

Zook, B. C., Carpenter, J. L., and Leeds, E. B.: Lead poisoning in dogs. J.A.V.M.A. 155:1329, 1969.

Zook, B. C., Kopito, L., Carpenter, J. L., Cramer, D. V., and Schwachman, H.: Lead poisoning in dogs: analysis of blood, urine, hair, and liver for lead. Am. J. Vet. Res. 33:903, 1972.

Zook, B. C., McConnell, G., and Gilmore, C. E.: Basophilic stippling of erythrocytes in dogs with special reference to lead poisoning. J.A.V.M.A. 157:2092, 1970.

SODIUM FLUOROACETATE (COMPOUND 1080) POISONING

W. EUGENE LLOYD, D.V.M.

Ames, Iowa

Sodium fluoroacetate (compound 1080) is a potent rodenticide that has been restricted to use by professional exterminators. Owing to its high toxicity in dogs and cats, it has been responsible for the deaths of these animals after they have ingested rodents killed by the compound. Fortunately, the use of compound 1080 and, therefore, the poisoning of pets have diminished during recent years. However, the practitioner should not rule out compound 1080 poisoning in carnivorous pet animals, even though there is no specific satisfactory treatment.

SOURCE AND TOXICITY

Fluoroacetic acid is produced by several toxic plants found in Africa, Australia, and Brazil. It is chemically synthesized for use in rodenticides, where it is present as either fluoroacetamide (CH_2FCONH_2) or sodium fluoroacetate, compound 1080 ($C_2H_2FNaO_2$). Fluoroacetate is mixed in baits, usually with a black dye, for rodents. The most recent federal regulations regarding fluoroacetate use are found in the 1978 Amendment of the Federal Insecticide, Fungicide, and Rodenticide Act. It essentially limits the use of the compounds to certified applicators for control of Norway rats, roof rats, and house mice around buildings and inside ships, but baits cannot be used inside occupied dwellings. It has not been used on public land since 1972. Four states allow the regulated use of compound 1080. California County Agricultural Commissioners can certify the use of compound 1080, largely for the control of ground squirrels. Colorado, Oregon, and Nevada also allow the restricted use of compound 1080 for the control of ground squirrels, meadow mice, and prairie dogs.

Dogs and cats are relatively sensitive to fluoroacetate, with lethal doses ranging from 0.05 to 1.0 mg/kg of body weight. Rodents such as rats and mice require doses of 2 to 8 mg/kg for lethal effects. Therefore, dogs and, to a lesser extent, cats and pigs have been poisoned by ingesting rodents and birds poisoned by compound 1080.

CLINICAL SIGNS

Biochemically, fluoroacetate acts by inhibiting the tricarboxylic acid (TCA) cycle, whereby it is incorporated into citric acid, forming fluorocitrate, which then inhibits aconitase and the oxidation of citric acid. The result is accumulation of citric and lactic acids. Fluoroacetate toxicosis elicits violent clinical signs in dogs, and the syndrome may appear similar to other convulsive diseases. Clinical signs occur from one-half to two hours after ingestion of compound 1080, beginning with restlessness and hyperirritability. The dog invariably vomits the gastric contents, usually early in the syndrome. However, this apparent protective mechanism is almost always too late to save the dog's life. There is hypermotility of the gastrointestinal tract, with tenesmus and resulting evacuation of the lower bowel and bladder. These phenomena occur during the early stage of intoxication. An affected dog then starts to walk in an aimless fashion, progressing to frenzied barking and running without apparent notice of physical barriers. The running and barking fits last for several minutes and terminate in a violent tonoclonic seizure, which usually lasts less than one minute. This is usually followed by paddling, after which the dog may rise to its feet. Following an apparent partial recovery the dog will appear exhausted and confused for several minutes. Thereafter, another running fit, terminating in opisthotonos and tonoclonic convulsions, will occur. After several episodes of remissions and exacerbations an affected dog will die during an extended tonic seizure. Depending on dose, death occurs within 2 to 12 hours after ingestion of compound 1080. Cats poisoned by compound 1080 may die in a seizure similar to that observed in dogs, but they do not display the marked excitement and running fits seen in dogs. Vocalization and cardiac arrhythmias are common in cats.

DIAGNOSIS

Diagnosis of fluoroacetate poisoning in dogs and cats may be quite difficult if clinical signs have not been observed and only the dead animal is presented to the veterinarian. One should first assess the likelihood of poisoning, especially by secondary intoxication, as related to the animal's exposure to areas where compound 1080 is used. These include shipyards, grain elevators, and meadows where burrowing rodents are prevalent. Rigor mortis occurs rapidly in animals poisoned by compound 1080, but distinctive post-mortem lesions have not been described. There is a generalized cyanosis, and the heart is usually noted in diastole with subepicardial hemorrhages. Most importantly, dogs and cats invariably have an empty stomach, colon, and urinary bladder.

Observations of clinical signs and reactions to outside stimuli are helpful in diagnosing compound 1080 toxicosis. Fluoroacetate-poisoned dogs do not respond to external stimuli, and seizures cannot be elicited by touch or loud noises in the way that strychnine convulsions can be induced. In fact, compound 1080–poisoned dogs and cats appear to be oblivious to their surroundings. Strychnine-poisoned dogs do not usually vomit or void the colon and urinary bladder nor do they have the running and barking seen with compound 1080 poisoning. Toxicoses due to the chlorinated hydrocarbon compounds also produce intermittent epileptiform convulsions, but vomiting, defecation, and running fits are not common. Hyperthermia occurs in both compound 1080 and chlorinated hydrocarbon poisoning. Lead poisoning may cause running fits in dogs, along with convulsions and vomiting. Lead-poisoned dogs may seem to have remissions, appearing more or less normal except for depression and anorexia between the convulsions and running fits. Confirmatory diagnoses of poisonings by strychnine, chlorinated hydrocarbons, and lead can be made by chemical analyses of proper specimens. The differential diagnosis should probably also include CNS diseases: distemper, rabies, pseudorabies, and epilepsy; and other diseases: heavy metal intoxication, hypercalcemia, and acute pancreatitis. Fluoroacetate compounds are stable in biologic tissue, so it is possible to confirm compound 1080 poisoning by analyzing vomitus or liver specimens for the presence of fluoroacetate. Diagnostic methods include the use of gas-liquid chromatography or a specific ion electrode, so few laboratories conduct the analyses. Moribund compound 1080–poisoned dogs and cats have elevated blood lactate and glucose values, but these findings are common in animals near death.

TREATMENT AND PROGNOSIS

There is no known specific antidote for compound 1080 poisoning. If a practitioner has the opportunity to treat an affected dog, the best that can be hoped for is palliation or symptomic relief. Intravenous injections of barbiturates q.s. to control convulsions have been used. Injections of calcium gluconate solutions have also been used to control tetany, which is probably caused by a lactic acidemia. Attempts have been made to decrease the concentration of citrate by the use of acetate. Monoacetin (glyceryl monoacetate) has been given intramuscularly in doses of 0.55 gm/kg. Solutions containing 50 per cent alcohol and 5 per cent acetic acid have been given orally in doses of 8.8 ml/kg. However, in practically all cases treatment is ineffective, and the prognosis of dogs poisoned with compound 1080 is grave.

SUPPLEMENTAL READING

Atzert, S. P.: A review of sodium monofluoroacetate (compound 1080). Its properties, toxicology, and use in predator and rodent control. United States Department of the Interior, Fish and Wildlife Service. Wildlife No. 146:1, 1971.

Buck, W. B., Osweiler, G. D., and Van Gelder, G. A.: *Clinical and Diagnostic Veterinary Toxicology*, 2nd ed. Dubuque, Iowa: Kendall/Hunt Publishing Co., 1976.

Cheng, S. C., Kumar, S., and Casella, G. A.: Effects of fluoroacetate and fluorocitrate on the metabolic compartmentation of tricarboxylic acid cycle in rat brain slices. Brain Res. 42:117, 1972.

Fanshier, D. W., Gottwald, L. K., and Kun, E.: Studies on specific enzyme inhibitors VI. Characterization and mechanism of action of the enzyme inhibitory isomer of monofluorocitrate. J. Biol. Chem. 239:425, 1964.

Federal Insecticide, Fungicide, and Rodenticide Act (FIFRA). Amendment 1978. Federal Register.

Guarda, F., and Dotta, R.: Experimental poisoning with sodium fluoroacetate in dogs: symptoms and lesions. Ann. Fac. Med. Vet. Torino 12:241, 1964.

Peters, P. A.: Organo-fluorine compounds present in certain plants and their effect on animals. Proceedings of the 49th Annual Meeting of the Biochemical Society. 8, 1963.

Peters, R. A., and Morselli, P. L.: Observations on the use and action of monacetin in fluoroacetate poisoning. Biochem. Pharmacol. 14:1981, 1965.

Roszkowski, A. P.: Comparative toxicity of rodenticides. Fed. Proc. 126:1082, 1967.

ETHYLENE GLYCOL (ANTIFREEZE) POISONING

FREDERICK W. OEHME, D.V.M.

Manhattan, Kansas

Antifreeze toxicity is a common poisoning in small domestic animals. The major toxic component is ethylene glycol, which constitutes 95 per cent or more of most commercial antifreeze preparations. Dogs and cats have frequently consumed radiator drainage containing antifreeze, probably owing to its sweet taste. The incidence of antifreeze poisoning increases significantly in the fall of the year, when radiators are being drained and new antifreeze is being incorporated into automobile– and other machinery–cooling systems. The toxic dose that has been reported in dogs varies from 4.2 to 6.6 ml of ethylene glycol/kg of body weight. Interestingly, the fatal dose of ethylene glycol in cats has been given as only 1.5 ml/kg.

CLINICAL SYNDROMES

The clinical diagnosis and treatment of ethylene glycol poisoning are difficult, since animals progress through varying stages of signs, and the clinician may be presented with the patient at any phase of the syndrome. The basis of ethylene glycol toxicity is twofold: (1) acute toxicity and acidosis due to rapid absorption of a large dose from the digestive tract, or, if the amount of ethylene glycol absorbed is small and time permits, (2) the metabolism of ethylene glycol through a series of metabolites to oxalic acid, which then combines with calcium to form a calcium oxalate complex that is deposited in the renal tubules, causing tubular epithelial damage, renal failure, and death due to uremia. Thus the clinician may be presented with dogs or cats in the acute acidotic phase or in the more chronic uremic syndrome resulting from renal failure.

ACUTE ETHYLENE GLYCOL POISONING

Absorbed ethylene glycol doses in excess of approximately 6 ml/kg of body weight characteristically produce an acute depression and death within 12 to 36 hours after ingestion. If observed, initial clinical signs of apprehension, moderate depression, and mild ataxia are seen 30 to 60 minutes after ethylene glycol ingestion. Vomiting frequently occurs, and progressive depression, incoordination, and ataxia are followed by paresis and coma. Coma usually occurs 6 to 12 hours after ingestion and progresses to death. Although convulsions are not common, some patients may display involuntary forced muscular activity ("paddling") in the terminal phases of poisoning.

Post-mortem examination predominantly reveals various degrees of digestive tract hyperemia. In addition, acute congestion of body tissues and swelling of the kidneys may be observed, but the latter is more common with animals surviving longer periods. Examination of urine sediments will show increasing numbers of oxalate crystals beginning approximately six hours after ingestion. Such crystals in the urinary sediment or those observed in kidney impression smears or on histopathologic examination of kidney tissue are useful diagnostic aids. However, the clinician should realize that small numbers of oxalate crystals may be observed in the urinary sediment of normal dogs.

CHRONIC ETHYLENE GLYCOL POISONING AND UREMIA

Dogs and cats surviving more than 24 hours exhibit increasing levels of blood urea nitrogen. The clinical signs described for the acute syndrome are present but in milder degrees. Vomiting and progressive depression with ataxia and eventual paresis may occur three to ten days following ingestion of ethylene glycol. Such animals may have ingested smaller amounts of ethylene glycol or may have vomited significant portions of the compound prior to absorption from the stomach. Increasing thirst is initially apparent, but renal failure results in small amounts of dark-colored urine being voided and eventual anuria. Blood urea nitrogen levels are often in excess of 200 mg/100 ml when coma develops. Muscle fasciculations, paddling of the limbs in slow running movements, occasional periods of diffuse and general muscle contractions, and neuromuscular manifestations of uremia may be seen. Terminal uremia leads to death.

Post-mortem examination of these animals reveals cachexia, dehydration, oral ulcerations, and a hemorrhagic gastritis. The kidneys may be swollen. Impression smears of the kidneys reveal abundant numbers of oxalate crystals; these are readily observed primarily in the proximal tubules when histopathologic examination utilizing polarized light is performed. In addition to the presence of oxalate crystals, cystic tubules, congestion, proteinaceous casts, and varying degrees of tubular epithelial damage are observed.

DIAGNOSIS

The clinical signs of ethylene glycol poisoning are predominantly vomiting, progressive depression, and coma with or without neuromuscular activity. These signs are extremely difficult to differentiate from similar signs arising from other causes during the acute syndrome, but the presence of numerous oxalate crystals in urinary sediment may be of value in making the diagnosis. Other intoxications, acute metabolic acidoses, and neuromuscular injuries and diseases must also be differentiated from ethylene glycol poisoning. Animals with rising blood urea nitrogen levels and the presence of abundant oxalate crystals in urinary sediment should be suspected of having ethylene glycol poisoning.

Commercial laboratories are capable of determining ethylene glycol or oxalate levels in whole blood samples. Practitioners with such facilities available may utilize them for diagnostic benefit. On histopathologic examination of kidney sections, the observation of abundant calcium oxalate crystals in the tubular lumen under polarizing light is characteristic.

TREATMENT

Successful therapy of antifreeze poisoning is based on a favorable combination of several factors:

(1) limited ingestion and absorption of ethylene glycol, (2) rapid diagnosis and initiation of treatment following poisoning, and (3) faithful application of a systematic therapeutic regimen of ethanol and sodium bicarbonate.

Animals receiving unusually large dosages of ethylene glycol (in excess of 10 ml/kg of body weight in dogs; in excess of 8 ml/kg of body weight in cats) are incapable of responding to any therapy. The rapid absorption and metabolic conversion of the ethylene glycol to a series of acids results in an acute acidosis and prompt death. Animals ingesting such large quantities of ethylene glycol are rarely seen except in a comatose condition, at which time diagnosis is extremely difficult and biologic response to antidotal therapy is improbable.

Animals receiving lethal amounts of ethylene glycol respond to therapy in direct relation to the promptness with which therapy is instituted. In general, dogs will recover from twice the lethal dose of ethylene glycol if treatment is instituted within 12 hours following ingestion. Cats respond to therapy for three times the lethal dose of ethylene glycol if therapy is instituted within eight hours following ingestion. This observation is logical when one realizes that the ethylene glycol, in itself, is relatively nontoxic; it is the metabolites that induce the toxicosis. Hence, the longer the time allowed for metabolism to occur before therapy is instituted, the less the chance of successful treatment and recovery.

Successful therapy of ethylene glycol poisoning in dogs and cats depends on the repeated systemic administration of solutions of 20 per cent ethanol and 5 per cent sodium bicarbonate. In dogs, the optimal dosage levels are 5.5 ml of 20 per cent ethanol/kg of body weight given intravenously and 8 ml of 5 per cent sodium bicarbonate/kg of body weight given intraperitoneally. This treatment level must be repeated every four hours for a total of five treatments and then every six hours for four additional treatments. In cats, lower enzyme levels require that the dosage be altered. Five milliliters of 20 per cent ethanol and 6 ml of 5 per cent sodium bicarbonate are given per kilogram of body weight, both intraperitoneally. This is administered every six hours for a total of five treatments and then given four more times at eight-hour intervals.

The treatment rationale is based on ethanol blocking the enzymes responsible for metabolizing the ethylene glycol to the more toxic end-products. Hence, only limited oxalic acid is produced, and reduced calcium oxalate formation and renal deposition of crystals occur. The administration of sodium bicarbonate prevents and reverses the acidosis, favors increased excretion of the unmetabolized ethylene glycol, and reduces calcium oxalate formation by altering urinary pH. Renal excretion of unchanged ethylene glycol is further enhanced by the volume of fluids being administered and the availability of frequent small amounts of drinking water to animals undergoing therapy.

Even though the amount of ethylene glycol ingested by spontaneously poisoned animals is often impossible to determine, clinical evaluation and prognosis is possible approximately 12 to 16 hours into the therapeutic regimen. Animals regaining consciousness, drinking water, and perhaps walking with difficulty after the third or fourth treatment may reasonably be estimated to have absorbed limited amounts of ethylene glycol. The prognosis for recovery with completion of the entire treatment schedule is fair to good. Aimals undergoing therapy that do not regain consciousness between treatments have a poor potential for recovery. Likewise, dogs presented in coma with suspected ethylene glycol ingestion must be given poor prognoses. Such animals are frequently in either a terminal state of acute intoxication or the more chronic renal syndrome with uremia. Such animals will not respond to ethanol-bicarbonate therapy.

Although not readily available under most clinical circumstances, hemodialysis and fluid therapy would be useful in comatose ethylene glycol–poisoned animals. Peritoneal dialysis is a practical compromise for hemodialysis, but it does not provide the effective cleansing of biologic fluids achieved by the latter. Until the current experimental resins and other techniques are further developed for practical "cage-side" use in dialyzing whole blood of foreign compounds, the prompt and conscientious application of ethanol and sodium bicarbonate remains the most effective treatment for antifreeze (ethylene glycol) poisoning in dogs and cats.

SUPPLEMENTAL READING

Beckett, S. D., and Shields, R. P.: Treatment of acute ethylene glycol (antifreeze) toxicosis in the dog. J.A.V.M.A. 158:472, 1971.

Kersting, E. J., and Nielsen, S. W.: Ethylene glycol poisoning in small animals. J.A.V.M.A. 146:113, 1965.

Kersting, E. J., and Nielsen, S. W.: Experimental ethylene glycol poisoning in the dog. Am. J. Vet. Res. 27:574, 1966.

Nunamaker, D. M., Medway, W., and Berg, P.: Treatment of ethylene glycol poisoning in the dog. J.A.V.M.A. 159:310, 1971.

Penumarthy, L., and Oehme, F. W.: Treatment of ethylene glycol toxicosis in cats. Am. J. Vet. Res. 36:209, 1975.

Sanyer, J. L., Oehme, F. W., and McGavin, M. D.: Systematic treatment of ethylene glycol toxicosis in dogs. Am. J. Vet. Res. 34:527, 1973.

ORGANOPHOSPHATE AND CARBAMATE INSECTICIDE POISONING

THOMAS L. CARSON, D.V.M.

Ames, Iowa

The organophosphate (OP) and carbamate insecticides have been widely employed for control of external parasites on companion animals and livestock and insect pests in the home and garden and have been used as agricultural insecticides for crop production. Usage of these insecticides has increased dramatically over the last few years as the more environmentally persistent chlorinated hydrocarbon insecticides have been restricted in usage.

Spilled or improperly stored insecticides, whether in the basement or the garage or on the farmstead, present a hazard of poisoning to companion animals. Dogs and cats have lapped up liquid concentrates and diluted sprays as well as dry powders intended for home and garden applications. Farm dogs have eaten granules of these insecticides that have been spilled on the ground or in farm vehicles. Leftover or improperly discarded insecticide preparations have also caused poisoning.

Miscalculation of insecticide concentrations in spraying or dipping procedures for external parasite control have also resulted in toxicosis. Re-treating animals with either external or oral OP or carbamate preparations within a few days may result in poisoning of these animals. In addition, some animals may be predisposed to poisoning because of concurrent or previous treatment with some anthelmintics and tranquilizers.

MECHANISM OF ACTION

The OP and carbamate insecticides are discussed together because their mechanisms of action are similar.

Cholinergic nerves utilize acetylcholine as a neurotransmitter substance. Under normal conditions, acetylcholine released at the synapses of parasympathetic nerves and myoneural junctions are quickly hydrolyzed by cholinesterase enzymes. When the hydrolyzing enzymes are inhibited, the continued presence of acetylcholine maintains a state of nerve stimulation and accounts for the clinical signs observed with poisoning from these insecticides. In general, inhibition of these enzymes by the OP insecticides tends to be irreversible, whereas inhibition by the carbamates is reversible.

CLINICAL SIGNS

The clinical syndrome produced by the OP and carbamate insecticides is similar in all species of animals and in general is characterized by overstimulation of the parasympathetic nervous system, skeletal muscle stimulation, and variable involvement of the central nervous system. The earliest sign of acute cholinesterase inhibitor poisoning in the dog is increased muscle stretching, an apparent early indication of skeletal muscle involvement. A state of uneasiness or apprehension may also be observed early in the course of the disease. An increase in salivation occurs at this time, but excess saliva may not be apparent because the dog is quite efficient at licking its lips and swallowing the excess secretions.

As the condition progresses, increased skeletal muscle tone becomes more pronounced and may be the only clinical sign observed at this time. The affected animal may walk with a stiff-legged gait, and muscle fasciculations may be observed. At this point urination, defecation, and/or emesis may occur.

In the more advanced stages slobbering may be more evident. The excess saliva, together with increased secretions in the respiratory system, often accounts for coughing and pronounced moist rales. Dyspnea and cyanosis can follow. Hypermotility of the gastrointestinal tract may result in diarrhea and straining. Excessive lacrimation, sweating, miosis, and urinary incontinence can be observed. Hyperactivity of the skeletal muscles is generally followed by muscular paralysis, as the muscles are unable to respond to continued stimulation.

Dogs and cats may exhibit increased central nervous system stimulation, which in some circumstances may lead to tonoclonic convulsive seizures. Many times, however, marked central nervous system depression can be observed.

Death usually results from hypoxia due to excessive respiratory tract secretions, bronchoconstriction, and erratic, slowed heartbeat. The onset of clinical signs in cases of acute poisoning may occur as soon as a few minutes or as late as several hours after exposure. Death can occur in severe poisoning at any time from a few minutes to several hours after the first clinical signs are observed.

NECROPSY LESIONS

Post-mortem lesions associated with acute OP or carbamate toxicosis are usually nonspecific. Excessive fluids in the mouth and respiratory tract as well as pulmonary edema may be observed.

DIAGNOSIS

A history of exposure to OP or carbamate insecticides associated with clinical signs of parasympathetic stimulation warrants a tentative diagnosis of poisoning with these compounds.

Chemical analyses of animal tissues for the presence of insecticides are usually unrewarding because of the rapid degradation of the OP and carbamate insecticides, resulting in low tissue residue levels. However, finding the insecticide in the stomach contents and in the suspect source material can be quite valuable in establishing a diagnosis.

The best method of confirming a diagnosis is to assess the degree of inhibition of cholinesterase enzyme activity in the whole blood and tissue of the suspected animal. A reduction of whole blood cholinesterase activity to less than 25 per cent of the normal is indicative of excessive exposure to these insecticides. Depending on the specific insecticide involved, blood cholinesterase activity in dogs may remain depressed for several days to several weeks following OP exposure. The variability of cholinesterase enzyme activity levels in clinically normal dogs may make interpretation of laboratory values difficult. In addition, it must be remembered that depletion of whole blood cholinesterase activity may not necessarily correlate with inhibition of cholinesterase at the parasympathetic synapses and myoneural junctions. Therefore, whole blood cholinesterase activity should be viewed as only an indication of the status of the cholinesterase enzymes in the body.

The cholinesterase activity can also be measured in brain tissue. The enzyme activity in brain tissue, especially the caudate nucleus, in animals dying from these insecticides will generally be less than 10 per cent of normal brain activity.

Whole blood and brain tissue samples should be well chilled but not frozen for best laboratory results. Samples of stomach contents as well as any suspect material should be submitted to a laboratory for chemical analyses.

TREATMENT

The treatment of animals poisoned by OP and carbamate insecticides should be considered on an emergency basis because of the rapid progression of the clinical syndrome.

Initial treatment for poisoned animals should involve administration of atropine sulfate at a dosage of approximately 0.2 mg/kg of body weight. This initial dose should be divided, and about one-fourth of the dose should be given intravenously and the balance subcutaneously or intramuscularly. Further treatment or handling should be withheld for several minutes or until respiratory distress has been alleviated. Atropine sulfate does not counteract the insecticide-enzyme bond but rather blocks the effects of accumulated acetylcholine at the nerve endings. Although a dramatic cessation of parasympathetic signs is generally observed within a few minutes after administration of atropine, it will not affect the skeletal muscle tremors. Repeated doses of atropine at approximately one-half the initial dose may be required but should be used only to counteract parasympathetic signs. Overatropinization should be avoided.

Orally administered activated charcoal in water slurry is helpful in reducing absorption following ingestion of these insecticides and may in some cases preclude the need for further atropine therapy.

The oximes, such as 2-PAM (Protopam chloride), are drugs that act specifically on the organophosphate-enzyme complex, freeing the enzyme. The oximes may supplement atropine therapy when used relatively early in the course of treatment. 2-PAM should be given either IV or IM at the dosage rate of 20 mg/kg of body weight. *The oximes are of no benefit in treating carbamate toxicosis.*

Dermally exposed animals should be washed with soap and water to prevent continued absorption of these compounds.

Morphine, succinylcholine, and phenothiazine tranquilizers should be avoided in treating OP or carbamate insecticide poisoning.

SUPPLEMENTAL READING

Buck, W. Osweiler, G. D., and Van Gelder, G. A.: *Clinical and Diagnostic Veterinary Toxicology.* Dubuque, Iowa: Kendall-Hunt Publishing Co., 1976.

Clarke, E. G. C., and Clarke, M. L.: *Garner's Veterinary Toxicology.* Baltimore: The Williams & Wilkins, Co., 1967.

Radeleff, R. D.: *Veterinary Toxicology,* 2nd ed. Philadelphia: Lea & Febiger, 1979.

Vestweber, J. G., and Krukenberg, S. M.: The effect of selected organophosphorous compounds on plasma and red blood cell cholinesterase in the dog. Vet. Med. Small Anim. Clin. 67:803, 1972.

SELECTED DRUG TOXICITIES

GEORGE E. BURROWS, D.V.M.

Stillwater, Oklahoma

Many of the drugs used in veterinary medicine have wide margins of safety with little likelihood of toxic reactions occurring. There are, however, a large number of drugs with low margins of safety that, for lack of alternative drugs or economic or other reasons, continue to be widely used. Fortunately in most cases, when indications of toxicity occur, withdrawal of the drug is followed by prompt recovery of the animal from the adverse effects. In a few cases drug toxicity may require therapeutic intervention and rarely may result in death of the animal. Although the frequency of serious adverse reactions that are either life threatening or of serious economic impact is relatively low, the extensive use of many classes of drugs, such as the antibacterials and anthelmintics, makes the occurrence of these reactions very possible. The ready availability of many drugs through retail over-the-counter outlets such as feed and pet stores contributes significantly to the potential for drug intoxication problems.

It is extremely important that individuals using drugs understand the possible side effects and hazards of use. This applies to both veterinarians and lay personnel caring for patients. Toxicity problems may occur by direct drug action or through indirect mechanisms such as an allergic reaction. All drugs should be considered capable of producing an allergic reaction. The expression of an allergic reaction may be quite variable in both the dog and the cat. These responses may range from peracute development of diarrhea, dyspnea, fever, chills, hypothermia, agitation, hyperesthesia, dermal changes, and CNS signs to more delayed dermal responses, anorexia, and depression. Peracute and acute allergic responses are not restricted to the gastrointestinal system in the dog and the respiratory system in the cat. Although these are considered the "shock organs" in these species, other systems may be affected and may present prominent clinical signs. In any such case of serious untoward response to a drug, assessment of the contribution of the drug should be made, with a view toward possible alternative therapy. The penicillins remain one of the most frequent causes of allergic reactions, many of which are serious and should be viewed with concern. Continued administration of a drug in light of some degree of allergic reaction, albeit minor, may produce serious consequences. Treatment of allergic reactions should include epinephrine IV (1:10,000) for acute anaphylaxis and antihistamines, corticosteroids, and/or nonsteroidal anti-inflammatories (e.g., phenylbutazone) as needed for acute or subacute reactions.

The following are summaries of possible reactions associated with various drugs and in some cases may represent only rare and unusual situations. These descriptions are meant only to indicate possible reactions and are not intended to dissuade use of the drugs. In the event a serious adverse reaction to a drug occurs, activated charcoal (Charcodote, Ormond Drug & Chemical) can be given as a nonspecific antidote at a dosage of approximately 1 to 2 gm/kg orally in a water slurry. Charcoal will markedly reduce absorption of many drugs and may also hasten elimination of drugs with a significant enterohepatic cycle such as nonsteroidal anti-inflammatory drugs. Additional information on drug intoxications may be found in the following article and in Section 13.

ANTIBACTERIALS

Aminoglycosides. This group of antibiotics includes dihydrostreptomycin, neomycin, kanamycin, gentamicin, tobramycin, and amikacin. These drugs are well recognized for their toxicity potentials. Most concern in veterinary medicine is focused on the nephrotoxicity potential of neomycin and gentamicin. The remaining four are less toxic, with amikacin the least toxic of all. The effects of these drugs are cumulative, and toxicity may occur with either prolonged use or high dosage. High dosage of gentamicin (10 mg/kg/day) will produce high serum levels and a high risk of nephrotoxicity if used longer than several days. A dosage of 3 to 5 mg/kg/day can be used for a week or longer; however, renal function should be monitored with long-term administration (one week or more). In the presence of pre-existing renal disease, even low dosage may produce clinical problems. This is particularly important because these drugs are excreted almost entirely by glomerular filtration and they may accumulate to high levels in the body when renal function is reduced. The renal tubular damage is reversible provided the animal survives the tubular regeneration period. Ototoxicity is another manifestation of aminoglycoside toxicity except for gentamicin and tobramycin, in which cases vestibular toxicity with incoordination may predominate. This type of toxicity may become irreversible and, in some cases, progressive. These drugs should be used with caution in pregnant animals, since the developing fetus (and the neonate) are very suscep-

tible to the ototoxic effects. Aminoglycosides such as gentamicin should also be used with caution for treatment of otitis externa, since ototoxic effects may occur in the presence of a perforated tympanum.

Parenteral use of any of these drugs may also produce neuromuscular blockade with respiratory paralysis. This condition is complicated by concurrent anesthetic or neuromuscular blocking relaxant use but is reversible with parenteral calcium preparations and/or acetylcholinesterase inhibitors (neostigmine). Aminoglycosides also produce some degree of cardiovascular depression, which in most situations is not clinically important. Oral usage is not accompanied by any significant systemic toxicity owing to very low absorption.

Chloramphenicol. The toxicity potential of this drug has been the subject of much concern because of the rare irreversible bone marrow depression which has been reported in humans. The marrow depression that occurs in dogs is usually mild and reversible and in most cases does not manifest unless the drug is used for several weeks. The marrow depression may be manifest as neutropenia, lymphocytopenia, or a slight reduction in platelet count. Reduced bone marrow cellularity and mitotic index may also be seen. The hematologic problems associated with chloramphenicol appear to be most important in cats, since they have a more limited capacity for hepatic metabolism of the drug. Although the bone marrow depression is considered reversible following discontinuance of the drug, some care should be taken when using it for longer than one week in any species. The more common side effects include anorexia, depression, vomition, and occasionally diarrhea. Some degree of incoordination may also be noted. The anorexia and depression may be quite severe at high dosage. Chloramphenicol use may increase the duration of barbiturate anesthesia, since it inhibits hepatic metabolism of many other drugs.

Chloramphenicol should be used with caution in all young animals, particularly puppies and kittens. In these animals chloramphenicol metabolism may not attain the adult rate for several months. Therefore, the drug sojourn in the body for a given dose may be increased as much as ten times, with a similar increase in toxicity potential—especially severe overall depression.

ANTHELMINTICS

Arsenamide (Caparsolate, thiacetarsamide). This drug is a trivalent arsenous acid derivative that may produce transient early vomiting and anorexia. More serious toxicity is evidenced by persistent vomiting several hours after drug administration. The drug is also potentially nephrotoxic and hepatotoxic, as evidenced by icterus, proteinuria, and elevated SGPT and BUN values in more serious intoxications. As a trivalent arsenical, the drug is capable of producing widespread capillary damage in the body in a manner similar to other arsenicals. A very serious respiratory reaction with polypnea, dyspnea, and collapse may also occur secondary to the lodging of the adult heartworm in the pulmonary vascular bed and the subsequent degeneration thereof.

Bunamidine (Scolaban). The toxic effects of this drug are usually limited by low absorption from the gut as long as the tablets are not crumbled. Most of the drug that is absorbed is cleared by the liver, the primary site of toxicity. Vomiting and transient diarrhea may be seen and rarely some depression of spermatogenesis. The lethal ventricular fibrillation that has been reported is extremely rare and has been associated with exercise stress within a few hours of worming. Therefore, exercise should be avoided for 24 hours following drug administration.

Dichlorophen (Dicestal). Vomiting, diarrhea, and abdominal pain may be associated with this drug. It uncouples oxidative phosphorylation in the tapeworm in a manner similar to niclosamide and may produce some untoward actions of a similar nature at high dosage in mammals (in a manner similar to disophenol; see hereafter).

Dichlorvos (DDVP, Task). This is a well-known organophosphate drug with pronounced cholinergic effects mediated by acetylcholinesterase inhibition. Vomiting in some animals and an increase in gut motility and fecal softening may be seen following normal dosage. More severe signs of intoxication include severe GI dysfunction such as diarrhea, salivation and colic. Additional signs of toxicity may include dyspnea, miosis, muscular fasciculation, severe weakness, and respiratory paralysis. Atropine in high doses (0.2 mg/kg parenterally as needed) alone or in combination with 2-PAM (20 mg/kg IM, b.i.d.) in severe cases is effective therapy. Two anticholinesterase inhibiting drugs should not be used concurrently as they may have additive or greater effects. Inadvertent administration of this drug or other organophosphate or carbamate drugs to microfilaria-infected dogs may result in a severe acute reaction of unknown etiology. The reaction occurs a few minutes to several hours after drug administration and has many symptoms characteristic of intoxication with anticholinesterase inhibitors such as salivation, vomiting, diarrhea, and dyspnea. However, atropine is of limited value as an antidote. The mortality is usually high, with terminal prostration and death occurring within a short time following onset of signs. Pathologic changes include hemorrhagic enteritis and some degree of hepatopathy including necrosis of hepatocytes. Therapy should proceed as for any nonspecific shock-like condition and in addition to atropine should include supportive use of fluids, electrolytes, corticosteroids, and possible nonsteroidal anti-inflammatories such as phenylbutazone or flunixin meglumine (Banamine, Schering).

Diethylcarbamazine (DEC) (Caricide). This is a drug of very low toxicity potential, especially when used at the low heartworm preventative dose. Higher doses may produce some gastric irritation with vomiting. The most serious problems are associated with apparent immune-mediated allergic-type reactions following inadvertent administration to microfilaria-infected dogs, somewhat similar to the reactions seen with organophosphate drugs. In this case the response is accompanied by evidence of disseminated intravascular coagulation (DIC) with an increase in fibrin split products and thrombocytopenia. The reaction occurs within 30 minutes of administration of the drug with clinical signs of a nonspecific shock-like condition with vomiting, salivation, weak pulse, dyspnea, and collapse. Mortality is very high, with death occurring in a few hours. Therapy, which is nonspecific, is similar to that for the preceding organophosphate/microfilaria reaction with the exception of atropine, but results have not been very successful.

Disophenol (DNP). This hookworm medicament may cause some vomiting and occasionally a transient lens opacity. This drug also uncouples oxidative phosphorylation with the resultant production of heat instead of useable energy from metabolism. At elevated dosages it may cause severe hyperthermia, polypnea, dyspnea, polyuria, polydipsia, tachycardia, and tetany. High environmental temperatures or exercise will worsen the condition. Therapy with ice baths, for example, is necessary to reduce the high temperatures. Prostaglandin inhibitors such as aspirin or phenylbutazone will not control the fever. Atropine and phenothiazine sedatives should not be used in therapy.

Dithiazanine Iodide (Dizan). This microfilariacide is well known for causing vomiting, diarrhea, and weakness as well as marked green to purple discoloration of the vomitus and feces. Nephrotoxicity or hepatotoxicity may also occur occasionally.

Drocarbil (Nemural). This is an arecoline (35 per cent) and acetarsone (65 per cent) combination that has the potential to produce either cholinergic alkaloid or arsenical intoxication. The cholinergic alkaloid may cause increased secretions (salivation and so on) and increased gut motility. The primary action is to promote expulsion of the tapeworm and may be associated with excessive diarrhea in some cases. Depression, polypnea, dyspnea, and ataxia may also occur. This drug should not be used in debilitated animals or in those with gastrointestinal, cardiovascular, or respiratory dysfunction. Atropine or related anticholinergic drugs are specific antidotes for the cholinergic effects.

Levamisole. This drug, although not approved

for use in dogs by the FDA, nevertheless remains a widely used microfilariacide in dogs. This nicotine-like drug activates acetylcholine receptors in both the nematode and the host and undergoes rapid hepatic metabolism. The acute toxic effects are similar to those produced by nicotine and include many signs similar to those seen with organophosphate intoxication such as salivation, excitability, increased gastrointestinal motility, and muscular tremors. Pupillary response is variable. In addition, prominent central nervous system and muscular effects may be noted. Fortunately the drug has a short half-life with rapid elimination, thus most side effects, including head shaking, are usually of short duration, subsiding in two to three hours. Anticholinergic drugs such as atropine are only partially effective as antidotes. Severe intoxication with arrhythmias and respiratory difficulties may require the use of a ganglionic blocking agent. If the toxicity progresses to the stage of ganglionic blockade with flaccid paralysis, drugs are useless and respiratory assistance should be given while the drug is metabolized. A preparation for humans, mecamylamine (Inversine, Merck) is the ganglionic blocker of choice. It should be given subcutaneously starting at 1 to 2 mg to effect.

Although there is little or no interaction between levamisole and organophosphates or other acetylcholinesterase inhibitor drugs, there may be potentiation of the toxic effects by pyrantel and perhaps even diethylcarbamazine, both of which may have nicotinic effects. These effects are probably dose related.

Other toxic effects reported rarely include a possible immune-mediated CNS reticuloproliferative disease, thrombocytopenia with hemorrhages and dependent edema, and hemolytic anemia. The hematologic problems occurred in dogs receiving 6 to 12 mg/kg for at least three to four weeks and were reversed with cessation of therapy.

Niclosamide. Some softening of the feces is the only common side effect of this drug, which has a very wide margin of safety. It acts to uncouple oxidative phosphorylation in the tapeworm and may produce similar actions in dogs at very high dosage.

Phthalofyne (Whipcide). Vomition is a common side effect, but more severe effects are unusual. Ataxia and depression occur only with large doses because of the low oral absorption.

Piperazine. This drug is rapidly excreted in the urine and is of low toxicity potential. In large doses it may cause some vomiting and diarrhea. It alters muscular polarization in ascarids, thereby producing flaccid paralysis of the helminth. Large doses may produce mild reversible neurotoxic effects such as transient incoordination.

Pyrantel (Nemex). This is a drug of low toxicity that is rapidly metabolized. It is, however, nicotinic in action and has cholinergic effects in both the nematode and the host. This may result in sweating, polypnea, and incoordination at high dosage. Severe toxicity is related to its nicotinic depolarizing neuromuscular blockade of skeletal muscle, resulting in muscular tremors and fasciculation. Atropine is not an effective antidote for the more severe signs, which are attributable to its predominant nicotinic effects. Effective antagonism requires the use of ganglionic blockers, as in levamisole intoxication, such as mecamylamine.

Thénium (Canopar). Vomition is the primary side effect of this poorly absorbed hookworm medicament. More severe toxicity is rare, but the toxic effects are similar to those of pyrantel and levamisole. High dosage or increased absorption due to gastrointestinal dysfunction may result in signs of excess cholinergic stimulation or a flaccid paralysis. Airedales and collies are reported to be more sensitive to the drug than other dog breeds. Therapy is similar to that for levamisole intoxication.

NONSTEROIDAL ANTI-INFLAMMATORY DRUGS

The gastrointestinal and other problems associated with aspirin are well known, being of greatest severity in cats, which have a more limited ability to metabolize the drug than dogs. Additional drugs that share prostaglandin synthesis inhibition activity with aspirin are also widely available and are often used in treatment of arthritic conditions. This group of drugs, commonly known as nonsteroidal anti-inflammatory drugs, includes phenylbutazone (Butazolidin), flunixin meglumine (Banamine), and meclofenamic acid (Arquel), all available as veterinary drugs. In addition, others such as naproxen (Naprosyn), ibuprofen (Motrin), tolmetin sodium (Tolectin), and sulindac (Clinoril) are available as human drugs.

The apparent common mechanism of action of these drugs is accompanied by one or more common side effects. The most important of these side effects are the gastrointestinal irritation and ulceration that occur. These may result in clinical problems such as vomition, anorexia, depression, diarrhea, abdominal pain, hypoproteinemia, weight loss, and death. The occurrence of persistent vomiting should be taken as an indication for discontinuation of drug use. Chronic intoxication may result in a wasting syndrome similar to protein loss enteropathy. Additionally, bone marrow depression has been described for several of these drugs including aspirin and phenylbutazone. The severe marrow depression (usually regenerative) with its accompanying anemia, neutropenia, and thrombocytopenia after prolonged drug use (weeks) may be manifest as a problem of hemorrhages and secondary infections in the skin, mouth, and so on.

The gastrointestinal toxicity, which is correlated with dosage, is of particular importance in the dog and cat because of the marked enterohepatic circulation of these drugs in these species. Because the drug concentrations in the enterohepatic circulation are higher in dogs and cats than in man, drug dosages cannot be safely extrapolated from man to dogs and cats. In general, dosages should be lower in cats than in dogs.

Treatment of the above disease problems is in general symptomatic and may include fluids (and/or blood), electrolytes, antibiotics, vitamins, iron, intestinal protectants, and soft, highly palatable foods. The last named is very important because while these animals are in poor condition they are very reluctant to eat.

SUPPLEMENTAL READING

Adams, H. R.: Acute adverse effects of antibiotics. J.A.V.M.A. 166:983, 1975.
Atkins, C. E., and Johnson, R. K.: Clinical toxicities of cats. Vet. Clin. North Am. 5:623, 1975.

Garlick, N. L., and Christy, K. E.: Microfiliaria-induced biochemical lesions in heartworm disease of canines. Vet. Human Toxicol. 19:14, 1977.
Hsu, W. H.: Toxicity and drug interactions of levamisole. J.A.V.M.A. 176:1166, 1980.
Kume, S.: Pathogenesis of allergic shock from the use of diethylcarbamazine in canine heartworm disease: A discussion of the current knowledge. In Bradley R. E. (ed.): 1st International Symposium, Canine Heartworm Disease. Gainesville: University of Florida Press, 1970, pp. 7–20.
Palumbo, N. E., Perri, S. F., Desowitz, R. S., Una, S. R., and Read, G. W.: Preliminary observations on adverse reactions to diethylcarbamazine (DEC) in dogs infected with Dirofilaria immites. Proceedings of the 1977 Heartworm Symposium. pp. 97–103.
Rew, R. S.: Mode of action of common anthelmintics. J. Vet. Pharmacol. Ther. 1:183, 1978.
Steel, R. J. S.: Suspected naproxen toxicity in dogs. Austr. Vet. J. 57:100, 1981.
Taylor, L. A., and Crawford, L. M.: Aspirin induced gastrointestinal lesions in dogs. J.A.V.M.A. 152:617, 1968.
Watson, A. D. J.: Further observations on chloramphenicol toxicosis in cats. Am. J. Vet. Res. 41:293, 1980.
Watson, A. D. J., Wilson, J. T., Turner, D. M., and Culvenor, J. A.: Phenylbutazone-induced blood dyscrasias suspected in three dogs. Vet. Rec. 107:239, 1980.
Williams, J. F., and Keahy, K. K.: Sudden death associated with treatment of three dogs with bunamidine HCl. J.A.V.M.A. 168:689, 1976.

ADVERSE DRUG REACTIONS

ARTHUR L. ARONSON, D.V.M.,
and J. EDMOND RIVIERE, D.V.M.

Raleigh, North Carolina

The value and benefit of drugs in modern therapeutics is unquestioned. Yet every pharmacologic substance has the potential to affect some individual patient adversely. Although there is no drug that is completely safe, the justification of using a given drug lies in the favorable ratio of anticipated benefits compared with potential risks.

A veterinarian ideally should be able to make a quantitative benefit-risk assessment for each drug that is used clinically. Although adverse drug reactions (ADRs) have been reported for drugs used clinically in veterinary practice, currently there is no detailed information available on their incidence. Thus it is not possible to make a quantitative benefit-risk assessment.

A brief consideration of ADRs will be made in this review, together with listings of selected ADRs in cats and dogs that have been reported to the Bureau of Veterinary Medicine (BVM) Drug Surveillance Program (Tables 1 and 2). These reports were obtained from BVM memos published since 1975 and updated yearly. In the preparation of these tables, drugs were listed only if they were judged primarily responsible for the ADR (neither drug interactions nor drug reactions secondary to pre-existing disease were included).

WHAT IS AN ADR?

Several definitions of ADRs have been advanced by various groups studying these reactions. It may be useful to consider some of these definitions.

An operational definition used by the Massachusetts General Hospital (Koch-Weser et al., 1969) is "any noxious change in a patient's condition which a physician believes to be due to a drug, which occurs at dosages normally used in man, and which (1) requires treatment, (2) indicates decrease or cessation of therapy with the drug, or (3) suggests that future therapy with the drug carries an unusual risk in this patient." This definition does not include as ADRs any trivial or expected side effects that do not require any change in therapy or noxious events due to deliberate or accidental overdosage.

The World Health Organization definition is similar (Venulet, 1977): "An ADR is one which is noxious and unintended and which occurs at doses used in man for prophylaxis, diagnosis, therapy, or modification of physiological functions."

The Bureau of Veterinary Medicine definition includes lack of drug efficacy as an ADR: "an unintended change in the structure, function and chemistry of the body including injury, toxicity,

Table 1. *Adverse Drug Reactions Reported in Cats*

Drug	Clinical Signs and Lesions
Analgesics	
Acetaminophen	depression, death
Acetaminophen/codeine	restlessness, excitement, fear, mydriasis, death
Aspirin	depression or excitability, ataxia, nystagmus, anorexia, emesis, weight loss, hyperpnea, hepatitis, bone marrow depression, anemia, gastric lesions, death
Phenylbutazone	inappetence, weight loss, alopecia, dehydration, emesis, severe depression, death
CNS Depressants	
Acetyl promazine	prolonged effect, cardiac arrest, hyperactivity, convulsions, death
Ketamine, ketamine/acetyl promazine	anoxia, apnea, hypopnea, ineffective and prolonged recovery, tremors, convulsions, excitement, hyperpyrexia, dyspnea, cardiac arrest, bladder and renal hemorrhage, nephrosis, fatty liver, lung edema, deafness, death
Halothane	cardiac arrest, apnea, shock
Methoxyflurane	ataxia, death
Thiamylal	cardiac arrest, respiratory arrest, apnea, prolonged anesthesia, ataxia, shock, death
Xylazine	prolonged anesthesia, apnea, convulsions
Proparacaine	mydriasis
Antiparasitics	
Bunamidine	seizures, coughing, dyspnea, pulmonary congestion, choking, lethargy, pallor, coma, hypersalivation, anorexia, fever, hypothermia, oral lesion, tongue edema, sudden death
n-Butyl chloride	emesis
Dichlorophene/toluene	ataxia, twitching, seizures, mydriasis, disorientation, posterior weakness, incoordination, hypersalivation, emesis, hyperpnea, tachycardia, death
Dichlorvos	death
Glycobiarsol	emesis, icterus, death
Levamisole	salivation, excitement, diarrhea, mydriasis
Niclosamide	depression, ataxia, hypothermia
Piperazine	emesis, dementia, ataxia, hypermetria, hypersalivation
Hormones	
Megestrol acetate	polyphagia, hydrometra, uterine rupture
Triamcinolone	nervousness, hypersalivation, disorientation, syncope
Antimicrobials	
Ampicillin	diarrhea
Amoxicillin	emesis
Amphotericin B	marked elevation of BUN and serum creatinine following single dose
Cephalexin	emesis, fever
Chloramphenicol	anaphylactoid-type reaction, anorexia, ataxia, emesis, depression, diarrhea, neutropenia, death
Gentamicin	pruritus, alopecia, erythema
Lincomycin	diarrhea, emesis, collapse and coma following IM injection
Tetracycline	malignant hyperthermia, emesis, dehydration
Tylosin	irritation at injection site
Hexachlorophene	anorexia, ataxia
Miconazole	erythema, alopecia
Sulfisoxazole	emesis
Procaine penicillin/dihydrostreptomycin	ataxia
Trimethoprim/sulfadiazine	emesis, hypersalivation, mydriasis, ataxia seizures
Miscellaneous	
Bethanechol	emesis

Table 2. *Adverse Drug Reactions Reported in Dogs*

Drug	Clinical Signs and Lesions
Analgesics	
Aspirin	bleeding disorders
Meclofenamic acid/corticosteroids	diarrhea, gastrointestinal bleeding, death
Phenylbutazone	anemia, leukopenia, thrombocytopenia, emesis, hemorrhagic enteritis, epistaxis, elevated liver enzymes, death
CNS Depressants	
Acetyl promazine	atypical behavior, aggression, apprehension, lameness of injected leg, prolonged effect, respiratory distress, bradycardia, pallor, seizures, syncope, weak irregular pulse, urination, defecation
Fentanyl/droperidol	behavior change, lameness, ataxia, hyperthermia, aggression, seizures, bradycardia, tachycardia, hyperpnea, apnea, tremors, hyperventilation, hyperexcitability, hyperkinesia, nystagmus, cardiac arrest, prolonged recovery, death
Ethylisobutrazine	hyperexcitability
Halothane	cardiac arrhythmia, malignant hyperthermia, nystagmus, torticollis, emesis
Ketamine	convulsions, cyanosis
Lidocaine	laryngeal and facial edema, respiratory arrest, seizures, ataxia, tremors
Methoxyflurane	cardiac arrest, hepatitis after 2 weeks, death
Oxymorphone	bradycardia
Prochlorperazine/isopropamide	tachycardia
Promazine	depression, hypotension, hyperthermia, death
Thiamylal	cardiac arrest, respiratory arrest, prolonged anesthesia, cyanosis, apnea, cardiac arrhythmias, bradycardia, temporary hearing loss, prolonged recovery, death
Thiopental	cardiac arrest, prolonged recovery, pulmonary edema, slough at injection site, death
Xylazine	viciousness, bradycardia, cardiac arrest, death
Anticonvulsants	
Phenytoin	ataxia, hepatotoxicity, leukopenia, emesis, coma, death
Primidone	liver failure, icterus, emesis, alopecia, polydipsia, polyuria, death
Antiparasitics	
Arecoline/tetrachlorethylene	mydriasis, ataxia, emesis, diarrhea, severe colic, inability to walk, depression, hypothermia
Bunamidine	dyspnea, ataxia, emesis, weakness, bloat, gastroenteritis, lung hemorrhage, seizures, sudden death
Butamisole	dyspnea, ataxia, muscle tremors, collapse, coma, depression, icterus, swelling at injection site, abscess formation, death
n-Butyl chloride	stupor, ataxia, death
Dichlorophene/toluene	incoordination, convulsions, emesis, disorientation, mydriasis, lethargy, anorexia, fever, death
Dichlorvos	diarrhea, emesis, ataxia, tremors, weakness, death
Diethylcarbamazine	pruritus, weakness, emesis, diarrhea, icterus, anaphylactoid reaction, death
Diethylcarbamazine/styrylpyridinium	diarrhea, emesis, sterilization, teratogenesis, death
Disophenol	hyperthermia, hyperventilation, ataxia, collapse, dyspnea, respiratory distress, swelling at injection site, death
Dithiazine iodide	emesis, diarrhea, depression, apprehension, hyperpyrexia, anorexia, lethargy, death
Glycobiarsol	emesis
Levamisole	dyspnea, pulmonary edema, emesis
Mebendazole	icterus, emesis, anorexia, diarrhea, lethargy, abnormal liver function tests, hepatotoxicity, death
Piperazine	paralysis, death
Metronidazole	lethargy, rear limb weakness
Phthalofyne	hepatitis, splenitis, ataxia, death
Pyrantel pamoate	emesis
Ronnel	emesis, twitching, depression
Thenium closylate	emesis, diarrhea, enteritis, anaphylaxis, hemorrhagic enteritis and liver, seizures, dyspnea, cyanosis, death
Thiacetarsamide	emesis, icterus, bilirubinuria, elevated liver enzymes, depression, anorexia, cough, renal failure, swelling at injection site, alopecia, dermatitis, bleeding disorders, death
Toluene	collapse
Trichlorfon	anorexia, weakness, lethargy
Uredofos	emesis, diarrhea, death
Hormones	
Betamethasone	shock, polydipsia, polyuria
Dexamethasone	polydipsia, polyuria, emesis, diarrhea, bloody diarrhea, melena, panting

Table 2.   *Adverse Drug Reactions Reported in Dogs (Continued)*

Drug	Clinical Signs and Lesions
Prednisolone	anorexia, polyphagia, pica, anemia, lethargy, diarrhea, polyuria, elevated liver enzymes
Methylprednisolone	disorientation, panting
Triamcinolone	Cushing's syndrome, emesis, depression, urticaria, dyspnea, seizures, shock
Estradiol cypionate	pain at injection site, pyometra
Megestrol acetate	polyphagia, hydrometra, uterine inertia, uterine rupture, anorexia, depression, death
Mibolerone	elevated liver function tests, icterus, vaginal discharge, behavioral changes, urinary incontinence
Antimicrobials	
Amoxicillin	skin rash, emesis
Ampicillin	wheals, injection site inflammation, emesis, diarrhea
Bacitracin/polymyxin B/neomycin (ophthalmic)	eye irritation
Cephalexin	panting, salivation, hyperexcitability
Chloramphenicol	emesis, depression, ataxia, diarrhea, death
Gentamicin	injection site inflammation, edema of lips, eyelids, and vulva; elevated BUN
Hetacillin	emesis
Lincomycin	emesis, soft stools, diarrhea, shock after IM injection, death
Nitrofurantoin	emesis
Potassium penicillin G	increased respiration and heart rate
Procaine penicillin G	ataxia, edema, dyspnea
Procaine and benzathine penicillin G	sterile abscess, anaphylaxis
Sulfachlorpyridazine	ataxia, hyperirritability
Sulfaguanidine	keratoconjunctivitis
Sulfamerazine/sulfapyridine	emesis, dyspnea
Tetracycline	emesis
Trimethoprim/sulfadiazine	emesis, diarrhea, anorexia, icterus, elevated liver function tests, bilateral keratoconjunctivitis
Trimethoprim/sulfamethoxazole	facial edema, depression
Miscellaneous	
Aminopropazine	injection site necrosis
Aminophylline	emesis, anorexia, polyphagia, polydipsia, polyuria, hyperexcitability
Asparaginase	ataxia, muscle weakness, lethargy
Atropine	paradoxical bradycardia, heart block
Calcium edetate	emesis, diarrhea, anorexia, depression
Copper naphthenate (topical)	skin burns
Dichlorphenamide	disorientation
Dinoprost tromethamine	panting, hypersalivation, discomfort, emesis
Digoxin	emesis, anorexia
Epinephrine/pilocarpine (ophthalmic)	conjunctivitis
Ibuprofen	depression, emesis, gastric ulcers, death
Metrizamide	seizures after myelogram
Neostigmine/physostigmine (ophthalmic)	emesis, diarrhea, bradycardia, pannus
Neostigmine methyl sulfate	apnea, cardiac arrest, death
Pyridostigmine	diarrhea, emesis
Sulfurated lime (topical)	skin burns, edema, dehydration
Theophylline	diarrhea

sensitivity reaction, or lack of efficacy associated with the clinical use of a drug."

Causes of ADRs.   ADRs associated with specific drugs are listed in Tables 1 and 2. Two basic causes of ADRs are *excessive drug use,* and *failure to establish a therapeutic endpoint.* It has been shown in several studies that the frequency of ADRs increases as the number of drugs used concurrently in a patient increases. These ADRs may or may not be due to drug interactions. Human patients receive an average of 14 different drugs during a normal stay in the hospital. The isolation and identification of an ADR for a specific drug in this situation is nearly impossible. Also, a toxic endpoint, if not predefined, may occur when toxicity is an extension of the pharmacologic action of a drug. For example, the maximal contractile force obtainable with digitalis glycosides occurs before alterations in cardiac conduction. ADRs to digitalis glycosides could be minimized by selecting improvement in hemodynamics or renal function as the therapeutic endpoint rather than changes in cardiac conduction or the onset of emesis. Failure to establish a therapeutic endpoint also may render it difficult to recognize lack of efficacy, and a useless but potentially toxic drug will continue to be given.

Recognition of ADRs. There are no unique clinical or laboratory findings that distinguish ADRs from the manifestations of concurrent disease. Thus, an accurate identification of an ADR often is difficult. An alert and suspicious clinician is of the utmost importance. It may be difficult to think of one's treatment as being responsible for the patient's disability. One should expect the unexpected. A suspicious reaction should not be dismissed because it is not described in a pharmacology textbook or on a drug package insert. ADRs may go largely undetected if the clinical signs they induce are indistinguishable from those of common disease syndromes. Drugs that induce a complex of rare clinical signs will attract more attention and will be identified, an example being chloramphenicol-induced aplastic anemia in humans or the teratogenic effects of griseofulvin in queens.

Comparisons of ADR evaluations among experienced observers reveal that the clinical identification of ADRs is complex and subjective. It is difficult to prove a cause-and-effect relationship, and there are differences in the subjective evaluations among individual investigators. The difficulties are compounded when combinations of drugs are administered to a patient.

Nevertheless, everyone does agree that ADRs do occur. The following guidelines may be helpful in identifying an ADR.

1. There is a plausible temporal relationship between administration of the drug and the ADR. Clinical signs develop while the drug is being taken. For example, if a patient goes into anaphylactic shock ten minutes following the injection of penicillin G, there is a strong likelihood that an ADR occurred. It must be remembered that some ADRs may occur long after the drug is administered. The occurrence of cervical cancer in teenaged girls whose mothers took diethylstilbestrol during pregnancy is a case in point.

2. There is improvement in the clinical syndrome when the drug is discontinued.

3. The ADR recurs if the patient is re-exposed to the drug.

Minimizing ADRs. Information relating to the frequency with which ADRs occur with drugs in clinical use would be most helpful. This would require a drug monitoring and reporting system that would document the frequency, kinds, and causes of ADRs to a specific drug in relation to the total use of the drug. A clinician then would have a basis for determining the possible benefits of a drug compared with its possible harmful effects under a given set of conditions. A study by Ndiritu and Enos (1977) involved a review of 39,541 cases presented to the University of California Veterinary Medical Teaching Hospital. Of these, 130 suspected ADRs were detected and 66 of these had sufficient data available to specifically identify the drug in-

volved. The following classes of drugs were involved (number of cases): anti-infective agents (21), antineoplastic agents (10), anesthetics and related drugs (20), cardiovascular drugs (2), ophthalmologic preparations (5), and miscellaneous drugs (8). Only four deaths were directly attributed to ADRs. It is worthwhile to emphasize that all drugs possess the potential for producing an ADR and that a drug should not be used unless there is a clearly defined therapeutic objective.

CLASSES OF ADRs

Side Effects. Side effects of drugs may be considered ADRs in that they lead to actions that are undesirable but inherent to the drug's action. For example, mydriasis produced when atropine is used as a preanesthetic is undesirable, but it must be accepted along with the desired tachycardia and decreased salivation, since atropine blocks muscarinic receptors nonselectively throughout the body. Similarly, anticancer drugs, by virtue of their ability to affect rapidly proliferating neoplastic tissues, also adversely affect normal tissues with rapid cell turnover, such as in the gastrointestinal mucosa and hematopoietic tissues. For the most part, ADRs related to side effects are predictable and expected, unlike the following classes of ADRs.

Disruption of Control Mechanisms. Two classes of drugs have a clearly established potential for disrupting control mechanisms in the body. Suprainfection has been associated with intensive antibacterial drug therapy, particularly when broad spectrum drugs or combinations of antibacterial drugs are used. Reduced resistance to infection and activation of latent infection have been associated with adrenocorticosteroids, especially during prolonged administration.

Drug Allergy. Certain ADRs have an immunologic basis. These types of reactions require previous exposure and sensitization to the drug. These drugs combine with protein, and antibodies are formed to the drug-protein complex. Subsequent exposure to the drug leads to a typical antigen-antibody reaction with the release of pathologic mediators (histamine, serotonin, bradykinin, and so on), which are responsible for inducing the pathologic effects. Although virtually any body system may be affected, ADRs of this type usually are manifested as abnormalities of the respiratory tract (rhinitis, asthma) and the skin (urticaria, hives) or as generalized systemic reactions (anaphylactic shock, interstitial nephritis). Penicillin and aspirin are examples of drugs that have been implicated in inducing these types of ADRs in humans. Drug allergies, although they undoubtedly occur, are not well documented in domestic animals.

Predisposition Due to Patient Status. Age, species, and concurrent disease can predispose a patient to an ADR. Very young as well as aged animals are more susceptible to ADRs than are middle-aged animals. Several weeks are required for a neonate to approach the capability of a young adult in drug biotransformation. The dosage schedule for drugs requiring drug biotransformation must be reduced in neonates, particularly if the drug has a high potential for producing toxicity. Chloramphenicol is an example of a drug requiring biotransformation, and it has the potential for producing bone marrow depression. The gray baby syndrome has resulted when the appropriate reductions in the adult dosage schedule of chloramphenicol were not made for human neonates.

There is very little information available on drug disposition in neonatal dogs and cats. As a consequence, drugs should be used sparingly and with caution in these groups. Another factor predisposing neonates to adverse drug effects is undeveloped renal and hepatic excretory mechanisms. As with drug biotransformation, several weeks are required for the excretory mechanisms of the neonate to become fully functional. Degeneration of organ function resulting in excessive drug accumulation may predispose older animals to ADRs. In humans, the risk of ADRs in patients over 60 years of age is about double that in young adults.

Veterinarians have long recognized that cats are more sensitive to many drugs than any other species. Some reasons for this include the following:

1. A slower rate of biotransformation for many drugs. Cats also cannot conjugate drugs with glucuronic acid because they have deficient glucuronyl transferase activity, a critical enzyme in this reaction.

2. Cats exhibit unusual receptor-site sensitivity to many drugs. For example, reserpine produces sedation, which persists for a week in cats, whereas a two-day period of tranquilization is characteristic of other species. Morphine, in high doses, produces excitation in cats, whereas sedation is characteristic in most other species.

3. The RBC of cats appears to be more susceptible to oxidative damage. Methemoglobinemia and Heinz bodies result.

4. The grooming habits of cats facilitate the ingestion of any substance falling on their fur. Thus, cats are likely to receive a larger internal dose than would other species of any substance being used in the area in the form of an aerosol or dust.

Concurrent disease can enhance the possibility of ADRs in several ways. Disease conditions characterized by depressed renal and/or liver function, dehydration, or acidosis may result in higher concentrations of drug in the body than would be expected following conventional drug doses. When the organ (kidney, liver) primarily involved in a

drug's elimination is diseased, dosage should be decreased in direct proportion to decreased function as described in the section "Checklist of Hazardous Drugs in Patients with Renal Failure." Shifts in the acid-balance associated with disease may alter the degree of ionization of the drug, which could affect its partitioning across biologic membranes, its degree of serum or tissue protein binding, or its rate of elimination from the body.

Drug Interactions. An ADR may stem from the concurrent use of another drug. These ADRs may occur either outside or within the body. Other possible interacting "drugs" include food additives, environmental contaminants, insecticides, and other exogenous chemicals or xenobiotics.

The practice of mixing drugs together in the same syringe or infusion solution prior to injection is risky, as the resultant mixture may be incompatible. Some drug incompatibilities include the inactivation of aminoglycoside antibiotics (e.g., gentamicin, kanamycin) by semisynthetic penicillins and the inactivation of penicillin G by solutions of high or low pH or those that contain vitamin B complex vitamins with vitamin C. It should be kept in mind that many drugs can alter the results of laboratory tests. Specimens should be taken for laboratory analysis before drugs are given to the patient.

A number of drug interactions can occur that involve the pharmacokinetic phase of drug action (e.g., absorption, distribution, biotransformation, and excretion) as well as the action at drug receptor sites. Some illustrative examples follow.

Tetracycline reacts with divalent metals to form insoluble complexes. The coadministration of Kaopectate, milk, or iron preparations has been shown to reduce markedly the intestinal absorption of tetracycline. When tetracycline and metal-containing preparations are administered orally, they should be given at least two hours apart.

Some drugs are potent inhibitors of the biotransformation of other drugs, including pentobarbital and phenytoin (Dilantin) in several species. Dogs remained anesthetized two times longer and cats three times longer when a therapeutic dose of chloramphenicol was given at the same time as phenobarbital. Signs of phenytoin toxicity (including ataxia, tremors, and incoordination) have been precipitated in dogs when chloramphenicol therapy was instituted to treat a concurrent infection. Signs of toxicity abated when the dosage of phenytoin was reduced by half.

Some drugs are potent stimulators of the biotransformation of other drugs. Phenobarbital has been shown to enhance the biotransformation of many drugs in several species. Phenobarbital has been reported to enhance the rate of biotransformation of digoxin in dogs. If these drugs are given together, more digoxin may be required to digitalize the dog. An ADR from digoxin could arise if the administration of phenobarbital ceased and the dosage of digoxin remained the same.

Finally, some drugs are capable of displacing other drugs from serum albumin binding sites with resultant increased biologic activity of the displaced drug. An example is the displacement of coumarin by some sulfonamide or salicylate, the result being an increased anticoagulant activity.

Human Errors. An adverse response resulting from human error perhaps should not be considered an ADR because the reaction may be expected to occur under the circumstances. Nevertheless, some human errors that can result in adverse responses include (1) dosage error due to miscalculation, (2) inappropriate route of administration, for example, a suspension designed for intramuscular or subcutaneous administration may produce a fatal embolism if administered intravenously, and (3) excessive rate of administration by the intravenous route, for example, meperidine can produce a fatal hypotensive collapse if a therapeutic dose is given by rapid intravenous administration. Meperidine, as with many drugs that are organic bases, is capable of effecting a rapid release of histamine in the body.

REFERENCES AND SUPPLEMENTAL READING

Jick, H.: The discovery of drug induced illness. N. Engl. J. Med. 296:481, 1977.

Koch-Weser, J., Sidel, V. W., Sweet, R. H., Kanarek, P., and Eaton, A. E.: Factors determining physical reporting of adverse drug reactions. Comparison of 2000 spontaneous reports with surveillance studies at the Massachusetts General Hospital. N. Engl. J. Med. 280:20, 1969.

Miller, R. R., and Greenblatt, D. T. (eds.): *Drug Effects in Hospitalized Patients.* New York: John Wiley and Sons, 1976.

Ndiritu, C. G., and Enos, L. R.: Adverse reactions to drugs in a veterinary hospital. J.A.V.M.A. 171:335, 1977.

Venulet, J.: Methods of monitoring adverse reactions to drugs. Prog. Drug Res. 21:231, 1977.

DEVELOPMENTAL AND GENETIC TOXICOLOGY

(Teratogenesis and Mutagenesis)

NORMAN R. SCHNEIDER, D.V.M.

Lincoln, Nebraska

Birth defects are a very real, unavoidable fact of life for both physician and practicing veterinarian. In the human population, birth defects have disastrous consequences for involved families and profound implications for society in general in terms of treatment and maintenance of afflicted individuals. This fact was thrust into worldwide perception two decades ago when the drug thalidomide, introduced as a treatment for anxiety in pregnant women, led to the birth of approximately 10,000 severely malformed children. Chemical agents are not unique in their ability to induce birth defects. The atomic explosions that successfully brought World War II to an end also exposed a large civilian population in Japan to high levels of intense ionizing radiation. The toll of genetic damage caused by this radiation was great and continues to grow. Another important cause of human birth defects is exposure of the pregnant mother to certain viral agents. Rubella infections in the first trimester of pregnancy have been responsible for a variety of congenital defects, frequently including blindness, deafness, and valvular heart lesions.

The same factors that adversely affect unborn offspring in the human population have the potential to induce similar genetic damage in the young of the family pet, whatever species it may be. It is hoped that birth defects in offspring of pets will not be due to inappropriate prenatal care, whether accidental or intentional. With normal precautions, it is unlikely that an animal could be exposed to and subsequently affected by the vast majority of potentially harmful agents, yet the hazard still exists. Every precaution should be taken to minimize the potential for inducing damaged offspring, since these can impose a difficult moral and ethical quandary to both the clinician and the owner. It is much easier to prevent developmental defects than to treat them post partum. Consequently, veterinary practitioners need to be aware of the etiologies and sequelae of abnormal development.

It is the express goal of this article to provide a current review of agents that have the potential to produce developmental or genetic defects in small animals, especially those species frequently seen in clinicial situations. The emphasis here is on information pertinent to dogs and cats. However, since laboratory animals are frequently maintained as pets, especially in urban areas where maintenance of larger animals is not feasible, data relating to rodents, lagomorphs, and primates are also included. Interspecies and intraspecies differences in metabolism and physiology make it highly unlikely that effects observed in one species can be presumed to occur in all untested species. Interspecies extrapolation of observed congenital deformities should be avoided, bearing in mind the possibility that an agent teratogenic in one species can be teratogenic in other species as well.

CURRENT CONCEPTS OF TERATOGENESIS AND GENETIC TOXICOLOGY

Teratology is the study of prenatal developmental abnormalities in structure or function that are related to the effects of intrinsic or extrinsic factors. Teratogens are those agents that can induce or increase the incidence of congenital maldevelopment when administered to or acting on the pregnant animal. These factors can be physical, nutritional, hereditary, chemical (including drugs and environmental pollutants), infectious, or metabolic (physiologic). Each of these factors will be discussed in this article.

Teratogenic changes are defined by some traditionalists to be only *generative* changes in development that are limited to the period of organogenesis. Developmental changes that occur during other periods of gestation are defined as toxicologic (rather than teratogenic) changes and are considered *degenerative*, since they affect biologic systems that are already partially or completely formed. Additionally, *in utero* deaths and resorptions are not regarded as specific teratogenic effects. Other experts in this field have promoted the broader concept of *developmental toxicology* and contend that exposure to potentially deleterious agents during the complete span of development can produce several different toxic effects on the developing conceptus, such as embryonic or perinatal death, structural malformations, growth retardation, postnatal functional or behavioral abnormality, and congenital neoplasia. This total concept of *embryotoxicity* includes, but is not limited to, teratogenic effects. It encompasses all various toxic effects mentioned previously.

Genetic disease is caused when errors occur in transmitting genetic material during cell division. Some investigators use the term "mutagenesis" in designating all genetic defects. A current and perhaps more accurate concept is to classify genetic lesions based on the molecular level of error in the transmission of genetic information. This classification system includes at least three separate modes of genetic failure that define specific structural changes in the cellular genetic complemenet: *mutagenesis, clastogenesis,* and *aneuploidization.*

Mutagenesis—specifically, mutations—involves chemical alterations in the DNA sequence within a gene only as gene-locus mutations or point mutations. Other investigators consider a mutation as *any* heritable macromolecular or micromolecular change in genetic material. *Clastogenesis* is genetic change that involves rearrangement, gain, or loss of pieces of chromosomes which may be microscopically visualized. Clastogenesis is alternately called *chromosomal mutation* by some scientists. *Aneuploidization* is gain or loss of one or more intact chromosomes.

Genetic defects can occur in any somatic or germ cell. Somatic defects are not transmitted but may result in neoplasia or teratogenesis. If the capacity for cellular division is unimpaired, germinal defects may be transmitted to descendant cells. Genetic changes may be so severe that cells involved will die. Results of genetic change are usually undesirable and may include embryonic death, abortion, congenital anomaly, genetic disease, lowered resistance to disease, decreased life span, infertility, behavioral aberration, and carcinogenesis.

Very few agents, and only a very limited number of the many therapeutic substances, have been demonstrated to be genetically active in animals. However, it behooves us as veterinarians to be aware of how heritable change in genetic material occurs, the agents that have the potential to induce genetic expression, and the possible consequences of genetic defects on animal health and breed characteristics. High neonatal mortality may result from inbreeding and may be caused by a recessive gene in homozygous offspring. The lethal factor may be perpetuated by the heterozygote. The X chromosome of dogs is thought to be the transmission site of familial amaurotic idiocy, hemophilia A and B, subluxation of the carpus, and cystinuria. In dogs, malformation of the mouth producing abnormal dentition usually occurs in toy breeds, especially those that are brachycephalic. Miniature poodles extensively inbred for color selection produced litters in which all the puppies exhibited dysgnathia, with severely undershot mandibles.

Some agents that cause genetic defects are also potential teratogens. However, there is not a high degree of correlation between teratogenicity and genetic expression. This may be related to the way these events are initiated in the biologic system. Adverse genetic activity implies action on a single cell, whereas teratogenesis requires interference with differentiation of many cells during organogenesis. However, teratogenic expression can result from, or can be accentuated by, genetically related events. For example, the urinary system is most frequently involved in autosomal chromosomal disorders in man. All known malformations of the urinary system in humans are observed in children with chromosomal diseases, except for infantile polycystic kidney, medullary spongy kidney, and embryonal nephroma.

There are a number of considerations in the teratogen-conceptus interaction that affect the actual production of terata in animals. Primary among these is that susceptibility of the unborn to teratogens or embryotoxic agents varies with (and depends on) gestational age at time of exposure. There are roughly three critical periods of development between conception and parturition: (1) the predifferentiation period prior to germ layer formation (pregastrulation stage), (2) the period of early differentiation and organogenesis (embryonic stage), and (3) the period of advanced organogenesis (fetal stage).

During the pregastrulation period, the mammalian conceptus is relatively refractory to teratogenesis. At this stage, all undifferentiated cells would be expected to react to a teratogenic agent in similar fashion. If the exposure affects a large enough portion of the cellular population, embryotoxicity rather than overt teratogenicity would be manifested, either as embryolethality or growth retardation. Prior to implantation, high concentrations of teratogenic or embryotoxic agents may also inhibit placentation, resulting in resorption of the zygote and cessation of pregnancy. Resorption of the developing organism from the uterus may simulate pregnancy. A 5 per cent fetal resorption rate after implantation is normal in dogs, but the causes of intrauterine deaths are not usually determined. Embryotoxic agents may not interfere with formation of the placenta, but they can still exert their effects.

Embryonic development is the period of greatest prenatal vulnerability to teratogenic agents. Mitotically active cells are uniquely susceptible to insult. This embryonic stage begins with implantation and germ layer differentiation and continues through organogenesis and the beginning of histogenesis. Organogenesis occurs at varying times during gestation, depending on the animal species (Table 1). Early in this period, the greater the teratogenic insult, the more likely that the effect will be manifested as embryolethality and resorption of the conceptus rather than by overt teratogenesis, especially if occurring soon after implantation and placentation. Embryos surviving the teratogenic insult are easily deformed and have the highest frequency of structural defects. Susceptibility to both teratogenicity and embryolethality declines as organogenesis advances. However, both types of responses can still occur if the insult is severe. Critical periods of increased sensitivity to harmful influences are also known to occur during relatively late stages of organ system development, and repeated exposure over the entire period of organogenesis may result in multiple malformations.

During the fetal stage of development, resistance

Table 1. *Organogenesis and Gestation in Various Mammals*

Species	Approximate Period of Organogenesis (Days)*	Average Duration of Gestation (Days)
Hamster	5–14	16–17
Mouse	5–16	19–21
Rat	6–17	21–23
Rabbit	6–20	30–32
Guinea Pig	6–25	65–68
Ferret	10–?	40–43
Pig	10–34	110–116
Sheep	10–35	145–152
Cat	10–30	60–65
Dog	13–30	58–63
Monkey (rhesus)	9–45	164–170
Baboon	9–47	172–178

*Implantation is considered the start of organogenesis for this compilation.

to teratogens and embryotoxic agents increases. Histogenesis, which began late in the embryonic stage, continues in the fetal stage to convert primordial organs into definitive ones through cellular and tissue differentiation. Functional activity and maturation continually progress throughout the fetal period. As embryos differentiate into fetuses, maldevelopment manifested by gross structural defects is less likely to occur, except in those structures undergoing growth and maturation, such as the palate, cerebellum, and some cardiovascular and urogenital structures. The effects of maldevelopment on structure may be detectable at only the microscopic level and may not be recognized in surviving young until well into the juvenile period, when behavioral and functional abnormalities such as learning and reproductive difficulties arise. The etiology of functional or behavioral aberrations may be due to interference with ongoing histogenesis or to prevention of final functional maturation. However, it is not always possible to determine which pathway was responsible.

A dose-response relationship prevails for teratogenic and embryotoxic effects just as it does for other toxic effects. Usually, there exists a relatively limited dose range in which terata are produced. Exposure above this teratogenic zone may result in embryolethality rather than congenital anomalies, and dosages below this zone are without detectable effect. Dosages within the upper limits of the embryolethal zone may also cause maternal death with the same dose-response relationship. The greater the dosage range over which terata are observed without death occurring, the more likely it is that a clearly graded response to the insult will result. If an agent is teratogenic over only a very limited dosage range and embryolethal above it, the teratogenic response may even appear all-or-none in character. The dosage below which no adverse effects are apparent is called the *no-effect dosage* or the *threshold dosage*. Even though no discernible effects occur at sub-threshold dosages, this may mean that damage has occurred but has subsequently been repaired. It may also mean that the biologic system can maintain homeostasis without repair. A reversible defect is defined as a *variation;* whereas *malformations* are those defects that are irreversible in the biologic system. As long as the final product does not differ appreciably from the usual product, no effects from the insult will be detected. Dosages of 1/10 to 1/100 of the threshold dosage are generally acceptable safety limits for exposure.

Teratogenic agents are thought to act via specific mechanisms on developing cells to cause abnormal development. A mechanism includes the entire series of events between a cause and an effect. Not all mechanisms that act to produce an abnormal offspring are clearly understood. However, mutation, metabolic changes, enzymatic inhibition, and other biochemical alterations are some of the cellular reactions thought to initiate events that culminate in developmental abnormalities. Pathogenesis of prenatal damage may be initiated by damage or destruction of primordial or precursor cells, which may subsequently result in failure of further development of an organ, tissue, or system. Secondary effects may be manifested in other organs or systems—CNS damage may cause failure of neurotropic stimuli and further result in failure of proper muscle, bone, and joint formation. Death, malformation, growth retardation, and functional disorders are the final manifestations of abnormal development.

Susceptibility to teratogenesis also depends on the animal genotype and the nature of the influencing agent. The same determinants that differentiate individuals, strains, and species in normal structure and function may also give varying degrees of sensitivity to deleterious influences. These factors include differences in metabolism, placentation, and morphology. They are related to both the host and the nature of the agent iself. There are only two ways in which an extrinsic factor can reach a developing conceptus to exert its influence: it can traverse the maternal body by direct penetration through organs and tissues (such as ionizing radiation), or it can be transmitted through it indirectly via the blood stream or other body channels (such as chemicals or infectious agents). Agents indirectly transmitted through the maternal body generally reach the conceptus in some fraction of the original concentration, the exact value of which is dependent on route of administration, absorption, metabolism, and resultant pharmacokinetics.

POTENTIAL CAUSES OF CONGENITAL MALDEVELOPMENT

GENERAL CONSIDERATIONS

The understanding of developmental and genetic toxicology should be related to one common goal, initiating and completing the gestational period with a minimum of risk to both the mother and her offspring, culminating in the delivery of normal, healthy neonates. This is true for both veterinary practitioners and the clients served. Relatively few agents are known to cause maldevelopment in dogs and cats, especially under other than experimental conditions. Agents shown to produce mammalian maldevelopment are usually administered under experimental conditions at higher dosages or exposures than would be normally expected, and species most often utilized are rodents and lagomorphs. Although the mutagenic, teratogenic, or embryotoxic effects of many of these agents have not been demonstrated beyond reasonable doubt, neither has adequate proof of their safety. Whereas predictive extrapolation between mammalian species is difficult at best, these agents still have demonstrated the potential to produce congenital defects in at least one species and should be managed accordingly.

HEREDITY

Since dogs, cats, and other companion animals inhabit an environment similar to that of their owners, they also share similar threats to their genetic health. Impaired genetic health can be caused by inheritance of genetic and chromosomal aberrations resulting from adverse genetic effects. Ionizing radiation is a potent mammalian mutagen, but a great number of suspected mutagens are found in the environment in addition to ionizing radiation.

The following agents have been tested for genetic effects and are referenced in the files of the Environmental Mutagen Information Center (EMIC) at the Oak Ridge National Laboratory. The presence of agents in this listing indicates *suspected,* not confirmed, mutagenicity. Although agents may belong to more than one category, they are listed only once for convenience.

AGENTS WITH SUSPECTED GENETIC ACTIVITY

1. **Agricultural chemicals.** This category is subdivided into various types of pesticides currently in use that are suspected of having mutagenic potential.

Herbicide	Fungicide	Insecticide	Chemosterilant	Rodenticide
2,4-D	cycloheximide	formaldehyde	triethylenemelamine	aminopterin

Herbicide	Fungicide	Insecticide	Chemosterilant
2,4,5-T	ethylene oxide	DDT	TEPA
	captan	dieldrin	metepa
	ethylene bromide	endrin	apholate
			hempa

2. **Industrial compounds and environmental pollutants.** These compounds have industrial application and are also released during the processing and combustion of fossil fuels.

dimethylnitrosamine	methylcholanthrene	Hg-, Pb-, and Cd-contain-
ethylenimine	benzene	ing compounds
benzo(a)pyrene	1,2-benzanthracene	

3. **Food additives.** These substances are intentionally added to foods during processing. However, residues (nonintentional additives) from other categories may also be present in animal diets.

sodium nitrite (nitrous acid)	EDTA
sodium cyclamate	sodium bisulfite

4. **Naturally occurring substances.** Coumarin is a plant alkaloid, found in sweet clover, that has anticoagulant properties. Aflatoxin B_1 is an extremely potent mycotoxin that is a metabolite of *Aspergillus flavus*, which is found as a contaminant of cereal grains and other foodstuffs.

5. **Drugs.** Compounds having a known use in veterinary medicine that were tested for genetic effects are listed below. Many of these are antibiotics and antineoplastic agents that have the ability to interfere with or suppress cellular function.

Drug	Use
caffeine	stimulant
colchicine	antineoplastic agent
actinomycin D	antibiotic
cyclophosphamide	antineoplastic agent
ethidium bromide	antiparasitic agent
urethane	anesthetic
hydrogen peroxide	topical antiseptic
cystosine arabinoside	antineoplastic agent
ethylene oxide	sterilizing surgical instruments
streptomycin	antibiotic
vincristine	antineoplastic agent
theophylline	muscle relaxant, diuretic, myocardial stimulant
hexachlorophene	bacteriocidal soap, antitrematodal agent
methylene blue	diagnostic dye, cyanide antidote
dichlorvos	antiparasitic agent
adriamycin	antileukemic agent
chlorpromazine	tranquilizer, antiemetic
carbaryl	antiparasitic agent
mercury chloride	disinfectant
griseofulvin	antifungal, antibiotic
phenylbutazone	analgesic, antipyretic
urea	antiseptic
lead acetate	astringent
erythromycin	antibiotic
gamma-lindane	scabicide, antiparasitic agent
dieldrin	antiparasitic agent
phenobarbital	sedative, anticonvulsant
mustard oil	counterirritant

6. **Biologic agents.** Viruses are capable of inducing genetic injury as well as potentiating damage induced by other agents. A large number of viral agents of importance to human medicine have been suspected of having genetic activity. Of these, the measles virus may be of some concern in veterinary medicine, since it is utilized in the immunization of dogs against canine distemper. The use of measles vaccine is contraindicated in breeding bitches.

RADIATION AND OTHER PHYSICAL AGENTS

Radiation can be either ionizing or nonionizing. Ionizing radiation is one of the most teratogenic agents known. Sources of ionizing radiation commonly utilized in veterinary medicine are x-rays and radioisotopes. The classic triad of radiation embryologic syndromes includes intrauterine or extrauterine growth retardation; embryonic, fetal, or neonatal death; and congenital malformations. The central nervous system is the structure most commonly affected in mammals. The veterinary practitioner should limit elective radiologic examinations or treatments of the pregnant bitch or queen until immediately prior to delivery.

Mammalian fetuses can also be malformed by microwave radiation, a nonionizing radiation used therapeutically in human medicine to raise the temperature of the pelvic organs. Hyperthermia is thought to be the primary effect of microwave radiation. The mammalian embryo, like the mammalian eye, is exquisitely sensitive to hyperthermia because of its relative inability to dissipate heat from its fluid compartments to the maternal circulation. Although microwave radiation is not routinely used in therapeutic regimens in veterinary medicine, it is mentioned here as a precautionary measure.

Hyperthermia can also result from other causes. Environmental causes, such as exposure to hot summer temperatures in conjunction with exercise or inadvertently locking a pregnant animal in a closed automobile in warm climates, can elevate deep-core body temperatures significantly. Febrile illnesses during pregnancy might also pose a significant risk of potential embryotoxicity owing to hyperthermia. The CNS is the primary target organ of hyperthermia effects, but brain growth retardation may be the only major manifestation. At the other end of the temperature scale, hypothermia during gestation in rats, mice, and hamsters caused increased embryonic mortality and developmental defects, which included skeletal and CNS abnormalities.

Ultrasound radiation is another form of nonionizing radiation that has application in veterinary medicine. Not only is ultrasonography used in obstetric procedures to determine fetal size and number, but it is also used in echocardiography and ocular examinations. Although diagnostic ultrasound in the milliwatt range has not been shown to be harmful to the mammalian embryo, it is suspected that ultrasonic radiation can produce tissue or cellular damage at any level of exposure. Therefore, the quantitative aspects are extremely important in considering embryotoxic effects on the developing conceptus. It is not certain what relationship the quantitative and qualitative aspects of ultrasonic radiation have on its interaction with the mammalian embryo, so the decision involving its elective use with pregnant animals should be made judiciously.

Hypoxia (anoxia) is one of the oldest known environmental teratogens and can produce a significantly frequency of structural and functional abnormalities in several species of animals including the cat. A number of conditions can lead to the hypoxic state: (1) inadequate oxygen in inspired air, such as from unaccustomed high altitude exposure or during anesthesia, (2) maternal or fetal anemia, or (3) chemically caused conditions such as methemoglobinemia, carboxyhemoglobinemia, or cyanide-induced inhibition of cellular respiration. *Excess* oxygen was also found to cause gross congenital abnormalities in mammals when pregnant females were exposed to hyperbaric conditions. This could occur during anesthesia. Common atmospheric pollutants that are also pulmonary irritants (ozone, nitrogen oxides, and sulfur dioxide) can have a physiologic effect by interfering with maternal breathing, and they are suspected of increasing prenatal mortality.

Trauma, such as a bad fall, cannot be overlooked as having possible deleterious effects during gestation, especially if severe. Osteogenic defects occurred following a traumatic incident with a resulting two-day coma in a pregnant bitch nearing the period of implantation. Abortions have also occurred in pregnant dogs following involvement in minor automobile accidents at days 32 to 35 of gestation.

INFECTIONS

Viruses are the most important etiologic agents in malformations caused by infectious agents, especially during the early stages of development (Table 2). The rubella (measles) virus, Venezuelan equine encephalitis virus, and mumps virus have been shown to cause congenital defects in the human fetus. Terata produced by viruses may resemble classic defects of embryogenesis, such as cerebellar degeneration and hypoplasia caused by the feline panleukopenia virus in cats. This virus has an affinity for dividing cells, making the CNS especially vulnerable to *in utero* or periparturient infections. In fact, the CNS is the organ system in which lesions and malformations due to viruses are most frequently described. The cerebellum is not fully developed and therefore is still susceptible at time of birth in kittens, puppies, and human infants. The feline viral rhinotracheitis (FVR) virus, also referred to as feline herpesvirus I, is implicated in abortion and embryolethality in natural and experimental infections in the pregnant queen. Canine herpesvirus (CHV) is species specific and has recently been more frequently reported as the etiologic agent responsible for abortions and fetal and early postnatal deaths in dogs. Nonsuppurative myocarditis in puppies has been attributed to intra-

Table 2. *Viral Teratology of Mammalian Species — Naturally Occurring and Experimentally Induced*

Viral Agent	Terata	Animal Species
Arbovirus		
Japanese encephalitis virus	Hydrocephalus, cerebromalacia	Swine
Arenavirus		
Lymphocytic choriomeningitis virus	Cerebellar hypoplasia, ataxia	Mouse, rat
Enterovirus		
SMEDI group viruses	Generalized edema, buffalo hump, cleft palate, atresia ani	Swine
Myxovirus		
Influenza virus	Hydrocephalus	Monkey, hamster
Oncornavirus		
Feline leukemia virus	Thymic atrophy	Cat
Orbivirus		
Bluetongue	Hydraencephaly, porencephaly	Lamb, mouse, hamster
Paramyxovirus		
Mumps virus	Hydrocephalus	Hamster
Parainfluenza virus type 2	Hydrocephalus	Hamster
Parvovirus		
Feline panleukopenia virus	Cerebellar hypoplasia	Cat, ferret
Rat virus	Cerebellar hypoplasia	Rat, hamster, cat, ferret
Minute virus	Cerebellar hypoplasia	Mouse
Reovirus		
Reovirus type 1	Hydrocephalus	Hamster, mouse, rat, ferret
Togavirus		
Bovine diarrhea-mucosal disease virus	Cerebellar hypoplasia, hydrocephalus, blindness, cerebral destruction	Calf, lamb
Hog cholera virus	Cerebellar hypoplasia, hypomyelinogenesis, microcephaly, hydrocephalus, small cerebral gyri, cerebellar agenesis, skeletal and urogenital defects, cleft palate, atresia ani	Swine
Venezuelan equine encephalitis virus	Cerebral cysts, microcephaly, cataracts, hydrocephalus	Monkey

Modified from Wilson and Fraser: *Handbook of Teratology*, 1977.

uterine exposure to canine parvovirus (CPV). Pregnant bitches or queens should not be vaccinated with untested modified live virus vaccines until the effects on the developing young have been adequately determined.

Infectious agents other than viruses can be teratogenic or embryotoxic. *Brucella canis* has been shown to cause early embryonic deaths in dogs. The protozoan agent causing toxoplasmosis, *Toxoplasma gondii*, has been responsible for structural and functional abnormalities of the CNS in human fetuses, but it is not known whether similar effects result from congenital infections in dogs and cats. Another infectious agent that is a human teratogen is *Treponema pallidum*, the human syphilis spirochete, which has caused CNS and skeletal developmental abnormalities in human neonates.

NUTRITION-RELATED DISORDERS

Maternal nutrition has an important effect on prenatal development. Although problems in nutrition are usually considered to be deficiency related, excesses of certain nutritional components can also have deleterious effects, especially concerning congenital abnormalities. Generally speaking, maternal malnutrition must be quite severe and prolonged to have an adverse effect on the developing fetus. This is because "Mother Nature" appears to make every effort to supply the intrauterine life at the expense of the dam's last reserves. However, malnutrition of the dam is very likely to prevent normal reproductive cycles, ovulation, or conception so that pregnancy fails to occur in the first place. Also, after parturition, malnutrition of the dam may take its toll on the newborn owing to inadequate milk supply.

In dogs, long-term maternal malnutrition can be one of the primary causes of puppy mortality in the neonate. Experimentally, malnutrition in pregnant rats produced no structural malformations in the young, but possible metabolic changes and less rapid development were the sequelae. Maternal undernutrition in pregnant queens caused abnormal brain development (decreased brain weights) and behavioral abnormalities in the kittens, but no gross defects were observed. Fasting for long periods during pregnancy was reported to have teratogenic effects in mice, but similar results have not been described in other species.

Improper dietary levels of nutritional factors can be deleterious to the developing young. Fat-soluble vitamins such as vitamin A can induce teratogenesis at either greater or less than dietary requirements. Congenital malformations due to vitamin A deficiency were initially reported in swine and later in rats and rabbits. The terata observed were ocular defects and anomalies of the urogenital and cardiovascular systems. Hypervitaminosis A also produces congenital malformations in various animal species—rat, guinea pig, hamster, rabbit, ferret, and swine. In pregnant bitches, vitamin A administration of 1,250-fold greater than the recommended daily intake of 100 IU/lb, when dosed from days 17 to 22 of gestation, produced abnormalities such as cleft palate, accessory auricles, and kinked tails in puppies that survived the embryotoxic effects. The minimal dosage of vitamin A known to produce teratogenic effects has not yet been identified.

Normal dietary levels of other fat-soluble vitamins are essential for normal mammalian prenatal development. Vitamin D deficiency results in skeletal defects and abnormal dentition, whereas hypervitaminosis D in rats and rabbits impairs fetal osteogenesis. Dicumarol, a vitamin K analog used in the prevention and treatment of thromboembolic disease, has been shown to cause decreased prothrombin levels in neonatal dogs and rabbits when administered at therapeutic dosages to pregnant females.

Experimentally induced deficiencies of B-complex vitamins in diets of pregnant rats have produced developmental abnormalities in their offspring. These effects ranged from increased embryotoxicity and low birth weight to skeletal and dental anomalies, CNS abnormalities, and soft tissue defects in the cardiovascular and urogenital systems.

Major mineral elements play an important role in proper fetal development and normal gestation. With a calcium-deficient maternal diet, fetal calcification and ossification can be normal at the expense of calcium removed from the maternal skeleton. Excess dietary calcium, however, has caused abnormal offspring in rats. Dietary magnesium deficiency in pregnant rats was more deleterious to fetal development, causing embryonic death and malformations. Pregnant rats maintained on a low sodium diet produced young not significantly different from controls with no abnormalities. However, hypernatremia in pregnant mice injected with high dosages of sodium chloride (2 gm/kg) contributed to increased fetal death and malformations.

Proper dietary levels of other minerals (trace elements) are important to prenatal development.

Iron, copper, iodine, manganese, and zinc deficiencies in maternal diets have all been implicated in developmental anomalies. Pregnant rats maintained on an iron-deficient diet had offspring that were severely anemic and nonviable. Copper deficiency in pregnant sheep produces a disease in their lambs called enzootic ataxia (swayback), characterized by abnormalities in development of the CNS. The guinea pig exhibits a similar syndrome, with marked agenesis of the cerebellum in the neonate. Rats on a copper-deficient diet produced offspring with skeletal anomalies and abdominal hernias. A characteristic ataxia in offspring of manganese-deficient animals due to failure of otolith development in the inner ear has also been reported. This syndrome has been described in the rat, pig, guinea pig, and mouse. Iodine deficiency in maternal diets is manifested as hypothyroidism in the fetus, producing a condition known as cretinism in humans. Excessive iodine in the mother's diet also produces cretinous children, and a cretinism-like condition has been produced experimentally in dogs with excess iodine in the diet of the dams. Malformations resulting from zinc deficiency in the pregnant rat affected every organ system, with a high incidence of CNS anomalies and hyperplasia of the esophageal mucosa.

METABOLIC AND ENDOCRINE FACTORS

Of the various syndromes in pregnant women that have the potential to induce teratogenic effects in the human fetus (diabetes, phenylketonuria, virilizing tumors), none are reported to produce abnormalities in pets as a result of naturally occurring conditions. Diabetic animals may become pregnant, but deliberate breeding obviously would be discouraged.

CHEMICAL AGENTS

This is by far the largest group of potential teratogens and includes both therapeutic agents and environmental chemicals. Many types of drugs and environmental chemicals have been reported or suspected as teratogenic in one or more species of mammals (Table 3). Few chemical agents are proven teratogens in dogs and cats, and teratogenic effects in experimental animals have usually been seen at dosages higher than recommended levels for therapeutic agents, or far above the usual exposure levels for environmental chemicals. Embryotoxicity other than teratogenesis is sometimes more subtle and difficult to detect or predict. Interactions with other compounds and other complicating factors may also be involved.

Many pesticides have been shown to be teratogenic in various species of animals. Carbaryl, a widely used insecticide that reversibly inhibits cholinesterase, caused multiple developmental abnor-

Table 3. *Potential Mammalian Teratogens*

Type of Compound	Specific Examples
Alkaloids	Caffeine, nicotine, colchicine
Alkylating agents	Busulfan, chlorambucil, cyclophosphamide
Analgesics	Aspirin (salicylates), morphine
Anesthetics	Halothane, urethane, nitrous oxide, pentobarbital
Antibiotics	Chloramphenicol, streptomycin, penicillin, tetracycline, dactinomycin, griseofulvin, streptonigrin, actinomycin D
Anticonvulsants	Diphenylhydantoin, phenobarbital, primidone
Antihistamines	Buclizine, meclizine, cyclizine, hydroxyzine, chlorcyclizine
Antimalarials	Chloroquine, quinacrine, pyrimethamine, quinine
Antimetabolites	Methotrexate and aminopterin (folic acid analogs), purine and pyrimidine analogs
Corticosteroids	Cortisone, triamcinolone, dexamethasone, hydrocortisone
Dyes	Trypan blue, FD & C red dye no. 2, Evans blue, Niagra sky blue 6B
Fungicides	Captan, methyl mercuric chloride, tetrachlorophenol
Heavy metals	As, Cd, Hg, Li, Ni, Pb, Tl, Sr, Se
Herbicides	MCPA (ethylester), paraquat
Hormonal agents	Progesterone plus norethinedrone, androgens, estrogens, vasopressin, insulin, thyroxine, epinephrine
Hypoglycemics	Carbutamide, tolbutamide, hypoglycins
Insecticides	Carbaryl, diazinon, lindane, aldrin, dieldrin, dichlorvos
Mycotoxins	Aflatoxin B_1, ochratoxin A, cytochalasin B, rubratoxin B, T-2 toxin, zearalenone, deoxynivalenol, ergot
Plants	*Astragulus* spp., *Lupinus* spp., *Datura stramonium, Lathyrus* spp., *Veratrum californicum, Conium maculatum, Prunus* spp., *Nicotiana* spp., *Colchicum autumnale, Podophyllum peltatum, Vinca rosea, Ricinus communis, Rauwolfia serpentina*
Solvents	Dimethylsulfoxide, chloroform, 1,1-dichloroethane, carbon tetrachloride, benzene, xylene, cyclohexanone, alkane, sulfonates, acetamides, formamides
Sulfonamides	Acetazolamide, sulfanilamide
Tranquilizers	Chlorpromazine, thalidomide, reserpine, meprobamate, diazepam
Other chemicals and drugs	Physostigmine, pilocarpine, saponin, thiadiazole, triazene, boric acid, hydroxyurea, triparanol (MER-29), serotonin, imipramine, EDTA, penicillamine, ethyl alcohol, opiates, mescaline, LSD, amphetamine, PCBs, glutethimide, barbital, TCDD, nitrosamines

malities in 21 of 181 beagle pups when administered in the diet to pregnant bitches throughout gestation. The teratogenic effects occurred at dosages as low as 3.125 mg/kg/day and were manifested as brachygnathia, ecaudate pups, failure of skeletal formation, superfluous phalanges, and abdominal-thoracic fissures with varying degrees of intestinal agenesis and displacement. Dystocia from uterine atony also occurred frequently.

The insecticides diazinon and dichlorvos have been shown experimentally to be teratogenic, and other insecticides have demonstrated embryotoxicity. In beagle dogs, diazinon-exposed pups had enlarged, pronounced fontanelles and dental agenesis. Dichlorvos, the active ingredient in flea collars and fly strips, was reported to produce malformations in the offspring of pregnant rats dosed on a single day of gestation with 15 mg/kg intraperitoneally. DDT was initially incriminated as an etiologic agent responsible for a number of biologically deleterious effects including teratogenesis, but extensive research recently conducted in a number of mammalian species has shown no conclusive teratogenic effects. Beagle dogs were chronically exposed to 1, 5, and 10 mg of technical DDT/kg/day with no effect on reproduction and no gross or

histologic findings in any of the 650 pups examined.

The phenoxy herbicide 2,4,5-T (and its related compound 2,4-D) also were incriminated as mammalian teratogens, especially as related to human exposure due to the utilization of 2,4,5-T as a defoliant (Agent Orange) in Vietnam. However, more recent works have shown that the teratogenic effects were due to dioxins (especially 2,3,7,8-tetrachlorodibenzodioxin: TCDD), which were contaminants associated with the manufacturing process. A change in manufacturing methods has reduced the dioxin content in 2,4,5-T to the parts per billion (ppb) range, but some experts feel this herbicide formulation may still be hazardous. By itself, 2,3,5-T is embryotoxic and fetotoxic at very high dosages. Other herbicides reported to cause mammalian malformations are paraquat and 4-chloro-2-methyl phenoxyacetic acid (MCPA, ethylester).

A number of fungicides have been shown experimentally to be teratogenic in dogs and cats as well as in other mammals. Pups from pregnant bitches receiving captan during gestation had crooked tails, gastroschisis, open fontanelles, and hydrocephalus. Offspring of pregnant bitches exposed to methyl mercury chloride (MeHgCl, a fungicide that is also an environmental contaminant) for 129 days before and during gestation at a dosage of 0.1 mg/kg developed congenital anomalies in one of ten litters, and these anomalies included cleft palate, patent fontanelles, superfluous phalanges, enlarged kidneys, and omphalocele. Fetal resorption and perinatal death were observed. Pregnant cats given MeHgCl at a dosage of 0.25 mg/kg/day had an increased incidence of abortions and increased cerebellar developmental defects in the surviving neonates. Pets should not be fed meat or fish suspected of containing excessive mercury residues, not only because of the teratogenic potential but also because it may cause irreversible neuropathy and blindness in the dam.

Griseofulvin, a systemic antifungal agent, is teratogenic in dogs, cats, and laboratory rodents. Cleft palate was present in six of seven pups from a golden retriever bitch treated with 750 mg griseofulvin per day for four weeks prior to pregnancy and throughout gestation. There was no history of abnormal litters from previous or subsequent matings, but the evidence is still circumstantial. Pregnant beagles given 35 mg/kg/day for periods as short as one week to as long as the entire gestation period delivered puppies that were small, weak, and short haired, with hemorrhages in the lumbar, cranial, and mandibular areas and in the extremities and abdomen. A large number of resorptions also occurred in the prenatal period.

Kittens from a pregnant cat receiving griseofulvin therapeutically have shown developmental anomalies such as shortened tails and hind limbs, absence of phalanges, and fused phalanges of the posterior limbs. Cleft palate was observed in one out of three kittens from an experimental queen given 35 mg/kg/day throughout pregnancy. Increased teratogenic effects of larger doses (500 to 1000 mg per animal), given at weekly intervals to three pregnant queens, included multiple congenital malformations of the brain and skeleton, specifically exencephaly, malformed prosencephalon, hydrocephalus, cranium bifidum, spina bifida, abnormal atlanto-occipital articulation, cleft palate, absence of maxillae, and lack of tail vertebrae. Cyclopia and anophthalmia with absence of optic nerves and rudimentary optic tracts were also reported. Other abnormalities present were atresia ani, atresia coli, lack of AV valves in the heart, and absence of external nares and soft palate.

Administration of hormonal agents to pregnant animals should be avoided, even late in gestation. Testosterone propionate, injected subcutaneously into a pregnant bitch between days 35 and 42 of gestation, is thought to have caused ovarian hermaphoditism in two pups and abnormal clitoral development in the third. Progesterone and norethindrone therapy, administered during the period of gestation when the external genitalia were being formed, resulted in the masculinization of the external genitalia (abnormal fusion of the labia) in female pups from a pregnant boxer.

Administration of corticosteroids during gestation results in congenital anomalies in laboratory rodents, especially certain strains of mice. Dogs are also affected, and clinical evidence indicates that the increase in anasarcous pups in the brachycephalic breeds may be related to corticosteroid therapy in the pregnant animal. Cleft palate was reported in five of five Great Dane puppies whelped after the dam was treated with betamethasone during pregnancy. The same anomaly occurred in all nine pups whelped after a golden retriever was orally dosed with dexamethasone during days 32 to 35 of gestation. Two normal litters had been whelped previously utilizing the same sire. Deformed forelegs, phocomelia, and ankylosed forelegs were observed in an entire litter of cocker spaniel pups after the dam had been treated with dexamethasone during the terminal half of gestation. However, these reports do not definitively prove teratogenicity.

Thalidomide, the notorious human teratogen, does not have the same teratogenic response of phocomelia in other mammals except for the simian primate. The dog is not a good model for thalidomide teratogenesis, but at high maternal dosages, the surviving neonates were weak, short haired, and had crooked tails, renal agenesis, patent fontanelles, and testicles attached near the kidneys. In cats, thalidomide teratogenesis was manifested primarily as cardiovascular defects such as ventricular septal defect, right atrial distention involving the coronary sinus, malpositioned great vessels, and narrowed left ventricular chamber with hypertrophied walls. Musculoskeletal and facial anomalies were also reported.

Other drugs shown to produce experimental teratogenesis in dogs are aminopterin, hydroxyurea, and hydroxyzine (Atarax). Atarax, in addition to being embryotoxic, produced pups with hooked, curved, and screw tails. Hydroxyurea, an antileukemia agent in humans, caused a wide variety of defects in pups of pregnant bitches given the drug. These developmental abnormalities included tail variants ranging from hooked tails to taillessness, hairlessness, hemorrhage in the muscles of the rear limbs, and agenesis; double cleft lip and palate; gastroschisis; scoliosis; patent fontantelles; and microphthalmia. In dogs, aminopterin caused no conclusive teratogenic response, but methotrexate, a similar compound that is also a folic acid antagonist, produced high frequencies of malformations in kittens when given to pregnant queens on days 11 to 14 and 14 to 17 at a dosage of 0.5 mg/kg. Reported defects included umbilical hernia and retarded ossification of the cranium. Resorptions and anomalies were observed in cats given α-methylfolic acid on days 5 to 11 or 10 to 25 of gestation. Multiple, severe malformations were observed in most of the kittens, and these included cleft palate, microphthalmia, celostomy or leg anomalies, and kidney agenesis.

Although salicylates such as aspirin are not ordinarily considered teratogenic in dogs and cats, they are potent teratogens in the rat, causing resorptions and malformations such as cleft lip, spina bifida, and other anomalies of the skeletal and vascular systems. Aspirin in dosages five to six times greater (500 mg/kg) than those effective in rats was found to be embryotoxic in monkeys. Acetylsalicylic acid was reported to have caused musculoskeletal anomalies in kittens when given to pregnant queens on days 10 to 20 of gestation.

The teratogenicity of diphenylhydantoin (phenytoin), an anticonvulsant, has been repeatedly demonstrated in mice and rats and is associated with a maternal plasma level of unbound drug that is only two to three times greater than normal therapeutic levels. Phenobarbital and primidone are suspected human teratogens, and the teratogenic potential of oxyzolidinedione anticonvulsants (trimethadione and paramethadione) must be considered before being used electively in the pregnant female.

Several antibiotics are teratogenic in rodents, whereas others are embryolethal. Tetracycline, streptonigrin, penicillin-streptomycin mixtures, and actinomycin D have been reported to cause malformations. Embryolethal antibiotics include those primarily inhibiting protein synthesis, such as puromycin, lincomycin, and streptomycin. Other antimicrobial agents, such as sulfonamides, would seem to be potentially deleterious to mammalian development owing to their mechanism of action. Yet, except for acetazolamide and sulfanilamide, these compounds have been reported to have little effect on development. Acetazolamide, a potent carbonic anhydrase inhibitor, caused uniquely localized malformation of the forelimbs in rodents.

Mycotoxins, the toxic fungal metabolites, are potential contaminants of both animal and human food supplies. Some mycotoxins are known teratogens, and may also have antigenetic activity. Mold or fungal invasion can occur in a variety of foodstuffs and under varying circumstances. Toxigenic genera of fungi most commonly isolated are *Aspergillus*, *Penicillium*, and *Fusarium*. Livestock and food animal production have been increasingly affected during recent years owing to changes in agricultural practices and unfavorable harvest conditions that have intensified exposure to toxigenic fungi. Cereal grains and other plant-related foodstuffs are utilized extensively in food animal production and may comprise a significant portion of the dietary constituents of companion animals and man. Dairy and meat products are also subject to fungal invasion and may serve as additional potential sources of contamination in pet foods. Almost all mammalian organ systems are subject to the toxic effects of mycotoxins. These toxic effects may be acute, chronic, or even subclinical in nature. Species, breed, and other variables play a significant role in both susceptibility and occurrence of toxic manifestations. Mycotoxins such as aflatoxin, ochratoxin, deoxynivalenol, and T-2 toxin are known for teratogenic or embryotoxic effects, but other mycotoxins (and possibly *all* mycotoxins) should be considered suspect. T-2 toxin is a trichothecene mycotoxin with reported radiomimetic effects. Diacetoxyscirpanol (DAS), another trichothecene mycotoxin, was detected in one brand of commercial dry dog food at concentrations ranging from 10 to 13 ppm. Hemorrhagic enteritis and death occurred in dogs consuming this ration, and the ration constituent source was apparently yellow corn contaminated with *Fusarium* spp.

Polychlorinated biphenyls (PCBs), industrial chemicals previously utilized in transformers and capacitors where heat resistant properties are required, have been involved in recent episodes of misuse or accidental contamination in food animals. By-products from slaughter or salvage animals could contain hazardous undetected PCB residues, which may enter or re-enter the animal food chain. FDA has established an action level of 3 ppm (fat basis) for unavoidable residues of PCBs in red-meat animals, but undetected levels in pet foods could be much higher. PCBs are reported to have teratogenic, fetotoxic, and other reproductive effects. The genetic activity of PCBs decreases with increasing chlorination. In one study, administration of PCBs as Aroclor 1254 to pregnant dogs at a dosage of 1.0 mg/kg/day resulted in puppies with a significantly higher incidence of patent fontanelles. This same anomaly was present in 50 per cent of puppies delivered from bitches administered a higher dosage of 5.0 mg/kg/day, and the fetal resorption rate was 45.5 per cent (a fourfold increase over controls). Female rhesus monkeys fed PCBs at rates of 2.5 and 5 ppm in the diet for six months prior to mating conceived with difficulty or aborted. Infant monkeys born alive were smaller than normal, and half died within six months. Surviving infants exhibited behavioral and learning defects.

SUMMARY AND DISCUSSION

Many agents affect the prenatal development of "experimental" animal species, but few are undisputed teratogens or mutagens for domestic animals. Expression of embryotoxicity involves many factors, some of which are known and some of which are as yet unresolved. The veterinary practitioner should establish a policy of minimizing the exposure of pregnant animals to potentially harmful agents during all phases of gestation.

Elective therapeutic, prophylactic, and diagnostic

procedures are contraindicated during pregnancy and should be avoided unless medical requirements dictate otherwise. However, one should not hesitate to risk potential prenatal damage to the unborn if the pregnant patient is in immediate need of medical attention, as long as the client is advised of the possibilities and agrees to the proposed treatment. Birth defects in animals do not involve the same magnitude of moral and legal implications for society as they do in humans. However, developmental defects in any mammalian species are far more easily prevented than they are corrected post partum, since by this time the response is irreversible.

The nutritional requirements of gestation should be met with an adequately fortified and properly balanced diet, but the client should be cautioned about excessive home-prescribed vitamin-mineral supplementation, however well intended. Immunization should be accomplished prior to breeding, and care should be taken to avoid exposure of pregnant females to infectious diseases during gestation. Extreme environmental temperatures, either heat or cold, should be avoided over prolonged periods, as should strenuous exercise or traumatic insult.

The veterinary practitioner will likely see terata in various species of animals. Clients should be asked for a careful history of treatments, illnesses, or unusual happenings during gestation, since cause may not be readily apparent. A breeding history of both sire and dam for three generations should be obtained to determine the incidence of previous developmental defects. Animals with defects of genetic origin should not be permitted to reproduce, but other anomalies may be surgically corrected if feasible. Even with all the scientific data at one's disposal, the etiology may be difficult to determine, requiring a judgemental decision.

SUPPLEMENTAL READING

Becker, B. A.: Teratogens. In Casarett, L. J., and Doull, J. (eds.): Toxicology—The Basic Science of Poisons. New York: Macmillan Publishing Co., 1975.

Earl, F. L.: Teratogenesis. In Kirk, R. W. (ed.): Current Veterinary Therapy VI. Philadelphia: W. B. Saunders Co., 1977.

Harbison, R. D.: Teratogens. In Doull, J., Klassen, C. D., and Amdur, M. O. (eds.): Casarett and Doull's Toxicology—The Basic Science of Poisons, 2nd ed. New York: Macmillan Publishing Co., 1980.

Robens, J. F.: Teratogenesis. In Kirk, R. W. (ed.): Current Veterinary Therapy V. Philadelphia: W. B. Saunders Co., 1974.

Thilly, W. G., and Liber, H. L.: Genetic toxicology. In Doull, J., Klassen, C. D., and Amdur, M. O. (eds.): Casarett and Doull's Toxicology—The Basic Science of Poisons, 2nd ed. New York: Macmillan Publishing Co., 1980.

Wilson, J. G.: Environmental and Birth Defects. New York: Academic Press, 1973.

Wilson, J. G., and Fraser, F. C. (eds.): Handbook of Teratology. Vols. 1–4. New York: Plenum Press, 1977.

Wilson, J. G., Kalter, H., Palmer, A. K., Hoar, R. M., Shenefelt, R. E., Beck, F., Earl, F. L., Nelson, N. S., Berman, E., Stara, J. F., Selby, L. A., and Scott, W. J., Jr.: Developmental abnormalities. In Benirschke, K., Garner, F. M., and Jones, T. C. (eds.): Pathology of Laboratory Animals. Vol. 2. New York: Springer-Verlag, 1978.

DRUGS OF ABUSE

H. DWIGHT MERCER, D.V.M.,
and STEPHEN P. STEPHEN, B.S. Pharm.

Mississippi State, Mississippi

The veterinarian, as a member of the health professions, often becomes the target for the experienced drug abuser. The veterinary clinic is often viewed as a potential source of a variety of drug and chemical substances. In fact, the veterinary clinic may be considered the sole source for unique drugs that are used in selective animal populations, e.g., wildlife. The veterinarian needs to have a knowledge of the broad spectrum of "drug abuse" and the potential common usage drugs that fall in this category. This brief discussion on drugs of abuse is not intended to be comprehensive. However, the information may serve as an overview of the topic from the veterinary medical viewpoint and, perhaps, a stimulus to further study.

The health professional, invested with a presumption of technical expertise and a degree of community leadership, must attempt to influence the development of attitudes toward users of both old and new drugs so that the damage from both drug effects and the social impact can be minimized.

The development of drug abuse seems to follow general patterns. These have been described (Meyers et al., 1978). Drug abuse patterns seem to imply a process of progression and relate drug use to other social and psychologic processes.

Experimental Use. Drug abuse generally begins with a desire to explore or experience something different. Experimentation with drugs may occur with the novice as a result of peer pressure, or the experienced drug user may be seeking new responses. This latter element must surely represent the motivation behind the reported abuses of veterinary drugs such as T-61 Euthanasia Solution.

In the case of the experimental uses of T-61, the consequences of acute toxic effects and death were the expected responses. Veterinarians need to be aware that these types of drugs have appeal to the community of drug abusers.

Social Use. The classic examples of social uses of alcohol, cigarettes, coffee, and soft drinks are generally of less concern to the veterinarian. He needs to be aware that this pattern of drug abuse may represent an intermediate stage of drug use, which may signal a drug misuse problem. This temperament and social behavior of employees and/or colleagues may be an indication that a more serious drug abuse pattern may exist or may potentially develop.

Episodic Abuse. This type of abuse pattern is still an elective rather than a compulsive one. Episodic drug abuse greatly resembles the experimentation phase except the drug selection may be of greater consequence. Alcohol and sedatives, when used to the extent that damage to self and others often occurs, may be a progressive indicator.

Compulsive Abuse. This stage, at which the use of a drug or drugs is no longer elective, results in a pattern of compulsion. There are many personalities and behaviors characteristic of this phase. Their complexities do not need total understanding, only a realization that the acquisition of the drug becomes of major importance. The veterinarian and his clinic, along with the common practice of large drug inventories, becomes an enviable "target" of drug users. The target may be the veterinary hospital employee, or an outright burglary of the facilities may take place. Some veterinarians prefer not to utilize many valuable therapeutic and controlled drugs because of this potential danger.

Drugs that are commonly abused fall into five general categories (Drugs of abuse, 1980). These are narcotics, depressants, stimulants, hallucinogens, and Cannabis. Each category will be discussed along with appropriate veterinary medical applications. The special category of drugs used for chemical restraint of wildlife will also be reviewed.

NARCOTICS

A summary of the types of compounds in this category can be found in Table 1. Morphine represents an excellent analgesic drug that has many applications in the practice of veterinary medicine. Many emergency practices consider morphine, or one of its congeners, essential. Codeine is often utilized for its antitussive effects, particularly in companion animal practices. Hydromorphone (Dilaudid) and oxymorphine HCl (Numorphan) are highly effective analgesic drugs in the horse as well as other species and are often utilized to manage the severe pain of equine colic. Fentanyl/droperidol (Innovar-Vet), propoxyphene (Darvon), pentazocine (Talwin), and diphenoxylate/atropine (Lomotil) are used routinely in veterinary practices, fentanyl probably being the most commonly used.

DEPRESSANTS

A list of commonly used depressant drugs is presented in Table 2. Chloral hydrate has long been used as an anesthetic agent for horses and cattle. The barbiturates and gaseous anesthetics have largely replaced chloral hydrate as an anesthetic agent. Preference for chloral hydrate still exists among some large animal practitioners because of the low cost of the drug. There is some concern that choral hydrate may still be found in significant quantities in old and unlabelled containers in many practices. The barbiturates represent the most highly visible and widely used of the potential abuse drugs in veterinary practices. The barbiturates remain a relatively safe and economical anesthetic. The remainder of this class of drugs has only limited application in veterinary medicine.

STIMULANTS

A review of these drugs may be found in Table 3. Cocaine and amphetamines represent a significant percentage of all the drugs of abuse. Recent court cases indicate that a few unethical veterinarians have been involved in the illegal trafficking of these drugs. Cocaine has several acclaimed beneficial uses in the horse, and a few veterinarians have become involved in concocting home remedy drugs containing cocaine. This is usually in response to overzealous and demanding equine trainers. The efficacy of many of the recommended topical uses for lameness in horses is unproved. Amphetamines and the other stimulant drugs have not attained the popularity they enjoy in human medicine for weight control. The unpredictable effects on a number of animal species have resulted in a limited use of amphetamines in veterinary medicine.

HALLUCINOGENS AND CANNABIS

The drugs in this classification do not have any approved clinical uses in veterinary medicine but are included in Table 4 for informational purposes. Some of the cannabinoids may have application for glaucoma in animals, but this indication has not yet received FDA approval.

CHEMICAL RESTRAINT OF WILDLIFE

There are a number of highly effective and potentially toxic chemical agents used for restraint of wildlife (Haigh, 1978). These drugs are tabulated in Table 5. Many of the drugs used to restrain wildlife

Table 1. Narcotics

Drug	Schedule	Trade and Other Names	Medical Uses	Probability of Use in Veterinary Practice
Opium	II, III, V	Dover's Powder, Paregoric, Parepectolin	Analgesic, antidiarrheal	Very little
Morphine	II, III	Morphine, Pectoral Syrup	Analgesic, antitussive	High probability in small animal analgesic
Codeine	II, III, V	Codeine, Empirin Compound with Codeine, Robitussin A-C	Analgesic, antitussive	High probability
Heroin	I	Diacetylmorphine, Horse, Smack	None	No use
Hydromorphone	II	Dilaudid	Analgesic	Analgesic for colic in horses — limited usage
Meperidine	II	Demerol, Pethadol	Analgesic	Very little
Methadone	II	Dolophine, Methadone, Methadose	Heroin substitute	No use
Other narcotics	I–V	LAAM, Leritine, Levo-Dromoran, Percodan, Tussionex, Fentanyl, Darvon, Talwin, Lomotil	Analgesic, antidiarrheal, antitussive	Several used routinely

Table 2. Depressants

Drug	Schedule	Trade and Other Names	Medical Uses	Probability of Use in Veterinary Practice
Chloral hydrate	IV	Noctec, Somnos	Hypnotic, anesthetic in bovine and equine	Used frequently by few practitioners
Barbiturates	II, III, IV	Amobarbital, Phenobarbital, Butisol, Phenoxbarbital, Secobarbital, Tuinal, Barbs, Blue Devils, Downers, Pink Ladies, Yellow Jackets	Anesthetic, anticonvulsant, sedative hypnotic	High probability
Glutethimide	III	Doriden	Sedative, hypnotic	Limited use
Methaqualone	II	Optimil, Parest, Quaalude, Somnafac, Sopor	Sedative, hypnotic	No use
Benzodiazepines	IV	Diazepam, Librium, Valium, Verstran	Antianxiety, anticonvulsant, sedative, hypnotic	Limited use
Other depressants	III, IV	Equanil, Miltown, Noludar, Placidyl, Valmid	Sedative, hynotic	No use

Table 3. Stimulants

Drug	Schedule	Trade and Other Names	Medical Uses	Probability of Use in Veterinary Practice
Cocaine	II	Coke, Flake, Snow, Girl, Heaven Dust, Lady, Nose Candy, Rock, White, Blow, "C," Coca	Local anesthetic, used in many veterinary home remedy and poltice applications for lame horses	Limited, but has on occasion served as a source for drug abuse
Amphetamines	II, III	Biphetamine, Dexedrine, Delcobese, Beans, Black Beauties, Co-pilots, Dexies, Meth, Speed, Uppers	Hyperkinesis, narcolepsy, and weight control	Very limited use
Phenmetrazine	II	Preludin	Hyperkinesis, narcolepsy, and weight control	Very limited use
Methylphenidate	II	Ritalin	Hyperkinesis, narcolepsy, and weight control	Very limited use
Other stimulants	III, IV	Adipex, Bacarate, Cylert, Didrex, Ionamin, Plegine, Pre-Sate, Sanorex, Tenuate, Tepanil, Voranil	Hyperkinesis, narcolepsy, and weight control	Very limited use

Table 4. Hallucinogens and Cannabis

Drug	Schedule	Trade and Other Names	Medical Uses	Probability of Use in Veterinary Practice
LSD	I	Acid, Microdot	None	None
Mescaline and peyote	I	Mese, Buttons, Cactus	None	None
Amphetamine variants	I	2, 5-DMA, PMA, STP, MDA, MMDA, TMA, DOM, DOB	None	None
Phencylidine analogs	I	PCE, PCPy, TCP	None	None
Other hallucinogens	I	Bufotenine, Ibogaine, DMT, DET, Psilocybin, Psilocyn	None	None
Marihuana	I	Pot, Acapulco Gold, Grass, Reefer, Sinsemilla, Thai Sticks	None	None

Table 5. Chemical Restraint of Wildlife

Drug	Schedule	Trade and Other Names	Medical Uses	Probability of Use in Veterinary Practice
Succinylcholine	None	Sucostrin	Neuromuscular blocking agent	Continues to be used for anesthetic
Nicotine sulfate	None	Black Leaf 40	Neuromuscular blocking agent, extremely toxic	Occasionally used by dog control officers
Morphine	I or II	Etorphine, M 99	Sedative, hypnotic, potent narcotic	Anesthetic, animal restraint
Diprenorphine	I or II	M50-50	Sedative, hypnotic, potent narcotic	Anesthetic, animal restraint
Fentanyl and droperidol	III	Innovar-Vet	Sedative, hypnotic	Primate and canine restraint
Phencyclidine	II	PCP, Angel Dust, Hog, Sernylan, Crystal, Supergrass, Tic-Tac, Rocket Fuel	Anesthetic	Animal restraint
Xylazine	None	Rompum	Mixed with narcotics to give sedation and anesthesia	Wildlife restraint
Ketamine	None	Ketaset, derivative of phencyclidine	May be combined with other drugs; "dissociative" anesthetic	Animal restraint

must be considered high on the list of potential abuse drugs. Succinylcholine is a hazardous drug even when used under controlled circumstances by experienced clinicians. Succinylcholine has been used on at least a few occasions for homicidal purposes. It continues to be a drug of choice for use by bow hunters as a "knock-down" agent delivered in "pod" arrows. Veterinarians are often requested to supply the drug. This drug has been reported to produce some bizarre effects in man and thus may qualify as a potential "new experience" sought by drug abusers. Despite the large number of undesirable properties of succinylcholine, both in mode of action and effect, the drug is still widely used in North America, not for wildlife immobilization but by dog control officers and even veterinarians for immobilization of large animals.

One of the objectives of an immobilizing drug intended for use in a projectile syringe is low volume–high potency. Etorphine (M 99) is a narcotic drug that fits this category. It is reported to be from 100 to 1000 times more potent than morphine, thus making it an extremely hazardous drug to handle.

The Drug Enforcement Agency (DEA) has established special guidelines for the acquisition of etorphine (M 99) and diprenorphine (M50-50). These guidelines include limited distribution to veterinarians engaged in zoo and exotic animal practices, wildlife management programs, and researchers; special registration and order forms; a class 5 security container for storage; complete and accurate usage records; amounts shipped and stored limited to minimum; and special shipping procedures. Veterinarians anticipating a need for these agents should contact their DEA regional office early in their planning.

In the cyclohexamine group, only phencyclidine hydrochloride and ketamine have been licensed for use in animals. Phencyclidine (Sernylan) is usually long acting, and ketamine is short acting. Owing to the abuse potential, phencyclidine is no longer marketed in the United States. Ketamine continues to be a valuable veterinary anesthetic drug.

With regard to the toxicity of these drugs in man, the items of major interest are the narcotics and cyclohexamines. Recent reports have documented the death of a veterinarian and the collapse of others who accidentally administered unknown but certainly minute quantities of etorphine to themselves. In a recent incident, a veterinarian pricked himself with a 23-gauge needle attached to an apparently empty syringe that had contained etorphine and acepromazine. The prompt administration of a specific antagonist following the onset of clinical signs of narcotic overdose may have prevented his death.

There is increasing documentary evidence of the lethal effects of cyclohexamines, in particular phencylidine. Both phencyclidine and, to a lesser extent, ketamine are available as street drugs under a variety of bizarre names. Because of the marked increase in phencyclidine abuse, the manufacturers and regulatory officials have drastically reduced its availability.

Even experienced professionals have encountered difficulties in the mixing or combining of many of these drugs. The potential results from the combination of these potent drugs and misuse by the drug abuser should be of great concern to the veterinarian.

Veterinarians who have access to and responsibility for drugs must take measures to assure that they do not become links to street use of drugs. When the veterinarian is faced with a potential drug abuse problem in connection with his practice, it is imperative that drug enforcement officials and local authorities be notified. The loss or theft of controlled substances must be reported to the DEA as required by law.

REFERENCES

Drugs of abuse. Reprinted from *Drug Enforcement*, Vol. 6, No. 2. Washington D.C.: Enforcement Administration, U.S. Department of Justice, 1980.

Haigh, J. C.: Use and abuse of drugs for chemical restraint in wildlife. Vet. Clin. North Am. 8:343, 1978.

Meyers, F. H., Jawetz, E., and Goldfion, A.: *A Review of Medical Pharmacology*, 6th ed. Los Altos, California: Lange Medical Publications, 1978.

POISONING AND INJURY BY PLANTS

ARTHUR A. CASE, D.V.M.

Columbia, Missouri

There are many reports of accidental poisoning of humans, usually children, from poisonous plants accessible to children (and also to dogs, cats, or other pets). Leaving a deadly poisonous plant where either a human or an animal can be exposed to it is a common but irresponsible act.

POISONING

No effort will be made here to provide a comprehensive coverage of all the possible toxic plant hazards that exist around homes, farms, or ranches. Several very toxic plants are commonly kept as ornamental shrubs, potted house plants, or garden flowers. Such showy flowers as monkshood, foxglove, larkspur, oleander, daphne, and castor beans and such poisonous plants as water hemlock and poison hemlock (*Conium*) are extensively grown as ornamentals. Yew, privet, and boxwood are very poisonous shrubs that are widely grown.

It is remarkable that so many persons seem to be unaware of the fact that puppies, kittens, and small children are likely to chew and attempt to eat vegetation of any kind. An owner recently stated that her cat would scratch to pieces and eat any potted plant that was brought into the house. Cats will also scratch toxic plants and then be poisoned by licking their claws. When such powerful irritants as the juice of large lilies or dumb cane; many spurges such as snow-on-the-mountain, dogbane, and oleander; or jessamine are involved, the cat may be seriously and acutely poisoned. Many families own pet ponies and horses, and such animals may be seriously poisoned, often fatally, if allowed access to oleander, yew, laurels, privet, boxwood (*Buxus*), black locust, castor beans, showy crotalaria, and other native or ornamental plants that are toxic.

Missouri has 195 genera of plants that are known to contain one or more toxic species. Those most likely to be involved in poisoning pets or children are summarized in Table 1. It lists plants that commonly grow about homes, farmsteads, and ranch headquarters and in yards and gardens. Some are tropical or subtropical plants grown in other areas, such as potted ornamentals in homes, greenhouses, and arboretums. Others are wild or domestic flowering species. A few toxic plants are important commercial crops that have toxic parts. The nightshades include potato, tomato, eggplant, garden huckleberry (black nightshade) as well as the groundcherries, or husk tomatoes, and Chinese lanterns. Onions of the lily family can poison dogs. Other lilies, such as death camas, jonquil, daffodil, and amaryllis, are quite toxic to many species of animals. There is no more picturesque plant than the large, brightly colored castor bean plant; the seed hull of this large spurge plant contains ricin, one of the most toxic of the phytotoxins. Most members of the euphorb family contain powerful poisonous principles, and the juice of many spurges is as caustic as branding fluid and has been used as such in earlier times. Table 1 lists such plants and their toxic parts.

INJURY

Table 2 outlines plants that have structures that may inflict physical or mechanical injuries of one type or another. Such injuries are seen and recognized much more frequently than are plant poisonings *per se*. Treatment of injury by plant structures consists of removing the offending awn, thorn, stem rachis, or other penetrating structure and applying appropriate therapeutic medical measures.

Inhaled plant structures may pose some real puzzles for the clinician, especially foreign bodies in the deeper air passages or actually within the lung (Fig. 1). Plant structures migrating into deeper recesses of the ear canal, urethra, nares, and conjunctival folds is a common occurrence in hunting dogs and other dogs that roam outdoors. Occasionally, a larger plant structure, such as a hickory nut, walnut, or a corncob (buttered roasting ear), may be swallowed and may lodge in the bowel, becoming an acute intestinal obstruction and, hence, an immediate emergency that threatens life. Figures 2 through 6 are examples of such foreign bodies. Pathologists may see similar lodging foreign bodies that proved lethal because of physical and mechanical effects rather than any particular toxic principle. As in many other situations involving dogs or cats, there is no reliable method of obtaining valid statistics on incidence. These situations are not reporta-

Table 1.   Common Poisonous Plants*

Plant	Toxic Part	Comments and Syndrome
Common lilies: amaryllis, daffodil, tulips, jonquil, narcissus, death camas, autumn crocus, star-of-Bethlehem, lily-of-the valley, others	Bulbs mostly	Violent gastrointestinal upsets, nausea, emesis, dyspnea, CNS excitement followed by depression, collapse, coma, and death. Young and very aged are most likely to be severely poisoned.
Tropical potted ornamentals: caladium, philodendron, dumbcane *(Dieffenbachia)*, elephant ear, and similar common house plants	Leaf, stem, stalk	Severe burning sensation in mouth and nasopharynx, swelling of oral passages and tissues, obstruction of air passage. Asphyxia and gastroenteritis the causes of death. Rich in oxalates.
Spring staggerweeds and cultivated ornamentals: *Dicentra* (bleeding-heart) and *Corydalis* spp.	Top growth, corms	Much as above plus powerful alkaloids, which produce CNS signs. Can be fatal to small pet or child.
Ornamental shrubs: often potted house, flowering, or decorative tropicals; *Daphne* spp., boxwood *(Buxus)*, *Nerium oleander* spp., yew *(Taxus)*, azalea, and other heath family shrubs; privet	All parts are poisonous. Fruit (berries) are attractive to children and pets of all kinds.	Many of this group have supertoxic cardiac principles, violent gastroenteritis, or CNS excitement or depressant active principles of complex nature.
Legumes: rosary pea *(Abrus precatorius)*	All parts of the seed	Supertoxic. Only one pea may be fatal if eaten. Abrin a supertoxic principle if given intradermally or subcutaneously.
black locust *(Robinia)*	Bark, green growth, and, likely, seeds	Robin produces intense gastroenteritis, cardiac effects, and CNS depression in any species.
wisteria, horse beans, java beans, loco weeds, and lupines have toxic principles; crotalaria may be ornamental	Seeds, especially	Toxic beans and peas have hepatoxic, teratogenic, and other poisonous properties.
Spurges and similar plants: poinsettia, snow-on-the-mountain; castor bean, and croton seeds	All parts, especially seeds	Only one leaf may be fatal to small pet or child. Hull of one castor bean may be lethal to adult human. Violent gastroenteritis and CNS shock; hepatoxic and nephrotoxic.
Buttercups: monkshood *(Aconitum)* foxglove *(Digitalis)*	All parts, seed is potent	CNS effects, intense GE upset, cardiotoxic effects, depression, collapse, coma, and death.
larkspur *(Delphinium)* peony *(officinalis)* buttercups *(Ranunculus)*, most species	Flowers and seeds Roots All top growth	As above, and CNS effects result in early impairment of judgment and walking syndrome. Severe GE upsets.
Nightshades; jimsonweed *(Datura* spp.)	All parts, seed very toxic	Narcotic alkaloids, GE upsets, abnormal thirst, delirium, coma, death.
eggplant, tomato, potato, ground cherry	Fruit and tubers edible; green growth and sprouts are toxic	Contain solanins.
nightshades *(Solanum* spp.) of many species	Variable, but toxic	Solanin principles.
tobacco	All parts	Alkaloid nicotine.
Parsleys: poison hemlock *(Conium maculatum)*	All parts	General CNS depressant from coniine.
water hemlock *(Cicuta maculata)*	Tubers mostly	Violent CNS convulsant.
Toxic Roots: may apple *(Podophyllum)*, poke weed *(Phytolacca)*	Roots	Violent GE syndromes, vomiting and purging, exhaustion, coma, death.
mistletoe	Berries	Fatal to both small pets and children; loss of cattle has also been reported from mistletoe.

*Reprinted with permission from Case: Norden News Winter: 10, 1973.

Table 2. *Plants that Cause Penetrating (Mechanical) Injuries**

Plant	Structure	Injury
Burdock (*Arctinum lappa*)	Hooked barbs of florets	Lacerations of eye, ears, nares, trachea and bronchus, subcutis
Rose, blackberry, dewberry	Hooked barbs of stems	Punctures and lacerations of eye, mouth, skin, feet
Quince, hawthorn, osage orange	Heavy spines on stems	Stab wounds of eye, skin, feet, legs
Honey locust (*Gleditsia triacanthos*)	Pronged spines	Eye lacerations and punctures; puncture wounds of skin
Cacti of a dozen types	Sharp spines of leaf	Multiple punctures with migrating spine fragments
Nettles (see Table 3)	Hollow hairs of stem	Hairs penetrate and break off under skin; chemical injection
Grasses—many species, (bromes, spear grasses, triple-awns, foxtails, bristle grasses, wheat, barley, rye, rice)	Awns, beards, barbs, fragmented seed heads	Barbs penetrate and migrate into ear canal, air passages, other natural body openings, into and under skin; into body cavities and internal organs

*These have been the common trauma-producing plants and plant structures seen in our veterinary clinics during the period 1948 to 1981. We have personal knowledge from having collected and identified the offending structures for the attending clinician, if we were not the actual veterinarians on the case. Most of the illustrations in this article are from our collection of artifacts.

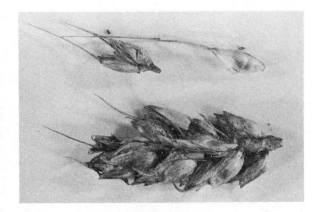

Figure 1. Fragment of wheat head, which was lodged in bronchus and removed via bronchoscope.

Figure 2. Juniper twigs removed from the ear canal of a beagle.

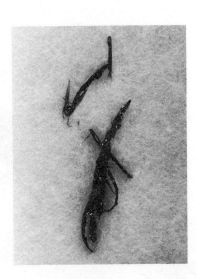

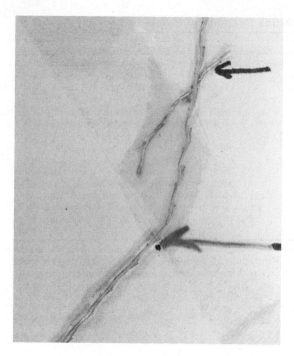

Figure 3. Crabgrass rachis: portion that was penetrating the eye beneath the third eyelid is indicated by arrows.

Figure 4. Hooked barbs become very aggressive, penetrating foreign bodies in eyes, ear and air passages and between digits of all species.

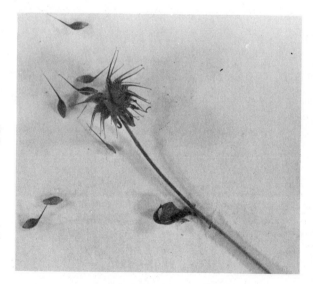

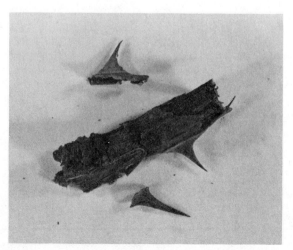

Figure 5. Rose thorns recovered from skin wounds in the flank of a foxhound. The "stab" was in an interdigital space.

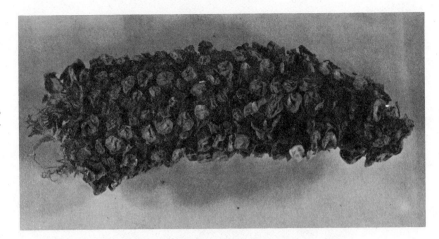

Figure 6. Fragment of corn cob from bowel obstruction. Patient recovered following surgical removal.

ble diseases, and there is no standard method of classification.

Personal observation and consultation with other veterinarians indicates that "primary" conditions, such as nocardiosis, may prove to be secondary to penetration by a foreign body, usually a plant structure of some kind. Kintner (1951–1981) has observed instances in which a foreign body was removed and the animal later died of pulmonary abscessation caused by another foreign body (part of a head of wheat) that was overlooked when the first foreign body was removed from deep in a bronchus. If all the foreign bodies had been successfully removed, the dog would probably have recovered and no significance would have been given to the incident.

Table 3 and Figures 7 through 10 provide additional possibilities of poisoning and injury by plants.

DIAGNOSIS AND TREATMENT

History is very important when poisoning or injury is a tentative diagnosis: the owner saw the dog (or cat) eat the mushroom, rodent bait, or yew leaf, and the presenting condition followed the ingestion within a short time period. The usual presenting signs of intoxication have been well discussed by Osweiler (1975), and the corrective procedures are outlined by other authors in this text.

Table 3. *Plants That Are Contact Irritants*

Plant	Active Part	Habitat
Spurges (Family Euphorbiaceae)	Milky sap, plant spines	Common ornamentals; fields; cultivars
Nettles (Family Urticaceae)*	Stinging hairs	Common flood plain wild plants
Nettle spurge, euphorb†	Spines, plant sap	Subtropics; ornamentals in warm house
Nettle amaranth, amaranth	Spines on mature plant	Common barnyard weed; pastures; fields
Bull nettle (nightshade family)‡	Spiny stems and leaves	Common perennial weed in most of US
Prickly nightshade ("do")	Spines over whole plant	Common annual weed in most of US

*Stinging nettles (*Urtica* spp.) may pose a lethal hazard to small breeds of young hunting dogs not previously exposed to these stinging plants. The hollow hairs of the nettles contain histamine, formic acid, acetylcholine, and serotonin. The anaphylaxis-like crisis, if not promptly treated, may result in sudden death to death within 48 hours for beagles and other smaller breeds. Clinicians use atropine to effect, plus a rapid-acting corticosteroid according to Digilio (1979–1981) and other veterinarians working with small animals.

†The euphorbs have such irritating sap that it can be used for cold branding fluid. Some hunting dogs show unusually severe scrotal dermatitis after hunting in heavy stands of snow-on-the-mountain, leafy spurge, three-seeded mercury, mat spurge, and similar spurges.

‡Some fair skinned dogs and many cats develop contact dermatitis following exposure to the parsley family plants, such as garden cultivars of parsnip and nightshades such as tomatoes (especially damp foliage). We have seen many such instances during the past 35 years in the central Missouri area.

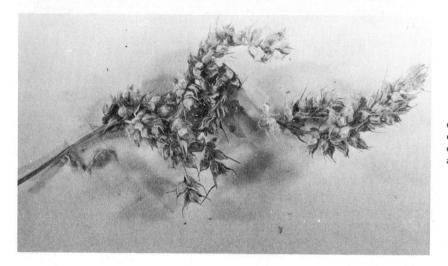

Figure 7. Barnyard grass is one of the most common traumatizers encountered by outdoor dogs and other animals in the late summer and fall.

Figure 8. Spanish needles are seed structures built on a needle with three barbed hooks. All species are vicious traumatizers.

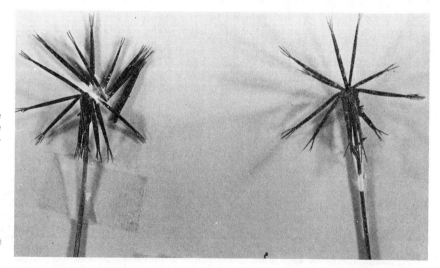

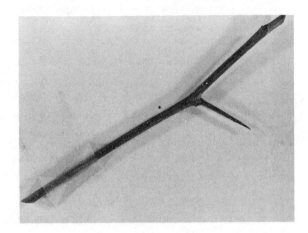

Figure 9. Rose, quince, hawthorn, and similar thorns often penetrate footpads and lacerate the cornea and oral mucosae of small animals.

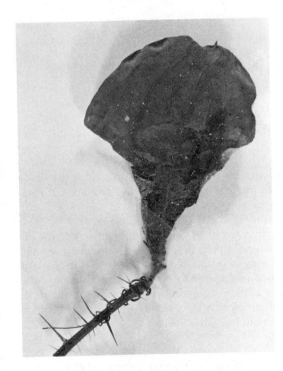

Figure 10. Smilax (greenbrier) spines penetrate the skin and break off in the wound, becoming migrating foreign bodies. This injury, which is very difficult to treat, occurs in dogs, cats, and man.

REFERENCES AND SUPPLEMENTAL READING

Atkins, C. E., and Johnson, R. K.: Clinical toxicities of cats. Vet. Clin. North Am. 5:623, 1975.

Bailey, W. S., and Groth, A. H., Jr.: Relationship of hepatitis X of dogs and moldy corn poisoning of swine. J. A. V. M. A. 134:514, 1959.

Barnes, B. A., and Fox, L. F.: Poisoning by *Dieffenbachia*. J. History Med. 10:173, 1955.

Bernard, M. A.: Mushroom poisoning in a dog. Can. Vet. J. 20:82, 1979.

Blood, D. V., Henderson, J. A., Radostits, O. M., Arundel, J. H., and Gay, C. C.: *Veterinary Medicine*, 5th ed. Philadelphia: Lea & Febiger, 1979, pp. 935–1034.

Case, A. A.: Beautiful but deadly. Norden News Winter:10, 1973.

Crane, S. (ed.): Symposium on trauma. Vet. Clin. North Am. 10:1, 1980.

Digilio, K.: Emergencies caused by ingestion or trauma by plants. Veterinary Clinics, University of Missouri-Columbia. 1979–1981. Personal communication.

Doull, J., Klaassen, C. D., and Amdur, M. O.: Casarett and Doull's *Toxicology, Basic Science of Poisons*, 2nd ed. New York: Macmillan Publishing Co., 1980.

Grain, E., Jr. and Evans, J. E., Jr.: What is your diagnosis. Case 2. J. A. V. M. A. 179:1024, 1981.

Greer, M. J.: Plant poisoning in cats. Mod. Vet. Prac. 42:62, 1961.

Hardin, J. W., and Arena, J. M.: *Human Poisonings from Native and Cultivated Plants*. Durham, North Carolina: Duke University Press, 1969.

Heister, C. B., Jr.: *Nightshades*. San Francisco: W. H. Freeman & Co., 1969.

Hendricks, H. V.: Poisoning by the false morel (*Gyrometra esculenta*). J. A. V. M. A. 114:1625, 1940.

Jones, I., and Lynn, E. V.: Differences in species of *Taxus*. J. Am. Pharm. Assoc. 22:528, 1933.

Kaplan, B.: Acute nicotine poisoning in a dog. V. M./S. A. C. 63:1033, 1968.

Kingsbury, J. M.: *Deadly Harvest, A Guide to Common Poisonous Plants*. New York: Holt, Rinehart and Winston, 1965.

Kintner, L. D.: Observations on penetrating plant structures at necropsy. College of Veterinary Medicine, University of Missouri-Columbia, 1951–1981. Personal Communication.

Lewis, W. H., and Elvin-Lewis, M. D. F.: *Medical Botany*. New York: John Wiley & Sons, 1977.

Litten, W.: The most deadly mushrooms. Sci. Am. 232:90, 1975.

Mushroom news. Sci. Am. 241:92, 1979.

Nelson, S. L.: Observations on penetrating plants structures at necropsy. College of Veterinary Medicine, University of Missouri-Columbia. 1961–1981. Personal communication.

Oehme, F. W. (ed.): Clinical toxicology for the small animal practitioner. Vet. Clin. North Am. 5:1, 1975.

Osweiler, G. D.: Common potential sources of small animal poisonings. In Kirk, R. W. (ed.): *Current Veterinary Therapy VII*. Philadelphia: W. B. Saunders, 1975, p. 149.

Poisonous Plants of the United States and Canada. Englewood Cliffs, New Jersey: Prentice-Hall, 1964.

Raisbeck, M. F.: Observations on poisoning and other injury by plants in small animals. College of Veterinary Medicine, University of Missouri-Columbia, 1979–1981. Personal communication.

Sebrell, W. H.: An anemia in dogs produced by feeding onions. U. S. Public Health Reports 24:1175, 1930.

Smith, H. A., Jones, T. C., and Hunt, R. D.: *Veterinary Pathology*, 4th ed. Philadelphia: Lea & Febiger, 1972, pp. 904–979.

Smith, J. D.: Experimental bluegreen algae poisoning in small animals. South Afr. Ind. Chem. 4:66, 1950.

Stauffer, V. D.: Poison caused by ingestion of chokecherry leaves in a dog. V. M./S. A. C. 76:1573, 1981.

Steyermark, J. A.: *Flora of Missouri*. Ames, Iowa: Iowa State University Press, 1972.

Toxic hazards around the home. Vet. News Notes 2:1, 1979.

West, J. L.: Lesions of gossypol poisoning in the dog. J. A. V. M. A. 96:74, 1940.

CARCINOGENESIS

JANE F. ROBENS, D.V.M.

Bethesda, Maryland

WHAT IS CARCINOGENESIS?

Carcinogenesis is characterized by a lack of control, e.g., the loss of one or more of the specific control mechanisms that characterize and regulate the activities of a normal cell or tissue. The most important of these mechanisms is the loss of control over cell division or cell replacement, that is, an alteration in the balance between cell division and cell death. Furthermore, the neoplastic state is inherited at the cellular level, and theories on the mechanism of carcinogenesis must ultimately explain how the effect becomes permanent. Some investigators believe the critical action to be the ability of the carcinogen to interact with DNA; thus they believe carcinogenesis to be fundamentally a mutagenic action. Others, however, have postulated that cellular proteins and RNA become permanently altered through epigenetic mechanisms of gene expression. In all probability, either or both mechanisms may apply to different chemicals. Although the term "carcinogen" literally means giving rise to carcinomas or epithelial neoplasms, it is generally used to include agents producing sarcomas of mesenchymal origin.

In spite of the diversity of cancers, that is, their many diverse causes and cellular manifestations, the critical underlying defect in cell biochemistry and physiology is probably very similar. Some facets of microscopic appearances are recognizable and common to all cancers, and common treatment regimens are often equally successful, or nonsuccessful, in diverse clinical situations.

TYPES OF CHEMICAL CARCINOGENS

A recent scheme classifies chemical carcinogens as genotoxic or epigenetic. Genotoxic carcinogens are those that interact with and alter DNA, and they can generally be identified through short-term *in vitro* tests for mutagenicity. The three categories of genotoxic carcinogens are the direct-acting or primary carcinogen, the procarcinogen requiring conversion through metabolic activation by the host, and the inorganic carcinogen, which changes DNA by selective alteration of the trueness of DNA replication. Direct-acting carcinogens are electrophilic reactants that interact with nucleophilic compounds. They include such compounds as beta-propiolactone, bischloromethyl ether, and probably ethylene dibromide and dibromochloropropane.

Procarcinogens need specific metabolic activation, and thus they generally produce tumors only under limited conditions at specific sites and not at the point of application. They are considered to be highly stereospecific. They include the polynuclear aromatic hydrocarbons such as benzpyrene, certain aromatic amines such as 2-naphthylamine, alkyl nitrosamines, mycotoxins such as aflatoxin B, plant toxins such as pyrrolizidine alkaloids found in plants of the *Senecio* genus and other plants, and the antimetabolite ethionine. Aflatoxin, the mycotoxin produced by *Aspergillus flavus*, has been shown to be highly carcinogenic in some laboratory animal species. It has also been associated with human tumors of the liver in Africa, although a cause-and-effect relationship has not been definitely established. Aflatoxin occurs in cottonseed, corn, and peanuts produced in the US, particularly when adverse weather conditions exist prior to harvesting. In particularly bad years when contamination is severe, aflatoxin has been implicated in clinical illness in dogs fed food produced by a local mill from largely local corn. Since aflatoxin is known to produce centrilobular parenchymal necrosis and biliary proliferation in dogs, the possibility exists that it could contribute to hepatic carcinogenesis in dogs.

The aromatic amine 2-naphthylamine has been demonstrated to be carcinogenic in several species, including the dog and humans, in which cancer of the urinary bladder is produced. Metals appear to be carcinogenic only under very specific conditions. Some, of course, have demonstrated carcinogenicity, attributed chiefly to their radioactive properties.

The epigenetic carcinogens usually lead to neoplastic change only following high and sustained exposure that predisposes to physiologic abnormalities, hormonal imbalances, or tissue injury. There is no direct evidence of their interaction with genetic material. These types of agents include hormones, asbestos in the lung, iron dextran complexes subcutaneously, and immunosuppressive drugs that allow the expression of oncogenic viruses.

Hormones can be carcinogenic when they are administered chronically at high dosages or are present chronically through disturbances of normal endocrine balance. In the dog the incidence of some tumors, such as the risk of tumor development in the mammary gland of the bitch, can be clearly associated with hormonal levels. Bitches neutered prior to any estrus have been shown to have a 200-fold less risk of developing mammary tumors than bitches not spayed. Those neutered after one cycle had a 12-fold less risk, and those neutered after maturity had no reduction in risk. Cats also had a reduction in risk when neutered after one or more cycles.

Cocarcinogens exacerbate the carcinogenic process of a genotoxic carcinogen when administered concomitantly and include the phorbol esters, catechol, and pyrene. Promoters increase genotoxic carcinogenic activity when applied after the carcinogen and include croton oil, bile acids, phenobarbital, and DDT. Large amounts of the possible promoter tryptophan when fed to dogs have resulted in hyperplasia but not tumors of the bladder.

BIOLOGIC CARCINOGENS

Although in humans the primary emphasis on the etiology of tumors has been environmental, an increasing number of tumors in animals are known to be caused by viruses. C-type RNA viruses have been shown to reproduce both malignant lymphoma and fibrosarcoma in the cat; however, the mode of transmission among cats in natural surroundings is still under study. No association has been found, however, between human cancer and cats with malignant lymphoma. In dogs, viruses are the cause of oral papillomas.

Esophageal fibrosarcoma of the dog has been related to *Spirocerca lupi*. Bile duct carcinoma in dogs and cats has been associated with the fluke *Clonorchis sinensis*.

PHYSICAL AGENTS

Irradiation is carcinogenic in all animal species in which it has been tested. Clinically, the risk of squamous cell carcinomas in a sun-exposed site on white cats has been shown to be much higher than the risk of developing oral squamous cell carcinomas. In a study of the effects of x-rays on the lifespan of female beagles, cancer appeared at an earlier age but not in excessive numbers in treated animals.

EVIDENCE OF CARCINOGENICITY

Evidence of the carcinogenicity of a given agent can be obtained from (1) epidemiologic evidence from exposed human or animal populations, (2) experimental evidence from long-term bioassays in laboratory animals, and (3) suggestive evidence derived from studies of chemical structure, reactivity, DNA damage and repair, mutagenicity, neoplastic transformation of cells in culture, and/or induction of preneoplastic changes *in vivo*. Because of both the difficulty in obtaining this evidence and the recognized limitations in applying it to other species, dosages, and environmental conditions, there are few known carcinogens among the multitude of suspected carcinogens for humans and even fewer for pet species.

Laboratory evidence using exaggerated doses cannot, of course, be tested in humans nor will it be tested in small pet species (with few exceptions). Extrapolation of results from one species to another is fraught with difficulties, and there even are known differences in the results from different rodent test species, i.e., rats and mice. All that can be concluded is that a compound that proves positive in all species tested and in the available *in vitro* tests is much more likely to be carcinogenic in humans (or in a pet species) than one that is negative in all but one test.

VARIATION IN OCCURRENCE

The difficulty in extrapolating from a test to a target species is emphasized by the difference in the incidence of various types of tumors as well as the sex and breed distribution found in dogs and cats. The dog has a high incidence of mammary tumors, but these are less common in the cat. In the dog one study found these tumors to be most frequent in pointers, poodles, and Boston terriers. In the cat, the Siamese breed carries twice the risk of developing mammary carcinoma compared with all other breeds combined. Lymphosarcoma is very common in the cat but appears with less frequency in the dog. Testicular tumors are common in the dog but rare in the cat. Chemoreceptor tumors, granulosa cell tumors, and hemangiopericytomas may be found in the dog but almost never in the cat. The overall incidence of tumors is greater in female dogs than in males; however, the reverse occurs in cats. Male dogs have been shown to have a slightly increased risk for primary carcinoma of the nasal cavity or paranasal sinuses. Boxers have been shown to be at high risk for many types of tumors.

EXPOSURE TO CARCINOGENS

The majority of human cancers, and presumably those of companion animals as well, are considered to be induced by chemicals in the environment. Individuals may be exposed through the atmosphere or from industrial operations or food. Although it is the food additives that have received the most attention from the regulatory agencies and the public, a far greater array of potentially harmful chemicals occur naturally in plant food products. Those with high intakes in humans include 3-hydroxyflavons, rutin, and pyrrolizidine alkaloids. Compounds formed during cooking, such as the yet unidentified hamburger mutagen, are believed by some researchers to be associated with cancer of the gastrointestinal tract. Fortunately, the plant-derived content of the diet of small animals comes primarily from commercially prepared pet foods utilizing grains of generally known composition.

The incidence of cancer in animals and humans has been shown to correlate with industry in a study that determined a significant positive correlation between canine bladder cancer and the overall industrial activity in the host county where detected.

SUPPLEMENTAL READING

Hayes, H. M., Jr., Hoover, R., and Tarone, R. E.: Bladder cancer in dogs: a sentinel for environmental cancer? Am. J. Epidemiol. 114:229, 1981.

Hayes, H. M., Jr., Milne, K. L., and Mandell, C. P.: Epidemiological features of feline mammary carcinoma. Vet. Rec. 108:476, 1981.

Interagency Regulatory Liaison Group: Scientific bases for identification of potential carcinogens and estimation of risks. J. Nat. Cancer Inst. 63:242, 1979.

MacVean, D. W., Monlux, A. W., Anderson, D. S., Silberg, S. L., and Roszel, J.: Frequency of canine and feline tumors in a defined population. Vet. Pathol. 15:700, 1978.

Schneider, R.: General considerations. *In* Moulton, J. E. (ed.): *Tumors in Domestic Animals*, 2nd ed. Berkeley, California: University of California Press, 1979.

Weisburger, J. H., and Williams, G. M.: Chemical carcinogens. *In* Doull, J. (ed.): Cassarett and Doull's *Toxicology: The Basic Science of Poisons*, 2nd ed. New York: Macmillan Publishing Co., 1980.

BITES AND STINGS OF VENOMOUS ANIMALS

G. L. MEERDINK, D.V.M.

East Lansing, Michigan

Many members of the animal kingdom produce toxins that are used offensively in the procurement of food, defensively for self-protection or protection of the colony, and occasionally as an aid in digestion. Venomous animals exist in essentially all parts of North America, although there is much variation in the venomous species that occur in specific regions of the country. The veterinarian should become familiar with the poisonous species of snakes and spiders in his area, since he will seldom know the identity of the perpetrator when presented with the bitten victim.

The therapeutic approach is stressed here through organization of the recommendations made by experts in the various areas. If further information regarding the toxic characteristics of a species is desired, a reading list is supplied for referral.

POISONOUS SNAKES

Many species of snakes exist in North America, but only a few are poisonous. These few are important, as an estimated 15,000 domestic animals are bitten annually in the United States, and rattlesnakes account for approximately 80 per cent of the deaths (Knowles et al., 1974). The poisonous snakes of the United States are the rattlesnake (*Crotalus* spp. and *Sistrurus* spp.), copperhead (*Agkistrodon* spp.), water moccasin or cottonmouth (*Agkistrodon piscivorous*), and coral snake (*Micrurus euryxanthus*). The California lyre snake (*Trimorphodon vandenburghi*) and mangrove snake (*Boiga dendrophila*) are also venomous but are of minor importance to domestic animals. The pit viper venoms (rattlesnake, copperhead, and water moccasin) are primarily necrotizing and hemolyzing; however, other body systems can certainly be affected. The venoms primarily contain proteinaceous and enzymatic toxins. Phospholipase A is a strong hemolytic agent; L-amino-oxidase and other homologous enzymes may be responsible for the activation of tissue peptidases. Hyaluronidase, or "spreading factor," enhances tissue penetration. Numerous other protein and nonprotein constituents have been detected that may produce deleterious biologic effects, and more than a single lethal component usually is included. The coral snake is a member of the elapid or cobra family, and its venom is primarily neurotoxic. Cholinesterase is present in high concentrations in some species; however, this enzyme has been shown not to be the neurotoxic factor and does not contribute significantly to the neuromuscular block produced by these venoms.

FACTORS THAT CONTRIBUTE TO THE SEVERITY OF THE BITE

The severity of the bite depends first on the type and size of the snake and the toxicity of the venom. Besides a species variation in venom potency, a wide variation in the volume of venom injected exists. The snake may be able to regulate the amount of venom injected (in fact, many bites may not be venomizing); more venom may be available if the snake has not eaten for some time.

The number of strikes and the degree of fang penetration are important considerations. When lost, fangs are replaced, and more than one fang may be present on each side. Thus, fang marks from pit viper bites may vary from one to as many as six from one bite. The coral snake, with relatively short, fixed fangs, must strike its victim squarely and securely to gain sufficient penetration for envenomation. On the other hand, the Eastern diamondback rattlesnake, with fangs of up to 2.4 cm, can readily penetrate into deeper, more vascular tissues. Fang length, overall size and strength, and the high yield of venom give the Eastern diamondback rattlesnake the dubious honor of being one of the most dangerous snakes in the United States.

Temperament as well as the local population of the species may affect the incidence of bites seen by the practitioner. The water moccasin is reputed to be quite aggressive and may attack with little provocation. Coral snakes are secretive and remain undercover and usually strike only if disturbed. Rattlesnakes, on the other hand, cause the majority of snakebites even though they sound due warning to the intruder. (They may not always sound off with rattle vibration if suddenly disturbed.) The copperhead has the least potent venom of the North American viperine snakes.

As would be expected, many host factors play a role in determining the severity of the bite including the site of the bite. Unfortunately, most snakebites in domestic animals occur around the head or neck area, increasing the chances of direct damage to vital structures and problems with treatment. Because of a lower venom/body weight ratio, increased severity would be expected in smaller animals, although cats are not often bitten and apparently have some increased resistance (Clarke and Clarke, 1974). Physical activity (which increases the uptake of venom into the circulation) and the length of time following the bite are also factors that the clinician must assess in his approach to treatment.

CLINICAL SIGNS AND DIAGNOSIS

Snakebite is not always easy to diagnose, particularly if heavy hair and swelling obscure fang marks. Other puncture-type wounds from sharp objects, fish spines, or other animal bites are usually more ragged and do not have the same progressive clinical signs. Wounds from arthropods are usually smaller and do not bleed as freely. Bites of nonpoisonous snakes cannot be differentiated reliably from those of poisonous snakes on the basis of puncture wound pattern. Any pattern may be observed with nonpoisonous snakes, from single punctures to rows of multiple punctures; palatine and molar teeth may cause puncture wounds in addition to the one or more venom fangs of the poisonous species. However, less pain, little swelling, and absence of the progressive clinical signs will aid in differentiating nonpoisonous from poisonous bites (Minton, 1974).

If venom is injected directly into the blood vascular system, severe systemic signs and sometimes death occur rapidly. Generally, however, the venom injected into tissues is transported via the lymphatics. Particularly with the pit vipers, the early signs are caused by the direct effects of the toxins on the local tissues. Pain, erythema, and edema develop as a result of the activation of histamine, bradykinin, and other tissue inflammatory agents. The swelling may become extensive and may be accompanied by petechiae, ecchymoses, and hematomas. Secondly in the clinical course, indirect effects from substances released from tissues because of the venom serve to enhance the local necrosis and promote the systemic effects of hypotension with tachycardia, pulmonary edema, salivation, diarrhea, and shock. After a few hours, hemolytic anemia, hemoglobinuria, and renal failure follow. In advanced cases, lethargy and paralysis develop; death is caused by respiratory and circulatory collapse (Knowles et al., 1974). If strikes occur in the head or neck area, swelling may rapidly cause respiratory distress.

Coral snake venom causes little local pain or swelling. Often, within a half hour, early neurotoxic effects can be observed, although a lag phase of several hours may elapse before the onset of signs. Difficulty in swallowing, depression, insensitivity of the limbs, and skeletal paralysis develop, leading to death by respiratory paralysis (Oehme et al., 1975).

TREATMENT

The bitten animal should be subdued and immobilized as much as possible to slow the uptake of venom. Basically, the objectives in the treatment of snakebite are: (1) prevent spread of the venom, (2) remove the venom, (3) neutralize the venom, (4) prevent shock, and (5) prevent infection. Knowles and colleagues (1974) proposed the following course of treatment after performing animal experimentation studies.

Incarcerate the Venom. In cases of wounds of the extremity, a flat tourniquet should immediately be applied proximal to the fang mark area. It should not be applied so tightly that the limb becomes ischemic but tight enough to impede superficial venous and lymphatic flow. Tourniquets of this sort may be left in place for as long as two hours without removal. A good rule to follow is to test the tightness by inserting a finger under the tourniquet band; if this can be done easily it is applied properly. The tourniquet should *not* be removed at intervals, because this will pump the venom from the initial site.

Remove the Venom. A continuous linear incision should be made through both fang mark perforations and should extend in depth to the fascia covering the muscle. Do not sever vital structures such as tendons, motor nerves, and major blood vessels. Do not use cruciate incisions, because the tips of the incision are subject to necrosis and such a wound is receptive to anaerobic contaminants and clostridial complications. Applying suction to the incision retrieves some of the venom and is advocated, although mouth suction is not recommended because two lives may be lost as a result. Elliptical excision of the fang marks, including skin and subdermal fat, is more efficacious than incision and suction in removing the venom in severe envenomation. The size of the area involved in the elliptical excision is dependent upon the fang marks but must extend at least ½ inch (1 cm) equidistant around the puncture wounds. This type of wound may be closed primarily at a later date.

Neutralize the Venom. Polyvalent antivenin should be used in every subject suspected of serpent envenomation (Antivenin, Fort Dodge Laboratories). The sooner the venom is neutralized, the better the therapeutic result. Because more time is required for the antivenin to reach the poisonous venom when given intramuscularly or into the bite area, we administer the antivenin intraarterially or intravenously. We believe that the arterial route produces a faster and more potent effect than the venous route because the drug is more concentrated and acts on the venom longer; antivenin given intravenously must traverse the cardiac-hepatic-pulmonary circulation before reaching the bite area.

The method of intra-arterial perfusion should be performed only by veterinarians and is as follows: Mix the contents of one vial of polyvalent antivenin into 100 ml of normal saline and, using a sphygmomanometer bulb, pump it into the regional artery with a tight tourniquet proximal to the arterial injection site. The tourniquet keeps the antivenin localized in the bite area, and direct neutralization of the venom takes effect. It requires about 20 minutes to pump the mixture into the area. If the patient has a history of allergic manifestations, 100 ml of hydrocortisone sodium succinate (Solu-Cortef) should be added to the intra-arterial solution. The regional arteries for infusion are the femoral artery for snakebites of the hind legs, the brachial artery for the forelegs, and the carotid artery for the head and neck. We are aware that complications can ensue from intra-arterial injection, but we have not observed any in our experience; on the other hand, we have observed death due to envenomation.

An antivenin is now available specifically for bites of coral snakes and may be ordered through the state boards of health.

Prevent Shock. When less than a 100 per cent lethal dose of moccasin venom is injected, pain is a significant factor in the onset of shock and in the longevity of the otherwise nontreated animal. Because morphine is excessively depressing to the respiratory mechanism, meperidine (Demerol) appears to be the drug of choice for pain control in snakebite. Dosage should be 1 mg/lb (2 mg/kg) of body weight initially, and it should be given as needed to alleviate pain. Meperidine administration should be continued until the pain has subsided.

Prevent Infection. Because snakes' mouths are frequently contaminated with pathogens, the skin in the bite area is not clean and massive tissue destruction with blood extravasation enhances bacterial activity; therefore, the administration of a broad spectrum antibiotic is mandatory. We recommend intramuscular or intravenous administration of cephaloridine (Loridine) initially every 12 hours, followed by oral administration of doxycycline (Vibramycin) every 12 hours.

Anaphylactoid Reactions. Specific anaphylactoid reactions, to either the venom or the antivenin, are rare in the dog. Corticosteroids should be given in ample dosage during the acute phase of this condition. Although they are not life saving, corticosteroids significantly increase longevity and may therefore enable other medicaments to exert their beneficial effects. They minimize pain, improve the patient's sense of well-being, promote the even distribution of edema, and hence minimize the possibility of slough. The snakebite victim that receives corticoids (prednisone, 1 mg/lb [2 mg/kg] of body weight initially and then 0.5 mg/lb [1 mg/kg] of body weight every 12 hours) is more likely to maintain a normal fluid balance by consuming larger quantities of water and a reasonable amount of food as compared with the noncorticoid-treated patient that usually will neither eat nor drink.

Lactated Ringer's solution or blood may be indicated to bolster fluid volume and electrolyte levels. The animal should be kept warm and quiet. Immobilization is the most effective mechanical means of combating envenomation. In our opinion, immobilization can best be accomplished under these circumstances by the judicious use of meperidine and quiet, comfortable quarters.

Ancillary Treatment. Calcium gluconate has been suggested to combat hemolysis and muscular twitching. Tetanus antitoxin is also indicated.

LIZARDS

The only species of poisonous lizards can be found in the Southwest—the Gila monster (*Heloderma suspectum*) and the Mexican beaded lizard (*H. horridum*). These lizards are lethargic and nonaggressive, and thus animal poisonings are rare. They do not have fangs *per se* but are armed with grooved teeth that are bathed in venom from modified salivary glands located on each side of the lower jaw. Lizards hold tenaciously on to the victim and, with chewing movements, increase the quantity of envenomation.

The teeth of these lizards usually produce simple puncture wounds, which may vary from one to as many as 18. If envenomation has taken place, pain will usually be present within several minutes. Intense pain may radiate from the periphery but seldom extends beyond the involved extremity. Some hemorrhage may occur at the site of the bite, but there is no clinical evidence, to date, to suggest that the venom alters blood coagulation. Most experimental evidence suggests that the venom affects the cardiovascular system, resulting in hypotension and shock. The mechanism of action has not been determined.

The bite of these lizards is persistent, and the reptile may have to be disengaged by sticking a prying instrument between the jaws and pushing against the back of the mouth. A flame to the underside of the jaw may also cause the lizard to loosen its grip. The teeth of the lizard can be broken and left in the wound, thus a forceful jerk of the reptile from the victim is not recommended.

Treatment is primarily symptomatic and can be managed clinically in a manner similar to that for snakebite therapy. Irrigation of the wound site is of value; the clinician should look for broken teeth. The victim should be monitored for signs of hypotension and shock, particularly during the first eight hours. Antihistamines and corticosteroids are not considered to be of value. Tetanus antitoxin (or toxoid) should be administered, along with antibiotics to control infection, and the wound can be soaked to enhance healing (Russell and Bogert, 1981).

BEES, WASPS, HORNETS, AND ANTS

The order *Hymenoptera* contains the important stinging insects—the bees, wasps, hornets, and ants. Many species of this order are more dangerous because of the colony's aggressive reaction to disturbance and its ability to inflict a multitude of stings within a few minutes. The venom apparatus is located on the terminal portion of the abdomen. In a few species, including the honey bee, the sting is barbed and the entire venom apparatus is torn from the insect's body and left attached to the victim. The venoms within this order vary among species but characteristically include proteinaceous compounds with histamine, hyaluronidase, and hemolyzing components. Insect stings are the leading cause of human deaths from venomous animals in the United States, primarily because of the hypersensitization properties of the venoms and anaphylactic deaths from subsequent exposure.

Stings of these insects cause painful local inflammation. The intensity of the reaction can be increased by multiple stings to the extent that shock becomes an important clinical problem. Deaths from multiple stings (hundreds) have been reported in dogs. If the victim has been previously exposed to the venom and hypersensitized, anaphylaxis can result from only one sting.

The first consideration in clinical management is the possibility of anaphylaxis or shock from multiple stings. The site of the bite(s) can be very important; asphyxiation may result from swelling of the buccal or pharyngeal area. If needed, 1 to 5 ml of a 1:10,000 aqueous solution of epinephrine should be injected subcutaneously in dogs and cats, as well as corticosteroids and antihistamines. (Antihistamines are of little value in fire ant stings.) The clinician must be alert to the fact that in some cases anaphylaxis may be delayed. Oxygen may be necessary if dyspnea is evident. Pain and swelling of local reactions can be reduced by cold packs (Minton, 1974; Oehme et al., 1975).

SPIDERS

Practically all spiders are venomous; however, severe reactions are limited to two genera: *Lactrodectus* spp. (black widow and red widow, female) and *Loxosceles* spp. (brown recluse and common brown). The infamous tarantula (*Eurytelma* spp.) is capable of a venomous bite, but serious reactions from natural bites in domestic animals have not been reported.

Spiders subsist on the body fluids of their prey and thus use their venom to immobilize the victim. Venom is injected through channeled bilateral head appendage fangs called *chelicerae*. Considering the inconspicuous size of the bite marks and animal hair cover, diagnosis of spider bites is difficult for the veterinarian unless, perhaps, the spider is located. The black widow is black (other species are brown to reddish) with red or red-yellow spots, the most common appearance being an hourglass shape on the ventral aspect of the abdomen. Brown recluse spiders are tawny to brown with a darker (often violin-shaped) mark on the dorsal cephalothorax. Because of its relatively long legs, the brown recluse is capable of quick movement.

Lactrodectus spp. venoms are highly toxic to mammals. The severity of the black widow bite may vary, but it is usually characterized by short-lived local pain. Neurotoxic manifestations soon follow and are characterized by muscle spasms, evidence of abdominal pain, ataxia, excessive salivation, tonic and clonic convulsions, and flaccid paralysis. Weakness with dyspnea followed by paralysis may occur within six hours in an acute case or not until several days later in a less severe envenomation. Increases in blood pressure and ECG abnormalities may be observed. Antivenin is available and, if used, should be administered as soon as possible. Corticosteroids, intravenous fluids, and prophylactic antibiotics should be administered. Methocarbamol, calcium gluconate, meperidine, and atropine may be used to control muscle spasms, pain, and excessive secretions. The prognosis is uncertain for several days (Minton, 1974; Clarke and Clarke, 1975; Oehme et al., 1975).

Loxosceles spp. are primarily found in the southern half of the US and are best known for the potent, enduring dermonecrotic effects of their toxin. The spider is often found in basements, storage areas, and other darkened areas and will not bite unless provoked. The initial reaction from the bite is evidently not painful. However, within a few hours, the hemolytic and necrotizing toxins cause local pruritus and swelling, which develops into focal erythema and the formation of a blister. Necrosis follows as a result of ischemia, and, by 7 to 14 days, the focal ulceration is evident. The lesion requires eight weeks or longer to heal. Depending on the particular *Loxosceles* species and the susceptibility of the animal, systemic signs of fever, weakness, vomition, convulsions, hemolysis, and thombocytopenia may also occur. Latest recommendations have advocated early excision of the affected tissue with primary repair. If not removed, the lesion has a tendency to spread, particularly into dependent areas. Corticosteroids and antibiotics should be administered, particularly if signs of systemic effects are detected (Oehme et al., 1975; Wasserman and Siegel, 1977).

SCORPIONS

Several genera of scorpions exist in North America, but the most dangerous species live in the arid climates of Mexico and Arizona. The last segment of the highly mobile tail of this eight-legged arthropod contains a hollow, curved stinging apparatus through which venom is injected. Scorpion bites are not uncommon in humans and do produce fatalities; however, the incidence of bites in domestic animals is not known. Difficulty in recognizing the condition may account for its relatively low recorded incidence in veterinary medicine. Scorpion stings usually produce severe immediate pain. The puncture is single, bleeds little if at all, and may be very difficult to differentiate from insect stings in the early stages.

Generally, the earliest sign of envenomation is intense local pain associated with erythema and edema. Although the stings of most species cause only local reactions that subside within a few hours, the more toxic varieties may cause systemic neurotoxic effects. Parasympathomimetic signs include excessive salivation, muscle fasciculations, and weakness. Generalized weakness and paralysis may lead to respiratory distress. The clinical condition generally improves within 24 hours.

If little time has elapsed since envenomation, the severity of the local reaction and the spread of the toxin can be partially prevented by prompt application of cold packs (without freezing of tissue) for up to two hours. Antivenins are available; one specific for the genus involved is best, although evidence exists of some cross protection. Atropine can be used to block the parasympathomimetic effects, and corticosteroids can decrease shock and edema. Meperidine and morphine derivatives are contraindicated, and intravenous fluids should be administered carefully because of the risk of pulmonary edema. Respiratory assistance may become necessary (Russell and Saunders, 1966; Minton, 1974; Oehme et al., 1975).

TICK PARALYSIS

Tick paralysis is an ascending afebrile motor paralysis that appears most commonly in children, cattle, sheep, and dogs. The offending ticks from paralyzed victims in North America are usually females of the *Dermacentor* or *Amblyomma* genera; their saliva contains hemorrhagic-neurotoxin elements that apparently interfere with acetylcholine synthesis or liberation at the neuromuscular junction. The tick may have been attached for several days. Ataxia is first observed, which soon develops into an ascending motor paralysis. Within 36 hours from onset, dyspnea may follow if paralysis proceeds to the respiratory center. The animal may demonstrate proprioception deficiency but maintain normal anal sphincter tone. Removal of the tick results in rapid recovery within hours, and the victim is usually completely asymptomatic within 48 hours. All ticks must be removed, as only one can cause the condition; the use of organophosphorus insecticide dips or sprays will aid in the removal process. Absence of fever, lack of abnormal spinal fluid findings, and evidence of normal sensory function will help differentiate this condition from central nervous system infections and other similar conditions.

REFERENCES AND SUPPLEMENTAL READING

Arnold, R. E.: *What to Do About Bites and Stings of Venomous Animals.* New York: Macmillan Co., 1973.

Brown, J. H.: *Toxicology and Pharmacology of Venoms from Poisonous Snakes.* Springfield, Illinois: Charles C Thomas, 1973.

Clarke, E. G. C., and Clarke, M. L.: *Veterinary Toxicology.* Baltimore: The Williams & Wilkins Co., 1975.

Frye, F. L.: Bites and stings of venomous animals. *In* Kirk, R. W. (ed.): *Current Veterinary Therapy VI.* Philadelphia: W. B. Saunders Co., 1977.

Huang, S. Y., and Perez, J. C.: Comparative study on hemorrhagic and proteolytic activities of snake venoms. Toxicon 18:421, 1980.

Knowles, R. P., Snyder, C. C., Glenn, J. L., and Straight, R. C.: Bites of venomous snakes. *In* Kirk, R. W. (ed.): *Current Veterinary Therapy V.* Philadelphia: W. B. Saunders Co., 1974.

Minton, S. A.: *Venom Diseases.* Springfield, Illinois: Charles C Thomas, 1974.

Oehme, F. W., Brown, J. F., and Fowler, M. E.: Toxins of animal origin. *In* Casarett, L. J., and Doull, J. (eds.): *Toxicology.* New York: Macmillan Co., 1975.

Russell, F. E., and Bogert, C. M.: Gila monster: Its biology, venom and bite—A review. Toxicon 19:341, 1981.

Russel, F. E., and Saunders, P. R. (eds.): *Animal Toxins.* New York: Pergamon Press, 1966.

Tu, A. T.: *Venoms: Chemistry and Molecular Biology.* Baltimore: John Wiley & Sons, 1977.

Wasserman, G. S., and Siegel, C.: Loxoscelism (brown recluse spider bites): a review of literature. Vet. Human Toxicol. 19:256, 1977.

TOAD POISONING

N. E. PALUMBO, D.V.M.,
and S. F. PERRI, B.A.

Honolulu, Hawaii

There is little question that the introduction during the past four decades of the giant tropical toad, *Bufo marinus*, into the southern states, and especially into Hawaii has paid great dividends in controlling undesirable insect pests. These toads, however, are capable of producing a potent toxin in their large, warty, paired parotid glands, which are roughly oval in shape, are situated behind the border of the tympanum, and extend backward over the shoulders. Numerous pinhole openings can be seen on the surface skin of these glands from which a thick, pasty, yellow-white toxin can be manually expressed. These toads therefore represent a threat to unsuspecting people who may mistake them for frogs and consume their skin, as has been documented in Hawaii, or who may be exposed to the toad's toxin through an open wound, as has been reported in Florida. More common, of course, is the threat of this potent toxin to animals mouthing the toads.

Although we have seen feline intoxications in rare instances, the principal cause for concern has been the threat to dogs. The lethargic hopping of the awkward toad will often attract dogs at dusk when other kinds of activity are minimal. These dogs will grasp the toad in their mouths, causing compression of the toad's parotid glands and expression of the toxin. Absorption of the toxin through the buccal and gastric mucosa apparently is quite rapid, resulting in a variety of symptoms that may culminate in death. The *Bufo marinus* in Florida, possibly because of diet, climate, or genetic factors, seems to produce a more potent toxin than that produced by the Hawaiian *Bufo marinus*. The death rate in Hawaii of exposed and untreated dogs is approximately 5 per cent as compared with nearly 100 per cent in Florida. In Texas, the death rate is also low.

The dog that mouths a toad will exhibit variable symptoms depending upon its age, concurrent disease, amount of toxin absorbed in relation to its total body weight, and length of time since exposure; the signs range from slight salivation to cyanosis and convulsive seizures. Obviously many other conditions could be confused with toad poisoning, and a history of having seen the dog mouth a toad will be sufficient evidence in a sick animal to warrant initiation of immediate antitoad-poisoning therapy.

COMPOSITION OF THE BUFO TOXIN COMPLEX

There are 12 species of *Bufo* toads distributed worldwide. The parotid gland secretions of all toads contain bufagins, bufotoxins, bufotenins, and other compounds. Bufotoxins are the conjugation product of the specific bufagin with one molecule of suberyl arginine. Bufotenins are organic bases containing an indole ring in the molecule. The action or effect of bufagins is described as digitalis-like, often resulting in ventricular fibrillation; the action of bufotoxin is similar. Bufotenins have, for the most part, an oxytocic action accompanied frequently by a marked pressor action.

Other compounds found in *Bufo marinus* toxin are epinephrine, cholesterol, ergosterol, and 5-hydroxytryptamine (5-HT). The last is also known as serotonin, or "serum vasoconstrictor." The highest biologic concentration of 5-HT occurs in the skins of certain toads. The physiologic role of 5-HT in bufo intoxication in the dog is not fully appreciated at this time. 5-HT is rapidly degraded in the gastrointestinal tract but might participate in the intoxication should some of the toxin be inspired via the respiratory tract.

PHARMACODYNAMICS OF BUFO INTOXICATION IN THE DOG

A syndrome resembling canine bufo intoxication was reproduced by giving ouabain and epinephrine intravenously in a rat study. A synergistic effect was found to exist between the glycoside and the catecholamine; sublethal doses of each given simultaneously were shown to be lethal.

When bufotoxin is given intravenously to a dog, the response is similar to that seen experimentally in the rat—a rapid rise in blood pressure, cardiac arrhythmias, and dyspnea. However, when the same amount of bufotoxin is given orally to the dog, the onset of signs is slower and there is no pressor effect. Following oral administration of a lethal dose of bufotoxin to an anesthetized dog, one finds a gradual deterioration of the ECG with progressive negative ventricular deflection, which eventually results in ventricular fibrillation and death if untreated. Respiratory rate and depth increase without any appreciable increase in blood pressure.

The fact that oral intoxication in the dog is not associated with increased blood pressure (and so is markedly different from the intravenous intoxication) is due to the inactivation of catecholamines by the digestive tract and liver. Toxic intravenous or oral doses of bufotoxin in the dog result in a moderate increase in packed cell volume, hemoglobin content, icterus index and concentrations of blood glucose, serum urea nitrogen, serum potassium, and serum calcium. The sedimentation rate increases. Serum sodium and chloride concentrations decrease slightly, but serum inorganic phosphorus content decreases markedly. Total protein usually decreases slightly owing to loss of albumin. The total white blood cell count decreases, principally because of neutropenia. After any initial spike in SGOT activity, which may be due to the stress and struggle associated with the intoxication, this enzyme tends to return slowly to baseline values. Neither the SGPT nor alkaline phosphatase levels change appreciably.

TRADITIONAL THERAPY: AN ANALYSIS OF THE RATIONALE

There is a wide range of preferred treatments for this kind of intoxication. Some of the preferred regimens of therapy reported to yield good rates of cure are actually conflicting. Not only is one confused by the conflicting recommendations of veterinary clinicians who have been intimately involved in solving the problem of bufo intoxication in sick pets, but there is much additional confusion to be found in the general scientific and veterinary literature.

In the past, preferred treatments for canine toad intoxication included atropine, prednisone, antihistamines, calcium gluconate, tranquilizers, and anesthesia (barbiturates).

Atropine is frequently used symptomatically to dry mucous membranes in the respiratory system and depress salivary secretions. Its action on the heart is to block the vagal effect, thus abolishing the normal slowing reflex. For these reasons, atropine may well be used in the treatment of bufo intoxication. It should be recognized, however, that atropine is not likely to produce any essential antitoxic effect on the myocardium and that swabbing may equally well accomplish drying of the mouth. Thus, atropine is not a specific antidote to the disease as we envision it. In animals that may have inspired foamy saliva containing the toxin into the respiratory tract, the 5-HT could conceivably cause bronchoconstriction. In these cases, the effect of atropine in clearing the airway will be desirable, but a specific antagonist of 5-HT would be more efficacious.

Calcium gluconate must be given intravenously, but some of its toxic side effects cause heart block

and ventricular fibrillation, the usual terminal events in bufo intoxication. One of the actions ascribed to calcium is the maintenance of membrane permeability. Digitalis intoxication inhibits ATPase activity in cell membranes, affecting the Na^+/K^+ pump and increasing Ca^{++} permeability. This effect is aggravated by giving additional Ca^{++} or by further depletion of K^+ and is improved by decreasing Ca^{++} or adding K^+. Calcium and digitalis have similar effects on the myocardium, and calcium may provoke arrhythmias and even ventricular fibrillation in the digitalized subject.

Antihistamines and steroids may also provide additional benefit by reducing the effects of bufotoxin on the mucous membranes of the mouth and other organs. Again, in this instance we do not envision these drugs as having any direct or vital beneficial effect.

Pentobarbital anesthesia increases canine tolerance to bufo intoxication. In one experiment, dogs given bufotoxin and anesthetized within five minutes could tolerate a dose that would prove fatal to nonanesthetized dogs. The major difference in the anesthetized animal's behavior seemed to be the marked decrease in the amount of mouthing, salivation, and labored respirations, Presumably this activity may increase absorption through the pharynx and mouth or perhaps even through the respiratory tract, where there could be the additional effect of serotonin and catecholamines. To a lesser extent, but possibly through the same general mechanisms of action, tranquilizers serve to protect animals soon after exposure. Thiamylal sodium, a short-acting barbiturate, is contraindicated, since its action is too brief and it may produce cardiac arrhythmias, which may predispose the dog to ventricular fibrillation.

The oldest and possibly one of the best ways of handling the early intoxication is to rinse the dog's mouth promptly with water. A garden hose serves well for this purpose. Inducing vomiting is another popular method of rendering first aid.

DISCUSSION

If propranolol HCl, a beta-adrenergic blocking agent, is given to a dog exposed to a lethal oral dose of bufotoxin prior to the onset of ventricular fibrillation or immediately following its onset, the ECG makes a spectacular reversal to normal.

Bufo intoxication in the dog is presumed to be due to the glycoside portion of the bufotoxin complex and is possibly potentiated by endogenous catecholamines. The mechanism of action of propranolol as an antidote is suspected to be due to this drug's ability to antagonize the glycosides' stimulatory effect on sympathetic nerves, thus blocking the release of endogenous catecholamines. This action then limits the intoxication essentially to a pure glycoside intoxication, which the dog can handle more effectively.

Propranolol effectively blocks the cardiac actions of catecholamines in dosages of 0.2 mg/kg; at the high dosages we used initially in our experiments (5 mg/kg), the drug still possesses its beta-adrenergic blocking action but presumably is exerting a quinidine-like action in reversing the arrhythmias associated with digitalis intoxication. D-Propranolol, which has no beta-blocking activity, is equally as effective as L-propranolol (a beta-adrenergic blocker) in antagonizing digitalis-induced arrhythmias. Another interesting hypothesis on the mechanism of action of propranolol as an antiarrhythmic agent is that it may act as a neurodepressant on cardiac sympathetic innervation.

Potassium administration is well established as standard therapy in glycoside intoxication. The danger of causing toxic side effects from improper administration of K^+ is also documented. Propranolol has been shown to cause massive leakage of K^+ from red blood cells, which results in an alteration of the Gibbs-Donnan equilibrium across the red blood cell membrane. Propranolol therapy results in elevated serum K^+ levels, which may also be of therapeutic value.

Elderly humans appear to be especially labile to digitalis intoxication, so if in the case of cardiac glycoside intoxication one may extrapolate from human to dog, then one may guess that old, sick dogs with pre-existing heart disease would be more susceptible to bufo intoxication than would be young, healthy dogs.

A NEW SUGGESTED THERAPEUTIC REGIMEN

On the basis of our observations and clinical experience, a new and more specific approach to the treatment of *Bufo marinus* intoxication in the dog is suggested:

1. Determine whether the history is compatible with toad intoxication.
2. Determine if there is a history of heart disease or asthma.
3. In the absence of any history of asthma or cardiac disease, proceed as follows:
   a. Place an intravenous catheter in the cephalic vein;
   b. Administer pentobarbital anesthesia intravenously, insert an endotracheal tube, wash out the mouth thoroughly;
   c. Administer propranolol intravenously at the

rate of 2 mg/kg body weight. With a stethoscope over the heart during propranolol administration, a return to a normal heart rate can be detected within 15 seconds;
   d. Monitor the patient using an oscilloscope, an ECG (lead II), or a stethoscope. Repeat propranolol administration after 20 minutes if necessary (2 mg/kg); and
   e. Administer fluids at a slow rate, if considered appropriate.
4. In the presence of a history of asthma or pre-existing cardiac disease, proceed as follows:
   a. Rinse the oral and buccal cavities well with water, using a wash cloth or toothbrush to clean all surfaces, because the toad toxin is waxy and tenaciously adheres to the teeth and mucosa;
   b. Place an intravenous catheter in the cephalic vein;
   c. Monitor the patient on an oscilloscope and administer propranolol intravenously slowly at the dosage of 0.5 mg/kg body weight until the cardiac rate returns to normal; and
   d. Administer fluids intravenously at a slow rate, if considered appropriate.

Note: Anesthetics may further compromise an already diseased myocardium and should be used with discretion. Asthmatic animals are dependent on endogenous catecholamines for bronchodilatation, just as animals with heart failure depend on these substances to drive the heart. When the beta-adrenergic drugs are administered, they block the host from the physiologic effect of these substances. In certain individuals this may cut the fragile last thread holding the animal to life. Although the drug has a wide margin of safety and is capable of correcting lethal toad intoxication, it should be used with caution and under close surveillance in older, asthmatic, or cardiac-diseased dogs.

SUPPLEMENTAL READING

Knowles, R. P.: The poison toad and the canine. V.M./S.A.C. Jan.: 38, 1964.
Otani, A. Palumbo, N., and Read, G.: Pharmacodynamics and treatment of mammals poisoned by *Bufo marinus* toxin. Am. J. Vet. Res. 30:1865, 1969.
Palumbo, N., Perri, S., and Read, G.: Experimental induction and treatment of toad poisoning in the dog. J. A.V.M.A. 11:1000, 1975.
Russell, R. L.: Toad poisoning. *In* Kirk, R. W. (ed.): *Current Veterinary Therapy III*. Philadelphia: W. B. Saunders Co., 1966, pp. 621–622.

GARBAGE-, FOOD-, AND WATER-BORNE INTOXICATION

R. W. COPPOCK, D.V.M.
Urbana, Illinois

Dogs, by virtue of their scavenging habits, are more prone to garbage-, food-, and water-borne intoxication than cats. This intoxication results from the ingestion of garbage, food, and water that contains toxic substances of biological origin. These toxins are produced by microorganisms growing in "food" and water and liberating the toxins either as toxic metabolites or by lysis of the microorganism and liberation of the toxic cellular components. Different species of microorganisms require different temperatures, oxygen tensions, and substrates for growth and toxin production. As a general rule, these conditions are met more frequently in warmer seasons and climates. The most common toxins involved in food and garbage poisoning are the enterotoxins, endotoxins, and mycotoxins. Water-borne intoxication is caused by the ingestion of water contaminated with toxins liberated during blooms of fresh water blue-green algae. Confirmed cases of botulism in dogs are rare but may occur more frequently than recognized.

MICROORGANISMS IN GARBAGE

SOURCES AND ETIOLOGY

Garbage is waste food materials, which is often highly contaminated with bacteria, especially those associated with man. Protein-rich garbage provides a favorable substrate for the growth of microorganisms and the liberation of toxins. The incidence of garbage poisoning is higher in the summer months and in warmer climates. Garbage is often contaminated with palatable refuse, such as meat packaging materials, and is a common source of foreign bodies that can obstruct the gut.

Food-borne intoxication is caused by the ingestion of animal food and table scraps contaminated with microbial toxins. The most common source of food poisoning in dogs is feeding leftovers from a picnic lunch, discarded food from the refrigerator, and other food that is considered unfit for human consumption. It is not uncommon to find that the dog has shared an episode of food poisoning with the human counterparts in its family. Owners are often surprised to find that dogs are susceptible to food poisoning. Forcing pets to eat animal food, especially those of high moisture content that have sat out at warm temperatures, is a frequent source of food poisoning.

Common enterotoxin-producing bacteria associated with enterotoxicosis in domestic animals are *Streptococcus* spp., *Salmonella* spp., and *Bacillus* spp. Enterotoxins are proteinaceous substances that produce their biologic effects by sorption with gastrointestinal epithelium. Enterotoxins as a general rule are strong irritants to the gastric epithelial cells and therefore are good emetics. Enterotoxins disturb the permeability of the gastrointestinal epithelial cells, causing fluid and electrolyte losses into the lumen and disruption of the absorptive mechanisms. Enterotoxins bind to the enteric epithelial cells and permanently disrupt their cellular functions. Resolution of this biochemical lesion is by necrobiosis of the affected cells and replacement with new cells migrating from the crypts, a process that generally requires three to five days. The irritation and other actions of the enterotoxins increase gut motility; however, this phase is often followed in 10 to 72 hours by dilation and stasis of the gut. The intestinal epithelium may be eroded, and hemorrhage into the intestinal tract may occur.

CLINICAL SIGNS

The first and often the only clinical sign of enterotoxicosis observed by the owner is vomiting, which generally occurs within 15 minutes to 3 hours following the ingestion of enterotoxins. In many cases vomiting removes sufficient toxin from the upper gastrointestinal tract to give complete remission of clinical signs. Because of the irritating properties of enterotoxins, vomiting and retching may persist and may require medical attention. Diarrhea, often bloody, is frequently observed 2 to 48 hours after exposure to enterotoxins. Abdominal tenderness over the anterior quadrant is a common clinical finding and may progress, becoming generalized over the entire abdomen within a few hours. Stasis and dilation of the gut often follows diarrhea, with gas accumulation in the gut, distention of the abdomen, and accompanying pain. Rebound tenderness of the abdomen may be observed. Appropriate radiographs are helpful in ruling out foreign body involvement. Stasis and dilation of the gut leads to an enteric environment, which favors rapid growth of bacteria, especially the gram negatives. Liberation of endotoxins often brings on shock and rapid deterioration of the patient.

A serious complication of food and garbage poisoning is stasis and dilation of the gut. When this phenomenon occurs, there is loss of gut tone and motility and stasis in the movement of ingesta through the intestinal tract. The ingesta generally provides a favorable environment for the growth of gram negative bacteria and the liberation of endotoxins. This leads to endotoxic shock, an anaerobic environment in the gut favoring growth, and toxin liberation by anaerobic bacteria. In many cases patients that develop stasis and dilation of the gut rapidly become critically ill and somewhat refractory to medical treatment.

TREATMENT

Treatment of enterotoxicosis has four major objectives. These are (1) removing the offending ingesta from the digestive tract; (2) controlling vomiting or retching and diarrhea if these conditions persist and present medical problems; (3) preventing ileus or dilation and stasis of the gut; and (4) planning a bland diet during healing of the gut and instructing the owner in preventing subsequent exposure to the offending "food" stuffs or garbage.

Vomiting is an efficient means of removing the offending ingesta from the stomach and duodenum. Enterotoxins are good emetics, and vomiting often removes sufficient toxin to give a spontaneous and complete recovery. Persistent irritations of the gastric mucosa after removal of the offending ingesta by the initial episode of vomiting often results in persistence of vomiting and retching. These cases generally require medical treatment. However, antiemetics should not be given until the clinician is confident that all of the offending ingesta, especially large pieces of bone and so on, has been removed from the stomach. Antiemetic drugs, such as Benadryl (0.5 to 2 mg/kg parenterally or 2 to 5 mg/kg PO) or Dramamine (1.0 to 1.5 mg/kg parenterally), are preferred over the narcotics, especially morphine. Stasis of the gut is a marked side effect of treatment with the morphinoids. Antiemetic drugs should always be followed by treatment with adsorbents such as ToxiBan (Table 1).

Diarrhea is also an efficient means of removing the offending ingesta from the gut. Antidiarrheal drugs should not be given until the clinician has sufficient evidence that the offending ingesta has been removed from the gut. Certain types of enterotoxins alter gut permeability, resulting in marked fluid and electrolyte losses into the gut lumen. In these cases fluid and electrolyte treatment should be initiated before marked dehydration and electrolyte and acid-base imbalances are observed. Antidiarrheal drugs, such as pectin U.S.P. (Table 1), are beneficial in the management of these cases, as they bind toxins and provide bulk in the gut. Parasympatholytic drugs such as atropine sulfate, methylscopolamine, and extracts of belladonna can bring on stasis and dilation of the gut. Combination antidiarrheal preparations that contain parasympatholytic drugs should not be prescribed early in the course of enterotoxicosis. Broad spectrum antibiotics should be given parenterally, especially to control proliferation of bacteria in the gut. Either chloramphenicol or gentamicin has a good spectrum of activity for this purpose. Adsorbents will bind orally administered drugs.

Table 1. *Dosage of Adsorbents for Dogs and Cats*

Drug	Dosage	Dosage Interval
Toxiban	12 to 24 ml/kg	q.i.d.
Pectin*	12 to 20 gm/kg	q.i.d.
Kaolin*	10 to 15 gm/kg	q.i.d.
Na bentonite†	15 gm/kg	q.i.d.
Activated carbon	10 to 20 mg/kg	q.i.d.

*Can be combined and the combination given at 10 to 18 gm/kg.

†The only ingredient in certain brands of cat litter.

ENDOTOXINS

SOURCES AND ETIOLOGY

Garbage, carrion, offal, and other decaying animal parts can serve as a favorable substrate for the rapid growth of gram negative bacteria and the liberation of endotoxins. Endotoxins are the lipopolysaccharide components of the cell walls of gram negative bacteria liberated upon bacteriolysis before or after ingestion of the offending substrate. Endotoxins are absorbed by the gastrointestinal epithelium and are biologically active through a number of different mechanisms: activation of certain inflammatory processes, cardiovascular insult and shock, alteration of the permeability of the gut epithelial cells, and interference with gut and other endocrine functions, especially those regulating intermediary metabolism.

Endotoxins are potent activators of the proteases and other enzymes necessary for the activation of autacoids (histamines, kinins) and in part induce shock by this mechanism. Endotoxins activate factor XII, which initiates the cascade reactions necessary for complement formation and blood coagulation. The autacoids alter capillary permeability and increase hepatic portal resistance to blood flow with splanchnic pooling of blood. Activation of clotting cascade reactions favors diffuse intravascular coagulation.

Endotoxins are also potent inducers of shock through insult to the cardiovascular system. Activation of the autacoids alters capillary permeability and increases the hepatic portal resistance to splanchnic circulation, with marked pooling of blood in the visceral vessels. The net results are hypovolemic shock and a decrease in cardiac output. Endotoxins uncouple oxidative phosphorylation in the myocardium with a net decrease in energy conversion in the heart, which is observed clinically as negative inotropism. Accompanying a decrease in cardiac output is a decrease in systolic blood pressure and renal blood flow. Endotoxic shock can progress very rapidly after the initial signs are observed.

Endotoxins alter the permeability of the gut epithelium with marked fluid and electrolyte losses into the lumen of the intestines. Erosions of epithelial cells may occur with frank hemorrhage. The permeability of the gut capillary bed appears to be altered with protein, especially the precursors of fibrin, leaking from the injured vessels.

Autoregulation of the gut is impaired by the endotoxins, apparently through a number of different mechanisms. It appears that endotoxins prevent the release of certain gut hormones and compete with others for the same receptors. The mechanisms for the emptying of the stomach are interfered with, and gastric emptying may be delayed over 72 hours. Digestive enzymes are not released by the pancreas, and clinical evidence suggests that endotoxins activate pancreatic zymogens, with acute pancreatitis being observed. Endotoxins compete with insulin for the same receptor. Clinical evidence suggests that repeated episodes of endotoxicosis in dogs result in permanent damage to the gut endocrine system.

CLINICAL SIGNS

Clinical features of endotoxicosis include fever, shivering, vomiting, diarrhea, abdominal tenderness, abdominal distention, twilight consciousness, and shock. Fever (102 to 103°F) generally is observed 2 to 24 hours after ingestion and is often accompanied by vomiting and diarrhea. Vomiting seldom leads to a spontaneous recovery. In cases in which vomiting does not occur the stomach is often distended with gas and contains the offending ingesta. The patient may have a watery diarrhea. The patient may be presented in twilight consciousness with a fragmentary history. The abdomen may be distended, with pain and rebound tenderness observed.

Concurrent with these clinical events, a transient leukopenia, especially a neutropenia, is observed and is often followed by a WBC count over 12,000 and a differential cell count consisteing predominantly of polymorphonuclear cells. Hyperglycemia

may be observed. As shock progresses there is loss of temperature in the body extremities, progressing to a generalized hypothermia. As cardiac output decreases there is a decrease in capillary filling time. Heart rate becomes rapid and has been referred to as thready. The liver becomes somewhat engorged and is enlarged on palpation. The patient may or may not be conscious.

TREATMENT

The primary objectives of treatment of endotoxemia are to prevent the onset of shock and remove the offending ingesta from the gastrointestinal tract. Prednisolone sodium succinate should be given at 5 to 7 mg/kg and repeated at one- to four-hour intervals. Appropriate fluid and electrolyte treatment should be initiated to maintain electrolyte and acid-base balance. The offending ingesta should be removed in cases in which spontaneous vomiting and diarrhea have not been sufficient to empty the gastrointestinal tract. Emetics (apomorphine 0.04 to 0.09 mg/kg subcutaneous, or ipecac, U.S.P. 2.2 ml/kg PO) may or may not be effective. Emetics should not be given to patients in twilight consciousness or shock. Gastric lavage is helpful; however, large pieces of ingesta are difficult to remove. Surgical removal of the ingesta may be necessary in certain cases. Adsorbents should be given to the conscious patient (Table 1). Chloramphenicol (25 mg/kg t.i.d.) should be given parenterally. The aminoglycosides are generally contraindicated, as they have the potential to act synergistically with the endotoxins in depressing the myocardium. Mannitol (1 to 3 gm/kg in 500 ml saline) should be given at a rate of 10 ml/min to oliguric patients to establish normal cardiac output and blood pressure. Alpha blockers generally are beneficial in the management of these cases.

Patients that recover from endotoxicosis may relapse. This is especially true of patients that retain much of the offending ingesta in the gastrointestinal tract. Relapses generally occur within the first 24 hours following the remission of clinical signs.

AUTOINTOXICATION

A phenomenon referred to as the "autointoxication syndrome" occurs when dogs and cats gorge on table scraps, pieces of horse hooves, spicy meats, spicy meat bones, chicken bones, meat trimmings, and other palatable items. Clinical signs of this syndrome are essentially identical to those described for endotoxicosis, and the patient is frequently presented in twilight consciousness. This syndrome occurs most frequently at the time of festive holidays, hunting seasons, horse ranch activities, home butchering, vacations, and fishing outings. Certain dogs appear to be predisposed to autointoxication and often develop malabsorption syndrome after repeated episodes. Strict control of the diet cannot be overemphasized in the management of these patients.

SECONDARY EFFECTS

Clinical evidence suggests that repeated exposure to certain endotoxins and enterotoxins will result in permanent damage to the mechanisms of autoregulation of the gastrointestinal tract. Practitioners have long associated acute pancreatitis with food and garbage intoxication. Malabsorption syndrome appears to develop in dogs after repeated exposure to enterotoxins and endotoxins.

UNDIGESTIBLE MATERIALS

Garbage often contains palatable but undigestible substances, such as meat packaging materials, which, when ingested, may result in foreign body obstructions of the intestinal tract. For example, strings used to tie rolled meats have been ingested by cats, with one end becoming looped under the tongue and the other end passing the entire length of the intestinal tract before the patient is presented to the veterinary hospital for diagnosis and treatment. Bologna ends attached by a string have obstructed the intestinal tract with the intestines puckering over the string to give a "string of beads" appearance on radiographs. In all cases of suspected garbage poisoning, appropriate radiographs of the abdomen should be taken to rule out foreign body obstruction of the intestinal tract.

WATER-BORNE TOXINS
(ALGAE)

Episodes of fresh water blue-green algae poisoning in dogs, although not common, do occur. Farm ponds, shallow lakes, and sewage lagoons that contain favorable concentrations of nutrients will have prolific growth of blue-green algae (algae blooms). Poisonings occur when dogs and other animals ingest this algae-contaminated water. However, the lethality of algal toxins in water is generally of short duration. The most common species of blue-green algae associated with this type of poisoning appears to be the *Anabaena* spp. The toxins of fresh water blue-green algae can be divided into the acute lethal toxins and the gastrointestinal irritants and hepatotoxins. The acute toxins generally produce death within 15 minutes to 2 hours after ingestion and appear to do so by inhibiting the release of acetyl-

choline from the nerve terminals. Vomiting may be observed, and the vomitus is often a pastel blue color. Treatment of acute algal toxicity includes maintenance of respiration, removal of the toxin from the stomach, and administration of adsorbents. Choline, D- and L-methionine, or acetylcystine (10 to 20 mg/kg t.i.d., PO) may be of benefit in preventing hepatic necrosis.

BOTULISM

Confirmed cases of botulism in dogs are rare. It appears that dogs are most susceptible to the serotype E botulism toxin. The most probable exposure of dogs to botulism toxins is from ingesting decaying water fowl and high protein garbage incubating under anaerobic conditions. Botulism toxins prevent the release of acetylcholine from the nerve terminals. Clinical signs observed include ascending flaccid paralysis. Treatment of botulism calls for maintenance of respiration, removal of the offending ingesta from the intestinal tract, and the administration of types C and E antisera unless the appropriate serotype is known. Botulism can be confirmed by submitting serum from the patient to the appropriate laboratory for mouse antitoxin protection tests. A therapeutic regimen of acetylcholinesterase inhibitors, such as physostigmine and neostigmine, can be administered with atropine sulfate to potentiate acetylcholine and block the muscarinic effects of acetylcholinesterase inhibitors. This regimen is similar to the management of myasthenia gravis.

MYCOTOXINS

Mycotoxins are the toxic metabolites of certain molds that are growing or have grown in animal and human foods. Cheese overgrown with mold has been a potent source of penitrem A in dogs. Discarded unprocessed animal hides may be the source of mycotoxins that are extremely irritable to the upper gastrointestinal tract. The use of self-feeders for dogs often creates a microenvironment that favors mold growth and the liberation of mycotoxins, especially aflatoxins. The reader is referred to the article on mycotoxicosis for additional information.

SUPPLEMENTAL READING

Arp, L. H., and Richard, J. L.: Intoxication of dogs with the mycotoxin penitrem A. J.A.V.M.A. 175:565, 1979.
Eberhart, G. W.: Garbage- and food-borne intoxications. *In* Kirk, R. W. (ed.): *Current Veterinary Therapy VI.* Philadelphia: W. B. Saunders, 1977, pp. 176–178.
Gentle, J. H.: Blue-green and green algal toxins. *In* Kadis, S. (ed.): *Microbial Toxins.* New York: Academic Press, 1971, pp. 27–63.

MYCOTOXICOSIS

STEVEN S. NICHOLSON, D.V.M.

Baton Rouge, Louisiana

Mycotoxins are metabolites of toxigenic fungi that grow on different feeds or foods. Thirteen mycotoxins have been associated with naturally occurring diseases in animals. Aflatoxins and tremorgens have been reported as causes of clinical entities in dogs presented to veterinarians and will be discussed here.

A specific hepatoxic disease of dogs and swine was recognized in the southeastern states prior to the discovery of aflatoxins. Termed "hepatitis X," it was later confirmed to be due to aflatoxin-contaminated peanut meal used in commercial dog food. Clinical signs included anorexia, icterus, dullness, melena, polyuria, polydipsia, and hemorrhagic diathesis. Greene (1977) described disseminated intravascular coagulation as a complication in several Walker hounds with chronic aflatoxicosis from contaminated commercial feed.

Necropsy lesions of icterus, hemorrhage, and toxic hepatic damage are observed in aflatoxicosis. Microscopic liver lesions include fibrosis and bile duct proliferation, which are said to be somewhat characteristic but not pathognomonic of subacute or chronic aflatoxicosis. Aflatoxins are potent carcinogens in mice and have been shown to impair the immune mechanism.

Arp and Richard (1979) confirmed two cases of penitrem intoxication in dogs that apparently ate moldy cream cheese discarded from a household. Produced by *Penicillium* spp., penitrem A induces muscle tremors, generalized seizures, intermittent opisthotonos, and ataxia. Pentobarbital sodium controls the seizures. *Penicillium crustosum* commonly grows on refrigerated food and produces considerable penitrem A at 4° C.

These and other mycotoxins may occur in commercial pet foods, but most people purchase pet foods weekly, so their animals are not likely to receive prolonged exposure if a specific lot is contaminated. Animals fed dry food bought in volume, such as at kennels or for packs of hounds, are exceptions.

REFERENCES AND SUPPLEMENTAL READING

Arp, L. H., and Richard, J. L.: Intoxication of dogs with the mycotoxin penitrem A. J.A.V.M.A. 175:565, 1979.
Greene, C. E.: Disseminated intravascular coagulation complicating aflatoxicosis in dogs. Cornell Vet. 67:29, 1977.
Pier, A. C., Richard, J. L., and Cysweski, S. J.: Implications of mycotoxins in animal disease. J.A.V.M.A. 176:719, 1980.

NEAR-DROWNING

(Water Inhalation)

CHARLES S. FARROW, D.V.M.

Saskatoon, Canada

Near-drowning is defined as survival, at least temporarily, following submersion in a fluid medium. Resultant pathophysiologic alterations may arise as a consequence of asphyxia owing to reflex laryngospasm or, more commonly, as a result of aspiration of the drowning fluid.

Experimental drowning of dogs has four distinct phases: (1) initial breath holding and automatic swimming movements, (2) aspiration of large amounts of water with associated choking and increasingly violent struggling, (3) explosive vomiting, and (4) cessation of all movement shortly followed by death (Loughkeed et al., 1939). Similar observations have been made in cats, rats, and guinea pigs. Although controlled observations are understandably lacking in man, reconstruction of the events closely parallels the animal data (Modell et al., 1976).

POPULATION AT RISK

Approximately 50 per cent of dogs and cats involved in immersion accidents are four months of age or less (AAHA Practitioner Survey, 1976). The most prominent factors in immersion incidents are owner carelessness, lack of close observation in potentially dangerous situations, and inadequate safety precautions.

LOCATION OF IMMERSION INCIDENT

In warmer climates the most common site for pet animal immersion incidents is the backyard swimming pool. Indoors, tubs, toilets, buckets, and other large, fluid-filled containers constitute high risk locations. Other common sites include canals, drainage ditches, rock pits, ponds, lakes, streams, and rivers. The last-named is of special concern, since rapid currents often delay, or even prevent, an animal from reaching shore once a problem develops.

PATHOPHYSIOLOGY OF DROWNING

The drowning victim first panics and struggles for freedom from the water while holding his breath. Carbon dioxide builds up, and the victim exhales air and begins to swallow water. In about 10 per cent of cases laryngospasm continues until breathing stops; no water is aspirated (dry drowning). In wet drowning—the majority of cases—the larynx relaxes before respiratory paralysis sets in, which allows aspirated vomitus and water with small suspended foreign bodies to enter the lungs and cause extensive pulmonary and alveolar damage. This, in turn, causes hypoxia, anoxic brain injury, loss of consciousness and reflexes, and finally convulsions and death. Dry-drowning victims have few primary pulmonary problems, but wet-drowning victims suffer extensive tissue and brain damage.

Fresh water invading the lungs inactivates the pulmonary surfactant. This leads to alveolar instability and collapse, resulting in decreased pulmonary compliance, a higher ratio of dead space to tidal volume, ventilation-perfusion imbalance, and intrapulmonary shunting. Water is hypotonic and crosses into the blood stream, which increases the blood volume and may cause temporary hyponatremia. It also makes the extracellular fluid space hypotonic, thus forcing equilibration of the intracellular fluids. This mechanism induces cellular and cerebral edema. Anoxia concomitantly increases the cerebral edema (Fig. 1).

In contrast, sea-water aspiration increases the volume of fluids in the air spaces within the lung. The hypertonic salt water in the alveoli attracts water from the blood, causing pulmonary edema. The extracellular fluid space is decreased, and solute concentration with hypernatremia follows (see Fig. 1).

The pulmonary edema from salt water aspiration may be accompanied by large losses of water and protein through the lungs, which necessitates the intravenous administration of colloids. Intrapulmonary shunting of blood often follows, similar to the perfusion through nonventilating alveoli that occurs in the adult respiratory distress syndrome. The fulminating pulmonary edema that occurs after successful initial resuscitation and clinical improvement is referred to as secondary drowning. Bronchospasm and pneumonitis from aspiration complicate matters, and the victim often dies from infection.

Anoxia produces acidemia, which in turn compromises the circulation and is the worst central nervous system insult. Experiments with dogs have shown that cerebral ATP, the primary source of energy in the brain, has a half-life of only four minutes after circulation stops. This initiates metabolic disruption that kills neurons and causes brain swelling, herniation, and death.

Water temperature is also an important consideration in cases of near-drowning. At temperatures much below 15°C, there is a rapid loss of body heat and a commensurate acceleration of fatigue. The ability to swim is greatly impaired. There is also a strong tendency to hyperventilate immediately upon entering the water. This reflex, which is mediated by widespread cutaneous receptors, often results in the inhalation of water in the event of an unexpected submersion. The same afferent impulses that cause the hyperventilation also result in a sensation of profound dyspnea. This often leads to a state of panic in the first moments of very cold immersions (Farrow, 1977).

Conversely, immersion in cold as opposed to warm water may prove lifesaving to the victim. There are reports of successful resuscitations with full recovery in persons who have been under cold water for 10 to 40 minutes. I know of a dog who recovered fully following an eight-minute immersion in an ice-covered river. These special situations are probably better explained by the mammalian diving reflex, which results in the shunting of oxygenated blood from all areas of the body to maintain a heart-to-brain perfusion circuit, which, together with the decreased metabolic levels of hypothermia, lessens the effects of short-term hypoxia.

Immersion syndrome is sudden death mediated by vagally induced cardiac arrest resulting from contact with extremely cold water.

Hyperventilation syndrome is the term applied to human swimmers who, in an effort to prolong their ability to remain under water, rapidly blow off their normal carbon dioxide load. This act eliminates the major physiologic stimulus to surface for air. Without warning, some such individuals have slipped into unconsciousness from hypoxia and have drowned.

Pail or bucket immersion accidents are relatively recent additions to the list of potential drowning

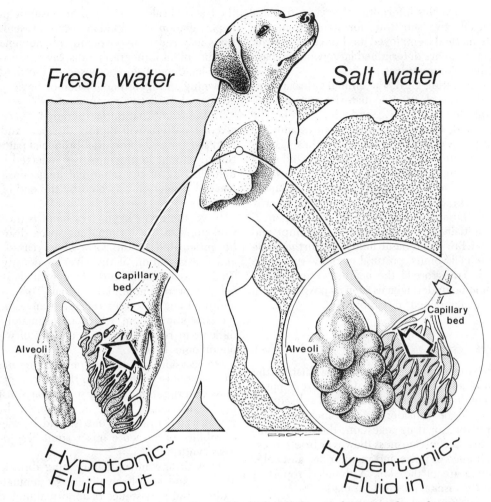

Figure 1. Pathologic changes in alveoli caused by fresh and salt water drowning and near-drowning.

situations. These unusual accidents may occur anywhere in which a pail of water may be found, indoors or out. In addition to the effects of the water, the adverse influence of the water content must also be considered, especially in light of possible systemic toxicity. Household detergents and disinfectants used in cleaning have widely differing systemic effects. Most household bleaches are benign in the usual concentrations employed in the home. Nonionic detergents (e.g., Purex) are not toxic when ingested. Anionic detergents (e.g., Cheer) are also low in toxicity, although vomiting and diarrhea may occur. On the other hand, cationic detergents and many disinfectants, especially those containing phenol, possess a high degree of local and systemic toxicity. Several liquid household cleaners contain hydrocarbons and pine oil, ingestion of which can lead to CNS depression and aspiration pneumonia. Low phosphate detergents have largely replaced high phosphate detergents, which contribute to water pollution. However, the low phosphate detergents are caustic and have caused esophageal injury.

The effect of these various materials on the tracheobronchial tree has not been documented, although it is assumed by many that they are harmful to varying degrees.

Standing water often harbors one or more bacterial populations as well as plant material such as algae. These elements, along with any inert particles such as mud, sand, or dirt, are likely to further complicate the pathologic picture.

On-Site Treatment

With the advent of numerous paraprofessional rescue units operating within or around most major population centers, it is entirely conceivable that a veterinary practitioner may be called upon to function as a remote medical advisor in a case of near-drowning involving a pet animal. Furthermore, it may be necessary to instruct a client directly in a similar situation.

Human cardiopulmonary resuscitation (CPR) techniques may easily be modified for veterinary field use. Clamping the animal's muzzle with both hands as one exhales intermittently via an oronasal seal is an effective substitute for standard mouth-to-mouth methods employed in humans. Specific patient positions are determined largely on the basis of individual circumstances.

Prior to initiating CPR, the animal's throat must be cleared of any obstructive material such as vomitus, plant material, clay, sand, or gravel. The tongue should then be drawn forward and the airways drained. The latter maneuver is best accomplished by holding the patient in the inverted erect position for approximately 30 seconds. Postural drainage is apt to be more productive in instances of saltwater immersion for the reasons previously mentioned. Drainage should not be dwelt upon. If it is not initially successful, halt the attempt and begin the CPR. If oronasal fluids are forthcoming or if the animal vomits, postural maneuvers may be reinitiated. Transport to the nearest veterinary facility should be undertaken as soon as possible, with CPR being maintained, if feasible.

Diagnosis

History is extremely important in evaluating the condition of a near-drowning patient. Every possible detail of the immersion incident and subsequent rescue should be considered. This includes prior hyperventilation or drug ingestion, duration of immersion, loss of consciousness (however brief), presence or absence of pulse and respiration, and color and temperature of the skin. A detailed report of rescue and resuscitation must be made.

A thorough physical examination must be done, and one should be sure to check body temperature. An arterial blood-gas determination is the most important laboratory examination. A thoracic radiograph is important but less urgent than a blood-gas determination. Findings may range from completely normal to mild perihilar or basilar infiltrates to diffuse pulmonary edema. The radiologic appearance of the lungs will not necessarily reflect the severity of the patient's condition, and there may be a delay of 24 to 48 hours before the appearance of roentgenographic evidence of pulmonary edema. A severely affected patient should have arterial and central venous lines inserted for continuous monitoring. Hemoglobin, hematocrit, and electrolyte determinations should be made, and plasma hemoglobin level should be measured.

Radiologic evaluation

The radiographic appearance of near-drowning in the dog is basically one of terminal air space disease. The alveolar pattern predominates during the early stages of the disorder, and it is usually accompanied by bronchial components. Increased ventilatory effort is often inferred, based on an enlargement of the tracheal caliber and a commensurate pulmonary hyperinflation. A reduction in cardiovascular dimensions may reflect hypovolemic phenomena.

This initial radiographic display is the result of a pathologic montage composed of the fluid of near-drowning and its attendant hemorrhagic, desquamative, and exudative components.

In the event that initial therapy is successful, the alveolar pattern will rapidly dissipate and leave in its place a mixed interstitial-bronchial pattern. Continued patient improvement is reflected by continued clearing of the abnormal lung densities, with marked resolution expected by the end of seven to ten days.

If, on the other hand, treatment is unsuccessful, worsening of the terminal air space disorder is to be anticipated in the form of increased intensity and dissemination of the alveolar density pattern. This radiographic picture strongly suggests the development of pneumonia, usually of a fulminant nature. Lung abscesses represent an additional potential complication, which unfortunately may be difficult to recognize in the context of widespread pneumonic disease.

On occasion, the radiographic picture may appear comparatively unchanged in the context of a precipitous deterioration. In this somewhat sinister situation, particularly when accompanied by severe dyspnea and cyanosis, one should be alert to the possibility of an acute onset adult respiratory distress syndrome.

As with any inflammatory lung disorder, intermediate and long-term progress examinations may indicate the persistence of abnormal lung densities. In the case of the completely recovered patient, the likelihood is greatest that these abnormal densities represent pulmonary scar formation. Specific radiographic appearances vary, depending on the degree and extent of the inflammatory process. The most commonly encountered scar pattern is one of heightened interstitial density, as indicated by blurring of the pulmonary vasculature. Pulmonary scar may also appear as a thin linear density resembling Kerley's lines in humans (Farrow, 1977).

On occasion, the initial thoracic radiographs may be entirely normal. Assuming the patient has indeed suffered a submersion accident, this finding most likely indicates that laryngospasm rather than inhalation has precipitated the acute asphyxia associated with near-drowning.

The presence of a "sand bronchogram" in the initial film series is a dire prognostic sign, and it indicates aspiration of clay, sand, or gravel into the tracheobronchial tree. The presence of such a sign is often associated with nonsurvival (Bonilla-Santiago and Fill, 1978).

The radiologic variants of near-drowning have been illustrated (Farrow, 1977). Figures 2 through 5 show a typical film series in a case of near-drowning in a dog.

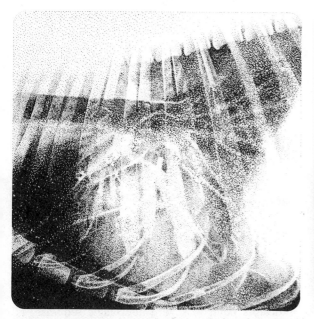

Figure 2. Illustration of a radiograph in the lateral projection made shortly following hospitalization for near-drowning. Severe widespread pulmonary edema is present, with distribution favoring the mid central and caudal lung fields. Much of the heart base along with the caudal mediastinum is obscured from view.

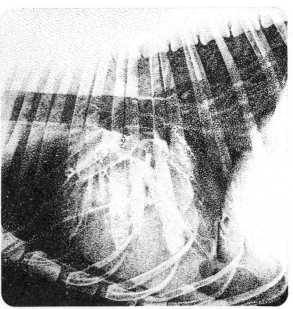

Figure 3. Illustration of a radiograph in the lateral view made 24 hours following hospital admission. The confluent air space density, indicative of extensive pulmonary edema, has undergone a dramatic improvement. Strong bronchial/peribronchial markings are now in evidence. The heart and associated pulmonary vasculature appear reduced in size.

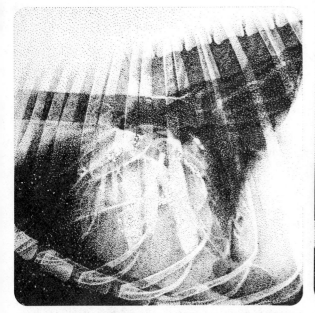

Figure 4. Illustration of a radiograph in the lateral view made two weeks following near-drowning. The radiographic picture continues to be one of gradual improvement. The heart margin now appears comparatively sharp, indicating the relative change that has occurred within the superimposed lung fields. A strong bronchial/peribronchial pattern persists.

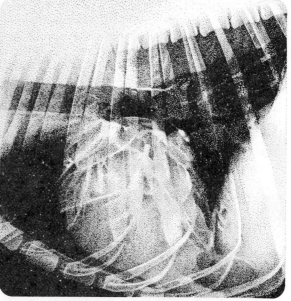

Figure 5. Illustration of a radiograph in the lateral view made one month following near-drowning. The lungs now appear relatively clear. Residual density within the interstitial and bronchial/peribronchial compartments of the lung is attributed to the aftermath of the near-drowning and is felt to be indicative of an active pathological process.

Hospital Management

Since hypoxia and acidosis are the causes of death, the veterinarian should direct treatment toward the correction of these biochemical lesions while awaiting the animal's recovery from the underlying pulmonary lesion. In an animal that is unconscious, has an altered sensorium, or is suffering from acute respiratory distress, it is probably prudent to administer bicarbonate (1 to 2 mg/kg) immediately on admission without awaiting the results of blood-gas determinations. Asphyxia leads to the rapid development of severe metabolic acidosis, and the need for prompt correction justifies this empirical treatment. Supplementary oxygen alone may be enough to achieve adequate oxygenation, or severe edema and pulmonary insufficiency may call for intubation and either positive end-expiratory pressure (PEEP) alone or intermittent positive-pressure ventilation (IPPV) with PEEP. PEEP may be started at 4 to 5 cm H_2O and adjusted according to blood-gas values. If IPPV is needed, a volume ventilator should be used. In cases of saltwater aspiration, PEEP alone may accomplish adequate oxygenation; mechanical ventilation may be needed in cases of fresh-water aspiration. Arterial blood-gas values and the patient's clinical condition, however, are the determinants in each case. The veterinarian must give careful attention to details of respiratory care including the administration of bronchodilators if there is wheezing, indicating an element of small airway obstruction. Weaning from ventilation should not vary markedly from that following other cases of pulmonary insufficiency. Steroids are ineffective in the treatment of aspiration (Calderwood et al., 1975), and antibiotics should be reserved until the development of secondary infection. Treatment of the sequelae of cerebral hypoxia may include dexamethasone, mannitol, fluid restriction, and hypothermia.

Fluid and electrolyte management is entirely dependent on the clinical condition and laboratory findings. Under no circumstance should hypo- or hypertonic fluids be administered on the basis of purely theoretical electrolyte changes. Administration of diuretics should be based on careful monitoring of urinary output and other clinical findings.

Complications of Therapy

In humans, there is a relatively high incidence of barotrauma (pneumothorax/pneumomediastinum) associated with the use of mechanical ventilation systems. This potential problem can be eliminated or minimized with constant patient supervision and periodic thoracic radiographs.

Gastrointestinal bleeding is also seen in one-third of all human patients maintained on ventilation systems and has been attributed to the presence of stress ulcers. The author has not encountered this complication in the dog.

Neurologic Sequelae

Neurologic sequelae may be predicted with a moderate degree of accuracy on the basis of one or more of the following presenting signs: the animal (1) arrived at the hospital unconscious or obtunded, (2) required prolonged CPR, (3) had an initial pH of less than 7, and (4) required mechanical ventilation to maintain minimal pO_2 levels. The likelihood of permanent neurologic deficit increases with the number of these indicators present.

Prognosis

The outcome as far as survival is concerned seems to be directly related to the patient's condition at the time of admission. Coma, a pH of less than 7, the need for cardiopulmonary resuscitation on admission, and the need for mechanical ventilation are all grim indicators. Subsequently, these same indicators point to severe neurologic sequelae, although the need for mechanical ventilation is a weaker indicator than the others.

Attention to oxygenation and correction of acidosis at all stages following the immersion incident will lead to a favorable outcome in patients who have not sustained irreversible hypoxic damage.

Psychosocial Considerations

In the majority of near-drownings, the owner either rescues the dog or is usually near the scene of the accident. In cases in which there is a prolonged period during which survival is questionable or in which there are severe neurologic sequelae, a significant psychologic burden is placed on the owner and other family members. Usually, the involved party experiences a tremendous feeling of guilt about the condition of the dog, which is not usually seen in other illnesses. The owner often expresses sentiments of remorse and negligence to the veterinarian as well as a profound sense of guilt for the near-drowning episode. "If only I had . . ." is a phrase repeated frequently during the clinician-client dialogue. These highly intense guilt feelings may also be expressed as criticism of the veterinarian involved in the care of the patient. Such psychologic "striking out" should be anticipated and countered with a controlled and uncomplicated explanation of the situation. Additional enlightenment of family members and friends may assist in palliating the involved party. It should be expected, however, that the majority of clients will bear their tragedy with resolution and will require no more (or less) than basic human concern and understanding.

PREVENTION

Drowning accounts for approximately 7 per cent of accidental deaths in the US and Canada annually, and it is the third most common cause of accidental death in children. Although comparable records are not maintained for pet animals, the figure is probably much lower owing to the reduced interaction between these animals and the aquatic components of their environment. Formal surveys conducted by the author among both Canadian and US veterinarians indicate that drownings and near-drownings do occur and most frequently involve dogs. Home swimming pools and recreational waters constitute the most common sites of involvement. It is therefore apparent that these accidents are preventable. Unsupervised poolside activity, particularly by the young, aquatically inexperienced pup, sets the stage for an immersion accident. The older dog, although wiser to poolside perils, may also meet an untimely end if encouraged to enter the pool by family members. Small-breed dogs with relatively poor swimming skills as well as short-legged dogs of any size tire rapidly while in the water and require a relatively higher water level to accomplish escape from the pool.

The hunting dog, on the other hand, is usually an excellent swimmer gifted with amazing endurance and strength. An injudicious challenge in the form of a ball or stick hurled from the shoreline of a rapidly flowing river or stream may result in a fatal misadventure. It is well to remember that the stamina of even the heartiest of dogs is quickly quenched in frigid waters, even over comparatively brief time spans.

Client counseling is therefore considered to be highly advisable in cases in which aquatic activities are anticipated. Owners of retriever breeds appear especially deserving of such advice, particularly if they are inexperienced in the training of such animals.

REFERENCES AND SUPPLEMENTAL READING

Bonilla-Santiago, J., and Fill, W. L.: Sand aspiration in drowning and near-drowning. Radiology 128:301, 1978.
Calderwood, H. W., Modell, J. H., and Rwiz, B. C.: The ineffectiveness of steroid therapy for treatment of fresh water near-drowning. Anesthesiology 43:642, 1975.
Farrow, C. S.: Near-drowning in the dog. J.A.V.R.S. 18:6, 1977.
Levin, D. L.: Near-drowning. Crit. Care Med. 8:590, 1980.
Loughkeed, D. W., Janes, J. M., and Hall, G. E.: Physiological studies in experimental asphyxia and drowning. Can. Med. Assoc. J. 40:423, 1939.
Modell, J. H., Graves, S. A., and Ketover, N.: Clinical course of 91 consecutive near-drowning victims. Chest 70:231, 1976.
Podolsky, M. L.: Action plan for near-drownings. Physician Sports Med. 9:45, 1981.
Walker, S., and Middelkamp, G. N.: Pail immersion accidents. Clin. Pediatr. 20:341, 1981.

INHALATION INJURY

CHARLES S. FARROW, D.V.M.

Saskatoon, Canada

Inhalation injury may be defined as the pathologic process that arises, directly or indirectly, subsequent to the exposure of one or more elements of the respiratory tract to the irritating or toxic constituents of a given gas or noxious fume.

When combined with burns, inhalation injury is invariably exacerbated. Carbon monoxide, although not a respiratory irritant, may prove a formidable clinical adversary in its own right by virtue of its strong avidity for hemoglobin binding and the consequent interference with oxygen carriage, ultimately leading to tissue hypoxia. In this regard the heart and brain are particularly sensitive.

Successful treatment of the inhalation injury patient is therefore predicated on both a clear understanding of the underlying pathophysiologic mechanisms, both short and long term, and a swift, carefully considered approach to patient care. Although it has perhaps attained cliché status in the modern medical literature, the term *aggressive patient management* seems nowhere more appropriate than in the case of the smoke inhalation victim.

HISTORICAL PERSPECTIVE

Smoke inhalation has been recognized for many years. Pliny the Elder reported that prisoners in the second Punic War were executed by placing them in cages above greenwood fires. Since then there have been many instances of smoke inhalation injuries.

The earliest well-documented cases of a pulmonary syndrome caused by smoke inhalation were those of the Cocoanut Grove fire in Boston in 1942. A large number of people died in this fire, but 39 survived long enough to obtain hospital treatment, and their clinical picture followed a set pattern. A few hours after admission, respiratory distress occurred, although all had been breathing easily at first. By the end of the first day, several patients became critically ill with dyspnea and cyanosis. They had copious secretions and often coughed up soot-stained plugs of mucus and bronchial casts. Laryngoscopy at this stage revealed severe laryngeal edema.

Post-mortem material available from several of the patients who died showed extensive necrotic lesions of the larynx, trachea, and primary bronchi, with formation of membranes that were either adherent or readily separable from the ulcerated wall underlying them. In these patients there was no correlation between the extent of surface burns and the severity of respiratory tract damage. Most of them showed burns around the mouth and nose, with singeing of nasal hair and reddening of the nasal mucosa.

These facts were taken up and stressed by Phillips and coworkers in a review of cases treated at the Massachusetts General Hospital between 1942 and 1962. Forty two per cent of the patients died of damage to the respiratory tract following inhalation of hot irritant fumes. Hence, respiratory injury should be suspected whenever there are deep flame burns around the nose and mouth, a history of burning in an enclosed space, or inhalation of smoke and products of incomplete combustion, even in the initial absence of respiratory signs and symptoms.

Physician scientists have carried out experimental research in which smoke inhalation injuries were produced in a number of different mammalian species including the mouse, rat, dog, goat, and monkey.

The earliest documented case of smoke inhalation in pet animals of which I am aware was reported in 1975. Subsequent veterinary publications have been largely of a review nature.

MECHANISMS OF INHALATION INJURY

Pathogenetically, inhalation injury may be the result of thermal as well as chemical influences, and its onset may be acute, delayed, or late.

Thermal injury mainly affects the upper respiratory tract and invariably results in some degree of pharyngolaryngeal inflammation. Commonly, the trachea and lobar bronchi are also involved, although often to a lesser extent, especially if laryngospasm is present.

In rare instances, inhalation of steam or still-burning oxygen or other combustibles may also damage the more distal branches of the bronchial tree. Edema, erosions, ulcers, sloughs, and abnormal luminal secretions usually follow. These destructive events usually produce a significant degree of upper and middle airway obstruction. This in turn results in varying degrees of hypoxemia and generalized respiration-oriented patient distress. Moreover, the associated increased work of breath-

ing will promote an increase in energy expenditure, thereby creating a concomitant demand for accelerated respiration. Thus, a self-sustaining pathophysiologic mechanism is created.

Chemical injury, in contrast to thermal injury, tends to damage the lower respiratory tract and lungs. Specific injury forms vary with the degree and duration of exposure, the extent of the entrapment, and the nature of the involved combustibles. Modern home furnishings incorporate numerous synthetics that, when pyrolyzed, produce highly toxic fumes containing not only carbon monoxide and irritant carbon particles but such substances as nitric, hydrochloric, and hydrocyanic acids. Even simple wood smoke contains comparatively high levels of toxic aldehydes.

These substances, singularly or in concert, produce a spectrum of pathologic changes incorporating some or all of the following elements: (1) bronchospasm, (2) ciliary paralysis (and, therefore, retardation or complete loss or the mucociliary clearance mechanism), (3) mucosal damage with sloughing, (4) luminal mucoid plugging, (5) atelectasis, (6) capillary instability, and (8) pulmonary edema. Further damage to the alveolar membrane, resulting in additional air space compromise, may occur under the influence of circulating "burn factor" (Fig. 1). The likelihood of this complication is directly related to whether or not there is an associated cutaneous burn injury. (The reader is advised to read further on the subject of thermal injuries, particularly with regard to how they may adversely affect the management of the inhalation injury patient. See article on Thermal Injuries.)

CLINICAL EVALUATION AND INITIAL TREATMENT

CLINICAL EVALUATION

Obviously, many degrees of inhalation injury may exist in a given patient. It therefore becomes imperative to determine the extent of respiratory tract injury before devising a specific therapeutic plan. Once treatment is under way, the patient's early response should be observed closely, with the intent of possible plan modification. Additionally, one must be constantly alert to the possible life-threatening sequelae that may develop, often in the face of an apparent recovery. Most importantly, these include post-inhalation pneumonia and the adult respiratory distress syndrome.

Table 1 indicates the author's preferred physical/biochemical/radiographic examination protocol for the inhalation injury patient. It is meant to serve as both a general guide and a checklist. Expediency is advised, although not at the cost of inadequate data acquisition. Flexibility is acceptable as regards the sequence of the individual examination components.

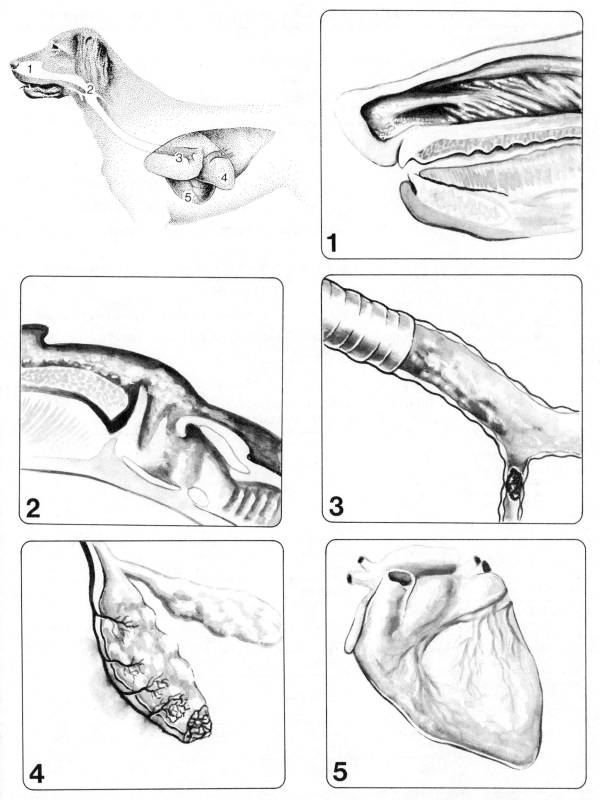

Figure 1. Anatomical levels of inhalation injury: potential areas of involvement. 1. *Nasal Passages:* generalized inflammation associated with variable degrees of discharge; both smell and breathing may be affected. 2. *Pharyngolaryngeal Cavity:* generalized inflammation often associated with swelling and laryngospasm. 3. *Tracheobronchial Tree:* mucosal damage, ciliary paralysis, edema, bronchospasm, sloughing, and pseudomembrane formation. The latter may be detached and coughed up as casts of the bronchi, sometimes leading to airway obstruction. 4. *Pulmonary Parenchyma:* atelectasis, surfactant disturbance, capillary instability, edema, and in more severe cases adult respiratory distress syndrome (ARDS). 5. *Heart:* hypoxic to some degree; may lead to decreased cardiac output, in turn affecting other highly sensitive tissues such as brain and kidney. Further compromise of the cardiovascular system occurs as a result of circulating "burn factor," a potent myocardial depressant.

Table 1. Recommended Physical Examination in Cases of Inhalation Therapy

PATIENT PRESENTED UNCONSCIOUS
1. Establish airway.
2. Begin breathing assistance using humidified high concentration oxygen.
3. Cardiac massage as required.
4. Drugs as needed (e.g., bicarbonate, epinephrine).
   Note: the mnemonic device "ABCD" is useful for remembering this vital resuscitative sequence.
5. Begin fluids.
   Note: central venous pressure monitoring aids in preventing pulmonary flooding.
6. Continue with the steps below.

PATIENT PRESENTED CONSCIOUS
1. Evaluate mental status (may range from unconscious to hyperactive).
   Note: a rapid evaluation of cerebral function should be included if patient was unconscious at time of rescue.
2. Evaluate respiratory status (consider rate, rhythm, character).
3. If present, evaluate extent and degree of associated burn injury (be particularly cognizant of orofacial burns and singed facial hair, coat, and whiskers).
4. Evaluate circulatory status: mucous membranes relative to color and perfusion (capillary refill time), heart and pulse (rate, rhythm, character).
5. Evaluate oral and pharyngeal cavities as much as possible for edema and swelling.
6. Obtain saliva or cough sample via laryngeal swab and microscopically examine for presence of: carbonaceous particles, cellular debris and frank tissue sloughs, red blood cells, neutrophils.
7. If CPR or respiratory assistance is required, bronchoscopy should be performed concomitantly.
   Note: flexible, "soft-headed" scope is advisable; use extreme caution not to rake tracheal lining.
8. Evaluate for presence of naso-ocular discharge and examine microscopically as in step 6 above. Take temperature and record body weight.
9. Obtain blood and urine sample for CBC, BUN, and urinalysis; obtain blood gases if available.
10. Make thoracic radiographs.

Table 2. Classification of Inhalation Injury
(BASED ON PRESENTING SIGNS)

CLASSIFICATION	CLASS I	CLASS II	CLASS III	CLASS IV
Extent of pulmonary injury (estimated)	Minimal	Slight	Moderate	Severe
State of consciousness	Alert, fully conscious	Distressed	Highly distressed	Unconscious
Respiratory rate	Normal or slightly increased	Mildly increased to moderately	Accelerated	Decreased or absent
Orofacial burns, singed whiskers, hair	Rarely present	Occasionally present	Often present	Usually present
Mucous membranes cherry-red (COHgb)	Not present	Rarely present	Occasionally present	Often but not necessarily present
pale (hypovolemia)	Rarely present	Occasionally present	Often present	Usually present
Carbonaceous particles present in cough products identified microscopically	Not present	Often present	Often present	Usually present
Naso-ocular discharge	Occasionally present	Usually present	Usually present	Usually present
Radiology	Normal	Usually normal	Variable—normal to consolidation	Variable—normal to consolidation
Bronchoscopy	Usually normal	Mild edema, increased mucus	Edema, mucous tissue sloughs, obvious luminal plugging	Usually as class III, except in flash fires where these may be normal to minimal findings
CBC, Chemistries, Urine	Usually normal	Highly variable depending largely on circulatory status of patient		
Hair coat smells of smoke	←————————————————NOT RELIABLE INDICATION————————————————→			

Table 3. *Initial Treatment of Inhalation Injuries*
(BASED UPON CLASSIFICATION PRESENTED IN TABLE 2)

CLASS I	CLASS II	CLASS III	CLASS IV
1. Symptomatically treat any minor burns and oculonasal discharge.	Inhalation injuries within these classifications are best managed on the basis of serial blood gas determinations. If unavailable, one must then rely more heavily on serial radiography and close clinical observation.		
2. Advise owner: complications unlikely, but phone back in 24–48 hours with progress report. Act on this information accordingly.	1. Place patient in low concentration (5–15%), humidified oxygen atmosphere for 4–6 hours and re-evaluate.	1. Place patient in intermediate concentration (15–30%) humidified oxygen atmosphere and re-evaluate every hour. Repeat blood gases frequently if available. Increase oxygen concentration if pO_2 continues to drop in the face of increasing oxygen concentration.	As in Class III, *note:* increase oxygen concentrations as necessary.
	2. Start fluids as circulatory status indicates but be extremely careful not to overload. If suspect the latter, repeat thoracic radiographs.		
	3. Start steroids: methylprednisolone, 2–4 mg/lb/BW initially; follow with longer acting drug such as dexamethasone, 4 mg/kg/BW, QID (non-divided) for 24–48 hours and re-evaluate.	2. Consider: suctioning upper airway if secretions become excessive.	
		3. Establish superficial and deep fluid lines to provide fluid routes and simultaneously monitor central venous pressure. CAUTION: avoid fluid overload.	
	4. Consider: use of morphine sulfate (0.1 mg/kg/BW) given S.Q. to alleviate pain and to decrease respiratory rate.	4. Start steroids as in Class II (#3).	
		5. Start morphine sulfate (0.2 mg/kg/BW) S.Q.	
	5. Withhold antibiotics until a proven need arises (e.g., pneumonia). Present evidence indicates little or no prophylactic capability.	6. Withhold antibiotics as in Class II (#5).	
		7. Consider: central antitussives if cough severe; discontinue as soon as possible.	
	6. Advise owner recovery likely (if no associated major cutaneous burn), although some degree of pneumonia will probably occur.	8. Advise owner recovery (if no associated burns) questionable. Complications likely. Play it day by day.	Advise owner recovery extremely questionable. Consider patient condition critical. Complications almost a certainty. If improving trend develops, exercise very cautious optimism.

Following the initial physical examination, it is recommended that the patient be placed in one of four major categories of inhalation injury according to the classification scheme proposed in Table 2.

Once this is accomplished, the patient may be treated in accordance with the recommendations presented in Table 3. A provisional prognosis may also be developed at this time, which should include a probability analysis relative to the development of delayed or late onset pulmonary distress syndrome. This information is provided in the following section dealing with sequelae to inhalation injury.

RADIOGRAPHIC DISPLAYS IN INHALATION INJURY

The radiographic display of an inhalation injury may change considerably, not only pathophysiologically but temporally as well. The author has found no strict correlation between the extent of abnormal thoracic signs (radiographic abnormalities) and the patient's respiratory status. This is not to say the radiographic examination is insensitive. On the contrary, radiographs may directly reveal pulmonary atelectasis, consolidation, effusion, and inflationary (volume) irregularities. Numerous *inferential* data

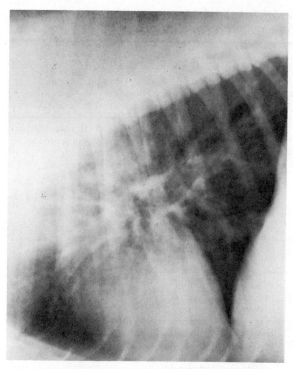

Figure 2. Lateral thoracic radiograph obtained two hours after smoke inhalation. Note the increased density and irregular profile of the bronchial tree. Peribronchial infiltrates compatible with interstitial and alveolar fluid accumulation are prominent. In the author's opinion, this is the most common radiographic display associated with acute inhalation injury. Remember, however, that the initial radiographic display may be normal, even though the lung is abnormal.

may be obtained from the static roentgen image including information on respiratory and cardiovascular dynamics. Sequential films often prove invaluable in determining trends of disease *activity, progression, resolution,* and *complication.* As a general rule, however, the greater the number of radiographic abnormalities encountered in the initial study, particularly consolidative alterations, the more guarded the early prognosis. For reasons to be described later, an initially clean lung does not preclude delayed sequelae.

The author has encountered four comparatively common radiographic displays in canine and feline patients suffering from acute inhalation injury at the time of initial examination. These include, in order of decreasing observed frequency, (1) diffuse bronchial-peribronchial line or ring densities, (2) diffuse patchy consolidation, (3) generalized hyperlucency and hyperinflation, and (4) diffuse (often massive) coalescive consolidation involving primarily the dorsal half of the thorax (Figs. 2 and 3). Less frequently seen abnormalities include localized or regional consolidation, moderate to marked mediastinal shift, and pleural effusion. The last-named is somewhat more common in the cat. As indicated earlier, these appearances need not and often do not correlate with the degree of existing pulmonary injury.

Hyperinflation is a radiographic feature of most inhalation injuries, although it may easily be missed if it coexists with a significant volume loss. This is especially true if there is an adjacent consolidation on the ipsilateral side. The trachea is often dilated, as are the primary conducting airways. Associated dyspnea often produces motion unsharpness, unless short exposure times are employed. This is a partic-

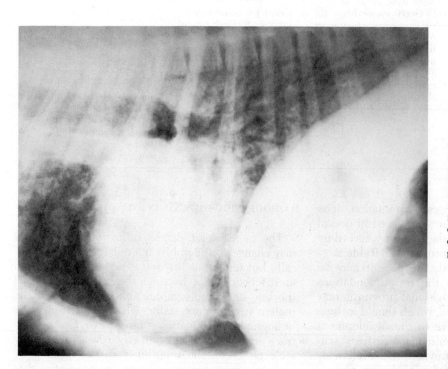

Figure 3. Lateral thoracic radiograph taken 16 hours after smoke inhalation. Multiple patchy densities compatible with severe pulmonary edema can be seen in the hilar and dorsal portions of the lung. Air bronchograms are numerous, and much of the pulmonary vasculature is obscured. The cardiac border is indistinct, and the caudal vena cava is small. Note the gas-distended stomach.

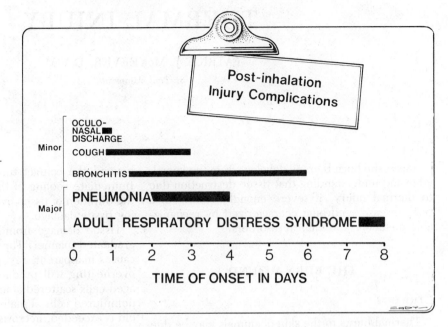

Figure 4. Post-inhalation injury complications.

ularly critical point to appreciate, since motion blur closely mimics abnormal bronchial-peribronchial density.

The radiographic appearances of delayed and late respiratory distress syndromes will be considered next.

INHALATION INJURIES AND THEIR SEQUELAE

As many as four distinct inhalation syndromes have been described in humans and experimentally reproduced in mice. In the latter instance, experimental variables included duration of smoke exposure, smoke temperature, presence or absence of associated poisonous gases, severity of cutaneous burn, airway infection (*Pseudomonas*), and treatment method. All were shown to influence recovery, although associated cutaneous burns appeared to be the most critical feature relative to both the development of complicating syndromes and, in many subjects, subsequent death.

In pet animals there appear to be at least four separate presentations of inhalation injury. Table 2 describes these potential patient profiles qualitatively. One can expect to encounter subsequent complications with any of these injury classifications. These sequelae may be of greater or lesser clinical consequence and may develop early or late relative to the time of original injury. Average onset times are presented in Figure 4.

Radiographically, it may be difficult to differentiate pneumonia from respiratory distress syndrome. Both are often characterized by a diffuse pulmonary disease pattern that has a strong tendency to undergo a rapid transition from the peribronchial-interstitial to the alveolar compartments of the lung. In the latter stages of either disease,

the air space pattern worsens precipitously, as evidenced by a marked tendency to coalesce and the development of numerous bronchogram signs.

When such radiographic alterations are viewed in the context of a patient whose clinical course is deteriorating swiftly as a result of an inability to maintain normal blood-gas levels, adult respiratory distress syndrome should be strongly considered. Differential and sometimes concomitant conditions in addition to pneumonia include pulmonary infiltrates with eosinophilia and disseminated intravascular coagulation.

Management of pneumonic complications presents no specific problems, except in patients who have previously been debilitated and probably immunocompromised. Tracheal wash combined with cultures and a sensitivity approach are strongly advocated.

Management of respiratory distress syndrome, on the other hand, is difficult without the proper equipment and monitoring capacity. The reader is referred to the supplemental reading list for further information on this subject.

SUPPLEMENTARY READING

Cudmore, R. E., and Vivori, E.: Inhalation injury to the respiratory tract of children. *In* Rickham, P. P., et al. (eds.): *The Management of the Burned Child, Progress in Pediatric Surgery,* Vol. 14. Baltimore-Munich: Urban and Schwarzenberg, 1981, pp. 173–188.

Farrow, C. S.: Smoke inhalation in the dog: current concepts of pathophysiology and management. V.M./S.A.C. 70:404, 1975.

Farrow, C. S.: Smoke inhalation. *In* Kirk, R. W. (ed.): *Current Veterinary Therapy VI.* Philadelphia: W. B. Saunders Co., 1977.

Farrow, C. S.: Thermal injuries. *In* Kirk, R. W. (ed.): *Current Veterinary Therapy VI.* Philadelphia: W. B. Saunders Co., 1977.

Powers, S. R.: Concensus summary on smoke inhalation. J. Trauma 19(Suppl.): 921, 1979.

Tams, T. R., and Sherding, R. G.: Smoke inhalation injury. Comp. Cont. Ed. 3:986, 1981.

THERMAL INJURY

PATRICK J. McKEEVER, D.V.M.

St. Paul, Minnesota

Successful burn therapy develops from the knowledge and understanding that tissue destruction due to thermal injury, if severe enough, results in a burn disease syndrome characterized by recognizable metabolic and clinical disorders.

THE BURN WOUND

ETIOLOGY

Thermal burns to the skin of animals may be due to friction, electric current, direct heat, or flame. Friction burns usually result from the animal being hurled or dragged over the pavement after being struck by an automobile. Electrical burns are generally seen in and around the oral cavity. They occur when a young dog chews an electrical cord. The most frequent direct heat burn is the "clipper burn," which results from holding a hot hair clipper in contact with the skin too long. Less frequently, direct heat burns result from situations such as cats walking over hot stove burners, poor supervision of paralytic animals on heating pads, hot liquids spilled on animals, and malfunction of hair drying equipment. Flame burns may result from fires of homes, apartments, or automobile accidents.

EXTENT OF TISSUE DAMAGE

The extent of a burn depends on the size of the area exposed to the heat source. The severity of a burn depends on the maximum temperature the tissue attains and the duration of overheating, both of which are dependent on such variables as the temperature and mass of the burning agent; the mass, specific heat, and thermal conductivity of the burned body; the temperature of the environment in which post-burn cooling takes place; and the amount of heat convection in the surrounding medium. Water and tissues, of which water is the main component, are characterized by high specific heat and low thermal conductivity. The term *high specific heat* implies that a large amount of heat is required to raise the temperature of tissue, and *low thermal conductivity* means the heat will be slow to dissipate. Accordingly, tissues become overheated slowly but are also slow in cooling. Therefore, the duration of tissue overheating extends beyond the contact time with the burning agent. Immediate cooling of the burned area can shorten the duration of tissue overheating, thereby decreasing tissue damage.

Tissue damage from overheating proceeds in a graduated manner. Threshold overheating of tissue causes inapparent, reversible cell damage. Further overheating will produce foci of irreversibly damaged cells scattered among reversibly damaged and noninjured cells. Finally, when the critical threshold is exceeded, necrosis of the entire tissue occurs.

Because transition from completely necrotic skin to completely healthy skin is gradual, regeneration of skin defects proceeds not from healthy tissue but from partly damaged tissue. This is thought to be one of the reasons why burn healing takes longer than mechanical injury healing of the same depth.

BURN CLASSIFICATION

Burns in humans have been classified as (1) first degree, with erythema and some damage to cells of the epidermis but no blistering; (2) second degree, with blistering and complete necrosis of epidermis with varying degrees of damage to the dermis; and (3) third degree, with total loss of all elements of the skin.

Application of this classification to dogs and cats in clinical situations is difficult because the thin skin of dogs and cats does not blister as easily as the skin of humans. Accurate evaluation may not occur until after separation of necrotic tissue is complete and the wound is healing. However, early assessment of burn depth is often required because of the need to excise necrotic tissue. For this determination, it is more practical to use a simplified classification that categorizes burns into two types. Partial thickness burns are characterized by incomplete destruction of the skin. Re-epithelization would be expected to occur from local epidermal elements with this kind of burn. Full thickness burns are characterized by complete destruction of all elements of the skin including skin adnexa and nerves. Re-epithelization would be expected to occur through migration of epidermal cells from the edges of the defect. Clinically, partial thickness burns are distinguished by erythema, local edema, small vesicles, evidence of persistent capillary circulation, and partial sensation to touch. Full thickness burns are distinguished by lack of superficial blood flow, insensitivity of the skin to touch, and easy epilation of hair.

BACTERIA

Acute infectious diseases that develop in previously healthy individuals usually are caused by microorganisms not normally present in the environment. In contrast, infections present in burn wounds are caused by microorganisms found in the normal microflora of the skin. They are opportunists in the burn wound because damaged tissue acts as a medium to support bacterial growth, and in severe burns the immunologic competency of the animal is impaired.

Bacteria most frequently reported to be found in burn wounds of humans are *Staphylococcus, Streptococcus, Proteus, Pseudomonas, Escherichia coli,* and *Klebsiella.* Too few cases of burn wounds in dogs and cats have been cultured and reported to confirm that these same bacteria are found. However, a small number of cases have been cultured and provide confirmatory evidence.

Systemic complications due to infection are rare in small- and medium-sized burns. In extensive burns, in which 15 to 30 per cent of the body is involved, septicemia and invasive spread of local infection are frequent complications. Septicemia results from extensive proliferation of microorganisms in the necrotic tissues of the burn wound and penetration of these microorganisms or their toxins into the circulation. Spread of local infection may convert superficial skin necrosis into a full thickness defect.

Qualitative bacteriologic analysis in humans has shown that neither systemic nor topical antibacterial treatment can sterilize a burn wound. However, quantitative methods show that topical antibacterial treatment, but not systemic antibacterial treatment, can significantly reduce the number of microorganisms in the burn wound. Systemically administered drugs apparently have limited or no access to necrotic tissues. Therefore, to minimize the complications of invasive spread and septicemia, topical antibacterial treatment is more appropriate.

PATHOPHYSIOLOGY OF BURNS

SHOCK

In accordance with current views, burn shock is defined as a set of events occurring when the autoregulative mechanisms of the body are unable to ensure normal blood flow in vitally important tissues and organs. These organs include heart, brain, lungs, liver, and kidneys. Hypovolemia be-

gins very soon after infliction of the burn and is typically most severe after several hours. The main eliciting factor is microvascular dilatation and permeability. Immediate transient vascular leakage occurs from venules owing to histamine liberated in response to the complement cascade, which is activated by heat-modified protein. Delayed, prolonged leakage also occurs, from either capillaries directly injured by heat or medium and small venules. The delayed permeability of venules is mediated by prostaglandins (PGE_2) and accounts for the majority of leakage. However, histamine and prostaglandins are probably not completely responsible for all changes in venules. This is because increased venule dilatation and permeability are found in areas remote from the burn even though serum levels of histamine and prostaglandins are not increased. Experimental evidence in dogs indicates that the central nervous system may also play a role. Despite lack of knowledge concerning complete mechanisms, it is clear that burn shock is a form of hypovolemic shock, and all ramifications of hypovolemia on other organs must be considered. For a complete discussion of shock see the article entitled Shock (The Pathophysiology and Management of the Circulatory Collapse States), page 2.

If over 15 per cent of the body surface area is burned, hypovolemic shock can be a serious problem in dogs and cats. It is probably not as severe as in humans, because less fluid and plasma protein is lost owing to the lack of development of vesicles and bullae in these species.

HEMOSTATIC DISORDERS

Capillary damage from burns results in aggregation of blood platelets on the damaged endothelium and exposed tissue. Adenosine diphosphate (ADP) released in the course of this process causes further recruitment and aggregation of platelets. Simultaneously, exposed collagen fibers activate the intrinsic coagulation system, leading to thrombin generation. Thrombin converts fibrinogen to fibrin strands, which stabilize the aggregated platelets. If damage is extensive, an initial phase of hypercoagulability evolves into a phase of hypocoagulability owing to exhaustion of clotting factors. This may lead to hemorrhagic diathesis.

LIVER DISORDERS

The central portion of the liver lobule is especially sensitive to anoxia. Hypovolemic shock leads to central lobular necrosis and depletion of glycogen stores. If hypovolemia persists, a state of systemic anoxia develops, manifested by metabolic disorders. These include elevated levels of ammonia, amino acids, phosphates, sulfates, and lipids.

KIDNEY DISORDERS

Abnormalities in kidney function occur, partially because of the hypovolemia and partially because of vasomotor-induced changes in intrarenal blood flow. Secretion of urine ceases when systolic blood pressure drops below 60 mm Hg. Therefore, oliguria or anuria may be an early sequela. Primary ischemic renal failure may develop if hypovolemia persists.

ERYTHRON DISORDERS

Evaluation of human burn patients and animals with experimentally produced burns reveals anemia to be an early phenomenon. However, anemia is often masked by hemoconcentration. The reduction in numbers of circulating erythrocytes parallels the severity of the burn. At first, anemia is due to a direct heat effect on red cells circulating in skin at the time of burning and accumulation of erythrocytes within the burn itself. The cause of anemia, which occurs later in the syndrome, is probably death of cells that suffered biochemical rather than morphologic damage.

RESPIRATORY DISORDERS

Severely burned patients often suffer from poor pulmonary ventilation. Ventilation is affected by inspiration of hot air and gases that may burn the upper respiratory tract and cause laryngeal and pharyngeal edema and bronchospasm. This may be followed by hypersecretion of the bronchi and plasma exudation, which obstructs respiration and reduces the vital capacity of the lungs. Later (five to six days), infectious pulmonary complications, focal atelectasis, and edema may appear (see page 174).

IMMUNOLOGIC DISORDERS

Severely burned animals are more prone to infections because of decreased immunologic capabilities. Immunoglobulin levels in serum are decreased, with the lowest values being found two days post burn. Decreased immunoglobulin levels may result from one or more of the following: leakage into burned areas, increased catabolism, or decreased synthesis.

Serious defects in polymorphonuclear leukocyte (PMNL) function, such as decreased chemotaxis, random migration, impaired phagocytic rate, and impaired bacteriocidal capacity, have also been observed in severely burned patients.

Humans with burns and severe sepsis have lymphocytes with a decreased ability to undergo transformation in response to phytohemagglutinin (PHA) and concanavalin A (ConA). As this depressed response predates clinical evidence of sepsis by two to four days, lymphocyte transformation studies are now used to predict sepsis.

TREATMENT

MINOR BURNS

Experimental studies in animals and clinical studies in humans have not demonstrated a particular treatment for minor burns that has distinct advantages. Accordingly, standard principles for the treatment of other small traumatic lesions of the skin may be applied to minor burns.

SEVERE BURNS

First Aid. If the burn has occurred within the preceding two hours and if the animal permits, icewater packs (ice and water in a plastic sack) may be applied to the burned areas. Exposed tissue, if present, may be gently overlaid or loosely wrapped with strips of old sheets or pillow cases. Owners should be instructed to spend minimal time on these endeavors, as they are not as critical as veterinary management of possible shock.

Shock. Initial evaluation and treatment of the burned patient should be similar to that used for other severe trauma. Airways should be examined to make sure they are patent, and any serious hemorrhage should be controlled; evaluation and, if necessary, treatment for shock can be started according to the principles outlined on page 8. If shock is not present, or once the animal is stabilized, evaluation and treatment of devitalized skin may be started.

Cooling. If the burn occurred within the preceding two hours, cooling of the affected areas should be done initially. Cooling reduces pain, depth of the burn wound, edema, and mortality. The affected area may be immersed in cold water, and cold compresses can be applied. The skin should be cooled for at least 30 minutes. In dogs, the optimal temperature for the water or compresses is 3 to 17° C.

Cleaning and Debridement. Contamination and debris may be removed from the burn wound by flushing with saline or washing with povidone-iodine soap. To facilitate evaluation of the wound, hair should be clipped from all affected areas. As indicated previously, determining the extent of burn wounds in dogs and cats is difficult, and in general the area of damaged skin is underestimated. Final confirmation of the extent of a burn may not be possible until about ten days post burn, when separation of normal and necrotic skin starts to occur. All tissue that is determined to be devitalized should be excised. Devitalized tissue and exudate provide a good growth media for bacteria. Baths are also helpful in removing necrotic tissue and surface exudates. Immersion of the affected areas in a whirlpool bath for 15 to 20 minutes, twice daily, is especially effective.

Topical Antibacterial Treatment. Silver sulfadiazine cream (Silvadene) is one of the most effective antibacterial drugs for topical therapy. Besides having antibacterial properties, it is nonirritating to exposed tissues, has no systemic side effects, and is easily applied to the wound. The exact technique for its use is as follows. After initial cleansing and debridement of burned skin, silver sulfadiazine cream is applied liberally to affected areas with a gloved hand or tongue depressor. Next, the area is bandaged with loose mesh gauze. Dressings are changed twice daily. During changes, necessary debridement is performed, old medication is removed, and the lesion is cleansed by irrigation with saline or immersion in a whirlpool bath.

Systemic Antibacterial Treatment. Although systemic antibiotics are used in the treatment of severe burns, their effectiveness is questionable. Studies on animal and human burn patients show that systemic antibiotic therapy does not favorably influence mortality, fever, or rate of healing. Its use should probably be limited to confirmed cases of bacterial septicemia. In these cases, antibiotic selection should be determined by sensitivity tests.

Skin Grafts. Severe burn wounds in dogs and cats should be treated as described previously until all necrotic tissue has been separated from the viable tissue, infection is controlled, and granulation tissue has developed. At this time, surgical procedures to decrease the wound size may be considered. Skin of dogs and cats is very elastic and has loose subcutaneous tissue that allows a marked amount of stretching. In many instances skin defects can be closed by either direct apposition or one of several reconstructive techniques utilizing skin flaps. If the defect is too large for these techniques, a free autogenous graft, either full or partial thickness, may be utilized.

SUPPLEMENTAL READING

Arthurson, G.: Pathophysiology of the burn wound. Ann. Chir. Gynaecol. 69:178, 1980.
McKeever, P. J., and Braden, T. D.: Comparison of full and partial-thickness autogenous skin transplantation in dogs: a pilot study. Am. J. Vet. Res., 39:1706, 1978.
Ofeigsson, O. J.: Water cooling: first aid treatment for scalds and burns. Surgery 57:391, 1965.
Rudowski, W., Nasitowski, W., Zietkiewiez, W., and Zietkiewiez, K.: *Burn Therapy and Research.* Baltimore: The John Hopkins University Press, 1976.

HEAT STROKE

(Heat Stress, Hyperpyrexia)

WILLIAM D. SCHALL, D.V.M.

East Lansing, Michigan

Heat stroke is encountered sporadically and is characterized by hyperthermia. The rectal temperature is usually 41 to 44°C (105 to 111°F). Heat stroke is often complicated by alterations in acid-base homeostasis, disseminated intravascular coagulation, and/or cerebral edema.

Several factors are necessary for, or may contribute to, the induction of heat stroke. A prerequisite is high ambient temperature that may be as low as 32°C (90°F) but is more often 38 to 46°C (100 to 115°F). Virtually all dogs in which the condition occurs are confined in some manner. In most instances, they are confined in an enclosure with poor ventilation, such as an automobile or a transporting crate. The condition can also occur in dogs confined by a chain outdoors. In these cases, excitement and exercise associated with animal fights appear to have precipitated heat stroke. Although exercise and excitement can significantly contribute to the induction of heat stroke in confined dogs, the condition is rare in dogs that run free, regardless of air temperature and exercise. High humidity contributes to the likelihood of heat stroke, because evaporation of water from the oral and nasal cavities is reduced in spite of maximal panting. Other predisposing factors are lack of available water, brachiocephalic anatomy, obesity, and decreased heat tolerance associated with youth and old age.

Cats apparently can tolerate higher temperatures than dogs. Heat stroke rarely occurs in this species.

PATHOPHYSIOLOGY

The initial compensatory response to increased ambient temperature is panting. This mechanism of dissipating body heat is efficient and involves the unidirectional flow of air into the nasal passages and out the oral cavity. This flow maximizes evaporation and heat loss because air is exposed to the greater evaporative surface area of the nasal turbinates. The process of panting, however, is not devoid of serious consequences. Significant pulmonary exchange takes place during panting and results in respiratory alkalosis. In dogs anesthetized with pentobarbital and subjected to an environment of 45.5°C (114°F) at 80 per cent relative humidity, respiratory alkalosis was documented 30 minutes after initiation of the experiment. Inasmuch as blood-gas determinations were not done between the time the dogs were subjected to the hot environment and 30 minutes later, the precise time of onset of respiratory alkalosis is not known. The magnitude of respiratory alkalosis in our experimental hyperthermic dogs was profound. Typically, one hour after entrance into the hot environment experimental dogs had an arterial blood pH of about 7.75 and a pCO_2 of less than 10 torr.

The respiratory alkalosis induced in pentobarbital-anesthetized dogs subjected to high temperature, however, eventually was modified by metabolic acidosis, presumably due to muscle activity associated with panting. Most dogs had an arterial blood pH of less than 7.3 three to four hours after experimental hyperthermia. The combination of respiratory alkalosis and metabolic acidosis was associated with cessation of panting and cerebral edema followed by death. Although the experimental hyperthermia that we induced may not be identical to naturally occurring heat stroke, it seems likely that when dogs with heat stroke are examined by the clinician they may have respiratory alkalosis or a combination of respiratory alkalosis and metabolic acidosis. The acid-base status of the individual patient can be determined only by blood-gas measurements.

Although serum electrolyte concentration assessments have not been done routinely on dogs with heat stroke, serum potassium concentration is known to increase in experimental canine and feline hyperthermia. The highest serum potassium concentrations coincide with the severest respiratory alkalosis. The increase in serum potassium concentration associated with experimental hyperthermia, however, is mild and may not be clinically significant. Typical serum potassium concentrations are about 5.0 mEq/liter.

Hypophosphatemia occurred in our experimental hyperthermic dogs approximately at the time of peak hyperkalemia and respiratory alkalosis. Most dogs had serum inorganic phosphorus concentrations of about 2.0 mg/dl compared with control values of 3.5 to 4.5 mg/dl. The mechanism of the hypophosphatemia is unknown.

Other alterations in serum electrolyte concentration known to be associated with experimental hyperthermia, and hence presumed to be typical of

heat stroke, have been minor and probably are the result of hemoconcentration.

The degree of hemoconcentration that occurs in heat stroke may be severe. Packed cell volumes (PCV) of 75 per cent have been reported. Whether hemoconcentration is mild, moderate, or severe is probably determined by environmental humidity and duration of the animal's exposure to the environment. In pentobarbital-anesthetized dogs subjected to 45.5°C (114°F) at 80 per cent relative humidity until rectal temperature reached 42.7°C (109°F), the PCV typically increased by 30 per cent and the serum osmolality increased by 10 per cent.

Disseminated intravascular coagulation (DIC) is known to occur as a result of heat stroke in humans and dogs. Experimental canine hyperthermia is also known to cause DIC and has been proposed as an experimental DIC model. The precise mechanism by which hyperthermia causes DIC is unknown but is characterized by progressive thrombocytopenia, increased activated clotting time, increased partial thromboplastin time, and the presence of fibrin (fibrinogen) degradation products in serum. The historical observation that some dogs with heat stroke die of a shock-like syndrome accompanied by hemorrhagic diathesis hours after seemingly complete recovery from heat stroke probably reflects the occurrence of DIC.

Another complication of heat stroke is cerebral edema. Although the mechanism by which hyperthermia induces cerebral edema is unknown, this complication is commonly present in heat stroke and experimental hyperthermia. Dogs with heat stroke–induced cerebral edema are initially stuporous. Involuntary paddling movements and coarse tremors are often present, and the dogs appear to be unaware of their surroundings. If the edema progresses, the menace reflex is lost and the dogs lapse into a coma. The panting reflex is abolished, the respiratory rate markedly decreases, and the dogs die of respiratory arrest.

CLINICAL FINDINGS

The physical findings in dogs with heat stroke vary, depending on the duration and severity of the disease. Initially, panting, tachycardia, bright red oral mucosa, and hyperthermia are the only findings. As the disease progresses, dogs become stuporous. The extremities become hot to the touch, and the bright red oral mucosa becomes pale because of decreased circulating blood volume and/or peripheral vasoconstriction. At this stage, dogs may involuntarily void watery diarrhea. If the diarrhea becomes bloody or if petechiae are present, DIC may be a complication. Finally, coma and respiratory arrest follow unless spontaneous recovery or medical intervention interrupts the pathophysiologic sequence.

Laboratory findings relate to the stage and severity of the disease and are considered in detail in the discussion of pathophysiology.

THERAPY

Our understanding of heat stroke pathophysiology remains incomplete, and the direct relevance of some experimental hyperthermia observations remains uncertain. For these reasons, some of the therapeutic recommendations are quasiscientific and based on inference.

The first objective of therapy is to lower body temperature. Experimental work supports the clinical observation that the chief determinants of survival are duration and degree of hyperthermia. An efficient method of lowering the rectal temperature is to submerge the trunk and limbs in a tub of cold or iced water. The rectal temperature should be taken at ten-minute intervals, and the dog should be removed when rectal temperature reaches 39.5°C (103°F), because further cooling may result in hypothermia. Since recurrence of hyperthermia is also possible, the rectal temperature should be determined at ten-minute intervals for a least 30 minutes after the dog is removed from the tub. Cold-water enemas have been suggested as a method of cooling but have the disadvantage of interfering with temperature monitoring. Evaporative methods of cooling, which are commonly used in humans, are ineffective in the dog because of the hair coat. Cold peritoneal lavage has been used to lower body temperature of experimental dogs, but the practicality and safety of this procedure have not been established. During the period of cooling, friction may be applied to the extremities to promote superficial circulation. Occasionally, severe shivering may hinder cooling. The intravenous administration of a phenothiazine tranquilizer such as chlorpromazine (1.0 mg/kg body weight) may be used to counteract shivering.

The second objective of therapy is to prevent cerebral edema. Dexamethasone should be administered intravenously in an antiedema dose (1.0 to 2.0 mg/kg body weight). This may also be helpful in preventing shock. Intravenous infusions of mannitol (2.0 gm/kg body weight as a 20 per cent solution over a ten-minute period) may be used if the patient is stuporous or comatose or if these develop during therapy. Mannitol should not be administered if serious blood loss complicates heat stroke. Mannitol should be administered cautiously if DIC is documented or suspected.

Intravenous fluids are indicated if hemoconcentration is documented or if peripheral circulation failure is suspected. Fluids are of potential benefit in preventing DIC and shock but must be administered with caution because of possible induction of pulmonary edema and aggravation of cerebral edema. In the absence of specific serum electrolyte determinations, individual electrolyte replacement is contraindicated; a balanced electrolyte solution such as Ringer's is the fluid of choice. Similarly, fluids that have little effect on acid-base balance should be administered unless blood-gas determinations are available.

If hemorrhagic diarrhea, excessive bleeding from venipuncture sites, or hemorrhage elsewhere is present, DIC may be a complication of heat stroke. Coagulation studies may help verify the presence of DIC and ideally should include one-stage prothrombin time, active partial thromboplastin time, activated clotting time, platelet count, and the detection of increased serum concentration of fibrin (fibrinogen) degradation products. If no facilities are available for these studies, the clinician should assume that DIC is present if bleeding tendencies are noted, and therapy for DIC should be initiated (see page 401).

SUPPLEMENTAL READING

Barry, M. E., and King, B. A.: Heatstroke. S. Afr. Med. J. 36:455, 1962.

Bova, C. M.: Heat illness. *In* Greenberg, M. I., and Roberts, J. R. (eds.): *Emergency Medicine.* Philadelphia: F. A. Davis, 1982.

Bynum, G. P., Patton, J., Bowers, W., et al.: Peritoneal lavage cooling in an anesthetized dog heat stroke model. Aviat. Space Environ. Med. 49:779, 1978.

Perchick, J. S., Winkelstein, A., and Shadduck, R. K.: Disseminated intravascular coagulation in heatstroke. J.A.M.A. 231:480, 1975.

Shapiro, Y., Rosenthal, T., and Sohar, E.: Experimental heatstroke. Arch. Intern. Med. 131:688, 1973.

Spurr, G. B., and Barlow, G.: Tissue electrolytes in hyperthermic dogs. J. Appl. Physiol. 28:13, 1970.

ACCIDENTAL HYPOTHERMIA

R. D. ZENOBLE, D.V.M.

Auburn, Alabama

There are numerous clinical settings in which hypothermia may be a consequence. Accidental hypothermia may be defined as a spontaneous decrease in core temperature, usually in a cold environment, associated with an acute problem without primary pathology of the temperature regulatory center. This is most commonly seen in old or unconscious animals, immobile animals (caught in leg traps), injured animals, and animals suffering from disease. Seldom will a healthy animal become hypothermic if it can seek shelter.

The physical findings of a patient with severe accidental hypothermia may be altered consciousness, unmeasurable blood pressure, a slow or absent pulse, and shallow, infrequent respirations. Heart sounds may be absent, pupils may be dilated, and reflexes may be delayed or absent. At temperatures less than 32°C (90°F), shivering will be absent and the patient may appear to be in rigor mortis because of increased muscle tone.

Management of the hypothermic patient presents the clinician with unique therapeutic challenges. Therapy may be divided into two categories: general supportive measures and specific rewarming techniques.

GENERAL SUPPORT

The first principle in dealing with hypothermia is recognition that it exists. This may seem self-evident, but many patients have been presented with hypothermia that was not diagnosed until a complication supervened. This problem is partly due to the fact that standard thermometers record only to 34.4°C (94°F). If the thermometer has not been shaken down initially, a hypothermic patient may not be identified. Glass thermometers recording to 27.8°C (82°F) are available for this purpose (Heart Thermometer, Becton-Dickinson Co., Rutherford, New Jersey) in addition to sophisticated thermocouple units with rectal probes. Handling of the patient should be minimal to avoid precipitation of ventricular fibrillation in the cold heart.

Continuous electrocardiographic monitoring is important for the severely hypothermic patient because of the frequency of rhythm disturbances. Atrial fibrillation and ventricular tachycardia are commonly seen with severe hypothermia but usually revert to normal as the patient is rewarmed. The hypothermic heart is relatively unresponsive to atropine or countershock. If ventricular fibrillation occurs, an attempt to reverse it with countershock is worthwhile. If this is unsuccessful, cardiopulmonary resuscitation should be instituted and continued until core temperature is raised. Most drugs will have little effect on the cold heart and may cause serious problems once the patient is rewarmed. This underscores the hazards of overmedication of these patients owing to delayed metabolism of drugs. Fluid replacement is essential; chronic hypothermia may lead to profound volume depletion. Intravenous fluids should be warmed prior to administration by passage through a hot-water bath. Fluid and electrolyte requirements for each patient must be assessed individually because of the effects of other associated diseases such as heart failure or diabetic ketoacidosis. If a central venous pressure line is used, it is important to avoid entrance into the heart to minimize myocardial irritability. Areas of frostbite should be treated separately once rewarming has been instituted. Close attention should be paid to chest radiographs during and after the rewarming period for signs of pneumonia, the most common sequela of hypothermia in humans.

SPECIFIC REWARMING TECHNIQUES

In conjunction with general resuscitative maneuvers, a mechanism for rewarming should be instituted. Rewarming methods remain a controversial area in hypothermia management (Table 1).

Table 1. *Rewarming Methods for Hypothermia*

PASSIVE REWARMING
1. Remove from environmental exposure
2. Apply insulating material (blankets)

ACTIVE EXTERNAL REWARMING
1. Apply heated objects (water bottle)
2. Apply electric heating pads
3. Immerse in heated water

ACTIVE CORE REWARMING
1. Peritoneal dialysis
2. Colonic irrigation
3. Mediastinal irrigation via thoracotomy
4. Hemodialysis
5. Intragastric lavage
6. Extracorporeal blood rewarming
7. Inhalation rewarming

186

The choice of method to be used should take into account the duration and degree of hypothermia, the available resources, and the time involved to mobilize resources. Methods of rewarming can be external (surface) or internal (core). Passive rewarming relies upon removing the patient from a cold environment and maximizing basal heat retention by use of insulating material such as a blanket. Many experts consider this to be the safest method of rewarming a mildly to moderately hypothermic patient.

Active external rewarming techniques are readily available and are advocated by some authors. Concern has been raised about actively rewarming the body surface because of inherent physiologic changes that may aggravate the effect of hypothermia on core tissues. The well-described "afterdrop" of core temperatures after removal of chronic cold stress may be exaggerated by the peripheral vasodilation associated with active external rewarming. This can cause paradoxic central cooling by shunting stagnant cold blood to the core, thus further chilling the myocardium and increasing the animal's vulnerability to ventricular fibrillation. Active external rewarming by immersion of the body in warm water may interfere with adequate monitoring of the patient and may precipitate ventricular fibrillation owing to excessive movement of the patient. Heating blankets carry a risk of causing thermal burns in underperfused areas.

Core rewarming techniques should be reserved for patients with severe (core temperature less than 32°C [90°F]) or prolonged hypothermia (> 12 hours). Core rewarming reduces the hazards of "afterdrop" and cardiac arrhythmias. Techniques for core rewarming useful for animals include high colonic lavage, administration of warmed intravenous fluids, direct mediastinal irrigation via thoracotomy, and peritoneal dialysis. Peritoneal dialysis has a high degree of success with minimum cost and special equipment. This makes it an excellent means of core rewarming in veterinary medicine. The dialysate is warmed to 43°C (109°F) and instilled into the peritoneal cavity. Rapid instillation and immediate removal are preferable, and normothermia usually is attained within six to eight exchanges. Other methods for core rewarming are used in human medicine but are impractical for veterinary medicine at the present time. These techniques include intragastric lavage with warm saline, extracorporeal blood rewarming, and inhalation of warmed oxygen.

In summary, passive external rewarming is the safest and easiest method of rewarming the mildly to moderately hypothermic patient. Active external heat is favored by some clinicians, but the rewarming must be slow to prevent "afterdrop" of the core temperature and precipitation of cardiac arrhythmias. Core rewarming should be reserved for severe or prolonged hypothermia. Peritoneal dialysis is the treatment of choice for severe hypothermia in veterinary medicine.

SUPPLEMENTAL READING

Reuler, J. B: Hypothermia: pathophysiology, clinical settings and management. Ann. Intern. Med. 89:579, 1978.

Reuler, J. B., and Parker, R. A.: Peritoneal dialysis in the management of hypothermia. J.A.M.A. 240:2289, 1978.

Zenoble, R. D., and Hill, B. L: Hypothermia and associated cardiac arrhythmias in two dogs. J.A.V.M.A. 175:840, 1979.

COLD INJURY

(Hypothermia, Frostbite, Freezing)

ROBERT A. DIETERICH, D.V.M.

Fairbanks, Alaska

Hypothermia, or lowering of body temperature, in domestic animals as a result of environmental exposure occurs more commonly in areas in the northern latitudes but is seen occasionally in other areas as a result of accidental cooling or freezing of a pet held captive in household refrigerators or freezers. Another frequently encountered cause of hypothermia is interference with thermoregulatory centers during surgery by anesthetics or sedatives. Hypothermia will be considered separately from freezing, even though both may be present in a patient at the same time. Treatment for each condition involves different principles, and they should be considered different entities.

HYPOTHERMIA

General hypothermia is defined as the condition produced by deep cooling from external cold, drugs, or failure of the temperature-regulating mechanisms, which results in a profound decrease in body temperature. Local hypothermia is also possible in the extremities but is without risk of damage unless freezing occurs. This definition does not include normal cooling due to circadian rhythms, which produce changes in body temperature of from 1 to 2°C. Mild hypothermia is characterized by body temperatures of 30 to 32C, moderate hypothermia by temperatures of 22 to 25°C, and profound hypothermia by temperatures of 0 to 8°C. These ranges vary according to the species being considered. The physiologic changes of hypothermia depend on the extent and duration of exposure. The duration of hypothermia can be characterized as acute (few hours), prolonged (several hours), or chronic (days).

Survival of animals suffering from hypothermia depends on the degree of cooling to which they are subjected. Moderate hypothermia allows survival for approximately 24 hours, whereas body temperatures of 15°C shorten survival time to five or six hours. Profound hypothermia narrows survival time still further to one to two hours.

TREATMENT

Treatment of hypothermia is directed toward rewarming and maintenance of vital body functions. A low-reading clincial thermometer is imperative for diagnosis and decisions on treatment. Rewarming may be accomplished by external (surface) means or internal (core) methods. External rewarming results in the body surface or shell being warmed first with the aid of warm-water immersion, water or electric heating blankets, hot-water bottles, or simply a warm room and blankets. Oxygen and appropriate intravenous fluid therapy may also be needed, depending on the degree of hypothermia being treated.

Internal rewarming is accomplished using peritoneal dialysis. The dialysate is heated to 50 to 55°C and is allowed to flow into the peritoneal cavity as fast as gravity permits. After flowing through the administration tubing, the dialysate fluid reaches the abdominal cavity at a temperature of approximately 45°C. Dialysis is continued until normal body temperature is reached. Methods of procedure to carry out peritoneal dialysis are described in the article on Peritoneal Dialysis.

The advantages of internal rewarming are several. Sometimes, when external rewarming is attempted, there will be vasodilation of surface vessels and a transfer of cooled blood to the body core, bringing about a further drop in internal temperature, which results in "rewarming shock." Normothermia can be achieved faster with peritoneal dialysis than with external rewarming methods. Cardiac output and electrocardiogram readings rapidly return to normal after rewarming by internal methods. When using either the external or the internal rewarming method, it is important to avoid overheating and resultant hyperthermia.

Resuscitation may still be possible in the deeply hypothermic patient even though there is no respiration or heart beat. Cardiac fibrillation is a risk in these circumstances. Ventilation of the lungs must be established before the heart restarts to stand any chance of success.

After a hypothermic patient is returned to normothermia, a complete examination should be carried out to determine whether another disorder led to the lowered body temperature. Renal failure, pneumonia, or malnutrition can easily lower an animal's resistance to cold exposure, and the resulting hypothermia may be only a secondary symptom.

FROSTBITE OR FREEZING

Frostbite, or freezing of tissue, is rare in animals that are healthy and well-nourished. Well-acclimatized, long-haired animals can remain exposed to temperatures of −50°C for indefinite periods with no ill effects. It is critical that animals exposed to very low environmental temperatures be fed adequate amounts of food to enable them to produce enough body heat to maintain normothermia. In cold regions, frostbite of the tips of the ears or tails of cats is perhaps the most common cold injury seen. This usually requires no treatment unless secondary infection is encountered. A bland ointment may be applied if needed. The scrotum of male dogs will sometimes be injured by cold from repeated contact with cold surfaces or deep snow. Erythema and scaliness or even minor sloughing of surface scrotal tissue can occur and is treated with ointments and reduced cold exposure. Continued contact with snow or cold surfaces will delay healing.

The deep freezing of tissues is seen in animals that have been physically injured or caught in various types of wildlife traps or other circulation-inhibiting situations. Recently, major advances have been made in the treatment of severe frostbite. The owner of the frostbite patient should be encouraged to bring the injured animal directly to a veterinarian and should attempt no home treatment unless an extended period would pass before the animal could reach a veterinary hospital. Tissue damage and tissue necrosis are increased greatly if thawing and subsequent refreezing occur (freeze-thaw-freeze-thaw syndrome). The frozen part should be kept frozen and protected to avoid trauma during transport or handling.

TREATMENT

Frozen tissue should be thawed rapidly in warm water (38 to 44°C) as soon as possible after it is known that refreezing can be prevented. The frozen part should not be massaged during warming. Previously thawed parts should not be subjected to rapid rewarming. The thawed part will soon become erythematous and edematous. Large blebs usually occur, and self-mutilation by the patient should be avoided. It is best to leave the injured tissue exposed rather than to use occlusive wet dressings or petrolatum gauze. Premature debridement or other surgical intervention should not be undertaken. Treatment should be confined to protection of the part from trauma and prevention of infection. Systemic antibiotics should be administered in severe cases.

Unnecessary debridement of necrotic tissue or amputation should be delayed as healing occurs. Irreversibly damaged tissues begin to demarcate in four to seven days. Often, 15 to 20 days are required for the injured tissue to reach a point at which there is a clear demarcation of the tissue to be lost, and therefore removed, and the tissue that is viable. Pads of frostbitten feet should be preserved if at all possible.

Fractures, dislocations, and extensive trauma of frozen tissue should not be repaired until after thawing is complete. Fracture treatment should be conservative. A high protein, high caloric diet with vitamin supplements is helpful, particularly in the malnourished patient that has suffered both hypothermia and frostbite.

SUPPLEMENTAL READING

Mills, W. J., Jr.: Frostbite and hypothermia, current concepts. Alaska Med. 15:27, 1973.

Petajan, J.: Prevention and treatment of frostbite. Report No. 103, Arctic Health Research Center, Fairbanks, Alaska, 1969.

Popovic, V., and Popovic, P.: *Hypothermia in Biology and in Medicine.* New York: Grune and Stratton, 1974.

Section 3

RESPIRATORY DISEASES

BRENDAN C. McKIERNAN, D.V.M.
Consulting Editor

CLINICAL RESPIRATORY PHYSIOLOGY

T. C. AMIS, B.V.Sc.

Davis, California

Diagnosis of disease in many organ systems is based on the recognition of patterns of clinical signs and the results of objective laboratory investigations. Clinical signs are an expression of the functional manner in which an organ system responds to physical or biochemical injury, i.e., pathophysiology. Diagnostic ability is greatly enhanced if clinical signs can be interpreted in terms of underlying pathophysiology. In clinical veterinary medicine the ability to undertake quantitative functional evaluation of the respiratory system has tended to lag behind advances made in the assessment of other organ systems. Evaluation of the functional nature of respiratory disease is largely confined to physical examination, chest radiography, and arterial blood gas analysis.

The aim of this article is to outline the manner in which the lung responds to injury and to show how the resultant functional disorders are translated into clinical signs. To approach this goal, we must, however, first discuss the normal structure, function, and physiology of the respiratory system.

STRUCTURE/FUNCTION OF THE RESPIRATORY SYSTEM

The primary function of the mammalian respiratory system is gas exchange; it provides the pathway whereby gases, principally oxygen and carbon dioxide, are exchanged between the metabolic machinery of the body and the environment. Its structure reflects this function by allowing air and blood to be brought to opposite sides of a gas-exchanging surface in the lungs.

It is important to remember that the lungs are not the whole of the respiratory system but represent only part of a complex integrated network that also includes the intracellular metabolic processes, the cardiovascular system, the chest wall, and the neural respiratory control structures. Failure of any link in this chain may result in respiratory failure and disruption of normal metabolic processes.

The anatomic pathway for inhaled air commences at the external nares, relatively narrow but variably sized orifices through which gas may flow into the *nasal passages*. A feature of the nasal passages is the convoluted bony turbinate structures covered

with a mucosa richly supplied with blood vessels, glandular structures, and a ciliated epithelium.

The nasal passages warm, humidify, and filter incoming air to protect the more delicate membranes in the lower part of the respiratory tract. The olfactory sensors are also located in the nasal passages. The paranasal sinuses, structures of questionable normal function but of considerable clinical significance, are associated with the nasal passages.

Leaving the nasal passages by the posterior nares, inhaled gases cross the *pharynx*. This area represents a crossroad of the alimentary and respiratory tract, a position demanding full functional integrity of deglutition and laryngeal processes. Failure of either of these may lead to aspiration of foreign material into the lungs. The pharynx is also an area where particles in the incoming airstream can be removed by impaction on the pharyngeal wall. This protective function is augmented by the presence of lymphoid tissue in the region.

The *larynx* is a complex cartilaginous and muscular structure that acts as a protective valve and pressure regulator for the lungs while also having important phonation functions. The mucous membrane lining of the larynx is richly endowed with receptors that detect the entry of large foreign particles and may initiate an explosive cough reflex designed to propel these materials out of the respiratory tract. Laryngeal spasm may also occur in response to stimulation of laryngeal irritant receptors.

Gas then flows through the *trachea*, a tubular structure allowing gas conduction while maintaining sufficient flexibility so that the animal is permitted a wide range of neck movements. This is achieved through a design of C-shaped cartilaginous supports lined with a mucous membrane and joined by a dorsal membrane containing the trachealis muscle. The tracheal lining consists of stratified ciliated columnar epithelium with numerous goblet cells and mucous secretory glands.

The trachea divides at the carina into right and left mainstem bronchi. *Division of the airways* is characterized by a dichotomous branching system: first lobar bronchi, then segmental bronchi, and on through succeeding branches to the bronchioles, which have no cartilage in their walls. The terminal bronchioles are the smallest airways that have no alveoli. The gas exchange area commences with the respiratory bronchioles, which are airways with scattered alveoli budding from their walls. Then follows the alveolar ducts, airways completely lined by alveoli, and the alveolar sacs, the final structures.

It is sometimes difficult to appreciate the prodigious effect of this branching system; in the dog lung it has been estimated that there are between 17,000 and 36,000 terminal bronchioles about 0.5 mm in diameter and 2.00 mm in length. Despite the fact that the diameter of the airways decreases toward the alveoli, the vast increase in the number of branches has a dramatic effect on the combined cross-sectional area. In the human lung there are 23 generations from trachea to alveolus, with the terminal bronchioles occurring at about generation 16. At this point the combined cross-sectional area of the airways increases dramatically because of the large number of airways. This has important effects on the dynamics of gas transport. Until the terminal bronchiole region, gas is transported largely by bulk conduction; beyond this point the cross-sectional area is so large that the linear velocity (movement) of the gas falls to very low levels and gas transfer is largely by diffusion. Because of this change in flow dynamics, inhaled particles tend to settle out in the terminal bronchiolar area, making it susceptible to damage. Low flow rates also make it exceedingly difficult to clear particles from the gas-exchanging zone of the lung by coughing.

The walls of the *alveoli* are lined by two types of cells, type I pneumocytes, which are the flat epithelial cells, and type II pneumocytes, which are more complex in structure and are thought to be the source of surfactant production. Surfactant is a phospholipid material that lowers the surface tension of the alveolus, thus promoting alveolar stability.

Gaps may be found in the walls of alveoli, known as pores of Kohn, that allow gas movement from one alveolus to another, a process known as *collateral ventilation*. Collateral ventilation can also take place via interconnections between bronchioles. Collateral ventilation is well developed in the dog and may be one reason why alveolar collapse (atelectasis) is less pronounced in association with pulmonary disease in this species than in animals that have well-developed fibrous septa between pulmonary lobules (e.g., bovine).

The alveolar walls are surrounded by a dense network of *pulmonary capillaries* carrying mixed venous blood from the right heart. The density of capillaries is such that some investigators regard the alveoli as being surrounded by a sheet of blood interrupted at intervals by posts of tissue.

Gas exchange takes place across the surfactant layer, alveolar epithelium, interstitium, capillary endothelium, plasma, and red cell interior. The presence of red blood cell hemoglobin is particularly important for the transport of oxygen. The maximum amount of oxygen that blood containing 15 gm of hemoglobin/100 ml can carry is about 20 ml O_2/100 ml blood. Without hemoglobin, only 0.3 ml O_2/100 ml of blood could be transported (dissolved in blood at a partial oxygen pressure of 100 mm Hg). The pulmonary capillaries empty blood into the pulmonary venules, pulmonary veins, left heart, and then into the systemic arterial system.

The pulmonary circulation, like the systemic, receives the whole of the cardiac output, but there are some important differences. The pulmonary circulation operates under very low pressure conditions, mean pulmonary artery pressure being about 15 mm Hg in the dog. This is a reflection of low resistance, pulmonary vascular resistance being only about one-tenth of that of the systemic circulation. Another feature is the collapsibility of pulmonary vessels, particularly capillaries, and the nature of the surrounding pressures. Since the alveoli are surrounded by capillaries, it follows that the capillaries are surrounded by alveoli and hence are exposed to alveolar pressure. This has important effects on the distribution of blood flow in the lung, as will be discussed later.

This brief introduction to structure/function correlations in the lung has been intended to highlight some points of interest and is by no means comprehensive. Structures not discussed include the bronchial circulation, pulmonary lymphatics, pleura, chest wall, and respiratory control structures.

RESPIRATORY PHYSIOLOGY

The process whereby gas reaches the alveolar spaces is known as ventilation. *Total ventilation or minute volume* is that volume of gas entering or leaving the lungs per minute and is equal to the product of *tidal volume* (V_T), the volume of gas in each breath, and the *respiratory rate* (f). Strictly speaking, the inspired and exhaled minute volumes are not equal because more oxygen is taken up from the inspired gas than is replaced by carbon dioxide. This may be seen from the *respiratory exchange ratio* (R), which is defined as the ratio between the rate of CO_2 excretion ($\dot{V}CO_2$) and the rate of oxygen uptake ($\dot{V}O_2$). Typically in mammals this is about 0.8, but it depends on metabolic factors. When an animal is utilizing an entirely carbohydrate diet for metabolism, R is closer to 1.0; when fats are being metabolized it may fall to 0.7.

Not all of the total volume of gas that enters the lung takes part in gas exchange. Some will not reach the alveolar membrane but will remain in the conducting airways of the lung. This volume of gas is known as *dead space*. Actually there are two components of dead space: *anatomic dead space* is the volume of gas contained in the conducting airways, whereas *alveolar dead space* is the volume of gas contained in the alveolar space of the lung but not participating in gas exchange. Alveolar dead space is a functional concept that regards any gas that does not exchange with the blood at peak efficiency (e.g., gas in an alveolus with reduced or no blood supply) as wasted ventilation. The sum of these two dead spaces is known as total or *physiologic dead space* (V_{DS}). Dead space is increased in many disease conditions, for example, in diseases that affect the blood flow to some lung units; increased dead space also usually results when an endotracheal tube is inserted during anesthesia.

Since we have introduced the concept of wasted ventilation, we can now concentrate on the effective ventilation of the lung. *Alveolar ventilation* ($\dot{V}_A$) is that portion of the total ventilation that takes part in gas exchange and is the difference between total minute ventilation and dead space ventilation. Adequate alveolar ventilation is very important for gas exchange. If the alveolar ventilation is low in relation to uptake of oxygen and production of carbon dioxide by the body, then the partial pressure of oxygen in the alveolar space ($P_{A_{O_2}}$) will fall and the alveolar partial pressure of carbon dioxide ($P_{A_{CO_2}}$) will rise. This will be reflected in the arterial partial pressures of oxygen ($P_{a_{O_2}}$) and carbon dioxide ($P_{a_{CO_2}}$) and is known as hypoventilation. Hyperventilation, on the other hand, occurs when alveolar ventilation is high in relation to carbon dioxide production and the arterial $P_{a_{CO_2}}$ falls. The tight bond between $P_{a_{CO_2}}$ and alveolar ventilation ($\dot{V}_A$) is such that if $\dot{V}_A$ is halved, for example, $P_{a_{CO_2}}$ will double. This is important in clinical practice in the interpretation of blood gas values, since if alveolar hypoventilation is present this will be reflected in an increase in $P_{a_{CO_2}}$.

It is well established in human pulmonary physiology that ventilation is not uniformly distributed even in normal lungs. This is thought to be related to differences in regional compliance (distensibility) associated with a nonuniform distribution of lung volume. The pressure in the pleural space is known to vary systematically in the vertical direction. Pleural pressure is more negative over superior lung regions than over inferior lung regions. In humans, pleural pressure varies by about 0.2 cm H_2O per cm descent in the thorax. In animals, the magnitude of the gradient may vary with body size and posture. In standing horses, vertical pleural pressure gradients of 0.3 to 0.4 cm H_2O per cm descent in the thorax have been reported, whereas in laterally recumbent dogs gradients of about 0.8 to 0.5 cm H_2O per cm descent have been described.

The origin of the *pleural pressure gradient* may lie in the weight of the lung. This can be viewed as the result of the lung having to be supported by the rib cage and diaphragm. Increasingly, other factors, including shape and mechanical properties of the chest wall and lung, are being suggested as playing a role.

Since alveolar pressure is the same throughout the lung, a systematic variation in pleural pressure results in a systematic variation in transpulmonary pressure. Thus, alveoli exposed to a more negative pleural pressure are more expanded than those exposed to a less negative pleural pressure. This leads to a *distribution of regional lung volume* and hence a distribution of compliance, since alveoli that are distended close to their maximum volume will be stiffer than less distended alveoli. During inspiration, when pleural pressure falls, the more compliant alveoli expand to a greater extent than the less compliant alveoli, resulting in a *distribution of ventilation* in the lung.

Regional ventilation can also be affected by the distribution of *time constants* in the lung. The time constant of any lung unit is defined as the product of its air flow resistance and compliance. Regions with a short time constant (i.e., low compliance and low resistance) should fill and empty faster than regions with a longer time constant. In normal lungs the dispersion of time constants is not large, and most alveoli fill and empty synchronously. In disease conditions there is considerably more range for a dispersion of time constants.

As was pointed out earlier, the pulmonary capillaries are surrounded by alveolar gas and are therefore exposed to alveolar pressure. Thus, the transmural pressure acting across the pulmonary capillaries is determined by the difference between alveolar pressure and pulmonary capillary pressure. This arrangement affects the *distribution of blood flow* in the lung. As we descend vertically in the lung, the mean pulmonary artery pressure increases by 1 cm water per cm descent because of the weight of the volume of blood in the chest. The alveolar pressure, however, remains constant. At the top of the lung the mean pulmonary artery pressure may be less than alveolar pressure, and under these conditions no flow is possible because the pulmonary capillaries will be collapsed. This has been referred to as zone 1 and probably does not exist in normal animals, the pulmonary artery pressure usually being sufficient to raise blood to the top of the lung. Zone 2 conditions are found when the pulmonary artery pressure is greater than alveolar pressure but alveolar pressure is greater than pulmonary venous pressure. Under these conditions blood flow is determined by the difference between pulmonary arterial and alveolar pressures. Blood flow increases vertically down this zone because the pulmonary artery pressure increases while the alveolar pressure remains constant. This results in the opening of some capillaries that would otherwise have been closed, a phenomenon known as *recruitment*. Below this zone, pulmonary artery pressure and pulmonary venous pressure are both greater than alveolar pressure; thus blood flow is controlled by the normal arterial-to-venous difference (Zone 3). Blood flow continues to increase down this zone because capillaries distend under the resulting increased capillary transmural pressure. Therefore, even in the normal lung blood flow is thought to be nonuniformly distributed. The pulmonary capillary bed has a great capacity to respond to the pressures acting upon it and under conditions of increased pulmonary artery pressure (e.g., exercise) is able to lower its already low resistance even further through capillary recruitment and distention.

Gas exchange itself takes place across the alveolar membrane, with oxygen diffusing from alveolar gas to blood and carbon dioxide moving in the opposite direction. Movement of these gases takes place by simple diffusion in response to a driving pressure equal to the difference between the partial pressure of the gas in the mixed venous blood and in the alveolar gas.

Diffusion reserves in the lung are large, and normally a red cell traversing the pulmonary capillary bed is almost fully loaded with oxygen by the time it is about one-third of the way along the capillary. Carbon dioxide is about 24 times as soluble as oxygen and therefore diffuses with even greater ease. Diseases that might be expected to impair diffusion by thickening the alveolar membrane or interstitium (e.g., pulmonary fibrosis) thus do not usually cause significant impairment of gas exchange in clinical practice.

We turn now from a consideration of the individual distributions of ventilation and perfusion to an examination of the role that the *relationship between pulmonary ventilation and perfusion* plays in determining the efficiency of gas exchange in the lung. Earlier it was pointed out that the rate of diffusion of oxygen or carbon dioxide between the alveolar gas and the pulmonary capillary blood depends on the partial pressure difference existing across the alveolar membrane. If we consider blood arriving in the lungs to have a fixed composition of oxygen and carbon dioxide, then gas transfer depends on the partial pressure of the particular gas in the alveolar space. This depends on the concentration of that gas in the alveolar space, which in turn is determined by the relationship between the rate of arrival of the gas in the alveoli (ventilation for oxygen, perfusion for carbon dioxide) and its removal (perfusion for oxygen, ventilation for carbon dioxide). Thus, the alveolar partial pressure of oxygen or carbon dioxide in any particular lung unit is uniquely determined by its ventilation-to-perfusion ratio ($\dot{V}A/\dot{Q}$). Since the distribution of ventilation and perfusion in the lung is not matched, there is also a nonuniform distribution of $\dot{V}A/\dot{Q}$, even in normal lungs.

Units with low $\dot{V}A/\dot{Q}$ ratios tend to have a low PA_{O_2} and a high PA_{CO_2}, since blood flow is high relative to ventilation. Correspondingly, units with high $\dot{V}A/\dot{Q}$ ratios tend to have a high PA_{O_2} and a low PA_{CO_2}. Mixed arterial blood consists of a mixture of blood from all units in the lung. Low $\dot{V}A/\dot{Q}$ units, however, contribute relatively more since their blood flow is high relative to their ventilation. This blood has a lower P_{O_2} and a higher P_{CO_2} than blood from higher $\dot{V}A/\dot{Q}$ units. Thus, the effect of a dispersion of $\dot{V}A/\dot{Q}$ ratios in the lung is to lower the Pa_{O_2} and raise the Pa_{CO_2}.

Increasing Pa_{CO_2}, however, stimulates ventilation, which tends to "blow off" carbon dioxide and return the Pa_{CO_2} to normal. This will not significantly raise the oxygen content of the blood, since it will, most likely, be already fully saturated. The sigmoid shape of the normal oxygen-hemoglobin dissociation curve means almost full saturation above a Pa_{O_2} of about 60 mm Hg. For this reason it is also not possible to "superload" blood from high $\dot{V}A/\dot{Q}$ units with oxygen to make up for the low oxygen content of blood coming from low $\dot{V}A/\dot{Q}$ units.

The concept of $\dot{V}A/\dot{Q}$ mismatch in the lung is a very important one, since there is considerable range for mismatch in almost any lung disease. A dispersion of $\dot{V}A/\dot{Q}$ ratios is probably the most important cause of arterial hypoxemia associated with respiratory disease. There are two reflexes that may come into play in disease situations in an attempt to maintain matching of ventilation and perfusion. Regions with impaired ventilation and therefore a low PA_{O_2} often also have reduced perfusion (*pulmonary hypoxic vasoconstriction*). A much less powerful reflex involves reduction of ventilation to lung regions where perfusion is reduced.

Impairment of gas exchange in the lung also occurs if mixed venous blood reaches the arterial system via a true *right to left shunt*, i.e., without passsing through ventilated regions of the lung. Many shunts are extrapulmonary, e.g., in some types of congenital heart disease. Another example of a shunt is the normal bronchial vein blood that drains into the left heart. However, shunting of blood may occur through arteriovenous fistulas or, more importantly, through unventilated but perfused alveoli. This latter situation can be often seen in association with pneumonia or pulmonary edema.

We are now in a position to list the *causes of arterial hypoxemia*: low inspired P_{O_2}, hypoventilation, diffusion impairment, ventilation-perfusion mismatch, and shunt.

Ventilation implies changes in lung volume. The major subdivisions of lung volume are as follows:

Total lung capacity: the volume of gas in the lung at the end of a maximal inspiration.

Functional residual capacity: the volume of gas in the lung at the end of a normal tidal expiration.

Residual volume: the volume of gas remaining in the lung at the end of a maximal expiration.

Tidal volume: the volume of gas inhaled or exhaled during breathing.

Vital capacity: the maximum volume of gas that can be exhaled after a maximum inspiration.

To change lung volume, a pressure difference must be established between the environment and the alveolar compartment. This is achieved by using the respiratory muscles, principally the diaphragm and intercostal muscles, to enlarge or reduce the size of the thoracic cavity, thus lowering or raising pleural pressure and, in turn, alveolar pressure. When these maneuvers are performed in a relatively slow manner, the amount of lung volume change per unit change in transpulmonary pressure is a measure of the elastic properties of the lung (compliance). Actually, *lung compliance* varies according to lung volume, since the lung becomes less distensible as it approaches maximum volume. In fact, the lung also becomes stiffer at very low volumes because closure of small airways may occur in response to large compressing pressures, thus trapping gas and preventing further change in lung volume. This is more likely to happen at the bottom of the lung, where pleural pressure is greatest, and is one of the mechanisms that may determine residual volume in older animals. In younger animals residual volume is probably reached when the rib cage cannot be made any smaller. The volume of gas that can still be exhaled from the point of commencement of airway closure until residual volume is reached is known as *closing volume*. This volume will be increased (i.e., airway closure occurs earlier during an expiration) by processes that decrease the elasticity of the lung (e.g., emphysema) or increase the resistance of small airways (e.g., chronic obstructive pulmonary disease). In some advanced disease situations closing volume may be so large that gas trapping occurs during tidal breathing.

Under higher flow conditions, such as during tidal breathing, the rate of gas flow in and out of the lung is markedly affected by the *resistance of the airways*. One would expect this to be greatest in the smaller airways; however, as pointed out earlier, the great number of small airways dramatically increases the total cross-sectional area and lowers airway resistance. Thus the small airways are thought to contribute only a relatively small percentage of the total airway resistance; this means that significant disease can occur in these airways before their resistance will be increased enough to produce clinical signs. This particularly applies to the dog, which has relatively large airways in relation to its size, and extensive collateral ventilation.

Airway resistance is affected by a number of factors even in normal animals. At higher lung volumes, for example, airways are pulled open (tethered) by the surrounding distended lung tissue. Contraction of bronchial smooth muscle, on the other hand, tends to decrease airway caliber. Obviously in diseases that affect bronchial smooth muscle contractility, considerable range exists for increasing airway resistance and impairing maximal gas flow rates.

Another important cause of flow limitation in both normal and diseased animals is *dynamic compression of airways*. During a forced expiration, gas flows out of the lung because of the pressure difference between alveolar pressure and atmospheric pressure. Alveolar pressure is the sum of pleural pressure and the elastic recoil pressure of the lung. Since airway pressure drops as we proceed from alveolus to mouth during expiration, a point will be reached at which airway pressure is equal to pleural pressure. This is known as the equal pressure point and represents that point along the airways where the elastic pressure generated by the lung has been dissipated. From this point on within the thorax there will be a pressure tending to compress the airways; they will narrow, thus limiting bulk gas flow. Outside of the thorax the pressure surrounding the trachea is atmospheric; intraluminal pressure remains greater than atmospheric pressure, so no tendency to collapse exists.

On inspiration the lowered pleural pressure tends to hold intrathoracic airways open, and the negative intraluminal pressures in the extrathoracic airways mean that they tend to be narrowed by the surrounding atmospheric pressure. In normal animals during tidal breathing these changes are minimal and are barely noticeable on inspiratory/expiratory radiographs. However, they are likely to be present during forced maneuvers such as coughing.

In disease situations in which airway resistance is increased (thus causing a greater drop in pressure along the airways) or airways are not as rigid, dynamic compression of airways can occur during tidal breathing and can impede either inspiration (e.g., laryngeal paralysis) or expiration (e.g., intrathoracic tracheal collapse).

The respiratory system has a complex control mechanism designed to ensure that oxygen uptake and carbon dioxide removal remain adequate to support metabolism. There are two main avenues for *regulation of ventilation:* chemical control and mechanical reflexes.

The levels of oxygen, carbon dioxide, and hydrogen ion in the arterial blood are monitored by both central and peripheral chemoreceptors, which in turn send signals to the respiratory center, a group of neurons located in the medullary area of the brain. The respiratory center is also influenced by signals from the pons, hypothalamus, and higher brain centers. Respiratory rate and tidal volume are controlled from the respiratory center via efferent nerve traffic to the muscles of respiration.

Carbon dioxide is the major chemical influence on breathing. Levels of carbon dioxide in the blood are detected primarily by receptors on the surface of the brain near the respiratory center. A rising level of carbon dioxide is a powerful stimulation for increased ventilation. Oxygen levels are sensed by carotid and aortic body receptors. Unlike carbon dioxide, however, the partial pressure of oxygen in the arterial blood has to fall to about 50 mm Hg before any appreciable increase in ventilation occurs. Thus, oxygen is thought not to contribute greatly to respiratory control under normal circumstances. The hypoxic drive to breathe, however, can be of particular importance in disease states. Animals with chronic obstructive pulmonary disease may tend to retain carbon dioxide, as they are unable to sustain adequate levels of ventilation because of the increased work of breathing. If such an animal becomes insensitive to carbon dioxide, it may rely substantially on its hypoxic drive to breathe. Removal of this drive by the administration of high levels of inspired oxygen may have disastrous consequences. Falls in arterial pH are also detected by peripheral chemoreceptors and stimulate ventilation.

A number of mechanical reflexes have been shown to be involved in respiratory control. The relative importance of these in animals is not well understood.

Some receptors in the airway epithelium respond to lung deflation. Stimulation of these receptors causes a relatively short, strong inspiratory effort and a rapid breathing frequency. This represents the deflation portion of the Hering-Breuer reflex. Stretching of the lungs, on the other hand, causes stimulation of inflation receptors, which tends to inhibit inspiration. These influences are mediated via the vagus.

Vagal transmission of afferent stimuli also occurs with stimulation of J receptors in the lung parenchyma, leading to increased ventilation. Mechanical or chemical stimulation of irritant receptors at various levels in the respiratory tract may lead to sneezing, coughing, increased ventilation, or bronchoconstriction.

Other reflex pathways involve receptors in the respiratory muscles that control strength of contraction and may be involved in the "sensation" of dyspnea. Receptors located in the joints are thought to be responsible for the increase in ventilation associated with the onset of exercise.

PULMONARY DEFENSE MECHANISMS

The respiratory surface represents an interface between the organism and the environment. As such it is continually exposed to a variety of injurious agents ranging from inanimate particulate matter to complex infectious agents. To protect the system from damage, the lung has developed a sophisticated defense system. When this defense system is breached, because of either the strength of the challenge or an inadequate response by the animal, respiratory disease results.

The *upper airway* design permits inspired air to be warmed and saturated with water vapor, thus protecting the lower respiratory tract membranes from drying. Bypassing this mechanism (e.g., tracheostomy) may predispose to respiratory tract damage unless sufficient precautions are taken (e.g., humidification).

Filtering hairs at the nares in some species, convoluted turbinate structures, mucous secretions, and the architecture of the nasopharynx serve to promote turbulence of inspired gas and particle filtration via impaction. In general, only particles less than about 3 μ in diameter reach the lower airways. Soluble gases also tend to be removed from the inspired air in the upper airways. Closure of the glottis during swallowing and on laryngeal stimulation also serves to restrict the passage of large particles into the lower respiratory tract.

If particles do enter the respiratory tract, a number of mechanisms promote their *clearance*. *Sneezing* forces gas at high velocity through the nasal passages, helping to remove particles entrapped in nasal mucus, whereas *coughing* is an important defense mechanism for the removal of particles in the lower airways.

The airway epithelium down to the respiratory bronchiole is supplied with *ciliated cells and mucus-secreting glandular structures*. Cilia beat in the direction of the pharynx, moving a fluid layer in which particles are entrapped. This layer has two components, a watery layer in which the cilia beat and a mucus layer in which particles are entrapped. This mucociliary escalator can move particles out of the major bronchi at rates of 1 to 2 cm per minute in the normal animal.

Foreign particles are removed from the respiratory bronchioles, alveolar ducts, and alveolar sacs by *alveolar macrophages*, monocytes that originate in the bone marrow. These cells migrate into the alveolar spaces from the interstitium of the lung and can phagocytose and detoxify particles and kill microorganisms. Macrophages laden with ingested particles may leave the lung via either the pulmonary interstitial fluid (and eventually the tracheobronchial lymph nodes) or the mucociliary escalator. Once an infection is established in the lung, large numbers of neutrophils may arrive to aid macrophages in the phagocytosis of infectious agents.

The lung can respond to the presence of an antigen through the *secretion of immunoglobulins* into the respiratory tract mucus as well as through the transudation of serum antibodies. The localization of these immune responses may be responsible for the variation in allergic responses in the respiratory tract. Thus, large particles that are filtered out in the nose may be responsible for allergic rhinitis syndromes, whereas smaller particles, reaching small airways, may cause bronchoconstriction, and still smaller particles, such as spores of certain fungi, may reach the alveolar regions and produce an acute alveolitis.

Secretory IgA is the predominant immunoglobulin in the upper airways and is important in resistance to respiratory viral infections. IgG is more important in the periphery of the lower respiratory tract, where it agglutinates particles, opsonizes bacteria, activates complement, neutralizes bacterial toxins and viruses, and lyses gram negative bacteria in the presence of complement.

IgM is also found in respiratory secretions, but its role is less well established. IgE is well known for its role in immediate hypersensitivity reactions in humans, but its role in respiratory diseases of small animals is not well understood.

Thymus-derived *lymphocytes* are found in the lymphoid tissue throughout the respiratory tract. Once sensitized, they produce a variety of proteins that inhibit macrophages from leaving the area, attract phagocytes, increase macrophage phagocytic and bacteriocidal activity, and stimulate the sensitization of still more T cells. They also lyse foreign and host cells with foreign antigen on their surface.

PATHOPHYSIOLOGIC CLASSIFICATION OF RESPIRATORY DISEASE

In approaching the differential diagnosis of respiratory disease, it is of some help to be able to categorize diseases on the basis of the nature of the pathophysiology that they produce. A classification system that has been widely used in human medicine for a number of years is outlined. This is presented with some trepidation, since it is not a complete system, not all diseases fit neatly into it, and considerable overlap can occur, with one disease producing clinical signs compatible with a number of different categories. It is also much more difficult in the veterinary clinical situation to apply this system, since many of the measurements on which its use in humans is based are not available. Its usefulness for the veterinary practitioner lies in the understanding it imparts of pathophysiologic processes in the lung and their relationship to clinical signs.

Obstructive respiratory diseases are characterized by airway (airflow) obstruction. This can be either endomural (e.g., mucus, foreign body in the airways), mural (e.g., airway wall edema, mucus hyperplasia, smooth muscle constriction), or extramural (e.g., dynamic compression of airways, impingement of mass on airways). Diseases such as chronic bronchitis, emphysema, and asthma fit into this category. Also included are upper airway obstructive diseases such as stenotic nares, elongated soft palate, and laryngeal paralysis.

The basic functional abnormality is limitation of inspiratory and/or expiratory gas flow. In humans this is documented through pulmonary function tests. In animals we usually have to rely on interpretation of clinical signs and chest radiographs.

Restrictive respiratory diseases are characterized by restricted expansion of the lung and/or chest wall, i.e., decreased compliance. Restrictive respiratory disease usually leads to decreased lung volume reserve (i.e., small lungs). This may be mediated by pathologic processes in the lung (e.g., fibrosis) or the pleural space (e.g., pleural effusion) or involving the chest wall (e.g., thoracic wall neoplasm). In general, airway caliber is appropriate for lung volume in these diseases; in fact, airways may be larger in diameter at the same lung volume in some restrictive diseases (e.g., fibrosis) because they are pulled open by increased lung elastic recoil.

Diffusion impairment respiratory disease tends to reduce gas exchange by thickening alveolar or vascular walls or the interstitium of the lung (e.g., interstitial fibrosis, pulmonary edema). However, as explained previously, "diffusion block" is usually not a clinical problem.

Pulmonary vascular diseases primarily affect the pulmonary vasculature (e.g., heartworms, pulmonary embolism).

Considerable overlap in the categorization of specific diseases can occur. For example, pulmonary edema is primarily a pulmonary vascular disease that can affect diffusion, cause a restrictive deficit by altering the elastic properties of the pulmonary interstitium, and finally cause an obstructive pattern when airways begin to fill with fluid.

CORRELATION OF CLINICAL SIGNS AND PATHOPHYSIOLOGY

Respiratory distress is a major clinical sign of respiratory disease in animals. It is often also referred to as dyspnea. However, this term is used in human medicine to describe a *sensation* of breathing difficulty experienced *by the patient* and communicated to the physician. As such, it is not really an appropriate term for use in veterinary medicine, and respiratory distress or respiratory difficulty seems more appropriate.

It is difficult, however, to accurately define respiratory distress in animals, although most clinicians have no difficulty in recognizing it. An inappropriate degree of breathing effort, based on an assessment of respiratory rate, rhythm, and character, seems to summarize what is recognized as respiratory distress.

The nature of respiratory distress can be used as an important clue to its etiology or at least to try to functionally characterize the pathophysiology involved. Animals with obstructive disease of the intrathoracic airways are likely to have more flow limitation on expiration than inspiration because of dynamic collapse of airways. Patients with chronic bronchitis or intrathoracic tracheal collapse are, therefore, more likely to have expiratory rather than inspiratory distress. On the other hand, if the site of airway obstruction is extrathoracic, dynamic compression occurs on inspiration rather than expiration. Thus, animals with extrathoracic tracheal collapse or laryngeal paralysis are more likely to have inspiratory rather than expiratory distress.

Fixed airway obstruction in either the upper or lower respiratory tract (e.g., intraluminal masses, extramural compression, bronchoconstriction) is present during both inspiration and expiration and may lead to both inspiratory and expiratory distress. Restrictive diseases usually inhibit expansion of the lungs and therefore lead most often to inspiratory distress (e.g., pleural effusion, diaphragmatic hernia).

As animals with intrathoracic airway obstruction have difficulty getting air out of the lungs, they are likely to spend more time on expiration than on inspiration. The reverse may occur in animals with upper airway obstruction or restrictive disease. Since the animal with restrictive disease has to do a greater amount of respiratory work to expand its lungs, a common strategy for maintaining adequate ventilation is to raise respiratory rate and lower tidal volume. Animals with obstructive disease would be more likely to maintain or increase tidal volume.

These patterns of breathing may be considerably affected by other factors. The need to maintain temperature control through ventilation in dogs may well influence respiratory rate and tidal volume in both obstructive and restrictive diseases.

When the amount of reduced hemoglobin in the capillary blood reaches approximately 5 gm/100 ml, a bluish color is imparted to the mucus membranes, known as *cyanosis*. Cyanosis is usually present when oxygen saturation is below 80 per cent, which with a normal oxygen-hemoglobin dissociation curve requires a Pa_{O_2} of less than 50 mm Hg. Hence, cyanosis is a late sign and considerable hypoxemia can be present without cyanosis; this is particularly true if the amount of hemoglobin in the blood is reduced by anemia. Cyanosis is also affected by blood flow; reduced local blood flow allows more oxygen extraction to occur and thus produces an increased amount of reduced hemoglobin.

Cough is an important protective reflex in the lung. The process of coughing commences with stimulation of receptors in the airways. A reflex pathway is then set in motion that first causes a deep inspiration; this increases lung volume, dilates airways, increases lung elastic recoil, and allows greater peak flows to be achieved. The glottis then closes while contraction of the abdominal and chest wall muscles raises pleural pressure. A sudden opening of the glottis is followed by rapidly accelerating expiratory flow. During this period dynamic compression expels gas from the large intrathoracic airways as a transient "spike" of gas flow while increasing the linear velocity of gas flowing through the compressed region. This high velocity gas stream shears mucus from the airway walls and carries it to the oropharynx, where it is swallowed or expectorated. As lung volume falls, smaller airways are compressed and cleared of mucus. Dynamic compression of airways is thought not to extend beyond segmental bronchi in the dog until lung volume is less than 25 per cent of the vital capacity; at lower lung volumes it could extend to airways of 0.5 to 1.0 mm in diameter. In the alveolar regions of the lung, gas flows are too low for cough to be an effective clearance method.

The differential diagnosis of cough is difficult, since it occurs in a wide variety of respiratory diseases. However, some broad generalizations may be possible; irritation of the larynx and large airways often results in a loud, harsh, dry cough of sudden onset, and chronic obstructive pulmonary disease with excess mucus production produces a chronic, productive cough. The cough associated with chronic mitral valve disease has been described as deep and resonant, first occurring in the early morning and then progressing to more frequent paroxysms of coughing. Attention to an accurate history concerning onset, nature, duration, and timing of cough may give the clinician some clues to its etiology.

A question that frequently arises is the desirability of suppressing coughing. Certainly when coughing is nonproductive, painful, exhausting, and annoying to both owner and patient cough suppression is probably indicated. However, it must be remembered that coughing is a lung defense mechanism that should not be indiscriminately removed. In other situations, notably when clearance of secretions from the respiratory tract is required but cough is ineffectual because of a variety of factors (e.g., neuromuscular weakness, pain, viscid secretions, bronchoconstriction, excessively collapsible airway segments, and so on), it may be necessary to facilitate coughing. This can be done with agents that improve mucus flow (e.g., hydration, inhaled mist, expectorants, mucolytics), gas flow (e.g., bronchodilators), or muscle power (e.g., manual compression of body wall, treatment of neuromuscular disease). Physiotherapy (e.g., percussion, chest vibration) may be particularly helpful in loosening secretions and promoting cough.

One of the most important diagnostic techniques

available to practitioners for the assessment of pulmonary disease is auscultation of the respiratory system using a stethoscope. A principal area of difficulty in attempting to discuss the normal and abnormal sounds heard over the chest is terminology. The literature and common usage abound with different terms that usually mean different things to different clinicians.

Lung sounds were first described by Laënnec in 1819. He proposed that all abnormal lung sounds be called *rales,* which could be divided into five groups: moist, mucous, sonorous, sibilant, and dry crepitant. Over the years the meaning of these terms has become altered and confused with the introduction of other terms such as *rhonchus*; this term originally had the same meaning as rale but was later changed to denote a musical-type sound, whereas rale was then applied to an interrupted nonmusical sound. In recent years attempts have been made to standardize nomenclature for lung sounds in human medicine. The approach described hereafter is largely based on recommendations by Forgacs.

Normal breath sounds include faint rustling sounds heard over areas of the chest away from large airways and are known as *vesicular sounds.* *Bronchial sounds* are louder, more tubular in quality, and have a wider range of frequencies than vesicular sounds. They are heard over the large airways. In regions where both types of normal sounds are heard the term *bronchovesicular* has been used.

Two types of *adventitious* or *abnormal* sounds are recognized: *wheezes* and *crackles.* Wheezes are musical sounds that are classified according to pitch (high and low), complexity (monophonic and polyphonic), duration (long and short), and timing (inspiratory and expiratory, early and late, random and sequential). Crackles are short, explosive nonmusical sounds that are classified according to pitch (high and low), number (scanty and profuse), and timing (inspiratory and expiratory, early and late).

A greater appreciation of the pathophysiologic meaning of the various lung sounds can be gained if the clinician has some understanding of the mechanisms that produce these sounds. Lung sounds are produced either by rapid fluctuations of gas pressure or by the oscillations of solid tissue. In most of the conducting airways of the lung gas flow is laminar and silent. Low flow rates in the terminal airways are one reason for the lack of detected sound over large areas of the normal lung.

Gas flow becomes turbulent above a critical flow velocity, resulting in rapid fluctuations in gas pressure, which produce noise. This is the sound heard over the large airways that becomes louder at higher gas flows (e.g., exercise, panting). If this mechanism produces large airway sounds, what process produces vesicular sounds? Some investigators feel that these sounds result from a low pass filter effect that occurs when sound passes through lung tissue and thus are only bronchial sounds with the higher frequencies removed.

Abnormal lung sounds are often associated with narrowing or closure of airways. If a region of an airway becomes narrowed (e.g., intraluminal mass, bronchoconstriction), then the linear velocity of gas will increase through the narrowed portion of the tube. Because of the Bernoulli or Venturi effect, lateral pressure decreases at such an obstruction and the airway tends to narrow further or close. If closure occurs, flow ceases and the airway re-opens. As this cycle repeats, the airway wall begins to oscillate, producing a musical sound, the wheeze. Similarly, dynamic compression of the airways also leads to airway wall oscillation and wheeze production. Loud, high-pitched, inspiratory wheezes heard without the aid of a stethoscope are often referred to as *stridor* and are most often generated by narrowing in the extrathoracic airways.

Crackles are thought to be produced by the sudden equalization of gas pressure, which occurs when previously closed airways re-open. Thus they are more commonly heard over dependent lung zones toward the end of inspiration as small airways re-open. Crackles may also be related to rupture of fluid films or bubbles in the airways. *Pleural crackles* may be heard when pleural surfaces roughened by fibrin deposits, inflammation, or neoplasia rub together. Note that pleural crackles will not be generated when pleural surfaces are separated, e.g., in pleural effusion.

PULMONARY FUNCTION TESTS

Pulmonary function testing consists of the quantitative assessment of aspects of respiratory physiology or pathophysiology. In human medicine many such tests are available and can be broadly divided into two groups: tests of ventilation and tests of gas exchange. Ventilatory assessment includes such approaches as measurement of lung volumes, maximal expiratory flow rates, ventilation distribution, and pulmonary compliance. Tests of gas exchange include the measurement of arterial blood gases and assessment of pulmonary diffusing capacity using carbon monoxide.

Some of these approaches have been modified for use with animals, but this has been confined to the research laboratory and has often involved general anesthesia. The goal of easily applied, everyday clinical pulmonary function testing in conscious dogs and cats has yet to be attained.

The major avenues available to the veterinary clinician for evaluation of the functional nature of respiratory disease involve interpretation of physical findings in terms of underlying pathophysiology, a subject already discussed in this article; pathophysiologic interpretation of chest radiographs, a subject beyond the scope of this discussion; and blood gas analysis.

Unfortunately, *blood gas analysis* does not allow early detection of respiratory disease, since the reserves for gas exchange in the lung are large. However, it is particularly useful in the assessment and monitoring of respiratory failure and can be used as an indication of the degree of gas exchange impairment present in lung disease. In addition, it provides an opportunity to determine which of the five causes of hypoxemia is dominating the clinical picture.

At first sight, Pa_{O_2} would seem to be a reasonable guide to gas exchange efficiency. However, consideration of Pa_{O_2} alone does not allow for the effect of ventilation; the Pa_{O_2} may be low if hypoventilation is present, and the patient's lungs may be normal.

One way to estimate the efficiency with which the lung is exchanging gas is to calculate the difference between alveolar P_{O_2} and arterial P_{O_2}. However, PA_{O_2} is difficult to measure in a lung with $\dot{V}A/\dot{Q}$ inequality, since there will be a wide spectrum of values of PA_{O_2}. It is also difficult to collect alveolar gas without contamination from dead space gas. To get around this problem, we can calculate what is called the *ideal alveolar* P_{O_2}. This is the PA_{O_2} that would be present in the lung if there were no $\dot{V}A/\dot{Q}$ abnormality. It is found by using the alveolar gas equation, a simplified form of which follows:

$$PA_{O_2} = PI_{O_2} - Pa_{CO_2}/R$$

where PI_{O_2} is the partial pressure of oxygen in the inspired gas and R is the respiratory exchange ratio.

The PI_{O_2} is calculated from the fractional concentration of oxygen in the inspired gas and the total *dry* gas pressure, i.e., barometric pressure minus water vapor pressure. Since we are now able to define alveolar gas in accurate physiologic terms, we have a reference point from which we can analyze deviations from the ideal. The difference between the ideal PA_{O_2} and the Pa_{O_2} is called the *alveolar-arterial difference for oxygen* ($PA_{O_2} - Pa_{O_2}$). This value can be as high as 20 mm Hg in normal animals, whereas in those with significant $\dot{V}A/\dot{Q}$ mismatch or physiologic shunt it is likely to be elevated. Note that the alveolar-arterial difference for oxygen is affected in normal animals by those factors that affect $\dot{V}A/\dot{Q}$ mismatch (e.g., body position, anesthesia, age) and also widens at higher levels of inspired oxygen.

It is possible to evaluate the amount of shunt present using the following equation:

$$\dot{Q}s/\dot{Q}T = Cc'_{O_2} - Ca_{O_2}/Cc'_{O_2} - C\bar{v}_{O_2}$$

where $\dot{Q}s$ is the blood flow through shunt channels, $\dot{Q}T$ is the total blood flow through the lung, Ca_{O_2} is the oxygen content of arterial blood, $C\bar{v}_{O_2}$ is the oxygen content of mixed venous blood, and Cc'_{O_2} is the oxygen content of end pulmonary capillary blood. This calculation requires measurement of both arterial and mixed venous (pulmonary artery) oxygen contents. Cc'_{O_2} is usually calculated from the ideal PA_{O_2} and the oxygen-hemoglobin dissociation curve. Note that this approach treats all depression of the Pa_{O_2} as if a certain amount of mixed venous blood were being added to end pulmonary capillary blood. Therefore, it includes the contribution of low $\dot{V}A/\dot{Q}$ units as well as true shunt. In this form it is known as *physiologic shunt* or venous admixture.

Depression of the Pa_{O_2} by true shunt can be separated from the effect of $\dot{V}A/\dot{Q}$ mismatch by giving the animal 100 per cent oxygen. Since shunted blood will not "see" the resulting increased PA_{O_2}, this maneuver will fail to significantly raise Pa_{O_2}.

The contribution of high $\dot{V}A/\dot{Q}$ units to inefficiency of gas exchange can be assessed by calculating physiologic dead space (VDS) using the Bohr equation:

$$VDS/VT = Pa_{CO_2} - PE_{CO_2}/Pa_{CO_2}$$

This measurement requires the collection of expired gas, for the assessment of the mixed expired gas partial pressure of CO_2 (PE_{CO_2}), as well as arterial blood for the measurement of Pa_{CO_2}.

From the preceding discussion, the following approach may be taken for an interpretation of arterial blood gas values. First, the oxygen tension of the inspired gas (PI_{O_2}) must be ascertained; without this knowledge no meaningful interpretation of Pa_{O_2} is possible. PI_{O_2} is calculated as follows:

$$PI_{O_2} = (PB - P_{H_2O}) \times FI_{O_2}$$

where PB is the barometric pressure, P_{H_2O} is the partial pressure of water vapor in the inspired gas at the animal's body temperature, and FI_{O_2} is the fractional concentration of oxygen in the inspired gas. An animal with a body temperature of 38°C breathing room air at sea level can be assumed to have a PI_{O_2} of about 149 mm Hg.

Second, check the Pa_{CO_2}; it may be within the normal range or greater than normal, indicating hypoventilation. If the Pa_{CO_2} is less than normal, hyperventilation is indicated. The Pa_{O_2} may also be within the normal range, less than normal (hypoxemia), or greater than normal (hyperoxemia).

The efficiency of gas exchange may then be assessed by calculating the $PA_{O_2} - Pa_{O_2}$. A value of less than 0 mm Hg is impossible and usually indicates a technical error, an error in calculation, or an incorrect assumption. A value of 0 to 15 mm Hg is normal; any hypoxemia is explained by hypoventilation. A $PA_{O_2} - Pa_{O_2}$ of greater than 15 mm Hg indicates the presence of $\dot{V}A/\dot{Q}$ mismatch and/or shunt. If the Pa_{O_2} remains less than 150 to 200 mm Hg during the administration of 100 per cent oxygen, significant shunt is present. The acid-base status of the animal may be assessed from the pH and Pa_{CO_2} (this subject is discussed elsewhere in this text).

SUPPLEMENTAL READING

Forgacs, P.: *Lung Sounds*. London: Bailliere Tindall, 1978.
Green, G. M., Jakab, G. J., Low, R. B., and Davis, G. S.: Defense mechanisms of the respiratory membrane. Am. Rev. Resp. Dis. 115:479, 1977.
Wanner, A.: Clinical aspects of mucociliary transport. Am. Rev. Resp. Dis. 116:73, 1977.
West, J. B.: Ventilation/Blood Flow and Gas Exchange, 3rd ed. Oxford: Blackwell Scientific Publications, 1977.
West, J. B.: *Respiratory Physiology—The Essentials*, 2nd ed. Baltimore: Williams & Wilkins, 1979.
West, J. B.: *Pulmonary Pathophysiology—The Essentials*, 2nd ed. Baltimore: Williams & Wilkins, 1982.

BLOOD GASES AND ACID-BASE BALANCE: CLINICAL INTERPRETATION AND THERAPEUTIC IMPLICATIONS

STEVE C. HASKINS, D.V.M.

Davis, California

INTRODUCTION

The appropriate application of pH and blood gas measurements to the clinical management of a patient is helpful and, in some cases, vital to a successful therapeutic endeavor. Access to these values, however, should not be used as a substitute for continuous clinical evaluation of the status of the patient. A particular patient could, for instance, maintain normal blood gases but only by exerting such an extreme amount of effort that he would become exhausted if left on his own. Lack of the ability to obtain pH and blood gas measurements, on the other hand, should not preclude concern for the existence of acid-base disturbances or the need for definitive therapy. It is, perhaps, necessary to have a better understanding of the nature and patterns of common disease processes when these measurements are not available.

Knowledge of the acid-base status of the patient seldom provides a diagnosis but often has important implications with regard to questions of when and what the treatment should be and how effective it is.

pH

pH is a logarithmic expression of hydrogen ion concentration and is the preferable unitage because it more accurately represents the *in vivo* chemobiodynamic activity of the hydrogen ion. The pH is the net result of the balance of all of the acidotic and alkalotic processes in the body. The general mechanism by which disease and therapy influence pH is via manipulation of carbonic acid, primarily by the respiratory component, and noncarbonic acids, by the metabolic component of the acid-base balance. This article is therefore broadly divided into a discussion of the respiratory and metabolic aspects of acid-base balance. Although the pH is a pawn of these two components, it is, nevertheless, the alteration of the hydrogen ion concentration that ultimately affects intracellular enzymatic homeostasis and causes harm to the organism.

The normal pH is usually considered to be within the range of 7.35 to 7.45 units. As a general rule, pH values between 7.2 and 7.6 are taken to be a quantitative measure of the severity of the disease process but are not assumed to represent an important stress to the patient *per se*. Values below 7.0 and above 7.8 are considered to be extreme threats to the welfare of the patient and are not conducive to prolonged survival. They mandate early definitive

Note: The author would like to express his appreciation to Dr. Elizabeth Hodgkins for help in preparing this manuscript.

therapy of the pH disturbance. Values between 7.0 and 7.2 and between 7.6 and 7.8 are severe alterations but exert an unknown and variable degree of impairment to homeostasis. Treatment of the pH disturbance in addition to the underlying disease process is usually indicated.

Buffer systems cushion the effect that an acid or alkali load has on the pH. They are very important in the stability of the pH of the internal milieu, but since they are not ordinarily accessible to clinical manipulation, except by alkali therapy, they will not be discussed further.

BLOOD CARBON DIOXIDE AND THE RESPIRATORY COMPONENT OF THE ACID-BASE BALANCE

The amount of carbon dioxide in the blood is determined by the balance between metabolic production and ventilatory elimination. Since metabolic production is reasonably constant under normal metabolic circumstances, the blood carbon dioxide level is primarily controlled by its rate of elimination through the lungs. CO_2 diffuses from the capillary venous blood into the alveoli of the lungs via a partial pressure gradient between these two areas. CO_2 is then removed from the alveoli by ventilatory exchange of atmospheric air with alveolar gases. The extent to which ventilation affects the alveolar partial pressure of carbon dioxide determines the amount of CO_2 diffusing from the capillaries and thereby establishes the partial pressure of carbon dioxide in the arterial blood (Pa_{CO_2}). If the blood carbon dioxide level is higher than normal, a decreased rate of elimination due to decreased alveolar minute ventilation (hypoventilation) is assumed to be the cause. An increased alveolar minute ventilation (hyperventilation) is cited if the measured blood carbon dioxide is low.

Most of the blood carbon dioxide is carried in the form of bicarbonate (HCO_3^-); the remainder is present in the form of carbonic acid (H_2CO_3) and as carbon dioxide gas (CO_2) dissolved in physical solution. The interrelationship between these three forms of carbon dioxide is expressed by the carbonic acid equilibration equation:

$$CO_2 + H_2O \rightleftharpoons H_2CO_3 \rightleftharpoons H^+ + HCO_3$$

An increase in any one of the components of the equation causes a proportionate increase in all of the others.

The normal Pa_{CO_2} in awake mammals is usually considered to range between 35 and 45 mm Hg. Hypoventilation causes an increase in Pa_{CO_2} (>45 mm Hg = hypercapnia), which increases the normal hydrogen ion/bicarbonate ion concentration ratio, resulting in an acidosis of respiratory origin. Hyperventilation causes a decrease in the Pa_{CO_2} (< 35 mm Hg = hypocapnia) and causes respiratory alkalosis.

BLOOD OXYGEN AND THE OXYGENATING EFFICIENCY OF THE LUNGS

Blood perfusing the alveolar capillary beds gathers oxygen from the alveoli (a process called arterialization) while simultaneously eliminating carbon dioxide. Diffusion of oxygen also occurs in response to a partial pressure gradient from the alveoli to the capillary blood. The partial pressure of oxygen in arterial blood (Pa_{O_2}) is an important index with regard to the functional efficiency of the lungs. The normal Pa_{O_2} is considered to range between 90 and 100 mm Hg.

There are two major reasons for the Pa_{O_2} to be lower than normal when a patient is breathing sea-level atmospheric air. The first is hypoventilation. In this case, atmospheric oxygen is simply not delivered to the alveoli in sufficient quantities to keep up with oxygen utilization by the tissues. The presence of hypercapnia substantiates the diagnosis of hypoventilation. The concomitant hypoxemia represents its major hazard.

The second cause of hypoxemia relates to the manner in which venous blood travels through the lungs. There are three ways for venous blood to get to the left ventricle without being properly oxygenated. (1) Blood may pass through anatomic venous-arterial shunts and never even get close to functioning alveoli (thebesian veins, congenital shunts, subpleural capillaries, or bronchial anatomoses). (2) Blood may pass through alveolar beds that are collapsed and nonfunctional (atelectasis, pulmonary edema, pneumonia, aspiration, or contusions). (3) Blood may pass through alveolar beds in which the alveoli are hypofunctional (hypoventilation) in proportion to the relative volume of blood flow. This ventilation-perfusion mismatching occurs to some extent in the ventral regions of normal lungs but is exaggerated by shallow breathing patterns and diseases that narrow bronchiolar lumen diameter and increase the resistance to air flow (pneumonia, bronchitis, or bronchospasm). Blood may pass through beds in which the respiratory membrane is thickened and oxygen diffusion is impaired (oxygen toxicity, interstitial edema, or neoplasia). Much of the diffusion of gases across the alveolar-capillary respiratory membrane occurs in regions where the basement membrane of the alveolar epithelium and of the capillary endothelium is fused (i.e., there is no space for the accumulation of interstitial fluids and cells). Therefore, the extent to which impaired diffusion interferes with proper oxygenation of the blood in atelectasis, pulmonary edema, pneumonia, aspiration, or contusions is probably minimal.

Venous admixture is the collective term for all of the previously mentioned mechanisms in which venous blood passes through the lungs without being properly oxygenated. This blood subsequently admixes with arterialized blood from normally functioning alveolar-capillary units and dilutes and decreases the P_{O_2} and oxygen content (hypoxemia). In contrast to patients exhibiting pure hypoventilation, patients with venous admixture often hyperventilate and exhibit normo- or hypocapnia along with the hypoxemia. In this situation, those areas of the lung that are functioning normally are able to compensate for the venous admixture in terms of carbon dioxide elimination but not the hypoxemia. The CO_2 dissociation curve is relatively straight, and the patient need only increase the alveolar minute ventilation in normal alveolar-capillary units to achieve a proportionate decrease in CO_2 content. Hyperventilation does not, however, proportionately increase the oxygen content of blood from normal alveolar-capillary units because of the horizontal position of the oxygen-hemoglobin dissociation relationship at P_{O_2} values greater than 90 mm Hg, and consequently the hypoxemia persists. Table 1, examples 2 and 3, summarize how consideration of the measured values for both Pa_{CO_2} and Pa_{O_2} shed light on the underlying pulmonary disturbance. It is, of course, entirely possible for hypoventilation and venous admixture to occur simultaneously in the same patient.

IDEAL ALVEOLAR P_{O_2} AND ALVEOLAR-ARTERIAL P_{O_2} GRADIENT

The normal Pa_{O_2} is 90 to 100 mm Hg when the Pa_{CO_2} is 35 to 45 mm Hg. Since variations in alveolar ventilation affect both alveolar and arterial P_{O_2} in the normal lung, it may be difficult to assess the oxygenating efficiency of the lungs by the Pa_{O_2} measurement alone when the patient is hyper- or hypoventilating. In this regard it would be helpful to be able to estimate the Pa_{O_2} value that would normally be associated with any given Pa_{CO_2}. First calculate the ideal alveolar P_{O_2} (PA_{O_2}) by this simplified version of the alveolar air equation:

$$PA_{O_2} = PI_{O_2} - Pa_{CO_2} (1.1)$$

where PI_{O_2} is inspired P_{O_2} and 1.1 is an average value for 1/respiratory quotient. PI_{O_2} is calculated by subtracting the saturated water vapor pressure (50 mm Hg at 38°C) from the barometric pressure and then multiplying this figure by 20.95%. PI_{O_2} is about 150 mm Hg at a barometric pressure of 765 mm Hg, and PA_{O_2} is therefore about 104 mm Hg at a Pa_{CO_2} of 40 mm Hg. Next, determine the difference between the calculated PA_{O_2} and the measured Pa_{O_2} (A-a D_{O_2}). The normal A-a D_{O_2} is about 10 mm Hg; a value greater than 15 mm Hg is indicative of a decreased oxygenating efficiency of the lungs (venous admixture). The following values for PA_{O_2}

and Pa_{O_2} can be calculated for specific Pa_{CO_2} values using the alveolar air equation:

Pa_{CO_2}	PA_{O_2}	Pa_{O_2}
40	106	96
20	128	118
65	79	69

The Pa_{O_2} values in Table 1, examples 2 and 4, reflect the normal variation expected during hypo- and hyperventilation, respectively. Examples 3 and 5 reflect hypoxemia due to venous admixture; the measured Pa_{O_2} is lower than the calculated Pa_{O_2} and the A-a D_{O_2} is higher than normal in both instances. The hypoxemia in example 6 is due to both hypoventilation and venous admixture. For practice, work through examples 6 to 8 and verify the interpretive comment.

Patients breathing an enriched oxygen mixture should be hyperoxemic. The PA_{O_2} may be approximated by using the alveolar air equation where PI_{O_2} = (barometric pressure − 50) × per cent oxygen inspired. If the inspired oxygen exceeds 90 per cent, the factor 1.1 may be ignored (Nunn, 1977). The A-a D_{O_2} is increased when a patient breathes an enriched oxygen mixture and is about 100 mm Hg with 100 per cent oxygen. An A-a D_{O_2} of greater than about 150 mm Hg is indicative of an increased venous admixture. The normal Pa_{O_2} during 100 per cent oxygen breathing should be about 575 mm Hg at a Pa_{CO_2} of 40 mm Hg at sea level; it should be about 260 mm Hg during 50 per cent oxygen breathing.

A more rapid, although less accurate, estimation of the expected Pa_{O_2} at any particular inspired oxygen concentration can be derived by multiplying the inspired per cent by 5; thus a Pa_{O_2} of 100 mm Hg would be expected when breathing 20 per cent oxygen, 250 mm Hg at 50 per cent, and 500 mm Hg at 100 per cent (Shapiro et al., 1977).

IMPORTANCE AND LIMITS OF PA_{CO_2} AND Pa_{O_2} ABNORMALITIES

Pa_{CO_2} measurements are an index of alveolar minute ventilation and have importance with regard to the effect that alterations in carbon dioxide concentrations have on pH. Pa_{CO_2} values of 22 and 70 mm Hg would be associated with a pH of 7.6 and 7.2, respectively, assuming no metabolic complications. Hypocapnia decreases cerebral blood flow and may impair adequate cerebral oxygenation at Pa_{CO_2} values of less than 20 mm Hg. Pa_{CO_2} levels of 60 to 70 mm Hg may be associated with severe hypoxemia when breathing room air (see Table 1), and values of 100 to 150 mm Hg may be associated with respiratory depression and narcosis. Pa_{CO_2} values above 60 mm Hg and below 20 mm Hg are

Table 1. *Meaningful Combinations of* Pa_{CO_2} *and* Pa_{O_2} *During Pulmonary Disease and Therapy*

Example	Inspired Oxygen Concentration (%)	Pa_{CO_2} (mm Hg)	Pa_{O_2} (mm Hg)	Interpretive Comment
1	20	38	96	Within normal range.
2	20	65	65	Hypoventilation; hypoxemia secondary to hypoventilation.
3	20	20	50	Hyperventilation; hypoxemia due to venous admixture
4	20	20	117	Hyperventilation; hyperoxemia secondary to hyperventilation.
5	20	38	55	Normoventilation; hypoxemia due to venous admixture.
6	20	65	40	Hypoventilation; hypoxemia due to hypoventilation and venous admixture.
7	100	30	250	Hyperventilation; hyperoxemia due to inhalation of 100 per cent oxygen but is not as high as expected; therefore some venous admixture persists.
8	40	30	100	Hyperventilation; normoxemia but lower than expected for inhaled oxygen concentration of 40 per cent, so some venous admixture persists. It is not necessary to further increase the inspired oxygen concentration since normoxia is the desired endpoint.

considered to represent an important imposition on patient homeostasis requiring early effective treatment of the underlying disease process and definitive supportive therapy, such as ventilatory support in the case of hypercapnia. Increasing the mechanical dead space or the inspired carbon dioxide concentration in the case of hypocapnia is seldom, if ever, indicated, since treatment of the underlying disorder is usually rapidly effective.

Unconsciousness occurs when the Pa_{O_2} decreases to about 36 mm Hg, in the absence of other cardiovascular abnormalities (Nunn, 1977). Although many compensatory mechanisms and hypothermia protect the brain from hypoxia, there are numerous cardiovascular and metabolic abnormalities that lower the threshold for hypoxemia-induced brain damage. Specific minimum values for P_{O_2} are therefore variable and difficult to predict. Hypoxemia becomes an important respiratory stimulant at Pa_{O_2} values below 60 mm Hg. Hemoglobin saturation and whole blood oxygen content are reasonably well maintained down to Pa_{O_2} values of 60 mm Hg (Table 2), and this is a commonly selected minimum value during respiratory therapy. It is assumed that values below 60 mm Hg represent a significant stress to the patient, and support procedures, such as enriching the inspired oxygen concentration and/or ventilation therapy, should be considered to maintain the Pa_{O_2} above 60 mm Hg.

Hyperoxia is not necessary, since it has minimal beneficial effects in terms of increasing the whole blood oxygen content and may cause pulmonary damage if exposure to 80 to 100 per cent oxygen is prolonged (for longer than 24 hours) (Morgan, 1968). Every attempt should be made to maintain the inspired oxygen concentration below 50 to 60 per cent (and the Pa_{O_2} above 60 mm Hg) when extended oxygen therapy is necessary.

P_{O_2} is only one of three measurements that can be made on blood oxygen. The extent to which the oxygen saturates the hemoglobin (per cent HbO_2) is another. The relationship between P_{O_2} and per cent HbO_2 is expressed by a sigmoid curve, and either value could be estimated from the other using published tables or charts with appropriate attention to temperature, pH, and P_{CO_2}-induced changes in the slope of the curve (Rossing and Cain, 1966). Slope changes secondary to alterations in intrared blood cell concentrations of 2,3 DPG and ATP are generally unknown and may detract from the accuracy of published P_{O_2}/per cent HbO_2 dissociation curves in some patients.

Oxygen content (Co) (ml O_2/100 ml whole blood)

Table 2. *Correlation Between* P_{O_2}, *Per Cent Hemoglobin Saturation* (S_{O_2}), *and Whole Blood Oxygen Content* (Co)*

P_{O_2} (mm Hg)	S_{O_2} (%)†	Co (ml/dl)‡
700	99.9	22.2
500	99.8	21.6
300	99.6	20.9
200	99.3	20.6
100	96.8	19.8
90	95.8	19.5
80	94.1	19.2
70	92.0	18.7
60	88.2	17.9
50	82.0	16.6
40	72.0	14.6
30	53.5	10.8
20	28.0	5.7

*At pH of 7.4, P_{CO_2} 40 mm Hg, temperature 37°C, and base excess/deficit 0 mEq/L.

†Per cent hemoglobin saturation with oxygen (Rossing and Cain, 1966; Kelman and Nunn, 1966).

‡Oxygen content per 100 ml whole blood calculated assuming: (1) that 1 gm of fully oxygenated hemoglobin binds 1.34 ml oxygen; (2) that oxygen in physical solution equals 0.003 ml/dl/ mm Hg; (3) a hemoglobin concentration of 15 gm/dl; and (4) the absence of carboxyhemoglobin.

is the third measurement of blood oxygen and is the most important of the three in terms of total oxygen available for delivery to the tissues. Oxygen content is difficult to measure and is commonly derived from simple* or complex (Kelman and Nunn, 1968) formulations based on human hemoglobin. There are some important aspects of the P_{O_2}/C_O interrelationship that should be noted (see Table 2). An increase in the P_{O_2} from 100 to 700 mm Hg does not result in a sevenfold increase in C_O. Changes in P_{O_2} cause larger changes in C_O in the lower P_{O_2} ranges. Assuming an oxygen consumption of 5 ml/dl, the venous P_{O_2} would be slightly above 40 mm Hg when the patient is breathing room air (Pa_{O_2} 100 mm Hg) but would only be 50 mm Hg when the patient breathes an enriched oxygen mixture (Pa_{O_2} 500 mm Hg). A P_{O_2} of 100 mm Hg is associated with an oxygen content of about 19.8 ml/dl when the hemoglobin is 15 gm/dl but only about 9.9 ml/dl when the hemoglobin is 7.5 gm/dl. A Pa_{O_2} measurement without reference to hemoglobin concentration may be misleading in terms of the amount of oxygen available for distribution to the tissues (even though lung oxygenating efficiency is satisfactory).

Oxygen content is, in turn, only one of the ingredients of oxygen delivery to tissues. Cardiac output, blood pressure, local tissue blood flow, and the extent of oxygen extraction are all important factors in this regard. It would be inappropriate to state that a patient is well oxygenated because of an existing normal Pa_{O_2} without reference to other cardiovascular parameters such as cardiac output, blood pressure, and amount of peripheral vasoconstriction. Calculated values of oxygen content ignore the potential for the accumulation of myoglobin, methemoglobin, and carboxyhemoglobin, the existence of which may detract from the accuracy of the calculated values in some patients.

Of the three parameters of blood oxygen, P_{O_2} is often easiest to measure; it relates directly to overall lung function and indirectly to blood oxygen content.

One method for evaluating the net efficiency of all of the factors that are involved in oxygen delivery to the tissues is to measure the P_{O_2} of a mixed venous (pulmonary artery or right ventricle) blood sample. The normal mixed venous P_{O_2} is 50 ± 5 mm Hg and will decrease secondary to diminished oxygen delivery to the tissues from any cause. The mixed venous P_{O_2} should be maintained above 30 mm Hg.

CAUSES AND TREATMENT OF HYPERCAPNIA AND HYPOXEMIA

There are many causes of inadequate alveolar ventilation, hypercapnia, and hypoxemia (Table 3).

All abnormalities must receive treatment appropriate to the specific underlying disease. Symptomatic treatment must provide, when necessary, for (1) an open airway, (2) adequate spontaneous or artificial ventilation, and/or (3) an enriched oxygen concentration in the inspired air.

Venous admixture during pulmonary parenchymal disease primarily involves ventilation-perfusion mismatching and physiologic shunting due to alveolar dysfunction. If the hypoxemia is predominantly due to ventilation-perfusion mismatching, enriching the inhaled oxygen mixture should be very beneficial in improving the alveolar oxygen concentration in the poorly ventilated alveoli. In most cases of alveolar dysfunction, fluids accumulate around the edges of the alveolus until the surface tension increases to some critical point, at which time the alveolus collapses. Since alveoli collapse rather than fill up, they can be re-inflated by positive pressure, restoring the functional status of the alveolar-capillary unit; this is the ideal treatment when alveolar dysfunction is the primary cause of the hypoxemia.

Venous admixture and alveolar dysfunction probably coexist in most cases of pulmonary parenchymal disease, and unfortunately, when a dyspneic patient is presented, it is difficult or impossible to differentiate the extent to which each of these two mechanisms is involved in the generation of the hypoxemia. Since it is considerably easier technically to enrich the inhaled oxygen mixture and since this does in fact compensate for hypoxemia due to mild degrees of alveolar dysfunction, it is convenient to start treatment with oxygen therapy. If provision of up to 100 per cent oxygen fails to provide symptomatic relief, positive pressure ventilation should be instituted.

Various techniques for oxygen therapy and methods of application of positive pressure ventilation are detailed elsewhere (Haskins, 1981; McKiernan, 1983). The effectiveness of therapy should be continuously monitored by observation of the progression of the physical signs of the patient, auscultation, radiography, and, when possible, arterial blood gas measurement. Pa_{CO_2} defines the ventilatory status of the patient and should be used to guide the ventilation therapy. Pa_{O_2} defines the oxygenating capabilities of the lung and should be used to guide the per cent inhaled oxygen concentration and the level of the end-expired airway pressure when this technique is used. The combination of all techniques should be sufficient to restore the Pa_{O_2} to at least 60 mm Hg. Example 3 (Table 1), for instance, requires oxygen therapy but not ventilation therapy.† Example 6 needs ventilation therapy as a first priority; the need for oxygen therapy should await the results of the ventilation therapy. If ventilation therapy converts example 6 to example 5, oxygen

---

*C_O (ml O_2/dl whole blood) = [Hb (gm/dl) × 1.34 (ml O_2/gm Hb) × % HbO_2] + [0.003 (ml/dl) × P_{O_2} (mm Hg)]

†Ventilation therapy is used here to imply correction of the underlying process that is impairing effective ventilation and/or positive pressure ventilation.

Table 3. *Causes of Inadequate Ventilation, Hypercapnia, or Hypoxemia*

Cause	Treatment
I. *Neuromuscular complication (bradypnea/apnea)* Temporary absence of chemical stimuli (hypocapnia) associated with hyperventilation or anesthetic induction agent. Inactivity of the central control unit due to organic lesions, cerebral edema, anesthetic depression, severe metabolic disturbances, hypothermia (mid 80s°F; 29 to 30°C), trauma, and hemorrhage. Interference with motor efferents: (a) spinal cord edema due to trauma of surgery, vertebral fractures, or disc prolapse; (b) neuromuscular blocking agents. **II. *Loss of integrity of the bellows*** Open pneumothorax, flail chest	Hypoventilate 1/30 sec until spontaneous ventilation begins. Weaning procedure should be limited to 10 to 15 minutes. Treat the primary disorder. Support ventilation.
III. *Upper airway obstruction* Laryngeal edema, foreign body Collapsing cervical trachea, laryngeal collapse Recurrent laryngeal nerve injury Brachycephalic syndrome Occluded endotracheal tube (endobronchial or esophageal intubation; dried lubricant occluding the lumen; occlusion of the end of the tube by the wall of the trachea at the carina; evagination of the inflated cuff over the end of the tube; accumulation of mucus, blood, and debris in the lumen; collapse of the tube by excessive cuff inflation or by tying the gauze roll too tightly; kinking of the tube; excessively small hole in the tracheal tube adaptor).	Remove or bypass obstruction.
IV. *Pleural filling defect* Hydrothorax, chylothorax, hemothorax Pneumothorax Diaphragmatic hernia **V. *Parenchymal disease*** Atelectasis, hypostatic congestion Pulmonary edema Pneumonia, aspiration, inhalation injury Neoplasia Trauma and hemorrhage Embolic phenomena Secondary to shock, intravascular coagulation, pancreatitis, uremia.	No treatment in absence of dyspnea. Thoracentesis. If fluid returns rapidly consider insertion of a chest drain. Avoid IPPV until after chest drain placement. Surgical repair; caution during anesthetic induction. Symptomatic treatment depends on the underlying disease mechanism, e.g., oxygen for V/Q mismatching, impaired diffusion, and small shunts, or IPPV for physiologic shunting due to atelectasis from any cause.
VI. *Apparatus-related problems* Excessive circuit resistance Exhausted soda lime or "channeling" of gas flow through the path of least resistance. Excessive dead space (e.g., improperly functioning unidirectional valves, insufficient flows with the nonrebreathing system or face masks, small patient/large machine).	
VII. *Apparent or associated problems to consider* Hypermetabolic states such as hyperthermia or hyperthyroidism cause hyperventilation. A false hypercapnia may result if blood sample is taken immediately following a large dose of bicarbonate, especially with a marginal ventilatory capacity. Failure to correct the measured value for hypothermia will cause an apparent increase in P_{CO_2}; for hyperthermia it will cause an apparent decrease in P_{O_2}. Drug-induced methoglobinemia causes cyanosis and a decrease in blood oxygen content without a decrease in Pa_{O_2}.	

Table 4.   Causes of Hypocapnia

Centrally mediated—hypoxemia, metabolic acidosis, anemia, hypotension, excitement, pain, exercise, CNS disease
Hypermetabolic states (hyperthermia, thyrotoxicosis, sepsis)
Intoxicants: salicylates
Cirrhosis

therapy is indicated in addition to ventilation. Causes of hypocapnia are listed in Table 4.

THE METABOLIC COMPONENT OF THE ACID-BASE BALANCE

The metabolic component of the acid-base equilibrium represents all of the noncarbonic acids. There are several methods of quantifying the metabolic contribution to the acid-base imbalance; base deficit/excess and bicarbonate concentration $[HCO_3^-]$ are the most common. Base deficit/excess is defined as the titratable acidity/alkalinity of a blood sample at 37°C, at complete hemoglobin saturation and a P_{CO_2} of 40 mm Hg, when titrated to a pH of 7.40 (Siggaard-Andersen, 1963). It can be estimated from the Siggaard-Andersen alignment nomogram (Fig. 1) and should be used when pH and P_{CO_2} measurements are available, since it is the more accurate of the two methods for quantifying the metabolic component. The normal base deficit/excess is 0 ± mEq/L. A base deficit greater than −4 mEq/L represents a metabolic acidosis; a base excess greater than +4 mEq/L represents a metabolic alkalosis.

Two economical instruments that estimate $[HCO_3^-]$ may be used when pH and P_{CO_2} measure-

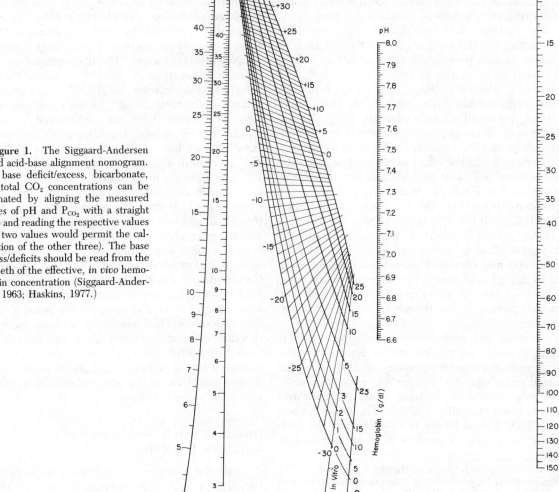

Figure 1. The Siggaard-Andersen blood acid-base alignment nomogram. The base deficit/excess, bicarbonate, and total CO_2 concentrations can be estimated by aligning the measured values of pH and P_{CO_2} with a straight edge and reading the respective values (any two values would permit the calculation of the other three). The base excess/deficits should be read from the isopleth of the effective, *in vivo* hemoglobin concentration (Siggaard-Andersen, 1963; Haskins, 1977.)

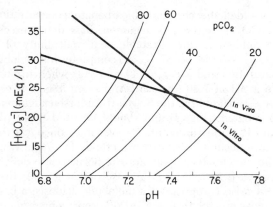

Figure 2. *In vivo* and *in vitro* carbon dioxide titration curves (slope of 30 and 12 slykes, respectively, and [Hb] = 15 gm/dl). The following P_{CO_2}/HCO_3^- relationship is taken from the *in vivo* curve:

P_{CO_2} (mm Hg)	20	40	60	80
$[HCO_3^-]$ (mEq/L)	21	24	25	26

ments are not available.*† The normal $[HCO_3^-]$ is 24 ± 3 mEq/L. A measured value below 21 mEq/ L is indicative of metabolic acidosis; a value above 27 mEq/L is indicative of metabolic alkalosis.

The carbonic acid equilibration equation illustrates that the $[HCO_3^-]$ is affected by variations in carbon dioxide (respiratory component) as well as by fluctuations in the metabolic component. The $[HCO_3^-]$, therefore, does not solely represent changes in the metabolic component. The normal $[HCO_3^-]$ is 24 mEq/L only when the P_{CO_2} is 40 mm Hg (Fig. 2). If the bicarbonate deficit is determined by subtracting the measured value from 24 without any reference to the effect of changes in P_{CO_2}, the usual error will be 0 to 3 mEq/L but may be as much as 5 to 6 mEq/L. If the P_{CO_2} is known, the baseline $[HCO_3^-]$ should be adjusted as indicated (see Fig. 2). If the P_{CO_2} is not known, the baseline $[HCO_3^-]$ could be adjusted upward if the patient is hypoventilating or downward during hyperventilation. You may choose to maintain a baseline value of 24 mEq/L and accept the aforementioned inaccuracies, since they are relatively minor in the overall picture of the disease/treatment interrelationship.

Accurate pH measurements utilizing commercially available pH probes and meters are not possible without proper temperature control and closed blood chambers. An inexpensive, easy-to-operate, accurate method of obtaining blood pH measurements is not currently available. The measurement of $[HCO_3^-]$ alone allows an estimation of the metabolic component. The effect of the measured met-

abolic change on pH and the interrelationship with P_{CO_2} would then need to be estimated by clinical reckoning.

UNMEASURED ANIONS AND THE ANION GAP

Many forms of endogenous and exogenous metabolic acidosis are associated with the accumulation of the anion of the added acid. Depending on the efficiency of the compensating mechanisms, the pH and even the base deficit value may be normal despite an existing acidosis. Indirect evidence of the presence of the acidosis can be determined by calculating the anion gap as follows:

$$\text{Anion gap} = [Na^+] - ([Cl^-] + [HCO_3^-])$$

The normal anion gap is about 10 mEq/L. A value greater than 15 mEq/L is assumed to represent an excess accumulation of unmeasured anions. The specific source of the metabolic acidosis must be determined from other laboratory measurements.

Since the concept of anion gap is important and has been confusing, this further explanation of its generation is offered. In shock, for example, there is an increased production of lactic acid (hydrogen cation and lactate anion). The hydrogen cation combines with bicarbonate (as well as other buffers), resulting in a decrease in $[HCO_3^-]$ and an accumulation of sodium lactate. In the anion gap equation $[Na^+]$ and $[Cl^-]$ are unchanged, whereas $[HCO_3^-]$ is decreased, resulting in an increase in the difference between $[Na^+]$ and $[Cl^- + HCO_3^-]$. The increased difference is made up by lactate, which is normally unmeasured.

The anion gap should be calculated whenever the necessary electrolyte concentrations have been measured, since it may signal the existence of an acidotic process even when there is no base deficit. It may be also help define the major source of the acidosis and/or serve as a guide to the severity of the disease process and the effectiveness of therapy. High anion gaps are invariably attributed to the accumulation of an acid in which the anion is other than chloride. When metabolic acidosis occurs in the absence of an increased anion gap, the cause is most likely attributable to disease associated with excessive loss of sodium bicarbonate, impaired hydrogen excretion, or the accumulation of an acid in which the anion is chloride (Table 5).

IMPORTANCE OF ABNORMALITIES IN THE METABOLIC COMPONENT

Metabolic acidosis or alkalosis is important for two reasons: first, as an index of the severity of the underlying disease process; and second, as a disease process in its own right when it is severe enough to cause the pH to fall below 7.2 or rise above 7.6

---

*Harleco Total CO_2 Apparatus, Harleco, Gibbstown, NJ. This apparatus actually measures total carbon dioxide, most of which is carried as bicarbonate. The total CO_2 measurement may be used as it stands as an estimate of the bicarbonate concentration or may be reduced by 1 mEq/L.

†Oxford Titrator, Oxford Lab, Foster City, CA.

Table 5.   *Causes of Metabolic Acidosis*

Increased Anion Gap
A. Endogenous addition of H^+
    Lactic and pyruvic acids
        Inadequate tissue oxygenation
    Ketoacids (hydroxybutyric, acetoacetic, acetic)
        Insulin deficiency, starvation
B. Impaired renal excretion of H^+
    Phosphoric and sulfuric acids
C. Exogenous addition of H^+
    Salicylate
    Ethylene glycol
    Methanol
    Paraldehyde
    Citrate anticoagulated blood
Normal Anion Gap
A. HCO_3^- loss
    Gastrointestinal
        Diarrhea, vomition
    Renal
        Proximal tubular acidosis
        Secondary to prolonged respiratory alkalosis
B. Impaired renal excretion of H^+
    Carbonic anhydrase inhibitors
    Distal tubular acidosis
    Hypoaldosteronism
    Impaired ammonia production
C. Exogenous addition of H^+
    Ammonium chloride
    Hyperchloremic intravenous solutions
    Cationic amino acid solutions

despite compensatory mechanisms. If the primary disease process can be readily treated, the pH is above 7.2, and the base deficit is not more negative than about −10 mEq/L, then serious consideration should be given to treatment of only the underlying disease process, allowing metabolic and excretory processes to correct the acidosis. If, on the other hand, the disease process is likely to be difficult to control, the pH is below 7.2, and the base deficit is more negative than about −10 mEq/L, then alkalinization therapy is indicated in addition to therapy directed at the underlying disease.

CAUSES AND TREATMENT OF METABOLIC ABNORMALITIES

The causes of metabolic acidosis can generally be grouped into those associated with an increased anion gap and those associated with a normal anion gap (see Table 5).

Effective therapy of the underlying disease process is the basis of successful treatment of metabolic acidosis. In metabolic acidosis associated with an increased anion gap, the aberrant anion and, in many cases, its associated hydrogen ion will be metabolized and/or excreted once the disease process has been controlled. If the pH is neutral prior to the metabolism of the lactate, ketoacids, or citrate, an alkalemia may develop. Alkalinizing ther-

apy should be conservative in these patients. Since an inadequate circulating volume is a common denominator in the origin or persistence of acidosis in many diseases, fluid administration (crystalloids containing lactate, acetate, or gluconate) should be considered.

Alkalinizing therapy (Table 6) should be considered only when the acidosis causes a severe disturbance in H^+ concentration as outlined previously or when effective therapy of the underlying disorder is not possible. Metabolism of the lactate, acetate, or gluconate anions in many replacement solutions has an alkalinizing tendency, but it is quantitatively insufficient in the treatment of serious degrees of acidosis.

Dosage of alkalinizing agent is ideally derived from actual measurements of the acid-base balance of the patient. When this is not possible, the magnitude of the acidosis is assumed to coincide with the extent of the involvement of the acidotic disease process, which is determined by other laboratory findings and the clinical signs of the patient. If the disease is advanced and the status of the patient is poor, then perhaps some alkali is indicated. Sodium bicarbonate (1 to 4 mEq/kg) is the most commonly used alkalinizing agent.

Very rapid alterations in pH with bolus dosages of alkalinizing drugs must be avoided. Severe hypotension, vomition, and cardiac arrest have been observed. The calculated dosage should be conservative and should be administered slowly, e.g., over 30 minutes or more. When possible, the progress of the disease and the alkali therapy should be monitored with serial measurements of acid-base status. Sufficient volumes of alkali should be administered to elevate the pH above 7.2 or to make the base deficit more positive than −10 mEq/L. Without knowledge of the acid-base status, the end point of alkali titration is rather nebulous, since the signs of acidosis (altered mentation and an unstable cardiovasculature) are nonspecific and most likely would be attributed to the primary disease process.

Metabolic alkalosis may be due to either excessive hydrogen loss or bicarbonate retention (Table 7). Effective therapy for metabolic alkalosis is usually limited to control of the causative process, with special reference to the nature of the administered fluids and to abnormalities in plasma chloride and potassium concentrations. Some advantage may be taken of the tendency for saline to cause a dilutional (of bicarbonate) acidosis when planning fluid therapy. Ammonium chloride and dilute solutions of hydrogen chloride (same dosage formula as for sodium bicarbonate) may be used, although they are seldom, if ever, necessary, since most alkaloses respond dramatically to control of the underlying process. Ammonium chloride should be avoided in renal and hepatic disease.

Table 6. *Alkalinizing Agents**

Generic Name (Trade Name)	Dosage	Mechanism of Alkalinization	Major Complications†
Sodium bicarbonate (MW = 84.0) 1.26% sol is isotonic 1.4% sol = 1.67 mEq HCO_3/L 7.5% sol = 0.89 mEq/ml 8.4% sol = 1 mEq/ml	mEq bicarbonate to administer = (1) base deficit‡ × 0.3 × kg bw (2) 1 to 4 mEq/kg	Bicarbonate combines with hydrogen ion and shifts the carbonic acid equilibration to the left	1. Hypercapnia in the face of marginal ventilation 2. CSF acidosis 3. Hyperosmolality (intracellular dehydration and intracranial hemorrhage)
Sodium lactate (MW = 112.1) 1.68% sol is isotonic 1.85% sol = 165 mEq/L	Same as for bicarbonate	Metabolized in liver to pyruvate, consuming a hydrogen ion in the process (requires an oxygenated, perfused liver and time)	Avoid in states of liver disease or dysfunction
Sodium acetate (MW = 82.0) 1.23% sol is osotonic	Same as for bicarbonate	Metabolized in liver and muscle and consumes a hydrogen ion in the process	1. Vasodilation and hypotension 2. Ketogenic
Trihydroxymethylaminomethane (THAM, TRIS, Tromethamine, Trometamol) (MW = 121.1) 3.6% sol is isotonic 3.6% sol = 300 mEq THAM/L	mEq THAM to administer = (1) base deficit × 0.4 (due to larger volume of distribution) × kg bw (2) 2 to 6 mEq/kg	Combines with hydrogen ion to form cationic buffer and shifts the carbonic acid equilibration to the right	1. Hypocapnia and apnea 2. Very irritating (avoid perivascular extravasation; administer in large veins in dilute solutions) 3. Osmotic diuresis

*All agents are available from one or several of the following manufacturers: Abbott, Bristol, Cutter, International Medication Systems, Ivnenex, Tera, McGaw, or Travenol.

†Alkalosis is an implied but not stated major complication of any alkali therapy, as is an increased hemoglobin affinity for oxygen and its tendency to reduce plasma potassium concentration.

‡Use bicarbonate deficit if base deficit is not available.

Table 7.   Causes of Metabolic Alkalosis

Hydrogen Loss
    Gastric
    Renal
        Mineralocorticoid excess
        Compensation for hypercapnia
        Hypokalemia
        Hypochloremia
        Diuretic therapy
        Hypoparathyroidism
    Movement of H^+ into cells
        Hypokalemia
Bicarbonate Retention
    $NaHCO_3$ administration
    Volume depletion
    Metabolism of organic anions (lactate, acetate,
        citrate, ketoacid anions)
    Secondary to prolonged respiratory acidosis
Contraction Alkalosis (HCO_3^- free fluid losses, e.g., diuresis)

INTERPRETATION OF MIXED DISTURBANCES

When evaluating a set of acid-base measurements, it is easiest to first consider the meaning of each of the values separately, without reference to one another or the patient. Interpret the following sets of values.

	Patient A	Patient B
pH	7.16	6.90
Pa_{CO_2} (mm Hg)	20	80
Base deficit (mEq/L)	−20	−15
Bicarbonate (mEq/L)	7	14

Patient A: the pH measurement indicates that the net effect of all processes in the body affecting the acid-base balance has resulted in an acidemia but does not indicate the origin. The Pa_{CO_2} measurement, by definition, indicates the presence of a respiratory alkalosis. The base deficit and the bicarbonate concentration indicate the presence of a metabolic acidosis. Patient B: acidemia; respiratory acidosis; and metabolic acidosis.

The second step in the interpretation process is to integrate each of the values with the others in the set to determine which of the two components is primarily involved in the generation of the hydrogen ion imbalance.

Patient A	Patient B
Acidemia	Acidemia
Respiratory alkalosis	Respiratory acidosis
Metabolic acidosis	Metabolic acidosis

As a general rule, the component that varies in the same direction as the pH aberration is the component that is primarily involved in the disturbance; components that vary in the opposite direction are probably compensatory to the primary disease process. Compensatory mechanisms do not overcompensate. The acid-base values for patient A indicate a primary metabolic acidosis and a secondary compensatory respiratory alkalosis, whereas the values for patient B indicate that both components are primarily involved in the acidemic process (neither is compensating in any way for the other).

The third and most important step in the evaluation process is the correlation of the acid-base picture with the patient's history, current clinical status, and other laboratory results. Patient A may represent a patient with ketoacidosis, hypovolemic shock, heat stroke, or a patient B that has just received positive pressure ventilation. Patient B may represent a deeply anesthetized or traumatized patient with primary metabolic and respiratory disorders. Measurements of the status of acid-base balance serve as a guide to the severity of the primary disease process, not as a diagnosis of the specific disease. Deviations in pH, P_{CO_2}, and base deficit represent signs of the primary disease and do not, in themselves, exert detrimental effects on homeostasis until the extremes of the respective ranges have been reached. If the acid-base values are not compatible with the clinical picture of the patient, it is prudent to remeasure the values prior to reformulating your judgments relative to the nature of the disease process.

Assessment of the quantitative extent to which compensatory events occur may be helpful in evaluating a patient's response to the primary disorder (Table 8). If, after a suitable period of time (assuming a stable equilibrium in the primary disease), compensating mechanisms have not had the expected effects, it would be appropriate to consider the existence of an additional disorder in the compensatory component. Metabolic compensation for a primary respiratory disorder is generally more complete than vice versa and should be maximal in three to five days in the dog. Respiratory compensation for metabolic disorders should be maximal in 8 to 12 hours but is limited by hypoxemia in compensatory respiratory acidosis (hypoventilation) and by cerebral effects and the work of breathing in compensatory respiratory alkalosis.

For ease of explanation of the various concepts, I have assumed the ideal central tendencies for normal acid-base values to be 7.4 ± 0.05 units for pH; 40 ± 5 mm Hg for P_{CO_2}; 95 ± 5 mm Hg for P_{O_2}; 0 ± 4 mEq/L for base deficit; and 24 ± 3 mEq/L for bicarbonate concentration. Actual reported values are listed for the dog (Table 9) and the cat (Table 10).

BLOOD SAMPLE COLLECTION, STORAGE, AND MEASUREMENT

Arterial blood should be used for pH and blood gas analysis when both the acid-base status and pulmonary function are to be evaluated. The dorsal

Table 8. *Ranges of Expected Acid-Base Values Without and With Compensation in Primary Metabolic and Respiratory Abnormalities*

Base Deficit/Excess (mEq/L)	Without Compensation			With Compensation		
	[HCO$_3$] (mEq/L)	P_{CO_2} (mm Hg)	pH	[HCO$_3$] (mEq/L)	P_{CO_2} (mm Hg)	pH
Metabolic acidosis						
−10	15.5	40	7.22	14 to 15	27 to 36	7.26 to 7.35
−15	12.0	40	7.10	9.5 to 10.5	20 to 29	7.21 to 7.31
−20	8.5	40	6.97	6 to 7	13 to 23	7.13 to 7.28
−25	5.5	40	6.78	3 to 5	9 to 14	7.04 to 7.15
Metabolic alkalosis						
+10	33.0	40	7.53	33 to 34	39 to 51	7.44 to 7.54
+15	37.5	40	7.58	38 to 39	41 to 56	7.46 to 7.58
+20	42.5	40	7.63	43 to 45	43 to 63	7.47 to 7.61
+25	48.0	40	7.68	44 to 50	48 to 66	7.49 to 7.65

P_{CO_2} (mm Hg)	Without Compensation			With Compensation		
	[HCO$_3^-$] (mEq/L)	BD/BE (mEq/L)	pH	[HCO$_3^-$] (mEq/L)	BD/BE (mEq/L)	pH
Respiratory acidosis						
60	26.0	0	7.26	30 to 37	+5 to +12	7.32 to 7.41
80	27.0	0	7.16	35 to 44	+9 to +19	7.27 to 7.36
100	28.0	0	7.08	40 to 49	+13 to +23	7.22 to 7.31
Respiratory alkalosis						
30	23.0	0	7.50	18 to 21	−2.5 to −7	7.38 to 7.46
20	21.5	0	7.64	11.5 to 14.5	−8.5 to −13	7.38 to 7.48
15	20.5	0	7.74	8.5 to 11.0	−10.5 to −16	7.38 to 7.48

Table 9. Normal pH and Blood Gas Measurements in Unanesthetized Dogs*

Reference	pH_a (units)	Pa_{CO_2} (mm Hg)	Pa_{O_2} (mm Hg)	HCO_3^- (mEq/L)	Base Deficit (mEq/L)	No. of Subjects	Age (yrs)	Location of Experiment	Altitude (meters)
Pickrell et al. 1971	7.44 ± 0.03	36.0 ± 3.1	73.7 ± 6.5	24†	0†	39	1.1	Albuquerque, NM	1511
Mauderly and	7.38 ± 0.03	41.0 ± 3.0	75.0 ± 5.0	23†	−1†	60	1.1	Albuquerque, NM	1511
Pickrell 1972	7.37 ± 0.03	42.0 ± 6.0	70.0 ± 10.0	23†	−1†	20	7–10	Albuquerque, NM	1511
Mauderly 1974	7.40 ± 0.04	37.0 ± 3.0	77.0 ± 5.0	22†	−2†	20	3–4	Seattle, WA	38
Feigl and D'Alecy 1972	7.414 ± 0.032	36.7 ± 2.6	89.1 ± 4.9	22.5†	−1†	30	NR‡	Charleston, SC	3
Wise 1973	7.453 ± 0.023	35.9 ± 2.4	90.9 ± 5.7	24.5 ± 1.5	+1†	11	NR	St. Paul, MN	266
Haskins 1977	7.402 ± 0.008	34.4 ± 0.9	98.5 ± 1.8	20.5	−3	12	adult	San Francisco, CA	19
Rodkey et al. 1978	7.416 ± 0.008	33.9 ± 1.2	82.7 ± 3.0	21.2 ± 0.7	−1.9 ± 0.6	6	NR	Davis, CA	15
Haskins et al. 1981	7.412 ± 0.042	34.9 ± 2.5	104.7 ± 8.7	20.9 ± 1.5	−2.0 ± 1.9	6	adult	Sydney, Australia	11
Rose and Carter 1979	7.411 ± 0.011	31.9 ± 0.7	97.1 ± 1.0	21.5 ± 0.6	−3.1 ± 0.6	12	NR	Athens, GA	238
Cornelius and Rawlings 1981	7.45 ± 0.03	31.0 ± 3.6	90.7 ± 8.8	20.9 ± 2.3	−2.5	38	NR		
Average§	7.407 ± 0.028	36.8 ± 3.0	92.1 ± 5.6‖	22.2 ± 1.7	−1.5 ± 1.1				

*pH_a is arterial pH; Pa_{CO_2} and Pa_{O_2} are partial pressures of carbon dioxide and oxygen, respectively, of arterial blood. Values represent mean ± 1 standard deviation. All reported values were corrected to body temperature.

†Values were not reported and were calculated for this summary by the Siggaard-Andersen alignment nomogram (Haskins, 1977).

‡NR = not reported.

§Average values represent subject-number weighted mean and standard deviations of the reported values from each study, excluding the study by Pickrell et al. (1971), the subjects of which are assumed to have been included in the report by Mauderly and Pickrell (1972).

‖Does not include first three references.

Table 10. Normal pH and Blood Gas Measurements in Unanesthetized Cats*

Reference	pH_a (units)	Pa_{CO_2} (mm Hg)	Pa_{O_2} (mm Hg)	HCO_3^- (mEq/L)	Base Deficit (mEq/L)	No. of Subjects	Age	Location of Experiment	Altitude (meters)
Haskins 1982	7.416 ± 0.024	29.2 ± 2.6	112.7 ± 6.5	18.1 ± 1.6	−5.5 ± 1.9	7	Adult	Davis, CA	15
Fink and Schoolman 1963	7.380 ± 0.06	28.0 ± 4.1	NR†	16.0‡	−0.8‡	12	Adult (?)	New York, NY	9
Herbert and Mitchell 1971	7.426 ± 0.005	32.5 ± 0.6	107.6 ± 2.7	21.0 ± 0.4	−3.0‡	10	Adult (?)	San Francisco, CA	19
Middleton et al. 1981	7.344 ± 0.052	33.6 ± 3.6	102.9 ± 7.6	17.5 ± 3.0	−6.4 ± 5.0	13	Adult	Sydney, Australia	11
Average§	7.386 ± 0.038	31.0 ± 2.9	106.8 ± 5.7	18.0 ± 1.8	−5.9 ± 3.9				

*pH_a is arterial pH; Pa_{CO_2} and Pa_{O_2} are partial pressures of carbon dioxide and oxygen, respectively, of arterial blood. Values represent mean ± 1 standard deviation. All reported values were corrected to body temperature.

†NR = not reported.

‡Values were not reported and were calculated for this summary by the Siggaard-Andersen alignment nomogram (Haskins, 1977).

§Average values represent subject-number weighted mean and standard deviations of the reported values from each study.

Table 11. ·*Correction Values for pH, P_{CO_2}, and P_{O_2} for Changes Due to in Vitro Metabolism During Storage*

Storage at Room Temperature (min)*	pH (add to measured value)	P_{CO_2} (mm Hg) (subtract from measured value)	P_{O_2} (mm Hg)† (add to measured value)
10	0.006	0.6	4
20	0.010	1.2	7
30	0.014	1.7	10

Storage in Ice Water (hr)‡	pH (add to measured value)	P_{CO_2} (mm Hg) (subtract from measured value)	P_{O_2} (mm Hg)† (subtract from measured value§)
1	.004	0	2.1
2	.009	0.4	2.6
3	.013	0.9	3.1
4	.017	1.4	3.7
5	.022	1.9	4.2
6	.026	2.4	4.7

*Human blood.

†P_{O_2} correction values apply only to the P_{O_2} range of 80 to 100 mm Hg. P_{O_2} values above 100 mm Hg or below 80 mm Hg will change more or less, respectively, than indicated in this table.

‡Dog blood (Haskins, 1977).

§The P_{O_2} increases during ice water storage, presumably because oxygen diffuses from the plastic syringe into the blood sample faster than it is metabolized by the white blood cells.

metatarsal and femoral arteries are readily accessible in the awake, minimally restrained dog; in addition, the radial, brachial, and lingual arteries are available in the anesthetized or cerebrally depressed patient. Restraint-induced patient excitement during the sampling process must be avoided

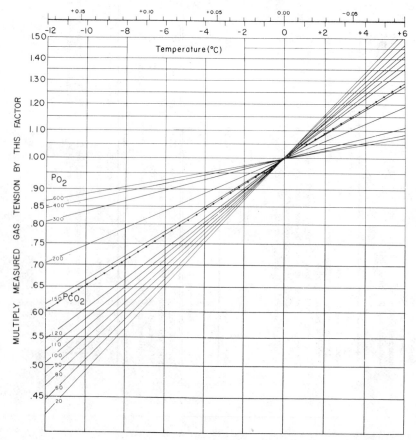

Figure 3. Correction chart for temperature differences between the patient and the water bath of the analyzer. Determine the difference between the temperature of the patient and the water bath and locate the point on the temperature scale. Add or subtract, as indicated, the adjacent pH correction factor to the measured pH value. Follow a vertical line from the temperature difference down to the point where it intersects with the P_{CO_2} isopleth (._._._.). Follow a horizontal line from the point of this intersection across to the left-hand axis of chart and determine the factor to be multiplied by the measured P_{CO_2} to obtain the temperature-corrected P_{CO_2}. Find the isopleth of the measured P_{O_2}; find the intersect point between this line and the vertical line of the temperature difference; follow a horizontal line to the left axis and determine the multiplication factor; multiply the measured P_{O_2} by this factor to obtain the temperature-corrected P_{CO_2}. Example: Determine the *temperature-corrected values* of a blood sample taken from a dog with a core temperature of 31°C and measured at 37°C. The measured values were: pH 7.20; P_{CO_2} 55 mm Hg; P_{O_2} 60 mm Hg. The temperature difference is 6°C. pH 7.200 + 0.088 = 7.288; P_{CO_2} 55 × 0.77 = *42.4 mm Hg*; P_{O_2} = 60 × 0.67 = *40.2 mm Hg.*

(and recorded if it occurs), since it will rapidly and dramatically alter blood gas values.

Venous and capillary blood provide rough screening values but are subject to considerable variation in some disease conditions and erroneous conclusions if the values are assumed to represent some consistent relation to arterial blood. For example, both anemia and hemorrhagic shock increase the arterial-venous difference in measured pH and blood gas values. In such cases, central venous blood may provide a better estimation of the status of the peripheral tissues than arterial blood. Calculated values of base deficit and bicarbonate concentration derived from venous blood, however, mirror those of arterial blood in virtually all cases. Measurements on free-flowing capillary blood may provide values representative of arterial blood if the technique is properly performed. The most important consideration in capillary collection techniques is that the blood be free flowing (there must be no stagnation due to tourniquets or vasoconstriction). This may be enhanced when necessary by warming of the appendage with hot water or heating blankets.

Heparin should be used as the anticoagulant (EDTA, ACD, CPD, sodium fluoride, and concentrated heparin anticoagulants may cause changes in the acid-base status of the blood). Only the dead space of the syringe should be filled with the heparin solution, and the syringe should be filled with consistent volumes of blood, since simple dilution of the blood sample by the anticoagulant solution will change the measured values.

The blood sample should be drawn anaerobically. One small air bubble will not cause important changes in the blood gas values, but many bubbles might and such samples should be discarded. The application of extreme negative pressure in the syringe should be avoided, since this may pull gases out of solution. The use of Silastic catheters for blood sampling is not recommended, since this material is very permeable to gases and samples may be altered between the patient and the syringe.

The most accurate measurements are obtained when the blood sample is analyzed immediately after being drawn. Storage of a blood sample allows *in vitro* metabolism, which changes the measured values. Oxygen consumption by the citric acid and cytochrome systems in leukocytes and reticulocytes varies with the concentration of these cell types. Glycolysis is the predominant metabolic process in mature red blood cells and is largely responsible for the measured rise in P_{CO_2}. If immediate analysis of the sample is not possible, it should be stored in ice water, since hypothermia decreases the metabolic rate (Table 11). The fact that pH and blood gas values change very little for several hours during ice water storage provides an opportunity for transport of the sample to a remote location for analysis.

The water bath of the blood gas analyzer is normally set at the normal body temperature for the species. If there is a difference between the temperature of the water bath and that of the patient when the sample is taken, the partial pressure of the gases in the blood will be altered. The measured values must be corrected for any temperature difference so that the reported values will reflect the true level at the temperature of the patient (Fig. 3) (Kelman and Nunn, 1966; Gabel, 1980).

REFERENCES AND SUPPLEMENTAL READING

Cornelius, L. M., and Rawlings, C. A.: Arterial blood gas and acid-base values in dogs with various diseases and signs of disease. J.A.V.M.A. 178:992, 1981.

Feigl, E. O., and D'Alecy, L. G.: Normal arterial blood, pH, oxygen, and carbon dioxide tensions in unanesthetized dogs. J. Appl. Physiol. 32:152, 1972.

Fink, B. R., and Schoolman, A.: Arterial blood acid-base balance in unrestrained waking cats. Proc. Soc. Exp. Biol. Med. 112:328, 1963.

Gabel, R. A.: Algorithms for calculating and correcting blood-gas and acid-base variables. Resp. Physiol. 42:211, 1980.

Haskins, S. C.: An overview of acid-base physiology. J.A.V.M.A. 110:423, 1977.

Haskins, S. C.: Sampling and storage of blood for pH and blood gas analysis. J.A.V.M.A. 110:429, 1977.

Haskins, S. C.: Standards and techniques of equipment utilization, *In* Sattler, F. P., Knowles, R. P., and Whittick, W. G. (eds.): *Veterinary Critical Care*. Philadelphia: Lea & Febiger, 1981.

Haskins, S. C.: Unpublished data (21 measurements of 7 cats), 1982.

Haskins, S. C., Munger, R. J., Helphrey, M. A., Gilroy, B. A., et al.: Effect of acetazolamide on blood acid-base and electrolyte values in dogs. J.A.V.M.A. 179:792, 1981.

Herbert, D. A., and Mitchell, R. A.: Blood gas tensions and acid-base balance in awake cats. J. Appl. Physiol. 30:434, 1971.

Kelman, G. R., and Nunn, J. F.: Normograms for correction of blood P_{O_2}, P_{CO_2}, pH and base excess for time and temperature. J. Appl. Physiol. 21:1481, 1966.

Kelman, G. R., and Nunn, J. F.: *Computer Produced Physiologic Tables*. Boston: Butterworths, 1968.

Mauderly, J. L.: Influence of sex and age on the pulmonary function of the unanesthetized beagle dog. J. Gerontol. 29:282, 1974.

Mauderly, J. L., and Pickrell, J. A.: Proceedings of the National Conference on Respiration in Animal Medicine, Washington, D. C., 1972.

McKiernan, B. C.: Principles of respiratory therapy. *In* Kirk, R.W. (ed.): *Current Veterinary Therapy VIII*. Philadelphia: W. B. Saunders, 1983.

Middleton, D. J., Ilkiw, J. W., and Watson, A. D. J.: Arterial and venous blood gas tensions in clinically healthy cats. Am. J. Vet. Res. 42:1609, 1981.

Morgan, A.P: The pulmonary toxicity of oxygen. Anesthesiology 29:570, 1968.

Nunn, J. F.: *Applied Respiratory Physiology*, 2nd ed. Boston: Butterworths, 1977.

Pickrell, J. A., Dubin, S. E., and Elliott, J. C.: Normal respiratory parameters of unanesthetized beagle dogs. Lab. Anim. Sci. 21:677, 1971.

Rodkey, W. C., Hannon, J. P., Dramise, J. G., White, R. D., Welsh, D. C., and Persky, B. N.: Arterialized capillary blood used to determine the acid-base and blood gas status of dogs. Am. J. Vet. Res. 39:459, 1978.

Rose, R. J., and Cater, J.: Some physiologic and biochemical effects of acetazolamide in the dog. J. Vet. Pharmacol. Therap. 2:215, 1979.

Rossing, R. G., and Cain, S. M.: A Nomogram relating P_{O_2}, pH, temperature and hemoglogin saturation in the dog. J. Appl. Physiol. 21:195, 1966.

Shapiro, B. A., Harrison, J. A., and Walton, J. R.: *Clinical Application of Blood Gases*. Chicago: Year Book Medical Publishers, 1977.

Siggaard-Andersen, O.: Blood acid-base alignment nomogram. Scales for pH, P_{CO_2}, base excess of whole blood of different hemoglobin concentrations, plasma, bicarbonate, and plasma total CO_2 Scand. J. Clin. Lab. Invest. 15:211, 1963.

Wise, W. C.: Normal arterialized blood gases and chemical components in the unanesthetized dog. J. Appl. Physiol. 35:427, 1973.

PRINCIPLES OF RESPIRATORY THERAPY

BRENDAN C. McKIERNAN, D.V.M.

Urbana, Illinois

The application of rational respiratory therapy requires the clinician to have a good understanding of normal pulmonary defense mechanisms and as specific and complete a diagnosis as possible. Although the pathophysiologic response of the respiratory system is limited compared with the many factors that may affect it, a specific etiologic diagnosis will allow the clinician to prognose, anticipate problems, and specifically treat the condition better.

There are three goals of respiratory therapy. The first is to control secretions and remove them from the respiratory tract. Second, alveolar ventilation must be kept at a level that maintains normal arterial blood gases and acid-base balance. Third, the control of normal reflexes, e.g., cough, sneeze, bronchomotor tone, must be ensured. The following article briefly discusses the normal pulmonary defense mechanisms and then reviews how these three goals are achieved in the clinical setting.

PULMONARY DEFENSE MECHANISMS

Various reflexes protect the respiratory system from injury and limit the penetration of and/or aid in the removal of foreign materials. Sneezing and coughing are violent and explosive, yet normal, reflexes that forcefully expel foreign materials and accumulated secretions from the larger nasal and lower airways, respectively. Interference with these reflexes may result in increased mucosal contact time for irritants; secretion retention; and increased risks of infection, airway obstruction, and ventilation-perfusion (V/Q) abnormalities.

Corticosteroids, cough suppressants, chest pain, dry gas administration, and tracheostomies may reduce the effectiveness of these reflexes. Mild exercise, chest percussion and vibration, aerosol therapy, nerve blocks, and adequate systemic hydration may facilitate these reflexes and are discussed hereafter.

Airway narrowing (bronchospasm) and closure (laryngeal spasm and closure during normal swallowing) function to limit or prevent the penetration of inhaled particulate matter and noxious gases into the lungs. Although important in limiting access to the respiratory tract, airway narrowing (especially bronchospasm and mucosal edema) often occurs secondarily to local inflammation and decreases the removal of secretions and alters regional ventilation while increasing the work of breathing (via airway resistance). Drugs may be chosen to specifically reduce the local inflammation (antibiotics, corticosteroids), the mucosal edema (decongestants), or the degree of bronchospasm (bronchodilators) in an attempt to improve secretion removal and regional ventilation.

The ciliated epithelial cells and the mucous secretions (together termed the "mucociliary blanket") function to trap and then remove debris from the tracheobronchial tree. Many clinical conditions and therapeutic interventions adversely affect mucociliary transport. Drying of the tracheobronchial secretions (through, e.g., dehydration, the administration of nonhumidified gases, improper tracheostomy care, or prolonged anticholinergic usage) must be avoided to ensure normal mucociliary function.

Alveolar macrophages are bone marrow–derived monocytes found in the respiratory bronchioles, alveolar ducts, and alveolar sacs. They function to engulf foreign particles and bacteria that have penetrated to this level within the lungs. Enzymatically potent lysosomes/phagosomes within the macrophage function to detoxify and/or destroy phagocytosed materials. As these cells represent the primary bacterial defense system in the resting lung, it is important that their function not be impaired. Viral infections directly alter macrophage function (and thereby allow for bacterial replication), but many clinical conditions and therapies may also adversely affect their function. Corticosteroids and other immunosuppressive/cytotoxic drugs, hypoxia, acidosis, uremia, starvation, and various aerosol pollutants (both particulate and gaseous) are examples.

It is obvious from this brief discussion that the clinician must exercise caution and care when recommending a given therapy so as not to adversely affect the respiratory system.

RESPIRATORY THERAPY GOALS

CONTROL OF SECRETIONS

A clean, patent tracheobronchial tree is necessary if normal gas exchange (ventilation and distribution) is to occur. The amount, type, and character of the secretions as well as the mechanisms for clearance such as coughing, mucociliary action, tracheobronchial suction, postural drainage, and maintenance of normal airway caliber are clinically important factors in the control of secretions.

SECRETION PRODUCTION

Epithelial goblet cells and submucosal mucous glands are the major sources of tracheobronchial secretions. They constantly secrete mucus. This mucus becomes part of the mucous blanket, which is swept toward the pharynx by the ciliated epithelium. Responding to irritation, these cells and glands can increase the amount of their secretions as well as change the actual physical properties of mucus, most importantly, viscosity and elasticity, as they are the main determinants of mucus transport. Obviously if the specific source of irritation can be determined and either removed or treated, the excess secretions can be limited.

SECRETION CLEARANCE

The removal of tracheobronchial secretions is dependent on many factors including a normal mucociliary blanket, cough reflex, airway caliber, and the character of secretions present. These items may be affected clinically—both favoring and, unfortunately, hindering clearance.

The mucociliary blanket is normally moved along at a moderate rate, 10 to 20 mm/min in the trachea. Many factors can affect the cilia and/or mucus and slow this process, such as drying, aerosol exposure (dusts, smoke, noxious gases), infectious agents, anesthesia, oxygen administration, and hypoxia, to name a few. Since mucus is approximately 95 per cent water, one of the major factors affecting its transport is the degree of mucus hydration. Any drying of these secretions will promote their retention and can potentially lead to airway obstruction. An important therapeutic regimen when trying to facilitate the clearance of secretions involves, therefore, optimal hydration of the mucociliary blanket. The best method is to ensure that the patient is systemically hydrated. *Aerosol therapy* has been recommended as a way of delivering fluid to the respiratory tract to thin secretions and facilitate their clearance. There is significant disagreement on this subject at present, yet the author has used it to treat selected cases (bronchopneumonia) with favorable results. It must be emphasized that this is not a substitute for systemic hydration.

Ultrasonic nebulizers and an enclosed cage are used most commonly for bland aerosol (0.45 to 0.9 per cent sterile saline) therapy. These nebulizers are capable of suspending a large number of very small particles of the solution in the air. Mean particle size with ultrasonic nebulizers is approximately 3 μ, with a range of 0.8 to 6.0 μ and greater. Although many of these particles "rain out" in the upper airways, the amount reaching the lower airways has clinically appeared to be helpful in loosening and clearing secretions. Patients are nebulized for 30 to 45 minutes three to six times a day. Mild exercise and chest percussion to encourage coughing are used after each treatment. The potential hazards of contamination, overhydration (especially in patients under 5 kg), bronchial irritation, and fever (inability to effectively dissipate heat by panting) must be avoided. Aerosol therapy utilizing antibiotics, mucolytics, or other drugs has not been proved efficacious and is not recommended. An exception to this is the face mask treatment of chronic *Bordetella bronchiseptica* airway colonization using some of the aminoglycoside antibiotics. Additional reading on the subject is available.

Expectorants are routinely included in most human respiratory preparations, even those containing antitussives and decongestants. They are, however, recognized to be ineffective in their ability to increase the rate of mucociliary clearance (at least at the routine dosages). The combination of these drugs, if used, with antitussives and antihistamine/decongestant products is irrational and is not recommended.

Coughing is probably not a necessary reflex in the normal animal. Rather, it functions when abnormalities exist such as excessive or dry secretions and poor ciliary function. It is, however, *the* major defense against retained secretions. The potential effects of retained secretions are dramatically shown in Figure 1. Many factors may be encountered clinically that interfere with effective coughing. Excessive dynamic airway compression (tracheal collapse), airway obstruction (hilar lymphadenopathy), muscular weakness (neuromuscular and electrolyte disorders), pain (fractured ribs, thoracic and especially anterior abdominal incisions, pleuritis, and peritonitis), tracheostomies, and drug usage (cough suppressants, corticosteroids, sedatives, and anesthetics) are common causes of an ineffective cough mechanism. Paricularly frustrating are acute, severe bronchopneumonia cases in which the inflammation and amount of retained secretions have obtunded the cough reflex. In two such cases, failure to cough resulted in a rapidly progressive condition and, essentially, the drowning of the animal in its own secretions.

Clinically, there are a number of important considerations. First, we must be cautious in the use of analgesics so as not to suppress the cough reflex or decrease ventilation. Totally abolishing pain may be a noble goal, but the adverse side effects of these drugs may cause greater harm. A degree of pain is actually good because the crying/vocalization that ensues requires an increase in ventilation, which is

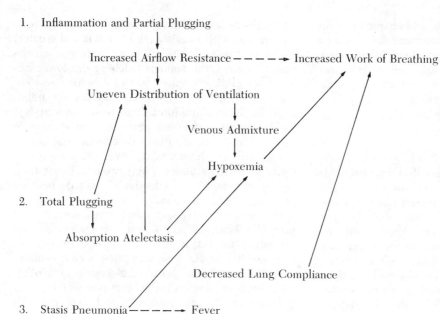

1. Inflammation and Partial Plugging

Increased Airflow Resistance – – – – → Increased Work of Breathing

Uneven Distribution of Ventilation

Venous Admixture

Hypoxemia

2. Total Plugging

Absorption Atelectasis

Decreased Lung Compliance

3. Stasis Pneumonia – – – – → Fever

Figure 1. Potential results of retained secretions. (Adapted from Shapiro, Harrison, and Trout: *Clinical Application of Respiratory Care.* Chicago: Year Book Medical Publishers, 1975.)

beneficial to the animal. Intercostal nerve blocks are not frequently used but represent a rational approach to eliminating pain without adversely affecting ventilation.

Second, *chest physiotherapy* should be employed, including chest wall manipulation (percussion, vibration), exercise-induced deep breathing, cough stimulation, and intermittent positive pressure breathing (IPPB) therapy. Since secretions tend to gravitate ventrally and ventral lung regions have less interdependence, allowing (encouraging) an animal to "rest and recuperate" may in reality promote poor ventilation and the pooling of secretions in ventral lung regions. Deep breathing must be encouraged through the use of mild forced exercise, limited by the patient's cardiorespiratory reserve.

Postural drainage is frequently used in human medicine, taking advantage of various positioning techniques to facilitate gravity drainage from the tracheobronchial tree. Because of the patient cooperation required for this technique, it is rarely applicable to veterinary patients.

Chest *percussion* or *vibration* (manually or with an electrical vibrator) is designed to transmit energy waves through the thoracic wall to theoretically loosen bronchial secretions, promoting better clearance and (often) inducing a normal cough reflex. Other methods of cough induction that may be employed are tracheal manipulation and the instillation (injection) of material into the trachea.

IPPB therapy may be administered to most dogs via face mask. The mask must be well sealed and the inspiratory effort sufficient to trigger the machine. In the author's experience dogs less than 8 to 10 kg may not develop enough inspiratory

pressure to routinely trigger the machine. IPPB treatments may be used to improve the distribution of ventilation, open collapsed airways/alveoli, improve the cough, and deliver specific medications (decongestants, bronchodilators, mucolytics). Although the clinical application of this form of therapy seems justified in selected cases, (e.g., those with poor regional ventilation), evaluation of this therapy based on large numbers of cases is still incomplete.

Airway caliber may significantly affect the flow of air and the clearance of secretions within the lungs. Methods of altering airway caliber are discussed hereafter.

Tracheostomized patients present unique problems to the veterinarian trying to clear tracheobronchial secretions. With the upper airways bypassed, normal filtration, warming, and humidification of inspired air as well as effective coughing are eliminated. These normal functions must be assumed by the clinician when a tracheostomy is performed.

Cuffed and cuffless tracheostomy tubes are available, and whatever type is chosen should include an inner cannula. Cuffed tubes are beneficial if any ventilation (IPPB, anesthesia) is to be performed. The inner cannula allows for the removal of secretions as they accumulate within the tube. Failure to use this type of tube or to routinely clean the cannula may result in complete airway obstruction secondary to secretion accumulation. Adequate hydration of the tracheobronchial epithelium is necessary to prevent cellular damage and drying of secretions. Routine nebulization (e.g., ultrasonic nebulization for 15 to 30 minutes every hour) of inspired air or the injection of small amounts of sterile saline into the tracheostomy tube will keep the secretions loose and will prevent epithelial desiccation.

Tracheobronchial suction is used in conjunction with physiotherapy and routine cleaning of the inner cannula to keep the large airways clear of secretions. Special tracheobronchial suction catheters have been developed that minimize or prevent mucosal invagination and trauma during the suction procedure.* The technique for proper airway suctioning includes (1) determination that secretions are present, (2) preoxygenation of the patient, (3) sterile insertion of the suction catheter through the tracheostomy tube and into the mainstem bronchi, (4) application of suction while the catheter is rotated and pulled out of the trachea (maximum suction application time should *never* exceed ten seconds), and (5) reoxygenation and repetition until the airways appear clear. Complications associated with tracheobronchial suctioning that have been reported in humans include hypoxemia, arrhythmias, hypotension, and lung collapse.

Sterile technique is absolutely essential when managing the tracheostomy patient. This pertains to insertion of the tube, at least daily changing of the dressings, and cleaning of the inner cannula as well as the suction technique and tracheostomy tube/cannula itself.

ALVEOLAR VENTILATION

Ensuring adequate and evenly distributed alveolar ventilation is a prerequisite for the maintenance of normal blood gases (oxygen and carbon dioxide) and acid-base balance. Clinically, the veterinarian can affect airway caliber to help ensure an even distribution of ventilation by preventing or treating bronchospasm, mucosal edema, and secretion accumulation. Oxygen and/or ventilatory support may be used to improve (normalize) arterial partial pressures of oxygen (Pa_{O_2}) and carbon dioxide (Pa_{CO_2}).

AIRWAY CALIBER

A decrease in airway caliber may increase the work of breathing (airway resistance), cause V/Q abnormalities, and potentially lead to secretion retention. External airway compression, an increased amount of endobronchial secretions, mucosal edema, and bronchospasm are examples of situations in which airway caliber may be reduced. The presence of a pronounced expiratory effort (e.g., prolongation or "heaving") and/or wheezing is a clinical finding consistent with a decrease in airway caliber. Other findings may include the presence of

*Aero-Flo Suction Catheters, Sherwood Medical Industries, St. Louis, MO.

crackles on auscultation (indicating the presence of secretions or the opening of closed airways) and grossly narrowed airways (visualized via radiography or bronchoscopy). Tracheobronchial inflammation may be expected to result in various degrees of mucosal edema. The functional importance of this edema and the other findings previously mentioned may be quantitated in humans through the use of specific pulmonary function tests. These, however, are not routinely available (or applicable) in veterinary medicine.

If a decrease in airway caliber is suspected, the cause should be determined and specifically treated if possible. Secretion retention is treated as described previously. Inflammation secondary to bacterial, allergic, or mechanical problems (e.g., foreign body) is usually reduced following appropriate therapy (e.g., antibiotics, corticosteroids, and physical removal, respectively).

Bronchospasm may subside after the inflammatory reaction is controlled or may be treated with a bronchodilator. Xanthines (e.g., theophylline) inhibit the degradation of cyclic 3', 5'-AMP (cAMP) by the enzyme phosphodiesterase. β-Adrenergics (e.g., Isuprel, isoetharine) promote bronchodilation by stimulating the conversion of ATP to cAMP via the enzyme adenyl cyclase. Increased levels of cAMP within the bronchial smooth muscle cell result in bronchodilation. The pharmacokinetics of theophylline in the dog and cat have been worked out, and these dosages are shown in Table 1. Various salts of theophylline exist (e.g., aminophylline dihydrate), each of which is equivalent to a different amount of the parent compound. It should be noted that the dosages given here are for aminophylline and may not be the same for other theophylline salts.

OXYGEN THERAPY

Due to differences in solubility, dissociation curves, and methods of transport in the blood, a decrease in Pa_{O_2} (i.e., hypoxemia) normally precedes any increase in Pa_{CO_2}. Arterial blood gas analysis is the definitive method of identifying changes in Pa_{O_2} and Pa_{CO_2}. Samples should be analyzed immediately if possible, although only minimal changes will occur if the sample is stored in an ice bath while being transported to a local lab or hospital for analysis. Additional information on hypoxemia, hypercapnia, sampling techniques, and the interpretation of blood gas analyses is available in the preceding article. In the absence of actual blood gas measurements, various clinical signs may be observed that are often associated with hypoxemia and the need for oxygen therapy. These include tachypnea, dyspnea, cyanosis, tachycardia, arrhythmias, and restlessness.

If hypoxemia is a problem, especially if it is due

Table 1.   Antitussives and Bronchodilators Commonly Used in Veterinary Medicine

Drugs	Dosage*	
	Dog	Cat
ANTITUSSIVES		
Narcotic		
Codeine (various)	1 to 2 mg/kg t.i.d.	Same
Hydrocodone bitartrate (Hycodan, Endo)	0.22 mg/kg s.i.d. to q.i.d.	—
Nonnarcotic		
Dextromethorphan hydrobromide (various)	2 mg/kg t.i.d. to q.i.d.	Same
Butorphanol tartrate (Torbutrol, Bristol)	0.055 to 0.11 mg/kg SC prn (1 ml/9 kg)	
BRONCHODILATORS		
Xanthines		
Aminophylline dihydrate (various)	11 mg/kg q.i.d.	5 mg/kg b.i.d. to t.i.d.
β agonists		
Isoetharine (β_2)	0.5 to 1.0 ml, 1:3 with saline by aerosol IPPB treatment (face mask or endotracheal tube)	—
Isoproterenol (β_1, various compounds and often in combination with other drugs)	0.44 ml/kg b.i.d. to q.i.d. as needed† (not recommended for dogs with advanced or acute heart failure)	—

*Dosages are *per os* unless otherwise indicated.
†Dosage given for Isuprel Compound Elixir, Breon.

to V/Q abnormalities, oxygen administration may be indicated. Pa_{O_2} values of less than 60 mm Hg usually warrant therapy. Methods of oxygen administration vary considerably depending on the size and condition of the patient as well as the available technical support and equipment. Oxygen therapy cages, which also control temperature, humidity, and CO_2 levels, are available. Although expensive, these cages are an excellent method of oxygen administration, since caging is not invasive or stressful to the animal and requires less technical support (supervision) than other methods. These cages are usually capable of achieving a 35 to 50 per cent oxygen concentration, which is adequate in all but the most severe cases of parenchymal disease. Other methods of oxygen administration include flexible, fenestrated catheters placed nasally or transtracheally, face masks, or direct delivery via an endotracheal tube. These methods limit the animal's freedom of motion; involve some degree of restraint, anesthesia, or invasiveness; and may not be well tolerated. Whichever method is chosen, it is important that the patient be re-evaluated frequently to determine if the hypoxemia is being reversed.

VENTILATORY ASSISTANCE

Intermittent positive pressure ventilation (IPPV) may be used in those cases that do not respond to routine oxygen administration. It is also indicated when alveolar hypoventilation (hypercapnia) occurs. Re-expansion of collapsed alveoli and the maintenance of small airway patency will facilitate/improve gas exchange. IPPV requires the placement of a cuffed endotracheal or tracheostomy tube. Tracheostomy care has been described previously. Pro-

longed endotracheal intubation is not possible in veterinary patients without some form of CNS depression, e.g., coma or narcosis. Low doses of morphine, however, often produce surprisingly good tube acceptance without severe CNS depression.

The application of positive end-expiratory pressure (PEEP) is reserved for those patients with severe parenchymal disease who do not respond to IPPV. Increasing the mean airway pressure via PEEP ensures that collapsed alveoli and small airways remain open and participate in the process of gas exchange. The adverse cardiovascular effects of positive pressure ventilation (IPPV and especially PEEP) can be severe, and patients undergoing these therapies must be carefully monitored. The principle adverse cardiovascular effect, decreased venous return to the heart and a subsequent decrease in cardiac output, can be particularly serious in shocky or hypovolemic animals. The clinician must be familiar with the effects as well as the equipment itself prior to using this form of therapy.

The metabolic components of *acid-base physiology* and the principle of *anion gap* are reviewed in the previous article.

NORMAL REFLEXES

Sneezing, coughing, and the protective airway reflexes (e.g., laryngeal spasm/closure, bronchospasm) are normal reflexes that function to protect the airways. In addition to avoiding particularly irritating substances, decreasing local inflammation, and taking care in manipulative procedures, little can be done to affect the sneezing and laryngeal reflexes. Bronchomotor tone and the cough reflex can be affected therapeutically.

Coughing, although a normal and important reflex, is a common presenting complaint in respiratory cases. Stimulation of subepithelial irritant receptors located primarily in the lower trachea and mainstem bronchi initiate this reflex. Extremely high airflow velocities and the "milking" action of peripheral airway collapse during a forceful cough act to propel secretions out of the lungs. Ineffective coughing (due to pain, debilitation, or tracheostomy) or the suppression of the cough (due to sedation or antitussives) may lead to secretion retention, especially when excessive secretions are present. Figure 1 reviews the potential effects of secretion retention. Coughing should not be suppressed when an increased amount of secretions is present; in fact, coughing should be encouraged, along with other methods of secretion removal. Inflammation and irritation of the tracheobronchial epithelium *not* associated with excessive secretion production may elicit a significant amount of nonproductive coughing. This type of "dry" coughing may be irritating in itself (e.g., the tracheal collapse or kennel cough case) and often is an indication for therapeutic intervention. Unchecked, nonproductive coughing may cause or produce cardiac problems (increased intrathoracic pressure → decreased venous return → decreased cardiac output with the potential for syncopal episodes and, if chronic, even cor pulmonale). It also may cause muscular fatigue and often interferes with rest of the owner as well as the animal. Cough suppression may then be warranted, but only if the *cause* of the cough cannot be eliminated and if the cough is not needed to facilitate the removal of secretions. For example, a tracheal foreign body will elicit a dry, nonproductive cough, but the correct treatment is to remove the foreign object, not to suppress the cough. Clinicians should take the time to explain to the client the importance of an effective cough reflex and the necessity of arriving at a specific diagnosis.

In addition to removing the cause of irritation, coughing may be controlled by interfering with the reflex, either locally at the irritant receptor site or centrally at the cough center in the medulla. Corticosteroids, as anti-inflammatory drugs, interfere with the local irritation in the tracheobronchial tree and, subsequently, the cough reflex. Short-term use of these drugs *is* effective in reducing the amount of coughing but may also suppress the normal pulmonary defense mechanisms and therefore may be detrimental to the patient. Both narcotic and non-narcotic cough suppressants are available for use in veterinary medicine. Table 1 lists the commonly used antitussives and their recommended dosages.

Bronchomotor tone is a balance between cholinergic and β-adrenergic stimulation. Increased amounts of cAMP within the bronchial smooth muscle (via increased production or decreased degradation) promote relaxation, i.e., bronchodilation. Increased amounts of cGMP (either via cholinergic stimulation or a relative decrease in cAMP) promote bronchoconstriction in susceptible fibers. β Blockade (through infection, a deficiency of adenyl cyclase, or the use of propranolol), α-adrenergic stimulation, and the prostaglandin $F_{2\alpha}$ promote bronchoconstriction. Prostaglandins E_1 and E_2 are released in the lung following antigen challenge and promote bronchodilation. Table 1 lists some of the commonly used bronchodilators. Additional information is given in the section on Alveolar Ventilation.

SUPPLEMENTAL READING

Davis, L. E.: Clinical pharmacology of the respiratory system. *In* Kirk, R. W. (ed.): *Current Veterinary Therapy* VII. Philadelphia; W. B. Saunders, 1980.

Haskins, S. C.: Standards and techniques of equipment utilization. *In* Sattler, F. P., Knowles, R. P., and Whittick, Wm. G., (eds.): *Veterinary Critical Care*. Philadelphia; Lea & Febiger, 1981.

McKiernan, B. C.: Principles of aerosol therapy—Applications in the canine. Proceedings of the Illinois Veterinary Respiratory Symposium, Champaign, Illinois, 1978.

Shapiro, B. A., Harrison, R. A., and Trout, C. A.: *Clinical Application of Respiratory Care*, Chicago: Year Book Medical Publishers, 1975.

DIAGNOSTICS FOR
RESPIRATORY DISEASES

PHILIP ROUDEBUSH, D. V. M.

Mississippi State, Mississippi

A comprehensive medical history, physical examination, careful auscultation, and radiography are all excellent routine tools for the detection of respiratory tract abnormalities. Often, however, these routine diagnostic procedures lack the specificity required for an etiologic diagnosis and the planning of a rational treatment protocol. The advent of special diagnostic procedures has helped practicing veterinarians expand their diagnostic approach to many respiratory problems. The following diagnostic procedures can be utilized in small companion animals showing signs of respiratory disease.

TRANSTRACHEAL WASHING AND ASPIRATION

A technique for bypassing the upper respiratory passages and obtaining secretions directly from the trachea of humans was originally described in 1963 and has since been modified for use in a wide variety of animals. Since animals are unable to expectorate sputum, transtracheal washing and aspiration is a safe, simple, and clinically valuable method for obtaining material from the tracheobronchial tree for microbiologic and cytologic examination. The technique is well tolerated by most small companion animals and requires only minimal restraint of the unanesthetized patient.

The indications for transtracheal washing and aspiration include a chronic cough (longer than four weeks duration) and pulmonary parenchymal disease of unknown cause. Transtracheal washing is also valuable in obtaining material for culture when airway infection is suspected. When compared with other airway culture techniques, transtracheal washing is preferred because it can be performed easily and it bypasses the oropharynx.

The equipment needed to perform a transtracheal washing and aspiration is relatively inexpensive and readily available. Local anesthestic, sterile saline, a 12-cc syringe, material for sterile preparation of the skin, and an 18-gauge needle-catheter device* are needed.

The animal is usually restrained in a sitting position or sternal recumbency. The ventral aspect of the neck over the larynx and proximal cervical trachea is clipped and prepared with an appropriate germicidal solution. The skin and subcutaneous tissue are infiltrated with 1 to 2 per cent lidocaine at the puncture site. A small wheal of anesthetic is usually adequate. The through-the-needle catheter is introduced into the tracheal lumen, either between cervical tracheal rings or, preferably, through the cricothyroid ligament of the larynx (Fig. 1). The cricothyroid ligament is an elastic ligament that extends from the rostral border of the cricoid cartilage to the body of the thyroid cartilage. With the neck extended, the cricothyroid ligament is located by moving the finger cranially (upward) along the trachea until the ridge of the cricoid cartilage is identified. Just cranial to this ridge is a small triangular depression, which is the location of the cricothyroid ligament.

The needle-catheter is advanced through the anesthetized skin and directed slightly caudad until the cricothyroid ligament or ventral tracheal wall is pierced (Fig. 2). Once the needle is positioned within the tracheal lumen, the catheter is advanced through the needle and down the trachea. The catheter should pass easily, and in most patients the irritation caused by the catheter induces coughing. The catheter is advanced until the tip reaches the distal trachea or mainstem bronchi. Inability to advance the catheter indicates that the needle either failed to enter the tracheal lumen or became embedded in the dorsal tracheal wall. In this case, the entire catheter and needle should be withdrawn and the procedure repeated. When the catheter has been properly positioned, the metal needle is withdrawn from the tissues of the neck so that only the catheter itself remains in the trachea. The catheter stylet is withdrawn and a syringe is attached (Fig. 3). If secretions are copious, they are aspirated directly. However, if no material is aspirated, then 2 to 5 ml sterile saline are introduced. The injected saline stimulates a cough and permits aspiration of secretions. Suction is immediately applied after the saline is injected and while the animal is coughing. When air alone is drawn into the syringe, it must be expelled so that adequate suction is maintained. This procedure of saline injection and immediate aspiration is repeated until an adequate sample is obtained.

---

*Venocath-18, Abbott Labs, North Chicago, IL.

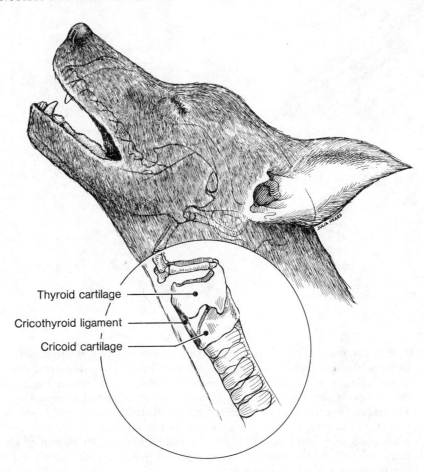

Figure 1. Diagrammatic representation of anatomic structures involved with transtracheal aspiration technique. The best landmark for percutaneous puncture is the cricothyroid ligament of the larynx, although the tracheal lumen can also be entered between cervical tracheal rings.

Thyroid cartilage

Cricothyroid ligament

Cricoid cartilage

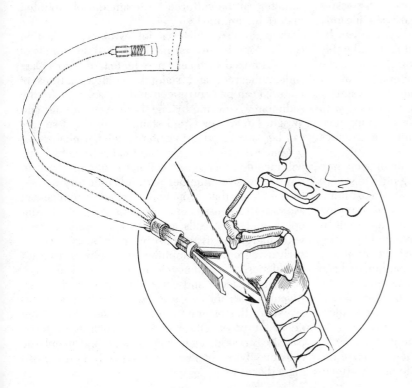

Figure 2. The needle is advanced and directed slightly caudal until the trachea is entered. Once the needle is positioned within the tracheal lumen, the catheter is advanced through the needle and down the trachea.

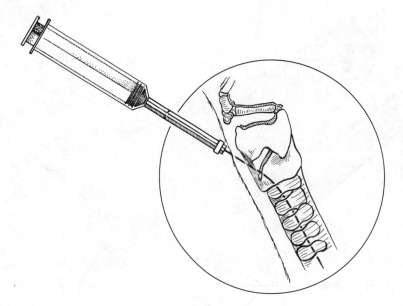

Figure 3. The indwelling catheter in the trachea with syringe attached. The needle has been withdrawn from the tissues of the neck and covered by the plastic needle guard. This prevents injury to cervical soft tissue structures or inadvertent severence of catheter during aspiration.

It is not unusual to infuse up to 30 ml of saline in large dogs to obtain an adequate sample. Most of the saline is not aspirated back into the syringe but is rapidly absorbed by the respiratory mucosa. The use of large volumes of saline is contraindicated only in cats, puppies, and small dogs. When an adequate sample has been obtained, the catheter is removed and gentle digital pressure applied over the puncture site for several minutes.

Although complications from transtracheal washing and aspiration are uncommon, the procedure is not without risk. As with the majority of invasive diagnostic procedures, the risks are significantly decreased with experience. The procedure can be performed in cats and small dogs but is considerably more difficult. Transtracheal washing should not be attempted in the fractious or uncooperative patient without adequate chemical and manual restraint.

The most common complication associated with transtracheal washing is subcutaneous emphysema. This occurs when persistent coughing or dyspnea causes air to leak from the puncture site into the cervical subcutaneous tissues. The air dissects into the fascial planes of the neck, causing mild to severe subcutaneous emphysema, pneumomediastinum, and rarely pneumothorax. Subcutaneous emphysema is most common in small patients, such as puppies and cats, but is usually prevented by maintaining gentle digital pressure over the puncture site after the procedure. Endotracheal hemorrhage may also occur owing to mucosal irritation from the needle, stylet, or catheter. This hemorrhage is usually minimal and rarely causes problems unless the animal is suffering from a bleeding diathesis. In the fractious or uncooperative patient, the needle may lacerate the trachea or sever the catheter if the head and neck are not restrained adequately. Infec-tion at the puncture site and cardiac arrhythmias in hypoxemic patients have been described as complications in humans but have not been observed in small companion animals by the author. Oxygen can be administered through a face mask during the procedure to a dyspneic or hypoxic patient.

An aliquot of the aspirated material can be cultured directly for aerobic and anaerobic bacterial organisms. Anaerobic culture is indicated only when aspiration pneumonia or pulmonary abscessation is suspected. Secretions that coat the distal end of the catheter can be cultured if the amount of aspirated material is minimal.

Preparation of material for cytologic evaluation can be done by several methods. Visible strands of mucous mixed with cells may be teased onto a glass slide, smeared, and stained. Small quantities of material can be centrifuged and smears made of the sediment. New methylene blue wet mounts and Wright-Giemsa or Gram stains of air-dried smears can be used for identification of cellular elements.

Material aspirated from the tracheobronchial tree will include mucous and cellular elements. Neutrophils increase in number with inflammatory disease to the point that bronchopneumonia produces an aspirate that consists entirely of neutrophils. Eosinophils and mast cells are recovered from animals with allergic or hypersensitive pulmonary diseases such as chronic eosinophilic bronchitis and occult dirofilariasis. Lymphocytes are seen in a wide variety of both acute and chronic pulmonary diseases. Alveolar macrophages are often identified and signify that the aspirate represents secretions from deeper airways. Other elements such as bacteria, parasite larvae or eggs, microfilaria, and neoplastic cells may be recognized and may help in establishing a diagnosis.

THORACOCENTESIS

Fluid in the pleural space detected by physical examination or radiography is an indication for diagnostic thoracocentesis. Analysis of aspirated material provides valuable information in the diagnostic approach to the patient with pleural space disease. (Pleural fluid analysis is reviewed in the article entitled *Pleural Diseases*.) In addition to the role of thoracocentesis as a diagnostic procedure, it is frequently used as a therapeutic tool, particularly when pleural effusions cause respiratory embarrassment.

The equipment utilized in performing thoracocentesis is inexpensive and readily available. Local anesthetic, syringes, three-way stopcock, material for sterile preparation of the skin, and a needle or needle-catheter device are all needed. An 18 to 20-gauge, 1- to 1½-inch needle usually suffices for an average small companion animal. Needle-catheter devices such as indwelling cephalic or jugular venous catheters* can also be utilized. Standard butterfly infusion sets† offer the advantages of convenience and greater safety than conventional needles. A three-way stopcock placed between the needle and syringe allows the aspirated fluid to be emptied without repeatedly removing the syringe from the needle (Fig. 4).

The patient with suspected pleural effusion should be thoroughly evaluated by physical exami-

---

*Venocath-18 or Sovereign Indwelling Catheter, Sherwood Medical Industries, St. Louis, MO.

†Argyle Medi-Wing Infusion Set, Sherwood Medical Industries, St. Louis, MO.

nation and radiography prior to thoracocentesis. Many patients with pleural effusion have compromised cardiopulmonary function, and care must be taken in restraining and positioning the patient for radiography or thoracocentesis. The patient frequently struggles when restrained in lateral recumbency but usually tolerates a standing or sternal position. An endotracheal tube, laryngoscope, and oxygen source should be immediately available in the event that asphyxia appears imminent.

The site of thoracocentesis is best determined after reviewing the thoracic radiograph. If pleural fluid accumulation is diffuse, then the seventh or eighth intercostal space is used. The puncture site is clipped and prepared with an appropriate germicidal solution. The skin, subcutaneous tissue, muscle, and parietal pleura are all infiltrated with 1 to 2 per cent lidocaine. The key to successful thoracocentesis and a comfortable patient is the proper and adequate use of a local anesthetic. Trauma to neurovascular structures can be avoided by advancing the needle through the chest wall on the cranial edge of the rib.

Once the needle penetrates the skin, slight negative pressure is placed on the syringe to prevent penetration into the lung parenchyma. Material will appear in the syringe when the needle enters the fluid-filled pleural space. Flexible indwelling catheters* will often slide into the pleural space and overcome the potential hazard of needles penetrating the lung or other vital structures. If thoracocentesis is performed solely for diagnostic purposes then 5 to 10 ml of fluid should be collected for appropriate cytologic and bacteriologic evaluation. Flexible catheters, three-way stopcocks, and large

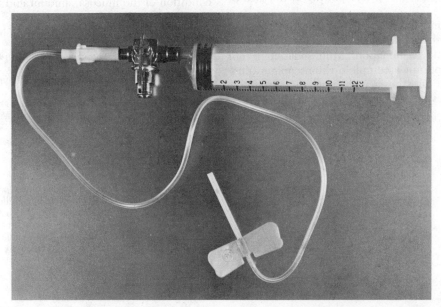

Figure 4.   A three-way stopcock, butterfly catheter, and syringe make a safe, convenient system for performing thoracocentesis.

syringes are often necessary to expedite the removal of large volumes of fluid. After thoracocentesis is completed, the needle or catheter is rapidly withdrawn while the puncture hole is occluded with digital pressure.

Complications of thoracocentesis usually result from trauma to vital thoracic structures. Iatrogenic pneumothorax and hemothorax may result from laceration or puncture of the lung. Infectious agents may also be introduced into the thorax if aseptic technique is not used. Pulmonary edema has been described in humans when large quantities of pleural fluid are quickly aspirated. Although this form of "re-expansion edema" has not been reported in animals, large quantities of pleural fluid should be removed with caution. The author has also experienced one case of fatal iatrogenic pericardial tamponade. An Irish wolfhound with massive cardiomegaly due to cardiomyopathy was found dead in her cage within 30 minutes after diagnostic thoracocentesis. Necropsy revealed that a coronary artery had been inadvertently punctured with a needle during thoracocentesis and pericardial tamponade ensued.

ENDOSCOPY

RHINOSCOPY

Endoscopic examination of the nasal passages can be used along with other diagnostic procedures to evaluate a wide variety of nasal problems in the dog and cat. Indications for rhinoscopy include chronic unilateral or bilateral nasal discharge, epistaxis, facial or nasal deformity, obstructed nasal or nasopharyngeal air flow (snorting, snuffling, or stertorous breathing patterns), and pawing at the face or nose.

The nasal mucosa is extremely sensitive, making general anesthesia necessary to allow a thorough and atraumatic examination. Mild sedation is not sufficient to permit a complete rhinoscopic evaluation. General anesthesia with inhalation agents or balanced anesthesia using muscle paralyzers like

succinylcholine plus narcotic analgesics is recommended.

Initially, the nasopharynx is examined using a mouth speculum, nasopharynx illuminator, dental mirror, and Allis tissue forceps. The forceps are used to grasp the posterior edge of the soft palate and retract it forward. A rotating nasopharyngeal illuminator* is available that incorporates a built-in lighted mirror that attaches to conventional otoscopic light handles.† This lighted mirror only allows a portion of the nasopharynx to be visualized but is relatively inexpensive (Fig. 5). A superior method of posterior rhinoscopy utilizes a flexible fiberoptic endoscope‡ to examine the entire nasopharynx including the choanae (Fig. 6).

Anterior rhinoscopy in the dog and cat is somewhat limited by the well-developed and convoluted nasal conchae (turbinates). A complete examination of the nasal cavity usually cannot be performed. The most convenient equipment for anterior rhinoscopy is a standard otoscopic light handle§ and otoscopic speculums. The disadvantage of using the otoscope is that only the rostral one-fourth to one-third of the nasal cavity can be examined. This type of examination may be adequate to rule out obvious foreign bodies but may not document such chronic nasal diseases as neoplasia, which usually arises in the caudal third of the nose. A more thorough examination of the nasal cavity is carried out using either a rigid or flexible fiberoptic endoscope. The rigid fiberoptic endoscope§ routinely used by the author for rhinoscopy has an outside diameter of 2.2 to 2.5 mm and affords an excellent view of a large portion of the nasal cavity. Flexible fiberoptic endoscopes‡ with an outside diameter of 4 to 6 mm are also used in larger breeds.

During endoscopy, the examiner should note the condition of the mucosa, amount and type of secre-

---

*Nasopharynx Illuminator, Welch Allyn Inc., Skaneateles Falls, NY.

†Halogen Diagnostic Otoscope, Welch Allyn Inc., Skaneateles Falls, NY.

‡Olympus BF-2TR Bronchofiberscope, Olympus Corp., New Hyde Park, NY.

§Needlescope, Dyonics Inc., Aurora, IL.

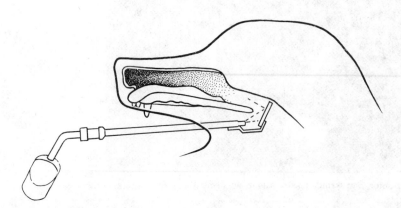

Figure 5. Schematic representation of using the nasopharyngeal illuminator (Nasopharynx Illuminator, Welch Allyn, Inc.). This built-in lighted mirror attaches to conventional otoscopic light handles and is utilized to examine the oropharynx and portions of the nasopharynx.

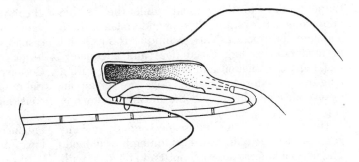

Figure 6. Schematic representation of using a flexible fiberoptic endoscope (Olympus BF-2TR Bronchofiberscope, Olympus Corp.) to examine the nasopharynx. This instrument is superior to the rigid nasopharynx illuminator because it allows examination of the entire nasopharynx and choanae.

tions, deviation of conchae and presence of abnormal tissue or foreign bodies. The normal nasal mucosa is the same color as the oral mucous membranes. A moderate amount of serous secretions is normal, but copious mucoid or mucopurulent exudate signals a nasal problem. Foreign bodies found during endoscopy are usually plant material such as grass awns. They may be readily visualized, or they may be obscured by mucopurulent exudate. Neoplastic tissue varies in color and consistency depending on the histologic type.

After the nasal cavity has been thoroughly examined, brush catheters and biopsy forceps* are used to obtain material for cytologic and histologic evaluation. Exudate and tissue obtained from nasal brushings are smeared directly onto glass slides, stained, and examined. Tissue obtained with the biopsy forceps is placed in formalin for submission to a pathologist.

Epistaxis is the major complication of rhinoscopy. It is rarely serious but makes further endoscopic evaluation difficult because the field of vision is obscured by the blood.

LARYNGOSCOPY

There is no substitute for direct laryngoscopy in animals suspected of having laryngeal disease. Clinical signs that should alert the veterinarian include noisy breathing (particularly upon exertion), significant change in sound production (bark, meow, or purr), inspiratory dyspnea, and stridor.

A mouth speculum and conventional intubating laryngoscope† are adequate for illumination and visualization of the larynx. Laryngoscopy is used to note abnormalities in the shape, color, and motility of the larynx. In assessing laryngeal function (i.e., arytenoid cartilage *abduction*), it is important to observe laryngeal movement with the animal under a light plane of anesthesia. Short-acting intravenous anesthetic agents allow the larynx to be examined closely for shape and color, and intrinsic laryngeal motor functions are assessed as the animal awakens. Subtle abnormalities in laryngeal function will be overlooked if the larynx is examined only under deep planes of anesthesia.

TRACHEOBRONCHOSCOPY

Tracheobronchoscopy is performed whenever it is necessary to directly visualize the tracheobronchial tree and obtain appropriate specimens. Major indications for diagnostic bronchoscopy include chronic persistent coughing, hemoptysis, suspicion of foreign body aspiration or obstructing secretions, and pulmonary parenchymal disease of unknown cause. Bronchoscopy is valuable in obtaining brush catheter specimens for cytologic examination and mucosal biopsies for histopathology.

Equipment may vary from moderately expensive rigid fiberoptic bronchoscopes‡ to the flexible fiberoptic bronchoscopes,§ which are often cost prohibitive for the veterinary practitioner. With the advent of newer, less expensive fiberoptic endoscopes, they will be used more routinely for diagnosis of respiratory problems. Brush catheters and biopsy forceps‖ are relatively inexpensive and are used with both rigid and flexible endoscopes.

Tracheobronchoscopy requires that the patient be maintained under general anesthesia. Intravenous anesthetic agents and a mouth speculum will allow a thorough tracheobronchial examination with a rigid bronchoscope passed through the mouth. The trachea, carina, mainstem bronchi, and, to a limited degree, the lobar bronchi can all be adequately examined with a rigid bronchoscope. Brush catheters, biopsy forceps, and suction cannulas may be passed through the lumen of the rigid bronchoscope to obtain specimens.

The transoral approach with a flexible fiberoptic bronchoscope inserted through an endotracheal tube is routinely used by the author. The patient is anesthetized using standard procedures, intubated, and maintained on inhalation anesthesia. An endotracheal tube "Y" adapter allows oxygen and anes-

---

*Medi-Tech, Watertown, MA.

†Hook-on Laryngoscope and Handle, Welch Allyn Inc., Skaneateles Falls, NY.

‡Holinger Ventilating Fiberoptic Bronchoscope, Pilling Co., Fort Washington, PA.

§Olympus BF-2TR Bronchofiberscope, Olympus Corp., New Hyde Park, NY.

‖Medi-Tech, Watertown, MA.

thetic to flow to the patient while the flexible endoscope passes through the endotracheal tube and into the trachea. This technique is successful in moderate- to large-sized dogs and adequately maintains oxygenation and anesthesia even during lengthy procedures. Smaller dogs are given an intravenous anesthetic, and the flexible endoscope is passed directly into the trachea.

The distal tip of the endoscope is gently maneuvered so that the entire tracheal lumen is examined. The normal mucosa appears moist and pinkish, with minimal mucous secretions. A network of fine, thread-like submucosal blood vessels and tracheal cartilage rings are readily visualized. The dorsal tracheal membrane is usually taut but may become pendulous in such diseases as tracheal collapse. In the distal trachea the carina is recognized as a sharp bifurcation, with the mainstem bronchi opening on either side. The right mainstem bronchus usually appears slightly larger than the left and serves as a landmark. A thorough systematic inspection is made of all accessible parts of the bronchial tree, beginning in the right side. If, however, the thoracic radiographs reveal that a disease process is confined to one side of the lung, then the normal side of the bronchial tree is examined first. Abnormalities in shape, size, and color of the airways and the absence or presence of secretions are noted. Brush catheters and biopsy forceps are passed through the biopsy channel of the endoscope to obtain specimens for further evaluation.

Tracheobronchoscopy can be performed in the cat but is more difficult than in the dog. Both short-acting intravenous anesthetics and ketamine are used for the procedure. The larynx is sprayed or swabbed with a local anesthetic because of the tendency for the cat to develop severe laryngospasm. A small diameter rigid fiberoptic endoscope* is used to examine the trachea and carina, but extensive examination of the lobar bronchi is difficult. Brush catheters are passed through an outer cannula that surrounds the endoscope to obtain specimens for cytology.

Complications of tracheobronchoscopy are minimal. During anesthesia, an adequate source of oxygen to the patient must be maintained at all times. Endobronchial hemorrhage caused by the biopsy procedures rarely is a serious problem.

The advantages of tracheobronchoscopy are numerous when compared with other diagnostic techniques. Endoscopy allows the direct visualization of the tracheobronchial tree and the lesions associated with various respiratory diseases. This evaluation allows a better assessment of the patient's clinical status and prognosis. The cytologic preparations obtained by mucosal brushings through the endoscope are superior to those obtained from transtra-

cheal washing and aspiration. This increases the value of cytology in the diagnosis of respiratory diseases. Endoscopy also allows specific mucosal lesions to be biopsied under direct observation. Because of passage through the oropharynx, bacterial cultures obtained via bronchoscopes have been considered unreliable in the past. A new commercially available catheter† has been developed that enhances the ability to obtain reliable cultures of lower airway secretions through a bronchoscope.

Interpretation of small mucosal biopsies from the respiratory tract is difficult. Specimens are best submitted to a commerical veterinary or human laboratory for evaluation.

LUNG BIOPSY

Five fundamental methods of pulmonary biopsy are currently available in human and veterinary medicine. These methods include (1) percutaneous transthoracic aspiration biopsy using a fine gauge needle; (2) percutaneous transthoracic punch biopsy using various cutting needles such as the Vim-Silverman, Franklin-Silverman, Tru-Cut,‡ and Lee§ soft tissue biopsy needles; (3) trephine biopsy using a high-speed air drill; (4) transbronchoscopic lung biopsy through a rigid or flexible bronchoscope; and (5) open thoracotomy. The choice of one of these methods depends primarily on the location and type of lesion, the clinical status of the patient, equipment availability, and expertise of the clinician.

Percutaneous fine needle aspiration biopsy of the lung has been used for many years in human medicine. The procedure was introduced by Leyden in 1883 for the diagnosis of bacterial pneumonia and expanded by Menetrier in 1886 with the diagnosis of a pulmonary carcinoma. The technique was reported in the English literature in 1909 as a valuable new application of clinical pathology. Since these early enthusiastic reports, there has been intermittent interest in this procedure. In the last two decades, interest in percutaneous aspiration biopsy as a routine diagnostic procedure has increased. Recent experience based on aspiration needle biopsy of a large series of human patients indicated the technique was 96 per cent successful in diagnosing malignant neoplasms and 77 per cent successful in culturing infectious agents from immunosuppressed patients with focal pneumonic infiltrates. This section will review the pulmonary fine needle aspiration biopsy technique and discuss the advantages, disadvantages, indications, contraindi-

---

*Needlescope, Dyonics Inc., Aurora, IL.

†Microbiology Specimen Brush, Medi-Tech, Watertown, MA.
‡Tru-Cut Disposable Biopsy Needle, Travenol Laboratories, Inc., Deerfield, IL.
§Lee Soft Tissue Biopsy Needle, Becton-Dickinson, Rutherford, NJ.

cations, and complications of this technique versus other forms of pulmonary biopsy.

Indications for fine needle aspiration biopsy are (1) investigation of solitary circumscribed nodular pulmonary lesions of unknown etiology; (2) confirmation of the presence of metastatic disease; (3) procurement of material for microbial culture; and (4) evaluation of diffuse or disseminated pulmonary parenchymal disease. These nodules and lesions may be associated with clinical signs or may appear on routine thoracic radiographs. Fine needle aspiration biopsy is best performed after other routine diagnostic procedures such as hematologic studies, thoracic radiographs, and transtracheal aspiration have proved negative. The procedure is also indicated in those patients who are considered poor surgical risks for open thoracotomy and biopsy.

Contraindications for the procedure are not numerous but are very important. The contraindications include any coagulopathy or bleeding diathesis, severe uncontrolled coughing, an uncooperative patient, pulmonary hypertension, pulmonary cysts, and severe bullous emphysema. Coagulopathies and pulmonary hypertension considerably increase the risk of serious intrapulmonary, intrapleural, or endobronchial hemorrhage. Coagulation tests and platelet counts should be performed prior to pulmonary biopsy procedures, as hemostatic abnormalities often accompany disseminated neoplasia or infection. The author has utilized the activated coagulation time (ACT) test as a simple, inexpensive coagulation test prior to a variety of biopsy procedures and believes that results obtained with ACT have correlated well with other coagulation tests. Even after correction of a coagulation abnormality, subsequent biopsies should be approached with marked caution. An uncooperative patient or one with an uncontrollable cough increases the chances of pulmonary laceration by the biopsy needle. Bullous emphysema may predispose the patient to severe pneumothorax.

The technique of percutaneous fine needle aspiration biopsy is initiated by localizing the lesion with appropriate lateral, ventrodorsal, and dorsoventral thoracic radiographs. The location of a focal lesion will determine where the needle will enter the thorax. In the presence of disseminated disease with diffuse lesions, biopsy of the thickest portion of the pulmonary parenchyma is advocated. This results in the greatest probability of obtaining material and the lowest likelihood of striking other vital structures. For these reasons, the caudal and dorsal lung lobe regions are recommended. The caudal lung lobes are entered in most dogs and cats between the seventh and ninth intercostal space approximately two-thirds of the distance from the costochondral junction to the vertebral bodies.

The patient should be in a lateral or sternal position for the procedure. It is important for the patient to remain calm yet alert. Heavy sedation may be necessary but is usually contraindicated because the sedated patient cannot clear respiratory secretions or endobronchial hemorrhage, which may result from the biopsy procedure. The use of a reversible narcotic-analgesic agent may be beneficial.

The biopsy site is clipped and prepared with an appropriate disinfectant or germicidal solution and is surgically draped. The skin, subcutaneous tissue, muscle, and parietal pleura are all infiltrated with 1 to 2 per cent lidocaine. The entire procedure should be performed aseptically. A small stab incision is made through the skin and subcutaneous tissue. The author generally uses a standard thin-walled 20- or 22-gauge diamond point spinal needle with stylet.* The biopsy needle is advanced through the chest wall on the cranial edge of the rib to avoid the intercostal vessels.

For a focal lesion, the needle (with stylet in place) is guided under fluoroscopic control to the margin of the lesion. For diffuse lesions, the needle is advanced into the pulmonary parenchyma of the caudal lobes approximately 1 to 3 cm. Once the lesion has been entered, the stylet of the needle is withdrawn and a 10- to 20-ml syringe is quickly attached to the needle. The gloved finger should always occlude the needle hub until the syringe is attached to prevent air-to-lung communication. While applying continuous suction, the needle tip is moved back and forth over a 0.5- to 1.0-cm distance several times using a jabbing and rotating motion. The simultaneous advancement and rotational movements cut a sharp core of tissue. An alternate method is to maintain the needle in one location and make several vigorous suction movements with the syringe. The needle is then withdrawn, maintaining moderate suction to hold the specimen in the needle and to avoid leaving the tissue along the tract. The skin and subcutaneous tissues are gently massaged to prevent air from entering the pleural space. After disconnecting the needle and refilling the syringe with air, the needle is reconnected and the aspirated material is blown onto clean glass slides, smeared, and stained for cytologic examination. When samples must be evaluated by an outside laboratory, it is best to check with the laboratory on their preferred submission format. If a small core of tissue is identified, it is transferred to 10 per cent formalin solution for subsequent histologic study. The needle may also be flushed with sterile saline for microbiologic culture.

The number of lung punctures is variable, usually ranging from one to five per patient or as many as are needed to obtain sufficient material. Most pa-

---

*Monoject Spinal Needle, Sherwood Medical Industries, St. Louis, MO.

tients require only one or two punctures. If several punctures fail to yield material, then a small amount of sterile saline is injected into the lesion before aspiration is performed. This is especially valuable when a culture is needed.

The patient should be observed closely for signs of pneumothorax or other complications. Routine thoracic radiographs immediately and 24 hours after the procedure are suggested. If a pneumothorax occurs after the first biopsy procedure, chest drainage should be considered before the procedure is repeated.

Complications of percutaneous fine needle aspiration biopsy of the lung in humans are common and are potentially serious. Complications reported in humans include hemoptysis, hemorrhagic pleural effusion, subcutaneous emphysema, pneumothorax, intrapulmonary hemorrhage and hematoma, fatal air embolism, fatal endobronchial hemorrhage, implantation of pulmonary tumor along the biopsy tract, and biopsy of an organ other than the lung.

In a series of several thousand cases, hemoptysis occurred in 0 to 35 per cent of human patients who underwent percutaneous needle aspiration. The hemoptysis was usually transient and self-limiting. Occasionally, intrapulmonary hemorrhage or hematomas were revealed on post-biopsy radiographs but never caused clinical signs. Hemorrhagic pleural effusion and subcutaneous emphysema are infrequent. Fatal endobronchial hemorrhage has also been reported as a complication in several human patients. Biopsy of another organ such as the diaphragm or spleen rarely occurs.

The primary complication of percutaneous fine needle lung biopsy is pneumothorax. Detectable pneumothorax has been reported to occur in 6.1 to 51 per cent of human patients during the post-biopsy period. Most of the pneumothoraces were small and asymptomatic and resolved spontaneously. Pneumothorax of a serious nature requiring insertion of a chest tube for drainage occurred in 1.5 to 14 per cent of human patients in these same clinical studies. Fatal air embolism has also occurred in human patients as a result of air-to-pulmonary vein communication when severe coughing occurs during the procedure. Empyema has never been a serious complication in aspiration of lobar pneumonia even before the advent of antibiotics.

Limitations of the fine needle aspiration technique include the inability to study parenchymal structures. The use of cutting needles increases the chance of obtaining a core of pulmonary tissue. Agreement on the value of cutting needle biopsies is lacking. Many believe that cutting needle biopsy should be abandoned altogether, whereas others continue to support its use. In the author's experi-

ence, cutting needle percutaneous biopsy has been associated with an increased incidence of serious complications including two cases of fatal tension pneumothorax. In general, cutting needle core biopsies are considered to have higher morbidity and mortality with essentially the same diagnostic accuracy as aspiration biopsy. *Percutaneous cutting needle biopsy should be restricted to large lesions adjacent to the thoracic wall when aspirations are inconclusive.*

The new technique of high speed trephine biopsy has been used in humans, horses, and dogs. It has the advantages of providing a fairly large and non-distorted tissue sample. Disadvantages include failure to obtain adequate tissue and unacceptably high morbidity and mortality rates. *The technique is not recommended for use in dogs.*

The newest pulmonary biopsy technique is the transbronchial biopsy obtained through the flexible or rigid fiberoptic bronchoscope. Special forceps are used to remove a section of the bronchial wall and underlying pulmonary parenchyma. Transbronchoscopic lung biopsy should present less hazard than percutaneous lung biopsy, since the pleural surface remains intact. However, the technique does require general anesthesia and special equipment. Complications in humans are apparently rare but include pneumothorax, hemoptysis, and fatal endobronchial hemorrhage. To the author's knowledge, no clinical studies of transbronchial biopsy have been completed in the dog or cat at this time.

Open thoracotomy should be reserved for those cases in which the lesion appears resectable, when large amounts of tissue need to be obtained under direct visualization, and when all other diagnostic tests have failed to supply a satisfactory diagnosis. Mortality with open lung biopsy in human patients ranges from 1.5 to 4.0 per cent.

In the author's experience, percutaneous transthoracic fine needle aspiration biopsy is a rapid and relatively safe method of obtaining material for further diagnostic study. The risk of the technique must be weighed against the risks of other biopsy alternatives and failure to establish a definitive diagnosis.

SUPPLEMENTAL READING

Creighton, S. R., and Wilkins, R. J.: Transtracheal aspiration biopsy: technique and cytologic evaluation. J. Am. Anim. Hosp. Assoc. 10:219, 1974.

Reif, J.S.: Lung and pleural biopsy. Vet. Clin. North Am. 4:363, 1974.

Roudebush, P., Green, R. A., and Digilio, K. M.: Percutaneous fine-needle aspiration biopsy of the lung in disseminated pulmonary disease. J. Am. Anim. Hosp. Assoc. 17:109, 1981.

Schall, W. D.: Thoracentesis. Vet. Clin. North Am. 4:396, 1974

Venker-van Haagen, A. J.: Bronchoscopy of the normal and abnormal canine. J. Am. Anim. Hosp. Assoc. 15:397, 1979.

MANAGEMENT OF CHRONIC
UPPER AIRWAY DISEASE

RICHARD B. FORD, D.V.M.

Raleigh, North Carolina

The upper respiratory tract of dogs and cats is a twisting, irregularly contoured conduit extending from the nares to the glottis. The nasal portion of the upper respiratory tract extends from the nares to the choanae and is divided into two symmetric chambers by a cartilaginous wall termed the "nasal septum." The two nasal chambers house the delicate turbinated bones or conchae. The frontal sinuses are paired, air-filled chambers that communicate with the corresponding nasal chamber by the small (nasofrontal) opening. The maxillary "sinus" of the dog and cat is, in fact, a maxillary recess. It is of minor clinical importance compared with the frontal sinuses. In addition to the frontal sinuses, the cat also has a sphenoid sinus.

Although the function of the paranasal sinuses is not precisely known, it has been suggested that the sinuses may enhance respiratory efficiency by dampening the surge of pressure within the nasal cavity twice during each respiratory cycle. It has also been suggested that the paranasal sinuses serve no purpose whatsoever.

The physiologic role of the nose should be more completely understood. Fundamentally, the nose functions (1) as a control mechanism for matching the supply of air with the need for alveolar ventilation, (2) to warm, humidify, and filter the inspired air, and, (3) to resist invasion by pathogenic organisms (Williams, 1973).

Perhaps the most notable trait for which the canine nose has been credited is olfaction. However, the nose merely houses the olfactory membrane in which bipolar nerve cells, the receptor cells for olfaction, are located. The anatomic relationship between the nose and the olfactory membrane has clinical implications that must not be overlooked in the small animal patient. Damage or destruction to the olfactory membrane subsequent to chronic upper respiratory disease can result in transient or even permanent anosmia. Loss of such a highly developed sense can be expected to have significant impact on normal behavior, e.g., breeding, hunting, and even appetite.

The approach to clinical management of upper respiratory diseases is largely determined by the duration and severity of clinical signs. Although both of these factors are subject to the client's ability to accurately observe and communicate historical information, the clinician should categorize as chronic any upper respiratory disease with clinical signs that persist in excess of four weeks. This necessarily includes animals that are reported to have intermittent, paroxysmal signs and animals that experience resolution during therapy only to relapse upon cessation of therapy. The clinician should not overlook the dog or cat that presents with episodic signs that have an apprently acute onset but are, in fact, of chronic duration.

SIGNS OF UPPER RESPIRATORY DISEASE

Certain clinical signs, whether observed by the owner or seen during physical examination, are unique to the upper respiratory tract. To the extent possible, clinical signs of upper respiratory disease should be used to localize the upper airway segment involved. Persistent sneezing with or without a nasal discharge is indicative of irritation to the nasal mucosa; the inciting cause may be primary intranasal disease or secondary to an active disease in a paranasal sinus or the oral cavity.

Stertor is an audible snorting sound for which an owner may seek veterinary attention. Paroxysms of stertorous breathing, occasionally referred to as reverse sneezing, may occur intermittently over several months. Signs are associated with the animal's attempt to displace the material from the nasopharynx into the oropharynx. A thorough examination of the oral cavity and pharynx is warranted in these patients.

Epistaxis is the visible manifestation of nasal bleeding and is commonly associated with chronic nasal disease. The absence of gross or historical evidence of epistaxis does not rule out nasal bleeding tendencies. Blood in the posterior nasal cavity or pharynx is likely to be swallowed; this may present as hematemesis or melena. Patients known to have epistaxis should receive a thorough visual and radiographic examination of the nose. Patients having severe or persistent epistaxis should be evaluated for a possible clotting disorder.

Sonorous, or noisy, respirations may result from partial obstruction of one or both nostrils. Most dogs and cats are unwilling to mouth breathe despite increased upper airway resistance, even to the point of becoming dyspneic. A visual examination of each nostril, rhinoscopy, nasal radiography, and contrast rhinography may be used to diagnose the cause of obstruction.

MODES OF THERAPY

AEROSOL THERAPY

The use of aerosol therapy in the treatment of respiratory disease in companion animals has only recently received attention in the veterinary literature. Aerosol therapy does permit the introduction of particulate suspensions of a liquid, such as saline or antibiotics, into the lower airways. The efficacy of aerosol therapy in treating specific respiratory diseases has not been established; however, it appears that it may have an important application in the adjunct therapy of lower respiratory tract diseases (see article entitled Principles of Respiratory Therapy).

The role of aerosol therapy in the treatment of *upper* airway disease has not been investigated. However, the inability to effectively distribute drugs onto the extensive surface area of the upper respiratory epithelium and the inability to transport particulate suspensions of liquid into or through an obstructed upper airway would appear to limit the routine application of aerosol therapy in management of upper airway disease.

Humidification of inspired air may, on the other hand, offer significant advantages in managing animals with chronic upper respiratory disease. This is particularly true when the absolute humidity of the inspired air is very low. Drying of the nasal respiratory epithelium results in impaired ciliary activity, increased viscosity of nasal secretions, and decreased resistance to bacterial invasion. It follows that humidification of dry air should not only enhance recovery of animals with upper respiratory infections but should also have a significant prophylactic effect. However, the role of humidification therapy in treating upper airway disease has not been established.

TOPICAL THERAPY

There are three classes of topical drugs commonly used in the treatment of upper respiratory disease in animals: nasal decongestants, corticosteroids, and antibiotics. Topical nasal decongestants have not been licensed for use in dogs or cats. Yet this class of topical drug does provide significant benefit in the management of chronic upper airway disease. The sympathomimetic action of nasal decongestants results in arteriolar vasoconstriction of the vessels supplying the nasal mucosa. Nasal congestion, or edema, is reduced as blood flow into the tissues decreases. The net effect is decreased resistance to air movement. Decongestion of nasal passages also

permits drainage of secretions from the frontal sinuses. Relief of clinical signs in animals with bilateral rhinologic disorders occurs rapidly whether the congestion is due to inflammation, infection, or trauma. Although topical nasal decongestants are of limited therapeutic value in small animals, they can substantially aid in the management of chronic upper respiratory disease.

Prolonged use of topical nasal decongestants can lead to chronic reactive hyperemia of the nasal mucosa, called *aftercongestion*. This problem can be avoided in animals by administering the drug into alternate nostrils at two- to three-day intervals.

Corticosteroid solutions can be absorbed from the nasal mucosa. However, the amount of steroid absorbed varies with the volume administered, concentration, potency, vehicle, duration and frequency of treatment, surface area of tissue treated, metabolism of the drug, and the integrity of the epithelial barrier. Although clinical hypercorticism is reportedly rare in humans treated with topical steroids, there are few, if any, indications for its use. Likewise, there are no known indications for the use of topical steroids in managing chronic upper respiratory disease in animals.

After a series of experiments in dogs, Wilson (1915) stated that (1) no chronic bacterial inflammation can occur in a sinus (or nasal chamber) unless its physiologic defense mechanisms are disturbed or destroyed; and (2) it is not the physical presence of bacteria in the lumen or even in its lymph or blood vascular system that induces chronic infection but the functional condition of the tissue on which the bacteria are implanted that influences the future course of disease. These axioms are applicable even today. Although chronic bacterial infections of the upper airways do occur, they should be considered secondary to one or more predisposing conditions, e.g., viral or fungal rhinitis. Intranasal antibacterial therapy may be effective in decreasing bacterial numbers and ameliorating clinical signs of upper respiratory disease during the course of treatment. Sustained improvement following cessation of treatment should not be expected. The extent of systemic penetration of intranasally administered antibiotics has not been fully evaluated. Antibiotics applied directly to the nasal epithelium do not have a significant effect on the course of chronic upper airway disease, even when mixed bacterial populations are present.

SYSTEMIC THERAPY

The most conventional method of managing upper respiratory disease is with parenterally or orally administered medications, particularly broad spectrum antibiotics. The high incidence of secondary bacterial infections in animals with chronic upper respiratory disorders justifies the use of antibiotics. Although the clinical signs are not likely to resolve subsequent to antibiotic therapy, the severity of associated clinical signs, the quantity of nasal discharge, and the risk of septicemia may be reduced.

Systemic therapy with corticosteroids often decreases or eliminates the signs of upper respiratory disease, at least transiently. Arbitrary administration of steroids to animals with undiagnosed fungal or viral disease is likely to have disastrous consequences. Furthermore, prolonged corticosteroid therapy may actually predispose an animal to chronic upper or lower respiratory disease. In humans, systemic and topical corticosteroids are used to treat allergic and vasomotor rhinitis and nasal polyps. At this time, the role of systemic corticosteroid therapy in the management of chronic upper respiratory disease of dogs and cats should be restricted to known noninfectious diseases, e.g., neoplasia and allergy.

DISEASES OF THE NASAL CHAMBERS AND FRONTAL SINUSES

NASAL TUMORS

In older dogs (average nine to ten years of age) signs of chronic rhinitis are most commonly associated with neoplasia. The incidence of nasal tumors is reportedly highest in dolicocephalic breeds and lowest in brachycephalic breeds. However, not all studies support this finding. Interestingly, nasal tumors are rarely reported in the giant and miniature breeds. Carcinomas are reported approximately twice as often as sarcomas.

Nasal tumors typically do not metastasize. Instead, invasion of turbinates, frontal sinuses, pharynx, and regional lymph nodes is more characteristic. Untreated, clinical signs are almost always progressive. When present, mucopurulent nasal discharges and epistaxis often resolve in response to systemic antibiotic therapy. This transient improvement may give the false impression of having effectively treated an undiagnosed rhinitis.

Since clinical signs may develop over a period of one to five months, early detection of nasal tumors is unlikely. Once the diagnosis has been confirmed, clinical management should consist of radical surgical curettage followed by cryosurgery or radiotherapy (Gillette, 1976). The role of immunotherapy and chemotherapy in the management of nasal neoplasia has not been completely established. It should be emphasized, however, that surgery alone is not effective in accomplishing long-term remissions.

MYCOTIC RHINOSINUSITIS

Several reports of mycotic rhinosinusitis have been published in the veterinary literature (Barrett and Scott, 1975). Colonization of *Aspergillus fumi-*

gatus in the nasal cavity and paranasal sinuses is the most common cause of mycotic rhinosinusitis in dogs. Clinical signs include unilateral or bilateral nasal discharge and paroxysmal sneezing. Signs are usually not responsive to systemic antibiotic therapy. Owing to the similarity of clinical signs, it is important that mycotic rhinitis be distinguished from neoplastic rhinitis. Although the clinical signs are similar, the treatment and prognosis are quite different. Canine aspergillosis is discussed in more detail in the following article.

Fatalities associated with pulmonary aspergillosis in cats have been reported. However, chronic rhinosinusitis caused by *A. fumigatus* has not been reported in cats.

Systemic *Cryptococcus neoformans* infection occurs in humans and in several species of animals. Cryptococcosis in dogs and cats characteristically involves the lung and central nervous system; localized infections of the nasal cavity, sinuses, and pharynx also occur (Barrett and Scott, 1975). Chronic, often copious, mucoid nasal discharges with sneezing and stertorous breathing are typical signs seen in dogs and cats with nasal and sinus infections. Lesions limited to the pharyngeal mucosa may not be associated with overt clinical signs. Cryptococcosis is the most common cause of mycotic rhinosinusitis in cats.

Two drugs, amphotericin B* and 5-fluorocytosine (5-FC),† have been used to treat nasal cryptococcosis in animals. 5-FC, an antimetabolite, inhibits nucleic acid synthesis in susceptible fungi but is not metabolized by mammalian cells. Unlike amphotericin B, 5-FC is readily absorbed from the intestinal tract and is not nephrotoxic. Dosages of 200 mg/kg/day, divided t.i.d. or q.i.d., are recommended for dogs and cats. However, relapses subsequent to the development of resistant organisms have been reported in animals and humans treated with 5-FC. Resistance may not be overcome by using larger dosages. In such cases, it has been necessary to change to amphotericin B. Amphotericin B is a polyene antibiotic that is effective in treating cryptococcosis as well as several systemic fungal infections. Despite its nephrotoxic properties, amphotericin B appears to be somewhat more effective in achieving cures than 5-FC. This is particularly true in cats.

Amphotericin B is given by either slow intravenous drip or rapid intravenous infusion. Combined with 5 per cent dextrose and water as a vehicle, the recommended dosage of amphotericin B is 0.5 mg/kg in dogs and 0.25 mg/kg in cats. The calculated dose is administered intravenously three days a week. Renal function should be monitored at least weekly throughout the course of therapy.

A stock solution is prepared by adding 10 ml of sterile water (without preservative) to a single 50-

---

*Fungizone, E. R. Squibb & Sons, Inc., Princeton, NJ.
†Ancobon, Hoffman-LaRoche, Inc., Nutley, NJ.

mg vial of crystalline amphotericin B. When reconstituted properly, the solution will be clear yellow. If the solution is too acidic or contains electrolytes (i.e., saline or lactated Ringer's solution), precipitation will occur. When not in use, the stock solution should be refrigerated and protected from direct light, thereby avoiding loss of potency and precipitation. If precipitation does occur, the solution should be discarded.

RAPID INTRAVENOUS INFUSION

This method is the most popular one for administrating amphotericin B. It is rapid, effective, can be completed on an outpatient basis, and is most economically feasible.

The entire stock solution (50 mg) of amphotericin B is added to 190 ml of 5 per cent dextrose and water, yielding a concentration of 0.25 mg/ml. In dogs, 1.0 ml/kg body weight of this solution (0.25 mg/kg amphotericin B) is given intravenously on day 1. The dose is administered over a three- to five-minute period. On day 3, 1.5 ml/kg body weight of stock solution (0.38 mg/kg amphotericin B) is similarly administered. On day 5, 2.0 ml/kg body weight of solution (0.5 mg/kg amphotericin B) is given. The last-named dose is administered three days a week until a minimum of 12 doses have been given. By gradually increasing the total daily dose for the first five days, azotemia may be avoided during the initial phase of treatment.

SLOW INTRAVENOUS DRIP

This method of treatment involves daily administration of amphotericin B at the same dosage levels as those described for the rapid intravenous infusion. However, the calculated daily dose is withdrawn from the stock solution and administered in 200 to 500 ml of 5 per cent dextrose in water. This is administered over a four- to six-hour period.

The rapid infusion technique is timely and cost efficient; however, the diluted stock solution (50 mg in 250 ml of 5 per cent dextrose and water) is more likely to precipitate during storage than is the undiluted stock solution (50 mg in 10 ml sterile water). The slow drip method requires hospitalization, thereby permitting closer monitoring of the patient during treatment. This advantage may be outweighed by the additional cost and prolonged catheterization. Neither method of administration has been shown to be more effective or safer than the other.

The same treatment regimen is used in treating cats with cryptococcosis; however, the total volume of solution should be adjusted so that the total maximum daily dosage of amphotericin B is 0.25 mg/kg.

With either 5-FC or amphotericin B, therapy typically continues for as long as two months. However, there are no rules that dictate when therapy should be discontinued. Treatment must be discontinued when evidence of impaired renal function exists. Resumption of therapy is based on the animal's physical appearance, willingness to eat, and a BUN of less than 75 mg/dl. Since secondary bacterial rhinosinusitis typically occurs in animals with nasal cryptococcosis, oral antibiotic therapy is justified.

Cryptococcosis may be predominantly a secondary disease. Chronic diseases (feline leukemia, lymphosarcoma) and immunosuppressive therapy may predispose an animal to infection with *C. neoformans*. Therefore, it is possible to successfully treat a patient for cryptococcosis only to have it succumb to a primary, underlying disorder. Furthermore, infections with *C. neoformans* are not restricted to the upper airways. Systemic infections are likely. Obviously, the prognosis for animals with cryptococcosis must be guarded.

DENTAL DISEASE

Clinical signs of chronic rhinitis may be caused by the extension of infections originating in the maxillary teeth. This is particularly true of the incisors and canine teeth of dogs with chronic periodontal disease. Subsequent to bacterial colonization in and around the periodontal ligament of the affected tooth, oronasal fistulas may develop secondary to osteomyelitis of the apical bone. Paroxysms of sneezing, sometimes associated with a blood-tinged serous nasal discharge, are characteristic signs. Fistulas are easily detected by probing the sulcus between the hard palate and the lingual side of the maxillary teeth. Using a polyethylene catheter as a probe, most animals may be examined without tranquilization or anesthesia. In the anesthetized patient, saline injected into the sulcus through the catheter can be seen as it drains from the nostril.

The most effective therapy entails extracting the affected tooth. Pre- and postoperative ampicillin (10 mg/kg) is prescribed orally, three times daily for a total of ten days. In lieu of extraction, curettage and vigorus flushing of the alveolus combined with a ten-day course of oral ampicillin can be attempted. If destruction of the periodontal ligament and surrounding tissue is not extensive, the periodontium will heal and the fistula will seal. The associated clinical signs will subsequently resolve.

CHRONIC FELINE SINUSITIS

Paroxysmal sneezing and a chronic bilateral mucopurulent nasal discharge, lasting months to years, in an otherwise healthy cat characterize chronic feline sinusitis. Clinical signs typically resolve during systemic antibiotic therapy only to reappear, unaltered, two to three days after discontinuing treatment. An impressive array of creative treatment regimens has been tried to put an end to this persistent catarrh. Yet, despite untold numbers of cats having been treated with intranasal antibiotics, steroids, astringents, enzymes, and so on, alone or in combination with systemic medications, we have given our clients and our patients little actual relief.

The clinical history of affected cats often includes previous experience with an acute onset, severe upper respiratory disease (Ford, 1979). With, and in some cases without, treatment the cat recovered only to develop signs of mild but chronic rhinosinusitis. Radiographs of the frontal sinuses show loss of the normal air density without bony destruction.

The nasal discharge of cats with chronic sinusitis is responsive to antibiotics; cytology reveals mixed bacterial populations and numerous neutrophils. However, it is unlikely that this condition is primarily bacterial in origin. Colonization of bacteria occurs in the nasal and sinus epithelium secondary to previous injury, either traumatic or viral. Cats recovered from viral upper respiratory disease are at greater risk of developing chronic rhinosinusitis.

Medical treatment is the recommended method for managing chronic feline rhinosinusitis. Ampicillin (20 mg/kg) is given three times daily for a minimum of three weeks. This is supplemented by a nasal decongestant (0.025 per cent oxymethazoline HCl: Afrin Pediatric Nasal Drops*). One or two drops are delivered into one nostril once daily for five days. If signs persist, the drops are continued for an additional five days in the other nostril.

The surgical approach to chronic feline rhinosinusitis offers no documented benefit over medical management. Surgery has been limited to exposing the frontal sinuses, removing the mucous membrane, and implanting autogenous fat into the sinus space. However, the syndrome of chronic frontal sinusitis in cats is not likely to be limited to the sinus membrane. Affected cats typically have involvement of the nasal epithelium and turbinate bones. In addition, otitis media may also be present.

The common term "chronic frontal sinusitis" may be somewhat of a misnomer. Chronic rhinosinusitis is more appropriate. This is supported by the fact that clinical signs persist in many cats following surgical obliteration of the frontal sinuses.

TRAUMA

Since the nose is the most prominent facial feature in most breeds, chronic rhinosinusitis secondary to trauma, particularly bite wounds and foreign bodies, is common in both dogs and cats. The clinical signs become chronic not as a result of improper treatment but as a result of failure of owners to seek veterinary attention soon after the injury is sustained. Fractures to bone and cartilage forming the nose and sinuses favor colonization of bacteria, with resultant sneezing and nasal discharge. The medical treatment for traumatic rhinosinusitis is similar to that outlined for feline rhinosinusitis. Malformations, sequestra, and obstructive sinus mucocele are complications stemming from facial fractures. Surgical exploration is warranted in these cases if response to systemic antibiotics and topical decongestants is not satisfactory.

DISEASES OF THE PHARYNX

The pharynx of the dog and cat has three anatomic subdivisions: (1) the nasopharynx, which lies directly behind the nasal cavities and above the soft palate, (2) the oropharynx, which lies posterior to the oral cavity beneath the lower margin of the soft palate, and (3) the hypopharynx, also called the laryngopharynx, which is a recess in the posterior pharyngeal wall that partially surrounds the larynx. The nasopharynx communicates with the oropharynx via the pharyngeal isthmus.

The pharynx communicates with the nasal cavities, the middle ear via the eustachian tubes, the oral cavity, the larynx, and the esophagus. As a common pathway for both respiration and alimentation, the pharynx is particularly subject to injury from ingested or inhaled foreign material. In addition to foreign bodies, congenital anomalies and neoplasia account for the majority of chronic pharyngeal disorders seen in small animals. Dysphagia, anorexia, drooling, and stertor are the most common clinical signs associated with pharyngeal disease. Animals with chronic pharyngeal diseases should be anesthetized for both visual and radiographic examination of the oral cavity and pharynx.

CONGENITAL ANOMALIES

Elongated soft palate is a common congenital anomaly causing signs of chronic pharyngeal disease. Signs are characterized by stertorous breathing and, occasionally, dyspnea. The condition is most common in brachycephalic breeds but can occur in mesocephalic breeds as well. The treatment for the elongated soft palate is surgery; the technique has been described (Knecht, 1979). Complete familiarity with the anatomic relationship of the soft palate with the larynx and the glottis of the normal dog is necessary before attempting any soft palate

---

*Schering Corp, Kenilworth, NJ.

surgery. During the examination, the patient should be anesthetized and placed in sternal recumbency. The pharynx should be thoroughly examined without the endotracheal tube in place. The neck should not be supported or handled during the examination. The elongated soft palate will tend to enter the glottis, particularly during inspiration. The normal soft palate should not contact the arytenoid cartilages of the larynx. Excessive shortening of the soft palate is likely to predispose the patient to aspiration pneumonia.

FOREIGN BODIES

A variety of foreign objects are capable of becoming lodged in the pharynx and retropharyngeal tissues of both dogs and cats. Occasionally, clinical signs become chronic. Visual and radiographic examination of the pharynx in the anesthetized patient usually yields the diagnosis. Careful extraction of the foreign material and adequate drainage of the site usually result in prompt resolution of clinical signs. Surgery is necessary on occasion to remove a foreign object from the retropharyngeal tissues (e.g., porcupine quills, needles). Systemic antibiotic therapy is indicated when deep penetration of the retropharyngeal tissues has occurred.

NEOPLASIA

In both dogs and cats, tumors of the pharynx are reported less often than tumors of the mouth and larynx. Squamous cell carcinoma appears as an ulcerated lesion of the pharyngeal epithelium. Occasionally, metastasis to regional lymph nodes occurs.

By the time pharyngeal tumors have been recognized, surgical excision may not be possible. Several regimens of therapy have been attempted with variable results. Cryotherapy has been used with some success in treating oral tumors. The feasibility of treating pharyngeal tumors with cryotherapy has not been described. Radiation therapy has been used with some success in treating squamous cell carcinomas in animals. Squamous cell carcinomas were controlled for at least one year in 34 per cent to 46 per cent of 52 dogs. Similar results were obtained in eight cats (Gillette, 1976). Results of chemotherapy in the treatment of oral pharyngeal neoplasia have not been favorable.

REFERENCES AND SUPPLEMENTAL READING

Barrett, R. E., and Scott, D. W.: Treatment of feline cryptococcosis: literature review and case report. J.A.A.H.A. 11:511, 1975.
Catter, S. M.: Oral pharyngeal neoplasms in the cat. J.A.A.H.A. 17:917, 1981.
Ford, R. B.: Feline viral upper respiratory disease: current concepts. Comp. Cont. Ed. Sm. Anim. Pract. 1:337, 1979.
Gillette, E. L.: Radiation therapy of canine and feline tumors. J.A.A.H.A. 12:359, 1976.
Knecht, C. D.: Upper airway obstruction in brachycephalic dogs. Comp. Cont. Ed. Sm. Anim. Pract. 1:24, 1979.
Williams, H. L.: Nasal physiology. *In* Paparella, M. M., and Shumrick, D. A.: *Otolaryngology*. Vol. 1. Philadelphia: W. B. Saunders, 1973, Chapter 9.
Wilson, J. G.: The etiology of pansinusitis. Laryngoscope 25:823, 1915.

NASAL ASPERGILLOSIS-PENICILLOSIS

COLIN E. HARVEY, M.R.C.V.S.,

and JOAN A. O'BRIEN, V.M.D.

Philadelphia, Pennsylvania

Aspergillosis and penicillosis are common and often severe diseases of the nasal cavity of the dog. Occasional cases have also been seen in cats. The diseases are almost always limited to the sinuses and nasal cavity in the dog; only 1 of 58 affected dogs was diagnosed as having disseminated aspergillosis at the Veterinary Hospital of the University of Pennsylvania (VHUP) between 1978 and 1981. Pulmonary or disseminated aspergillosis has been reported occasionally in cats. Nasal aspergillosis was first diagnosed in the 19th century and has been recognized worldwide. Penicillosis is less common and was documented only recently (Harvey et al., 1981). The two diseases can be separated only by culture or serologic testing, and both organisms may be grown from the same dog.

The following diagnoses were made in dogs presented at VHUP between 1978 and 1981 for investigation of the cause of their nasal discharge: nasal tumor in 42 per cent, confirmed or suspected aspergillosis and penicillosis in 34 per cent, other confirmed diagnoses in 10 per cent, and unknown diagnosis in 14 per cent.

Nasal and sinus aspergillosis in humans is usually associated with diseases or treatment methods that cause immune suppression. Immune suppression, usually T-cell deficiency, has been reported in dogs with nasal aspergillosis (Barrett et al., 1977). It has been found in most, although not all, dogs with aspergillosis tested at VHUP. However, there is usually no history in affected dogs of concurrent disease or treatment known to cause immune suppression. Fungal infections may cause immune suppression. Less than 10 per cent of dogs with aspergillosis-penicillosis seen at VHUP have a total lymphocyte count of less than 700, suggesting that immune suppression may be caused by the disease rather than existing as a primary abnormality with secondary infection by opportunistic fungal elements. There is no evidence that infected dogs endanger humans or other animals.

HISTORY AND CLINICAL SIGNS

Aspergillosis and penicillosis have been diagnosed in dogs of a wide variety of ages, from less than 1 year to more than 15 years. The range of breeds affected is equally wide, although brachycephalic breeds are infrequently represented, and collies are over-represented. Owners reported trauma to the nasal or head area prior to the onset of clinical signs in 19 per cent of affected dogs seen at VHUP.

Nasal discharge of some type is the only clinical sign common to all affected dogs and is usually the first sign noted by the owner. The discharge is unilateral throughout the course of the disease in about one-third of affected dogs and bilateral in the other two-thirds. In 10 per cent of dogs, the discharge is bloody only, sometimes presenting as profuse episodic epistaxis. Blood mixed with other kinds of discharge is seen in 45 per cent of cases. The nature and volume of the discharge may change, particularly with administration of antibiotics, as secondary bacterial infection is common. However, the beneficial effect of antibiotic administration is short-lived.

Other clinical signs, seen in about 50 per cent of affected dogs, are sneezing and noisy, snorting, or open-mouth breathing. Less common are cough, ocular discharge, exophthalmos, and facial or palatal swelling. Less than 10 per cent of affected dogs show signs of systemic illness such as loss of appetite and lethargy. An occasional animal presents with erosion of the frontal, nasal, maxillary, or palatine bones and a discharging skin or oral fistula.

With the exception of facial or palatal swelling present in 50 per cent of dogs with nasal tumors but in only 5 per cent of aspergillosis-penicillosis dogs seen at VHUP), the clinical signs in dogs with nasal tumors and aspergillosis-penicillosis are indistinguishable. Nasal discharge and sneezing caused by nasal irritation and snorting or mouth breathing due to nasal airway obstruction are nonspecific signs.

PHYSICAL EXAMINATION

With the exception of inspection and palpation for facial or palatal swelling, physical examination rarely provides information of value in the differential diagnosis. Discharge is usually obvious or may be seen following sneezing. Because of the slow growth of fungi on culture, it is advantageous to submit a sample of the discharge for fungal culture immediately. The nose may be painful, particularly the area of the external nares, because of crusting or excoriation associated with the discharge. The external shell of the nose and the palate are palpated for symmetry and areas of softness. The nasopharynx can be palpated through the soft palate in a cooperative dog. Both eyes are retropulsed to check for orbital encroachment.

Airflow through the nasal cavities is examined by looking for misting on a glass slide or movement of hair strands held in front of one nostril while the other is occluded and the mouth is held closed. A normal resting dog can breathe comfortably through one nostril. Percussion of the nasal cavity and sinuses is possible, although because of the wide variety of sizes and shapes of the face comparisons are rarely of benefit and gross dissimilarities between the two sides are the only observations that can be made. Auscultation of the nasal cavity may also show obvious differences between the two sides. The merit of evaluation of nasal airflow, percussion, and auscultation is mainly in establishing whether bilateral disease exists in a dog presented with a history of unilateral discharge.

Auscultation of the lower airway and lungs may be made difficult by the rattling noises referred from the pharynx and nose. Mandibular and cervical lymph nodes are enlarged and painful in a few cases. Rectal temperature varies from normal to 104°F, although persistent pyrexia is rare.

DIAGNOSIS

History and physical examination of a dog with nasal discharge usually suggest that the disease is limited to the nasal area but in the absence of facial swelling do not provide specific information with which to differentiate between neoplasia and fungal disease. In an occasional case, the history or type and periodicity of the discharge may suggest an alternative diagnosis such as allergic rhinitis. Occasionally, diagnosis is made easy because the owner brings in a piece of tissue that the animal has sneezed or coughed on.

Complete examination of the nose requires anesthesia. Diagnostic tests that do not require anesthesia include culture and serology. If tests of immune competence are to be run, the samples should be obtained prior to anesthesia or medical treatment. A therapeutic trial with antifungal medications may provide a presumptive diagnosis in some cases. Antibiotics often provide temporary benefit for an animal with nasal discharge of whatever cause but needlessly delay definitive diagnosis.

CULTURE

Bacterial culture of nasal discharge or the nasal cavity very rarely provides useful information. The nasal cavity of the normal dog often contains organisms considered pathogenic when cultured from other areas (staphylococci, streptococci, *E. coli*, *Proteus*, *Pseudomonas*, *Klebsiella*, and so on); bacterial culture is rarely negative, and often two or three organisms are isolated. Time is then lost while the dog is treated by antibiotics chosen by sensitivity testing, only to have the discharge recur shortly after cessation of treatment. Bacterial culture of nasal discharge may be indicated if a persistent purulent discharge develops following nasal surgery, as infection may have developed in connective tissues from contamination during surgery, although this is more likely to be due to a bone sequestrum or suture foreign body reaction that requires further surgical management.

Fungal culture is more useful, although *Aspergillus* or *Penicillium* spp. can be cultured from the nose of 30 to 40 per cent of normal dogs and dogs with nasal neoplasia. Fungal culture of dogs with aspergillosis-penicillosis may be negative, because of both failure to obtain an appropriate specimen and bacterial overgrowth, particularly *Pseudomonas* spp., which actually inhibit *Aspergillus* spp. hyphal growth.

Discharge is collected on a sterile dry swab, or a sterile swab moistened with sterile saline is inserted into the affected nasal cavity. The swab is planted on Sabouraud's agar containing antibacterial agents and incubated at room temperature. Growth of *Aspergillus* and *Penicillium* spp. is usually evident within one week, although fungal cultures are not reported as negative until four weeks. Sensitivity testing is not routinely available for fungi.

SEROLOGY

The agar gel double diffusion test has been available for several years (Lane et al., 1974; Lane and Warnock, 1977; Poli et al., 1981). The test is avail-

able at many institutional veterinary hospitals, human hospitals, and commercial or state public health laboratories. The test requires approximately 5 ml of serum, which can be mailed; refrigeration is unnecessary. Most laboratories normally test with *Aspergillus* spp. antigens only; additional examination for *Penicillium* spp. should be specifically requested. False negative tests are rare, although the antigen should be tested periodically against a known positive control. The test may be negative early in disease and positive subsequently. A positive serologic test for aspergillosis or penicillosis does not rule out other causes of nasal disease. Fifteen per cent of dogs with nasal tumors tested at VHUP were serologically positive for aspergillosis or penicillosis.

The immunodiffusion test is not quantitative. An equally reliable test requiring a smaller sample and providing a quantitative result is the enzyme-linked immunosorbent assay (ELISA). Samples (3 ml or more of separated serum) can be sent to: Clinical Immunology Laboratory, Veterinary Hospital of the University of Pennsylvania, 3850 Spruce Street, Philadelphia, PA. 19104.

OTHER CLINICAL LABORATORY EXAMINATIONS

Even if anesthesia is not considered, a complete blood count should be performed, particularly on animals with profuse epistaxis. Nasal hemorrhage is often spectacular but rarely life-threatening. A sample should be submitted for a clotting profile if the hematocrit is less than 30 to 35 per cent or if the platelets are decreased. The total white blood cell count may indicate the severity of the infection, and a low absolute lymphocyte count (< 600/cu mm) may indicate a primary immune deficiency. Serologic examination for *Ehrlichia canis* infection should be considered in animals with epistaxis and decreased platelet and white blood cell counts.

Lymphocyte transformation and other immune system tests require fresh blood in a sterile heparin container taken at a time convenient for the incubation process and before administering medication or anesthesia. Arrangements should be made in advance with the clinical immunology laboratory.

RADIOLOGY

Because of the bony detail of the nose, accurate radiographic interpretation requires that nasal radiographs be made with the patient under anesthesia. An occlusal view of the symmetric nasal cavity is the most useful projection, although lateral, open mouth, and frontal sinus projections are also usually made. Radiographic features of intranasal disease in the dog have recently been reviewed in detail (Gibbs et al., 1979; Harvey et al., 1979). Radiographs of some dogs with aspergillosis-penicillosis are normal. Most dogs show areas of increased intranasal density and loss of turbinate detail, although gross erosion of the nasal, maxillary, or palatine bones is unusual. A characteristic radiographic sign in approximately 50 per cent of aspergillosis-penicillosis cases is large areas of increased intranasal radiolucency. This sign is uncommon in dogs with nasal neoplasia. Nasal radiographs should be made before the nose is flushed.

RHINOSCOPY, NASAL FLUSH, BIOPSY

Crusted nasal discharge will often have to be removed, and the nasal cavities may require flushing before the nasal chambers can be directly examined (samples of discharge should be obtained for fungal culture prior to flushing the nose). An otoscope, or fiberoptic telescope, if available, is used. Atrophied turbinates or a white plaque lining the nasal mucosa may be seen occasionally in dogs with aspergillosis-penicillosis, although more usual findings are inflamed turbinates and nasal air spaces clogged with discharge. Indirect rhinoscopy, using a laryngeal mirror with the soft palate reflected, is rarely useful in dogs with aspergillosis-penicillosis.

Nasal flush serves to obtain specimens for biopsy and to clear nasal passages that are obstructed with discharge. A pack is placed beneath the neck, with the head placed so that fluid from the nostrils or pharynx is strained through a sponge. The endotracheal tube cuff is inflated and checked for gas leaks. A rubber ear syringe filled with saline is inserted firmly into one external naris, and fluid is vigorously flushed into the nasal cavity several times until fluid draining from the pharynx is clear. The opposite nasal cavity is then flushed. Samples caught on the sponge are submitted for microscopic examination. The usual findings in animals with aspergillosis-penicillosis are strings of mucus and blood clots.

If vigorous flushing does not provide a suitable sample, tissue can be obtained for biopsy by one of two methods. Long-handled uterine biopsy or laryngeal cup forceps are inserted to a length indicated from radiographic examination; the forceps jaws are opened and pushed into the tissue, then closed, and the forceps removed. Alternatively, a sharp pointed stiff plastic tube (cut to a length to avoid penetration of the cribriform plate) is thrust into the turbinates and the area penetrated is flushed (Withrow, 1977). With either method, a subsequent attempt can be made to obtain a sample by vigorous flushing of the entire nasal cavity. Blind biopsy is often satisfactory in obtaining neoplastic tissue but rarely provides a diagnostic sample in dogs with aspergillosis-penicillosis. Chronic rhinitis, often with a plasma cell infiltrate, and seromucinous gland hyperplasia are frequent pathologic diagnoses from biopsy specimens in dogs with aspergillosis-penicillosis but are not helpful to the clinician. Special stain examination for fungal elements is also rarely helpful.

Definitive diagnosis requires microscopic demonstration of hyphal invasion of bone or the finding of a gross hyphal mat or caseous clump at surgery, both of which require surgical intervention, which may not be necessary or permitted. A strong presumptive diagnosis of aspergillosis-penicillosis can be made if serologic examination and culture are positive and radiographs and blind biopsy do not indicate neoplasia.

THERAPY

Four forms of therapy are currently in use for aspergillosis-penicillosis: local antifungal medication, systemic antifungal medication, surgical nasal curettage, and immune stimulant therapy.

Surgery is usually reserved for those dogs in which turbinate destruction is visible radiographically or when there is poor response to medical therapy.

LOCAL MEDICAL TREATMENT

In animals in whom aspergillosis-penicillosis is suspected, medical treatment commences immediately following diagnostic flush. Several fungicidal agents are available for local use, including Lugol's iodine, povidone-iodine solution, and amphotericin B. Thiabendazole is available as a suspension but may dry out and cause post-flushing obstruction in a nose with an intact turbinate system. We currently use povidone-iodine solution,* diluted 1:10 with water, flushed vigorously through the nose several times.

Natamycin is a new antifungal agent that has been used in Europe by Venker-van Haagen (1981) with good short-term results even in severe cases. Under anesthesia, a 0.1 per cent solution is infused into the nasal cavities over a 15- to 25-minute period twice weekly for two to three weeks. This drug is presently unavailable in the U.S.

SYSTEMIC MEDICAL TREATMENT

For the last several years, the treatment of choice at VHUP for aspergillosis-penicillosis has been thiabendazole,† given usually for six-week periods at a dose rate of 20 mg/kg/day in a single dose or divided

---

*Betadine Solution, Purdue-Frederick Co., Norwalk, CT.
†Mintezol, Merck Sharp and Dohme, West Point, PA.

doses. Thiabendazole is an anthelmintic; however, it also reaches *Aspergillus*-inhibiting levels in dog serum when given at 20 mg/kg/day. It frequently causes some initial loss of appetite, and less commonly, vomition; when this occurs, administration of the drug is stopped, then restarted in two to three days at half dosage and gradually increased to the full dose. It is available as tablets and suspension. In dogs with mild disease visible radiographically, complete cessation of discharge is obtained in 50 to 60 per cent of dogs, although 30 per cent show little or no improvement. Intermittent administration of thiabendazole is necessary in some animals to maintain control of the disease.

Other oral medications that have been used, with mixed results, include nystatin-tetracycline and 5-fluorocytosine (5-FC),* an antifungal drug with immune stimulant properties but that causes an ulcerating pruritic dermatitis in some dogs (Barrett et al., 1977).

A new oral fungicidal agent, ketoconazole,† is available that may be more effective and cause less gastrointestinal abnormality than thiabendazole. Results of treatment of canine aspergillosis-penicillosis are unavailable. Short-term results of treatment (10 mg/kg daily for six weeks) are encouraging.

Treatment of aspergillosis-penicillosis by intravenous administration of amphotericin B‡ has been described in several case reports with mixed results. When an alternative is available, the use of amphotericin B is generally avoided because of nephrotoxicity and phlebitis at the injection site.

SURGICAL TREATMENT

Dogs with obvious turbinate destruction visible radiographically or that do not respond to an initial course of medical treatment are treated surgically. The object of surgery is to remove the entire affected area, which occasionally is just one or both frontal sinuses but more often one or both nasal cavities. Thus, the procedure performed is usually a unilateral or bilateral complete turbinectomy. Anesthetic and surgical management, control of hemorrhage, and postoperative care are described in detail elsewhere (Harvey, 1982). During surgery, a tube is placed through the skin into the frontal sinus through which 20 mg/kg thiabendazole suspension is injected into the nasal cavity each day for ten days. Following injection, saline is injected to clean the tube. During the thiabendazole injection, the dog often gags or sneezes and much of the thiabendazole is swallowed. The dog is then given a six-week course of oral thiabendazole at the same dose level. Long-term results following treatment by surgery, thiabendazole flush, and oral thiabendazole are cessation of nasal discharge in 10 to 15 per cent, improvement in 40 per cent, and little or no improvement in 45 per cent of dogs.

IMMUNE STIMULANT THERAPY

When an animal with aspergillosis-penicillosis is known to be (from lymphocyte transformation testing) or suspected of being (from lymphocyte count) immune suppressed, immune stimulants are indicated. Thiabendazole and 5-FC are both considered to be immune system potentiators in normal dogs; however, the immunologic evidence is insufficient to judge their effect in immune-suppressed dogs with nasal fungal infections. Levamisole§ (2 to 5 mg/kg every other day) is a nonspecific immune stimulant in dogs; however, results of treatment of a few dogs with aspergillosis-penicillosis at VHUP were not encouraging. Indomethacin‖ is a potent *in vitro* stimulant of lymphocytes in T cell–deficient dogs with chronic nasal disease; however, as yet there is insufficient experience *in vivo* to suggest a safe and effective dose. Complications include gastric ulceration and hemorrhage. It is rarely possible to provide a completely satisfactory immune system work-up and follow-up for these cases because of expense and availability of the patient at times dictated by test methodology.

NURSING CARE

The external nares of affected dogs should be gently cleansed once or twice a day. The epithelium below the external nares is coated with petrolatum to reduce excoriation. Because the sense of smell is severely restricted in many of these dogs, appetite is poor and is often worsened by thiabendazole therapy. Hot water mixed with dry dog food will increase the aroma, or a rich gravy or sauce can be mixed with the dog food. In severe cases, food may have to be placed in the mouth to stimulate the taste buds.

Nose drops (Neo-Synephrine, 0.25 per cent, two to four drops two to three times a day, alternating one side without medication each day) are helpful in some dogs in reducing discharge and making the dog more comfortable. Some dogs may tolerate the regular instillation of povidone-iodine solution (diluted 1:10 with water) into the nose.

A seven- to ten-day course of broad spectrum antibiotics will often temporarily improve a depressed dog with copious purulent discharge.

---

*Ancobon, Hoffman-LaRoche, Nutley, NJ.
†Nizoral, Janssen Pharmaceutica Inc., New Brunswick, NJ.
‡Fungizone, E.R. Squibb & Sons, Princeton, NJ.

§Ripercol-L, Cyanamid Agric. de Puerto Rico, Inc., Manati, PR.
‖Indocin, Merck Sharp and Dohme, West Point, PA.

REFERENCES AND SUPPLEMENTAL READING

Barrett, R. E., Hoffer, R. E., and Schultz, R. D.: Treatment and immunological evaluation of 3 cases of canine aspergillosis. J.A.A.H.A. 13:328, 1977.

Gibbs, C., Lane, J. G., and Denny, H. R.: Radiological features of intranasal lesions in the dog: Review of 100 cases. J. Small Anim. Pract. 20:515, 1979.

Harvey, C. E.: Nasal and sinus surgery. In Bojrab, M. J. (ed.): Current Techniques in Small Animal Surgery II. Philadelphia: Lea & Febiger, 1982.

Harvey, C. E., Biery, D. N., Morello, J., and O'Brien, J. A.: Chronic nasal disease in the dog: Its radiographic diagnosis. Vet. Radiol. 20:91, 1979.

Harvey, C. E., O'Brien, J. A., Felsburg, P. J., Izenberg, H. L., and

Goldschmidt, M. H.: Nasal penicillosis in six dogs. J.A.V.M.A. 178:1084, 1981.

Lane, J. G., Clayton-Jones, D. G., Thoday, K. L., and Thomsett, L. R.: The diagnosis of and successful treatment of Aspergillus fumigatus infection of the frontal sinuses and nasal chamber of the dog. J. Small Anim. Pract. 15:79, 1974.

Lane, J. G., and Warnock, D. W.: The diagnosis of Aspergillus fumigatus infection of the nasal chambers of the dog with particular reference to the value of the double diffusion test. J. Small Anim. Pract. 18:169, 1977.

Poli, G., Ponti, W., Balsani, A., Addis, F., and Mortellaro, C. M.: Aspergillus fumigatus and specific precipitins in dogs with turbinate changes. Vet. Rec. 108:143, 1981.

Venker-van Haagen, A. J.: Personal communication, 1981.

Withrow, S.: Diagnostic and therapeutic nasal flush in small animals. J.A.A.H.A. 13:704, 1977.

PARASITIC DISEASES OF THE RESPIRATORY TRACT

JEANNE A. BARSANTI, D.V.M.,

and ANNIE K. PRESTWOOD, D.V.M.

Athens, Georgia

Numerous helminths of dogs and cats are transient inhabitants of the respiratory tract during migration; however, comparatively few are permanent residents of the respiratory system. This discussion will concentrate on those parasites that reside and reproduce within the air passages or pulmonary parenchyma and, in particular, those parasites that produce significant pulmonary disease. The parasites will be discussed according to their location within the host, since location frequently governs the clinical signs presented by the patient.

NASAL PASSAGES

Clinical signs are seldom associated with parasites of the nasal passage. In some severely affected animals, however, sneezing and nasal discharge may be present. Diagnosis is made by cytologic examination of the nasal discharge or observation of the parasite as it emerges from the nose during anesthesia or within the nasal passage with the aid of an otoscope or a rigid or flexible endoscope. Two arthropods have been reported emerging from the nasal passages of dogs, Pneumonyssus caninum and Linguatula serrata.

Nasal mites, P. caninum, are found in the nasal passages primarily on the mucous membranes of the turbinates or the paranasal sinuses. They do not usually occur deeper within the respiratory system. The mites are barely visible with the unaided eye.

Female mites are viviparous or ovoviviparous, giving birth to larvae. The mode of transmission is unknown, but it is probably by way of direct contact, since mites have been observed crawling from the nares of dogs. Organophosphates in the form of flea collars or resinous fly strips placed in the dog house have been suggested control measures.

The pentastome nasal worm, L. serrata, attaches to the mucosal surface of the nasal passages and frontal sinuses or occasionally the eustachian tube and middle ear. Adults appear segmented and may attain a maximum length of about 13 cm. Females produce eggs that are passively ingested by an intermediate host, which is usually a small herbivorous mammal, e.g., cottontail rabbit. Here larval pentastomids burrow through the abdominal viscera, undergoing nine nymphal stages. Dogs and other mammals become infected by ingesting infected intermediate host tissues. Up to 15 months are required for females to become gravid and shed eggs. Clinical signs are rare, but sneezing, coughing, and occasionally epistaxis have been observed. Eggs may be found in the nasal discharge, or the adult may be visualized with an otoscope or endoscope. Parasites must be removed surgically if clinical signs warrant treatment.

TRACHEA AND MAJOR BRONCHI

The primary clinical sign caused by parasites of the major bronchi is a dry, harsh cough that can be elicited by tracheal palpation. The cough is similar to that associated with infectious tracheobronchitis (kennel cough) in dogs. Occasionally a white foamy mucus may be produced by coughing. The presence of parasites in the trachea or bronchi may predispose the animal to secondary bacterial pneumonia, which makes clinical signs more severe. Diagnosis may be difficult, and frequently a combination of one or more diagnostic procedures such as fecal examination, transtracheal washing, and bronchoscopy may be necessary.

Three helminths are located in the trachea and bronchi: *Capillaria aerophila, Oslerus (Filaroides) osleri*, and *Crenosoma vulpis*. The threadworm, *C. aerophila*, infects dogs, cats, and a variety of wild carnivores; *O. osleri* infects dogs and coyotes; and *C. vulpis* parasitizes dogs and foxes.

C. aerophilia is the most commonly encountered lungworm infecting dogs and cats in North America. Adult worms, 12 to 38 mm long, are located immediately beneath the epithelium of the trachea, bronchi, and occasionally the nasal passages and frontal sinuses. Earthworms serve as intermediate hosts, and dogs or cats become infected upon ingestion of earthworms containing infective larvae. The prepatent period is approximately one month. Infected animals often are asymptomatic, since usually only a few worms are present. The infection is most commonly diagnosed by finding yellowish, unembryonated, double operculated eggs (60 × 35 μm) (Fig. 1) in fecal samples or in a transtracheal washing. Bronchoscopy may reveal an inflamed bronchial epithelium. Therapy has not been evaluated for *C. aerophila* infections. Levamisole (dogs) and albendazole (dogs and cats) may be tried if clinical signs warrant treatment.

O. osleri are nematodes 5 to 10 mm long located in tough fibrous polypoid nodules near the tracheal bifurcation of dogs, coyotes, and related canids. Nodules contain masses of immature and adult worms. Females are ovoviviparous, and larvated eggs or free larvae may be shed. The life cycle is direct, and first-stage larvae are directly infective. Infected dogs may have a chronic cough, although wheezing and dyspnea occur if nodules are sufficiently extensive to occlude an air passage. Eosinophilia may occur.

Diagnosis by fecal examination is difficult even if a Baermann technique is used, since eggs or larvae are shed erratically. Larvae may be found by transtracheal washing, or nodules may be seen on bronchoscopy. Results of drug trials in *O. osleri* infections have been variable. Dorrington (1968) concluded that only thiacetarsamide (0.22 ml of a 1 per cent solution/kg IV every 24 hours for 21 days) had activity against *O. osleri*. Thiacetarsamide was not completely effective, so surgery was also necessary six weeks later for most satisfactory results. Thiabendazole (30 to 70 mg/kg per os every 12 hours for 21 to 23 days) and levamisole (7.5 mg/kg per os every 24 hours for 10 to 30 days) have been reported effective in some cases. Thiabendazole has been used most often in the few cases treated at the University of Georgia. Vomiting is a frequent side effect. Symptomatic therapy includes bronchodilators such as aminophylline.

Crenosoma vulpis are relatively small nematodes, 8 to 16 mm long, found in the lumen of the

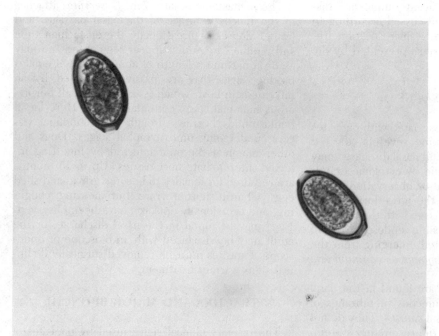

Figure 1. *Capillaria* eggs. Notice the asymmetric placement of the polar plugs.

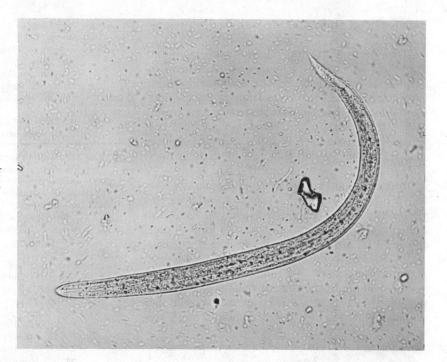

Figure 2. First-stage larva of *Crenosoma*. Note the absence of a cuticular spine on the tail.

bronchioles. Females are ovoviviparous, and motile, first-stage larvae without a dorsal cuticular spine (Fig. 2) are shed in the feces. Terrestrial snails and slugs serve as intermediate hosts, and dogs and foxes become infected upon ingestion of snails or slugs. The prepatent period is approximately three weeks. Active larvae are found in a transtracheal washing or by the Baermann technique on feces. Diethylcarbamazine at a dose rate of 80 mg/kg every 12 hr for three days or levamisole at a rate of 8 mg/kg given once orally was highly effective in eliminating infections.

LUNG PARENCHYMA

The clinical signs elicited by parasites that live in the lung parenchyma vary from none to coughing to tachypnea and dyspnea and rarely to respiratory failure and death. Fulminating disease is probably related to immunoincompetence. Bacterial pneumonia may secondarily complicate lung damage initiated by the parasite and may exacerbate clinical signs. Diagnosis may require fecal examination, transtracheal washing, and thoracic radiographs. The cat lungworm, *Aelurostrongylus abstrusus*, and the lung fluke, *Paragonimus kellicotti*, have been studied extensively. Recent emphasis has been placed on *Filaroides hirthi* infections in dogs, both naturally occurring and experimentally induced. Occasional infections by *Andersonstrongylus (Filaroides) milksi* occur in dogs and skunks. The migrating larvae of *Toxocara* and *Strongyloides* spp. may adversely affect respiratory function.

The feline lungworm, *A. abstrusus*, is a small nematode, 5 to 10 mm long, that lives in terminal bronchioles and alveolar spaces. Eggs are deposited in clusters by the female; they embryonate *in situ* and hatch. First-stage larvae are swept up the bronchial tree, swallowed, and eliminated in the feces. Larvae actively penetrate the foot of terrestrial snails or slugs. Cats become infected by ingesting snails or slugs containing infective larvae or by ingesting paratenic hosts such as amphibians, reptiles, small mammals, or birds. The prepatent period ranges from about four to six weeks. There is no correlation between number of larvae observed in the feces and the number of worms harbored by the cat. In some cats experimentally infected with 1000 larvae, an apparent intense immune response occurred that effectively blocked development of eggs and subsequent release of larvae. Radiographic lesions remained for over a year, indicating the presence of living worms. Most infections with *A. abstrusus* are asymptomatic and self-limiting. When clinical signs occur, they usually manifest as occasional coughing. The cough may be induced by tracheal palpation and is often dry and nonproductive. Harsh lung sounds may be auscultated. More severe signs, such as dyspnea, may be present in immunosuppressed cats.

Thoracic radiographs may show indistinctly circumscribed small nodules through all lung fields but most numerous in the caudal lobes. Histologically, the nodules are masses of developing ova and larvae surrounded by an inflammatory reaction with neutrophils, eosinophils, plasma cells, and lymphocytes. An alveolar, bronchial, interstitial, vascular, or mixed radiographic pattern may be present. We have had one infected cat that presented with pneumothorax. Infected cats may have an eosinophilia.

Diagnosis of aelurostrongylosis is made by finding larvae by cytologic examination of a transtracheal washing or by a Baermann fecal examination (Table 1). Eosinophils are also often found in the transtracheal washing. Larvae of *A. abstrusus* float readily in Sheather's sugar solution, but they are distorted. Larvae have characteristic dorsal and ventral cuticular spines on the tail that can be demonstrated after immobilization with heat (Fig. 3).

Most infections by *Aelurostrongylus* do not warrant treatment since they are asymptomatic. In cats presenting clinical signs attributable to lungworm infections, supportive therapy in the form of antibiotics to combat secondary infection and glucocorticoids to reduce inflammation should be administered as indicated. The lungworm infection is usually self-limiting owing to the development of an immune response. Although tetramisole has been advocated to eliminate feline lungworms, this

Table 1.   *Fecal Flotation/Sedimentation Techniques**

I. Sheather's Sugar Centrifugal Flotation Technique
This technique reveals most nematode eggs and protozoan cysts. Fluke eggs are not demonstrated well nor are tapeworm eggs. Most nematode larvae are distorted.
A. Sheather's sugar solution

sugar (regular table sugar)	500 gm
distilled water	320 ml
phenol crystals	6.5 gm
(melt in hot water bath)	

B. Procedure
1. Soften feces with water to a soft, fluid consistency.
2. Pass aqueous suspension through a tea strainer or two layers of gauze.
3. Thoroughly mix 1 part aqueous fecal suspension with 2 parts of Sheather's sugar solution. Pour into a centrifuge tube and add sufficient solution to bring a meniscus to the tube. Place a coverslip on top. Centrifuge at 1500 rpm for ten minutes.
4. Remove coverslip and place on a slide. Examine at ≥ 200× magnification for sporocysts of *Sarcocystis* or *Toxoplasma* oocysts. These organisms adhere to the bottom of the coverslip, so it is necessary to focus there.

II. Formalin-Ether Sedimentation of Fluke Eggs
This technique is used for the recovery of fluke eggs from feces. Formalin-ether sedimentation offers two advantages over the usual fecal flotation procedures used to diagnose fluke infections (sucrose and $NaNO_3$): (1) more fluke eggs can be recovered, increasing the chances of detecting an infection, and (2) the fluke eggs recovered are less distorted and, therefore, more easily identified.
A. Procedure
1. Comminute the entire stool specimen, or a large portion of it, in enough saline solution so that 10 to 12 ml of the emulsion will, when centrifuged, contain 1 to 2 ml of fecal sediment. Strain 10 to 12 ml of the emulsion through two layers of gauze into a 15-ml centrifuge tube.
2. Centrifuge and decant supernatant. The fluke eggs will be in the sediment. Additional washings with saline are of advantage in removing finer debris.

3. Add 10 ml of 10 per cent formalin to the sediment, stir, and allow five minutes for the formalin to fix the fluke eggs. Then add 3 ml ether, stopper the tube, and shake vigorously. Centrifuge at low speed for two minutes, loosen the debris plug with an applicator stick, and decant ether, debris, and formalin.
4. Mix the sediment with the few drops of fluid that drain from the wall of the tube and pour onto a slide. Add a drop of 2 per cent iodine solution to one edge of the drop, cover with coverslip, and examine.

III. Zinc Sulfate Centrifugal Flotation Technique
This procedure reveals most nematode eggs and protozoan cysts without distortion. It is the only technique that will demonstrate *Filaroides hirthi* larvae.
A. Zinc sulfate, sp gr 1.18
    Mix 330 gm dry zinc sulfate in 670 ml distilled water. Use a hydrometer and adjust specific gravity to 1.18.
B. Procedure
1. Mix 1 gm feces with 1 to 2 ml water. Comminute thoroughly and place in a test tube. Fill test tube to within 2 to 3 mm of top with water.
2. Centrifuge for one minute at 1500 rpm and discard supernatant.
3. Add 1 to 2 ml zinc sulfate; mix thoroughly.
4. Fill tube to within 2 to 3 mm of top with additional $ZnSO_4$ and strain suspension through gauze into a beaker. Discard gauze and return suspension to centrifuge tube. A few drops of Lugol's iodine may be added at this time or later on.
5. Centrifuge for one minute at 1500 rpm. Allow centrifuge to come to a stop without disturbance.
6. Place a small drop of iodine or water on a slide.
7. Without removing the centrifuge tube from the centrifuge and using a freshly flamed and cooled 5- to 7-mm wire loop, remove one or two drops from the surface film and add them to the drop of iodine or water on the slide.
8. Add coverslip and examine the preparation microscopically.

IV. Baermann Technique
This procedure will concentrate living larvae of lungworms, hookworms, and *Strongyloides*.
A. Equipment
    6″ funnel
    rubber tube
    wire gauze (4″ circle)
    cheesecloth or Kimwipes
    pinch clamp or Mohr clamp
    water
    ring stand
B. Procedure
1. Slip rubber tube on the funnel and attach pinch clamp. Place wire gauze within funnel and fill funnel with water until it slightly covers the wire gauze. Place funnel on ring stand. Cover wire gauze with two layers of cheesecloth or two Kimwipes.
2. Place fecal sample on top of gauze. Be sure water is touching the bottom of the fecal sample. Allow to stand at least two hours in a warm room.
3. Withdraw 10 ml of fluid from the tube and place in a centrifuge tube. Centrifuge for five to ten minutes at 1500 rpm. Pour off supernatant and discard.
4. Examine sediment for larvae. If larvae are present, gently heat the slide with a match or cigarette lighter to immobilize larvae for morphologic study. Do not boil liquid.

*Modified, in part, from Garcia and Ash: *Diagnostic Parasitology. Clinical Laboratory Manual*, 2nd ed. St. Louis: C. V. Mosby, 1979.

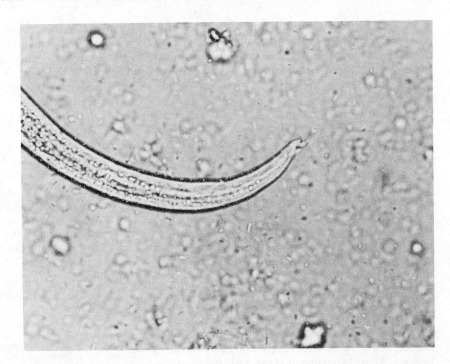

Figure 3. Tail of first-stage larva of *Aelurostrongylus*. Notice the presence of both dorsal and ventral cuticular spines.

drug is often toxic to cats. Fenbendazole at a dosage of 50 mg/kg/day for three days showed partial activity against *A. abstrusus* in experimentally infected cats.

Lung flukes, *Paragonimus kellicotti*, occur as pairs within cysts in the lungs of dogs, cats, and numerous wild carnivores. Adult flukes are reddish brown and measure 8 to 12 mm × 4 to 6 mm. Yellow-brown operculated eggs measure 80 to 115 × 40 to 65 μm and are shed in the feces. Two intermediate hosts are required, aquatic snails and crayfish. Crayfish limit the geographic distribution of this parasite to the Great Lakes region and the Midwest and Southern United States. Animals become infected by ingesting the metacercaria in the crayfish. The prepatent period is five to six weeks. Within the lungs, trematodes are walled off by a fibrous capsule, but a tract remains for exit of eggs. Infections may be asymptomatic or may manifest as coughing, wheezing, or, exceptionally, dyspnea. The cough can be elicited by tracheal palpation. Occasionally animals may cough up blood. Harsh vesicular sounds most prominent in the caudal lung lobes may be heard, especially after a coughing episode. Pneumothorax and bacterial pneumonia are potential secondary complications. Thoracic radiographs show solid or cavitated spheroid parenchymal densities, most commonly in the right caudal lung lobe. The number of lesions is variable but averaged three to four in one study. Other considerations for such lesions are primary or metastatic neoplasia, abscesses, and granulomas. Secondary radiographic findings in *Paragonimus* infections include interstitial infiltrates, bronchial thickening, patchy alveolar disease, and atelectasis. Eosinophilia may be present.

Diagnosis of *Paragonimus* infection is confirmed by finding eggs in a transtracheal washing or in feces. Fluke eggs may be recovered by routine fecal flotation procedures using zinc sulfate or sodium nitrate. Early, light infections are best diagnosed by sedimentation techniques (see Table 1). Clinical signs and radiographic lesions may be present prior to patency by the parasite. Diagnosis in this case must be presumptive, based on, history, physical examination, and radiographs.

There is no approved drug for this infection. Bithionol (100 mg/kg every 48 hours for 30 days) has been used in one dog without adverse side effects. At higher dosages, the drug is not well tolerated and may cause diarrhea. It is also a phenol derivative and as such may be more toxic to cats than dogs. Albendazole (25 mg/kg every 12 hours for 10 to 21 days) was effective experimentally in cats. Mild lethargy and hypersalivation were reported side effects. Anorexia usually develops after eight to ten days of therapy. Treatment is stopped when no eggs are found in feces or when anorexia occurs. Fenbendazole (25 mg/kg every 12 hours for 10 to 14 days) was effective in dogs. No adverse effects were reported.

Filaroides hirthi are exceeding small nematodes, 0.5 to 2.0 mm long, found in the alveolar spaces and terminal bronchioles of dogs. The life cycle is direct with a 32- to 35-day prepatent period. First-stage larvae are directly infective, and autogenous reinfection occurs. Infections with *F. hirthi* have been most frequent in research beagle colonies. *F. hirthi* most often produces mild granulomatous inflammation in the lungs of dogs without associated clinical signs. It is important mainly because these lesions may be confused with pathologic changes induced by drugs, oncogenic influences, and other pathologic processes in research animals. Fatal cases due to respiratory failure have been reported in two pet dogs that were immunosuppressed by glucocorticoids or by trauma requiring several surgical procedures.

Diagnosis of *F. hirthi* infection is difficult, since eggs or larvae are not usually recovered by flotation or Baermann techniques. Approximately 20 per cent of infections may be demonstrated by flotation with zinc sulfate (specific gravity 1.18). Examination of fluid obtained by transtracheal wash may reveal larvated eggs, or adult worms may be found by aspiration or biopsy of the lung. Linear and miliary interstitial parenchymal infiltrates of all lung lobes may be demonstrated radiographically. These may coalesce to radiodense parenchymal lesions approximately 1 cm in diameter.

Albendazole (50 mg/kg per os every 12 hours for 5 days; repeated in 21 days) was effective in killing or sterilizing the parasite in experimental infections. Treatment is therefore useful in controlling or eliminating infection in breeding colonies of research beagles. However, clinical signs and pathologic lesions are exacerbated by treatment. This is apparently due to an immune response to dead and dying worms. Dogs treated with albendazole should not be stressed during or after therapy until granulomatous lesions resolve.

Andersonstrongylus (*Filaroides*) *milksi* is somewhat larger than *F. hirthi* (3 to 10 mm). It also lives in alveolar spaces and terminal bronchioles of dogs. Its life cycle is unknown. Clinical signs are rare, but occasionally polypnea and dyspnea are observed. Thoracic radiographs may show a bronchial and interstitial pattern. Diagnosis is made by finding embryonated eggs or larvae in a transtracheal wash or larvae in sediment obtained via the Baermann technique. The absence of nodules at bronchoscopy differentiates *A. milksi* infection from *O. osleri* infection. No effective therapy has been reported. Levamisole has been recommended, but one animal treated with levamisole died, perhaps due to antigen release from rapid parasite destruction. Since *A. milksi* is usually an incidental finding unassociated with clinical signs, treatment is usually not warranted.

Owing to prenatal infection, larval stages of *Toxocara canis* may be present in the lungs of newborn pups. Larval *T. cati* may be present in the lungs of kittens five days after ingestion of embryonated eggs. Heavy infections by migrating larvae may produce pneumonia owing to physical damage and, possibly, a hypersensitivity response. Pulmonary hemorrhage may occur. Migration of *Toxocara* larvae is one postulated cause of eosinophilic lung disease in dogs and cats. Definitive antemortem diagnosis is difficult. Occasionally, migrating larvae may be demonstrated by examining sediment from a transtracheal wash. Fenbendazole (25 mg/kg per os every 12 hours for 14 days) is reportedly effective against tissue stages of *T. canis*.

Larvae of *Strongyloides stercoralis* penetrate the skin and travel to the lungs. Here they break out of alveolar capillaries and are swept up the bronchial tree and swallowed. A cough and anorexia, therefore, may precede gastrointestinal signs. Diagnosis is made by recovering larvae by the Baermann technique from fresh feces. Treatment of the migratory phase of strongyloidiasis has not been reported.

REFERENCES AND SUPPLEMENTAL READING

August, J. R., Powers, R. D., Bailey, W. S., and Diamond, D. L.: *Filaroides hirthis* in a dog: fatal hyperinfection suggestive of autoinfection. J.A.V.M.A. 176:331, 1980.

Bennett, D., and Beresford-Jones, W. P.: Treatment of *Filaroides osleri* infestation in a 16-month-old male Yorkshire terrier with thiabendazole. Vet. Rec. 93:226, 1973.

Craig, T. M., Brown, T. W., Shefstad, D. K., and Williams, G. D.: Fatal *Filaroides hirthi* infection in a dog. J.A.V.M.A. 172:1096, 1978.

Dorrington, J. E.: Studies in *Filaroides osleri* infestation in dogs. Onderstepoort J. Vet. Res. 35:225, 1968.

Dubey, J. P.: Effect of fenbendazole on *Toxocara canis* larvae in tissues of infected dogs. Am. J. Vet. Res. 40:698, 1979.

Dubey, J. P., Hoover, E. A., Stromberg, P. C., and Toussant, M. J.: Albendazole therapy for experimentally induced *Paragonimus kellicotti* infection in cats. Am. J. Vet. Res. 39:1027, 1978.

Dubey, J. P., Miller, T. B., and Sharma, S. P.: Fenbendazole for treatment of *Paragonimus kellicotti* infection in dogs. J.A.V.M.A. 174:835, 1979.

Garcia, L. S., and Ash, L. R.: *Diagnostic Parasitology. Clinical Laboratory Manual*, 2nd ed. St. Louis: C. V. Mosby, 1979, p. 174.

Georgi, J. R.: *Filaroides hirthi*: Experimental transmission among beagle dogs through ingestion of first-stage larvae. Science 194:735, 1976.

Georgi, J. R., Georgi, M. E., Fahnestock, G. R., and Theodorides, V. J.: Transmission and control of *Filaroides hirthi* lungworm infection in dogs. Am. J. Vet. Res. 40:829, 1979.

Georgi, J. R., Slauson, D. O., and Theodorides, V. J.: Anthelmintic activity of albendazole against *Filaroides hirthi* lungworms in dogs. Am. J. Vet. Res. 39:803, 1978.

Hill, B. L., and McChesney, A. E.: Thiabendazole treatment of a dog with *Filaroides osleri*. J. Am. Anim. Hosp. Assoc. 12:487, 1976.

Hoskins, J. D., Malone, J. B., and Root, C. R.: Albendazole therapy in naturally occurring feline paragonimiasis. J. Am. Anim. Hosp. Assoc. 17:265, 1981.

Johnson, K. E., Kazacos, K. R., Blevins, W. E., and Cantwile, H. D.: Albendazole for treatment of *Paragonimus kellicotti* infection in two cats. J.A.V.M.A. 178:483, 1981.

Rendano, V. R., Georgi, J. R., Fahnestock, G. R., and King, J. M.: *Filaroides hirthi* lungworm infection in dogs: its radiographic appearance. J.A.V.R.S. 20:1, 1979.

Roberson, E. L., and Burke, T. M.: Evaluation of granulated fenbendazole (22.2%) against induced and naturally occurring helminth infections in cats. Am. J. Vet. Res. 41:1499, 1980.

Scott, D. W.: Current knowledge of aelurostrongylosis in the cat. Cornell Vet. 63:483, 1973.

Stockdale, P. H. G., and Smart, M. E.: Treatment of crenosomaisis in dogs. Res. Vet. Sci. 18:178, 1975.

PNEUMONIA

GARY W. THAYER, D.V.M.

Athens, Georgia

Dogs and cats exhibiting signs of lower airway disease constitute a significant part of small animal practice. Many of these animals, dogs more often than cats, have pneumonia. Pneumonia requires rapid diagnosis and specific therapy to prevent loss of life, or irreversible parenchymal or airway damage. *Pneumonia* is defined as inflammation of the lungs and is used specifically to describe exudative disease processes affecting alveolar spaces. *Pneumonitis* is used to describe a cellular infiltration or proliferation of cells lining the alveolar wall. These anatomic classifications share the same etiologies, and pneumonia and pneumonitis may only be different stages in the progression of the disease process (Jubb and Kennedy, 1970). In this article, the inflammatory diseases of the lung will be divided into infectious and noninfectious categories.

DIAGNOSTIC PLAN

Dogs and cats with pneumonia usually exhibit one or more of the following clinical signs: cough, tachypnea, hemoptysis, fever, and restrictive dyspnea (e.g., rapid, shallow respirations). Those animals presented with an acute cough and for no other abnormalities are usually given symptomatic therapy without further diagnostic evaluation. Animals with an acute cough and abnormal lung sounds, a cough that has been unresponsive to previous therapy, a chronic cough (persisting for more than 14 days), tachypnea, or dyspnea require expansion of the data base to further define the problem. Following the history and physical examination, thoracic radiographs, complete blood counts, microfilaria determination, and transtracheal aspiration for bronchial cytology and culture may be indicated. Fecal examinations, including a Baermann procedure in cats, should be done when animals reside in areas where pulmonary parasites are endemic. In tachypneic or dyspneic animals, arterial blood gas determinations are helpful in assessing the severity of pulmonary insufficiency. If a definitive diagnosis cannot be made after assessing the data from the previously stated procedures, more invasive procedures, such as bronchoscopy with selective bronchial washing or transbronchial lung biopsy, needle aspiration of the lung, or open thoracotomy and lung biopsy, should be considered.

INFECTIOUS PNEUMONIAS

BACTERIAL PNEUMONIA

A retrospective study of 51 consecutive patient records of dogs with bacterial pneumonia presented to the Veterinary Teaching Hospital at the University of Georgia was performed. It was found that 41 of the 51 dogs were sporting breeds, working breeds, mixed breeds weighing more than 12 kg, or hounds. Pneumonia in small dogs was rare. Twenty-four dogs were less than one year of age, and 37 dogs were less than five years of age. Male and female dogs were represented in about equal numbers. Dogs with bacterial pneumonia as a result of aspiration of food or stomach contents secondary to an anesthetic episode or esophageal dysfunction were not included in the study. Predisposing conditions previously reported include inadequate vaccination programs for canine distemper, parainfluenza virus, and canine adenovirus. Viral infections as a result of poor vaccination protocols may compromise mucociliary transport or alveolar macrophage activity. Compromise of these host defense mechanisms allows for airway colonization and infection by pathogenic bacteria. Animals with bronchiectasis as a result of previous pulmonary disease or pulmonary neoplasia are also predisposed to bacterial pneumonia.

DIAGNOSIS

Patients with bacterial pneumonia may be presented for any one or a combination of the following clinical signs: anorexia, depression, weight loss, nasal discharge, cough, tachypnea, or dyspnea. Abnormalities found during physical exmination may include fever, tachypnea, purulent nasal discharge, restrictive dyspnea, dehydration, and a moist productive cough. Normal lung sounds can be auscultated in only a small number of dogs or cats with bacterial pneumonia. Abnormal lung sounds in animals with bacterial pneumonia include crackles, increased breath sounds, silent areas, and wheezes. Crackles are nonmusical explosive sounds caused by delayed opening of small airways. They are usually heard in the ventral lung fields and are generated by the sudden equalization of pressure that follows removal of a barrier separating two compartments of air at widely different pressures.

In bacterial pneumonia these barriers are purulent exudates or infiltrations of inflammatory cells into the walls of small airways. Increased breath sounds are due to an increased velocity of inspired and expired air or consolidation of an area of lung between an open large airway and the chest wall, which creates a more efficient medium for sound transmission. Silent areas are present over areas of consolidated lung where large airways are filled with exudates. Wheezes are occasionally heard and are the result of air passing through severely stenosed airways under tension, probably as a result of tenacious secretions or bronchoconstriction (Forgacs, 1978).

Radiographic signs include an increased alveolar opacity seen in the ventral portions of the cranial lobes, right middle lobe, and intermediate lobe, with occasional involvement of the ventral portion of the caudal lobes. Air bronchograms are commonly seen. A small amount of pleural effusion is sometimes observed.

The complete blood count is characterized by a leukocytosis with a neutrophilia or neutrophilic left shift and monocytosis. Measurement of arterial blood gases may reveal hypoxemia. When present, hypoxemia is a result of ventilation-perfusion mismatching and pulmonary arterial-venous shunting (Light et al., 1981). Bronchial cytologic examination reveals either mucopurulent or septic purulent exudate.

Bacterial culture of 51 consecutive specimens collected from dogs at the University of Georgia resulted in isolation of primarily gram negative organisms, including *Pseudomonas* sp., *Escherichia coli, Klebsiella* sp., and *Bordetella bronchoseptica*. Bacterial culture of 30 specimens from dogs presented to the Angel Memorial Hospital revealed primarily gram positive organisms including alpha-hemolytic and beta-hemolytic *Streptococcus* spp., *Staphylococcus aureus, Enterococcus* spp., and *Diplococcus* spp. (Harpster, 1981). The difference in the results of these two series of bacterial isolations emphasizes the importance of planning antibiotic therapy based on results of bacterial isolation and antibiotic sensitivity testing.

THERAPY

Therapy should be designed to eliminate the bacteria and inflammation from the lung as rapidly as possible. This will prevent irreversible change in the pulmonary parenchyma and ineffective restoration of pulmonary defense mechanisms. In addition, hypoxemic patients must be supplied with oxygen until antibiotic therapy improves pulmonary function. Specific antibiotic therapy determined by antibiotic sensitivity testing is mandatory. Until results of such therapy are available, broad spectrum antibiotic therapy with gentamicin and penicillin, chloramphenicol, ampicillin, or tetracycline should be instituted. Therapy should be altered in response to the results of the antibiotic sensitivity test and changes in clinical and radiographic signs. Some improvement in clinical signs should be seen in 24 to 72 hours and in radiographic signs in 48 to 96 hours. Antibiotic therapy should be continued for at least ten days after clinical and radiographic improvement is achieved.

Removal of exudates from the lung is necessary for effective recovery. This is accomplished by effective cough and mucociliary transport mechanisms. Therefore, antitussives are contraindicated. Cough should be encouraged by mild exercise, such as leash walking, or chest percussion. Mucociliary transport functions best when secretions are of an optimal viscoelasticity. Drying of secretions significantly alters these properties. Adequate systemic hydration is, therefore, very important in the removal of exudates from the respiratory tract. If adequate fluids are not being taken voluntarily, parenteral fluid therapy should be instituted. The use of cold or steam vaporizers will prevent drying of secretions of the upper airway but will have little effect on small airways. Aerosols produced by jet or ultrasonic nebulizers are capable of depositing fluids and medication in small airways (see Principles of Respiratory Therapy). Objective evidence is not available to substantiate the claim that the use of aerosol therapy results in a more rapid or complete recovery, with the exception that *Bordetella bronchoseptica* is eliminated from the upper respiratory tract with an aerosol of gentamicin (Bemis and Appel, 1977).

Oxygen therapy can be accomplished with an oxygen cage or by tracheal cannula. When using a tracheal cannula, it is necessary to set flow rates at 4 to 6 L/min to achieve an inspired oxygen concentration of 30 to 40 per cent. Oxygen cages should be operated according to the manufacturer's instructions. If therapy is to continue beyond two to four hours, oxygen should be humidified prior to administration.

In patients in whom disease is localized to one or two lobes and antibiotic therapy is not effective or in whom pneumonia recurs after therapy is stopped, lobectomy may be necessary for cure.

COMPLICATIONS

Complications of bacterial pneumonia include pulmonary abscess or granuloma formation, lung necrosis, suppurative pleuritis, pneumothorax, bacteremia, and toxemia. These can be prevented by early diagnosis and identification of the bacteria followed by specific and aggressive antibiotic therapy.

PROGNOSIS

The prognosis is good in animals that are not dyspneic and in whom the bacteria are susceptible to available antibiotics. The prognosis is guarded in those patients that do not show partial resolution of clinical signs in 24 to 48 hours after initiation of therapy.

PREVENTION

Prevention of bacterial pneumonia is best accomplished by eliminating predisposing factors. Therefore, adequate vaccination against canine distemper, parainfluenza, and canine adenovirus is important. Vaccination against *Bordetella bronchoseptica* should also be considered in show animals or those in kennels.

Careful adherence to a reliable anesthesia protocol, including fasting patients prior to anesthesia and proper endotracheal intubation procedures, will prevent aspiration and secondary bacterial pneumonia.

FUNGAL PNEUMONIA

When considering a diagnosis of fungal pneumonia, it is helpful to establish that the dog or cat has (sometime during its life) resided in an area where these pathogenic organisms are endemic. Blastomycosis and histoplasmosis are endemic to the Mississippi and Ohio River valleys and their bordering states. Coccidioidomycosis is endemic to the arid Southwest.

Dogs affected with blastomycosis generally have one or a combination of the following clinical signs: chronic persistent cough, weight loss, persistent or intermittent fever, depression, anorexia, lameness, draining skin lesions, generalized lymphadenopathy, and ocular lesions (anterior uveitis, retinal detachment). Blastomycosis is rare in cats. Lung auscultation is frequently normal; sometimes increased normal breath sounds are heard. In animals with marked pulmonary involvement, severe dyspnea may be observed. Thoracic radiographic signs include diffuse nodular interstitial opacification and occasional mild hilar lymphadenopathy. Definitive diagnosis is established by observing multiple thick-walled, budding organisms, 8 to 15 μ in diameter, in body fluids, pus, or cytologic preparations from percutaneous fine needle lung aspirations (see Diagnostics for Respiratory Diseases). Culture of the same specimens will yield the organisms. Fungal organisms can be seen in hematoxylin and eosin–stained histologic sections, but Gomori's methenamine silver makes identification easier. A fourfold increase in serum antibody titer over three to four weeks indicates active infection.

Histoplasmosis is the most common deep fungal disease of the dog. It is uncommon in the cat. The majority of infections are asymptomatic or present as low-grade respiratory infections with a mild cough. Some dogs are unable to eliminate the organism, and pneumonia develops, characterized by persistent cough, pyrexia, tachypnea, or dyspnea. The organisms sometimes disseminate from the lung and may affect the small intestines, liver, adrenal glands, colon, spleen, kidney, meninges, and various lymph nodes. Thoracic radiographic signs of the pulmonary form include hilar lymphadenopathy, miliary interstitial opacification, and occasionally mild pleural effusion. In acute histoplasmosis, alveolar opacification similar to that present in bacterial pneumonia may be seen.

DIAGNOSIS

A definitive diagnosis is made by finding the organism in a cytologic examination of material from a transtracheal aspiration, lymph node aspiration, or fecal smear. Culture may reveal the organism, but specimens must be inoculated into the culture medium within one hour after collection. Organisms can be seen in hematoxylin and eosin–stained histologic sections. A complement fixation serum antibody titer of 1:8 is indicative of active disease and is usually present by 21 days after the observation of clinical signs.

Coccidioidomycosis is also more common in the dog than in the cat. It is usually a self-limiting pulmonary infection. Most animals are asymptomatic. Others develop a dry cough and pyrexia. Dissemination to bone, liver, pericardium, skin, and urinary tract occurs but is not common. The most common radiographic sign of pulmonary infection is hilar lymphadenopathy. A definitive diagnosis is made by cytologic examination and culture of aspirates from affected areas of lung or lymph node.

THERAPY

Traditional therapy for deep fungal infections is amphotericin B.* Its major disadvantage is its nephrotoxicity. Other toxic effects include suppression of the erythropoiesis (more commonly seen in cats), weight loss, hypokalemia, perivascular irritation, nausea, vomiting, and cardiac arrhythmias, which may result if amphotericin B is administered rapidly. At The University of Georgia, amphotericin B is administered in a dose of 0.15 to 0.5 mg/kg IV in two to five minutes every other day in a small volume (5 to 10 ml) of 5 per cent dextrose or sterile

---

*Fungizone, E. R. Squibb & Sons, Inc., Princeton, NJ.

water.* Therapy is started at the lower end of the dose range and increased until an increase in blood urea nitrogen (BUN) is observed. BUN is evaluated every other day before administration of amphotericin B, and therapy is stopped if the BUN is greater than 40 ml/dl. Fluid therapy is instituted if azotemia ensues. Amphotericin B therapy is resumed when the BUN is normal. Therapy is continued for several weeks after remission of clinical signs. The total cumulative dose over two to four months should be 5 to 25 mg/kg, depending on the patient's response. Absolute rest during and for several weeks after termination of therapy may be helpful.

Cats are given amphotericin B 0.1 to 0.5 mg/kg IV every other day. BUN is monitored as in the dog. For cats, amphotericin B is diluted in 10 ml of 5 per cent dextrose and administered intravenously over two to five minutes. Simultaneous subcutaneous administration of an isotonic, balanced electrolyte solution at the rate of 20 ml/kg may reduce renal toxicity. The total effective cumulative dose in the cat appears to be about 4 mg/kg.

Ketoconazole,† a synthetic water-soluble imidazole, has potent activity against dermatophytes, yeasts, and pathogenic fungi after oral administration. Clinical evaluation of this compound in the dog and cat is under way.

A dog with osseous blastomycosis was treated with ketoconazole (30 mg/kg PO daily for 61 days). During this time, no clinical or laboratory evidence of toxicity or adverse reactions were noted. The dog was clinically normal six months after therapy was stopped (Dunbar and Pyle, 1981). Recently, a dog with disseminated coccidioidomycosis was treated at the Veterinary Teaching Hospital at The University of Georgia with ketoconazole 7.5 mg/kg PO daily for 120 days. No adverse reactions were observed. Clinical signs resolved by the sixtieth day of therapy. Long-term follow-up was not available. Ketoconazole's apparent low toxicity and ease of administration will make it an important agent in the therapy of fungal pneumonia if further evaluation proves its efficacy. Early reports appear very encouraging.

PROGNOSIS

The prognosis is guarded in all patients with deep fungal disease. Dogs and cats with widely disseminated disease and severe systemic signs have the poorest prognosis. Those patients with disease localized to the thorax that are still eating and drinking have a more favorable prognosis if they tolerate drug therapy without uncontrollable adverse side effects.

PROTOZOAN PNEUMONIA

Pneumonia due to infection with *Toxoplasma gondii* occurs in both the dog and cat but is more common in the cat. It can occur as an acute infection or as a stress relapse several years after the initial infection. Clinical signs of acute toxoplasma pneumonia in the cat include lethargy, anorexia, fever, dyspnea, and increased breath sounds. Cough is uncommon. These respiratory signs occur in only 25 per cent of cats with chronic infections. In dogs the usual presentation is an acute self-limiting cough. In severe cases fever, depression, anorexia, tachypnea, and dyspnea are reported. Crackles are heard during auscultation of the lungs. Thoracic radiographic findings in the cat consist of ill-defined, mottled coalescing alveolar opacities. Thoracic radiographic signs in the dog are variable and include focal alveolar opacifications, lobar consolidations, and multiple nodular opacities.

DIAGNOSIS

A definitive clinical diagnosis in the cat of toxoplasma pneumonia is made by finding oocysts in the feces and or by a rising antibody titer from two serum samples taken a week or more apart. In the dog, serology alone must be used because oocysts are not found in the feces. If both serum samples are negative for toxoplasma antibody or if the titer is stable, the pneumonia is not due to toxoplasmosis.

THERAPY

The purpose of therapy is to prevent further damage to the patient until immunity is acquired. Treatment is accomplished by interference with sequential steps of dihydrofolate synthesis within the toxoplasma organism. Patients are treated with a combination of sulfadiazine at a dose of 60 mg/kg PO daily divided every four to six hours and pyrimethamine‡ at a dose of 0.5 to 1 mg/kg/day PO.

If animals are to be treated for more than two weeks, WBC and platelet counts should be done. If hematology results are less than one-fourth to one-half of reported normal values for the species, antagonist therapy should be instituted with folinic acid at a dose of 1 mg/kg daily and baker's yeast at a dose of 100 mg/kg daily. These can be administered along with the antidihydrofolate treatment, because mammalian cells utilize the folinic acid,

---

*Editor's Note: Controversy exists regarding the most efficacious method of administering amphotericin B, e.g., slow versus rapid IV infusion. Additional views on the subject are available in the articles entitled Management of Chronic Upper Airway Disease and Subcutaneous and Opportunistic Mycoses (Sec. 14).

†Janssen Pharmaceutica, Inc., New Brunswick, NJ.

‡Daraprim, Burroughs Wellcome Co., Research Triangle Park, NC.

whereas the toxoplasma organisms do not. Treatment should be continued beyond resolution of clinical signs for at least two weeks. Improvement in clinical signs should be seen two or three days after initiation of therapy. If no response is seen, the prognosis is poor or an error was made in diagnosis. The drug combination is inhibitory but does not eradicate the infection. In pregnant animals, the antagonists should always be administered with the therapeutic agents to prevent harm to the embryo (Frenkel, 1977). Toxoplasmosis in pets represents a potential public health hazard, and the treatment of these animals must be questioned.

NONINFECTIOUS PNEUMONIAS

PULMONARY INFILTRATION WITH EOSINOPHILIA

Pulmonary infiltration with eosinophilia (PIE) is characterized by pulmonary infiltrates and peripheral eosinophilia. The etiology is unknown but is thought to be hypersensitivity to an antigen. Usually, no specific antigen is identified. Clinical signs vary from a mild chronic dry cough to tachypnea and dyspnea. Fever is usually absent. Auscultatory findings vary from normal to the presence of increased breath sounds, crackles, or wheezes. Radiographic signs are also variable and include increased interstitial opacity, bronchial or peribronchial opacity, alveolar opacity, or a mixed pattern. An absolute peripheral eosinophilia (2000 to 50,000 eosinophils/mm^3) is usually present. Cytologic specimens from the bronchial tree reveal the eosinophil as the predominant cell. Bronchial culture is usually negative.

THERAPY

Therapy consists of systemic corticosteroids. Initially 2 mg/kg of prednisolone is administered daily until the clinical signs resolve. This is followed by a decreasing dosage schedule. Therapy should continue for 90 days. Some dogs require long-term maintenance therapy to prevent relapse. Supportive oxygen therapy may be needed in dyspneic patients. Dogs that present with acute signs generally respond to therapy within hours. Those with more chronic disease do not respond as rapidly.

The prognosis for PIE is good with proper steroid and supportive therapy.

ASPIRATION PNEUMONIA

Aspiration pneumonia is the result of some other underlying disease. Acute aspiration pneumonia usually results from the animal being in a reduced state of consciousness because of sedation, anesthesia, or trauma. Chronic aspiration pneumonia is usually the result of megaesophagus, pharyngeal dysphagia, or abnormalities of the larynx resulting in improper protection of the airway against food and body secretions. Studies in humans have shown that aspiration of oral and gastric secretions commonly occurs during sleep without adverse effects. Aspiration pneumonia only occurs with frequent or large volume aspirations or when secretions of low pH are aspirated. Most aspirations are probably self-limiting, and no clinical disease is observed.

When severe pneumonia develops, clinical signs include tachypnea, dyspnea, cyanosis, and shock. Fever is present when secondary bacterial pneumonia develops. Auscultation of the lungs reveals crackles in the area of the aspirated material, increased breath sounds, and wheezes. Radiographic signs, if present, develop as alveolar infiltrates and follow the onset of clinical signs by several hours. Arterial blood-gas assessment reveals moderate to severe hypoxemia and a decrease in blood pH. Definitive diagnosis is based on the history of an underlying disease process or actual observation of a reduced state of consciousness that could result in aspiration pneumonia.

THERAPY

There is no widely accepted therapeutic plan for aspiration pneumonia. If the animal is hypoxic, oxygen therapy is indicated. Some authors recommend immediate initiation of positive end-expiratory pressure (5 to 10 cm H_2O), which decreases the amount of hemorrhage and congestion within the lung. Saline bronchial lavage is effective only if performed immediately after the aspiration episode. Some authors feel this may expose a greater area of lung to gastric acid, resulting in a more severe pneumonia. If particulate matter was known to be aspirated, large particles can be removed with a bronchoscope.

There are no convincing data to show that administration of corticosteroids are of any benefit. If they are given, they should be administered immediately after the aspiration episode and then discontinued. Antibiotics should be administered only after evidence appears that a secondary bacterial pneumonia is developing, e.g., finding a septic purulent exudate or a positive bacterial culture on transtracheal aspiration.

PROGNOSIS

The long-term prognosis depends on correction of the underlying cause. The short-term prognosis depends on the effectiveness of supportive therapy to alleviate the hypoxemia until pulmonary function improves. Shock and hypoxemia with apnea immediately after aspiration suggest a guarded prognosis.

REFERENCES AND SUPPLEMENTAL READING

Bemis, D. A., and Appel, M. J. G.: Aerosol, parenteral and oral antibiotic treatment of *Bordetella bronchoseptica* infections in dogs. J.A.V.M.A. 170:1082, 1977.

Dunbar, M., and Pyle, R. L.: Ketoconazole treatment of osseous blastomycosis in a dog. V.M./S.A.C. 76:1593, 1981.

Forgacs, P.: The functional basis of pulmonary sounds. Chest 73:399, 1978.

Frenkel, J. F.: Toxoplasmosis. *In* Kirk, R. W. (ed.): *Current Veterinary Therapy VI.* Philadelphia: W. B. Saunders, 1977, pp. 1318–1324.

Harpster, W. K.: The effectiveness of the cephalosporins in the treatment of bacterial pneumonias in the dog. J.A.A.H.A. 17:764, 1981.

Jubb, K. V. F., and Kennedy, P. C. (eds.): The respiratory system. *In Pathology of Domestic Animals*, 2nd ed. New York: Academic Press, 1970.

Light, R. B., Mink, S. N., and Wood, L. D.: Pathophysiology of gas exchange and pulmonary perfusion in pneumococcal lobar pneumonia in dogs. J. Appl. Physiol. 50:524, 1981.

PULMONARY EDEMA

TIMOTHY G. BAUER, D.V.M.,

Seattle, Washington

and WILLIAM P. THOMAS, D.V.M.

Davis, California

As with the body's extrathoracic vascular beds and surrounding tissues, the air space and interstitium of the lung are kept dry by three major physiologic mechanisms: (1) the balance between capillary and interstitial hydrostatic and oncotic pressures (Starling's forces), which tends to limit the transcapillary extravasation of fluid from vascular to interstitial spaces, (2) the integrity of the normal capillary wall ultrastructure, which limits the transcapillary movements of solutes such as protein, and (3) the integrity of normal lymphatic function, which plays a major role in the removal of interstitial fluid from the lungs. Under normal physiologic conditions, small amounts of fluid and protein move continuously from the pulmonary capillaries into the interstitial space, where they are rapidly removed by peribronchial and perivascular lymphatics, which drain via the hilar lymph nodes into the thoracic duct. Significant aberrations of one or more of these mechanisms can cause the accumulation of excessive fluid in the pulmonary interstitium and air spaces, which manifests as pulmonary edema.

Although the most common cause of pulmonary edema in dogs and cats is increased capillary hydrostatic pressure secondary to pulmonary venous hypertension (most often due to left ventricular failure), there is a diverse group of conditions that causes pulmonary edema by this or another mechanism. It is convenient to group these disorders etiologically on the basis of their primary physiologic effect into (1) pulmonary edema with elevated pulmonary venous pressure, (2) pulmonary edema with normal pulmonary venous pressure (increased capillary permeability), and (3) pulmonary edema with both elevated pulmonary venous pressure and increased capillary permeability, as shown in Table 1.

Table 1. ***Causes of Pulmonary Edema***

I. Elevated pulmonary venous pressure
  A. Cardiogenic pulmonary edema
    1. Myocardial failure: congestive cardiomyopathy
    2. Chronic pressure or volume overload: mitral regurgitation, congenital heart disease (patent ductus arteriosus [PDA], subaortic stenosis, etc.)
    3. Obstruction to ventricular filling: hypertrophic cardiomyopathy, mitral stenosis, left atrial thrombus or neoplasm
  B. Neurogenic pulmonary edema: seizures, trauma, other CNS disorders
  C. Post-pericardiocentesis
II. Normal pulmonary venous pressure with altered membrane permeability
  A. Aspiration syndromes
    1. Gastric contents
    2. Near-drowning
    3. Hypertonic material
  B. Inhalation injury: oxygen, smoke, chlorine, ammonia, etc.
  C. Endogenous and exogenous toxicosis: snake venom, alphanaphthylthiourea (ANTU), paraquat, monocrotaline, uremia, pancreatitis
  D. Hypoxemia: high altitude disease
  E. Lung re-expansion
III. Elevated pulmonary venous pressure with altered membrane permeability
  A. Adult respiratory distress syndrome (ARDS, shock lung): sepsis, trauma, surgery, etc.
  B. Electric shock injury

PULMONARY EDEMA WITH ELEVATED PULMONARY VENOUS PRESSURE

CARDIOGENIC PULMONARY EDEMA

Disorders that affect the left heart and progress to left ventricular failure cause elevated pulmonary venous and capillary hydrostatic pressure. Pulmonary edema occurs when pulmonary venous pressure reaches about 25 mm Hg (normal < 10 mm Hg). The development of pulmonary edema in the dog has three progressive phases. When lymphatic capacity is exceeded, fluid accumulates first in the interstitial spaces. It tends to migrate to the perivascular and peribronchial interstitial spaces, which become distended along with associated lymphatics. Continued fluid accumulation results in edema of alveolar walls and ultimately alveolar edema. The edema may fill some alveoli and leave adjacent ones air filled. Although these phases can be identified histologically, it is likely that most clinical cases represent a mingling of interstitial and alveolar (air space) edema. The terms are used to indicate the predominant radiographic appearance and clinical significance.

The radiographic progression of cardiogenic edema follows a predictable sequence, particularly in the dog. Progressive elevation of pulmonary venous pressure results in pulmonary venous engorgement (congestion) and perivascular and interstitial clouding, which tends to obscure the pulmonary vasculature. This is followed by air space edema with the appearance of coalescing fluffy densities and air bronchograms. The edema consistently appears first in the central perihilar region in the dog and progresses outward, sparing the periphery of the lungs until the condition is advanced. In the cat, the distribution of cardiogenic edema is less consistent, often occurring in a patchy, irregular pattern, particularly in the caudal lobes.

NEUROGENIC PULMONARY EDEMA

Pulmonary edema is occasionally seen in patients with elevated intracranial pressure and following generalized seizures or central nervous system (CNS) trauma. Although precise mechanisms have not been proved, experimentally produced cerebrospinal fluid (CSF) pressure elevation in animals has been shown to result in elevations of pulmonary venous pressure. The mechanism is believed to involve direct (CNS) and indirect (catecholamine) adrenergic stimulation, which causes vasoconstriction. The result of pulmonary venous constriction and elevation of pulmonary venous pressure is pulmonary edema without evidence of left ventricular failure.

Patients most likely to develop neurogenic pulmonary edema are those suffering from multiple or prolonged seizures or major CNS trauma. The development of edema is often gradual. The radiographic appearance is variable and may be confused with pulmonary contusion sustained from the initial trauma. Some of these patients have derangements of consciousness and are susceptible to aspiration,

positional atelectasis, and centrally mediated apnea, all of which may complicate their pulmonary disorder.

POST-PERICARDIOCENTESIS

Mild pulmonary edema is frequently observed in dogs following pericardiocentesis for relief of cardiac tamponade. Following drainage of a large, chronic pericardial effusion, widespread but mild interstitial and air space edema has been observed on survey thoracic radiographs. The cause is believed to be cardiogenic, but this is poorly documented. In the authors' experience, dogs with this type of edema rarely become symptomatic or require therapy. The pulmonary density may affect the interpretation of post-drainage radiographs and pneumopericardiograms.

PULMONARY EDEMA WITH NORMAL PULMONARY VENOUS PRESSURE

A large and diverse group of etiologies produce their effect primarily by altering alveolar–capillary membrane permeability. Many also produce damage to conducting and respiratory areas of the lung. The majority of the agents described hereafter reach the exchange areas via the airways rather than via the vascular bed.

ASPIRATION SYNDROMES

These disorders result from the inhalation of noxious materials into the tracheobronchial tree. The range of potential offending materials is broad (see Table 1). Although the course of these disorders may be complicated by pulmonary infection, hemorrhage, or airway obstruction, the principal pathologic effect is pulmonary edema. Although the dependent regions of the lung are usually the most severely affected, many patients present acutely with widespread edema throughout both lungs. Aspirated materials are often spread throughout the lungs by coughing and hyperventilatory effort following the initial aspiration. The materials are distributed to the periphery of the lungs, where edema results from direct injury to alveolar-capillary membranes with increased permeability. Hypertonicity may also favor vascular to alveolar movement of fluid.

ASPIRATION OF GASTRIC CONTENTS

Experimental aspiration of acidic liquids, particularly those with a pH of 2.5 or less, results in severe alveolar damage and pulmonary edema. Aspiration of gastric secretions is a relatively frequent complication of general anesthesia and consciousness disorders, and is seen with certain anatomic abnormalities such as megaesophagus. The severity of the pulmonary reaction and the resulting radiographic appearance depend on the volume and nature of the aspirated material and the anatomic distribution of the aspirate. The acute edema is frequently complicated by infection, resulting in aspiration pneumonia.

NEAR-DROWNING

Aspiration of either fresh or salt water without immediate asphyxiation may be fatal in the hours following the initial event. Although early reviews of the subject attributed death to electrolyte alterations, recent studies in dogs clearly demonstrate that the principal abnormality is profound hypoxemia and that electrolyte abnormalities play a minor role. The volume of aspirated water rarely exceeds 10 ml/kg. Tonicity determines the pathophysiology of the pulmonary injury.

Sea water is hypertonic relative to plasma and contains mechanical irritants such as sand and plankton. Direct alveolar injury and an osmotic gradient result in extravasation of fluid and protein from the vascular compartment into the alveoli. Hypoxemia and acidemia result from diffusion impairment, and hypotension may result from intravascular volume reduction. Inhalation of other hypertonic agents, such as radiographic contrast material, probably causes pulmonary edema by similar mechanisms.

In fresh-water aspiration, the osmotic gradient in exchange areas is opposite that seen with salt water. Absorption of the hypotonic water may cause modest hemodilution. Besides alveolar injury, loss of pulmonary surfactant predisposes to collapse of air spaces at the exchange level. The result is severe hypoxemia.

Although there are pathophysiologic differences between fresh and salt water, the aspiration of either probably results in alveolar-capillary injury and similar clinical syndromes that require similar medical management.

INHALATION OF IRRITANT OR TOXIC GASES

A number of industrial and environmental gases are known to cause pulmonary edema of acute or gradual onset. The most common mechanism for the pulmonary injury is oxidative damage to alveolar-capillary membranes. Oxidant gases interfere with microstructural enzyme systems, and ultrastructural damage occurs from protein disruption caused by the formation of free radicals and the consumption of sulfhydryl bonds. The severity and distribution of the pulmonary injury depend on (1) the toxicity of the agent, (2) the inhaled concentration and exposure time, and (3) the presence of any

pre-existing lung disease. The solubility of the gas is important in determining the concentration reaching the exchange areas. More soluble gases are absorbed in the conducting airways, resulting in more airway than exchange area disease.

HIGH ALTITUDE PULMONARY EDEMA

Although incompletely understood, this type of edema appears to occur in association with pulmonary hypertension. In susceptible individuals inhalation of air with a low P_{O_2} causes pulmonary arterial constriction and pulmonary hypertension. Pulmonary capillary hypertension and edema probably result from either intrapulmonary shunting or direct capillary vasoconstriction. Experimental production of this type of hypertension and edema in the dog requires a 75 per cent reduction in vascular cross-sectional area, which can only be achieved in a small percentage of normal dogs. Compared with animals such as cattle, dogs are relatively resistant to this form of edema.

LUNG RE-EXPANSION

Rapid reduction of a large pleural effusion or pneumothorax may result in pulmonary edema. Although not precisely understood, this syndrome is believed to result from one of several mechanisms, including (1) primary hypoxic injury to pulmonary capillaries from lung collapse, (2) the acute effects of exaggerated negative intrapleural pressure, and (3) alterations in pulmonary veins and lymphatic stasis. Several criteria appear to be important in this syndrome: (1) the effusion or pneumothorax must be large, causing collapse of 80 per cent of the lung, (2) the disorder must be present for several days, and (3) the pleural drainage and lung re-expansion must be performed rapidly. Edema is much less common when drainage is accomplished gradually by tube thoracostomy and waterseal drainage.

Although physical examination and thoracic radiography may indicate the presence of an air space disorder in these patients, they rarely become symptomatic. This probably reflects the degree of respiratory embarrassment caused by the pleural disorder and its relief by drainage. The pulmonary density must be recognized on radiographs obtained following pleural drainage.

PULMONARY EDEMA WITH ELEVATED PULMONARY VENOUS PRESSURE AND INCREASED MEMBRANE PERMEABILITY

ADULT RESPIRATORY DISTRESS SYNDROME

Improved critical patient care and survival in patients with major injury or illness have resulted in the emergence of secondary pulmonary disorders, especially acute respiratory failure, as important medical syndromes. This group of related disorders is collectively termed the *adult respiratory distress syndrome* (ARDS). ARDS can occur in patients without pre-existing pulmonary disease secondary to a wide variety of medical and surgical disorders, including sepsis, major trauma, major surgery, aspiration, pancreatitis, hematologic disorders (disseminated intravascular coagulopathy [DIC], transfusion reactions) and shock.

Although it is incompletely understood, the pathogenesis of the illnesses predisposing to ARDS is believed to be similar, despite their diversity. There is alveolar-capillary membrane damage, often with concurrently elevated pulmonary venous pressure (due to myocardial failure). Histologic examination reveals edema and hemorrhage in both the interstitium and alveoli. The result is a stiff, noncompliant lung; major gas diffusion impairment; and a wide arterial-alveolar O_2 tension difference due to widespread intrapulmonary shunting. (Refer to the article on Blood Gases and Acid-Base Balance for additional information on arterial-alveolar O_2 differences.)

The clinical presentation of ARDS consists of a patient with (1) a history of predisposing illness or injury, (2) no history of pre-existing pulmonary disease associated with illness (pneumonia, and so on), (3) a rapidly progressive air space disorder with hypoxemia and loss of lung compliance, and (4) thoracic radiographs showing diffuse air space disease involving most of the lungs.

ELECTRIC SHOCK

Patients who survive a major electric shock injury often develop respiratory distress due to pulmonary edema within hours of the event. Although traditionally considered to be noncardiogenic, there is ample pathologic and experimental evidence of major myocardial damage resulting from electric shock. Edema probably results from direct capillary injury coupled with elevated pulmonary venous pressure due to myocardial failure. Until the pathogenesis is clarified, the authors recommend that treatment of these patients be similar to that for others with cardiogenic edema or ARDS.

TREATMENT OF PULMONARY EDEMA

Essential to the treatment of pulmonary edema is an accurate diagnosis. Physical examination, particularly thoracic auscultation, and thoracic radiography are most important in distinguishing pulmonary edema from other disorders causing dyspnea and tachypnea, including pleural disorders (effusion, pneumothorax, diaphragmatic hernia), conducting airway disorders (collapse, perforation,

Table 2. *Drug Dosages Used in the Treatment of Canine Pulmonary Edema*

Aminophylline: 11 mg/kg IV, SC, PO q6h
Morphine sulfate: 0.2 to 0.5 mg/kg IV, IM, SC
Furosemide: 2 to 4 mg/kg IV, IM, SC, PO, repeat as needed
Digoxin: 0.02 to 0.04 mg/kg IV in divided 1/4 to 1/2 doses over
    two to six hours
    0.06 to 0.15 mg/kg orally in divided doses over 24 to 48
    hours
Dopamine: 5 to 10 μg/kg/min constant-rate infusion
Dobutamine: 5 to 10 μg/kg/min constant-rate infusion
Sodium nitroprusside: 5 to 20 μg/kg/min constant-rate infusion
*Prazosin: 0.5 to 1.0 mg t.i.d. initially up to 10 to 15 mg t.i.d.
    PO
*Hydralazine: 6.25 to 25 mg t.i.d. PO
Nitroglycerine ointment (2 per cent): 1/4 to 1/2 inch on the
    abdominal skin q6 to 8h

*These doses are based on limited clinical trials. Hemodynamic studies documenting the effectiveness of these oral vasodilators in animals with different types of heart disease have not been reported.

obstruction), and other pulmonary disorders (pneumonia, mass lesions or metastatic infiltration, pulmonary thromboembolism). Once a diagnosis is reached, the aggressiveness of its treatment depends on the severity, including the degree of respiratory distress exhibited by the patient, and the underlying etiology.

The principal objectives in the treatment of pulmonary edema include the following: (1) decrease oxygen demands, (2) improve alveolar oxygen delivery, (3) decrease the amount of excess pulmonary fluid, (4) support and maintain adequate pulmonary circulation, and (5) treat underlying or complicating disorders, including shock and myocardial failure, sepsis, pulmonary infection, renal failure, and so on. The emphasis placed on each of these objectives depends on the severity and etiology of the edema. Two major categories requiring different approaches will be considered. Drug dosages are listed in Table 2.

PULMONARY EDEMA WITH ELEVATED PULMONARY VENOUS PRESSURE (CARDIOGENIC EDEMA)

Accurate diagnosis is important, since many patients, especially older dogs with acquired mitral valve disease, develop pulmonary complaints in the absence of congestive heart failure, including acute or chronic tracheobronchitis and tracheobronchial collapse. Fine inspiratory crackles, other physical signs of cardiac disease, radiographic signs of cardiac disease, and a centrally distributed pulmonary density support a diagnosis of cardiogenic edema.

In patients not receiving prior treatment, the objectives in treating cardiogenic edema are to (1) decrease oxygen demands and myocardial work, (2) improve oxygen delivery if dyspnea and discomfort are severe, (3) lower pulmonary venous pressure to enhance reabsorption of edema, and (4) improve myocardial performance by enhancing contractility and reducing ventricular preload and afterload.

The simplest means of reducing oxygen demands and myocardial work is to restrict physical activity to a small cage. Sedation using narcotics or tranquilizers in low doses is usually reserved for patients who remain active or anxious despite restriction to a cage. If dyspnea and discomfort are severe, an oxygen cage that can maintain a 40 to 50 per cent oxygen concentration is very valuable. Oxygen tents are acceptable if temperature, humidity, and CO_2 levels can be controlled. Administration of a bronchodilator such as aminophylline may help reverse the small airway constriction and collapse associated with interstitial edema in the presence of preexisting small airway disease.

In cardiogenic edema, the safest and most rapidly effective means of reducing pulmonary venous pressure and edema formation is to reduce the intravascular volume with a potent diuretic. Furosemide is administered in doses of 2 to 4 mg/kg intravenously as soon as the diagnosis is made. This can be repeated, if required, in two to four hours. In new patients with only modest discomfort and in cardiac patients already receiving oral maintenance medications, this may be the only therapy needed to eliminate the edema within 6 to 12 hours. The overzealous use of diuretics can cause severe volume depletion and hypotension, particularly in patients with severely depressed myocardial function. In both dogs and cats with left ventricular failure due to congestive (dilated) cardiomyopathy, aggressive diuresis should be accompanied by inotropic support in the form of digitalis, dopamine, or dobutamine to prevent the development of cardiogenic shock.

When cardiogenic pulmonary edema results from myocardial failure, acute or chronic pressure, or volume overload, inotropic therapy is indicated. Oral digitalization using digoxin is used in patients with mild edema, which responds rapidly to diuretic therapy. In acute congestive left ventricular failure and cardiogenic shock, digoxin is administered intravenously over two to eight hours, depending on the urgency. Intravenous infusions of dopamine or dobutamine are usually reserved for critically ill patients with severe acute heart failure or cardiogenic shock. These interventions require careful monitoring of the ECG, heart rate, blood pressure, and cardiac output in an intensive care setting.

Another approach to improving cardiac output and lowering pulmonary venous pressure is the administration of vasodilators. In left ventricular failure, increased adrenergic tone and arterial vasoconstriction act to maintain blood pressure at the expense of ventricular output. Controlled arterial dilation improves forward cardiac output and helps lower ventricular diastolic pressure in a ventricle capable of responding. Venous dilation also helps lower pulmonary venous pressure and edema formation. Since the principal side effects of these drugs are hypotension and reflex tachycardia, they should only be administered when the patient can be appropriately monitored and observed. Oral hydralazine or prazosin may be given to patients who are not critically ill. Intravenous infusion of sodium nitroprusside, a potent arterial and venous vasodilator, is reserved for patients with critical left ventricular failure unresponsive to other measures.

In summary, mild cardiogenic edema is usually managed by a combination of enforced rest, oral or parenteral furosemide or another diuretic, and oral digitalization. Severe, acute cardiogenic edema is managed by a combination of enforced rest (with or without sedation) and the administration of oxygen, intravenous furosemide, and digoxin. Infusions of dopamine, dobutamine, and nitroprusside are reserved for unresponsive patients. The value of oral vasodilators in dogs and cats with mild cardiogenic edema remains to be studied.

PULMONARY EDEMA WITH NORMAL PULMONARY VENOUS PRESSURE (NONCARDIOGENIC EDEMA)

The key to successful treatment of severe, noncardiogenic edema is early diagnosis and aggressive medical management. Mild edema may not require treatment, or it may respond adequately to simple diuretic therapy. The severity of the disorder is assessed by means of physical examination, thoracic radiography, and arterial blood gas analysis, performed serially as the disorder is managed. Once the condition is recognized, the objectives are to (1) improve oxygen delivery to maintain a Pa_{O_2} above 60 mm Hg, (2) decrease the amount of excess pulmonary fluid, and (3) manage and prevent underlying disorders or complicating sequelae, including shock and myocardial failure, sepsis, DIC, uremia, hepatic failure, CNS disorders, hypoventilation, and pulmonary infections. Localized or systemic infections must be aggressively diagnosed by cultures of blood, urine, airway secretions, and so on, and specific antimicrobial therapy must be instituted as soon as possible. This is especially important in patients with acquired, resistant nosocomial infections. In the absence of demonstrable infection, there is little evidence supporting the prophylactic use of antibiotics in these patients.

Although still controversial, there is evidence that corticosteroids may be useful in reversing the microcirculatory injury characteristic of ARDS. Administration of one or two doses of methylprednisolone or dexamethasone, four to six hours apart, has been beneficial in humans with septic shock and ARDS.

The administration of diuretics in noncardiogenic edema should be considered only after evaluation of the patient's cardiac function and state of hydration. In normotensive, normovolemic patients, intravenous furosemide may be as beneficial as in cardiogenic edema. However, since many of these patients may already be hypovolemic and marginally hypotensive, especially following trauma, surgery, or sepsis, diuretic therapy may further compromise intravascular volume and cardiac output, resulting in hypovolemic shock. Depending on the patient's hydration, cardiac output, and blood pressure, measured directly or indirectly from the evaluation of arterial pulses and peripheral perfusion, a choice must be made between volume depletion using diuretics and volume expansion using intravenous fluids. If hypotension and shock are present, intravenous fluid therapy and inotropic support with dopamine, dobutamine, or digoxin are indicated despite the presence of pulmonary edema.

Maintenance of adequate oxygenation is critical. In mild cases, oxygen administration at 40 to 50 per cent concentration in a tent or cage may be adequate. When severe lung involvement with loss of compliance, edema, and terminal airway collapse occurs, maintenance of Pa_{O_2} above 60 mm Hg may require ventilatory support. The early use of mechanical ventilation has become the most common means of treating humans with these disorders. In the authors' experience, mechanical ventilation and the use of positive end-expiratory pressure have also been extremely valuable in small animals with these disorders. The principles of mechanical ventilation are discussed in detail elsewhere in this text and are only briefly mentioned here.

Although dogs and cats usually require heavy sedation with or without paralyzation to tolerate prolonged endotracheal intubation and ventilation, mechanical ventilation by means of a tracheostomy is tolerated with only mild sedation. It has the further advantage of allowing intermittent spontaneous breaths and permits the animal to remain in an upright posture. Ventilation is usually begun using 100 per cent oxygen, which is reduced as soon as possible to the minimal level that maintains the Pa_{O_2} above 60 mm Hg. Positive end-expiratory pressure of 5 to 15 cm H_2O may be used to prevent airway collapse. The concentration of inspired oxygen is decreased progressively as Pa_{O_2} improves. Nursing care of the tracheostomy tube is critical to prevent infection and obstruction. Particular attention to circulatory function is required, especially in critically ill patients, as positive pressure ventilation can interfere with venous return and can adversely affect cardiac output.

In summary, mild noncardiogenic edema may be managed using parenteral furosemide and oxygen administration. Progressive, severe noncardiogenic edema with dyspnea, hypoxemia, and shock usually requires artificial ventilation and circulatory support. Even with aggressive management, the mortality of severe, noncardiogenic edema is high if treatment is begun late in the course of the disorder. Early diagnosis and aggressive management have been associated with increased survival in both humans and small animals.

SUPPLEMENTAL READING

Ayres, S. M.: Mechanisms and consequences of pulmonary edema: Cardiac lung, shock lung, and principles of ventilatory therapy in adult respiratory distress syndrome. Am. Heart J. 103:97, 1982.
Staub, N. C.: Pulmonary edema. Physiol. Rev. 54:678, 1974.
Staub, N. C.: State of the art review: Pathogenesis of pulmonary edema. Am. Rev. Resp. Dis. 109:358, 1976.

PULMONARY THROMBOEMBOLISM

MARK G. BURNS, D.V.M.

New York, New York

Pulmonary artery *thrombosis* is the formation of clot material within the pulmonary arterial vasculature. It may involve the main pulmonary artery, one of its branches, or one of the smaller lobar arteries and may or may not be occlusive. Pulmonary *thromboembolism* is the obstruction or occlusion of the pulmonary vasculature by clot material originating at some distant site in the body and usually entering the pulmonary arterial circulation as a "shower" of clot fragments. These showers of fragments tend to settle in the smaller diameter pulmonary vessels and capillary systems and are usually occlusive at these sites. However, some regions of the pulmonary vasculature may be less severely affected than others. Thrombosis and thromboembolism as well as embolism with fat or vegetative or foreign matter and parasites may also occur at other sites within the body. This article, however, is limited to a discussion of thrombosis and thromboembolism within the pulmonary arterial circulation, which will be referred to collectively as pulmonary thromboembolism.

In human medicine, acute pulmonary thromboembolism is estimated to be the sole or major contributing cause of death in 5 to 15 per cent of adults dying in acute-care general hospitals. These may be tumor, air, or fat emboli, but 90 per cent are thromboemboli resulting from thromboses in the deep venous system of the pelvis and thighs. Patients are predisposed to these deep venous thromboses by many factors, including prolonged bed rest, congestive heart failure, malignant disease, various shock syndromes, pregnancy, obesity, trauma, and surgery, especially pelvic and orthopedic procedures. It is estimated that 10 per cent of patients with acute pulmonary thromboembolism die within one hour and that of the remainder (approximately 563,000 each year), two-thirds go undiagnosed and one-third die. There are no historical, physical, or laboratory findings allowing for rapid, accurate diagnosis. If rapid, effective diagnostic procedures were available, 50,000 to 100,000 deaths might be prevented in the United States each year (Rosenow et al., 1981).

Pulmonary thromboembolism exists as a clinical entity in veterinary medicine. However, the condition is not well-recognized and its overall incidence is unknown. It has been seen in association with hyperadrenocorticism, with endocarditis secondary to heartworm disease, in hypothyroidism (experimentally in dogs on a high-fat, high-cholesterol diet), and as a post-operative complication. It has also been noted in post-mortem studies of dogs with renal amyloidosis, dogs and cats with membranous nephropathy, and in cases of acute unexplainable death. A cause-and-effect relationship has not always been established in these cases.

Before the incidence, predisposing factors, and causes of pulmonary thromboembolism in companion animals can be ascertained, we must recognize it as a clinical entity. We can best do this by having an understanding of thrombogenesis and its related pathophysiology, a high level of suspicion, and a means of diagnosing the condition. Efficacious means of therapy may then be established.

THROMBOGENESIS/FIBRINOLYSIS AND PATHOLOGIC THROMBOSIS

Within the blood vascular system, a dynamic balance exists between those naturally occurring factors that promote clot formation (procoagulants) and those that inhibit clot formation (anticoagulants).

Central to the mechanism of clotting is the formation of thrombin. Trauma to the vascular wall or extravascular tissues results in activation of the extrinsic clotting mechanism; tissue factor, tissue phospholipid, calcium, and clotting factors V, VII, and X react to form prothrombin activator. Alternatively, injury to the blood itself results in the release of platelet thromboplastin and activation of the intrinsic clotting pathway. After the classical interaction of clotting factors IV (calcium), V, and VIII through XII, prothrombin activator is similarly formed. Prothrombin activator is capable of catalyzing the conversion of prothrombin to thrombin. Thrombin acts as an enzyme, converting fibrinogen to a fibrin monomer, which polymerizes to form long fibrin threads. These threads then bond, "stabilizing" the clot, when fibrin-stabilizing factor (from platelets) is activated by thrombin. Thrombin, in addition to its previously mentioned functions, also promotes further clot formation by stimulating further platelet aggregation, promoting the further conversion of prothrombin to thrombin and accelerating the activation of clotting factors VIII through XII. It is easy to see that this mechanism, if left unchecked, would lead to a vicious cycle of clot growth.

Fortunately, several mechanisms are present to prevent an unhindered proliferation of the developing clot, thus preventing thrombotic vessel obstruction. First, a critical concentration of procoagulants is necessary to overcome the naturally occurring anticoagulants. As the clot grows into the more rapidly flowing stream of blood in the center of the vessel, the excessive concentrations of thrombin and other procoagulants present within the core of the clot are swept away, diluted in the general circulation, and rapidly destroyed by the liver. Second, 85 to 90 per cent of formed thrombin is bound to the fibrin threads that form the meshwork of the clot, thus preventing thrombin from entering the circulation. Third, the remainder of the thrombin is bound and rendered inactive by antithrombin III (antithrombin-heparin cofactor), a naturally occurring anticoagulant. Last, activation of the fibrinolytic system plays a major role in controlling an unmitigated activation of the clotting mechanism. In this system, plasminogen is converted to plasmin, a proteolytic enzyme, by either lysosomal enzymes from destroyed tissue, thrombin, or activated clotting factor XII. Plasmin has the ability to enzymatically destroy the fibrin threads, fibrinogen, prothrombin, and clotting factors V, VIII, and XII, thus inhibiting clot growth and promoting clot lysis. The fibrinolytic system is most important in removing clots from the very small peripheral vessels. Many other factors play a role in maintaining a balance between coagulation and fibrinolysis, but their discussion is beyond the intent of this article.

Classically, three factors have been associated with "tipping the scales" in favor of pathologic thrombosis. First, local endothelial injury of a chronic nature, whether infectious, immunologic, mechanical, or chemical, will promote a persistent activation of the clotting mechanism. A thrombus (clot) may eventually grow to the extent that it may obstruct the involved vessel. Second, changes in the blood flow, especially those favoring turbulence or stasis, favor thrombosis. Activated procoagulants are allowed to accumulate locally rather than being diluted in the general circulation, thus favoring pathologic clot growth. Also, turbulent blood can cause chronic endothelial injury. The third factor is an increased tendency of the blood to clot. This relative increase of procoagulant factors (or decrease in anticoagulant factors) has been associated with many diverse diseases and is generally referred to as a "hypercoagulable state" (Mobin-Uddin, 1975; Moser and Stein, 1973).

PATHOPHYSIOLOGY OF GAS EXCHANGE—VENTILATION/PERFUSION MISMATCHING

Normal respiratory function is dependent on adequate alveolar *ventilation* as well as *perfusion* of these alveoli with pulmonary capillary blood. In the normal state, in fact, ventilation ($\dot{V}A$) and perfusion ($\dot{Q}$) maintain a fairly constant relationship (Fig. 1, A), allowing for the normal diffusion of oxygen (O_2) and carbon dioxide (CO_2) between the alveoli and the pulmonary capillary circulation. This relationship is called the *ventilation/perfusion ratio* ($\dot{V}A/\dot{Q}$). The ventilation/perfusion ratio is altered in many pulmonary diseases; two extreme situations exist.

As ventilation decreases and eventually reaches 0, the $\dot{V}A/\dot{Q}$ becomes 0 (Fig. 1, B). In this situation the partial pressures of O_2 and CO_2 in the alveolus would equilibrate with the partial pressures of O_2

and CO_2 in the venous blood, after which no further diffusion of O_2 or CO_2 would take place. The partial pressures of O_2 and CO_2 in the alveoli and in the arterial blood would approach those of venous blood, and a right-to-left shunt would develop. If perfusion is increased relative to ventilation, shunting of venous blood might also occur; however, in this situation there is a large reserve capacity to maintain normal gaseous exchange.

In the other extreme, as perfusion decreases and eventually becomes 0, the $\dot{V}A/\dot{Q}$ approaches infinity (Fig. 1, C). In this situation the normally ventilated air would not have a pulmonary blood supply with which to exchange O_2 and CO_2. The partial pressures of O_2 and CO_2 in alveolar air would equilibrate with the partial pressures of O_2 and CO_2 in inspired, humidified, atmospheric air. Inspired air would not undergo gaseous exchange with venous blood, and a state of increased respiratory dead space would develop.

Obviously neither of these extremes is compatible with life; however, many degrees of change may be seen within these limits, or these changes may occur locally.

In thromboembolism there is a lack of perfusion to the involved lung areas. This lack of perfusion may be acute or chronic. In those areas of the lung undergoing thrombosis, ventilation may be normal, but there is an interruption of perfusion. A *ventilation-perfusion mismatch* occurs and a state of increased respiratory dead space develops. The $\dot{V}A/\dot{Q}$ increases in these areas. In response, pulmonary blood will be directed to those pulmonary vessels that remain open, and reserve pulmonary vessels and alveolar capillaries will come into use. Pulmonary blood will flow through these patent vessels more rapidly than normal, thus increasing perfusion relative to ventilation. The $\dot{V}A/\dot{Q}$ will tend to decrease in these areas. Normally, however, O_2 and CO_2 diffuse within the first third of the capillary-alveolar interface, and there is a large reserve for O_2 and CO_2 exchange as perfusion increases. Since

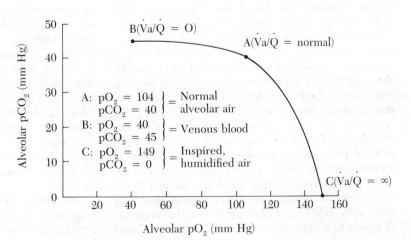

Figure 1. The normal pO_2-pCO_2, $\dot{V}A/\dot{Q}$ diagram. (Modified from Guyton: *Textbook of Medical Physiology*, 6th ed. Philadelphia: W. B. Saunders, 1981).

A: $pO_2 = 104$ $pCO_2 = 40$ } = Normal alveolar air

B: $pO_2 = 40$ $pCO_2 = 45$ } = Venous blood

C: $pO_2 = 149$ $pCO_2 = 0$ } = Inspired, humidified air

B($\dot{V}a/\dot{Q} = 0$)

A($\dot{V}a/\dot{Q} =$ normal)

C($\dot{V}a/\dot{Q} = \infty$)

Alveolar pCO_2 (mm Hg)

Alveolar pO_2 (mm Hg)

O_2 is less soluble and therefore diffuses less rapidly than CO_2 and as perfusion continues to increase in the nonthrombosed areas, hypoxemia develops. The respiratory rate increases in response to hypoxemia in an attempt to rematch ventilation with perfusion. When this reflex tachypnea occurs, hyperventilation leads to an increased loss of the more highly soluble and diffusible CO_2. Hypoxemia and hypocarbia coexist, and there is a tendency toward respiratory alkalosis. If the condition worsens there will be a failure of CO_2 exchange. Pathologic shunting with hypoxemia, hypercarbia, and respiratory acidosis will then develop.

Another compensatory mechanism for thrombosis is mediated by the left and right bronchial branches of the bronchoesophageal artery. These bronchial arteries are the chief *nutritional* blood supply to the lung, and they account for the low incidence of pulmonary infarction in cases of pulmonary thromboembolism. At the level of the respiratory bronchioles the bronchial arteries terminate in capillary beds that are capable of acting as reserve areas for O_2 and CO_2 exchange.

When hypoxemia becomes severe (less than 60 mm Hg), tissue hypoxia develops and the cells begin to rely more on anaerobic glycolysis for energy production. The end-product of anaerobic glycolysis is lactic acid, and a mild to severe metabolic acidosis may develop. Regarding acid-base balance, then, one would expect to see metabolic acidosis with a respiratory alkalosis (which may or may not be compensatory) and, terminally or in severe cases, a respiratory acidosis.

PATHOPHYSIOLOGY OF PULMONARY HEMODYNAMICS—COR PULMONALE

Cor pulmonale refers to those changes in right ventricular function that develop owing to hypertension in the pulmonary vascular system occurring secondary to pulmonary disease. As thromboembolism ensues, the total number of pulmonary blood vessels available for blood flow decreases, total pulmonary resistance increases, and pulmonary hypertension develops. Hypoxemia also causes pulmonary vasoconstriction, as do elevated levels of serotonin released from degranulating platelets, thus aggravating hypertension. Several mechanisms compensate for thromboembolism and thus retard the development of hypertension, including the "opening up" of previously dormant pulmonary alveolar capillaries. It is known that 25 to 50 per cent of the cross-sectional area of the pulmonary vasculature must be obstructed before hypertension develops. As hypertension develops, the right ventricle initially dilates and hypertrophies and may ultimately fail. The overall cardiovascular response depends to a large degree on the status of the heart

pump prior to thromboembolism. Degrees of pulmonary hypertension are less predictable, and right heart failure is more likely to occur when underlying heart disease is present.

DIAGNOSIS OF PULMONARY THROMBOEMBOLISM

The diagnosis of pulmonary thromboembolism depends, to a large degree, on a high level of suspicion.

CLINICAL SIGNS

In humans, pulmonary thromboembolism results in three different clinical syndromes: (1) acute dyspnea with normal thoracic radiographs, (2) dyspnea with abnormal thoracic radiographs due to pulmonary hemorrhage/infarction, and (3) acute cor pulmonale. Most cases probably start as acute dyspnea without radiographic changes and progress with subsequent embolism to pulmonary hemorrhage/ infarction or acute cor pulmonale.

There are no historical or physical findings that are accurate enough for the certain diagnosis of pulmonary thromboembolism. However, certain findings are consistently seen and can be divided into those resulting from the pathologic exchange of O_2 and CO_2 and those resulting from pulmonary hypertension. In addition, predisposing factors and underlying diseases should be considered.

CLINICAL SIGNS RELATED TO PATHOLOGIC GAS EXCHANGE

The most consistent historical and physical finding in pulmonary thromboembolism is *severe intractable dyspnea* unresponsive to rest, oxygen, diuretics, thoracocentesis, or other conventional means of therapy. Dyspnea results from several factors. Bronchoconstriction occurs in the obstructed regions of the lung for several reasons, including the local release of humoral factors, such as serotonin and histamine from platelets within the thrombus, as well as the airway hypocarbia that occurs in dead space respiration. Bronchoconstriction tends to return the $\dot{V}_A/\dot{Q}$ toward normal in these thrombosed areas. Even though this has the effect of decreasing dead space respiration, lung volume is reduced in these areas and dyspnea is the "price" that the patient must pay. Dyspnea also occurs as a result of hypoxemia, pleural effusion, pleuritic pain, pulmonary edema, and psychological stress.

Orthopnea (positional dyspnea) is manifested by reluctance on the part of the patient to assume certain positions; if the patient is placed in one of these positions, dyspnea (often severe) may result. The positions that cause dyspnea vary greatly from patient to patient and probably depend on which lung areas are involved.

In severe cases there may be a history of syncope, and cyanosis may be noted. Less commonly seen clinical signs include restlessness, cough, hemoptysis, and crackles.

CLINICAL SIGNS RELATED TO PULMONARY HYPERTENSION

Cor pulmonale may be detected clinically by noting a prominent or split second heart sound, a gallop rhythm, or a right-sided systolic murmur occurring secondary to tricuspid valvular insufficiency. If right-sided congestive heart failure develops, a pendulous abdomen associated with ascites may be part of the history. Physical findings include distended jugular veins and a jugular pulse, hepatomegaly, and, rarely, peripheral edema. Heart sounds may become muffled owing to a pleural or pericardial effusion. These changes are inconsistent and nonspecific in humans with pulmonary thromboembolism, and the same may be true in companion animals.

PREDISPOSING FACTORS AND UNDERLYING DISEASES

Several factors are known to predispose to thrombosis in humans as mentioned earlier. These factors are not known in companion animals, but many possibilities might be considered. Major surgical procedures, especially with long periods of postoperative cage confinement, or situations in which the patient is unable to stand or walk for prolonged periods of time may predispose to thrombosis. Various shock syndromes, whether endotoxic, hypovolemic, cardiogenic, or neurogenic, may predispose to thrombosis and may be associated with trauma, surgery, systemic diseases, and prolonged cage confinement. Congestive heart failure may lead to stasis of blood and a tendency for thrombosis. Malignant disease may result in the local stasis of blood, sequestration of clotting factors, and activation of the clotting mechanism secondary to the destruction of vascular endothelium and the alteration of blood elements. Also, certain paraneoplastic syndromes have been associated with hyperviscosity, blood stasis, altered clotting ability, and protein dyscrasias, all of which have been incriminated in hypercoagulable states. Pregnancy and obesity in animals might also predispose to thrombosis, especially in those animals that have prolonged periods of inactivity.

Dyspnea is usually the only historical finding that is directly associated with pulmonary thromboembolism. There may be other major historical findings related to an underlying and perhaps primary disease. Conditions most commonly associated with pulmonary thromboembolism in companion animals have been renal amyloidosis, dirofilariasis, hyperadrenocorticism, hypothyroidism, membranous nephropathy, and postoperative states. Pulmonary thrombotic events have also been seen as a cause of acute death.

LABORATORY FINDINGS

Hematologic and biochemical studies may be normal or may be a nonspecific reflection of tissue damage occurring secondarily to tissue hypoxia. In pulmonary thromboembolism in humans, a generalized inflammatory response to cellular damage may occur, resulting in leukocytosis and neutrophilia. Eosinophilia may occasionally be seen. Other changes may be those of an underlying or primary disease.

BLOOD GAS AND ACID-BASE MEASUREMENTS

As discussed previously, oxygen tensions will usually be below normal. If hypoxemia becomes severe (less than 60 mm Hg), tissue hypoxia and anaerobic energy production may result in a mild to severe metabolic acidosis. Respiratory alkalosis will usually exist and may or may not compensate for a metabolic acidosis. If thrombosis is severe and there is a failure of CO_2 exchange, respiratory acidosis may develop. In three dogs with pulmonary thrombosis and hyperadrenocorticism, all had hypoxemia (pO_2 = 64.6 to 67.2 mm Hg). One dog had metabolic acidosis and a partially compensating respiratory alkalosis, another dog had a mild respiratory alkalosis, and a third dog had a normal blood pH with insignificant changes in the HCO_3^- and pCO_2 (Burns et al., 1981).

HEMODYNAMIC STUDIES

In an experimental study in dogs, obstruction of 25 to 50 per cent of the pulmonary arterial circulation was necessary to induce pulmonary artery hypertension. With obstruction of greater than 40 per cent of the cross-sectional area of the pulmonary vasculature, concurrent pressure elevations were also seen in the right ventricle, right atrium, and cranial vena cava. In humans, alterations in systemic blood pressure, cardiac output, cardiac index, and heart rate are uncommon. When they do occur it is usually a result of acute massive obstruction with resultant cardiovascular collapse.

Pressure studies in three dogs with pulmonary artery thrombosis showed elevated central venous pressures (three out of three), elevated right ventricular systolic pressures (two out of two), and elevated pulmonary arterial systolic and diastolic pressures in the one dog in which these were measured.

ELECTROCARDIOGRAPHIC FINDINGS

Electrocardiographic changes may be seen and are those of right heart dilatation, hypertrophy, and failure. Deviation of the mean electrical axis to the right with P (pulmonale) and S waves in leads I, II, and III have been associated with cor pulmonale. Conduction defects may occur, and a depression of the ST segment may be associated with tissue hypoxia. In three dogs shown to have pulmonary artery thrombosis, a left-axis shift was seen in one dog. In humans, electrocardiographic changes are seen in 85 per cent of patients, but these changes are often transient and nonspecific.

RADIOGRAPHIC STUDIES

Routine thoracic radiographs can be normal, or they may demonstrate increased radiolucency due to decreased vascular filling of the obstructed lung lobes (oligemia or Westermark's sign). Hypervascularity of the unobstructed, hyperperfused areas may be noted. These findings are confusing, however, when obstruction is diffuse or involves several lobes. An enlarged pulmonary artery segment and right heart enlargement may be present but can be somewhat obscured by the presence of pleural fluid. In humans, bronchoconstriction leads to a decreased lung volume in obstructed areas and an elevation of the hemidiaphragm on the side of the obstruction. This is difficult to interpret in cases of bilateral obstruction. Abdominal radiographs may demonstrate hepatomegaly or ascites if right heart failure exists.

PULMONARY ANGIOGRAPHIC STUDIES

Pulmonary angiography is the definitive study in the diagnosis of pulmonary thromboembolism. It should be performed in the following situations: (1) when an animal that is predisposed to pulmonary thromboembolism is experiencing dyspnea, (2) in cases of intractable dyspnea when the cause of this dyspnea cannot be ascertained with certainty on routine thoracic radiographs, (3) when the clinical picture is suspicious for pulmonary thromboembolism, and (4) prior to therapy. Angiography should be performed early for rapid diagnosis and before 24 to 72 hours, after which resolution of clot material may hinder interpretation of the angiogram. To be interpreted as positive, the angiogram should show intraluminal filling defects created by the presence of clot material or "cutoffs," well-demarcated interruptions in the pulmonary arterial blood flow, or both. The pulmonary arterial vasculature in the nonobstructed areas may be dilated and tortuous due to overcirculation. Asymmetry of blood flow and lack of perfusion of certain areas are seen but are not specific for pulmonary embolism. Nonselective pulmonary angiography was performed on three dogs with pulmonary artery thrombosis, and selective angiography was performed on one of these dogs (Fig. 2). An intravenous catheter was passed

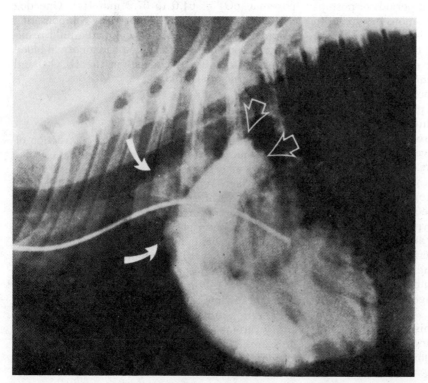

Figure 2. Nonselective angiogram taken three seconds after injection of contrast media into the right atrium. The pulmonary artery is blunted or "cut off" (open arrows), and the caudal lobe arteries do not opacify. The right ventricle is dilated and the aorta has already opacified (closed arrows). (Reprinted with permission from Burns et al.: J.A.V.M.A. 178:390, 1981.)

into the jugular vein so that the tip of the catheter was positioned in the right atrium. An injection of 1 to 2 ml/kg of contrast media (Renografin-60)* was made. In the nonselective studies, optimal visualization of the obstructed areas occurred 3 seconds after the start of the injection. In the selective study, contrast media flowed from the right atrium to the aorta in 1.5 seconds (normal = 5 seconds), demonstrating extremely rapid transit time through the nonoccluded portions of the pulmonary vasculature. Nonselective angiography is easy, rapid, inexpensive, relatively safe, and the only means of definitively diagnosing pulmonary thromboembolism.

VENTILATION/PERFUSION SCANNING

In human medicine, lung scanning has become a useful noninvasive technique in the diagnosis of pulmonary embolism. As nuclear medicine facilities become available in veterinary teaching hospitals, these techniques will become important in the diagnosis of many diseases including pulmonary thromboembolism.

Perfusion lung scanning is accomplished by the intravenous injection of technetium-99m labeled albumin complexes. Imaging with a gamma camera will then demonstrate the functional pulmonary blood flow. In human medicine, a normal perfusion scan is highly specific in ruling out pulmonary embolism; however, an abnormal perfusion scan does not constitute a positive diagnosis. When combined with ventilation lung scanning, effective diagnosis of pulmonary thromboembolism is possible.

Ventilation lung scanning is performed using a radioactive inert gas such as xenon-133. The lung is scanned as the patient takes a first breath, as xenon-133 reaches equilibrium in the alveoli, and during a five-minute washout period. A normal scan will show uniform wash-in and wash-out periods.

In pulmonary thromboembolism, areas of abnormal perfusion will have normal ventilation, that is, ventilation-perfusion mismatching. Other conditions will result in areas of both abnormal ventilation and abnormal perfusion, or ventilation-perfusion matching.

TREATMENT OF PULMONARY THROMBOEMBOLISM

There are no existing guidelines for antithrombotic therapy in veterinary medicine. One dog with pulmonary artery thrombosis in association with hyperoadrenocorticism was treated initially with heparin at a dose of 100 mg/kg (3900 mg), q.i.d., IV for three days. Thereafter, heparin was discontinued and the dog was given 10 mg (0.25 mg/kg)

of crystalline warfarin sodium (Coumadin†) once daily PO. Warfarin therapy was continued until the prothrombin time (PT) was 1.5 times the pretreatment baseline value. Therapy was monitored by clinical evaluation and by checking the prothrombin time, the activated partial thromboplastin time (APTT), and the platelet count. Gingival bleeding was noted on the seventh day of therapy, and the dosage was decreased to 2.5 mg (0.06 mg/kg) daily PO for several weeks. Even though a subsequent pulmonary angiographic study showed a dissolution of the pulmonary thromboemboli, the weaknesses of this therapy become apparent after studying the therapeutic procedures used in human medicine.

THERAPY IN HUMAN MEDICINE

HEPARIN

Heparin has been shown to be effective in the prevention and treatment of pulmonary thromboembolism. It is derived from porcine intestinal mucosa or beef lung and is metabolized by the liver and excreted by the kidney. Heparin combines with and profoundly augments the action of antithrombin III (heparin cofactor) to inactivate thrombin and thus prevent the conversion of fibrinogen to fibrin. Heparin inhibits the reactions that lead to clotting without actually depleting the levels of clotting factors present in blood. The clotting time may be prolonged, although the bleeding time is usually unaffected. One microgram of antithrombin III will neutralize 32 units of active thrombin but will prevent the formation of 1,600 *new* units of thrombin. It is easy to see that it takes much less heparin to prevent clotting than to treat it. Heparin has no fibrinolytic activity, but by shifting the procoagulant-anticoagulant balance, anticoagulation may be achieved if the fibrinolytic system is intact. Other effects of decreasing thrombin levels include decreased attraction of platelets to the clot and therefore decreased clot growth and decreased thrombin-stimulated platelet degranulation and therefore decreased levels of vasoactive and bronchoconstrictive substances in the lung.

Different dosage regimens for heparin are used for the prevention and treatment of thromboembolism. It has been estimated in humans that 4000 to 8000 deaths per year from pulmonary thromboembolism could be prevented if low-dose heparin therapy were used in all hemostatically competent patients over the age of 40 years undergoing abdominothoracic surgery. The recommended dose is 5000 units (USP) subcutaneously two hours preoperatively and then 5000 units every 12 hours until the patient is either dismissed or fully ambulatory. The

---

*E. R. Squibb and Sons, Princeton, NJ.

†Endo Laboratories, Inc., Garden City, NY.

incidence of deep venous thrombosis from hip surgery was reduced from 48 to 13 per cent when 5000 units were given every 8 hours instead of every 12 hours. There was an increased incidence of wound hematomas at this dose, and the APTT rose slightly.

When deep venous thrombosis or pulmonary thromboembolism has already occurred, large-dose heparin therapy is given. Fifteen thousand units are given initially and 40,000 to 60,000 units are given over the first 24 hours. After the first 24 hours, 25,000 to 35,000 units per 24 hours are given intravenously. When constant infusion of heparin was given there was a lower incidence of bleeding complications, and the dose of heparin required was reduced by 25 per cent. Large-dose heparin therapy should be continued until the patient is on oral anticoagulant therapy for three to eight days at a level sufficient to raise the PT to at least 1.5 times the baseline value.

The APTT should be 1.5 to 2.5 times normal and the Lee-White clotting time 2 to 3 times normal to be certain that *enough* heparin is being given. These tests are done before the next scheduled dose. Bleeding occurs in 3 to 8 per cent of most patients receiving heparin therapy. Protamine sulfate neutralizes heparin if bleeding occurs but may have anticoagulant action itself if overdosed. Aspirin or any other antiplatelet drugs are contraindicated within five to seven days of heparin usage.

COUMARIN DERIVATIVES

Also available for anticoagulation are the coumarin derivatives dicoumarol and crystalline warfarin sodium (Coumadin), among others. These drugs work by inhibiting the liver synthesis of the vitamin K–dependent clotting factors II (prothrombin), VII, IX, and X. Their use results in the actual depletion of these clotting factors in the blood. They have no fibrinolytic activity but, like heparin, shift the procoagulant-anticoagulant balance in favor of anticoagulation. Their effect requires two to seven days, and heparin should be continued until this effect is achieved. The coumarin derivatives are metabolized by the liver and excreted by the kidneys.

Factor IX is the only affected clotting factor in the intrinsic clotting mechanism, and factor VII is the factor most subject to depletion. As factor VII decreases, the risk of bleeding increases even though a significant antithrombotic effect is not achieved. Factor X shows the lowest activity after several days. The dose of coumarin derivatives is adjusted to achieve a PT that is two times baseline (pretreatment) values. If heparin is being given along with coumarin derivatives, the PT should be checked prior to the next heparin treatment. Coumarin derivatives should be used for six weeks to six months or longer, depending on whether the initial problem is self-limiting or recurrent.

Bleeding occurs in about 3 per cent of human patients. When it occurs, discontinuation of therapy is all that is needed if bleeding is not serious. When bleeding is serious, vitamin K_1 may be used to restore the depleted clotting factors to their normal levels. However, vitamin K_1 may maintain its effects for one to three weeks, thus hindering resumption of antithrombotic therapy. Fresh frozen plasma returns the PT to normal rapidly and allows for the rapid resumption of anticoagulation therapy using lower doses. Coumarin derivatives are teratogenic and have a large number of drug interactions.

FIBRINOLYTIC THERAPY

Streptokinase (from cultures of group C beta-hemolytic streptococci) and urokinase (from pooled human urine or cultured human embryo kidney cells) have the ability to enzymatically convert plasminogen to plasmin, which promotes active clot lysis. The major complication of fibrinolytic therapy is hemorrhage. The list of contraindications to the use of these drugs is extensive and includes any surgery or invasive procedure involving arterial needle punctures, hepatic or renal biopsies, gastrointestinal ulceration, atrial fibrillation, or any hemorrhagic diathesis. For these reasons the major indication for their use is acute massive thromboembolism with a deteriorating hemodynamic situation within the first 24 hours. After 24 hours, heparin is just as effective and does not carry the risks of these enzymes. In addition, fibrinolytic agents are extremely expensive.

Other therapeutic techniques include (1) interruption of the inferior vena cava by surgical ligation, plication, or the placement of intravenous umbrellas to trap emboli migrating from the deep venous areas of the lower limbs and pelvis to the lungs, (2) transvenous interruption with filters or balloons, (3) surgical embolectomy, a procedure that is associated with a 30 to 60 per cent mortality rate, and (4) various physical therapy techniques.

RECOMMENDATIONS FOR THERAPY OF PULMONARY THROMBOEMBOLISM IN COMPANION ANIMALS

There are currently no existing guidelines for therapy of pulmonary thromboembolism in companion animal medicine. Before therapeutic principles can be established, we must be able to recognize the condition and predict diseases or situations that may result in pulmonary thromboembolism. Even though much information is available in the research literature, controlled studies need to be done relating the use of available drugs in various doses to predictable changes in clotting factors, tests of coagulability, and potential drug toxicities, side effects, and adverse reactions.

If we can anticipate situations that are likely to result in venous thrombosis and pulmonary thromboembolism, preventive therapy is then indicated. Heparin would seem to be the drug of choice in these situations. Drawing from the human literature and very limited experience in veterinary medicine, a preoperative dose of 75 mg/kg subcutaneously two hours before surgery would be indicated. Postoperatively, 75 mg/kg every 12 hours subcutaneously until the patient is ambulatory would seem appropriate. The dose should be adjusted so that the APTT is 1.5 to 2.5 times normal.

At this stage of our recognition of situations that result in thrombosis or thromboembolism, it is quite likely that we will be confronted with a dyspneic, perhaps unstable patient who has already developed pulmonary thromboembolism. After the diagnosis has been made by pulmonary angiographic procedures, the patient should be given strict cage rest in an intensive care area. This will decrease oxygen demands by the body and may prevent or slow the further showering of emboli that may occur if deep venous thrombosis exists. If possible, this should be in a cage where 40 per cent oxygen can be provided. Blood gas studies, if not done previously, will provide information regarding the oxygenation status of the blood as well as acid-base data. Heparin should be given intravenously. An initial dose of 200 to 225 mg/kg and a total dose of 500 to 750 mg/kg over the first 24 hours should be given in boluses every four hours. Thereafter, 350 to 500 mg/kg per 24 hours can be given in boluses every six hours. If given by continuous drip, these dosages should be decreased by 25 per cent (except for the initial treatment). When the APTT is stabilized at 1.5 to 2.5 times baseline, treatment with oral anticoagulants can begin. The initial dose of crystalline warfarin sodium should be 0.2 mg/kg PO once daily. Subsequent doses should be 0.05 to 0.1 mg/kg once daily but must be adjusted so that the PT is 1.5 to 2.5 times the baseline normal. When this has been achieved, heparin therapy may be stopped.

Until further guidelines are established, the patient should be kept under strict cage confinement until there is clinical resolution of dyspnea. At this time, the patient may be transferred from the intensive care area or sent home. Conscientious client education and communication should be undertaken, and the patient should be examined no less frequently than every three to five days initially. The PT should be checked on these occasions. If the patient continues to do well, the PT remains stabilized, and the client has a good understanding of his pet's condition, these intervals may be lengthened. Once the patient is clinically normal, repeat angiographic studies should be done at two-month intervals; when patency of the pulmonary circulation has been re-established, therapy may be stopped. If the PT becomes greater than two times the baseline value, the dose of anticoagulant should be cut in half. If bleeding develops, anticoagulants should be stopped, the patient hospitalized, and treatment with fresh frozen plasma or vitamin K_1 instituted promptly.

If moderate to severe pleural effusion is present, thoracocentesis should be undertaken. Care should be taken to avoid stress. If sedation is required for thoracocentesis or any other procedure, a product should be chosen that has a minimal effect on respiratory function.

Treatment of underlying or primary disease problems may be started when the patient is stabilized unless these conditions are life-threatening. If congestive heart failure is present, the use of digitalis agents should be undertaken with caution because hypoxemia and acidosis predispose these patients to the arrhythmogenic effects of these drugs. If right-sided heart failure is present, diuretics and salt restriction are indicated.

Until we have a better understanding of pulmonary thromboembolism, the prognosis remains guarded or poor.

REFERENCES AND SUPPLEMENTAL READING

Bell, W. R., and Meek, A. G.: Guidelines for the use of thrombolytic agents. N. Engl. J. Med. 301:1266, 1979.

British Medical Bulletin 34:1978.

Burns, M. G., Kelly, A. B., Hornof, W. J., and Howerth, E. W.: Pulmonary artery thrombosis in three dogs with hyperadrenocorticism. J.A.V.M.A. 178:388, 1981.

Cherniak, R. M.: Ventilation, perfusion and gas exchange. *In* Frolich, E. D. (ed.): *Pathophysiology*, 2nd ed. Philadelphia: J. B. Lippincott, 1976, pp. 149–166.

Guyton, A. C. (ed.): Physical principles of gas exchange. *In Textbook of Medical Physiology*, 6th ed. Philadelphia: W. B. Saunders, 1981, pp. 491–503.

Hood, D. M., Hightower, D., and Tatum, M. E.: Lung perfusion imaging in the dog. J. Am. Vet. Radiol. Soc. 18:124, 1977.

Migaki, G., and Casey, H. W.: Conditions associated with thrombosis in animals. *In Animal Models of Thrombosis and Hemorrhagic Diseases*. Bethesda: National Academy of Sciences, National Institutes of Health, 1975, pp. 55–60.

Mobin-Uddin, K. (ed.): *Pulmonary Thromboembolism*. Springfield: Charles C Thomas, 1975, pp. 5–15.

Moser, K. M., and Stein, M. (eds.): *Pulmonary Thromboembolism*. Chicago: Year Book Medical Publishers, 1973.

Rosenow, E. C., Osmundson, P. S., and Brown, M. L.: Subject review. Pulmonary embolism. Mayo Clin. Proc. 56:161, 1981.

Slawson, D. O., and Gribble, D. H.: Thrombosis complicating renal amyloidosis in dogs. Vet. Pathol. 8:352, 1971.

PLEURAL DISEASES

KENNETH G. KAGAN, V.M.D.,

and MARILYN E. STIFF, D.V.M.

Gainesville, Florida

The pleural space, a potential space between the visceral and parietal pleura, has two functions. First, it provides a slippery interface between the lungs and the adjacent thoracic structures. The low friction of the pleural space allows opposing pleural surfaces to glide over each other without distorting the lung as pulmonary expansion and deflation occur during respiration. Second, the pleural space is an area of negative pressure, maintained by Starling's forces of equilibrium of capillary exchange governing the formation and absorption of pleural fluid (Fig. 1). This negative pressure is needed to keep the lungs expanded and acts as a pump, aiding venous and lymphatic flow into the thorax. Certain pleural and systemic diseases may alter the forces governing fluid balance, resulting in fluid accumulation, an increase in the volume of the pleural space, and subsequent partial collapse of the lungs.

Pleural fluid originates from the subpleural capillaries of the parietal pleura. The sum of Starling's forces favors a net movement of fluid into the interstitial space surrounding these capillaries and across the mesothelial lining into the pleural space. The pleural fluid contains electrolytes, a small amount of protein, and a few cells. Fluid is absorbed by the venous and lymphatic capillaries of the visceral pleura, which have a much lower hydrostatic pressure. Protein, cells, and particulate matter are taken up by the lymphatics of the caudal mediastinal and costal pleura. Pleural effusions, which are due to decreased plasma oncotic pressure (e.g., hypoproteinemia) or increased venous hydrostatic pressure (e.g., congestive heart failure), initially are without significant protein or cellular components and are termed *transudates*. Disease and trauma of the pleura may cause fluid accumulation with significant quantities of cells and protein. These types of effusions may result from inflammation of the pleura or local vascular inflammation, obstruction, or disruption. Such fluid may be classified as modified transudates or exudates.

If sufficient amounts of effusion accumulate in the pleural space, the lungs collapse and respiration becomes labored. When the visceral and parietal pleurae are separated by fluid, the lungs are no longer tethered to the chest wall and torsions of lung lobes may occur.

The parietal pleura is well innervated, especially on the diaphragm. Therefore, some diseases of the parietal pleura may be painful. The visceral pleura is not innervated.

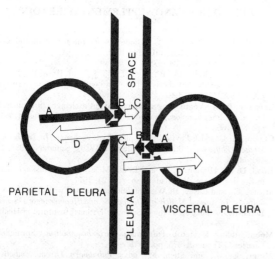

Figure 1. Formation and absorption of pleural fluid. Parietal capillary hydrostatic pressure (A), pleural space "negative" pressure (B), and osmotic pressure (C) tend to move fluid into the pleural space because, combined, they exceed the opposing colloid osmotic pressure (D). Fluid tends to move from the pleural space into the visceral pleural capillaries because the hydrostatic pressure (A'), the "negative" pleural space pressure (B), and osmotic pressure (C) combined are less than the colloid osmotic pressure (D') (lengths of arrows are proportionate to the pressure.) (Reprinted with permission from Lowell: *Pleural Effusions, A Comprehensive Review.* Baltimore: University Park Press, 1977.)

DIAGNOSIS OF PLEURAL DISEASES

Since most pleural diseases cause an increase in the pleural volume at the expense of lung volume, the most frequent and earliest presenting complaint is dyspnea. Other presenting signs may be depression, fever, anorexia, or a dry, nonproductive cough. History should include questions relating to possible penetrating wounds of the thorax or lower neck. Dogs that run through weeds, brush, and shrubs may inhale a foreign body, which can migrate down a bronchus, through the pulmonary parenchyma, and into the pleura. Penetrating wounds caused by sticks or twigs may go unnoticed by an owner.

Physical findings vary according to the type and

extent of pleural disease. Respiratory difficulty ranges from increased rate and decreased tidal volume to severe orthopnea. Auscultation of the heart and lungs may reveal sound patterns characteristic of certain diseases. Effusions cause muffled heart sounds without displacement. Lung sounds are heard well on the dorsal areas of the thorax and are reduced or absent in dependent areas with accumulations of free fluid. Trapped or loculated areas of exudate or fluid cause irregular distributions of breath sounds and occasional shifts in heart sounds. Free pleural air causes reduced vesicular sounds dorsally and variable degrees of sound reduction in dependent areas. Fibrinous pleuritis may auscultate as a friction rub. Percussion of the thorax can be helpful in assessing the pleural space when the thoracic wall is intact and stable. The examiner places the palmar surface of an open hand to the thoracic wall. The index or middle finger, the plessimeter, is extended and nestled in an intercostal space, pressed slightly against the muscles. The tips of the index and middle fingers of the opposite hand, the plessor, are held tightly together and are used to strike the midpoint of the plessimeter. The hands are moved dorsally and ventrally along succeeding intercostal spaces to define the patterns of resonance or dullness of each hemithorax. With experience one can recognize normal resonance of air-filled lungs and the dullness of the cardiac and hepatic (diaphragm) regions. Free air in the pleural space is hyper-resonant when compared with pulmonary parenchyma. Pleural effusions are hyporhesonant (dull), similar to the cardiac and diaphramatic regions.

In most cases a tentative diagnosis of pleural disease is established on the basis of the history and physical examination. Confirmation can be obtained through radiography. A definitive diagnosis is established by pleurocentesis and the identification of air or through the analysis of an effusion.

If an animal is severely dyspneic and pneumothorax or hydrothorax is suspected, pleural drainage may be required to stabilize the patient before radiography. In such a patient with decreased pulmonary reserve, the stress of manipulation and radiographs may be fatal. Initially, pleurocentesis is performed with a needle and syringe to confirm the presence of air or fluid. If the tap is positive, drainage of the thorax may proceed.

When the animal's condition is stable, thoracic radiographs are taken. Two views are made whenever possible. Radiographic findings relative to pleural disease include the following: presence of fluid or air; displacement of structures, e.g., diaphragmatic hernias; rib fractures; tumors; thickening of the pleura, e.g., fibrosis. With small amounts of freely movable fluid, the lung margins are separated from the parietal pleura by fluid density, and the edges of the lungs appear scalloped. The sepa-

rations between lung lobes fill with fluid and are seen as fissure lines. The cardiac silhouette is obscured on both lateral and dorsoventral views. In horizontal beam projections, the lungs appear to float on the fluid. Larger amounts of fluid allow more retraction of the lungs and obscure most, if not all, of the cardiac silhouette and mediastinal structures. Pneumothorax causes similar retraction of the lung lobes; however, they are surrounded by air rather than fluid density.

Diaphragmatic hernia is an important differential diagnosis in pleural effusion cases. Visualization of bowel loops on thoracic radiographs establishes the diagnosis; however, this is not always seen. Radiographic assessment of the continuity of the diaphragm usually requires pleural drainage.

Traumatic pleural disease, such as pneumothorax, rib fractures, pulmonary contusions, or diaphragmatic hernias, can often be diagnosed through history, physical examination, and radiology. Similarly, radiographs may identify neoplasia or congestive heart failure as a source of pleural effusion. Frequently, pleural drainage is necessary for optimal radiographic interpretation.

If radiographs are not diagnostic, analysis of the pleural effusion may be necessary to identify the disease process. The pleural fluid must first be categorized as either a transudate or an exudate. Many criteria are used to separate transudates from exudates (Table 1). Protein content has been used. A rule of thumb is that fluids with a protein content of less than 3.0 gm/dl are transudates and fluids with a protein content of greater than 3.0 gm/dl are exudates. Actually, there is a considerable overlap in protein concentration for the various effusions. In fact, none of the criteria used to evaluate pleural fluids are diagnostic in themselves.

FLUID TYPES

TRANSUDATES

Transudates are effusions of low protein and cellular content. They result from alterations in the normal mechanisms of pleural fluid formation, such as with hypoproteinemia or right heart failure. In such cases, the diagnosis and treatment are directed toward the underlying disease process. If treatment is successful, the pleural effusion will resolve.

MODIFIED TRANSUDATES

Transudates that have been in the pleural space for an extended period of time contain nucleated cells and erythrocytes. As these cells degenerate, cellular contents are released that are chemotactic to neutrophils and macrophages. With increasing concentration of cells or protein, the fluid loses the characteristics of a transudate and is called a modi-

Table 1. *Analysis of Pleural Effusions*

	Transudates		Exudates				
	Transudates	Modified Transudates	Nonseptic Exudates	Septic Exudates	Chylous Effusions	Pseudochylous Effusions	Hemorrhagic Effusions
Color / Transparency	Pale yellow / Clear	Yellow-pink / Clear to cloudy	Yellow-pink / Cloudy	Yellow / Cloudy to flocculent	White-pink / Opaque	White-pink / Clear to opaque	Red / Opaque
Protein (gm/dl) / RBC	<2.5 / Absent to rare	>2.5 / Variable	>3.0 / Variable	>3.0 / Variable	>2.5 / Variable	>2.5 / Variable	>3.0 / Acute: high number Chronic: moderate number
Nucleated cells/μl	<500	>200	>2000	>4000	>400	>100	>1000
Neutrophils	Rare	Variable number Nondegenerative	Moderate number Nondegenerative	Moderate to high number Nondegenerative* to degenerative	Acute: low number Chronic: moderate number Nondegenerative	Variable number Nondegenerative	Variable number Nondegenerative
Lymphocytes	Rare	Variable	Variable	Variable	Acute: high number Chronic: low number	Variable	Variable
Macrophages	Occasional	Variable	Increased number Contain ingested debris	Increased number Contain ingested debris	Present	Present	Chronic: moderate number Contain ingested RBCs
Mesothelial cells	Occasional	Occasional	Rare	Rare	Occasional	Occasional	Chronic: present
Fibrin / Bacteria	Absent / Absent	Absent / Absent	Present / Absent	Present / Present intra- and extracellularly	Chronic: present / Absent	Chronic: present / Absent	Variable / Absent
Lipid	Absent	Absent	Absent	Absent	High triglycerides, low cholesterol, positive to lipotrophic stains	Low triglycerides, high cholesterol, negative to lipotrophic stains	Absent
Etiology	Right heart failure Hypoproteinemia	Chronic transudates Diaphragmatic hernia	Neoplasia Feline infectious peritonitis Chronic diaphragmatic hernia Lung torsions	Foreign body Penetrating wound	Ruptured thoracic duct	Neoplasia Feline cardiomyopathy	Trauma Neoplasia Bleeding disorders Lung torsions

Nocardia and Actinomyces spp.

fied transudate. As these changes occur, interpretation of the cytology of the fluid becomes more important. The predominant cell types in a modified transudate are nondegenerative neutrophils and mesothelial cells.

EXUDATES

Exudates are classified as septic and nonseptic and result from alteration of the pleura. Examples of nonseptic exudates are neoplastic effusions, chylous effusions, pseudochylous effusions, and hemorrhage. Hemorrhagic exudates may be associated with trauma, lung torsion, or neoplasia. Penetrating wounds, foreign bodies, and infectious pleuritis are causes of septic exudates. Exudates typically have high cellular and protein contents. As with transudates, changes occur with time such that the results of analysis vary and lead to difficulty in interpretation.

CELL TYPES

Neutrophils. In transudates, neutrophils number less than 500/μl and appear similar to neutrophils seen in peripheral blood. With chronicity, neutrophils may increase to 10,000/μl and morphology may change to reactive nondegenerative cells with nuclear hypersegmentation and pyknosis. Neutrophils in nonseptic exudates appear similar to those in modified transudates but may reach numbers of 20,000 to 40,000/μl. Neutrophil morphology becomes degenerative in septic exudates, with toxic changes such as cytoplasmic vacuolization and disintegration of the nuclei (karyorrhexis). The neutrophil count can rise to 100,000/μl or more. Bacteria may be seen in the cytoplasm of neutrophils or free in the fluid.

Mesothelial Cells. The presence of fluid in the pleural space causes the mesothelial lining cells to hypertrophy and exfoliate into the effusion. These free-floating cells have a deep-blue cytoplasm and coarse, granular nuclear chromatin. Multiple nucleoli and mitotic figures are commonly seen. Fine cytoplasmic processes develop around the cell margin, giving a "brush border" or "sunburst" appearance. Cells with these characteristics are termed *reactive mesothelial cells*. They are most frequently seen in modified transudates and are rarely found in exudates. The presence of nucleoli, occasional mitotic figures, and multinucleation of these reactive mesothelial cells necessitates differentiation from neoplastic cells.

Lymphocytes. Lymphocytes are rare in pleural fluid except for chylous effusions, lymphosarcoma, and chronic inflammatory processes. In the early stages of chylothorax, lymphocyte numbers vary from 10,000 to 40,000/μl or higher. Chylous effusions contain primarily mature small lymphocytes. This is in contrast to the predominance of immature lymphocytes seen in lymphosarcoma.

Macrophages. Macrophages are seen most often in transudates and chronic exudates. They may arise from peripheral blood monocytes or more commonly from transformation of reactive mesothelial cells. Macrophages are characterized by light-blue vacuolated and granulated cytoplasm. Phagocytized neutrophils, with or without bacteria, fungal elements, and debris may be seen within the cytoplasm.

Erythrocytes. Many pleural effusions appear bloody. One milliliter of peripheral blood in 500 ml of fluid (10,000 RBC/μl) will give an effusion a grossly bloody appearance yet is of little diagnostic significance. Only when the RBC count exceeds 100,000/μl is hemorrhage suspected secondary to trauma, neoplasia, or pulmonary infarction.

Neoplastic Cells. In the dog and cat, cytology of a modified transudate or nonseptic exudate secondary to the presence of a tumor is usually unrewarding. The most easily recognized neoplastic cell of pleural effusions is the lymphoblast of malignant lymphoma. Another exfoliative pleural neoplasm that has been diagnosed is the mast cell tumor.

PNEUMOTHORAX

Owing to the high incidence of blunt trauma in small animals, pneumothorax is the most common pleural disease of dogs and cats. When air disrupts the seal between the parietal and visceral pleura, negative pressure diminishes and the lungs partially collapse. Ventilation is impaired since maximal expansion of the lungs is not possible. To compensate, the animal must increase ventilatory rate, maximize rib expansion, and retract the diaphragm. With slight or moderate cases of pneumothorax, increasing ventilatory rate is usually sufficient. With more severe pneumothorax, the animal must devote more effort to ventilation.

The animal compensates for the presence of pneumothorax by reducing activity and assuming a posture that makes breathing easier. Animals are reluctant to move and prefer to remain in a sternal position. The more severely affected animals sit or stand, refusing to eat or sleep in order to breathe. The same pattern of compensation occurs in all forms of pleural disease when the pleural space expands at the expense of lung volume.

Air in the pleural space reduces the negative pleural pressure. If atmospheric pressure is reached in the pleura, no ventilation will be possible. Also, loss of this negative pressure reduces the effectiveness of the thoracic pump and venous return. Air can enter the pleural space from a penetrating wound of the thorax, laceration or rupture of the lung or airways, or rupture of the esophagus. Lung or airway rupture is the most common cause of pneumothorax. The source of the air, the severity of the ventilatory compromise, and the extent of other injuries must be considered when treating the patient.

Tension pneumothorax can occur secondary to penetrating wounds or pulmonary lacerations if a tissue flap is created that acts as a one-way valve. During inspiration the negative pleural pressure draws air into the space, but during expiration the tissue flap seals the wound and traps the air. As the animal tries to breathe harder, more air is pumped into the pleural space, until intrapleural pressure becomes positive and complete collapse of the lungs and distention of the thorax ensue. This is a life-threatening situation that calls for immediate treatment.

Since most cases of pneumothorax are due to accident, the duration of the pneumothorax can often be established in the history. By the time animals with pneumothorax are presented to the veterinarian, the critical period has usually passed. However, because of the ventilatory compromise, these patients do not tolerate manipulation. The physical exam should be as complete and thorough as possible without stressing the patient. The initial differential diagnosis for a dyspneic patient with a recent history of trauma should include pneumothorax, diaphragmatic hernia, hydrothorax, and pulmonary contusion. By auscultation, percussion, and palpation, the clinician should be able to recognize a severe pneumothorax. The diminished lung sounds and hyper-resonance on percussion tend to rule out diaphragmatic hernia and hemothorax. Evidence of a penetrating thoracic wound does not eliminate the possibility of other internal sources of air. Observation of the character and frequency of respiration gives a good estimation of the severity of the problem. The majority of pneumothorax cases do not require pleural drainage. A conservative approach with continued observation and definitive treatment for other injuries are usually sufficient. However, if the animal becomes cyanotic and has labored respiration, a diagnostic needle pleurocentesis should be done and a pleural drain placed immediately if the diagnosis of a pneumothorax is confirmed.

Once the patient is stabilized, thoracic radiographs are taken to evaluate the extent of pneumothorax and lung contusions. The position of the pleural drain can also be evaluated. Initial radiographs serve as baseline for evaluation of response and resolution of the pneumothorax. The decision to drain the pleural space is based on the clinical evaluation of the patient and not the radiographic appearance of the pneumothorax. Rib fractures are frequently observed in thoracic trauma cases. Radiodense foreign material (such as projectiles) may be visualized. Pulmonary contusion, displacement, and atelectasis are patterns of pulmonary damage and may indicate the source of pneumothorax. Rupture of the airways or esophagus causes pneumomediastinum. Visualization of mediastinal structures such as the brachiocephalic trunk or the tracheal and esophageal walls is possible when air surrounds them. Esophageal perforation should always be considered when pneumomediastinum is detected.

Subcutaneous emphysema is seen in some cases of pneumothorax. Air may enter the subcutaneous tissues from the pleural space, mediastinum, or an external wound. Subcutaneous emphysema that starts at the thoracic inlet and spreads over the chest, back, and neck is suggestive of pneumomediastinum. If emphysema is detected over the ribs with no evidence of laceration, it is probably due to pneumothorax with damage to both the visceral and parietal pleurae.

TREATMENT OF PNEUMOTHORAX

Most cases of pneumothorax respond to conservative management. If the animal is stable, there is no need to drain the pleural cavity. Air leakage from the lung diminishes or stops as the lung collapses from the pneumothorax. By draining the pleural space and expanding the lungs, further air leakage may occur. As a general guide, if an animal is comfortable and able to eat and sleep with a respiratory rate < 60/min, pleural drainage is not necessary. When the leak seals, the air will be absorbed and the lung will expand. However, if the animal's respiratory rate is > 80/min or the animal is in moderate to severe distress, pleural drainage should probably be initiated. In all cases, clinical evaluation of the patient is the deciding factor, not the respiratory rate.

Pleural drainage can be performed on an intermittent or continuous basis. Intermittent drainage is the most practical method in veterinary medicine. Either needle or tube drainage can be performed. If needle drainage is repeated more than three times a day, a tube should be placed. A pleural drain gives dependable access to the pleural space without the risk of pulmonary laceration from repeated needle insertions and the stress of restraint for each procedure.

The upper third of the seventh to ninth intercostal spaces is the preferred site for pleural insertion. Air is removed until the animal is comfortable. Attempting complete drainage may dislodge a fibrin seal from a pulmonary laceration and is not advisable. By using a three-way stopcock and syringe rather than a suction pump, the volume of air removed can be recorded. Repeat drainage is done only if

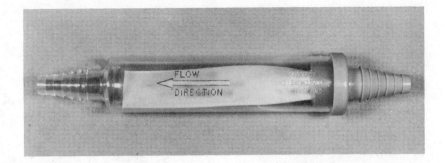

Figure 2. The latex tube inside the plastic case of the Heimlick valve functions as a low-resistance, one-way valve for pleural drainage.

respiratory distress returns. When an air leak continues and prevents stabilization of the patient, a decision must be made either to continue drainage or attempt surgical repair of the leak. Shock, blood loss, and other effects of trauma may dictate the advisability of surgery. If the facilities for close, constant monitoring and patient support are available, surgical intervention can be delayed for 24 to 48 hours while waiting for a leak to seal. The technique of pleural drainage is reviewed at the end of this article.

When large volumes of air are drawn off of the pleural space, constant drainage is advisable. Passive devices for constant pleural drainage such as the Heimlick valve* (Fig. 2) and the waterseal bottle (Fig. 3) do not work well in the dog and the cat. These devices depend on a brief period of positive pleural pressure developing during expiration to evacuate the air from the thorax. Cats and most dogs do not develop a high enough positive pleural pressure long enough to allow air to escape from the thorax. Also, animals do not voluntarily perform a Valsalva maneuver to raise pleural pressures.

Continuous pleural drainage requires a regulated constant negative pressure source or suction system (Fig. 4). Limiting the suction to 5 to 10 cm of water will evacuate the pleura well enough to improve ventilation and may limit the expansion of the lung to allow the leak to seal. Furthermore, a low suction pressure source prevents pulmonary damage to tissue caught in the catheter openings. Passing the pleural drainage system through a waterseal bottle allows a semiquantitative evaluation of the amount of air being evacuated by the rate of bubble formation. Long periods without bubbles indicate that the air leak has stopped or the catheter is obstructed. If the animal's condition is stable and the bubble rate is low or stopped, the pneumothorax is responding.

Animals with pleural tubes should be under continuous observation. Any malfunction of the drainage system may allow open communication of the pleural space with the outside, which is rapidly fatal. Covering tubes with wraps and bandages cannot be depended upon to maintain the tubes in

an uncooperative patient. When pneumothorax is treated conservatively without pleural drainage, continuous observation should be maintained for at least four to eight hours initially until the patient is stable; sudden changes are not likely. Thereafter,

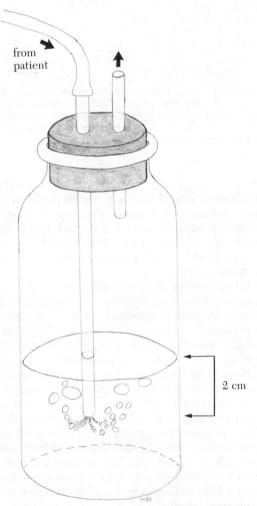

from patient

2 cm

Figure 3. The waterseal bottle acts as a low-pressure one-way valve. The tube on the left is connected to the thoracic catheter. When the interpleural pressure exceeds 2 cm of water (the depth that the tube is submerged), pleural air will force the water out of the tube and is observed as bubbles. The patient must be elevated 3 ft above the water level so that negative pleural pressure cannot aspirate water into the pleural space.

*Heimlick Chest Drain Valve, Bard Parker, Rutherford, NJ.

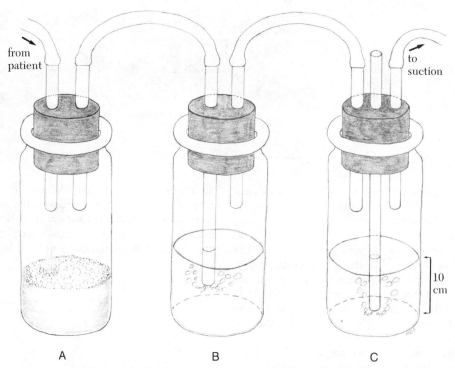

from
patient

to
suction

10
cm

A   B   C

Figure 4. Three-bottle system for pleural drainage. Bottle A acts as a trap for collecting and measuring pleural effusion if present. This bottle is optional in cases of pneumothorax. The waterseal bottle (B) prevents the entrance of air into the pleural space if there is a break in the suction line. Bottle C regulates the amount of suction in the system. When the vacuum (measured in cm of H_2O) exceeds the length of the center tube below the water level, room air is drawn into the system, preventing high negative pressures in the thoracic catheter.

observation should be on a regular and frequent basis as clinical judgement dictates. Unobserved intervals should probably not exceed 1 to 2 hours for the first 24 hours. Once the air leak has ceased, resorption of the residual pneumothorax may take up to two weeks.

When stability does not occur within 24 to 48 hours or if the severity of the pneumothorax and respiratory distress increases, surgical intervention is indicated. Selection of the surgical approach is critical, since lobectomy is required for most massive air leaks. Certain physical and radiographic findings help to localize the site of the air leak. They are: external signs of thoracic trauma, more air in one hemithorax, and a consolidated or malpositioned lung lobe. If the leak cannot be localized, a sternal splitting approach would give good exposure to both sides of the thorax. If the leak is amenable to partial resection or suturing, this approach will be quite satisfactory; however, a lobectomy will be difficult because of the distance to the pulmonary hilus.

INFECTIOUS PLEURITIS (Pyothorax, Empyema)

Pleural infection may result from penetrating wounds, foreign bodies, or an extension of sub-

pleural infections such as pneumonia. An example of a foreign body that can cause pleural disease is the foxtail (*Hordeum* sp.), a plant awn of the Western United States. These awns can lodge in the pleural space following inhalation and airway migration or direct penetration of the skin. Penetrating bite wounds frequently produce pyothorax in cats.

Clinical signs of an animal with infectious pleuritis may be due to the volume of pleural exudate, the infectious (toxic) process itself, or both. Some animals are presented for depression, anorexia, and loss of condition, although owners may note a shallow respiratory pattern or report a nonproductive cough. Other animals, with a large amount of exudate, present with acute dyspnea and exercise intolerance. They may or may not be febrile. Physical examination may reveal loss of breath sounds, muffling of the heart, and dullness on percussion. However, the thoracic examination may seem normal in many cases.

Thoracic radiographs will demonstrate a pleural effusion. Because of the fibrin content of the exudate, adhesions and loculations of fluid may occur. The loculations are recognized as irregular fluid densities that do not shift when radiographs are taken in different positions. Fibrinous encapsulation of fluid may even lead to a unilateral pleural effusion.

Thoracocentesis with fluid analysis and culture is

diagnostic. Fluid is usually thick, cloudy, and foul smelling and often contains flocculent debris composed of bacteria and degenerating leukocytes. The color may vary from yellow to brown and may be bloody. The protein concentration is usually greater than 4.5 gm/dl. The cell types encountered in a septic exudate are neutrophils, macrophages, and red blood cells. The predominant cell is the degenerating neutrophil. These cells have poorly defined, disintegrating nuclei that stain a pale pink. Some neutrophils may be observed with a fragmented, pyknotic nucleus. Toxic granulation and vacuolization are seen in the cytoplasm. Occasional macrophages are found, and red blood cell numbers vary greatly. Microorganisms may be seen extracellularly, within neutrophils and macrophages, or clumped in colonies (i.e., sulfur granules). The volume of fluid in cases of septic exudates tends to be less than that found in transudates and nonseptic exudates.

Treatment of infectious pleuritis involves (1) elimination of the source of infection, (2) pleural drainage and lavage, and/or (3) antimicrobial therapy. If a foreign body of any type is suspected, surgical exploration is indicated. A lateral thoracic approach is preferred if localizing signs are present, e.g., unilateral effusion or external wounds. When no such evidence is available, a sternal-splitting approach is used. In cases of migrating plant awns, the search for the foreign body is tedious and often frustrating owing to a fibrinous proliferation of the mediastinal and diaphragmatic pleura. As much of the fibrinous pleura is excised as possible. The ventral sections of the mediastinum are usually the most severely affected and are removed to the level of the phrenic nerve. Penicillin-sensitive organisms such as *Actinomyces* sp. and *Pasturella* sp. are usually associated with plant awn–induced pleural infections.

If foreign bodies are not suspected in cases of septic pleural effusion, treatment consists of systemic antibiotics with or without pleural drainage or lavage. The decision to drain the pleura is based on the character and cytology of the fluid. Septic exudates with rare microorganisms, low fibrin content, and low to moderate cell counts are treated with systemic therapy. If satisfactory progress does not occur or bacterial and cell counts are elevated, pleural drainage in conjunction with antibiotics is needed. In cases of frank pyothorax with thick purulent exudate, pleural lavage (pleuroclysis) is added to the treatment regimen. A pleural tube is placed on one or both sides of the thorax as indicated. The pleural cavity is drained and lavaged two or three times daily. The lavage solution is composed of warmed isotonic saline or Ringer's solution (1 to 2 mg/kg) and antibiotics. If the exudate is loculated, proteolytic enzymes are added to the lavage solution. The solution is drained after five to ten minutes. Serial radiographs are useful to evaluate the effectiveness of therapy.

Feline infectious peritonitis causes a distinctive pleural effusion. It is typically thick and amber colored. The high protein content (av. 6.2 gm/dl) gives the fluid its characteristic stringy appearance when dropped from a syringe. The cytology is that of a nonseptic exudate or modified transudate with low numbers of nondegenerative neutrophils and macrophages.

CHYLOTHORAX

The lymphatic system is an auxilliary route by which fluid, protein, cells, and particulate debris from the interstitial spaces are transported to the general circulation. The lymphatic capillaries from various regions gradually coalesce into larger lymphatic vessels, which eventually empty into the great veins at the thoracic inlet. The largest lymphatic vessel is the thoracic duct, which carries the majority of body lymph. However, the right lymphatic duct drains the head and right front limb. The confluence of the lymphatic vessels from the rear legs, the caudal trunk, and the abdominal viscera is the cisterna chyli. Originating from the cisterna chyli, the thoracic duct carries body tissue and intestinal lymph through the mediastinum to the thoracic inlet.

After digestion and absorption most dietary fats, except for the short– and medium–chain fatty acids, are transported from the intestines via the lymphatics in the form of chylomicrons. The lymph is a creamy fatty fluid postprandially owing to the high concentration of chylomicrons.

Chylous pleural effusion is a well-recognized clinical entity. Effusions containing thoracic duct lymph (chyle) may occur secondary to trauma, neoplasia. obstruction, inflammation, or congenital abnormalities. However, the greatest percentage of cases have no easily identifiable cause and are, thus, classified as idiopathic. A possible congenital form of chylothorax occurs in young Afghan hounds. Studies of these dogs have demonstrated abnormal patterns of the anterior mediastinal lymphatic vessels. It is suspected that these lymphatics either are easily disrupted by minor trauma or exude chyle transmurally owing to lymphatic hypertension.

Animals with chylothorax usually are presented because of dyspnea from pleural effusion. Since chyle accumulates slowly, the animals are able to compensate for a period of time until their pulmonary reserve is exhausted. As with any patient with respiratory compromise, manipulations should be minimal. Thoracocentesis will yield a creamy or milky fluid that may contain blood.

The diagnosis of chylous effusion is based on the demonstration of chylomicrons in the fluid. Several drops of the effusion are mixed with an equal amount of lipotropic stain (Sudan III or IV or oil red 0) and examined microscopically for the presence of orange- or pink-stained fat globules. A new methylene–blue stained smear of the sediment will show chylomicra as tiny refractile bodies ringing erythrocytes. True chyle will clear with ether. Two equal volumes of supernatant from the effusion are mixed separately with 1 or 2 drops of 1 N sodium hydroxide. An equal volume of ether is added to one sample and water to the other. If the effusion is chyle, the sample receiving the ether will become clear after mixing. An *in vivo* test for chyle consists of feeding the animal a lipophilic dye, such as D and C (Drugs and Cosmetics) Green number 6, mixed with butter or oil. Within one hour after ingestion, a chylous effusion will be stained green. If these tests are equivocal or negative, the levels of triglycerides and cholesterol in the pleural fluid should be compared with those in the serum. Chyle has a higher triglyceride and lower cholesterol level than serum. In humans, pleural fluids with a triglyceride level greater than 110 mg/dl are chylous, whereas those with a level of less than 50 mg/dl are nonchylous.

Pseudochylous effusions containing lecithin and cholesterol resulting from chronic inflammation and cellular degeneration resemble true chyle. Pseudochylous effusions have been seen with cardiomyopathy in the cat. Occasionally, a pseudochylous effusion may appear to contain chylomicrons when examined microscopically; however, the triglyceride levels will be lower and the cholesterol levels higher than those in serum. Pseudochylous effusions do not clear with ether.

The cytology of chylous effusions shows high lymphocyte counts early in the course of disease. With time, inflammation of the pleura modifies the character of the effusion. Nondegenerative neutrophils will then predominate, with the addition of macrophages and mesothelial cells. Because of the bacteriostatic effect of chyle, bacteria are rarely seen and chylous effusions are usually sterile. Thoracic radiographs demonstrate the degree of pleural effusion. When the chylous effusion has been removed, radiographs should be repeated to rule out other pleural or thoracic diseases such as mediastinal masses or cardiac enlargement.

Treatments for chylothorax are dietary management with pleural drainage, thoracic duct ligation, and pleurodesis. A practical approach to the treatment of chylothorax is to attempt conservative management initially with dietary modification and pleural drainage. The flow of lymph in the thoracic duct is related to food and water intake as well as physical activity. Absorption of fatty acids greater than ten carbon atoms is by way of the intestinal lymphatics. Limiting oral intake, especially fats, and reducing exercise will theoretically decrease the flow of chyle and the volume of pleural effusion. An example of a homemade low-fat, high-quality protein diet is boiled chicken, potatoes, and honey. An alternative is the commercially available veterinary

reducing diet for dogs.* Concurrent pleural drainage may allow adhesions of the pleura to seal any leaking lymphatics. Pleural drainage is performed via an indwelling thoracic catheter. If the patient is cooperative and facilities are available, continuous suction drainage is used. However, an alternative is intermittent aspiration with a stopcock and syringe repeated three or four times daily.

Successful resolution of chylothorax may require two or three weeks of medical therapy. However, the majority of cases do not respond, and owners should be informed of this possibility before beginning treatment. Some animals may be severely debilitated and cachexic as a result of the chronic loss of protein, fats, and vitamins in the chyle during medical management. Close monitoring of serum protein levels is important. Some patients may require plasma transfusions or intravenous alimentation during extended periods of conservative treatment. If an animal is debilitated, there is a risk that further loss of condition may increase the risk at surgery.

The surgical treatment of chylous effusion is thoracic duct ligation. The pleural effusion in chylothorax is thoracic duct lymph. If the thoracic duct is occluded by ligation at the diaphragm, the flow of chyle into the pleura should be eliminated. The lymphatic system will open another anastomosis to the venous system caudal to the diaphragm after such a ligation is made in normal animals.

When surgery is performed, radiographic contrast studies of the thoracic duct system (lymphangiograms) are recommended preoperatively to attempt identification of the site of leakage and to demonstrate the anatomy of the thoracic duct in the caudal mediastinum. Unfortunately, the site of leakage has rarely been demonstrated radiographically. Recently a technique for cannulation of intestinal lymphatic trunks through a laparotomy has been developed for improving the lymphangiographic study. Also, by infusing small amounts of diluted methylene blue dye into the lymphatic system with the same catheter, visualization and identification of the thoracic duct and collaterals at surgery are improved.

The thoracic duct is approached through the ninth or tenth intercostal space. In the dog the thoracic duct lies on the right side of the mediastinum on the dorsolateral surface of the aorta and ventral to the azygos vein. In the cat the thoracic duct is on the left side of the mediastinum. There are usually multiple collateral branches of the thoracic duct widely distributed in the mediastinum. These branches are identified and ligated close to the diaphragm.

The success rate using this treatment method is approximately 50 per cent. The variation in collat-

---

*R/D, Hills Pet Products, Inc., Topeka, KS.

eral lymphatics probably accounts for the poor results. If any unidentified collateral lymphatic circumvents the ligature, flow through the thoracic duct will be re-established. Preoperative lymphangiography and interoperative dye infusion may help the surgeon identify all of the collateral lymphatics.

When other means of therapy for chylothorax have been unsuccessful, pleurodesis may be attempted. Pleurodesis involves the instillation of irritants or sclerosing compounds into the pleural space to produce adhesions between the parietal and visceral pleurae. By obliterating the pleural space, the accumulation of chyle should be eliminated. This technique has been used extensively in humans for both unresponsive pneumothorax and pleural effusions; however, it has not been evaluated in veterinary medicine. In addition to chylothorax, pleurodesis may be of value in patients with nonseptic exudates secondary to neoplastic processes or idiopathic effusions that have not responded to other modes of therapy.

Pleurodesis is accomplished by infusing an irritating substance through a thoracic catheter into the pleural space bilaterally after complete pleural drainage. Tetracycline hydrochloride has been used at 15 mg/kg (maximum 500 mg) diluted in 2 to 4 ml/kg of saline. Other cytotoxic agents, such as nitrogen mustard, have been used in humans. The catheters are then clamped, and the animal is placed in various positions (sternal, left and right lateral recumbency, dorsal recumbency) for approximately ten minutes in each position to distribute the drug in the thoracic cavity. Constant suction drainage of the pleural space is then necessary to maintain apposition of the pleural surfaces. Adhesions should occur in 24 to 48 hours. Pain is controlled with narcotics or non-narcotic analgesics as necessary. The requirements for continuous pleural drainage may make pleurodesis an impractical technique for many private practices.

PLEURAL DRAINAGE

Continuous or intermittent pleural drainage and pleuroclysis is accomplished through a catheter inserted into the pleural space. Special thoracic catheters with stylets are manufactured for this purpose; however, soft urethral catheters or Silastic tubing function quite well. The seventh to ninth intercostal spaces are generally used as a site for catheter placement since this area is caudal to the heart and cranial to the diaphragm. The dorsal third of the thorax is selected for removal of air. To remove fluid, the catheter can be placed ventrally, at the costochondral junction; however, subcutaneous leakage of the fluid may occur, especially if large volumes of effusions are present. Dorsal placement of the catheter can be used for fluid drainage if the

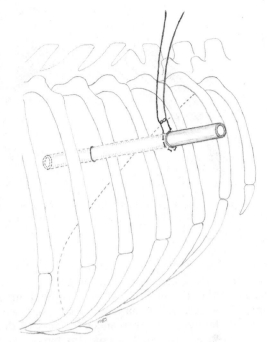

Figure 5. The skin incision for thoracic drain placement with a purse string suture opens into a subcutaneous tunnel two intercostal spaces in length.

patient is positioned in lateral and dorsal recumbency during aspiration.

The thoracic tube can be inserted under local anesthesia if two assistants are available to restrain the animal. The animal is usually placed in lateral recumbency; however, if there is severe dyspnea, a sternal or sitting position is adequate. The catheter will be tunneled subcutaneously for one or two rib spaces caudally or cranially from the skin incision prior to entering the pleural space to create a tissue seal around the tube. The area is clipped and scrubbed, and the surgical site is infiltrated with lidocaine. Then a final surgical scrub is performed, and the field is draped. A purse string suture of 2-0 or 3-0 nylon is placed around the site of the skin incision. A single throw is made in the suture but is not pulled taut. The ends of the suture are left long and tagged with a clamp. A stab incision is made in the center of the purse string suture. A subcutaneous tunnel is bluntly dissected to the appropriate intercostal site from the stab incision (Fig. 5). If a urethral catheter or tubing is used, four to six side holes are cut in the distal 2 or 3 cm.* The holes should be one-quarter to one-third the diameter of the catheter. The length of the fenestrated section of the catheter should not be longer than the length of the subcutaneous tunnel.

---

*Fenestrations are made by folding the tube and cutting the edge of the fold with scissors. This produces a hole with a smooth border, which is less likely to damage the lung than those made with a scalpel blade.

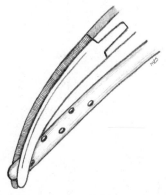

Figure 6. The catheter is held in the jaws of a hemostat ready to be passed through the subcutaneous tissue and into the pleural space. Note the multiple fenestrations in the distal end of the tube.

The catheter is crossclamped or plugged prior to insertion. The tip of the catheter is held in a hemostat or forceps of an appropriate size and advanced through the subcutaneous tunnel to the intercostal space (Fig. 6). The tip of the forceps and catheter are bluntly forced into the thorax in the caudal half of the intercostal space to avoid the intercostal vessels. The catheter is then quickly advanced into the thorax as the forceps is withdrawn. Traction exerted on the purse string suture prevents air from entering the thorax. The catheter is advanced so that the fenestrations are well within the pleural space. The patency of the catheter should be checked, and the positioning can be adjusted to ensure a steady flow of fluid or air. The first throw on the purse string suture is tightened, and a bow is tied to complete the knot. An adhesive tape butterfly is attached to the catheter at the point

where it enters the skin and is sutured to the skin to secure the catheter against motion (Fig. 7).

A special thoracic catheter with stylet* (Fig. 8) can be used to simplify the procedure. Since the stylet is straight, the technique is slightly modified. The skin incision, purse string suture, and subcutaneous tunnel are created as previously described, but the skin is then advanced so that the incision is situated directly over the intercostal space by elevating the catheter and stylet to a perpendicular position. The catheter and stylet are held in position with one hand and forced through the muscles into the space with the other. Once the catheter enters the pleura, it is advanced slightly, the stylet is withdrawn, and the catheter is crossclamped or occluded. Positioning of the catheter in the thorax is performed as described previously. These catheters have a raised radiopaque strip that can be used to suture the catheter directly to the skin.

_____

*Trocar Catheter, Deknatel, Floral Park, NY.

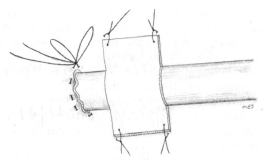

Figure 7. An adhesive tape butterfly is sutured to the skin to hold the thoracic tube in place, and the purse string suture is tied in a bow.

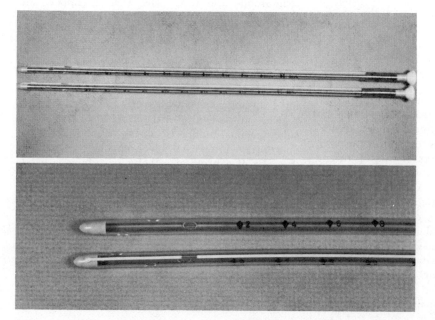

Figure 8. The specially designed thoracic catheter has several important features. The trocar tip is covered by the plastic on the end of the tube to minimize the chance of lacerating the lung. Markings indicate the distance to the most proximal side hole. The radiopaque marking strip is raised and can be used to suture the tube to the skin.

An antibacterial or povidone iodine ointment and dressing are applied to the incision, and the catheter is covered with a bandage. The bandage and dressing should be changed daily. Animals with chest drains may have potentially fatal complications if the catheter becomes open to room air. Thus, animals with chest drains should be under constant supervision.

When the thoracic catheter is removed, the skin sutures are removed and the purse string bow is untied but left in place. The catheter is pulled with a rapid motion to avoid introducing pneumothorax. As the tip of the catheter is extracted, the purse string suture is tightened to seal the incision, and a square knot is tied. The incision is covered with a sterile dressing for 24 hours.

SUPPLEMENTAL READING

Bessome, L. N., Ferguson, T. B., and Burford, T. H.: Chylothorax. Ann. Thorac. Surg. 12:527, 1971.

Fox, R. E.: Refractory and recurrent spontaneous pneumothorax—a medical or surgical disease? Medical management with intrapleural tetracycline. J. Am. Osteopath. Assoc. 78:882, 1979.

Kagan, K. G., and Breznock, E. M.: Variations in the canine thoracic duct system and the effects of surgical occlusion demonstrated by rapid aqueous lymphography, using an intestinal lymphatic trunk. A.J.V.R. 40:948, 958, 1979.

Light, R. W.: Pleural effusions. Med. Clin. North Am. 40:1339, 1977.

Lord, P. F., et al.: Lung lobe torsion in the dog. J.A.A.H.A. 9:473, 1973.

Lowell, J. R.: *Pleural Effusions: A Comprehensive Review.* Baltimore: University Park Press, 1977.

Staats, B. A., et al.: The lipoprotein profile of chylous and nonchylous pleural effusions. Mayo Clin. Proc. 55:700, 1980.

Suter, P. F., and Green, R. W.: Chylothorax in a dog with abnormal termination of the thoracic duct. J.A.V.M.A. 159:302, 1971.

Section

4

CARDIOVASCULAR DISEASES

JOHN D. BONAGURA, D.V.M.
Consulting Editor

Additional Pertinent Information found in **Current Veterinary
Therapy VII:**

CONCEPTS AND THERAPEUTIC STRATEGIES IN THE MANAGEMENT OF HEART FAILURE

MARK KITTLESON, D.V.M.

East Lansing, Michigan

CHRONIC HEART FAILURE

Heart failure is the general term indicating conditions that interfere with the heart's ability to pump adequate quantities of blood to the tissues (forward failure) or that result in elevated venous pressures behind the affected heart chambers (backward failure). Since most chronic heart failure patients show evidence of both forward and backward heart failure, both of these hemodynamic problems must be treated.

Heart failure can be divided pathophysiologically into (1) myocardial failure, (2) volume or pressure overloaded failure, and (3) compliance failure. Ideally, each type of failure should be treated differently.

Myocardial failure is caused by an inability of the myocardium to contract normally (primary systolic dysfunction) and relax normally (primarily diastolic dysfunction). The decreased contractility results from dysfunction of the sarcoplasmic reticulum, which loses its ability to bind and release calcium (Fig. 1). This results in fewer calcium ions available for interaction with cardiac muscle proteins during systole. It may also cause higher intracellular calcium concentrations during diastole, which may lead to poor myocardial relaxation. Mitochondria attempt to lower the intracellular calcium concentration by binding additional calcium. This causes

mitochondrial damage and decreases cellular energy production, further reducing cardiac function. The basic sarcoplasmic reticulum abnormality can be primary (e.g., congestive cardiomyopathy) or secondary to prolonged hemodynamic overload (e.g., aortic stenosis, ventricular septal defect, mitral insufficiency).

Reduced myocardial contractility results in an inadequate ventricular stroke volume. Numerous humoral and neurogenic mechanisms attempt to compensate for reduced contractility through increases in heart rate and venous return. Many of the signs of heart failure are the result of these compensatory responses. Venous return is increased by expanding the plasma volume through renal sodium and water retention and decreasing vascular space through vasoconstriction. Although the increased venous return increases myocardial fiber stretch (preload) and initially improves stroke volume, this mechanism also fails with time. The increased venous return combines with reduced diastolic relaxation and compliance to elevate ventricular and atrial diastolic pressures, which leads to signs of venous congestion and edema.

Heart failure is also caused by *pressure* or *volume overloads* that are so severe that the ventricle cannot compensate for them. Severe volume overloads (e.g., mitral regurgitation, patent ductus arteriosus) are more common. Although a hemody-

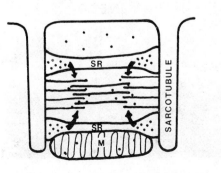
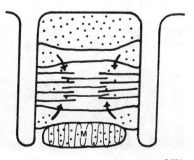

NORMAL   **MYOCARDIAL FAILURE**

Figure 1. Schematic diagram of systolic calcium ion movements and sarcoplasmic reticulum function in normal cells and in myocardial failure cells. During myocardial failure, the sarcoplasmic reticulum loses its ability to bind and release calcium. Black dots represent calcium. SR = sarcoplasmic reticulum; M = mitochondrion.

namic overload can eventually lead to myocardial failure, heart failure frequently occurs before myocardial decompensation can be demonstrated. At Michigan State University, more than 50 per cent of the dogs with mitral regurgitation and severe heart failure have no echocardiographic evidence of myocardial failure. Echocardiographically, these patients have large ventricular end-diastolic diameters but normal end-systolic diameters (Fig. 2). The result is a dilated but hyperfunctioning left ventricle, which, because of severe mitral regurgitation, ejects up to 90 per cent of the total stroke volume backward, into the left atrium. This results in elevated left atrial pressures and reduced stroke volume. Thus, patients may have clinical signs of heart failure without demonstrable *myocardial* failure.

Compliance failure is present when a ventricle is unable to distend properly during ventricular filling. This can be caused by massive ventricular hypertrophy with normal contractility (e.g., hypertrophic cardiomyopathy), ventricular destruction and fibrosis (e.g., restrictive cardiomyopathy), or a diseased pericardium limiting diastolic filling (e.g., constrictive pericarditis, cardiac tamponade). In each case diastolic blood pressures are elevated owing to poor ventricular compliance, not as the result of myocardial failure.

Heart failure therapy is based on the severity of the failure. Therefore, it is useful to separate patients into classes based on their degree of physical impairment. Heart failure severity and degree of physical impairment generally correlate well. The classification system developed by the New York Heart Association is useful in veterinary medicine.

Class I heart failure patients have cardiac disease but are compensated so that there is minimal evidence of myocardial dysfunction and no clinical signs of heart failure. Frank-Starling (ventricular function) curves can be utilized to illustrate the myocardial function of the class I patient (Fig. 3).

These curves plot preload (atrial pressure) against cardiac function (cardiac index). The curve of a class I patient is normal. As atrial pressure increases, cardiac index increases appropriately. *Class II* patients exhibit signs of heart failure during exercise because tissue oxygen demands are not met or because pulmonary congestion is produced by exercise-induced increases in venous return to the diseased heart. *Class III* individuals have signs at night (orthopnea) or during normal activity (Fig. 4). *Class IV* patients have clinical signs at rest (Fig. 5).

Frank-Starling curves are useful for illustrating the various stages of myocardial failure and the responses to therapy. As contractility decreases and resistance to myocardial fiber shortening (afterload) increases, the curves shift downward; that is, greater elevations in filling pressures are needed to increase cardiac output. Frank-Starling curves are less useful for depicting changes in volume-overloaded heart failure, such as mitral insufficiency, because contractility may be normal. Volume-overloaded patients with mitral regurgitation may have a normal Frank-Starling relationship, but they operate on the outermost portions of the curve (Fig. 3, point E). Although such patients have greatly increased cardiac outputs, most of the blood goes into the left atrium. To maintain this high cardiac output, these patients must have very large diastolic

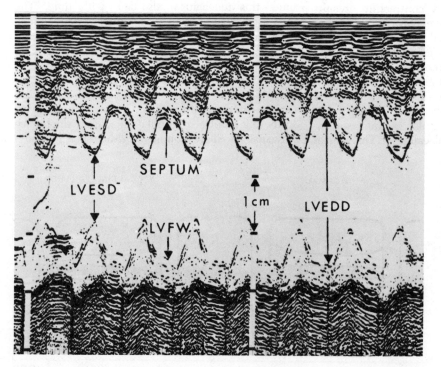

Figure 2. Echocardiogram (left ventricular position) from a dog with mitral regurgitation and class IV heart failure. The left ventricular free wall and septal motions are excellent. Estimated end-systolic volume index is 10 ml/m², indicating myocardial failure is not present. LVEDD = left ventricular end-diastolic diameter; LVESD = left ventricular end-systolic diameter; LVFW = left ventricular free wall.

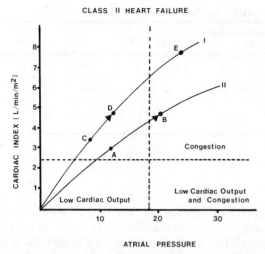

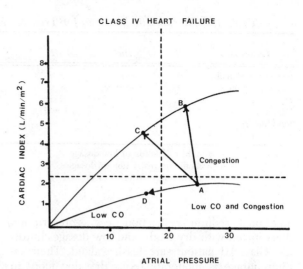

Figure 3. Relationship between cardiac index and left atrial pressure (Frank-Starling curve) in classes I and II myocardial failure. Points A and C represent cardiac function at rest, and points B and D represent function during exercise. In class II myocardial failure, cardiac output increases with exercise to an appropriate level, but at the expense of developing pulmonary congestion. Point E represents class IV volume overloaded failure. Point D can also represent class IV volume overloaded failure after large doses of a diuretic have been administered.

Figure 5. Frank-Starling curve of class IV myocardial failure. Point A is resting cardiac function. Cardiac output is inadequate even at rest (i.e., venous Po_2 <30) and congestion is present. Point B represents cardiac function after digitalis or an arteriolar dilator. Point C is cardiac function after digitalis and diuretics or after a combination vasodilator. Point D is after diuretics alone or after digitalis and diuretics in a patient refractory to digitalis.

volumes and, subsequently, high filling pressures. These pressures predispose to edema.

Myocardial failure can only be distinguished from other types of heart failure by echocardiography, angiography, radionuclide studies, or cardiac catheterization. Echocardiographically, left ventricular myocardial failure is characterized by poorly moving ventricular walls, a shortening fraction of less than 25 per cent, and large end-diastolic and end-systolic

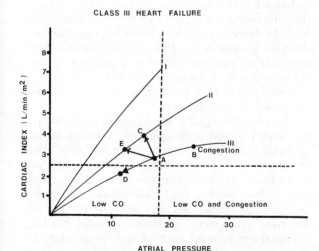

Figure 4. Frank-Starling curves of classes I, II, and III myocardial failure. Point A represents a patient in class III failure at rest. During normal activity, cardiac function moves to point B, where congestion develops and cardiac output is inappropriately low. Point C represents the patient's cardiac function after digitalis and point D is after diuretics. Point E is after digitalis and diuretics.

dimensions. When mitral regurgitation is present, only the end-systolic volume index is valuable in identifying myocardial failure. This index is estimated in humans by cubing the end-systolic diameter obtained from the echocardiogram or angiocardiogram. When it is less than 30 ml/m², myocardial function is normal. When it is greater than 90 ml/m², severe myocardial failure is present. Our findings with dogs have been similar to these data. If an objective means of characterizing the type of heart failure is not available, however, the clinician must make *clinical assumptions* regarding the type of heart failure present. As examples, congestive cardiomyopathy patients always have myocardial failure; based on our studies, most patients with mitral regurgitation do not.

The treatment for patients with *myocardial failure* (e.g., congestive cardiomyopathy) is outlined in Table 1 according to the functional class. Classes IIa, IIIa, and IVa are added to represent patients currently receiving appropriate medication for their degree of failure but continuing to show clinical signs of heart failure. The treatments listed include conventional management with exercise and sodium restriction and the administration of diuretics and digitalis and also indicate the role of vasodilator and dobutamine therapy. Class I patients are not treated. Previously untreated class II patients respond well to mild exercise (i.e., no hunting, confinement to the yard) and sodium restriction. They should not receive treats that contain salt (e.g., pretzels, potato chips). Animals that still show signs of heart failure during exercise (class IIa) are given further exercise restriction (e.g., leash walks only),

Table 1.   *Therapeutic Strategy for Treating Myocardial Failure Based on Functional Class*

Treatment	Functional Class						
	II	IIa	III	IIIa	IV	IVa	IVb
Exercise restriction	+	+ +	+ +	+ +	+ + to + + +	+ + +	+ + +
Salt restriction	+	+ to + +	+ +	+ + +	+ + +	+ + +	+ + +
Diuretics		+	+ +	+ + to + + +	+ + to + + +	+ + +	+ + +
Digitalis			+ + +	+ + +	+ + +	+ + +	
Vasodilators						+ + +	+ + +
Dobutamine							+ + +

Notes: + = mild restriction or low dosage.
          + + = moderate restriction or dosage.
          + + + = maximum restriction or dosage.

additional sodium restriction (e.g., prescription diets mixed with dry food), and low-dosage diuretics. Class III patients are leash walked. Their sodium intake is moderate (e.g., dry dog food) to maximally restricted (e.g., prescription low-sodium diet or home-cooked low salt diet [see CVT VI, page 61]), and moderate dosages of diuretics are administered. These patients are also digitalized to increase myocardial contractility, and they generally respond well to digitalis. Class IIIa patients should receive maximal salt restriction and increased doses of diuretics. Additional symptomatic therapy, such as bronchodilator and cough suppressant therapy, may be useful.

Class IV patients with myocardial failure need cage rest, a salt-free diet, and moderate to maximal dosages of diuretics. These patients are also digitalized. However, in severe myocardial failure, cardiac contractility does not increase in 50 to 60 per cent of the patients given digitalis; in these cases, cardiac output may not increase or can actually decrease owing to digitalis-induced decreases in heart rate and diuretic-induced decreases in venous return. Since backward heart failure signs tend to improve (e.g., decreased pulmonary edema, reduced amount of ascites) because of diuretic administration, the patient's condition appears to improve; however, cardiac output can still be inadequate with clinical signs of weakness, azotemia, or low venous P_{O_2}. Therefore, if the patient does not respond appropriately to digitalis and diuretics (class IVa), an arteriolar dilator is administered to improve cardiac output. The adequacy of the cardiac output can be monitored by measuring cardiac output or venous oxygen tensions or by evaluating the capillary refill time and mucous membrane color, as discussed hereafter.

Class IVb consists of patients with life-threatening signs requiring emergency therapy. They are treated as per subset IV patients, described in the following section on Acute Heart Failure, using additional drugs like dobutamine.

Treatment for severe *ventricular volume overload* secondary to mitral regurgitation or left-to-right shunts is similar to that for myocardial failure, except that digitalis may not be indicated as initial therapy since myocardial contractility is usually normal. However, digitalis is used to slow the heart rate when sinus or supraventricular tachycardias are present. Arteriolar dilators are indicated for the therapy of class IV volume-overloaded patients. These agents reduce the amount of regurgitation in mitral insufficiency patients and decrease the magnitude of left-to-right shunting in patients with congenital heart disease. Thus, they decrease volume overload, increase cardiac output, and relieve congestion. Diuretics can effectively control congestive signs in class III and IV patients. However, since diuretic administration to class IV patients can decrease cardiac output (see Fig. 3), an arteriolar dilator may also be prescribed.

Hypertrophic cardiomyopathy is the only type of *compliance failure* treated medically. Pericardial disease is best managed by surgical techniques (see CVT VII, page 321). Hypertrophic cardiomyopathy is characterized by massively hypertrophied left ventricular walls. Ventricular stiffness, plus the tachycardias that are often present, causes reduced diastolic function (i.e., poor ventricular filling). This leads to decreased stroke volume because the end-diastolic volume is less than normal. Outflow tract obstructions may also be present and may further decrease stroke volume. Contractility is normal or supernormal in such patients, so positive inotropic agents are contraindicated.

The ideal therapy for hypertrophic cardiomyopathy would consist of blocking the stimulus for hypertrophy. Since this therapy is not available, other drugs are used. Propranolol, a beta-blocking drug, slows heart rate and depresses contractility, which may reduce outflow tract obstruction. It does not improve compliance but does increase diastolic filling time. Verapamil, a calcium channel blocking agent, shows promise for treating hypertrophic cardiomyopathy. It depresses contractility, reduces heart rate, and increases compliance. However, it can reduce arterial blood pressure and increase outflow tract gradients. Therefore, the demonstration of its usefulness in the dog or cat awaits the results of clinical trials. The pharmacokinetics of

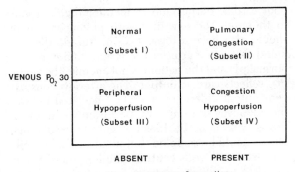

	Normal (Subset I)	Pulmonary Congestion (Subset II)
VENOUS P$_{O_2}$ 30	Peripheral Hypoperfusion (Subset III)	Congestion Hypoperfusion (Subset IV)
	ABSENT	PRESENT
	Pulmonary Congestion	

Figure 6. Amended version of Forrester and Waters' classification of acute heart failure based on hemodynamic subset identification.

propranolol and verapamil are discussed in the section on Therapy of Cardiac Arrhythmias (page 360).

ACUTE HEART FAILURE

In veterinary practice, acute heart failure is most commonly caused by acute myocardial failure secondary to either metabolic abnormalities that directly depress myocardial contractility (e.g., hypoxia, acidosis, myocardial depressant factors) or drug administration (e.g., halothane, barbiturates). However, acute heart failure may also be due to acute volume overload (e.g., ruptured chordae tendinae) or cardiac arrhythmias. In addition, a patient with chronic compensated heart failure may experience an acute cardiovascular insult and may be presented in fulminant heart failure (class IVb). Knowledge of the precipitating factors and the patient's hemodynamic status is essential before therapy can be instituted.

Forrester and Waters (1978) have identified four "subsets" of *acute* heart failure based on cardiac output, blood pressure, and the presence of pulmonary congestion (Fig. 6). Identifying the subset gives the clinician a guide to therapy (Fig. 7). We have found that low cardiac output, which leads to

	No Cardiovascular Therapy	Diuretic Venodilator
VENOUS P$_{O_2}$ 30	Volume Infusion	Positive Inotropic Agent, Arteriolar Dilator if BP Normal Diuretic
	ABSENT	PRESENT
	Pulmonary Congestion	

Figure 7. Therapeutic strategy of acute heart failure based on Forrester and Waters' hemodynamic subset classification.

peripheral hypoperfusion, is indicated by a venous P$_{O_2}$ <30 mm Hg (providing that arterial P$_{O_2}$ and hemoglobin concentration are not severely abnormal). Pulmonary congestion or edema is determined by the typical changes in thoracic radiograms.

If examination reveals neither congestion nor hypoperfusion (subset I), the patient is monitored and the initial diagnosis reassessed. When congestion is present and perfusion is normal (subset II), *diuretics* or a *venodilator* such as nitroglycerine is given. In this case, the venous P$_{O_2}$ is monitored frequently, since peripheral perfusion may decline as the therapy reduces effective blood volume and ventricular filling. If hypoperfusion is present but congestion is absent, as in some forms of shock (subset III), the initial therapy is the *infusion of fluids* while checking frequently for pulmonary congestion by auscultation, radiography, and, preferably, the measuring of venous pressure. A central venous or Swan-Ganz catheter can be placed to monitor right and left ventricular filling pressures. If congestion develops or ventricular filling pressures rise above normal during volume expansion, fluid administration is discontinued. If venous pressures rise with volume infusion but hypoperfusion persists, the treatment is the same as for subset IV described hereafter.

Both hypoperfusion and congestion are present in subset IV. It is preferable to obtain an index of myocardial contractility in patients in this group (e.g., an echocardiogram) prior to initial therapy. This helps to determine if myocardial failure is present and if there is a need for positive inotropic agents. If echocardiography is unavailable, myocardial failure is assumed and initial therapy includes dobutamine, a positive inotropic agent, and the diuretic furosemide. If positive inotropes are not indicated or if there is an inadequate response to dobutamine, vasodilator therapy is given. Intravenous nitroprusside is recommended but requires blood pressure monitoring. Intravenous or oral hydralazine or intravenous nitroglycerin is also available. Oral hydralazine acts within 30 to 60 minutes. Topical nitroglycerin can be used as a venodilator, but it is less potent than the other agents. Patients receiving vasodilators should have their arterial blood pressure monitored, particularly when potent intravenous agents such as nitroprusside or IV nitroglycerin are given.

MONITORING THERAPEUTIC TRENDS:
NEW IDEAS

To objectively assess the therapeutic effects of a particular drug, hemodynamic monitoring is necessary. Although cost may prevent veterinarians from using Swan-Ganz thermodilution catheters, adequate monitoring can be done relatively noninvasively and inexpensively. Left-sided backward failure can be monitored radiographically. Right-sided backward failure can be assessed by hepatic size and abdominal girth, but central venous pressure measurements provide a more objective means of monitoring right-sided filling pressures.

Clinical signs of backward failure (congestion, edema) usually dominate the clinical picture of a heart failure patient, so therapy is frequently aimed at relieving these signs. Signs of forward failure (low cardiac output) are usually less apparent unless they are severe (i.e., shock) and are frequently overlooked. Chronic low cardiac output states probably contribute to long-term mortality. Certainly chronic myocardial hypoperfusion causes myocardial deterioration, so greater attempts should be made to improve hypoperfusion in heart failure. Since clinical signs of low cardiac output are subtle, an objective means of monitoring cardiac output must be used. We have found that venous PO_2 determination is a simple, inexpensive way to monitor cardiac output. This test is readily available in most commercial laboratories and many veterinary hospitals.

Central venous oxygen tension ($P\bar{v}O_2$) is an excellent indicator of adequate peripheral oxygen delivery. Peripheral oxygen delivery depends on the cardiac output, the per cent oxygen saturation of hemoglobin, the hemoglobin concentration, and the number and size of peripheral arteriovenous shunts. Derangement of any one factor may decrease O_2 delivery to peripheral tissues. When oxygen delivery is inadequate, the cells attempt to extract the same quantity of oxygen from the capillary blood and cause the O_2 content of venous blood to be lower. Since the per cent oxygen saturation of hemoglobin and the venous PO_2 are linearly related on the venous portion of the oxyhemoglobin dissociation curve, venous PO_2 correlates well with venous oxygen content.

The PO_2 within the capillary is the factor that determines O_2 delivery into the cell. Based on previous studies, the venous PO_2 falls below 30 mm Hg when cardiac output and tissue oxygen delivery are low enough to be clinically significant. Therapeutic interventions (e.g., oxygen inhalation, arteriolar dilator) are warranted at this time. When the venous PO_2 falls below 20 mm Hg, the peripheral cells are unable to extract enough oxygen to meet their metabolic demands and they switch to anaerobic metabolism. Shock or impending circulatory collapse may be evident at this time.

In resting heart failure patients without severe arterial hypoxemia or anemia, the venous PO_2 correlates significantly with the cardiac output. Although many patients have mild arterial hypoxemia, this must be severe to compromise peripheral oxygen delivery.

The venous PO_2 can be used to detect patients with inadequate tissue oxygen delivery owing to poor cardiac output and to monitor their response to therapy. Those with severe pulmonary edema should also have arterial PO_2 measured. We have found that when arterial PO_2 is above 65 mm Hg at normal pH and the patient is not anemic, the venous PO_2 reflects cardiac output. The arteriovenous oxygen content difference must be calculated to assess the adequacy of peripheral perfusion when arterial PO_2 is < 65 mm Hg. Ideally, central mixed venous blood should be sampled, but jugular blood samples correlate well with central samples and are more practical to obtain. Venous flow must not be occluded for longer than five to ten seconds when sampling or the venous PO_2 will be falsely low. When a sample is taken for blood gas analysis, it should be collected in an air-free syringe, corked, and stored on ice. This sample is then good for one to two hours and can be transported to a hospital or commercial laboratory.

As an example, thoracic radiograms and a venous PO_2 are obtained in patients with class IV left-sided myocardial failure. Generally, pulmonary edema is present and the venous PO_2 is <30 mm Hg. Digitalis, diuretics, and a low-sodium diet are administered. Thoracic radiograms and venous PO_2 are obtained every 24 hours. If pulmonary edema decreases and venous PO_2 improves, maintenance therapy is instituted. If edema improves but the low venous PO_2 remains static or further decreases, an arteriolar dilator is administered to increase cardiac output. A venodilator is also given when no improvement in pulmonary edema occurs. Responses to these agents are monitored.

The only clinical, noninvasive alternative to measuring venous PO_2 is to assess capillary refill time and mucous membrane color. These perfusion monitoring methods are subjective and prone to error, and the clinician must attempt to standardize all variables to reduce error.

REFERENCES AND SUPPLEMENTAL READING

Borow, K. M., Green, L. H., Mann, T., et al.: End-systolic volume as a predictor of postoperative left ventricular performance in volume overload from valvular regurgitation. Am. J. Med. 68:655, 1980.

Braunwald, E.: Clinical manifestations of heart failure. *In* Braunwald, E. (ed.): *Heart Disease: A Textbook of Cardiovascular Medicine.* Philadelphia: W. B. Saunders, 1980.

Clemmer, T. P.: Oxygen transport. Int. Anesthesiol. Clin. 19:21, 1981.

Forrester, J. S., and Waters, D. D.: Hospital treatment of congestive heart failure. Management according to hemodynamic profile. Am. J. Med. 65:173, 1978.

Katz, A. M.: Congestive heart failure: Role of altered myocardial cellular control. N. Engl. J. Med. 293:1184, 1975.

Kittleson, M.D., Eyster, G. E., Anderson, L. K., et al.: Myocardial function in dogs with spontaneous chronic mitral regurgitation and severe congestive heart failure. Proceedings of the Annual Meeting of The American College of Veterinary Internal Medicine, Salt Lake City, Utah, 1982.

Rosing, D. R., Kent, K. M., Borer, J. S., et al.: Verapamil therapy: a new approach to the pharmacologic treatment of hypertrophic cardiomyopathy. Circulation 60:1201, 1979.

Smith, T. W., and Braunwald, E.: The management of heart failure. *In* Braunwald, E. (ed.): *Heart Disease: A Textbook of Cardiovascular Medicine.* Philadelphia: W. B. Saunders, 1980.

DRUGS USED IN THE MANAGEMENT OF HEART FAILURE

MARK KITTLESON, D.V.M.

East Lansing, Michigan

The veterinarian has a variety of drugs available to him for the pharmacotherapy of cardiac failure. Most of these agents are extremely potent, with a narrow therapeutic index. Thus the clinician must be familiar with their cardiac and extracardiac effects, the adverse effects that can result from their use, and their potential for drug interaction. This familiarity can only be achieved through an understanding of the clinical pharmacology of these agents. Subsequent articles describe the specific utilization of cardiac drugs in the management of cardiomyopathy, valvular heart disease, congenital heart disease, and cardiopulmonary arrest. This article provides information that is important for proper drug therapy in the medical management of patients with these disorders.

DIGITALIS GLYCOSIDES

Although digitalis glycosides have been used as cardioactive drugs for the last 200 years, they are often used inappropriately, ineffectively, and in improper doses. Toxicity occurs in 18 to 23 per cent of human patients treated with digitalis, and the same holds true for veterinary patients. However, digitalis remains a valuable drug in certain types of cardiovascular therapy. To use the drug correctly one must know the indications, contraindications, pharmacokinetics, and pharmacodynamics of the drug as well as the many factors that alter these properties. Even with this knowledge toxicity occurs, so the clinician must know how to recognize and treat toxicity.

PHARMACODYNAMICS

Digitalis (digoxin, digitoxin, and other related glycosides) increases the rate and force of myocardial contraction in both the normal and mildly to moderately failing myocardium by nonspecifically increasing intracellular calcium concentration. The mechanism for this action is incompletely studied, but the prevailing theory is that digitalis inhibits the myocardial cell membrane Na^+-K^+ ATPase

pump. This inhibition results in increased intracellular sodium concentrations. The sodium must exit by exchanging with extracellular calcium. In the normal to moderately failing myocardial cell the sarcoplasmic reticulum binds the excess calcium and uses it to increase contractility. In severe myocardial failure digitalis is often ineffective because the sarcoplasmic reticulum has lost its ability to bind and release calcium. Since intracellular calcium concentration is already high in severe myocardial failure, an attempt to force it higher with digitalis may be ineffective or may produce cardiac toxicity (Fig. 1).

The antiarrhythmic properties of digitalis are mostly confined to the atria and A-V node, although digitalis may also benefit ventricular arrhythmias. The atrial antiarrhythmic effects are mediated by enhanced parasympathetic nerve activity, which decreases atrial automaticity, depresses atrial conduction, and increases the effective and functional refractory periods. Digitalis' direct effects on the atria are contrary to its parasympathetic effects, so that, in toxic concentrations or when the parasympathetic nerves are blocked, atrial arrhythmias can occur. Digitalis also increases parasympathetic

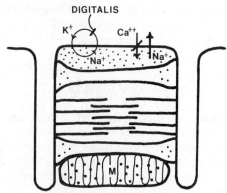

Figure 1. The effect of digitalis on calcium movements in a severely failing myocardial cell. Diastolic intracellular calcium concentration is elevated because of ineffective binding by the sarcoplasmic reticulum. Inhibition of the Na^+-K^+ ATPase pump may result in further calcium loading, which either enhances toxicity or does not result in calcium influx because of the concentration gradient. M = mitochondrion.

285

nerve activity to the A-V node and directly decreases conduction through the node, resulting in a slowed ventricular response to atrial fibrillation and flutter.

CLINICAL USES

Digitalis glycosides are indicated in the treatment of heart failure–induced sinus tachycardia, atrial tachyarrhythmias, and myocardial failure. Sinus tachycardia increases myocardial oxygen consumption, and this can be deleterious in heart failure patients. Digitalis is the drug of choice for heart failure–induced sinus tachycardia because it does not decrease contractility. It also slows the ventricular rate reponse to atrial flutter and fibrillation and thus may decrease myocardial oxygen consumption and increase ventricular filling.

Atrial tachyarrhythmias may be suppressed by digitalis' vagomimetic effects; however, the drug may also induce atrial or junctional arrhythmias at higher plasma levels.

Digitalis is generally indicated for the therapy of myocardial failure (see previous article). Without sophisticated studies, it is difficult to determine if myocardial failure is manifest when a heart failure patient is first presented. However, some generalizations are useful. Patients with congestive (dilated) cardiomyopathy have a contractile defect with sinus tachycardia or atrial fibrillation and should initially be treated with digitalis. However, myocardial contractility may not increase in all patients with class IV myocardial failure. Therefore, arteriolar vasodilators may also be needed for this group. Up to 90 per cent of mitral regurgitation patients have normal or mild depression of myocardial function. In my experience, the drugs of choice are diuretics and arteriolar dilators such as hydralazine. Since a major side effect of vasodilators is sinus tachycardia, digitalis is still indicated for heart rate control. Digitalis is contraindicated in compliance failure caused by pericardial disease or hypertrophic cardiomyopathy.

PHARMACOKINETICS

Digitoxin and digoxin are the two most commonly used digitalis glycosides. There are no differences in their cardioactivity despite a minor difference in molecular structure. However, this structural difference changes the pharmacokinetics of the two drugs.

Digoxin is a moderately polar compound that binds well to the Na^+-K^+ ATPase pump and increases parasympathetic activity. It is well absorbed (60 to 75 per cent) from the intestinal tract. About 20 per cent of the drug is bound to serum proteins (with the balance free in the serum), which explains the lower serum concentrations of digoxin needed for therapeutic effect as compared with digitoxin. This property does not change bioavailability, action, or toxicity of the drug. The serum half-life of digoxin varies in dogs from 24 to 36 hours. Since it takes two to three half-lives to achieve 75 to 88 per cent of steady state serum concentrations on a maintenance dosage schedule, it takes two to four days to achieve therapeutic serum levels. If toxicity occurs, it also takes at least 24 to 48 hours to reduce serum concentrations to nontoxic levels. Digoxin's half-life in the cat is still a matter of controversy, but the mean half-life appears to be between 33 and 58 hours.

Approximately 15 per cent of digoxin is metabolized in the liver, and the remainder is excreted unchanged in the urine. Renal clearance rate depends on glomerular filtration rate. Since renal failure reduces renal clearance, these patients have higher serum digoxin concentrations. As a result, either digoxin cannot be utilized in renal failure patients or the dosage must be reduced. No studies have been done to correlate serum digoxin concentration with renal function in the dog. Dosing a dog with renal failure with digoxin is, therefore, very difficult. It appears that digitoxin is a better choice in dogs with renal failure, but widespread clinical experience with digitoxin is still very limited.

Digitoxin is less commonly administered to small animals. Recent studies show its half-life in the dog to be 8 to 12 hours, indicating that therapeutic serum concentrations can be obtained on a maintenance schedule in 24 to 36 hours and that toxicity will diminish in 8 to 12 hours. The half-life of digitoxin in cats is greater than 100 hours; therefore it is not used in this species.

Digitoxin is well absorbed (95 to 100 per cent) from the gastrointestinal tract, and 90 per cent is protein bound. Most digitoxin is eliminated by the liver, but a small amount is metabolized to digoxin. Hepatic failure in the dog does not influence its half-life.

DIGITALIS PREPARATIONS

Digoxin is supplied in elixirs, tablets, and intravenous preparations. Whereas all forms can be used in the dog, the elixir is unpalatable for cats. Bioavailability differs among the preparations: 100 per cent of the IV form, 75 per cent of the elixir, and 60 per cent of the tablet are available. Bioavailability of the tablets may also differ among manufacturers. Lanoxin* has been shown to be reliably uniform in bioavailability.

Digitoxin intravenous and oral preparations are available (Crystodigin, Foxalin†).

---

*Burroughs Wellcome Co., Research Triangle Park, NC.
†Standex Laboratories, Inc., Columbus, OH.

DOSAGES AND METHODS OF ADMINISTRATION

The accepted digoxin dosages (0.011 mg/kg b.i.d. in dogs; 0.008 mg/kg b.i.d. in cats) and digitoxin dosage (0.033 mg/kg t.i.d. in dogs) are derived from studies on normal young animals weighing 5 to 20 kg. As such, these dosages are considered too high for most clinical heart failure cases and need to be adjusted downward depending on such factors as body size, age, presence of obesity, electrolyte disturbances, thyroid function, concomitant administration of other drugs, and type of digitalis preparation.

Body size or compartment size into which a drug will diffuse is usually estimated by body weight. Body weight dosages work well for most drugs because their toxic/therapeutic ratio is high, but those with low toxic/therapeutic ratios (e.g., cancer chemotherapy agents, digitalis) must be given in dosages based on body surface area estimates, which more closely predict volume of distribution. Because large dogs have a lower body surface area/body weight ratio, they require less digitalis than small dogs to produce the same therapeutic effects or toxicity. Figure 2 shows a comparison of digoxin dosage and body weight based on a dosage of 0.22 mg/m^2 b.i.d. assuming that digoxin kinetic studies have been done on 10- to 20-kg dogs (0.5 m^2). Since cats vary little in body size, this conversion is not needed in that species. Since digitoxin is supplied only in 0.1- and 0.25-mg capsules, it is inconvenient to use in large dogs; a 100-lb dog requires 12 0.25-mg capsules t.i.d. For convenience, digoxin is recommended for large dogs.

Age also decreases standard digitalis dosage because geriatric dogs or cats have less skeletal muscle mass/body weight. Since most digoxin and digitoxin is bound in skeletal muscle, older dogs have smaller volumes of distribution. Glomerular filtration rate also decreases with age, so digoxin excretion is slower. These two factors often necessitate dose *reductions up to 50 per cent* for digoxin.

Obesity is important because digoxin has poor lipid solubility; dosages must be based on lean body weight estimates. Because digitoxin is lipid soluble, dosage is unchanged.

Electrolyte disturbances alter dosage. Potassium competes with digitalis for binding sites on the Na$^+$-K$^+$ ATPase pump, so hypokalemia leaves more binding sites, whereas hyperkalemia leaves fewer.

Hypokalemic animals require either less digitalis or correction of potassium deficit. Hypercalcemia potentiates digitalis' cellular calcium loading, so hypercalcemic animals require less digitalis. Hypernatremia potentiates the cellular sodium loading seen with digitalis; again, dosage must be reduced.

Animals with hypothyroidism excrete digitalis at a slower rate; hyperthyroidism increases cellular sensitivity to digitalis. Reduced dosages of digitalis are required in both states.

Concomitant drug administration also affects digitalis pharmacokinetics. Furosemide decreases renal blood flow and glomerular filtration rate by decreasing circulating blood volume. This may require a decreased digoxin dosage when furosemide is administered, especially when administered at its maximum therapeutic dose. Quinidine reduces the volume of digoxin distribution by displacing it from skeletal muscle and reduces renal clearance. Serum digoxin concentrations rise when quinidine is added to a therapeutic regimen; thus, the digoxin dose is usually decreased by 50 per cent. This effect does not occur with digitoxin in the dog.

Drugs that induce hepatic microsomal enzymes (e.g., barbiturates, phenylbutazone) may increase the elimination rate of digoxin, whereas drugs that are microsomal enzyme inhibitors (e.g., chloramphenicol, tetracycline) may decrease the rate of elimination and produce higher serum concentrations. These drugs should be avoided when digoxin is being used. The effects of these drugs on digitoxin kinetics are not known.

Patients with myocardial failure or hypoxemia are more sensitive to the effects of digitalis and need lower dosages. In severe myocardial failure, cells are calcium loaded, and the addition of digitalis may result in further calcium loading, which may lead to an increase in abnormal automaticity and arrhythmias. Digitalis must be used very cautiously in these patients. Acute or chronic hypoxemia may also enhance digitalis-induced arrhythmia formation by an unexplained mechanism.

The route or form of administration does not affect digitoxin dosage because it is 90 to 100 per cent absorbed. It does affect digoxin administration, since the tablets are 60 per cent absorbed and the elixir is 75 per cent absorbed. The dosages in the literature have generally been derived from kinetic studies using tablets; therefore the dosage should be decreased by 20 per cent when using the elixir

Body Weight (Kg)

BID Digoxin dosage (mg/Kg)	10	20	30	40	50
	.011	.009	.008	.007	.006

Figure 2. Digoxin dosage calculated for body weight from a body surface area dosage of 0.22 mg/m^2.

and by 45 per cent when using the intravenous preparation.

Previous recommendations for digitalis in loading doses are no longer tenable because production of toxicity is consistent and predictable. This has been proved in healthy dogs, in dogs with heart failure, and in a mathematical model of digitalis kinetics. The possible exception to this is the patient with life-threatening supraventricular tachyarrhythmia. In addition, it has been proved that digoxin plasma levels are in the therapeutic range after two to three half-lives, i.e., a patient can be "digitalized" within two to four days. Digitoxin, because of its short half-life, reaches therapeutic concentrations within 24 to 48 hours. Most dogs or cats needing inotropic support can be treated effectively with digitalis on a maintenance schedule because their condition does not demand more rapid intervention. Patients that need more acute intervention usually require intravenous treatment (e.g., dobutamine, nitroprusside). Rapid intravenous digitalization is generally contraindicated because of potential toxicity and deleterious hemodynamic effects. Intravenous digitalis may increase peripheral vascular resistance and afterload and may initially reduce cardiac output.

A patient that requires digitalis therapy should be carefully evaluated physically and biochemically prior to the institution of therapy. A maintenance dosage should be calculated, keeping in mind all the aforementioned factors, and administered while the patient is monitored. The therapeutic endpoint for digitalis administration is clinical improvement, not toxicity, EKG changes, or reductions in heart rate. These signs are either dangerous or unreliable. Clinical improvement means improvement of backward failure (i.e., decreased congestion/edema) and forward failure (i.e., increased venous oxygen tension, increased cardiac output, improved perfusion). Clinical improvement dictates that maintenance therapy should be continued. Toxicity, because of its associated mortality, should be avoided at all costs. If signs of mild toxicity develop, digoxin should be discontinued for 24 hours (digitoxin for 12 hours) and maintenance therapy given at 50 per cent of the initial level.

Digitalis serum concentrations can now be readily analyzed at most commercial laboratories. They are helpful in documenting toxicity and identifying low serum concentrations in patients that apparently are not responding to the drug. Serum samples should be collected eight hours after the last digitalis dosage for consistent analysis. Therapeutic serum concentrations of digoxin fall between 1.0 and 2.5 ng/ml; concentrations of 2.5 to 6.0 ng/ml are considered moderately toxic and concentrations greater than 6.0 ng/ml are highly toxic. Digitoxin concentrations between 15 and 35 ng/ml are therapeutic; toxicity occurs above 40 ng/ml. Differences in patient sensitivity to digitalis glycosides exist (e.g., myocardial failure patients are more sensitive), so clinical signs are still the standard for assessing toxicity.

TOXICITY

Digitalis glycosides are associated with a high morbidity, and digitalis intoxication is associated with a high mortality. Mild digitalis toxicity generally affects the central nervous system, where it stimulates the area postrema in the medulla, inducing anorexia and vomiting and increasing gastrointestinal vagal tone, which increases gastrointestinal motility, leading to diarrhea. Intoxication is benign at this stage. If unrecognized, it can rapidly progress if additional dosages are given.

Moderate to severe digitalis intoxication produces potentially fatal arrhythmias through complex electrophysiologic changes in the heart. Sympathetic tone to the heart is increased by digitalis, which increases normal automaticity. Abnormal automaticity (late afterdepolarizations) occurs because of cellular calcium overloading. Digitalis also enhances ventricular re-entrant arrhythmia formation by slowing Purkinje fiber conduction, decreasing the ventricular refractory period, and enhancing the formation of unidirectional blocks. Any rhythm disturbance may occur including supraventricular and ventricular tachyarrhythmias and bradyarrhythmias. The more common rhythm disturbances include isolated ventricular or junctional premature beats, nonparoxysmal nodal or ventricular tachycardia, paroxysmal ventricular tachycardia, atrioventricular block, and junctional escape rhythms.

Digitalis toxicity must be recognized early for successful therapy, since severe cardiac toxicity is often fatal, even with aggressive therapy. When toxicity is recognized early, digitalis withdrawal only is required. Bradyarrhythmias may be controlled with atropine, but patient referral for electrical pacing may be needed in the unresponsive case. Tachyarrhythmias, especially ventricular tachycardia, have a high mortality and must be treated aggressively. Phenytoin and lidocaine are the drugs of choice because they reduce automaticity, disrupt re-entrant pathways, and reduce sympathetic tone (see following article). Potassium supplementation is necessary if hypokalemia is present in a patient intoxicated with digitalis. Propranolol, which blocks sympathetic nerve activity and exerts some direct myocardial effects, is the second drug of choice. Quinidine and procainamide are less effective. Cholestyramine binds digitalis glycosides in the intestinal tract and can be especially useful in digitoxin intoxication because of digitoxin's enterohepatic circulation. With early administration it may also be useful in binding an inadvertently large dose of digoxin. Cardiac glycoside-specific antibodies represent a possible future treatment to directly reduce free serum digitalis concentrations.

AMRINONE

Amrinone and its derivatives are new positive inotropic, mild vasodilating agents that have not as yet received FDA approval. Initial clinical trials of one of the derivatives look promising.

Amrinone is a bipyridine derivative that increases myocardial contractility, but its actions are unlike those of sympathomimetics or digitalis glycosides. Its mechanism of action is unknown, but it probably improves intracellular calcium kinetics. Amrinone is equipotent with dobutamine and much more potent than digitalis. It is very safe in dogs and has a large therapeutic range. When used in myocardial failure in humans, amrinone increases cardiac index and decreases left ventricular filling pressures, peripheral vascular resistance, blood pressure, and myocardial oxygen consumption. Patients do not develop tolerance to the drug as with catecholamines. A small percentage of human patients have developed thrombocytopenia while receiving amrinone, but this does not appear to occur in the dog. This drug and its analogues are now in the clinical trial phase in veterinary medicine. It is an exciting drug with significant potential for replacing other oral, long-term inotropic agents.

DIURETICS

Diuretics act by reducing plasma volume in the heart failure patient, thereby reducing venous return and ventricular filling volumes and pressures. In chronic heart failure venous return is elevated because of renal sodium and water retention and venoconstriction. In left-sided heart failure systemic venoconstriction shifts blood volume from the systemic to the pulmonary circuit, which increases venous return to the left ventricle. Venous return is elevated in an effort to maintain or increase cardiac output by placing more stretch on myocardial fibers (preload). In myocardial failure the stiff ventricular myocardium is unable to dilate adequately in response to the increased preload. This results in elevated diastolic pressures in the affected chambers and congestion/edema behind them (backward failure). In volume-overloaded failure the myocardium is still compliant, but the body overzealously increases venous return to a point where pressures rise above the tolerable level.

Diuretics alleviate the clinical signs of congestion and edema associated with backward failure but may also affect forward flow. In the normal animal diuretic-induced decreases in venous return are compensated for by increases in contractility and heart rate. These compensatory mechanisms are already utilized in heart failure, so that decreases in venous return can directly decrease cardiac output. This is especially true in primary mitral regurgitation because muscle failure may not be present;

the normal relationship between filling pressures and cardiac output exists. Small decreases in atrial pressure can markedly reduce cardiac output. The situation is not as critical in myocardial failure because it takes large decreases in atrial pressure to significantly decrease cardiac output. However, since these patients may have marginal cardiac output, even small decreases in forward flow can markedly affect their resting tissue oxygen delivery. Therefore, when diuretics are given to a class IV heart failure patient, cardiac output or tissue oxygen delivery (i.e., venous P_{O_2}) should be monitored carefully, since other medications (digitalis, vasodilators) may need to be given concurrently to improve forward flow.

There are a myriad of diuretics available for veterinary use, but only three groups are needed for routine clinical therapy of congestion. The thiazides can routinely be used in class II or III patients to relieve congestive signs. They may also be used in class IV patients, but generally the loop diuretics, such as furosemide, are preferred because they are capable of promoting greater sodium excretion than the thiazides. Potassium-sparing diuretics are used concurrently with either thiazides or loop diuretics in patients that become hypokalemic or that are refractory to the other diuretics because of high aldosterone levels.

THIAZIDES

Thiazide diuretics act in the distal tubule, probably by reducing membrane permeability to sodium and chloride. Potassium secretion is promoted in the distal tubule, so potassium loss is comparable with that seen with furosemide even though urine flow is less. Thiazide diuretics are moderately effective in heart failure. They promote large increases in urine sodium concentrations but only mild to moderate increases in urine volume. The urinary sodium excretion rate is determined by multiplying urine sodium concentration by urine volume. When compared in this manner the loop diuretics promote two to two and one-half times the sodium excretion that the thiazides do. The thiazides, on the other hand, induce about two times the sodium excretion of the potassium-sparing diuretics. Since the thiazides work in a different area than other diuretics, they can be used in combination with other diuretics in refractory congestive patients to promote additional natriuresis. Along with their diuretic effects, thiazides reduce renal blood flow, particularly after IV administration; therefore, they should not be used in patients with renal failure or compromised renal perfusion.

The thiazides are well absorbed after oral administration. The older thiazides (chlorothiazide, hydrochlorothiazide) are predominantly water soluble. The newer ones (methyclothiazide, cyclothiazide) are more lipid soluble, are highly protein bound, and have a large volume of distribution and a longer duration of action. All thiazides have similar dose-response curves and similar maximal effects. The newer thiazides have not been studied in the dog or cat.

Chlorothiazide (Diuril)* is supplied as 250- and 500-mg tablets; hydrochlorothiazide (Hydro-Diuril)* is supplied as 25- and 50-mg tablets. Both are administered orally.

Chlorothiazide dosage is 20 to 40 mg/kg PO b.i.d. in the dog and cat. Its action begins within one hour after administration, with peak effect at 4 hours and duration extending from 6 to 12 hours. Hydrochlorothiazide dosage is 2 to 4 mg/kg PO b.i.d. in the dog and cat, with onset of action within 2 hours, peak effect at 4 hours, and a 12-hour duration of effect.

POTASSIUM-SPARING DIURETICS

This group (spironolactone, triamterene) inhibits the effect of aldosterone in the distal nephron. These diuretics promote only mild increases in sodium and water excretion in normal animals but may cause larger increases in heart failure patients because of higher circulating aldosterone levels. Their major benefit is prevention of potassium loss associated with the administration of other diuretics.

Spironolactone is structurally related to aldosterone and competitively inhibits its action in the distal tubule. Triamterene competitively displaces aldosterone and directly inhibits distal tubular transport.

Spironolactone (Aldactone)† is supplied in 25-mg oral tablets. Oral spironolactone dosage in dogs is 2 to 4 mg/kg/day. Its onset of action is gradual, with peak effect two to three days after therapy is initiated and duration of effect extending for two to three days after drug administration is discontinued. Serum detection of spironolactone is impossible because it is so rapidly metabolized. Metabolites, especially conrenone, are thought to account for the drug's pharmacologic activity.

Triamterene (Dyrenium)‡ is marketed in 100-mg capsules. Oral triamterene dosage is 2 to 4 mg/kg/day, with its action beginning within 2 hours, peak effect at 6 to 8 hours, and duration of effect extending from 12 to 16 hours. Because of its more reasonable pharmacokinetics it may be preferred over spironolactone.

LOOP DIURETICS

The loop diuretics (furosemide, ethacrynic acid) promote profound sodium and water excretion by inhibiting chloride reabsorption in the thick portion of the ascending loop of Henle. They also redistribute renal blood flow from juxtamedullary to outer cortical regions. Furosemide may also act as a venodilator, increasing systemic and/or pulmonary venous capacitance. Both drugs are highly protein bound and are not extensively metabolized in the dog and cat. A small fraction of the drug is filtered by the glomerulus, and the rest is secreted into the proximal tubules. Initially the loop diuretics decrease renal vascular resistance and increase renal blood flow. With chronic use vascular volume is decreased, as is renal blood flow.

Furosemide (Lasix§) is supplied as 12.5-, 20-, 40-, and 50-mg tablets; as an elixir (10 mg/ml); and as a preparation for parenteral administration containing 50 mg/ml.

Furosemide has a half-life of 15 minutes. It is effective when administered parenterally or orally but has an onset of action within five minutes intravenously and one hour orally. Peak effect occurs one to two hours after oral administration and within 30 minutes of intravenous administration. Effects last for six hours after oral use and for two hours when given intravenously. The oral dose in dogs and cats is 2 to 4 mg/kg and may be repeated up to every 8 to 12 hours or as infrequently as every two to three days. The intravenous dose of 2 to 4 mg/kg may be repeated every four hours in patients with severe cardiogenic pulmonary edema.

The major complications of loop diuretic use are abnormalities of fluid and electrolyte balance, including dehydration, decreased perfusion, hypokalemia, and hypochloremic alkalosis. Complications occur more readily during intensive diuresis induced by high-dose therapy. The loop diuretics can be used safely as maintenance dose therapy in class IV heart failure patients over extended periods of time, but perfusion and electrolyte levels should be monitored regularly, especially when maximum dosages are being employed.

VASODILATORS

Vasodilators were first used to treat heart failure in 1957 but did not become popular in human medicine until the 1970s. In the last ten years their use has become widespread for human heart failure therapy. These agents are starting to be used in veterinary medicine, but little is known about the pharmacology of most of the particular agents. Only hydralazine has been studied clinically in the dog.

Vasodilators relax the smooth muscle of arterioles or veins and so promote decreases in peripheral vascular resistance or increases in venous capacitance. The smooth muscle relaxation may be due to either direct drug effects or indirect blockade of alpha receptors or angiotension II formation. Arter-

---

*Merck Sharp and Dohme, West Point, PA.
†Searle Laboratories, Chicago, IL.
‡Smith Kline & French Laboratories, Philadelphia, PA.

§Hoechst-Roussel Pharmaceuticals Inc., Somerville, NJ.

iolar dilators (hydralazine) decrease the resistance against which the failing ventricle has to pump, allowing an increase in myocardial fiber shortening and stroke volume.

Peripheral vascular resistance is increased in heart failure so that mean systemic blood pressure is maintained at 90 to 110 mm Hg when cardiac output is low according to the following formula:

Mean pressure drop across the systemic circuit = cardiac output × peripheral vascular resistance

This increased resistance increases ventricular afterload and depresses cardiac output further (Fig. 3). The decreased stroke volume and cardiac output can be increased by either increasing contractility with a positive inotrope or decreasing resistance with an arteriolar dilator.

As for other physiologic systems, arterial blood pressure has a relatively large reserve in that no regional vascular bed needs 100 mm Hg pressure to maintain adequate blood flow. The cerebral, myocardial, and renal vascular beds require the highest pressures but function normally at mean pressures of 60 to 70 mm Hg. Arteriolar dilators exploit this reserve. They increase the cross-sectional area of the systemic arteriolar bed and so reduce peripheral vascular resistance. The decreased resistance and decreased impedance result in a lowered arterial pressure and an increased flow according to the following formula:

$$\text{peripheral vascular resistance} = \frac{\text{aortic pressure}}{\text{cardiac output}}$$

Decreased arterial blood pressure coupled with the usual decrease in ventricular size results in a decreased afterload (mean circumferential wall stress). Wall stress is the force opposing myocardial fiber shortening. When wall stress decreases, fiber shortening and velocity of fiber shortening increase and end-systolic volume decreases. The net result is an increase in stroke volume. The stroke volume is generated at the same or a lesser filling pressure, therefore myocardial performance is improved. Tissue perfusion is augmented, tissue oxygen delivery is increased, and the patient's status improves.

In addition to improving patients with myocardial failure, arteriolar dilators also decrease backward flow and improve forward flow and backward failure in volume-overloaded heart failure caused by mitral regurgitation or left-to-right shunts. The amount of mitral regurgitation depends on the systolic pressure gradient across the mitral valve and the impedance to flow. Impedance is primarily governed by the size of the mitral regurgitant orifice. Arteriolar dilators reduce systolic intraventricular pressure, which in turn reduces the systolic pressure gradient across the valve. They also reduce ventricular end-diastolic circumference by allowing the ventricle to better "unload" itself. In doing so the mitral annulus circumference reduces and the mitral orifice size decreases. The net results are decreased regurgitant flow, reduced left atrial pressure, and increased forward (aortic) flow.

Since arteriolar dilators are used to increase cardiac output and improve tissue oxygen delivery, they should be used in patients with poor perfusion at rest (venous P_{O_2} < 30 mm Hg); i.e., class IV patients. They are generally used in myocardial failure only when the myocardium is refractory to digitalis. In mitral regurgitation and some left-to-right shunts, they are the treatment of choice since surgical correction frequently cannot be performed.

Since arteriolar dilators reduce blood pressure and increase cardiac output, both parameters should ideally be monitored during initial therapy. Although blood pressure can be measured in the dog, most veterinarians do not have the equipment necessary. If blood pressure cannot be measured, dosage titrations must be given slowly and carefully to prevent hypotension, weakness, and fainting. Cardiac output can be evaluated indirectly by venous P_{O_2} measurements or mucous membrane perfusion.

Arteriolar dilator dosages must be titrated to a therapeutic endpoint (Table 1). Using blood pressure measurements, most oral arteriolar dilators are given every one to two hours until a cumulative dose is reached that drops pressure to the desired level. When only venous P_{O_2} measurements are used, the titration schedule should be slower, giving

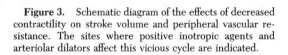

Figure 3. Schematic diagram of the effects of decreased contractility on stroke volume and peripheral vascular resistance. The sites where positive inotropic agents and arteriolar dilators affect this vicious cycle are indicated.

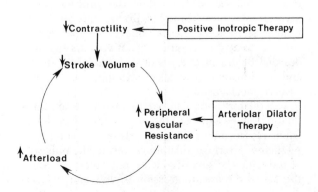

the drug every two to three hours. When only capillary refill time is evaluated, the drug dosages should be gradually and cautiously increased every three to five hours.

The obvious complication of arteriolar dilator therapy is systemic hypotension, which produces depression, weakness, and syncope from poor cerebral blood flow. This complication is infrequent if dosage titration is done properly. If hypotension does occur, no therapy is advised if mean systemic blood pressure does not drop below 50 mm Hg; however, if blood pressure is below 50 mm Hg or if urine production diminishes, dopamine should be given to increase myocardial contractility, cardiac output, and peripheral vascular resistance.

Venodilators (nitroglycerin, isosorbide dinitrate) produce the same net results as diuretics but by an alternate mechanism. They increase systemic vascular space, reduce venous pressures, and ultimately reduce venous return by pooling blood peripherally. In left-sided failure they allow blood to be distributed back into the systemic circuit so that venous return to the left ventricle is diminished and pulmonary capillary pressure decreases. In right-sided failure, venodilators reduce systemic venous pressure, reducing edema or ascites formation. When used alone, venodilators, like diuretics, may decrease cardiac output by decreasing cardiac filling.

Venodilator effects can be monitored radiographically in left-sided failure. Central venous pressure measurements or subjective evaluation of peripheral edema or ascites is used in patients with right-sided failure.

Most patients with severe myocardial failure have both congestive signs and low cardiac output. Therefore they may require both an arteriolar dilator and a venodilator. Alternatively, a "balanced" vasodilator (captopril, prazosin), which dilates both veins and arterioles, may be given. A combination of drugs may provide more finite control, but using one "balanced" drug improves owner compliance because fewer drugs need to be administered.

Vasodilators initially were expected to prolong the life of the myocardial failure patient. Theoretically, the reduction in cardiac size and systolic pressure should decrease myocardial oxygen demands and should help slow the progression of myocardial failure. However, preliminary studies in humans show no increased longevity compared with patients treated conventionally. It appears that myocardial failure progresses at its own inherent rate and vasodilators only take advantage of the last reserve mechanism.

Vasodilator therapy in patients with mitral regurgitation can be expected to improve longevity. Since valve replacements are not feasible in veterinary medicine, arteriolar dilators represent the only way of reducing the severity of the regurgitation. Since the actual disease progression is slow and myocar-dial contractility is frequently normal, reduction in lesion severity should prolong life.

HYDRALAZINE

Hydralazine is the only vasodilator that has been studied clinically in veterinary medicine. Hydralazine dilates arterioles either by elevating local concentrations of PGI_2 or by inhibiting calcium influx into vascular smooth muscle cells. The arteriolar dilation is not the same in all vascular beds. Resistance to cerebral, coronary, renal, and splanchnic flow decreases more than does resistance to skeletal muscle and skin flow. Since skeletal muscle blood flow is not markedly augmented, exercise capacity may not be increased. The increased renal blood flow produces an increased glomerular filtration rate if it is depressed initially, decreases filtration fraction toward normal, and increases total cation excretion. Hydralazine directly releases histamine, which in turn releases norepinephrine, increasing heart rate and automaticity. Autonomic reflexes remain intact so that postural changes do not usually occur, although the author has seen postural hypotension in one dog.

Hydralazine is used clinically to increase cardiac output in patients with myocardial failure and to increase cardiac output and lower atrial pressures in patients with volume-overloaded heart failure. Concomitant diuretic and/or venodilator administration is often required in either situation, especially after prolonged administration. Hydralazine lowers blood pressure, thereby stimulating the renin-angiotensin-aldosterone system. Angiotensin is generally unable to reverse the arteriolar dilating effects, but high aldosterone levels may cause refractory edema in some patients. If this occurs, diuretic combinations, including spironolactone or triameterene, may be beneficial. Because of its ability to decrease peripheral vascular resistance without decreasing venous return, hydralazine is the vasodilator of choice for mitral regurgitation.

Hydralazine is rapidly absorbed after oral administration in the dog. Its onset of action occurs within one hour. The drug is metabolized in the liver by acetylation and undergoes fairly extensive hepatic metabolism during initial passage through the liver in the portal blood (first pass effect). The drug is not excreted by the kidney, but uremia affects biotransformation of hydralazine, so that serum concentrations may rise in renal failure.

Hydralazine hydrochloride (Apresoline)* is available in 10-, 25-, 50-, and 100-mg tablets for oral administration and in 1-ml ampules, which contain 20 mg of drug, for intravenous or intramuscular injection. In dogs, the initial oral hydralazine dosage is 1 mg/kg, which can be titrated upwards to a

---

*Ciba Pharmaceutical Company, Summit, NJ.

***Table 1.** Hydralazine Titration Protocol*

1. Obtain baseline chest radiograph, venous oxygen tension or capillary refill time, and systemic arterial blood pressure, if available.
2. If the venous oxygen tension is <30 mm Hg or the capillary refill time is >2 seconds and the mean blood pressure is >80 mm Hg, administer 1 mg/kg hydralazine orally.
3. Repeat blood pressure measurement in one hour, venous oxygen tension measurement in two to three hours, or capillary refill time in three to five hours.
4. If the mean blood pressure is 70 to 80 mm Hg and/or the venous oxygen tension is >30 mm Hg or the capillary refill time is <1 second, do not administer any more drug. Repeat this dosage every 12 hours.
5. If an adequate response is not seen, administer another 1 mg/kg dose and repeat number 3. If the criteria in number 4 are still not met, give another 1 mg/kg dose.
6. Do not exceed 3 mg/kg.

maximum of 3 mg/kg (see Table 1). Cats require an initial oral dose of 2.5 mg, which may be titrated upwards to 10 mg. Drug effect lasts 11 to 13 hours; therefore the effective dose is given b.i.d. Onset of action after oral administration is within one hour, and peak effects occur at three to five hours. Intravenous hydralazine dosages have not been established for the dog and cat.

A common complication associated with hydralazine is increased heart rate, but this can usually be controlled with concurrent digitalis administration. An alternative is beta-receptor blockade with propranolol, but this method must be carefully monitored because of possible decreases in cardiac output. Other complications include anorexia and vomiting, probably from local gastrointestinal irritation. This occurs infrequently in dogs but frequently in cats. Often digestive upsets cannot be eliminated, precluding the further use of hydralazine. Increased automaticity, stimulated by hydralazine, has the potential of exacerbating existing arrhythmias. If arrhythmias exist, an electrocardiogram should be monitored during initial therapy.

NITROPRUSSIDE

Nitroprusside is a potent hypotensive agent that acts specifically on vascular smooth muscle by an unknown mechanism. It dilates both systemic arterioles and veins and also appears to increase ventricular compliance, reducing diastolic intraventricular pressures. Since it has an ultrashort half-life, nitroprusside must be given intravenously, which limits its use to acute heart failure.

Nitroprusside reduces diastolic pressures and increases cardiac output, therefore it is limited to patients in subset IV of Forrester and Waters' classification (see Fig. 6 of previous article, page 283). Since it is a potent drug that can easily induce pronounced hypotension, it should only be given when blood pressure can be monitored.

Infusion rates up to 25 µg/kg/min have been given to normal dogs, but infusion rates in dogs generally should be from 1 to 5 µg/kg/min. Nitroprusside therapy has not been studied in dogs or cats with heart failure. Nitroprusside produces pronounced decreases in end-diastolic pressures and increases in cardiac output in human myocardial failure patients. It produces variable cardiac output responses in patients with mitral regurgitation.

The most important complication of nitroprusside therapy is hypotension, but because of its short half-life this effect is reversed within ten minutes after the drug is discontinued. Other important complications are cyanide and thiocyanate poisoning. Nitroprusside is metabolized to cyanide in red cells and tissues, and circulating cyanide is converted to thiocyanate in the liver. High doses of nitroprusside or prolonged administration produces toxicity in dogs. Concomitant hydroxocobalamin use can prevent toxicity by combining with cyanide to form cyanocobalamin.

Sodium nitroprusside (Nipride)* is marketed as 50 mg of powder in a 5-ml vial. The powder is reconstituted with and diluted into 5 per cent dextrose and water. Generally 50 mg of drug is placed in 1 liter of fluid. The drug is unstable once it is reconstituted, and solutions older than four hours should not be used. The compound decomposes in light, so an opaque wrapping is provided with the drug to cover the bottle. Continuous monitoring of blood pressure and venous P_{O_2} is essential. The infusion rate can be varied to produce any desired blood pressure.

NITRATES

The nitrates are potent venodilators and mild to moderate arteriolar dilators depending on their route of administration. Generally they reduce preload more than afterload and so do not increase stroke volume as much as nitroprusside or hydralazine. They may be helpful in treating backward failure.

Nitroglycerin is both a coronary and a systemic vasodilator that, in oral and parenteral forms, has a very short half-life, making it unacceptable for long-term heart failure therapy. However, 2 per cent topical nitroglycerin creams are available that have a three-hour duration of action. They are effective when applied to hairless or shaved areas. The cream can be applied to the medial surface of the pinna of the dog, where the drug can be slowly absorbed through the skin and the cream cannot be licked off. Protective gloves should be worn when applying the cream.

Isosorbide dinitrate (Isordil)† is a nitrate that is

---

*Roche Laboratories, Nutley, NJ.
†Ives Laboratories Inc., New York, NY.

absorbed orally and that has a longer duration of action than nitroglycerin. Neither isosorbide dinitrate nor topical nitroglycerin has been studied in veterinary heart failure patients. Isordil is supplied in 10-, 20-, and 30-mg scored tablets.

Nitroglycerin can be used intravenously in acute heart failure situations, where it is generally administered at rates of 5 to 20 µg/kg/min. Topical nitroglycerin is dosed to effect, generally 1/4 to 3/4 inch cutaneously, q4 to 6h.

PRAZOSIN

Prazosin is an orally effective alpha$_1$-adrenergic receptor blocking agent that dilates both systemic veins and arterioles. Since the drug does not block presynaptic alpha$_2$ receptors, norepinephrine release functions normally to exert its negative feedback and control its own release so that tachycardia is generally not seen. Renin release is not stimulated by prazosin's hypotensive effects; however, fluid retention has been reported with chronic administration. Besides its alpha$_1$ blocking effects, prazosin also directly relaxes vascular smooth muscle through phosphodiesterase inhibition.

Although prazosin is used clinically in veterinary medicine, no studies have been reported on its pharmacology or toxicity in veterinary heart failure patients. In humans, the drug decreases congestion and edema and increases stroke volume. However, this effect may be short-lived in some patients since tolerance to the drug can develop. If it is used in a veterinary patient, the dosage should be titrated as for other vasodilators, and therapy should be monitored over time to determine duration of effect. In dogs, an initial dose is generally 1 mg of drug given t.i.d. Dogs larger than 15 kg are given 2 mg t.i.d.

Prazosin hydrochloride (Minipress)* is available in capsules containing 1, 2, and 5 mg.

ANGIOTENSIN–CONVERTING ENZYME INHIBITORS

Captopril, a drug that inhibits the action of the angiotensin-converting enzyme peptidyl dipeptidase, has recently been released for commercial use. It decreases circulating levels of angiotensin II and aldosterone (Fig. 4). Angiotensin II is a potent vasoconstrictor whose levels are elevated in heart failure; blocking its formation results in arteriolar and venous dilation. Blockage of aldosterone release results in a decrease in renal salt and water retention. The net effect in patients with myocardial failure is decreased congestion and edema, decreased peripheral vascular resistance, and increased stroke volume. Stroke volume may increase or decrease in volume-overloaded failure.

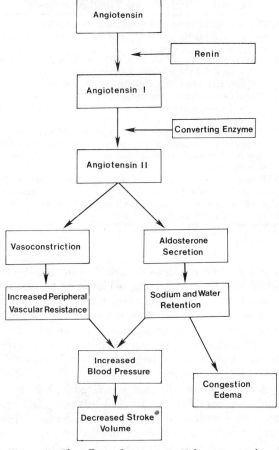

Figure 4. The effects of angiotensin II formation in chronic heart failure and the site of converting enzyme action.

Captopril (Capoten)† is supplied as 25-, 50-, and 100-mg tablets for oral use. Preliminary studies by the author in canine congestive cardiomyopathy patients are encouraging. Peripheral vascular resistance and plasma aldosterone levels have decreased and pulmonary edema or ascites has diminished. Dogs with mitral insufficiency have experienced a decrease in pulmonary edema, but cardiac output has also decreased in some patients because of the decrease in preload. The drug effect lasts about eight hours in the dog. Dosage information is not yet available, although 1 to 2 mg/kg orally t.i.d. has been used with success. As for any other vasodilator, an initial low dosage must be given and the dosage titrated upwards until a clinical or hemodynamic response is seen. Along with the parameters given previously, plasma aldosterone levels can be monitored to document efficacy.

Captopril is renally excreted, so renal failure may increase blood levels. Since the drug inhibits aldosterone secretion, hyperkalemia is a potential side effect, especially if potassium-sparing diuretics are used concomitantly. Gastrointestinal disturbances have been noted in some dogs.

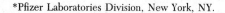

*Pfizer Laboratories Division, New York, NY.

†E.R. Squibb and Sons Inc., Princeton, NJ.

SYMPATHOMIMETICS

Adrenergic receptors are prevalent in the heart, blood vessels, bronchioles, gastrointestinal tract, and brain where they have varying and often opposite effects. Alpha$_1$ receptors are post-synaptic and are located on vascular smooth muscle, where they produce vasoconstriction. Alpha$_2$ receptors are presynaptic and lie on the sympathetic neurons, where they inhibit norepinephrine release. There are also alpha receptors in the brain that mediate reflex sympathetic arcs and so mediate vasoaction. Beta$_1$ receptors are located exclusively in the heart, where their stimulation causes increased heart rate, contractility, and myocardial cellular energy production. Stimulation of beta$_2$ receptors causes relaxation of vascular and bronchial smooth muscle. Dopaminergic receptors are located in the renal and mesenteric vessels. They are stimulated by dopamine to produce vasodilation, resulting in increased blood flow.

Sympathomimetics differ in their potency and action on adrenergic receptors. Only those sympathomimetics relevant to current cardiovascular therapy are presented.

ISOPROTERENOL

Isoproterenol is a synthetic catecholamine with almost pure beta-adrenergic stimulating properties; thus it increases cardiac contractility and heart rate and decreases peripheral vascular resistance. It is a potent arrhythmogenic agent that increases myocardial oxygen consumption. High doses may provoke systemic arterial diastolic hypotension.

Isoproterenol is indicated in atropine refractory bradycardia, but electrical pacing is more effective and has fewer side effects. It is also used to provoke outflow tract gradients in hypertrophic cardiomyopathy for diagnostic purposes. The lowest effective dosage should always be given because of the risk of producing ventricular arrhythmias, including ventricular fibrillation.

Isoproterenol (Isuprel Hydrochloride)* is supplied in 0.2-mg vials. Intravenous infusion rates vary from 0.045 to 0.09 µg/kg/min. Generally, 0.2 mg is mixed with 1 liter of 5 per cent dextrose in water to a concentration of 0.2 µg/ml. An oral form is available but is ineffective.

DOBUTAMINE

Dobutamine is a synthetic catecholamine with balanced adrenergic vascular effects and beta$_1$-stimulating properties. Because it weakly stimulates both beta$_2$ and alpha$_1$ receptors in the peripheral vasculature, dobutamine does not change arterial blood pressure. It increases contractility two to three times that of digitalis, is relatively nonarrhythmogenic, and does not increase heart rate as much as other catecholamines. When given to human heart failure patients it increases cardiac output, decreases intraventricular diastolic pressures, and does not increase myocardial oxygen consumption. In contrast to dopamine, dobutamine favors cardiac output redistribution to coronary and skeletal muscle beds. Renal and mesenteric flow also increase owing to the total increase in cardiac output.

Dobutamine is the drug of choice for increasing contractility in patients with subsets III and IV acute heart failure and those in class IVb (page 282) except when atrial fibrillation is present, in which case it increases heart rate. When given to chronic myocardial failure patients it is only used to immediately stabilize the patient until other longer-action drugs can take effect.

Dobutamine (Dobutrex)† is packed in powder form, with 250 mg to be reconstituted in 5 per cent dextrose in water (Fig. 5A). Infusion rate is 5 to 40 µg/kg/min. Drip rate must be determined once drug concentration and infusion rate are known (Fig. 5B).

Dobutamine administration can induce tachyarrhythmias, especially at infusion rates above 20 µg/kg/min. Heart rate usually increases at higher infusion rates but may increase even at low infusion rates in anesthetized dogs.

DOPAMINE

Dopamine is a naturally occurring precursor of norepinephrine. In the dog, dopamine stimulates beta$_1$ receptors, increasing contractility. Heart rate is also increased, but less than with most other catecholamines. Dopamine produces a biphasic change in the peripheral vasculature, i.e., within the first 15 to 45 seconds it produces vasoconstriction through alpha$_1$-receptor activation and an increase in arterial blood pressure. Following that, it decreases resistance, especially in mesenteric and renal vascular beds, through direct action on dopaminergic receptors. At high infusion rates it continuously increases resistance by stimulating norepinephrine release.

Dopamine is indicated in acute myocardial failure when inotropic support is indicated (subsets III and IV) and is especially useful in shock when renal and mesenteric flow is reduced from vasoconstriction.

Dopamine (Intropin)‡ is supplied in 5-ml ampules containing 200 mg of powdered drug. The infusion rate starts at 1 µg/kg/min, with a maximum rate of around 10 µg/kg/min.

---

*Breon Laboratories Inc., New York, NY.

†Eli Lilly and Company, Indianapolis, IN.
‡American Critical Cure, McGaw Park, IL.

Weight (Kg)

	10	20	30	40	50
low dose (5 µg/Kg/min)	150/1000	200/1000	250/1000	250/1000	250/1000
high dose (20 µg/Kg/min)	250/500	250/500	250/250	250/250	250/250

A

µg/Kg/min x Kg = µg/min.

µg/min ÷ µg/ml = ml/min.

B

Figure 5. *A,* A chart for determining the dobutamine concentration when body weight and anticipated infusion rate are known. The first number represents the mg of drug; the second number represents the ml of 5 per cent dextrose in water into which the drug is mixed. *B,* The formula for determining infusion rate of a solution when drug concentration and body weight are known.

Dopamine is less effective than dobutamine in chronic heart failure. It may increase ventricular diastolic pressures through venoconstriction and may increase venous return. It increases heart rate more than dobutamine and is more arrhythmogenic. Therefore it is only indicated for acute heart failure therapy.

EPINEPHRINE

Epinephrine is an endogenous catecholamine with both alpha- and beta-stimulating properties. It should not be used to treat heart failure because it is very arrhythmogenic. It is the catecholamine of choice for cardiac arrest.

During cardiac arrest, the beta-stimulating properties of epinephrine increase automaticity and excitability of cells in the conduction system. It also converts fine, low-amplitude fibrillation to coarser, high-amplitude fibrillation, which is more susceptible to conversion by electrical countershock. When the heart contracts again, epinephrine increases the force of contraction. Its alpha-stimulating properties may help augment cerebral, myocardial, and renal perfusion by raising arterial pressure.

Epinephrine (Adrenalin Chloride Solution)* is supplied in 1-ml ampules containing 1 mg (1:1000 dilution) or as prefilled syringes with 1 mg in 10 ml solution (1:10,000 dilution). Epinephrine dosage is 0.5 cc/10 kg of a 1/10,000 solution (5 µg/kg) IV (or 2 µg/kg IC) during resuscitation, repeated every five minutes if necessary. When no vein is available, epinephrine (1.0 cc/10 kg) may be injected into the trachea to be absorbed by the pulmonary circula-

tion. Proper epinephrine doses must be given, since overdosed patients usually cannot be resuscitated. Since epinephrine is usually supplied in a 1:1000 dilution, a common mistake is to inject ten times the proper dose, which can be lethal.

SUPPLEMENTAL READING

Braunwald, E.: Vasodilator therapy—a physiologic approach to the treatment of heart failure. N. Engl. J. Med. 297:331, 1977.

DeRick, A., Belpaire, F. M., Bogaert, M. G., and Matteeuws, D.: Plasma concentrations of digoxin and digitoxin during digitalization of healthy dogs and dogs with cardiac failure. Am. J. Vet. Res. 39:811, 1978.

Hahn, A. W.: Digitalitis glycosides in canine medicine. *In* Kirk, R. W. (ed.): *Current Veterinary Therapy VI.* Philadelphia: W. B. Saunders, 1977.

Hamlin, R. L.: Basis for selection of a cardiac glycoside for dogs. Proceedings of the 1st Symposium on Veterinary Pharmacology and Therapeutics, Baton Rouge, Louisiana, 1978.

Kittleson, M. D.: Dobutamine. J.A.V.M.A. 177:642, 1980.

Kittleson, M. D., and Eyster, G. E.: Using hydralazine in dogs with congestive heart failure. Acad. Vet. Cardiol. Newsletter 3:3, 1981.

Kittleson, M. D., Eyster, G. E., Knowlen, G. G., et al.: The effect of digitalis glycosides on peripheral tissue oxygen delivery and myocardial function in dogs with congestive cardiomyopathy. Proceedings of the Annual Meeting of the American College of Veterinary Internal Medicine, Salt Lake City, Utah, 1982.

Kittleson, M. D., and Hamlin, R. L.: Hydralazine therapy in a canine heart failure model. Proceedings of the Annual Meeting of the American College of Veterinary Internal Medicine, Salt Lake City, Utah, 1982.

Kittleson, M. D., and Hamlin, R. L.: Hydralazine pharmacodynamics in the dog. Am. J. Vet. Res. in press, 1982.

Kullberg, M. P., Dorrbecker, B., Lennon, J., et al.: High performance liquid chromatographic analysis of amrinone and its N-acetyl derivative in plasma. Pharmacokinetics of amrinone in the dog. J. Chromatogr. 187:264, 1980.

LeJemtel, T. H., Keung, E., Ribner, H. S., et al.: Sustained beneficial effects of oral amrinone on cardiac and renal function in patients with severe congestive heart failure. Am. J. Cardiol. 45:123, 1980.

Pedersoli, W. M.: Serum digoxin concentrations in healthy dogs treated without a loading dose. J. Vet. Pharmacol. Therap. 1:279, 1978.

Smith, T. W., and Braunwald, E.: The management of heart failure. *In* Braunwald, E. (ed.): *Heart Disease: A Textbook of Cardiovascular Medicine.* Philadelphia: W. B. Saunders, 1980.

Weidler, D. J., Jallad, N. S., Movahhed, H. S., et al.: Pharmacokinetics of digoxin in the cat and comparisons with man and dog. Res. Commun. Chem. Pathol. Pharmacol. 19:57, 1978.

*Parke-Davis, Morris Plains, NJ.

DRUGS USED IN THE THERAPY OF CARDIAC ARRHYTHMIAS

MARK KITTLESON, D.V.M.

East Lansing, Michigan

Antiarrhythmic therapy is based on a number of factors, but essential considerations include an appreciation of the clinical and electrophysiologic basis of cardiac rhythm disturbances and a thorough knowledge of the clinical pharmacology of antiarrhythmic agents. Cardiac arrhythmias are caused by disturbances of automaticity and by abnormal conduction in the heart. These alterations are the result of changes in the electrophysiologic characteristics of cardiac cells and are predisposed by myocardial disease, heart failure, cardiac chamber enlargement, hypoxia, ischemia, electrolyte disturbances, acidosis, abnormal autonomic tone, drugs, and other factors.

The cellular mechanisms responsible for ectopic complexes and tachyarrhythmias include (1) increased normal automaticity, (2) abnormal automaticity, and (3) re-entry. *Normal automaticity* is a property inherent in the sinoatrial node and the subsidiary pacemaker cells in the specialized atrial fibers, the distal region of the atrioventricular node, the bundle of His, and the ventricular Purkinje fibers. In these tissues, the normal transmembrane potential spontaneously drifts to a less negative potential. When a critical voltage (threshold) is encountered, the cell depolarizes. Normally the sinoatrial node depolarizes at a rate faster than other subsidiary pacemakers and so controls the cardiac rhythm. When automaticity in a subsidiary pacemaker increases, the rate of this automatic focus may predominate, causing premature complexes or tachyarrhythmias. Such normal automaticity can be enhanced by cellular injury, increased endogenous or exogenous catecholamines, and digitalis. From a therapeutic standpoint, it should be remembered that depression of normal automaticity is a property common to all antiarrhythmic drugs except bretylium.

Abnormal automaticity is a myocardial cell's ability to reach threshold by a means other than slow diastolic depolarization. This can occur in any cell in the heart when the cell membrane is unstable, allowing the transmembrane voltage to fluctuate. If this fluctuation reaches threshold, a premature beat or, if repetitive, a tachycardia may occur. Abnormal automaticity is enhanced by myocardial cellular damage, low serum potassium, high serum calcium, myocardial failure, and digitalis glycosides. Certain drugs appear to blunt or abolish such abnormal automaticity.

Re-entrant tachyarrhythmias are generated when a depolarization wave traverses regions of nonuniform conduction and excitability. Conditions necessary for re-entry include (1) a damaged region of myocardium that creates a unidirectional block to conduction, (2) slow conduction of the depolarization wave in another direction, (3) the ability of the region that was initially refractory to conduction to conduct the impulse when it is re-encountered by the depolarization wave, and (4) adequate time for the normal tissue to repolarize so it can conduct the depolarization wave again (Fig. 1). Disruption of any of these factors will result in abolition of the tachyarrhythmia. Since many antiarrhythmic drugs either enhance or delay cardiac conduction and prolong refractoriness, pharmacotherapy may be effective in the treatment of cardiac re-entrant arrhythmias.

A detailed account of the electrophysiologic changes responsible for cardiac arrhythmias and their pharmacologic treatment is beyond the scope of this textbook; however, the clinician should rec-

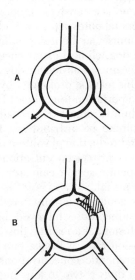

Figure 1. Schematic representation of the re-entry theory of arrhythmia formation. *A*, Normal conduction. *B*, A site of abnormal conduction (crosshatched area) is present, causing a unidirectional block. It subsequently conducts slowly (unsteady line), allowing a re-entrant pathway to form.

ognize that the ability of a drug to reverse an abnormal cardiac rhythm is related to electrophysiologic effects mediated at the cellular level. Since antiarrhythmic agents differ in their electrophysiologic and extracardiac actions, each drug has specific indications, contraindications, and toxicity. The purpose of this article is to review the clinical pharmacology of common antiarrhythmic drugs and emphasize factors that are of clinical relevance. Additional information concerning clinical causes of cardiac rhythm disturbances and the specific use of the agents described herein can be found in Therapy of Cardiac Arrhythmias (page 360).

LIDOCAINE

Lidocaine is an antiarrhythmic drug capable of abolishing both automatic and re-entrant *ventricular arrhythmias*. It may also decrease sympathetic nerve discharge or abnormal automatic rhythms caused by digitalis toxicity. In arrhythmias generated by increases in normal automaticity, lidocaine decreases the slope of phase 4 and increases threshold voltage but has no effect on the resting membrane potential. Unless the sinoatrial node is diseased, lidocaine has no effect on its automaticity. Lidocaine can abolish ventricular re-entrant arrhythmias either by increasing or decreasing conduction velocity or by prolonging the refractory period. Lidocaine has little effect on atrial conduction or refractoriness and is not used for atrial arrhythmias. Lidocaine produces very few electrocardiographic changes except for a possible shortening of the Q-T interval.

Lidocaine is given parenterally because it has a short half-life and is extensively metabolized by the liver to toxic metabolites after oral administration. Although intramuscular lidocaine administration is feasible in the dog, clinical experience is limited at this time. Lidocaine's half-life in dogs is 90 to 100 minutes, but this may be prolonged by liver disease or poor hepatic perfusion (e.g., heart failure, shock, propranolol administration). Heart failure may also reduce the volume of distribution. Both half-life prolongation and reduction of volume of distribution result in higher serum concentrations for a given dosage. Therapeutic serum concentrations are between 2 and 6 µg/ml.

Lidocaine is generally administered as an initial intravenous loading dose followed by a constant intravenous infusion. If a loading dose is not given, maximum infusion rates will take one to two hours to achieve therapeutic concentrations. The initial loading dose in dogs is two to four mg/kg, followed by an infusion of 25 to 80 µg/kg/min. In cats the initial dose is 0.25 to 0.75 mg/kg, followed by an infusion given at 10 to 40 µg/kg/min. Half the initial loading doses may need to be repeated in 20 to 40 minutes.

Lidocaine is used clinically to treat acute life-threatening arrhythmias in many different clinical settings. Its rapid onset of action, effectiveness, safety, and short half-life make it ideal for acute interventions. Its short half-life also allows rapid changes in serum concentration so that lidocaine's effects can be titrated quickly.

Lidocaine exerts toxic effects on the central nervous system, producing signs of drowsiness, emesis, nystagmus, muscle twitching, and seizures. These toxic effects can be particularly severe in the cat. Treatment for toxicity is lidocaine withdrawal and, when necessary, diazepam or barbiturates administered to effect for seizure control. Lidocaine can depress ventricular function in severe myocardial failure, produce AV block in conduction system disease, and exacerbate sinus bradycardia and arrest in patients with sick sinus syndrome. It must be used with care in dogs with AV or ventricular conduction disorders. Prolonged lidocaine infusions during concurrent propranolol administration prolong lidocaine's half-life.

PHENYTOIN

Phenytoin, when used as an antiarrhythmic, shares many properties with lidocaine. It reduces normal automaticity in Purkinje fibers, abolishes abnormal automaticity due to digitalis intoxication, and has effects identical to those of lidocaine on re-entrant arrhythmias. It can repolarize abnormal, depolarized cells, reduces sympathetic nerve effects, and may modify parasympathetic nerve activity in digitalis toxicity.

Phenytoin can be effective in treating *ventricular arrhythmias* due to many causes, but because of dosing difficulties, lidocaine is generally preferred. Phenytoin, however, is useful for treating *digitalis intoxication*. Because it can be given orally, phenytoin can be administered prophylactically to patients that may be easily intoxicated with digitalis (e.g., severe myocardial failure patients).

Oral phenytoin dosage is 30 to 35 mg/kg t.i.d. Phenytoin absorption is erratic, slow, and incomplete from both the gastrointestinal tract and intramuscular injection sites. Half-life is three to four hours. Serious arrhythmias require intravenous treatment in intermittent doses of 2 mg/kg given over three to five minutes to prevent hypotension and cardiac arrest from the propylene glycol vehicle. Total dose should not exceed 10 mg/kg. Because phenytoin solution has a pH of 11.0, phlebitis will occur unless a large vein is used and flushed immediately with normal saline.

Phenytoin is metabolized by the liver; any drugs affecting microsomal enzymes will, therefore, also affect phenytoin metabolism. Phenytoin may also decrease quinidine concentrations.

QUINIDINE

Quinidine is effective against automatic and re-entrant *supraventricular* and *ventricular tachyar-rhythmias*. It acts to decrease phase 4 slope and increase the threshold potential towards 0. In doing so it suppresses normal automaticity in the atria and Purkinje fibers. Sinus node automaticity is unchanged or may even increase owing to decreasing vagal tone. Quinidine has little effect on abnormal automaticity, although it can suppress triggered premature depolarizations. Quinidine slows conduction and prolongs the refractory period in atrial, ventricular, and Purkinje cells, effectively interrupting re-entrant pathways.

Quinidine is most commonly most used for the long-term suppression of *ventricular premature depolarizations* and *tachyarrhythmias*. It can also be used acutely to abolish ventricular arrhythmias and is occasionally effective in the control of atrial premature depolarization and paroxysmal supraventricular tachycardia. However, other drugs (e.g., digitalis, propranolol, verapamil) are generally more effective in the dog for supraventricular arrhythmias. Quinidine is relatively ineffective in the dog with atrial fibrillation except in special circumstances (see Therapy of Cardiac Arrhythmias, page 369).

Quinidine is about 85 per cent protein bound and has a half-life of five to six hours in the dog. Pharmacokinetics have not been studied in cats. It is metabolized in the liver to some cardioactive and some inactive metabolites and is also excreted by the kidneys. Renal disease and heart failure may elevate serum concentrations. Microsomal enzyme–inducing drugs, such as anticonvulsants, may shorten the half-life of quinidine. Quinidine displaces digoxin from skeletal muscle binding sites and reduces digoxin renal clearance, resulting in higher digoxin serum concentrations. This is an important drug interaction and can lead to digitalis intoxication.

In dogs, the oral dose of quinidine is 6 to 16 mg/kg given every six hours. This results in therapeutic concentrations within 12 to 24 hours. Quinidine sulfate is more rapidly absorbed than quinidine gluconate. Quinidine may also be given parenterally, but rapid intravenous injections may cause dangerous hypotension.

Although gastrointestinal disturbances do occur, the majority of toxic quinidine effects are cardiovascular. Quinidine toxicity is manifest as QRS and Q-T interval prolongation. A 50 per cent increase in QRS duration necessitates prompt drug withdrawal. Patients with evidence of conduction system disease should be treated cautiously, if at all, with quinidine since it can produce varying degrees of sinoatrial and atrioventricular block or asystole. Toxic concentrations of quinidine can also induce ventricular arrhythmias by increasing Purkinje fiber automa-ticity and decreasing conduction velocity. If conduction is severely impaired, catecholamines are used to improve it.

Quinidine is available as quinidine gluconate, quinidine sulfate, and quinidine polygalacturonate. Quinidine sulfate (Cin-Quin*, Quinora†) is available as 100-, 200-, and 300-mg tablets and as an injectable solution containing 200 mg/ml. Quinidine polygalacturonate (Cardioquin)‡ tablets contain 275 mg, which is equivalent to 200 mg of quinidine sulfate. Quinidine gluconate comes as an extended-release capsule (Duraquin§) containing 324 mg or as a solution for parenteral use (Quinidine Gluconate Injection‖) containing 80 mg/ml. Extended-release forms of quinidine have not been studied in the dog or cat.

DISOPYRAMIDE

Disopyramide is a recently approved oral antiarrhythmic agent with properties almost identical to those of quinidine and procainamide. In the dog, disopyramide has a half-life of only one to two hours, which makes effective dosing very difficult. When used as an antiarrhythmic in dogs, 7 to 30 mg/kg is administered every four hours. It is not used in cats and is contraindicated in heart failure patients because it decreases myocardial contractility and increases peripheral vascular resistance, a potentially lethal combination. Disopyramide possesses significant anticholinergic properties that may produce toxic effects.

Disopyramide phosphate (Norpace**) is available in 100- and 150-mg capsules.

PROCAINAMIDE

Procainamide is an antiarrhythmic agent with properties very similar to those of quinidine. It is effective against *ventricular tachyarrhythmias* and may be effective against supraventricular tachyarrhythmias in high doses. Procainamide suppresses phase 4 diastolic depolarization, depresses conduction, and lengthens the refractory period. Indications for procainamide use are essentially the same as those for quinidine, although individual patients may improve with one drug and not the other.

Procainamide has a short half-life of 2.5 to 4.7 hours in the dog. Parenteral and oral routes of administration are used, but intravenous injections must be given slowly to prevent circulatory collapse

---

*Rowell Laboratories, Inc., Baudette, MN.
†Key Pharmaceuticals, Inc., Miami, FL.
‡Purdue Frederick Co., Norwalk, CT.
§Parke-Davis, Morris Plains, NJ.
‖Eli Lilly and Co., Indianapolis, IN.
**Searle Laboratories, Chicago, IL.

from peripheral vasodilation and decreased cardiac contractility. When given intravenously, intermittent boluses of 2 mg/kg should be given slowly (over two minutes) up to a total dose of 12 to 20 mg/kg until the arrhythmia is controlled. This can be followed by a constant rate infusion of 10 to 40 μg/kg/min. The intramuscular and oral doses are 12 to 20 mg/kg q.i.d. Procainamide pharmacokinetics have not been studied in the cat.

Procainamide cardiotoxicity is similar to that of quinidine in that high concentrations can cause QRS and Q-T interval prolongation. It can also stimulate ventricular tachyarrhythmias. Toxic concentrations depress myocardial contractility and produce hypotension. The same rules that apply to quinidine therapy also apply to procainamide use.

Procainamide hydrochloride (Pronestyl*) is available for oral administration in tablets or capsules containing 250, 375, or 500 mg and for parenteral administration in 10-ml vials containing 100 mg/ml and 2-ml vials containing 500 mg/ml. A sustained-release preparation (Procan SR†) is available in 250- and 500-mg tablets.

PROPRANOLOL

Propranolol is the prototype beta-receptor blocking agent. Other beta blockers have been recently introduced, but their pharmacokinetics have not been studied in the dog and cat.

Propranolol has antiarrhythmic effects that depend on its ability to block beta-receptor stimulation. It reduces catecholamine–dependent automatic (normal and abnormal) rhythms and slows conduction in abnormal ventricular myocardium. Propranolol also increases the refractory period of A-V nodal tissues, which slows the ventricular response to atrial fibrillation and flutter and effectively abolishes supraventricular arrhythmias due to A-V nodal re-entry. By reducing contractility, propranolol reduces myocardial oxygen consumption, which may reduce myocardial hypoxia and arrhythmia formation. Propranolol is used in treating *digitalis-induced tachyarrhythmias* when no conduction blocks are present because it decreases sympathetic discharge and may reduce the ability of afterdepolarizations to reach threshold by decreasing calcium influx. Propranolol also abolishes *supraventricular* and *ventricular arrhythmias* due to pheochromocytoma and thyrotoxicosis.

Oral propranolol is almost completely absorbed and undergoes variable but extensive first pass hepatic metabolism. As a result, its bioavailability ranges from only 2 to 17 per cent for oral administration (with a half-life of about one hour in the dog), and relatively high oral doses are administered. Chronic oral dosing increases bioavailability and half-life to about two hours and results in serum concentrations 1.25 to 10 times greater than after initial doses. In dogs, the initial oral dose is from 0.1 to 0.3 mg/kg t.i.d. This dose may be gradually increased up to a maximum of 1 mg/kg. Very low doses may be needed to slow the ventricular response to atrial fibrillation, whereas higher doses are generally needed to control ventricular tachyarrhythmias. The feline oral dose is 2.5 to 10 mg t.i.d. Duration of drug effect is longer than the drug's half-life because of active propranolol metabolites and receptor binding of the drug. The intravenous dose in dogs is given as intermittent boluses to effect. The initial IV dose of 0.02 mg/kg is much lower than an oral dose, and the total dose should not exceed 0.1 mg/kg. Oral or intravenous doses of propranolol must be given cautiously to heart failure patients because a decrease in contractility may acutely worsen hemodynamics. The therapeutic endpoint for propranolol is abolition or improvement of an arrhythmia or slowing of the ventricular response to a supraventricular tachyarrhythmia.

Toxicity of propranolol is related to its beta-blocking actions. Patients with myocardial or volume-overloaded failure may have their failure state exacerbated by propranolol, especially if it is given intravenously. These patients usually receive propranolol for control of heart rate, and only low oral doses generally are needed. If acute heart failure is precipitated, catecholamines cannot reverse the problem, so calcium or digitalis must be used. Digitalis plus propranolol can cause varying degrees of A-V block.

Propranolol should not be used in patients with asthma or chronic lower airway disease, as increases in lower airway resistance may occur with beta blockage. Propranolol should also be used with caution in diabetic patients receiving insulin because propranolol reduces sympathetic compensation for hypoglycemia. Acute propranolol withdrawal may exacerbate the orginal problem for which the drug was being administered, so gradual withdrawal should be performed in any situation.

Propranolol hydrochloride (Inderal‡) comes as 10-, 20-, 40-, and 80-mg tablets for oral administration and in 1-ml ampules containing 1.0 mg for intravenous administration. When administered intravenously for therapy of acute arrhythmias, ECG and blood pressure should be monitored and the drug should be given slowly.

VERAPAMIL

In humans, calcium channel blockers are highly effective for paroxysmal supraventricular tachycar-

---

*E. R. Squibb & Sons, Inc., Princeton, NJ.
†Parke-Davis, Morris Plains, NJ.

‡Ayerst Laboratories, New York, NY.

dia and are useful in slowing ventricular response to atrial flutter and fibrillation.

Calcium channel blocking agents block the slow inward calcium current during phase 2 of the cardiac cell action potential. Since fast sodium channel (phase 0) activity is absent in the sinus node and in portions of the A-V node, slow calcium channel activity is responsible for depolarization in these areas. Calcium channel blockers decrease sinus rate, prolong A-V conduction, slow the ventricular response to supraventricular tachyarrhythmias such as atrial fibrillation, and abolish supraventricular arrhythmias when caused by re-entry through the A-V node. Verapamil may be useful for treating ventricular re-entrant arrhythmias and enhanced abnormal automaticity.

Verapamil has been studied in normal dogs, but there are no reports of its clinical use. In dogs, verapamil is absorbed well (more than 90 per cent) but undergoes extensive first pass hepatic metabolism so that bioavailability is only 10 to 23 per cent. Most of the metabolites are excreted in the bile. The half-life of verapamil is three to seven hours, and effective plasma concentrations are 50 to 200 ng/ml. Only intravenous dosing has been studied in the dog. The initial intravenous dose ranges from 0.05 to 0.15 mg/kg; this is followed by infusion of 2 to 10 µg/kg/min or repeated slow injections in 30 minutes.

Verapamil can depress cardiac contractility and cause peripheral vasodilation and should not be used in severe myocardial failure patients unless hemodynamic monitoring can be done. In mild to moderate myocardial failure patients, verapamil may increase cardiac output by dilating arterioles. Verapamil and propranolol must not be used together. Verapamil should be avoided in patients with sick sinus syndrome and A-V block and may cause sinus bradycardia. Adverse effects can be reversed by calcium or catecholamine administration.

Verapamil hydrochloride (Calan*, Isoptin†) is supplied for intravenous use in a 2-ml ampule containing 5.0 mg and in 80- and 120-mg tablets for oral administration.

---

*Searle Laboratories, Chicago, IL.
†Knoll Pharamaceutical Co., Whippany, NJ.

SUPPLEMENTAL READING

Bigger, J. T., Jr., and Hoffman, B. F.: Antiarrhythmic drugs. *In* Gilman, A. G., Goodman, L. S., and Gilman, A. (eds.): *The Pharmacological Basis of Therapeutics.* New York: Macmillan Publishing Co., 1980.

Karim, A., Kook, C., Novotny, R. L., et al.: Pharmacokinetics and steady-state myocardial uptake of disopyramide in the dog. Drug Metab. Disp. 6:338, 1978.

Kates, R. E., Keene, B. W., and Hamlin, R. L.: Pharmacokinetics of propranolol in the dog. J. Vet. Pharmacol. Therap. 2:21, 1979.

Mangiardi, L. M., Hariman, R. J., McAllister, R. G., Jr., et al.: Electrophysiologic and hemodynamic effects of verapamil. Circulation 57:366, 1978.

Muir, W., and Sama, R.: *Pharmacodynamics of Cardiac Drugs.* Columbus: Ohio State University Press, 1978.

Neff, C. A., Davis, L. E., and Baggot, J. D.: A comparative study of the pharmacokinetics of quinidine. Am. J. Vet. Res. 33:1521, 1972.

Saunders, J. E., and Yeary, R. A.: Serum concentrations of orally administered diphenylhydantoin in dogs. J.A.V.M.A. 172:153, 1978.

Walsh, R. A., and Horwitz, L. D.: Adverse hemodynamic effects of intravenous disopyramide compared with quinidine in conscious dogs. Circulation 60:1053, 1979.

White, R. D.: Cardiovascular pharmacology. *In* McIntyre, K. M., and Lewis, A. J. (eds.): *Textbook of Advanced Cardiac Life Support.* Dallas: American Heart Association, 1981.

CONGENITAL HEART DISEASE

WILLIAM P. THOMAS, D.V.M.
Davis, California

Although congenital heart disease accounts for less than 10 per cent of the diagnoses in small animal patients with clinically significant cardiac disease, it is the most common cardiac disease encountered in dogs and cats less than one year of age. Congenital heart disease is also occasionally diagnosed in middle-aged and aging animals, requiring differentiation in these circumstances from the more common acquired diseases. The veterinarian should be familiar with the common congenital heart defects of the dog and cat and should be prepared to make a preliminary evaluation of the type and severity of the defect. The therapy of congenital heart disease, when indicated, is surgical correction, with medical treatment limited to therapy for congestive heart failure, reduction of polycythemia and hypoxemia, and control or prevention of associated arrhythmias. Therapy will, therefore, be discussed only briefly (see CVT VII for discussions of therapy). Instead, this article emphasizes the differential diagnosis of congenital heart disease in the dog and cat, based on results of the nonin-

Table 1.　Diagnostic Characteristics of Common Canine Congenital Heart Defects

Heart Defect	Physical Examination	Electrocardiogram	Thoracic Radiographs	Other Characteristics
Innocent (functional) murmur	Murmur usually soft, <grade 3/6, short, early to mid systolic, loudest on left side but variable with position, heart rate, etc. All else normal.	Normal	Normal	Common in puppies, kittens, and animals < six months of age.
Patent ductus arteriosus (PDA)	Continuous murmur loudest in aortic area at left base. May radiate widely; often accompanied by thrill. Exaggerated (bounding, water hammer) arterial pulses. R → L type usually has no murmur, accentuated and split S_2, normal arterial pulses, and differential cyanosis.	LV enlargement patterns (↑ QRS amplitudes with normal mean axis) usually present. Left atrial enlargement pattern (↑ P duration) often present. Advanced cases with heart failure often develop arrhythmias, including atrial fibrillation. RV hypertrophy pattern always present in R → L type.	Enlargement of left atrium, left ventricle, aortic arch, main pulmonary artery, and pulmonary arteries and veins proportional to shunt magnitude. DV view shows dilatation of aorta and main pulmonary artery at site of ductus. R → L type usually shows RV enlargement, prominent main pulmonary artery (±), and normal to slightly enlarged pulmonary arteries.	Polygenic inheritance proven in poodles. Poodles, Pomeranians, collies, German shepherds, and shelties are predisposed. 2:1 ratio of incidence of females to males.
Pulmonic stenosis	Systolic ejection murmur loudest in pulmonic area near left cranial sternal border or slightly more dorsal. Often equally loud along right cranial sternal border. Arterial pulses normal.	RV hypertrophy pattern nearly always present, even in mild cases (may require thoracic leads to be seen). Right atrial enlargement (↑ P amplitude) is inconsistent.	RV enlargement and post-stenotic dilatation of main pulmonary artery usually seen. Pulmonary vasculature appears normal to slightly diminished.	Polygenic inheritance in beagles. Beagles, bulldogs, fox terriers, miniature schnauzers, Chihuahuas, and Samoyeds predisposed.
Subaortic stenosis	Systolic ejection murmur loudest in aortic area at left base and/or cranial right thorax. May radiate cranially to thoracic inlet and carotid arteries in neck. Arterial pulses have diminished amplitude and delayed upstroke.	May be normal. LV enlargement pattern often present but not striking. ST depression may be present at rest or postexercise. Ventricular premature beats are common in severe cases.	May be normal. LV enlargement often present but not striking. Post-stenotic dilatation of aorta may be visible in lateral view, especially in dogs >6 months of age. Left atrial enlargement is variable. Pulmonary vasculature is normal.	Polygenic inheritance in Newfoundland retrievers. Newfoundlands, boxers, German shepherds, German short-haired pointers, and golden retrievers predisposed. Syncope and sudden death are common sequelae.

Ventricular septal defect (VSD)	Harsh, regurgitant holosystolic murmur loudest in right 2 to 4 intercostal spaces. Often heard well on cranial left thorax. Arterial pulses are normal or brisk and short with larger shunts.	May be normal with small shunts. LV enlargement pattern may develop with larger shunts. Partial or complete right bundle branch block may occur.	May be normal with small shunts. Enlargement of left atrium, left and right ventricles, and pulmonary vasculature proportional to shunt magnitude.	Small defects may close within the first year of life. English bulldogs predisposed.
Atrial septal defect (ASD)	Soft, mid systolic ejection murmur loudest in pulmonic area on left cranial thorax. Split S$_2$ is audible and helps distinguish ASD from pulmonic stenosis. Arterial pulses are normal in most cases.	May be normal. Partial or complete right bundle branch block is common and may be confused with RV hypertrophy.	May be normal with small shunts. Left and right atrial, right ventricular, and pulmonary vascular enlargement proportional to shunt magnitude. Left ventricle is normal, and left atrium may also appear normal in some cases.	This defect is infrequently diagnosed in the dog. Samoyeds may be predisposed.
Mitral valve dysplasia	Harsh, regurgitant holosystolic murmur loudest in mitral area at left apex. Arterial pulses are normal or brisk with significant regurgitation.	Left atrial enlargement pattern (↑P wave duration) is almost always present. LV enlargement pattern varies with severity.	Moderate to marked left atrial enlargement is consistently present. Left ventricular enlargement usually present. Pulmonary veins often enlarged, but pulmonary arteries are normal.	Medium to giant breeds most often affected. Great Danes and German shepherds predisposed. Higher incidence in males.
Tricuspid valve dysplasia	Harsh, regurgitant holosystolic murmur loudest over tricuspid area on right mid thorax. May radiate well to left side. Arterial pulses are usually normal. Jugular distention and pulse may occur with significant regurgitation.	Right atrial enlargement pattern (↑P wave amplitude and often duration) usually present. RV enlargement pattern variable and inconsistent.	Moderate to marked right atrial enlargement and right ventricular enlargement consistently present and may produce ovoid or globular cardiac silhouette. Left atrium and ventricle are normal. Pulmonary vasculature normal or slightly diminished. Caudal vena cava often enlarged.	Medium to giant breeds most often affected. Great Danes, German shepherds, and Weimaraners predisposed. Higher incidence in males.
Tetralogy of Fallot	Systolic ejection murmur of pulmonic stenosis loudest in pulmonic area. Murmur may diminish in intensity with pulmonary hypoplasia. Symmetric cyanosis at rest or after exercise. Arterial pulses are usually normal.	RV hypertrophy pattern is always present.	Cardiac size is often normal and may appear small due to lucent, hyperinflated lungs. RV enlargement usually recognized. Main pulmonary artery may or may not show poststenotic dilatation. Pulmonary vasculature consistently diminished. Malpositioned aorta.	Polygenic inheritance in keeshonds. Keeshonds and English bulldogs predisposed.

Table 2.   Diagnostic Characteristics of Common Feline Congenital Heart Defects

Heart Defect	Physical Examination	Electrocardiogram	Thoracic Radiographs
Ventricular septal defect (VSD)	Holosystolic murmur is loudest on the right cranial thorax or is equal bilaterally.	Frequently normal with small defects. With larger shunts LV enlargement pattern may develop.	Generalized cardiomegaly, left atrial enlargement, and prominent pulmonary vasculature proportional to shunt magnitude.
Aortic stenosis	Ejection systolic murmur at the heart base, loudest on the left or bilaterally. S_4 may be audible. The femoral pulse strength is diminished.	Increased QRS amplitudes (LV enlargement) are common but variable.	Mild to moderate cardiomegaly with LV and left atrial enlargement. Poststenotic dilatation of aorta is often difficult to recognize. Pulmonary vasculature normal.
Patent ductus arteriosus (PDA)	Continuous murmur loudest at the heart base bilaterally and often widespread. Femoral pulses are brisk and bounding.	LV enlargement consistently present with significant shunts. Increased P wave duration (left atrial enlargement) variable.	Cardiomegaly with left atrial and ventricular enlargement and pulmonary hypervascularity proportional to shunt magnitude. On DV view the heart may appear elongated and prominent pulmonary artery and aortoductal aneurysms are visible.
Endocardial fibroelastosis	Signs of dyspnea and heart failure usually occur at an early age (<16 weeks). Tachycardia and mitral systolic murmur most common.	Variable. LV enlargement (increased QRS amplitude and duration) is common.	Generalized, marked cardiomegaly without pulmonary hypervascularity. Pulmonary edema and pleural effusion are often present.
Tetralogy of Fallot	Fatigue, tachypnea, and cyanosis are common, but congestive heart failure is rare. Systolic ejection murmur audible at left base.	Right ventricular hypertrophy pattern usually present.	Cardiomegaly is usually mild. Right ventricular enlargement and pulmonary hypovascularity common. Post-stenotic dilatation of pulmonary artery may not be obvious.
Mitral and tricuspid valve dysplasias	Systolic murmurs over left and/or right thorax consistently present. Advanced tricuspid insufficiency may cause jugular vein distention and ascites.	Variable. Enlarged P waves often found. The signs of ventricular enlargement are inconsistent.	Mitral: left atrial enlargement consistently present; more difficult to recognize than in dogs. Cardiomegaly may be slight to severe. Tricuspid: marked right atrial enlargement often appears as generalized cardiomegaly with normal pulmonary vasculature. Caudal vena cava often enlarged.
Endocardial cushion defect (atrial septal defect or atrioventricular canal)	Fatigue and dyspnea often occur at an early age. Loud systolic murmur over left thorax from mitral insufficiency or VSD.	Variable. Atrial enlargement common. QRS changes of ventricular enlargement or partial or complete right bundle branch block often present.	Cardiomegaly is usually marked and generalized. Pulmonary hypervascularity helps distinguish this defect from other nonshunting defects.

vasive examinations available to the practicing veterinarian, including history, physical examination, electrocardiography, and survey thoracic radiography. The use of specialized studies such as echocardiography, cardiac catheterization, and angiocardiography are discussed in other texts.

There are several reasons for attempting to identify the specific heart defect and assess its severity. First, *prognosis* depends on the type and severity of the defect, and this may be important to an owner from both emotional and financial standpoints. Potential sequelae, such as heart failure and sudden death, should be anticipated and the owner advised accordingly. Second, a *genetic basis* has been proved for several congenital heart defects in the dog and is suspected in others, and breeding of affected animals should be discouraged. This is often very important to owners of expensive, purebred animals. Third, an early, precise anatomic diagnosis is essential when *surgical correction* is contemplated. Finally, when indicated and desired by an owner, the veterinarian should be able to identify patients requiring *referral* to specialists for consultation, specialized diagnostic studies, or surgery.

Although the list of potential cardiac defects is long, relatively few are regularly encountered in veterinary practice. The most commonly diagnosed congenital heart defects in the dog and cat and their typical diagnostic characteristics are listed in Tables 1 and 2. Defects that usually do not produce signs

of cardiac disease, including vascular ring anomalies, other vascular anomalies such as persistent left cranial vena cava, and peritoneopericardial hernia, are not included here. In considering a patient with potential congenital heart disease, certain *acquired* cardiac diseases that occasionally affect young animals, including pericardial effusion, primary myocardial disease (cardiomyopathy or myocarditis; see Canine Myocardial Diseases, page 321), and infectious endocarditis, must also be considered as well as the frequent occurrence of innocent murmurs in young animals.

The diagnosis of congenital heart disease is a challenging exercise in clinical logic and is based on a knowledge of normal cardiac anatomy, the anatomy of the common defects, the physiologic alterations associated with each defect, and their resulting clinical manifestations. Diagnosis can often be made by combining information derived from the history, physical examination, electrocardiographs, and thoracic radiographs. Newer noninvasive studies, such as echocardiography, are also extremely useful in obtaining information on intracardiac anatomy and physiology. Cardiac catheterization and angiocardiography, the definitive methods of cardiac diagnosis, are indicated to establish a diagnosis when other noninvasive methods are inadequate, to obtain anatomic or hemodynamic information that may affect prognosis or surgical treatment, and for clinical research. They are *not* routinely indicated

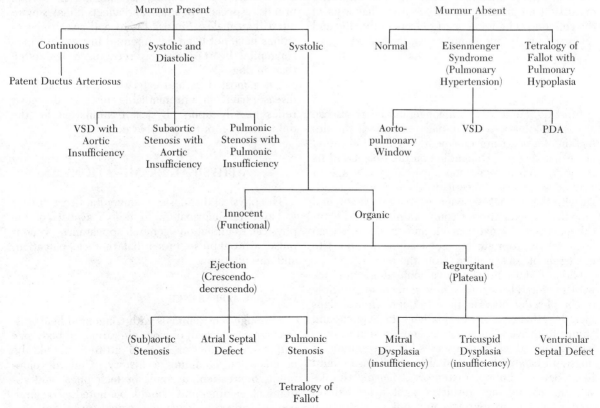

Figure 1. Classification of heart murmurs in congenital heart disease.

in patients in which an adequate diagnosis can be obtained by noninvasive methods, e.g., puppies with patent ductus arteriosus. Because there is considerable individual variation in the clinical manifestations of congenital heart disease in dogs and cats (only the typical characteristics are listed in Tables 1 and 2 and Fig. 1), it must be emphasized that diagnosis rarely depends on a single finding. Rather, information from all sources is combined to make a tentative diagnosis.

Since the common simple congenital heart defects produce their effects by causing either an increased pressure load (pulmonic stenosis, subaortic stenosis) or a volume overload (mitral and tricuspid dysplasia, patent ductus arteriosus [PDA], ventricular septal defect [VSD], atrial septal defect [ASD]) on the heart, a physiologic approach to differential diagnosis is most appropriate in an attempt to answer the following questions:

1. What is the character of the murmur? (physical exam)

2. Does the lesion originate in the right heart, left heart, or both? (physical exam, ECG, radiographs)

3. Is pulmonary blood flow increased, decreased, or normal (evidence of a shunt)? (radiographs)

4. Is there cyanosis? (physical exam)

5. Is there evidence of pulmonary hypertension? (physical exam, ECG, radiographs)

Accurate answers to these questions will usually allow a correct anatomic diagnosis. The following discussion emphasizes the differential diagnosis of the common congenital heart defects in the dog and cat based on routine, noninvasive evaluation.

HISTORY

Most dogs and cats with congenital heart disease are asymptomatic when initially examined, the detection of a heart murmur being the first indication of cardiac disease. Depending on the defect and its severity, clinical signs may develop at any age or may never appear. Since many owners are unfamiliar with the normal behavior, exercise capacity, and growth characteristics of young animals, mild clinical signs may be overlooked, and the veterinarian must ask appropriate but not leading questions to elicit reliable observations from the owner.

Clinical signs usually develop in dogs and cats with moderately severe simple defects or multiple or complex defects. The most frequent clinical signs include lethargy, exertional fatigue, tachypnea, and failure to thrive. Coughing, a common sign in dogs with acquired cardiac diseases, is uncommon in dogs and cats with congenital heart disease. Right heart defects (pulmonic stenosis, tricuspid dysplasia, and so on) may result in right heart failure, ascites, and a presenting complaint of abdominal

swelling. Exertional syncope (fainting), an infrequent sign, may occur with defects involving right-to-left shunting and cyanosis (tetralogy of Fallot, Eisenmenger-type defects) or with severe obstructive lesions (pulmonic stenosis, subaortic stenosis) and is an ominous sign. When queried, some owners indicate that they have noticed a very strong heartbeat or vibration (thrill) on the chest when lifting the animal. Seizures and/or posterior weakness may occur with defects involving right-to-left shunting, polycythemia, and hypoxemia (tetralogy of Fallot, Eisenmenger-type defects), especially in animals that survive past one year of age. Significant growth impairment (stunting) usually occurs only with severe defects, especially those causing cyanosis.

The sex and breed of the dog may suggest the type of defect. Although any defect can occur in any animal, certain breed predispositions (which are characteristic of inherited disorders) have been reported in canine congenital heart disease (see Table 1). For example, Newfoundland retrievers are predisposed to subaortic stenosis, whereas other defects are uncommon in this breed. Both mitral and tricuspid valve dysplasias tend to occur in large breeds and are more common in males than in females. Tetralogy of Fallot is most common in keeshonds, whereas atrial and ventricular septal defects do not have strong breed predilections. Patent ductus arteriosus, the most commonly diagnosed defect in the dog, is common in several breeds, especially poodles, and affects females more often than males. Similar breed and sex predispositions have not been documented in cats, in which congenital heart disease is recognized less often than in dogs.

Since most dogs and cats with congenital heart disease have an unremarkable history, diagnosis relies heavily upon physical examination for the differentiation of the possible defects.

PHYSICAL EXAMINATION

The physical diagnosis of congenital heart disease is based on information from five aspects of the physical examination: general appearance, venous pulse, arterial pulse, precordial (thoracic) palpation, and auscultation.

GENERAL APPEARANCE

Although most animals with congenital heart disease appear normal, obvious alterations in body size and conformation or general attitude should be noted when obtaining a history. Underdevelopment, depression, dyspnea or tachypnea, and abdominal enlargement should be noted. The oral, ocular, and posterior (anal, vaginal, preputial) mucous membranes and footpads should be observed at rest and, if a right-to-left shunt is suspected, following mild exercise, which increases right-to-left shunting. Symmetric cyanosis (cranial and caudal membranes equally affected) indicates a right-to-left shunt at the level of the atria, ventricles, or roots of the great vessels. Differential cyanosis (caudal membrane cyanosis greater than cranial membrane cyanosis) is characteristic of a right-to-left shunt into the descending aorta at the level of the ductus arteriosus. A pale or muddy mucous membrane color may develop if congestive heart failure complicates any defect. Most dogs and cats with congenital heart disease have normal mucous membranes.

VENOUS PULSE

Examination of the jugular veins may be difficult in some endomorphic dogs but is usually possible in mesomorphic and ectomorphic dogs and most cats. In most cases the jugular veins are unremarkable. Venous distention and exaggerated venous pulses, either visible or palpable, occur with defects that affect the right heart (pulmonic stenosis, tricuspid dysplasia, ASD, VSD, tetralogy of Fallot), especially when right ventricular failure develops. With defects that primarily affect the left heart (PDA, subaortic stenosis, mitral dysplasia), systemic veins remain normal.

ARTERIAL PULSE

Variations in body size, conformation, and pulse character among breeds may make subtle alterations in pulse strength and shape difficult to detect in small animals. In contrast to venous pulse abnormalities, alterations in the femoral pulses occur mainly with defects that affect left ventricular function, although a diminished pulse amplitude may occur with congestive heart failure from any cause. The widened pulse pressure of a left-to-right shunting PDA, caused by diastolic run-off from the aorta into the pulmonary artery, causes a brisk, bounding (water hammer) arterial pulse in both dogs and cats. A similar pulse occurs with significant aortic valve regurgitation (which occasionally complicates VSD or aortic stenosis) for the same reason. Significant aortic stenosis results in a pulse of diminished amplitude (stength) with a delayed upstroke. The pulse is normal or brisk (sharp upstroke) with mitral dysplasia and VSD. Defects that mainly affect the right heart (pulmonic stenosis, tricuspid dysplasia, ASD, tetralogy of Fallot) usually result in normal arterial pulses. These changes are often detectable in dogs, but because normal femoral pulses may be barely palpable in some normal cats, they may be difficult to appreciate in affected cats.

PRECORDIAL PALPATION

Thoracic deformities, the strength and location of the cardiac impulse, and the presence of abnormal impulses or vibrations (thrills) should be noted by palpation prior to auscultation. Significant cardiomegaly often results in a more diffuse and sustained cardiac impulse. A thrill indicates a murmur of grade 5/6 or louder as well as the point of maximum intensity of the murmur. A thrill with PDA is maximal in the aortic region and high on the cranial left thorax and is usually transystolic (extending into diastole); other defects produce a systolic thrill at the point of maximum intensity of the murmur. Cardiac arrhythmias may also be initially detected by palpation. Differentiation between left and right heart enlargement by palpation is unreliable in dogs and cats because of the mobility of the heart within the thorax.

AUSCULTATION

Most congenital heart diseases in small animals are detected by the presence of a heart murmur, and emphasis is placed on diagnosis based on the timing, location, and character of the murmur. Before discussing the typical heart sound alterations associated with congenital heart defects, it is important to make the following points regarding the reliability of the murmur in diagnosis:

1. Innocent (functional) murmurs of uncertain origin are common in young animals, especially dogs, and may be misinterpreted as representing significant heart disease. These innocent murmurs are typically soft (< grade 3/6), short, early to mid systolic ejection murmurs that may be difficult to localize but are loudest between base and apex on the left side. The first and second heart sounds remain clearly audible. An important characteristic of such murmurs is their variability with body position and heart rate. All other aspects of the cardiac examination are normal. When there is uncertainty about the origin or significance of a soft murmur, further studies can be performed or the animal can be re-evaluated at a later date to note any change in the murmur.

2. Serious congenital heart disease can occur without an audible heart murmur. In particular, defects associated with pulmonary hypertension and right-to-left shunting (Eisenmenger-type defects) often produce no murmur; instead, accentuation and/or splitting of the second heart sound (S_2) may be the only auscultatable feature. Severe tetralogy of Fallot with pulmonary artery hypoplasia may result in little or no systolic murmur, especially if polycythemia develops. The character of the murmur and other physical findings often change dramatically when congestive heart failure develops in animals with congenital heart disease. Medical treatment of the heart failure is often necessary

before the murmur can be properly evaluated. Most importantly, the intensity of the murmur *cannot*, in most cases, be used to predict the severity of the defect.

3. Since the majority of congenital heart defects produce systolic murmurs, timing of the murmur is of limited value in diagnosis (except when the murmur is continuous). Location and character (harsh versus blowing, ejection versus regurgitant) are more important, but variations are common, and these characteristics alone are often not definitive. The real challenge in evaluation of congenital heart disease in dogs and cats is the differentiation of defects associated with systolic murmurs. The ECG and thoracic radiographs are very important in this differentiation.

The typical auscultatory features of the common congenital defects are described in Tables 1 and 2, and a flow chart of the major types of murmurs is shown in Figure 1.

A *continuous murmur* is characteristic of an AV fistula or aortopulmonary communication. When heard over the left heart base, PDA can be easily and reliably diagnosed. The murmur is occasionally soft and localized to this area, but it often radiates widely and there may be a palpable thrill. When aortic or pulmonic valve insufficiency complicates defects such as VSD, subaortic stenosis, and pulmonic stenosis, both systolic and diastolic murmurs may be heard and may be misinterpreted as the continuous murmur of PDA.

Systolic murmurs are differentiated by location and character (shape and frequency characteristics). Ejection murmurs are typically crescendo-decrescendo and mid to holosystolic, whereas regurgitant murmurs are plateau- or band-shaped and usually holosystolic. The systolic ejection murmur of pulmonic stenosis is typically smooth and is either loudest on the left cranioventral thorax or equal on both sides. The murmur of tetralogy of Fallot is identical to that of pulmonic stenosis (flow through the large VSD in this instance produces no murmur, owing to equalization of ventricular pressures). The murmur of ASD is an early to mid systolic ejection pulmonic murmur caused by increased flow through a normal pulmonary valve (flow through the ASD does not produce a murmur). It is distinguished from the murmur of pulmonic stenosis and innocent murmurs by the preservation of audible first and second heart sounds and the presence of a distinctly split S_2. Aortic stenosis produces a harsher systolic ejection murmur loudest in the aortic area on the left and/or cranial right thorax. In some cases (but not all) it may radiate well to the carotid arteries in the neck. Mitral and tricuspid dysplasias usually cause valvular insufficiency and regurgitant holosystolic murmurs over their respective valve areas. The murmur of VSD varies from regurgitant to ejection in quality and is usually loudest on the cranial right thorax or equally loud bilaterally.

The most difficult murmurs to differentiate by auscultation because of their similar timing and location are those of pulmonic stenosis, aortic stenosis, and VSD. These can usually be differentiated by using other aspects of the physical examination and findings from the ECG and thoracic radiographs.

ELECTROCARDIOGRAM

In congenital heart disease, the ECG is principally used to identify cardiac chamber enlargement, although other measurements are also important. The ECG is generally more reliable in the dog than in the cat for this purpose. ECG readings may be normal with mild forms of the simple defects, and abnormalities are variable and are never pathognomonic. The ECG is particularly useful in helping to differentiate systolic murmurs, which are difficult to identify. It is very important to obtain a *complete* ECG, including accurately positioned thoracic leads. Typical ECG findings for the common defects are summarized in Tables 1 and 2.

P wave changes indicative of atrial enlargement occur most consistently with mitral and tricuspid dysplasias, in which marked atrial dilatation occurs. The P wave is often increased in both amplitude and duration with these defects. Evidence of left atrial enlargement is also common with PDA and is less common with aortic stenosis and VSD. Evidence of right atrial enlargement may be present, although infrequently, with pulmonic stenosis, ASD, and tetralogy of Fallot.

Right ventricular hypertrophy (RVH) (right axis deviation; S waves in leads I, II, III, and aVF; and deep S waves in CV_6LU and CV_6LL) is consistently present in tetralogy of Fallot and Eisenmenger-type defects in dogs. It is consistently present but variable with pulmonic stenosis, even in mild cases, although changes may only be observed in thoracic leads. It is often present, though not striking, in tricuspid dysplasia. Left ventricular enlargement (normal mean electrical axis and increased QRS amplitude and/or duration) is present in most cases of PDA and mitral dysplasia. It is often minimal with a small VSD and in subaortic stenosis, even some advanced cases. A partial or complete right bundle branch block pattern occurs in some cases of ASD and VSD, particularly in cats, requiring differentiation from true right ventricular hypertrophy. The presence of an obvious systolic murmur and a normal ECG is most compatible with a small VSD or aortic stenosis.

Other ECG abnormalities include ST segment depression, either at rest or following exertion, in some dogs with subaortic stenosis, and cardiac arrhythmias. Supraventricular arrhythmias, including atrial fibrillation, may occur with PDA and mitral or tricuspid dysplasia. Ventricular arrhythmias are common in severe forms of subaortic stenosis in dogs. Arrhythmias are less frequently detected with most other defects.

THORACIC RADIOGRAPH

In congenital heart disease, radiographic changes reflect the *response* of the heart and associated vessels to the defect rather than the defect itself. Attention should be given to (1) the degree of cardiac enlargement, (2) signs of individual chamber or great vessel enlargement, and (3) the pulmonary vasculature (arteries and veins). As with the ECG, radiographic changes are generally easier to interpret in dogs than in cats, although the principles of interpretation are similar. In general, shunting lesions (PDA, ASD, VSD) are characterized by enlargement of those cardiac chambers and vessels that must handle the shunted blood. Obstructive lesions (pulmonic stenosis, aortic stenosis) are characterized by enlargement (often slight) of the affected ventricle and a variable degree of post-stenotic dilatation of the artery distal to the obstruction. Valvular insufficiencies (mitral and tricuspid dysplasias) result in enlargement of the affected atrium and ventricle. Shunts are recognized by increased (left to right) or decreased (right to left) size of the pulmonary vasculature. When combined with the ECG, the radiographs may indicate the severity of the defect. As with the physical examination and ECG, variations are common. Typical radiographic features of the common defects are summarized in Tables 1 and 2.

Left-to-right shunting defects are distinguished by differences in the cardiac silhouette. In PDA, enlargement may be slight to severe and involves the left atrium and left ventricle. In the dorsoventral (DV) view the heart often appears narrow and elongated, and the characteristic prominence of the main pulmonary artery and aneurysmal bulge in the aorta at the site of the ductus in the 1 to 2 o'clock position allows the diagnosis to be made with confidence. With a small VSD and a small shunt, the radiographs may appear normal. With larger shunts, generalized cardiomegaly develops, including the left atrium and both left and right ventricles. The main pulmonary artery may be prominent on the DV view, but the aorta is normal. In ASD, the enlargement mainly involves the right heart, including the right atrium and ventricle, whereas the left atrium and ventricle appear normal or near normal. The pulmonary artery may enlarge, but the aorta remains normal.

The most prominent radiographic feature of the AV valve dysplasias is enlargement of the respective atrium with normal or near-normal pulmonary vasculature (which distinguishes them from the shunting defects). In mitral dysplasia, striking left atrial enlargement is seen in both views, whereas the

degree of left ventricular enlargement is considerably less but variable. Marked right atrial enlargement with tricuspid dysplasia may be seen on the DV view but often produces an ovoid or globular silhouette, which may be confusing, particularly in the lateral view. Generalized cardiomegaly may be suspected, but left atrial enlargement is conspicuously absent. The caudal vena cava may appear widened, whereas the pulmonary vasculature appears normal or slightly diminished.

Obstructive lesions generally cause lesser degrees of cardiomegaly than shunting or AV valvular lesions. In pulmonic stenosis, the rounded right ventricle and post-stenotic dilatation of the main pulmonary artery are seen best in the DV view. The pulmonary vasculature appears normal or slightly diminished, whereas the left heart is normal. In aortic stenosis, radiographic changes are often minimal. Cardiomegaly, when present, is usually mild, and post-stenotic dilatation of the ascending aorta is often slight, especially in very young animals. When present, it is best seen as an anteroventral bulge in the cardiac silhouette on the lateral view. On the DV view, the heart may appear somewhat narrow and elongated, as with PDA, and the cardiac apex is often shifted to the left in young dogs. The pulmonary vasculature and right heart are normal. As on the ECG, the presence of an obvious systolic murmur and a normal thoracic radiograph is most compatible with a small VSD or aortic stenosis.

Right-to-left shunting defects are characterized by minimal cardiomegaly with right ventricular enlargement, seen best as rounding on the DV view and apex elevation on the lateral view. In tetralogy of Fallot, the heart often appears diminished in size because of the appearance of hyperlucent, hyperinflated, hypovascular lungs. The main pulmonary artery may show post-stenotic dilatation on the DV view in the 1 to 2 o'clock position, but this is frequently absent in severe cases. The misplaced aorta may result in widening of the mediastinal shadows. The hyperinflated, hypoperfused lungs are characteristic of a right-to-left shunt at the atrial or ventricular level without pulmonary hypertension. In defects associated with pulmonary hypertension (Eisenmenger-type defects), the pulmonary vasculature may appear nearly normal or diminished less than with tetralogy of Fallot. The pulmonary arteries may appear irregular, tortuous, or blunted, although this is usually difficult to recognize without contrast angiography. The left heart remains normal with these defects.

The differentiation of congenital heart defects in dogs and cats is straightforward if information from all noninvasive studies is synthesized in a logical fashion. The majority of these patients are asymptomatic and have a systolic murmur that requires identification. When combined, the following information usually allows a tentative diagnosis to be made: (1) location and character of the murmur, (2)

ECG and radiographic signs of specific chamber and great vessel enlargement, and (3) presence or absence of radiographic signs of shunting. Such information allows the practicing veterinarian to make logical recommendations concerning suitability of the dog or cat as a pet, necessity for further study by referral, potential surgical correction, prognosis, and appropriate follow-up.

TREATMENT OF CONGENITAL HEART DISEASE

As mentioned at the outset, the ideal treatment of significant congenital heart disease is surgical correction. Patent ductus arteriosus is a readily correctable defect. Several techniques have been described for the surgical relief of pulmonary stenosis, repair of atrial or ventricular septal defects, and palliative relief of tetralogy of Fallot (see CVT VII). Artificial valve implantation and other open heart procedures are performed regularly in humans with these and other heart defects, and the reader is referred to human and veterinary surgery texts for discussions of such techniques.

Several circumstances may warrant medical therapy in dogs and cats with congenital heart disease. Whenever congestive heart failure complicates any of the described defects, medical therapy with cardiac glycosides, diuretics, and so on is indicated, following the same principles as those used for acquired heart diseases (see Drugs Used in the Management of Heart Failure, page 285). In general, heart failure resulting from uncorrectable congenital heart disease is often difficult to control medically for more than a few months without frequent relapses. Hypoxemia and polycythemia (particularly a packed cell volume > 65 per cent), which result from chronic right-to-left shunting, may aggravate the condition of patients with these severe defects. Temporary relief of severe dyspnea, exertional fatigue, and syncope may be obtained by phlebotomy, with the goal of maintaining the animal's packed cell volume in the range of 45 to 50 per cent. Arrhythmias that complicate congenital heart disease are treated the same as those seen in acquired heart diseases (see Therapy of Cardiac Arrhythmias, page 360).

The frequency of syncope and sudden death in dogs with subaortic stenosis is believed to be caused by left ventricular ischemia and the development of fatal ventricular arrhythmias. Although there are no reports of the prophylactic use of antiarrhythmic drugs in such dogs, such action would seem to be justified. Propranolol, a beta-adrenergic blocker, in doses of 2.5 to 10 mg t.i.d. in cats and 10 to 80 mg t.i.d. in dogs may both provide antiarrhythmic activity and reduce myocardial oxygen demands. It may reduce the tendency for such arrhythmias to develop in dogs and cats with obstructive congenital heart disease, especially aortic stenosis. Its use has also been advocated for the symptomatic relief of severe tetralogy of Fallot by reducing myocardial oxygen consumption and right-to-left shunting. Such therapy has provided clinical improvement in dogs; however, its use in this setting has not been studied thoroughly in dogs and cats.

Vasodilators such as hydralazine may prove useful in the treatment of left-to-right shunts by decreasing arterial resistance and lowering the pressure gradient between systemic and pulmonary circulation.

SUPPLEMENTAL READING

Bolton, G. R., and Liu, S.-K.: Congenital heart diseases of the cat. Vet. Clin. North Am. 7:341, 1977.

Ettinger, S. J., and Suter, P. F.: *Canine Cardiology*. Philadelphia: W. B. Saunders, 1970.

Harpster, N. K.: Cardiovascular diseases of the domestic cat. Adv. Vet. Sci. Comp. Med. 21:39, 1977.

Mulvihill, J. J., and Priester, W. A.: Congenital heart disease in dogs: epidemiologic similarities to man. Teratology 7:73, 1973.

Patterson, D. F.: Canine congenital heart disease: epidemiology and etiological hypotheses. J. Small Anim. Pract. 12:263, 1971.

Patterson, D. F.: Pathologic and genetic studies of congenital heart disease in the dog. Adv. Cardiol. 13:210, 1974.

Patterson, D. F.: Congenital defects of the cardiovascular system of dogs: studies in comparative cardiology. Adv. Vet. Sci. Comp. Med. 20:1, 1976.

Perloff, J. K.: *The Clinical Recognition of Congenital Heart Disease*, 2nd ed. Philadephia: W. B. Saunders, 1978.

Thomas, W. P.: The differential diagnosis of congenital heart disease in the dog. Small Anim. Vet. Med. Update Ser. 2: No. 12, 1979.

VALVULAR HEART DISEASE

BRUCE W. KEENE, D.V.M.,

and JOHN D. BONAGURA, D.V.M.

Columbus, Ohio

Valvular heart disease can be either congenital or acquired in origin. Dysplasias of the semilunar and atrioventricular valves are common congenital heart defects and are described elsewhere (see Congenital Heart Disease, page 301). Atrioventricular (AV) valvular insufficiency is frequently associated with ventricular dilatation and thus complicates the clinical course of canine and feline cardiomyopathies, dirofilariasis, and congenital heart disease. Since ventricular disease leads to atrial and valve annulus dilatation or papillary muscle dysfunction, the resultant AV insufficiency is labile and potentially reversible. Acquired *structural* valvular disease of the canine heart encompasses two major disorders: chronic degenerative valvular disease and bacterial endocarditis. These lesions also occur sporadically in the cat but are of lesser clinical significance. Other acquired valvular lesions, such as traumatic disruption of a valve, are quite rare.

CHRONIC VALVULAR DISEASE IN THE DOG

INCIDENCE AND PATHOLOGY

Chronic valvular disease (CVD) is the most common cardiovascular lesion of the dog and is a major cause of disability and death in geriatric patients. This disorder has been studied by different investigators who have identified the degenerative valvular lesions as endocardiosis, mitral valve fibrosis, or chronic valvular-myocardial heart disease. Various epidemiologic studies have estimated the overall incidence of CVD to range from 17 to 40 per cent. Since normal aging also leads to valve thickening and the incidence of CVD increases with age, the different data most likely reflect the population studied and the criteria used for diagnosis. Whitney found that 58 per cent of dogs nine years of age and older had severe lesions of CVD. Clinical and pathologic studies suggest that males are affected more often than females (1.5:1) and that small breeds have a higher incidence than large breed dogs.

The principal lesions of CVD are degenerative and predominantly affect the atrioventricular (AV) valves. Buchanan found that 62 per cent of 230 dogs

had mitral involvement only and 32.5 per cent had both mitral and tricuspid valve disease. Isolated tricuspid valve disease is rare, and aortic and pulmonic valve involvement is insignificant. The histologic changes include thickening of the valve spongiosa caused by edema and deposition of acid-staining mucopolysaccharide, with degeneration and interruption of collagen in the valve–supporting fibrosa layer. Gross alterations include valve contraction, thickening, nodularity, and "rolling" of the free border of the cusps. These changes lead to the AV valvular regurgitant murmurs that are the hallmark of this syndrome. The chordae tendineae are also affected and may rupture, a catastrophic clinical event that leads to fulminant congestive heart failure.

Other lesions are the result of AV valvular regurgitation or associated myocardial disease. Advanced cases of CVD have significant atrial and ventricular dilatation with eccentric hypertrophy, changes that are easily recognized by radiography. The mitral and tricuspid valve rings can dilate, leading to further valve insufficiency. Severe mitral regurgitation (MR) causes sclerosis (jet lesions) or linear tearing of the left atrium. Rupture of the atrial wall with cardiac tamponade is an infrequent complication of these lesions. Additional abnormalities may be found in the ventricular myocardium. These consist of small areas of myocardial fibrosis, caused by hyalinization of intramural coronary arteries, and ischemic infarction of the ventricle. The incidence and overall significance of such lesions are unknown. Advanced chronic valvular disease can cause congestive heart failure (CHF) with generalized cardiomegaly, pulmonary venous distention, and pulmonary edema as characteristic necropsy findings. Dogs with right ventricular failure have dilation of the caudal vena cava, hepatic congestion, ascites, and pleural effusion. Small transudative pericardial effusions are occasionally observed.

In spite of considerable clinical experience with this disorder and numerous correlative pathologic studies, the etiology of CVD is elusive. It is interesting to note that CVD frequently occurs with other connective tissue problems including rupture of the cruciate ligaments and intervertebral disc disease; however, a unifying hypothesis for these problems has not evolved. The clinician can be assured, however, that with better overall veteri-

311

nary care, CVD will continue to be a major clinical problem in geriatric small animal practice.

PATHOPHYSIOLOGY: MECHANISMS OF CLINICAL SIGNS

Chronic valvular heart disease is an example of a systolic hemodynamic volume overload. Atrioventricular valvular insufficiency reduces cardiac output. Since more than half of the ventricular stroke volume can be regurgitated into the atrium, this chamber enlarges owing to the increased pressure and volume. To maintain an adequate cardiac output, the heart must increase its stroke work, and this is accomplished through ventricular and atrial dilatation and hypertrophy. Other compensatory mechanisms, including renal retention of sodium and water and activation of the sympathetic nervous system, act to augment ventricular filling and increase contractility, heart rate, and peripheral resistance. As a result of these mechanisms, ventricular diastolic, mean atrial, and venous pressures rise. Forward stroke volume and arterial blood pressure are supported by these reserve mechanisms; however, the elevated venous pressures cause edema and congestion.

These circulatory changes can occur with only minimal alterations in the ventricular myocardial function, an indication that the initial disorder, AV valve regurgitation, is mechanical (see Concepts and Therapeutic Strategies in the Management of Heart Failure, page 279). However, myocardial contractility may deteriorate with protracted volume overload and is further compromised by myocardial fibrosis, inadequate coronary perfusion, and cardiac rhythm disturbances. Thus the signs of congestive heart failure (pulmonary edema, pleural effusion, ascites) are actually manifestations of cardiac and circulatory compensations in response to inadequate cardiac output. Low-output signs of heart failure (weakness, depression, azotemia) result from reduced forward stroke volume, arrhythmias, and, in severe cases, myocardial failure. Syncope may occur from diverse causes, including (1) inadequate ventricular output during exercise, (2) paroxysmal cardiac arrhythmias, and (3) abnormal pulmonary function, including coughing. Although most patients have left heart failure, ascites and other clinical signs of right ventricular failure are also common. Severe right ventricular failure often seems to occur secondary to left heart failure, and this may be related to the increased pressure work necessary to pump blood against a hypertensive pulmonary venous circulation. Dogs with progressive right ventricular dilatation and tricuspid regurgitation (TR) can develop severe biventricular failure and experience marked reductions in cardiac output.

CLINICAL SYNDROME

It has long been recognized that clinical signs are not helpful in the early diagnosis of mitral or tricuspid regurgitation. Mild degrees of valvular insufficiency can be tolerated for years owing to circulatory compensation and myocardial reserves. In practice, MR and TR are usually diagnosed during a routine physical examination conducted for unrelated purposes or complaints. The auscultation of a systolic murmur or a high-pitched mid systolic click in a middle-aged or older dog should alert the clinician to the possibility of CVD. Although the typical murmur of MR is heard best at the left fifth intercostal space, a dorsal, cranial, or caudal radiation of the regurgitant jet is common, and the murmur may be very loud at the left base. A decrescendo murmur is typical of mild MR, but with progressive insufficiency the murmur becomes holosystolic. Murmur intensity or frequency is not a good indicator of the severity of MR, and a spectrum of auscultatory features may be detected, ranging from a harsh mixed-frequency murmur to a high-pitched musical systolic "whoop." Determination of the hemodynamic significance of MR and TR thus must rely on supporting clinical and radiographic data.

The clinical documentation of TR can be difficult, as mitral insufficiency is usually present, and this murmur frequently radiates to the tricuspid area. Clinical findings that support a diagnosis of TR include (1) prominent jugular pulsations, (2) precordial thrill at the right fourth intercostal space, and (3) marked differences in frequency of the murmurs at the right and left hemithoraces.

Dogs with symptomatic CVD generally are presented because of tiring, coughing, restlessness, dyspnea, syncope, or ascites. Physical examination of symptomatic dogs usually reveals an elderly, small breed dog with normal arterial pulses, the previously described murmurs, inspiratory and expiratory dyspnea, pulmonary crackles or rales, and possibly an S_3 gallop. Premature beats, paroxysmal tachycardia, or atrial fibrillation may be auscultated in some cases. Caudoventral displacement of the cardiac apex beat suggests ventricular dilatation, whereas ascites and prominent jugular venous pulsations are indications of right ventricular failure. In many cases there is a gradual progression of clinical signs, beginning with exertional cough and ending with intractable biventricular failure.

Thoracic radiographs illustrate varying degrees of cardiomegaly and extracardiac signs of heart failure. In typical cases there is significant dilatation of the left atrium and ventricle. If the left atrium is particularly compliant, there may be massive atrial enlargement with no evidence of pulmonary edema. A frequent finding is compression of the left mainstem bronchus caused by the expanding left atrium. Right heart enlargement is common and results from TR, pulmonary venous hypertension, or concurrent chronic obstructive pulmonary disease. Pulmonary venous distention and pulmonary edema are radiographic correlates of left heart failure. Engorgement of the caudal vena cava, hepatomegaly, and pleural effusion indicate right ventricular failure.

Electrocardiographic abnormalities include widening of the P waves owing to left atrial enlargement, augmentation of the QRS voltages suggesting left ventricular dilatation, and ST-T segment coving, a nonspecific sign of cardiac enlargement. Notching and widening of the QRS complexes to greater than 65 msec are suggestive of myocardial disease.

The majority of untreated patients exhibit a normal sinus rhythm or sinus tachycardia; however, sinus arrhythmia is occasionally found and may be associated with concurrent obstructive lung disease. Supraventricular premature complexes are typical and are suggestive of underlying atrial enlargement. Serious supraventricular rhythm disturbances, including paroxysmal supraventricular tachycardia, atrial tachycardia, and atrial flutter or fibrillation, are recognized in some patients. Ventricular premature complexes are common, and their genesis may be myocardial ischemia, ventricular dilatation, increased ventricular wall tension, or hypoxia. Digitalis intoxication is a frequent cause of iatrogenic rhythm disturbances, which include atrioventricular block; sinus arrest; premature atrial, junctional, and ventricular complexes; and junctional or ventricular tachycardia.

Other studies are useful in the diagnosis and assessment of dogs with CVD. *Serum biochemical profiles* are essential in guiding cardiac drug therapy, with particular attention directed to renal function, serum electrolytes, and serum protein determinations. Hypokalemia and renal failure predispose to digoxin toxicity. Renal failure, a potential sequela to low cardiac output, may also result from the volume contraction associated with diuretic therapy or digitalis intoxication. Other disorders that complicate CHF, such as anemia, hypothyroidism, and infections, must be identified and managed.

Ultrasonic studies are useful in the identification of structural lesions of advanced CVD but are less valuable in the assessment of ventricular function. Left ventricular dilatation, left atrial enlargement, right ventricular dilatation, and thickening of the mitral valve can be imaged by echocardiography. Unfortunately, left ventricular systolic function is difficult to assess. The left atrium provides a "pop-off" valve that permits the ventricle to shorten normally and eject against a low-pressure resistance. This results in a hyperdynamic left ventricle despite potential underlying myocardial dysfunction.

The *differential diagnosis* of CVD is important,

since the clinical significance of valvular insufficiency is often overemphasized. Chronic obstructive pulmonary disease must be ruled out as the cause of clinical signs in any mature dog with coughing, dyspnea, and auscultatable pulmonary crackles or rales. A cardiac murmur is not definitive evidence of heart failure but may merely be an incidental finding. Suitable diagnostic tests including thoracic radiographs, ECG, and other studies are performed to rule out chronic bronchitis, pulmonary fibrosis, and collapsing trachea or bronchus. Other causes of pulmonary disease including pneumonia, allergic pneumonitis, dirofilariasis, pulmonary neoplasm, and systemic mycosis are eliminated before therapy for cardiac failure is initiated.

PRINCIPLES OF THERAPY

The ideal treatment for CVD is surgical replacement of the diseased valve apparatus. However, such therapy is, at this time, impractical. Therefore, management is directed toward the following: (1) reduction of venous pressure and alleviation of edema and effusions, (2) reduction of cardiac work-

Table 1. *Principles of Therapy in Chronic Valvular Disease*

Therapeutic Goal	Treatment
Reduce venous pressure	Dietary sodium restriction
	Diuretic therapy (furosemide, thiazides)
	Vasodilators (nitroglycerin, prazosin, hydralazine, captopril)
Reduce cardiac workload	Enforced rest
	Weight reduction, vasodilator therapy (decreased preload and afterload)
Maintain sufficient cardiac output	Digitalis glycosides (digoxin, digitoxin)
	Vasodilators
	Dobutamine
Reduce mitral regurgitation	Arterial vasodilators (hydralazine, prazosin, captopril)
Control cardiac arrhythmias, supraventricular arrhythmias, and ventricular arrhythmias	Antiarrhythmic drugs (digitalis, propranolol, procainamide, quinidine, lidocaine, phenytoin)
Reduce clinical signs	Successful management of cardiac failure
Improve exercise capacity	Bronchodilators (aminophylline, theophylline)
	Cough suppressants (Hycodan, Tussionex)
Alleviate pleural and abdominal effusions	Diuretics and management of heart failure
	Captopril
	Thoracocentesis, abdominal paracentesis
Avoid complications	Manage extracardiac disorders
	Prevent drug toxicosis

Table 2.   Drugs Commonly Used in the Management of Chronic Valvular Disease

Drug	Beneficial Effects	Common Adverse Effects	Approximate Dose
Digoxin (Lanoxin: 0.05 mg/ml elixir, 0.125-, 0.25-, 0.5-mg tablets; Cardoxin: 0.05, 0.15 mg/ml elixirs)	Increases myocardial contractility, decreases heart rate, treats supraventricular tachyarrhythmias	Anorexia, depression, vomiting, diarrhea, AV block, ectopia, junctional tachycardia	Oral maintenance: 0.01 to 0.02 mg/kg divided b.i.d. Rapid oral digitalization: 0.02 to 0.06 mg/kg divided b.i.d. for one day
Digitoxin (Foxalin: 0.1-, 0.25-mg tablets; Crystodigin: 0.1-, 0.2-mg tablets)	Same as digoxin Useful in renal failure due to hepatic elimination	Same as digoxin	Oral maintenance: 0.04 to 0.1 mg/kg divided b.i.d. to t.i.d.
Dobutamine (Dobutrex)	Increases myocardial contractility	Sinus tachycardia at high doses, ectopia	2 to 15 μg/kg/min, constant rate infusion
Furosemide (Lasix: 50 mg/ml injection, 10 mg/ml syrup, 12.5-, 20-, 40-, 50-mg tablets)	Reduces blood volume, venous pressure, edema, and ascites	Dehydration, azotemia, electrolyte imbalance, loss of compensatory increases in ventricular preload	2 to 4 mg/kg (IV, IM, SC, oral); repeat b.i.d. or t.i.d. if needed
Hydrochlorothiazide (Hydro-Diuril: 25-, 50-mg tablets, combined with 25 mg spironolactone as Aldactazide: 50-mg tablet)	Same as furosemide Potassium-sparing with spironolactone	Same as furosemide	2 to 4 mg/kg b.i.d. 2 mg/kg b.i.d. (Aldactazide)
Hydralazine (Apresoline: 10-, 25-, 50-mg tablets)	Arterial vasodilator, decreases regurgitant fraction, increases cardiac output, reduces myocardial tension and preload	Weakness, depression, hypotension, fainting, emesis, sinus tachycardia	0.5 to 3 mg/kg b.i.d. to t.i.d.
Prazosin (Minipress: 1-, 2-mg capsules)	Arterial and venodilator, reduces afterload and preload, other effects as per hydralazine	Same as hydralazine	1 to 2 mg b.i.d. to t.i.d.
Captopril (Capoten: 25-mg tablets)	Arterial vasodilator, venodilator, angiotensin-converting enzyme inhibitor (decreases aldosterone)	Same as hydralazine	1 to 2 mg/kg t.i.d.

Drug	Action	Side effects	Dosage
Nitroglycerine ointment 2% (Nitrol, Nitro-Bid)	Vasodilator, primarily venous, reduces venous pressure, decreases myocardial oxygen consumption	Hypotension, weakness, depression, sinus tachycardia	1/4 to 3/4 inch cutaneously every 4 to 8 hours
Procainamide (Pronestyl: 100 or 500 mg/ml, Injection, 250-, 500-mg tablets; Procan-SR: 250-, 500-mg sustained-release tablets)	Ventricular premature complexes, ventricular tachycardia	Weakness, hypotension, decreased contractility, gastrointestinal side effects, widening of QRS-T complex	6 to 8 mg/kg IV over 5 min, 8 to 20 mg/kg IM q4 to 6h; Tablets: 8 to 20 mg/kg q6h q8h for Procan-SR
Quinidine sulfate, gluconate, polygalacturonate[b] (Quinidine Gluconate USP: 80 mg/ml injection; Quinidine Sulfate USP: 200-mg tablets; Quinaglute Dura-Tabs[d]: 324 mg-tablets; Cardioquin[b]: 275-mg tablets)	Ventricular premature complexes, ventricular tachycardia, acute atrial fibrillation, refractory supraventricular tachycardias	As per procainamide, drug interaction with digoxin	6 to 20 mg/kg IM, q6h; 6 to 16 mg/kg orally q6h (sulfate); 8 to 20 mg/kg orally q6 to 8h[a,b] dogs only
Propranolol (Inderal: 10-, 20-, 40-mg tablets)	Beta-adrenergic blocker, antiarrhythmic, slows response to atrial fibrillation, decreases myocardial oxygen consumption	Reduces myocardial contractility, bronchial constriction, hypotension, loss of compensatory mechanisms	0.1 to 1.0 mg/kg (oral) t.i.d
Theophylline (Aminophylline: 100-, 200-mg tablets; Elixophyllin elixir)	Bronchodilation, mild increase in myocardial contractility	Emesis, excitement, urticaria	Aminophylline: 6 to 10 mg/kg (IV, SC, oral), repeat q6 to 12h; Elixophyllin: 0.3 to 0.4 ml/kg b.i.d. to t.i.d. Lower dose if concurrent renal failure is present.

load, (3) maintenance of a cardiac output that is sufficient to prevent low-output signs of muscle weakness, syncope, and azotemia, (4) reduction of mitral regurgitant fraction, (5) normalization of cardiac rate and rhythm, (6) control of clinical signs of cough and dyspnea, (7) improvement of exercise capacity, and (8) prevention of complicating factors, including adverse or toxic drug effects (Tables 1 and 2). The practical attainment of these goals requires the use of potent and potentially dangerous drugs such as furosemide, digoxin, and vasodilators. Effective utilization of these pharmacologic agents is contingent on the clinician's knowledge of pharmacology and pharmacokinetics. Inadequate and inappropriate use of cardiac drugs is one of the most frequent causes of clinical failure. Therefore, it is imperative that the veterinarian be familiar with the indications, uses, and adverse effects of any drug before it is administered to a patient. The reader is directed to pages 279 to 301 of this volume for a discussion of the clinical pharmacology of these agents.

Reduction of venous pressure is accomplished initially by dietary sodium restriction and diuretic therapy, both of which act in concert to decrease plasma volume. Dogs with congestive heart failure (CHF) have a diminished capacity to excrete a sodium load; thus dietary salt restriction, but not water restriction, is indicated to minimize fluid retention by the kidney. Mild to moderate sodium restriction includes elimination of salt-containing treats and mixing the usual diet with low–sodium prescription diets such as H/D or H Diet. Some hard vegetables can be substituted for dog biscuits and rawhide bones. Strict sodium restriction requires the elimination of all food except prescription diets or specially formulated diets prepared by the owner. Such diets should limit total sodium intake to 12 mg/kg/day (see CVT V).

Of the diuretics employed, hydrochlorothiazide and furosemide are the most commonly administered. Appropriate treatment with diuretics is probably the most effective method of controlling pulmonary edema and ascites. However, overzealous use commonly leads to dehydration, volume contraction, prerenal azotemia, hypokalemia, and digitalis intoxication. Because of these adverse effects, serum creatinine and electrolyte levels are evaluated periodically in dogs receiving diuretic agents.

Other methods available for reducing venous pressure include the administration of drugs that increase stroke volume and reduce ventricular diastolic size and pressure and the use of agents that directly dilate systemic veins, increase venous capacity, and lower venous pressures. Arterial vasodilators such as hydralazine (Apresoline) and prazosin (Minipress) and the digitalis glycosides are examples of drugs that may increase left ventricular stroke volume and cardiac output. Venodilators such

as nitroglycerin ointment (Nitro-Bid, Nitrol) and prazosin increase venous capacitance, shift blood volume away from the pulmonary vascular bed, and lower venous pressures (Fig. 1). Captopril (Capoten), an angiotensin-converting enzyme inhibitor, is an effective vasodilator that also inhibits the release of the sodium-conserving hormone aldosterone. If these pharmacologic measures fail to control pleural effusion or ascites, mechanical removal of fluid is indicated when the patient experiences significant restriction of ventilation.

Reduction of cardiac workload is achieved through enforced rest, minimum exercise, control of obesity, and vasodilator therapy. Simple cage (or room) rest promotes a diuresis of retained fluid and is mandatory for dogs with moderate to severe heart failure. Vasodilators in particular have the capacity to reduce left ventricular work by decreasing afterload, preload, myocardial tension, and ventricular size (see Fig. 1).

Maintenance of a sufficient *cardiac output* is difficult when diuretic or venodilator therapy decreases ventricular filling pressures below a critical level. For this reason, clinical and laboratory indicators of cardiac output such as muscle strength, capillary refill time, serum creatinine level, pulmonary vascularity, and venous P_{O_2} (see page 284) are determined periodically to assess cardiac output and the need for additional therapy. Drugs that may increase ventricular stroke volume and cardiac output include arterial vasodilators (see Fig. 1), digitalis glycosides, and antiarrhythmic agents.

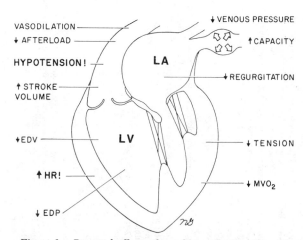

Figure 1. Potential effects of vasodilator therapy. Venodilators reduce venous pressure and edema by increasing systemic venous capacity. Arterial vasodilators reduce arterial impedance (afterload), permitting the ventricle to eject a larger stroke volume at a reduced tension. As stroke volume increases, left ventricular volume (EDV) and end-diastolic pressure (EDP) are reduced. Vasodilators also reduce the amount of blood regurgitated back into the left atrium, decrease intramyocardial tension, and may reduce myocardial oxygen consumption (MVO_2). Important adverse effects of vasodilators include arterial hypotension and reflex tachycardia. (Reprinted with permission from Bonagura: Vet. Clin. North Am. 11:705, 1981.)

Since severe cardiac muscle failure is not an initial feature of cardiac failure caused by CVD, the authors reserve *digitalization* for advanced heart failure, heart failure that is refractory to diuretics and vasodilators, right ventricular failure, and the treatment of persistent sinus tachycardia and atrial arrhythmias (see page 368).

A *reduction of mitral regurgitation* may occur with the administration of arterial vasodilators such as hydralazine or prazosin (see Fig. 1). There is considerable experimental evidence to suggest that reducing arterial peripheral resistance decreases left ventricular afterload and facilitates ejection of blood into the aorta. The authors have achieved clinical success with such therapy and routinely administer these agents to dogs with advanced mitral disease (functional classes III and IV) and with atrial compression of the mainstem bronchus. These drugs are administered cautiously, since serious weakness and syncope occur in some patients, particularly when they are volume contracted from diuretic therapy. Reflex sinus tachycardia can result from the administration of these agents; therefore, digitalization may be needed to control cardiac rate.

Cardiac rhythm disturbances complicate advanced CVD, and it is important to *control serious arrhythmias*. Most dogs experience mild sinus tachycardia and occasional atrial or junctional premature complexes. Maintenance digitalization may be adequate to control these. Repetitive supraventricular premature beats, paroxysmal supraventricular tachycardia, and atrial fibrillation are more serious dysrhythmias and, if not controlled by digitalis glycosides, necessitate additional therapy with propranolol (see page 369). Occasional ventricular premature complexes may not require antiarrhythmic therapy; however, repetitive complexes or paroxysmal ventricular tachycardia is treated with oral procainamide or quinidine (see page 369). Since cardiac glycosides can cause any of these arrhythmias, digitalis therapy is temporarily suspended and serum drug levels determined when a new rhythm disturbance develops.

The client often equates the success of cardiac therapy with *reduction of coughing and dyspnea*. These results are best obtained through medical management of pulmonary edema; however, additional measures can be useful. Dogs with signs of cardiac "asthma," including wheezing and dyspnea, frequently benefit from the bronchodilators aminophylline or theophylline. Such therapy is particularly useful in dogs with concurrent chronic obstructive pulmonary disease. Since coughing and dyspnea are barometers of the success of therapy for cardiac failure, the use of cough suppressants such as Hycodan and Tussionex is discouraged unless heart failure is unresponsive to other therapy or there is concomitant tracheal or bronchial collapse. Supplemental oxygen therapy is an important adjunct to the treatment of severe pulmonary edema.

The *improvement of exercise capacity* provides important emotional benefits to the client and, presumably, the patient. Whereas strenuous exercise is discouraged in animals with CHF, mild leash exercise appears valuable. To achieve this aim, pulmonary edema must be controlled and cardiac output maintained or increased as previously described. Exercise capacity is another benchmark of the efficacy of treatment.

In the therapy of dogs with CVD, the *prevention of complications* such as drug toxicity is essential to the comfort of the dog and the attitude of the client. Many dogs have clinical signs of mild to moderate CHF, are administered toxic dosages of digitalis, and become acutely ill to the distress and discouragement of the client. The authors are reluctant to use the suggested maximum doses of any drug unless combinations of agents at moderate dosages have failed to produce the desired clinical effect. This is an individual decision, of course, and one that must be tempered by the ability of the owner to administer multiple treatments and to bear the cost of such therapy.

SPECIFIC THERAPY

Dogs with objective signs of CVD are classified by their functional status as previously described on page 280. Asymptomatic patients with cardiac murmurs *(Class I)* are not treated; however, the owner is advised of the natural history of CVD and is instructed to return at the earliest sign of cardiac failure. Weight reduction and elimination of high-sodium treats are encouraged, if appropriate, at this time. Neither digitalis glycosides nor rigid sodium restriction is advocated for this class of patient. Regular follow-up examinations are advised.

Dogs with clinical signs of cardiac failure during exercise *(Class II)* are managed medically provided other causes of coughing or exertional dyspnea have been discounted by a thorough radiographic evaluation. Following a clinical evaluation that includes thoracic radiography, electrocardiography, and serum biochemical determinations, initial cardiac therapy consists of moderate sodium restriction and the administration of a diuretic. Either hydrochlorothiazide or furosemide is given twice daily for the first one or two days of treatment. The dose is then reduced to the longest consistent interval (e.g., once every other day, once a day, b.i.d., and so on) that keeps the dog free of pulmonary congestion. This type of therapy is highly effective in dogs with mild to moderate congestive heart failure, and an inadequate clinical response should prompt a reassessment of the diagnosis. Occasionally, dogs with marked left atrial distention will continue to cough, apparently from compression of the mainstem bronchus. In such cases, hydralazine is given to decrease mitral regurgitant fraction and is continued if there is clinical improvement. Some dogs also benefit from bronchodilator therapy; however, this is delayed until the efficacy of diuresis or vasodilators can be evaluated. Following these determinations, a trial course (one week) of theophylline or aminophylline can be administered, assessed for favorable effects on pulmonary function, and continued if clinically useful. Digitalis glycosides are not routinely given to dogs with Class II CHF unless serious supraventricular tachyarrhythmias are present.

Dogs with advanced heart failure often develop clinical signs with routine activities such as walking or awaken coughing from pulmonary edema. They are considered functional *Class III* patients. Treatment for this group consists of strict sodium restriction, exercise restriction, and daily administration of diuretics. If furosemide therapy (2 to 4 mg/kg b.i.d.) is not adequate to ameliorate clinical signs, the arterial vasodilator hydralazine or the "balanced" vasodilator prazosin is given to increase cardiac output, lower venous pressures, and reduce mitral regurgitant fraction.

Digoxin is administered, if needed, to treat sinus tachycardia or supraventricular arrhythmias or to manage congestive heart failure that is refractory to the previously mentioned measures. Loading doses of digoxin are not advocated, and the clinician is advised to use daily doses that approach the lower end of the dosage range (see Table 2). Therapy must be *individualized*. If azotemia is present, either the dose of digoxin is reduced by 25 to 50 per cent or digitoxin is administered. Since digitoxin is eliminated by the liver, this preparation is recommended when there is concurrent primary renal disease. After five to seven days of administration, serum digitalis concentrations are determined by drawing 5 ml of blood eight to ten hours after the previous dose and submitting the serum to a commercial laboratory for radioimmunoassay. This evaluation is simple and practical and permits accurate calculation of daily maintenance doses. Suggested therapeutic serum drug concentrations are 1 to 2 ng/ml for digoxin and 15 to 35 ng/ml for digitoxin. Digoxin values greater than 2.5 ng/ml are frequently associated with clinical toxicity.

Additional therapy may be needed for this group of patients. The administration of bronchodilators or cough suppressants is guided as previously described for Class II patients. Modifications in the drug dosages are necessary for some patients to relieve progressive CHF or reduce adverse drug effects. For example, digitalization must be individualized to minimize toxicity, vasodilator dose and frequency of administration corrected to avoid weakness or lethargy, and the daily diuretic dose adjusted to prevent dehydration and hypokalemia.

When clinical signs of cardiac failure are obvious at rest, the patient has progressed to functional *Class IV*. Dogs in this group either have severe cardiac failure that requires emergency therapy or progress to this class by becoming refractory to conventional therapy. The therapeutic approach depends in part on the clinician's ability to monitor the patient, the severity of CHF, and the previous medication history. Of particular concern are factors that had previously been well controlled but that now may lead to the sudden demise of the dog. Complications such as ruptured chordae tendineae, rupture of the left atrium, development of atrial fibrillation, progressive myocardial failure, digitalis intoxication, lack of owner compliance, oral sodium loads, pulmonary infection, bronchitis, environmental stress (heat, smoke), and anemia (blood loss) are recognized causes of cardiac decompensation in dogs with CVD.

Principles of management of *fulminant functional Class IV heart failure* caused by CVD include (1) improvement of tissue oxygenation using supplemental inspired oxygen (40 to 50 per cent) and parenteral aminophylline, (2) reduction of pulmonary edema with parenteral furosemide and nitroglycerin ointment, (3) relief of anxiety with morphine sulfate (0.2 mg/kg SC), (4) continuation or initiation of maintenance digitalization, with frequent ECG evaluations of cardiac rhythm, (5) control of cardiac arrhythmias, (6) mechanical removal of large pleural or abdominal effusions, (7) correction of dehydration and maintenance of hydration using intravenous 5 per cent dextrose in water, (8) absolute cage rest, and (9) administration of additional inotropic agents such as dobutamine if the patient is refractory to the previously mentioned treatment.

The majority of dogs respond to these measures within one to two days; however, a small percentage continue to have refractory pulmonary edema or ascites, low cardiac output, azotemia, or weakness. In these dogs, dobutamine (Dobutrex) is administered by constant rate intravenous infusion for 12 to 36 hours in an effort to increase ventricular contractility. We generally reserve this therapy for patients with intractable right ventricular failure or echocardiographic evidence of reduced left ventricular contractility. It is also important to correct and prevent dehydration in nonalimentative dogs. Although diuretics are effective in mobilizing edema, they also lead to cellular dehydration and azotemia. These are treated with (sodium free) 5 per cent dextrose solution supplemented with potassium chloride (0.5 to 2.0 mEq/kg/day) at the usual maintenance rate of 40 to 60 ml/kg/day. We find it useful to measure central venous pressure (or pulmonary capillary wedge pressure) when possible to keep the CVP at less than 14 cm H_2O (or the pulmonary wedge pressure between 14 and 18 mm Hg). Although the intercurrent therapy of IV fluids, diuretics, and vasodilators may seem inexplicable, there appears to be clinical value in shifting fluid volumes from the lung while preventing marked reductions in ventricular filling pressures, dehydration, and renal failure.

Many patients with CVD *progress* to functional Class IV by becoming *refractory to conventional treatment* with digitalis, furosemide, and sodium restriction. If vasodilators are already being used, the possibility of increasing the daily dose of digitalis, furosemide, or vasodilator drug is considered. If the serum digoxin concentration is less than 1.0 ng/ml, the daily maintenance dose is increased cautiously by 15 to 25 per cent, while watching for toxic signs. Furosemide is administered at 4 mg/kg b.i.d or t.i.d. The vasodilator drug dose is also increased, if the dog can tolerate it without untoward effects (weakness, depression). If a vasodilator has not yet been administered, either hydralazine, prazosin, or captopril is prescribed to increase cardiac output and reduce edema (see page 293). Serious arrhythmias are treated as described on page 360.

Refractory pulmonary edema or ascites occasionally is amenable to therapy with combinations of diuretics. The use of hydrochlorothiazide or Aldactazide (hydrochlorothiazide-spironolactone) alternated with furosemide is helpful in some patients. In other cases, substituting the vasodilator angiotensin-converting enzyme inhibitor captopril (Capoten) for other vasodilators has led to dramatic diuresis and mobilization of edema. We then continue captopril therapy in place of hydralazine or prazosin. Thoracocentesis or paracentesis is necessary in selected patients. Some dogs are refractory to maximum tolerated dosages of cardiac medications and symptomatic therapy. Such patients are candidates for euthanasia.

BACTERIAL ENDOCARDITIS

Bacterial endocarditis (BE) is a serious systemic disorder resulting from infection of the heart valves or mural endocardium. Clinical signs of BE are related to cardiac lesions, bacteremia, arterial embolization, metastatic infection, and host responses to infection. Endocarditis in the dog and cat generally involves the mitral and aortic valves. Principal etiologic agents are the streptococci, *Staphylococcus aureus*, *Aerobacter aerogenes*, *Escherichia coli*, *Pseudomonas aeruginosa*, and *Erysipelothrix rhusiopathiae*.

Bacterial endocarditis occurs most often in larger breed male dogs older than four years of age. The German shepherd is frequently affected. The source of infection can be normal bacterial flora of the alimentary tract or skin or a localized infection of the subcutis, bone, lung, urogenital tract, oral cavity, or perianal tissues. Previous antibiotic or im-

munosuppressive drug therapy, intravenous catheters, surgery, and invasive medical procedures predispose to BE. Certain cardiac lesions, such as congenital subaortic stenosis, are associated with a higher than usual incidence of BE. However, chronic degenerative valvular disease apparently does not increase the incidence of valve infection.

Valvular infection is acute or subacute, although the distinction may not be clinically apparent. Highly virulent organisms can invade a valve, leading to ulceration and destruction of the affected tissue. In subacute BE, normal body flora colonizes a valve that has been previously injured. Factors important to this type of invasion include hemodynamic or endogenous stress causing valve injury, a sterile platelet fibrin thrombus, bacteremia, and host agglutinating antibody.

The *cardiac manifestations* of BE are varied and lead to diverse clinical findings (Fig. 2). Despite valvular lesions, there may *not* be a cardiac murmur; however, most cases are characterized by a "new" systolic murmur of MR or the diastolic murmur of aortic regurgitation (AR). Functional systolic murmurs may be present during febrile episodes. With AR, the arterial pulse is hyperkinetic. Extension of the infection into the myocardium, pericardium, or cardiac conduction system or embolization of a coronary artery can result in auscultatable cardiac arrhythmias. Ventricular premature complexes, ventricular tachycardia, and atrioventricular blocks are the most commonly recognized rhythm disturbances. Significant valvular regurgitation leads to increased cardiac size, which is evident on thoracic radiographs. Cardiac failure and congestive heart failure are present in some cases.

The *extracardiac manifestations* of BE can dominate the clinical picture, leading to clinical signs of fever, shaking (chills), muscle stiffness, lameness, cutaneous petechial hemorrhages, seizures, or depression. These clinical signs occur secondary to (1) bacteremia, (2) metastatic infection of the joints, kidney, muscle, central nervous system, or lung, (3) embolism, or (4) host immunologic responses (see Fig. 2). Clinical and laboratory evidence of pyelonephritis, meningitis, inflammatory arthritis, or hematogenous pneumonia is suggestive of BE. Subacute BE can mimic immunologic disorders and result in positive immune tests. Hematologic responses are common and include mild nonregenerative anemia, leukocytosis, and monocytosis.

The definitive diagnosis of BE may be elusive. In suspected cases, blood cultures are obtained, and other cultures (urine, cerebrospinal fluid, joint fluid) may be useful. Multiple blood cultures should be obtained using at least 5 to 10 ml of blood, aseptically collected and incubated in appropriate aerobic and anaerobic media. Echocardiography is very useful for the detection of moderate sized (3 mm) to large vegetations; however, this test is not uniformly available. If acute BE is suspected, blood

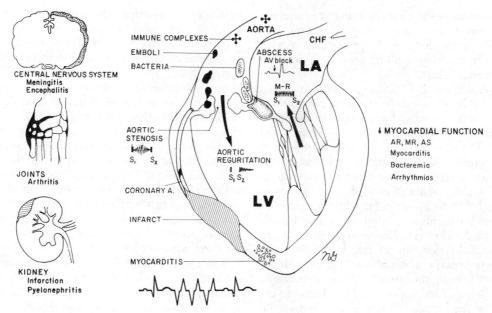

Figure 2. Pathogenesis of clinical signs in bacterial endocarditis. This drawing illustrates important features of bacterial endocarditis. Damage to the mitral or aortic valves leads to cardiac murmurs of valvular insufficiency. Large vegetations are capable of producing obstruction and associated murmurs such as aortic stenosis. Bacteria and parts of the vegetation are shed into the blood stream. Emboli may lodge in major vessels, producing infarction and necrosis in organs such as the heart, kidney, and brain. Septic emboli or recurrent bacteremia leads to fever, infectious myocarditis, and seeding of other tissues with infection. Prominent organs of involvement include the brain and meninges, joints, and kidneys. Immune complexes may form and may result in immunologic injury in joints or glomeruli. Cardiac failure may result from a variety of factors including increased work from valvular disease, inflammation and necrosis of myocardium, bacteremia, and cardiac rhythm and conduction disturbances. (Reprinted with permission from Bonagura *in* Ettinger: *Textbook of Veterinary Internal Medicine*, 2nd ed. Philadelphia: W. B. Saunders, 1983.) The medical illustrations of Nancy Goldschmidt are acknowledged.

should be cultured and therapy instituted without delay.

THERAPY

The principles of treatment of BE include the use of (1) high doses of antibiotic (up to 20 times MIC) and protracted therapy, (2) bacteriocidal antibiotics, (3) antibiotics that penetrate fibrin, and (4) the narrowest spectrum antibiotic capable of inhibiting the organism *in vitro*. However, if BE is suspected but blood cultures are sterile, broad spectrum antibiotic therapy is utilized. Sodium or potassium penicillin G (40 to 60,000 units/kg IV q6h), procaine penicillin G (40 to 80,000 units/kg IM b.i.d.), and ampicillin (20 to 40 mg/kg IV or IM t.i.d.) can be effective against streptococci and anaerobic bacteria; however, these drugs have limited efficacy against penicillinase-producing staphylococcus, coliforms, and some gram negative organisms. The addition of aminoglycosides to the treatment regimen widens the antibiotic spectrum but increases cost and the potential for toxicosis. Inappropriate antibiotic combinations such as penicillin and chloramphenicol may be ineffective.

Parenteral treatment is used initially, and either intravenous infusions or boluses are preferable to intramuscular injection. The ultimate choice of antibiotic therapy is based on the clinical situation, results of culture and sensitivity, patient serum bacteriocidal tests, and feasibility of parenteral therapy. The combination of ampicillin and gentamicin (2 mg/kg t.i.d.) is recommended by the authors when blood cultures are negative or cannot be obtained. Antibiotics are given for four to six weeks, although it is unusual to continue parenteral treatment (e.g., gentamicin) for more than 14 days. At that time, a suitable oral antibiotic such as ampicillin or Keflex (20 mg/kg, t.i.d.) is chosen for the duration of therapy. Supportive care, such as intravenous fluid therapy, diuretics for congestive heart failure, and medical or surgical management of the precipitating cause, is important. Following release from the hospital, the patient is re-examined at frequent intervals.

SUPPLEMENTAL READING

Buchanan, J. W.: Chronic valvular disease (endocardiosis) in dogs. Adv. Vet. Sci. Comp. Med. 21:75, 1977.
Whitney, J. C.: Observations on the effect of age on the severity of heart valve lesions in the dog. J. Small Anim. Pract. 15:511, 1974.

CANINE MYOCARDIAL DISEASES

GARY L. WOOD, D.V.M.

Portland, Oregon

Myocardial diseases of dogs vary greatly in their etiology, presentation, and clinical management. The myocardium is affected by apparently diverse disease states. In its own primary disease form, it causes dysfunction in many other organs. A dog presenting with myocardial disease may or may not appear as a typical "heart case." The veterinarian must have a high index of suspicion for myocardial involvement to recognize its frequent occurrence secondary to other disorders. The most frequent clinical finding associated with myocardial disease is cardiac arrhythmia. Signs of congestive heart failure also occur frequently. When either of these occurs, the veterinarian is then challenged to rule out myocardial disease.

In this article, a clinical approach to myocardial diseases (see also page 329), and specific myocardial disorders and their management will be described. Myocardial diseases are broadly divided into those of known etiology and those of unknown etiology, i.e., the cardiomyopathies. After discussing the cardiomyopathies, myocardial diseases associated with infectious agents, infiltrative processes, ischemia, metabolic defects, and physical and toxic agents will be described.

APPROACH TO MYOCARDIAL DISEASES

DIAGNOSIS

The approach to canine myocardial diseases must be guided by the whole animal concept. Knowledge of the cardiovascular effects on other organs, particularly the nervous, respiratory, and urinary systems, is called upon in each case. Table 1 lists some of the clinical signs that may be associated with myocardial diseases and many other diseases. When a dog presents with one or more of these signs, a minimum data base should be collected and evaluated. After all information is evaluated, additional items are added until the problem is defined sufficiently for clinical management. Frequently the dog with myocardial disease requires treatment before the minimum data base is complete. Or the stress of collecting data may be harmful or fatal if done before clinical signs are controlled.

Table 2 lists the minimum data base used in the author's clinic for dogs with suspected myocardial disease. "History" and "Physical examination" call for a different emphasis from that for other problems. Much time is spent with the owner defining the presenting complaint by confirming or eliminating the items in Table 1. In addition to the complete routine physical exam, special emphasis is placed on color and refill time of mucous membranes; auscultation of heart and lung sounds; character of veins and arteries and their pulses; and palpation of the thorax, abdomen, and subcutaneous tissues. The synchrony of the heart rate and rhythm with that of the femoral pulse is noted. Often, by the time the examination is completed, a tentative diagnosis can be made.

The rest of the data base is then used in a confirmatory manner, which may give the veterinarian confidence to begin specific therapy sooner. The minimum data base is still collected for concurrent diseases or organ dysfunction may be present. The emphasis of the history and physical findings may be misleading, and baseline information is needed to later evaluate the success of treatment.

Table 1. *Frequent Presenting Signs in Myocardial Diseases*

Tachypnea	Syncope
Dyspnea	Seizures
Wheezing	Sudden death
Cough	Fever
Orthopnea	Diarrhea
Cyanosis	Cyanosis
Anorexia	Restlessness
Weight loss	Subcutaneous edema
Cachexia	Abdominal distention
Depression	Abdominal pain
Weakness	Pink fluid in nose and mouth
Exercise intolerance	Chest wall heave

Table 2. *Minimum Data Base for Suspected Myocardial Disease*

Signalment
History
Physical examination
Hemogram
Blood chemistry profile
Microfilaria check
Electrocardiogram
Dorsoventral and lateral thoracic radiographs
Cardiac enzymes
Transudate fluid analysis

TREATMENT

In treating dogs with myocardial disease, it is helpful to keep the following therapeutic principles in mind. The first principle is that client education and cooperation will affect the outcome more than any other factor. It is the client who will actually treat the patient. The more educated and cooperative the client, the more rewarding clinical management will be. Of course, this means spending more time initially to give the client the knowledge he needs to care for the dog.

Another therapeutic principle is the classic adage of medicine "first, do no harm." Dogs with myocardial disease are often severely ill, and the clinician may be tempted to try anything. It must be remembered that many drugs are potentially dangerous.

The third principle for treating dogs with myocardial disease is to define the severity of the disease and match treatment intensity to it. For example, dogs with cardiomyopathy are often in phase IV (class IV, New York Heart Association scheme) congestive heart failure and need very intensive treatment. They are not likely to survive with mere sodium restriction and slow oral digitalization. Change in therapeutic intensity must be guided by careful re-evaluation of the patient.

A fourth principle is that successful management of dogs with myocardial disease depends, to a great degree, on the recognition and control of cardiac arrhythmias. Arrhythmias frequently signal myocardial involvement, and they may actually pinpoint affected areas of the heart. The goal of arrhythmia therapy is to find and treat the cause. Antiarrhythmic drugs are often necessary. See other articles in this section for details.

MYOCARDIAL DISEASES OF UNKNOWN ETIOLOGY

CONGESTIVE (DILATED) CARDIOMYOPATHY

Cardiomyopathy means degenerative disease of the heart muscle. This suggests, but does not require, a generalized malady of the muscular tissue of the heart.

In congestive cardiomyopathy, degenerative changes are apparent biochemically, ultrastructurally, microscopically, and grossly. The significant gross change from a clinical point of view is marked generalized dilatation of all cardiac chambers. Hypertrophy is also present but is masked by the severity of chamber dilatation. The dilatation is associated with severe hypokinesis, which may be recognized by fluoroscopy, echocardiography, or angiocardiography. Contractility is greatly reduced, causing a decreased cardiac output and eventual severe congestive heart failure despite compensatory mechanisms. Usually atrial dilatation and degenerative changes become severe enough to cause atrial fibrillation, which further reduces cardiac output and worsens congestive heart failure. Although many etiologies have been suggested, the cause of congestive cardiomyopathy in dogs (and most animals) remains obscure.

HISTORY

Dogs of any age over about 15 to 20 kg body weight of either sex may be affected by congestive cardiomyopathy. However, the typical presentation is a young to middle-aged, male, large or giant breed dog with sudden onset of severe congestive heart failure. Frequently, the only prior suggestion of illness is weight loss or subtle premonitions of the impending heart failure. Other abnormalities are occasionally observed (see Table 1). It is probable that subclinical disease exists for some time, with sudden decompensation at the onset of atrial fibrillation.

PHYSICAL FINDINGS

Physical examination reflects any combination of signs of congestive heart failure. Signs of left or right heart failure may occur first. Often generalized heart failure is evident at presentation. Clinical signs include venous distention, fatigue, weakness, dyspnea, orthopnea, cough, abdominal distention, or, more rarely, peripheral edema. Most signs are caused by fluid transudation into body cavities or organ parenchymas and inadequate tissue perfusion. Ascites, hepatomegaly, pleural effusion, or pulmonary edema often results.

Auscultatory findings vary from muffled respiratory and cardiac sounds to loud, harsh, and moist respiratory sounds and a pounding heart. Heart sounds are difficult to characterize owing to masking respiratory noise, rapid heart rate, and an often irregular rhythm. Frequently an S_3 gallop is audible. Owing to dilatation of the atrioventricular rings, grade 1 to 3/6 soft systolic murmurs are usually audible over the mitral and tricuspid valves. However, murmurs may initially be inaudible owing to tachycardia and interfering respiratory sounds. The heart rate is usually between 150 and 250 beats per minute. A pulse deficit of 20 to 100 signals atrial fibrillation, premature arrhythmias, or both. The heart and pulse rates are hard to count because they vary greatly in amplitude and frequency owing to atrial fibrillation. Sometimes sinus rhythm is present. If so, tachycardia without a pulse deficit or irregularity is noted.

ECG, X-RAY, LABORATORY FINDINGS

The most frequent electrocardiographic finding is atrial fibrillation with signs of generalized cardiomegaly (Fig. 1). In atrial fibrillation, P waves are absent and R-R intervals vary in a random manner.

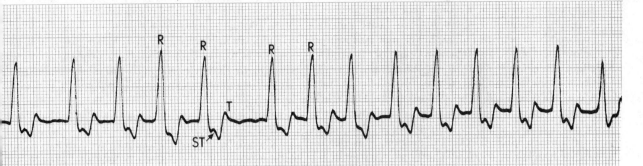

Figure 1. Lead II electrocardiogram from a six-year-old Great Dane with severe generalized congestive heart failure. The rhythm is atrial fibrillation. Note absence of P waves and irregular R-R intervals. The heart rate is about 200 bpm. There is evidence of left ventricular enlargement and myocardial ischemia. Note tall, wide QRS complexes and depressed ST segments. Paper speed = 50 mm/sec. ½ cm = 1 mV.

QRS complexes may exceed 0.06 sec in duration or 3 mV in amplitude, suggesting left ventricular enlargement. The mean electrical axis in the frontal plane is normal. As stated previously, the heart rate is excessive. Myocardial ischemia and congestive heart failure may be associated with ST segment and T wave changes or ventricular premature complexes.

Radiography is usually best delayed until the stress involved is not endangering. If not obscured by pleural fluid, the cardiac silhouette is very large in all dimensions. In addition, caudal vena caval distention, pulmonary vascular prominence, or the interstitial and alveolar density of pulmonary edema may be present in any combination. Large pleural effusions are not uncommon. Hepatomegaly or poor abdominal detail from ascites may be present on abdominal films. Fluoroscopic or echocardiographic examination usually shows marked hypokinesis.

Laboratory findings only confirm the presence of severe congestive heart failure. Mild to moderate hypoproteinemia, azotemia, and elevation of liver enzymes occur. Elevation of aspartate aminotransferase (SGOT) or lactate dehydrogenase (LDH) probably reflects liver congestion rather than myocardial disease. Analysis of pleural or abdominal fluid is compatible with a true or modified transudate. Chylothorax is a rare finding. A disproportionate number of dogs with congestive cardiomyopathy show laboratory evidence of hypothyroidism. The significance of this finding is not understood.

MANAGEMENT

Clinical management of congestive cardiomyopathy involves controlling severe congestive heart failure. Success can usually be measured by the degree to which the excessive ventricular rate is reduced. Exercise reduction and sodium restriction are important. Dry or moist low-sodium prescription diets such as H/D* or homemade meat-rice-vegetable diets are recommended. When guided by informational handouts, it is surprising how many dog owners are willing and able to prepare special diets.

Digoxin,† because it slows atrioventricular nodal conduction, is used to slow the ventricular rate. Furthermore, it increases myocardial contractility. For their size, large and giant breed dogs do not tolerate as much glycoside as smaller dogs, frequently requiring a daily maintenance dose of 0.375 to 0.75 mg divided b.i.d. Tablets are preferred to elixirs for large dogs. It may be necessary to rapidly digitalize initially.‡ A loading dose is calculated using 0.06 to 0.1 mg/kg. This total dose is given to effect in four to six divided oral doses over 48 hours. If adequate clinical response or clinical or electrocardiographic signs of toxicity develop before the entire loading dose is given, subsequent doses are delayed for 12 to 24 hours and maintenance levels started. The maintenance dose is ⅒ to ¼ the total loading dose, which is usually 0.375 to 0.75 mg divided b.i.d.§ Frequent electrocardiograms may be necessary initially, since the heart rate and especially the rhythm are difficult to determine when atrial fibrillation is present as the initial rhythm.

Furosemide‖ mobilizes retained transudates and pulmonary edema and prevents continued fluid accumulation. Initial doses may be given intravenously, intramuscularly, or orally, depending on the severity of congestive heart failure. A dose of 2 to 4 mg/kg should be given two to four times the first day, followed by 0.5 to 2 mg/kg once or twice daily as clinical signs improve. If frequent or higher doses are necessary, serum electrolyte and urea nitrogen or creatinine determinations should be repeated.

---

*H/D, Hills Division Riviana Food, Inc., Topeka, KS.

†Lanoxin, Burroughs Wellcome Co., Research Triangle Park, NC.

‡Editor's Note: Loading doses are advocated only in severe CHF.

§Editor's Note: Some giant breed dogs (particularly Doberman pinschers) may require 0.25 mg/day.

‖Lasix, Hoechst-Roussel Pharmaceuticals, Inc., Somerville, NJ.

Lower doses of furosemide or potassium chloride supplementation may become necessary.

If, after acute management, the heart rate (as assessed by electrocardiography) cannot be lowered below the 150 to 170 range, propranolol* is used to effect. Beginning with 10 mg t.i.d., the dose is titrated until the desired slowing of heart rate occurs. It is unusual to need more than 40 mg t.i.d. Because it is a beta-adrenergic blocking agent, propranolol has negative inotropic as well as negative chronotrophic effects. In addition, it is potentially bronchoconstrictive. Therefore, it should be used cautiously and dosed on an individual basis in congestive heart failure. At this writing there is no information about the use of other beta blockers in the treatment of canine congestive cardiomyopathy.

It is usually fruitless to attempt electric or pharmacologic conversion of atrial fibrillation to normal sinus rhythm, except when it occurs in a dog with only mild atrial enlargement, which is rare. Synchronized electrical cardioversion is necessary, followed by quinidine.† The vast majority of dogs with cardiomyopathy return to atrial fibrillation within a few days to a few weeks of cardioversion.

In recent years, the use of vasodilating agents for congestive heart failure has received much attention in human and veterinary medicine. More information is necessary before the routine use of vasodilators can be recommended in canine cardiomyopathy. However, in those animals that do not respond to the regimen previously outlined, the use of these agents is recommended. The veterinarian must thoroughly understand the pharmacophysiology and rationale of vasodilator therapy and the individual agents to be used (see Drugs Used in the Management of Heart Failure, page 297).

In limited studies, several vasodilating agents have been shown to have beneficial effects in canine congestive heart failure. The author uses hydralazine‡ in refractory cases. The usual initial dose is 0.5 to 1 mg/kg. This dose is then continued or titrated upward until either the desired response or side effects occur. In the acute situation another dose is given as often as every two hours to a maximum of 6 mg/kg/day. Close attention is paid to the character and rate of pulses, membrane color and capillary refill time, and degree of dyspnea. When pulses become stronger, capillary refill time shortens, and dyspnea wanes, the desired level has been reached. If adverse effects such as depression, weakness, disorientation, weakened pulses, syncope, or worsening of heart failure occur, hydralazine is tried at a lower dose or another agent is substituted. Titration is made easier if indirect blood pressure and venous oxygen tension can be monitored. The b.i.d. maintenance dose is 50 to 100 per cent of the total titration dose needed to achieve improvement. In typical cases, this is usually between 1 and 3 mg/kg b.i.d. An alternate vasodilator that is particularly useful for refractory ascites or edema is captopril (Capoten§), 1 to 2 mg/kg t.i.d.

Even with successful treatment, it is hard to predict the outcome in individual cases. Some do not survive the initial visit; others live several years. Although the prognosis must be guarded to poor, it is best based on regular clinical re-evaluation and not on the severity of the initial presentation. A complete re-evaluation should be repeated at three-month intervals or more often if problems develop.

HYPERTROPHIC CARDIOMYOPATHY

Hypertrophic cardiomyopathy occurs in several species including dogs. In this condition the ventricular wall becomes thickened and stiff by inappropriate muscular hypertrophy. This process involves the left ventricle more than the right and may occur symmetrically or asymmetrically. In symmetric hypertrophy both the free wall and ventricular septum are equally involved. In asymmetric hypertrophy, which is apparently more common in dogs, the ventricular septum is disproportionately thickened.

Hypertrophic cardiomyopathy in dogs is difficult to recognize ante mortem, as there may be no clinical signs prior to sudden death. Whenever unexplained death occurs, especially during general anesthesia, hypertrophic cardiomyopathy should be ruled out. If clinical signs do appear, syncope, behavioral changes, arrhythmias, and evidence of congestive heart failure may be observed. German shepherds may be predisposed. Electrocardiography may reveal evidence of left ventricular enlargement or conduction disturbances such as first degree atrioventricular block, complete heart block, or bundle branch block. Or ECG findings may be normal. Thoracic radiographs may suggest cardiomegaly, especially of the left heart, and pulmonary congestion or edema. Experience with clinical management is limited. In those cases recognized in time, control of congestive heart failure with diuretics, low-sodium diet, and perhaps venodilators is indicated. Use of digitalis glycosides may be contraindicated in the face of atrioventricular conduction disturbances or obstructive hypertrophy. Experience with other species suggests that propranolol and calcium antagonists (verapamil) should be helpful.

---

*Inderal, Ayerst Laboratories, New York, NY.
†Quinidine Sulfate, Eli Lilly and Co., Indianapolis, IN.
‡Apresoline, Ciba Pharmaceutical Co., Summit, NJ.

§E. R. Squibb & Sons, Inc., Princeton, NJ.

OTHER MYOCARDIAL DISEASES OF UNKNOWN ORIGIN

BOXER MYOCARDITIS

A syndrome of myocarditis occurs in the boxer breed. For a complete discussion of this condition see the following article.

DOBERMAN CARDIOMYOPATHY

As veterinary cardiologists become more skilled in recognizing differences in animals with myocardial diseases, additional distinct varieties will become apparent and may parallel those in other species. A variety of cardiomyopathy different from that seen in other dogs occurs in Doberman pinschers. This disorder may be familial.

These dogs present with severe left ventricular failure, sometimes without atrial fibrillation (Fig. 2). Electrocardiographically, we may find atrial fibrillation or sinus tachycardia, sometimes interrupted by premature ventricular complexes or ventricular tachycardia. Evidence of severe ventricular degenerative disease, conduction disturbances, or ventricular enlargement is suggested by very wide QRS complexes, slurred ST segments, and large T waves. Radiographically, the size of the cardiac shadow, and especially that of the left atrium and ventricle, may be large. However, cardiac size is often not as great as expected. The alveolar pattern associated with pulmonary edema is accompanied by additional mixed pulmonary densities, giving the lung fields an unusually dense appearance. Low-output heart failure, shock, and prerenal azotemia are common.

The prognosis in these cases is worse than in other dogs with cardiomyopathy. Clinical management is similar to that outlined previously for congestive cardiomyopathy, except that ventricular arrhythmias may not improve with digitalization. Additional antiarrhythmic therapy such as procainamide or propranolol may be required (see page 369). Diuretic doses are high. The use of vasodilators may be called for earlier. Fluid therapy may be indicated if there is low cardiac output (see page 283).

MYOCARDIAL DISEASES OF KNOWN ETIOLOGY

INFECTIOUS AGENTS

Infectious agents may affect the myocardium directly or indirectly. Until recently, primary inflammatory disease of the myocardium associated with an infectious agent was considered rare in dogs.

PARVOVIRUS MYOCARDITIS

In 1978, a viral myocarditis associated with the previously unrecognized canine parvovirus was seen in several parts of the world. It appeared that a truly new disease entity had developed. Typically, the disease affects pups four to eight weeks of age, although the real age limits of infection are not clear. Infection probably occurs *in utero* or in the first few weeks of life. It is thought that the virus invades myocardial cells during a narrow period of susceptible myocardial proliferation. Typically this virus attacks more rapidly proliferating cells, such as those of the gastrointestinal or lymphoid system. Some litters may be affected by both the gastrointestinal and myocardial forms of the disease; however, in the four- to six-week age group, myocardial disease alone is more typical.

Any number in the litter may be affected. The most frequently observed clinical sign is sudden

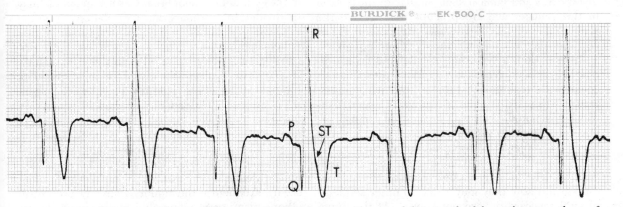

Figure 2. Lead II electrocardiogram from a five-year-old Doberman with severe left ventricular failure. There is evidence of generalized cardiomegaly and partial left bundle branch block. Note wide P waves, deep Q waves, tall R waves, wide QRS complexes, slurred ST segments, and large T waves. This dog developed atrial fibrillation and died after a short clinical course despite vigorous therapy. Paper speed = 50 mm/sec. 1 cm = 1 mV.

death, often with no premonitory signs. Some pups show dyspnea, depression, anorexia, crying out, vomiting, or convulsive movements a few minutes to several hours before death. Often the opportunity for veterinary examination is lost owing to early death. Those pups that are examined ante mortem may show dyspnea, tachycardia, systolic cardiac murmurs, ventricular gallop rhythms, arrhythmias, or pink fluid in the nose and mouth. Electrocardiograms may show small R waves, ST segment elevation, QRS notching, or ventricular tachycardia. Small R waves indicate a poor prognosis, as Robinson and associates (1979) found that five of seven pups with R waves less than 0.4 mV in lead II died, whereas four of four pups with R waves greater than 0.5 mV in lead II survived. Treatment with oxygen, diuretics, antiarrhythmics, and supportive care usually causes temporary improvement. However, many pups will die despite vigorous treatment.

At necropsy, evidence of congestive heart failure of varying degrees may be seen. Heavy, wet lungs, frothy fluid in airways, fluid in pleural or peritoneal cavities, or hepatomegaly may be found. The heart may not show any gross abnormalities; however, pale streaks or engorged epicardial vessels may be noted. The myocardium and endocardium may be marked by varying degrees of gray, brown, or white discoloration. There may or may not be dilatation of either ventricle or the left atrium. The most distinguishing histopathologic finding, when present, is large, dense intranuclear myocardial inclusion bodies. Other microscopic changes mirror the gross findings of chronic passive congestion or edema in affected organs.

The maximum age that dogs may be affected by myocardial parvovirus is not known. In addition, the spectrum of sequelae in surviving pups is not well understood, nor is how these sequelae may be altered by vaccination or treatment. Some pups in the 8- to 16-week age group may continue to have myocarditis and clinical signs similar to those seen in the younger age group. Pups that survive the acute phase of the disease may suffer sequelae at any later date with a wide variety of consequences.

In some dogs a syndrome of post-viral myocardiopathy has been recognized. Various presentations occur, with weakness, waxing and waning murmurs, tachycardias, arrhythmias, or congestive heart failure being noted. Serologic testing for canine parvovirus sometimes suggests previous infection, but titers are difficult to interpret in this age group. Cardiac dysfunction may continue or may be self-limiting. The long-term consequences of this condition, and how they may relate to other sequelae of viral myocarditis, are not known. At this time, symptomatic therapy of these disorders includes digitalization, diuretics, and antiarrhythmic drugs.

It has been speculated that the idiopathic varieties of cardiomyopathy are long-term consequences

of viral myocarditis in many species, including dogs. This connection has been reiterated with the advent of canine parvovirus, even though cardiomyopathy was a well-established canine disease entity before parvovirus appeared. It will be interesting to observe whether cardiomyopathy incidence increases following parvovirus outbreaks.

OTHER INFECTIOUS AGENTS

Bacteria that affect the myocardium may spread there hematogenously or may spread from the endocardium or valves in animals with bacterial endocarditis. Myocardial involvement is usually signaled by tachyarrhythmias. Management consists of appropriate antimicrobial therapy, control of arrhythmias, and prevention of congestive heart failure and thromboembolism.

A wide variety of other infectious agents may cause myocarditis. Any of the so-called deep funguses or other fungal agents, such as *Aspergillus* sp., may involve the heart. *Toxoplasma gondii* preferentially encysts in the myocardium, brain, and skeletal muscle, but the clinical significance of this is unknown. *Trypanosoma cruzi*, causative agent of Chagas' disease in humans in South America, may affect dogs in the southwestern United States. This organism primarily attacks myocardial cells. Myocarditis occurs secondary to exerimental distemper virus infection. As immunosuppressive agents are used more commonly in veterinary medicine, we can expect unusual cardiac infections to increase in incidence.

INFILTRATIVE MYOCARDIAL DISEASES

Diseases that result in the invasion of the myocardium by abnormal substances or cells are called *infiltrative myocardial diseases*. The most common of these in dogs is neoplasia. Cardiac neoplasia may be divided into primary and metastatic varieties.

The most common primary cardiac tumor in dogs is hemangiosarcoma. This neoplasm may arise primarily in the heart, most often in the right atrium. It may arise multicentrically, or it may spread to the heart from other locations, such as the spleen, liver, or lungs. Older German shepherds are predisposed to develop cardiac hemangiosarcoma. The most frequent presentation is sudden collapse, dyspnea, and weakness, often associated with acute or chronic hemorrhage into the pericardium. Supraventricular and ventricular arrhythmias often occur. Frequently the tumor is already present in other organs or is inoperable in the heart by the time of diagnosis. However, pericardiocentesis followed by exploratory pericardectomy should be considered in those cases in which multiple organ involvement is not demonstrated. Nonselective angiocardiography, pneumopericardiography, or echocardiography may help to define the extent of disease, but surgery should not be long delayed. Solitary right atrial masses may be amputated successfully. The client should be warned that metastasis is likely and that chemotherapy has been disappointing.

Another neoplasm that invades the heart is the chemodectoma, or heart base tumor. This tumor arises from the aortic body chemoreceptor cells and grows between and into the aorta, the pulmonary artery, and the base of the heart. Nearly all affected dogs are of brachiocephalic breeds. The tumor is usually slow to enlarge but invades vital structures so that curative operation is usually impossible by the time of diagnosis. Frequently, pericardial effusion, various arrhythmias, and signs of congestive heart failure appear. Accordingly, treatment consists of pericardiocentesis, pericardiectomy, appropriate antiarrhythmic therapy, or congestive heart failure management. Again, chemotherapy has been unsatisfactory.

A wide variety of other primary and metastatic neoplasms, such as lymphosarcoma and thyroid carcinoma, rarely invade the myocardium. Arrhythmias are the usual signals of myocardial involvement. Angiocardiography and echocardiography are helpful diagnostic aids. Management consists of controlling abnormal rhythms and reducing tumor size without disrupting cardiac function. Surgery may be more useful than anticipated. It is important to get a cell type diagnosis, as some tumors, particularly lymphosarcoma, respond to multi-drug chemotherapy or immunotherapy.

Invasion of the myocardium with amyloid material is rare. It may or may not be accompanied by invasion of other organs such as the kidneys. The prognosis is poor.

ISCHEMIC MYOCARDIAL DISEASE

MYOCARDIAL INFARCTION

Naturally occurring major coronary artery disease is rare in dogs. "Heart attacks" are diagnosed much more often than they occur. Dogs with hypothyroidism may rarely have coronary atherosclerosis and infarction. The most frequent causes of coronary obstruction in dogs are embolization from bacterial valvular vegetations or neoplasms and septicemic conditions. Angina is apparently rare; however, electrocardiographic and enzymatic changes may parallel the findings in humans with coronary obstruction. Unfortunately, no data exist with which to develop pathognomonic clinical findings for infarction in dogs. When serial electrocardiograms are available and sudden changes in ST segments, T waves, or mean electrical axis occur; or when Q waves, bundle branch block, atrioventricular block, low voltage QRS complexes, or ventricular arrhythmias suddenly develop, infarction may be suspected.

One can be more certain of infarction when electrocardiographic signs are accompanied by myocardial muscle enzyme elevations. When myocardial cell injury is sufficient, creatinine phosphokinase (CPK), SGOT, and LDH may be released into the blood stream and measured at abnormally high levels. Cardiac trauma or severe myocarditis may also cause these elevations. Disease or injury in many other tissues, such as skeletal muscle, liver, and brain, may cause serum elevations of these enzymes. Sometimes the enzyme absolute values are within normal limits, but elevated levels of the cardiac isoenzymes of CPK (MB CPK) and LDH (LDH 1) may be present. Unless these are measured, myocardial cell damage may be undetected. Isoenzyme and total enzyme values are almost always normal in noninflammatory myocardial disease such as cardiomyopathy, atrioventricular valve insufficiency, and microscopic intramural myocardial infarction.

Since most myocardial infarctions in dogs are secondary, the most important factor in treatment is to define and control the primary disease. Frequent re-evaluation and monitoring are necessary. Good supportive care, arrhythmia control, and prevention of congestive heart failure are important. For its antiplatelet-aggregation effects, aspirin may be empirically given at a dose of 10 mg/kg b.i.d. Aspirin is contraindicated in thrombocytopenia, which occurs in some bacterial infections. Nitroglycerine ointment may have a role in the treatment of dogs with concurrent CHF.

MICROSCOPIC INTRAMURAL MYOCARDIAL INFARCTIONS

Microscopic intramural myocardial infarctions occur as a part of the acquired atrioventricular valve insufficiency syndrome. Small intramural coronary arteries, particularly in and near the left ventricular papillary muscles, undergo intimal and medial hyaline degeneration and progressive occlusion. Nearby myocardium undergoes necrosis and ultimate fibrosis. These changes are microscopic in size yet possibly cause significant functional changes. Reduction in myocardial contractility, genesis of supraventricular or ventricular tachyarrhythmias, and impairment of mitral valve apparatus function are potential sequelae. These dogs may be more prone to syncope due to cardiac arrhythmias. This disorder may be suspected when tachyarrhythmias occur and when electrocardiograms show marked slurring or notching of the downstroke of the QRS complex. Essentially, management of dogs with microscopic intramural myocardial infarctions parallels that for other dogs with atrioventricular valve insufficiency.

SUBAORTIC STENOSIS

Focal areas of necrosis, fibrosis, and calcification seen in the hypertrophic myocardium of dogs with congenital subaortic stenosis probably are also ischemic in origin. Syncope and sudden death are commonly observed in these dogs. Propranolol may be useful for both its antiarrhythmic properties and its ability to reduce left ventricular oxygen consumption.

METABOLIC MYOCARDIAL DISEASES

The myocardium may be adversely affected by a wide variety of metabolic conditions. A complete discussion is impossible, but a partial list includes myocardial depressant factors in shock and pancreatic disease, endotoxins, electrolyte imbalances, anemia, adrenal dysfunction, renal disease, obesity, pyometra, systemic lupus erythematosus, diabetes mellitus, hypertension, acidosis, and pregnancy. Only thyroid dysfunction and gastric dilatation and volvulus will be discussed here.

THYROID DYSFUNCTION

Myocardial performance may be adversely affected by either excessive or inadequate thyroid function. In hyperthyroidism, the heart is stimulated to beat more rapidly and more forcibly, with a subsequent increase in cardiac output. Over time, as the cardiac workload increases, compensatory hypertrophy occurs. If the potential for compensation is exceeded, congestive heart failure may occur. Pregnancy or anemia may have similar effects. Unless digitalis-sensitive arrhythmias are present, the use of digitalis glycosides in this so-called high-output failure is not indicated. When euthyroidism is achieved, progression toward normal occurs. In the meantime, propranolol and furosemide are indicated.

Hypothyroidism may complicate congestive heart failure by decreasing myocardial contractility. Sinus bradycardia and low amplitude ECGs may be associated with hypothyroidism. Hypothyroid animals also require lower doses of digitalis glycosides, as they eliminate them more slowly. When the dog is rendered euthyroid by treatment, management becomes easier. As stated previously, hypothyroidism may be seen in dogs with cardiomyopathy or ischemic heart disease secondary to atherosclerosis.

GASTRIC DILATATION AND VOLVULUS

In acute gastric dilatation or volvulus reduced cardiac output, hypoxemia due to shock, release of cardiodepressant peptides, and dysautonomia can cause ventricular arrhythmias. Premature ventric-

ular complexes, ventricular tachycardia, or other ventricular arrhythmias may arise at any time from presentation to a few days after the acute episode. As arrhythmias are often the cause of death in these cases, their control becomes an important part of clinical management in the syndrome.

Physical examination for evidence of arrhythmias and electrocardiographic monitoring should be routine. Premature ventricular complexes and ventricular tachycardia are treated initially with intravenous lidocaine* (without epinephrine). A dose of 2 to 4 mg/kg is given in one to two minutes. A beneficial effect is usually obvious almost immediately and lasts 10 to 30 minutes. Recurrence of arrhythmias is prevented by an intravenous drip of lidocaine, 1 to 2 mg/ml, at whatever rate is necessary to maintain sinus rhythm. Periodically stopping the drip will help determine the minimum amount of necessary drug. Depression, tremors, or convulsions signal toxicity, requiring a decreased dose and, ocasionally, the administration of 5 to 15 mg intravenous diazepam.† Lidocaine is only maintained until intramuscular or oral treatment is possible, at which time quinidine gluconate‡ or sulfate is used. The initial dose is 10 mg/kg q.i.d. (range from 5 to 20 mg/kg). This dose may be altered if initial therapy is ineffective. Available longer-acting quinidine products in equal tablet doses to quinidine sulfate can be given b.i.d. to t.i.d. Gastrointestinal problems are frequently reported side effects of quinidine products. If ineffective, they may be combined with or replaced by procainamide,§ 125 to 500 mg orally t.i.d. to q.i.d., or lidocaine as mentioned previously. Gradual weaning from antiarrhythmic therapy is done over a period of 7 to 21 days if abnormal rhythms do not recur.

TOXIC AND PHYSICAL MYOCARDIAL DISEASES

TOXINS

A wide variety of toxic substances, including drugs, anesthetic agents, heavy metals, alcohol, and venoms, are known to be injurious to the myocardium in humans and animals. The degree to which many of these affect dogs is unknown. Ironically, iatrogenic causes are the most commonly recognized cardiac toxicities.

The antineoplastic antibiotic doxorubicin‖ may cause cardiomyopathy and profound congestive heart failure. The mechanism is not clear; however, the drug binds to myocardial DNA and later causes marked biventricular failure. This effect is more

---

*Xylocaine, Astra Pharmaceutical Products, Inc., Worcester, MA.
†Valium, Roche Products, Inc., Manati, Puerto Rico.
‡Quinidine Gluconate, Eli Lilly and Co., Indianapolis, IN.
§Pronestyl, American Pharmaceutical Co., Passaic, NJ.
‖Adriamycin, Adria Laboratories, Inc., Columbus, OH.

likely at cumulative doses exceeding 160 to 250 mg/M^2. However, its occurrence cannot be predicted accurately in individual cases. Atrioventricular and fascicular blocks may occur. The combined use of digitalis glycosides, diuretics, and vasodilators is useful for medical therapy. The prognosis is poor.

TRAUMA

Penetration or blunt trauma to the heart often causes contusion, laceration, or infarction of the myocardium. These injuries may easily go unnoticed. In addition, cardiac arrhythmias may occur in dogs with trauma not obviously involving the chest. Arrhythmias secondary to brain and spinal cord trauma, possibly mediated by the autonomic nervous system, have been reported. For these reasons, electrocardiograms and thoracic radiographs should be taken often in trauma cases. Anesthesia should be delayed until the effects of cardiac dysfunction are assessed and controlled. Usually, with proper supportive therapy, myocardial injuries heal completely in a matter of days. Sometimes antiarrhythmic therapy as outlined under gastric dilatation and volvulus is necessary.

ELECTRIC SHOCK

Electric shock can have peracute or acute adverse effects on the myocardium. The immediate danger is ventricular fibrillation or cardiac arrest. Those dogs, usually pups, that survive immediate electrocution often develop acute left ventricular failure. The pathogenesis is not understood. Treatment includes 2 to 4 mg/kg furosemide intravenously, 10 mg/kg aminophylline* slowly intravenously, and 10 mg/kg prednisolone sodium succinate† intrave-

---

*Aminophyllin, Searle Laboratories, Chicago, IL.
†Solu Delta Cortef, The Upjohn Co., Kalamazoo, MI.

nously. Narcotic sedation, oxygen, or vasodilators may be needed. Digitalis glycosides are infrequently used.

The canine myocardium can be affected by a wide variety of apparently unrelated conditions. The incidence of any single disease is low. Taken together, however, they account for frequent myocardial involvement. The myocardium responds to adversity in limited ways. The majority of cases have clinical signs attributable to arrhythmias or congestive heart failure. Even though these signs may vary widely, if the veterinarian maintains a high index of suspicion for myocardial disease, it can be recognized and treated appropriately.

SUPPLEMENTAL READING

Bonagura, J.: Acute heart failure. *In* Kirk, R. W. (ed.): *Current Veterinary Therapy VII.* Philadelphia: W. B. Saunders, 1980, pp. 359–367.

Carpenter, J. L., Roberts, R. M., Harpster, N. K., and King, N. W., Jr.: Intestinal and cardiopulmonary forms of parvovirus infection in a litter of pups. J.A.V.M.A. 176:1269, 1980.

Hayes, M. A., Russell, R. G., and Babiuk, L. A.: Sudden death in young dogs with myocarditis caused by parvovirus. J.A.V.M.A. 174:1197, 1979.

Hurst, J. W. (ed.): *The Heart*, 4th ed. New York: McGraw-Hill, 1978.

Jezyk, P. F., Haskins, M. E., and Jones, C. L.: Myocarditis of probable viral origin in pups of weaning age. J.A.V.M.A. 174:1204, 1979.

Liu, S. K., Tilley, L. P., and Maron, B. J.: Canine hypertrophic cardiomyopathy. J.A.V.M.A. 174:708, 1979.

Mulvey, J. J., Bech-Nielsen, S., Haskins, M. E., Jezyk, P. F., Taylor, H. W., and Eugster, A. K.: Myocarditis induced by parvoviral infection in weanling pups in the United States. J.A.V.M.A. 177:695, 1980.

Robinson, W. F., Huxtable, C. R. R., Pass, D. A., and Howell, J. McC.: Clinical and electrocardiographic findings in suspected viral myocarditis of pups. Aust. Vet. J. 55:351, 1979.

Thomas, W. P.: Long-term therapy of chronic congestive heart failure in the dog and cat. *In* Kirk, R. W. (ed.): *Current Veterinary Therapy VII.* Philadelphia: W. B. Saunders, 1980, pp. 368–376.

Tilley, L. P.: *Essentials of Canine and Feline Electrocardiography.* St. Louis: C. V. Mosby, 1979.

Wood, L., Hirsh, D. C., Selcer, R. R., Rinaldi, M. G., and Boorman, G. A.: Disseminated aspergillosis in a dog. J.A.V.M.A. 172:704, 1978.

BOXER CARDIOMYOPATHY

NEIL K. HARPSTER, V.M.D.

Boston, Massachusetts

Over the past 15 years, a primary myocardial disorder has been recognized in the boxer breed. Unlike the majority of primary myocardial disorders that have been identified in large and giant breed dogs and are characterized by biventricular dilatation, atrial fibrillation, biventricular failure, and a paucity of microscopic myocardial changes, boxer cardiomyopathy is distinguished by an absence of similar degrees of ventricular dilation, infrequent occurrence of atrial fibrillation, and extensive histologic myocardial alterations.

Until recently, this disorder has been considered to have unique features not seen in other breeds. However, a similar condition has now been identi-

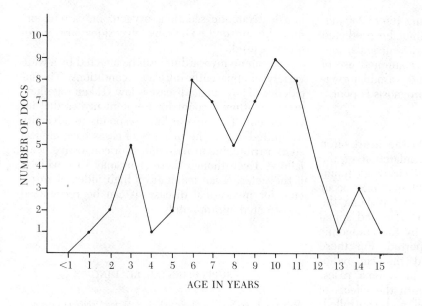

Figure 1. The age distribution in boxer cardiomyopathy (64 cases).

fied in a small number of Doberman pinschers. This article will deal with our observations and experience in 64 dogs with boxer cardiomyopathy.

ETIOLOGY

A specific cause of boxer cardiomyopathy has not been established. Therefore, by the accepted standards in humans (Oakley, 1974), this myocardial disorder fulfills the criteria for a primary cardiomyopathy. Based on the high incidence of this disorder among dogs in New England and its occurrence in a group of closely related dogs, an inherited origin must be strongly considered. An in-depth survey of affected dogs and their relationships is currently in progress.

INCIDENCE

The actual incidence of this disease in the boxer breed has not been defined. It is unquestionably of greater prevalence in some breeding lines than others, and multiple affected littermates from a single mating have been observed. In a group of 64 dogs with either proven cardiomyopathy or clinical findings strongly suggestive of that diagnosis, males (57.8 per cent) were more commonly affected than females. Although the ages of affected dogs ranged from 1 to 15 years, only 10 (15.6 per cent) were under six years of age, whereas 16 dogs (25 per cent) were older than ten years of age. The average age of affected dogs at the time of initial diagnosis was 8.2 years, with a median of 8.5 years. Figure 1 presents the age distribution in this group of 64 dogs.

CLINICAL FEATURES

The clinical signs in dogs with boxer cardiomyopathy can be nearly equally divided into three distinct categories. First, some dogs are presented with signs suggestive of syncope or episodes of weakness, usually related to stressful environmental conditions. In between these episodes the dogs are generally felt to be completely normal without other overt clinical signs. Second, some dogs are presented with clinical signs associated with heart failure. Left heart failure with its accompanying signs usually predominates, but biventricular failure may occur. Isolated right heart failure is unusual. Dogs in the third category do not evidence any clinical signs related to heart disease. These dogs are presented for routine office visits or for other unrelated complaints, and cardiac arrhythmias are found on physical examination. Table 1 summarizes the clinical signs in 64 dogs with boxer cardiomyopathy.

The most characteristic finding on physical examination is the presence of cardiac arrhythmias. Occasional to frequent premature beats are the

Table 1. *Clinical Signs in Boxer Cardiomyopathy (64 Cases)*

Presenting Sign	Number	Per Cent
Collapsing spell (syncope)	22	34.3
Coughing	15	23.4
Difficulty breathing	8	12.4
Weight loss	7	10.9
Abdominal enlargement	5	7.8
Generalized weakness	5	7.8
Hindleg weakness	4	6.2
None attributed to heart disease	21	32.8

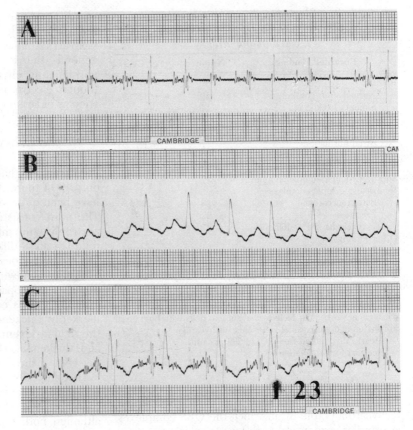

Figure 2. Single channel phonocardiographic (PCG) recording from a five-year-old female boxer with cardiomyopathy. *A*, The PCG alone is recorded and identifies the presence of three distinct heart sounds. *B*, A lead II electrocardiographic recording. When the PCG and electrocardiogram (ECG) are superimposed *(C)*, the relationship of the abnormal heart sound to the ECG can be defined. The abnormal third heart sound (3) occurs during the period of passive ventricular filling, characteristic of an S_3 gallop. 1 = first heart sound; 2 = second heart sound. Recordings were made at 50 mm/sec.

predominant finding, but paroxysmal tachyarrhythmias and a totally irregular ventricular rhythm also may be found on auscultation. These arrhythmias are frequently accompanied by a pulse deficit as well as a variability in the strength of the femoral pulse.

The second most common finding in boxer cardiomyopathy is the presence of a systolic or holosystolic murmur over the mitral area. The prevalence of mitral insufficiency tends to increase with disease severity, although the murmur never becomes as loud as those typically heard in dogs with chronic valvular heart disease. Auscultation of a diastolic gallop rhythm is a significant finding (Fig. 2). However, this is detected infrequently (Table 2). Other clinical findings that are commonly present but are nonspecific for boxer cardiomyopathy are those related to the heart failure state. Polypnea, dyspnea, moist rales, hepatomegaly, and peritoneal effusion may all be found, depending on the characteristics and the severity of heart failure.

The thoracic radiographic findings in boxer cardiomyopathy are quite variable and nonspecific. In the majority of the asymptomatic dogs (category 1) and in nearly 50 per cent of the dogs with syncopal episodes (category 2), the thoracic radiographs are within normal limits. In more advanced stages of the disease, varying degrees of generalized heart enlargement accompanied by mild to moderate left atrial enlargement are the expected findings. When left heart failure is present, pulmonary venous distention and pulmonary edema will be visualized. Pleural effusion is an uncommon finding.

In boxer cardiomyopathy the electrocardiographic findings are almost pathognomonic. Ventricular premature beats of variable frequency, which occur singly, in pairs, and in runs, are the most common finding. Somewhat less common, but of equal diagnostic importance, are paroxysms of ventricular

Table 2. *Abnormal Cardiovascular Findings in Boxer Cardiomyopathy (64 Cases)*

Physical Finding	Number	Per Cent
Polypnea/dyspnea	11	17.2
Cyanotic mucous membrane	8	12.5
Cardiac rhythm		
Regular	19	29.6
Regular with premature beats	31	48.4
Totally irregular	14	21.8
Tachycardia (HR >160/min)	24	37.4
Murmur of mitral insufficiency	32	50.0
Gallop rhythm	8	12.5
Abnormal lung sounds	14	21.8
Hepatomegaly	10	15.6
Ascites	7	10.9
Pulse deficit	16	25.0

Table 3. *Electrocardiographic Findings on Admission in 63 Dogs With Boxer Cardiomyopathy*

Recorded Finding	Number	Per Cent
Rhythm		
Normal sinus rhythm	20	31.7
Sinus tachycardia†	11	17.5
Paroxysmal supraventricular tachycardia	4	6.3
Atrial fibrillation	7	11.1
Paroxysmal ventricular tachycardia	22	34.9
Supraventricular ectopic complexes	7	11.1
Ventricular ectopic complexes		
Rare to occasional	23	36.5
Frequent	22	34.9
Tachycardia (HR >160/min)	27	42.9
Other findings		
Prolongation of QRS interval (>0.07 sec)	9	14.3
LVH pattern‡	7	11.1

*Predominant recorded rhythm on admission. Includes three dogs with both paroxysmal supraventricular tachycardia and paroxysmal ventricular tachycardia and two dogs with both atrial fibrillation and paroxysmal ventricular tachycardia.

†Heart rates ranged from 160 to 200 per min.

‡See text for explanation.

tachycardia (Table 3), in which the QRS complexes are similar or identical to the ventricular premature beats (Fig. 3). In the great majority of affected dogs the ventricular ectopic beats appear to arise from the right ventricle, resulting in upright, widened, and bizarre QRS complexes (left bundle branch block pattern) in leads I, II, and III. In rare instances, multiform ventricular complexes and fusion beats have been observed (Fig. 4). Less commonly, supraventricular tachyarrhythmias (i.e., atrial fibrillation, paroxysmal supraventricular tach-

ycardia) are the predominating arrhythmias. In a few dogs, both supraventricular and ventricular tachyarrhythmias have been recorded (Fig. 5). In general, the P, QRS, and T complexes during normal sinus rhythm are within normal limits, although electrocardiographic evidence of left ventricular enlargement is found occasionally.*

POST-MORTEM FINDINGS

Although we have had the opportunity to examine only 18 of these dogs at post mortem, the findings have been quite similar and unique for this disease. The most consistent gross findings were mild hypertrophy and dilatation of the left ventricle and mild left atrial dilatation, along with occasional pale foci in the endocardium and myocardium. In addition, the atrioventricular valves were thickened, nodular, and opaque in 50 per cent of the dogs examined. Less commonly, the aortic valves were markedly thickened, opaque, and immobile, and the right atrioventricular valves were mildly nodular and thickened. Hepatomegaly was present in 41 per cent of the dogs.

Histologically, diffusely distributed and severe myocardial changes were found routinely. These could be divided into active and chronic changes, although both types could be found in all hearts examined. Active myocardial disease was characterized by focal areas of myocytolysis, myofiber necrosis, hemorrhage, and a mild cellular infiltration. A mononuclear cell infiltration was the major response, with macrophages, lymphocytes, and plas-

---

*Electrocardiographic criteria for left ventricular enlargement include R wave amplitudes exceeding 3.0 mV in leads II and V_4 (CV_6LL) and prolongation of the QRS interval in lead II to beyond 70 msec.

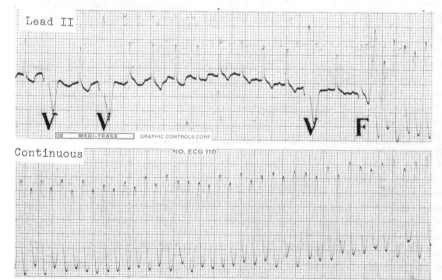

Figure 3. A continuous lead II tracing from a six-year-old spayed female boxer with cardiomyopathy. In the upper strip sinus tachycardia (182/min) is sporadically interrupted by single unifocal ventricular ectopic beats (V). Near the termination of the upper strip a single fusion beat (F) is followed by a prolonged period of ventricular flutter. This latter tachyarrhythmia is most likely the mechanism responsible for the observed collapsing episodes. Recorded at 25 mm/sec. 1.0 cm = 1.0 mV.

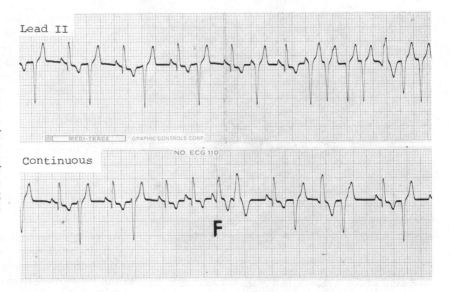

Figure 4. A continuous lead II tracing from a seven-year-old spayed female boxer with cardiomyopathy. A mixed bag of arrhythmias is seen, including ventricular bigeminy, multifocal ventricular ectopic beats, and a short burst of ventricular tachycardia. In addition, a single fusion beat (F) is recorded. There is prolongation of the P wave with slurring on the downstroke (P mitrale), suggesting left atrial enlargement. Recorded at 25 mm/sec. 0.5 cm = 1.0 mV.

ma cells predominating. Less commonly, a polymorphonuclear leukocyte infiltration was found, but usually in combination with a mononuclear cell response. Chronic myocardial changes were far more frequent than active lesions in all the hearts examined. These changes consisted of myofiber atrophy, characterized by marked variation in size and shape of individual myofibers; fibrosis; extensive fatty infiltration; and fatty change (Fig. 6).

Evidence of chronic myocardial changes was present in nearly all sections of myocardium examined.

The alterations that were observed grossly in the left and right atrioventricular valve leaflets were histologically similar to those found in dogs with chronic valvular heart disease (Buchanan, 1977). Whether this myxomatous transformation is unrelated to the myocardial disease or is the result of increased stress placed on the mitral apparatus by

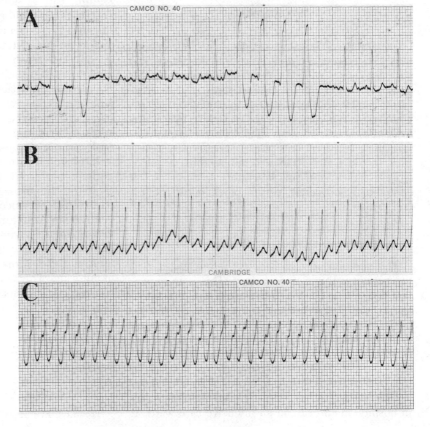

Figure 5. Sustained supraventricular and ventricular tachycardias recorded in a three and one half-year-old male boxer with cardiomyopathy within 24 hours following admission. *A,* Normal sinus rhythm is sporadically interrupted by repetitive ventricular arrhythmias, first by a pair of ventricular ectopic beats and then by a short burst of ventricular tachycardia (1.0 cm = 1.0 mV). *B,* A supraventricular tachycardia can be seen, occurring at a rate of approximately 320/min (1.0 cm = 1.0 mV). *C,* Ventricular tachycardia is present at 370/min (0.5 cm = 1.0 mV). Notice the differences in the rate and the QRS configurations between the supraventricular and ventricular tachycardias. All tracings were recorded at 25 mm/sec.

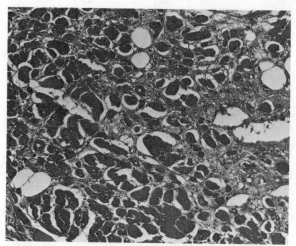

Figure 6. Photomicrograph taken of the left ventricle of an eight-year-old spayed female boxer that died of cardiomyopathy. Myocardial atrophy is characterized by marked variation in size and shape of individual muscle cells. This is accompanied by extensive fibrosis and fairly diffuse fatty infiltration. Many myocytes contain small clear areas, suggesting fatty change (hematoxylin-eosin × 150).

alterations in its myocardial components has not been established (Perloff and Roberts, 1972). The changes seen histologically in affected aortic valvulae consisted of both myxomatous transformation and proliferation of collagenous fibers.

MANAGEMENT

Treatment of dogs with boxer cardiomyopathy must be tailored to the individual needs of the patient. Thus it will be determined, in part, by the presence or absence of clinical signs, the electrocardiographic characteristics of the arrhythmia, and whether or not congestive heart failure exists. An in-depth patient work-up should be performed before final decisions on optimal therapy are made. This should include thoracic radiographs, an electrocardiogram, and full laboratory testing (i.e., a complete blood count, serum biochemical profile, and urinalysis).

The asymptomatic dog (category 1)

The question here is when is therapy justified in the patient without clinical signs. This is an important decision, as the long-term use of antiarrhythmic agents can cause further compromise of cardiac performance. Our approach in the asymptomatic dog has been to avoid therapy when infrequent (<20/min), singly occurring premature beats alone are recorded. However, a more critical decision in this patient can be made following a 24-hour monitoring period, either with a Holter monitor or by in-hospital monitoring in an intensive care ward. If

this monitoring period does not identify the occurrence of more serious arrhythmias, a program of frequent (i.e., every two to four weeks) outpatient monitoring is recommended. When isolated, premature beats occur more frequently (>20/min), arise from more than a single ectopic focus, or occur in pairs or runs, when paroxysmal or sustained tachyarrhythmias are recorded, antiarrhythmic therapy is indicated. These dogs are managed similarly to those in which clinical signs are present (see hereafter).

Ventricular arrhythmias without congestive heart failure (category 2)

As ventricular tachyarrhythmias predominate in the majority of dogs with syncopal episodes, dogs in this category require frequent attention. Hospitalization with constant or frequent ECG monitoring is preferred to obtain optimal results in the shortest period of time.

When recurring bursts of paroxysmal ventricular tachycardia or sustained ventricular tachycardia are present, the use of intravenous antiarrhythmic agents is indicated. Lidocaine hydochloride,* 2 per cent *without* epinephrine, or procainamide hydrochloride† is the drug of choice. For sustained ventricular tachycardia a bolus of lidocaine can be given at 2 to 4 mg/kg, intravenously. If this proves effective, a constant infusion of lidocaine, 30 to 60 μg/kg/min, can be administered to maintain constant control. This should be accompanied by ECG monitoring. The advantages of lidocaine over procainamide in this setting include a shorter duration of action and fewer myocardial depressant effects. However, these advantages may be overshadowed by certain drawbacks, including a less consistent and predictable response, the frequent occurrence of central nervous system (CNS) depression and seizures, and the eventual need to change to an orally administered antiarrhythmic agent.

Intravenous procainamide is a reasonable and perhaps preferred alternative to intravenous lidocaine in the management of recurring bursts of paroxysmal ventricular tachycardia and sustained ventricular tachycardia in boxer cardiomyopathy. Procainamide is administered by adding 500 to 1000 mg to 500 ml of 5 per cent dextrose in water and infusing this mixture to effect with continuous ECG monitoring. The rate of infusion should not exceed 30 mg/kg/hr for more than three hours; toxic manifestations are likely to occur with higher doses (also see pages 370–371). These may include CNS and myocardial depression, hypotension, prolongation of the QRS and Q-T intervals, and even ventricular arrhythmias. When control of the tachycardia is

*Xylocaine, Astra Pharmaceutical Products, Inc., Worcester, MA.

†Pronestyl, E. R. Squibb & Sons, Princeton, NJ.

accomplished with intravenous procainamide, the rate of infusion is slowed, and intramuscular or oral procainamide is initiated at 8 to 17 mg/kg every six hours.

Although in the great majority of dogs with boxer cardiomyopathy the ventricular arrhythmias can be controlled with intravenous procainamide infusions, control may not be maintained with oral administration. In these dogs, alternative antiarrhythmic agents or combinations of antiarrhythmic drugs should be tried. Propranolol* alone at 0.6 to 2.0 mg/kg every eight hours has been effective in some dogs. In other dogs, combinations of antiarrhythmic drugs, such as procainamide (8 to 17 mg/kg every six to eight hours) and propranolol (0.6 to 1.4 mg/kg every eight hours) or quinidine sulfate (6 to 10 mg/kg every eight hours) and propranolol (0.6 to 1.4 mg/kg every eight hours), have been required for effective, long-term control. Dosages of quinidine sulfate in excess of 10 mg/kg every eight hours should be avoided owing to the risk of fatal arrhythmias. In our experience, disopyramide phosphate† does not appear to offer any advantages over quinidine sulfate.

In dogs with less serious ventricular arrhythmias, the initial use of oral antiarrhythmic agents is an effective and rational approach. As mentioned previously, the importance of hospitalization and frequent or constant monitoring should be emphasized. Those agents and the dosages listed in the preceding paragraph are recommended, with lower dosages of single agents being tried before higher dosages or combinations of drugs. Although the optimal goal of therapy is complete elimination of all arrhythmias, this cannot always be accomplished. An acceptable end point is the termination of all repetitive (i.e., paired) arrhythmias.

CONGESTIVE HEART FAILURE IN ASSOCIATION WITH CARDIAC ARRHYTHMIAS (CATEGORY 3)

Boxers having both congestive heart failure and cardiac arrhythmias present the greatest problems in management. The proper approach to these dogs will depend to a large extent upon the type of arrhythmia or tachyarrhythmia that exists. The severity of the heart failure also plays a role, but to a lesser extent. For these reasons dogs falling into this category must be separated into subgroups, which are discussed individually.

Atrial Fibrillation. When the predominating tachyarrhythmia is atrial fibrillation (AF), therapy is similar to that recommended for dogs with AF due to other causes. Digoxin‡ is administered at 0.0175 mg/kg/day, divided every 12 hours, to slow atrio-

---

*Inderal, Ayerst Laboratories, New York, NY.

†Norpace, Searle Laboratories, Chicago, IL.

‡Lanoxin, Burroughs Wellcome Co., Research Triangle Park, NC.

ventricular conduction and the ventricular rate and to improve myocardial contractility. Diuretics are administered in dosages sufficient to resolve the excess fluid state. In addition, a low-salt diet is recommended. If congestive heart failure (CHF) proves difficult to control by these standard approaches, then vasodilator agents should be tried (Cohn and Franciosa, 1977; McIntosh, 1981) (see page 290). When the CHF is well controlled but the ventricular rate remains excessively rapid at rest (i.e., >140/min), propranolol should be added. A conservative starting dose for propranolol is 0.2 to 0.3 mg/kg every eight hours. If this does not result in the desired reduction in the ventricular rate, the dosage should be doubled. Additional increases in propranolol can be attempted, provided undue fluid retention does not result.

Supraventricular Tachycardia. When the major arrhythmia is either paroxysmal supraventricular tachycardia (PSVT) or sustained supraventricular tachycardia (SVT) (see page 368), the initial approach is similar to that discussed for atrial fibrillation. But an attempt should be made to control the excess fluid state as quickly as possible, as volume overload (i.e., increased preload) and associated cardiac dilation may be significant contributing factors to the tachyarrhythmia. The addition of digoxin alone may be effective in terminating the supraventricular tachycardia. This may be accomplished by an increase in vagal tone or by a direct effect on the electrophysiologic mechanism responsible for the tachyarrhythmia (i.e., digitalis glycosides cause a shortening of the action potential and a more rapid recovery time). Every effort should be made to terminate the tachyarrhythmia as rapidly as possible. The rapid heart rates that are typically found in both PSVT and SVT cause a marked reduction in cardiac performance and may contribute significantly to the heart failure state. This is one of the rare instances in which intensive methods of digitalization can be justified, provided constant or frequent ECG monitoring is performed. A method that is frequently effective in terminating SVT but that avoids the inherent problems encountered with toxicity is the administration of digoxin at 0.0175 mg/kg intravenously every two to four hours (maximum total dose 0.07 mg/kg). Maintenance dosages of digoxin are then continued. When SVT is resistant to these approaches, other therapeutic methods may be effective (Table 4).

Ventricular Tachyarrhythmias. The combination of serious ventricular arrhythmias and congestive heart failure is very dangerous and is one of the most difficult cardiac disorders to manage successfully. The simultaneous resolution of both the excess fluid state and the tachyarrhythmias needs to be accomplished, since each represents a potentially life-threatening problem. The administration of intravenous diuretics is preferred. The absorption

Table 4. *Approach to the Termination of Sustained Supraventricular Tachycardia**

1. Perform vagal maneuver
   A. Carotid sinus massage
   B. Eyeball pressure
2. Administer vagal stimulants
   A. Morphine sulfate—0.2 mg/kg IM
   B. Digoxin—½ TDD† IV over two- to four-hour period
3. Repeat vagal maneuver
4. Control congestive heart failure, if present
   A. Furosemide (Lasix)—4 mg/kg IV; repeat every two hours or as needed
5. Repeat vagal maneuver
6. Administer propranolol
   A. 1.0 mg IV over a three-minute period
   B. 0.6 to 2.0 mg/kg PO
7. Repeat vagal maneuver
8. Administer quinidine sulfate‡
   A. 6 to 10 mg/kg PO every two hours
   B. Should not exceed four doses§
9. Perform cardioversion

---

*Only indicated for sustained supraventricular tachycardia, not the paroxysmal variety. However, the drugs listed are frequently effective for both.

†TDD = total digitalization dose.

‡When quinidine sulfate is effective in terminating the arrhythmia, maintenance therapy should be started eight hours later at 6 to 10 mg/kg t.i.d.

§Dosages in excess of this have commonly been associated with sudden death.

of drugs administered by other routes may be less than optimal owing to a reduction in peripheral circulation. Furosemide* is the diuretic of choice and may need to be administered in dosages greater than 4 mg/kg to effect an adequate response. (Renal blood flow is substantially decreased in this situation, the result of both the heart failure state and the reduction in blood pressure caused by the tachyarrhythmia.)

Antiarrhythmic agents with short serum half-lives and minimal myocardial depressant effects should be used to control the arrhythmias. Although it is generally agreed that antiarrhythmic agents with these ideal properties are not currently available, lidocaine and procainamide most closely approach these optimal properties when administered in the dog. The intravenous infusion of these agents in 5 per cent dextrose in water, as discussed previously, must be performed cautiously to prevent additional circulatory volumes and worsening of the heart failure state. This can be accomplished by adding larger quantities of lidocaine or procainamide to 500 ml of 5 per cent dextrose in water so that less fluid is given per milligram of active drug administered. Constant ECG monitoring is extremely helpful in evaluating the response. Alternatively, procainamide may be administered intramuscularly at 4 to 8 mg/kg every six hours. Lower dosages than those recommended previously are given initially to minimize depressant effects on the myocardium. Fol-

lowing antiarrhythmia therapy, a low maintenance dose of digoxin (i.e., 0.008 to 0.0125 mg/kg/day, divided every 12 hours) may be useful to treat heart failure. Although relatively contraindicated for ventricular arrhythmias, some dogs tolerate digitalization without a worsening of the cardiac rhythm.

With the judicious use of digoxin, diuretics, and antiarrhythmic agents, the majority of these dogs can be stabilized. The long-term outlook is better when the arrhythmias are effectively controlled by low dosages of antiarrhythmic drugs. When high dosages of antiarrhythmic agents are required, heart failure is generally more difficult to control. It is preferable to attempt control of repetitive tachyarrhythmias, but not complete termination of all arrhythmias, if these prove difficult to resolve.

PROGNOSIS

As might be expected in a myocardial disorder characterized by extensive structural changes and serious unifocal or multifocal tachyarrhythmias, the long-term prognosis is poor. This is particularly true in the boxer presented with both congestive heart failure and ventricular tachyarrhythmias. In the majority of dogs in category 3, a comfortable existence can rarely be maintained for more than six months. Many of these patients die suddenly during attempts to stabilize their condition. However, the prognosis for dogs in categories 1 and 2 tends to be better than that seen in other forms of cardiomyopathy, provided congestive heart failure does not intervene. We have followed a number of dogs in category 1 for more than two years. The majority of dogs in category 2 can be managed successfully for more than one year but usually develop congestive heart failure in the second year.

Inability to stabilize heart failure and sudden death due to fatal arrhythmias are the major complications that have been encountered in boxer cardiomyopathy. The former is seen most commonly in the dog with serious tachyarrhythmias that are difficult to manage. The myocardial depressant effects of aggressive antiarrhythmic therapy, plus the severe underlying myocardial pathology, are probably the reasons for the resistance to management of heart failure in the majority of dogs with boxer cardiomyopathy. Less commonly, recurring pleural effusion is seen in the boxer with chronic atrial fibrillation, similar to that seen in other forms of cardiomyopathy.

CONCLUSIONS

In many ways the disease described as boxer cardiomyopathy differs considerably from that reported previously as both hypertrophic and dilata-

---

*Lasix, Hoechst-Roussel Pharmaceuticals Inc., Somerville, NJ.

tive cardiomyopathy in the dog. These differences encompass the clinical manifestations as well as the histologic changes that are observed. Although the microscopic alterations in the myocardium are somewhat similar to those described for primary xanthomatosis and Hand-Schüller-Christian disease in humans, the absence of fatty infiltration in other body organs makes these possibilities unlikely.

Until recently, this disease, with its characteristic and unique histologic changes, had been recognized only in the boxer breed. However, over the past two years a condition with similar clinical and histologic findings has been seen in Doberman pinschers. Whether these findings represent inborn metabolic abnormalities or degenerative processes has not been established. Investigative studies are currently in progress to better define the etiology of these diseases.

REFERENCES AND SUPPLEMENTAL READING

Buchanan, J. W.: Chronic valvular disease (endocardiosis) in dogs. Adv. Vet. Sci. Comp. Med. 21:75, 1977.
Cohn, J. N., and Franciosa, J. A.: Vasodilator therapy of cardiac failure. N. Engl. J. Med. 297:27, 254, 1977.
Liu, S. K., Maron, B. J., and Tilley, L. P.: Canine hypertrophic cardiomyopathy. J.A.V.M.A. 174:708, 1979.
McIntosh, J. J.: The use of vasodilators in treatment of congestive heart failure: A review. J. Am. Anim. Hosp. Assoc. 17:255, 1981.
Oakley, C. M.: Clinical recognition of the cardiomyopathies. Circ. Res. 35(Suppl.):152, 1974.
Perloff, J. K., and Roberts, W. C.: The mitral apparatus. Circulation 46:227, 1972.
Van Fleet, J. F., Ferrans, V. J., and Weirich, W. E.: Pathologic alterations in congestive cardiomyopathy of dogs. Am. J. Vet. Res. 42:416, 1981.

FELINE MYOCARDIAL DISEASES

PHILIP R. FOX, D.V.M.
New York, N.Y.

Feline myocardial diseases comprise a diverse group of pathologic forms and clinical expressions. Etiologies may be varied, and the specific inciting cause is often obscure. Increased awareness of these conditions combined with improved diagnostic techniques allows the recognition of myocardial disorders as significant causes of morbidity and mortality.

Cardiomyopathies are disease processes in which the basic cardiac pathology resides in the heart muscle (Fig. 1). Myopathic changes involving or resulting predominantly from valvular, ischemic, pericardial, or congenital abnormalities or arising secondary to disease in other organ systems are excluded. Cardiomyopathy constitutes the major proportion of feline cardiovascular abnormalities and has been recorded in 8.5 per cent of 4,933 cats consecutively autopsied during a 14-year period at The Animal Medical Center.

Cardiomyopathies can be classified based on various schemes. These are determined by etiologic, clinical, pathologic, or functional characteristics or whether the heart is the sole site of disease manifestation or is involved secondary to multi-organ involvement (Table 1). No one method totally defines all features of a given form. Feline myocardial diseases are most commonly divided into (1) primary cardiomyopathies (signifying idiopathic, primary myocardial diseases without coexisting or pre-existing disease of other cardiovascular structures or systemic abnormalities), and (2) secondary myocar-diopathies (including those afflictions of the heart muscle caused by known systemic abnormalities). Primary cardiomyopathies are subdivided into hypertrophic, dilated, restrictive, and excessive left ventricular moderator band forms according to their anatomic, functional, and pathophysiologic characteristics. This permits attention to be focused on common clinical features and hemodynamic patterns. It must be remembered that functional categories are not absolute, and a particular designation may be appropriate only for a given time. Very early stages of myocardial disease may not be distinctive, and characteristic features of different forms may overlap. Thus, diagnostic and therapeutic intervention may change during the natural history of a given disease process.

PRIMARY CARDIOMYOPATHIES (PRIMARY MYOCARDIAL DISEASES)

HYPERTROPHIC CARDIOMYOPATHY (HCM)

This heterogeneous group of cardiac muscle diseases is represented by pathologic abnormalities characterized by marked increases in myocardial mass, a small left ventricular cavity, a dilated and often hypertrophied left atrium, restriction of ventricular filling, and, occasionally, dynamic left ventricular outflow obstruction. Septal myocardial cel-

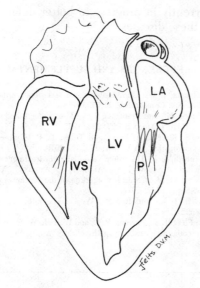

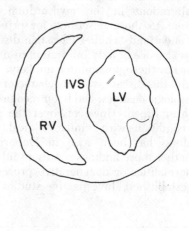

Figure 1. Normal feline heart. RV = right ventricle; LV = left ventricle; IVS = interventricular septum; P = papillary muscles; LA = left atrium.

lular disorganization and asymmetric septal hypertrophy occur in one-fourth of affected cats (Fig. 2), whereas the majority have symmetric, concentric ventricular hypertrophy (Fig. 3) with normally arranged cellular architecture. Numerous terms have been employed to describe these disease processes, including asymmetric septal hypertrophy, hypertrophic obstructive cardiomyopathy (HOCM), idiopathic myocardial hypertrophy, obstructive cardiomyopathy, and idiopathic hypertrophic subaortic stenosis. The designation "hypertrophic cardiomyopathy" (HCM) is preferred, since it does not imply left ventricular outflow obstruction.

The etiology of HCM is unknown. The inference of a heritable basis is suggested from accounts of affected related cats and persuasive human data of genetic transmission. Other etiologies have been proposed.

Table 1. *Classification of Cardiomyopathies*

Primary Cardiomyopathies
    Hypertrophic cardiomyopathy
    Dilated cardiomyopathy
    Restrictive cardiomyopathy
    Cardiomyopathy associated with excessive left ventricular
        moderator bands
Secondary Myocardiopathies
    Infectious
        Bacterial
        Fungal
        Viral
        Protozoal
    Noninfectious
        Toxins
        Chemicals
        Drugs
        Hypersensitivity
        Physical agents
    Metabolic
        Uremia
        Nutritional
    Endocrine
        Hyperthyroidism (thyrotoxicosis)
    Infiltrative
        Neoplasia
        Amyloidosis

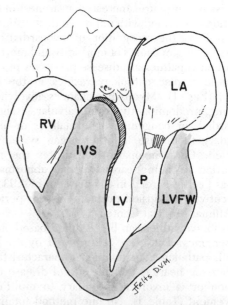

Figure 2. Asymmetric hypertrophic cardiomyopathy. The interventricular septum (IVS) is disproportionately thicker than the left ventricular free wall (LVFW). Endocardial fibrosis (hatch-marked area) is present in the left ventricular outflow tract. RV = right ventricle; LV = left ventricle; LA = left atrium; P = papillary muscles.

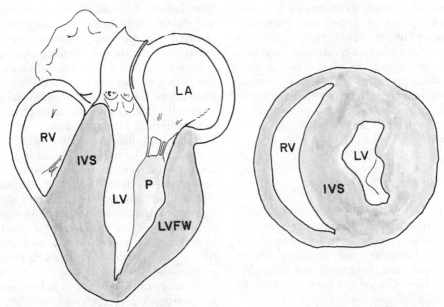

Figure 3. Symmetric, hypertrophic cardiomyopathy. The left ventricular free wall (LVFW), interventricular septum (IVS), and papillary muscles (P) are uniformly hypertrophied. The left atrium (LA) is hypertrophied and severely enlarged. RV = right ventricle; LV = left ventricle.

Clinical manifestations are seen in middle-aged cats (range 8 months to 16 years) of all breeds. Males are over-represented. The most striking clinical sign is *acute dyspnea* resulting from pulmonary edema (left heart failure). Paresis from *aortic thromboembolism* often accompanies congestive heart failure. Sudden death is occasionally the only witnessed clinical event.

Physical examination in asymptomatic cats may be unremarkable. More commonly, a gallop rhythm (usually fourth heart sound) is heard best at the left base (but often audible at the left apex) and a systolic murmur of mitral regurgitation of low to moderate intensity may be present at the left apex or between the apex and the sternum. An exaggerated left apical impulse may be readily palpated. In symptomatic cats, fine to coarse rales (crackles) and arrhythmias may be auscultated. Dyspnea and tachypnea accompany advanced decompensation.

Electrocardiographic abnormalities have been observed in approximately two-thirds of affected cats. Prolonged P-wave and QRS duration and amplitude occur frequently. Left axis deviation, presumably caused by left anterior fascicular block, is a common and highly specific indicator of HCM. Ventricular and atrial arrhythmias may be recorded, but absence of electrocardiographic abnormalities is not uncommon.

Thoracic radiographs are variable but usually represent cardiomegaly, especially left atrial enlargement. This is most readily distinguished on the dorsoventral view where left atrial enlargement may contribute to a "valentine"-shaped cardiac silhouette or "biatrial" enlargement. Both terms are mis-

nomers, however, since the right atrium is usually normal or only minimally enlarged and the "valentine"-shaped appearance is not a reliable diagnostic sign. Right atrial enlargement, when present, is usually associated with chronic, severe left heart failure. Moderate to severe pulmonary edema is a hallmark of decompensated HCM. Mild to moderate pleural effusion is a frequent accompanying sign. Angiocardiography is necessary to form a diagnosis in many instances. Nonselective studies are easily performed using an injection of contrast media into a jugular or cephalic vein. Sequential, multiple exposures are facilitated by manually advancing cassettes through a cassette tunnel using a push stick. Relative changes in chamber size and wall thickness are then compared during systolic and diastolic phases. Characteristic signs include moderate to severe left atrial enlargement, tortuous pulmonary veins, increased left ventricular posterior wall thickness with decreased left ventricular chamber dimension, hypertrophied left ventricular papillary muscles, normal to shortened circulation time, and good aortic opacification.

Echocardiographic changes may include hypertrophy of the left ventricular posterior wall and sometimes of the interventricular septum, decreased left ventricular chamber dimension, left atrial enlargement, and occasionally systolic anterior motion of the mitral valve (contributing to left ventricular outflow obstruction).

Hemodynamic consequences of HCM relate to diastolic dysfunction. This is associated with decreased left ventricular compliance due to hypertrophy. As a result, left ventricular diastolic pressure is greatly elevated, leading to increased left atrial and pulmonary venous pressures and pulmonary edema (left heart failure). Mitral regurgitation results from papillary muscle hypertrophy, and subsequent geometric alteration of the mitral valve apparatus. Systolic pressures are generally normal. Occasionally, a functional left ventricular outflow obstruction and pressure gradient are present. Right heart failure may become severe following chronic left heart failure.

THERAPEUTIC STRATEGY

Treatment is directed toward increasing ventricular distensibility and filling; decreasing contractility, left ventricular outflow obstruction, and pulmonary venous pressure; and reducing clinical signs. Diuretics, oxygen, cage rest, and beta-adrenergic blockers have formed the basic approach for treatment of HCM.

Diuretics represent the initial therapeutic step. Furosemide* is the most effective and most commonly used agent. As a result of diuresis, blood volume and pulmonary capillary pressures are reduced and pulmonary edema is diminished. Maximal effects may occur within 30 minutes of intravenous administration and may persist for three hours. Cats are very sensitive to its effects, and overzealous administration may cause hypovolemia, reduced cardiac output, or hypokalemia with weakness (head hanging).

In severe left heart failure, furosemide in an initial intravenous bolus of 1 to 2 mg/kg is given, followed by 1 mg/kg IV or IM b.i.d. to t.i.d. Pronounced improvement during the first 24 to 36 hours is common, at which time the drug may be administered once or twice daily. The initial intravenous bolus is omitted if left heart failure is mild. Route of administration may then be IM or PO. After improvement of clinical signs and resolution of pulmonary congestion radiographically, furosemide is reduced to the lowest effective dose. Ideally this is 1 mg/kg every second or third day, but progression of the disease process or exacerbations of heart failure may necessitate once or twice daily administrations.

Oxygen and cage rest are important adjuncts to diuretic therapy in severe heart failure. Oxygen-enriched inspired gas (40 to 60 per cent) is administered during the first 18 to 24 hours in an effort to improve gas exchange by increasing the driving force for diffusion into the alveolar capillary. Improved myocardial oxygenation reduces ventricular irritability. Restricted physical activity (cage rest) is critical during the stages of fulminant congestive

heart failure. Because stress can precipitate dyspnea and death, techniques requiring excessive animal manipulation are best minimized or delayed until initial stabilization can be accomplished.

Beta-adrenergic blockade is employed once a compensated state has been achieved. It is intended to improve left ventricular compliance and filling, diminish left ventricular outflow obstruction (which can accompany stress), and exert an antiarrhythmic action. Propranolol,† a nonselective beta blocker, is used most commonly. Because it is thought to improve left ventricular compliance in obstructive and nonobstructive HCM, it is advocated in symptomatic but compensated cats and as prophylactic therapy in asymptomatic cats. Propranolol has negative inotropic and chronotrophic effects that accentuate heart failure or provoke cardiac decompensation in cats with early heart failure. Therefore, propranolol therapy should be avoided in these circumstances. Other contraindications for therapy are recognized. Propranolol may increase airway resistance in the presence of chronic obstructive lung disease or feline asthma. It may augment insulin's hypoglycemic action (in diabetes mellitus) by decreasing the compensatory effects of sympathoadrenal action. Propranolol should be used with caution in the presence of atrioventricular block or acute aortic thromboembolism. Gastrointestinal disturbances, weakness, and anorexia are uncommon toxic manifestations.

Propranolol (10-mg tablet) is dosed at 2.5 mg b.i.d. to t.i.d. for cats less than 6 kg body weight and 5.0 mg b.i.d. to t.i.d. for cats more than 6 kg. Dosage adjustments may be necessary to attain the therapeutic end points of relief of clinical signs and elimination of arrhythmias. ECG monitoring of heart rate is useful in determining if propranolol has a therapeutic effect, since most cats experience moderate reductions in heart rate with therapy.

The use of more cardioselective, longer-lasting beta-blocking drugs may offer advantages over propranolol. The efficacy of these agents has not been suitably evaluated in cardiomyopathic cats.

Other therapeutic principles have recently been added to the treatment strategies for HCM. Diuretics, while reducing pulmonary capillary pressure, do little to increase cardiac output. *Vasodilators* may be selected to (1) produce venodilation, reduce preload, and decrease pulmonary capillary pressure and/or (2) cause arteriolar dilation and lower systemic vascular resistance and afterload, thereby augmenting cardiac output. Their use may be hazardous, however, if not properly monitored. Untoward effects include hypotension. Since most cats respond to previously described therapy, vasodilators are reserved for fulminant or intractable heart failure.

---

*Lasix, Hoechst-Roussel Pharmaceuticals, Inc., Somerville, NJ.

†Inderal, Ayerst Laboratories, New York, NY.

Calcium channel blockers such as verapamil* are being evaluated in human studies because of the poor efficacy of beta blockers in nonobstructive HCM. Improvement of left ventricular relaxation and filling and reduced left ventricular outflow obstruction are among the beneficial effects recorded with this class of drugs. Their effectiveness and safety in feline HCM has not yet been studied.

Bronchodilators such as the theophyllines (4 to 8 mg/kg b.i.d. to t.i.d.) can be administered in states of severe left heart failure to help counteract bronchospasm and bronchiolar narrowing accompanying pulmonary edema. They have mild positive inotropic, venodilative, and diuretic effects. Routine use is not advocated, because most cats respond to diuretics and cage rest. Untoward effects (gastrointestinal and neurologic) have been observed with excessive dosages.

Fluid therapy may be required to satisfy replacement or maintenance needs. Although intravenous administration may be necessary, the subcutaneous route will often suffice with mild left heart failure.

Aspirin is advocated for all cats with HCM that have evidenced clinical signs (see Arterial Thromboembolism).

Digitalis glycosides increase myocardial contractility and left ventricular outflow obstruction. They are thus contraindicated in the state of supernormal left ventricular contractility and ejection fraction usually characteristic of HCM. Digoxin† is reserved for treating atrial fibrillation or advanced right heart failure when decreased right ventricular contractility may be an end-stage finding. Mild pleural effu-

---

*Isoptin, Knoll Pharmaceutical Co., Whippany, NJ; Calan, Searle Pharmaceuticals Co., Chicago, IL.
†Lanoxin, Burroughs Wellcome Co., Research Triangle Park, NC.

sion accompanying severe left heart failure does not warrant digitalization.

In cats presenting initially for left heart failure, clinical signs can usually be controlled within one to two days. The cat is then maintained in a compensated state indefinitely with propranolol, furosemide, aspirin, sodium restriction (feline H/D), and rest. The prognosis is favorable. Survival times of up to three or more years are possible. The natural history, however, is quite variable. Exacerbations of left heart failure are not uncommon. Often they are associated with aortic thromboembolism. Atrial fibrillation is a rare but ominous complication. Occasionally, severe right heart failure will become the predominant clinical affliction. Sudden death commonly interrupts an otherwise stable, compensated course.

DILATED (CONGESTIVE) CARDIOMYOPATHY

Dilated cardiomyopathy (CM) represents a variety of pathologic processes characterized by impaired systolic pump function and increased end-systolic and end-diastolic volumes. Cardiomegaly and biventricular congestive heart failure (predominantly right sided) result. Affected hearts display globoid cardiomegaly owing to extreme ventricular dilation and moderate atrial enlargement. Ventricular wall thickness may be normal, increased, or decreased. Papillary muscles and trabeculae are atrophied (Fig. 4).

The etiology of this syndrome (also referred to as congestive cardiomyopathy or idiopathic congestive cardiomyopathy) is unknown. It has been speculated that dilated CM may represent a final pathway for some types of myocardial injury or cardiomyopathy.

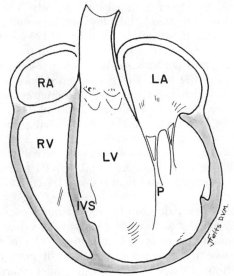
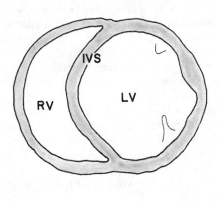

Figure 4. Dilated cardiomyopathy. All four chambers are dilated, giving a rounded, globoid shape to the heart. Papillary muscles (P) are atrophied. RA = right atrium; LA = left atrium; RV = right ventricle; LV = left ventricle; IVS = interventricular septum.

In addition, a possible role of viral infection (feline infectious peritonitis—FIP) linking the kitten mortality complex with dilated CM has been suggested but not substantiated.

Clinical manifestations of dilated CM are observed in predominantly middle-aged (range 5 months to 16 years) male cats. All breeds are affected, although Siamese and Burmese are more highly represented. Presenting signs may consist of gradual onset of lethargy and anorexia, but more commonly these symptoms have progressed to include dyspnea, depression, dehydration, hypothermia, shock, and paresis (related to aortic thromboembolism).

Physical examination performed on cats with mild symptoms may reveal a low to mid intensity systolic murmur loudest at the mitral and/or tricuspid area. This atrioventricular valvular regurgitation is a result of distortion of subvalvular geometry caused by ventricular dilation. A gallop rhythm is usually present. Mild hypothermia and slightly muffled heart sounds may be noted. More advanced symptoms include dyspnea with profoundly muffled heart sounds, hypokinetic pulses, pulmonary rales, hypothermia (less than 35.5°C), paresis (from thromboembolism), and, very occasionally, hydroperitoneum. Pericardial effusion is rare.

The electrocardiogram may be unremarkable but frequently displays sinus bradycardia. First-degree atrioventricular block and wide QRS complexes (greater than 0.04 sec) are common findings. R waves may occasionally be taller than normal (greater than 0.9 mV in lead II), and ventricular premature complexes may be present.

Generalized cardiomegaly (especially a globoid, rounded apex on the dorsoventral view) and transudative pleural effusion are radiographic hallmarks. Angiocardiography, although not performed during acute, decompensated states, shows left and right ventricular dilation, mild to moderate atrial enlargement, small papillary muscles, decreased to slightly hypertrophied left ventricular posterior wall thickness, delayed circulation time, and a poorly opacified, thin, ascending aorta. Echocardiographic changes include increased left atrial and ventricular internal dimensions, reduced ejection fraction and fractional shortening, diminished left ventricular wall motion, and, occasionally, abnormal mitral valve motion. Hemodynamically, elevated left ventricular end-diastolic pressure occurs in conjunction with elevation of right ventricular filling pressures. Central venous pressure may exceed 16 cm H_2O. Ventricular performance may also be profoundly compromised by arrhythmias. Prerenal azotemia is frequently observed.

THERAPEUTIC STRATEGY

Cardiogenic shock is common in cats with severely decompensated dilated CM. Several factors contribute to decreased cardiac output in this situation. Impaired myocardial contractility decreases stroke volume. Diminished preload can result from relative or absolute hypovolemia (i.e., lack of fluid intake, fluid sequestration in the pleural space, excessive use of diuretics) and arrhythmias. Objectives underlying therapeutic management include (1) improving myocardial function and ventricular performance while reducing or avoiding elevated myocardial oxygen requirements, (2) reducing cardiac workload, (3) controlling sodium intake and extravascular fluid retention while carefully expanding the intravascular blood volume, and (4) preventing secondary myocardial and organ injury. Therapy must be individualized, but a basic strategy underlies management.

Mechanical removal of fluid from the thoracic cavity is performed initially to reduce extrapulmonary constraints on respiration and to minimize stress during further diagnostic testing. Severe dyspnea with muffled heart and lung sounds are definite indications for thoracocentesis.

Digitalization is employed to improve cardiac contractility. Intravenous administration of digoxin is selected in severely ill cats. A total calculated dose of 0.005 mg/kg lean body weight is given over four divided doses or to effect. One-half of the calculated dose is injected. One hour later, one-quarter of the calculated dose is given and is repeated one hour later, if necessary. This final dose is omitted if ECG changes of pronounced bradycardia, progressively diminished atrioventricular conduction, or digoxin-related arrhythmias or clinical signs appear. Oral maintenance digoxin is started immediately after the last intravenous dose.

Oral maintenance digoxin may be given in the elixir or tablet form. Although higher plasma levels and more accurate dosing can be attained with the elixir, this form is unpalatable to cats. The tablet form is more readily tolerated and is recommended. The major disadvantage of tablets (0.125 mg) is their small size, which makes them difficult to accurately divide into portions smaller than one-quarter of a tablet (0.031 mg). The maintenance dose is highly individualized and may vary with progression of the disease. Based on a calculated dose of 0.005 to 0.01 mg/kg lean body weight, the following guidelines are suggested: cats weighing 1.9 to 3.2 kg, 1/4 of 0.125-mg digoxin tablet every second day; cats weighing more than 3.2 to 6.0 kg, 1/4 tablet daily; cats weighing more than 6.0 kg, 1/4 tablet daily or b.i.d.

Males may develop higher plasma digoxin levels than females at the same body weight dose. Food should not be given in conjunction with oral digoxin because it decreases absorption. In most clinical settings, treated cats tend to suffer more from digoxin toxicity than inadequate digitalization. Extracardiac signs of toxicity (anorexia, lethargy, vomiting) almost always precede electrocardiographic changes. Azotemia, especially when complicated by excessive diuretic dosage, can impair digoxin excretion and lead to toxic manifestations.

Diuretics are used to reduce pleural effusion and pulmonary edema. Excessive diuresis may decrease cardiac output. Furosemide for CM therapy is dosed similarly to the regimen discussed for HCM.

Sympathomimetic amines are being increasingly used during initial management of congestive heart failure. Dopamine hydrochloride,* a sympathomimetic amine precursor, stimulates myocardial contractility directly by affecting beta-1-adrenergic myocardial receptors and indirectly by releasing norepinephrine from sympathetic nerve terminals. Dobutamine hydrochloride,† a synthetic catecholamine, directly stimulates adrenergic myocardial receptors. It has less propensity to cause tachyarrhythmias or vasoconstriction. These drugs require careful infusion and close monitoring (see page 295).

Vasodilators may inprove cardiac performance and clinical status. Arterial dilators decrease impedance to arteriolar flow, decrease afterload, and improve cardiac output. Venous dilators reduce preload by increasing venous capacitance and lowering ventricular filling pressures, which relieves pulmonary edema. The use of 2 per cent nitroglycerin ointment‡ (1/4 inch cutaneously t.i.d. to q.i.d.) in combination with digoxin and furosemide has produced subjectively favorable clinical responses. Hydralazine§ and prazosin‖ are other potentially useful vasodilators. Guidelines for use of vasodilators are not yet established. Hypotension is a potential complication.

Beta-blocking agents have been reported to have a salutary effect in human dilated CM, although these claims are now highly debated. Because of the potential detrimental hemodynamic effects of propranolol in congestive heart failure and the lack of demonstrated efficacy in feline dilated CM, their routine use is not recommended.

Fluid therapy with central venous pressure monitoring should be initated in hypothermic and shock patients and balanced to optimize cardiac output without inducing or exacerbating pulmonary edema. The rate of fluid replacement varies with each patient and is dependent upon cardiovascular status, state of hydration, and degree of oral fluid intake. When inotropic therapy and diuretics are administered in conjunction with fluids, the central venous pressure may not change or may actually fall in spite of volume loading. Although subcutaneous administration of fluids is adequate in some instances, significant dehydration and hypovolemia (from diuretic therapy, pooling, and inadequate consumption) make intravenous administration necessary in severely affected cats. To avoid excessive sodium retention, 0.45 per cent NaCl in 2.5 per cent dextrose is given during the first 24 to 48 hours. Potassium supplementation may eventually be necessary; however, cats that initially are oliguric may be hyperkalemic. When heart failure precludes satisfying actual replacement and maintenance requirements, a modified dose of 20 to 35 ml/kg/day is administered slowly in three divided treatments. The development of moist lung sounds or further elevations of central venous pressure indicate fluid overload. This warrants cessation or reduction of infusion or diuresis with intravenous furosemide.

Aspirin should be administered indefinitely to dilated cardiomyopathic cats that have had heart failure (see Arterial Thromboembolism).

Once clinical signs have appeared, the prognosis for cats with dilated CM is generally poor. Death within 24 to 48 hours after presentation or shortly after hospital discharge is not uncommon. Aortic thromboembolism or intractable arrhythmias worsen the prognosis. Cardiac compensation for one to three months is possible using maintenance dosages of digoxin, furosemide, and nitroglycerin ointment (1/4 inch b.i.d. to t.i.d.), and occasionally cats will survive six to nine months.

RESTRICTIVE CARDIOMYOPATHY

Of the three major functional categories of primary cardiomyopathy, restrictive cardiomyopathy (RCM) is the least common. Diastolic dysfunction results from reduced ventricular compliance, whereas systolic function is not severely impaired. Endocardial fibrosis and impeded ventricular filling cause this increased ventricular stiffness. The hemodynamic consequence is an elevated left ventricular filling pressure.

Endomyocardial fibrosis is the classic form of RCM (Fig. 5). Affected cats are predominantly mature males (range 1 to 15 years), and there is no breed predilection. A variety of pathophysiologic processes may result in RCM, although the etiology is usually unknown. Autopsy findings include severe left ventricular endocardial thickening, endomyocardial fibrosis involving and distorting the mitral valve apparatus, extreme left atrial enlargement, and dilation of the right atrium and ventricle.

Dyspnea is the most common clinical sign, followed by anorexia and paresis (from aortic thromboembolism). Systolic murmurs (especially those of mitral insufficiency), a gallop rhythm (usually fourth heart sound), pulmonary rales, or muffled heart and lung sounds may be detected during physical examination. Electrocardiographic abnormalities include atrial or ventricular premature complexes, atrial fibrillation, conduction disturbances, and P-mitrale. Thoracic radiographs usually display severe left atrial enlargement and pulmonary edema.

---

*Intropin, Arnar-Stone Laboratories, Inc., McGaw Park, IL.
†Dobutrex, Eli Lilly and Co., Indianapolis, IN.
‡Nitrol Ointment, Kremers-Urban Co., Milwaukee, WI.
§Apresoline, Ciba Pharmaceutical Co., Summit, NJ.
‖Minipress, Pfizer Laboratories Div., New York, NY.

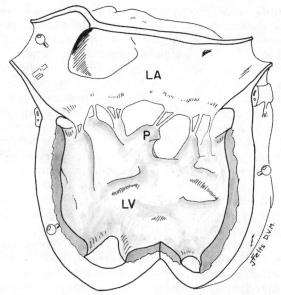

Figure 5. Restrictive cardiomyopathy. Extensive endocardial fibrosis involves the left ventricle (LV), papillary muscles (P), left ventricular outflow tract, chordae tendineae, and mitral leaflets. The left atrium (LA) is hypertrophied.

Prominent, tortuous pulmonary veins can occasionally be detected in the perihilar region on lateral view. Pleural effusion may be present. Angiocardiography may illustrate an irregular left ventricular chamber, mid ventricular stenosis, left ventricular hypertrophy, mitral regurgitation, and extreme left atrial enlargement.

Therapy is often unrewarding, since the majority of decompensated cats have end-stage disease. Lanoxin is used to control the ventricular rate with atrial fibrillation or when severe right-sided heart failure develops. Diuretics and vasodilators are employed to control pulmonary edema. Death is due to progressive myocardial failure, often combined with sudden onset of arrhythmia.

CARDIOMYOPATHY ASSOCIATED WITH EXCESSIVE LEFT VENTRICULAR MODERATOR BANDS

This newly described syndrome represents a family of myocardial abnormalities in which abnormal and excessive moderator bands bridge the left ventricular septum and free wall, entangling papillary muscles (Fig. 6). Although gross and histologic changes are distinctive, functional and hemodynamic characteristics are not well elucidated. They may represent a spectrum of functional stages resembling restrictive and dilated forms of cardiomyopathy.

Affected cats are mature (range 1.5 to 13 years), with slightly more males than females reported. There is no breed predisposition.

Clinical findings may be similar to those of HCM,

dilated CM, or RCM. They include anorexia, lethargy, dyspnea, pleural effusion, pulmonary edema, cardiomegaly, systolic heart murmurs (mitral and sometimes tricuspid insufficiency), gallop rhythm, hypothermia, and paresis (associated with aortic thromboemboli). Thoracic radiographs indicate cardiomegaly, pulmonary edema, and/or pleural effusion. Angiocardiographic evidence of left atrial and, often, left ventricular enlargement may be present, although left ventricular dimensions may be normal. Left ventricular filling defects are only occasionally detectable.

A number of cats have been successfully managed with digoxin, furosemide, and vasodilators. Some affected cats respond to furosemide alone.

ARTERIAL THROMBOEMBOLISM

All forms of primary cardiomyopathy may lead to spontaneous thromboembolism. The event is usually associated with cardiac decompensation, resulting in congestive heart failure. Although thrombi may originate from the left atrium or ventricle, these sites are usually devoid of such lesions at necropsy. Thrombus formation is thought to involve hemodynamic abnormalities associated with cardiomyopathy, especially in the decompensated state.

The terminal aorta is the most common site of enlodgement. A "saddle thrombus" may form where the abdominal aorta bifurcates into the external iliac arteries. Occasionally, an extensive thrombus may occlude the aorta more proximally, blocking the caudal mesenteric and renal arteries. Less com-

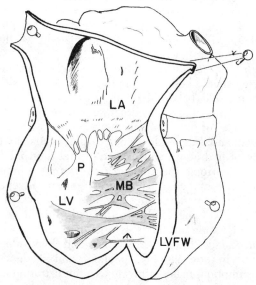

Figure 6. Excessive left ventricular moderator band cardiomyopathy. Abnormal, excessive moderator bands (MB) bridge the interventricular septum (IVS) and the left ventricular free wall (LVFW) and the papillary muscles (P) and the LVFW. The left atrium (LA) is extremely enlarged.

monly, a brachial or pulmonary artery will sustain thromboembolization. It is probable that vasoactive compounds released from the thrombus cause failure of collateral circulation and are more significant than mechanical occlusion by the thrombus itself in reducing circulation.

Clinical signs include acute lower motor neuron (flaccid) paraparesis or occasionally paraplegia; cold, pulseless distal limbs; and cyanotic nail beds. Motor ability distal to the stifle is most severely impaired, and one leg is often more profoundly affected. The condition is initially very painful, with soft muscles, but shortly thereafter they become firm (especially the anterior tibial group and the gastrocnemius). Ischemic neuromyopathy results. As a consequence, affected cats can flex and extend their hips but are unable to adequately flex the hocks; thus, they "walk" on the dorsum of their hind paws.

Serum lactic acid dehydrogenase (LDH), creatine phosphokinase (CPK), and asparate aminotransferase (SGOT) levels are greatly elevated. Renal, pulmonary, or intestinal infarction with associated clinical laboratory abnormalities may occur concomitantly. Coagulation assays may reveal chronic disseminated intravascular coagulation. Nonselective angiocardiography can locate the site and anatomic extent of distal aortic and pulmonary arterial thromboemboli.

Surgery is not recommended. Ischemic neuromyopathy has usually occurred prior to surgery. The decompensated state (congestive heart failure) makes these cats poor surgical risks for embolectomy, and the underlying condition (cardiomyopathy) may cause future thrombotic events. Measures are directed instead toward stabilizing the cardiovascular status, using aspirin for antiplatelet aggregation and allowing time for recannulization of the thrombus. Aspirin with an antacid* is administered at a dose of ¼ of a 5-gram tablet every second to third day. All cardiomyopathic cats that have presented for heart failure and/or thrombi are treated with aspirin indefinitely because of the high incidence of recurrence. Recannulization or lysis of a distal aortic thromboembolism can occur in two to four days in some cases, with return of femoral pulses and warm limb extremities. In other cats it takes longer. Improved motor function is common in two to three weeks as evidenced initially by increased flexion and extension of the hips. Improved tarsal flexion follows. Four to seven weeks may be required for maximal clinical recovery. Retention of a conscious proprioceptive deficit is common. When a thrombus occurs in a front leg, recovery is usually more rapid.

Other drugs with the potential for direct antithromboembolic activity include antiserotonergics, nonspecific activators of thrombolysis (streptoki-

nase, urokinase), and prostacyclins. These have not been studied in cats. The use of anticoagulants, such as sodium heparin, has been advocated by some clinicians.

SECONDARY MYOCARDIOPATHIES

Conditions in which myocardial disease results from other cardiovascular abnormalities or is a manifestation of a systemic disease process are referred to as secondary myocardiopathies. It is possible that some of the primary cardiomyopathies are caused by various myocardial insults or stimuli. When the offending stimuli can be defined (e.g., viral myocarditis or adriamycin myocardiopathy), the process is classified as secondary myocardiopathy. An overlap may occur between functional categories, however, since neoplastic or fungal myocardial infiltration causes restrictive features and doxorubicin† toxicity results in a state similar to congestive cardiomyopathy.

Myocarditis denotes inflammation of the myocardium involving the myocytes, interstitium, and/or vessels. The term is sometimes used loosely, however, to include degenerative as well as inflammatory myocardial disease. Cardiac inflammation may occur in a variety of systemic diseases, but it is generally not a primary event. Histologic characterization depends largely on the inciting cause. Myocarditis may be acute or chronic. The process may become chronic following an acute phase, or it may be subacute and chronic from the onset. Lesions may persist following resolution of inflammation, leaving myocardial structural or functional impairment.

The incidence of myocarditis is difficult to assess, since most cases probably have mild or no clinical signs, resolve spontaneously, or are masked by more severe systemic abnormalities. Myocardial disease may be suspected when comprehensive patient evaluation and diagnostic tests suggest a disorder that also causes myocarditis. In some cases, the etiology of myocardial disease remains obscure.

Clinical expressions of myocarditis include congestive heart failure, arrhythmias, and lack of discernible signs. Electrocardiographic abnormalities, if present, may be transient and nonspecific. Alterations of the ST segment and T wave may be difficult to appreciate because of the small feline P-QRS-T complexes and rapid heart rate. Atrial or especially ventricular arrhythmias may be noted, and conduction defects can occur. Electrocardiographic abnormalities without concurrent clinical or diagnostic evidence of congenital cardiac anomalies or primary cardiomyopathy raise the index of

---

*Ascriptin, Rorer, Inc. Ft. Washington, PA.

†Adriamycin, Adria Laboratories Inc., Dublin, OH.

suspicion of myocarditis or myocardial degeneration.

Therapy is often supportive or tailored toward the more dominant systemic disease and its manifestations. Heart failure and arrhythmias are treated according to the nature of their specific circumstances. Recognized causes of secondary myocardiopathy follow.

Bacterial endomyocarditis may result from septicemia or other suppurative conditions. Bacterial myocarditis is generally the result of extension from an infective valvular lesion. Nonspecific clinical signs such as weight loss and lethargy can be evident. Pyrexia is uncommon. Heart murmurs are present only if there are significant vegetative valvular lesions.

Electrocardiography may reveal atrial or ventricular ectopia. Progressive left heart enlargement detected by radiography and leukocytosis with a left shift may occur with vegetative endocarditis. The sudden onset of an arrhythmia accompanying refractory suppurative disease should prompt consideration of endomyocarditis. Therapy requires prolonged antibiotic treatment employing blood culture and sensitivity data when possible. Unsatisfactory response to antibiotics when blood cultures are negative may suggest bacterial resistance or mycotic infections.

Myocardial fungal infections are usually a secondary manifestation of disseminated mycotic disease. Systemic mycosis often occurs in conjunction with reduced host defense from infection, metabolic or neoplastic disease,or immunosuppressive therapy. Diagnosis of myocardial involvement may be difficult and of secondary importance compared with the generalized disease process.

Viral myocarditis is described in the dog but has not been well documented in the cat. Kitten mortality complex involves multiple problems in kittens and adults including dilated CM. A possible association with feline infectious peritonitis has been suggested, although conclusive evidence is lacking.

Protozoal myocarditis may be caused by the obligate intracellular coccidian parasite *Toxoplasma gondii*, a widely endemic zoonotic agent of birds and mammals. Asymptomatic infection, as detected by serologic studies, is relatively common in certain areas of the United States. Acute infection with myocardial necrosis, demonstrable *T. gondii* tachyzoites, and clinical manifestations are rare. More often, immunity develops as bradyzoites encyst in various tissues, including the heart. This characterizes chronic infection and induces minimal myocardial injury. Rupture of cysts with release of bradyzoites elicits a hypersensitivity response or induces a rapid proliferative phase of tachyzoites. Myocarditis can ensue. Immune suppression from drugs (glucocorticosteroids) or disease (feline leukemia

virus—FeLV) may result in proliferation of released bradyzoites and myocardial injury.

Cardiac signs of protozoal myocarditis are often less pronounced than those associated with multisystemic infection. Arrhythmias may occasionally be significant. Fecal oocyst identification, rising serologic titers, and organism identification are helpful in confirming a clinical diagnosis. In addition to supportive therapy, folic acid inhibitors such as pyrimethamine and sulfadiazine or trimethoprim and sulfadiazine* are utilized to inhibit *Toxoplasma* multiplication until the cat can mount a favorable immune response.

Noninfectious agents (drugs, toxins, chemicals) may cause acute or chronic myocardial injury. Myocardial response is correlated with dose and rate of exposure. Inflammation, fibrosis, or myocardiopathy can result. Many stimuli induce cardiotoxicity in humans and are therefore potentially injurious to animals. Such examples include doxorubicin, heat stroke, hypothermia, and myocardial allergic responses to certain drugs.

Feline hyperthyroidism (thyrotoxicosis) may cause clinical, electrocardiographic, and radiographic changes that resemble those seen with primary cardiomyopathies. Therefore, hyperthyroidism should be considered in the differential diagnosis of mature and aged cats with suspected cardiomyopathy. Excessive triiodothyronine (T_3) and thyroxine (T_4) produced by a hyperfunctioning thyroid adenoma (hyperfunctional thyroid carcinomas are rare) can cause gallops, cardiomegaly, arrhythmias, conduction disturbances, and, occasionally, congestive heart failure. Clinical signs of thyrotoxicosis in order of decreasing frequency may include weight loss, polyphagia, hyperexcitability, tachycardia, polydipsia, polyuria, diarrhea, voluminous stools, emesis, dyspnea, and congestive heart failure. Biochemical and hematologic testing is not usually of diagnostic value. Diagnosis is facilitated by history and physical examination (i.e., palpation of thyroid gland enlargement) and is confirmed by a demonstration of elevation of serum T_4 (usually > 6.0 μg/dl) and T_3 (usually > 300 μg/dl).

Thoracic radiographs are generally unremarkable, although cardiomegaly and occasionally pulmonary edema or pleural effusion may appear. Angiocardiography may fail to display abnormalities or illustrate mild to moderate hypertrophy of the left ventricular posterior wall. Echocardiography may demonstrate increased ejection fraction and velocity of fiber shortening and a hypercontractile left ventricle. Sinus tachycardia (greater than 240 beats/min) and increased R wave amplitude (greater than 0.9 mV in lead II) are common electrocardiographic

---

*Tribrissen, Burroughs Wellcome Co., Research Triangle Park, NC.

abnormalities. Other changes include atrial and ventricular premature complexes and tachycardias, ventricular bigeminy, prolonged QRS duration, and shortened QT interval. Intraventricular conduction disturbances are rare. Normal ECGs may be present.

Therapy is directed toward both the underlying endocrine abnormality and cardiovascular manifestations. Beta-adrenergic blockade (propranolol, 2.5 mg t.i.d.) is used to counter the tachycardia and cardiac hypercontractility preoperatively but has no effect on the underlying disease process or the accompanying elevated metabolic rate. Antithyroid drugs (i.e., propylthiouracil,* 50 mg orally t.i.d.) should be given concurrently in an effort to achieve euthyroidism, which may take one to three weeks. If congestive heart failure develops, a furosemide may reduce or eliminate pulmonary edema or pleural effusion. Beta-blockers must be administered with caution. Although they lower the heart rate, the decreased contractility they cause may be detrimental. Hyperthyroidism can also develop with concurrent primary cardiomyopathy.

Surgical thyroidectomy is the favored strategy for managing hyperthyroidism. Hypoparathyroidism, a potential postoperative complication of bilateral thyroidectomy, may cause hypocalcemia, tetany, and QT segment prolongation as accompanying signs. In most successful surgically managed cases, electrocardiographic abnormalities undergo resolution.

Cardiovascular abnormalities associated with other disease processes are numerous, and several warrant discussion. The normal heart can augment its output in response to many systemic insults. High-output states (e.g., hyperthyroidism, anemia) by themselves rarely produce heart failure. But the development of these conditions within the setting of underlying heart disease may precipitate cardiac decompensation. *Chronic anemia* causes cardiac output to rise (predominantly as a function of increased heart rate with little change in stroke volume). With chronic severe anemia, heart rate may be only minimally affected, and elevated cardiac output is due primarily to increased stroke volume associated with cardiac dilation and hypertrophy. Increased R wave voltage may be recorded electrocardiographically. In anemia (PCV < 20 per cent) secondary to FeLV infection, cardiovascular changes can include tachycardia, soft systolic heart murmurs, gallop rhythms, and generalized cardiomegaly. *Chronic renal failure* may also be associated with systolic murmurs, gallop rhythms, cardiomegaly, arrhythmias, and, rarely, pulmonary edema or pleural effusion. Systemic hypertension and effects of chronic anemia are proposed mechanisms for these cardiovascular manifestations.

---

*Propylthiouracil, Eli Lilly and Co., Indianapolis, IN.

REFRACTORY HEART FAILURE WITH MYOCARDIAL DISEASE

Heart failure is refractory when it resists all therapeutic regimens or when the clinical condition worsens. The first step in treating refractory heart failure is to re-evaluate the cat and identify any underlying reversible disease.

1. Could hyperthyroidism be present? Tests of thyroid function (T_3, T_4) should be performed in cats with appropriate signalments or histories.

2. Is there evidence of vegetative endocarditis? Blood cultures should be taken and appropriate diagnostic tests carried out.

3. Does a congenital cardiovascular anomaly exist? Patent ductus arteriosus and pulmonic stenosis are surgically correctable.

4. Are there primary or metastatic cardiac tumors? An evaluation of body systems and a FeLV test should be made. Lymphosarcoma is potentially a treatable disease.

5. Does the cat have heartworms? Tests for microfilaremia and serologic assay (ELISA, IFA) can be performed. A nonselective angiocardiogram may detect heartworms in pulmonary arteries.

Precipitating causes of heart failure may have been missed or undiagnosed. Although these conditions would not normally affect a healthy animal, their additional burden in a baseline state of myocardial function contributes to decompensation. They must be elucidated.

1. Is severe anemia present?

2. Could underlying chronic renal failure be associated with systemic hypertension?

3. Could excessive use of diuretics have severely reduced preload and, subsequently, cardiac output?

4. Could azotemia have precipitated digoxin toxicity and severe clinical signs, interfering with therapy and recovery?

5. Are there systemic disease processes exerting secondary cardiac abnormalities (e.g., toxoplasmosis, mycoses)?

6. Is current therapy inadequate? Are optimal levels of pharmacologic agents being used? What is the serum digoxin level?

7. Has the client been complying with the prescribed dosage regimen?

8. Are other metabolic or systemic factors contributing to cardiac decompensation?

Sometimes the diagnosis of the suspected cardiomyopathic process can be incorrect or the underlying condition has significantly changed.

1. Should additional or more advanced diagnostic tests (e.g., angiocardiography, echocardiography, catheterization) be performed or repeated?

2. Have any routine diagnostic procedures been omitted?

3. Should this case be referred?

REFERENCES AND SUPPLEMENTAL READING

Bonagura, J. D., Myer, C. W., and Pensinger, R. D.: Angiocardiography. Vet. Clin. North Am. 12:239, 1982.

Bond, B. R., and Tilley, L. P.: Cardiomyopathy in the dog and cat. *In* Kirk, R. W., (ed.): *Current Veterinary Therapy VII.* Philadelphia: W. B. Saunders, 1980.

Fox, P. R., Tilley, L. P., and Liu, S. K.: Cardiovascular system. *In* Catcott, E. J. (ed.): *Feline Medicine.* Santa Barbara: American Veterinary Publications, Inc., in press.

Harpster, N. K.: Feline cardiomyopathy. Vet. Clin. North Am. 7:355, 1977.

Liu, S. K.: Pathology of feline heart diseases. Vet. Clin. North Am. 7:323, 1977.

Liu, S. K., and Tilley, L. P.: Animal models of primary myocardial diseases. Yale J. Biol. Med. 53:191, 1980.

Liu, S. K., Fox, P. R., and Tilley, L. P.: Excessive left ventricular moderator bands in the cat. J.A.V.M.A. 180:1215, 1982.

Liu, S. K., Maron, B. J., and Tilley, L. P.: Feline hypertrophic cardiomyopathy. Am. J. Pathol. 102:388, 1981.

Peterson, M. E., Keene, B., Ferguson, D. C., and Pipers, F. S.: Electrocardiographic findings in 45 cats with hyperthyroidism. J.A.V.M.A. 180:934, 1982.

Tilley, L. P., Liu, S. K., Gilbertson, R. S., Wagner, B. M., and Lord, P. F.: Primary myocardial disease in the cat. Am. J. Pathol. 87:493, 1977.

Weneger, N. K.: Infectious myocarditis. *In* Burch, G. E. (ed.): *Cardiomyopathy*, Vol 4, No. 1. Philadelphia: F. A. Davis, 1972.

Wynne, J., and Braunwald, E.: The cardiomyopathies and myocarditides. *In* Braunwald, E. (ed.): *Heart Disease*, Vol. 2, Philadelphia: W. B. Saunders, 1980.

DIAGNOSIS AND MANAGEMENT OF CANINE HEARTWORM DISEASE

CLAY A. CALVERT, D.V.M.,

and CLARENCE A. RAWLINGS, D.V.M.

Athens, Georgia

Canine heartworm disease has been endemic in the coastal areas of the southeastern United States for at least 50 years. The highest incidences are still along the southeastern Atlantic and Gulf coasts as far west as Texas. *Dirofilaria immitis* has gradually spread to most of the eastern United States and the Midwest. In the Midwest, the highest incidence is found in the large river valleys, including most of Illinois, Indiana, southern Michigan, and in Minnesota and Wisconsin along the Mississippi River Valley. *D. immitis* is reported to occur in 1 to 5 per cent of the dogs throughout Texas, Oklahoma, Kansas, and Nebraska. Infection also occurs in northern California and in the Denver, Colorado area. Various parts of southern Canada report infections, usually in southeastern Ontario adjacent to Michigan and in Winnipeg, Manitoba, bordering Minnesota.

Dirofilaria immitis infects dogs of any age, but most infections occur in dogs between four and seven years of age (range 1 to 15 years of age). The male dog appears to be infected approximately twice as often as the female, although some reports have cited a 4:1 male to female ratio of infection. In general, large dogs are infected more often than small dogs, and dogs housed outside are four to five times more likely to become infected. The increased risk of infection in large dogs may be a reflection of

their greater likelihood of being outside. At the University of Georgia Veterinary Teaching Hospital, the most commonly infected breeds are the German shepherd, English pointer, setters, retrievers, and beagles. Length of haircoat has not been shown to be of great importance in determining the risk of infection.

The canine heartworm (*Dirofilaria immitis*) is usually found in the pulmonary arteries and the right ventricle. Although the dog is the most important host, *D. immitis* may infect numerous mammalian species. It is a long (12 to 30 cm) nematode whose larvae are transmitted by the bite of various mosquitoes. Another filaroid nematode, *Dipetalonema reconditum*, is important because its microfilariae may be confused with those of *D. immitis*.

Mosquitoes ingest the microfilariae (L_1) of *D. immitis* from the peripheral blood of infected dogs. The microfilariae migrate to the malpighian tubules, where they develop through the L_2 to L_3 (infective larvae) stages. Infective larvae enter the dog through the cutaneous puncture wound produced by the mosquito and migrate to subcutaneous or subserosal tissues, muscle, or adipose tissue. The L_3 molts to L_4 at approximately two weeks post infection. Further development to L_5 occurs by 80 days post infection, and the young adult (L_5) *D. immitis* arrives in the right ventricle in 90 to 100 days. Female *D. immitis* are gravid by 5 to 6 months, and circulating microfilariae are detected six to seven months post infection.

Although the microfilariae of *D. immitis* have been known to gain transplacental access to the fetal circulation, the L_3 to L_5 stages have not been shown to cross the placental barrier. The presence of microfilariae in puppies less than six months of age is possible but rare. Most likely, such infections in puppies are not due to patent infections and adulticide treatment is not indicated. However, microfilaricide therapy would be indicated.

DISEASE MECHANISM AND DEVELOPMENT

The typical clinical signs of chronic coughing, dyspnea, decreased exercise tolerance, syncope, hemoptysis, and congestive heart failure are produced by the disease mechanisms initiated by the adult heartworm parasite. The time course and severity of illness depend on the relative numbers of heartworm parasites, duration of infection, and host-parasite interaction. Immature adult heartworms are initially found within the small pulmonary arteries, particularly those of the caudal lung lobes, at 90 to 100 days after infection. Over the next three to six months these worms develop to mature adult size within the pulmonary arteries. When the number of mature heartworms exceeds 25 in a 25-kg dog, heartworms are commonly found extending from the pulmonary arteries into the right ventricle. Dogs with more than 50 heartworms commonly also have them in the right atrium, and if greater numbers are present they may obstruct the caudal vena cava.

The disease mechanisms have been traced to changes on the endothelial surface of the pulmonary arteries in response to the adult heartworms within their lumina. Endothelial cells swell, develop wider intercellular junctions, have activated leukocytes adhering to them, and slough longitudinal strips within three days of the arrival of adult heartworms into these pulmonary arteries. Activated platelets adhere to the focal areas of exposed subendothelium and appear to release a trophic factor, platelet–derived growth factor (PDGF). Intimal smooth muscle cells beneath these activated platelets multiply rapidly and migrate toward the surface. These cells, and the collagen that they produce, result in the pathognomonic villus proliferation from the pulmonary arterial surface. The de-endothelialized areas of the villi eventually develop an endothelial type of covering. Villi are present within three weeks of heartworm infestation and progressively increase in size and severity. Villi are distributed throughout the pulmonary arterial tree from the pulmonary valves to arteries as small as can accommodate a heartworm. Smaller pulmonary arteries also have medial hyperplasia that tends to obstruct their lumina to blood flow.

The lesions on the pulmonary arterial surface are associated with the gross pathognomonic changes seen on pulmonary arteriograms. All large arteries, especially the caudal lobar arteries, dilate, become tortuous, develop aneurysms, and lose their normal tapering and arborization. The linear lucencies of adult heartworms may be seen by angiography, and small arterial disease is recognized as an abrupt "pruning" of peripheral arteries. Flow of contrast media may be negligible or delayed through these lung regions, with poor small vessel circulation. Alveolar consolidation is present radiographically as a focal area about the caudal lobar arteries. The consolidation is due to focal edema and inflammatory reaction, which are extensions of changes occurring on the endothelial surface. These lung lesions probably involve the associated airways enough to initiate the coughing reflex.

Morphologic changes in the small pulmonary arteries increase pulmonary arterial resistance and pressure, leading to increased right ventricular afterload. The changes in the walls of larger arteries increase their "stiffness" and the pulse pressure within the pulmonary arteries. Pulmonary hypertension develops within a few months of adult heartworm infestation and appears to be produced by the morphologic changes. Pulmonary hypertension results from these vascular changes, not from the physical presence of adult or microfilarial *D. immitis*. The pulmonary hypertension that causes difficulties in propelling blood through the lungs can lead to decreased exercise tolerance and right-side congestive heart failure. Decreased exercise tolerance occurs when the infected dog can no longer increase cardiac output in response to the increased metabolic requirements during physical exertion. Inability to increase blood flow through the pulmonary vessels is due to hypertensive characteristics and the inability to collaterally recruit and dilate small pulmonary arteries.

The right heart initially can respond to the increased right ventricular afterload. As the afterload increases and stroke volume declines, the right ventricle compensates with right ventricular dilatation. Right atrial and systemic venous distention occur as a result of ventricular dilatation, activation of the sympathetic nervous system, and renal retention of sodium. Stretching of the right ventricle during diastole by the Frank-Starling mechanism can increase the force of right ventricular contraction and thus respond to the increased right ventricular afterload. As the hypertensive disease progresses, however, the work and metabolic requirements of the right ventricle increase and the right ventricle begins to hypertrophy. Electrocardiographic signs of right ventricular hypertrophy usually coincide with the onset of right ventricular failure and signs of congestive heart failure.

Although considerable morphologic changes are initiated by the presence of live heartworms, this host-parasite interaction is less severe than those changes initiated by the death of the heartworm. Extensive pulmonary changes are produced when heartworms die owing either to adulticide treatments or following a natural life course. These changes are most obvious during the first three to six weeks following heartworm death; the host's disease processes then begin to reverse to preinfection normalcy. The death of heartworms eliminates their protective mechanisms against the host defense mechanism. Severe thrombosis and a granulomatous inflammatory response are initiated. The most characteristic response of the arterial wall lining is an exaggerated development of the same myointimal proliferation into rugose villi as is produced in response to live heartworms. These arterial walls have areas with focal loss of endothelium and an increased protein permeability. Coagulation is initiated and the coagulation fibrinolysis may be severe enough to initiate either a local or systemic disseminated intravascular coagulopathy. The villus proliferation and thrombosis are typically so severe that flow is obstructed through the caudal lobar and intermediate arteries. Flow obstruction increases pressure sufficiently to distend the large pulmonary arteries and increases right ventricular afterload. The characteristic radiographic sign of worm embolism after therapy with an adulticide is the development of a focal area of increased alveolar density in the caudal and accessory lung lobes. These alveolar changes frequently involve whole lobes. The density may be produced by either edema or blood. The caudal airways of some dogs may fill with blood, and hemoptysis can occur. The radiographic and arteriographic changes produced by dead heartworms are usually resolved within three to four weeks after adulticide treatment.

Resolution of the changes in the surface of the proximal pulmonary arteries can be detected as early as six weeks after the adulticide treatment. The villi are either markedly reduced in size or absent. The cellular axis remains disoriented, and there is a swirling appearance to the endothelium. Villi are uncommon findings in arteries one year after treatment. Pulmonary hypertension, a reflection of small arterial disease, can revert to normal pulmonary artery pressure as soon as six months after successful adulticide treatment. The larger arteries decrease in size and tortuosity as the hypertension resolves. The aneurysms and dilation in the small arteries also tend to resolve but frequently retain more abnormalities. The parenchymal lesions about these arteries should be markedly resolved two to three months after adulticide treatment.

D. immitis infection in dogs without circulating microfilariae (*occult infection*) is relatively common and may come about by several mechanisms. Prepatent infections may produce clinical signs and demonstrable pulmonary changes. Occasionally a unisex infection occurs. Thiacetarsamide may fail to kill all adult worms but may render female worms sterile. If microfilaricide therapy is effective, adult worms will persist in the absence of circulating microfilariae.

Probably the most common cause of occult heartworm disease is an immune-mediated reaction. Antimicrofilarial antibodies develop against circulating microfilariae. The microfilariae are rapidly removed from the circulation within the lungs, and as a result multiple pulmonary granulomas are produced.

PRETREATMENT EVALUATION

Each heartworm-infected patient must be thoroughly evaluated prior to treatment. Documentation of a *Dirofilaria immitis* infection requires only the detection of their circulating microfilariae or the diagnosis of occult infection. The patient evaluation should include the severity of the heartworm disease and should detect other diseases. Diagnostic procedures include history, physical examination, thoracic radiography, complete blood count, blood urea nitrogen, urinalysis, liver enzymes, sulfobromophthalein (BSP) retention, and electrocardiography. To justify the expense of a specific diagnostic procedure, it must have a significant likelihood of providing useful information for either modifying the treatment regimen or altering the treatment prognosis. The cost of these procedures must be put into perspective with the client's and practitioner's desire for a particular quality of patient care. An algorithm (Fig. 1) has been developed in an attempt to categorize the diagnostic needs of various dogs with a circulating *D. immitis* microfilaria.

All dogs suspected of having heartworm infection should have a thorough history and physical examination. Asymptomatic dogs over five years of age should have a complete blood count, urinalysis, and blood urea nitrogen determination. Heartworm positive dogs of any age that are either coughing or dyspneic should be examined by thoracic radiography. The coughing dog with parenchymal disease and an inflammatory leukogram should have a transtracheal wash for cytology and bacterial culture. Dogs with signs of heart failure or marked enlargement of the right heart as viewed on thoracic radiographs should have the previously mentioned tests plus an electrocardiogram.

Dogs that are microfilaria negative but that have typical clinical signs of heartworm disease are usually presented for coughing and dyspnea, congestive heart failure, or the vena caval syndrome. Any dog

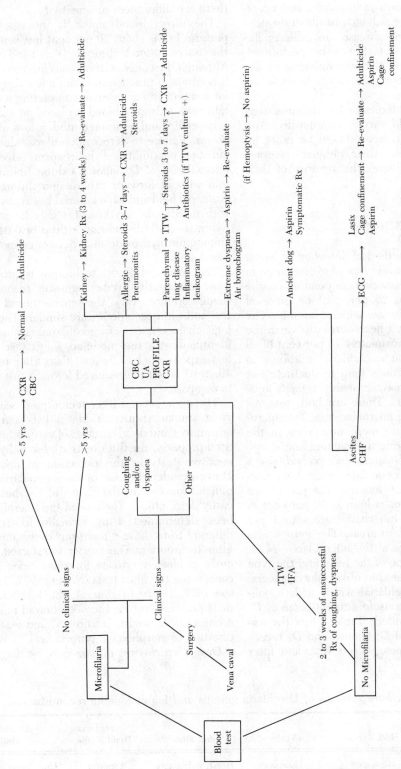

Figure 1. Algorithm for the management of canine heartworm disease. TTW = transtracheal wash, culture, and sensitivity; CXR = thoracic radiograph; IFA = indirect fluorescent antibody test; CHF = congestive heart failure.

with a history of coughing and dyspnea that has been nonresponsive to symptomatic treatment of two to three weeks duration should be studied via transtracheal wash, thoracic radiographs, and a complete blood count. If the radiographs illustrate signs suggestive of heartworm disease, an indirect fluorescent antibody (IFA) test may be performed. Electrocardiography and thoracic radiography are performed on dogs with signs of either heart failure or vena caval syndrome.

The age factor as an indicator for vigorous diagnostic evaluation should vary geographically. Animals in highly endemic areas should be more intensely evaluated, as their higher average heartworm burden increases the severity of their disease.

DIAGNOSIS

The most practical method of detection of heartworm disease is the identification of microfilariae in the peripheral blood. However, depending on the geographic area, up to 25 per cent or more of heartworm-infected dogs are amicrofilaremic. The overall incidence of occult heartworm disease in the continental U.S. is approximately 15 per cent of all infections. The fact that microfilarial numbers in dogs with chronic infections tend to fluctuate but do not continually increase probably reflects antigen-antibody interaction. There are both seasonal and diurnal variations in microfilaremia. The microfilariae of *D. immitis* are more numerous in the warmer months and during the evening hours.

The microfilariae of *Dipetalonema reconditum*, a nonpathogenic filaroid nematode, must be differentiated from those of *D. immitis*. The prevalence of the former varies from as high as 50 per cent in the southeastern and Gulf coastal areas to 1 per cent or less in the eastern areas. The most useful diagnostic characteristics of the microfilariae of *D. reconditum* are the shape of the head and the type of movement demonstrated in direct blood smears. Determination of microfilarial width with a calibrated lens may also be useful (microfilariae of *D. immitis* are generally wider). Table 1 lists the important characteristics of *D. immitis* and *D. reconditum*. Direct blood smear, Knott test, and filter techniques are all efficient in detecting high levels of microfilaremia. However, when there are only a few microfilariae per milliliter of peripheral blood, there are differences in sensitivity.

The direct blood smear is the easiest test to perform but is about 10 per cent less sensitive than the concentration techniques (Knott and filter tests). Although the concentration tests are recommended, it is common practice to retain a few drops of blood for a direct smear prior to completing a concentration test. A drop of blood is placed on a slide under a coverslip and examined under low microscopic power. Failure to detect microfilariae does not rule out the possibility of heartworm infection. The microfilariae of *D. immitis* exhibit undulating motion without forward progression through the microscopic field and have tapered heads. Interference with motility by erythrocytes may be reduced by lysing the cells by adding a drop of 0.04 per cent ammonium hydroxide or 2 per cent saponin to the blood smear.

The modified Knott technique is probably the most commonly used diagnostic technique. Although opinions vary, the sensitivities of the Knott test and filter techniques are similar. The morphologic characteristics of microfilariae are more easily identified with the modified Knott test, and it is less expensive (1 to 5¢/test) than filter tests (20 to 40¢/test). The time required for each test is difficult to compare.

There are several filter techniques available that yield similar results. Table 2 lists some of the advantages and disadvantages of various tests. When used properly, the filter tests are felt to be the most sensitive tests in the detection of microfilariae. However, identification of the microfilariae is more difficult since only the shape of the head can be easily determined. The size of the microfilariae has been determined using formalin fixative and is different from those dimensions determined by the filter techniques. The reader is referred to previously published articles for more specific details concerning the filter tests (Noyes, 1977, 1978; Jackson 1977, 1978). In general, the Knott test is the most practical test for the detection of microfilariae if one considers cost, sensitivity, and ease in identification of morphologic criteria.

Occult heartworm disease may be diagnosed by

Table 1. *Characteristics of* Dirofilaria immitis *and* Dipetalonema reconditum

Species	Host Range	Vector	Adult Sites	Microfilaria Head Shape	Microfilaria Motility
Dirofilaria immitis	Dog, cat, marine mammals, humans	Mosquitoes	Heart, pulmonary artery	Tapered	Undulation without progression
Dipetalonema reconditum	Dog	Fleas, ticks	Connective tissue	Blunt	Serpentine progressive movement

Table 2. *Advantages and Disadvantages of Various Microfilariae Detection Methods*

Direct Smear
   Less sensitive than concentration tests
   Least expensive and least time-consuming test
   Motility can be evaluated
Modified Knott Test
   Morphologic criteria identifiable
   Less expensive supplies than filter techniques
   Cross-contamination possible if centrifuge tubes
      improperly cleaned
   Microfilariae stick to centrifuge tube walls
Filter Tests
   Cross-contamination possible via lysing solution or
      dispenser nozzle
   Cross-contamination possible if filter housing or re-used
      syringes improperly cleaned
   Loss of some microfilariae possible
      Wrinkle in filter
      Through 8-μ pore-size filters
      Removal of excess fluid from edge of coverslip
      Improper assembly
      Slick-surfaced filter
   Morphologic criteria difficult to assess
   Microfilariae difficult to see on opaque filter
   Must examine edge of some filters
   More expensive
   Most sensitive of tests (?)

CLINICAL PATHOLOGY

The hematologic abnormalities in dogs with heartworm disease vary widely. A normocytic normochromic anemia is sometimes present in severely affected dogs. At the University of Georgia Veterinary Teaching Hospital, approximately 10 per cent of all heartworm-infected dogs have hematocrits of 27 to 36 per cent at the time of diagnosis. Ninety-five per cent of these anemic dogs are symptomatic for heartworm disease. Approximately 60 per cent of severely affected dogs are anemic, but severe anemia is uncommon. When a regenerative anemia occurs, poikilocytes are usually present, suggesting erythrocyte fragmentation. Erythrocyte fragmentation is a special contributing factor to anemia in the vena caval syndrome.

Although the total neutrophil count is usually

means of an IFA test. This test detects IgG directed against *D. immitis* microfilarial antigens. Approximately 20 per cent of dogs with occult heartworm disease do not have detectable antimicrofilarial antibody. The reasons for these false negative tests include (1) low levels of circulating antibody (early infections), (2) lack of free circulating antibody, and (3) lack of microfilariae production. Most dogs with occult heartworm infections have radiographically detectable pulmonary vascular and parenchymal changes that are consistent with heartworm disease and that permit a diagnosis to be made.

normal, the total band or juvenile neutrophil count tends to increase slightly with chronic infection. Approximately 20 per cent of the heartworm-infected dogs seen at this hospital have a neutrophilia, with a left shift in approximately 20 per cent of these cases. There is little correlation between neutrophilia and mild to moderate clinical signs. Neutrophilia is present in approximately 75 to 80 per cent of the dogs with concomitant right-side congestive heart failure.

A mild to moderate lymphopenia is present in almost all heartworm-infected dogs and probably reflects a stress response. When a marked eosinophilia exists, there is an increase in the number of blast-transformed lymphocytes in response to immune stimulation.

Approximately 85 per cent of microfilaremic and 95 per cent of amicrofilaremic (occult) infected dogs diagnosed at this hospital have an eosinophilia. Heartworm disease is probably the most common cause of basophilia in the dog. Approximately 50 per cent of the heartworm-infected dogs at this hospital have a basophilia at the time of diagnosis. This basophilia is almost always associated with an eosinophilia. Approximately 70 per cent of dogs with occult heartworm disease have a basophilia. In general, the mean and median eosinophil and basophil counts are highest in dogs with occult heartworm disease. In endemic areas, owing to the high incidence of intestinal and ectoparasites, eosinophil and basophil counts are of little diagnostic value unless the counts are very high. Marked eosinophilia may also be detected in dogs with *D. reconditum* infections.

The serum alkaline phosphatase (SAP) and glutamic pyruvate transaminase (SGPT) levels are normal in most dogs with heartworm disease. Approximately 5 per cent of the dogs have elevated enzyme levels. The severity of disease or likelihood of post-adulticide complication, even in dogs with severe pulmonary pathology and/or right-side congestive heart failure, does not correlate with elevations of liver enzymes. BSP retention is elevated in about 20 per cent of heartworm-infected dogs. There is a lack of correlation between clinical severity and the likelihood of abnormal BSP retention, except in dogs with right-side congestive heart failure, in which 40 to 50 per cent of the dogs have BSP retention of 8 to 15 per cent at 30 minutes. Less than 5 per cent of all heartworm-infected dogs are azotemic at the time of diagnosis. When azotemia is encountered, it is usually in dogs with moderate to severe heartworm disease.

Serum beta globulin levels are elevated in both symptomatic and asymptomatic heartworm-infected dogs. Dogs with more severe clinical signs often have low serum albumin levels. Approximately 20 per cent of the asymptomatic dogs have proteinuria compared with a 30 per cent incidence in mildly and moderately symptomatic dogs. The majority of dogs with concomitant heart failure are proteinuric. The proteinuria is due primarily to albumin and is usually of a mild degree. Some dogs have a severe proteinuria and a nephrotic syndrome due to amyloidosis.

Arterial blood gas tensions are normal in most heartworm-infected dogs. Approximately 15 to 20 per cent of the dogs have a mild, compensated metabolic acidosis. Mild hypoxia is observed in approximately 30 per cent of our cases and is attributed to severe obstructive pulmonary arterial disease. Most hypoxic dogs have normal acid-base values, but occasionally a metabolic acidosis occurs that is probably due to lactic acidosis.

THORACIC RADIOGRAPHY

In many dogs, particularly in endemic areas, the possibility of heartworm infection is first considered when radiographic changes consistent with the disease are encountered. Thoracic radiographic changes most often seen with heartworm disease are enlargement of the right ventricle, main pulmonary artery, and parenchymal pulmonary arteries. At the University of Georgia Veterinary Teaching Hospital, 86 per cent of 200 dogs seen consecutively with heartworm disease with microfilaremia had radiographic abnormalities consistent with dirofilariasis. One-third of these dogs had enlargement of the right ventricle, main pulmonary artery, and right cranial lobar pulmonary artery. Approximately 60 per cent had enlargement of the right ventricle, with severe enlargement seen in 20 per cent. Two-thirds of the dogs had enlargement of the main pulmonary artery. The absence of enlargement of the right cranial lobar pulmonary artery is a poor indicator of the absence of heartworm disease. Enlargement of the right caudal pulmonary artery occurs earlier; however, the caudal lobar arteries are difficult to evaluate unless the dorsoventral position is utilized.

Dogs with the greatest enlargement of the right ventricle also have the greatest enlargement of the main pulmonary artery. As the radiographic signs of heartworm disease worsen, abnormal pulmonary arterial tortuosity worsens and parenchymal lung disease develops, primarily in the caudal lung lobes. By the time right ventricular hypertrophy (RVH) can be identified electrocardiographically, 50 per cent of the dogs have obvious excessive pulmonary artery tortuosity and 75 per cent have parenchymal lung disease. When the right ventricle is normal electrocardiographically, there is no radiographic evidence of enlargement in 70 per cent of the dogs (severe enlargement is always absent), and only 10 per cent have parenchymal lung disease.

ELECTROCARDIOGRAPHY

The electrocardiogram (ECG) is normal in most dogs with heartworm disease, and ECG criteria of RVH are seen only with advanced heartworm disease. The ECG criteria that are most sensitive to RVH are listed in Table 3. When any three of these criteria are present, the diagnosis of increased right ventricular free wall weight as compared with total ventricular weight and body weight can be made with greater than 90 per cent accuracy. RVH is suspected when two criteria exist. RVH is unlikely to be present when none or one criterion exists.

In dogs with heartworm disease, approximately 80 per cent of those with three or more ECG criteria of RVH have right-side congestive heart failure. The rest develop heart failure within two months, particularly if they continue to exercise. When there are less than three criteria of RVH present, fewer than 5 per cent of the dogs will be in heart failure.

Table 3.   *Individual and Combined ECG Criteria of RVH**

Radiographic Evaluation of Right Ventricle	No. of Dogs With ECG Criteria of RVH (%)								
	≥ 3	S_1	S_{v2}	S_{v4}	MEA_f	MEA_x	S_{II}	R/S_{v4}	$+T_{v10}$
Normal (n = 53)	4(7)	3(6)	9(18)	6(11)	4(7.5)	3(6)	1(2)	0	1(2)
Severe enlargement (n = 44)	37(84)	30(68)	36(82)	34(77.5)	32(75)	16(36)	17(32)	7(13)	3(6)

*Observed in dogs with normal or severely enlarged right ventricles as assessed radiographically.
$S_1 > 0.05$ mV.
$S_{v2} > 0.8$ mV.
$S_{v4} > 0.7$ mV.
MEA_f = frontal plane mean electrical axis $> +103°$.
MEA_x = transverse plane mean electrical axis $> +90°$.
$S_{II} > 0.35$ mV.
$R/S_{V4} < 0.87$.

PREADULTICIDE MANAGEMENT OF OCCULT HEARTWORM DISEASE– ASSOCIATED ALLERGIC PNEUMONITIS

An allergic pneumonitis occurs in some dogs with occult heartworm disease. The reasons for this reaction are unclear but are probably related to microfilarial antigen-antibody interaction. Affected dogs are usually three to eight years of age, and there is no sex predilection. Observed clinical signs are coughing, dyspnea, orthopnea, wheezing, moist rales or crackles, and exercise intolerance. Although concomitant right-side congestive heart failure may exist, the clinical signs are usually disproportionate to the degree of pulmonary arterial pathology. The electrocardiogram of affected dogs is normal unless heart failure coexists; however, there are characteristic radiographic pulmonary changes. There is a diffuse alveolar pattern resembling pulmonary edema along with a diffuse linear interstitial infiltrate.

Transtracheal lavage usually reveals an eosinophilic exudate (20 to 60 per cent eosinophils) with macrophages and nondegenerative neutrophils. Occasionally, culture of the transtracheal exudate yields bacteria. When bacteria are cultured, antibiotic therapy alone may produce a transient, partial improvement of clinical signs. However, glucocorticosteroids or glucocorticosteroids plus an appropriate antibiotic should be administered.

The salient clinical pathologic findings in dogs with heartworm disease–associated allergic pneumonitis are eosinophilia (1,500 to 10,000/mm³), basophilia (150 to 2000/mm³), marked hyperglobulinemia, a negative Knott's test, and a positive occult microfilaria test.

Dogs affected with this allergic pneumonitis may be treated with prednisone (2 mg/kg, once or twice daily). The clinical and roentgenographic signs improve dramatically, usually within one to two days. Occasionally, improvement is gradual over a seven- to ten-day period. Adulticide therapy is given following improvement of clinical signs. Prednisone is continued for three to four weeks and may be discontinued one to two weeks prior to microfilaricide treatment.

ADULTICIDE THERAPY

Thiacetarsamide sodium has been an effective drug in the treatment of infestation by the adult *D. immitis* organism for over a quarter of a century. The currently recommended regimen has been in use for almost 20 years (Table 4). The drug may produce renal and hepatic toxicity. Following injection, gravid female *D. immitis* organisms expel their microfilariae. A few adults are killed within a few

Table 4. Summary of Drug Dosages and Schedules for Management of Canine Heartworm Disease

Adulticide
Thiacetarsamide (Caparsolate, Abbott; Filaramide, Fromm)
0.22 ml/kg, IV, b.i.d., for two days
Treatment interval: minimum of six hours, maximum of 15 hours

Microfilaricide
Dithiazanine (Dizan, Pitman-Moore)
1. 8.8 mg/kg, PO, for seven days
2. Microfilaria test on day 8
3. If microfilaremic, 13 to 14 mg/kg daily for ten days maximum
4. Microfilaria test between days 12 and 17
Levamisole (Ripercol L, Capri)
1. 11 mg/kg, PO, for seven days
2. Microfilaria test on day 7
3. If microfilaremic, 11 mg/kg daily for five days
4. Microfilaria test on day 12
5. Repeat microfilaria test three months after successful microfilaricide therapy

Prophylaxis
Diethylcarbamazine
1. 5.5 to 6.5 mg/kg (citrate), PO, daily
2. Microfilaria test biannually
3. Microfilaria test three months post-microfilaricide therapy

Thiacetarsamide
0.22 ml/kg, IV, b.i.d., for two days every six months

days, but most die slowly over a two- to three-week period.

Pretreatment administration of ascorbic acid, glucocorticoids, and "liver-sparing" drugs is not indicated. Feeding one-half to one hour prior to each adulticide injection may have a protecting effect on the liver.

Thiacetarsamide is available as a 1 per cent solution in a multiple-dose vial that should be stored under refrigeration. The dosage (0.22 ml/kg b.i.d. for two days) is given intravenously, with extreme caution to avoid extravasation. Swelling, inflammation, and tissue necrosis may occur if more than a few drops are extravasated. Should extravasation occur, the tissues should be infiltrated with sterile saline, dexamethasone, and DMSO applied topically.

About 50 per cent of the dose of thiacetarsamide is excreted in the first 24 hours. At least 6 and not more than 15 hours should elapse between doses. No dosage adjustments are made for size of dog. Deviation from this regimen results in decreased efficacy or increased toxicity. If the previously mentioned dosage is given b.i.d. for three days, excessive post-therapy pulmonary pathology without increased adulticide activity results. Thiacetarsamide appears to be less effective against young, female adult *D. immitis* organisms, therefore persisting microfilaremia may result. A 100 per cent kill of adult worms may not be attained. Although pulmonary and cardiac performance will improve substantially, microfilaremia will persist or recur under these circumstances, and adulticide therapy should be repeated.

Levamisole has been employed as an adulticide. However, the dosage schedules utilized have yielded erratic results. The drug may be active against male *D. immitis* organisms but may be much less effective against females. It is not indicated for adulticide treatment.

ADVERSE REACTIONS TO THIACETARSAMIDE

Prior to each dosage, it is recommended that the dog be fed and evaluated for overt signs of illness. Occasionally, vomiting, which is the most common adverse effect of thiacetarsamide, will occur following the first or second dose. Vomiting is not an indication to stop therapy unless (1) it is persistent, (2) the dog is also anorexic and depressed, or (3) icterus or azotemia develops. The last-named complication is unusual. Mild prerenal azotemia may result from persistent vomiting, anorexia, and dehydration. If the dog is dehydrated owing to vomiting and anorexia, fluid therapy is given and the animal discharged from the hospital when these problems are resolved, usually in 24 to 48 hours. Urine examination is recommended prior to each dose of thiacetarsamide, particularly in older or more clinically affected dogs.

The earliest sign of hepatotoxicity is bilirubinuria. However, bilirubinuria (regardless of severity) is not an indication to stop treatment if only one dose remains and there are no other signs of illness. If bilirubinuria develops after the first or second dose, therapy may be terminated. Icterus, on the other hand, is an indication to stop therapy. If adulticide treatment is stopped, it should be repeated in four weeks and usually is then completed without complication. No specific therapy is recommended for dogs in which adulticide therapy is terminated owing to adverse reactions. Rest and a high-carbohydrate diet are recommended. Steroids, vitamins, and "liver-sparing" agents such as inositol, choline, and methionine are of no proven value.

About 20 per cent of all dogs with normal SGPT and SAP values prior to thiacetarsamide treatment will develop abnormally elevated enzyme levels post treatment. These values become abnormal one to two days after the first injection of the drug but decrease within seven days. Less than 10 per cent of these dogs have elevated SGPT or SAP values six weeks post treatment. Thiacetarsamide does not cause abnormal BSP retention.

Pre-existing elevations of SGPT, SAP, or BSP are not indications to delay adulticide treatment, and microfilaricide treatment prior to adulticide treatment is not indicated. The best treatment for elevated liver enzymes is to eradicate the heartworm infection. The likelihood of thiacetarsamide toxicity causing renal failure is increased if pre-existing renal insufficiency is not detected. Thus, in older or symptomatic dogs, the BUN and urine specific gravity should be determined prior to adulticide treatment.

It is rare that a delay in adulticide treatment of four to six weeks will worsen the prognosis for successful therapy. Therefore, adulticide therapy should not be continued in the face of signals indicating discontinuation. If the dog also suffers from congestive heart failure, cage rest should be enforced for at least one week and severe exercise restriction enforced for two to three additional weeks until adulticide treatment can be repeated. Furosemide and a low-sodium, high-carbohydrate diet are also provided.

Post-adulticide pulmonary arterial obstructive lung disease is the most dangerous sequela of adulticide therapy. The adult worms die as early as a few days after the start of thiacetarsamide treatment and continue to die over a three-week period. Mild febrile reactions are first detected from five to eight days after the start of treatment, and periodic fever continues for approximately three weeks. Additional clinical signs are detected 10 to 14 days after the start of treatment. Although it is not always possible to predict which dogs will experience severe obstructive pulmonary disease, pre-existing radiographic evidence of obstructive lesions and advanced arterial pathology increase the likelihood of complications.

Fever, coughing, and, in more severe cases, dyspnea and hemoptysis are the typical signs of pulmonary thromboembolism. Mild reactions require no therapy other than enforced exercise restriction, although glucocorticoids will reduce febrile reactions. Dogs that become dyspneic or hypoxemic, or that have hemoptysis should be hospitalized and cage confined. Bronchodilators, glucocorticoids, and antibiotics are usually prescribed but are of no proven value. Cage confinement is the most important treatment. Disseminated intravascular coagulopathy occurs in many dogs with severe clinical signs. The prognosis is poor in the presence of pre-existing congestive heart failure, epistaxis, other signs of hemorrhage, and clinical and biochemical data substantiating disseminated intravascular coagulopathy. Therapy of advanced coagulopathy with heparin and clotting factors is usually unrewarding.

MICROFILARICIDE THERAPY

Treatment to eradicate microfilariae is indicated (1) to eliminate the carrier dog as a source of infection (of questionable significance), (2) because microfilariae can result in renal, hepatic, and pulmonary pathology, (3) to allow prophylactic chemotherapy, and (4) to enable verification of effective adulticide therapy. Both dithiazanine and levamisole cause expulsion of microfilariae from the gravid female worms. If adulticide therapy is less than 100 per cent effective, microfilaremia may recur following effective microfilaricide therapy.

Microfilaricide therapy is begun four to six weeks following adulticide therapy (see Table 4). Dithiazanine (8.8 mg/kg) is given daily for seven days. On day 8, a microfilariae test is performed. If positive, the dose of dithiazanine may be increased to 13 to 14 mg/kg daily for a maximum of ten days. Vomiting and diarrhea are common side effects of dithiazanine, especially at higher doses. The stools of dogs on dithiazanine will have a purple stain. Although dithiazanine has been reported to be a nephrotoxic drug, there is little or no documentation of such toxicity. Dithiazanine may fail to kill all of the microfilariae.

Levamisole (11 mg/kg daily) is an effective microfilaricide. A microfilariae check is performed on day 7 and, if positive, the same dose schedule is continued on days 7 through 12. A microfilariae check is performed on day 12. At least 70 per cent of the dogs will be microfilariae negative on day 7 and over 90 per cent by day 12. Levamisole should be administered as a single daily dose following a small meal. Because of its short half-life, dividing the daily dose will decrease efficacy. Levamisole given on an empty stomach often results in vomiting, the most common side effect. When vomiting occurs, therapy is temporarily halted and the treatment regimen re-evaluated. Vomiting can be prevented or diminished by premedication with an antiemetic. Continued therapy in the face of vomiting may result in more serious signs such as central nervous system toxicity. Panting, nervousness, and shaking are the most commonly observed neurologic signs. The therapeutic index of levamisole is narrow. Doses of less than 11 mg/kg are less effective, and doses greater than 15.5 mg/kg usually result in toxicity.

Fenthion, an organophosphate, is a microfilaricide. Fenthion is not currently FDA approved for use in dogs. When given at a dosage of 15 mg/kg subcutaneously every two weeks, 60 per cent of the dogs may be cleared after one treatment and 95 per cent cleared after two treatments. Significant side effects were noted in 3 of 45 dogs in one study (Jackson, 1969). Organophosphate– or carbamate–containing flea collars, dips, and dusts should not be administered two weeks prior to, during, and two weeks following completion of fenthion treatment. The simultaneous action of two such agents may produce as much as 50 times the effect of either alone. Fenthion (13.8 per cent solution) may also be applied topically every 14 days for three treatments. Microfilarial counts decrease sharply after three weeks. Topical fenthion application for flea control also eradicates microfilariae. For that reason, the heartworm status must be determined prior to fenthion application. If the dog is amicrofilaremic, diethylcarbamazine prophylaxis is instituted. Anorexia, vomiting, fever, and other signs of organophosphate toxicity may be observed but are uncommon.

Ivermectin, one of the avermectin compounds produced by the actinomycete *Streptomyces avermitilis*, has shown good microfilaricide activity. A single dose of 0.25 mg/kg orally two weeks after adulticide therapy was found safe and effective. Minor reactions were occasionally observed. The avermectin compounds have not yet received FDA approval (Jackson, 1981).

Dithiazanine and levamisole are the agents most often used as microfilaricides. In the event of microfilaremia following the use of either, the alternate drug protocol is given. If microfilaremia persists, it is recommended that adulticide therapy be repeated. An additional microfilariae test should be repeated two months after microfilaricide therapy is completed to detect those instances in which live adults persist.

There is no therapeutic advantage to administration of microfilaricide before an adulticide. Experience at the University of Georgia has failed to reveal any benefit in severely affected dogs. The theoretical concept that pathophysiologic responses due to microfilariae increase thiacetarsamide toxicity is unproved. In fact, the pathophysiologic responses from thiacetarsamide are independent of microfilariae.

HEARTWORM DISEASE AND CONCOMITANT RIGHT-SIDE CONGESTIVE HEART FAILURE

Heartworm disease with concomitant right-side congestive heart failure is common in endemic areas. The diagnosis of heart failure is based on the presence of a jugular pulse, distended jugular veins, and ascites. The ECG of these dogs almost always reveals three or more criteria of RVH (see Table 3). Thoracic radiographs reveal severe pulmonary vascular changes.

Dogs with heartworm disease and concomitant right-side congestive heart failure are usually three to eight years of age, male (75 per cent), large breeds, and, usually, amicrofilaremic. The appropriate treatment for these dogs is (1) cage rest seven to ten days prior to and two to three weeks post-adulticide treatment, (2) furosemide, (3) aspirin (10 mg/kg) daily until three weeks post-adulticide treatment, (4) a low-sodium diet, and (5) the standard adulticide protocol administered after seven to ten days of cage confinement. Twenty-three (82 per cent) of 28 dogs treated in this manner survived with few severe complications. Four dogs died within seven days of adulticide treatment owing to disseminated intravascular coagulopathy. Therapy for heart failure can be withdrawn in four to eight weeks. Dogs treated with aspirin or cage confinement as described previously were statistically more likely to survive than those dogs not given aspirin or cage confinement for seven to ten days prior to and three weeks post-adulticide treatment. Digitalization usually is unnecessary, and digoxin toxicity can complicate therapy. That adulticide therapy is indicated is demonstrated by the fact that ten dogs treated only for heart failure failed to improve significantly and died or were euthanized within 30 days.

Occasionally, gastrointestinal bleeding may complicate aspirin therapy. For that reason we suggest that cimetidine* (20 mg/kg divided t.i.d.) be given during aspirin treatment.† Significant blood loss can be detected by monitoring the hematocrit.

VENA CAVAL SYNDROME

The vena caval syndrome usually occurs in dogs three to five years of age in highly endemic areas. The affected dog apparently receives a large exposure to infected mosquitoes during a short period of time. Occasionally, the syndrome is seen in older dogs. There are no prior signs of heartworm disease. There are usually over 100 worms present, the majority located in the right atrium and vena cava. In asymptomatic and chronic heartworm disease there are usually 25 to 30 and 50 to 60 worms, respectively, with greater than 85 per cent located in the right ventricle and pulmonary artery.

The vena caval syndrome is characterized by the sudden onset of anorexia, severe depression, dyspnea, collapse, pale mucous membranes, and a weak thready pulse. Azotemia, hemoglobinuria, bilirubinuria, elevation of liver enzymes, abnormal BSP retention, and anemia are typically present. Without therapy, death usually occurs in 24 to 72 hours. Disseminated intravascular coagulation (DIC) is an inherent phenomenon in the syndrome. DIC probably is initiated by (1) the intravascular destruction of erythrocytes that contact the worms and (2) the liver's inability to remove procoagulants from the circulation.

The only effective treatment of the vena caval syndrome is to remove as many worms as possible

---

*Tagamet, Smith Kline & French Laboratories, Philadelphia, PA.

†Editor's Note: Cimetidine has been found to reduce the clearance of many drugs. The clinician must be alert to potential drug interactions that may occur and may be reported in future literature.

from the right atrium and post cava. Jackson has described a procedure whereby the worms are removed, under local anesthesia, with a long alligator forceps passed through the right jugular vein. Eighty-five per cent of the dogs treated in this way were saved. The forceps are repeatedly passed into the right atrium and post cava until five to six successive attempts fail to retrieve worms. From none to 12 worms may be retrieved during any one attempt, but usually 1 to 4 are retrieved. Many worms are removed, but marked clinical improvement may result from removal of only 25 to 30 worms.

Following removal of the worms, a jugular catheter is placed and intensive fluid therapy is given. The central venous pressure is monitored to avoid excessive fluid administration. An indwelling urinary catheter is placed and the bladder emptied. The volume and character of urine is monitored to assess renal function and hemoglobinuria. The BUN and hematocrit are monitored post-surgically. Following recovery, thiacetarsamide is administered to kill the adults in the right ventricle and pulmonary artery. The dog's appetite, mucous membrane color, heart rate, respiratory rate, and BUN should be normal prior to adulticide therapy. The hematocrit should be greater than 35 per cent. Chemotherapy may be given, even in the presence of seven- to eightfold elevations of SAP and SGPT and BSP retention of up to 10 to 15 per cent.

HEARTWORM DISEASE PROPHYLAXIS

Diethylcarbamazine (DEC) is administered daily to dogs at risk of developing heartworm disease. DEC prophylaxis is particularly important in endemic areas. In warmer climates, such as the southeastern United States, DEC is given year round. In other areas, DEC prophylaxis is begun simultaneously with the appearance of mosquitoes and is continued for two months after the mosquito season. DEC is the only drug with a proven, well-tested record of efficacy against the larvae of *D. immitis*. DEC is primarily effective during the L_3 (infective larvae) to L_4 molt (approximately 15 to 17 days post infection).

Because of its short half-life and lack of residual activity, DEC should be given daily. It is imperative that DEC not be given to microfilaremic dogs, as it often produces an anaphylactic shock syndrome (type I hypersensitivity, immediate hypersensitivity). Hypovolemic shock of variable degree occurs. The clinical signs may include vomiting, diarrhea, tachycardia, dyspnea, pale mucous membranes, incoordination, weakness, and collapse. Hepatic congestion with variable degrees of centrilobular necrosis occurs. Pooling of blood in the splanchnic vessels results in decreased circulating blood volume and splanchnic hypertension. The decreased blood flow causes intestinal hypoxia and hemorrhage into the intestinal lumen. The hematocrit increases, as do the SGPT and SAP values. The platelet and WBC counts decrease significantly within one hour but rebound to produce a leukocytosis and neutrophilia within six hours.

The specific antigen mediating the anaphylaxis has not been identified. It is postulated that prior IgE production and mast cell sensitization occur in response to microfilarial antigen. Subsequently, DEC may combine with the microfilaria-related antigen, resulting in mast cell degranulation. Alternatively, DEC may trigger the release of large amounts of the antigen, which attach to IgE, resulting in mast cell degranulation. The mast cell mediators decrease circulating blood volume, blood pressure, and vasodilation of capillary beds. Also, platelet activation and release of coagulation factors may initiate disseminated intravascular coagulation.

When microfilariae are detected in dogs on DEC prophylaxis, DEC should not be discontinued but continued during adulticide and microfilaricide therapy. It is unlikely that low numbers of circulating microfilariae will incite untoward reactions in response to DEC prophylaxis. Since L_4 and prepatent adult *D. immitis* organisms may be present prior to DEC prophylaxis, adult worms may develop as late as six months after the start of DEC administration. Therefore, microfilaria tests should be performed every six months after DEC prophylaxis is started. This is particularly important in highly endemic areas.

The recommended dose of DEC (5.5 to 6.5 mg/kg daily) rarely produces untoward effects, but anorexia or vomiting may occur. Occasionally, daily DEC prophylaxis is not practical. In such cases, implementation of the adulticide protocol every six months will prevent the development of heartworm disease.

There have been anecdotal reports of impaired fertility caused by DEC and DEC-styrylpyridinium chloride (DEC-SC). Although both sexes of a variety of breeds have been reported to be affected, the problem has been reported most often in male greyhounds. Normal libido with low sperm counts was observed, and sperm counts returned to normal following the withdrawal of DEC or DEC-SC. Subsequent controlled experiments in dogs using DEC and DEC-SC have failed to detect abnormalities in semen quality or decreased reproductive efficiency. However, the possibility of idiosyncratic effects in individual dogs or breeds exists. The clinician should keep in mind that one semen sample following a long period of sexual inactivity may be of inferior quality.

As many as 20 per cent of the clients starting DEC prophylaxis may fail to continue owing to the necessity for daily administration. Proper client education is a vital factor in overcoming this problem. Underdosing DEC may be a problem, usually in puppies when the dose is not increased as the dog grows.

Ivermectin administered orally on a monthly basis is an effective prophylactic agent that has not yet received FDA approval. This compound affects the L_4 and L_5 stages. Ivermectin prophylaxis has the advantage of monthly versus daily administration. Ivermectin has been shown to be safe and produces only mild side effects at dosages much higher than those needed for prophylaxis against infective larvae (McCall, 1980).

REFERENCES AND SUPPLEMENTAL READING

Jackson, R. F.: Complications during and following chemotherapy of heartworm disease. J.A.V.M.A. 154:393, 1969.

Jackson, R. F.: The venae cavae syndrome. *In* Morgan, H. C (ed.): *Proceedings of the Heartworm Symposium.* Bonner Springs, KS: Veterinary Medicine Publishing Co., 1975, pp. 48–50.

Jackson, R. F.: Studies on the filter techniques for the detection and identification of canine microfilariae. *In* Morgan, H. D. (ed.): *Proceedings of the Heartworm Symposium.* Bonner Springs, KS: Veterinary Medicine Publishing Co., 1978, pp. 38–44.

Jackson, R. F., and Seymour, W. G.: Efficacy of avermectins against microfilariae of *Dirofilaria immitis. In* Morgan, H. D. (ed.): *Proceedings of the Heartworm Symposium.* Edwardsville, KS: Veterinary Medicine Publishing Co., 1981, pp. 131–136.

Jackson, R. F., Seymour, W. G., Growney, P. J., and Otto, G. F.: Surgical treatment of the caval syndrome of canine heartworm disease. J.A.V.M.A. 171:1065, 1977.

McCall, J. W., Lindemann, B. A., and Porter, C. A.: Prophylactic activity of avermectins against experimentally induced *D. immitis* infections in dogs. *In* Morgan, H. D. (ed.): *Proceedings of the Heartworm Symposium.* Edwardsville, KS: Veterinary Medicine Publishing Co., 1981, pp. 126–130.

Morgan, H. C. (ed.): Proceedings of the Heartworm Symposium 1974. Bonner Springs, Kansas: VM Publishing Co., 1975.

Morgan, H. C. (ed.): Proceedings of the Heartworm Symposium 1977. Bonner Springs, Kansas: VM Publishing Co., 1978.

Morgan, H. C. (ed.): Proceedings of the Heartworm Symposium 1980. Edwardsville, Kansas: VM Publishing Co., 1981.

Noyes, J. D.: Comparison of Knott and filter techniques. *In* Morgan, H. C. (ed.): *Proceedings of the Heartworm Symposium.* Bonner Springs, KS: Veterinary Medicine Publishing Co., 1978, pp. 34–37.

Otto, G. F., and Jackson, R. F.: Heartworm disease. *In* Ettinger, S. (ed.): *Textbook of Veterinary Internal Medicine.* Philadelphia: W. B. Saunders, 1975. pp. 1014–1038.

Rawlings, C. A., Keith, J. C., and Schaub, R. G.: Development and resolution of pulmonary disease in heartworm infection: Illustrated review. J. Am. Anim. Hosp. Assoc. 17:711, 1981.

Rawlings, C. A., Losansky, J. M., Lewis, R. E., and McCall, J. W.: Development and resolution of the radiographic lesions in canine heartworm disease. J.A.V.M.A. 178:1172, 1981.

Rawlings, C. A., McCall, J. W., and Lewis, R. E.: The response of the canine heart and lungs to *Dirofilaria immitis.* J. Am. Anim. Hosp. Assoc. 14:17, 1978.

Wong, M. M., and Suter, P. F.: Indirect fluorescent antibody test in occult dirofilariasis. Am. J. Vet. Res. 40:414, 1979.

THERAPY OF CARDIAC ARRHYTHMIAS

JOHN BONAGURA, D.V.M.

Columbus, Ohio

Cardiac arrhythmias are disturbances in the rate, rhythm, and conduction of the electrical activity of the heart. Arrhythmias (dysrhythmias) are caused by heart disease or extracardiac disorders that affect the cardiac rhythm. The normal heartbeat is initiated by the spontaneous depolarization of pacemaker cells in the sinoatrial (SA) node. This impulse is rapidly and sequentially distributed through the heart by an elaborate conduction system of specialized myocardial cells (Fig. 1). Disruptions of this normal activation process result in cardiac rhythm disturbances that can be detected on the electrocardiogram (ECG). The basic cellular mechanisms responsible for abnormal cardiac automaticity or conduction are beyond the scope of this article. However, the resultant cardiac arrhythmias are of great clinical importance and are the focus of this article.

Abnormal cardiac rhythms are associated with a wide variety of disorders (Table 1), including heart disease, acid-base and electrolyte imbalances, ischemia, autonomic imbalance, endocrinopathies, metabolic disease, and pulmonary disease, and with the administration of certain drugs. Although it may be impossible to determine the precise cellular electrophysiologic mechanism responsible for a particular dysrhythmia, a knowledge of the *clinical disorders* that are associated with certain rhythm

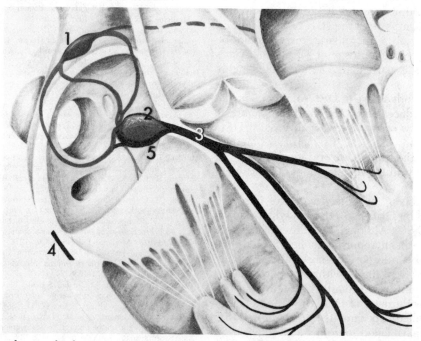

Figure 1. The cardiac impulse forming and conduction system. The sinoatrial node (1) initiates the cardiac electrical activity. The impulse is rapidly transmitted to the atrioventricular node (2) via specialized internodal pathways. Depolarization of the atrial muscle results in the P wave of the ECG. During conduction across the AV node, bundle of His (3), and ventricular bundle branches, the PR interval of the ECG is inscribed. Activation of the ventricular myocardium leads to the QRS complex, whereas the genesis of the ST-T segment is repolarization of the ventricular muscle mass.

Ectopic rhythms can develop in the atrium, AV junctional region, and ventricular specialized conduction system. These can be associated with altered automaticity of the heart or abnormal conduction through the major or minor portions of the cardiac conduction system. Major conduction blocks, such as complete atrioventricular block, may occur, resulting in dissociation between the atrial (P) and ventricular (QRS) complexes. Abnormal conduction pathways can lead to ventricular pre-excitation or re-entrant supraventricular tachycardias via accessory Kent (4) or James (5) pathways. Atrial or ventricular myocardial fibrillation can result from abnormal conduction and nonuniform cell recovery.

Table 1. *Clinical Associations of Common Cardiac Arrhythmias*

Rhythm	Clinical Setting
Sinus Rhythms	
Normal sinus rhythm	Normal rhythm; can be associated with abnormal conduction
Sinus arrhythmia	Normal rhythm; uncommon in the cat
Sinus bradycardia	Increased vagal tone; elevated cerebrospinal fluid pressure; brain stem lesions; head trauma; hypothermia; hypothyroidism; hyperkalemia; administration of propranolol, digitalis, or inhalation anesthetics
Sinus tachycardia	Increased sympathetic tone; fear; excitement; pain; hypovolemia; hypotension; anemia; heart failure; hyperthyroidism; administration of vagolytic drugs, such as atropine, or sympathomimetics
Sinoatrial arrest and sick sinus syndrome (SSS)	High vagal tone; digitalis, surgical manipulation; SSS can alternate with supraventricular tachycardia; breed predilection in miniature schnauzers, pugs, dachshunds, cocker spaniels
Supraventricular Arrhythmias	
Supraventricular (atrial and junctional) premature complexes	Atrioventricular valve regurgitation; cardiomyopathy; congenital heart diseases; chronic obstructive pulmonary disease; hypoxia; anemia; digitalis intoxication; increased sympathetic tone; administration of anesthetic agents; "toxemia"; hypokalemia; atrial tumors
Supraventricular (atrial, junctional, re-entrant) tachycardia	Causes of supraventricular premature complexes; atrial septal defect; tricuspid valve dysplasia; accessory atrioventricular pathway; electrocution; hyperthyroidism; cardiac catheterization
Atrial flutter and fibrillation	Atrial dilatation; cardiomyopathy; AV valvular insufficiency; untreated congenital heart disease; cardiac catheterization; trauma; drug administration
Junctional escape rhythm	A protective rhythm associated with sinus bradycardia, sinus arrest, and atrioventricular block
Ventricular Arrhythmias	
Ventricular premature complexes, idioventricular tachycardia, and ventricular tachycardia	Cardiomyopathy; heart failure; endomyocarditis; chronic valvular heart disease; pericarditis; cardiac tumor; congenital heart disease; hypoxia; anemia; acidosis; hypokalemia; autonomic imbalance; thoracic and abdominal trauma; gastric dilatation-volvulus; sepsis; pyometra; pulmonary disease; digitalis intoxication; hyperthyroidism, administration of anesthetics or sympathomimetics
Ventricular escape rhythm	As per junctional escape rhythm
Conduction Disorders	
Atrial standstill	Hyperkalemia; hypoadrenocorticism; urinary obstruction; if persistent (silent atria), due to muscular dystrophy
Incomplete atrioventricular block (1°, 2°)	Normal variant; increased vagal tone; administration of digitalis glycosides or xylazine; AV nodal disease; cardiomyopathy; doxorubicin cardiotoxicity
Complete atrioventricular block (3°)	AV nodal or junctional disease including infarction, replacement with connective tissue, and neoplasia; severe drug toxicity (digitalis, xylazine, doxorubicin); aortic valve bacterial endocarditis
Intraventricular conduction defect (fascicular and bundle branch blocks)	Congenital or acquired heart disease including atrial and ventricular septal defects, pulmonary stenosis, AV valve insufficiency, patent ductus arteriosus, and cardiomyopathy; smoke inhalation; acute cor pulmonale; digitalis intoxication; doxorubicin toxicity

disturbances is important and influences both therapy and prognosis.

The significance of a cardiac arrhythmia depends on both the type of rhythm disturbance and the associated clinical setting (Table 2). Many arrhythmias do not require therapy or prove to be self-limiting when the underlying disorder is treated. Serious arrhythmias, such as atrial tachycardia, atrial fibrillation, and ventricular tachycardia, can lead to decreased cardiac output, inadequate coronary perfusion, venous congestion, and hypotension. Weakness, syncope, deterioration of the cardiac rhythm, reduced myocardial performance, congestive heart failure, and sudden death are potential sequelae to serious cardiac arrhythmias.

This article describes the clinical management of patients with cardiac rhythm disturbances, which is predicated on the prior determination of the cardiac rhythm diagnosis (Fig. 2, Table 3). Inasmuch as an accurate rhythm diagnosis is essential for successful therapy, the reader is thereby encouraged to refer to the supplemental reading list found at the end of this article. The specific clinical uses of antiarrhythmic drugs are outlined here. However, the reader is directed to Drugs Used in the Therapy of Cardiac Arrhythmias (page 285) for a description of the clinical pharmacology of these agents.

Table 2. *Evaluation of the Patient With a Cardiac Arrhythmia: A Checklist*

Electrocardiography
    Rhythm diagnosis: underlying and abnormal
    Ventricular rate/atrial rate
    Atrioventricular synchronization
    Number of ectopic complexes per minute
    Timing of ectopic complexes
    Effect of therapy on rhythm and duration of complexes
       and intervals
Hemodynamic State
    Level of consciousness
    Arterial blood pressure
    Capillary refill time
    Muscle weakness
    Syncope
    Urinary output
    Central venous pressure
    Thoracic radiographs: cardiomegaly, venous congestion,
       edema
Fluid, Electrolyte, and Acid-Base Status
    Blood pH
    Serum bicarbonate, potassium, sodium, chloride, calcium
    Renal function
    Hepatic function
    Level of hydration, adequate venous pressure
Drug Therapy
    Response to previous medication
    Current medication, dose, and frequency of administration
    Adverse effects
    Potential for reduced hepatic or renal clearance
    Potential drug interactions

SUPRAVENTRICULAR ARRHYTHMIAS

SINUS RHYTHMS

The normal cardiac rhythm originates in the sinoatrial (SA) node; is spread through specialized atrial conduction pathways to the atrioventricular node, bundle of His, bundle branches, and fascicles; and is distributed to the ventricular myocytes via a network of Purkinje cells (see Fig. 1). The ECG correlates to these processes are P wave (atrial activation), PR interval (primarily atrioventricular conduction), QRS complex (ventricular activation), and ST-T wave (ventricular repolarization). The SA node is richly innervated by sympathetic and parasympathetic fibers and is also affected by body temperature, metabolic state, serum electrolyte concentrations, and drugs. As a result of these influences, the SA discharge rate may vary considerably.

Normal sinus rhythm (regular sinus rhythm) and irregular sinus rhythm (*sinus arrhythmia*) are normal cardiac rhythms in the dog. Sinus rhythm and sinus tachycardia are normal rhythms for cats under examination, whereas sinus arrhythmia is quite unusual in this species. The SA rate varies significantly in dogs, with normal rates as low as 60 and as high as 180 bpm. The normal SA rate for awake cats is higher, generally from 160 to 240 bpm. Sinus arrhythmia is mediated by the vagus nerve. Waxing and waning of vagal tone changes SA nodal discharge rate, alters the atrial depolarization process ("wandering pacemaker"), and may cause slight variations in the P-R interval (see Fig. 2). In some resting dogs, an occasional nonconducted P wave may be recorded (second degree AV block) as a normal finding.

Pronounced sinus arrhythmia is often observed in animals with disorders that increase parasympathetic tone, including diseases of the respiratory, nervous, and gastrointestinal systems. Drugs that increase vagal effects or that withdraw sympathetic tone can also lead to marked sinus arrhythmias. Pilocarpine (for glaucoma), xylazine sedation, and pyridostigmine bromide (for myasthenia gravis) are examples of drugs related to sinus arrhythmia. In some dogs, sinus arrhythmia may be so pronounced as to mimic the sick sinus syndrome (SSS). Sinus arrhythmia is not treated unless it is complicated by sinus bradycardia (Tables 4 and 5).

Sinus bradycardia is associated with numerous clinical disorders including SSS, increased vagal efferent traffic, central nervous system disease, endocrinopathies such as Addison's disease and hypothyroidism, and hypothermia and with drug administration (see Table 1). In most cases sinus bradycardia is self-limiting, resolving with correction of the underlying disorder. In dogs with oth-

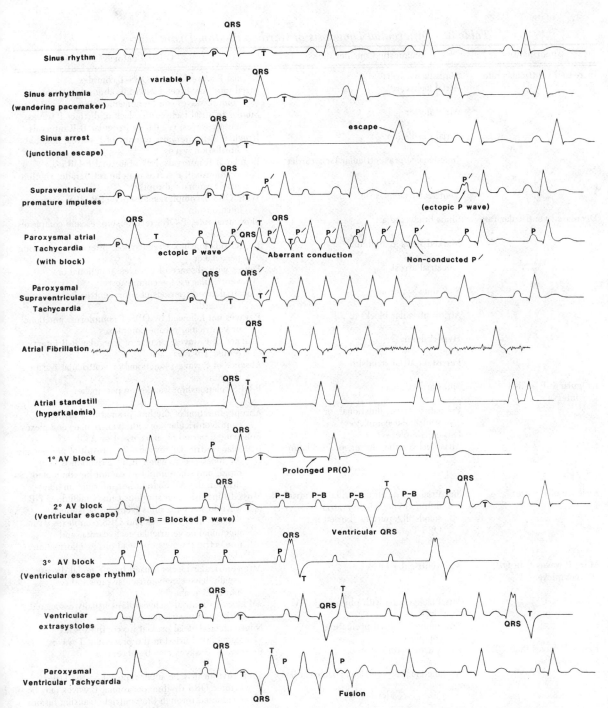

Figure 2. Essential features of common cardiac rhythm disturbances in the dog and cat. (Reprinted with permission from Bonagura and Berkwitt *in* Fenner: *Quick Reference to Veterinary Medicine.* Philadelphia: J.B. Lippincott, 1982.)

Table 3. *Differential Diagnosis of Cardiac Rhythm Disturbances*

Abnormality	Diagnostic Considerations	Other Features*
Increased ventricular rate	Sinus tachycardia	Normal P wave for each QRS-T complex
	Atrial tachycardia	Atrial rate may exceed 240/min; abnormal P waves; some P waves can be nonconducted
	Atrial flutter	Similar to atrial tachycardia; lack of distinct P waves; flutter waves; regular or irregular R-R intervals
	Atrial fibrillation	Irregular R-R intervals; absence of P waves; possible fibrillation waves
	Junctional/supraventricular tachycardia	Regular R-R intervals; lack of normal P-QRS relationship; P waves may be retrograde, rhythm may terminate abruptly
	Ventricular tachycardia	Wide QRS-T complexes; absence of P-QRS relationship
Decreased ventricular rate	Sinus bradycardia	Slow atrial rate; P-QRS relationship; escape complexes possible
	Marked sinus arrhythmia	P-QRS relationship; irregular P-P intervals; wandering pacemaker
	Sinoatrial arrest	Pauses with absence of P waves; junctional or ventricular escape complexes
	Sick sinus syndrome	Sinoatrial arrest; periods of supraventricular tachycardia
	Atrioventricular blocks (2°, 3°)	P waves not followed by QRS-T complexes; junctional or ventricular escape complexes
	Hyperkalemia	Absence of P waves; regular or irregular R-R intervals; tented T waves
	Persistent atrial standstill	Absence of P waves; junctional or ventricular escape rhythm
Irregular P-P or R-R intervals	Sinus arrhythmia	P-QRS relationship; wandering pacemaker
	Premature atrial, junctional, or ventricular complexes	Abrupt alteration of rhythm; premature narrow (supraventricular) or wide (ventricular) complexes
	Escape complexes	Following a period of sinus arrest or AV block
	Atrial tachycardia, flutter, or fibrillation	Irregular ventricular response as a result of physiologic AV block occurs when atrial activation is very rapid, and some impulses cannot be conducted through the AV node (other information above).
Absence of P waves	Sinoatrial arrest, atrial fibrillation, atrial flutter, hyperkalemia, atrial standstill, spurious (buried in QRS-T)	Must distinguish from spurious causes including T-P wave fusion with sinus tachycardia, super imposition of P waves and QRS complexes with junctional or ventricular tachycardia, and isoelectric P waves in a lead (other information above)
More P waves than QRS complexes	Atrioventricular block	Atrioventricular blocks caused by AV nodal disease usually have slow ventricular rates (other information above)
	Atrial tachycardia with physiologic AV block	AV block with atrial tachycardia is usually associated with rapid ventricular rates
	Nonconducted atrial premature complexes	Nonconducted atrial premature complexes are frequently buried in the preceding T waves.
Fewer P waves than QRS complexes	Sinus arrest with escapes	Retrograde P waves may be observed
	AV junctional or ventricular tachycardia	Sinus rhythm may be superimposed on the faster ectopic QRS rhythm; occasional P waves may be conducted through the ventricle, causing fusions or normal (narrow) capture complexes

*These are typical features; other variations or combinations can occur.

erwise normal hearts, ventricular rates as low as 40 to 50 bpm may still supply a normal cardiac output at rest. However, when this degree of bradycardia is dangerous (as with anesthesia or hypovolemia) or if the animal is symptomatic for bradycardia, therapy is given. Treatment for sinus bradycardia includes correction of the underlying disorder. This is particularly important in hypothermia, hypothyroidism, and anesthetic- (halothane) induced bradycardia, since these conditions may be refractory to treatment with atropine. Symptomatic sinus bradycardia is treated with parenteral atropine or glycopyrrolate. The intramuscular (IM) or subcutaneous (SC) route of administration is used in most cases since the initial autonomic effect of these drugs, when given intravenously, may be *increased* vagotonia, further slowing of the rate, or incomplete AV block. Sympathomimetic agents such as epinephrine, isoproterenol, and dopamine can also be used to initiate or maintain sinus rhythm in emergency situations (see page 381). These agents have significant extracardiac effects and may lead to other arrhythmias. Blood volume expansion with isotonic crystalloids is useful adjunctive therapy in symptomatic bradycardia.

Sinus tachycardia is a secondary rhythm disturbance. Consequently, the underlying cause of the increased sympathetic tone must be identified and treated (see Table 1). Specific antiarrhythmic therapy is not indicated except in heart failure or hyperthyroidism, in which digitalization or beta-adrenergic blockade might be useful in slowing the heart rate.

The *sick sinus syndrome* (SSS) is a term used to describe a complex of arrhythmias that primarily affect miniature schnauzers, pugs, dachshunds, and cocker spaniels. Electrocardiographic abnormalities include sinus bradycardia, sinus arrest, SA exit block, supraventricular tachycardia, and supraventricular premature complexes. Frequently there is evidence of AV nodal and intraventricular conduction disease. These arrhythmias predispose the animal to hypotension, weakness, and syncope, although sudden death is unusual. A small percentage of these dogs also have congestive heart failure owing to chronic valvular myocardial heart disease.

Asymptomatic dogs are not treated. Symptomatic patients are arbitrarily divided into group I (dogs predominantly showing sinus bradycardia and sinus arrest) or group II (dogs showing bradycardia-tachycardia syndrome). As a general rule, digitalis glycosides are not given to group I dogs. However,

Table 4. *Treatment of Cardiac Arrhythmias in the Dog*

Rhythm	Acute Therapy*	Chronic Therapy†
Sinus Rhythms		
Sinus bradycardia	Atropine or glycopyrrolate; dopamine; epinephrine	Pacemaker
Sinus tachycardia	Treat underlying cause	Digitalis glycosides if CHF‡ or SSS is present
Sinoatrial arrest, sick sinus syndrome (SSS)	Atropine or glycopyrrolate	Pacemaker; oral anticholinergic therapy
Supraventricular Arrhythmias		
Atrial and junctional premature complexes	Digitalis; propranolol; quinidine	Same as for acute therapy
Atrial, junctional, and supraventricular tachycardia	Vagal maneuver; digitalis; propranolol; verapamil; quinidine	Digitalis, propranolol, or quinidine (consider response to acute therapy); verapamil (?)
Atrial fibrillation or flutter	Quinidine if indicated (see text); digitalis	Digitalis; propranolol
Ventricular Arrhythmias		
Ventricular premature complexes; ventricular tachycardia	Lidocaine; procainamide; propranolol; aprindine; quinidine	Procainamide, quinidine, propranolol, phenytoin (consider response to acute therapy)
Conduction Disturbances		
Atrial standstill (hyperkalemia)	Sodium bicarbonate; intravenous saline; calcium gluconate; Rx primary disorder	Treat the primary disorder
Persistent atrial standstill	Atropine or glycopyrrolate; transvenous pacemaker	Pacemaker
Atrioventricular blocks	Transvenous pacemaker; atropine or glycopyrrolate; infusion of isoproterenol	Cardiac pacemaker; oral isoproterenol

*The usual agent of choice is listed first. See text for details.
†Chronic therapy varies with etiology and response to acute therapy.
‡Congestive heart failure.

Table 5. *Drugs Used in the Therapy of Cardiac Arrhythmias*

Generic Name	Commonly Used Preparations	Indications	Adverse Effects	Approximate Dosage
Atropine	Atropine sulfate injection USP 0.4 mg/ml	Sinus bradycardia; sinoatrial arrest; incomplete AV block	Sinus tachycardia; ectopic complexes; ocular, gastrointestinal, and pulmonary side effects; paradoxic vagomimetic effects	0.01 to 0.02 mg/kg IV, IM 0.02 to 0.04 mg/kg SC
Digitoxin*	Crystodigin injection 0.2 mg/ml; 0.1-, 0.2-mg capsules Foxalin 0.1-, 0.25-, 0.5-mg capsules	Supraventricular premature complexes; supraventricular tachycardia; atrial flutter/fibrillation	Anorexia; depression; vomiting; diarrhea; AV block; ectopia; junctional tachycardia	Oral maintenance: 0.04 to 0.1 mg/kg divided b.i.d. to t.i.d. Rapid IV digitalization: 0.01 to 0.03 mg/kg; administer 1/2 of calculated dose IV, wait 30 to 60 min and administer 1/4 of dose, wait 30 to 60 min and administer remaining dose if necessary
Digoxin*	Lanoxin elixir 0.05 mg/ml; 0.125, 0.25, 0.5-mg tablets Cardoxin elixir 0.05, 0.15 mg/ml	Same as digitoxin	Same as digitoxin	Oral maintenance: 0.01 to 0.02 mg/kg divided b.i.d. Rapid IV digitalization: 0.01 to 0.02 mg/kg IV as per digitoxin Rapid oral digitalization: 0.02 to 0.06 mg/kg divided b.i.d. for one day
Glycopyrrolate	Robinul injection 0.2 mg/ml	Sinus bradycardia; sinoatrial arrest; incomplete AV block	As per atropine	0.005 to .01 mg/kg IV, IM 0.01 to .02 mg/kg SC
Isopropamide	Darbid 5-mg tablets	Sinoatrial arrest	As per atropine; keratoconjunctivitis sicca	2.5 to 5.0 mg b.i.d. to t.i.d.

Drug	Preparation	Indications	Toxicity	Dosage*
Isoproterenol	Isuprel HCl injection 0.2 mg/ml; 1- and 5-ml ampules; Proternol 20-, 40-mg tablets; Isuprel 10-mg glossets	Sinoatrial arrest; sinus bradycardia; complete AV block	CNS stimulation; ectopic complexes; tachycardia; emesis	Isuprel: 0.4 mg in 250 ml D₅W; drip slowly to effect; Proternol: 10 to 20 mg q4 to 6 h; Isuprel glossets: 5 to 10 mg per rectum q4 to 6h
Lidocaine HCl	Xylocaine (*without* epinephrine) 2 per cent (20 mg/ml)	Ventricular premature complexes; ventricular tachycardia	CNS excitation; seizures; tremors; emesis (Rx with diazepam); other rhythm disturbances	2 to 4 mg/kg IV slowly, repeat to maximum of 8 mg/kg; For the *cat*: 0.25 to 1.0 mg/kg IV over five min; Constant rate infusion (CRI)† for the *dog*: 25 to 75 µg/kg/min
Procainamide	Pronestyl injection 100, 500 mg/ml; 250-, 500-mg tablets; Procan sustained release (SR) 250-, 500-tablets	Ventricular premature complexes; ventricular tachycardia	Weakness; hypotension; decreased contractility; anorexia; vomiting; diarrhea; widening of QRS and QT interval; AV block	6 to 8 mg/kg IV over 5 min; CRI: 25 to 40 µg/kg/min; 6 to 20 mg/kg IM q4 to 6h (see text); Tablets: 8 to 20 mg/kg q6h; Procan SR: 8 to 20 mg/kg q6 to 8h; *dogs only*
Propranolol HCl	Inderal 1 mg/ml vials; 10-, 20-, 40-, 80-mg tablets	Supraventricular premature complex and tachyarrhythmias; atrial fibrillation; ventricular premature complexes	Decreased contractility; bronchoconstriction; loss of compensatory mechanisms	0.02 to 0.06 mg/kg IV slowly; 0.2 to 1.0 mg/kg orally t.i.d.
Quinidine sulfate	Quinidine sulfate USP 200-mg tablets, 300-mg Quinidine Extentabs	Ventricular premature complexes; ventricular tachycardia; acute atrial fibrillation; refractory supraventricular tachycardias	As per procainamide; drug interaction with digoxin	6 to 16 mg/kg PO, q6h (sulfate), q8h Extentabs
gluconate	Quinidine gluconate USP injection 80 mg/ml			6 to 20 mg/kg IM, q6h (gluconate) (see text)
	Quimaglute Dura Tabs 324 mg			8 to 20 mg/kg PO, q6 to 8h
polygalacturonate	Cardioquin 275-mg tablets			8 to 20 mg/kg PO, q6 to 8h; *dogs only*

*Canine doses; see page 342 for feline doses.

†Formula for CRI: bodyweight (in kg) × dose (in µg/kg/min) × 0.36 = total dose in mg to administer IV over six hours (do *not* include units; see example.) Example: CRI for a 50 µg/kg/min infusion for a 20-kg dog: 20 × 50 × 0.36 = 360 mg over six hours.

digoxin may be useful in controlling bouts of tachycardia in group II patients and is given to these dogs as a therapeutic trial. The author conducts an atropine response test in group I dogs by administering 0.04 mg/kg IM and recording an ECG 15 to 30 minutes later. Dogs that develop a regular sinus rhythm or sinus tachycardia may benefit from oral anticholinergic therapy and are given Darbid tablets* (2.5 to 5 mg b.i.d. to t.i.d.) or Pro-Banthine† (7.5 mg b.i.d. to t.i.d.). Dogs that fail to respond to vagolytic therapy or that cannot tolerate anticholinergic side effects are treated with a permanent pacemaker (see page 373). The prognosis with pacemaker therapy is excellent. The response to medical therapy is inconsistent, and some dogs may faint frequently in spite of medical treatments.

ATRIAL AND JUNCTIONAL RHYTHMS

Supraventricular (atrial and junctional) premature complexes often indicate underlying cardiac disease and are associated with chronic valvular heart disease, cardiomyopathy, viral myocarditis, congenital heart disease, and cor pulmonale. Other causes include hypoxia, electrolyte disturbances, administration of anesthetic agents, digitalis intoxication, "toxemias," and sympathetic stimulation. The significance of these complexes relates to their frequency and the underlying clinical condition. In animals with severe myocardial disease, these arrhythmias can be harbingers of serious electrical disorders such as atrial tachycardia, atrial flutter, and atrial fibrillation.

Infrequent or isolated premature complexes are not treated. The author currently uses the following criteria for initiating antiarrhythmic therapy: clinical signs of low output (e.g., syncope), repetitive complexes (pairs, paroxysmal tachycardia), or frequent occurrence of premature complexes (greater than 20/min). Principles of therapy include control of heart failure when present, administration of digoxin, and the potential use of other antiarrhythmic agents. Treatments for heart failure, such as diuretic and vasodilator therapy, may lower the incidence of premature complexes by decreasing cardiac size. The effect of digoxin is variable, and it must be monitored since the frequency of premature complexes can actually increase with digitalization. Patients that are refractory to digitalis may benefit from the use of propranolol, given in graded doses to achieve an antiarrhythmic effect. In selected cases, the administration of oral quinidine is effective in controlling refractory atrial premature complexes.

Supraventricular tachycardia (SVT) is a serious rhythm disturbance, and patients with this disturbance are difficult to manage. The clinician must not confuse SVT with the more common sinus tachycardia. Supraventricular tachycardia is a general term used here to describe atrial and junctional "automatic" tachycardias and tachyarrhythmias that use atrium or AV junction as part of a re-entrant loop. ECG abnormalities can include a rapid atrial rate (often greater than 300/min) with irregular ventricular response; lack of the normal P-QRS relationship with regular, narrow QRS complexes; or paroxysms of closely linked narrow QRS-T complexes (see Fig. 2). The nonparoxysmal form of SVT is particularly serious and constitutes a medical emergency. Animals with sustained SVT usually have serious underlying myocardial disease, and a rapid ventricular rate, with loss of atrial synchronization, can lead to hypotension, venous congestion, and death.

The therapy for *paroxysmal* SVT is similar to that for supraventricular premature complexes as outlined previously. Initial therapy for *sustained* (nonparoxysmal) SVT includes (1) cage rest and supplemental oxygen, (2) intravenous furosemide (2 to 4 mg/kg) if congestive heart failure (CHF) is present, (3) intravenous fluid therapy if the patient is hypotensive, with monitoring of the central venous pressure (keep below 12 cm H_2O), (4) administration of morphine sulfate (0.2 mg/kg SC) if the dog is anxious or difficult to handle, and (5) a vagal maneuver (gentle pressure on the eyeballs or carotid sinus for 30 seconds), which may abruptly terminate a re-entrant SVT.

If a vagal maneuver is ineffective, intravenous digoxin is given. Although digitalization may not convert the arrhythmia, it can slow the ventricular response; therefore, in the case of atrial tachycardia, the rapid and regular atrial rhythm will continue, whereas the ventricular response will become slower and erratic. If digitalization is unsuccessful, the use of intravenous propranolol or verapamil is suggested, but these drugs must be administered with caution. Both agents are potent negative inotropes and can result in serious myocardial dysfunction. Verapamil (Calan, Isoptin: 1 to 5 mg IV slowly) holds promise for the treatment of re-entrant SVT, but more experience is needed before its use can be routinely advocated. The author has treated dogs in which refractory atrial tachycardia converted to normal sinus rhythm (NSR) after the intramuscular use of quinidine gluconate.

Atrial flutter is relatively uncommon in dogs but has been observed in association with serious myocardial disease and atrial enlargement. Atrial flutter is similar to other supraventricular tachycardias, since the rapid and regular activation of the atria results in a rapid but often irregular ventricular response. Therapy for atrial flutter is similar to that for sustained SVT as described previously. In addition to drugs such as digitalis, quinidine, and propranolol, direct current (DC) countershock can be employed to convert this arrhythmia to sinus rhythm. This requires special equipment and train-

*Smith Kline & French Laboratories, Philadelphia, PA.
†Searle & Co., San Juan, PR.

ing. Atrial flutter is a short-lived rhythm disturbance in many dogs and often spontaneously reverts to sinus rhythm or proceeds to atrial fibrillation.

Atrial fibrillation (AF) is a common arrhythmia and complicates the clinical course of cardiomyopathy, advanced atrioventricular valvular disease, and untreated congenital heart disease. Although unusual causes of AF have been recognized, including thoracic trauma and anesthesia, the clinician should always suspect serious underlying heart disease whenever AF is diagnosed in a dog or cat. Since most animals with AF have progressive myocardial disease and enlargement, only exceptional cases are converted from AF to normal sinus rhythm. For example, the author administers intramuscular quinidine gluconate to convert dogs with acute AF and no other clinical or radiographic evidence of cardiac enlargement or CHF. However, patients with cardiomegaly or CHF are neither given quinidine nor are subjected to DC countershock, since reversion to AF occurs within a short period of time.

Principles of therapy of AF include the following: (1) control congestive heart failure if present, (2) slow the ventricular response with digitalis glycosides, and (3) administer beta-adrenergic blocking drugs such as propranolol if the ventricular rate is not adequately reduced with digitalis. The administration of digitalis may be salutary, since it increases myocardial contractility and blocks cardiac impulses in the AV node, thereby slowing the ventricular rate and increasing ventricular filling time. Unfortunately, the majority of dogs with AF caused by cardiomyopathy cannot tolerate the dose of digitalis needed to slow the ventricular rate to less than 140 per minute. In these cases, the administration of propranolol in incremental doses is effective in slowing the ventricular response. Propranol is not given until digitalis glycosides have been administered for at least 36 hours. Initial doses of 0.2 mg/kg t.i.d. are increased by 0.1 to 0.2 mg/kg each day to a maximum of 1 mg/kg t.i.d. In clinical practice, most giant breed dogs require from 20 to 50 mg of propranolol t.i.d. to maintain the ventricular response at or below 140 bpm. It is imperative that propranolol be given in graded dosages, with frequent ECG monitoring of cardiac rate and rhythm, and that the lowest daily dose needed be utilized. This is essential to minimize the negative inotropic effects of this drug. Additional therapeutic measures are required in the treatment of atrial fibrillation caused by cardiomyopathy, and these are described on pages 323 to 324.

VENTRICULAR ARRHYTHMIAS

VENTRICULAR PREMATURE COMPLEXES

Ectopic ventricular complexes are characterized by the appearance of wide, bizarre QRS-T complexes on the ECG (see Fig. 2). Ventricular premature complexes (VPC) abruptly break the sinus rhythm. A ventricular complex that rescues the heart from a period of ventricular asystole is termed an "escape" (see Fig. 2). VPCs are generally considered to indicate heart disease or a noncardiac disorder that is affecting the cardiac rhythm. Noncardiac causes of ventricular ectopia include electrolyte disturbances, autonomic imbalance, hypoxia, ischemia, trauma, and other disorders. Although myocardial inflammation can cause VPC, these terms are not synonymous, and most dogs with ventricular arrhythmias do *not* have myocarditis. Owing to the multiple potential causes of VPC, a thorough physical, radiographic, and laboratory evaluation of the patient is needed to properly assess the significance of VPC (see Table 2). The clinician must also be aware that *supraventricular* ectopic rhythms with aberrant ventricular conduction (e.g., bundle branch block) can result in QRS complexes that appear to be ventricular in origin (see Fig. 2).

Ventricular premature complexes are common but are not always treated with antiarrhythmic agents. Major concerns with VPC are hemodynamic embarrassment and ventricular electrical instability. Although it is impossible to accurately gauge these problems in all patients, the author administers antiarrhythmic agents when any of the following occur: (1) frequent VPC (greater than 20/min), (2) repetitive complexes (pairs, paroxysms), (3) multiform (multifocal) QRS configurations, (4) short coupling intervals (the VPC occurs on the T wave of the previous complex), and (5) appearance of clinical signs of decreased cardiac output (weakness, depression, syncope). Ventricular escapes are *never* suppressed. The therapy of VPC is discussed hereafter.

VENTRICULAR TACHYCARDIA

Ventricular tachycardia (VT) is a serious arrhythmia that demands immediate medical attention. As with supraventricular tachycardia, VT can be paroxysmal or sustained. Paroxysmal ventricular tachycardia (PVT) is a frequent cause of weakness and syncope in dogs (see page 330) and occurs in a variety of clinical settings (see Table 1). Sustained VT can lead to hypotension, myocardial ischemia, and electrical instability and may be a harbinger of ventricular fibrillation. These are particularly evident when there is reduced myocardial contractility or hypovolemia or when VT occurs at rates of greater than 140 bpm in the dog.

Most animals with ventricular rhythms are treated with antiarrhythmic drugs; however, there are some exceptions to this rule. Ventricular escape rhythms occur as protective mechanisms during sinus bradycardia and AV block, and these foci are never suppressed, since asystole could occur. Some dogs with pronounced sinus arrhythmia and other medical problems, such as hypokalemia, digitalis intoxication, and dysautonomia (with gastric dilation volvulus), develop a *slow*, competing, ventricular rhythm (60 to 120 bpm) that is best termed an *idioventricular tachycardia*. Such rhythms are clinically benign. Correction of the underlying problem usually results in spontaneous disappearance of this dysrhythmia. However, when in doubt about the clinical significance of a ventricular rhythm, the clinician is best advised to administer antiarrhythmic therapy and seek consultation.

INITIAL THERAPY

Drugs useful in the treatment of ventricular arrhythmias include lidocaine, quinidine, procainamide, propranolol, phenytoin, aprindine, and, occasionally, digitalis (see Tables 4 and 5). It should be emphasized that patients with VPC or VT should NOT be given digitalis glycosides unless myocardial failure or a supraventricular tachyarrhythmia is also present. In such cases, the use of digitalis must be accompanied by frequent ECG monitoring and, possibly, the concurrent use of other antiarrhythmic drugs. Many dogs with CHF and occasional unifocal VPC can be safely digitalized. In most cases, the frequency of VPC either decreases or remains the same. If the frequency of VPC increases, however, or if repetitive ventricular complexes are present, antiarrhythmic drugs are given *prior* to digitalization.

Antiarrhythmic drug therapy can be given by the intravenous, intramuscular, or oral route. The method of administration depends on the clinical circumstances. The IV route is obviously preferred in the anesthetized or critical patient, whereas the IM or oral route is appropriate for animals without clinical signs of hemodynamic or electrical instability.

In most situations, lidocaine HCl is the intravenous agent of choice for immediate control of VPC or VT. Lidocaine has minimal adverse hemodynamic effects, and the neurotoxic signs associated with higher doses are readily controlled by IV diazepam. Initial doses of 2 to 3 mg/kg IV for dogs (lower for cats) are usually effective within two to three minutes of administration. An initial total dose of 8 mg/kg can be given to dogs with refractory arrhythmias; however, many dogs exhibit toxicity at this dosage level. Lidocaine is injected slowly over one to two minutes and must be used with caution in cats, since they are particularly susceptible to neurotoxic effects (see Table 5). Owing to the rapid redistribution and clearance of lidocaine, the antiarrhythmic effect is short-lived unless repeated boluses or an IV constant rate infusion (CRI) is administered. If IV boluses achieve sinus rhythm, then a CRI is usually effective in maintaining the normal rhythm. Since it takes four to five hours for lidocaine to attain a steady state plasma concentration when administered by CRI, supplemental IV bolus injections (0.5 to 1.0 mg/kg) may be needed to control arrhythmias during the initial infusion period. Infusions can be given for two to three days, if necessary, or replaced with IM or orally administered agents (quinidine, procainamide) after the patient has been stabilized. Serum potassium concentration must be monitored and kept within the normal range for lidocaine to exert its full effect. Hypokalemia is a frequent cause of therapeutic failure.

When parenteral therapy is indicated and lidocaine is ineffective in controlling ventricular ectopia, procainamide, quinidine, or propranolol is administered. These drugs have significant cardiodepressant effects when given intravenously; therefore, they must be injected slowly and carefully, with attention directed to cardiac rhythm and arterial pulse pressure. Procainamide, the first drug chosen when lidocaine is ineffective, is particularly versatile since it also can be given by IM and oral routes. In patients needing long-term antiarrhythmic therapy, procainamide is ideal (except for its short three- to four-hour half-life), since the initial IV bolus (if effective) can be followed with a CRI, IM injections, and eventual administration of an oral preparation.

The IV use of propranolol, quinidine, and phenytoin is limited. The electrophysiologic effects of quinidine are similar to those of procainamide; therefore, if procainamide is ineffective, quinidine is unlikely to convert the arrhythmia. Propranolol is occasionally successful in treating VT, particularly when the administration of other antiarrhythmic drugs has preceded its use. The experimental antiarrhythmic drug aprindine is highly effective in converting refractory VT to sinus rhythm when given slowly to dogs at a dose of 0.5 to 2.0 mg/kg IV. Phenytoin demonstrates efficacy in the treatment of digitalis-induced ventricular arrhythmias, but lidocaine is still the preferred intravenous agent since it is safer to administer than phenytoin to dogs and cats. Electrocardioversion can be utilized to treat VT; however, the equipment needed is not routinely available to veterinarians.

When IV bolus or CRI therapy is unnecessary or not feasible, the use of *intramuscular* quinidine or procainamide can be successful in controlling VPC and VT. The hypotensive effects of these agents are minimized by IM use, and if they are given every four to six hours the animal may achieve and maintain normal sinus rhythm. The author generally gives the initial IM dose of 12 to 20 mg/kg and subsequent doses of 6 to 12 mg/kg at the appropriate dosing intervals.

MAINTENANCE THERAPY

Certain dogs require long-term antiarrhythmic therapy for ventricular arrhythmias. These animals must be managed with available oral preparations of quinidine, procainamide, or propranolol (see Tables 4 and 5). The choice of an oral drug depends on numerous factors including efficacy of parenteral therapy, dosing frequency, owner compliance, elimination half-life, concurrent drug administration, efficacy of oral therapy, and adverse drug effects. Quinidine and procainamide are the two most frequently used oral agents. Disopyramide (Norpace) does not appear to offer any advantage over quinidine and has a very short half-life (one to two hours) in the dog. Since the elimination half-lives of quinidine (six to eight hours) and procainamide (four hours) in the dog are also relatively short, t.i.d. to q.i.d. drug administration is required. Sustained-release preparations of these drugs (Quinaglute and Quinidex, and Procan-SR, respectively) are prescribed with the intent that serum concentrations will be maintained with the recommended dosages. However, critical pharmacodynamic and clinical studies of these drugs have not been performed in dogs.

Follow-up evaluation is essential in the management of patients with persistent ventricular arrhythmias. The dog must be examined and the owner questioned about adverse drug effects or lack of drug efficacy. The author obtains a long ECG rhythm strip at the end of a dosing interval (when plasma drug concentrations should be at the nadir). Antiarrhythmic therapy frequently reduces the number of repetitive complexes or VPC per minute but may not totally abolish the ectopic beats. In such cases, the current clinical signs and daily drug dosage must be weighed against the possibility of drug toxicity if the dose is increased. The total daily drug dose is increased if the dog is symptomatic or the VPCs are repetitive. If this therapy is inadequate, propranolol may be effective in controlling the rhythm. Although there are theoretical disadvantages to using antiarrhythmic drug combinations, the author has successfully administered propranolol in combination with procainamide or quinidine for refractory arrhythmias.

Therapy of other ventricular dysrhythmias such as ventricular standstill, flutter, and fibrillation are discussed on pages 377 to 387.

CONDUCTION DISTURBANCES

ATRIAL CONDUCTION DISTURBANCES

In addition to atrial tachyarrhythmias, which can result from abnormal cellular conduction, other atrial conduction disorders can be diagnosed from the ECG. Atrial standstill, an inexcitability of the atrial muscle, can be caused by hyperkalemia or muscular dystrophy. In both situations, there is a lack of demonstrable P waves on the ECG.

Hyperkalemia, the most common cause of temporary atrial standstill, is frequently caused by hypoadrenocorticism and acute renal failure (e.g., urinary obstruction). In addition to atrial inexcitability, intraventricular conduction may be prolonged, resulting in widening of the QRS complexes, and ventricular repolarization can be shortened, leading to tented T waves (see Fig. 2). The ventricular rate is usually slow and can be regular or irregular. Immediate therapy consists of the IV administration of sodium bicarbonate (1 mEq/kg slowly over three to four minutes) to drive potassium into the cell. This is repeated in ten minutes if there has been no ECG improvement. Correction of the primary problem and intravenous therapy with normal saline are important parts of adjunctive therapy. Hyperkalemia can cause cardiac arrest. If bicarbonate therapy is ineffective, the slow IV administration of calcium gluconate (1 ml of a 10 per cent solution of calcium gluconate per 10 kg body weight) is used to antagonize the effects of potassium on the heart.

Persistent atrial standstill ("silent atria") is a congenital muscle disorder observed in cats and dogs (primarily springer spaniels) and is characterized by absence of P waves, normal serum potassium level, slow junctional or ventricular escape rhythm, and radiographic evidence of biatrial and ventricular enlargement. Histologic lesions include loss of SA and atrial muscle and replacement by fibrous tissue. The dog develops clinical signs owing to decreased myocardial function and bradycardia. Initial therapy consists of oxygen, furosemide (2 to 4 mg/kg) if there is congestive heart failure, and cage rest. Definitive treatment requires placement of a ventricular pacemaker (page 373). Initially, a transvenous pacemaker is inserted to stabilize the dog. Following implantation of a permanent artificial pacemaker, the prognosis is guarded to good, with some dogs living more than two years.

ATRIOVENTRICULAR BLOCK

Atrioventricular block can be incomplete (1°, 2°) or complete* (3°) (see Fig. 2). Increased vagal tone, primary myocardial diseases, electrolyte disorders, and drug therapy cause AV blocks. Most cases of incomplete AV block do not result in clinical signs and are either physiologic or self-limiting when the cause (e.g., digitalis) is eliminated. High-grade second degree AV block (P:QRS >3:1), and complete AV block generally indicate a severe drug toxicity or conduction system disease. High-grade second degree AV block type II (constant PR interval) associated with widening of the conducted QRS

---

*Some authors consider the atrioventricular dissociation associated with persistent ventricular and junctional tachycardia to be an example of a third degree AV block. As these are examples of physiologic block caused by increased automaticity below the AV node, they will not be considered here. The current discussion pertains to complete dissociation caused by anatomic disruption of the AV conduction pathways.

complexes frequently progresses to complete AV block. Syncope and CHF are common sequelae of complete AV block.

Treatment of AV block requires an appreciation of the underlying cause. Incomplete AV block is normal in some resting dogs and may be abolished simply by exercise. AV block caused by xylazine or digitalis glycosides is usually abolished by vagolytic agents such as atropine. However, such therapy is only indicated for symptomatic bradycardia. Withdrawal of the drug is the treatment of choice. High-grade second degree and complete AV blocks are usually refractory to therapy with atropine or isoproterenol (although this may increase the ventricular escape rate) and require pacemaker therapy. Although some clinicians have treated symptomatic bradycardia with high doses of oral isoproterenol (Proternol), this type of treatment is usually ineffective and unnecessarily prolongs the period before diagnosis and implantation of a pacemaker.

Pacemaker therapy for symptomatic bradycardia caused by AV block is effective and results in a median survival of about one and one-half years. Prior to implantation of a permanent pacemaker, a temporary transvenous pacemaker is utilized to increase cardiac output and stabilize the patient. Syncope, weakness, and signs of CHF should abate after 24 to 48 hours of pacing, and patients that do not respond to this type of treatment are suspected of having serious underlying myocardial failure. Such dogs are poor candidates for permanent pacing. Following implantation of a permanent pacemaker, immediate and long-term complications may be encountered. Many of these can be managed medically as described on page 376.

VENTRICULAR PRE-EXCITATION

Examples of ventricular pre-excitation include the Wolff-Parkinson-White (W-P-W) and the Lown-Ganong-Levine (L-G-L) syndromes. Both of these conditions are characterized by an accessory atrioventricular pathway that permits early depolarization (pre-excitation) of the ventricle. These syndromes are unusual but have been reported in the dog and cat. The hallmark of these disorders is a consistent but short PR interval. In the L-G-L syndrome, the AV node is completely bypassed and the P wave is followed immediately by a narrow QRS-T complex (see Fig. 1). The W-P-W bypass tract permits early depolarization of part of the ventricles; however, the latter portions of the ventricular activation process follow normal conduction pathways. Thus, the initial portion of the QRS is widened and slurred (delta wave), resulting in a wider than normal QRS-T.

These conditions predispose to syncope owing to re-entrant supraventricular tachycardia. Successful management of the syndromes consists of antiarrhythmic therapy designed to inhibit re-entrant conduction through the accessory pathway. Digitalis and verapamil should not be given to such patients, since these drugs can block normal AV nodal transmission and facilitate conduction through the accessory pathway. Quinidine and procainamide have been used in a few cases to block re-entrant tachyarrhythmias in dogs.

INTRAVENTRICULAR CONDUCTION DISTURBANCES

Intraventricular conduction disturbances are common. Fascicular and bundle branch blocks produce significant complex widening and deviation of the QRS axis. These changes can be confusing and can lead to an erroneous diagnosis of ventricular ectopic rhythm if the relationship of the preceding P waves to the abnormal QRS-T is unobserved. Although intraventricular conduction disturbances may indicate underlying myocardial disease, they do *not* require antiarrhythmic therapy. If congestive heart failure is present the patient should be treated with appropriate therapy.

SUPPLEMENTAL READING

Bolton, G. R.: *Handbook of Canine Electrocardiography.* Philadelphia: W. B. Saunders, 1975.
Mandel, W. J.: *Cardiac Arrhythmias.* Philadelphia: J. B. Lippincott, 1980.
Tilley, L. P.: *Essentials of Canine and Feline Electrocardiography.* St. Louis: C. V. Mosby, 1979.

PACEMAKER THERAPY

MELVIN L. HELPHREY, D.V.M.,

Seminole, Florida

and MICHAEL SCHOLLMEYER, D.V.M.

Minneapolis, Minnesota

Artificial pacing of the heart has been standard therapy for bradycardia in humans since the late 1950s when external cardiac pacemakers were first used. Since that time, biomedical manufacturers have made tremendous strides in producing small pacemakers that can be implanted subcutaneously and that have an effective life of up to ten years. Pacemaker therapy has been effective in the management of complete heart block and other symptomatic bradycardias and the termination of ectopic tachycardias. Although pacemakers have been available for over 20 years, the veterinary profession has been slow to adopt this technology for the treatment of symptomatic bradycardia. The main drawback has been the high cost of equipment. Although there are no accurate records available, it is estimated that approximately 20 to 30 pacemakers are implanted each year in small animal patients. This estimate is based on the records of manufacturers who have donated pacemakers to veterinarians.

INDICATIONS FOR PACEMAKER THERAPY

Pacemaker therapy is indicated for animals that have symptomatic bradycardia caused by defects in the atrioventricular conduction system. It should be used when an adequate heart rate cannot be maintained with drug therapy. The most common conditions are high-grade second degree AV block (Mobitz type II), complete AV block (Fig. 1), the sick sinus syndrome (including sinus bradycardia, sinus arrest, S-A block, and the bradycardia-tachycardia syndrome), and persistent atrial standstill (see page 371) (Table 1). The use of cardiac pacing therapy has yielded dramatic results in these disorders and is the treatment of choice for animals as well as humans.

EQUIPMENT

A pacing system consists of the lead (heart wire) and the pacemaker (pulse generator). The pacemaker produces a small electrical current that is sent to the heart via the lead and causes the myocardium to contract. Early implantable pacemakers put out a continuous pulse at a fixed rate and had a battery life of 16 to 24 months. These generators were called asynchronous pacemakers and were effective albeit short-lived treatments; however, they were not synchronized with the underlying intrinsic rate of the heart.

Most modern pulse generators are synchronous with the intrinsic cardiac rhythm. Instead of a continuous output, the pacemaker has a sensing circuit that detects spontaneous ventricular activity via the lead. If ventricular (R wave) activity is sensed, the generator's pulsing circuit remains off. If the generator does not sense ventricular activity within a specific period of time, the pulsing circuit discharges a short burst of current to the heart. This advancement in pacemaker technology has permitted synchronous pacing of the heart and increased longevity of the pacemaker by decreasing the current drain from the batteries.

Table 1. Indications for Cardiac Pacemakers

High grade 2° AV block
Complete AV block
Sick sinus syndrome
Sinus bradycardia
Sinus arrest
SA block
Bradycardia-tachycardia syndrome
Persistent atrial standstill

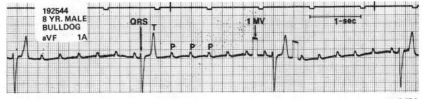

Figure 1. Typical electrocardiogram of a dog in complete AV block. Notice P waves (P) are not followed by a QRS-T complex, indicating obstruction of the electrical impulse to traverse the A-V node.

Pacemakers are given a three-letter code based on (1) which chamber is paced (atrium = A, ventricle = V, or both = D), (2) which chamber is sensed (A, V, or D), and (3) whether that information triggers (T) or inhibits (I) the pacemaker or serves a dual (D) function. Thus, VVI (a demand synchronous pacemaker) has ventricular pacing and ventricular sensing, and the sensed signal inhibits the pacemaker from discharging an electrical impulse. Sophisticated pacemakers (DDD) are available that sense and pace both the atria and ventricles of the heart. This provides a more physiologic myocardial contraction sequence and increases cardiac output. These pacemakers (DDD) may also be computer programmed to function in a variety of modes. To date, such units are too expensive for routine use in veterinary medicine.

Although the pacemaker is the primary functional part of the pacing system, the lead also plays an important role. Pacemaker leads are basically of two types, endocardial and epicardial. Endocardial leads are implanted in the right ventricle from a peripheral vein in the upper extremities, neck, or chest. This method of lead implantation is popular in humans because of the ease of implantation under local anesthesia. Fluoroscopy is necessary for correct placement of the leads. A disadvantage of endocardial leads in veterinary therapy is the greater chance of dislodgement following placement. The easiest route for endocardial lead placement in the dog is via the external jugular vein. However, owing to the wide range of head and neck movements, considerable strain is placed on the lead. This can cause dislodgement of the lead tip from the heart. Unless a veterinarian has considerable experience in cardiac catheterization and permanent endocardial lead placement, this method is not recommended.

Epicardial leads are implanted on the epicardial surface near the apex of the heart. Implantation does not require fluoroscopy, but instead requires a major surgical operation. Although there is greater intraoperative risk, the results of epicardial implantation in the dog are superior.

SURGERY

The preoperative implantation of a temporary right ventricular transvenous pacemaker is necessary to ensure continued ventricular electrical activity during induction of anesthesia. If congestive heart failure is present, a transvenous pacemaker lead is placed two to seven days in advance of general anesthesia and surgical implantation of a permanent epicardial lead. A lack of clinical response to pacing in such patients is indicative of severe myocardial disease and militates against permanent pacemaker implantation.

The most critical part of the procedure is induc-

tion and maintenance of anesthesia. The dog is preanesthetized with diazepam (0.1 to 0.25 mg/kg) or morphine (0.2 to 0.5 mg/kg IM), and the skin over the jugular vein is clipped, surgically prepared, and blocked with 2 per cent lidocaine. The jugular vein is penetrated with a 10-gauge needle, and a bipolar transvenous pacing wire is inserted through the trochar. A modified Seldinger technique using a catheter introducer can also be employed. Fluoroscopy may be used to confirm placement of the lead wire in the right ventricle, or premature ventricular contractions arising from the right ventricle may be visualized on the electrocardiogram. The lead wire is then connected to the temporary pacemaker.

To test the function of the lead and generator, the rate is set 10 to 20 beats/min faster than the intrinsic ventricular rate, and the paced rhythm is confirmed via the electrocardiogram. General anesthesia is induced with thiamylal sodium (4 to 6 mg/kg, IV), and the dog is maintained on halothane.* The dog is clipped and surgically prepared for a ventral midline abdominal exploratory celiotomy and caudal median sternotomy.

The linea alba is opened to the umbilicus, and the incision is carried through the caudal third of the sternum. The pericardium may be opened over the apex of the left ventricle to better visualize the coronary vessels. A corkscrew lead wire is inserted into the apex of the left ventricle, avoiding the coronary vessels. The lead wire is twisted so the Dacron collar is fitted tightly against the ventricle. If it is too loose, excessive motion may cause scar tissue to form under the lead, resulting in impulse exit block. If the lead is screwed in too tightly, it may actually "core" out the left ventricle. The number of turns on the corkscrew indicates the number of turns necessary to properly insert the lead (usually three turns). The collar is not sutured to the epicardium. The lead wire is then passed around the diaphragm and through the peritoneum caudal to the left lobe of the liver. The generator is connected to the lead wire and checked for continuity by placing the ground plate of the generator (+ charge) against the peritoneal surface. The set screw is tightened to secure the lead wire to the generator.

To prevent a competitive rhythm, the rate of the temporary pacemaker is decreased. The electrocardiogram should demonstrate that the permanent pacemaker is discharging at its programmed rate (usually 80 to 100/min) and that the ventricle is depolarizing accordingly. A polypropylene mesh pouch† is sutured with nonabsorbable material to the left lateral peritoneal surface caudal to the liver to store the generator. The ground plate of the

---

*Enflurane or isoflurane is preferred, if available.
†Prolene mesh, Ethicon, Summit NJ.

Figure 2. Postoperative lateral radiograph of a dog following implantation of a permanent pacemaker and epicardial lead electrode. The pulse generator, is situated in the left lateral abdomen. The lead wire extends cranially from the pulse generator and enters the thorax through a small opening lateral to the diaphragm. The corkscrew epicardial electrode is embedded in the apex of the left ventricle. A transvenous pacing wire is also visible extending from the jugular vein, through the cranial vena cava, and into the lumen of the right ventricle. (Reprinted with permission from Bonagura et al.: J.A.V.M.A. 182:149, 1983.)

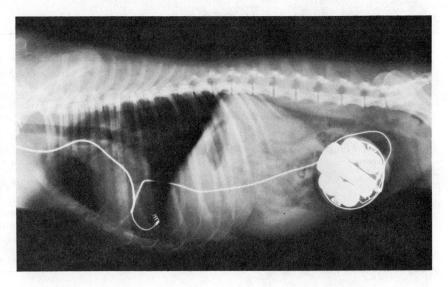

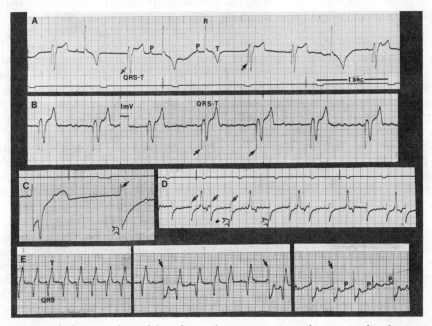

Figure 3. Typical electrocardiograms obtained from dogs with permanent pacemakers. *A*, Reading from a properly functioning demand pacemaker. In this dog, a demand pacemaker discharges following a period of sinus arrest or sinus bradycardia. When the sinus rhythm (PRT) is inadequate to maintain a heart rate of 100/min, the demand pacemaker discharges the ventricle. Stimulus artifacts (arrows) are followed by a wide QRS-T complex of left ventricular origin (lead V₃, 50 mm/sec, 1 cm = 1 mV). *B*, An ECG from a dog 27 months after implantation of a pacemaker. The atrial rhythm is atrial fibrillation, however, the ventricular rate is slow owing to complete AV block. A paced ventricular rhythm is evident with stimulus artifacts (arrows) preceding ventricular QRS-T complexes (lead aVF, 50 mm/sec). *C*, Epicardial lead exit block recorded in a dog. Two complexes are shown. The first complex is a ventricular QRS-T initiated by the pulse generator and associated with a femoral pulse (closed arrow). The second complex is a local electrical response (open arrow) that follows the stimulus artifact. This was not associated with mechanical activation of the ventricle (lead aVF, 100 mm/sec, 1 cm = 1 mV). *D*, The results of lead wire dislodgement are evident. In this dog, the pacemaker continues to discharge at regular intervals; however, it neither senses the ventricular escape rhythm nor captures the ventricle. Local electrical responses (open arrows) can be observed following the regular stimulus artifacts (arrows). The ventricle is discharged by a slow right ventricular escape rhythm that regularly activates the ventricles but is unrelated to the artificial pacemaker impulses. Atrial fibrillation is also present (lead aVF, 25 mm/sec, 1 cm = 1 mV). *E*, Sequential ECG traces from a dog following implantation of a pacemaker. The initial recording demonstrates ventricular tachycardia (QRS-T). The middle tracing reveals nonconducted sinus impulses (small P waves) and two paced complexes following stimulus artifacts (arrows). The final recordings, taken after treatment with lidocaine, demonstrate both paced ventricular beats and one conducted sinus impulse. P waves are labelled. (Reprinted with permission from Bonagura et al.: J.A.V.M.A. 182:149, 1983.)

Table 2.   *Complications of Pacemaker Therapy*

Clinical Setting	Resulting Complication	Management
Organic heart disease	CHF	Temporary pacing; cage rest; furosemide; digitalis; vasodilators
Cardiac arrhythmias	Ventricular asystole; atrial fibrillation; ventricular tachycardia; ventricular fibrillation	Antiarrhythmic drugs; CPR; defibrillation
Administration of drugs and anesthesia	Cardiac arrest upon induction	Prevent with transvenous pacer; avoid high doses of inhalation anesthesia
Surgery	Infection	Meticulous surgical technique; broad spectrum antibiotics
Pacemaker and lead implantation	Lead dislodgement; migration; generator failure; exit block; failure to pace	Screw in epicardial electrode; prevent unnecessary tension on wire; insert Prolene mesh pouch; evaluate for lead disruption (x-ray), exit block (ECG), or pulse generator failure; replace pacemaker or lead wire

generator is placed in contact with the peritoneum. To avoid its dislodgement postoperatively, sufficient lead wire is left in the thoracic cavity. The sternotomy incision is closed with wire, the diaphragm securely closed, and the abdominal incision closed routinely.

Postoperatively, radiographs are taken to confirm the location of the generator and lead wire (Fig. 2). These are useful when evaluating the placement of the implants or the type of generator implanted. Electrocardiograms are obtained frequently for the first 72 postoperative hours (Fig. 3). Myocardial irritation from the placement of the epicardial lead wire frequently results in ventricular premature contractions. If persistent or severe ventricular tachycardia occurs, intravenous boluses (2.0 to 4.0 mg/kg) and constant intravenous administration of lidocaine (see page 298) may be needed. Care is taken to avoid excessive administration of lidocaine, which could result in fatal suppression of the myocardial response to the generator's electrical impulse. Because of the foreign material that has been implanted, broad spectrum antibiotic therapy is indicated.

COMPLICATIONS

The incidence of complications associated with pacemaker implantation is high, but perioperative mortality is low. Complications are associated with organic heart disease, cardiac arrhythmias, drugs, surgery, and pulse generator and pacemaker lead malfunction (Table 2). Congestive heart failure may result from bradycardia or underlying myocardial disease. Initial therapy consisting of cage rest, sodium restriction, and furosemide, plus therapy to increase heart rate including atropine, isoproterenol, or transvenous pacing, is instituted to manage edema and ascites. Halothane-induced ventricular asystole and fibrillation can be fatal if not identified immediately and are best prevented by temporary

transvenous pacing. Atrial fibrillation secondary to atrial dilatation and congestive heart failure related to underlying myocardial disease are potential long-term complications. These are treated with digitalis, diuretics, vasodilators, and reprogramming of the pacemaker to a slightly higher heart rate.

Surgically related infections can be difficult to treat because of the implanted foreign material. Special care should be taken to avoid surgical contamination. Lead dislodgement from the ventricle may occur if sufficient lead wire is not left in the thoracic cavity. Migration of the generator has been eliminated with the use of synthetic mesh to position the generator against the peritoneal surface. Muscle twitching is also less noticeable with intra-abdominal placement of the generator. Exit block can occur when scar tissue develops under the epicardial lead, thereby preventing propagation of the electrical impulse. If the lead wire is not secured against the epicardium, there may also be excessive movement and formation of scar tissue. Pulse generator failure may require replacement but is easily accomplished through a routine abdominal celiotomy. The new pacemaker is attached to the previously implanted lead wire.

SUPPLEMENTAL READING

Bonagura, J. D., Helphrey, M. L., and Muir, W. S.: Complications associated with permanent pacemaker implantation in the dog. J.A.V.M.A. in press.

Buchanan, J. W., et al.: Medical and pacemaker therapy of complete heart block and congestive heart failure in a dog. J.A.V.M.A. 152:1099, 1968.

Lombard, C. W., Tilly, L. P., and Yoshioka, M. M.: Pacemaker implantation in the dog. Survey and literature review. J. Am. Anim. Hosp. Assoc. 17:751, 1981.

Muir, W. W.: Anesthesia for the dog with heart disease. *In* Kirk, R. W.: *Current Veterinary Therapy VI.* Philadelphia: W. B. Saunders, 1977, pp. 388–392.

Sykes, F. P.: Pacemaker and sutureless lead implantation in a dog with third-degree heart block. V.M./S.A.C. 74:1463, 1979.

Yoshioka, M. M., et al.: Permanent pacemaker implantation in the dog. J. Am. Anim. Hosp. Assoc. 17:746, 1981.

CARDIOPULMONARY RESUSCITATION

STEVE C. HASKINS, D.V.M.

Davis, California

Cardiac arrest, or the absence of cardiac output, is usually considered a three-minute emergency. Hypoxic central nervous tissue deterioration ensues after this period of time in the normothermic patient and may occur sooner in patients with serious systemic debilitation prior to the arrest. Successful resuscitation requires early, vigorous, and effective therapy. This article will discuss the multiple components of successful cardiopulmonary resuscitation and suggest guidelines and priorities for a coordinated effort.

CAUSES

Cardiac arrest may be caused by severe abnormalities in electrical or mechanical functioning of the heart or in the oxygenating and decarboxylating efficiency of the lungs. Fluid volume and electrolyte, red cell, protein, caloric, amino acid, carbohydrate, fatty acid or mineral imbalances may also cause cardiac arrest. Maldistribution of blood to and from the tissues is also a contributing factor. Cardiac arrest may be caused by an inability of the liver and other organs to metabolize and process foodstuffs properly or an inability of the kidney and gastrointestinal tract to excrete metabolic products. Abnormalities in the integrated function of the central and peripheral nervous systems may also cause cardiac arrest. Effective treatment of these primary changes is likely to be the most successful approach to the therapy of cardiac arrest.

CLASSIFICATION

There are four major categories of cardiac arrest: (1) ventricular asystole, (2) ventricular fibrillation, (3) cardiovascular collapse, and (4) electrical-mechanical dissociation. It is important to differentiate between the four categories because the emphasis of therapy is different for each (Table 1).

Each form of arrest may occur during a single episode of cardiopulmonary resuscitation, and it may be necessary to repeatedly change the focus of therapy.

There is an absence of electrical activity and myocardial contractions in *ventricular asystole*. Beta-receptor stimulants (epinephrine) are used to elicit pacemaker activity.

Ventricular fibrillation is usually diagnosed by electrocardiography or direct cardiac visualization. Other methods include (1) palpation of a coarsely fibrillating myocardium through the chest wall (this is rarely possible), (2) insertion of a hypodermic needle through the chest wall (location of the needle in the heart can be ascertained by the aspiration of blood through the needle) and observation of a nonrhythmic wiggling of the hub, and (3) indirect suspicion of the existence of ventricular fibrillation

Table 1. Categories of Cardiac Arrest

Classification	Electrical Activity	Coordinated Mechanical Contraction	Visual Appearance of the Heart	Treatment
Ventricular asystole	None	No	Standstill	Catecholamines to stimulate pacemaker activity
Ventricular fibrillation*	Chaotic	No	Fine to coarse myocardial rippling, like a "bag of worms"	Defibrillation to create simultaneous asystole
Cardiovascular collapse due to excessive vasodilation	Normal	Yes	Normal contractions	Rapid fluid administration; alpha-receptor agonists
Electrical-mechanical dissociation	Normal	No	Standstill	Calcium (?); catecholamines (?); bicarbonate (?)

*In some cases of ventricular fibrillation or asystole, the atria will contract rhythmically, but this must not obscure the ongoing ventricular activity.

by virtue of the passage of time and lack of response to support and drug therapy. The fibrillating heart must be defibrillated (simultaneous depolarization of all automatic pacemaker cells) to asystole prior to resumption of a normal sinus rhythm. Cats may be capable of spontaneous defibrillation; however, this possibility should not be relied on for successful resuscitation efforts.

In *cardiovascular collapse* the vascular system fails to return a sufficient volume of blood to the heart. This may be due to anesthetic-induced vasodilation, peripheral pooling of blood in the irreversible stages of shock, or hypovolemia from any cause. Complete absence of a stroke volume is the terminal event in the continuum of decreasing cardiac output associated with any of the previously mentioned conditions. Equally important and much more common is a severely deficient cardiac output (near cardiovascular collapse), which, if recognized prior to complete cardiovascular collapse, is usually correctable with appropriate fluid or drug therapy.

Electromechanical dissociation (normal electrical activity without mechanical contraction) may be due to failure to conduct the action potential from the sarcolemma through the T system, failure of the depolarized T system to cause calcium release from the sarcoplasmic reticulum, or failure of the released calcium to elicit myofibril contraction. The treatments listed in Table 1 are speculative.

Clinical signs

The signs of cardiac arrest are (1) unconsciousness, (2) absence of an auscultable heart beat, (3) absence of a palpable pulse, (4) gray or cyanotic discoloration of the mucous membranes, (5) dilated pupils, and (6) absence of ventilatory attempts. Each sign may occur by itself in a variety of diseases, and it is important to verify the presence of all of them prior to establishing a diagnosis of cardiac arrest. If a conclusive decision cannot be made, artificial ventilation and cardiac compression should commence and should continue until adequate and stable cardiovascular functioning can be positively affirmed.

The color of the mucous membranes is usually dishwater gray (indicating the presence of unoxygenated hemoglobin). It may approach a navy blue in primary respiratory arrest. The color may be white in hypovolemic patients if the blood volume pooled ventrally after the arrest. The membrane color may also be pink or pale pink if there has not been enough time for it to turn gray or if effective artificial ventilation and cardiac compression have been initiated.

Coordinated ventilation will cease when medullary blood flow stops. The agonal gasps that occur as a terminal event some time after cessation of perfusion are probably mediated by primitive inspiratory and spasmodic respiratory centers in the medulla and should not be interpreted as true ventilation.

The capillary refill time of most arrested patients is between one and two seconds, much faster than during the vasoconstrictive phase of hypovolemic shock. Capillary refill time is a good indicator of the extent of vascular constriction or dilation but has no particular usefulness as a sign of cardiac arrest.

CARDIOPULMONARY SUPPORT

Cardiopulmonary resuscitation has two very different objectives, which, of necessity, are pursued simultaneously. The first, and most important, is the effective support of the cardiopulmonary system by cardiac compression, artificial ventilation, and fluid administration. The second goal is to restart a normal sinus electrical rhythm and an effective mechanical contraction with drug and electroshock therapy. For conceptual purposes it is helpful to discuss the techniques and protocols for achieving each goal separately. The ABCs (and DEFs) of cardiopulmonary resuscitation are outlined in Table 2.

ESTABLISHMENT OF AN AIRWAY

Establishment of an airway normally involves the placement of an endotracheal tube or a reasonable facsimile. If an emergency tracheostomy is indicated

Table 2. *Multiple Objectives of Cardiopulmonary Resuscitation*

Airway
  Establish and maintain an open airway via endotracheal intubation

Breathing
  Begin intermittent positive pressure ventilation; one ventilation per five seconds

Circulation
  Begin external cardiac compression; 60 to 80 compressions per minute
  Evaluate the effectiveness of cardiac compression continuously
    If external technique is ineffective:
      Alter external technique
      Perform thoracotomy for internal cardiac compression

Drugs
  Epinephrine: 0.1 to 0.5 mg
  Sodium bicarbonate: 1.0 mEq/kg/5 min of cardiac arrest
  Calcium solution: 1.5 to 2.0 ml of 10% $CaCl_2$
              6.0 to 8.0 ml of 10% CaGluc
  Fluids (lactated Ringer's): 40 ml/kg in the dog
              20 ml/kg in the cat
  Atropine: 0.01 to 0.02 mg/kg

Electrocardiographic monitoring
  Electroshock therapy when necessary

Follow-up monitoring and support
  Cardiovascular, pulmonary, and CNS function
  CNS dehydration therapy

it must be done as an orderly, albeit hurried, surgical procedure. Rapid surgical exposure of the trachea can cause such untoward events as cutting of the jugular vein and carotid sheath, placement of the tracheostomy tube so close to the thoracic inlet that the sternocephalicus muscle mass causes dislodgement of the tube, pneumothorax, infection, and a traumatic or malpositioned tracheal incision (which predisposes to future tracheal stenosis).

In the absence of a tracheal tube of any kind, the head and neck should be extended to open the pharyngeal airway in preparation for mouth-to-nose ventilation.

BREATHING (EFFECTIVE VENTILATION)

Positive pressure should be applied to the endotracheal tube by any method available (e.g., mouth-to-tube, a self-inflating resuscitation bag, the reservoir bag on an anesthetic machine or nonrebreathing circuit, a T piece via a compressed oxygen source) when there is an absence of effective spontaneous ventilation. One deep ventilation should be administered every five seconds, approximately every fifth chest compression. Any pause in the compression cycle to allow time for ventilation must be as brief as possible. The tidal volume should be deftly administered between cardiac compressions. This coordination of cardiac compression and ventilation is not necessary during open-chest cardiac compression, since the lungs are not being compressed by this procedure.

When the resuscitation is being performed by one person, i.e., the chest compression procedure must be interrupted to ventilate the patient, the best combination is 2 to 3 large, rapid ventilations for every 15 chest compressions. With only one person, a ventilation every five seconds takes too much time away from artificial circulation. A method of coordinating artificial ventilation with cardiac compression has been described. In this technique, a nonrebreathing valve from a self–reinflating resuscitation bag is attached to the endotracheal tube, which is connected via a segment of corrugated tubing to the resuscitator via a mouthpiece (Blum, 1968). The resuscitator can inflate the patient's lungs with his exhaled air whenever desired. Automatic ventilators may be used for ventilation purposes. An inspiratory cycle can be triggered by compression of the chest wall, and a short pause in the compression sequence allows for a full tidal volume. Since the ventilator is triggered every time the chest is compressed, the subsequent inspiratory cycle and chest compression will frequently coincide. Although this may impair direct cardiac compression, it may also improve artificial blood flow by increasing the overall intrathoracic pressure.

Mouth-to-nose ventilation can be achieved by grasping the muzzle with one or both hands so that an airtight seal of the lips is created. The head and neck are extended to provide an open pharyngeal airway. Air is then blown through the nose. Care should be taken not to inflate the stomach since this may impede full lung excursions and may predispose the animal to regurgitation or vomition. If the stomach is being inflated, gently compress the larynx (not the trachea) dorsally so that it compresses the esophagus, and make certain that the head and neck are extended maximally. It may also be helpful to try a different flow pattern during the inspiratory effort.

Although it is not effective ventilation in terms of carbon dioxide removal, the insufflation of oxygen via a catheter or needle placed into the trachea through the cricothyroid membrane or between tracheal rings will temporarily support oxygenation by mass flow of oxygen to the alveoli. This technique is not a substitute for ventilation and is limited by the accumulation of systemic carbon dioxide and chest compression–induced atelectasis. However, it may serve as a stopgap procedure in certain circumstances.

Chest compression *per se* will not suffice as effective ventilation. The tidal exchange of the expiratory reserve capacity, especially in the presence of atelectasis, does not constitute enough volume to provide for adequate blood oxygenation and carbon dioxide removal.

CIRCULATION (ARTIFICIAL CARDIAC COMPRESSION)

An artificial stroke volume can be achieved by either compression of the heart from outside the chest or compression of the ventricles directly via a thoracotomy. The very best mean blood pressure and mean blood flow that can be achieved with effective external or internal cardiac compression is minimal when compared with normal, so it is important to re-establish normal electrical and mechanical activity as quickly as possible. Under controlled experimental circumstances, internal cardiac compression is often more effective than external compression, but clinically there is great individual variation. In barrel-chested breeds of dogs, large breeds of dogs, farm animal species, and patients with severe pneumothorax, external chest compression will never be effective, and it is wise to move on to an internal cardiac compression technique. In most other cases it is prudent to first attempt external chest compression since it can usually be expected to work reasonably well, requires no special preparation, can be rapidly applied, and avoids the hazards associated with emergency thoracotomy if the heart resumes spontaneous activity. If an effective stroke volume cannot be generated with several different external chest compression techniques, internal cardiac compression is indicated.

External cardiac compression should not be continued for more than about 10 to 20 minutes, even if it is effective, because of trauma to the chest wall, lungs, and other thoracic and abdominal organs.

Regardless of the mode of cardiac compression, it is imperative that the effectiveness of the procedure be continuously evaluated throughout the resuscitation procedure until a spontaneous and effective heart beat returns. There are no precise ways to determine this in the emergency situation, but it is an evaluation that must be made. If the artificial circulation procedure is effective, there will be an improvement in mucous membrane color, a reduction in pupil size, and a palpable pulse with each compression. If the technique is judged to be ineffective at any point, a different compression technique (external or internal) should be utilized until effective artificial circulation is achieved.

Drugs and techniques that increase diastolic and mean blood pressure during the resuscitation procedure improve survival. A continuous compression procedure maximizes diastolic pressure and mean blood pressure and should never be interrupted unless absolutely necessary and then for as brief a period as possible.

An absolute or relative hypovolemia resulting in the lack of venous return and diastolic ventricular filling is a common cause of ineffective compression. Therefore, a loading dose of fluids (20 to 40 ml/kg) should be administered early in the resuscitation procedure to supplement the venous return.

Impeding blood flow to the lower half of the body by applying a tight abdominal binding or by clamping the descending aorta (following a thoracotomy) may increase diastolic blood pressure and coronary and cerebral circulation, improving the chance for survival.

EXTERNAL CARDIAC COMPRESSION

Compression of the chest should be applied directly over the heart and with a force that is appropriate for the size of the patient. The compression should not be a jerky or stabbing motion. The compression should be held for a brief period of time to maximize the elimination of blood from the heart and chest, but it should not be excessively prolonged. Time must be allowed between compressions for diastolic filling of the ventricles. A general rule is to compress the heart for about one-third of a cycle and release for about two-thirds of a cycle at a minimum rate of 60 cycles per minute. If the initial technique does not generate acceptable results (improvement in color, reduction in pupil size, and a palpable pulse with each compression), try something different: more force, less force, a new location for the compression, a different position for the patient, a shorter or longer

compression technique, a longer interval between compressions to allow for greater diastolic ventricular filling, or a bolus of fluids to improve venous return.

In small to medium-sized dogs, direct external cardiac compression is often effective. However in large or barrel-chested breeds in which direct external cardiac compression is limited by the size, shape, or rigidity of the chest wall, it may be useful to take advantage of the thoracic pump mechanism of artificial blood flow. In this technique, when pressure is applied to the thorax by external compression, blood is squeezed out of all intrathoracic vessels as well as the ventricles of the heart. A competent tricuspid valve, pressure-induced collapse of the great veins in the chest, and peripheral venular valves act to prevent retrograde flow of blood from the chest.

Adjunctive procedures can increase intrathoracic pressure during chest compression. These include simultaneous ventilation, end-inspiratory airway occlusion, and abdominal binding (decreases paradoxical diaphragmatic motion). Perfusion pressures (arterial minus venous pressure) and blood flow improve dramatically when these combined techniques are utilized as compared with external chest compression alone (Chandra et al., 1980; Rudikoff et al., 1980). When the thoracic compression is released, the elastic rebound of the chest wall draws blood into the thorax from the periphery.

INTERNAL CARDIAC COMPRESSION

Internal cardiac compression is indicated any time the external technique is ineffective. Three minutes are allowed at the beginning of a resuscitation to establish an effective artificial circulation: one to two minutes to position the patient (including endotracheal intubation and ventilation) and to evaluate the efficacy of external compression, and, if necessary, one minute to perform the thoracotomy and start direct cardiac compression. The decision to do internal cardiac compression must not be delayed for 10 or 20 minutes and then performed "because everything else has failed." It is a procedure that should be performed immediately in those patients in which external massage is not likely to be effective, within three minutes following cardiac arrest if the external technique is judged to be ineffective, or at any time during the resuscitation endeavor when the external technique becomes ineffective. Internal cardiac compression is also indicated if the chest wall is already open or if it is badly deformed by injury. This technique may be appropriate following prolonged (but effective) external compression to minimize further chest wall and lung trauma.

Direct visualization of the heart permits the detection of (1) insufficient venous return as evidenced by absent or poor filling of the ventricles between compressions (a bolus of fluids should be administered), (2) pre-existing or developing pericardial tamponade (secondary to direct cardiac and/or coronary vessel punctures), which impedes diastolic filling (the sac must be opened for decompression), and (3) ventricular fibrillation when an electrocardiograph is not available. Direct visualization also permits compression of the descending aorta with a clamp or the index finger of the opposite hand to aid perfusion of the brain and heart.

Thoracotomy is an emergency procedure, and no time should be taken to aseptically prepare the patient or the clinician. The incision should be made approximately at the fifth intercostal space. Several guidelines apply when making the incision: (1) Keep the incision in the middle of the intercostal space to avoid the intercostal arteries, which lie on the caudal edge of each rib (avoid the common tendency to make a straight incision; the ribs are concave anteriorly). (2) Avoid the internal thoracic artery, which runs parallel and approximately 0.5 to 1.0 cm lateral to the sternum in the dog (resist the temptation to extend the incision down to the sternum). (3) Avoid incising the lung parenchyma by incising only partially through the intercostal muscles with the scalpel. Puncture through the remaining muscles and pleura with blunt scissors, allow the lungs to fall away, and extend the incision dorsally and ventrally with scissors. The incision should be long enough to provide a convenient entrance of the hand, or two fingers in the case of small patients, into the chest. It is usually recommended that the pericardial sac be opened with a longitudinal incision below the phrenic nerve and that the heart be removed. This will maximize diastolic filling and prevent pericardial tamponade from the accumulation of blood or transudate. Following successful resuscitation, the heart may be placed back into the pericardial sac, but the sac should not be closed, since transudate may continue to exude from the traumatized epicardium.

Direct cardiac compression should be applied with a force that is appropriate to the size of the heart. It should only be applied for the time that it takes to expel the blood from the ventricles. The compression may be repeated as soon as the ventricles have refilled.

Following successful re-establishment of stable mechanical heart function, the hair around the edges of the incision should be carefully clipped and the skin aseptically prepared. The chest should be cleaned and flushed of all hair and debris. The thorax should be flushed with an antibiotic solution and closed in a routine manner. The patient should be placed on systemic antibiotics for several days.

DRUGS

Effective cardiac compression and ventilation may be all that are needed to restart the heart. If the heart is not started by these techniques, drug therapy should be instituted (Table 3). The order in which the drugs are given varies with the needs of each patient. Ideally, cardiotonic drugs like catecholamines and calcium should be administered as close to the coronary arteries as possible, i.e., into the left ventricle. In small patients such as the cat, the heart can be palpated through the chest wall. In medium-sized patients such as the dog, the heart may be rapidly located at its normal position adjacent to the fourth through sixth intercostal spaces in the lower third of the thorax by bringing the point of the elbow back to the costochondral line while maintaining the shoulder in its normal relaxed location. This is the point at which external cardiac compression should be centered and where intracardiac injections can be made.

The farther away from the left ventricle the drugs are given, the greater will be their dilution prior to reaching the coronary microcirculation, the more that will be taken up by cells and receptors along the way, and, depending on the adequacy of the circulation, the less that will reach the heart. When the desired effect is peripheral or when large volumes of drug are to be administered (fluids, sodium bicarbonate), it is not necessary to expose the myocardium to the risk of repeated needle punctures. Drugs can be administered intravenously. When no intravenous catheter is in place, catecholamines may be diluted and administered intratracheally, where they have been reported to be as effective as intracardiac administration for vasoconstrictive purposes (Redding et al., 1967).

Epinephrine is an ideal sympathomimetic for cardiac arrest because it is both a potent inotropic and chronotropic myocardial stimulant and a potent peripheral vasoconstrictor. As such, it is the most effective agent for increasing cerebral and coronary blood flow during resuscitation. Much of the beneficial effect of epinephrine is due to peripheral vasoconstriction. Experimental studies have shown that the alpha-receptor agonists, such as phenylephrine, methoxamine, and metaraminol, are as effective as epinephrine in restarting the hypoxic-arrested heart, whereas the beta-receptor agonist isoproterenol and alpha-receptor blockade prevent resuscitation (Pearson and Redding, 1965; Yakaitis et al., 1979). These findings underscore the importance of maximizing diastolic pressure during cardiac resuscitation, define a role for peripheral vasoconstrictors, preclude the use of isoproterenol during the acute phase of the resuscitation, and warn against the preanesthetic use of phenothiazines in cardiovascularly debilitated patients.

Table 3. Drugs Used During and After Cardiac Resuscitation

Drug (Receptor Activity)	Trade Name (Manufacturer)	Myocardial Chronotropy and Inotropy	Peripheral Vasomotor Tone	Major Indication	Dosage (IV)
Catecholamines					
Epinephrine (α + + +; β + + +)	Adrenalin (Parke-Davis; Vitarine; Bristol)	Increased	Increased	Cardiac arrest	0.05 to 0.5 mg (0.5 to 5 ml 1:10,000 solution) for average-sized dog (15 kg)
Norepinephrine (α + + +; β +)	Levophed bitartrate (Breon)	Variable	Increased	Vasoconstriction	0.01 to 0.1 mg for average-sized dog
Dopamine (dopa and β + + +; α + +)	Intropin (Arnar-Stone)	Increased	Variable	↑Visceral perfusion Blood pressure support	0.1 to 1.0 mg for average-sized dog 80 to 200 mg in 500 ml D5W (to effect; start 2.5 μg/kg/min)
Isoproterenol (α0; β + + +)	Isuprel (Winthrop)	Increased	Decreased	Cardiac stimulation	0.4 to 1.0 mg in 500 ml D5W (to effect; start 0.01 μg/kg/min)
Noncatecholamines					
Mephentermine (α +; β + +)	Wyamine (Wyeth)	Increased	Variable	Blood pressure support	0.1 to 0.5 mg/kg
Metaraminol (α + + +; β +)	Aramine (Merck, Sharp & Dohme) Metaraminol bitartrate (Bristol; Invenex)	Variable	Increased	Vasoconstriction	0.1 to 0.2 mg/kg
Methoxamine (α + + +; β0)	Vasoxyl (Burroughs Wellcome)	None	Increased	Vasoconstriction	0.1 to 0.2 mg/kg
Phenylephrine (α + + +; β0)	Neo-synephrine (Winthrop)	None	Increased	Vasoconstriction	0.01 to 0.1 mg/kg

Agent	Trade name (manufacturer)			Indication	Dosage
Dobutamine (α+; β+++)	Dobutrex (Lilly)	Increased	Variable	Blood pressure support	100 to 400 mg in 500 ml D5W (to effect; start 5 μg/kg/min)
Calcium	(Bristol; Invenex; Vitarine)	Increased	Variable	Increase cardiac output	10% CaCl 1.5 to 2.0 ml 10% CaGluc 6 to 8 ml for average-sized dog
Sodium bicarbonate				To prevent the severe acidosis associated with extremely poor tissue perfusion	0.5 to 1.0 mEq/kg per 5 minutes of arrest 0.1 to 0.25 mEq/kg per bolus
Sodium-containing replacement solutions	(Abbott; Cutter; McGraw)			To fill the increasing capacity of the vascular compartment and generate a suitable venous return	40 ml/kg (dog); 20 ml/kg (cat) of lactated Ringer's or equivalent solution very rapidly, then slow drip
Atropine				To minimize parasympathomimetic influences on the heart	0.01 to 0.02 mg/kg
Lidocaine	Xylocaine (Abbott; Astra; Bristol; Invenex)			To stabilize excitable cell membranes and depress ectopic ventricular pacemaker activity (class II)	1 to 5 mg/kg Mix 1 to 2 mg/ml D5W; administer 10 to 50 μg/kg/min (to effect)
Procainamide	Pronestyl (Squibb)			To stabilize excitable cell membranes and depress ectopic ventricular pacemaker activity (class I)	1 to 5 mg/kg 10 to 50 μg/kg/min (to effect)
Propranolol	Inderal (Ayerst)			Beta-receptor blocking agent	0.05 to 0.3 mg/kg
Mannitol	(Travenol; Merck, Sharp & Dohme)			Osmotic reduction in perivascular cellular and interstitial edema and diuresis	1 to 2 gm/kg

Beyond the conclusive requirement for peripheral vasoconstriction during cardiac resuscitation, there is no way to predict which of the catecholamines is best for a particular patient. Epinephrine or dopamine should be used when cardiac stimulation is desirable, but these drugs may cause ventricular fibrillation. This tendency to cause fibrillation may be minimized by starting at the low end of the suggested dose range and increasing dosage with each administration until the desired effect is achieved. Lidocaine may decrease the tendency for ectopic pacemaker activity or ventricular fibrillation. Those events that predispose to catecholamine-induced arrhythmias, such as halothane anesthesia, hypoxia, acidosis, or myocardial trauma, preclude the use of epinephrine when myocardial stimulation is not needed. However, they do not contraindicate its use when myocardial stimulation is desirable. Other sympathomimetics may be efficacious under certain circumstances either during or following resuscitation. Isoproterenol (with fluid volume expansion) for bradycardia and dopamine, dobutamine, or mephentermine for hypotension may be useful in the post-resuscitation period because of their greater ability to support myocardial contractility and blood pressure with the least impairment of peripheral organ perfusion.

Sodium bicarbonate is used to combat the severe metabolic acidosis that occurs when tissue perfusion is grossly inadequate. Marked acidemia may lower the threshold for ventricular fibrillation, and, in general, recovery is faster and more complete with appropriate alkali therapy (Lendingham and Norman, 1962; Stewart, 1974). Bicarbonate administration is probably not necessary if the heart is restarted within five minutes of the arrest (assuming the patient was not profoundly debilitated and acidotic prior to the arrest). The accumulated lactic acid will be rapidly metabolized by the liver. Bicarbonate should not be used to compensate for respiratory acidosis; this should be prevented with adequate ventilation. Adequate ventilation is even more important following bicarbonate administration because the conversion of bicarbonate to water and carbon dioxide can cause dramatic elevations in the partial pressure of carbon dioxide (P_{CO_2}).

Calcium administration stabilizes the surface of excitable cells and improves muscle tone and contractility by increasing the calcium concentration in the sarcoplasma. It is primarily indicated for the flabby or weakly beating heart and may be useful in electrical-mechanical dissociation. Excessive dosages may cause tachycardia and ventricular arrhythmias; hyperstabilization of the surface membrane, which makes depolarization difficult or impossible; or sustained myocardial tetany. Calcium very effectively antagonizes the effect of hyperkalemia on electrically excitable cells and should be the first drug administered if this is the cause of the arrest or near arrest. The calcium dosage should be reduced or its administration avoided in known cases of digitalis toxicity.

Perhaps the most common cause of unsuccessful resuscitation is the lack of an effective functional circulating blood volume and venous return. The longer the duration of the cardiopulmonary arrest, the greater will be the hypoxic vasodilation and the increase in vascular volume and the greater will be the need for fluid loading. Possibly the next most common causes for resuscitation failure are excessive fluid administration (either in terms of rate or volume) and precipitous serosanguineous pulmonary edema. The suggested fluid dosage (see Table 3) is one that we have found to be generally acceptable. During internal cardiac compression the dose can be accurately tailored to obtain the desired rate and volume of diastolic filling. During external chest compressions, start with the suggested dosage. If the combination of fluid volume and compression does not generate an effective circulation, internal cardiac compression is indicated and fluid volume requirements can then be more accurately gauged. If the fluid volume initially provides for effective external cardiac compression but the effect subsequently diminishes, suspect a progressive increase in the vascular volume capacity and/or redistribution of fluids out of the vascular compartment and administer another loading dose of fluids. Depending on the hemoglobin concentration prior to the arrest or the amount of hemorrhage during the resuscitation, whole blood administration may be warranted. The hemoglobin concentration should be maintained above 6.0 gm/dl (PCV > 18 to 20 per cent).

Vagal tone is increased during cardiac arrest, and small doses of atropine may be useful in cardiac arrest therapy. Care must be exercised by utilizing appropriate dosing intervals. The combined use of parasympatholytics and sympathomimetics predisposes to severe tachycardia and may predispose to ventricular fibrillation.

Xylocaine is indicated for the treatment of frequent ectopic ventricular pacemaker activity or when the heart is exhibiting such poor electrical stability that it is in danger of fibrillating. Excessive doses of xylocaine may cause hypotension or cardiovascular collapse, myocardial depression or arrest (asystole), CNS excitation, and nausea and vomiting. A recently resuscitated heart that has been traumatized from compression, defibrillation, and intracardiac injections is expected to exhibit multi-focal pacemaker activity. These are often self-limiting within several hours. Xylocaine should not be routinely administered unless the arrhythmias are serious.

ELECTROSHOCK THERAPY (DEFIBRILLATION)

The fibrillating heart must be converted to asystole before the previously mentioned methods of cardiopulmonary support and cardiac stimulation can be effective. DC current defibrillation is the most reliable method of defibrillation (Table 4). The energy necessary for external defibrillation is 0.5 to 10 watt-sec/kg body weight for externally applied electrodes and approximately 0.2 to 0.4 watt-sec/kg for internally applied electrodes (Geddes et al., 1974a and b). There is considerable variation among patients with regard to the amount of energy necessary for successful defibrillation. This may be due to different degrees of acidosis or hypoxia, previous or concurrent drug therapy (Xylocaine decreases susceptibility to defibrillation, whereas digitalis increases the incidence of post-shock arrhythmias), or progressive deterioration of organ function in general. Progressively longer periods of fibrillation require increased countershock energies and are associated with fewer successful defibrillations. The fibrillating heart should be defibrillated as early as possible.

Excessive countershock energies may cause postshock arrhythmias by persistent myocardial cell depolarization (Jones and Jones, 1980) or myocardial damage including cellular necrosis (Van Vleet et al., 1978). Both decrease the frequency of successful defibrillation. Countershock energies should be appropriate for the size and condition of the patient, and settings should initially be on the low side of the suggested ranges.

The procedure for defibrillation of the heart is as follows:

1. Provide adequate support therapy to help assure that conditions are optimal for the heart to establish a normal sinus rhythm once it is defibrillated with (a) prior oxygenation and ventilation, (b) administration of appropriate amounts of sodium bicarbonate and calcium, and (c) enhancement of the coarseness of the fibrillation pattern with epinephrine.

2. Apply a liberal amount of contact paste to the paddles as well as the chest wall over the heart. (If external, use commercial EKG gels, PHisohex soap, or K-Y jelly and salt. Do not use alcohol, because it is flammable. For internal defibrillation use saline.)

3. Apply the electrodes firmly to the chest wall or heart. If the electrodes are not firmly in contact, the shock will pass through small cross-sectional areas of the chest wall and/or heart rather than being diffusely distributed. This decreases the defibrillation efficiency and increases the tissue damage associated with the procedure. Be sure that the electrodes are not in contact with each other either directly or via a bridge of electrolyte solution.

4. Make sure that all personnel are clear of the patient, the table, the anesthetic machine, the EKG machine, and the defibrillator. Then discharge the machine.

5. Check for cardioversion and re-institute cardiopulmonary support therapy. Repeat the process at a higher power setting if the heart did not defibrillate the first time.

Table 4. Methods of Defibrillation

DC Current Defibrillation

	Power Settings (watt-seconds)	
	Internal	External
Plan A		
Small patient	10 to 25	100 to 150
Large patient	100 to 150	400

	Internal	External	
		Weight (kg)	Energy (watt-sec)
Plan B*	0.2 to 0.4 watt-sec/kg	<7	2/kg
		8 to 40	5/kg
		>40	5 to 10/kg

AC Current Defibrillation

	Power Settings (volts)	
	Internal	External
Small patient	50	100
Large patient	100	150 to 200

Pharmacologic Defibrillation

1. Potassium chloride (20 to 30 mEq) for an average-sized dog (15 kg) followed by 2 ml calcium chloride or 8 ml calcium gluconate
2. Potassium chloride (1 mEq/kg) and acetylcholine (6 mg/kg)†

*Geddes et al., 1974a and b.
†Breznock et al., 1978.

FOLLOW-UP MONITORING AND SUPPORT

Once an effective heart beat is re-established, continued ventilatory support and continuous observation of the electrical and mechanical functioning of the heart are important. The duration and extent of the monitoring and support vary greatly from patient to patient. As a rule, monitoring should be continued until the patient is stable and able to maintain homeostasis.

Hypoxic central nervous system damage is common following cardiopulmonary arrest (persistent blindness in otherwise normal patients or persistent coma in the presence of well-regulated cardiovascular and respiratory function and body temperature). Support measures that may be helpful in minimizing post-resuscitation neurologic deficits include the following: (1) Controlled ventilation to prevent further hypoxia and hypercapnia and cause moderate hypocapnia. This will decrease flow to brain areas with normal circulatory autoregulation and, it is hoped, increase flow to damaged areas with the greatest need. Controlled ventilation should be continued until the patient no longer tolerates the endotracheal tube. (2) Moderate hypertension to maximize the re-establishment of perfusion of damaged areas (Ames et al., 1968). (3) Avoidance of extracranial complications such as hypoxemia, hypercapnia, hypotension, severe hypertension, hyperthermia, uremia, or sepsis. (4) Perivascular cellular swelling and "blebs" from endothelial cells are responsible for the no-reflow phenomenon (Chiang et al., 1968), and an increased brain sodium and water content occurs after periods of prolonged cerebral ischemia (Zimmerman and Hossmann, 1975). To combat these events, CNS dehydration therapy is instituted using mannitol (1.0 gm/kg administered over 30 minutes and repeated in three to four hours) and anti-inflammatory therapy with large pharmacologic doses of corticosteroids: dexamethasone (4 to 6 mg/kg) or prednisolone or methylprednisolone (30 mg/kg). (5) Barbiturate loading (large anesthetizing doses) may decrease the extent of the brain damage due to global ischemia by decreasing metabolic rate and oxygen consumption, but the efficacy of the technique is subject to considerable controversy (Michenfelder, 1981). The new benzodiazepine derivative, midazolam, also decreases cerebral metabolic rate more than it decreases cerebral blood flow (similar to the barbiturates) and is not associated with the severe cardiovascular depression seen with the barbiturates. Heparinization and systemic hemodilution do not improve neurologic survival, except as they would treat primary extracranial complications. The efficacy of hypothermia is unknown at this time.

SUMMARY

The resuscitation procedure has been divided into its component parts for discussion and conceptualization. In reality all of the various procedures should be accomplished simultaneously. The following outline is offered as an example of a resuscitation effort. Patients are presented under a variety of circumstances. The flow of treatment should be adjusted and tailored to the specific needs of each one.

Time (min)	Event
0	Cardiac arrest occurs. Airway secured and external cardiac compression and ventilation is instituted.
0.5	Determine whether the heart has started beating. If not, continue cardiac compression and ventilation and assure that the compression technique is effective.
1.0	Determine whether the heart has started beating. If not, apply abdominal wrap and continue cardiac compression and ventilation (continuously evaluating its effectiveness).
1.5	Determine whether the heart has started beating. If not, administer epinephrine and continue cardiac compression and ventilation.
2.0	Determine whether the heart has started beating. If not, administer bicarbonate and atropine. If external chest compression has been effective, continue the cardiac compression and ventilation. If not, perform a thoracotomy for internal massage. Determine if the heart is fibrillating (the EKG should be attached by this time); if yes, defibrillate. Rapid fluid administration should be instituted by this time.
3.0	Determine if the heart started beating. If not, repeat the epinephrine, and continue effective cardiac compression and ventilation.
4.0	Determine whether the heart has started beating? If not, administer calcium, continue effective cardiac compression and ventilation.
Appropriate intervals	Continue to evaluate effectiveness of the cardiac compression procedure. Defibrillate when necessary. "Fluidate" as necessary. Repeat drug therapy as necessary.

A comprehensive resuscitation effort requires substantial preplanning and a coordinated group effort. Necessary equipment and drugs should be organized and set up in advance. Protocols and drug dosages should be posted in plain view. And most importantly, *all* persons in the area should be trained to be a functional part of the resuscitation team.

The resuscitation effort should continue for as long as there is any hope of successfully restarting the heart. Most resuscitations that lead to complete recovery of cardiovascular and cerebral function are accomplished within 5 to 10 minutes of the arrest, but successful resuscitations have been known to occur after as long as 30 to 40 minutes in the dog. Maximally dilated pupils, lack of return of mucous membrane color, and persistent lack of electrical or mechanical activity of the heart represent poor prognostic signs. Early return of ventilatory efforts, pupillary light reflexes, lacrimation, stable electrical and mechanical activity of the heart, electrocortical activity, definitive responses to pain, and normal levels of consciousness represent favorable prognostic signs.

Prevention of the cardiac arrest is considerably

easier than its treatment. Tranquilizers and anesthetics cause vasodilation and hypotension and can unmask an existing preanesthetic hypovolemia. Fluid preloading in any patient at risk for cardiovascular collapse (dehydration, shock, general debilitation from any cause) with a crystalloid sodium replacement solution (10 to 40 ml/kg in the dog; 5 to 20 ml/kg in the cat) is recommended. The intraoperative use of automatic, continuous, audible monitors of mechanical heart and lung function and body temperature is encouraged.

REFERENCES

Ames, A., Wright, R. L., Kowada, M., Thurston, J. M., and Majno, G.: Cerebral ischemia II. The no-reflow phenomena. Am. J. Pathol. 52:437, 1968.

Blum, L. L.: A method for concurrent artificial ventilation and cardiac massage by the same individual. Anesthesiology 29:841, 1968.

Breznock, E. M., Kagan, K. G., and Attix, E. S.: Chemical cardioversion of electrically induced ventricular fibrillation in dogs. Am. J. Vet. Res. 39:971, 1978.

Chandra, N., Rudikoff, M., and Weisfeldt, M. L.: Compression and ventilation at high airway pressure during cardiopulmonary resuscitation. Lancet 1:175, 1980.

Chiang, J., Kowada, M., Ames, A., Wright, R. L., and Majno, G.: Cerebral ischemia III. Vascular changes. Am. J. Pathol. 52:455, 1968.

Geddes, L. A., Tacker, W. A., Rosborough, J. P., Moore, A. G., and Cabler, P. S.: Electrical dose for ventricular defibrillation of large and small animals using precordial electrodes. J. Clin. Invest. 53:310, 1974a.

Geddes, L. A., Tacker, W. A., Rosborough, J., Moore, A. G., Cabler, P., Bailey, M., McCrady, J. D., and Witzel, D.: The electrical dose for ventricular defibrillation with electrodes applied directly to the heart. J. Thorac. Cardiovasc. Surg. 68:593, 1974b.

Jones, J. L., and Jones, R. E.: Postshock arrhythmias—a possible cause of unsuccessful defibrillation. Crit. Care Med. 8:167, 1980.

Lendingham, I. M., and Norman, J. N.: Acid-base studies in experimental circulatory arrest. Lancet 2:967, 1962.

Michenfelder, J. D.: Cerebral protection and resuscitation. Refresher Course Proceedings of the American Society of Anesthesiologists. Lecture 124, 1981.

Pearson, J. W., and Redding, J. S.: Influence of peripheral vascular tone on cardiac resuscitation. Anesth. Analg. 44:746, 1965.

Redding, J. S., Asuncion, J. S., and Pearson, J. W.: Effective routes of drug administration during cardiac arrest. Anesth. Analg. 46:253, 1967.

Rudikoff, M. T., Maughan, W. L., Effron, M., Freund, P., and Weisfeldt, M. L.: Mechanisms of blood flow during cardiopulmonary resuscitation. Circulation 61:345, 1980.

Stewart, J. S. S.: Management of cardiac arrest, with special reference to metabolic acidosis. Br. Med. J. 1:476, 1964.

Van Vleet, J. F., Tacker, W. A., Geddes, L. A., and Ferrans, V. J.: Sequential cardiac morphologic alterations induced in dogs by single transthoracic damped sinusoidal waveform defibrillator shock. Am. J. Vet. Res. 39:271, 1978.

Yakaitis, R. W., Otto, C. W., and Blitt, C. D.: Relative importance of alpha and beta adrenergic receptors during resuscitation. Crit. Care Med. 7:293, 1979.

Zimmerman, V., and Hossmann, K. A.: Resuscitation of the monkey brain after one hour's complete ischemia. II. Brain water and electrolytes. Brain Res. 85:1, 1975.

Section
5

HEMATOLOGY— ONCOLOGY— IMMUNOLOGY

ARTHUR I. HURVITZ, D.V.M.
Consulting Editor

Additional Pertinent Information found in Current Veterinary Therapy VI:
Hurvitz, Arthur I., D.V.M.: Gammopathies, p. 451.

Hematology

THROMBOCYTOPENIA

JUDITH S. JOHNESSEE, D.V.M.,
and ARTHUR I. HURVITZ, D.V.M.
New York, New York

Thrombocytopenia, defined as a platelet count of less than 200,000 cells/μl, is characterized clinically by petechiae and ecchymoses, which occur with or without other signs such as hematuria, melena, hyphema, epistaxis, and bleeding at venipuncture sites. Normal platelet counts in the dog and cat range from 200,000 to 500,000 cells/μl; however, bleeding is not usually clinically significant until the platelet count falls below 50,000 cells/μl, unless there are concomitant platelet function or vessel wall defects. Since bleeding may not be clinically apparent, thrombocytopenia may be found inadvertently during routine hematologic testing.

Thrombocytopenia does not occur as a primary disease entity but is the result of one of a number of disease processes. The cause must be determined in each case for treatment to be effective. Abnormally low platelet numbers are the result of decreased production, abnormal distribution, or increased destruction of cells (Table 1).

Table 1. *Diagnostic Scheme for Differentiating Causes of Thrombocytopenia in Dogs and Cats*

Suppression of Platelet Production
    Scan peripheral blood smear for platelet size
    Check bone marrow for thrombopoiesis
    Look for evidence of other disease—carcinoma, leukemia, fungal infection, *Ehrlichia* spp.

Platelet Sequestration
    Examine for splenic masses via palpation and abdominal radiography
    Look for evidence of liver disease via biochemical testing, prothrombin time, and BSP retention

Enhanced Platelet Destruction
    Take drug history
    Look for evidence of other disease—disseminated intravascular coagulation, thrombosis, infection (*Ehrlichia*, rickettsia-like organisms)
    Check for autoimmune phenomena—platelet factor 3, antinuclear antibody, rheumatoid factor, Coombs' test

DISORDERS OF DECREASED PRODUCTION

DIAGNOSIS

To determine if there is adequate platelet production, a peripheral blood smear should be examined. If the smear reveals few platelets of varying sizes with large ones predominating, the bone marrow is probably producing platelets in adequate numbers. However, if all the platelets are small and of uniform size, there is probably inadequate platelet production. If there is still doubt as to platelet production after examining the smear, a bone marrow sample should be examined for the number and maturation sequence of megakaryocytes. Absence of megakaryocytes in the bone marrow sample indicates that lack of production is the cause of the thrombocytopenia.

CAUSES

Common causes of decreased platelet production include neoplasia, infectious disease, and drug toxicity. Neoplasia causes crowding of the bone marrow by aberrant cells or general bone marrow suppression. Infectious agents such as *Ehrlichia* spp. may suppress the bone marrow as well as cause increased peripheral destruction of blood cells (Huxsoll and Hildebrandt, 1977). In cases of decreased platelet production for which a cause cannot be determined, the serum should be tested for the presence of an antibody titer against *Ehrlichia* spp. (Huxsoll and Hildebrandt, 1977.) Many viruses have a specific tropism for megakaryocytes and may cause transient thrombocytopenia. This is true of many live virus vaccines (lowest platelet count occurs seven to ten days post-vaccination), but rarely is this clinically significant unless surgery is performed during this period.

Drug toxicity is an important cause of bone marrow suppression. Suppression caused by estrogens, either exogenously administered or produced by Sertoli cell tumor of the testes, is the most thoroughly documented bone marrow suppression in animals. Estrogens typically produce (in order of occurrence) leukocytosis, thrombocytopenia, anemia, leukopenia, and, terminally, complete bone marrow aplasia. In rare cases, estrogens may also cause drug-induced antiplatelet antibody production, resulting in thrombocytopenia via immune-mediated mechanisms. Other drugs may be more difficult to incriminate, but careful historical examination may reveal use of an exogenous agent that could be associated with bone marrow suppression.

TREATMENT

In cases of decreased platelet production, treatment is supportive: administer platelet-rich plasma (Wilkins and Dodds 1977) or whole fresh blood (O'Rourke, 1983) to control life-threatening bleeding. Estrogen-producing tumors should be removed, but recovery may take several months. In cases in which the cause of decreased platelet production cannot be identified, prednisolone (1 to 3 mg/kg, divided b.i.d. to t.i.d., PO) may be administered for several weeks as a therapeutic trial to rule out the possibility to immune destruction of megakaryocytes. Alternatively, vincristine (Oncovin, Eli Lilly) (.01 to .025 mg/kg, once weekly IV) may be administered in an attempt to stimulate platelet production. Treatment, however, generally consists of supportive care while waiting for bone marrow regeneration. The prognosis is guarded in these cases.

DISORDERS OF ABNORMAL DISTRIBUTION

If the bone marrow contains adequate numbers of megakaryocytes, an abnormality in platelet distribution or life span must be considered. In disorders of distribution the platelet life span is normal, and the number of platelets in the body may actually be increased above normal, but very few are seen in the peripheral circulation. Normally one-third of the platelets pass through the splenic pulp at one time. If the transit time is prolonged, up to 80 per cent of the platelets may be sequestered. Severity of sequestration is more closely associated with the vascularity rather than the size of the spleen. Common causes of splenomegalic thrombocytopenia in dogs are advanced liver disease and splenic neoplasia. There is no treatment for thrombocytopenia associated with liver disease except for supportive care and administration of vitamin K to prevent further bleeding caused by decreased liver production of the prothrombin complex of clotting factors.

If a splenic mass is present and there is no evidence of metastasis, whole fresh blood or platelet-rich plasma should be given and the mass removed, if possible.

DISORDERS OF INCREASED DESTRUCTION

DIAGNOSIS

If adequate platelets are being produced and there is no evidence of splenomegalic thrombocytopenia, shortened platelet life span must be considered as the cause. Hemorrhage alone is rarely enough to cause significant thrombocytopenia unless consumptive coagulopathy or massive thromboses are present, which should be evident from clinical signs. Infectious agents that can cause increased peripheral removal of platelets by the reticuloendothelial system are *Ehrlichia* spp. and a rickettsia-like organism reported in dogs in Florida (Harvey et al., 1976). The peripheral blood should be examined carefully for these organisms. Although there is a serologic test available for *Ehrlichia* spp. (Huxsoll and Hildebrandt 1977), one is not available for the rickettsia-like organism.

Increased peripheral platelet destruction is most frequently mediated immunologically through one of three mechanisms: production of specific antiplatelet antibody (autoimmune thrombocytopenic purpura, AITP); induction of antibody production against a hapten-platelet membrane complex; or passive absorption of preformed antigen-antibody complexes onto the platelet surface and consequent incidental removal of the platelet when the antigen-antibody complexes are removed by the reticuloendothelial system. If antibody is produced in response to a drug-platelet membrane complex, the disease process should stop when the drug is discontinued. Therefore, only drugs that are essential to therapy should be administered to thrombocytopenic patients. Table 2 lists drugs that have been shown to cause immune-mediated thrombocytopenia in animals. However, all drugs should be considered to have the potential to cause thrombocytopenia.

If it is suspected that the thrombocytopenia is produced by an autoimmune process, a platelet

Table 2. *Drugs That Cause Immune-Mediated Thrombocytopenia in Dogs**

Phenylbutazone
Styrid caracide (American Cyanamid)
Amphetamines
Dilantin
Estrogens

*Data from Jean Dodds, D.V.M., New York Department of Health, Division of Laboratories and Research, Albany, N.Y., Dec., 1981. Personal communication.

factor 3 release assay can be performed. The test is positive in the presence of specific antiplatelet antibody and negative in drug-induced and antigen-antibody complex–mediated disease. If the thrombocytopenia is autoimmune in nature, efforts to identify other autoimmune phenomena should be made to rule out polysystemic autoimmune disease.

TREATMENT

Because of the different modes of therapy available to the clinician for the treatment of immunologically mediated platelet destruction, it is important to understand the platelet kinetics involved. The major site of removal of antibody-labelled platelets is the spleen owing to slow rate of flow through the sinusoids, locally high levels of antibody (most antiplatelet antibody is produced in the spleen), and the presence of large numbers of macrophages, which engulf and remove antibody-coated platelets. Only in the presence of extremely high numbers of antibody molecules does the liver become important in removing coated platelets.

The modes of therapy used to treat thrombocytopenia (splenectomy, administration of steroids and chemotherapeutic agents) have different mechanisms of action, and several therapies can be combined effectively if the rationale for the use of each is understood. Corticosteroids work by inhibiting the removal of platelets by the reticuloendothelial system and probably by interfering with the attachment of antibodies to platelets; suppression of antibody production is not a major reason for efficacy. The dosage range for prednisolone is 1 to 3 mg/kg, divided b.i.d. to t.i.d., PO. Intramuscular injections should be avoided. It has not been documented that added benefit is derived from increasing the dosage of prednisolone; in fact, side effects worsen. If other steroids are used, dosages should be calculated according to relative potency compared with prednisolone. No randomized clinical trials have been performed to support the use of one steroid over another.

The platelet count should begin to rise within two to four days, after which the dosage of prednisolone may be tapered by 50 per cent every week or every two weeks. Prolonged use of high dosages of steroids ultimately suppresses the bone marrow. To avoid toxicity, alternate-day therapy should be instituted as soon as the disease process is well controlled. Toxicity is exhibited by hind limb weakness, profound polyuria and polydipsia, muscle wasting, and hepatomegaly. These signs resolve as steroid administration is tapered. The reduction should be slow, with the dosage regimen extended over several months. If the initial therapy is effective, the platelet count usually rises to greater than 200,000 cell/μl. Lower counts are acceptable as long as the animal is asymptomatic. Those animals that

show only a mildly elevated platelet count (less than 100,000 cells/μl) in response to initial steroid therapy may show a delayed response after several weeks of administration of high dosages of steroids. In animals that do not respond at all to steroids alone or that cannot tolerate high levels of steroids, other therapy modalities, such as splenectomy, should be considered.

Splenectomy removes the major site of antibody production as well as the main site of platelet removal. Before undertaking splenectomy it is critical to eliminate all nonimmunologic causes of thrombocytopenia such as neoplasia or infectious disease. Be certain that the bone marrow is functional. Prior to surgery, the patient should undergo transfusion with platelet-rich plasma or fresh whole blood (if red blood cells are necessary), and prednisolone should be administered (1 to 3 mg/kg, daily PO). Even if splenectomy does not effect a remission, it may still allow for reduction of the maintenance steroid dosage. After surgery, the corticosteroid dosage should be tapered as described previously.

An alternative to splenectomy is the administration of chemotherapeutic agents. The most specific drug for thrombocytopenia is vincristine, which should be given at a low dosage (.01 to .025 mg/kg, IV once weekly). Vincristine is usually effective within two to four days and may be repeated once weekly as necessary. Since the mechanism of action of vincristine is increased platelet *production*, administration of steroids should be continued at a dosage of 1 to 3 mg/kg daily to decrease platelet *destruction* until the platelet count begins to rise. Vincristine may then be discontinued and steroids tapered as previously discussed. Occasionally an animal does well on periodic vincristine given alone, administered as dictated by recurrence of thrombocytopenia. This may be attempted in animals that react adversely to corticosteroid administration.

The administration of immunosuppressive drugs such as cyclophosphamide (Cytoxan, Mead Johnson) and azathioprine (Imuran, Burroughs Wellcome) is generally the last choice of therapy for immune-mediated thrombocytopenia. Since these drugs suppress the bone marrow, the white blood cell count must be monitored carefully during their administration. Cyclophosphamide also causes hemorrhagic cystitis, and therefore its usefulness in long-term control is limited. Cyclophosphamide is given orally four consecutive days out of seven for a maximum of three weeks. The dosages are 2.50 mg/kg (1.25 mg/lb) for cats and dogs under 5 kg, 2.2 mg/kg (1 mg/lb) for dogs 5 to 25 kg, and 1.50 mg/kg (.75 mg/lb) for dogs over 25 kg (Pederson, 1976). Cyclophosphamide may also be given intravenously at a dosage of 7 mg/kg once a week. Alternatively, azathioprine (2.2 mg/kg, s.i.d. PO) may be given indefinitely as needed as long as the white blood cell count remains normal. Results of the use of azathioprine in cats are unpredictable. The dosages of both cyclophosphamide and azathioprine should be decreased by 25 per cent if the white cell count falls between 5000 to 7000 cells/mm³ and stopped if the white count falls below 5000 cells/mm³ (Pederson, 1976). During therapy with these immunosuppressive chemotherapeutic agents, corticosteroids are continued at a dosage of 1 to 3 mg/kg daily to decrease reticuloendothelial removal of antibody-coated platelets. In rare cases in which administration of steroids and vincristine or splenectomy have not controlled thrombocytopenia, cyclophosphamide and azathioprine have been used together to keep the platelet count at an acceptable level. These difficult cases must be monitored very carefully, because such animals are rendered immunologically incompetent as a result of this therapy. Prophylactic antibiotics are not necessary, but infection should be treated vigorously if it occurs.

Once control is established, relapse must be anticipated. Relapse must be treated vigorously with the same drugs and dosages used for initial therapy. Recurrence of thrombocytopenia is often more difficult to control. Common causes of relapse are live virus vaccination, infection, estrus, and pregnancy. If at all possible, the animal should undergo ovariohysterectomy. Administration of steroids should be reinstituted or the dosage increased prior to elective surgery or the stress of surgery may also cause a relapse. Administration of any other medications should be kept to a minimum, especially if the cause of the thrombocytopenia has not been firmly established.

REFERENCES AND SUPPLEMENTAL READING

Erslev, A. J., and Gabuzda, T. G.: *Pathophysiology of Blood.* Philadelphia: W.B. Saunders Co., 1979, pp. 157–172.
Harvey, J. W., Simpson, C. F., and Gaskin, J. M.: Cyclic thrombocytopenia induced by a rickettsia-like agent in dogs. J. Infect. Dis. 137:182, 1978.
Huxsoll, D. L., and Hildebrandt, P. K.: Tropical canine pancytopenia (ehrlichiosis). *In* Kirk, R. W. (ed.): *Current Veterinary Therapy V.* Philadelphia: W.B. Saunders Co., 1977, pp. 369–371.
Karpatkin, S.: Autoimmune thrombocytopenic purpura. Blood 56:329, 1980.
Koller, C.A.: Immune thrombocytopenic purpura. Med. Clin. North Am. 64:761, 1980.
McMillan, R.: Chronic idiopathic thrombocytopenic purpura. N. Engl. J. Med. 304:1135, 1981.
O'Rourke, L.: Blood transfusion. *In* Kirk, R. W. (ed.): *Current Veterinary Therapy VIII.* Philadephia: W.B. Saunders Co., 1983.
Pedersen, N. C.: Canine joint disease. Proceedings of the 43rd Annual Meeting of the American Animal Hospital Association. 351, 1976.
Wilkins, R. J., and Dodds, W. J.: Idiopathic (immunologic) thrombocytopenic purpura. *In* Kirk, R. W. (ed.): *Current Veterinary Therapy V.* Philadelphia: W.B. Saunders Co., 1979, pp. 365–367.

MANAGEMENT OF THE ANEMIC CAT

SUSAN M. COTTER, D.V.M.

Boston, Massachusetts

Management of anemia in cats can be frustrating to the veterinarian. However, a systematic approach to these patients allows for relative ease of classification and determination of prognosis. A complete physical examination and history may give clues as to underlying disease or environmental causes of anemia in cats. Blood should be drawn for proper evaluation. The packed cell volume (PCV) is used to determine if an immediate transfusion is necessary. Most cats become anemic gradually, compensate for their hypoxic state, and remain comfortable until the PCV drops below 10 per cent. If severe weakness is present with a PCV of greater than 10 per cent, it is an indication of acute blood loss, hemolysis, or other underlying infection or organ failure.

Examination of red cell morphology gives a quick indication as to the type of anemia. Polychromasia and anisocytosis may indicate regenerative anemia. Hypochromasia indicates chronic blood loss. Fragmented cells indicate microangiopathic hemolysis or disseminated intravascular coagulation. Heinz bodies in large numbers may indicate exposure to oxidant drugs, such as methylene blue, acetaminophen, or phenazopyridine. Anemia without change in red cell morphology is frequently nonregenerative. Nucleated red cells are not a good prognostic sign unless accompanied by marked reticulocytosis. White cell and platelet counts give clues as to marrow activity. Increased counts often indicate active marrow response, whereas leukopenia and thrombocytopenia often occur in aplastic anemia. A well-made and well-stained blood smear should be scanned for atypical white cells suggestive of leukemia. Red cell parasites such as *Haemobartonella* may be a primary or secondary cause of anemia.

In addition to the blood count, a reticulocyte count is important in the evaluation of anemia. This test is critical in separating regenerative and nonregenerative anemias. One must remember that cat reticulocytes mature over approximately one week so that immature and mature reticulocytes differ in significance. Immature (aggregate) reticulocytes occur in acute anemias with marked bone marrow response. A test for feline leukemia virus (FeLV) should be done on every anemic cat, since FeLV positive cats (naturally and experimentally) may suffer from either hemolytic or nonregenerative anemia. Approximately 70 per cent of all anemic cats carry FeLV, which can cause anemia in the absence of leukemia. No specific treatment is successful in eliminating FeLV; so the prognosis is less favorable than for a FeLV negative anemic cat.

The initial step in laboratory evaluation of an anemic cat should be classification of either regenerative or nonregenerative anemia. The presence or absence of blood loss usually can be decided clinically. Hemolytic anemia may be divided into chemical (e.g., Heinz body), immune-mediated, or parasitic (e.g., *Haemobartonella*) categories. A positive Coombs' test indicates that the hemolysis is immune-mediated. Coombs' positive anemia may be caused by a primary anti–red cell antibody, or another antibody directed to an organism such as *Haemobartonella* or FeLV may attach to a red cell and cause immune-mediated hemolysis. Blood loss anemia does not require specific treatment except volume replacement in acute hemorrhage or transfusion if loss is massive or if the cat is severely anemic from chronic blood loss. Hemolytic anemia, if Coombs' positive, is treated with prednisone at 2.0 mg/kg/day PO. If a Coombs' test is not available or if it is negative, the initial treatment can be tetracycline 25 mg/kg t.i.d. for 10 days, as in cases of hemobartonellosis. *Haemobartonella* organisms may be found only transiently in peripheral blood. If there is no response to tetracycline, prednisone can be given as previously mentioned. Prednisone may allow for longer survival of red cells because of decreased extravascular removal. Prednisone should be avoided in cases of hemobartonellosis because it may suppress the immune response to the organism.

There is no added benefit with the use of arsenicals to treat hemobartonellosis since they have been shown to be no more effective than tetracycline in eliminating the carrier state. Hemolytic anemia caused by oxidant drugs (Heinz body anemia) can usually be managed by elimination of the drug and support with transfusions if needed. If methemoglobinemia is also present, as in acetaminophen toxic-ity, supportive care becomes more difficult and liver toxicity is an added problem. Intravenous fluids, transfusion, and possibly even exchange transfusion may be needed. Acetylcysteine, a compound similar to glutathione, has been used to facilitate conjugation and inactivation of acetaminophen, thus reducing methemoglobin formation and hepatic toxicity. The dose utilized in experimental toxicosis is 140 mg/kg (14 per cent solution by gavage).

TREATMENT OF NONREGENERATIVE ANEMIA

An anemic cat with a low reticulocyte count and normal red cell morphology can be classified as having a nonregenerative anemia. This carries a less favorable prognosis than regenerative anemia. The most common cause of nonregenerative anemia in the cat is FeLV. A bone marrow aspirate should be part of the work-up of every cat with nonregenerative anemia. This is done primarily to rule out early leukemia, which can occur occasionally in the absence of peripheral blast cells. Examination of the marrow may also give clues as to asynchronous maturation of red cells, as seen in some myeloproliferative disorders. The most typical marrow finding is erythroid hypoplasia. A careful search for underlying infection or other disease should be made in any cat with nonregenerative anemia. If the underlying disorder can be resolved, the anemia may improve spontaneously. This phenomenon has been observed repeatedly in FeLV positive cats that develop an infection such as an upper respiratory virus or infected bite wound. Anemia may complicate the illness, but as the infection subsides the PCV may rise. Any anemic cat with known infection or with a fever of unknown origin should be treated initially with antibiotics but no corticosteroids.

Transfusion is the primary treatment for nonregenerative anemia and is given whenever the PCV drops below 10 per cent. This relieves clinical signs and allows time for further treatment or work-up as indicated. Prednisone (2.0 mg/kg PO) appears to be beneficial in some cats with nonregenerative anemia. It may help by prolonging the life span of cells or by blocking some as yet undefined immune-mediated injury, perhaps to early erythroid precursors.

Testosterone derivatives and anabolic steroids have been advocated in the treatment of nonregenerative anemia. The mechanism of action is thought to be through stimulation of erythropoietin production. The role of these drugs in treatment of feline anemia is still not certain, but their effect seems to be minimal. Hematinic drugs containing iron, folic acid, or B_{12} have no role in the treatment of anemic cats except in special circumstances of chronic blood loss. Folate and B_{12} deficiencies are almost impossible to produce in the cat, even with experimental diets.

MECHANICS OF BLOOD TRANSFUSION (SEE ALSO PRACTICAL BLOOD TRANSFUSIONS)

Veterinary hospitals giving few transfusions probably should keep a donor cat. This cat should not be allowed to mingle with hospital patients and should have periodic blood counts and *Haemobartonella* and FeLV checks. If blood is donated more than once monthly, an iron supplement can be given. Whenever blood is needed the cat is sedated and bled from the jugular vein into heparinized syringes. Approximately 75 cc can be taken from a large cat every two weeks. The circulating volume can be immediately restored by giving 100 cc of an intravenous fluid such as lactated Ringer's. In veterinary institutions giving frequent transfusions, blood can be banked for later use. In this case several donor cats are needed. If stray cats are available, they can be tested as described for the resident donor and then anesthetized and exsanguinated into 250-cc acid citrate dextrose (ACD) bottles. In this case, two cats could benefit from the blood of a single donor and a larger volume of blood could be given to each. Blood collected in this manner can be stored in the refrigerator for as long as three weeks without significant loss of viability. Platelets can be supplied in limited numbers only if blood is collected in plastic bags and transfused within six to eight hours without prior refrigeration. White blood cells cannot be supplied by routine transfusion, as their life span is too short.

Crossmatching is not required for transfusion of anemic cats. Blood types have been described in cats, but isoantibodies apparently do not occur. One published report (Auer et al., 1982) described "shock-like" reactions to incompatible feline blood transfusions in one patient and several experimental cats. This type of reaction has not been observed by the author, and acute hemolytic reactions are almost unheard of in cats, even those receiving multiple transfusions. One might argue against multiple transfusions from the same donor since a cat might develop antibodies against the donor's red cells. The use of multiple unrelated donors over a period of time appears safe in the cat, but not in the dog. *Under no circumstance should dog blood be given to cats.* Any immediate volume benefit is outweighed by delayed hemolysis.

Sedation of the cat receiving the transfusion should be avoided if possible. Most anemic cats will sit quietly if a butterfly needle or IV catheter is used. Transfusion reactions of any type are uncommon. Vomiting during transfusion occurs occasionally and usually can be controlled by temporarily stopping the drip and restarting at a slower rate. Acute left-sided congestive heart failure due to volume overload has occurred occasionally in chronically anemic cats that are not dehydrated. This is treated by temporarily stopping the infusion and giving IV furosemide. Contamination of the blood by bacteria can be avoided by aseptic technique. Spread of disease such as hemobartonellosis or FeLV can usually be avoided by selection of the donor. One must also be careful in collecting blood to avoid a large excess of anticoagulant. Although unlikely, it may be possible to cause hypocalcemia or coagulation difficulties.

Most anemic cats that recover do so within the first month of therapy. Those persistently anemic after that time have a poor prognosis. Many chronically anemic cats may be kept alive and comfortable for months with periodic transfusions if that is what the owner desires. The transfusion is repeated whenever the PCV drops below 10 per cent. This typically occurs approximately every three weeks in a cat with red cell aplasia without hemolysis. After a period of time most observant owners can predict the need for a transfusion, and frequent visits to the hospital to monitor the PCV can be avoided. If these cats are stressed by some concurrent disease the frequency of transfusion may need to be increased. Some spontaneous partial remissions may also occur, thus lengthening the time between transfusions. Eventually the interval between transfusions becomes shortened, probably because of an immune response to repeated transfusions. At this point euthanasia is the only remaining option.

Recovery rates for anemic cats differ with the type of anemia. The prognosis is relatively good for cats with regenerative anemia. Even cats with nonregenerative anemia have a chance of recovery. In one study of FeLV positive anemic cats, 8 out of 100 recovered to normal PCV, although only one converted to FeLV negative and 71 cats were destroyed within the first two weeks for various reasons. Cats with anemia secondary to infiltration of the marrow with leukemic cells will not improve without chemotherapy. Anticancer drugs are not indicated in FeLV positive cats with primary nonregenerative anemia.

REFERENCES

Auer, L., Bell, K., and Coates, S.: Blood transfusion reactions in the cat. J.A.V.M.A. 180:729, 1982.

Cotter, S. M.: Anemia associated with feline leukemia virus. J.A.V.M.A. 175:1191, 1979.

Cotter, S. M.: Disorders of the hematopoietic system. *In* Holzworth, J. (ed.): *Feline Medicine and Surgery.* Philadelphia: W.B. Saunders, in press.

Jain, N. C., and Zinkl, J. G. (eds.): Symposium on clinical hematology. Vet. Clin. North Am. 11:1, 1981.

Schalm, O. W.: Heinz body hemolytic anemia in the cat. Fel. Prac. 7:30, 1977.

Schalm, O. W., Jain, N. C., and Carroll, E. J.: *Veterinary Hematology,* 3rd ed. Philadelphia: Lea & Febiger, 1975.

MANAGEMENT OF THE ANEMIC DOG

BERNARD F. FELDMAN, D.V.M.

Davis, California

Anemia is a sign of disease, not a specific disease entity. However, anemia is a diagnostically rewarding sign because, with basic information, a cause may be ascertained and specific therapy initiated. In the clinical evaluation special attention is given to history, especially exposure to toxic agents and drugs. Signs related to other disorders that are commonly complicated by varying degrees of anemia, such as bleeding, malaise, fever, or weight loss, should be considered. In practice, the initial judgment is based on a combination of clinical data, kinetic analysis, and morphologic clues. Clues to the mechanism of anemia may be provided by physical examination, findings of infection, blood in the stool or urine, lymphadenopathy, splenomegaly, or petechiae. As examples, lymphadenopathy may suggest lymphoma, whereas petechiae suggest that more than one cell line—red cells and platelets—is involved in the pathologic process.

KINETIC ANALYSIS

A brief kinetic analysis is made to determine whether hypoproliferation (peracute or chronic blood loss, impaired production), maturation abnormality, or hemolysis is the major cause of anemia (Table 1). Red blood cell production can be quickly assessed by performing a reticulocyte count and correcting for the erythrocyte count and the degree of anemia (Table 2). For example, if a dog with a hematocrit of 15 per cent and a red blood cell count of 1.5 million/μl has a reticulocyte count of 6 per cent, the corrected number of reticulocytes is 36,000/μl, a low normal value. Because this patient is profoundly anemic, as shown by the hematocrit and red blood cell count, and shows no compensatory increase in erythropoiesis, a severe hypoproliferation or maturation abnormality exists. Only patients responding to hemorrhage or hemolysis will have a corrected reticulocyte number that exceeds the reference range. This calculation is not useful when myeloid metaplasia exists because of irregular shift of cells from the bone marrow to peripheral blood.

Table 1. *Clinical Classification for Evaluation of Anemia**

Hypoproliferation (reticulocyte numbers within reference range)
    Iron deficiency
        Acute and severe blood loss (first one to four days)
        Chronic blood loss
        Anemia of inflammatory disease (AID)
    Decreased erythropoietin
    Marrow damage
Maturation abnormality (reticulocyte numbers within reference range and macrocytosis or microcytosis)
    Vitamin B_{12} deficiency
    Folate deficiency
    Intrinsic marrow disease (e.g., erythemic myelosis)
    Severe iron deficiency
Blood loss/hemolysis (reticulocyte numbers greater than reference range)
    Monocyte macrophage phagocytosis
    Fragmentation hemolysis
    Intravascular hemolysis
    Response from acute blood loss
    Hemangioma (rare)

*Modified from Feldman: Vet. Clin. North Am. 11:277, 1981.

STUDY OF CELL MORPHOLOGY

Examination of the blood smear by a veterinarian who knows the patient clinically is a central part of the laboratory evaluation of anemia. When a blood smear is inspected as part of a routine examination, even highly proficient laboratory personnel may overlook abnormalities that are apparent to an examiner who is familiar with the clinical background. Red cells are examined for size, shape, and hemoglobin concentration, distribution, and staining properties. Although red cell indices provide useful information regarding morphology, they are measurements of mean red cell size and hemoglobin concentration. This information is inadequate when there is a mixed red cell population, as in the presence of prominent anisocytosis or poikilocytosis. Some inclusions can be demonstrated only by supravital staining. These include reticulocytes and Heinz bodies. Examination of a smear should always include a rough estimate of platelet numbers. On

Table 2. *How To Estimate RBC Production From a Reticulocyte Count**

1. Formula for calculation

$$\text{Corrected number of reticulocytes} = \frac{\text{reticulocyte count} \times \text{RBCs/μl}}{\text{maturation time of peripheral blood reticulocytes (days)}}$$

2. Reticulocyte maturation factor*

Hematocrit	Maturation Time (Days) of Reticulocytes in Peripheral Blood
45	1.0
35	1.5
25	2.0
15	2.5

3. Examples of calculations
   A. Normal dog

Reticulocyte count	1.5 ± 0.5%
RBC count	7,000,000
Hematocrit	45
Maturation time	1 day

   $$\text{Corrected number of reticulocytes (reference range)} = \frac{0.01 \pm 0.005 \times 7,000,000}{1}$$
   $$= 70,000/\mu l \ (35,000 \text{ to } 105,000/\mu l)$$

   B. Anemic dog

Reticulocyte count	6%
RBC count	1,500,000
Hematocrit	15
Maturation time	2.5 days

   $$\text{Corrected number of reticulocytes} = \frac{0.06 \times 1,500,000}{2.5}$$
   $$= 36,000/\mu l$$

*Extrapolated from studies in humans, this table is quite applicable to the dog.

the average, the ratio of platelets to red cells is between 1:10 and 1:20.

RED CELL INDICES

With electronic counting of red cells, standardized procedures for hemoglobin determination, and microhematocrit technique, red cell indices provide useful and reliable information for the morphologic classification of anemia when they are abnormal. The indices are generally consistent with the findings on examination of the blood smear. However, as was previously noted, they may be misleading in the presence of mixed red cell morphology since they represent mean values. Mean corpuscular volume (MCV) is a measure of red cell size, and mean corpuscular hemoglobin concentration (MCHC) is a measure of hemoglobin concentration. Since mean corpuscular hemoglobin (MCH) reflects both size and hemoglobin concentration, it is the least useful of the indices. A low MCV indicates microcytosis, and a high MCV indicates macrocytosis. A low MCHC indicates hypochromia, but a low MCH indicates hypochromia and/or microcytosis. A high MCH is always seen with a high MCV, reflecting the presence of macrocytosis. A high MCHC is seen only with prominent spherocytosis and reflects the

increased hemoglobin volume associated with decreased red cell membrane.

The following discussion will consider the basic management of the anemic dog. It assumes that the anemia has been categorized after a thorough history, physical examination, kinetic analysis, examination of the blood smear, and evaluation of the red blood cell indices.

ACUTE BLOOD LOSS

Usually acute blood loss is dramatic and there is no difficulty in identifying the site of bleeding. Occasionally, however, the origin of blood loss is hidden. Deep tissue bleeding into the thigh and pelvis in a patient with a fractured pelvis may account for severe blood loss. Similar cryptic blood loss may occur in retroperitoneal hemorrhage. The dominant feature in massive acute blood loss is a decrease in blood volume that results in shock and death if replacement is not undertaken. The mechanisms for restoring plasma volume operate slowly, and it has been shown that the hematocrit does not drop to its "true" plateau value for as long as 24 to 48 hours after the acute blood loss.

Volume replacement must be prompt. After plasma volume and electrolytes have been restored, the clinician can turn to red cell replacement. Although estimates of the amount of blood loss may be difficult to make, an approximation is necessary to avoid fluid underreplacement or overloading. A discussion of replacement therapy will be found in the article on transfusion (p. 408). Central venous pressure and clinical indices of adequacy of replacement are ambiguous.

CHRONIC BLOOD LOSS

Iron deficiency anemia is usually caused by chronic blood loss from the gastrointestinal tract or urinary tract or into the lungs. As iron deficiency progresses, conversion of erythrocyte protoporphyrin to heme stops, hemoglobin synthesis is impaired, and anemia develops. Only severe iron deficiency anemia will be revealed in microcytic, hypochromic red cell indices. The usual clinical presentation is normal red cell morphology and indices. Prussian blue staining of bone marrow spicules will reveal iron deficits. A marked decrease in serum iron concentration and an increase in transferrin (total iron binding capacity, TIBC) concentration are diagnostic.

The proper management of iron deficiency anemia requires correction of the underlying disorder. If this is achieved, iron replacement therapy may be initiated. Ten to twenty milligrams of oral ferrous sulfate is administered once a day for one week. An additional dose is given during the second week and a third dose during the third week. If gastrointestinal signs of vomiting or diarrhea develop, the dosage is reduced. The patient should respond with a marked hemoglobin rise and reticulocytosis. If there is no response several possibilities should be considered: the diagnosis is wrong; the patient is continuing to bleed; a concurrent inflammatory disorder is blocking red cell production; or there is lack of client compliance.

ANEMIA OF INFLAMMATORY DISEASE (AID)

Anemia associated with inflammation usually is a complication of infection, inflammation, and disseminated or necrotizing neoplasms. However, it is clinically innocuous except when it complicates reovery from chronic hemorrhage. The laboratory findings document decreases of serum iron *and* TIBC. However, iron is found in marrow spicules stained with Prussian blue. Supplying additional iron will simply result in increased sequestration of iron in the already overloaded iron storage compartments. Alleviating the underlying disorders is most fruitful in correcting this anemia. Therapy using hematinics is unnecessary in AID and should be avoided unless the anemia becomes symptomatic.

DECREASED ERYTHROPOIETIN ANEMIAS

The causes for anemia in *renal disease* include erythropoietin deficiency, decreased red cell life span, and red cell loss due to gastrointestinal hemorrhage. The anemia is normocytic, normochromic, and hypoproliferative owing to the inhibition of bone marrow erythroid precursors by toxic uremic metabolites.

Once the acute phase of the disease is controlled, androgens are reported to be beneficial. Oral androgens (e.g., oxymetholone) may be administered at a rate of 2.5 mg/kg daily. Weekly intramuscular injections of 100 mg of nandrolone decanoate (Deca-Durabolin) are also effective. It may take several months before the red cell mass changes. These drugs are effective only if some renal tissue is present. They may not be effective in severely azotemic, nondialyzed patients. If evidence of iron deficiency due to gastrointestinal hemorrhage is present, oral iron therapy may be instituted (see Chronic Blood Loss).

Lead poisoning results from the ingestion of lead pigment house paints and putty and from industrial exposure (smelting, storage battery). Anemia is mild to moderate and the red cells are normochromic, normocytic, or slightly hypochromic and microcytic. Basophilic stippling is often striking but not invariably present. Reticulocyte counts are low or slightly increased, and nucleated red cell counts are increased. Lead inhibits sulfhydryl-dependent enzymes, which leads to impaired heme and cyto-

chrome production. The diagnosis of chronic lead poisoning is established by finding increased blood and urinary lead concentrations and increased urinary excretion of delta-amino-levulinic acid and coproporphyrin. Treatment with 0.25 to 0.5 g/day of calcium sodium ethylene diaminetetraacetic acid (CaEDTA) intravenously leads to chelation and urinary excretion of lead with symptomatic improvement within several days.

Hypothyroidism is associated with mild anemia, but the mechanism and incidence appear variable. Included are decreased marrow stimulation and deficiencies of iron and vitamin B_{12}. The anemia is hypoproliferative, but peripheral blood findings are nonspecific. Diagnosis depends on specific hormone assay and response. Treatment of the anemia of hypothyroidism is hormone replacement. If iron deficiency is present or vitamin B_{12} deficiency is suspected, supplementation should be started to achieve complete recovery.

With *adrenal insufficiency* there is a reduction in red cell production. Anemia is rarely seen as the reduced cell mass is masked by a reduction in plasma volume. No therapy other than recognition of the deficient state and hormone replacement is required.

Iatrogenic estrogenic hormones or Sertoli cell tumor may cause a normocytic, normochromic, hypoproliferative anemia. Removal of the offending drug or tumor and concurrent administration of testosterone propionate often has a salutary effect.

MARROW DAMAGE

Anemia associated with foreign cells in the bone marrow (myelophthisis) results in a hypoproliferative anemia and may affect other cell lines, causing leukopenia and/or thrombocytopenia. Pancytopenia and a leukoerythroblastic blood picture (left shift in the neutrophil series and nucleated red cells noted in peripheral blood) develop in patients with advanced myelophthisis. Diagnosis requires a bone marrow *biopsy*. Treatment with hormones (see Renal Disease) and chemotherapy may cause hematologic improvement. High dose androgen therapy has occasionally produced improvement in anemia. Symptomatic improvement may be achieved with red cell and platelet transfusions, but a poor prognosis must be given to clients with animals refractory to chemotherapy and hormone therapy.

APLASTIC PANCYTOPENIA

The finding of aplastic marrow from a bone marrow *biopsy* establishes the diagnosis of aplastic pancytopenia. This disease may be caused by infection, neoplasia, or drugs. Treatment involves removing the identified offending agent and providing support in the form of transfusion therapy. In humans, serum inhibitors to the various poietins have necessitated immunosuppressive therapy.

PURE RED CELL APLASIA (PRCA)

PRCA is a condition in which patients cease producing red blood cells but continue to have normal or near normal white blood cell and platelet production. Despite severe anemia, reticulocytes are virtually absent from blood, and red cell precursors are virtually absent from the marrow. Acquired PRCA may be idiopathic or may be caused by immune marrow inhibition, thymoma, infections, drugs or chemicals, systemic lupus, severe renal failure or lymphoid malignancy, or it may be a preleukemic event. Diagnosis requires a bone marrow *biopsy*. Patients with PRCA generally respond to corticosteroids. Treatment should begin with daily doses of prednisone (2 mg/kg), which is slowly decreased to the minimum dose sufficient to maintain a normal hematocrit. Infections must be diagnosed and treated. Blood cultures may be necessary. Tumors should be resected when possible. Androgens have been successful in very few cases of PRCA. Oxymetholone, 50 mg orally three times daily, or nandrolone decanoate (Deca-Durabolin), 100-mg weekly intramuscular injections, may be used. If the disease does not respond to glucocorticoids, cytotoxic drugs such as cyclophosphamide may be added.

VITAMIN B_{12} AND FOLATE DEFICIENCY

Anemia with reticulocytopenia may be seen in spite of intense erythroid hyperplasia in the marrow. This paradoxic situation occurs when there is ineffective erythropoiesis with intramedullary hemolysis. The underlying defect may cause generalized impairment of the erythroid line or it may be characteristic of specific subpopulations of developing erythroid precursors. Some of these subpopulations escape death in the marrow, but the remaining mature erythrocytes are so severely damaged that they are rapidly removed from the circulation, giving the picture of peripheral hemolysis. Megaloblastic anemia is a disease that produces significantly ineffective erythropoiesis. This anemia is characterized by macrocytosis and hypersegmented neutrophils. The underlying defect involves a lack of DNA synthesis while RNA production and protein synthesis continue, thus producing larger cells, or megaloblasts. This clinical picture is produced by vitamin B_{12} or folic acid deficiencies and by drugs that interfere with the synthesis of DNA or the absorption of vitamin B_{12}. The specific diagnosis depends on morphologic clues on blood smears, finding a disease that involves the stomach and duodenum, and decreased serum B_{12} concentrations. Other more specific diagnostic laboratory tests are not practical. Specific replacement therapy consists of 500 to 1000 μg of parenteral vitamin B_{12} weekly followed by a monthly parenteral dosage of 1000 μg for as long as necessary. In cases of megaloblastic anemia resulting from pancreatic insufficiency, vitamin B_{12} may be given as previously described. Administration of pancreatic enzymes in pancreatic insufficiency will alleviate megaloblastosis of vitamin B_{12} or folate deficiency. Replacing folic acid with 1 mg orally per day is effective. Megaloblastosis and severe marrow depression secondary to drugs that block dihydrofolate reductase (such as methotrexate) may be treated with 5-formyltetrahydrofolate (folinic acid). A single milligram-for-milligram dose (folinic acid for methotrexate) intramuscularly will be effective.

HEMOLYTIC ANEMIA

In general, the extent of the anemia is determined by the rate of red blood cell destruction and by the marrow's capacity for erythroid production. Erythrocytic survival time may be reduced to one-sixth of normal without accompanying anemia but with substantial reticulocytosis. Conversely, severe hemolysis may exist without reticulocytosis, as is seen when marrow compensation is impaired.

Most forms of hemolysis are extravascular. The damaged cell signals its changed status to the monocyte macrophage system via its membrane. Intravascular hemolysis is due to complement-mediated lysis or fragmentation or to circumstances in which the monocyte-macrophage system cannot cope with the burden of damaged cells. Intravascular hemolysis leads to hemoglobinemia. Intravascular hemolysis is important because it provides dramatic evidence of erythrocyte destruction and because erythrocyte membrane particles released into the plasma may act as potent stimuli for disseminated intravascular coagulation.

Since a decrease in the production of red blood cells leads to a gradual fall in hemoglobin concentration, a rapid fall in hemoglobin concentration is the result of either bleeding or hemolysis. It takes time for the marrow to establish a heightened level of erythropoiesis in response to anemia, so reticulocytosis may be modest in the first days after an acute hemolytic event. After several days, calculation of the corrected number of reticulocytes will usually show increased reticulocyte numbers. Note, however, that in some patients in which inflammatory suppression of erythropoiesis coincides with a hemolytic process (such as microangiopathic hemolytic disease associated with inflammatory disorders or cancer), the corrected reticulocyte count may be within the reference range.

Once hemolytic anemia is deduced by the absence of blood loss and the presence of elevated reticulocyte numbers, the blood smear should be studied for clues to the mechanism of the hemolytic process. The mechanism may be evident from the predominant abnormal red cell shape. Spherocytes may indicate immune hemolytic anemia, and schistocytes may indicate disseminated intravascular coagulation. For more information on the management of these two processes see Management of DIC and Thrombosis, and Therapy of Immune-Mediated Diseases.

SUPPLEMENTAL READING

Feldman, B. F.: Hypoproliferative anemias and anemias caused by ineffective erythropoiesis. Vet. Clin. North Am. 11:227, 1981.

Jain, N. C., and Zinkl, J. G. (eds.): Clinical hematology. Vet. Clin. North Am. 11:2, 1981.

Mohler, E. R.: Evaluation of anemia in adults. In Hartmann, P. M. (ed.): Guide to Hematologic Disorders. New York: Grune and Stratton, 1980, pp. 29–44.

Schrier, S. L.: Anemia: hemolysis. In Rubenstein, E., and Federman, D. D. (eds.): Scientific American Medicine, Vol. IV. New York: Scientific American Illustrated Library, 1981, pp. 1–31.

DIPHACINONE COAGULOPATHY (TOXICITY) IN DOGS

BERNARD F. FELDMAN, D.V.M.,
and MICHAEL E. MOUNT, D.V.M.

Davis, California

Coumarin and indandione anticoagulant drugs are widely used for control of small mammal pests. Included are 3-alpha-phenyl-beta-acetylethyl-4-hydroxycoumarin (warfarin), 2-pivalyl-1,3-indandione (pindone), and 2-diphenylacetyl-1,3,indandione (diphacinone; diphenadione). Diphacinone is a potent hypoprothrombinemic, anticoagulant agent that has been utilized as a rodenticide since the 1950s. This rodenticide has become more widely used in recent years, with increasing morbidity and mortality in nontarget mammals. Canine patients known to have ingested diphacinone have responded to fresh frozen plasma, vitamin K_1 (phytonadione), and oral vitamin K_1 only to relapse, often fatally, one to three weeks after cessation of therapy.

MECHANISM OF ACTION

It has been proposed that coumarin and indandione anticoagulants inhibit clotting protein synthesis by preventing the regeneration of vitamin K_1 from its 2,3 epoxide metabolite. Experimentally, diphacinone caused a delayed inhibition of prothrombin synthesis, which correlated with a delayed inhibition of the epoxide-K_1 conversion in vitro. Diphacinone is readily absorbed from the gastrointestinal tract but is not significantly absorbed through intact skin or the respiratory tract. It is a potent and long-acting depressant of prothrombin complex activity. The peak effect of diphacinone occurs within 48 to 72 hours. Prothrombin depression may persist for 20 days.

TOXICOLOGY

The LD_{50} for dogs ingesting diphacinone is 8 mg/kg (cats 15 mg/kg). Ramik Green,* the commercially available form of diphacinone used by professional exterminators, is weather resistant. It is formulated as apple- (green), meat- or fish- (red), or peanut- (brown) flavored pellets and bars. Diphacinone is particularly concentrated in the liver of animals and appears to be more potent than warfarin in single- or multiple-dose exposures. Dogs poisoned with diphacinone die of tissue hypoxia resulting from massive internal bleeding due to increased capillary permeability and decreased plasma coagulability. An added problem with diphacinone is the long hepatic half-life, which may exceed 20 days. Depression of vitamin K–dependent coagulation proteins may persist for at least 20 days.

CLINICAL DIAGNOSIS

Dogs known to have ingested diphacinone are presented in an anorexic, weak, depressed, and febrile state. Nonlocalized abdominal pain is also a common finding. Not all dogs will have hemorrhagic manifestations. Those that do have oral cavity hemorrhage and evidence of gastrointestinal hemorrhage. Gross necropsy findings include hemorrhage in the pleural cavity, pericardium, and retroperitoneum.

---

*Velsicol Chemical Corp., Chicago, IL.

LABORATORY DIAGNOSIS

Vitamin K is necessary for the hepatic synthesis of coagulation proteins II, VII, IX, and X. Vitamin K completes the final step in biosynthesis of these coagulation proteins by converting glutamic acid residues on precursor molecules into γ-carboxyglutamic acid residues, thus producing functionally normal procoagulant factors. In the absence of vitamin K or in the presence of vitamin K antagonism, as occurs with diphacinone toxicosis, these precursor proteins are functionally inactive, and prolongation of prothrombin time (PT) and activated partial thromboplastin time (APTT) results. Since factor VII has the shortest half-life (four to six hours), the PT (affected by factors VII, X, V, II, and I; extrinsic and common coagulation pathways) will be prolonged before the APTT (affected by factors XII, XI, IX, VIII, X, V, II, and I; intrinsic and common coagulation pathways). To diagnose diphacinone toxicosis, the PT and APTT are the tests of choice. Prolongation of these screening tests is considered significant when the patient's test time is 25 per cent greater than the high value of the reference range. Platelet counts are variable. It is noteworthy that the activated coagulation time (ACT), which tests for the same coagulation patterns as APTT, will be normal until significant factor reduction has occurred. This is because the ACT is relatively insensitive to decreasing coagulation protein concentrations, prolonging only after the APTT is prolonged.

CLINICAL COURSE OF SEVEN CASES

Dogs known to have ingested diphacinone had significant increases in the PT within 24 hours. The PT tripled entry values within 72 hours. Significant increases in the APTT occurred within 48 hours. The APTT tripled entry values within 96 hours. Factor II concentrations were found to be less than 10 per cent of normal within 24 hours of diphacinone ingestion; factor X concentrations were found to be less than 10 per cent of normal within 48 to 72 hours; factors II and IX were reduced to less than 30 per cent of normal after 72 hours, by which time hemorrhage was evident. Dogs were treated with subcutaneous injections of vitamin K_1 at a dose rate of 5.0 mg/kg twice daily. Fresh plasma was administered equivalent to 10 per cent of total blood volume (total blood volume for the dog is calculated based on 90 ml/kg body weight). Oral vitamin K_1 was administered at 5 mg/kg in three divided doses daily for five days. Screening PT and APTT returned to baseline times within 24 hours. After the five-day course of therapy all treatment was discontinued. All patients appeared alert, active, playful, and nonfebrile. However, within 48 to 72 hours after cessation of therapy the PT had tripled baseline times and the APTT had doubled baseline times with evidence of hemorrhage (dropping hematocrit and plasma proteins). This pattern was repeated for a period of three weeks, at which time the dogs maintained their PT and APTT within the reference range.

Several dogs exhibited neurologic signs during periods of hemorrhagic diatheses. Transient sensory and proprioceptive deficits were noted in the hind legs. The etiopathogenesis of these findings is unknown at this time.

MANAGEMENT

Vitamin K_1 should be administered (5.0 mg/kg) subcutaneously twice daily for 24 to 48 hours. In an emergency, *fresh* plasma equivalent to 10 per cent of the total blood volume (see Clinical Course) may be administered intravenously. There is no reason to give vitamin K_1 intravenously. It may produce anaphylaxis and is not effective for two to three hours. Oral administration of vitamin K_1 (5.0 mg/kg twice daily) should be continued for a minimum of 16 to 21 days. Coagulation screening tests (PT, APTT) should be performed at weekly intervals for at least three weeks. Client education is critical for patients returned to the home environment. Patients that appear febrile or reluctant to move or those that are vomiting or have diarrhea should be returned to the hospital immediately. Because of the rapidity with which diphacinone toxicosis can cause hemorrhage and death, clients must be able to monitor their dogs continually during the posttoxicosis period (one to three weeks).

SUPPLEMENTAL READING

Buck, W. B., et al.: *Clinical and Diagnostic Veterinary Toxicology*, 2nd ed. Dubuque, IA: Kendall-Hunt, 1976.

Feldman, B. F.; Coagulopathies in small animals. J.A.V.M.A. 179:559, 1981.

Feldman, B. F., Mount, M. E., et al.: Diphacinone (2-diphenylacetyl-1,3 indandione; diphenadione) coagulopathy in California dogs. Calif. Vet. 35:15, 1981.

Registry of Toxic Effects of Chemical Substances. National Institute for Occupational Safety and Health 2:485, 1977.

Suttie, J. W.: The metabolic role of vitamin K. Fed. Proc. 39:2730, 1980.

MANAGEMENT OF DIC AND THROMBOSIS

CRAIG E. GREENE, D.V.M.

Athens, Georgia

Intravascular coagulation, with or without gross or microscopic thrombus formation, is a pathophysiologic event that complicates many disease processes. Considerable controversy exists regarding the diagnosis and treatment of hypercoagulable states. The confusion exists because of oversimplification of the complex interplay between coagulation pathways and opposing anticoagulatory mechanisms. Activated clotting factors are utilized during coagulation or are activated and subsequently removed by the mononuclear-phagocyte system. Fibrinolysis, which dissolves formed fibrin, is accelerated in a magnitude proportional to the degree of hypercoagulability. The initial fibrinolytic response is beneficial for resolving thrombi and antagonizing hypercoagulability; however, in excess it can contribute to the development of a hemorrhagic diathesis. Products of enhanced fibrinolysis interfere with platelet function, thrombin action, and fibrin polymerization. Described interactions of the coagulation, fibrinolytic, complement, and kallikrein-kinin systems through the central mediator of the Hageman factor (factor XII) are presently being elucidated, which complicates our understanding of the coagulation mechanism.

Disease processes known to initiate coagulation do so through activation of intrinsic or extrinsic pathways or by direct conversion of prothrombin by proteolytic pathways. Hypercoagulability can also result from conditions of stagnant flow or increased viscosity of blood. Decreased clearance of activated coagulation factors and decreased coagulation inhibitor activity are less commonly recognized but important contributors to the thrombotic process.

The spectrum of clinical signs and laboratory abnormalities associated with intravascular coagulation is a result of the intensity and localization of the coagulatory process. Intravascular coagulation may present as an acute, subacute, or chronic process, localized or diffuse. *Disseminated* or *excessive intravascular coagulation* (DIC) is a term reserved for intravascular coagulation that occurs beyond physiologic needs and to the detriment of the affected animal. A presumptive diagnosis of DIC should be entertained when a sudden onset of shock, hemorrhage, hemolysis, or organ failure occurs alone or in combination in a previously diseased animal.

Localized thrombosis (regional intravascular coagulation) is less commonly recognized in the dog and cat as compared with human patients. Specific diseases associated with localized thrombosis in dogs and cats include bacterial endocarditis, feline cardiomyopathy, canine heartworm disease, and canine renal amyloidosis. The diagnosis and management of disseminated and localized intravascular coagulation syndromes will be discussed separately.

DIC

There are no specific values for coagulation tests that alone are diagnostic of DIC. Although coagulation factors and platelets are consumed in the coagulation process, their measured concentration in the blood only decreases when coagulation is extensive. DIC can be divided into three arbitrary stages based upon the severity and extent of laboratory abnormalities. Such a separation allows a more rational therapeutic approach to a disease with a variable spectrum of clinical signs.

A platelet count and activated coagulation time (ACT) test can be used as rough guidelines to separate DIC into (1) chronic or low-grade, (2) acute, and (3) end-stage (Table 1). These two tests have the advantages of being simple to perform and being readily available to most veterinary practitioners. They may be used as a screening procedure in evaluating the stage of intravascular coagulation. Additional diagnostic tests such as the activated partial thromboplastin time (APTT), prothrombin time (PT), thrombin time (TT), fibrin degradation products (FDPs), antithrombin III, plasminogen, and factor analysis may be used when available or for subsequent confirmation of the coagulation disorder.

Platelet counting is performed indirectly by estimating platelet numbers relative to leukocytes on stained smears or by direct counting with a hemocytometer using commercially available diluting-lysing solutions.* Appropriate clinical pathology

---

*Unopette Microcollection System No. 5855, Becton Dickinson Co., Rutherford, NJ.

Table 1. *Laboratory Findings in Stages of DIC*

Stage of DIC	Platelet Cells/mm³ × 10³	Activated Coagulation Time (sec)*	Other Coagulation Test Findings	Clinical Signs
Normal values	150 to 500†	<120 (dog) <75 (cat)	FDP <30 μg/ml (dog) <8 μg/ml (cat)	
Early, low-grade, or chronic	Decreased ≤100	Normal <120 (dog) <75 (cat)	FDP, PT, PTT, TT: normal Plasminogen, antithrombin III: normal to decreased Coagulation factors‡: normal to increased	Petechial hemorrhages, hemolysis
Acute	Decreased <100	Slightly to moderate prolongation 120 to 200 (dog) 75 to 120 (cat)	FDP: moderate increase PT, PTT, TT: moderate prolongation Plasminogen, antithrombin III, coagulation factors: marked decrease	Variable, organ dysfunction, hemorrhagic diathesis, hematomas, petechiae, hemolysis
End-stage	Decreased <75	Marked prolongation >200 (dog) >120 (cat)	FDP: marked increase PT, PTT, TT: marked prolongation Plasminogen, antithrombin III, coagulation factors: marked decrease	Severe hemorrhagic diathesis, petechiae, hematomas, body cavity effusions, frank hemorrhage

*ACT values are a rough guideline and should not be taken as absolutes.
†Values apply to dogs and cats unless specified.
‡Factors XIII, XII, XI, VIII, V, II, and I.

texts should be consulted for proper techniques. A rough screening of platelet number can be made by looking at a stained blood smear with a microscope for three to five platelets per high power (400×) field. Platelet morphology should also be evaluated at this time, since large forms appear in the blood during consumptive coagulatory states. Blood smears can also be evaluated for erythrocyte morphology, since fragmented or distorted erythrocytes (schistocytes) are suggestive of ongoing intravascular coagulation.

ACT is a relatively reproducible measure of the intrinsic and common coagulation pathways. The ACT is more rapid and less variable than standard whole blood coagulation time tests. The presence of a surface activator in the tube produces more consistent coagulation times. ACT is relatively easy to perform and offers an immediate assessment of coagulation status. It is more readily available to veterinarians on an emergency basis than other laboratory tests of intrinsic coagulation such as the APTT. The evacuated tubes, which are commercially available,* should be kept at 37° C just prior to and during the test procedure. Blood is taken by clean venipuncture with rapid aspiration from a large vein. Blood may be collected directly in the tube or quickly transferred from a syringe. Whatever method is used, it should be consistent every

time. The time interval from injection of 2 ml of blood into the ACT tube until the first visible appearance of clot formation is determined to be the ACT. Differences between various manufactured tubes and existing conditions require each hospital to establish its own normal range. Using the previously mentioned materials and methods, the author has determined a normal ACT to be <120 sec in dogs and <75 sec in cats.

The ACT progressively prolongs and the platelet count decreases as DIC goes from a low-grade or chronic to an acute and finally end-stage process (Table 1). The ACT is generally not as sensitive as the platelet count in detecting intravascular coagulation. It is rarely prolonged with chronic or low-grade (mild) intravascular coagulation. The platelet count, in contrast, is decreased because of the inability of the bone marrow to replace platelets as fast as they are consumed. The ACT is prolonged moderately to markedly in acute and end-stage DIC, respectively, and clinically overt bleeding tendencies are usually noted. Marked prolongation of the ACT under the latter circumstance may be caused by coagulation factor consumption or anticoagulant activity from increased FDP concentration. The contribution of either of these two processes to the incoagulability can be assessed by simultaneously mixing 1-ml volumes of freshly drawn blood from a normal dog and the diseased animal in an ACT tube. A normal or mildly prolonged ACT value is found with coagulation factor

*Activated coagulation time tubes No. 6522, Becton Dickinson Co., Rutherford, NJ.

depletion, but moderate prolongation persists with circulating anticoagulants such as FDPs.

The ACT and platelet count can also be used to distinguish between DIC (chronic, acute, or end-stage), vitamin K deficiency, and primary thrombocytopenia. These three syndromes probably account for 90 per cent of the acquired bleeding disorders seen in small animal practice. Primary thrombocytopenia is characterized by a low platelet count (<100,000) and normal ACT, whereas vitamin K deficiency is characterized by a normal platelet count with a prolonged ACT. The major confusion comes in distinguishing between low-grade or chronic DIC and primary thrombocytopenia. Both are characterized by a reduced platelet count and a normal or slightly prolonged ACT. Here clinical observation is helpful, since hemorrhage is the main clinical abnormality noted with most primary thrombocytopenias. In contrast, DIC is usually associated with clinical abnormalities of an underlying disease process. The slight prolongation of the ACT (never >10 to 20 sec), which may occur in marked primary thrombocytopenia (<20,000 cells/mm³), results from a deficiency in platelet phospholipid required in the coagulation reaction.

Specific or more complex laboratory tests can be used to confirm the diagnosis of DIC. These are not always readily available to many practicing veterinarians. Fibrinolytic activity may be measured simply, but relatively inaccurately, by observation of whole blood clot lysis in the ACT tube maintained at 37°C. Clot lysis is frequently difficult to determine with severe hypofibrinogenemia and thrombocytopenia because of insufficient or absent clot formation and retraction. Decreased plasminogen in extensive or severe intravascular coagulation may be responsible for erroneously prolonged *in vitro* clot lysis times despite the presence of activated fibrinolysis *in vivo*.

Estimation of serum FDPs has been established as a clinical and sensitive indication of fibrinolysis. FDPs are not in themselves specific for DIC. They can be falsely elevated by improper sampling techniques, physiologic stresses, and surgical manipulations. They may be increased in conditions other than DIC and thus should be evaluated only in the presence of other coagulation tests. A commercial latex agglutination test* developed for use with human serum has been adapted for use in the dog and cat. Increased FDP concentrations should only be expected in acute or end-stage DIC when FDP production exceeds mononuclear-phagocyte clearance mechanisms. Increased concentrations are greater than 20 to 30 μg/ml in dog serum and 8 to 10 μg/ml in cat serum.

Specific coagulation tests, including the PT,

APTT, and TT, may be performed in an attempt to confirm a diagnosis of DIC. Progressive prolongation in these times is expected with more severe and extensive DIC. Decreases in coagulation factors, antithrombin II, plasminogen, and complement component 3 have been used to establish the presence of ongoing DIC, but their use has been confined to research laboratories. Coagulation factors I, II, V, VIII, X, XI, XII, and XIII may be decreased from consumption in the clotting process or from their removal following activation.

THERAPY

The initial plan for management of DIC involves removal of procoagulant stimuli and correction of the primary disease process. The underlying disease should be managed vigorously, including correction of hypotension and volume deficits with fluid therapy, hypoxemia with ventilatory assistance and oxygen, sepsis with appropriate antimicrobial drugs, and acidosis with alkalinizing agents. Supportive care is also essential for organ systems that are compromised by the coagulation process. Adequate diuresis is essential to prevent renal shutdown.

The most controversial aspect concerning DIC centers around the recommendation for restoring the hemostatic balance. A rational therapeutic approach depends on the stage at which DIC is identified. This variability in appropriate therapy explains the present controversy. Each case should be evaluated independently prior to anticoagulant therapy with a platelet count and ACT. Prophylactic or mild anticoagulation is recommended in early or low-grade DIC in which the procoagulatory stimulus is weak. This consists of the administration of thrombocytopathic drugs (aspirin) or low dose subcutaneous heparin therapy (Table 2).

Table 2. *Summary of Therapeutic Regimens for DIC*

Stage of DIC	Therapy

Early, low-grade (mild), or chronic	Platelet inhibitor
	  Aspirin
	    Dog: 5 to 8 mg/kg b.i.d.
	    Cat: 25 mg/kg twice weekly
	  Low dose heparin
	    Dog: 150 to 250 U/kg SQ t.i.d.
	    Cat: 50 to 100 U/kg SQ t.i.d.

Acute	Intermediate dose heparin
	  Dog: 500 U/kg SQ t.i.d.
	  Cat: 250 to 375 U/kg SQ t.i.d.

End-stage	Low dose heparin
	  Dog: 150 to 250 U/kg SQ t.i.d.
	  Cat: 100 U/kg SQ t.i.d.
	Plus immediate factor replacement
	  (10 ml/lb/24 hours of blood or
	  plasma maximum if
	  normovolemic)

---

*Thrombo-Wellcotest, Burroughs Wellcome Labs, Research Triangle Park, NC.

More potent anticoagulant therapy should be considered in acute DIC when the predisposing disease cannot be readily eliminated or effectively treated. Heparin is considered the anticoagulant of choice under such circumstances because of its rapid onset of action and inhibitory effect on activated clotting factors. The subcutaneous route for heparinization is recommended because it offers the most consistent and predictable response. Intermittent or continuous intravenous heparin therapy causes either extreme fluctuations or too high a heparin concentration.

Anticoagulation is not the only therapeutic measure in end-stage intravascular coagulation. Heparin causes further bleeding when used alone in the presence of high circulating FDP concentrations, decreased coagulation factor activity, severe thrombocytopenia, and marked prolongation of coagulation time tests. Heparinization will only be beneficial under such circumstances if it is accompanied by immediate replacement therapy with fresh blood or plasma transfusions. The danger of accelerating the clotting process is outweighed by the immediately prior (15 min) and continued administration of low or prophylactic dosages of subcutaneous heparin.

Several important points should be discussed concerning heparin therapy in dogs and cats. Subcutaneous administration appears superior to intravenous therapy because it is associated with more gradual elevations and reduced fluctuations in coagulation times than intravenous therapy. Heparin dosages should not be taken as absolute guidelines, since heparin may vary slightly depending on its lot and source (beef lung or hog intestine). Heparin is also less effective in the presence of acidosis and with severe or prolonged thrombotic episodes. Decreased antithrombin III (heparin cofactor), which occurs with the latter circumstance, alters the sensitivity of coagulation mechanism to a given heparin dosage. The effectiveness of heparin can be modified by concurrent disease and may also vary with respect to numerous factors including its absorption and elimination. Studies on the coagulation times following heparin dosages have only been performed in healthy animals, making absolute guidelines in diseased animals impossible. Appropriate monitoring of heparin therapy by coagulation times is essential because of these variations.

The effects of heparin on blood coagulation are most accurately followed by intrinsic coagulation tests including ACT and APTT. These values reflect the overall influence of the anticoagulant on the coagulation pathway but unfortunately require normal baseline preheparin data for accurate interpretation. Ideally, heparin should be administered during acute DIC so that the APTT is prolonged one and one-half– to twofold normal. Prolongation of ACT parallels that of APTT so that it may be used

as an appropriate indicator. Unfortunately, the correlation is logarithmic and the ACT is prolonged in progressively smaller increments compared with the APTT as the absolute value of the APTT increases.* Furthermore, the ACT usually has a finite endpoint even in the presence of high heparin concentration (>1 U/ml of plasma) when the APTT cannot even be measured. The ACT also remains slightly prolonged for longer periods than the APTT once heparin therapy has been discontinued.

There is also ambiguity in monitoring anticoagulant therapy by strict use of clotting function tests. Prolongation of the ACT or APTT may indicate further coagulation factor depletion or increased FDPs rather than effective anticoagulation. The heparin dose should be reduced under any circumstance that prolongs the ACT greater than twice its normal maximum. An increase in coagulation factors or platelets in the circulation following the deceleration of coagulation is the most reliable indicator of adequate therapy in the control of consumptive coagulopathies. Fibrinogen and other coagulation factors will be rapidly synthesized in the absence of severe hepatic disease. Unfortunately, the measurement of coagulation factors other than fibrinogen is not only difficult but is interfered with by heparin. New platelets are synthesized more slowly (five to ten days) as compared with coagulation factors (five to ten hours), so that an immediate increase in the platelet count is not a requirement for successful therapy. Furthermore, heparin at higher dosages is known to lyse platelets, a phenomenon that may temporarily slow down the expected increase in platelet numbers. A rise in the platelet count may be more dramatic in chronic or mild DIC following therapy because of accelerated megakaryocyte synthesis in the bone marrow. An increase in platelets usually occurs within 24 to 48 hours after consumption ceases.

If the platelet count and fibrinogen concentration are increasing but the ACT, PT, and PTT remain prolonged, then excessive heparinization is present. There may be a delay of two to four days before the bleeding stops and laboratory values become normal. If the bleeding stops or thrombotic complications decrease, then dramatic clinical improvement can be expected. Mere correction of abnormal coagulation tests has not always resulted in survival of the patient. Animals with fewer abnormalities in their clotting function at the time of initial diagnosis and treatment usually respond more favorably.

Heparin therapy should always be maintained when active or predisposing causes of DIC are still present and tapered gradually in cases of low-grade DIC or resolved DIC to avoid rebound hyperco-

---

*A prolongation of the APTT of 1.5 to 2.0 normal baseline for the dog and cat corresponds to an ACT prolongation of 15 to 20 and 10 to 15 sec, respectively.

agulability from too rapid withdrawal of the drug. Administration of thrombocytopathic drugs such as aspirin is frequently indicated, as heparin therapy is reduced or discontinued in cases of DIC when ongoing disease processes have not been resolved. Aspirin therapy should only be used in combination with a reducing dosage of heparin after the platelet count and ACT have returned to normal.

Additional means of anticoagulant therapy have not been well-documented as being efficacious in the treatment of DIC. The use of adjunctive measures to control thrombosis will be discussed under the management of localized thrombotic syndromes.

LOCALIZED THROMBOSIS

Dogs and cats with valvular endocarditis are predisposed to organ embolization through the formation of septic and/or fibrin thrombi. Systemic arterial embolization is more common with left heart valve involvement. Pulmonary and systemic arterial embolization have also been reported with *Dirofilaria* infections in dogs. Pulmonary thrombi are most common in severely infested dogs or following arsenical treatment. Systemic arterial thrombosis is a rarer event when the worms migrate ectopically into the left side of the heart. Arterial thromboembolism is a commonly observed complication of feline cardiomyopathy. Thrombi in this disease probably originate from the left atrium and lodge most commonly in the caudal aortic bifurcation. Occlusion of other vessels has been reported. Pulmonary and systemic arterial thromboembolism also appears to be a significant pathophysiologic complication of renal amyloidosis in dogs or, less commonly, with other protein-losing nephropathies. The exact mechanism for increased embolic tendency in the nephrotic syndrome is uncertain. A multiplicity of factors probably accounts for the hypercoagulable state.

The clinical signs of localized thromboembolic phenomena in dogs or cats reflect the severity and distribution of the ischemia produced. Cardinal symptoms of pulmonary embolism include dyspnea, cyanosis, tachycardia, hypotension, cyanosis, and fever. Peripheral arterial occlusion will result in pain, coolness, lower motor neuron paralysis, and swelling or loss of palpable pulses in the affected extremity. Thrombosis of the vascular supply to a particular organ will result in the sudden onset of dysfunction and clinical signs related to that organ system.

Diagnosis of localized embolic phenomena is primarily based on historical and physical findings. Specific laboratory tests are not available to detect the presence of vascular insufficiency in a particular organ system. Contrast angiography may be helpful in delineating large vessel occlusion. Standard coagulation tests performed by sampling jugular venous blood are usually unrewarding in detecting a localized thrombotic process because the correction of limited clotting abnormalities is within the compensatory limits of the body. Selective sampling of venous effluent from an infarcted region will be more revealing.

Anticoagulant therapy for localized thrombotic processes is administered similar to that for mild or chronic DIC. Low dose subcutaneous heparin or aspirin therapy may be instituted. There is some evidence in human medicine to suggest that thrombocytopathic drugs such as aspirin are more effective in treating or preventing systemic arterial occlusion by thrombi, whereas heparin is more effective on venous thromboembolism. Either drug may be used with pulmonary embolism. Propranolol, which is recommended in the treatment of hypertrophic cardiomyopathy, has established antiplatelet effects.

Additional medical therapy proposed for treating localized thromboembolic phenomena comes from experimental studies in animals. The use of alpha-adrenergic agents has been proposed for minimizing vasoactive changes that occur following thrombus formation. Antiserotonin drugs such as cyproheptadine, hydroxyzine, and diazepam have been suggested because vasoactive amines are released from platelets and mast cells during coagulation as a result of kinin and complement activation. Streptokinase and urokinase are fibrinolytic agents used in human medicine to accelerate the breakdown of formed blood clots. Urokinase is more effective and less antigenic than streptokinase, but its high cost makes it impractical in veterinary medicine. Instead of modifying fibrinolysis directly, most attempts are made to block further coagulation with anticoagulants and allow endogenous fibrinolysis to dissolve already formed clots. Low molecular weight dextran has been recommended as a substitute for urokinase therapy. Dextrans are somewhat inferior unless they are combined with fibrinolytic drugs. Unfortunately, they are also very expensive.

SUPPLEMENTAL READING

Feldman, B. F.: Disseminated intravascular coagulation. Comp. Cont. Ed. 3:46, 1981.

Green, R. A.: Activated coagulation time in monitoring heparinized dogs. Am. J. Vet. Res. 41:1793, 1980.

Greene, C. E.: Disseminated intravascular coagulation in the dog: A review. J. Am. Anim. Hosp. Assoc. 11:674, 1975.

Greene, C. E., and Meriwether, E.: The activated partial thromboplastin time and activated coagulation time in monitoring heparinized cats. Am. J. Vet. Res. 43:1473, 1982.

Kociba, G. J.: Disseminated intravascular coagulation. *In* Kirk, R. W. (ed.): *Current Veterinary Therapy VI.* Philadelphia: W. B. Saunders Co., 1977, pp. 448–451.

DIAGNOSIS AND TREATMENT
OF POLYCYTHEMIA

MARK E. PETERSON, D.V.M.,
New York, New York
and JOHN F. RANDOLPH, D.V.M.
Ithaca, New York

Polycythemia is characterized clinically by an increase in red blood cell (RBC) count, hemoglobin concentration, and packed cell volume (PCV). Based on the pathogenesis, polycythemia can be classified into three groups including relative polycythemia, secondary polycythemia, and primary polycythemia (polycythemia vera) (Table 1).

Relative polycythemia is characterized by an elevated venous PCV in the presence of normal total RBC mass. Relative polycythemia usually occurs secondary to a disturbance in fluid balance leading to diminished plasma volume, as with severe dehydration or extensive burns; therefore, elevated RBC count or PCV does not necessarily signify true increase in the RBC mass. Direct measurement of total RBC mass must be performed to differentiate absolute from relative polycythemia, especially with only modest increases in PCV (55 to 65 per cent).

The absolute polycythemias, characterized by both increased PCV and total RBC mass, include primary (polycythemia vera) and secondary polycythemia. Absolute secondary polycythemia results from excessive production of erythropoietin, a hormone that stimulates RBC production. If erythropoietin is secreted in response to systemic hypoxia, as in cardiac disease, pulmonary disease, or hemoglobinopathy, the polycythemia represents an appropriate, compensatory response to the tissue hypoxia. Inappropriate secondary polycythemia, on the other hand, is associated with increased erythropoietin secretion without systemic tissue hypoxia. In humans, a variety of neoplasms including renal tumors, hepatomas, uterine leiomyomas, and cerebellar hemangioblastomas have been associated with inappropriate production of erythropoietin and secondary polycythemia. Non-neoplastic renal abnormalities have also been reported to cause secondary polycythemia and include renal cysts, hydronephrosis, and polycystic kidneys. In both humans and dogs, Cushing's syndrome may also produce mild secondary polycythemia. In the dog, tumor-related secondary polycythemia has been reported only in association with renal carcinoma and renal lymphosacoma.

Primary polycythemia, or polycythemia vera, is a myeloproliferative disorder; in the dog and cat, it is a disease of young to middle-aged adult animals, without apparent predilection for breed or sex. Polycythemia vera is currently thought to result from clonal proliferation of erythroid precursors that require little to no erythropoietin for differentiation. In primary polycythemia, serum and urinary erythropoietin concentrations are usually undetectable, in contrast to increased concentrations found in appropriate or inappropriate secondary polycythemia.

The clinical signs of both primary and secondary polycythemia may include erythema of mucous membranes, polydipsia, polyuria, bleeding diatheses (epistaxis, hematemesis, melena, and hematuria), or neurologic disturbances (lethargy, ataxia, weakness, dementia, convulsions, and blindness). Many of these clinical manifestations, including hyperemic mucous membranes, hemorrhagic complications, and neurologic disturbances, are related

Table 1. *Classification of Polycythemia*

Type	Cause
Relative	Dehydration
Absolute	
Primary (polycythemia vera)	Myeloproliferative disorder
Secondary	
Physiologically appropriate (decreased tissue oxygenation)	Pulmonary disorder Cardiac disorder Venoarterial shunt Hemoglobinopathy
Physiologically inappropriate (normal tissue oxygenation)	
Inappropriate erythropoietin production group	Renal tumor Miscellaneous tumor
Hormonal stimulus to erythropoiesis	Cushing's syndrome Administration of high dosage adrenocortical steroids

to increased RBC mass resulting in increased blood viscosity. This hyperviscosity slows blood flow, distends capillaries and small vessels, and increases the likelihood of hypoxia, thrombosis, and rupture of these vessels.

DIAGNOSIS

The first step in determining the cause of polycythemia is to exclude relative polycythemia. Since acute dehydration is readily assessed, relative polycythemia can usually be determined clinically. In some cases with only mild increases in PCV (55 to 65 per cent) and no obvious evidence of fluid loss, direct measurement of RBC mass may be necessary to differentiate relative from absolute polycythemia.

Once absolute polycythemia is established, the next step is to differentiate primary and secondary causes for the erythrocytosis. Urine or serum erythropoietin determinations are useful in distinguishing the two types of absolute polycythemia: in secondary polycythemia, elevated erythropoietin concentrations are present, whereas such concentrations are undetectable in primary polycythemia. Since erythropoietin assays are not routinely available, however, other laboratory tests and clinical signs must be used to make the differentiation. Many of the clinical and laboratory features of human primary polycythemia, including hepatomegaly, splenomegaly, leukocytosis, and thrombocytosis, are rare in dogs and cats with the disorder; therefore, the absence of these features does not exclude primary polycythemia in these animals. In addition, examination of bone marrow aspirates, useful in humans, is of limited value in differentiating canine and feline primary and secondary polycythemia. In most cases, a diagnosis of primary polycythemia is made by excluding the common causes of secondary polycythemia.

The determination of arterial blood oxygen saturation is useful in assessing the state of tissue oxygenation. A level less than 92 per cent reflects tissue hypoxia and warrants a diagnosis of secondary polycythemia; examination of cardiac and pulmonary systems by means of electrocardiography and chest radiography usually reveals the cause. If arterial oxygen saturation is normal, high oxygen affinity hemoglobinopathies can be excluded by measurement of the oxygen pressure at which hemoglobin is 50 per cent saturated (P_{50}). Low values for P_{50} indicate decreased release of oxygen to tissue as a result of high-affinity hemoglobin. Once hypoxia is excluded as the cause of erythrocytosis, conditions causing inappropriate erythropoietin production should be considered. Results of physical and neurologic examination, plain radiography, and intravenous pyelography will identify most of these conditions.

TREATMENT

The cause of polycythemia determines treatment. In secondary polycythemia, therapy should be directed toward the underlying cause. Erythropoietin-secreting tumors should be surgically removed; preoperative phlebotomy to decrease the PCV to within normal range reduces morbidity and mortality associated with postoperative hemorrhage and thromboembolism. In polycythemia secondary to systemic hypoxia, as in cardiac or pulmonary disease, phlebotomy is contraindicated since the polycythemia represents a compensatory response to tissue hypoxia. If the PCV reaches levels that increase blood viscosity and compromise blood flow, however, judicious phlebotomy may be of clinical benefit.

In primary polycythemia, the goal of therapy is to reduce and maintain the PCV within the normal range, thereby alleviating clinical signs and preventing the serious thrombotic and hemorrhagic complications associated with this disorder. The optimal therapy for primary polycythemia is unknown; in the dog, the disease has been treated with phlebotomy, radioactive phosphorus (^{32}P), or chemotherapeutic agents such as chlorambucil, busulfan, and melphalan. Phlebotomy is relatively safe but must usually be repeated at frequent intervals to maintain the PCV within normal range. Radioactive phosphorus induces prolonged remission and reduces the morbidity of primary polycythemia but may increase the risk of leukemia and myelofibrosis. In human polycythemia vera, chlorambucil and other alkylating agents have also proved to be leukemogenic.

Hydroxyurea (Hydrea, Squibb) can also be used to manage primary polycythemia. Hydroxyurea causes reversible bone marrow suppression; it inhibits DNA synthesis without affecting RNA or protein synthesis. In the dog and cat, side effects of hydroxyurea may include anorexia, vomiting, spermatogenic arrest, bone marrow hypoplasia, and sloughing of the nails. No carcinogenic effects have yet been related to hydroxyurea administration.

Hydroxyurea should first be given at a loading dosage of 30 mg/kg, PO daily for seven to ten days, followed by 15 mg/kg, PO daily in single or divided doses. The effects of hydroxyurea are enhanced by first reducing the PCV to less than 50 per cent with successive phlebotomies (20 ml/kg) and simultaneous fluid replacement. Complete blood and platelet counts should be monitored at 7- to 14-day intervals until the PCV has normalized. Subsequent blood counts and examinations should be scheduled at three- to four-month intervals. If leukopenia, thrombocytopenia, or anemia develops, hydroxyurea should be discontinued until the blood count returns to normal; hydroxyurea therapy should then be resumed at a lower maintenance dosage. If relapse occurs, the daily dosage of hydroxyurea should be increased for seven to ten days and blood count monitored until normal; in some dogs, a higher maintenance dosage may be required to prevent further relapse. The hydroxyurea dosage must be individualized for optimal control of primary polycythemia.

SUPPLEMENTAL READING

Golde, D. W., Hocking, W. G., Koeffler, H. P., et al.: Polycythemia: Mechanisms and management. Ann. Intern. Med. 95:71, 1981.

Hoffman, R., and Wasserman, L. R.: Natural history and management of polycythemia vera. Adv. Intern. Med. 24:255, 1979.
Peterson, M. E., and Randolph, J. F.: Diagnosis of canine primary polycythemia and management with hydroxyurea. J.A.V.M.A. 180:415, 1982.
Peterson, M. E., and Zanjani, E. D.: Inappropriate erythropoietin production from a renal carcinoma in a dog with polycythemia. J.A.V.M.A. 179:995, 1981.
Scott, R. C., and Patnaik, A. K.: Renal carcinoma associated with secondary polycythemia in the dog. J. Anim. Hosp. Assoc. 8:275, 1972.

PRACTICAL BLOOD TRANSFUSIONS

LAURIE G. O'ROURKE, D.V.M.
Davis, California

INDICATIONS AND GOALS OF THERAPY

Blood and blood products can be lifesaving. Blood transfusion, however, is substitution therapy that provides temporary support. Therapeutic goals include restoration of the oxygen carrying capacity, volume replacement, and coagulation factor replacement.

Whole blood is indicated whenever an animal presents with hypovolemia, anemia, or dyspnea. Give red cell concentrates to normovolemic but anemic patients when the oxygen carrying capacity needs improvement, as this meets the animal's needs but reduces the risk of circulatory overload.

Plasma therapy may be used for volume restoration and coagulation factor replacement. Plasma is indicated for volume restoration in the nonanemic, hypovolemic patient and may be used to supplement whole blood transfusions. Large quantities of plasma are necessary to elevate plasma protein concentrations measurably. Fresh plasma or fresh frozen plasma may be used in therapy of coagulation disorders, including coumarin toxicity, disseminated intravascular coagulopathy, and other factor deficiencies.

Platelet-rich plasma is indicated in thrombocytopenic patients. Unfortunately, transfused platelets have a short half-life. The functional capacity of the platelets may be further diminished in animals with diseases that have immune activity against platelets.

CONTRAINDICATIONS

The etiology and degree of anemia must be assessed before the administration of blood or blood components. Give careful consideration to all the advantages and consequences. Blood therapy may be contraindicated in an immune-mediated hemolytic crisis, since supplying more red cells may only result in continued and more rapid hemolysis. Adequate crossmatching may be impossible when autoagglutination occurs. However, transfusion must be considered if the anemia becomes life-threatening in these cases.

Incompatible blood is contraindicated. Rare exceptions are those instances in which the emergency does not allow time to assure compatibility. *Interspecies transfusions are always contraindicated.*

DONOR SELECTION

Maintaining donor dogs and cats in the veterinary hospital ensures that the donor will be a healthy and disease-free animal. (In emergencies, and *only* with owner agreement, patients with good dispositions may be typed and used as donors.) To ensure donor blood quality, hemograms and plasma protein concentrations should be performed whenever blood is collected. Regular screening for *Dirofilaria immitis* in the dog and *Haemobartonella felis* and feline leukemia virus in the cat should be performed and recorded. Compatibility will depend on donor typing, crossmatching, and previous transfusion history. Approximately 60 per cent of the canine population carry hemolytic antibody to the A antigen, making an A negative donor preferable. The pleomorphic antigen system of the cat is currently the subject of intensive study; however, definitive typing is not available, leaving crossmatch as the only screening method.

Crossmatching for major and minor histocompatibility should be performed to screen for any agglutinating antigen-antibody incompatibility (Table 1). The procedure is performed using a 2-ml EDTA sample from the recipient and a 2-ml sample from the donor. If the donor blood sample is drawn from stored blood, it is important to thoroughly mix the blood before the sample is obtained.

In animals, hemolysis is the major incompatibility reaction. Agglutination is a lesser problem. *A crossmatch between an A positive donor and a sensitized A negative recipient will not show agglutination.* To determine the hemolytic nature of this incompatibility, complement lysis with positive control cells is required, thus placing it out of the realm of the veterinary practice. Although this point may be used as an argument against the value of crossmatching, at the University of California Veterinary Medical Teaching Hospital it is felt that crossmatching is a valid screening test for potential incompatibilities.

The transfusion history of the patient must be investigated. Prior transfusions, even though typed and crossmatched, may have sensitized the recipient and may result in a subsequent reaction. Patients with such histories should be carefully monitored for adverse reactions (see Complications).

Table 1.   Crossmatching

1. Centrifuge samples at 3400 × G for 1 minute. Remove and retain plasma.

2. Wash red cells three times in isotonic saline: resuspend, centrifuge, and discard supernatant, retaining packed RBCs.

3. Prepare 2 per cent red cell saline suspension: 0.02 ml washed packed red cells plus 0.98 ml of 0.85 per cent saline.

4. Major crossmatch:
   2 drops donor red cell suspension
   2 drops recipient plasma

5. Minor crossmatch:
   2 drops recipient red cell suspension
   2 drops donor plasma

6. Control:
   2 drops recipient red cell suspension
   2 drops recipient plasma

7. Incubate major, minor, and control at 25°C for 30 minutes.

8. Centrifuge all tubes at 3400 × G for 1 minute.

9. Positive test = agglutination.

COLLECTION AND STORAGE

The three anticoagulants commonly employed are heparin, acid citrate dextrose (ACD), and citrate phosphate dextrose (CPD). ACD and CPD are also red cell preservatives and should be used if the blood is to be stored for any length of time. Surface contact with plastic bags or containers is less likely to activate platelets or coagulation factors than is glass, making plastic preferable for collection and storage purposes. Whole blood or red cell concentrates may be maintained at a temperature between 1 and 6°C (32 and 43° F) for 21 days with ACD and 28 days with CPD. At the end of the storage time, 70 to 75 per cent of the red cells will remain viable. Among the clinical concerns when using stored blood for transfusion purposes is the decreased concentration of red cell 2,3 diphosphoglycerate (2,3-DPG) and the increased acidity of the stored blood. The effect of the lowered 2,3-DPG is transitory and does not appear to be of clinical significance. The pH of stored blood may fall to 6.5 after three weeks of storage. Citrate is taken up rapidly by the liver, with a net effect of alkalosis. Thus, bicarbonate administration with the transfusion is contraindicated.

Red cell concentrates can be prepared by centrifugation or sedimentation of the units over 24 hours and withdrawal of the plasma supernatant, giving a concentrate of 60 to 80 per cent red blood cells. Alternatively, units may be stored in an upside-down position to allow direct administration of the sedimented red cells, leaving the plasma in the container.

To obtain viable platelets, animals must be transfused immediately with fresh whole blood or platelet-rich plasma. Functional platelets are almost nonexistent in two- to three-day-old blood. Platelet-rich plasma is obtained by centrifuging blood at 210 × G for 15 minutes and withdrawing plasma with a plasma extractor, taking care to avoid leukocyte contamination from the buffy coat.

Fresh or fresh frozen plasma can be used for coagulation factor replacement therapy and volume replacement. When red cell concentrates are prepared, the extracted plasma can be frozen immediately at −70°C. The cyclic nature and relatively warm temperature of refrigerator freezers will cause factor deterioration. Albumin is more stable, and plasma for this purpose can be stored in conventional freezers for one year. Coagulation factors can be preserved for one year by freezing and storing at −70°C.

Blood collected in heparin is considered usable for only 48 hours. This is because heparin, a natural anticoagulant, is slowly reversed, so small but significant clotting takes place by 48 hours.

Banked blood should be carefully examined for discoloration and hemolysis. Any questionable blood must be discarded to avoid the risk of transfusion reactions.

ACD and CPD vacuum glass containers and plastic bags can be used for collection. Vacuum containers will draw blood quickly and only require gentle rotation throughout collection. However, blood drawn under negative pressure may be subjected to excessive stress, resulting in damaged red cells or hemolysis. The passive gravitational flow of blood into plastic bags is slower and requires frequent gentle mixing but results in less erythrocyte damage. Containers with anticoagulants are available that will collect a total of 250 or 500 ml. For cats, a syringe with 10 ml of standard CPD can be used to draw 50 ml of blood, for a total of 60 ml. Donor animals may have 20 per cent of their blood withdrawn safely. Blood volume is estimated to be 85 to 90 ml/kg body weight in the dog and 65 to 75 ml/kg body weight in the cat.

Collection must be aseptic. Blood may be collected from the jugular vein or by intracardiac puncture. The collection site should be clipped, scrubbed and prepped with a skin antiseptic for sterile technique. A jugular venipuncture using a large gauge needle (16 to 18 gauge) and collection set works well in the dog. Use a large syringe with an 18-gauge butterfly catheter to manually draw blood from anesthetized donor cats. Dogs should not donate blood more frequently than every 14 days. Cats may be bled every 21 days.

ADMINISTRATION

The clinical cause of anemia and the physical condition of the patient will determine the plan of therapy. Subjective clinical judgement should determine how aggressive the therapy will be.

Blood and blood components should be warmed before administration to prevent hypothermia. Thawing and warming can be done in a warm water bath ($< 42°C$).

Administer blood and blood products through an indwelling catheter into the cephalic, jugular, or lateral saphenous vein. When peripheral routes are used, support the limb in extension with a splint to help keep the catheter patent. Catheter placement should always be preceded by surgical preparation of the skin. Although intraperitoneal administration is possible, absorption is slow and some cells are not recovered. This route should be reserved for animals that do not need an immediate increase in their red cell mass. Intramedullary transfusion may be the preferred route in kittens or puppies. A needle is placed in the trochanteric fossa of the femur and directed into the medullary cavity. A 20-gauge needle with stylet should be used to prevent a core of bone from occluding the needle lumen.

The rule of thumb for administration of blood for medical purposes is 10 ml/kg body weight/hr. The

Table 2. *Example of Estimating Volumes in Blood Therapy*

30-kg dog with PCV = 10%; desired PCV = 18%; anticoagulated donor blood with PCV = 50%
1. Total blood volume = (90 ml/kg)(30 kg) = 2700 ml
2. Existing red cell mass = (2700 ml)(10%) = 270 ml
3. Desired red cell mass = (2700 ml)(18%) = 490 ml
4. Required red cell mass = 490 ml − 270 ml = 220 ml
5. Required blood volume = (220 ml)/(50%) = 440 ml

maximum amount safely given is 20 per cent of the estimated normal volume per 24 hours. The amount of blood needed can be estimated from the recipient's hematocrit and weight, the hematocrit of the donor blood with anticoagulant, and the lowest acceptable hematocrit post therapy. Normal blood volume is 85 to 90 ml/kg for dogs and 65 to 75 ml/kg for cats. An example of a typical calculation is given in Table 2.

The full effect of the transfusion will be realized 12 to 24 hours after fluids have been redistributed. The initial portion of a transfusion should always be given slowly. Signs of a transfusion reaction during this period may signal a serious incompatibility (see Complications). After the initial period the rate of administration may be increased. Remember, however, that rapid transfusions often cause vomiting.

The blood administration set must include a filter that will remove most of the aggregated debris. During the transfusion the patient should be checked regularly for vomiting, coughing, or respiratory embarrassment. Modified administration sets can be made to adapt to a syringe for use in cats, kittens, and puppies: (1) The tubing at either end of the filter is shortened to approximately 12 cm. (2) A three-way valve is attached to the inflow. (3) A female Luer lock is attached to the outflow tubing. The entire set can then be gas sterilized. Administration is accomplished by attaching the syringe to the three-way valve and the Luer lock to the catheter or needle hub. Blood is then slowly infused. It may be necessary to use a Y connector to piggy back the blood administration set to a pediatric drip set of an isotonic crystalloid solution. Fluids can be given at a rate that will keep the catheter patent and allow a slow administration of blood.

Much has been written on the concurrent administration of calcium when citrated blood is given. Empirical use of calcium may result in hypercalcemia as citrate is removed from the system. It is safest to monitor the recipient for clinical signs of hypocalcemia and then treat accordingly. The acid-base status of the patient may be monitored using blood gases or by calculating the anion gap.

COMPLICATIONS

Antibody to the A antigen in the dog is a potent hemolysin. When an A negative dog receives A positive blood, any one of several responses may occur: (1) no reaction, but the dog will be sensitized to A positive blood, (2) a delayed response resulting in sensitization and hemolysis of the transfused cells at 12 to 14 days, or (3) erythroblastosis fetalis (hemolytic disease of the newborn). A previous transfusion that caused sensitization allows an anamnestic response, resulting in immediate, rapid hemolysis.

True transfusion reactions are not common in the dog or cat. Urticaria, fever, hemolysis with hematuria, and anaphylaxis are all indications of incompatibility. Hemolysis may be the result of incompatibility or improper storage and administration. Forcing blood through a small needle lumen may rupture cells. Bacterial contamination or poor storage conditions may cause cells to lyse. Hemolysis is a serious complication because of the nephrotoxic effects of free erythrocyte membranes and hemoglobin casts. In these cases diuresis must be employed to protect the kidney. When complications are arrested, administration may be reinstituted provided compatible donor blood is available.

Though transfusion reactions are dramatic, the most common complication is circulatory overload created by giving blood too quickly or in too great a quantity. Early signs of circulatory overload include vomition and a dry cough. Continued administration may cause pulmonary edema.

Blood improperly collected, stored, or handled may serve as an ideal culture medium for bacteria, producing lethal endotoxins. Administration of contaminated blood may result in endotoxic shock and disseminated intravascular coagulation. If you suspect that this has happened, perform Gram stains and cultures of the donor blood, and institute immediate therapy.

SUPPLEMENTAL READING

Byars, T. D., and Divers, T. J.: Clinical use of blood transfusion. Calif. Vet. 35:14, 1981.

Conrad, M. E. (ed.): Transfusion problems in hematology. Semin. Hematol. 18:79, 1981.

Dodds, W. J.: Bleeding disorders. *In* Ettinger, S. J. (ed.): *Textbook of Veterinary Internal Medicine*, Vol. II. Philadelphia: W. B. Saunders, 1975.

Dodds, W. J.: Inherited hemorrhagic defects. *In* Kirk, R. W. (ed.): *Current Veterinary Therapy VI*. Philadelphia: W. B. Saunders, 1977.

Haskins, S. C.: Blood volume support. Vet. Clin. North Am. 6:265, 1976.

Hollan, S. R.: Controversial and changing trends in blood transfusion. Vox Sang. 40:309, 1981.

Norsworthy, G. D.: Blood transfusion in the cat. Feline Pract. 7:29, 1977.

Schall, W. D., and Perman, V.: Diseases of red blood cells. *In* Ettinger, S. J. (ed.): *Textbook of Veterinary Internal Medicine*, Vol. II. Philadelphia: W. B. Saunders, 1975.

Sheldon, G. F.: Blood from bag through patient. Emerg. Med. 12:36, 1980.

Oncology

CARE OF THE FELINE LEUKEMIA VIRUS POSITIVE NORMAL CAT

AUDREY A. HAYES, V.M.D.

New York, New York

Many clients are reluctant to accept euthanasia in response to the diagnosis of feline leukemia in an asymptomatic cat. In order for the veterinarian to offer the client a viable alternative it is necessary to consider several aspects of feline leukemia virus (FeLV) infection.

CONTAGION TO OTHER CATS

Owners intending to keep their FeLV test positive (FeLV+) cats must be advised that the FeLV is contagious to susceptible cats in close contact with positive cats. Viral intermediaries include urine, blood, milk, and saliva. One milliliter of saliva from an FeLV+ cat may contain as many as 1×10^6 viral particles. Therefore, if there are FeLV− cats in the household, the FeLV+ cats and their food dishes, water bowls, and litter pans must be separated from the FeLV− cats. Confining the positive cats to one room of the house constitutes effective isolation. To further limit the spread of FeLV, FeLV+ normal cats should be kept inside.

Confinement limits contagion to outside cats by eliminating exposure through breeding or fighting.

PUBLIC HEALTH SIGNIFICANCE

Clients' questions regarding the public health significance of the FeLV should be answered by addressing the following points:

1. The FeLV will infect and replicate in human fibroblast cells in tissue culture (*in vitro*). The FeLV does not, however, transform these cells into cancer cells.

2. A recent epidemiologic survey of 19,000 American veterinary school graduates resulted in the observation that there was an excessive number of leukemia-related deaths in graduates 45 years of age and older when compared with the American general population and physician mortality data. However, as stated by the authors of this recent study, the data may not be valid since the study failed to differentiate among occupational categories within veterinary medicine, geographic location, and service in the armed forces. In particular, the study did not allow for either the increased exposure to x-rays or the variable degree of adherence to radiation safety standards in the older age group.

3. Several seroepidemiologic studies have attempted to detect evidence of FeLV infection in high-risk human population groups. These investigations have failed to find any evidence of FeLV antigen or antibody in the more than 2000 sera drawn from owners of FeLV + cats; veterinarians, researchers, and laboratory personnel exposed to FeLV; and in human patients with a variety of malignant tumors.

To date, the results of more than 20 epidemiologic and serologic studies have been published and new investigations are under way. No conclusive evidence exists to indicate that the human population is at any increased risk of developing leukemia or other neoplasms as a result of exposure to FeLV + cats.

FeLV IMMUNOSUPPRESSION

FeLV infection suppresses and alters the host's natural immune response to disease. The p15 envelope antigen of the FeLV causes immunosuppression. Owners must be informed that FeLV + cats have an increased incidence of systemic viral, mycotic, and bacterial infections. FeLV + cats should never be exposed to cats suffering from contagious diseases such as upper respiratory tract infections or feline infectious peritonitis (FIP) virus. Indoor confinement of the positive cat also decreases the possibility of bacterial infection due to bite wounds. Bite wound abscessses are often slow to heal in FeLV + cats. Any illness in an FeLV + normal cat necessitates prompt and aggressive veterinary therapy and conscientious nursing care by the owner if the patient is to make a complete recovery.

RESPONSE TO STRESS

A stressful event may precipitate the onset of one of the FeLV-related diseases (e.g., panleukopenia-like syndrome) in an FeLV + normal cat. Elective surgical procedures are both immunosuppressive and stressful. Ovariohysterectomy, castration, declawing, and dentistry should be avoided unless necessary. The owner must be advised of the possibility of postoperative complications. However, spraying behavior, aggression, and constant estrus cycles in intact FeLV + confined cats often become stressful for both the cat and the owner. It is sometimes possible to avoid ovariohysterectomy and castration by using megestrol acetate tablets (Ovaban, Schering). During winter months in northern latitudes of the United States a dose of 2.5 mg will control sexual activity for seven to ten days. The dosage must be increased to effect in warmer climates and as the hours of daylight extend.

Greater than 50 per cent of the FeLV + cats that develop a panleukopenia-like syndrome associated with stress can survive one crisis if they receive immediate and conscientious treatment. In addition to supportive care a blood transfusion may be indicated.

Other stressful situations that may adversely affect FeLV + normal cats include the owner's absence, travel, relocation, loss of a companion, or the addition of another FeLV + cat to the household.

PROGNOSIS FOR FeLV + NORMAL CATS

Owners want to know if it is possible for their FeLV + cats to reject the FeLV. Less than 5 per cent (approximately 3 per cent) of persistently FeLV-infected cats will subsequently mount an immune response, produce FeLV neutralizing and feline oncornavirus cell–associated membrane antigen (FOCMA) antibodies, and reject the virus. In general, the longer a cat remains FeLV infected, the less likely it is that it will reject the virus. It is not possible, however, to predict the outcome of FeLV infection in a particular cat.

What is the life expectancy for a FeLV + normal cat? One group of investigators followed 96 FeLV + normal cats for three and one-half years. Within this period 80 of the 96 cats (83 per cent) died of leukemia, lymphosarcoma, FeLV-related diseases, or FIP. Since October 1974 the staff of the Donaldson-Atwood Cancer Clinic of the Animal Medical Center has followed the course of FeLV infection in 98 normal cats. During this seven-year observation period 41 per cent died of FeLV-associated illnesses or FIP.

An FeLV+ normal cat, then, may reject the virus, may live only months, or may live for many years. It is not possible to predict the outcome of FeLV infection in an otherwise normal cat.

ROUTINE CARE OF THE FeLV+ NORMAL CAT

FeLV+ normal cats should be examined by a veterinarian every three months to detect early signs of leukemia, lymphosarcoma, or one of the FeLV-related diseases. During physical examination special attention should be given to the color of the mucous membranes, the size of the peripheral lymph nodes, auscultation and compressibility of the thoracic cavity, and palpable abnormalities of the liver, spleen, kidneys, intestinal tract, and abdominal lymph nodes. A complete blood count and differential white blood cell count may reveal incipient leukopenia, anemia, or leukemia. The FeLV test should be repeated periodically.

Thymic, alimentary, and renal lymphosarcomas respond well to chemotherapy, especially if disease is diagnosed in the early stages. The staff of the Donaldson-Atwood Cancer Clinic has treated 106 cats with various forms of lymphosarcoma. Their median survival time is 5.5 months, but 33 per cent of these cats have lived eight months or longer. A few cats are alive and doing well three or more years after diagnosis.

An owner's decision to keep an FeLV+ normal cat is a commitment. The owner must be informed of the danger to other cats, the public health controversy, and the prognosis for FeLV-infected cats. The owner must have the facilities to isolate the positive cat from susceptible FeLV− cats, must be able to devote more time to caring for this cat, and must be able to afford the expense of the required additional veterinary care. Most important is the owner's ability to cope emotionally with the instability inherent in a guarded prognosis. These dedicated owners are entitled to all the veterinary assistance available to keep their FeLV+ cats in good health for as long as possible.

SUPPLEMENTAL READING

Blair, A., and Hayes, H. M., Jr.: Cancer and other causes of death among United States veterinarians, 1966–1977. Int. J. Cancer 25:181, 1980.
Gutensohn, N., Essex, M., Francis, D. P., and Hardy, W. D., Jr.: Risk to humans from exposure to feline leukemia virus: Epidemiological considerations. In Essex, M., Todaro, G., and ZurHausen, H. (eds.): Viruses in Naturally Occurring Cancers. Cold Spring Harbor, New York: Cold Spring Harbor Laboratory, 1980, pp. 699–706.
Hardy, W. D., Jr.: Hematopoietic tumors of cats. J.A.A.H.A. 17:921, 1981.
Hardy, W. D., Jr.: Feline leukemia virus non-neoplastic diseases. J.A.A.H.A. 17:941, 1981.
Hardy, W. D., Jr.: The feline leukemia virus. J.A.A.H.A. 17:951, 1981.
Hardy, W. D., Jr., Old, L. J., Hess, P. W., Essex, M., and Cotter, S. M.: Horizontal transmission of feline leukemia virus. Nature 244:266, 1973.
Mathes, L. E., Olsen, R. G., Hebebrand, L. C., Hoover, E. A., Schaller, J. P., Adams, P. W., and Nichols, W. S.: Immunosuppressive properties of virion polypeptide, a 15,000 dalton protein, from feline leukemia virus. Cancer Res. 39:950, 1979.
McClelland, A. J., Hardy, W. D., Jr., and Zuckerman, E. E.: Prognosis of healthy feline leukemia virus infected cats. In Hardy, W. D., Jr., New York: Elsevier/North Holland, 1980, pp. 121–126.

TRANSMISSIBLE VENEREAL TUMOR IN THE DOG

CLAY A. CALVERT, D.V.M.
Athens, Georgia

Transmissible venereal tumor (TVT) is a naturally occurring tumor of the dog that usually affects the external genitalia. Although transmission of the tumor usually occurs during coitus, licking and biting may also result in transmission. Extragenital sites of TVT include the face, buccal cavity, nasal passages, and skin. Synonyms of TVT include "Sticker tumor," venereal granuloma, transmissible sarcoma, contagious venereal tumor, and transmissible lymphosarcoma.

The TVT is a naturally occurring allograft that results from transplantation of tumor cells to susceptible hosts. Despite reports of virus or viral-like cytoplasmic inclusions in TVT cells, the tumor has not been consistently transmitted by cell free extracts.

TVT has a worldwide distribution but is more prevalent in temperate zones, especially where dog populations are large. Young, sexually active, unconfined dogs are largely responsible for transmission of TVT. The mean age of 71 consecutive cases of TVT seen at the University of Georgia Veterinary

Teaching Hospital and the Animal Medical Center was 4.2 years (range 2 to 10 years). Only 8 of 71 dogs (13 per cent) were over five years of age. German shepherds accounted for an unusually high proportion of cases (30 per cent), and only 12 dogs (17 per cent) weighed less than 20 kg. There was nearly equal distribution between male and female dogs. Tumors occurred in eight ovariohysterectomized dogs as late as eight months after surgery. The clinical signs observed in 64 dogs with genital TVT almost always included a serosanguineous or hemorrhagic vaginal or preputial discharge. Occasionally, particularly in the female, a protruding mass was observed. TVT in the nasal passages resulted in sneezing and epistaxis. Metastasis was detected in only two dogs. In the female, regional metastasis was to the internal iliac lymph nodes and in the male to the superficial inguinal and lumbar lymph nodes. Although the reported metastasis rate is less than 5 per cent, metastases to most organs, including the eye and central nervous system, have been reported.

The gross appearance of TVT is rather consistent. Tumors are cauliflower-like, pink to red, friable masses that may be solitary or multiple. In the male, the tumors are often located near the bulbus glandis but may be anywhere on the penis and prepuce. Multiple genital tumors are more common in the male. In the female, tumors are located in the caudal vagina and frequently encroach upon the urethral orifice. Although a presumptive diagnosis can usually be made from the gross appearance and location of the tumor, specimens for microscopic examination can be obtained from the discharges and/or tumor fragments.

The TVT is an undifferentiated round cell tumor of reticuloendothelial origin. The cells are round to oval with prominent nucleoli and scant cytoplasm. The cells are usually seen in clusters, and mitotic figures are common. Plasma cells, lymphocytes, and macrophages are often present among the tumor cells. The TVT cell usually has 59 chromosomes (57 to 64) compared with the normal of 78. However, the DNA content of TVT cells is near normal, and cells from naturally occurring TVT from widely separated geographic areas reveal almost identical karyotypes and histocompatibility antigens (Cohen, 1978).

Although spontaneous remission of the experimentally transplanted TVT is well-documented, spontaneous remission of the naturally occurring TVT is poorly documented. Although uncommon, it is probable that spontaneous remission of naturally occurring TVT does occur.

The goal of therapy of TVT is to eradicate the tumor and possible metastases as quickly as possible with minimal cost and untoward effects. Although surgical resection may be curative, 18 of the 71 cases (25 per cent) in our series relapsed following one to three surgeries. Most other reports have also cited a relatively high incidence of post-surgical relapse. Surgery should be limited to those dogs with solitary, small tumor nodules.

Radiotherapy resulted in cures in 18 of 18 cases using orthovoltage radiation (Thrall, 1981). In most cases a single dosage of 1000 rads was curative. The primary limitation of radiation therapy is the availability of radiation facilities.

Various forms of passive and active immunotherapy have been employed with variable results in the treatment of naturally occurring and experimentally induced TVT. A practical immunotherapy might be the intralesional injection of the bacillus Calmette-Guerin (BCG) or other active nonspecific immunotherapeutic agents. Both injected and noninjected experimentally induced tumors have been reported to regress within 63 days of BCG therapy (Hess et al., 1977). However, BCG therapy of naturally occurring TVT has not been reported.

Overall, the most effective and practical therapy is chemotherapy. In the presence of metastatic disease, chemotherapy is the only reasonable choice. The most effective chemotherapeutic agents are vincristine (Oncovin, Eli Lilly Co.) and doxorubicin (Adriamycin, Adria Lab.). Results of treatment with cyclophosphamide, methotrexate, or cyclophosphamide plus prednisone have been inconsistent. Owing to increased cost, doxorubicin should be reserved for the occasional tumor that is refractory to vincristine.

Combination chemotherapy utilizing vincristine, cyclophosphamide, and methotrexate resulted in complete remission, without relapse, in 93 per cent of 30 consecutive cases treated at the University of Georgia and the Animal Medical Center (Brown et al., 1980). However, single agent vincristine (0.8 mg/m², IV, weekly) is just as effective as combination therapy and is associated with fewer side effects. Table 1 lists the results of 41 consecutive cases treated with vincristine. Complete remission occurred in 39 of 41 dogs. A complete blood count is recommended prior to each treatment, but platelet counts are unnecessary. When the pretreatment WBC count is below 4000/mm³, treatment should be delayed for three to four days, at which time the

Table 1. *Results of Vincristine Treatment of 41 Consecutive Cases of TVT*

Duration of Observed Signs (Days) Prior to Therapy		Onset of Tumor Regression*	No. of Weekly Treatments Until NED†	Complete Remission
Mean	125	7 days: 39 dogs	Mean 3.3	39/41
Median	60	14 days: 41 dogs	Range 2–7	
Range	1–510			

*Days following first injection of vincristine.
†No evidence of disease in 38 dogs undergoing complete remission.

Table 2. *Side Effects of Vincristine Treatment of TVT*

Effect	No. of Dogs With Effect	Onset (Days After Vincristine)	Duration of Effect (Days)	Severity of Effect
Diarrhea	1	1	1	Bloody
Vomiting	3	1	1,3,1,3	1 to 6 Vomitions
Lethargy	3	1	1,2,2	Mild
Anorexia	3	1	2,2,5	Partial
Weakness, constipation	1	3	3	
Leukopenia	2	3	3	WBC count: 3000 to 4000/mm³
Total	9			

WBC count should be repeated. Further doses of vincristine may remain at 0.8 mg/m² or may be reduced to 0.5 mg/m.² Nine dogs in our study experienced side effects. Three dogs vomited, and two developed transient leukopenias (Table 2). In all instances the degree of untoward effects was mild.

Chemotherapy has been effective against primary and metastatic TVT. TVT involving the central nervous system may be treatable with intrathecal cytosine arabinoside, or methotrexate. Alternatively, drugs that cross the blood-brain barrier such as the nitrosourea compounds may be useful. Intraocular metastases may be effectively treated with systemic vincristine. However, severe uveitis secondary to tumor necrosis and/or release of tumor antigens frequently results in glaucoma and blindness. Aggressive glucocorticoid treatment should begin prior to chemotherapy and should continue throughout the treatment regimen.

REFERENCES AND SUPPLEMENTAL READING

Brown, N. O., Calvert, C. A., and MacEwen, E. G.: Chemotherapeutic management of transmissible venereal tumors in 30 dogs. J. A. V. M. A. 176:983, 1980.

Brown, N. O., MacEwen, E. G., and Calvert, C. A.: Transmissible venereal tumor in the dog. Calif. Vet. 35:6, 1981.

Cohen, D.: The transmissible venereal tumor of the dog—A naturally occurring allograft? A review. Israel J. Med. Sci. 10:565, 1978.

Hess, A. D., Catchatourian, R., et al.: Intralesional *Bacillus Calmette-Guerin* immunotherapy of canine venereal tumors. Cancer Res. 37:3990, 1977.

Richardson, R. C.: Canine transmissible venereal tumor. Comp. Cont. Ed. 3:951, 1981.

Thrall, D. E.: Orthovoltage radiotherapy of canine transmissible venereal tumor. Vet. Radiol., 1982.

MANAGEMENT OF SOLID TUMORS

NANCY O. BROWN, V.M.D.

Plymouth Meeting, Pennsylvania

Solid tumors include a variety of tumors in both the sarcoma and carcinoma classes. Some oncologists include all solid malignant tumors in this category except for hematopoietic and lymphoid cancers. To others, these tumors represent solid masses exclusive of tumors in specific organs. For the purpose of this discussion, solid tumors will include connective tissue tumors and superficial carcinomas.

The annual incidence of both connective tissue tumors and malignant skin tumors is higher in dogs and cats than in humans (Dorn, 1976). The rate in dogs in both instances is higher than in cats (Dorn, 1976). The major connective tissue tumors in the dog are fibrosarcoma, hemangiosarcoma, and hemangiopericytoma, whereas in the cat they are fibrosarcoma and hemangiosarcoma (Dorn, 1976). The major malignant skin tumors in the dog are mastocytoma, adenocarcinoma, and squamous cell carcinoma, and in the cat, squamous cell carcinoma (Dorn, 1976).

The treatment of solid tumors has lagged behind that of hematopoietic and lymphoid cancers, and this can be attributed to several factors. With sarcomas, the wide variety of histologic types and the rapid development of metastases preclude adequate controlled trials to prove the efficacy of various therapies (Wilbur, 1975). Solid tumors have a slower doubling time as compared with leukemias and lymphomas, making them more resistant to drugs (Sonntag and Brunner, 1975). It is also thought that solid tumors develop primary and secondary resistances to drugs earlier than other neoplasms (Sonntag and Brunner, 1975).

Sarcomas tend to spread by hematogenous routes, bypassing regional lymph nodes and thus making staging systems difficult (Bramwell and Pinedo, 1979). In humans it has been shown that the location, that is, proximal or distal (Simon et al., 1979), the histologic grade (Bramwell and Pinedo, 1979; Simon et al., 1979; Sears et al., 1980), the adequacy and type of initial surgical procedure (Simon et al., 1979), and the size of the primary tumor (Bramwell and Pinedo, 1979; Sears et al., 1980) affect the

prognosis more than histologic subtype. In agreement with this is one veterinary report of fibrous connective tissue sarcomas (Bostock and Dye, 1980), in which the mitotic index was found to affect prognosis. Adequate staging systems in veterinary medicine must include tumor, node, metastasis (TNM) classification, tumor grade, tumor size, and location as well as histologic subtype.

The goals of treatment of solid tumors are to determine the extent of disease and to treat as adequately as possible to prevent recurrence or metastasis. Surgical excision remains the most effective treatment, and other therapies, alone or in combination, are often given empirically. Surgery must be extensive and may involve removing muscles from their origin to their insertion and/or removing entire fascial sheaths. Amputation is often done in preference to excision.

The use of chemotherapy shows promising results in humans and awaits randomized trials in dogs and

Table 1. *Drugs Used to Treat Solid Tumors in Dogs and Cats*

Drug	Suggested Dosages
Plant Alkaloids	
Vincristine (Oncovin, Eli Lilly), 1- and 5-mg vials	0.5 mg/m² weekly or biweekly, IV 0.0125–0.025 mg/kg weekly, IV
Vinblastine (Velban, Eli Lilly), 10-mg vials	2 mg/m² weekly or biweekly, IV 0.05–0.1 mg/kg every 7 to 10 days, IV
Antimetabolites	
Methotrexate (Lederle Labs), 2.5-mg tablets, 5- and 10-mg vials	0.06 mg/kg daily, per os (may vomit) 2.5 mg/m² daily, per os (may vomit) 5–10 mg/m² once per day × 4 days weekly, per os or IV 0.3–0.8 mg/kg weekly, IV 15 mg/m² for dogs ≤15 kg or 20 mg/m² for dogs ≥16 kg IV every 3 weeks in combination therapy
5-Fluorouracil (Roche Labs), 500-mg vials	DO NOT USE IN CATS 100–200 mg/m² weekly, IV 2–5 mg/kg weekly, IV
Alkylating Agents	
Cyclophosphamide (Cytoxan, Mead Johnson), 25- and 50-mg tablets; 100-, 200- and 500-mg vials	50 mg/m² once per day × 3 to 4 days, weekly, IV or per os 10 mg/kg every 7 to 10 days, IV 200 mg/m² or 10 mg/kg, every 3 weeks, IV, in combination therapy
n,n',n'' Triethylenethiophosphoramide (thio-TEPA, Lederle Labs), 15-mg vials	9 mg/m² as single dose or as 2 to 4 divided doses on successive days, IV or intracavitary 0.2–0.5 mg/m² as single dose repeated weekly, IV or intracavitary 0.2–0.5 mg/kg daily × 5 or 10 days, repeat every 3 weeks
Antibiotics	
Actinomycin D (Cosmegan, Merck, Sharp, and Dohme), 500-µg vials	0.015 mg/kg every 3 to 5 days, IV, wait 3 weeks for marrow recovery 1.5 mg/m² once weekly
Doxorubicin hydrochloride (Adriamycin, Adria Labs), 10- and 50-mg vials	30 mg/m² every 21 days, IV, maximum cumulative dose 300 mg/m², dose every 5 weeks in cats
Bleomycin (Blenoxane, Bristol Labs), 15 units/vial	10 mg/m² once per day × 3 to 4 days, IV or SQ, repeat weekly, maximum cumulative dosage 200 mg/m² 0.3–0.5 units/kg weekly, IM
Hormones	
Adrenal corticosteroids (prednisone)	0.5–1.0 mg/lb divided b.i.d., per os 10–40 mg/m² daily, per os, gradually change to 10–20 mg/m² every 2 days 30 mg/m² once per day, per os, decreasing weekly
Miscellaneous	
Dacarbazine (DTIC, Dome Labs), 100- and 200-mg vials	100 mg/m² IV, days 1 to 5 every 3 weeks in combination therapy 200 mg/m² × 5 days every 3 weeks, IV 300 mg/m² IV, every 3 weeks

Table 2. *Chemotherapy Protocols for Soft Tissue Sarcomas*

Institution	Protocol
The Animal Medical Center*	Adriamycin: 30 mg/m² IV every 3 weeks DTIC: 100 mg/m² IV, days 1 to 5; repeat every 3 weeks
University of Pennsylvania†	Day 1: vincristine sulfate, 0.03 mg/kg IV Adriamycin, 30 mg/m² IV (20 mg/m² in cats) Days 3 to 6: cyclophosphamide, 100 mg/m² once per day, per os
Michigan State University‡	Vincristine sulfate: 0.5 mg/m² IV, day 1 NaHCO₃ in D₅W: 2 mEq/kg in 250 to 500 cc infused over 1 hour Methotrexate: 15 mg/m² IV, 30 minutes after vincristine Cyclophosphamide: 50 mg/m² per os, days 2 to 5 Repeat every 14 days for 12 weeks. Then switch to every 21 days for 12 weeks.
Purdue University§	Adriamycin: 30 mg/m², days 1/21 If cost prohibitive, use vincristine sulfate at 0.5 mg/m², days 1/7 as substitute for Adriamycin If partial response, add in cyclophosphamide at 50 mg/m² per os, days 4 to 7/7 If no response, use DTIC at 200 mg/m² IV, days 1 to 5/21 for cyclophosphamide

*Courtesy of Dr. E. G. MacEwen, Head, Donaldson-Atwood Cancer Clinic, The Animal Medical Center, 510 East 62nd Street, New York, New York 10021.
†Courtesy of Dr. A. Jeglum, Associate in Oncology, Department of Clinical Studies, School of Veterinary Medicine, University of Pennsylvania, Philadelphia, Pennsylvania 19104.
‡Courtesy of Dr. S. E. Crow, Assistant Professor, Department of Small Animal Surgery and Medicine, Michigan State University College of Veterinary Medicine, East Lansing, Michigan 48824.
§Courtesy of Dr. R. C. Richardson, Associate Professor, Department of Small Animal Clinics, Purdue University School of Veterinary Medicine, West Lafayette, Indiana 47907.

cats. Chemotherapeutic drugs used in humans include doxorubicin (Adriamycin), cyclophosphamide, dacarbazine (DTIC), vincristine, dactinomycin, mitomycin, actinomycin D, phenylalanine mustard, and chlorambucil (Leukeran) (Morton, 1974; Wilbur, 1975). The combination of cyclophosphamide, dacarbazine, vincristine, and doxorubicin has been shown to be one of the most effective combination chemotherapy approaches in the treatment of sarcomas (Bramwell and Pinedo, 1979; Yap et al., 1980). Additional drugs used in the treatment of patients with carcinomas include methyl-CCNU and bleomycin (Livingston et al., 1975).

The chemotherapeutic agents currently under evaluation in veterinary medicine for the treatment of solid tumors are summarized in Table 1 (MacEwen, 1980; Madewell and Thielen, 1979; Hess, 1977; Hess et al. 1976). The drugs can be used singly or in combination. Dosage schedules that have been used are listed to serve as a guideline for those persons interested in treating these tumor types.

Table 3. *Chemotherapy Protocols for Carcinomas*

Institution	Protocol
The Animal Medical Center*	Adriamycin: 30 mg/m² IV, every 3 weeks Cyclophosphamide: 75 to 100 mg/m², days 3 to 6, per os, every 3 weeks (every 5 weeks in cats)
Michigan State University†	5-Fluorouracil: 200 mg/m² IV once weekly × 6 weeks; then every 2 weeks × 18 weeks Cyclophosphamide: 50 mg/m² per os × 4 days for 6 weeks; then, × 4 days every other week for 18 weeks
University of California‡	5-Fluorouracil: 150 mg/m² IV, day 1 of weeks 1 to 5 Cyclophosphamide: 50 mg/m² per os, days 2 to 5 of weeks 1 to 5 No therapy on week 6. Then repeat cycle.
Purdue University§	Cyclophosphamide: 50 mg/m², days 4 to 7/7

*Courtesy of Dr. E. G. MacEwen, Head, Donaldson-Atwood Cancer Clinic, The Animal Medical Center, 510 East 62nd Street, New York, New York 10021.
†Courtesy of Dr. S. E. Crow, Assistant Professor, Department of Small Animal Surgery and Medicine, Michigan State University College of Veterinary Medicine, East Lansing, Michigan 48824.
‡Courtesy of Dr. G. H. Theilen, Department of Surgery, University of California, Davis School of Veterinary Medicine, Davis, California 95616.
§Courtesy of Dr. R. C. Richardson, Associate Professor, Department of Small Animal Clinics, Purdue University School of Veterinary Medicine, West Lafayette, Indiana 47907.

Protocols used to treat dogs and cats with solid tumors vary among veterinary institutions (Tables 2 and 3). No results have been published to date, but the dosage schedules can serve as guidelines for the practitioner treating an animal with an appropriate tumor type. Dosages are given in either kg or m². Conversion tables are available in standard texts. Toxicities associated with the various drugs are also well recognized and can be found in the references cited at the end of this article.

Randomized trials in the treatment of malignant tumors involve prospective design, control of as many variables as possible, unbiased assignment to a treatment group, and complete follow-up. By definition, these are difficult to accomplish in a clinical setting and involve a follow-up period of many months for dogs and cats. Most of the trials that have been reported are retrospective analyses of case materials.

Classification and results of therapy have been reported for 23 cats with soft tissue sarcomas (Brown et al., 1978). Results showed that radical excision was the most effective treatment modality. Results of chemotherapy and immunotherapy were inconclusive. In a second study, 13 cats with nonresectable solid tumors were evaluated as to their response to combined modality therapy (Brown et al., 1980). After biopsy or partial excision, all cats received mixed bacterial vaccine, cyclophosphamide, vincristine, and methotrexate. Eight cats (61 per cent) had a measurable reduction in tumor volume. More clinical trials are necessary to compare and evaluate therapeutic efficacies.

Ancillary therapy involves general medical care and treatment of any illness associated with the primary tumor as well as concurrent disease, if present. Frequent blood screens and radiographs are necessary to monitor progression of the disease and response to therapy. Complications include debilitation from the primary tumor or its metastatic foci, the development of paraneoplastic syndromes, and failure of organ systems as a result of advancing age, the tumor, or the treatment. Appropriate therapy must be instituted as necessary.

The treatment of solid tumors represents a relatively unexplored area in veterinary medicine. In animals with lymphomas and leukemias, protocols are designed for induction and maintenance. In animals with solid tumors, protocols are still being investigated for inducing remission. In the treatment of soft tissue sarcomas in humans, surgical excision remains the only curative treatment, with response rates of 40 to 50 per cent after various polychemotherapies (Beretta et al., 1980). Results of treatment of soft tissue sarcomas and other solid tumors in veterinary medicine do not compare with these figures. Additional trials are warranted to evaluate the relevance of various treatment regimens. Additional and as yet totally unexplored areas include irradiation of cancer foci before surgical closure, preoperative chemotherapy, evaluation and treatment of steroid receptors, and hyperthermic perfusion. As veterinary oncology advances, the benefits of combined modality therapy as well as the relevance of other, more experimental, approaches in the treatment of solid tumors will be determined.

REFERENCES AND SUPPLEMENTAL READING

Beretta, G., Fraschini, P., and Tedeschi, L.: Chemotherapy of soft tissue sarcomas. Oncology 37:92, 1980.

Bostock, D. E., and Dye, M. T.: Prognosis after surgical excision of canine fibrous connective tissue sarcomas. Vet. Pathol. 17:581, 1980.

Bramwell, V. H. C., and Pinedo, H. M.: Bone and soft tissue sarcomas. In Pinedo, H. M. (ed.): *Cancer Chemotherapy 1979*. New York: Elsevier/North Holland, Inc., 1979.

Brown, N. O., Hayes, A. H., Mooney, S., et al.: Combined modality therapy in the treatment of solid tumors in cats. J. Am. Anim. Hosp. Assoc. 16:719, 1980.

Brown, N. O., Patnaik, A. K., Mooney, S., et al.: Soft tissue sarcomas in the cat. J.A.V.M.A. 173:744, 1978.

Dorn, C. R.: Epidemiology of canine and feline tumors. J. Am. Anim. Hosp. Assoc. 12:307, 1976.

Hess, P. W.: Principles of cancer chemotherapy. Vet. Clin. North Am. 7:21, 1977.

Hess, P. W., MacEwen, E. G., and McClelland, A. J.: Chemotherapy of canine and feline tumors. J. Am. Anim. Hosp. Assoc. 12:350, 1976.

Livingston, R. B., Einhorn, L. H., Bodey, G. P., et al.: COMB (cyclophosphamide, Oncovin, Methyl-CCNU, and Bleomycin): A four-drug combination in solid tumors. Cancer 36:327, 1975.

MacEwen, E. G.: Cancer chemotherapy. In Kirk, R. W. (ed.): *Current Veterinary Therapy VII*. Philadelphia: W. B. Saunders Co., 1980.

Madewell, B. R., and Thielen, G. H.: Chemotherapy. In Thielen, G. H., and Madewell, B. R. (eds.): *Veterinary Cancer Medicine*. Philadelphia: Lea & Febiger, 1979.

Morton, D. L.: Soft tissue sarcomas. In Holland, J. F., and Frei, E. (eds.): *Cancer Medicine*. Philadelphia: Lea & Febiger, 1974.

Sears, H. F., Hopson, R., Inouye, W., et al.: Analysis of staging and management of patients with sarcoma: A ten-year experience. Ann. Surg. 191:488, 1980.

Simon, M. A., Spanier, S. S., and Enneking, W. F.: Management of adult soft tissue sarcomas of the extremities. Surg. Ann. 11:363, 1979.

Sonntag, R. W., and Brunner, K. W.: The chemotherapy of other solid tumors. In Bagshawe, K. D. (ed.): *Medical Oncology*. London: Blackwell Scientific Publications, 1975.

Wilbur, J. R.: Sarcomas. In Greenspan, E. M. (ed.): *Clinical Cancer Chemotherapy*. New York: Raven Press, 1975.

Yap, B. S., Baker, L. H., Sinkovics, J. C., et al.: Cyclophosphamide, vincristine, Adriamycin, and DTIC (CYVADIC) combination chemotherapy for the treatment of advanced sarcomas. Cancer Treat. Rep. 64:93, 1980.

ADVERSE EFFECTS OF CHEMOTHERAPY

BRUCE R. MADEWELL, V.M.D.

Davis, California

Anticancer chemotherapy (as surgery, radiotherapy, and immunotherapy) is a treatment modality aimed at destroying malignant cells. With solid tumors, surgery and/or radiotherapy is the traditional method used when the tumor is confined to a specific tissue or organ site. Neither modality, however, can be considered curative once disease has metastasized beyond the local region. Chemotherapy is relegated almost exclusively to secondary treatment of solid tumors, i.e., when primary methods of therapy fail. Conversely, in hematologic malignancies—diseases usually disseminated from the very beginning—chemotherapy is the treatment of choice from the onset.

The response of hematologic neoplasms in dogs to chemotherapy has been well established; treated dogs achieve relief from clinical signs and prolonged survival times compared with those not given treatment. Tumors most responsive to chemotherapy include lymphoid and plasmacytoid types, and preliminary data indicate that chemotherapy also has a palliative role in the management of nonlymphocytic leukemias. For leukemias and lymphomas, drugs, dosages, and intervals between dosages of drugs used to induce clinical remission, maintain remission (disease-free interval), and reinduce remission after clinical relapse of signs have been summarized in earlier editions of Current Veterinary Therapy and elsewhere.

Data describing the response of solid tumors to chemotherapy in veterinary medicine are scant; problems encountered in generation of data have included nonuniformity in clinical staging and histologic grading methods, absence of nontreated concurrent (control) animals, ignorance of appropriate drug dosages, and failure to achieve long-term follow-up of animal patients. Nevertheless, chemotherapy has an established role in the palliative management of solid tumors in humans, and has also been used in curative programs adjuvant to surgery or irradiation. We feel that it is only a matter of time before anticancer drug therapy for solid tumors is optimized in veterinary clinical practice.

In addition to their cytotoxic effect, most anticancer drugs by virtue of their mechanism of action are also immunosuppressive. Thus, these drugs are also used in clinical practice for the management of immunologically mediated diseases such as autoimmune hemolytic anemia, immunologically mediated thrombocytopenia, systemic lupus erythematosus, rheumatoid arthritis, pemphigus, and others.

The purposes of this article are to review the adverse effects and complications of anticancer chemotherapy and to offer methods of management for those untoward effects. Drugs reviewed include those that have been used in veterinary settings, some of which have had considerable toxicologic evaluation in normal beagles. The drug toxicities are categorized (Table 1) and discussed individually.

ALLERGIC REACTION

The occurrence of hypersensitivity reactions after administration of some drugs, such as antimicrobial agents, is a well-recognized phenomenon. Several cytotoxic drugs have been reported to cause allergic problems, and certain drugs, such as L-asparaginase, cause such reactions with considerable frequency. Because L-asparaginase is a parenterally administered polypeptide, one would anticipate that it would be immunogenic. Signs of L-asparaginase hypersensitivity include urticaria, agitation, abdominal cramps with vomiting and diarrhea, dyspnea, hypotension, pruritus, and loss of consciousness. Most animals recover after cessation of the drug therapy and treatment with epinephrine and a glucocorticoid. Veterinarians must be prepared to deal

Table 1. *Adverse Effects of Chemotherapy*

Allergic reactions
Alopecia
Bone marrow toxicity
Cardiac toxicity
CNS toxicity
Coagulation defects
Cystitis
Dermatologic toxicity
Endocrine-metabolic toxicity
Gastrointestinal toxicity
Hepatic toxicity
Immune suppression
Pancreatitis
Peripheral neuropathy
Pulmonary toxicity
Renal toxicity

419

with anaphylactic reactions and shock whenever this agent is used, particularly if the drug has been given repeatedly. The problem is minimized if the drug is used in combination with a corticosteroid. Also, intraperitoneal or intramuscular administration as opposed to intravenous administration appears to decrease the likelihood of acute allergic reactions.

Adriamycin-induced allergic reactions have also been reported in dogs. Dogs react with cutaneous hyperemia, head shaking, and vomiting immediately after adriamycin injection. Treatment for allergic reactions is similar to that for reactions caused by L-asparaginase. Another reaction associated with adriamycin is the so-called flare or localized urticaria in the area of drug injection. It is characterized by erythematous areas along the course of the vein, which develop soon after the drug is given. The reaction may be histamine mediated, for it has been shown that adriamycin administration can increase serum histamine levels in dogs. Premedication with corticosteroid and antihistamine is useful in preventing repeat episodes.

Less frequently encountered drug-induced allergic reactions are associated with bleomycin, cytosine arabinoside, and procarbazine.

ALOPECIA

The hair follicle has rapid metabolic and mitotic activities. Many of the antimitotic agents used in cancer chemotherapy reduce or arrest both activities, resulting in hair loss. Epilation begins within one month after chemotherapy is instituted and is most severe in dogs with continuously growing haircoats such as poodles and Kerry blue terriers. Hair regrowth starts within one to three months after the course of therapy is completed. Chemotherapeutic agents most likely to cause alopecia include cyclophosphamide, methotrexate, 5-fluorouracil, vincristine, vinblastine, adriamycin, the nitrosurea drugs, and imidazole carboxamide.

BONE MARROW TOXICITY

Hematopoietic toxicosis is the most common adverse effect of anticancer chemotherapy. Aregenerative states are characterized by bone marrow hypoplasia of myeloid and erythroid cell lines. Because most chemotherapeutic agents act on rapidly dividing cells, those cells having long life spans (erythrocytes) often will not decrease in numbers in blood, whereas those with short life spans (granulocytes, platelets) will decrease rapidly. Thus it may be erroneous to attribute anemia to chemotherapy if platelet and leukocyte counts are normal. However, anticancer drugs such as nitrosureas and alkylating agents, which act primarily on stem cell components of marrow, may cause anemia without leukopenia and thrombocytopenia.

A major cause of morbidity and death in cancer patients is infection, attributed at least in part to myelosuppression. Neutropenia is associated with a high risk of infection. In humans, and presumably in animals, the risk of infection correlates inversely with the neutrophil count, and serious infections are likely to ensue when the count falls below 1000/µl. For animals, temporary cessation of drug administration is advised when neutrophil counts fall below 2500/µl.

Virtually all of the anticancer drugs cause myelosuppression. Notable exceptions are the glucocorticoids, and only minimal myelosuppression has been attributed to vincristine, L-asparaginase, and bleomycin.

CARDIAC TOXICITY

Adriamycin has shown considerable clinical promise in the treatment of solid, slow-growing tumors, but cardiotoxicity is a serious complication of therapy. Serious toxicities in the form of a dose-dependent congestive cardiomyopathy and non dose-dependent dysrhythmias are well known in humans and have been described in dogs. Dysrhythmias include atrioventricular dissociation, ventricular tachycardia, atrial fibrillation, and second degree A-V block, and there is evidence that ventricular dysrhythmias may antedate cardiomyopathy. Therapy calls for discontinuation of the drug, but congestive heart failure nonresponsive to digitalis may ensue if cardiomyopathy is severe. M-mode echocardiography to evaluate left ventricular contractility may be a useful method to detect adriamycin cardiotoxicity before the appearance of overt congestive heart failure.

CNS TOXICITY

Numerous antineoplastic drugs have neurologic side effects in human cancer patients, but few of these syndromes are described in veterinary practice. Cerebellar dysfunctions have been induced in dogs and cats using the antimetabolite drug 5-fluorouracil. Signs included dementia, agitation, tremors, and ataxia, followed later in some dogs by opisthotonus, tonic-clonic seizures, and death. In most cases, however, cerebellar signs induced by 5-FU are transitory and disappear after treatment is discontinued. Owing to its severe neurotoxicity in cats, 5-FU is contraindicated in this species.

COAGULATION DEFECTS

Coagulation abnormalities frequently complicate neoplastic disease. Serious defects, including disseminated intravascular coagulation, may result upon entrance of foreign material into the circulation or exposure of abnormal vascular surfaces.

Rapid cell destruction in leukemias from intensive chemotherapy has been incriminated as a precipitating factor of disseminated intravascular coagulation. Also, a specific toxicity of L-asparaginase is coagulation abnormality, characterized by low fibrinogen levels and prolonged thrombi, prothrombin, and partial thromboplastin times. Bleeding may also occur secondary to drug-induced thrombocytopenia.

Cystitis

Cyclophosphamide is excreted in feces and urine. In the urinary bladder, activated metabolites of cyclophosphamide may cause ulceration of the mucosa, hemorrhage and edema in all tissues, and necrosis of smooth muscle and small arteries. Urinary bladder complications that have been reported with use of cyclophosphamide include acute hemorrhagic cystitis, chronic cystitis, urine cytologic abnormalities, interstitial fibrosis, and transitional cell carcinoma.

When using cyclophosphamide, an adequate fluid intake must be maintained and urinary tract infections treated promptly. Acute hemorrhagic cystitis may be managed palliatively by the intravesical instillation of dilute (1 per cent) formalin solution.

Dermatologic toxicity

Several of the anticancer drugs are so cytotoxic that they destroy cells on contact in confined areas. These drugs include adriamycin, actinomycin D, vincristine, and vinblastine. Localized cellulitis follows extravasation of drugs into subcutaneous tissues from intravenous sites. The reaction presents as regional phlebitis with pain, redness, and swelling of the overlying skin and evolves into desquamation, necrosis, and slough. The tissues often become secondarily infected. Drugs must be injected carefully (best into the tubing of an intravenous infusion set) to avoid infiltration of perivascular spaces. Although there are no specific antidotes to prevent cellulitis should extravasation occur, several measures have been empirically employed to decrease the severity of the local reaction. When an extravasation is noted, the injection should be stopped immediately, but the needle should not be removed. With the needle still in place, withdraw 3 to 5 ml of blood to remove some of the drug. Using a 27-gauge needle and tuberculin syringe, aspirate the bleb to withdraw as much of the remaining solution as possible. Instill an appropriate antidote (i.e., for adriamycin, use sodium bicarbonate 8.4 per cent [5 ml] and dexamethasone 4 mg/ml [2 ml]; for vincristine or vinblastine, use sodium bicarbonate as previously mentioned and/or hyaluronidase 150 μ/ml [1 ml]). Following these meas-

ures, remove the butterfly needle and apply warm compresses at the extravasation site for 60 minutes. As an alternative to dexamethasone, give hydrocortisone (25 to 50 mg) locally.

A serious complication of drug extravasation is deep ulceration causing exposure of underlying structures such as tendons or bone. These ulcers are indolent and neither develop a granulation tissue response nor epithelialize; surgical excision and skin grafting may be required for healing if the animal has a life expectancy that justifies the procedure.

Hyperpigmentation may occur following chemotherapy. Adriamycin is reported to cause an increase in melanin pigmentation in dogs following chronic (four to six weeks) administration. Other agents associated with hyperpigmentation in humans, and possibly in animals, include busulphan, cyclophosphamide, methotrexate, and bleomycin.

Other dermatologic effects of chemotherapy are petechiae and ecchymoses from thrombocytopenia associated with myelosuppression and cutaneous infections attributed to myelosuppression and immunosuppression.

Endocrine-metabolic toxicity

The use of hormonal agents for treatment of tumors derived from endocrine-dependent tissues may cause endocrine abnormalities, most notably, Cushing's syndrome and feminization from glucocorticoids and estrogenic steroids, respectively. Metabolic effects of estrogenic steroids include hypercalcemia and fluid retention. A syndrome of inappropriate secretion of antidiuretic hormone and clinical signs of water intoxication has been described in association with cyclophosphamide and vincristine use, and there is evidence that cyclophosphamide may alter insulin requirements in diabetic patients. Although these syndromes were described in human patients receiving chemotherapy, there is preliminary evidence of similar adverse effects in dogs.

Gastrointestinal toxicity

The most frequent toxicity of antitumor agents as a class is related to their primary action on rapidly dividing tissues. Thus, gastrointestinal toxicities, including vomiting and diarrhea, are common side effects of many antineoplastic agents. Vomiting may follow oral or intravenous administration of drugs, suggesting a centrally mediated response. When severe signs of vomiting or diarrhea appear, treatment should be discontinued temporarily. If the drug is continued, extensive ulcerations develop in the esophagus, small intestine, and colon, and sepsis may ensue.

HEPATIC TOXICITY

Hepatotoxic drugs include methotrexate, 6-mercaptopurine, cytosine arabinoside, L-asparaginase, and imidazole carboxamide. Long-term use of high doses of glucocorticoids consistently induces hepatopathy; the severity of liver disease can be mitigated by alternate-day administration of the drug. Pre-existing hepatic disease may preclude use of hepatotoxic anticancer drugs. Adriamycin is primarily metabolized in the liver, and its metabolites are excreted in the bile. Animals with elevated serum bilirubin levels circulate the drug for prolonged periods, which augments its toxicity. Also, cyclophosphamide requires conversion to its metabolically active metabolites by the liver, necessitating adequate liver function for effective utilization of this alkylating agent.

IMMUNE SUPPRESSION

Oncologists are using drugs identical or analogous to immunosuppressive drugs, and anticancer chemotherapy can effect an immunosuppressive influence. Methods of discontinuous or fractionated courses of therapy, in contrast to continuous application, decrease the immunologic impairments. Nevertheless, in some animal cancer patients, immunosuppression in concert with drug-induced leukopenia favors superinfection. Specific anti-infectious therapy is used when the etiologic agent is known. For cancer patients with neutropenia and fever, infection is suspect, and treatment may be given empirically based on clinical considerations and corrected after return of further laboratory results. Broad spectrum cytocidal antibiotics are used, such as aminoglycosides, penicillins, and their derivatives.

PANCREATITIS

Corticosteroids can induce clinical pancreatitis in dogs, most often when the dose exceeds one milligram per pound of body weight. L-Asparaginase has also been incriminated as a cause for pancreatitis in man.

PERIPHERAL NEUROPATHY

Neurotoxicity is a side effect of vincristine; vincristine does not cross the blood-brain barrier, and its toxicity is usually limited to peripheral nerves. Vincristine blocks the formation of neurofilaments, disrupts those already formed, and impairs axoplasmic transport. Clinically, vincristine neurotoxicity is manifested by decreased sensory and motor function, usually involving extremities. Vincristine-induced neuropathy is slowly reversible after drug discontinuation.

PULMONARY TOXICITY

Administration of a number of cytotoxic agents has been associated with interstitial pneumonitis, alveolitis, and pulmonary fibrosis. Bleomycin, busulphan, and methotrexate are the commonest cytotoxic drugs to cause interstitial pneumonitis in man. Clinical signs include cough, dyspnea, and, at times, low-grade fever. Although lung damage from cytotoxic drugs has not been described in veterinary clinical settings, many of the drug-toxicity studies for the aforementioned drugs were done in dogs, and the dog is particularly susceptible to bleomycin-induced lung disease. Awareness of this complication may reduce severe morbidity in clinical practice.

RENAL TOXICITY

Methotrexate is excreted principally by the kidneys, and its use in the presence of impaired renal function may result in the accumulation of toxic amounts of drugs and additional renal damage. The animal's renal status should be monitored prior to and during methotrexate therapy.

Adriamycin has been associated with nephrosis in dogs, but to date there is no evidence of consistent adriamycin nephrotoxicity. Streptozotocin, an antitumor antibiotic that causes destruction of pancreatic beta cells, has been used in humans for the treatment of pancreatic islet cell carcinomas. Severe renal tubular damage followed use of streptozotocin in several dogs, and nephrotoxicosis appears to preclude its clinical use.

SUMMARY

The aim of optimum anticancer chemotherapy is to give drugs at appropriate dosages and intervals to reduce the number of tumor cells to zero (theoretically) without host toxicity. In practice, however, anticancer drugs are generally used for palliation rather than cure, and because of the nonspecificity of drugs used, some normal tissue damage occurs. Awareness of drug toxicities, however, as well as specific and supportive measures may minimize these adverse reactions. For example, the cytotoxicity of methotrexate has long been known to be reversible with leucovorin. Adequate hydration and renal function will decrease the risk for methotrexate toxicity and cyclophosphamide-induced hemorrhagic cystitis. The rational use of drugs in combination is based in part on selection of agents with different dose-limiting toxicities. A fractionated course rather than a continuous course of chemotherapy will minimize immunosuppression and risk of superinfection. Simultaneous use of synergistic treatment methods such as irradiation or hyperthermia may enhance tumor cell death and decrease the risk for drug toxicity through use of lower dosages of drugs.

Until cancer-specific drugs are developed, clinicians will use less specific agents to provide palliation from suffering and useful prolongation of life, i.e., use the best methods of treatment that are currently available. Although drug toxicity is real, judicious use of drugs and knowledge of their adverse effects will optimize patient care.

SUPPLEMENTAL READING

Armstrong, U., Hoerni, B., Lacut, J. Y., and Durand, M.: *Opportunistic Infections in Cancer Patients*. New York: Masson Publishing, 1978.

Carter, S. K., Bakowski, M. T., and Hellmann, K.: *Chemotherapy of Cancer*. New York: John Wiley and Sons, 1977.

Collis, C. H.: Lung damage from cytotoxic drugs. Cancer Chemother. Pharmacol. 4:17, 1980.

Dreizen, S., Bodey, G. B., and Rodriquez, V.: Oral complications of cancer chemotherapy. Postgrad. Med. 58:75, 1975.

Dreizen, S., Bodey, G. P., Rodriquez, V., and McCredie, K. B.: Cutaneous complications of cancer chemotherapy. Postgrad. Med. 58:150, 1975.

Hildebrand, J.: Neurotoxic effects of drugs used in cancer chemotherapy. In Hildebrand, J. (ed.): *Lesions of the Nervous System in Cancer Patients*. New York: Raven Press, 1978.

Ignoffo, R. J., and Friedman, M. A.: Therapy of local toxicities caused by extravasation of cancer chemotherapeutic agents. Cancer Treat. Rev. 7:17, 1980.

MacEwen, E. G.: Cancer chemotherapy. In Kirk, R. W. (ed.): *Current Veterinary Therapy VII*. Philadelphia: W. B. Saunders Co., 1980.

Madewell, B. R., and Theilen, G. H.: Chemotherapy. In Theilen, G. H., and Madewell, B. R. (eds.): *Veterinary Cancer Medicine*. Philadelphia: Lea & Feiger, 1979.

Van Vleet, J. F., and Ferrans, V. J.: Clinical observations, cutaneous lesions, and hematologic alterations in chronic adriamycin intoxication in dogs with and without vitamin E and selenium supplementation. Am. J. Vet. Res. 40:691, 1980.

Weiss, R. B., and Bruno, S.: Hypersensitivity reactions to cancer chemotherapeutic agents. Ann. Intern. Med. 94:66, 1981.

Weller, R. E.: Intravesical instillation of dilute formalin for treatment of cyclophosphamide-induced hemorrhagic cystitis in two dogs. J.A.V.M.A. 172:1206, 1978.

HYPERTHERMIA — AN OLD CANCER THERAPY REVISITED*

RALPH C. RICHARDSON, D.V.M.

West Lafayette, Indiana

One physical modality of cancer therapy not commonly utilized in veterinary medical oncology is hyperthermia. The term "hyperthermia," as utilized in cancer management, refers to tissue temperatures between pyrexia (41.1°C) and cautery. Most effective therapeutic temperatures are between 42 and 50°C. Hyperthermia has been used since before 2000 BC, when red-hot irons were applied to fungating growths and palliative remissions were observed. In the early 1900s antitumor effects of hyperthermia were demonstrated by the deliberate infection of human patients with erysipelas and later with the injection of patients with bacterial toxins to induce fever. Local hyperthermia was subsequently attempted, but interest declined because application of heat was (and still is) technically difficult. In the 1970s and early 1980s hyperthermia was reinvestigated, and today there is a significant amount of knowledge about the application of hyperthermia to treat cancer.

Little doubt exists that hyperthermia is more damaging to tumors than to normal tissues. Tumor cells in culture, experimental tumors, and spontaneous tumors are consistently killed at temperatures 1 to 1.5°C lower than their normal counterparts. Such selective thermosensitivity seems to be most evident at 42 to 44°C. At temperatures of 45°C or higher, the threshold of thermal pain in man, the differential sensitivity between tumor and normal tissue is lost as changes take place within both tumor and normal cells. Heat destroys tissue by coagulation necrosis and vascular thrombosis and possibly by inducing immune response. Normal cellular enzyme systems are disrupted, and lysosomal membranes become more permeable. Such changes are most profound in a hypoxic, acidotic, poorly nourished environment. Heating times required to produce such irreversible changes vary with the temperature. Some tumors heated to 42°C require more than 30 hours to produce thermal death, whereas only minutes of heating are necessary at 50°C for death to occur. Surface tumors generally slough in response to adequate heating. Deep tumors of humans are reported to undergo replacement with fibrous tissue even though the tumors might appear unchanged in size.

One important reason for the selective heat sensitivity of tumors is that they are poorly vascularized compared with the surrounding normal tissue. They

*Supported in part through the Purdue Comparative Oncology Program and the Showalter Trust, Indianapolis, IN.

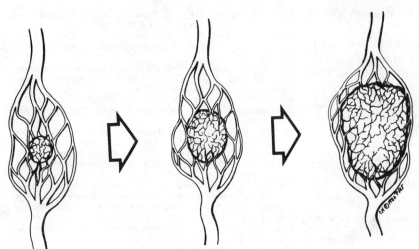

Figure 1. Tumor growth begins in preformed vascular beds. The tumor pushes the vessels away and develops primitive capillaries within the center of the tumor, which have sluggish blood flow and are nonresponsive to vasoactive drugs. (Drawing by Veterinary Medical Illustration, School of Veterinary Medicine, Purdue University, Lafayette, Indiana. Reprinted with permission.)

cannot eliminate heat as well as normal tissues by blood perfusion, nor can they tolerate heat stress, which increases oxygen demand. Blood vessels in normal tissue are laid down during embryologic development. Cancer begins in tissue supplied by preformed blood vessels and usually grows away from a vascular supply. Angiogenesis does occur in tumor masses; however, new capillaries are formed in a random manner so that blood flows as if through sinuses rather than through normal capillaries. Total blood flow through tumors is therefore very sluggish (Fig. 1), and transport of heat away from the center of a tumor is compromised. Another reason for the lack of blood flow through the center of a heated tumor is that normal capillaries around the periphery of a tumor dilate in response to applied heat and shunt blood away from the tumor parenchyma. However, primitive tumor capillaries do not dilate under the influence of heat because they lack the smooth muscle in their walls that is necessary for vasomotor activity. A slight cooling effect may even be noted on the periphery of a heated tumor owing to increased blood flow through normal capillaries.

WHOLE BODY VERSUS LOCAL HYPERTHERMIA

Clinical applications of hyperthermia fall into two broad categories: whole body hyperthermia and localized hyperthermia. During whole body hyperthermia patients are maintained with a core body temperature of 41.8 to 42°C. Therapeutic temperatures are produced by reducing heat losses and introducing thermal energy. Techniques utilized include wax baths, hot air cabinets, water blankets, space suits, and extracorporeal heat exchange. In humans, complications including fatigue, extremity edema, diarrhea, nausea and vomiting, and respiratory depression have been observed. Sudden myelopathy secondary to whole body hyperthermia after spinal cord irradiation has also been reported.

Laboratory abnormalities include hypocalcemia, hypophosphatemia, hyperglycemia, and elevated LDH and SGOT levels. The heart and liver seem to be the organs most easily damaged by whole body hyperthermia. Nevertheless, objective tumor remission has been observed in a significant number of patients. Very little information is available regarding whole body hyperthermia in veterinary medicine. Dogs with osteogenic sarcoma that were treated with whole body hyperthermia failed to live longer compared with dogs treated with amputation alone. However, atypical metastatic patterns were noted.

Local hyperthermia offers a wide range of treatment possibilities without the morbidity of whole body hyperthermia. When local hyperthermia is utilized, tissue temperatures above 45°C are easily achieved. Heating techniques are intended to selectively elevate tumor temperature while sparing normal surrounding tissue. Care must still be taken to preclude raising body core temperatures above 42°C. Local heating methods that have the greatest promise of clinical application involve acoustic waves (therapeutic intensity ultrasound) or electromagnetic waves (microwaves or radiofrequency waves). Energy transferred into the tissue by focused waves causes oscillation of ions or creates magnetic reorientation of molecules. If local cooling effects are insufficient to carry the generated heat from the area, local hyperthermia occurs.

ULTRASOUND

Ultrasound at 0.5 to 2.0 megahertz (MHz) is more able to be focused than any other wave form used in hyperthermia. The precision of local heat placement is limited by intervening air spaces (e.g., lung, gut) or firm substances (e.g., bone), which reflect the beam. Ultrasound has been useful for treating superficial tumors. Considerable technical expertise is needed to assure good penetration and focusing of acoustic waves to the desired site.

MICROWAVES

Microwaves at 434, 915, and 2,450 MHz provide excellent heating for superficial tumors. The ability to focus the beam is reasonable, and intense local heat (46 to 50°C) may be obtained. Microwave therapy is best suited to superficial tumors. Sloughing routinely occurs at the heated site; however, healing by second intention is uneventful. Antibiotic support is frequently necessary during wound slough periods. Apparent pain is demonstrated while patients are undergoing microwave heating, so chemical restraint is required. Little discomfort is demonstrated following therapy, in fact patients frequently show less discomfort following therapy than before.

RADIOFREQUENCY WAVES

Radiofrequency hyperthermia offers, perhaps, the most effective form of local heating. The two forms of radiofrequency hyperthermia are inductive heating and conductive (dielectric) heating. Wavelengths of 13.56 and 27.12 MHz are most frequently used in inductive or conductive heating to allow deep penetration into tissues. *Inductive heating* generates electric currents only in tissue electrolytes (muscle, blood, and proteinaceous tissue). Fat and air-containing tissues are warmed secondarily by thermal diffusion. Radiofrequency current used in inductive heating flows in a coil that generates a rapidly changing magnetic field near the portion of the body to be heated. The field induces eddy currents in the nearby tissue, which produce resis-

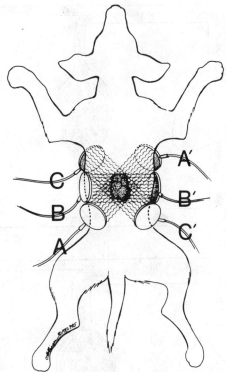

Figure 3. A deep tumor may be heated through sequentially activated skin portals. The tumor receives continuous therapy, whereas each skin contact point is only intermittently heated. (Drawing by Veterinary Medical Illustration, School of Veterinary Medicine, Purdue University, Lafayette, Indiana. Reprinted with permission.)

tive heating. *Conductive heating* involves placing that portion of the body to be heated between two electrodes or capacitor plates. The body acts as a conductor for the radiofrequency current, and heat is generated. Skin cooling techniques must be utilized for such heating because considerable dissipation of energy (heat) occurs during conductive heating as current is forced through the skin.

The focusing of waves to heat a desired portion of the body has been a difficult task. Inductive heating has been focused using two coils arranged as in Figure 2. Such coils, known as Helmholtz coils, produce an approximately uniform alternating magnetic field throughout most of the area between the coils. LeVeen and coworkers (1980) have proposed focusing of conductive heating by sequentially activating multiple electrode pairs, each of which pass waves through the tumor (Fig. 3).

ENHANCEMENT OF THERAPEUTIC EFFECTS

Aggressive local hyperthermia requires selective heating of tumor tissue and protection of normal tissue. Because of the differences between blood vessel development in tumors and normal tissues, vasodilator drugs have been effective in allowing such selective tumor heating. Blood flow through normal tissues is enhanced and flow through tumor tissue is impeded by a shunting action (Fig. 4),

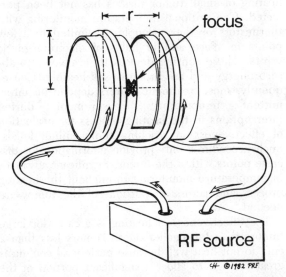

Figure 2. Helmholtz coils allow inductive heating focused in the area between the coils. (Drawing by Veterinary Medical Illustration, School of Veterinary Medicine, Purdue University, Lafayette, Indiana. Reprinted with permission.)

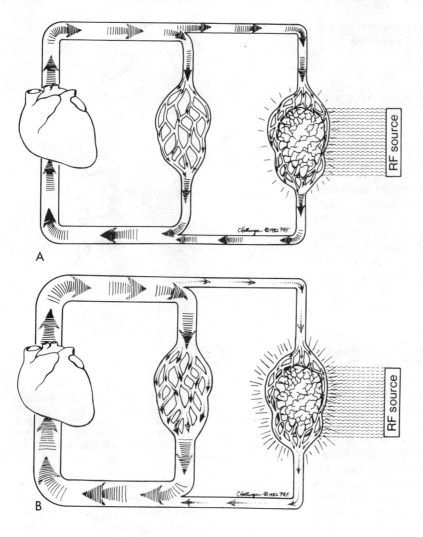

Figure 4. As vasodilator drug causes greater blood flow in normal tissue, blood is shunted away from the tumor, resulting in greater cooling of normal tissue and selective tumor heating. *A*, Normal flow. *B*, Blood flow under the influence of vasodilator drugs. (Drawing by Veterinary Medical Illustration, School of Veterinary Medicine, Purdue University, Lafayette, Indiana. Reprinted with permission.)

since only normal vasculature is responsive to vasodilators. Enhanced cooling of the surrounding normal tissue is achieved through a radiator-like effect. Hydralazine at 0.5 mg/kg IV is very effective in causing increased normal tissue blood flow (Fig. 5) as well as enhanced tumor heating (Fig. 6). We have observed temperature differentials of greater than 10°C in implanted tumors (e.g., transmissible venereal tumors) as well as in spontaneous tumors (e.g., canine hemangiopericytoma, feline fibrosarcoma) during inductive heating after hydralazine pretreatment.

PROBLEMS IN CLINICAL APPLICATION

Instrumentation for generating therapeutic hyperthermia is being developed rapidly. Commercial devices are available, ranging from small hand-held veterinary units to computerized models in sophisticated hyperthermia treatment centers. Despite the fact that treatment units are readily available, two major problems have not been resolved, keeping hyperthermia as an experimental mode of cancer therapy. Accurate temperature monitoring devices

for scanning cross sections or volumes of the treated region have not been developed; and thermistor heating of small tumor masses has not been perfected. Conventional temperature monitoring with thermistors or thermocouples is limited to a few points in space and in fields of electromagnetic waves. These sensing devices themselves also absorb energy and are prone to self-heating. Consequently, most treatment centers depend on intermittent temperature measurement during interruptions in the heating process for evaluation of effectiveness in reaching tumor-killing levels. Such procedures only provide information for discrete points within the tumor. Significant advances in temperature monitoring throughout the heating process and across all portions of the tumor are needed.

The effectiveness of heating is greater for large tumors than for smaller ones. Tumors less than 2 cm³ do not heat well because peripheral cooling is great enough to affect a significant portion of the tumor. Many tumors have a hyperperfused outer shell, an underperfused mantle layer, and a necrotic center. If heat is deposited uniformly in the tumor

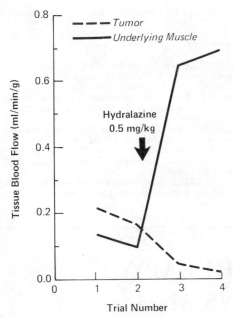

Figure 5. Tissue blood flow in an experimental transmissible venereal tumor and underlying muscle as influenced by hydralazine. Each trial determined blood flow with radioactive microspheres at approximately ten-minute intervals. (Data from Babbs: Med. Instrument. 16:23, 1982.) (Graph by Veterinary Medical Illustration, School of Veterinary Medicine, Purdue University, Lafayette, Indiana. Reprinted with permission.)

and surrounding tissue, the cooling effects of normal blood flow limit the temperature rise within the outer shell, and it may never reach tumor-killing levels. Following heating, some residual viable tumor cells are likely to remain near the periphery of the tumor and must be dealt with by other methods.

COMBINATION THERAPIES

Radiation therapy, chemotherapy, and immunotherapy have been combined with hyperthermia to accomplish total destruction of tumor tissue within the treatment field. Radiation therapy with hyperthermia provides an additive or synergistic effect. When hyperthermia is supplied at a sufficiently low level so that there is little or no observable heat damage (less than 43°C), the effectiveness of radiation, as measured by tumor regression, nearly doubles. As previously noted, hyperthermia is most effective in a hypoxic environment, whereas radiation is most effective in a well-oxygenated setting. Combination therapy may be the solution to killing viable tumor cells resistant to either treatment method alone.

Hyperthermia coupled with chemotherapy may provide enhancement over either mode of therapy alone. Increased membrane permeability induced by heat has stimulated research in this area. *In vitro* data and clinical trials are supportive of continued efforts in this field.

Hyperthermia/immunotherapy is an area of continued investigation. Because heat therapy is immunogenic (rather than immunosuppressive as chemotherapy, radiation therapy, and surgery are), immune stimulants (e.g., BCG) have been used as an adjunct to heat therapy with promising results.

At present, hyperthermia in the treatment of cancer is experimental, and it should not be used in lieu of standard forms of effective therapy. As instrumentation for heating and temperature monitoring improves, there is little doubt that this treatment modality will take an important role in

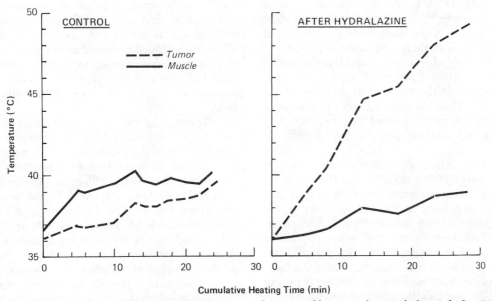

Figure 6. Inductive radiofrequency heating of an experimental transmissible venereal tumor before and after IV hydralazine (0.5 mg/kg). Differences of more than 10°C between normal and tumor tissues are observed. (Data from Babbs: Med. Instrument. 16:23, 1982.) (Graph by Veterinary Medical Illustration, School of Veterinary Medicine, Purdue University, Lafayette, Indiana. Reprinted with permission.)

the management of cancer in both animals and humans.

REFERENCES AND SUPPLEMENTAL READING

Babbs, C. F.: Biology of local heat therapy for cancer. Med. Instrument. 16:23, 1982.

Babbs, C. F., and DeWitt, D. P.: Physical principles of local heat therapy for cancer. Med. Instrument. 15:367, 1981.

Field, S. B., and Bleehen, N. M.: Hyperthermia in the treatment of cancer. Cancer Treat. Rev. 6:63, 1979.

Grier, R L., Brewer, W. G., Paul, S. R., and Theilen, G. H.: Treatment of bovine and equine ocular squamous cell carcinoma by radiofrequency hyperthermia. J.A.V.M.A. 177:55, 1980.

Grier, R. L., Brewer, W. G., and Theilen, G. H.: Hyperthermic treatment of superficial tumors in cats and dogs. J.A.V.M.A. 177:227, 1980.

Kainer, R. A., Stringer, J. M., and Leuker, D. C.: Hyperthermia for treatment of ocular squamous cell tumors in cattle. J.A.V.M.A. 176:356, 1980.

LeVeen, H. H., Obrien, P., and Wallace, K. M.: Radiofrequency thermotherapy for cancer. J. S. C. Med. Assoc. 76:5, 1980.

Ostrow, S., VanEcho, D., Whitacre, M., Aisner, J., Simon, R., and Wiernik, P. H.: Physiologic response and toxicity in patients undergoing whole-body hyperthermia for the treatment of cancer. Cancer Treat. Rep. 65:323, 1981.

Song, C. W., Rhee, J. G., and Levitt, S. H.: Blood flow in normal tissues and tumors during hyperthermia. J.N.C.I. 64:119, 1980.

Storm, F. K., Harrison, W. H., Elliott, R. S., and Morton, D. L.: Hyperthermic therapy for human neoplasms: Thermal death time. Cancer 46:1849, 1980.

Thrall, D. E.: Clinical requirements for localized hyperthermia in the patient. Radiat. Environ. Biophys. 17:229, 1980.

RADIATION THERAPY: APPLICATIONS AND AVAILABILITY

DANIEL A. FEENEY, D.V.M.,
and GARY R. JOHNSTON, D.V.M.
St. Paul, Minnesota

Radiotherapy is the administration of ionizing radiation to a specific location in the body (field) and the absorption of this energy by the normal and neoplastic tissues in the irradiated field. The intracellular target of the ionizing radiation is DNA. The damage to the DNA molecule takes the form of chemical alteration of the purine and pyrimidine bases or breaking of the phosphodiester strands of the DNA helix. With therapeutic doses of radiation, immediate cell death is uncommon, but the potentially lethal damage, if not repaired, becomes evident during one of the subsequent divisions of the irradiated cell. Thus, damage to rapidly proliferating cell systems can be recognized much earlier than damage to cell systems dividing less rapidly or rarely.

Terminology in radiation therapy is potentially confusing, necessitating definition of the terms radiosensitive, radioresponsive, and radiocurable. *Radiosensitive* is defined as the susceptibility of the cells or tissues to the killing effects of absorbed radiation. *Radioresponsive* is the degree to which a normal or neoplastic tissue visibly changes following (or during) a radiotherapy regimen. *Radiocurable* is defined in veterinary medicine as a two-year patient survival following radiotherapy with no further tumor progress and no subsequent metastases. From a clinical standpoint the radiosensitivity of tumors varies considerably and has not been quantitated. However, as defined previously, a tumor may be radiocurable without being radioresponsive. The outcome of radiotherapy must be judged by periodic reassessment of the patient to determine if tumor growth is continuing. A failure to decrease the size of the tumor, during or shortly after the radiation dose regimen is completed, does not constitute a radiotherapy failure provided tumor growth ceases. Connective tissue tumors or tumors with much connective tissue stroma typically respond (if they do respond) much more slowly than epithelial tumors.

In general, the radiation doses administered to treat tumors are limited by the tolerance of the normal tissues in the irradiated field. Simply stated, radiation therapy is most effective for those tumors more susceptible to the killing or sterilizing effect of ionizing radiation than the adjacent normal tissues. Those tumors that do not respond to radiotherapy at dose levels that can be tolerated by the local normal tissues are considered radioresistant. During and for varying periods of time following the administration of radiation, some reaction of the normal tissues is expected. In small animals this frequently involves the skin in the form of epilation, hyperemia, and dry or moist desquamation. The degree of involvement of internal organs, most notably the lung, kidney, and intestine, varies with the type of radiation used and the purpose for the irradiation field in the thoracic and abdominal regions. The results of overtreatment of normal tissues include fibrosis, necrosis, loss of parenchymal function, and possibly patient death, depending on the tissue or organ involved and the volume treated. The differential effects of radiotherapy on tumors (more damaged) versus normal tissues are achieved (if at all) by a variation in the responses of neoplastic and normal cells to the following processes. These are the so-called 4 Rs of radiotherapy and are the reasons why the radiation doses from external beam sources (away from the body) are divided into several treatments (fractions).

Tumors commonly contain varying proportions of poorly oxygenated cells owing to the potential for cell proliferation to exceed the available blood supply. These hypoxic cells are more resistant to radiation effects than are normally oxygenated cells. *Reoxygenation* has the potential to occur during a fractionated radiotherapy regimen owing to the killing of the well-oxygenated cells in close proximity to the blood supply. This affords greater oxygen availability to cells previously hypoxic, thus making them more radiosensitive. Between radiation treatments, sublethal damage is *repaired*, and this process is thought to be more efficient in normal cells than in neoplastic cells. As cells (both normal and neoplastic) die, they are usually replaced, and this *repopulation* is thought to be more readily achieved by normal cells than by neoplastic cells, especially in response to irradiation. The final "R" is *redistribution*, which implies that cells in the mitotic and early synthetic phases of the cell cycle, which are more easily injured by radiation, will be selectively killed. Theoretically this should result in population uniformity within the cell cycle and subsequent fractions could be given at optimal times for maximum effect. However, at present the high variability in and general lack of knowledge of specific tumor cell cycles preclude using cell cycle synchronization and specific fractionation regimens to any clinical advantage.

Failures in radiotherapy are based on evaluation of the whole patient and the purpose for which the patient was treated. If the therapy was intended to be curative, the discovery of metastases as well as local recurrence constitutes a failure. The metastatic potential of a particular tumor should be assessed and a search for macroscopic metastases initiated before the tumor is irradiated. Obviously if the metastatic potential is high, the likelihood of patient cure is low even if localized radiotherapy is successful. Local recurrences or continued growth following radiotherapy may be attributed to three causes. First, recurrence may be due to the presence of the hypoxic, radioresistant tumor cells as discussed previously. Second, the tumor cell type

(i.e., connective tissue) may not have been sensitive to the dose administered. (It is assumed that the dose given was at the level of local normal tissue tolerance.) Finally, an inadequate irradiation field size may have been used, leaving some tumor cells unirradiated. In general, a 2.0-cm field width beyond the clinically detectable tumor mass is used to decrease the likelihood of residual, unirradiated cells.

METHODS OF RADIOTHERAPY

There are three basic methods of radiotherapy, based on the location of the radiation source relative to the patient. These methods are external beam therapy (source at a distance from the patient), brachytherapy (source in or on the patient), and systemic therapy (source administered and distributed throughout the body). External beam therapy and brachytherapy are administered in such a manner as to keep the maximum dose localized as near as possible to the tumor.

External beam therapy is typically given in a multiple treatment (fractionated) protocol. Low- to medium-energy x-radiation (orthovoltage) is the external beam source most often available in veterinary medicine. Orthovoltage, however, has the disadvantage of limited depth penetration, precluding its use on deep-seated (more than 5 to 6 cm) tumors except where multiple fields involving different surface fields can be used to "crossfire" the deep tumor. High-energy x- or gamma-irradiation (supervoltage) is only available on a limited basis in veterinary institutions but can be used to treat deep-seated tumors. External beam supervoltage sources include ^{60}Co, ^{137}Cs, and linear accelerators. High-energy electrons from linear accelerators may be used to treat superficial lesions, but at present only one veterinary institution has such capability.

Treatment schedules for external beam therapy varied among veterinary institutions, but three fractions per week (Monday, Wednesday, Friday) was the most common. The number of fractions ranged from 5 to 15 (most often 10) with a total dose of from 3000 to 6000 rads (most often 3500 to 5000) for neoplasms. However, schedules of one or two fractions per week for five to ten treatments with a total dose of 1500 to 5400 rads were also used for treatment of neoplastic conditions. The treatment of non-neoplastic conditions (i.e., canine lick granulomas) followed the same general pattern except that fewer fractions (usually two to six) with lower total doses (usually 900 to 3000 rads) were utilized. Specifics on the radiotherapy protocols used by each institution must be obtained from the staff radiotherapist, preferably prior to referral.

Brachytherapy is typically given in one prolonged (hours, days, weeks) treatment. Brachytherapy sources (radioisotopes) should be removed and reused if the half-life of the isotope is long or permanently implanted if the half-life is short. Brachytherapy sources are usually in the form of surface applicators, needles, or seeds but may be in suspension for distribution throughout serosal cavities. Specific methods of brachytherapy include interstitial (source within the tumor), pliesotherapy (sources on patient surface), and intracavity (solid source placed through body openings or liquid source instilled into body cavities). Strontium 90 (^{90}Sr) applicators are most commonly used for ophthalmic radiotherapy because the penetration of the beta-radiation is limited to a few millimeters. ^{90}Sr has been used for non-neoplastic conditions such as pannus as well as small, superficial ocular tumors.

Systemic therapy is used for only specialized tumor types that have the potential to concentrate the administered isotope, resulting in higher doses to neoplastic tissues. An example of this is ^{131}I treatment for disseminated thyroid carcinoma. It must be noted that animals implanted or infused with radioactive sources must be hospitalized or equivalently confined until the sources have been removed or decayed and must be monitored for loss of nondecayed radioactive sources. In addition, animal excrement must be treated as radioactive waste if the patient was given a nonencapsulated source of radioactive material.

Other modalities often used in conjunction with radiotherapy include hyperthermia, hypoxic cell sensitizers, and radioprotective agents. Hyperthermia (42 to 48°C) may be used alone or in combination with radiation. Higher temperatures are usually used clinically if heat is used as a primary therapeutic agent versus a radiosensitizer. Hyperthermia may be applied locally, regionally, or to the whole body depending on the type and distribution of the neoplasm and the facilities available. Hypoxic cell sensitizers are currently undergoing clinical trials at selected veterinary institutions. Chemically these are systemically administered nitroaromatic compounds with high electron affinity. They are used to enhance the response of the radioresistant hypoxic cells within tumors to radiotherapy. These compounds are toxic when used in optimum therapeutic doses, and extensive investigations are underway to improve the therapeutic ratio of these compounds. Radioprotective agents are being used for clinical trials or have been incorporated into oncologic protocols at selected veterinary institutions. Chemically, these are systemically administered compounds with a free sulfhydryl group at one end of the molecule, which theoretically serves as a scavenger for the highly reactive free radicles formed as a result of intracellular water ionization. These compounds are used clinically for x- or gamma-radiation to decrease radiation reaction in well-vascularized, normal tissues. Potentially, these compounds may improve the therapeutic ratio for radiotherapy if full expectations are realized.

SOURCE OF SPECIFIC DATA

A questionnaire was sent (Summer-Fall, 1981) to all major veterinary institutions employing a Diplomate of the American College of Veterinary Radiology. The information solicited included (1) the availability (and types) of radiotherapy routinely offered to small animal clients, current radiotherapy protocols employed, and tumor cell types routinely treated with radiotherapy (alone or in combination with other modalities); and (2) the probability of a two-year cure and the availability of other modalities used specifically with radiotherapy. The data in Tables 1 and 2 represent the responses obtained.

APPLICATIONS OF RADIATION THERAPY

Before radiotherapy is considered, a histologic diagnosis as to tumor cell type involved is mandatory. Knowledge of the neoplastic cell type aids in determining if radiotherapy is applicable or if additional modalities may increase the likelihood of cure or long-term palliation and aids in making an estimate of the prognosis based on available data. The data obtained from the previously described questionnaire regarding the probability of cure for specific tumors and the modalities utilized in combination with radiotherapy (if any) are listed in Table 1.

Before radiotherapy is begun, the patient must be evaluated for any concurrent disease that may result in the patient's death during or shortly after the radiotherapy regimen. This is particularly important because patients must be sedated or anesthetized for each treatment. In our experience evaluation of a complete blood count, serum chemistry profile, urinalysis, and a test for microfilaria of *Dirofilaria immitis* in addition to a complete physical examination are adequate. A definitive search for metastases should be initiated based on the specific cell type of the neoplasm as determined by histologic evaluation of the tumor tissue. A special effort should be made to examine common routes of metastases including local and regional lymph nodes and organs downstream (arterial or venous) from the neoplasm (i.e., lung-thoracic radiographs). Patients with tumors with the potential for detectable circulating metastatic cells (i.e., mast cell tumor) should have a buffy coat cytologic examination and possibly a bone marrow evaluation. If metastases are identified, curative radiotherapy should not be considered, and alternate applicable therapeutic measures should be employed such as chemotherapy or immunotherapy. Radiotherapy might still be employed, but strictly for local palliation. Specific tumor types viewed by some radiotherapists/oncol-

Table 1. *Probability of Cure for Neoplasms When Radiotherapy Was Incorporated in Treatment**

Tumor	Probability of Cure (%)†				
	0–29	*30–49*	*50–69*	*70–89*	*90–100*
Perianal gland adenoma			RS, RC	R(2), RS(2), RSCCh	R, RS(2)
Perianal gland adenocarcinoma	R, RS	RS, RSC	R, RS, RSCCh	RS(2)	
Squamous cell carcinoma (excluding nasal)		R(2), RSC	R(4), RS(4), RC, RSChH	R, RS, RSCH	
Adenocarcinoma (excluding nasal)	RSC	R	R, RSC		R
Tooth: germ neoplasms			R, RS	R(5), RS	R, RS
Fibrosarcoma (see references)	RS, RSI	R	R(4), RSChH	RH	
Malignant melanoma	RSI	RS, RSCCh	RS		
Chondrosarcoma	R		R, RSC, RSH		
Intranasal adenocarcinoma	RS		R	R	
Intranasal neoplasms (mostly epithelial origin)	R, RS	RS	R, RS, RSC	RS	
Transmissible venereal tumor					R(3)
Mast cell tumors	RS, RCh	RS	R(2), RS(2), RSC	RSC	
Hemangiopericytoma	RH		RS	RS	
Osteosarcoma	RI				

*Based on a survey of the veterinary institutions listed in Table 2. Cure defined as a two-year survival, no continued growth, and no subsequent metastases.

†Number in parentheses indicates number of institutions responding using that therapeutic mode. No number indicates one (1) institution responding using that method.

Notes: Each abbreviation represents a response by an institution and the mode(s) of therapy utilized. Data in this table do not take into account size, local invasion, etc. These criteria may vary among institutions when tumors are selected for treatment.

R	=	radiotherapy alone
RH	=	radiotherapy + hyperthermia
RS	=	radiotherapy + surgery (includes castration, if applicable)
RC	=	radiotherapy + cryosurgery
RCh	=	radiotherapy + chemotherapy
RI	=	radiotherapy + immunotherapy
RSC	=	radiotherapy + surgery + chemotherapy
RSH	=	radiotherapy + surgery + hyperthermia
RSI	=	radiotherapy + surgery + immunotherapy
RSCCh	=	radiotherapy + surgery + cryosurgery + chemotherapy
RSCH	=	radiotherapy + surgery + cryosurgery + hyperthermia
RSChH	=	radiotherapy + surgery + chemotherapy + hyperthermia

ogists as exhibiting only a palliative response to radiotherapy include osteosarcoma, chondrosarcoma, fibrosarcoma, melanoma, and mammary carcinoma, prostatic adenocarcinoma, and adenocarcinomas in general. However, the probability of cure for these tumors as described in Table 1 should be considered, especially for fibrosarcoma and nasal epithelial tumors including adenocarcinoma.

As described in Table 1, radiotherapy may be combined with other modalities. However, caution should be exercised when combining concurrent radiotherapy and chemotherapy or sequential radiotherapy and cryotherapy, as radiation tolerance may be decreased. The chronologic sequence of surgery and radiotherapy may vary, but surgery followed by radiotherapy is the most common protocol. Radiotherapy should be initiated either immediately postoperatively or following a three-week postoperative delay to avoid wound dehiscence. Preoperative radiotherapy may be used in selected instances to decrease the size and extent of a tumor, to convert an inoperable tumor to an operable tumor, and possibly to decrease distant metastases. However, surgery following radiation (to tissue tolerance) may be complicated by poor healing. Intraoperative radiotherapy has been employed to irradiate and potentially sterilize the remaining nests (after major mass removed) of tumor cells by a massive single radiation dose during the surgical procedure. Unique problems with a high potential

Table 2.   Availability of Radiotherapy Among North American Veterinary Institutions

Institution	Location	External Beam Therapy				Brachytherapy			Miscellaneous		No Radiation Therapy
		Orthovoltage	Cesium-137	Cobalt-60	Linear Accelerator	Interstitial	Intracavitary	Pliesotherapy	Systemic Isotopes	Other	
Animal Medical Center	New York, NY										X
Angell Memorial Hospital	Boston, MA										X
Auburn University School of Vet. Med.	Auburn, AL	X		X			^{198}Au	^{90}Sr			
University of California-Davis, School of Vet. Med.	Davis, CA	X		X		^{137}Cs, ^{125}I, ^{192}Ir		^{137}Cs, ^{90}Sr	^{131}I		
Colorado State University, College of Vet. Med.	Fort Collins, CO			X	6 MeV			^{90}Sr			
Cornell University, New York State College of Vet. Med.	Ithaca, NY		X					^{90}Sr	^{131}I		
University of Florida, College of Vet. Med.	Gainesville, FL										X
University of Georgia, College of Vet. Med.	Athens, GA	X						^{90}Sr			
University of Illinois, College of Vet. Med.	Urbana, IL	X						^{90}Sr	^{131}I		
Iowa State University, College of Vet. Med.	Ames, IA	X						^{90}Sr			
Kansas State University, College of Vet. Med.	Manhattan, KS	X				^{137}Cs		^{90}Sr			
Louisiana State University, School of Vet. Med.	Baton Rouge, LA	X				^{137}Cs		^{90}Sr			
Michigan State University, College of Vet. Med.	East Lansing, MI	X						^{90}Sr*			
University of Minnesota, College of Vet. Med.	St. Paul, MN	X		*		^{222}Rn		^{90}Sr	^{131}I*		
Mississippi State University, College of Vet. Med.	Starkeville, MS										X

Institution	Location						Neutrons (cyclotron produced)
University of Missouri-Columbia, College of Vet. Med.	Columbia, MO	^{131}I, ^{32}P	^{137}Cs, ^{90}Sr	^{32}P	^{137}Cs	X	†
Ohio State University, College of Vet. Med.	Columbus, OH	^{131}I	^{90}Sr		^{198}Au, ^{192}Ir, ^{222}Rn	X	
Oklahoma State University, College of Vet. Med.	Stillwater, OK		^{90}Sr			X	
Ontario Veterinary College, University of Guelph	Guelph, ON, CANADA					X	‡
University of Pennsylvania, School of Vet. Med.	Philadelphia, PA		^{90}Sr			X	
Purdue University, School of Vet. Med.	West Lafayette, IN		^{90}Sr		^{222}Rn	X	
University of Saskatchewan, Western College of Vet. Med.	Saskatoon, SK, CANADA						
University of Tennessee, College of Vet. Med.	Knoxville, TN	^{131}I	^{90}Sr		^{125}I, ^{222}Rn	X	
Texas A & M University, College of Vet. Med.	College Station, TX	^{131}I, ^{32}P	^{137}Cs, ^{90}Sr	^{198}Au, ^{32}P	^{198}Au, ^{137}Cs	X	X
Tufts University, School of Vet. Med.	Boston, MA					X	
Tuskegee Institute, School of Vet. Med.	Tuskegee, AL						N/R
Virginia-Maryland Regional College of Vet. Med.	Blacksburg, VA						
Washington State University, College of Vet. Med.	Pullman, WA		^{90}Sr		^{137}Cs	X	X
Yale University School of Medicine, Section of Comparative Medicine	New Haven, CT					X	

*Soon to be available.
†Available and *routinely used* at a *local* hospital or medical school.
‡In process of development; date of availability uncertain.
N/R No response.

for introduction of pathogens are associated with intraoperative radiotherapy unless optimum facilities are available. The specific radiotherapy protocol to be used and the modalities to be combined with radiation are decisions based on the combined knowledge of a radiotherapist, a medical oncologist, and a surgeon and must be evaluated for each case individually. Alternatively, patients may be empirically assigned to routine oncologic protocols. Each individual and institution may vary in the specifics of treatment.

AVAILABILITY OF RADIATION THERAPY IN NORTH AMERICA

The North American veterinary institutions with radiologists on staff and the available radiotherapeutic modalities are summarized in Table 2. For the applicability of these modalities to a specific patient, consultation with the radiologist in charge of radiotherapy at the institution is advised.

Intraoperative, external beam radiotherapy is currently offered, when applicable, by the radiotherapists at the University of California, Davis; Colorado State University, Fort Collins; and the University of Pennsylvania, Philadelphia. Consultation with the staff radiotherapist is recommended when the applicability of this procedure is under consideration prior to referral.

Hyperthermia as an adjunct to radiotherapy is available for selected neoplasms at several institutions. Regional hyperthermia is currently available at the University of California, Davis; Colorado State University, Fort Collins; Purdue University, West Lafayette; and Texas A & M University, College Station. Regional hyperthermia is available on a limited basis through the University of Minnesota, St. Paul, by arrangement with an allied institution. Whole body hyperthermia is currently available at Colorado State University, Fort Collins; and Yale University, New Haven. Consultation with staff radiotherapists as to specific tumor cell types on which this modality may be used is recommended prior to referral.

Hypoxic cell sensitizers are currently being used in selected patients at the University of California, Davis; and Yale University, New Haven. Radioprotective agents are used in selected patients at Colorado State University, Fort Collins; and the University of Pennsylvania, Philadelphia. Applicability and risk versus benefit must be assessed by the radiotherapist for each patient.

CONCLUSION

The methods and modalities described here are highly complex and have been superficially summarized to provide potential users with some insight as to what to expect if radiotherapy is performed and where it can be obtained. Only those individuals with specific training and appropriate isotope licensure should perform these treatments. Those veterinarians with patients that may benefit from radiotherapy should contact a staff radiologist or oncologist at the institutions described in Table 2.

SUPPLEMENTAL READING

Abe, M., Takahashi, M., Yabumoto, E., et al.: Clinical experiences with intraoperative radiotherapy of locally advanced cancers. Cancer 45:40, 1980.

Banks, W. C., and Morris, E.: Results of radiation treatment of naturally occurring animal tumors. J.A.V.M.A. 166:1063, 1975.

Gillette, E. L.: Radiation therapy. *In* Kirk, R. W. (ed.): *Current Veterinary Therapy VI*. Philadelphia: W. B Saunders Co., 1977, pp. 479–482.

Gillette, E. L.: Radiation therapy. *In* Gillette, E. L. (ed.): *Carlson's Veterinary Radiology*, 3rd ed. Philadelphia: Lea & Febiger, 1977, pp. 477–489.

Gillette, E. L.: Radiotherapy. *In* Theilen, G. H., and Madewell, B. R. (eds.): *Veterinary Cancer Medicine*. Philadelphia: Lea & Febiger, 1979, pp. 85–94.

Gillette, E. L.: Large animal studies of hyperthermia and irradiation. Cancer Res. 39:2242, 1979.

Hilmas, D. E., and Gillette, E. L.: Radiotherapy of spontaneous fibrous connective-tissue sarcomas in animals. J. Natl. Cancer Inst. 56:365, 1976.

Silver, I. A.: Use of radiotherapy for the treatment of malignant neoplasms. J. Small Anim. Pract. 13:351, 1972.

Thrall, D. E.: Orthovoltage radiotherapy of oral fibrosarcomas in dogs. J.A.V.M.A. 179:159, 1981.

Thrall, D. E., and Biery, D. N.: Principles and application of radiation therapy. Vet. Clin. North Am. 7:35, 1977.

TREATMENT OF LYMPHOSARCOMA*

K. ANN JEGLUM, V.M.D.
Philadelphia, Pennsylvania

Lymphosarcoma (LSA), also known as lymphoma, is a lymphoproliferative disease arising from lymphoid tissue and involving any tissue or organ. The most common anatomic forms are (1) multicentric or generalized lymphadenopathy, (2) anterior mediastinal, (3) alimentary, (4) cutaneous, and (5) other extranodal forms. True leukemia is distinguished from LSA because it arises in the bone marrow and then is manifested in peripheral blood. Leukemias in the dog and cat can be more difficult to treat than LSA due to infections, bleeding, and central nervous system involvement.

MEDICAL WORK-UP

Prior to therapy, all animals should undergo a medical work-up including (1) physical examination, (2) complete blood count, (3) biochemical profile, (4) chest and abdominal radiographs, (5) urinalysis, (6) bone marrow aspirate or biopsy, and (7) lymph node biopsy. Systemic complications called paraneoplastic syndromes associated with neoplasms require supportive care during remission induction with chemotherapy. Paraneoplastic syndromes associated with LSA include pseudohyperparathyroidism or hypercalcemia, fever, anemia, thrombocytopenia, disseminated intravascular coagulation, gammopathies, and hypoglycemia. These syndromes have been discussed extensively in the literature.

CLINICAL STAGING AND PROGNOSIS

Animals can be clinically staged according to the classification adopted by the World Health Organization (WHO) and Veterinary Cancer Society. This aids in determining prognosis and allows for comparisons of treatment protocols (Table 1). Recent data in canine LSA from the Veterinary Hospital at the University of Pennsylvania (VHUP) correlated the effectiveness of chemotherapy with the clinical stage of disease based on the WHO classification. Dogs in stage III (15 dogs) had a median survival

time of 9 months, stage IV (15 dogs) correlated with a survival time of 8 months, and stage V (12 dogs) correlated with a survival time of 4.3 months. Clinically ill dogs (29 dogs) as determined by subclassification (b) had a median survival time of 5 months, whereas clinically normal dogs, i.e., those in subclassification (a), had a median survival time of 9.1 months. Other prognostic factors that have been determined in canine LSA are anatomic type and body weight. Dogs with bone marrow involvement, diffuse alimentary LSA, or a cutaneous form have a poorer prognosis with treatment. One report states that cats with generalized lymphadenopathy or the anterior mediastinal form respond better than alimentary cases. Lighter dogs have longer survival times with chemotherapy than heavy dogs. At VHUP, cats with generalized lymphadenopathy respond significantly better than cats with any other form of LSA. The feline leukemia virus status does not seem to affect prognosis.

TREATMENT

The goal of treating canine and feline LSA is to induce a clinical remission with minimal side effects. The animals should return to a normal quality of life. The veterinarian and owner must be aware that individual animals differ in regard to response, side effects, and length of survival. The modalities used to treat any form of cancer include surgery, radiation therapy, chemotherapy, and immunotherapy.

Surgery and radiation therapy are used primarily to treat local disease and regional metastases in veterinary medicine. The primary application of surgery in LSA is biopsy for histopathologic diagnosis. Some rare solitary forms or extranodal forms of LSA such as the alimentary or anterior mediastinal form may be treated surgically followed by systemic therapy. One must assume systemic involvement in the majority of cases of LSA and treat accordingly. In the presence of massive splenomegaly, splenectomy or radiation therapy has been advocated in humans as a debulking procedure. The effects of splenectomy in canine and feline LSA have not been examined adequately.

Lymphocytes are radiation-sensitive cells. Total body irradiation with autologous bone marrow trans-

*This work is supported by the American Kennel Club Research Fund for Canine Oncology at the University of Pennsylvania.

435

Table 1.   *Clinical Staging of Lymphosarcoma**†

Lymphosarcoma and Lymphatic Leukemia in Domestic Mammals	Case number _____ Date _____

Lymphosarcoma and Lymphatic Leukemia in
    Domestic Mammals

Clinical Stages   Species _____

Final Histologic Diagnosis _____

Case number _____ Date _____
Name of owner _____
Age _____ Sex _____ Breed _____
Body weight _____ lbs _____ kgs
(1 kg = 2.2 lbs)

1. ANATOMIC TYPE
   A. Generalized
   B. Alimentary
   C. Thymic
   D. Skin
   E. Leukemia (true)‡
   F. Others (including solitary renal)
2. STAGE (to include anatomic type)
   I. Involvement limited to a single node or lymphoid tissue in a single organ§
   II. Involvement of many lymph nodes in a regional area (± tonsils)
   III. Generalized lymph node involvement
   IV. Liver and/or spleen involvement (± Stage III)
   V. Manifestation in the blood and involvement of bone marrow and/or other organ systems (± Stages I–IV)
   Each stage is subclassified
      (a) without systemic signs
      (b) with systemic signs

*Excluding myeloma.
†Approved by World Health Organization, Geneva, April 1978.
‡Only blood and bone marrow involved.
§Excluding bone marrow.

plantation has been suggested as an alternative form of treatment in canine LSA. This is obviously not a practical modality. Surgery and/or radiation therapy may induce long-term remission in stage I disease. However, stage I LSA is rare. Regional radiation therapy offers rapid relief of problems caused by regional lymphadenopathy. Examples of such applications are lymphedema due to lymphatic obstruction, respiratory distress due to mediastinal masses or cervical lymphadenopathy, and obstruction due to external iliac lymphadenopathy.

Chemotherapy using cytotoxic or antitumor drugs is most successful and is the treatment of choice for canine and feline LSA. Cytotoxic drugs act primarily by killing the most rapidly dividing cells in the body. Few drugs are specific for normal tissue types or tumor cells. Therefore, normal cells (including bone marrow, gastrointestinal mucosal cells, germinal cells, and hair follicle cells) can be killed. Side effects result from this effect on normal cells. Specific toxicities and management of the animal are discussed hereafter.

Historically, single drug therapy or single sequential drug protocols have proved less effective than combination chemotherapy. In canine LSA, the overall survival time improved as increased numbers of sequential drugs were used. Drug resistance and toxicity were reasons for discontinuing each drug. More recent studies have reported the superiority of combination chemotherapy with drugs used effectively as single agents. Drugs that have antitumor effects when used in canine and feline LSA are vincristine (Oncovin), cyclophospha-

mide (Cytoxan), L-asparaginase (Elaspar), doxorubicin HCl (Adriamycin), and prednisolone. Chlorambucil (Leukeran), antimetabolites including methotrexate and cytosine arabinoside (Cytoxan), 6-mercaptopurine (Purinethol), and 6-thioguanine (Tabloid) have been advocated in combination protocols but have not shown antitumor activity as single agents. Other drugs have been used in drug-resistant or relapsed LSA cases. These include dacarbazine (DTIC), procarbazine (Matulane), CCNU (Lomustine), Cis-platinum, and bleomycin sulfate (Blenoxane). Attempts to reinduce remission with these drugs have been discouraging. The protocol we recommend is presented in Table 2.

COMMON PROBLEMS IN MANAGEMENT OF LSA
(see page 419)

Myelosuppression. This is most often associated with cyclophosphamide administration. The nadir (lowest blood count) occurs seven days after the start of therapy. Rebound can occur within 24 hours. If the WBC count is decreased, other side effects, such as fever, vomiting, diarrhea, and hemorrhagic cystitis, may be manifested. Use antibiotics (e.g., ampicillin 10 mg/kg t.i.d.) if the animal is symptomatic with a WBC count of less than 3000 or leukocytosis with a left shift. If the WBC count is less than 1000, support with fluids and continuous infusion of cephalothin and gentamicin IM. Also set up a whole blood transfusion.

Hemorrhagic Cystitis. This problem is commonly associated with cyclophosphamide and a low

Table 2. *Combination Chemotherapy for Canine and Feline Lymphosarcoma*

Protocol*

Vincristine (Oncovin) 0.025–0.05 mg/kg IV, week 1
Cyclophosphamide (Cytoxan) 10 mg/kg IV, week 2
Vincristine (Oncovin) as above, week 3
Methotrexate 0.8 mg/kg IV or PO, or cytosine arabinoside
Begin cycle again at week 5 with vincristine

Specific Drug Side Effects

Vincristine—perivascular irritation, constipation, neurologic signs
Cytoxan—myelosuppression, hemorrhagic cystitis
Methotrexate—myelosuppression, GI signs (vomiting, diarrhea)

"Rescue" Measures

Prednisolone 0.5–1 mg/lb PO div. b.i.d.
  1. Add to protocol following one cycle if remission is not attained.
  2. Add to protocol when animal begins to come out of remission.
  3. Use in felines with anterior mediastinal masses at dose of 2.5 mg PO b.i.d. (in addition to regular protocol).
L-asparaginase 200–400 IU/kg
  1. Use to rescue remissions.
  2. May give IV the first time, then give IP every time thereafter owing to anaphylaxis.
  3. Use no more often than once every four weeks.
  4. Maximum dose 10,000 IU.
  5. Watch for anaphylaxis; treat with hydrocortisone.
Adriamycin 30 mg/m² IV using intracatheter and slow IV drip
  1. Use to rescue remissions when L-asparaginase not effective.
  2. Monitor EKG; prolongation of QRS and ST segment, heightened QRS.
  3. Perivascular irritation; be sure of venipuncture, use catheter.
  4. Use no more often than once every three weeks.
  5. Immediate reaction: pruritus (use hydrocortisone).
  6. Side effects: GI signs, myelosuppression, cardiotoxicity.
Radiation therapy

*This protocol is used widely. At the VHUP recently it is being changed by deleting methotrexate or cytosine arabinoside because of low efficacy and a high incidence of side effects. Use of L-asparaginase is recommended in their place.

WBC count. Salting the animal's food to increase thirst may help to prevent hemorrhagic cystitis. Prednisolone can be given to induce polydipsia and polyuria. Diuretics, such as furosemide (Lasix), and antispasmodics, such as sulfisoxazole (Gantrisin), can also be administered. This is a sterile cystitis, therefore no antibiotics should be given.

Vomiting/Diarrhea. These complications are associated with methotrexate and doxorubicin HCl therapy. They should be treated symptomatically with antiemetics. Avoid phenothiazine derivatives if the animal is thrombocytopenic. Watch for blood in the feces or vomitus. This is especially important with doxorubicin HCl therapy, which can cause hemorrhagic enterocolitis. If the animal is dehydrated with increased packed cell volume and total solids, treat with fluid therapy. These symptoms may appear to be caused by hemorrhagic gastroenteritis, and the animal may die without aggressive treatment. Therefore, it is imperative that the correct diagnosis be made as soon as possible. Prophylactic prochlorperazine (Darbazine, Compazine) should be included in all combination drug therapy programs for LSA, especially those using methotrexate and doxorubicin HCl.

Hair Loss. This side effect is breed related and is seen most commonly in poodles and terriers. Increased shedding can lead to patchy hair loss. Hair loss changes the texture of feline haircoats and leads to loss of whiskers in both cats and dogs.

Fever. This sign appears during tumor breakdown and in the presence of interstitial lung LSA. Use antibiotics and treat the tumor. Always check the WBC count; it may signal myelosuppression.

Resistance to Chemotherapy Drugs. Resistance occurs with antimetabolites, such as methotrexate, and L-asparaginase.

At VHUP we have compared the previously described cyclic combination protocol of vincristine-cyclophosphamide-methotrexate (VCM) versus these three drugs and "rescue" drugs (L-asparaginase and doxorubicin HCl) for treatment of canine LSA. Following enlargement of lymph nodes after initiating and maintaining remission with VCM, "rescue" drugs were used to reinduce remission. L-asparaginase (L-aspar) was used as a first rescue, whereas doxorubicin HCl (Adria) was used after resistance to L-aspar developed. Dogs were returned to the VCM protocol as maintenance after remission was reinduced. The median survival time for VCM alone (23 dogs) was 3.25 months, for VCM-L-aspar (22 dogs), 7.5 months, and for VCM-L-aspar-Adria (33 dogs), 9.75 months. The improvement in survival with "rescue" drugs was statistically significant. The remission duration of VCM alone was nine weeks. With addition of both "rescue" drugs, the remission duration was prolonged to 18.5 weeks.

Based on these data, we have undertaken a phase I trial of chemoimmunotherapy using VCM-L-aspar-Adria and intralymphatic (IL) autochthonous tumor cell vaccine. The autochthonous tumor cell vaccine is a viable cell preparation that is irradiated prior to administration via the lymphatic vessels in the extremities. Thirty dogs have been entered on the chemoimmunotherapy protocol. Eighteen of the thirty dogs have received three or more IL vaccines. The median survival time of the 18 dogs is currently 10.5 months, with 13 of 18 dogs still alive (range 5.5 to 17 months). The induction of remission with combination chemotherapy followed by maintenance therapy with IL tumor cell vaccine will allow dogs to discontinue chemotherapy and may improve long-term survival as well as quality of life.

SUPPLEMENTAL READING

Jeglum, K. A.: Malignant lymphoma in the dog. Comp. Cont. Ed. 1:503, 1979.

Juillard, G. J., Boyer, P. J. J., Yamashiro, C. H., Snow, H. D., Weisenburger, T. H., McCarthy, T., and Miller, R. J.: Regional intralymphatic infusion of irradiated tumor cells with evidence of distant effects. Cancer 39:126, 1977.

MacEwen, E. G.: Canine lymphosarcoma. In Kirk, R. W. (ed.): Current Veterinary Therapy VII. Philadelphia: W. B. Saunders Co., 1980.

MacEwen, E. G., Brown, E. O., Patnaik, A. K., Hayes, A. A., and

Passe, S.: Cyclic combination chemotherapy of canine lymphosarcoma. J.A.V.M.A. 178:1178, 1981.

Mangan, C., Jeglum, K. A., Sedlacek, T. V., Guintoli, P. L., Wheller, J. E., Rubin, E., and Mikeeta, J. J.: Intralymphatic BCG in the treatment of gynecologic malignancies: A phase 1 study. Cancer 40:2933, 1977.

Theilan, G. H., and Madewell, B. R. (eds.): Veterinary Cancer Medicine. Philadelphia: Lea & Febiger, 1979.

Weller, R. E., Theilan, G. H., Madewell, B. R., Crow, S. E., Benjamini, E., and Villalobos, A.: Chemoimmunotherapy for canine lymphosarcoma: A prospective evaluation of specific and nonspecific immunomodulation. Am. J. Vet. Res. 41:516, 1980.

PHOTOTHERAPY

RICHARD E. THOMA, D.V.M.
Cheektowaga, New York

Phototherapy is a new concept for the treatment of solid malignant tumors in domestic pets. It was developed at Roswell Park Memorial Institute (RPMI), in Buffalo, New York, by Dougherty, Weishaupt, and Boyle.

The term "phototherapy" is used to describe a method of treating malignant tumors using a photosensitizing drug. An ideal photosensitizer for this treatment would be one that has no systemic toxicity, is taken up and retained only by malignant tissue, and is efficient at destroying malignant tissue at light wavelengths not absorbed by the tissue. Currently there is no such ideal photosensitizer.

The theory of drugs causing a photosensitive reaction is not new. In 1902 eosin and topical sunlight were used to treat cancer, and although some favorable responses were noted, the project was discontinued. Interest was revived in the early 1970s when researchers at RPMI tried to develop a drug to aid in x-irradiation therapy. Since tumors that are oxygen poor are radioresistant, Dougherty was trying to find a drug that would localize in the tumor and produce oxygen when x-irradiated. He noted that cell cultures with fluorescein were destroyed when exposed too long to room light. Further research led to the porphyrins and then to hematoporphyrin derivative (Hpd).

Having obtained a therapeutically useful level of a photosensitizer in a tumor, it is desirable to be able to activate it using light wavelengths not absorbed or greatly modified by the tissue. Since tissue components, e.g., melanin, hemoglobin, and oxyhemoglobin, absorb throughout the visible spectrum, this requirement is not completely obtainable, although it is approachable, at least in some tissues. Visible wavelengths greater than 600 nm are least absorbed by the skin and other tissue

components and would, therefore, be least attenuated if light were applied through the skin to treat these lesions. In this regard, the porphyrins are most useful since nonmetallic porphyrins demonstrate weak absorption in the red part of the spectrum (600 to 700 nm). The porphyrins do absorb more strongly in the blue-green part of the spectrum, but these wavelengths are unable to sufficiently penetrate the tissues (skin, muscles, and so on) to be useful. When concentrated in cells, the Hpd used by Dougherty absorbs between 620 and 640 nm.

This is extremely beneficial, because wavelengths in the red part of the spectrum penetrate tissue better and deeper than other wavelengths. Hpd was also concentrated, or at least was selectively retained, in malignant tissue. The RPMI scientists spent many months trying to optimize this unique combination of tissue cellular biology, drugs, and photoenergy.

Phototherapy takes advantage of the favorable tissue distribution of Hpd: a higher concentration in tumorous tissue than in the surrounding normal tissue. A high therapeutic ratio can often be achieved, provided the light is applied after the skin level of Hpd has dropped below a certain critical level. This has been determined empirically in all cases. A therapeutic ratio for curability (no tumor regrowth) has yet to be determined, since it apparently varies in the different histopathologic types of tumors. There is a fine line between light delivery low enough to preserve normal tissues and light delivery high enough to destroy the tumor.

Early preclinical tests and trials on segments of advanced-stage cancer patients were very encouraging. Drug toxicity studies proved a very wide margin of safety, fiftyfold over therapeutic dose. US human medicine is conservative, and years would pass before this could be tried on spontaneous primary tumors. An alternative source of these tumors was necessary. Privately owned pet dogs and cats with otherwise incurable spontaneous primary tumors provided the answer. These pets were treated at RPMI before the equipment was installed in a veterinary hospital. After treatment the pets were returned to their owners for convalescence and follow-up. Referrals from New York, Michigan, and Connecticut provided a good early base for trials.

Developing good sources of light has taken many hours of thought and many trials. The initial light source was a 5-kw xenon arc lamp with filtration for producing the correct wavelength of 625 to 635 nm. This was good for superficial tumors. Deeper tumors were beyond the range of the light waves. Other sources were tried including laser equipment. Our current source of light is a laser system (Fig. 1) consisting of a 5- to 19-watt argon ion laser to produce the amount of light needed. This light is used to activate a dye laser (using rhodamine B dye) to change the wavelength of the beam to 632 ± 2 nm. The red laser beam emitted from the dye laser is then split equally into (four) beams of 150 to 500 mW each. The final power is dependent on the size of the ion laser, the type of dye laser, the efficiency of the beam splitters and couplers, and the length of the fibers. These beams are then coupled or optically transmitted into quartz fibers, which are the same as those used in telephone line transmissions. These fibers are flexible and are efficient light transmitters. They permit the light to be "carried" from the laser to the treatment area or into surgical suites. The fibers are small enough to pass through an 18- to 19-gauge hypodermic needle. Skin absorption and reflection and refraction of the light are bypassed because the light tip can be introduced directly into the tumor via needles; this is interstitial application of the light. The shape of this light tip varies with the tumor shape, but if the volume allows, a tetrahedronal arrangement with 1-cm sides gives the best apparent tissue-drug reaction.

The drug reaction is the key to this method of therapy. Hpd is a compound drug, and the active component is being researched. The component is light sensitive. When it is photoradiated it becomes very excited and has excess electronic energy. Enough of this energy is available to excite the tissue oxygen into singlet oxygen. Singlet oxygen is very unstable and must oxidize what it can. Within microseconds it oxidizes whatever is nearby; i.e., cell membranes within the tumor structure. The tumor, which is rich in Hpd, is oxidized and destroyed. There is very little Hpd in the adjacent normal tissue, so the normal tissue is spared. This selectivity for tumor tissue, especially along the microvascular bed, makes it an excellent therapeutic tool.

TECHNIQUE

The Hpd is given by intravenous injection at a rate of 2 to 5 mg/kg. Twenty four to seventy two hours are allowed to elapse, ensuring drug concentration in the tumor and maximal normal tissue clearance. We have found 72 hours to be optimal in the dog and cat and 24 hours in mice. There will be some minimal amounts of the drug in all tissues

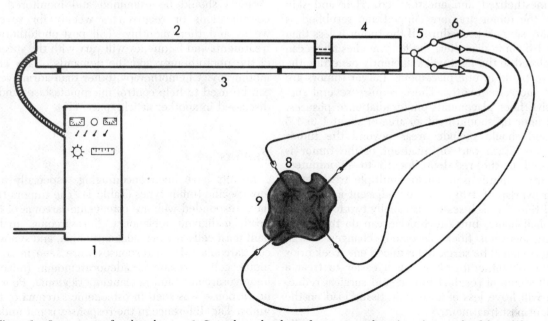

Figure 1. Laser system for phototherapy. *1,* Control panel and transformer; *2,* ion laser (argon); *3,* steel rail for stability; *4,* dye laser (rhodamine B dye); *5,* optical beam splitters; *6,* couplers (beam into fibers); *7,* four quartz fibers; *8,* 18-gauge needles in place to carry fibers into tumor; *9,* red light dispersed in tumor tissue.

for a few weeks. Because of this, a photosensitive skin reaction can occur after exposure to sunlight or other very bright light. This is a transient sunburn-erythema-edema reaction that is reversible with antihistamines. Avoidance of bright light is recommended for three to four weeks after injection in dogs and cats. Their haircoats and pigmentation have minimized these problems.

The technique is simple, making it a good one for practitioners. The cost of the equipment necessitates that therapy be done on a regional basis. Each metropolitan area with a population of over 750,000 people could generate enough cases to justify the cost of a phototherapy unit. Lower cost light sources are being developed and will allow more widespread use of this modality.

Definite procedures and protocols are being developed for phototherapy treatment of cancer in animals. Prudent medicine should prevail on the initial and pretreatment examinations and tests. Biopsy should confirm the diagnosis. Hemograms and chemistry profiles should define the animal's internal status. Ancillary tests such as electrocardiograms, urinalysis, and chemistry panels should be done as needed. Radiographic examination is necessary to determine the size and extent of the lesion and to aid fiber placement, which will ensure adequate light exposure beyond the limits of the tumor. A heavy metastatic load would alter the prognosis. Body weight is used to calculate the dose of Hpd. Intravenous administration is set up at the rate of 5 mg/kg. The long period of avoidance of bright light is then begun.

Seventy two hours after drug administration, the patient is ready for phototherapy. The patient is preanesthetized and anesthetized. Hair and skin over the tumor area are clipped and scrubbed as for any surgical procedure. If the tumor is less than 1 to 1.5 cm in diameter, the four needles/fibers can be placed so the light will sufficiently penetrate the entire tissue in one placement. Larger tumors are seen more frequently. These require several successive fiber placements/photoradiation exposures. The fiber tip should light an area of about 1 to 1.5 cc and should include areas beyond the tumor margins. Each part or quadrant of the tumor is exposed to the red light for 15 to 45 minutes. Twenty minutes is usual for multiple treatments, with overlap of 4 to 5 mm on adjacent areas. The total time for each session is usually two to two and one-half hours, but a technician can do the monitoring between fiber placement changes. Large tumors should be surgically reduced one week prior to the phototherapy; it is much easier to treat a small stump of residual tumor, and surgical reduction will leave less of a necrotic tissue load on the patient post treatment.

As the phototherapy proceeds, the tumor usually becomes much larger because of edema and the reaction to cell necrosis. Superficial tumors with a thin mucous membrane covering also develop a darkening or discoloration that coincides with the necrosis. This edema is usually transitory, subsiding after 48 hours. Necrosis of superficial tumors is evident by some tissue and fluid drainage or by frank necrosis and slough. Underlying granulation and healing then should proceed at a normal pace. Within two to three weeks enough healing will occur to allow determination of tumor regrowth so further treatments can be scheduled. There are no contraindications to repeated treatments at whatever frequency is deemed safe for the administration of anesthesia. Particularly large tumors that cannot be surgically reduced may be treated at close intervals, but the second dose of drug (if within four to six days of the previous injection) should be reduced by one-third to one-half.

Occasionally some hemorrhage will occur when the needles are inserted in the interstitial fibers. This usually will not interfere with the light transmission unless it is excessive. Any interference will be obvious, since the light in the tumor is visible and will be dimmed by a blood clot over the tip of the fiber. The fiber is removed from the needle, cleaned, and reinserted. Treatment proceeds as planned unless hemorrhage recurs. Then the needle and fiber are removed and replaced in an adjacent and less hemorrhagic spot in the tumor.

Post-treatment care is supportive. The only known drug to be contraindicated with Hpd is adriamycin. Topical or parenteral antibiotics, steroids, topical antiseptics and washes on sloughs, vitamins, anabolic steroids, fluids, diuretics, and so on can all be used at the clinician's discretion. Patients should be examined and monitored for complications or recurrences weekly for several weeks and then monthly. The post-phototherapy treatments and frequency will vary with the success of the phototherapy and the demands of any chemotherapy. Chemotherapy, other than adriamycin, can be used to help control micrometastases and is discussed in another article (page 415).

RESULTS

Results have been encouraging, especially in a few specific tumor types (Table 1). The tumors that have responded well are osteogenic sarcoma of the head, malignant melanoma, fibrosarcoma, malignant mast cell sarcoma, adamantinoma, and synovial cell sarcoma. Mixed responses were seen in squamous cell carcinoma, adenocarcinoma (mixed), leiomyosarcoma, and hemangiopericytoma. Poor or no response was seen in osteogenic sarcoma of the limbs. The difference in the responses is not understood, but several theories are being tested. These differences and rates of response are similar to those

Table 1. Current Statistics for Tumor Responses to Phototherapy

Tumor	No.	Current	Complete†	Partial	None	No Follow-up
Adenocarcinoma (differentiated)	4		1	1	2	
Adenocarcinoma (mammary, cat)	2		2			
Adenocarcinoma (undifferentiated)	1			1		
Adamantinoma	2		2 (2)			
Eosinophilic granuloma	1			1		
Fibromatous epulis	1		1			1
Acanthomatous epulis	1		1			
Fibroma	1		1			
Fibrosarcoma	6	1*	2 (1)	2	1	
Hemangiopericytoma	1			1		
Leiomyosarcoma	1			1		
Liposarcoma	1		1			
Malignant mast cell	5		4 (2)	1		
Malignant melanoma, melanotic	5	1*	3 (2)	1		
Malignant melanoma, amelanotic	2		1 (1)	1		
Myxoma	2			1	1	
Osteosarcoma, head	5		3 (2)	2		
Osteosarcoma, limb	3			1 ?	2	
Sarcoma (undifferentiated)	1	1				
Sebaceous gland carcinoma	1			1		
Sebaceous gland sarcoma	2		1 (1)	1		
Squamous cell carcinoma	4		1 (1)	3		
Synovial cell sarcoma	3		1 (2)	2		
Total types: 23	56	3	25	21	6	1
Percentage		5	45	38	11	2

83% total positive responses

*Indicates partial response or better currently seen.
†Number in parentheses indicates complete remission for more than one year.

seen in humans. The variables that can affect therapy include the following:

1. The amount of circulation in the tumor can alter the amount of Hpd delivered to the area.

2. The permeability of the vessels in the tumor can affect the drug delivery into and the clearance out of the tumor and surrounding tissues.

3. The tissue density can alter the penetrability of light, i.e., bone and melanin granules.

4. Other less understood variables can alter therapy such as osteogenic sarcoma of the head, which is more osteoblastic, and osteogenic sarcoma of the limbs, which is more lytic.

The overall picture for phototherapy is bright (no pun intended). There are several histopathologic tumor types that should respond well. Some of them are unresponsive to presently available types of therapy. The clinical simplicity and safety of this therapy make it very appealing. When the light source becomes less expensive, its availability to the practitioner will be more practical.

SUPPLEMENTAL READING

Dougherty, T. J., Thoma, R. E., Boyle, D. G., and Weishaupt, K. R.: Interstitial photoradiation therapy for solid primary tumors in pet cats and dogs. Cancer Res. 41:401, 1981.

Dougherty, T. J., Weishaupt, K. R., and Boyle, D. G.: Photoradiation therapy of malignant tumors. *In Principles and Practice of Oncology.* Philadelphia: J. B. Lippincott Co., 1982, pp. 1837–1843.

Weishaupt, K. R., Gomer, C. J., and Dougherty, T. J.: Identification of singlet oxygen as the cytotoxic agent photoactivation of a murine tumor. Cancer Res. 36:2326, 1976.

Immunology

INTENSIVE THERAPEUTIC PLASMAPHERESIS IN VETERINARY MEDICINE

ROBERT E. MATUS, D.V.M.

New York, New York

Plasmapheresis is a modified blood-letting procedure in which autologous cells are returned to the donor. Therapeutic plasmapheresis is useful in disease processes characterized by circulating toxins, humoral mediators, altered viscosity, and abnormal hemostasis. Plasmapheresis and selective immunoadsorption, which uses columns or filters to remove specific plasma components, represent major breakthroughs in the investigation and therapy of primary immune-mediated disease and disease processes associated with secondary immunologic responses.

Technical advances in the last decade have made the procedure of plasmapheresis less time consuming and have minimized potential complications inherent in the manual procedure, which necessitated sequential phlebotomy, fractionation, plasma extraction, and retransfusion of suspended cells. The advent of the cell separator has enabled withdrawal, collection, and return of blood components to be done simultaneously, minimizing blood volume deficit.

The major difficulty in the application of continuous plasmapheresis is developing a technique for adequate venous access to the blood supply for large volume withdrawal and replacement of fluid and cells. Several methods have been devised including surgical creation of arteriovenous shunts. We have developed a procedure in which percutaneous catheters are placed in the external jugular and cephalic veins, making access less invasive and less time consuming than previously published methods. Another important consideration is that application of plasmapheresis must be monitored immunologically to define the mechanism of action of the procedure and to confirm the clinical response of the patient.

INDICATIONS

Absolute indications for intensive therapeutic plasmapheresis include hyperviscosity syndrome associated with paraproteinemia (in which the procedure may be life-saving) and immune complex disease associated with systemic lupus erythematosus refractory to standard immunosuppressive therapy. Relative indications for plasmapheresis include autoimmune hematologic disease such as immune-mediated thrombocytopenia and hemolytic anemia, acquired myasthenia gravis, pemphigus syndrome, acute immune-mediated glomerulonephritis, rheumatoid arthritis, and vasculitis. These disease entities all have in common a pathophysiologic process in which antibodies or antigen-antibody complexes initiate leukoclastic and/or complement-mediated end-organ injury. Plasmapheresis alters this pathologic process, and the mechanism by which it does so is currently under intense investigation. Two theories have been proposed: plasmapheresis may work by correcting a reticuloendothelial cell defect, which blocks the clearance of immune complexes that eventually deposit in blood vessel walls and initiate immune-mediated vasculitis in various end-organs; or it may work by removing circulating factors responsible for immunosuppressor activity as the primary pathologic etiology.

Plasmapheresis and selective immunoadsorption are presently considered palliative therapeutic measures. We have used plasmapheresis as part of the therapeutic regimen to successfully treat hyperviscosity syndrome and systemic lupus erythematosus in dogs, and in one case of canine lupus, selective immunoadsorption of immune complexes was performed. Currently we and others are investigating the use of *Staphylococcus* immunoadsorption both as primary therapy and as an adjuvant to chemotherapy in the treatment of canine mammary cancer and lymphosarcoma.

AVAILABILITY

Plasmapheresis and selective immunoadsorption, although not available as routine therapeutic modalities because of high costs and unavailability of equipment, are rapidly emerging as useful clinical and research tools. With continuing technical advances, facilities for application of plasmapheresis will become more readily available to practitioners at large veterinary referral centers and teaching institutions. Currently, The Animal Medical Center, New York, New York; The University of Minnesota, College of Veterinary Medicine, St. Paul, Minnesota; and The Hutchison Cancer Research Center, University of Washington, Seattle, Washington, are conducting controlled clinical trials incorporating therapeutic plasmapheresis and immunoadsorption.

SUPPLEMENTAL READING

Behan, P. O., Shakir, R. A., and Simpson, J. A.: Plasma-exchange combined with immunosuppressive therapy in myasthenia gravis. Lancet II:438, 1979.

Terman, D. S., Durante, D., Buffaloe, G., et al.: Attenuation of canine nephrotoxic glomerulonephritis with an extracorporeal immunoadsorbent. Scand. J. Immunol. 6:195, 1977.

Terman, D. S., Yamamoto, T., Tillquist, R. L., et al.: Tumoricidal response induced by cytosine arabinoside after plasma perfusion over protein A. Science 209:1257, 1980.

Wenz, B., and Barland, P.: Therapeutic intensive plasmapheresis. Sem. Hematol. 18:147, 1981.

THERAPY OF IMMUNE-MEDIATED DISEASES

NIELS C. PEDERSEN, D.V.M.

Davis, California

THE RATIONALE AND OBJECTIVES OF IMMUNOSUPPRESSIVE DRUG THERAPY

Disorders of an immunopathologic nature are being recognized with increasing frequency in the dog and cat. It seems that analogues will eventually be recognized for most of the immunologic diseases of humans. With this increasing recognition of immunologic diseases, more information is required on the best ways to treat these disorders.

The standard treatment for immunologic diseases of dogs and cats has been glucocorticoids. Even with advances in glucocorticoid pharmacology and the use of alternate-day therapy, many immunologic disorders remain difficult to treat with steroids alone. Recently, cytotoxic drugs have been used to treat a wide range of immunopathologic disorders in dogs and cats. The use of these agents in veterinary medicine is based on over a decade of experience with the treatment of similar disorders in humans.

The various cytotoxic agents produce their anti-inflammatory and immunosuppressive effects in a number of different ways. Furthermore, their immunosuppressive effects are far more potent and specific than are the immunosuppressive effects of glucocorticoids. By combining these drugs with glucocorticoids, it is possible to produce potent and broad spectrum anti-inflammatory and immunosuppressive effects. When several drugs are used in combination, the effective dose of each drug is often reduced. This reduces toxicity while retaining therapeutic efficacy.

Cytotoxic agents are usually used in the treatment of immunologic diseases in conjunction with glucocorticoids, hence the term "combination immunosuppressive therapy." They are used alone only in cases in which animals show adverse reactions to steroid therapy. Cytotoxic agents are generally added to the regimen when steroids alone prove inadequate, when the dosage of steroids necessary to control signs is excessive, or when a more rapid remission of symptoms is considered desirable. The question always asked is, "When should combination immunosuppressive drug therapy be used and when should glucocorticoids alone be used?" This cannot be answered completely, but from clinical experience it is apparent that many veterinarians rely on high dosages of glucocorticoids to control conditions that are better treated with combination therapy or accept partial control of the disease when better control could be achieved by the addition of cytotoxic agents.

GLUCOCORTICOIDS

Prednisone, prednisolone, and dexamethasone are the most commonly used glucocorticoids in combination immunosuppressive drug therapy. The main differences among these glucocorticoids are in their relative potencies, sodium-retaining effects, and biologic half-lives (Table 1).

Table 1. *Comparison of Commonly Used Glucocorticoid Preparations**

Compound	Equivalent Potency (mg)	Sodium-Retaining Effect	Biologic Half-life (min)
Cortisone	25	2+	30
Cortisol	20	2+	90
Prednisone	5	1+	60
Prednisolone	5	1+	200
Dexamethasone	0.75	0	200

*These are values determined for humans. The biologic half-life for dogs is about one-third of the value given for humans. The equivalent potencies and sodium-retaining potentials are similar in humans and dogs.

Glucocorticoids exert their immunosuppressive effects in various ways. Glucocorticoids are not highly suppressive to normal primary and secondary antibody responses at therapeutic dosages, although they do seem to markedly depress abnormal autoantibody formation (i.e., Coombs' antibody, antiplatelet antibodies, antinuclear antibodies, and so on). In this regard, they appear to have a favorable regulating effect on events leading to abnormal antibody production. Glucocorticoids cause a pronounced lymphopenia, which limits the number of these cells available for participation in cell-mediated processes. Glucocorticoids may reduce specific antigen-induced blastogenesis of lymphocytes. These drugs produce a monocytopenia and diminish the response of these cells to some inflammatory mediators. Monocyte function *in vitro* and *in vivo* is decreased. This effect is manifested systemically by a decrease in the uptake of opsonized and nonopsonized materials by the reticuloendothelial system and locally by a decreased influx of monocytes into inflammatory sites. The reticuloendothelial blockade effect has obvious benefits in the control of red cell and thrombocyte destruction in autoimmune hemolytic anemia and thrombocytopenia.

Glucocorticoids also effect neutrophils. They increase blood neutrophil levels by stimulating their release from the marrow; paradoxically, glucocorticoids inhibit the migration of neutrophils from the blood into the inflammatory site. They also impair neutrophil chemotaxis, adhesiveness, bacterial killing, and lysosomal enzyme secretion *in vivo*. Glucocorticoids greatly reduce the number of circulating eosinophils.

There are several miscellaneous effects of glucocorticoids that may be of benefit in the treatment of immunologic diseases. Glucocorticoids appear to depress serum complement levels. They also interfere with the passage of immune complexes through basement membranes. Both of these effects have obvious benefits in the treatment of immune complex–mediated disorders.

There is a great deal of confusion surrounding the use of glucocorticoids for the treatment of immunologic disorders. The following are guidelines that may be of some help:

1. Use corticosteroids whose side effects, dose responses, and therapeutic efficacy are well-documented. Prednisone and prednisolone are the glucocorticoids of choice. Because prednisone has a shorter half-life and in this respect more closely resembles endogenous cortisone (Table 1), it is theoretically more suitable for alternate-day therapy. In clinical practice, however, there is no difference between the two drugs. Dexamethasone can be substituted for prednisone or prednisolone. It is seven times more potent than these two agents, so it should be given at one-seventh the dosage recommended for prednisone and prednisolone. It is available in both oral and injectable forms, which is an added benefit. Because of its longer biologic half-life, dexamethasone does not lend itself to alternate-day therapy.

2. Use the highest dosage levels during the first few days to control the disease and then decrease the dosage as rapidly as possible when clinical signs abate. The initial dosage should not exceed 2.0 to 4.0 mg/kg PO per day, except in very small dogs and cats, in whom the dosage may be greater. When giving these initial high levels, it is beneficial to administer the drug in divided daily doses.

3. Once the clinical signs have disappeared, glucocorticoid levels should be decreased over several weeks to maintenance levels. Maintenance levels of prednisone or prednisolone should be approximately 1.0 mg/kg PO every other day, or lower if possible.

4. Do not discontinue glucocorticoid therapy for at least two to three months after the disease is in remission. If drugs are discontinued too soon the disease is more likely to recur and the disease-free interval will often be shorter.

CYTOTOXIC DRUGS

In combination immunosuppressive drug therapy, glucocorticoids are used in conjunction with any one of a number of different cytotoxic drugs. The term "cytotoxic drug" refers to the drug's ability to kill cancer cells, for which most of them were initially developed. Cytotoxic drugs also have potent effects on the immune system and are often antiinflammatory as well. Cytotoxic immunosuppressive drugs used in veterinary medicine belong to three basic groups: alkylating agents, thiopurines, and vinca alkaloids. Folic acid antagonists, such as methotrexate, compose a fourth group. Methotrexate, however, is too toxic to be considered for routine use.

Alkylating agents have been found to be among the most potent immunosuppressive drugs available. Alkylating agents work by crosslinking the DNA of both dividing and resting cells. They produce most of their effects, therefore, by interfering with cell division.

Cyclophosphamide (Cytoxan) and chlorambucil (Leukeran) are the most potent immunosuppressive agents in this group. Alkylating agents act against many arms of the immune response. They inhibit normal primary and secondary responses as well as delay hypersensitivity reactions. They prolong the survival of organ grafts, decrease the production of interferon, diminish antigen trapping in lymph nodes, and inhibit local inflammatory responses. Alkylating agents act on lymphoid cells by killing slowly proliferating antigen reactive cells as well as rapidly proliferating specifically stimulated cells. As such, they inhibit antibody synthesis from 48 hours before to a week or more after antigen administration.

Cyclophosphamide is the most popular of the alkylating agents. It is usually given at a dosage based on the body surface area rather than on body weight. This is also true of the other cytotoxic drugs that will be discussed. Larger dogs require less of the drug per kilogram of body weight than small dogs and cats. Cyclophosphamide is given at a dosage of 1.50 mg/kg PO daily for dogs greater than 25 kg, 2.0 mg/kg PO daily for dogs 5 to 25 kg, and 2.50 mg/kg PO daily for dogs under 5 kg and cats. Cyclophosphamide is given daily for four consecutive days of each week, followed by three days with no drug; this is referred to as one cycle of therapy. Cyclophosphamide can also be given at the previously mentioned dosage on an alternate-day basis.

Chlorambucil has been much less utilized than cyclophosphamide for the treatment of immunologic diseases. In humans it has been most effective in the treatment of a number of glomerulonephritides, such as lupus nephritis, and idiopathic nephrotic syndrome of children. In these diseases of humans, chlorambucil has been shown to be much more effective than cyclophosphamide and has fewer side effects. We have used it instead of cyclophosphamide in several dogs and cats, and it has proved in these cases to be as effective as cyclophosphamide. This drug will probably see increasing usage in veterinary medicine for the treatment of immunologic diseases as clinicians learn to use it to treat more conditions.

Chlorambucil is given at a dosage of around 1 mg/15 kg (.07 mg/kg) PO, once daily, for animals in the 15- to 30-kg weight range. Smaller dogs and cats should receive about 0.08 mg/kg and larger dogs around .06 mg/kg PO once daily. After remission is achieved, the drug should be administered at the previously mentioned dosage once every other day.

Cyclophosphamide and chlorambucil have several potential side effects at the prescribed dosages (see page 419). They can be bone marrow suppressive in some animals. For this reason, blood counts should be done every week or two for the first two months of therapy and monthly thereafter. The white blood cell counts should not go lower than 5,000/µl. If this occurs, the drug should be briefly discontinued and reinstituted at three-fourths the original dose. A sterile hemorrhagic cystitis is a common side effect of chronic cyclophosphamide therapy. For this reason cyclophosphamide should not be used for longer than four to five months. If cytotoxic drug therapy is required after this period of time, chlorambucil or azathioprine should be substituted for cyclophosphamide. Neither of these drugs induces sterile hemorrhagic cystitis. Cyclophosphamide and chlorambucil retard new hair growth in shaved areas.

Thiopurines achieve their effect by competing with adenine in the synthesis of nucleic acids. The net result of the substitution of nucleic acids with these "nonsense" bases is an inoperable nucleic acid strand. Thiopurines, therefore, prevent the proliferation of rapidly dividing cell populations. This differs from the effect of cyclophosphamide, which works against resting and slowly dividing cells as well.

Azathioprine (Imuran) and 6-mercaptopurine (Purinethol) are the most widely used of the thiopurine compounds. Azathioprine is cleaved in the body to two molecules of 6-mercaptopurine, which is the active moiety. These two drugs can, therefore, be used interchangeably.

The thiopurines strongly inhibit T lymphocyte–related functions such as cell-mediated immunity and T lymphocyte–dependent antibody synthesis. For optimum effect they must be given during the stage of the immune response in which cells are rapidly dividing. The thiopurines have been useful in preventing allograft rejection and have a particularly strong inhibitory effect on the expression of delayed hypersensitivity. They also have a potent inhibitory effect on the nonspecific inflammatory response, which may be due in part to inhibition of the influx of mononuclear cells into the site. The thiopurines are potent inhibitors of the primary humoral antibody response. Inhibition of the secondary antibody response requires higher levels of the drugs.

The thiopurines have been used successfully to treat many autoimmune disorders of humans. These drugs have been beneficial in the treatment of autoimmune hemolytic anemia, pure red cell aplasia, Crohn's disease, pemphigus vulgaris, systemic lupus erythematosus, lupoid hepatitis, chronic active liver disease, Goodpasture's syndrome, allergic vasculitis, Wegener's granulomatosis, polyneuritis, and rheumatoid arthritis. We have had experience with the thiopurines in a number of diseases of dogs, such as idiopathic polyarthritis, systemic lupus

Table 2. *Immunologic Diseases and Their Treatment With Immunosuppressive Drug Therapy*

Immunologic Disorder	Suggested Treatment
I. Hematologic	
a. Autoimmune thrombocytopenia or idiopathic thrombocytopenia of apparent immunologic origin (megakaryocytes present in normal or increased numbers in bone marrow).	Prednisone or prednisolone alone. If no favorable response in one to two weeks, add cyclophosphamide or vincristine. Discontinue cytotoxic drugs when platelet count returns to normal, usually within three weeks. If there is severe bleeding associated with the initial episode, vincristine should be used earlier.
b. Pure thrombocyte aplasia (thrombocytopenia with no megakaryocytes in bone marrow; all other blood and bone marrow cells normal).	Prednisone or prednisolone in combination with cyclophosphamide. Discontinue cytotoxic drugs when platelet count returns to normal.
c. Autoimmune hemolytic anemia	Prednisone or prednisolone alone. If no favorable response in five to seven days, add cyclophosphamide. Discontinue cytotoxic drugs when RBC count approaches normal.
1. Associated with Coombs' antibodies of the IgG class with or without complement fixation.	
2. Associated with complement on RBCs, but not IgG. No cold agglutinins present.	
3. Cold agglutinin disease (Coombs' antibodies of cold reactive IgM type, complement present on RBCs at body temperature).	Prednisolone or prednisone in combination with cyclophosphamide. Discontinue cyclophosphamide when cold agglutinins disappear and PCV approaches normal.
d. Pure red cell aplasia (hypoplastic anemia with decreased red cell precursors in bone marrow; all other blood cell and marrow elements normal).	Prednisone or prednisolone for two to four weeks. If partial or unfavorable response occurs, add cyclophosphamide. Discontinue cyclophosphamide when RBC count approaches normal.
II. Musculoskeletal	
a. Nonerosive polyarthritis (associated with SLE or idiopathic).	Prednisone or prednisolone alone. If unfavorable or partial response, add cyclophosphamide, chlorambucil, or azathioprine.
b. Erosive polyarthritis (rheumatoid arthritis).	Prednisone or prednisolone with cyclophosphamide or chlorambucil. Full remission may take four months or longer.
c. Polyradiculoneuritis.	Prednisone or prednisolone alone. The use of cyclophosphamide and azathioprine should be considered in steroid unresponsive or partially responsive cases. Although not used for these disorders in dogs, their therapeutic effectiveness in human cases is documented.
d. Polymyositis, myositis of immunologic cause.	
e. Polyneuritis of immunologic cause.	
III. Ophthalmologic	
a. Steroid refractory uveitis.	Cyclophosphamide has been used successfully in some cases in humans. We have had dramatic effects with cyclophosphamide in one dog.
IV. Dermatologic	
a. Pemphigus vulgaris.	Prednisone or prednisolone alone. If response is poor or disease cannot be controlled with lower drug levels, add azathioprine, chlorambucil, or cyclophosphamide. Disease suppression may be slow and difficult in many cases. Alkylating agents have been reported to be inadequate in controlling active disease but may be extremely useful in maintaining a steroid-induced remission without the further use of steroids.
b. Pemphigus foliaceus.	
c. Pemphigus vegetans.	
d. Bullous pemphigoid.	Glucocorticoids used in combination with azathioprine have been particularly useful for bullous pemphigoid.
V. Miscellaneous	
a. Systemic lupus erythematosus.	Prednisone or prednisolone alone. If response is poor, add cyclophosphamide, chlorambucil, or azathioprine.
b. Glomerulonephritis (lupus, idiopathic, nonsteroid, or poor steroid response).	Prednisone or prednisolone in combination with chlorambucil. Monitor daily urine total protein loss. If therapy is effective, proteinuria should begin to steadily decrease after two to four weeks.

erythematosus, and bullous pemphigoid. Generally speaking, the thiopurines are not as effective as the alkylating agents in controlling immunologic diseases. They are less toxic, however, than the alkylating agents, and for diseases not requiring vigorous immunosuppression, the thiopurines are preferable.

The dosages for azathioprine and 6-mercaptopurine are the same, around 2.0 mg/kg PO once daily. When the disease is under control, alternate-day therapy is used at the dosage previously mentioned. With alternate-day therapy, the glucocorticoids and the thiopurines are given on consecutive days.

Used at the recommended dosages, azathioprine and 6-mercaptopurine are safe drugs. They are potentially bone marrow suppressive and gastrointestinal toxic at higher levels. As with the use of all cytotoxic drugs, it is recommended that the white blood cell counts be monitored and not allowed to fall below 5000/µl. Like the alkylating agents, the thiopurines retard hair growth.

Vinca alkaloids are used for the treatment of certain cancers in animals and humans. Vincristine (Oncovin) is the most widely used drug of this group. Vincristine inhibits the formation of the cytoplasmic microtubular network and prevents cell division by interfering with the formation of the mitotic spindle. Since phagocytosis also involves the cytoplasmic endoskeleton, this is also affected. The vinca alkaloids have been reported to have only 1/10 to 1/100 the immunosuppressive effect of drugs such as cyclophosphamide. Their most potent immunosuppressive effect is at nearly toxic levels. The sole use of vincristine in immunologic disorders is the treatment of autoimmune thrombocytopenia in humans and animals. In addition to its effect on phagocytosis of abnormal platelets, the drug has a curious thrombocytotic property that actually increases the production of platelets.

The dosage of vincristine for dogs and cats is about 0.02 mg/kg IV once a week. If it is going to be effective, a dramatic rise in the platelet count will occur within two to four days after the first or second injection. Therapy is discontinued if no response is seen after the second dose. Vincristine is recommended for use in cases of thrombocytopenia in three situations: (1) in animals with severe blood loss; vincristine often gives a much more rapid response than prednisone or prednisolone alone; (2) in animals with a poor or negligible response to glucocorticoids; or (3) in animals that fail to respond to glucocorticoids and splenectomy. Vincristine and splenectomy have an apparent additive effect, even if no response was seen to splenectomy alone. Most cases of thrombocytopenia of immune origin respond well to glucocorticoids alone and do not require vincristine therapy. Even when vincristine is used, it should be combined with glucocorticoid therapy to facilitate and maintain remission once it is achieved.

GENERAL CONSIDERATIONS

Cytotoxic drugs should be withdrawn once the disease is in complete remission for at least one month or more. During the same period the glucocorticoid dosage also should be incrementally decreased as clinical improvement occurs. When complete remission of disease occurs, the glucocorticoids should be administered every other day at maintenance levels. At this stage it usually is possible to maintain the disease in remission on alternate-day steroid therapy alone. If signs reappear when the animal is receiving glucocorticoids alone, re-establish remission with combination therapy, then maintain remission with the lowest possible dosages of glucocorticoid and cytotoxic drug. If the disease remains in remission for at least two to three months on steroids alone, the glucocorticoids can be withdrawn. The biggest mistake made is to decrease drug dosages too rapidly and to follow a rigid time schedule for treatment. As long as steady, albeit slow, improvement is seen, vigorous therapy should be continued. Decreased levels or discontinuation of drugs should only follow substantial degrees of improvement. Therapy should never be completely discontinued when there is active disease present, even though it appears slight.

Table 2 lists a range of immunologic diseases that have been successfully managed with combination immunosuppressive drug therapy. Included in the table are suggestions on treatment protocols for these various disorders.

CHRYSOTHERAPY

(Gold Therapy)

DANNY W. SCOTT, D.V.M.

Ithaca, New York

Chrysotherapy refers to the therapeutic use of gold compounds. Chrysotherapy has been used successfully for the treatment of rheumatoid arthritis in humans for about 50 years. More recently, chrysotherapy has been used for the treatment of other autoimmune or immune-mediated disorders in dogs, cats, and humans.

MECHANISM OF ACTION

The exact mechanism of action of gold compounds in the diseases for which they are prescribed is unknown. *In vitro* and *in vivo* studies in humans and various laboratory animals have shown that gold compounds have a multitude of effects (Table 1). Clearly, gold compounds are capable of modulating virtually all phases of immune and inflammatory responses.

METABOLISM

The metabolism and distribution of gold compounds have been studied in humans and laboratory animals but *not* in dogs and cats. Injectable gold compounds are rapidly absorbed following intramuscular injection. With weekly injections, plasma gold concentrations rise gradually during the first six to eight weeks and then plateau. The majority (about 90 per cent) of plasma gold is protein bound.

Gold excretion is primarily renal and fecal. From 30 to 50 per cent of an administered gold dose is excreted each week. Of the fraction excreted, 50 to 85 per cent is eliminated in the urine and 15 to 50 per cent in the feces.

The highest gold concentrations are found in the lymph nodes, adrenal glands, liver, kidneys, bone marrow, and spleen. Gold concentrations in the skin are very low, with about 97 per cent of the total present in the dermis, particularly within the lysosomes of dermal histiocytes. Gold appears to be preferentially concentrated in the phagolysosomes ("aurosomes") of mononuclear phagocytic (reticuloendothelial) cells.

CLINICAL USE

Chrysotherapy has been most frequently used for the management of salicylate- and glucocorticoid-unresponsive rheumatoid arthritis in humans and dogs, and glucocorticoid-unresponsive pemphigus in humans, dogs, and cats. Two injectable gold compounds are presently available in the United States: aurothioglucose (Solganol, Schering) and gold sodium thiomalate (Myochrysine, Merck, Sharp, and Dohme). Neither product is licensed for use in dogs and cats. Aurothioglucose is the recommended product because its use is accompanied by a much lower incidence of the nitritoid reaction (an acute, shock-like vasomotor reaction).

Table 2. *Chrysotherapy for the Management of Canine and Feline Pemphigus*

Canine Pemphigus	
Pemphigus foliaceus	2 cases in remission, no Rx for 2½ years
	1 case in remission, monthly Rx for 1½ years
	1 case in remission, monthly Rx for 2 years
	1 case in remission for 6 months, euthanized owing to unrelated pododermatitis
Pemphigus erythematosus	1 case in remission, monthly Rx for 1½ years
Pemphigus vulgaris	2 cases in remission for 1 year, monthly Rx
Feline Pemphigus	
Pemphigus foliaceus	2 cases in remission, monthly Rx for 1 year
	1 case in remission for ½ years (monthly gold and twice monthly dexamethasone)
Pemphigus erythematosus	1 case in remission for 1½ years, euthanized owing to dermatophytosis
Pemphigus vulgaris	1 case in remission, monthly Rx for 1½ years

Table 1. In Vitro *and* In Vivo *Effects of Gold Compounds*

Stabilization of lysosomal membranes
Enzyme inhibition
Decreased migration and phagocytic activity of macrophages and neutrophils
Inactivation of complement
Inhibition of prostaglandin synthesis
Inhibition of antigen- and mitogen-induced lymphocyte responses
Suppression of immunoglobulin synthesis
Increased stability of collagen

Table 3. *Side Effects of Chrysotherapy in Humans*

Dermatitis
Stomatitis
Proteinuria (severe nephrotoxicity is rare)
Eosinophilia
Leukopenia*
Thrombocytopenia*
Pulmonary reactions*
Gastrointestinal reactions*
Ocular reactions*
Neurologic reactions*
Hepatic reactions*
Nitritoid (anaphylactoid) reaction (rare with aurothioglucose)

*These reactions are rare.

Because metabolic studies with gold compounds have not been conducted on dogs and cats, presently recommended regimens for chrysotherapy in these species are totally empirical. Cats and small dogs (less than 10 kg body weight) are initially given two test doses (1 mg, then 2 mg total dose) of aurothioglucose intramuscularly at weekly intervals. Dogs over 10 kg are given test doses of 5 mg, then 10 mg. Induction therapy is then continued with weekly intramuscular injections of 1 mg/kg until remission is achieved. The lag effect with chrysotherapy is about six to twelve weeks.

After remission is achieved, injections are administered bimonthly for one month, then once monthly. Since 1978, eight dogs and five cats with various forms of pemphigus have been managed with chrysotherapy (Table 2). Chrysotherapy was utilized when glucocorticoids had been ineffective or had produced unacceptable side effects. The first two dogs (pemphigus foliaceus) treated received chrysotherapy for six to seven months and have been in complete remission for about two years since therapy was stopped.

SIDE EFFECTS

Side effects are reported to occur in up to 30 per cent of all humans treated with gold compounds (Table 3). The most common side effect is some type of cutaneous eruption. The cutaneous eruptions are quite variable in morphologic appearance (eczematous, macular, lichenoid, nodular, and so on) and are pruritic. Oral reactions (ulcerative sto-matitis, gingivitis, or glossitis) are seen less commonly. These reactions usually clear within a few weeks to three months after treatment is stopped. Human patients who have experienced cutaneous reactions to gold compounds are at no increased risk of suffering a second occurrence when chrysotherapy is restarted at a lower dose.

Proteinuria occurs in 2 to 10 per cent of the humans receiving chrysotherapy. However, this usually regresses when therapy is stopped and often does not recur when therapy is restarted at a lower dose. Severe nephrotoxicity is rare. Hematologic side effects (leukopenia, anemia, thrombocytopenia) occur in 1 to 3 per cent of the humans receiving chrysotherapy.

In dogs and cats, no side effects attributable to chrysotherapy with aurothioglucose have been reported. One dog with pemphigus erythematosus developed an unexplained eosinophilia, which spontaneously regressed after six weeks. It is recommended that a hemogram be checked every two weeks and a urinalysis every week during induction (weekly) therapy and then every one to two months during maintenance therapy.

SUPPLEMENTAL READING

Frost, P., and Gomez, E.: *Recent Advances in Dermatopharmacology.* Jamaica: Spectrum Publications, Inc., 1978, pp. 161–174.
Gibbons, R.: Complications of chrysotherapy. Arch. Intern. Med. 139:343, 1979.
Gottlieb, N. L.: Metabolism and distribution of gold compounds. J. Rheumatol. 6:2, 1979.
Lorber, A., Simon, T. M., Leeb, J., Peter, A., and Wilcox, S. A.: Effect of chrysotherapy on parameters of immune response. J. Rheumatol. 6:82, 1979.
Manning, T. O., Scott, D. W., Kruth, S. A., Sozanski, M., and Lewis, R. M.: Three cases of canine pemphigus foliaceus, and observations on chrysotherapy. J.A.A.H.A. 16:189, 1980.
Newton, C. D., Schumacher, R., and Halliwell, R. E. W.: Gold salt therapy for rheumatoid arthritis in dogs. J.A.V.M.A. 174:1308, 1979.
Penneys, N. S.: Gold therapy: Dermatologic uses and toxicities. J. Am. Acad. Dermatol. 1:315, 1979.
Penneys, N. S., Ackerman, A. B., and Gottlieb, N. L.: Gold dermatitis. Arch. Dermatol. 109:372, 1974.
Penneys, N. S., Eaglstein, W. H., and Frost, P.: Management of pemphigus with gold compounds. A long-term follow-up report. Arch. Dermatol. 112:185, 1976.
Penneys, N. S., Eaglstein, W. H., Indgin, S., and Frost, P.: Gold sodium thiomalate treatment of pemphigus. Arch. Dermatol. 108:56, 1973.
Scott, D. W., Miller, W. H., Lewis, R. M., Manning, T. O., and Smith, C. A.: Pemphigus erythematosus in the dog and cat. J.A.A.H.A., 16:815, 1980.
Scott, D. W., Manning, T. O., Smith, C. A., and Lewis, R. M.: Observations on the immunopathology and therapy of canine pemphigus and pemphigoid. J.A.V.M.A. 180:48, 1982.

IMMUNOTHERAPY

E. GREGORY MacEWEN, V.M.D.

New York, New York

Each of the currently used methods of cancer therapy—surgery, chemotherapy, and radiation therapy—continue to have severe limitations in controlling many neoplasms and the most devastating aspect of neoplasia, metastasis. As a result of experimental and clinical investigation in tumor immunology, immunotherapy or "biologic response modifier therapy" is considered a potentially valuable approach to the treatment of cancer. All attempts to modify the immunologic response to cancer are based on the assumption that cancer cells can be distinguished from normal cells by the presence of distinctive antigens on their surfaces. This concept of distinct tumor antigens represents the cornerstone of cancer immunology. For immunotherapy to be effective, the animal must have minimal residual disease and the animal's host defense system must be intact or able to respond to immunologic manipulation. In addition, patient selection is important; those patients having tumors with the greatest "relative immunogenicity" are the best candidates for immunotherapy.

The purpose of this article is to review the current approaches to the treatment of cancer, i.e., methods to modify the immunologic functions of the host.

Clinical investigations of immunotherapeutic agents have centered around the use of crude microbial adjuvants such as bacillus Calmette-Guerin (BCG), *Corynebacterium parvum*, and mixed bacterial vaccine (MBV). Studies conducted to date are only preliminary indicators for further research; they are not definitive proof that any of these agents are effective in the treatment of spontaneous malignancies. In spite of these reservations, immunotherapy or biologic response modifier therapy has high priority in research because of the promising positive data yielded by clinical trials in both animals and humans.

Biologic response modifiers are agents or approaches that modify the relationships between tumor and host by altering the host's biologic response to tumor cells with resultant therapeutic benefit. Biologic response modifiers can be grouped as follows: (1) immunoaugmenting agents, (2) immunomodulating treatments, (3) immunorestorative agents, (4) interferon inducers and interferon,

(5) thymic hormones and factors, and (6) tumor specific treatments.

IMMUNOAUGMENTING AGENTS

The agents in this group, which includes BCG, methanol extract residue of BCG (MER), muramyl dipeptides (MDP), *C. parvum*, and MBV, act by stimulating macrophage and reticuloendothelial system function. Numerous studies have been performed on the use of these agents in humans, and additional studies have been performed on the use of these agents in dogs and cats with spontaneous neoplasms. To date there is only suggestive positive evidence that these crude bacterial components possess any significant anticancer activity in spontaneous cancers.

An area of intense interest and potential in regard to augmentation of the immune system involves methods of activating macrophages. The ability of activated macrophages to recognize and destroy neoplastic cells while leaving normal cells unharmed has led to studies of the activation of macrophages *in vivo*. Macrophages can be activated by a lymphokine referred to as macrophage activation factor (MAF), which is released from stimulated lymphocytes. Attempts to administer MAF *in vivo*, however, have not resulted in any significant tumorcidal effects. Recently, Fidler (1980) found that encapsulating macrophage activating agents such as MAF and MDP into lipid vesicles called liposomes greatly enhances the delivery of this agent into the macrophage, resulting in regression of lung metastasis in experimental animals.

Another important area of clinical research in regard to augmenting the immune system involves the removal of circulating immune complexes (blocking factors) from the blood of tumor-bearing animals. Studies show that these immune complexes inhibit the cell-mediated response against tumor cells. Recent studies also show that immune complexes can be absorbed from the plasma of both dogs and cats using *Staphylococcus aureus* Cowan I strain (*S. aureus*), which has protein A or covalently immobilized protein A on its surface. The passage or incubation of plasma results in the lowering of circulating immune complexes and tumor necrosis.

IMMUNOMODULATING TREATMENTS

Studies are now under way to determine the effect of agents on the balance of the immune response. Augmentation of responses through inhibition of T-cell suppression function has only recently been studied. Examples include cimetidine, which blocks H2 receptors on suppressor cells, and indomethacin, which interferes with prostaglandin synthesis by suppressor macrophages. There is considerable evidence that suppressor cells may be activated by the systemic administration of immunotherapeutic agents. Antisuppressor cell therapy may greatly augment the activity of these immunomodulating agents.

IMMUNORESTORATIVE APPROACHES

It has been shown that immunologic reactivity is decreased in aged patients and in patients with widespread malignancy. One drug that has been studied extensively for antitumor activity is levamisole. Levamisole, of the class of agents known as imidathiazole compounds, increases phagocytosis by polymorphonuclear cells and macrophages and enhances T-cell responses to mitogens but does not seem to affect B-cell responses. Studies also demonstrate that levamisole helps to abrogate the immunosuppressive effects of radiation and chemotherapy. Studies to evaluate levamisole for its antitumor effects have yielded variable results. Some beneficial results have been reported in human patients with lung and breast cancers. Studies of canine and feline mammary cancer have shown levamisole to be ineffective when used in combination with surgery.

A potent antitumor factor has been identified in normal plasma. Normal plasma infused into mice, cats, and dogs has been shown to have striking antitumor effects in leukemia and lymphosarcoma. Recently we have found that purification of a plasma protein called fibronectin or cold insoluble globulin (CIg), when infused into leukemic cats, produced insignificant regressions of disease in 50 per cent of the cats treated. Further studies are in progress to determine the mechanism of action of purified fibronectin on animals with leukemia.

INTERFERONS

Interferons are inducible secretory glycoproteins that are produced both *in vivo* and *in vitro* by eukaryotic cells in response to viral infection and other stimuli. Interferons are essentially species specific. The antitumor mechanisms of interferons have not been elucidated but seem to be mediated through immunomodulation of the immune system and direct antiproliferative action on the tumor cell. The mechanisms by which interferon-treated cells inhibit virus replication are both multiple and complex; much evidence indicates that interferon inhibits translation of viral protein. Interferon also inhibits the multiplication of tumor cells. These cells do not appear to be blocked in any particular phase of their cell cycle but exhibit a lengthening of each phase.

Interferon inducers such as poly I-C and poly-L-lysine exhibit prophylactic and therapeutic activities agains many viral, localized, and systemic infections as well as antitumor and immunomodulatory activities in mice. Antitumor effects have been seen in human patients with multiple myeloma, non-Hodgkins lymphomas, and lymphocytic leukemia. The number of cancer patients studied thus far is very small and the possible therapeutic benefit has yet to be evaluated.

LYMPHOKINES

Lymphokines are glycoproteins in the 15,000- to 75,000-dalton range. Produced by activated T-lymphocytes, lymphokines obtained from lymphoid tissue can be directly cytocidal or can affect cell proliferation. Some lymphokines exert selective regulatory effects on various components of immune response, and others effect bone marrow proliferation, ossification, or vessel proliferation. One major lymphokine that has been studied is called tumor necrosis factor (TNF). TNF, which is released from host cells, most likely macrophages, is produced in mice treated with BCG or *C. parvum* and then endotoxin. Unlike endotoxin, TNF is toxic *in vitro* for neoplastic murine cells but is nontoxic for normal cells. It is thought that TNF enhances the action of lipopolysaccharides (LPS) on tumors; it may be the mediator of LPS-induced hemorrhagic necrosis.

THYMIC HORMONES AND FACTORS

Several factors have been identified that have thymic hormone–like activity. The importance of these thymic hormones as biologic modifiers lies in the potential usefulness of chemically defined hormones to increase host resistance by accelerating the maturation of T cells from precursor cells. Theoretically, this represents an immunoaugmenting effect, which should be helpful to some patients with cancer, particularly those with T-cell deficiencies. Clinical studies are now under way to evaluate the antitumor effects of these various thymic factors.

TUMOR SPECIFIC TREATMENTS

Some therapeutic studies have centered around the use of tumor cell antigens to evoke a specific antitumor immunologic reaction. The use of anti-tumor antibodies and immune cells shows promise in the field of immunotherapy. In veterinary medicine, the use of specific tumor cell vaccines has been studied in canine lymphosarcoma combined with chemotherapy and in feline mammary adeno-carcinoma combined with mastectomy. The results in the lymphosarcoma study showed that dogs given the autologous tumor cell vaccine had a significantly longer remission time than dogs given chemotherapy alone. The study in cat mammary cancer is still under way; results are not yet available.

Specific antibody therapy has been used in cats with lymphosarcoma. Much is known about the immunology of feline leukemia virus and the response of cats to FeLV infection. Studies show, for example, that FeLV–transformed feline lymphosarcoma cells express an antigen, the feline oncorna-virus-associated cell membrane antigen (FOCMA) on their surface; FOCMA appears to be a tumor-associated antigen. Moreover, it has been shown that some cats with high titers of naturally occurring antibodies of FOCMA are protected from the development of lymphosarcoma. Since FOCMA is only expressed on FeLV– and feline sarcoma virus (FeSV)–induced tumor cells, and since antibody to FOCMA lyses tumor cells in tissue cultures, the effectiveness of FOCMA antibody as a therapeutic agent has been tested in cats with LSA. In a recent study 8 of 15 cats treated showed a response characterized by complete regression of disease.

In conclusion, further experimental and clinical studies need to be done to determine how and under what conditions immunotherapy can be effective in the control of cancer. A greater understanding of the immune system must be obtained in order that its intricate regulating network can be controlled and manipulated so that tumor cells do not escape immunologic destruction.

REFERENCES AND SUPPLEMENTAL READING

Fidler, I. J.: Therapy of spontaneous metastases by intravenous injection of liposomes containing lymphokines. Science 208:1469, 1980.

Hardy, W. D., Jr., MacEwen, E. G., and Hayes, A. A.: FOCMA antibody as specific immunotherapy for lymphosarcoma of pet cats. *In* Hardy, W. D., Essex, M., and McClelland, A. J. (eds.): *Feline Leukemia Virus.* New York: Elsevier North Holland, Inc., 1980, pp. 227–233.

Kassel, R. L., Old, L. J., Day, N. K., et al.: Plasma-mediated leukemia cell destruction: Current status. Blood Cells 3:605, 1977.

Krown, S. E.: Prospects for the treatment of cancer with interferon. *In* Burchenal J. H. and Oettgen H. F. (eds.): *Cancer: Achievements, Challenges, and Prospects for the 1980s,* Vol. I. New York: Grune & Stratton, 1981, pp. 367–379.

Terman, D. S., Yamamoto, T., Mattioli, G. C., et al.: Extensive necrosis of spontaneous canine mammary adenocarcinoma after extracorporeal perfusion over *Staphylococcus aureus* Cowans. J. Immunol. 124:795, 1980.

Section

6

DERMATOLOGIC DISEASES

ROBERT W. KIRK, D.V.M.

Consulting Editor

Additional Pertinent Information found in **Current Veterinary Therapy VII:**

Eyre, Peter, M.R.C.V.S.: Pharmacology of Antipruritic Drugs, p. 497.
Kunkle, Gail A., D.V.M.: The Treatment of Canine Atopic Disease, p. 453.
Kunkle, Gail A., D.V.M.: Zinc-Responsive Dermatoses in Dogs, p. 472.

McKeever, Patrick J., D.V.M., and Dahl, Mark V., M.D.: Subcorneal Pustular Dermatosis and Dermatitis Herpetiformis, p. 443.
Reedy, Lloyd M., D.V.M.: The Diagnosis of Canine Atopic Disease, p. 450.
Scott, Danny W., D.V.M.: Canine Pododermatitis, p. 467.
Scott, Danny W., D.V.M.: Drug Eruption, p. 458.

SYSTEMIC THERAPY OF SKIN DISORDERS

ROBERT W. KIRK, D.V.M.

Ithaca, New York

ANTIBIOTICS

Antibiotic agents for systemic use in skin disorders have rather special and specific indications. More general details of antibiotics and their specific doses are covered on pages 41 and 1216. Antibiotics are used only to kill bacteria. Since the overwhelming majority of skin infections are caused by *Staphylococcus aureus* coagulase-positive bacteria, antibiotics that affect these organisms and that concentrate in the skin are of primary interest. Occasionally *Proteus* sp., *Pseudomonas* sp., and coliform bacteria are involved as secondary invaders in deeper skin infections.

On an empirical basis, erythromycin, lincomycin, oxacillin, and chloramphenicol are the drugs of choice for therapy of skin disorders. The cephalosporins, e.g., cephalexin, are excellent but expensive. Gentamicin is useful for short periods, especially if gram negative organisms are involved. The trimethoprim-sulfadiazine combination is also useful, but for pyodermas the dosage must be increased 50 to 100 per cent above the routine dose. Most antibiotics do not distribute as well to the skin as to other tissues; therefore higher doses are needed for optimum effect. Duration of therapy is also important. Once antibiotic therapy is started for a skin infection, it should always be continued for *at least* ten days. If the problem is chronic, relapsing, or complicated, a *minimum* duration for therapy is 30 days. Deep folliculitis and other deep pyodermas may require several months of vigorous treatment.

Because many of the common skin pathogens (staphylococci) are penicillinase producers, penicillin, ampicillin, and other antibiotics inactivated by those enzymes are ineffective and should not be used unless specific tests dictate otherwise.

Although initial therapy of simple pyodermas and superficial folliculitis may be guided by a Gram stain of the exudate, culture and inhibition studies should guide the therapy in more complex infections.

Sulfonamides, except in the combination noted previously, have little use in a dermatologic formulary.

ANTIMYCOTICS

Systemic antifungal agents are now used effectively for many severe fungal diseases. Newer agents have broad spectrum antimycotic effects.

Ketoconazole (Nizoral, Janssen Pharmaceutica) is a broad spectrum antimycotic that is an almost white, tasteless, odorless powder. It is practically insoluble in water, soluble in acids, and stable under normal room storage for two years. It is a dioxolone imidazole, structurally related to miconazole and clotrimazole. It impairs synthesis of ergosterol, which alters the integrity of the fungal cell membrane. Fortunately, this mechanism is not important to mammalian cell walls.

Ketoconazole is rapidly absorbed following oral administration, reaching peak levels in one to two hours with a plasma half-life of eight hours. Because it requires acidity for dissolution, ketoconazole should be given with meals. The tentative dose for dogs is 10 mg/kg every 8 to 12 hours (Wolfe and Poppagianis, 1981).

Effective blood levels depend on the organism and its sensitivity. Maximum levels reached are 3.5 μg/ml. It is present (in rats) in high levels in the lung, liver, kidney, bladder, connective tissue, and bone marrow. In dogs it passes the placenta and is present in milk. Very little of the drug enters the CNS or brain. It is teratogenic in rats at a dose comparable to ten times the maximum human dose. It is detoxified in the liver, and 20 per cent of a single dose is excreted in 24 hours. Minor side effects demonstrated in humans are gastric irritation, photophobia, and pruritus. Combination therapy with amphotericin B seems to enhance the antimycotic activity of both drugs (Attleberger, 1983).

Ketoconazole has been used on canine blastomycosis (Attleberger, 1983; Wolfe and Poppagianis, 1981) and dermatophytosis. In humans and experimental animals, it produced good results in treating candidiasis, dermatophytosis, histoplasmosis, and paracoccidioidomycosis; moderate results with coccidioidomycosis, chromomycosis, and aspergillosis; but poor response with mycetomas, aspergillomas, and phaeohyphomycosis (Symoens et al., 1980). *In vitro* activity has been shown against *Cryptococcus*, *Sporothrix schenckii*, *Actinomyces*, *Phycomycetes*, and various other yeasts and fungi, but the clinical significance is unknown (Restrepo et al., 1980). Treatment length varied from 7 to 10 days for candidiasis, 6 to 8 weeks for dermatophytosis, and up to 12 months for onychomycosis. A minimum treatment course for systemic mycoses is six months. This drug is extremely expensive, so it should be used only when griseofulvin or other therapy fails. Initial experience showed some incidence of relapse following premature cessation of therapy. However, resistance to ketoconazole has not been reported. Ketoconazole is not currently licensed for use in dogs and cats.

Griseofulvin (Fulvicin P/G, Schering Corp.) is a fungistatic antibiotic obtained by fermentation from several species of *Penicillium*. It is a white crystalline powder with a bitter taste. It acts by inhibiting DNA synthesis in susceptible fungi. Absorption following oral dosage is greatly enhanced if the ultra microcrystalline form is used and if it is given with food of high fat content. This also helps alleviate the gastrointestinal distress that may be a side effect. Active griseofulvin is deposited in the horny layer within eight hours after oral administration (Epstein et al., 1972). Skin levels begin to decline in 24 hours and are 0 in 48 to 72 hours. The drug remains in a state of flux in the skin; therefore, once or twice daily administration is indicated. It should be given for six to eight weeks for dermal infections and for up to six months for nail infections (or until cultures are negative). Once weekly dosage is not appropriate. Daily doses of 50 mg/kg are suggested (Scott, 1980a).

Griseofulvin has a rather narrow spectrum but is used against all known species of *Microsporum*, *Trichophyton*, and *Epidermophyton*. It is not effective against bacteria, yeasts (such as *Candida* or *Malassezia*), or the systemic fungi. Topical applications of griseofulvin are ineffective. This drug should not be prescribed haphazardly. It should only be given to treat positively diagnosed cases of dermatophytosis. Griseofulvin must be given for long treatment periods. It is expensive and has a toxic potential. It may cause severe vomiting and is highly teratogenic, especially in the early weeks of gestation. Thus it is important not to give it to pregnant females or females that may become pregnant during the prolonged period of therapy.

Flucytosine (Ancobon, Roche), a fluorinated pyrimidine, is an antifungal agent whose exact mode of action is not known. It is not metabolized significantly when given orally. Its use is indicated only in the treatment of serious infections caused by susceptible strains of *Candida* or *Cryptococcus*. Only about one-half of the originally isolated strains of *Candida* are susceptible, and resistance by *Candida* and *Cryptococcus* organisms readily develops during treatment. About one-half of the organisms will develop resistance within three weeks. Toxic effects include hepatotoxicity, bone marrow suppression, and skin and gastrointestinal disturbances. Animals under treatment should have 10- to 14-day evaluations of BUN, CBC, and liver enzyme (SGPT) levels.

The dosage of flucytosine is 60 mg/kg every eight hours. Combining this drug with amphotericin B is now the therapy of choice for cryptococcal infections. With such a combination, the dose of amphotericin B is reduced by one-half, which reduces its toxicity while maintaining its efficiency. Flucytosine is not currently licensed for use in dogs and cats.

Amphotericin B (Fungizone, E. R. Squibb) is a fungicidal antibiotic agent that ionically binds to acid phospholipids in the bacterial (and fungal) cell membrane and exerts a detergent-like action. It also binds to mammalian cell membranes and so is relatively toxic to mammals. It is probably most effective for blastomycosis, histoplasmosis, coccidioidomycosis, cryptococcosis, and candidiasis (in the last two cases when combined with flucytosine).

Amphotericin B must be given by injection, and the powder must be dissolved *only* in 5 per cent dextrose and water. In dogs, 0.15 mg/kg is given IV in 20 to 30 ml of diluent over a period of 20 to 30 minutes. Dosage is increased gradually to 0.20 to 0.25 mg/kg per injection after the second or third week. The injections are given every other day for a total of 20 to 22 injections. Dosage for cats is 0.8 mg in 10 ml of 5 per cent dextrose and water given IV every third or fourth day. Use a 25-gauge needle and inject as rapidly as possible. Attleberger (1983) has not seen severe toxicity with the above schedules (page 1180), but animals should have a high caloric diet and should be treated as outpatients and monitored with once or twice weekly urinalysis and BUN evaluations. If proteinuria develops or BUNs exceed 40 for dogs or 60 for cats, therapy should be discontinued until normal levels return.

Complications of therapy include nephrotoxicity, anemia, phlebitis, and hypokalemia. In addition, resistant strains may develop easily.

ANTI-INFLAMMATORY AGENTS

Dapsone (Avlosulfon, Ayerst) is an anti-inflammatory, antibacterial chemical (4-4′ diaminodiphenyl sulfone) whose mechanism of action is unknown. Its anti-inflammatory activity does not involve the adrenal glands, however. It is rapidly absorbed orally and reaches peak concentration in four to eight hours. Its serum half-life varies from 10 to 50 hours (average 28) in humans. It is indicated for leprosy, dermatitis herpetiformis, subcorneal pustular dermatosis, and glucocytoclastic vasculitis in humans and has been used effectively for the last three disorders in dogs. Dosage in dogs is 1 mg/kg t.i.d. orally. This is continued for two to three weeks or until the lesions clear, at which time dosage can be reduced to twice daily. Further reductions to once or twice weekly may be possible for maintenance, and in some cases the drug may be withdrawn without a relapse. Adverse effects include blood dyscrasias (granulocytopenia, anemia, thrombocytopenia), drug sensitization skin reactions, and hepatotoxicity. These usually occur early in therapy and are reversible, but periodic CBC and SGPT values should be monitored. Dapsone is not presently cleared for use in dogs and cats.

BACTERIAL ANTIGENS

Several agents may be used to hyposensitize patients who are thought to have type III hypersensitivities to staphylococcal antigens from bacteria cell walls or exotoxins. Autogenous bacterins are expensive and difficult to obtain (MacDonald et al., 1972). Staphoid A-B* overcomes these problems and has been effective in special cases. It is a commercial staphylococcal cell wall antigen and toxin mixture. Table 1 lists the Staphoid A-B administration schedule.

Staphylococcal phage lysate products have been reported effective by several clinicians (Anderson, 1980; Kunkle, 1980; Rosser, 1982). The antigens are prepared by lysing parent cultures of *S. aureus*, serologic types I and III, with a polyvalent *Staphylococcus* bacteriophage. After ultrafiltration the lysates contain antigenic fractions of *S. aureus* and active bacteriophage. The phage is polyvalent and has lysed *in vitro* a significant proportion of field

---

*JenSal Labs, Division of Burroughs Wellcome, Research Triangle Park, NC.

Table 1.   *Staphoid A-B Schedule**

Day	ID Administration (ml)	SQ Administration (ml)	Total Dose (ml)
1	0.1	0.15	0.25
2	0.1	0.40	0.50
3	0.1	0.65	0.75
4	0.1	0.90	1.00
5	0.1	1.15	1.25
12	0.1	1.40	1.50
19	0.1	1.65	1.75
26	0.1	1.90	2.00
Monthly	0.1	1.90	2.00

*Staphoid A-B is mixed with equal parts of saline. Data from Baker: Vet. Clin. North Am. 4:107, 1974.

Table 2.   *Staph Lysate Schedule*

Week	Staph Lysate (ml, SC)
1	0.1
2	0.2
3	0.3
4	0.4
5*	0.5

*Continue 0.5 ml every seven days or as needed for life.

strains of staphylococci. Its ability to lyse staphylococci *in vivo* has been shown in experimental animals. Clinical benefits following vaccination have been attributed to stimulation of antibacterial antibodies. However, benefit is now understood to result from a favorable effect on the state of cellular sensitivity to staphylococci.

Rosser (1982) has shown a positive effect on T-cell depression (measured by lymphocyte blastogenesis) of staph pyoderma folliculitis patients treated with staph lysate products. For superficial infections he used the subcutaneous injection schedule advocated by Anderson (1980) (Table 2). The protocol for deep pyodermas can be found in Table 3.

Bacterial antigens should be reserved for patients with a history of pyodermas that responded to long-term antibiotic therapy followed by relapse when therapy was discontinued. Antibiotic therapy is used in addition to the antigen injections for the first month. Then phage lysate is used alone. STAPHPHAGE LYSATE† is not currently licensed for use in dogs and cats.

HYPOSENSITIZATION

Hyposensitization is a biologic therapy for atopic patients that involves giving multiple increasing doses of reactive agents (allergens) parenterally. The patient responds by forming IgG antibodies against each specific antigen. These circulating antibodies are protective since they bind with invading allergens before the allergens reach tissue-fixed IgE.

---

†Delmont Labs, Swarthmore, PA.

Table 3.   *Staph Lysate Schedule for Deep Pyodermas*

Week	Staph Lysate (ml, SC)*
1	0.25
2	0.50
3	0.75
4	1.00

*Can be increased to 2.0 ml weekly if necessary.

This blocking antibody theory is now being questioned and may be only a partial explanation of hyposensitization, since a decrease in cellular sensitivity and a long-term diminution of the reaginic antibody available to sensitize mediator-releasing cells are also proposed mechanisms.

Hyposensitization can be used when there is good correlation between the clinical history and correctly run positive intradermal skin tests. No more than ten allergens should be used in any series. Ideally, hyposensitization should be started when the environmental allergen load is low and should reach maintenance dosage levels several weeks before the clinical exposure or signs should start.

There are two basic methods of hyposensitization (Kunkle, 1980). One uses aqueous extracts, which are rapidly absorbed. Therefore, frequent, low-dose injections are required (Table 4). The other uses alum precipitated extracts, which are slowly absorbed, requiring fewer, high-dose injections (Table 5). Response to therapy is gradual and may not be evident for four to six months. Maintenance injections, if needed, must be tailored to the individual case. In all instances hyposensitization should fit in with a total program of exclusion and the judicious use of antihistamines or corticosteroids when needed.

IMMUNE MODULATORS

Levamisole is a simple chemical, first introduced as a broad spectrum anthelmintic, that is an im-

Table 4. *Aqueous Schedule For Hyposensitization**

Day	Vial 1 (100–200 PNU/ml)	Vial 2 (1000–2000 PNU/ml)	Vial 3 (10,000–20,000 PNU/ml)
0	0.1 cc		
2	0.2 cc		
4	0.4 cc		
6	0.8 cc		
8	1.0 cc		
10		0.1 cc	
12		0.2 cc	
14		0.4 cc	
16		0.8 cc	
18		1.0 cc	
20			0.1 cc
22			0.2 cc
24			0.4 cc
26			0.8 cc
28			1.0 cc
38			1.0 cc
48†			1.0 cc

*Data from Kunkle *In* Kirk: *Current Veterinary Therapy VII.* Philadelphia: W. B. Saunders, 1980.

†Thereafter, repeat injections (1.0 cc) every 20 to 40 days for the next 18 months.

Injections are given by subcutaneous administration. The extracts must be kept refrigerated.

Table 5. *Alum Precipitated Schedule* Allpyral (Dome Laboratories) and Centeral (Center Laboratories)*

Week	Vial 1 (100–200 PNU/ml)	Vial 2 (10,000–20,000 PNU/ml)
1	0.1 cc	
2	0.2 cc	
3	0.4 cc	
4	0.8 cc	
5		0.1 cc
6		0.2 cc
7		0.4 cc
8		0.8 cc
9		1.0 cc
12		1.0 cc
16		1.0 cc
20		1.0 cc
24		1.0 cc
28		1.0 cc
32		1.0 cc

*Data from Kunkle *In* Kirk: *Current Veterinary Therapy VII.* Philadelphia: W. B. Saunders, 1980.

Injections are given by subcutaneous administration. The extracts must be kept refrigerated. Shake well.

munotherapeutic compound with anti-anergic properties (Symoens and Rosenthal, 1977). Although the exact mechanism of action is unknown, studies on isolated cells and experimental animals suggest that levamisole restores to normal functions of phagocytes and lymphocytes from compromised hosts. The effects are most pronounced in increasing the numbers and function of T lymphocytes from old, diseased, or immunosuppressed donors. There is no direct effect on B lymphocytes. Therapeutic doses of levamisole do not seem to increase immune responses above normal levels. There is little or no effect on healthy young people, but the drug restores to normal a variety of immunologic functions in older people (Symoens and Rosenthal, 1977).

Although levamisole does not consistently repress a primary invasion by virulent bacteria, viruses, or tumor cells, it may increase the protective effect of some vaccines and stabilize tumor remission. The *in vivo* effect may be due to a serum factor that appears in responding animals and that can be transferred to other animals by serum injections. The drug is a potent anthelmintic but is not toxic to bacteria, viruses, protozoa, fungi, or normal or tumor cells.

Levamisole is well absorbed following oral dosage with peak levels in 2 hours, a half-life of 4 hours, and virtual elimination via the urine in 48 hours (humans). The dosage is critical as there is a so-called window effect (Rosser, 1982). Doses higher or lower than optimum may produce immunosuppression rather than stimulation. Currently an immunomodulating dose for levamisole in small animals is not well worked out. Clinicians presently use 0.5 to 2.0 mg/kg repeated three times *weekly.*

Indications for levamisole include chronic or recurrent infections involving skin or soft tissues and primary and secondary immune deficiency states. It has also been used in rheumatic, allergic, and neoplastic diseases in humans. Adverse effects may include granulocytopenia, allergic skin reactions, and immune suppression.

Thiabendazole is an immunostimulant used in a manner similar to levamisole in doses of 5 to 10 mg/kg orally three times weekly.

CHRYSOTHERAPY

Chrysotherapy is the use of *gold* as a therapeutic agent in disease. The mechanism of action of gold compounds in controlling a variety of inflammatory disorders is unknown. The therapeutic effects develop slowly, and maximal immunosuppression may not be attained for several months or even years. Gold compounds may act at various levels of the immune and inflammatory responses. Studies have shown that gold therapy causes decreases in blood levels of rheumatoid factor, antiepithelial antibodies, circulating lymphocytes, IgM, and IgA. Other mechanisms of action may include enzyme inhibition, collagen and lysosomal stabilization, anti-infective activity, phagocytosis inhibition, alteration of reticuloendothelial cell function, and interference with prostaglandin biosynthesis.

The only indication for chrysotherapy in veterinary medicine is the pemphigus complex. A sterile suspension of *aurothioglucose* (Solganal, Schering) is given once weekly by intramuscular injection (Scott et al., 1982). Since there is concern about adverse reactions (common in humans but, so far, rare in animals), small test doses are given (Table 6). When remission occurs, doses are scheduled biweekly, then monthly or are discontinued. In some cases prolonged remission follows cessation of several months of therapy (Scott et al., 1982).

Adverse reactions occur more commonly in humans during induction and only rarely during maintenance therapy. These may include cutaneous reactions, stomatitis, nephrotoxicity, blood dyscrasias, gastrointestinal upsets, hepatitis, and anaphylactoid reactions. Reactions have not been a problem in animals; however, animals should be carefully observed, and hemograms and urinalysis should be evaluated weekly or monthly as needed during treatment. A few patients have proteinuria while on gold therapy. Chrysotherapy is contraindicated in patients with diabetes mellitus, systemic lupus erythematosus, or hematologic, renal, hepatic, or cardiac disorders. Solganal is not presently licensed for use in dogs and cats.

HORMONAL THERAPY

Hormonal medications are an enigma. Dosage levels are critical, and maintenance of constant, uniform levels or planned fluctuating levels by replacement therapy may be crucial to a proper response. Only a few preparations are prescribed effectively for specific skin effects.

Thyroid hormone can be replaced successfully by oral medication, although four to six weeks are needed to obtain the initial response. Usually, it must be given for the duration of the patient's life. There is great individual variation in dosage response, and proper dosage is best monitored by post-pill testing. In general the dosage varies inversely with the size of the patient. Synthetic thyroid hormones, sodium 1-thyroxine (T_4) and/or sodium triiodothyronine (T_3), are strongly recommended for routine therapy. Initial canine doses may be 20 μg/kg every 12 hours for T_4, and 4 μg/kg every 8 hours for T_3. See page 854 for complete details on hypothyroidism and its treatment (Rosychuk, 1983).

Glucocorticoid hormones have potent effects on the skin and are commonly prescribed in dermatologic therapy. The most obvious effects are a reduction in itching, which is accomplished by inhibition of antigen-antibody reactions, and a decrease in inflammation (Fine, 1973; Scott, 1980b). This symptomatic treatment removes one of the major complaints of the patient (and its owner), but the drug is too often abused by overuse. Iatrogenic hyperadrenocorticism commonly occurs from long-term, constant use of repositol or long-acting corticosteroids. Corticosteroid use should be strictly regulated; it should be administered for as short a time as possible and in as low a dose as possible (Storrs, 1979). *Once the initial response is obtained, glucocorticoids should be withdrawn or continued when necessary using only alternate-day therapy with short-acting oral medications* (Chastain and Graham, 1979). For complete details of glucocortical therapy, see page 869 (Rosenthal and Wilcke, 1983).

Sex hormones are useful in special cases. The principal effects of sex hormones may be known, but the clinical effects are often unpredictable. Androgenic hormones have a tendency to increase sebum production and the formation of comedones. Therefore they are contraindicated in the presence

Table 6.   Dosage Schedule for Aurothioglucose

Week	Dog Over 20 lb	Cat and Dog Under 20 lb
1 (test)	5 mg	1 mg
2 (test)	10 mg	2 mg
3 to 8	1 mg/kg	1 mg/kg

Injections are given intramuscularly.

of seborrhea. It is useful in the male feminizing syndrome of dogs and in combination with estrogen in feline endocrine alopecia. Testosterone repositol injections at a dose of 1.0 to 2.0 mg/kg (up to a maximum of 50 mg) are given once every ten days, or testosterone in oil at one-half this dose is given every other day to effect, then once weekly. Testosterone cyclopentylpropionate (TCP) for injection and fluoxymesterone (Halotestin, Upjohn) tablets for oral use are alternative androgenic preparations. When available or when mixed for each patient, a combination of 12 mg repositol testosterone and 0.6 mg diethylstilbestrol is effective as an intramuscular injection once every four to six weeks for feline endocrine alopecia.

Estrogens or diethylstilbestrol tend to reduce sebum production, but their use in skin disease is highly unpredictable. Diethylstilbestrol given orally is effective for ovarian imbalance type II. It is administered daily in doses of 0.1 to 1.0 mg/dog for three weeks; after one week of rest the dosage is repeated. When response is noted, the dosage should be given only once or twice a month for maintenance. Constant long-term estrogen therapy may produce bone marrow suppression (in dogs) or hepatic damage (in cats).

PROGESTATIONAL COMPOUNDS

Megestrol acetate (Ovaban, Schering), repositol progesterone, and medroxyprogesterone acetate (Depo-Provera, Upjohn) are compounds that have been used extensively for skin diseases in the cat (Scott, 1980a). They have been a mixed blessing. These agents have several actions: they suppress gonadotropin release and androgenic and/or estrogenic effects on target organs, induce growth hormone release, and affect hypothalamic functions. They have few direct glucocorticoid or mineral corticoid effects, but they markedly suppress adrenal response to ACTH. This occurs in one week with doses of only 2.5 mg megestrol acetate every other day, and suppression is severe by three weeks (Chastain and Graham, 1979; Scott, 1980a). The clinical implications of this adverse effect can be unfortunate. In addition, there is the possibility of immunosuppression (T cells), which is of concern in patients with infections and neoplasia. Suppression of fibroblast function may delay wound healing. The inhibition of collagenolytic enzymes may explain the beneficial effects seen in treating eosinophilic granulomas and pruritus.

Side effects vary from inconvenient polyphagia, polydipsia, and weight gain to a happy change in behavior. A few cats become tigers. These effects are the result of action on the hypothalamus and limbic system. More serious effects include a fairly high incidence of mammary hyperplasia or neoplasia (adenocarcinoma) in either sex and a transient occurrence of diabetes mellitus. Injections of progestational compounds may produce temporary local alopecia, cutaneous atrophy, and pigmentary disturbances in which a dark cat's skin and hair turn white. Pyometra is well documented following the injudicious use of repositol progestational products. Therefore, care should be taken when prescribing oral forms to intact females; these compounds should only be given for short periods, or better, not at all. These drugs depress testosterone production and spermatogenesis, so they should not be used in breeding males.

Progestational agents have been used effectively in treating feline endocrine alopecia, eosinophilic granuloma complex, psychogenic alopecia and dermatitis, miliary dermatitis, and "stud tail." They should be used with due caution, as they are not cleared for use in cats. Scott (1980a) has suggested dosage of megestrol acetate at 2.5 to 5.0 mg/cat every other day until lesions respond and then once weekly or biweekly. Repositol progesterone 2 to 20 mg/kg or medroxyprogesterone acetate 50 to 175 mg/cat IM or SC is given once and then only as needed (which may be only every few months or for life).

NUTRITION

Nutritional factors that influence the skin are exceedingly complex. It is obvious, however, that for proper skin health and function the diet must be complete in all essential nutritional factors. When deficiencies are produced experimentally they often result in cutaneous disorders; but these are seldom characteristic enough to allow specific diagnosis. Furthermore, the interaction of nutrients is such that a deficiency of one item may upset delicate balances, and the skin manifestation may be the result of the imbalance rather than the initial deficiency. For these reasons it is felt that a complex diet of well-balanced, wholesome, and fresh ingredients is the proper approach to providing adequate nutrition for skin health. It is necessary in some cases to modify the diet or use nutritional supplements to improve skin health, but the cliche "add more fat to the diet" is overworked and seldom helpful.

> Nutritional factors influencing the skin are complex. There is no simple supplementation program that cures a skin disease.

General overeating leads to obesity, which may cause intertriginous dermatitis and bacterial infections or, by increasing the fat layer, may make heat dissipation more difficult.

General malnutrition, on the other hand, causes

the skin to become dry, inelastic, and scaly. It may become more susceptible to infection and may show hemorrhagic tendencies and pigment disturbances. Undernourishment can develop through interference with intake, absorption, or utilization; through increased requirements or excretion; or through inhibition by antisubstances.

Specific nutritional factors are most difficult to evaluate; a great number of nutrients have been determined to have an influence on skin health. These include essential fatty acids, amino acids, proteins, vitamins, and minerals.

FATTY ACIDS

The polyunsaturated fatty acid linoleic acid is an essential element in the diet of all animals. Arachidonic and linoleic acids are also necessary, but except for arachidonic acid in the cat they can be synthesized from linoleic acid. Fatty acid deficiency causes dry, lusterless hair, fine scaling, thickened skin, alopecia, and later pruritus, acute moist dermatitis, and greasy skin and hair from excess sebaceous activity (Lewis, 1982). This deficiency is rare, but it may result from feeding dry food stored more than six months, oxidized (rancid) fat, or food with inadequate antioxidants such as vitamin E. These signs are also suggestive of riboflavin and zinc deficiencies, but these disorders are often associated with erythema on the thighs, chest, and abdomen. Vitamin A deficiency may have similar manifestations but is also characterized by follicular lesions and centrally keratinized papules. Vitamin A toxicity has characteristics similar to those seen in vitamin A deficiency, but a history of vitamin A supplementation should be diagnostic. The fatty acid deficiency responds within one month to the daily administration of 2 teaspoonfuls of vegetable oil (corn or soybean) per cup of dry food. Because the clinical syndrome can be caused by several deficiencies, supplements of fatty acids, vitamin A, zinc, and riboflavin assure that the skin condition will be adequately treated (Lewis, 1982). There is no controlled data to support claims that extra fatty acid supplementation promotes a glossy coat.

PROTEIN AND AMINO ACIDS

Hair is 95 per cent protein with a high percentage of sulfur–containing amino acids. The normal growth of hair (total of 100 feet per day) and the keratinization of skin require 25 to 30 per cent of the animal's daily protein requirement (Lewis, 1982). Animals with protein deficiency have hyperkeratosis, epidermal hyperpigmentation, and loss of hair pigment. There is patchy alopecia with hairs

that become thinner, rough, dry, dull, and brittle; they are easily broken and grow slowly. These lesions, together with scales and crusts, may appear symmetrically on the head, back, thorax, and abdomen. Lesions are more prominent in young, growing dogs, in which protein needs are higher. In humans, a mean hair root of less than 0.06 mm diameter suggests protein deficiency. Similar data are not available for animals. Analysis of the diet and provision of a protein content of at least 25 per cent on a dry matter basis for the dog and 33 per cent for the cat should be therapeutic. High-quality protein from eggs, meat, or milk is important.

VITAMINS

Vitamin A maintains healthy skin and epithelial cells. Signs of deficiency or toxicity (similar) are manifested cutaneously. There is keratinization of the epithelial surfaces. Hyperkeratitis occurs in the ducts of the sebaceous glands, occluding their ducts and blocking secretion. Firm papule-like eruptions with a firm center are formed, which may be local or general. There is also alopecia, scaling of the skin, and an increased susceptibility to infection. A single injection of 6000 IU aqueous vitamin A solution/kg body weight is adequate therapy for two months for a serious deficiency. Overtreatment can easily produce vitamin A toxicity.

VITAMIN DEFICIENCIES

Deficiencies of single B vitamins are very rare, and the signs of many of the avitaminoses are similar (dry, dull hair; scaly, nonpruritic dermatosis; decreased food intake). Therapy for any of these conditions or a suspected deficiency of any of the B vitamins should consist of the use of preparations containing the entire complex of B vitamins. At least five times the minimum daily requirement of each should be given, since they are water soluble; excesses are easily excreted without toxicity (Lewis, 1982).

Biotin deficiency results from prolonged oral antibiotic therapy or excess feeding of raw egg whites. Riboflavin deficiency in pet animals is almost unheard of if *any* meat or dairy products are fed.

Niacin deficiency is manifested as pellagra and is characterized by ulcerated mucous membranes, diarrhea, and emaciation. To produce a deficiency, diets must be low in animal protein and high in corn, which is low in tryptophan. Except for the cat, animals convert tryptophan to niacin. Commercial pet diets have more than enough niacin, so a deficiency is a rarity today.

Ascorbic acid deficiency (scurvy) causes hemorrhage in many body tissues including skin and mucous membranes, broken "corkscrew" hairs, and follicular hyperkeratosis. Although dogs can synthesize ascorbic acid, a secondary deficiency may occur during stress or disease. Fifty milligrams of ascorbic acid daily is adequate supplementation.

Vitamin E in doses of 400 IU b.i.d. has been used successfully in treating discoid lupus, epidermolysis bullosa, systemic lupus erythematosus, and disorders involving the basement membrane.

Doses of 10 mg/kg daily are used as an antioxidant and for the therapy of pansteatitis in cats (excess tuna or fat in the diet).

Sheffy (1979) found that a vitamin E deficiency combined with a high polyunsaturated fatty acid intake caused the development of a severe dermatosis. This could not be distinguished clinically from the dermatosis seen with an essential fatty acid deficiency. However, analysis of serum from vitamin E–deficient dogs revealed *elevated* levels of the essential fatty acids linoleic and arachidonic acids. Sheffy suggested that the skin disease is related to increased synthesis of prostaglandins (Sheffy, 1979).

MINERALS

A copper deficiency should never affect small animals on good commercial diets. Animals on a diet of unbalanced homemade rations or on excessive zinc supplementation may develop a deficiency. This results in a lack of pigmentation and faulty keratinization of the skin and hair follicles. The hair is dull and rough. An adequate intake is 4 mg copper/lb of dry matter.

Two zinc–responsive deficiency syndromes occur in dogs. One is caused by excess calcium supplementation in growing puppies. Calcium in the diet decreases zinc absorption and results in deficiency. Reduction of calcium supplements and addition of zinc sulfate at a rate of 10 mg/kg body weight brings improvement in 10 to 14 days. Clinically, the pups are small, with thick, fissured footpads. There are crusted, scaly lesions on the body, especially on the face and extremities.

The second syndrome occurs primarily in huskies and malamutes. The onset occurs during puberty, although older dogs can be affected. Some individuals have decreased zinc absorption. Absorption is increased by a high-protein diet and is decreased by a high-calcium or plant diet, which binds zinc. Some dogs show lesions only with stress. The coat may be rough, and there are scales and crusts, which may be thick, around the eyes, mouth, chin, ears, extremities, scrotum, prepuce, and vulva. There may be local hyperpigmentation. Zinc sulfate supplementation at 10 mg/kg may be needed for the rest of the dog's life, since many animals relapse within six weeks if supplementation is stopped.

Lewis (1982) has suggested feeding the supplements in the formula given hereafter to correct most skin conditions caused by nutritional deficiencies. If the condition persists in spite of the supplementation, it undoubtedly does not have a nutritional origin.

Supplement formula:
  1 tsp vegetable cooking oil
  2 to 3 oz raw liver
  100 mg zinc sulfate
  1 drop tincture of iodine

Add to the diet daily for a 20- to 30-lb dog. This supplement provides fat, protein, vitamins A and E, biotin, riboflavin, niacin, iodine, and zinc.

REFERENCES AND SUPPLEMENTAL READING

Anderson, R. K.: Canine pododermatitis. Comp. Cont. Ed. 11:361, 1980.

Attleberger, M. H.: The systemic mycoses. *In* Kirk, R. W. (ed.): *Current Veterinary Therapy VIII*. Philadelphia: W. B. Saunders, 1983, pp. 1180–1184.

Baker, E.: Staphylococcal disease. Vet. Clin. North Am. 4:107, 1974.

Chastain, C. B., and Graham, C. L.: Adrenocortical suppression in dogs on daily and alternate prednisolone administration. Am. J. Vet. Res. 40:936, 1979.

du Vivier, A., and Stoughton, R. B.: Tachyphylaxis to the action of topically applied corticosteroids. Arch. Dermatol. 111:581, 1975.

Epstein, W. L., Shah, V. P., and Riegelman, S.: Griseofulvin levels in stratum corneum. Arch. Dermatol. 106:344, 1972.

Fine, R. M.: Physiologic effects of systemic corticosteroids in dermatology. Cutis 11:217, 1973.

Goette, D. K., and Odom, R. B.: Adverse effects of corticosteroids. Cutis 23:477, 1979.

Ihrke, P. J.: Antibiotic therapy in canine skin disease—dermatologic therapy III. Comp. Cont. Ed. 11:177, 1980.

Kunkle, G. A.: The treatment of canine atopic disease. *In* Kirk, R. W. (ed.): *Current Veterinary Therapy VII*. Philadelphia: W. B. Saunders, 1980, pp. 453–458.

Lewis, L. D.: Cutaneous manifestation of nutritional imbalances. Lecture notes, 1982.

MacDonald, K. R., Greenfield, J., and McCausland, H. R.: Remission of staphylococcal dermatitis by autogenous bacteria therapy. Can. Vet. J. 13:45, 1972.

Mailbach, H. I., and Stoughton, R. B.: Topical corticosteroids. Med. Clin. North Am. 57:1253, 1973.

Mulnix, J. A.: Corticosteroid therapy in the dog. Proceedings of the 44th Annual Meeting of the American Animal Hospital Association, 1977.

Reedy, L. M.: The role of staphylococcal bacteria in canine dermatology. Proceedings of the Annual Meeting of the American Animal Hospital Association, Atlanta, 1982, pp. 71–73.

Restrepo, A. K., Stevens, D. A., and Utz, J. P. (eds.): First international symposium on ketoconazole. Rev. Infect. Dis. 2:519, 1980.

Rosenthal, R. C., and Wilcke, J. R.: Glucocorticoid therapy. *In* Kirk, R. W. (ed.): *Current Veterinary Therapy VIII*. Philadelphia: W. B. Saunders, 1983, pp. 854–863.

Rosser, E.: Presentation at the 49th Annual Meeting of the American Animal Hospital Association, 1982.

Rosychuk, R. A. W.: Management of hypothyroidism. *In* Kirk, R. W. (ed.): *Current Veterinary Therapy VIII*. Philadelphia: W. B. Saunders, 1983, pp. 869–876.

Scott, D. W.: Hyperadrenocorticism. Vet. Clin. North Am. 9:3, 1979.

Scott, D. W.: Feline dermatology 1900–1978. J. Am. Anim. Hosp. Assoc. 16: May/June 1980a.

Scott, D. W.: Systemic glucocorticoid therapy. *In* Kirk, R. W. (ed.): *Current Veterinary Therapy VII*. Philadelphia: W. B. Saunders, 1980b, pp. 988–994.

Scott, D. W.: Dermatologic use of glucocorticoids. Vet. Clin. North Am. 12:19, 1982.

Scott, D. W., and Green, C. E.: Iatrogenic secondary adrenocortical insufficiency in dogs. J. Am. Anim. Hosp. Assoc. 10:555, 1974.

Scott, D. W., Lewis, R. M., Manning, T. O., et al.: Observations on the immunopathology and therapy of canine pemphigus and pemphigoid. J.A.V.M.A. 180:48, 1982.

Sheffy, B. E.: Report of Veterinary Virus Research Laboratory, Cornell University, 1979.

Storrs, F. J.: Use and abuse of systemic corticosteroid therapy. J. Am. Acad. Dermatol. 1:95, 1979.

Symoens, J., et al.: An evaluation of two years of clinical experience with ketoconazole. Rev. Infect. Dis. 2:674, 1980.

Symoens, J., and Rosenthal, M.: Levamisole in the modulation of the immune response: The current experimental and clinical state. J. Reticuloendothel. Soc. 21:176, 1977.

Wolfe, A. M., and Poppagianis, D.: Canine coccidioidomycosis, treatment with a new antifungal agent, ketoconazole. Calif. Vet. 5:25, 1981.

TOPICAL THERAPY

THOMAS O. MANNING, D.V.M.
Raleigh, North Carolina

Veterinary dermatology has not made the progress in topical therapy that it has made in systemic therapy or diagnostics. Standards for assessment of a new topical treatment still fall far below those that would be acceptable in other specialties. This problem also relates to dermatologic and pharmaceutical colleagues, on whom we rely heavily for innovations in topical therapy. Even when a drug may have a known pharmacologic effect on the skin, there may be little concrete evidence of the best way to use a particular drug or group of drugs.

In spite of this, the treatment of patients with skin disease may be a rewarding experience. A few simple drugs may often produce great results. Unfortunately, topical therapy is often considered a mystery revealed only to specialists.

All patients must be treated as individuals. No list of useful drugs, however thoughtfully compiled, can be a substitute for judgment and experience. Because of the chronicity of many skin diseases, the supportive role of the sympathetic veterinarian is as important as the medication prescribed.

This article will review previous papers published on the basic principles of veterinary topical therapy and then outline the author's experiences with topical therapy.

I am not a strong advocate of topical therapy, but it does play an important role in dermatologic therapy. I listed all of the products I use daily for topical therapy. I found 24 products in our pharmacy that I frequently prescribe. They illustrate the two dozen ways I treat skin topically.

LITERATURE REVIEW

Schwartzman (1977) introduced topical dermatologic therapy as an "art as much as . . . a science." Topical therapy may be used to treat a particular disease (e.g., scabies) or in a way that serves to (1) abate or control a dermatosis until specific measures can be employed, (2) facilitate healing in conjunction with specific internal medication, or (3) control or cure a problem of unknown cause.

Particular difficulties are related to understanding dermatologic therapy because the modes of action of many topical drugs are not known. Veterinary literature dealing with topical therapy does not have in-depth studies that allow critical evaluation of specific medicines. We have to rely on data dealing with laboratory animals or humans, and these data do not necessarily apply to domestic animals.

Schwartzman's general principles of topical therapy are as follows:

1. Correct treatment depends on the definitive diagnosis. However, in the absence of etiologic information, topical therapy is an important aspect of the therapeutic management of the patient.

2. The choice of topical measures is determined largely by the presenting morphologic characteristics and the stage and site of the eruption.

3. Topical remedies are chosen to produce specific effects according to the characteristics of the lesion. Rather than be confused by numerous dermatologic drugs, use few remedies but know everything about them.

4. A remedy may harm rather than help. When in doubt, begin with the mildest and most nonaggressive medicine. Do not practice polypharmacy.

5. When a remedy disagrees with the patient, discontinue it at once.

6. The action of topical remedies depends to some degree on the mode of application and removal, so adequate instructions to the client (often in the form of demonstrations) are essential.

Percutaneous absorption is important. There are two routes of passage by which an agent may penetrate the skin: transepidermal and transappendicular. The actual ability to penetrate the skin seems to be an inherent quality of the particular agent. A vehicle may facilitate absorption, but it cannot force penetration of an agent that is not capable of passing through the skin. Ihcreasing the concentration of a particular medicament does not facilitate penetration. Occlusion, however, has a dramatic effect on cutaneous absorption and leads to hydration of the stratum corneum, which promotes softening and maceration of the epidermal barrier.

Cleansing Methods. Before initiation of specific dermatotherapy, the presenting lesion should be cleaned. Surface debris tends to trap and retain inflammatory and/or infectious material. Surface debris also may absorb or inactivate an active agent applied to the skin and may possibly prevent contact between the topical agent and the skin.

Scott (1979) presented topical cutaneous medicine as not only what we "put on" but also what we "take off" the involved skin. Thus, topical therapy must include the removal of all external factors that may initiate, prolong, or complicate cutaneous reactions.

Ihrke (1980a, b, and c) compiled a three-part series on topical therapy aimed at stressing the principles of proper therapy and the comparison of medications useful in various diseases and in different stages of disease.

WATER

Plain tap water is one of the most effective agents in the therapy of skin diseases. Depending on how it is managed, hydrotherapy may be used to hydrate or dehydrate skin. Damp compresses applied once an hour for 15 minutes stimulate evaporation of water from the skin, compress nonspecifically, and are drying. Because of easier application, the frequent use of whirlpools or water baths is preferred in veterinary dermatology. Alternately wetting and drying the coat (use room air or a blow dryer) will quickly dry any acute moist dermatosis. On the other hand, if water is maintained on the skin for longer periods the skin will rehydrate as water is absorbed by the hair and keratin. If a film of oil or humectant (Alpha Keri, Domol, HyLyt EFA bath oil, Humilac) is applied immediately after soaking, evaporation is stopped or slowed and the skin will remain moist.

Wet dressings (compresses, soaks, lotions) and medicated baths are indicated for acute eruptions. Different methods of application have increased their clinical use. Compresses should be sufficiently thick and pinned snuggly above the affected area with or without an occlusive wrap. They should be kept constantly wet. They are difficult to maintain properly and require extensive nursing care and patient cooperation. For this reason, compresses are rarely used in veterinary dermatology. However, compresses do maintain drainage. They are efficient in cleansing and help prevent rapid temperature changes in the skin.

Soaks are the most satisfactory method of handling localized acute eruptions. They may be applied with moist towels. Alternatively, the animal may be placed in a water-filled pail or pan or a large bath tub. Soaks for local acute dermatoses of skin should be applied for 10 to 15 minutes three or more times daily. The wrapping or area should be kept constantly moist at a temperature of approximately 100°F. Soaks act in a manner similar to compresses and therefore are an excellent substitute for wet compresses in veterinary medicine. Some of the more common solutions used for wet dressings are *pure water* (so often forgotten); *aluminum acetate* (Burow's solution, Domeboro); *subacetate or chloride* (1:10 to 1:20 solution in water); *magnesium sulfate* (1:65 solution in water, 1 tbs/liter); and *physiologic or hypertonic saline* (1 tsp table salt/pt water).

Astringents are mild protein precipitants that form a thick coagulum on the surface of an area of acute damage or coagulate and remove overlying debris. These agents do not penetrate deeply. The permeability of the surface cell membrane is reduced without the loss of cell viability. Astringent drugs include the salts of heavy metals such as silver, mercury, zinc, and aluminum.

Aluminum acetate, besides making a fine solution for wet soaks, is an excellent mild astringent for acute or subacute dermatoses.

A separate group of astringents of vegetable origin owe their activity to tannic acid. Tansal (5 per cent tannic acid, 5 per cent salicylic acid) in 70 per cent alcohol is a potent astringent to be used only once. It is especially good for localized acute moist dermatitis (hot spots).

Cleansing baths are used to remove dirt, debris, scale, and so on. Most cleansing soaps are strongly alkaline in reaction and may be used in the more chronic dermatoses. Soluble soaps are sodium (hard) or potassium (soft) salts of high molecular weight monobasic aliphatic acids. The irritation of soaps is caused by the mechanical effect of the foam, the emulsification of skin oils and sebum, and the softening of the epidermis. No matter how soft the soap, it should always be thoroughly rinsed out of the coat. Vegetable oil soaps (coconut oil) are the most bland. Mild, balanced pH soaps are also available and include products such as HyLyt EFA Shampoo and Johnson's Baby Shampoo.

Soap substitutes in the form of detergents are commonly used. Because these products do not foam vigorously, they seem to work better in areas with less hair. They cause little irritation to sensitive skin and are particularly effective in removing greasy films or glandular secretions. Phisoderm, a hypoallergenic formulation, is an example of an aqueous detergent cleanser.

Among the best mild cleansing soaps or detergents for practical cleaning are the mild dishwashing detergents or soaps, e.g., Joy Dishwashing Soap and Palmolive Liquid. Mycodex Shampoo is also a fine cleaning detergent.

Whirlpool baths with or without Nolvasan or Betadine whirlpool solution are the best methods for gentle, effective cleansing. The whirlpool may be used to remove crusts and scales, rehydrate the skin, cleanse wounds and draining fistulas, and prevent decubital problems. Adequate therapy usually requires ten minutes of whirlpool bathing once or twice daily.

A medicated bath is applied as a shampoo or a rinse poured on the animal. After being rubbed in, it should remain on the skin for a period of time. The individual response to the medicated bath determines the required frequency of application. Since body odor is associated with bacterial growth on the skin, odor can be used as an indication of the need for a bath. Odor is a practical sign that owners can utilize for determining home maintenance therapy. Medicated baths contain ingredients that enhance other actions of the cleansing shampoo. Soap should remove substances from the skin; therefore it is essential that medicated shampoos be lathered into the coat for 10 to 15 minutes. This allows the medication in the soap time for effect or limited absorption. We have found three types of medicated baths helpful: (1) colloidal oatmeal (Aveeno, 2 cups powder per bath tub) for its soothing and antipruritic action, (2) tar-sulfur shampoos (Sebaffon, Mycodex Tar and Sulfur, LyTar) and selenium sulfide shampoos (Selsun Blue) for their use in dry, flaky seborrheic conditions, and (3) Oxydex shampoo with 2½ per cent benzoyl peroxide for its use in treating acne, hyperkeratosis, and oily seborrheic conditions.

Dips or rinses utilize water as a vehicle for assorted antifungal, antiparasitic, and antipruritic agents. Effective rinses may carry residual effects (if dipped regularly). They are a reliable technique for the treatment of mite infestations. Unfortunately, they may also be a toxic form of therapy.

With the emphasis on new drugs, we sometimes forget that sulfur and its derivatives are excellent parasiticides. Commercial lime sulfur solutions, when used correctly, are safe for dogs and cats and are an inexpensive, effective treatment for several mite infestations (*Sarcoptes, Cheyletiella*). They are also fungicidal, bacteriocidal, and antipruritic.

Organochlorides (chlorinated hydrocarbons) tend to persist in the environment and in animal tissues. They are contact and ingested poisons, and their primary site of action is the nervous system. The mechanism of action of chlorinated hydrocarbons is still unknown. They act on the central nervous system and chronically cause both hepatic and renal degeneration. Organochlorides can be especially toxic to cats. Organochlorides "tend not to decompose" and "persist" in the environment. Some have been legally restricted (chlordane, DDT, lindane). Of the chlorinated hydrocarbons, 0.05 per cent lindane dips are useful for sarcoptic mange, lice, fleas, and ticks. We recommend lindane only if lime sulfur has failed in cases of canine scabies.

Organophosphates are cholinesterase inhibitors and do not persist in the environment. These drugs have the highest potential for toxicity, especially in cats. Organophosphates may be divided into two groups: quick knockdown organophosphates (DDVP, malathion) and residual-acting organophosphates (e.g., ronnel, ciodrin).

Examples of dips containing organophosphates are Ectoral, Paramite, and Dermaton II. An interesting and important point is that every dip has specific efficacy against each type of parasite. This may vary owing to factors such as technique of dipping, regional resistance, and parasite resistance. Be sure to read all literature pertaining to parasiticide products carefully and critically and follow the directions.

Carbamates are broad spectrum, residual, moderate-acting contact poisons that have little environmental persistence. They are cholinesterase inhibitors but have lower toxicity than the organophosphates. Carbamates can be toxic if used in too concentrated a solution or if used on puppies and kittens. There are many carbamate derivatives. Para Dip is an example of a carbamate dip that is effective against fleas, ticks, lice, and *Cheyletiella*. This dip is not effective against sarcoptic mange, even though it does contain lindane.

Generalized demodicosis deserves special attention. Ectoral is temporarily unavailable for veterinary use. We are searching for a reliable replacement. Neguvon Pour-On, another organophosphate, has been used as an alternative to Ectoral 4 per cent. It is employed for those animals in which Ectoral 4 per cent is unacceptable. Neguvon's major attraction is that it can be mixed with water rather than propylene glycol.

Three per cent Neguvon solution is used as a full-body dip every three days or as a one-third body dip daily. This solution may produce considerable irritation and toxicity, especially with the full-body protocol.

Amitraz (N'-2, 4-dimethylphenyl)-N-([2, 4-diethyl phenyl] imino methyl)-N-methylmethanimidamide) (Mitaban) is a new product. The experimental therapeutic protocol consisted of whole-body clipping and shampooing followed by an amitraz full-body rinse and sponging (five to ten minutes). Amitraz, 6.25 ml of concentrate, was diluted in one gallon of warm water. Dips were performed every 14 days for six dips, followed thereafter with once a month dips for four months. The author used a commercial orchard spray (BAAM) in the above protocol.

All dogs responded well to the initial two to three dips. However, only 1 of 16 dogs was totally cured. Most dogs improved in appearance but were found to be consistently positive (large numbers of mites at all stages), especially during the one-month dip regimen. The most common recurrence was a pododermatitis. Some dogs never became negative on skin scrapes, even during the biweekly dips.*

In summary, we need a suitable topical dip for generalized demodicosis in the adult dog. Both Neguvon and Mitaban are possible alternatives. They are attractive because they are formulated in water. Both these dips seem to be attractive for use in the young dog (less than one year of age) with generalized demodicosis. They may offer the young animal temporary relief and a decreased parasite load until natural cure occurs.

Neguvon is not licensed for veterinary use as a dip for demodicosis. Therefore, a consent form for experimental use is required.

OINTMENTS, CREAMS, AND OILS

Ointments are thicker than creams and when applied leave the skin feeling greasy. Because they contain little water, they are occlusive and increase the penetration of active constituents. They usually do not require the addition of preservatives.

Ointments and creams function to soften, lubricate, and protect and facilitate the removal of scales and crusts. They form a protective seal, which decreases contact with the environment. Certain formulations may reduce water loss. Ointments or creams may be emulsified with water into oil-in-water (vanishing cream) emulsions or water-in-oil (cold cream) emulsions.

Natural-mineral and synthetic greases and oils (petrolatum, mineral oil, polyethylene glycol) are superior to animal and vegetable fats or oils because they do not become rancid and are more resistant to microbial growth. Common applications for ointments or creams are as follows:

1. Petrolatum or baby oil is used for softening and hydrating nasal hyperkeratosis or noninfected elbow or sternal callosities.

2. Antibiotic or antiseptic ointments are used in one-day occlusive wraps for postoperative pododermatitis therapy. These packs are removed the following day, and the feet are whirlpooled or soaked.

3. Antibiotic-corticosteroid combination topicals have been shown to be superior to either agent alone in many dermatoses. This can be explained by the fact that *Staphylococcus aureus* can significantly contribute to the severity of a chronic inflammatory skin disorder without gross infection.

The author believes these agents (ointments, creams, or lotions) are of limited value except in otic preparations. The very nature of ointments, creams, and oils requires that the area for treatment be small for economical and practical reasons, clipped or hairless, and protected from instant removal by licking. Tresaderm and Panalog cream or ointment are most practical. Remember that creams and ointments are occlusive and are not indicated for draining or exuding lesions.

POWDERS

Powders may be used in shake lotions or pastes or by themselves. They are primarily drying agents but are also used for areas of friction and as parasiticides (flea powder–carbamates 5 per cent). Different substances are selected for particular qualities; e.g., zinc oxide and talcum for their absorbency; boric acid for its mild disinfectant properties; tannic acid for its astringency; and sulfur for its antimicrobial, antiparasitic, and antipruritic properties. The author finds very few indications for powders. They should be applied one to three times daily but must be removed prior to each new application.

Carbaryl powders (5 per cent) are perhaps the most practical means of maintaining flea control in both the cat and dog. These powders are readily accessible at local farm stores and garden stores under the trade name of Sevin. One must be sure that the product label mentions that the product is safe for cats and dogs. Powdering should be done more frequently than once a week. The powder must be worked down into the coat to prevent toxicity and increase the parasiticidal effect.

ANTIFUNGALS

Dermatophytosis is a commonly misdiagnosed or overdiagnosed disease. It is often self-limiting, and therefore many topical products seem to be effective. Antifungal products may be applied as the only type of therapy or as an adjunct to oral griseofulvin.

Topical creams or lotions must be restricted to small lesions owing to practical factors and expense. The most effective and available topical agents for use in localized lesions include miconazole, haloprogin, and thiabendazole.

Since local therapy (ointment) for dermatophyto-

---

*Note: These results should not be equated with those that might be obtained with Mitaban. Clinicians should recommend neutering all animals with generalized demodicosis.

sis in dogs and cats is often insufficient in treating or preventing reinfection, rinses or dips are important.

Clipping of the hair and the use of liquid vehicles are helpful in obtaining more penetration in animals with thick keratin scales and crusts. In these cases, multiple medicated shampoos or whirlpools may be advantageous prior to each medicated rinse. Three iodine solutions for surface therapy are fungicidal. These may be irritating if used repeatedly. Sodium hypochlorite solution (0.5 per cent), diluted 1:20 in water, may be used safely on all animals. Nolvasan solution is fungicidal when used at recommended dilutions.

Captan is a garden fungicide that is a safe and highly effective product for generalized ringworm infestation. One ounce of the liquid or powder is mixed with one gallon of water. Captan has been reported to be a contact sensitizer in humans. Therefore, the person applying the rinse should wear gloves and a plastic apron.

Two per cent lime sulfur is also an effective fungicide. Owners must be warned in advance about its odor and staining characteristics.

Currently, creams and rinses are the author's choice of treatment vehicles for dermatophytosis.

TOPICAL STEROIDS

Topical corticosteroid agents have revolutionized the local treatment of skin diseases. Used sensibly, they represent an essential part of the management of many conditions. Used indiscriminately for undiagnosed disorders, they can cause great harm.

Hydrocortisone was the first corticosteroid used topically. The formulation of even more potent steroids (fluorinated) can cause extensive and dangerous side effects.

The choice of formulation is as important as the type of steroid. Dry, lichenified conditions respond better with an ointment. The occlusive base helps the stratum corneum retain water and so maintain its plasticity. Creams and lotions are less effective in water retention, but since they vanish they are less messy and have high patient/owner acceptability.

Topical corticosteroids can be combined with antibiotics or antiseptics. In using combination therapy remember the following points. (1) Combinations should not be used if steroid or antibiotics would be equally effective alone. (2) A corticosteroid may aggravate infected disorders even when combined with an antiseptic or antibiotic. (3) The presence of a steroid in the formulation may not prevent the expression of hypersensitivity to another ingredient in the medication.

The initial topical treatment of a glucocorticoid-responsive dermatosis is most satisfactorily accomplished with a potent fluorinated glucocorticoid. A fine example of this type of product is the betamethasone-17-valerate (Valisone) line of topical glucocorticoids. They are available in an aerosol spray, lotion, cream, and ointment. This allows the clinician to select the best formulation for the individual case.

When a chronic dermatosis is managed exclusively with topical glucocorticoid therapy, it is best to avoid prolonged use of potent glucocorticoids owing to the increased risk of side effects (skin thinning, iatrogenic Cushing's syndrome). Topical hydrocortisone is the agent of choice in such cases. The generic ½ or 1 per cent hydrocortisone available from medical laboratories may be sufficient for this particular need.

OTIC PREPARATIONS

Otitis externa is most likely due to a combination of events that result in changes in the physiologic, anatomic, and microbiologic state of the ear. The etiology is often obvious. When a specific diagnosis is made, specific treatment is essential. If any underlying factors are recognized, an attempt should be made to correct them.

Several techniques are used to clean the ear canals. The choice of one depends on the type of material to be removed, the amount of inflammation present, and the preference of the clinician. Sedation or general anesthesia usually is necessary to provide restraint for proper examinations and cleansing of the ear canal.

The ear canal is cleaned by trimming and plucking any hair. When exudate, wax, and/or debris is present, the ear canal must be flushed. Cleaning is often facilitated by instilling softening ceruminolytic agents (Seb-U-Sol, Surfak) into the ear canal. These agents are best applied the day prior to the otic examination. Once the ceruminolytics have softened the wax or debris, the ear can be carefully cleaned with a Water Pic or cotton swabs or flushed with a bulb syringe. The canal should be dried with astringents such as aluminum acetate solution.

Many otic products are available with combinations of drugs. Most contain antibiotics, parasiticides, antifungals, and anti-inflammatory agents.

Simple otitis externa, with no severe skin changes, is usually adequately treated with gentle ear cleaning and a combination otic preparation.

Most formulations (ointments, creams, or lotions) contain various combinations of antibiotics, parasiticides and anti-inflammatory and antifungal agents. Topical antibacterial agents are indicated whenever infection is present. Chloramphenicol and the aminoglycosides (neomycin, polymyxin, and Gentocin) are reliable topical antibiotics. Aminoglycosides have been reported to cause ototoxicity when used for prolonged periods in cases of tympanic membrane rupture. Corticosteroids have been recommended on the basis that they decrease inflammation, exudation, and globular excretion. Antifungals are indicated for dermatophytes, *Malassezia pachydermitis (Pityrosporum)*, and the rare *Candida* infection. Thiabendazole and miconazole are excellent for dermatophytes and *Malassezia pachydermitis*. Nystatin is effective for *Candida* infections.

Acetic acid (vinegar 5 per cent diluted to a 1 per cent solution), Domeboro Otic, and Domeboro Tablets (at 1 to 2 per cent) lower the pH and are very effective in controlling *Pseudomonas*, *Proteus*, and *Staphylococcus* infections. Acetic acid solutions are excellent for controlling "summer ear" *Malassezia pachydermitis*. Acetic acid would also help treat *Pseudomonas*-related problems. However, one must remember not to mix acetic acid (low pH) and Gentocin (it may be inactivated by the low pH). Gentocin is also inactivated by pus; prior cleaning, therefore, is essential.

The author has found a mixture of Nolvasan solution, 1½ per cent, and propylene glycol to be useful for the treatment of otitis externa due to bacteria (*Staphylococcus*, *Streptococcus*, *Pseudomonas*, *Proteus*) or yeasts (*Malassezia pachydermitis*) or secondary bacterial and/or yeast problems

due to chronic moisture (anatomic or due to swimming), allergy-associated otitis (atopy), or seborrheic otitis (primary or secondary). Control of the primary problem is the best treatment. In allergic or seborrheic otitis, a two-week course of Nolvasan propylene glycol followed by Synotic once daily to once weekly has often worked wonders.

Parasiticides such as rotenone (Canex) in oil and thiabendazole (Tresaderm) are indicated in *Otodectes* otitis. Results are best appreciated if the entire animal is also treated with an effective insecticide (carbaryl, Dermaton II), because the mites may be found virtually anywhere on the coat.

REFERENCES AND SUPPLEMENTAL READING

Ihrke, P. J.: Dermatologic therapy. I. Uses, principles and vehicles of topical therapy. Comp. Cont. Ed. 2:28, 1980a.
Ihrke, P. J.: Dermatologic therapy. II. Specific topical pharmacologic agents. Comp. Cont. Ed. 2:156, 1980b.
Ihrke, P. J.: Dermatologic therapy. III. Antibiotic therapy in canine skin disease. Comp. Cont. Ed. 2:177, 1980c.
Muller, G. H., and Kirk, R. W.: *Small Animal Dermatology*, 2nd ed. Philadelphia: W. B. Saunders, 1976.
Schwartzman, R. M.: Topical dermatologic therapy. *In* Kirk, R. W. (ed.): *Current Veterinary Therapy VI.* Philadelphia: W. B. Saunders, 1977, pp. 506–512.
Scott, D. W.: Topical cutaneous medicine. Proceedings of the 79th Annual Meeting of the American Animal Hospital Association, New Orleans, 1979, pp. 89–104.

AUTOIMMUNE DERMATOSES

DANNY W. SCOTT, D.V.M.

Ithaca, New York

The autoimmune dermatoses of dogs and cats are rare. In dogs, these disorders account for about 0.6 per cent of all the canine dermatoses seen at the New York State College of Veterinary Medicine between 1974 and 1980. Too few cases have been documented in cats to allow reliable comments on exact frequency of occurrence.

The autoimmune dermatoses often present with strongly suggestive historical and clinical findings. However, the differential diagnosis is still lengthy, and definitive diagnosis cannot be made without adequate biopsy and immunologic evaluation.

The biopsy is usually the key to specific diagnosis. Pemphigus, pemphigoid, and occasionally systemic lupus erythematosus have as their primary skin lesions vesicles, bullae, and vesicopustules. Intact primary lesions are critical to histopathologic diag-

nosis. Because these primary lesions are so fragile and transient in the thin canine and feline epidermis, it may be necessary to hospitalize suspect animals so that they can be carefully scrutinized every two to four hours for the presence of primary lesions. Multiple biopsies and serial sections will greatly increase the likelihood of demonstrating diagnostic histologic changes. In addition, because canine and feline blisters often fill rapidly with leukocytes, they may be grossly and microscopically pustular, thus confusing both clinician and pathologist.

Immunofluorescence testing of cutaneous or mucosal lesions and serum is also an integral diagnostic procedure in documenting autoimmune disorders. Direct immunofluorescence testing of skin and/or mucosa is vastly superior to indirect immunofluorescence testing of serum when checking for pemphigus or pemphigoid antibodies. Intact primary lesions and perilesional tissue are biopsied and either (1) quick frozen in isopentane at −160°C and held at −70°C until tested, or (2) placed in a special preservative transport media (Michel's fixative) and tested within 7 to 14 days.

PEMPHIGUS

Pemphigus is a group of rare autoimmune vesicobullous, erosive to ulcerative disorders of the skin and/or oral mucosa. Pemphigus is characterized histologically by intraepidermal acantholysis and immunologically by the presence of an autoantibody ("pemphigus antibody") against the glycocalyx of keratinocytes. Pemphigus antibody–induced acantholysis is not dependent on complement or inflammatory cells and is thought to represent a type II hypersensitivity reaction.

PEMPHIGUS VULGARIS

Pemphigus vulgaris has been recognized in dogs and cats with no age, breed, or sex predilection. In dogs, it is a vesicobullous, erosive to ulcerative disorder that may affect the oral cavity, mucocutaneous junctions (lips, nostrils, eyelids, prepuce, vulva, anus), skin, or any combination thereof. About 90 per cent of the dogs have oral lesions at the time of diagnosis, and oral involvement is the initial clinical sign in about 50 per cent of cases. Cutaneous lesions occur most commonly in the axillae and groin. Dogs with this distribution of skin lesions may have been previously misdiagnosed as having "hidradenitis suppurativa." Onychomadesis may be seen. Pemphigus vulgaris limited to the skin is rare. The Nikolsky sign may be present, pruritus and pain are variable, and secondary pyoderma is common. Severely affected animals may be anorectic, depressed, or febrile. In the cat, pemphigus vulgaris is a vesicobullous disorder of the oral cavity, lips, nostrils, and nasal philtrum.

PEMPHIGUS VEGETANS

Pemphigus vegetans has been recognized only in dogs. It is the rarest form of pemphigus and appears to have no age, breed, or sex predilection. Pemphigus vegetans is a vesicopustular disorder that evolves into verrucous vegetations and papillomatous proliferations, which ooze and are studded with pustules. The Nikolsky sign may be present. Pruritus and pain are variable, and affected dogs are usually otherwise healthy. Pemphigus vegetans is thought to represent a more benign or abortive

form of pemphigus vulgaris in a patient that has more "resistance" to the disease.

PEMPHIGUS FOLIACEUS

Pemphigus foliaceus has been recognized in dogs and cats with no age, breed, or sex predilection. It is characterized by a vesicobullous or pustular dermatitis. Mucocutaneous orientation is uncommon, and oral cavity involvement is rare. Pemphigus foliaceus usually begins on the face and ears; commonly involves the feet, footpads (villous hyperkeratosis or "hard pad"), and groin; and usually becomes multifocal or generalized within days to weeks. The Nikolsky sign may be present, pruritus and pain are variable, and secondary pyoderma is frequent. Severely affected animals may be anorectic, depressed, or febrile.

PEMPHIGUS ERYTHEMATOSUS

Pemphigus erythematosus has been recognized in dogs and cats with no age, breed, or sex predilection. It is characterized by a vesicobullous or pustular dermatitis of the face and ears. The Nikolsky sign may be present, pruritus and pain are variable, and affected animals are usually otherwise healthy. The nose frequently becomes depigmented, whereupon photodermatitis may become an aggravating factor. If the nasal region is primarily involved, the dogs are often worse in sunny weather and may be misdiagnosed as having "nasal solar dermatitis" (collie nose). Oral cavity involvement has not been recognized. Pemphigus erythematosus is thought to represent a more benign or abortive form of pemphigus foliaceus and possibly a crossover syndrome between pemphigus and lupus erythematosus.

DIAGNOSIS OF PEMPHIGUS

Microscopic examination of direct smears from intact vesicles or pustules or from recent erosions often reveals numerous neutrophils (nondegenerative), occasionally numerous eosinophils, few to no bacteria, and numerous acantholytic keratinocytes. Histologic examinations reveal the following: (1) *pemphigus vulgaris*: suprabasilar acantholysis with resultant cleft and vesicle formation; (2) *pemphigus vegetans*: epidermal hyperplasia, papillomatosis, and intraepidermal microabscesses containing predominantly eosinophils and acantholytic keratinocytes; and (3) *pemphigus foliaceus and pemphigus erythematosus*: intragranular or subcorneal acantholysis with resultant cleft and vesicle or pustule formation.

Direct immunofluorescence testing reveals the diffuse intercellular deposition of immunoglobulin (usually IgG), and occasionally complement, within the epidermis or mucosa. Indirect immunofluorescence testing is rarely positive in canine and feline pemphigus. In pemphigus erythematosus, direct immunofluorescence testing often reveals the deposition of immunoglobulin, with or without complement, at the basement membrane zone in addition to the intercellular spaces of epidermis. These patients usually have a positive antinuclear antibody test as well.

TREATMENT OF PEMPHIGUS

Large doses of systemic glucocorticoids (1 to 3 mg/kg prednisolone or prednisone, given orally b.i.d.) are usually listed as the initial treatment of choice. In many instances, however, glucocorticoid therapy is unsuccessful or intolerable side effects develop. In one study of 22 dogs with pemphigus, the following observations were made: (1) 1 mg/kg prednisolone, given orally b.i.d., was ineffective in controlling the disease, and (2) 3 mg/kg prednisolone, given orally b.i.d., was effective in controlling the disease in 17 of 22 dogs. However, at the higher dose, 2 of the 17 dogs were euthanatized owing to unacceptable side effects, and 5 dogs had to be managed with additional immunomodulating drugs, as glucocorticoid side effects were unacceptable. Thus, systemic glucocorticoids were unacceptable in 12 of 22 dogs (54.5 per cent).

When systemic glucocorticoids are unsatisfactory, the addition or substitution of other immunomodulating drugs may allow significant reduction or termination of glucocorticoid dosage and superior patient management. Drugs that may be useful include aurothioglucose (Solganol, Schering: see page 448, (2) azathioprine (Imuran, Burroughs Wellcome: 2.2 mg/kg orally s.i.d.), (3) chlorambucil (Leukeran, Burroughs Wellcome: 1 mg/kg orally every 48 hours), and (4) cyclophosphamide (Cytoxan, Mead-Johnson: 50 mg/m² BSA orally every 48 hours).

In animals in which significant nasal depigmentation has occurred and photodermatitis has become an aggravating factor, photoprotection is an important therapeutic adjunct. Avoidance of sunlight between 8 AM and 5 PM is helpful. The use of sunscreens containing para-aminobenzoic acid (Sundown, Johnson & Johnson) is mandatory.

PEMPHIGOID

Bullous pemphigoid is a rare vesicobullous, ulcerative disorder of skin and/or oral mucosa. It has been recognized only in dogs. Bullous pemphigoid is characterized histologically by subepidermal vesicle formation and immunologically by the presence of an autoantibody ("pemphigoid antibody") against antigen at the basement membrane zone of the skin and oral mucosa. It is thought to represent a type II hypersensitivity reaction.

Canine bullous pemphigoid has no age or sex predilection. However, collies appear to be a predisposed breed. Bullous pemphigoid is a vesicobullous, ulcerative disorder that may affect the oral cavity, mucocutaneous junctions, skin, or any combination thereof. About 80 per cent of the dogs have oral lesions at the time of diagnosis. Cutaneous lesions occur most commonly in the axillae and groin. Dogs with this distribution of skin lesions may previously have been misdiagnosed as having "hidradenitis suppurativa." The Nikolsky sign is usually absent, pruritus and pain are variable, and secondary pyoderma is common. Severely affected dogs may be anorectic, depressed, and febrile.

Histologically, bullous pemphigoid is characterized by subepidermal cleft and vesicle formation. Acantholysis is *not* seen. Direct immunofluorescence testing reveals the linear deposition of immunoglobulin, and usually complement, at the basement membrane zone of skin or mucosa. Indirect fluorescence testing is rarely positive.

Mild cases of bullous pemphigoid may be successfully managed with relatively low doses of systemic glucocorticoids (1 mg/kg prednisolone or prednisone orally b.i.d.), and therapy may occasionally even be terminated. However, most cases require aggressive chemotherapy. In one study of nine dogs with bullous pemphigoid, the following observations were made: (1) 1 mg/kg prednisolone given orally b.i.d. was ineffective in controlling the disease, and (2) 3 mg/kg prednisolone given orally b.i.d. was effective in controlling the disease. However, at the higher dose, two of the nine dogs were euthanatized because of unacceptable side effects, and another two died after seven to ten days of therapy (acute pancreatitis). Thus, systemic glucocorticoids were unsatisfactory for treatment in four of nine dogs (44 per cent).

When systemic glucocorticoids are unsatisfactory, the addition or substitution of other immunomodulating drugs may allow significant reduction or termination of glucocorticoid dosage and superior patient management.

LUPUS ERYTHEMATOSUS

Lupus erythematosus is an autoimmune disorder that is traditionally divided into two subsets: (1) *systemic lupus erythematosus*: a multisystemic disorder with frequent cutaneous involvement, and (2) *discoid lupus erythematosus*: a cutaneous disorder without systemic involvement.

The etiology of lupus erythematosus appears to be multifactorial, with genetic predilection, immunologic disorder (suppressor T–cell deficiency, B-cell hyperactivity), viral infection, and hormonal and ultraviolet light modulation all playing a role. Tissue damage in lupus erythematosus appears to be due to a type III hypersensitivity reaction.

SYSTEMIC LUPUS ERYTHEMATOSUS

Systemic lupus erythematosus is rare in dogs and cats. In dogs, there is no age predilection, but females and German shepherds may be predisposed. In cats, no age, breed, or sex predilections are apparent.

The clinical signs associated with systemic lupus erythematosus are varied and changeable. Because of this phenomenal clinical variability and ability to mimic numerous diseases, systemic lupus erythematosus has been called the "great imitator." In a compilation of 68 canine cases reported in the literature, lameness due to polyarthritis (71 per cent of the cases), hematologic disorders (anemia, thrombocytopenia, leukopenia) (57 per cent), fever (47 per cent), proteinuria due to glomerulonephritis (40 per cent), and skin lesions (35 per cent) were the most common clinical disorders. Other syndromes reported in association with canine systemic lupus erythematosus include muscular disorders (polymyositis, myocarditis), peripheral lymphadenopathy, splenomegaly, oral ulcers, pleuritis, neurologic disorders (seizures, meningitis, myelitis), and lymphedema. In the cat, skin lesions, persistent skin infections, fever, peripheral lymphadenopathy, hemolytic anemia, oral ulcers, and glomerulonephritis have been recognized in association with systemic lupus erythematosus.

The cutaneous manifestations of canine and feline systemic lupus erythematosus are extremely diverse and include seborrheic skin disease, cutaneous or mucocutaneous vesicobullous and ulcerative disorders, refractory secondary pyodermas, panniculitis (lupus profundus), and nasal dermatitis (nasal solar dermatitis or "collie nose"). Skin lesions may be multifocal or generalized; commonly involve the face, ears, and distal extremities; and may be exacerbated by exposure to sunlight. Pruritus is variable.

The definitive diagnosis of systemic lupus erythematosus is often one of the most challenging accomplishments in medicine. The clinicopathologic abnormalities demonstrated will depend upon the organ system involved. The *lupus erythematosus* (LE) cell test may be positive in up to 60 per cent of the patients. However, the test is variable from day to day and steroid labile and lacks sensitivity and specificity. The antinuclear antibody (ANA) test is presently considered the most specific and sensitive serologic test for systemic lupus erythematosus and is positive in about 90 per cent of the active cases. Great caution is warranted in the interpretation of ANA results. In general, results from different laboratories cannot be compared. In addition, positive ANA results may be seen in a number of other conditions.

Skin biopsy findings vary with the type of gross morphologic lesions and are thus often quite nondiagnostic. The most characteristic finding is interface dermatitis (hydropic and/or lichenoid). These findings are often not present until the clinical lesions are four to six weeks old.

Direct immunofluorescence testing reveals the deposition of immunoglobulin and/or complement at the basement membrane zone ("lupus band"). Contrary to the situation in humans, normal skin in dogs and cats is rarely positive. Indirect immunofluorescence testing is negative.

The prognosis in systemic lupus erythematosus is, in general, unpredictable. In dogs, it appears that patients with joint, skin, and/or muscle disease respond more reliably to medication and are maintained in relatively long periods of clinical remission. On the other hand, dogs with hemolytic anemia and/or thrombocytopenia often do not respond well to systemic glucocorticoids and require other immunomodulating drugs and/or splenectomy. Animals with glomerulonephritis regularly develop progressive renal failure in spite of therapy.

Therapy of systemic lupus erythematosus must be individualized. The initial agent of choice is probably large doses of systemic glucocorticoids (1 to 2 mg/kg prednisolone or prednisone orally b.i.d.). When systemic glucocorticoids are unsatisfactory, other immunomodulating drugs may be useful. Splenectomy may be needed for patients with severe hemolytic anemia and/or thrombocytopenia.

Several reports have recently shown that people in close contact with dogs with systemic lupus erythematosus or high titer ANA have *no* increased clinical or serologic evidence of systemic lupus erythematosus when compared with nonexposed humans.

DISCOID LUPUS ERYTHEMATOSUS

Discoid lupus erythematosus is thought to be a benign variant of systemic lupus erythematosus in which systemic involvement is absent. The disorder is confined to the skin. It has been reported in dogs with no age or sex predilection. Discoid lupus erythematosus may be more common in collies and Shetland sheepdogs.

Clinical signs initially include depigmentation, erythema, and scaling of the nose. Erosion, ulceration, and crusting commonly develop, and the disorder often spreads up the bridge of the nose.

Less frequently, lesions may be seen periocularly and on the ears and distal limbs. The lips may also be involved, and small ulcers may be seen in the oral cavity. Pruritus and pain are variable, and scarring is common. Canine discoid lupus erythematosus is frequently exacerbated by ultraviolet light and is, thus, worse in summer. It is very likely that the disorder previously referred to as nasal solar dermatitis (collie nose) was, in many cases, discoid lupus erythematosus.

The diagnosis of discoid lupus erythematosus is based on biopsy and immunofluorescent testing. LE cell and ANA tests are almost always negative. Skin biopsy reveals interface dermatitis (hydropic and/or lichenoid). Focal hydropic degeneration of basal epidermal cells, pigmentary incontinence, focal thickening of the basement membrane zone, and marked accumulations of mononuclear and plasma cells are important histopathologic findings.

Direct immunofluorescence testing of lesional skin reveals the deposition of immunoglobulin and/or complement at the basement membrane zone. Indirect immunofluorescence testing is negative.

The prognosis for discoid lupus erythematosus is usually good. However, marked depigmentation predisposes to sunburn and squamous cell carcinoma.

Treatment of canine discoid lupus erythematosus must be individualized. Mild cases may be controlled by, and all cases will benefit from, avoidance of exposure to intense sunlight (8 AM to 5 PM) and the use of topical sunscreens (Sundown, Johnson & Johnson) and topical glucocorticoids (Valisone, Schering). For more severe or refractory cases, systemic glucocorticoids (1 mg/kg prednisolone or prednisone orally b.i.d.) are often effective. When systemic glucocorticoids are contraindicated or unsatisfactory, vitamin E (dl-α-tocopherol acetate) given orally at 400 IU b.i.d. may be effective. Vitamin E appears to have a one- to two-month lag phase before its benefit is recognized clinically, and it must be given on an empty stomach.

SUPPLEMENTAL READING

Drazner, F. H.: Systemic lupus erythematosus in the dog. Comp. Cont. Ed. 2:243, 1980.

Halliwell, R. E. W.: Skin diseases associated with autoimmunity part I. The bullous autoimmune skin diseases. Comp. Cont. Ed. 2:911, 1980.

Halliwell, R. E. W.: Skin diseases associated with autoimmunity part II. The nonbullous autoimmune skin diseases. Comp. Cont. Ed. 3:156, 1981.

Manning, T. O., Scott, D. W., Kruth, S. A., Sozanski, M., and Lewis, R. M.: Three cases of canine pemphigus foliaceus, and observations on chrysotherapy. J.A.A.H.A. 16:189, 1980.

Manning, T. O., Scott, D. W., Smith, C. A., and Lewis, R. M.: Pemphigus diseases in the feline: seven case reports and discussion. J.A.A.H.A. 18:433, 1982.

Monier, J. C., Dardenne, M., Rigal, D., Costa, O., Fournel, C., and Lapsas, M.: Clinical and laboratory features of canine lupus syndromes. Arthritis Rheum. 23:294, 1980.

Scott, D. W., and Lewis, R. M.: Pemphigus and pemphigoid in dog and man: comparative aspects. J. Am. Acad. Dermatol. 5:148, 1981.

Scott, D. W., Manning, T. O., Smith, C. A., and Lewis, R. M.: Observations on the immunopathology and therapy of canine pemphigus and pemphigoid. J.A.V.M.A. 180:48, 1982.

Scott, D. W., Miller, W. H., Lewis, R. M., Manning, T. O., and Smith, C. A.: Pemphigus erythematosus in the dog and cat. J.A.A.H.A. 16:815, 1980.

Walton, D. K., Scott, D. W., Smith, C. A., and Lewis, R. M.: Canine discoid lupus erythematosus. J.A.A.H.A. 17:851, 1981.

PANNICULITIS

DANNY W. SCOTT, D.V.M.
Ithaca, New York

Panniculitis is defined as inflammation of the subcutaneous fat (panniculus adiposus). Steatitis refers to inflammation of all adipose tissue. Panniculitis is rare in dogs and cats.

ETIOLOGY

The lipocyte (fat cell, adipocyte) is particularly vulnerable to trauma, ischemia, and neighboring inflammatory disease. In addition, damage to lipocytes results in the liberation of lipid, which undergoes hydrolysis, forming glycerol and fatty acids. Fatty acids are potent inflammatory agents and incite further inflammatory and/or granulomatous tissue reactions.

There are multiple etiologic factors involved in the genesis of panniculitis (Table 1). Many of these factors have yet to be recognized in dogs and cats, but this may only reflect lack of awareness. Infectious and nutritional causes of canine and feline panniculitis (deep mycosis, pansteatitis) will not be addressed here. This article will concentrate on sterile forms of panniculitis.

"Nodular panniculitis" refers to sterile subcutaneous inflammatory nodules and is *not* a specific

Table 1. *Differential Diagnosis of Panniculitis (Humans)*

Infectious
    Bacterial,* mycobacterial,* actinomycetic,* fungal,*
        chlamydial, viral
Immunologic
    Lupus erythematosus,* rheumatoid arthritis, drug
        eruption
Physicochemical (factitial)
    Trauma, pressure, cold, foreign body* (e.g., post-
        subcutaneous injection of bulky, oily, or insoluble
        liquids)
Pancreatic disease
    Inflammation, neoplasia
Post-glucocorticoid therapy
Vasculitis
    Leukocytoclastic, periarteritis nodosa, thrombophlebitis,
        embolism
Nutrition
    Vitamin E deficiency*
Enteropathies
Idiopathy*

*Recognized in the dog and cat.

disease. It is purely a descriptive term representing the clinical end result of several known and unknown etiologic factors. The term "Weber-Christian panniculitis" has been frequently misused and should be reserved only for patients with both subcutaneous nodular lesions and systemic features. In dogs and cats, the majority of sterile nodular panniculitis cases have been idiopathic in origin. A few cases of lupus erythematosus panniculitis have been recognized in dogs.

CLINICAL SIGNS

Panniculitis is manifested clinically as deep-seated cutaneous nodules. The lesions may occur singly or in groups, either localized to specific areas or generalized, and vary in size from a few millimeters to several centimeters in diameter. Nodules may be firm and well-circumscribed or soft and ill-defined. They are initially subcutaneous but may fix the overlying skin as they progress. The lesions may become cystic and/or ulcerate and/or develop draining tracts, which discharge an oily, yellowish brown to bloody substance. The lesions may or may not be painful and often heal with depressed scars. In dogs and cats, the nodular lesions associated with panniculitis are usually multiple and have a predilection for the trunk.

In a study of 22 dogs (14 reported in the literature, 8 seen by the author), idiopathic sterile nodular panniculitis was found to occur most commonly in the dachshund (13 cases). Other breeds represented included the miniature poodle, wire-haired fox terrier, Manchester terrier, boxer, collie, Old English sheepdog, and Weimaraner. There was no sex predilection. Ages of affected dogs varied from 10 weeks to 11 years, with 13 of the 22 dogs first developing lesions at less than six months of age. In cats, sterile nodular panniculitis has no reported breed or sex predilection and occurs between five and nine years of age.

Many cases of canine and feline idiopathic sterile nodular panniculitis are associated with constitutional signs, including poor appetite, depression, lethargy, and pyrexia. These signs are usually intermittent and often herald a new crop of skin lesions. If the panniculitis is associated with lupus erythematosus (lupus erythematosus panniculitis, lupus panniculitis, lupus profundus), concurrent signs of this disease may also be present.

DIAGNOSIS

Sterile nodular panniculitis is most commonly misdiagnosed as deep pyoderma, systemic mycoses, cutaneous cysts, or cutaneous neoplasms. Aspirates from intact lesions usually reveal numerous neutrophils, "foamy" macrophages, and no microorganisms. Sudan stains may reveal extra- and intracellular lipid droplets.

The diagnosis of panniculitis can only be made by biopsy. Excision biopsy is the *only* biopsy technique that is satisfactory for subcutaneous nodules. Punch biopsies fail to deliver sufficient tissue to be of diagnostic value in about 75 per cent of the cases. Most panniculitides are characterized by varying degrees of fat necrosis, acute inflammation, pyogranulomatous to granulomatous inflammation, and fibrosis. It is imperative to realize that most panniculitides, regardless of cause, look identical histologically. Thus, one cannot diagnose sterile nodular panniculitis from a biopsy specimen. Special stains and cultures are *always* indicated to rule out infectious agents, and polarization is indicated to rule out foreign bodies.

If the panniculitis is predominantly lymphohistioplasmacytic or if other clinical signs suggest lupus erythematosus, other diagnostic tests may include ANA and LE cell tests and direct immunofluorescence testing of lesional skin. If a vasculitis is present, diagnostic tests indicated may reflect the differential diagnosis of vasculitis. If the panniculitis is persistent and refractory or if the patient shows concurrent signs of gastrointestinal disease, pancreatic disease should be ruled out.

TREATMENT

Sterile nodular panniculitis responds well to systemic glucocorticoids. Prednisolone or prednisone may be given orally at 1 mg/kg b.i.d. (dog) or 2 mg/kg b.i.d. (cat) until the lesions have regressed (7 to 14 days). Therapy should be stopped at this point, as many dogs, especially young dogs, will go into long-term or permanent remission. In recurrent cases, alternate-day steroid therapy may be required for prolonged periods.

In a few canine and feline cases, the author has had good results with oral vitamin E (dl-α-tocopherol acetate), 400 IU b.i.d. The vitamin E must be given at least two hours before or after a meal for maximum effectiveness. In humans, oral potassium iodide has been used successfully in cases of sterile nodular panniculitis.

SUPPLEMENTAL READING

Baker, B. B., and Stannard, A. A.: Nodular panniculitis in the dog. J.A.V.M.A. 167:752, 1975.

Baker, K., and Howlett, C. R.: Nodular panniculitis in a Dachshund dog. Aust. Vet. Pract. 9:159, 1979.
Beaumont, P. R., and Glauberg, A. F.: Nodular panniculitis in a Dachshund dog. Canine Pract. 7:27, 1980.
Fitzpatrick, T. B., Eisen, A. Z., Wolff, K., Freedberg, I. M., and Austen, K. F.: Dermatology in General Medicine, 2nd ed. New York: McGraw-Hill, 1979.
Ringheim, H. P.: Idiopathic panniculitis in a dog. Canine Pract. 4:42, 1977.
Rook, A., Wilkinson, D. S., and Ebling, F. J. G.: Textbook of Dermatology, 3rd ed. Oxford: Blackwell Scientific Publications, 1979.
Scott, D. W.: Immunologic skin disorders in the dog and cat. Vet. Clin. North Am. 8:641, 1978.
Scott, D. W.: Feline dermatology 1900 to 1978: a monograph. J.A.A.H.A. 16:331, 1980.
Winkelmann, R. K., and Tucker, S. B.: Biopsy in diagnosis of inflammatory nodules of the leg. Cutis 21:183, 1978.

NECROTIZING SKIN DISEASES

VALERIE A. FADOK, D.V.M.
Knoxville, Tennessee

A wide variety of dermatoses can produce necrosis and ulceration of the skin and mucous membranes. Etiologic factors include drug reactions, immunologic disorders, chemical irritants, ischemia secondary to pressure, ionizing radiation, dermonecrotic toxins from venomous snakes and spider bites, and temperature-related injuries. Identification of the underlying cause is vital to the appropriate treatment of these disorders.

DRUG ERUPTION

Drug reactions may injure any organ system; however, drug reactions that result in skin eruptions are more often identified because of their visibility. Drug eruptions may result from any route of administration, including oral, injectable, topical, and even topical ocular routes. A drug eruption may present as exfoliation, bullae, purpura, alopecia, and necrosis, thereby mimicking almost any skin disease. The lesions may be localized or generalized. There are no typical reactions associated with particular drugs in veterinary medicine. Virtually any drug may cause an eruption; however, antibiotics such as penicillin, ampicillin, tetracycline, neomycin, and the sulfonamides are most commonly implicated in drug reactions in animals. Drugs may cause skin eruptions through both immunologic and nonimmunologic mechanisms.

Drug eruption should be considered in necrotic skin lesions of animals not exposed to necrotizing physical or chemical agents. A thorough drug history should be obtained. Owners should be questioned extensively to ensure that medications such as a heartworm preventative, vitamins, and recent vaccinations have not been excluded. Biopsies may be helpful in ruling out other dermatoses, but there is no characteristic histologic pattern for drug eruption. Necrotizing drug eruptions are accompanied by epidermal necrosis and ulceration. Diagnosis is established by withdrawing the offending drug, with subsequent resolution of the skin lesions, usually within one to two weeks. In rare cases, the lesions may take weeks to months to heal. Provocative exposure to reproduce the skin lesions is not recommended and may be life-threatening.

Treatment involves withdrawing the suspected drug and supportive therapy. Soaks and compresses with astringent solutions such as aluminum acetate (Domeboro Tablets, Dome Laboratories) are comforting and drying. Oral corticosteroids may be indicated, particularly if pruritus is a significant component. Although corticosteroids are widely used for drug eruptions in both humans and animals, especially in inflammatory and exudative reactions, their efficacy is still unsubstantiated. The offending drug and chemically related compounds should be avoided in the future. The prognosis is usually very good, with the exception of toxic epidermal necrolysis (see hereafter), which can be fatal.

TOXIC EPIDERMAL NECROLYSIS

Toxic epidermal necrolysis (TEN, Lyell's disease) is an uncommon disease characterized by full thickness necrosis and sloughing of the epidermis. The disease is often fatal. Rapid diagnosis and aggressive supportive therapy are essential to the survival of the patient.

Several clinical settings have been associated with the development of this disease in humans, including drug reactions; viral, bacterial, and fungal infections; vaccination; neoplasia; and idiopathy. Drug reactions, chronic infections, and neoplasia have been associated with TEN in the dog and cat. The true pathogenesis of this disorder is unknown; however, immune mechanisms have been proposed. TEN may represent a severe variant form of erythema multiforme, a skin disorder characterized by macules, papules, vesicles, bullae, and target lesions. Erythema multiforme (central red or bullous area surrounded by a pale zone, which is surrounded by an erythematous ring) shares similar causes, such as drug reactions or infections. Early histopathologic changes of TEN are identical to those of erythema multiforme. Since immune complexes have been associated with the development of cutaneous lesions in erythema multiforme, they may also play a role in the development of TEN. In addition, direct immunofluorescence of skin biopsies from drug-induced TEN in some human patients demonstrated deposits of immunoglobulin and complement around basal cells (Rasmussen, 1980).

TEN represents one of the few dermatologic emergencies. Diagnosis is made from clinical signs, history, and biopsy. The clinical signs usually appear suddenly. The early erythema is followed by sloughing of affected skin, leaving a lesion resembling a scald. Multiple individual erosions may coalesce to denude large areas of the skin surface. The skin is often very painful. The oral and ocular mucous membranes are frequently affected. Fever, anorexia, and malaise often accompany the onset of the dermatologic signs. Secondary infection of the exposed dermis is common.

A complete drug history should be obtained; drugs commonly associated with this disorder include penicillin, tetracycline, sulfonamides, barbiturates, phenylbutazone, and gold salts. The patient should be thoroughly evaluated for any underlying disease. Early histopathologic changes include necrosis of basal cells with subsequent dermoepidermal cleft formation. Later, full thickness necrosis of the epidermis is found. The epidermis separates easily from the dermis of the biopsy specimen; therefore, biopsies should be handled with care. Inflammatory infiltrates in the dermis increase with the duration of the lesion.

Treatment of patients with TEN requires aggressive supportive care similar to that given burn patients. Considerable fluid loss occurs through the exposed dermis. Animals should be given intravenous fluids based on maintenance needs and estimated losses. Fluid requirements can be estimated using formulas developed for burn patients: body weight (in kilograms) × per cent of area affected × 4 ml = volume of fluids required in the first 24 hours (Davis, 1979). A balanced electrolyte solution such as lactated Ringer's solution is best. Hematocrit, total protein, and electrolyte values should be monitored regularly.

Topical therapy for TEN is also similar to that for burn patients. Silver sulfadiazine cream (Silvadene, Marian Laboratories, Inc.) has been used successfully in human burn and TEN patients. It is antibacterial, antifungal, water miscible, and nonirritating. It has no systemic side effects, as it is poorly absorbed from wounds. Application is relatively painless. The cream is applied with gloved hands. Occlusive dressings reduce the frequency of administration to once a day and also decrease evaporative loss from the exposed dermis. Exposed areas, such as the head, require more frequent application.

The use of systemic corticosteroids is controversial, as the exact cause of TEN is unknown. Corticosteroids are recommended, however, in both human and veterinary medicine for use early in the course of the disease. Prednisone or prednisolone should be used at a dosage of 2 to 4 mg/kg divided and given every 12 hours, but this dosage should be rapidly reduced. Extended use of corticosteroids suppresses wound healing and increases susceptibility to infection through damaged skin. Systemic antibiotics should be used only when signs of systemic infection, such as pyrexia or sudden development of leukocytosis, appear. Involvement of ocular mucous membranes may result in keratoconjunctivitis sicca, corneal ulcers, and synechia. Topical corticosteroids and ocular lubricants reduce the severity of these signs. If possible, the underlying cause of TEN should be determined and corrected; offending drugs should be discontinued and underlying diseases treated.

Prognosis is related to the extent of skin involvement. Diffuse sloughing of the skin is associated with a higher mortality. Pemphigus vulgaris and bullous pemphigoid should be differentiated from TEN. These dermatoses rarely have the sudden onset and rapid progression seen in TEN.

CUTANEOUS VASCULITIS

The vasculitides comprise a group of inflammatory disorders of blood vessels that often result in vascular necrosis. Necrotizing vasculitis is associated with the deposition of immune complexes within vessel walls, subsequent complement activation, and chemotactic attraction of neutrophils. The neutrophils invade the vessel walls and release lysosomal enzymes. These enzymes damage and may cause necrosis of the vessel wall. Vascular damage results in thrombosis and hemorrhage, which contribute to the development of ischemia in the surrounding tissue.

Cutaneous leukocytoclastic vasculitis (hypersensitivity vasculitis, allergic vasculitis) has been identified in the dog. Post-capillary venules of the superficial dermis are affected, causing ulceration of the overlying epidermis. Precipitating factors most commonly associated with leukocytoclastic vasculitis in humans include drugs (sulfonamides, penicillins), viral infections, bacterial infections, neoplasia, and connective tissue diseases such as systemic lupus erythematosus and rheumatoid arthritis. Necrotizing vasculitis of small veins and arterioles, with infiltrates of neutrophils, has been produced in dogs experimentally infected with *Rickettsia rickettsii*, the etiologic agent of Rocky Mountain spotted fever. Approximately 50 per cent of the cases in humans are idiopathic, as are the few cases identified in the dog.

Diagnosis of cutaneous leukocytoclastic vasculitis is made by clinical appearance, history, and biopsy. The clinical appearance is characterized by ulcers of the mucocutaneous junctions of the oral cavity, the aural pinnae, pressure points, and footpads. Fever, anorexia, depression, and lymphenadopathy may be associated symptoms. The identification of leukocytoclastic vasculitis should be followed by a search for an inciting cause. A good drug history should be obtained as well as a history of any recent infectious problems. CBCs, chemistries, and radiographs may contribute to the identification of the underlying problem, which should be corrected. Biopsy of the lesions shows involvement of the vessels of the superficial dermis. Endothelial swelling, neutrophil accumulation within and around vessel walls, nuclear dust (neutrophil pyknotic nuclei, leukocytoclasis), and extravasation of red blood cells are prominent histopathologic features. Fibrinoid necrosis also may be seen.

Specific treatment for idiopathic vasculitis in humans has been difficult to evaluate, as the disease is often self-limiting. The cases identified in the dog have been refractory to corticosteroids. Dapsone has been used successfully to induce remission. Initial dosage is 1 mg/kg three times a day until the lesions are healed. The dosage is slowly reduced until the animal is maintained on 1 mg/kg two to three times a week. If the disorder remains quiescent for several weeks the medication can be discontinued. If relapses occur dapsone therapy should be resumed. Hemograms and hepatic enzyme determinations should be done weekly initially. Potential side effects of dapsone include hemolytic anemia, methemoglobinemia, hepatopathy, peripheral neuropathy, and drug eruption. Signs of toxicity respond well to discontinuation of therapy.

Sulfasalazine (Azulfadine, Pharmacia Laboratories) has also been used successfully in one case of canine idiopathic leukocytoclastic vasculitis at an initial dosage of 45 mg/kg t.i.d. When the lesions were healed the dosage was reduced to once daily administration. Sulfasalazine may produce keratoconjunctivitis sicca and other less common side effects such as blood dyscrasias, hepatopathy, drug eruption, and drug fever in the dog. The dosage of sulfasalazine for canine dermatoses has not been established. Other possible therapeutic agents include immunosuppressive drugs such as cyclophosphamide or azathioprine. These drugs have not been evaluated for the treatment of leukocytoclastic vasculitis in the dog.

Other forms of vasculitis also have been identified in the dog. Polyarteritis nodosa, documented in the beagle, is characterized by neutrophilic infiltration of medium-sized arteries. Cutaneous lesions are uncommon but occur as ulcerating subcutaneous nodules. Corticosteroids and cyclophosphamides are recommended for the treatment of polyarteritis nodosa in humans.

COLD HEMAGGLUTININ DISEASE

Cold hemagglutinin disease (cold agglutinin syndrome) is characterized by the development of cyanosis and necrosis of extremities secondary to the occlusion of vessels by clumped red blood cells. The presence of cold-acting antibodies directed against red blood cells causes this intravascular clumping. These antibodies are of the IgM class of immunoglobulins and interact with red cells only at temperatures below 37°C. Production of these antibodies occurs secondary to abnormalities of the immune system, infection, or lymphoreticular neoplasm. These antibodies are most active at 0 to 4°C; however, activity can persist up to 30°C.

Clinical signs consist of acrocyanosis (gray-blue discoloration of the skin, which does not blanch), necrosis, and ulceration of extremities such as the nose, ears, digits, tip of the tail, and prepuce. There may be mild to moderate anemia in this condition. Skin lesions result from intracapillary hemagglutination and stasis of blood flow in extremities where the temperature is lower than that of the body core. The clinical signs are induced by exposure to cold.

Diagnosis is made by history, physical examination, and demonstration of the cold hemagglutinins. Blood should be collected for a Coombs' test, which should be run at 37 and 0°C. The IgM autoantibody may be evaluated from the red cells at 37°C, giving a negative result. A drop of blood can be placed on a slide, mixed with an equal volume of physiologic saline, and placed in an ordinary refrigerator for a few minutes. Autohemagglutination under these conditions can be diagnostic for cold-acting antibodies. Autohemagglutination may also be present at room temperature and is reversed by warming the blood to 37°C. Treatment of this disorder involves finding and correcting the underlying cause if possible. Avoidance of cold temperatures is beneficial. In humans glucocorticoids are not helpful in this disorder; however, immunosuppressive drugs such as cyclophosphamide are recommended.

IRRITANT CONTACT DERMATITIS

Primary irritant contact dermatitis differs from allergic contact dermatitis in that the offending substance causes an inflammatory reaction in the skin of most animals without an underlying allergic mechanism. Many chemical agents are potent irritants, causing vesiculation and epidermal necrosis. These include soaps, detergents, insecticidal sprays and dips, solvents, fertilizers, and corrosive substances such as strong acids and alkalis. Organophosphate–impregnated flea collars have also been associated with a contact dermatitis, especially in the cat.

Clinical signs of severe irritant contact dermatitis appear shortly after exposure to the offending agent and consist initially of erythema and variable pruritus, followed by vesiculation, necrosis, and sloughing. Pain and discomfort may become marked. Relatively hairless areas, such as the ventral surfaces of the feet and abdomen, are affected most commonly. The scrotal skin and tip of the prepuce are especially sensitive. The entire body may be affected if the causative agent is applied as a cleansing agent, dip, or spray.

The diagnosis is made by history of exposure to an irritant substance and by the clinical signs. The pain and discomfort associated with necrosis help differentiate primary irritant contact dermatitis from allergic contact dermatitis, which is marked by signs of erythema and pruritus. Subsequent ulceration and necrosis are less common in allergic contact dermatitis. Biopsy of affected skin in primary irritant contact dermatitis reveals epidermal vesiculation, necrosis, and ulceration accompanied by a predominantly neutrophilic inflammatory infiltrate in the dermis.

Treatment involves gently clipping and cleansing the affected areas with astringents. Aluminum acetate soaks and packs (Burow's solution; Domeboro Tablets, Dome Laboratories) three times a day are soothing and effective. Depending on the extent of involvement and degree of discomfort, topical and/or parenteral corticosteroids may be indicated. Many topical corticosteroid preparations are available. Ideally, an ointment should not be used. Ointments are occlusive to ulcerated and exudative lesions. Oral prednisone or prednisolone at 1.0 mg/kg divided b.i.d. may be used initially and then reduced over 10 to 14 days. Systemic antibiotics may be required to combat secondary infections.

The most important component of treatment is the identification of the offending substance. This may be difficult in the free-roaming animal, as it may contact many substances in its environment of which the owners are unaware. It may be necessary to confine the animal on a bedding such as newspaper until the lesions are completely healed. Thorough questioning of the owner may identify exposure to the causative agent such as caustic detergents or fertilizers used in and around the home. Once the offending agent is identified, avoidance will prevent recurrences of the dermatologic lesions.

DECUBITAL ULCERS

Decubital ulcers occur as a result of compression of the soft tissues of the subcutis and skin between a bony prominence and the surface on which the patient lies. Animals with neurologic and/or orthopedic problems are most commonly affected. A lack of sensory innervation or inability to change body positions leads to prolonged pressure on a small focal area of skin. Circulation to the area is impaired, resulting in ischemia, necrosis, and subsequent ulceration. Local acidosis, increased capillary permeability, and thrombosis result in impaired cellular metabolism. Several factors predispose the skin to the development of decubital ulcers. Decreased padding may result from loss of fat owing to debilitating diseases or atrophy owing to disuse. Loss of tissue elasticity, as is seen with hyperadrenocorticism, may contribute to the development of ulcers. Laceration, friction, and burns from heating pads may contribute to the development of decubital ulcers, as does irritation from fecal and urine contamination. Malnutrition of tissues secondary to inadequate diet, anemia, hypoproteinemia, and poor circulation associated with stasis of blood and lymph flow promote necrosis and ulceration.

Clinical signs of decubital ulcers begin with hyperemia that progresses to necrosis and ulceration if pressure is not relieved. Sites predisposed to the development of ulcers include the scapular acromion, the lateral epicondyle of the humerus, the tuber ischii, the tuber coxa, the trochanter major of the femur, the lateral condyle of the tibia, and the lateral sides of the fifth digits of the fore- and hind limbs. Secondary infection may develop, leading to considerable undermining of the skin beyond the ulcer edges. Osteomyelitis may occur in exposed bones.

The treatment of decubital ulcers requires maximizing conditions for wound healing. The animal should be placed on a padded surface such as an air or water mattress, foam pads, or thick fleece bedding, and its position should be changed frequently. The ulcerated areas should be kept free of fecal and urinary contamination. Daily whirlpool baths or soaks remove contaminating debris and necrotic skin as well as promote circulation to affected areas. The animal should be fed a well-balanced high protein diet. Specific topical therapy for ulcers has included the application of protamine zinc insulin and nitrofurazone (Swaim, 1980), topical enzyme ointments and sprays, and antibiotic ointments.

Surgical treatment of ulcers has been recommended to promote primary healing in the affected area. The necrotic tissue of the ulcer and surrounding skin should be debrided and the wound closed to heal by primary intention. Sliding skin flaps may be required to provide enough tissue to close the wound. Large ulcers can be managed medically until they are small enough to repair surgically.

Ideally, decubital ulcers should be prevented. Frequent examination of the skin overlying pressure points is mandatory in recumbent patients. Frequently changing the animal's position, padding the surface on which it lies, and scrupulously maintaining good skin hygiene assist in the prevention of decubital ulcers. A well-balanced diet is as important to prevention as it is to treatment.

Necrosis and ulceration of the skin and subcutis may result from pressure due to improperly padded casts and restrictive bandages. The pathophysiology is similar to that of decubital ulcers: restricted blood supply leads to ischemia and subsequent necrosis and ulceration. Animals that lick and chew at their bandages may be indicating that they are too tight. Prevention is best accomplished by meticulous application of casts and bandages and frequent observation. Any indication of an impending problem such as excessive licking and chewing or swelling of exposed digits necessitates removal and examination. If pressure necrosis occurs, reconstructive skin surgery is usually required.

RADIATION INJURY

With the increasing use of radiation therapy for the treatment of skin tumors in small animals, the veterinarian may be called upon to treat local radiation injuries. Ionizing radiation is absorbed by the cell nucleus and deposited as energy, resulting in direct or indirect injury to DNA. DNA synthesis and cell division are impaired. This damage may be reversible or irreversible. Regularly proliferating cells are most sensitive to radiation effects. The total therapeutic radiation dose is therefore fractionated and given over several weeks to maintain function of normal tissue and allow for repair. Radiation injuries may be acute or chronic. The severity and course of both acute and chronic radiation injuries depend on the type of radiation, the radiation dose as it relates to tissue volume (field volume × depth) and frequency of administration, and the tissue's sensitivity to radiation. Increasing the volume of tissue irradiated lowers its tolerance to radiation. The total dose of radiation is divided into fractions, and the frequency of administration alters the radiation response. Decreasing the time period over which the total dose is administered increases tissue damage. Young skin, unpigmented skin, and skin exposed to repeated friction, such as skin in intertriginous areas, are more radiation sensitive.

Acute radiation dermatitis occurs days to weeks after exposure. The lesions are characterized by progression from erythema to vesiculation and erosion. If the tissue tolerance is exceeded, necrosis and ulceration will occur. The lesions may be extremely pruritic or painful, and secondary infection is common. Hyperpigmentation and scarring follow healing. The healed area is more susceptible to physical and chemical damage than is normal skin. Treatment includes gentle cleansing with astringents and lukewarm compresses for the acute exudative phases. Topical antibiotic and corticosteroid creams are used once the exudation is controlled. The ability of corticosteroid creams to reduce radiation-induced inflammation is disputed; however, the lubricating effects of the cream may be beneficial. Analgesics may be required if pain is severe. The healing skin should be protected from self-inflicted trauma with Elizabethan collars if necessary. If ulceration does occur, wide excision and full thickness grafting are recommended.

Chronic radiation dermatitis occurs weeks to months after radiation exposure and is characterized by necrosis and ulceration within an area of atrophic skin. Initial lesions of acute radiation dermatitis develop including epidermal lysis and sloughing. Although the injury initially heals, the scar degenerates and becomes extremely atrophic. Ulceration may occur in severe cases of chronic radiation dermatitis. The area is extremely sensitive to trauma of any kind. Chronic radiation dermatitis is always progressive and irreversible. Treatment includes protection of the areas from trauma and use of topical lubricating creams and ointments as needed.

Envenomation by snakes and spiders and thermal injuries are covered more extensively (pages 155 and 180) but will be mentioned briefly here.

SNAKE BITES

Envenomation by crotalid snakes or pit vipers, including rattlesnakes and moccasins, can result in significant necrosis and sloughing of skin. The degree of damage is affected by many variables, such as the species and size of the snake and the virulence and volume of venom injected. The injection of bacteria with the venom further complicates the victim's response to the bite. The venom of pit vipers contains a variety of enzymes and toxins that produce hemolysis, intravascular coagulation, hemorrhage, and necrosis. Necrosis is enhanced by activation of bradykinin and release of other vasoactive substances from injured tissues.

Pit viper bites produce immediate swelling, erythema, pain, and serous transudation from the punctures. Swelling extends rapidly into surrounding tissues, causing severe distention of the skin. Laryngeal edema and respiratory distress may accompany bites on the head and neck. Petechiae, ecchymoses, and frank hemorrhage occur in the swollen areas. Systemic signs of shock may accompany the local signs.

Treatment of pit viper envenomation varies with the severity of clinical signs and the duration of time since the bite. Initially the patient should be kept quiet and the affected part should be immobilized. The use of tourniquets, incision, and suction is controversial. Application of a broad, flat tourniquet such as a belt or band of cloth is recommended within one hour of envenomation for wounds on the extremities. It should compress only lymphatic and superficial venous flow and should be released every 30 to 45 minutes. Incision and suction were ineffective in the dog when applied more than 30 minutes after venom injection (Van Mierop, 1976).

In humans, the mainstay of the treatment of pit viper envenomation is the use of polyvalent antivenin. Methods for its use in the dog have been described (Frye, 1977). Detailed brochures accompany the antivenin. Anaphylactic shock is possible; therefore, epinephrine should be available. Antivenin should be administered in adequate amounts within 24 and preferably within 4 hours of the bite. It can be administered in intravenous fluids such as normal saline, lactated Ringer's, or 5 per cent dextrose and water through an intravenous catheter. The dosage for the dog has not been determined; however, the smaller the body of the victim the larger the initial dose required. Severe envenomation in humans often requires 10 to 20 vials.

The use of glucocorticoids is controversial. Some human medical journals maintain that they are detrimental to the patient (Van Mierop, 1976); however, most veterinary sources recommend their use (Frye, 1977). Because the wounds are often contaminated secondarily with both aerobic and anaerobic bacteria, broad spectrum bactericidal antibiotics, such as ampicillin or the cephalosporins, should be used. Necrotic wounds should be kept clean. Any abscesses should be drained. Whirlpool therapy may be indicated once the patient can tolerate it. Debridement of necrotic tissue will facilitate granulation and healing.

SPIDER BITES

The two significant species of spiders causing necrotizing skin disorders (necrotic arachnidism) are the brown recluse spider, *Loxosceles reclusa,* and the common brown spider, *Loxosceles unicolor.* These spiders inhabit undisturbed indoor environments, where large populations can build up, and outdoor environments under stationary objects. They are not aggressive and will usually bite only when disturbed. These spiders inject a potent dermonecrotic toxin when they bite. The pathogenesis of the resulting lesion is related to both the enzymatic properties of the venom and the immune response of the envenomated animal. Initially the bite is not painful. Pain and pruritus appear with the development of erythema within two to eight hours. Vesicle formation is followed by hemorrhage and subsequent necrosis and ulceration. The ulcer may require several weeks to heal. A depressed scar often remains. Associated systemic signs may include pyrexia, malaise, vomition, arthralgias, seizures, and, rarely, intravascular hemolysis and thrombocytopenia.

Diagnosis is made on the basis of clinical signs and a history supportive of exposure to these spiders. Early excision of the bite wound is recommended to prevent the toxin from spreading because antivenin and drug therapy will not inhibit local necrosis. Corticosteroids and supportive care are recommended for patients showing systemic signs. The development of intravascular hemolysis, with associated hemoglobinuria and renal failure, is a grave prognostic sign.

TEMPERATURE-RELATED INJURIES

FROSTBITE

Frostbite most commonly affects the tips of the ears and the tail in cats. Scrotal dermatitis in the dog, ranging in severity from erythema to sloughing of epidermis, may result from exposure to cold surfaces. Severe frostbite rarely occurs in normal, well-nourished animals. Debilitated or injured animals are more likely to develop severe frostbite of the extremities. The pathogenesis involves direct cold injury to the cell, indirect cold injury by formation of ice crystals, and impaired circulation with hypoxia. Vasoconstriction occurs both as a local response to cold on the vasculature and as a centrally mediated response to conserve body heat.

Treatment depends on the severity of the injury. Mild cases of frostbite manifesting as only hyperemia and edema, such as those involving cats' ears and dogs' scrotum, may require no treatment. Reducing exposure to cold will prevent these lesions from occurring. In cases of severe frostbite, the affected extremities should be kept frozen until the animal can be treated by a veterinarian. If the limb thaws and refreezes, damage is more severe. Rapid rewarming of the extremity, although more painful, has been shown to be considerably more effective in preserving tissue than slow rewarming. The affected part should be immersed in a warm water bath (40 to 42°C). Whirlpool therapy is especially beneficial. Rewarming will be accompanied by erythema, vesiculation, and edema. The pain associated with rewarming should be managed with an analgesic, such as meperidine, as needed. If self-trauma can be prevented, it is best to allow the lesions to remain uncovered during healing. Systemic antibiotics are indicated only when severe secondary infection is present. Secondary infection can be prevented by cleansing the lesion gently with a topical germicide such as chlorhexidine. Surgical debridement should be postponed for several days, as tissue loss is extremely difficult to predict initially.

BURNS

Although infrequent in small animals, major burns can cause significant necrosis and loss of skin tissue as well as distinct pathophysiologic changes systemically. Burn injuries may result from direct heat, flames, scalding liquids, friction, and electricity. Burns are usually classified according to depth and extent. First degree burns involve the epidermis and present as painful, erythematous lesions that heal rapidly. Second degree burns involve the epidermis and variable depths of the dermis and present as painful, erythematous and vesiculated lesions that heal with some scarring within two to four weeks. Third degree burns imply complete full thickness destruction of the epidermis, dermis, and appendages. No pain is associated with the white or charred centers of the lesions. A major burn covers greater than 20 per cent of the body and may involve second or third degree depths.

The pathophysiology and treatment of the systemic signs associated with major burns have been discussed more completely elsewhere. In brief, problems requiring management include shock, pulmonary damage, protein and electrolyte loss, reduced immunocompetence, cardiovascular and hepatic dysfunction, and malnutrition. The treatment of the skin itself depends on the depth and extent of the injury. Minor superficial burns should be managed immediately at home with ice water packs and soaks to decrease pain and reduce injury. If the patient is brought to the veterinarian, the burned area should be gently clipped and cleansed with a cool isotonic solution such as physiologic saline or lactated Ringer's solution. Any devitalized tissue can be debrided and a topical preparation such as silver sulfadiazine cream (Silvadene, Marian Laboratories, Inc.) applied. A sterile bandage may be applied to protect the wound.

Major burns require intensive and aggressive topical therapy. Because burns cause coagulation necrosis of the epidermis and dermis, the protective barrier against bacterial invasion is lost. In addition, burn–induced neutrophil dysfunction contributes to the likelihood of infection. Sepsis of the burn area and septicemia are frequent complications of major burns. The initial treatment of major burns involves relieving pain with an analgesic such as meperidine and flushing the wound with a cool isotonic fluid. Necrotic tissue should be debrided. A topical antibacterial cream such as silver sulfadiazine is applied and the wound is closed with sterile dressings. Silver sulfadiazine is antibacterial, antifungal, and nonpainful and is not significantly absorbed systemically. Nitrofurazone and gentamicin creams have been recommended also. Dressings should be changed twice daily. Mafenide (Sulfamylon, Winthrop Laboratories) is antibacterial but is extremely painful when applied and is absorbed systemically, causing respiratory alkalosis. Topical silver nitrate solution (0.5 per cent) is very beneficial in controlling sepsis and is relatively inexpensive. Considerable leaching of sodium and chloride occurs from the burn wound, and therefore electrolyte values must be frequently monitored. Loose gauze dressings are applied to the wounds and are kept continually saturated with silver nitrate. Dressings are changed twice daily until the wound heals. Frequent debridement of necrotic debris from wounds will remove ideal media for bacterial growth. Ideally, burn patients should be handled as aseptically as possible. Wounds should be cultured twice a week to monitor for sepsis. Bacteria commonly isolated from burn wounds in humans include *Pseudomonas aeruginosa* and staphylococcal species. *Candida* sp. may be found as well. *Pseudomonas* sp. has been isolated from animal burn patients. Systemic antibiotics are not used unless septicemia develops; therefore, temperature and hemograms should be monitored frequently. Successful management of burn wounds is enhanced by early wound closure with biologic dressings such as lyophilized pig skin as well as definitive closure with autografts.

Oral and topical aloe products (Dermaide Aloe tablets and 80% cream*) have been used successfully in patients with major burns. Extracts of aloe vera kill bacteria associated with burns and decrease tissue thromboxane levels, reducing vasoconstriction. Please see references for more information.

The treatment of major burns in the small animal requires a major commitment on the part of both the veterinarian and the owner. The staff at human burn centers are often enthusiastic about giving advice and should be consulted whenever the opportunity to treat a burn patient arises.

---

*Dermide Corp., Chicago, IL.

REFERENCES AND SUPPLEMENTAL READING

Burke, J. F., and Bandoc, C. C.: Burns: the management and evaluation of the thermally injured patient. *In* Fitzpatrick, T. B., et al.: *Dermatology in General Medicine*, 2nd ed. New York: McGraw-Hill, 1979, pp. 931–936.

Cera, L. M., et al.: The therapeutic efficacy of *Aloe vera* cream (Dermaide Aloe) in thermal injuries: Two case reports. J.A.A.H.A. 16:768, 1980.

Cera, L. M., et al.: Therapeutic protocol for thermally injuried animals and its successful use in an extensively burned Rhesus monkey. J.A.A.H.A. 18:633, 1982.

Davis, L. E.: Thermal burns. *In* Catcott: *Canine Medicine*. Santa Barbara, CA: American Veterinary Publications, 1979, pp. 188–203.

Fauci, A. S., et al.: The spectrum of vasculitis. Clinical, pathologic, immunologic, and therapeutic considerations. Ann. Intern. Med. 89(Part 1):660, 1978.

Foil, L. D., and Norment, B. R.: Envenomation by *Loxosceles reclusa*. A review article. J. Med. Entomol. 16:18, 1979.

Frye, F.: Bites and stings of venomous animals. *In* Kirk, R. W. (ed.): *Current Veterinary Therapy VI*. Philadelphia: W. B. Saunders, 1977, pp. 166–173.

Manning, T. O., and Scott, D. W.: Cutaneous vasculitis in a dog. J.A.A.H.A. 16:61, 1980.

Muller, G. H., and Kirk, R. W.: *Small Animal Dermatology*. Philadelphia: W. B. Saunders, 1976, pp. 413–419.

Rasmussen, J.: TEN, cutaneous signs of systemic disease. Med. Clin. North Am. 64:901, 1980.

Scott, D. W.: Immunologic skin disorders in the dog and cat. Practical immunology. Vet. Clin. North Am. 8:641, 1978.

Swaim, S. F.: *Surgery of Traumatized Skin: Management and Reconstruction in the Dog and Cat*. Philadelphia: W. B. Saunders, 1980, pp. 60–62, 199–201, 347–354.

Urbach, F.: Reactions to physical agents. *In* Moschella, S. L., Pillsbury, D. M., and Hurley, H. J., Jr. (eds.): *Dermatology*, Vol. 2. Philadelphia: W. B. Saunders, 1975, pp. 1441–1455.

Van Mierop, L. H. S.: Poisonous snake bite: a review. J. Fla. Med. Assoc. 63:191, 1976.

Wintroub, B. U., et al.: Adverse cutaneous reactions to drugs. *In* Fitzpatrick, T. B., et al.: *Dermatology in General Medicine*, 2nd ed. New York: McGraw-Hill, 1979, pp. 555–567.

Wiskemann, A.: Effects of ionizing radiation on the skin. *In* Fitzpatrick, T. B., et al.: *Dermatology in General Medicine*, 2nd ed. New York: McGraw-Hill, 1979, pp. 936–941.

DIFFERENTIAL DIAGNOSIS OF NASAL DISEASES

C. E. GRIFFIN, D.V.M.

Garden Grove, California

The differential diagnosis of facial dermatitis has been reviewed by several authors. The discussions are primarily concerned with those diseases that predominantly or initially affect the face (Table 1). The facial disorders can be further differentiated by the presence or absence of nasal planum lesions. By considering nasal planum involvement, the differential diagnosis is narrowed from 20 to 12 diseases (see Table 1). Even more important is the finding that up to 68 per cent of nasal planum involvement appears in one of three diseases (Table 2). This article will cover the diseases that involve the nasal planum. For complete descriptions of the other diseases affecting the face, see the supplemental reading list.

DISCOID LUPUS ERYTHEMATOSUS

Discoid lupus erythematosus (DLE) is a recently recognized immune-mediated disease that is seen predominantly in collies and German shepherds and their crosses. Age of onset has varied from 11 months to 10 years, with no sexual predilection. In contrast to systemic lupus erythematosus (SLE), canine DLE is relatively benign with no systemic involvement.

Cutaneous lesions consist of erythema, depigmentation, scaling, erosions, ulcers, crusts, alopecia, and scarring. Lesions are most prominent on the nasal planum and bridge of the nose. Involvement of the lips, ears, oral cavity (especially the tongue), and eyelids may also occur. Chronic atrophic lesions frequently have the appearance and texture of parchment paper. In some cases, hemorrhage may be induced by relatively minor trauma, and up to one-half of patients with DLE have a history of exacerbation following exposure to sunlight. The lesions of canine DLE usually differ from those of pemphigus foliaceus/erythematosus by the absence of pustules and vesicles in DLE and the more prominent crusting found in pemphigus foliaceus/erythematosus.

A presumptive diagnosis is based on history and physical examination. The diagnosis can be confirmed by demonstrating characteristic histopathology and/or by direct immunofluorescence. Characteristic histopathology includes focal intracellular edema of the basal cell layer (liquefaction degeneration) and a periadnexal lymphocytic/plasmacytic infiltrate. Direct immunofluorescence of involved skin usually reveals the presence of immunoglobu-

The author acknowledges with deep gratitude the extensive help of A. A. Stannard and P. J. Ihrke in the preparation of this paper.

Table 1.   *Differential Diagnosis of Facial Dermatitis*

Diagnosis	Nasal Planum Involvement		
	Commonly Seen	Sometimes Seen	Never or Rarely Seen
Discoid lupus erythematosus	+		
Nasal dermatitis	+		
Pemphigus foliaceus/erythematosus	+		
Nasal depigmentation	+		
Nasal hyperkeratosis	+		
Trauma		+	
Dermatophyte		+	
Allergic contact dermatitis ("plastic dish syndrome")	+		
Zinc-responsive dermatitis		+	
Neoplasia		+	
Drug eruption		+	
Systemic lupus erythematosus		+	
Pyoderma			+
Food allergy			+
Atopy			+
Demodicosis			+
Dermatophilosis			+
Seborrhea			+
Subcorneal pustular dermatosis			+
Epidermolysis bullosa simplex			+

lins and/or complement in the basal laminar region. Direct immunofluorescence on uninvolved skin should be negative.

Initial treatment should include vitamin E, 200 to 400 IU given twice daily. If vitamin E is not effective, oral administration of corticosteroids is necessary (prednisone 2.2 mg/kg/day). Once a response is seen, prednisone should be given on an alternate-day basis. Every effort should be made to reach the lowest dose possible that retains a state of remission. Vitamin E therapy may be helpful in reaching the lowest possible dose of prednisone. Use of topical vitamin E and sunscreens containing para aminobenzoic acid (PABA) and avoidance of direct sunlight may be helpful.

NASAL DERMATITIS

The author acknowledges that the term "nasal dermatitis" has been applied only when a more

Table 2.   *Diagnosis of Nasal Planum Involvement*

Diagnosis	No. Cases/35
Discoid lupus erythematosus	12
Nasal dermatitis	7
Pemphigus foliaceus	5
Dermatophytosis	2
Trauma	2
Mycosis fungoides	2
Miscellaneous*	5

*Diseases with only one case diagnosed.

specific diagnosis was not obtainable. These cases present with lesions typical of DLE and are characterized by negative fungal cultures, nonspecific dermatopathology, and negative or unusual direct immunofluorescence. The author believes that most or all of these cases represent DLE or possibly pemphigus foliaceus and that the specific criteria for diagnosis were not obtained. The lack of a more specific diagnosis may reflect the selection of biopsy sites that were chronic or inactive at the time of sampling. In addition, concurrent or prior corticosteroid therapy may have altered laboratory results.

Nasal dermatitis has been successfully treated by following the treatment regimen described for DLE.

PEMPHIGUS FOLIACEUS/ERYTHEMATOSUS

Pemphigus foliaceus (PF) and pemphigus erythematosus (PE) are autoimmune diseases characterized by acantholysis, which is a result of the action of antibodies and complement on the epidermal intercellular cement substance (ICS). These diseases in humans are also characterized by circulating antibodies against the ICS, although in the dog these antibodies are frequently absent or difficult to demonstrate.

No age or sex predilections have been noted. Akitas and Dobermans are predisposed, and German shepherds and their crosses appear to be predisposed. Lesions consist of erythematous macules rapidly progressing to pustules and crusts overlying erosions. Lethargy, anorexia, pyrexia, and peripheral edema may be seen intermittently in these cases. Usually the systemic signs will be seen during an acute flare-up characterized by erythematous macules and pustules. Following the wave of pustules, the involved areas will be covered with crusts. The crusting nature of this disease must be stressed, as it is the most prominent clinical feature and helps to differentiate PF from DLE. Although vesicles occur microscopically, they are rarely seen grossly.

Lesions are usually not limited to the nasal planum. Other frequent sites include the bridge of the nose, periocular region (especially the dorsal medial canthus), pinna, external ear canal, and the footpads. Lesions can generalize over the whole body.

Diagnosis is usually based on the history, physical examination, and biopsies. Dermatopathology may demonstrate the classic subcorneal pustules and acantholysis. Direct immunofluorescence may reveal the presence of immunoglobulin and/or complement in the intercellular space. Indirect immunofluorescence may reveal circulating immunoglobulins against ICS. Smears from pustules usually reveal combinations of neutrophils, eosinophils, and acantholytic cells, both singly and in clusters.

In humans, PE is felt to be a benign variant of PF, with lesions usually being limited to the face, head, and neck. With the advent of immunofluorescence, other differentiating features of PE have been described. These include the presence of circulating antinuclear antibodies and basal laminar fluorescence. The finding of antinuclear antibodies and basal laminar fluorescence has also led to the belief that PE is a combination of PF and lupus erythematosus. Dogs with PE have been seen with all of the previously mentioned features found in humans.

Therapy should start with prednisone 1.1 mg/kg twice daily. The dose is increased to 2.2 mg/kg/day in the morning and is then tapered to an alternate-day maintenance dose.* If alternate-day therapy is not obtainable or if undesirable side effects occur, other immunosuppressives such as chrysotherapy 1 mg/kg/wk and azathioprine 50 mg/m² every other day may be added, allowing a decreased dose or discontinuation of prednisone.

Prior to starting chrysotherapy, the author suggests reviewing the discussion on page 448 or the articles in the supplemental reading list.

NASAL DEPIGMENTATION

Nasal depigmentation is a syndrome of unknown etiology seen in various breeds, although golden

retrievers, German shepherds, poodles, Siberian huskies, and Samoyeds are most commonly involved. These dogs are born with a pigmented nasal planum, which slowly fades until a light gray to pink color remains. This may be a cyclic problem, with the lighter color being more prominent in winter. Some animals will remain permanently depigmented, whereas others will repigment and remain that way. Haired regions are spared, although the lips are occasionally involved. The cyclic nature in some cases and repigmentation in others suggest that melanocytic destruction does not occur.

There is no known effective therapy. Tattooing may mask the lesions, but a question of ethics is involved, as the lack of pigmentation is a show ring fault. Some animals with noncyclic depigmentation may be prone to sunburn, which may be helped by the application of topical sunscreens and limited exposure to direct sunlight.

NASAL HYPERKERATOSIS

Nasal hyperkeratosis is an entity of unknown etiology. It must be differentiated from the nasodigital hyperkeratosis associated with canine distemper. Dermatophytes have also been found to rarely cause hyperkeratosis of the nasal planum. Owing to the nature of the disease, one might suspect a keratinization abnormality. However, little work has been done on this disease.

Diagnosis is based on history, physical examination, and a negative fungal culture. Therapy includes topical application of keratolytics and corticosteroids.

ALLERGIC CONTACT DERMATITIS

A specific type of allergic contact dermatitis called "plastic dish syndrome" has been described in the dog. This is felt to be a delayed hypersensitivity reaction to various ingredients found in certain red flexible plastic dishes. Lesions are limited to the nose, lips, and chin and are more prominent anteriorly, as contact with the dish is necessary. Lesions consist of erythema, edema, depigmentation, and alopecia. Pruritus is usually present. Interestingly enough, the classic human lesion of contact dermatitis, the vesicle, has not been described in these cases. It is the author's opinion that this is a rare cause of nasal disease.

Diagnosis is based on the history, physical examination, and, most importantly, the response to removal of the offending allergen by substituting a stainless steel or ceramic dish for the plastic dish. Removal of the plastic dish is also the most effective treatment.

---

*Editor's Note: This dose is correct for the author's method. Some clinicians use higher doses but often have more side effects.

TRAUMA

Trauma may be responsible for the development of focal lesions involving the nasal planum and bridge of the nose. Trauma-related nasal disease is usually seen in dogs that are kept in a chain link enclosure or that have a habit of rooting. Lesions consist of erythema, erosions, and ulcers. Secondary infection may occur, causing a purulent exudate and crusting.

Diagnosis is based on the history and physical examination. Effective treatment is based on correcting the underlying problem, such as changing the enclosure to a solid wall or modifying the behavior of a rooting dog. When secondary infection is present, topical or systemic antibiotics should be used. Mild soaps and cleansers may be applied to the lesions. Topical corticosteroids are not indicated and may slow the normal healing process.

DERMATOPHYTOSIS

Dermatophytes, especially *Trichophyton mentagrophytes*, may produce lesions of the nasal planum, including erythema, alopecia, scaling, and crust formation. Lesions will very rarely be limited to the nasal planum; in most cases there will be involvement of other areas as well.

Diagnosis is based on history, physical examination, fungal cultures, and, in some cases, dermatopathology. Treatment includes topical antifungals such as Captan (2 tbs/gal H_2O), 2 per cent lime sulfur, or miconazole. The choice depends on the extent of the disease. Topical agents should be applied daily for two weeks and then two times per week thereafter. Treatment should be continued for at least one week following clinical remission. Oral griseofulvin is also effective at doses ranging from 90 to 150 mg/kg/day. However, in larger dogs this is an expensive, although convenient, method of treatment.

ZINC-RESPONSIVE DERMATOSIS

A clinicopathologic entity of unknown pathogenesis that frequently responds to zinc supplementation has been recognized in Siberian huskies and Alaskan malamutes. The disease usually occurs in dogs less than two years of age. No sex predilection has been determined. Occasionally, the disease is seen in older dogs. When the disease is seen in older dogs (older than four years of age), other breeds appear to be at risk.

Lesions consist of thick, tightly adherent crusts that may be associated with alopecia and erythematous borders. Lesions most commonly involve the skin adjacent to commissures of the lips, eyes, and ears. Lesions may also be found on the scrotum, footpads, nasal planum, elbows, and hocks.

Diagnosis is based on history, physical examination, histopathology, and response to zinc supplementation. Histopathology reveals marked parakeratosis, serum exudation, and acanthosis. Treatment with oral zinc sulfate 220 mg once daily usually results in a complete response. Occasionally the dose has to be increased to 220 mg twice daily.

NEOPLASIA

It has been reported that chronic nasal solar dermatitis (NSD) may progress to a squamous cell carcinoma, although the author considers this a very rare complication. Treatment for squamous cell carcinoma includes surgery and radiation therapy.

Two cases of mycosis fungoides with nasal planum lesions have been seen. In both cases, lesions were present on most regions of the body. In one case, the lips and nasal planum lesions were noticed very early in the progression of the disease. Mycosis fungoides may be helped by prednisone. Topical nitrogen mustard is also beneficial in the treatment of mycosis fungoides; however, the disease is eventually fatal.

DRUG ERUPTIONS

Drug eruptions result from allergic or nonallergic reactions to systemically administered chemical compounds. Usually the eruptions occur following oral or parenteral administration, although they can be seen following systemic absorption of topical or inhaled chemicals. Drug eruptions are relatively common in humans and are infrequently reported in dogs. The low incidence of diagnosed drug eruptions may reflect a low index of suspicion, difficulty in proving the diagnosis, or the pleomorphic nature of the disease.

Virtually any lesion or pattern of disease can result from a drug eruption. Ulcerative nasal planum lesions have been described in dogs as a result of drug eruption.

A high index of suspicion is essential if one expects to diagnose drug eruptions. A presumptive diagnosis is based on the history, physical examination, elimination of other differentials, and resolution following discontinuation of the suspected compound. Subsequent challenge with the suspected chemical may substantiate the diagnosis. However, subsequent reactions may be more severe, and this risk is not warranted.

Treatment consists of discontinuing and avoiding future exposure to the suspected and closely related drugs. Systemic corticosteroids may be indicated, especially in cases involving a systemic reaction to the drug.

SYSTEMIC LUPUS ERYTHEMATOSUS

Systemic lupus erythematosus (SLE) is an immune-mediated disease characterized by multiple organ involvement and the presence of abnormal serum antibodies. There is a tendency for the disease to appear in young to middle-aged female dogs. The skin may be involved in 20 to 30 per cent of the cases, although these percentages may partially reflect the bias of the investigators.

Cutaneous lesions and their distribution are extremely variable and may be limited to patches of scaling, alopecia, or generalized erythema. Some animals have lesions similar to those seen in DLE.

Diagnosis is based on history, physical examination, and the presence of abnormal antibodies. A high-titer antinuclear antibody is usually present in addition to positive basal laminar zone fluorescence from affected skin. In humans, 50 to 70 per cent of samples from uninvolved skin demonstrate basal laminar fluorescence on direct immunofluorescence, in contrast to the negative findings in human and canine DLE.

Treatment involves the long-term use of immunosuppressive drugs such as corticosteroids, cyclophosphamide, and azathioprine (see page 416).

CONCLUSION

Facial dermatitis can be a challenging and rewarding diagnostic problem. Successful treatment is best achieved by first establishing an accurate diagnosis. This discussion has tried to demonstrate the value of differentiating cases of facial dermatitis based on the presence or absence of nasal planum lesions. Although the reported incidence of these diseases reflects the author's type of practice (100 per cent dermatology, mostly referral), it is evident that the common causes of nasal dermatitis are limited to a few diseases.

SUPPLEMENTAL READING

Griffin, C. E., Stannard, A. A., Ihrke, P. J., et al.: Canine discoid lupus erythematosus. Vet. Immunol. Immunopathol. 1:79, 1979.
Miller, W. H.: Canine facial dermatoses. Comp. Cont. Ed. 1:640, 1979.
Manning, T. O., Scott, D. W., Kruth, S. A., et al.: Three cases of canine pemphigus foliaceus and observations on chrysotherapy. J.A.A.H.A. 16:189, 1980.
Muller, G. H., and Kirk, R. W.: *Small Animal Dermatology II.* Philadelphia: W.B. Saunders, 1976.
Scott, D. W.: The differential diagnosis of facial dermatitis. *In* Kirk, R. W. (ed.): *Current Veterinary Therapy VII.* Philadelphia: W.B. Saunders, 1979.
Walton, D. K., Scott, D. W., Smith, C. A., et al.: Canine discoid lupus erythematosus. J.A.A.H.A. 17:851, 1981.

CANINE DEMODICOSIS

STEPHEN D. WHITE, D.V.M.

Boston, Massachusetts

and ANTHONY, A. STANNARD, D.V.M.

Davis, California

Canine demodicosis (demodectic mange) is a skin disease of dogs caused by the follicular mite *Demodex canis.*

ETIOLOGY AND PATHOGENESIS

D. canis is found in small numbers on normal canine skin. The mites reside in the hair follicles and occasionally in the sebaceous and apocrine sweat glands. The mite progresses through four stages during its life cycle: egg, six-legged larvae, eight-legged nymph, and finally eight-legged adult. Details of the life cycle are poorly understood. The mites are transmitted from bitch to nursing pups during the first two to three days of life. Pups delivered by cesarian section and raised away from the dam do not have demodex mites. With the exception of this mother-neonate transmission, the entire life cycle is spent on the host.

Many theories have been advanced as to why this normal skin resident produces disease in certain dogs. The most likely reason is an aberration of the immune response that compromises the dog's ability to limit the mite population on its skin. Scott and colleagues (1974, 1976) demonstrated a serum factor in dogs with generalized demodicosis that suppressed T lymphocytes' ability to respond in *in vitro* lymphoblastogenesis tests. Demodicosis has also been noted in dogs given immunosuppressive agents such as high-dose corticosteroids, antineoplastic drugs or antilymphocyte serum.

A definite hereditary predilection for demodicosis has been observed. The disease is most commonly seen in purebred dogs. Demodicosis is often seen in littermates and related dogs. Frequently a clinically normal bitch will produce several litters in which all or most of the pups will develop demodicosis.

Most cases of demodicosis occur in young dogs less than one and one-half years of age. Occasionally the disease appears spontaneously in an older dog (senile demodicosis). When this occurs the clinician is obligated to look for an underlying immunosuppressive disease, such as neoplasia or Cushing's syndrome (endogenous or iatrogenic). However, in the authors' experience, an underlying disease is rarely determined.

CLINICAL SIGNS

Demodicosis occurs in two forms: localized and generalized. The appearance, prognosis, and therapy of the two forms are quite different. The localized form is characterized by one or more focal areas of alopecia. Scaling, erythema, papules, pustules, and pruritus may be present. These lesions most commonly involve the face but may appear anywhere on the body. A high percentage of localized demodicosis will resolve spontaneously within six to eight weeks.

Generalized demodicosis initially resembles localized demodicosis. Owners should be advised that a small percentage of apparent localized demodicosis will progress to generalized demodicosis. The progression may be gradual, over the course of several weeks, or quite rapid, over a few days. Alopecia, papules, pustules, erythema, scales, crusts, ulcers, or fistulous tracts may be seen involving large areas of the dog's body. The face, feet, and ventral neck are frequently the most severely affected areas. Pruritus is variable and when present is usually associated with a secondary pyoderma. In very severe cases, a septicemia may be noted. Generalized demodicosis is a potentially life-threatening disease owing to sepsis, debilitation, or euthanasia by disconsolate owners.

DIAGNOSIS

Skin scrapings are diagnostic. The area to be scraped should be clipped, gently squeezed to facilitate extrusion of the mites from the follicles, and scraped deep enough to draw blood. The scraped material should be placed in a drop of mineral oil on a slide and examined microscopically using a coverslip under low-power magnification (40×). Finding many live (moving) mites, often in various life cycle stages, is diagnostic of the disease. One or two adult mites are occasionally seen on scrapings from normal dogs. In those cases repeated scrapings should be done to effectively eliminate or substantiate demodicosis as a diagnosis.

Rarely, dogs with severe pyogranulomatous pododermatitis secondary to demodicosis may have such extensive thickening and scarring of the paws that the clinician may not be able to scrape deep enough to demonstrate the mites. In those cases a biopsy for histopathologic evaluation is indicated. Histopathology of canine demodicosis either shows the mites confined to the follicles with minimal inflammatory cell infiltrate, or the mites may be released into the dermis following follicular rupture, with an extensive cellular response.

THERAPY

Therapy is usually not necessary for localized demodicosis owing to the high rate of spontaneous remission. Topical benzyl peroxide shampoo (OxyDex, DVM) may be used when a secondary pyoderma is present. Topical acaricidals (Goodwinol, Goodwinol Co.; Canex, Pitman-Moore; Benzyl-Hex, Evsco) may also be used. However, there is no evidence that these medications penetrate into the follicle where the mites are located. In addition, their application may be irritating to the skin and may cause the clinician and the owner to believe the condition is worsening.

There are many drugs and substances that have been used unsuccessfully in the past to treat generalized demodicosis (see CVT VI, page 531). It has been estimated that 40 per cent of generalized demodicosis cases may eventually resolve spontaneously. Thus, most reported "cures" must be viewed with suspicion. At this time only two protocols of effective therapy are known to the author. These are outlined hereafter.

It should be emphasized that an important aspect of any successful therapy is the treatment of the secondary pyoderma, which is a frequent complication of the disease. Whirlpool bathing in dilute povidone-iodine (Betadine, Purdue-Frederick) or chlorohexidine (Nolvasan, Fort Dodge) solution, 15 to 20 minutes once or twice daily, is helpful in healing ulcerated areas and fistulous tracts. This should be done prior to initiating topical acaricidal therapy to minimize systemic absorption and potential toxicosis.

A bacteriocidal antibiotic should be chosen based on culture and sensitivity tests. Until the results are known, penicillin-resistant *Staphylococcus aureus* should be assumed to be the bacterial pathogen and an appropriate antibiotic regimen should be initiated (see page 505). The isolation of *Pseudomonas* sp. warrants a poorer prognosis. If septicemia is suspected, blood cultures are indicated.

Corticosteroids suppress the immune system. Dogs with generalized demodicosis are already immunosuppressed. It therefore must be stated that corticosteroids are strictly contraindicated in demodicosis and have no place in the therapy of this disease *whatsoever*.

The therapeutic protocol that offers the greatest chance of clinical cure is the topical use of ronnel. This protocol was initially reported by Scott, Farrow, and Schultz in 1974. The dog's entire haircoat is clipped. A 4 per cent solution* of ronnel (Ectoral Emulsifiable Concentrate, Pitman-Moore) in propylene glycol is applied to one-third of the dog's body every day. The authors have used an 8 per cent solution in refractory cases. The person applying the solution should wear protective gloves, and the procedure should be done outside or in an area with good ventilation to minimize human exposure. The solution should be shaken prior to application, as the ingredients tend to separate. The solution is allowed to dry on the dog. No other baths or dips should be used once therapy is initiated. It should be stressed that the entire dog must be treated, not just the areas that grossly appear to be involved. Spot treatment is not effective and may result in poor response once the correct protocol is initiated.

Every two to three weeks the dog is re-evaluated and skin scrapings are performed. These should always include scrapings from the face and feet. A decrease in the number of live mites and immature stages is indicative of a favorable response to therapy. When all scrapings are negative for mites, the treatment is continued for another three weeks. If numerous scrapings are again negative, therapy is discontinued with a prognosis of a 90 per cent cure. Since the stability of ronnel in propylene glycol is unknown, replenishment of the owner's stock is generally done at the re-evaluation appointments.

Most dogs will have slight to moderate weight loss and an increased amount of scaling on the protocol. If scaling and weight loss are not seen, the clinician should be suspicious of improper compliance. Owners sometimes report that the solution appears to irritate the dog when the treatment is initiated. This problem may be circumvented by feeding or exercising the dog immediately after treatment in an attempt to preoccupy the animal until the irritation, which is generally of short duration, ceases. Occasionally signs of organophosphate toxicity may be seen. These may include salivation, lacrimation, vomiting, diarrhea, and trembling. In severe cases, hepatotoxicity and central nervous system signs such as head pressing and seizures may be seen. If mild lacrimation and salivation occur only during application, no change in the protocol is advised. If more severe signs develop, the dog should be washed in water and supportive care given. Ronnel, like other organophosphates, is an acetylcholinesterase inhibitor, and atropine is the indicated antidote. Dogs who manifest toxic signs on the previously described regimen may be managed with alternate-day application of ronnel to one-third of the body following a 48-hour recovery from toxic signs. To minimize toxic reactions, phenothiazine derivatives, inhalant anesthetics, and endoparasiticides (including levamisole) should be avoided. The use of ronnel tablets has no beneficial effect on the previously described protocol but will increase the potential for organophosphate toxicity.

This treatment is time-consuming, messy, potentially hazardous, and somewhat expensive. The treatment period is usually two to five months, and owner understanding, compliance, and communication are essential. Despite its potential side effects, this protocol is the authors' treatment of choice.

As stated previously, older dogs with spontaneously occurring demodicosis should be evaluated for underlying causes of immune suppression. When no primary disease is found, the ronnel protocol may be used. A cure may be effected in these older dogs; however, the treatment period is generally longer and the overall rate of success lower.†

Over the past several years, the Upjohn Company has been investigating an experimental drug for canine demodicosis and scabies. The drug, known as U-36,059 or Mitoban, is a monoamine oxidase inhibitor with amitraz as the active ingredient. The precise mechanism of its acaricidal action is not known. The drug was made available to the dermatology service, Veterinary Medical Teaching Hospital, School of Veterinary Medicine, University of California at Davis, for therapeutic trials. Thirty-four dogs with generalized demodicosis were treated. The haircoat was clipped before therapy was initiated. Twelve milliliters of Mitoban were diluted in two gallons of water, and the solution was applied to the entire dog and left to dry. The treatments were given every two weeks for six treatments. (If the patient had negative skin scrapings after the third treatment, the therapy could be discontinued.) The regimen was repeated for those dogs that failed to respond to six dips or those in which the disease recurred.

Three years after the dogs had been treated, their status was investigated. Clinical success or cure was defined as no *clinical* evidence of demodicosis. The results are shown in Table 1.

The clinical success rate of these dogs was 18/34 or 53 per cent. The authors have thus concluded

---

*90 ml of Ectoral (33 per cent ronnel) in 500 ml propylene glycol.

†Editor's Note: Ronnel products have been withdrawn from the market.

Table 1. *Dogs Treated with Mitoban for Generalized Demodicosis—Evaluation Three Years After Therapy*

No. of Treatments	Total No. of Dogs	Clinical Successes	Clinical Failures
Less than six	6	5	1
Six	16	4	12
More than six	12	9	3
Totals	34	18	16

that Mitoban, with this protocol, does not have the efficacy of the ronnel regimen. Clinical progress and prognosis were difficult to monitor using skin scrapings or clinical appearance. Some dogs, clinically normal with negative skin scrapings after six treatments, had relapses as late as ten months post therapy. The drug does have its advantages in that it requires only twice monthly application, and when effective it rapidly improves the appearance of the patient. Mitoban has a place in the therapy of demodicosis, particularly in those dogs (or owners) who cannot tolerate the toxic side effects of ronnel or those dogs in which therapy may be prolonged, such as older dogs or dogs on immunosuppressive therapy for other diseases.

The Upjohn Company also produces BAAM, an agricultural product for the treatment of pear tree pests. Although BAAM also contains amitraz, it is not as pure a grade as Mitoban and is highly inflammable as packaged. Its use on dogs is potentially dangerous and illegal. Any veterinarian using BAAM would be open to litigation.

PROPHYLAXIS

As stated previously, there is a strong hereditary predisposition for the generalized form of demodicosis. Certain breeds and lines within those breeds have a high incidence of the disease. It is the recommendation of the authors (as well as the American Academy of Veterinary Dermatology) that animals with a generalized demodicosis be neutered and sires and dams of offspring with generalized demodicosis not be used for future breeding.

REFERENCES AND SUPPLEMENTAL READING

Scott, D. W.: Canine demodicosis. Vet. Clin. North Am. 9:79, 1979.
Scott, D. W., Farrow, B. H., and Schultz, R. D.: Studies on the therapeutic and immunologic aspects of generalized demodectic mange in the dog. J. Am. Anim. Hosp. Assoc. 10:233, 1974.
Scott, D. W., Schultz, R. D., and Baker, E.: Further studies on the therapeutic and immunologic aspects of generalized demodectic mange in the dog. J. Am. Anim. Hosp. Assoc., 12:203, 1976.

FELINE DEMODICOSIS

GEORGE H. MULLER, D.V.M.

Walnut Creek, California

Feline demodicosis is a rare skin disease; only a few cases have been reported. As clinicians become more aware of the existence of feline demodicosis and make more skin scrapings, the number of cases diagnosed may increase.

Most textbooks report the feline mite to be *Demodex cati*. However, the author obtained mites from a domestic short-haired cat with generalized demodicosis in 1979 expecting to find *Demodex cati*. Nutting examined the specimens and reported them not to be *Demodex cati* (1979). Apparently, a second, still unnamed, mite exists on cats. In 1982, Conroy and coworkers also found a similar mite (1981).

As in dogs, there are two types of demodicosis: localized and generalized. Although the clinical cases show some similarities to the canine disease, feline demodicosis is unique and different in many respects.

Localized feline demodicosis occurs most commonly on the eyelids and periocular area. The next most common area is the chin; a skin scraping for demodectic mites should be made in all cases of feline acne. This is especially important if the chin and skin posterior to the chin are alopecic, scaly, erythematous, and hyperpigmented. The affected skin will be sharply demarcated and usually bilaterally symmetric. Other suspicious alopecic areas on the face may also be demodicosis and should be checked with a skin scraping.

Treatment for localized demodicosis may not be necessary, as it is self-limiting (as it is in dogs). However, a rotenone ointment (Goodwinol)* can be used. All cats with localized demodicosis seen by the author healed in a short time when treated with rotenone.

---

*Goodwinol Products Co.

Generalized feline demodicosis is very rare and is never as severe as the canine form (Stogdale and Moore, 1982). The condition may be more common in purebreds such as Siamese and Burmese cats. It has been seen in two long-haired cats (Scott, 1980). Scaly, crusted, alopecic patches are most common on the head. Hemorrhagic crusts are matted with hair, and the lesions do not resemble demodectic lesions until the hair is clipped away. Then, slightly raised erythematous papules and plaques become visible and are easily accessible for adequate skin scrapings. The mites are primarily found on the head but may spread from there to the neck and legs. A few lesions may extend to the trunk. Always make skin scrapings from scaly and pigmented patches on the skin of cats. The ear canals, if affected, should also be examined as demodectic mites have been found in large numbers in otic exudates (Desch and Nutting, 1979).

Although the data are scarce in such a rare disease, clinicians should be aware of the possible association of generalized feline demodicosis with serious systemic disease. Of the few cases seen, one cat had feline leukemia (Scott, 1980), another had diabetes mellitus (Nutting, 1976), and a third had severe lymphopenia associated with long-term therapy for a respiratory infection.

Feline generalized demodicosis is mildly pruritic but does not turn pustular as in the canine form.

Secondary infection with *Staphylococcus aureus* is mild and not deep as in dogs.

Generalized feline demodicosis can be treated with topical lime sulfur dips or rotenone in mineral oil (Canex). Since the few cats reported so far have all recovered, treatment is not as great a problem as it is in dogs.

Although amitraz is not approved for use in cats in the U.S., Wilkinson has reported its success in treating feline scabies (notoedric mange). He used a single application of 0.025%. It may have future use in feline demodicosis, although further tests are needed.

REFERENCES AND SUPPLEMENTAL READINGS

Conroy, J. D., Healey, M. C., and Bane, A. G.: New *Demodex* sp. infesting a cat: a case report. J.A.A.H.A. 18:405, 1982.

Desch, C., and Nutting, W. B.: *Demodex cati*, Hirst, 1919. A redescription. Cornell Vet. 69:280, 1979.

Muller, G. H., and Kirk, R. W.: *Small Animal Dermatology*, 1st ed. Philadelphia: W. B. Saunders, 1968.

Nutting, W. B.: Hair follicle mites *(Demodex spp.)* of medical importance. Cornell Vet. 66:214, 1976.

Nutting, W. B.: Personal communication, 1979.

Scott, D. W.: Feline dermatology. 1900–1978: A monograph. J.A.A.H.A. 16:367, 1980.

Stogdale, L., and Moore, D. J.: Feline demodicosis. J.A.A.H.A. 18:427, 1982.

Wilkinson, G. T.: An overview of feline skin diseases in Australia. Proceedings for the University of Sydney, Postgraduate Committee, Veterinary Science 57:277, 1981.

ECTOPARASITES

J. M. MacDONALD, D.V.M.

Auburn, Alabama

Depending on the geographic region of practice, ectoparasites may represent the major cause of dermatologic problems in the dog and cat. This is particularly true in endemic areas. Ectoparasitic diseases are associated with pruritus and must be strongly considered when one is confronted with a scratching animal. Dermatologic diagnosis is predicated on a complete and thorough history and clinical examination. These two elements account for 80 per cent or more of the criteria necessary for a diagnosis. Historoclinical findings should be used to develop a realistic differential diagnosis and formulate a diagnostic plan. The minimum data base should include multiple skin scrapings. Too often, despite overt manifestations of an ectoparasitic problem, a diagnosis of endocrinopathy is proposed because lesions include bilateral symmetrical alo-

pecia, hyperpigmentation, lichenification, crusts, and scales.

A prerequisite for successful treatment is a rational diagnostic approach. The first pitfall is an inadequate history and dermatologic examination. Treatment is attempted without a definitive or even presumptive diagnosis. Glucocorticoids are often administered as an alternative to appropriate therapy for a specific disease.

Client education is paramount when treating ectoparasitic problems. The "rest of the story" is frequently omitted, assuring failure of even the best therapeutic regimens. There is no substitute for good communication.

The array of commercial products makes selection of parasiticides a confusing issue for the practitioner. Products highly efficacious in one locality may have little effect in another. Many veterinarians innocently accept the manufacturer's claims or diligently record the findings of an esteemed colleague who is reporting experiences based on completely different circumstances.

The following is a general presentation of selected ectoparasitic diseases important to the practicing veterinarian.

FLEA INFESTATION

Fleas are insects of the order Siphonaptera. They are well-adapted parasites, obtaining blood meals from the host as their source of nutrition. *Ctenocephalides canis* and *C. felis* are the two species most often encountered on the dog and cat, although they are not host specific.

In many parts of the country the flea is the major source of dermatologic problems, particularly in the southeastern U.S., where environmental conditions enhance their survival and reproduction. Increased resistance to insecticides has accentuated the problem.

LIFE CYCLE

Small white spherical eggs are laid by the adult and hatch in the environment in four to seven days. The first-stage larva feeds on organic material and fecal pellets and within a week molts to the second-stage larva. Within seven days the second-stage larva molts to the third and final larval stage. This larval form spins a cocoon shortly after molting and enters the pupal stage. The adult flea emerges from the pupa in several days to two weeks. The time required to complete the life cycle depends on environmental conditions but is usually 18 to 21 days. High temperature and humidity accelerate the cycle. Only adult fleas parasitize the host. The life span of the flea is also influenced by environmental conditions but will not exceed one year even under optimum conditions and may be less than six months.

Fleas cannot live at high altitudes (greater than 5000 ft) and are quite susceptible to desiccation in low humidity. The flea spends the majority of its life away from the host, making the environment the prime target for control measures. Blood meals are taken at intervals, and the adult flea can withstand prolonged periods (several months to one year) without nourishment. Hungry fleas are more apt to seek nourishment from humans.

CLINICAL SIGNS

The effects of flea infestation are variable and, for the most part, depend on the reactivity of the host. Some animals can tolerate a large flea population with minimal signs. Cats are notorious asymptomatic carriers.

Pruritogenic substances in flea saliva or the focal inflammatory response to the flea bite elicits the irritative phenomenon observed in the nonallergic animal. Clinical signs are variable, and pruritus is usually of mild to moderate intensity. Lesions are typically distributed over the lower back and caudomedial thighs. Erythema and papular eruption may be observed along with secondary lesions consisting of crusts, scales, and excoriations. Alopecia is variable and proportional to the extent of pruritus. Sensitization may occur, resulting in an allergic state.

Flea allergy dermatitis (FAD) is by far the most common allergic dermatosis in the dog and cat and merits far more discussion than is possible in this article (see following article). FAD lesions are more profound and pruritus more intense in the allergic animal than in the nonallergic animal. Early FAD presents with minimal lesions that are proportional to the severity of pruritus. FAD has been recognized in dogs as young as three months of age. Lesions are typically observed on the dorsal lumbosacrum and tailhead and on the caudal and medial thighs. The disease in the untreated or uncontrolled animal becomes generalized as distribution of the lesions progresses cranially from the lower back and inguinal region. Involvement of the caudal third of the body is most severe and ultimately results in hyperpigmentation and lichenification in addition to papules, erythema, and alopecia. Scales and crusts become more prominent, and owners often report an offensive odor. Excoriations and fractured hairs result from the animal's chewing and scratching. Poor response to systemic glucocorticoid therapy is observed without concomitant control of the flea.

DIAGNOSIS

History and clinical findings are highly suggestive of FAD. Classic lesions of FAD are frequently seen if the disease has not become generalized but are commonly overlooked in many pruritic dogs. Nonallergic dogs will frequently be infested with fleas but will have no signs of FAD. Fleas or flea dirt may not be present on some animals with FAD, as owners often bathe the dog prior to examination despite instructions to the contrary. Also, the flea may spend only short intervals feeding on the host and may return to the environment, making detection difficult.

Careful examination for fleas is essential, particularly in long-haired dogs. Placing particles collected from the coat on a piece of moist cotton or filter paper will aid in identification of flea dirt, since it dissolves and turns red. Segments of *Dipylidium caninum* around the anus or in the area are indirect evidence of flea infestation. Intradermal skin testing with a nonglycerinated antigen is a beneficial diagnostic aid. Injecting 0.05 ml of 1:1000 w/v antigen extract* intradermally (with a histamine

---

*Flea Extract 1:100, Greer Laboratories, Lenoir, NC.

[1:100,000 w/v] and a saline control) will produce a positive "wheal and flare" reaction within 15 minutes in approximately 90 per cent of FAD cases.

The reluctance of owners to accept a diagnosis of FAD is generally overcome by observation of a positive skin test. Although a positive reaction does not always indicate flea allergy, correlation with a positive history and clinical signs is usually excellent. Sites of flea antigen injection should be re-examined at 24 and 48 hours for a delayed reaction. A small percentage of animals with signs suggestive of FAD will not demonstrate any reaction, and other differentials may need to be pursued more vigorously. Delayed reactions may be observed alone or in combination with an immediate reaction. Previous therapy with corticosteroids, antihistamines, or phenothiazine tranquilizers may cause false negative reactions.

Many animals with FAD have concurrent hypersensitivity to inhalant or ingestant allergens or both, requiring further investigation of those suspected cases. Seasonal exacerbation of signs may occur in animals with FAD, particularly in cooler climates where the environmental flea population is naturally controlled. A dietary allergy may produce clinical signs that mimic those of FAD. Scabies must always be considered in the intensely pruritic animal, and treatment with an appropriate scabicide may be indicated.

TREATMENT

Treatment for fleas is one of the greatest challenges facing the practicing veterinarian in the Southern US. Client communication must be excellent for successful management. The affected animal, in-contact animals, and the environment must all be treated. Only insecticides with proven efficacy should be used. In the author's experience, flea collars, medallions, and oral preparations (cythioate)* are usually inadequate and, furthermore, provide a false sense of security for the owner. Most flea shampoos, either over the counter or prescription varieties, offer little more than a detergent effect. Antiseborrheic shampoos such as Sebbafon† or Allergroom‡ are somewhat more helpful, as they reduce scale and crusts. Intermittent use of a humectant such as Humilac‡ is helpful.

INSECTICIDAL DIPS

Aqueous insecticidal dips provide the most reliable flea-killing effect but have little residual repellent or killing capability. Organic phosphorus com-

pounds such as phosmet,§ malathion,‖ Adams Flea-Off Dip,** or Dermaton II Dip†† are successful when applied at weekly intervals. In cases of coexisting seborrheic conditions, emollients may be added to the insecticidal solution. Both Para-Mite§ and Ectocide‖ may be used on cats at the recommended dilutions. Products containing lindane (Gamma-Rx‡‡ and Kil-A-Mite††) should be avoided in cats but are satisfactory for use in dogs. Carbamates are cholinesterase inhibitors that are effective against many parasites. However, increased flea resistance has been reported in certain geographic regions. VIP Flea and Tick Dip§§ and F-T Sevin Dip‡‡ are suitable in areas where fleas are nonresistant. Alternating insecticides every three to four weeks may help prevent the development of resistance.

DUSTS AND SPRAYS

Intermittent use of dusts and sprays between dips provides additional killing effects as well as offering some repellent activity. Pyrethrin combined with piperonyl butoxide‖‖ is available in hand–pump spray bottles and does not leave an oily residue following treatment. This product is safe for cats and dogs but should not be used on animals less than four weeks of age. Daily or alternate-day application may be needed for continued insecticidal activity owing to poor residual properties. Para-Mite*** and Dermaton II Dip†† are available in a dust as well as a dip. Malathion has been used successfully in a spray. A combination of carbamate and pyrethrin is used in the formulation of some sprays (e.g., DFT Spray‡‡).

Shampoos and sprays containing newer synthetic insecticides may prove to be superior to many currently in use. Examples include: Durakyl††† (which contains resmethrin, a synthetic pyrethroid) and Duocide‡ (which contains D-transallethrin and sumithrin, synthetic pyrethrins).

Fenthion‡‡‡ is a potent organophosphorus compound that is not approved for use in the dog or cat. Adverse reactions (acute organophosphate intoxication in animals and humans, permanent CNS disorders and death in animals) have made this

---

*Proban, American Cyanamid, Princeton, NJ.
†Winthrop Laboratories, New York, NY.
‡ Allerderm Inc., Hurst, TX.

§Para-Mite, Vet-Kem, Dallas, TX.
‖Ectocide, Hart-Delta, Inc., Baton Rouge, LA.
**Adams Veterinary Research Labs, Inc., Miami, FL.
††Burroughs Wellcome Co., Research Triangle Park, NC.
‡‡Carson Chemical Co., New Castle, IN.
§§Pet Chemicals Inc., Miami Springs, FL.
‖‖Adams Flea-Off Mist, Adams Veterinary Research Labs, Inc., Miami, FL.; ParaPyrethrin Mist, Haver Lockhart, Bayvet Div., Cutter Labs, Inc., Shawnee, KS.
***Vet-Kem, Dallas, TX.
†††Dermatologics for Veterinary Medicine, Miami, FL.
‡‡‡Spotton, Cutter Lab, Inc., Shawnee, KS.

product highly controversial. All potential risks should be reviewed before considering use of this product as a form of flea therapy. It should *not* be considered a substitute for more traditional forms of treatment. The dosage and regimen are outlined on page 498.

ENVIRONMENTAL CONTROL

The success of any attempt to control fleas depends on the extent of environmental control. Regular use of insecticides both indoors and outdoors is essential and may need to be continued year round in warm climates. Commercial foggers are available for indoor use. Methoprene* is an effective flea larvicide but does not affect the egg or adult stage. When combined with an adulticide such as Vet-Fog,† extended flea control may be achieved if adults do not repopulate the area. Rigorous vacuuming of carpets to remove eggs should be encouraged. Professional exterminators should be employed when clients are reluctant to diligently work on the environment or when a large area is involved. Microencapsulated, synergized, natural pyrethrin‡ is available to veterinarians in concentrated and ready-to-use forms. The solution may be sprayed on floors, walls, carpeting, and so on. The manufacturer claims that controlled release of pyrethrin maintains residual insecticidal activity for up to 60 days. It should not be sprayed on pets. Adams Anti-Crawl§ is another product designed for environmental flea eradication.

Outside areas should be periodically treated and may require insecticide application as frequently as every two weeks. The best control is achieved with fenced-in backyards where restriction from reinfestation is possible. Fifty per cent malathion can be diluted and applied as a 0.75 to 1.0 per cent solution. Ectocide,‖ a commercial malathion spray, can also be used for environmental control.

Ten per cent methylcarbamate dust** has been highly effective in some areas and ineffective in others, suggesting increased resistance of fleas in certain regions. Dermaton II Dip†† also includes dilutions for environmental use. Regardless of the product used, control programs are only as effective as client compliance. Parasitic control of the affected animal, in-contact pets (including cats), and the environment cannot be overemphasized.

Hyposensitization and antipruritic therapy are covered on page 499.

---

*Siphotrol 10, Vet-Kem, Dallas, TX.
†Vet-Kem, Dallas, TX.
‡Sectrol, S. Jackson Inc., Alexandria, VA.
§Adams Veterinary Research Labs, Inc., Miami, FL.
‖Hart-Delta Inc., Baton Rouge, LA.
**Sevin Dust, Stauffer Chemical Co., Westport, CT.
††Burroughs Wellcome Co., Research Triangle Park, NC.

CANINE SCABIES

Scabies has recently become a serious problem in veterinary dermatology because of its increased prevalence, contagious nature, and public health significance. The disease is characterized by an intense pruritus and is often confused with allergic dermatoses and is inappropriately treated. In humans, scabies has been observed in epidemics that last about 15 years and recur every 30 years. The recent increase in prevalence began in the 1960s. A comparable rise has been observed in canine scabies in the last decade.

ETIOPATHOGENESIS AND EPIDEMIOLOGY

Sarcoptes scabiei is a permanent parasitic mite that is reported to infest 40 different species of mammals. It has been proposed that humans are the original or primary host and that domestic animals acquired the mites from humans. Adaptation has led to host specificity.

Sarcoptes scabiei was first discovered in 1687, and scabies was the first disease in humans with a recognized cause. Acceptance of this finding took a mere two centuries. There has been considerable debate about the classification of the genus *Sarcoptes*. Although 30 species and 15 varieties have been recognized, it is now believed that there is only a single, variable and adaptable, species. Only three morphologic variations have been observed. Each host has a high proportion of one variety of mites, although smaller numbers of the other variants may be present. Adaptation to any host group may be accomplished by modifying the proportion of a given variant in the infesting population. Therefore, it is postulated that the dog *Sarcoptes* mite could adapt to humans and, by the process of selection, become morphologically similar. This process would require several generations, and the mite would likely be rejected before this could occur. However, the dog scabies mite will transiently infest humans and other animals.

Sarcoptes scabiei variety *canis* is the mite responsible for scabies in the dog. The adult female is twice as large as the male, measuring 400 microns. The body is rounded and has no distinct head. The four pairs of legs are short and are characterized by long, unjointed stalks with suckers on the anterior legs in both the male and female. The male also has suckers on the fourth pair of legs, whereas the female has long trailing bristles. The mite possesses spines with sharp points, triangular scales, and a few bristles on its dorsal surface.

The complete life cycle of the mite takes place on the dog. Once fertilization is completed, the adult female burrows into the superficial layers of the skin, producing a tunnel at the boundary of the stratum corneum and stratum granulosum, where she feeds on cellular particles and fluid. Shortly after starting the burrow, the female deposits two to three eggs per day while she tunnels. The female remains in the skin for the duration of her three- to four-week life span. The eggs hatch in several days, releasing the first larval stage. The first-stage larva has an adult appearance but possesses only three pairs of legs. The newly hatched larva soon migrates to the skin surface and forms a new burrow of its own where it is protected and where it begins to feed. Here the larva molts and becomes a nymph, which possesses four pairs of legs. The nymph lives on or beneath the skin and molts into a second nymphal stage or an adult. An estimated 10 per cent or less of the eggs develop into adult mites. The total life cycle is about 17 to 21 days.

Pathomechanisms of the disease are not completely understood. Much of the research has been performed in humans, particularly during World War II when conscientious objectors were used for experimental infestation. Individuals infested for the first time required over four weeks before clinical signs developed. When reinfestation was attempted, the incubation period was much shorter, and pruritus was immediately observed in some individuals. Reinfestations were successful in only 40 per cent of the subjects. An average of 11.3 adult female mites were found per infected individual.

Crusted, or Norwegian, scabies is a severe variant characterized by a large population of mites. This manifestation has been observed in mentally retarded and physically or immunologically debilitated humans. These individuals fail to react positively to intradermal injection of crude mite extract and may have minimal pruritus. A delayed reaction to intradermal testing has been observed in humans having scabies for six months or longer. Immediate and delayed reactions to intradermal injection of mite extract in pigs developed within seven weeks of experimental infestation.

The intense pruritus associated with clinical scabies is undoubtedly the result of several factors. Evidence of hypersensitivity exists in humans and some animals. Mechanical irritation produced by the burrowing female and the immature forms also must be considered. Pruritogenic substances from the mite or as the result of a focal inflammatory response are also involved in the pathogenesis.

Human infestations with canine *Sarcoptes* are generally considered self-limiting, although lesions and pruritus may continue for several weeks and may persist until treatment is initiated. Clinical signs may be observed after a very short incubation period. Lesions are located on body areas that have been in contact with the animal. Burrows are not found and mites are generally rare, although they have been found on humans four to seven days after contact with an infested animal. Thirty per cent or less of in-contact humans will develop clinical signs. Consultation with a dermatologist should be advised.

Scabies is highly contagious among dogs and has no age, breed, or sex predilection. Infested asymptomatic dogs have been identified by skin scrapings and biopsy. Occasionally only one dog in a kennel or household will have clinical signs. Transmission is primarily by direct contact with affected animals.

CLINICAL SIGNS

The hallmark of scabies is an intense pruritus that may persist from weeks to years. Animals in the early stages of infestation may be remarkably free of lesions in proportion to the intensity of pruritus. Erythema and a papular eruption may be the first lesions observed followed by excoriations, alopecia, crusts, and scales with or without hyperpigmentation and lichenification. Classical areas affected include the pinnae, elbows, hocks, ventral thoracoabdominal region, and the extremities. Initially, lesions may be restricted to the ears and elbows. The facial area and distal extremities are affected as the disease progresses. Crusting of the ear margins and an easily elicited scratch reflex when the ear is rubbed are highly suggestive of scabies but are not pathognomonic. Lesions on the extremities may be restricted to the medial and lateral surfaces, sparing the interdigital spaces and dorsum of the feet. Involvement of the trunk is not typical unless the disease is chronic and generalized or of the crusted (Norwegian) form. Insecticidal shampoos or dips with limited scabicidal activity and corticosteroid therapy will modify the clinical signs.

The term "scabies incognito" has been used to describe cases with profound pruritus but minimal clinical lesions because of ineffective therapy. Lesions of coexisting bacterial pyoderma may be observed. Moderate to severe seborrhea is seen in chronic cases, and a peripheral lymphadenopathy is a consistent finding.

DIAGNOSIS

HISTORY AND CLINICAL SIGNS

Scabies may be a diagnostic challenge. The majority of cases are diagnosed by history, clinical findings, and response to specific scabicidal therapy. Only 10 per cent of the animals observed by the author had *not* received prior treatment for the problem. Response to empirical corticosteroid therapy may entice the clinician into a misdiagnosis of other pruritic diseases. Although corticosteroids may diminish the itching, there is *never* complete relief. Affected in-contact animals or humans should arouse suspicions of scabies. A history of recent boarding or other activity outside the animal's regular environment should be determined. It is essential to inquire about the response to previous therapy. Description of the disease progression may be most helpful in diagnosis, since the appearance and distribution of *early* lesions may be more typical of scabies. A detailed clinical examination usually reveals lesions highly suggestive of scabies.

ANCILLARY DIAGNOSTIC AIDS

Finding a single scabies mite, egg, or immature form is diagnostic. Multiple skin scrapings should be performed on nonirritated areas, particularly where excessive crusting is observed. Ear margins should always be scraped. Each scraping should cover a reasonably large area and should continue until capillary bleeding is produced. Twenty-five diligently performed skin scrapings per animal will be diagnostic in only 40 to 50 per cent of scabies cases. Fewer scrapings will yield a lower positive percentage. Negative scrapings *do not* rule out scabies. The number of scrapings obtained from one animal before finding a mite may exceed 80.

Other diagnostic findings are controversial. A circulating eosinophilia is observed only if there is concurrent disease such as endoparasitism and/or *Dirofilaria immitis*. *Most* animals without other parasitic disease have normal leukograms. Dermatohistopathology usually shows a nonspecific inflammatory infiltrate consisting of neutrophils, plasma cells, and lymphocytes. An eosinophilic infiltrate is less common. It is rare to find a mite in the tissue except in heavy infestations. In those cases, demonstration of the mite by skin scraping is relatively easy. Lymph node aspirates show evidence of a reactive node.

TREATMENT

If scabies is suspected from the historical and clinical findings, even if skin scrapings are negative, the animal should be treated for scabies. A scabicide with recognized effectiveness should be used at weekly intervals for six to eight treatments. Keratolytic and antiseborrheic shampoos are frequently indicated when secondary seborrhea is present. The skin should be shampooed before applying the scabicide solution. Client education is paramount. Detailed instruction should be given, proper technique described, and the scabicide dilution emphasized. In-contact dogs should be treated and regular bedding discarded. Every square inch of the dog should be treated and allowed to "drip dry" without rinsing. Lime sulfur (either 2 per cent generic or scented preparations such as Lym Dip*) is a proven

scabicide. Disadvantages include odor and discoloring qualities. It is the most innocuous preparation available and an excellent choice for small or young animals. Phosmet (Para-Mite†) and malathion (Ectocide‡) are organophosphates appropriate for the treatment of scabies. Lindane (Gamma Rx§) is also highly effective. Manufacturers' claims that only a single application is necessary to eradicate the mites should be viewed with skepticism. Marked clinical improvement is usually seen by the third weekly treatment. As a rule of thumb, treatment should be continued through clinical remission plus two additional applications.‖

Corticosteroid therapy should *only* be used in confirmed cases (i.e., following a positive skin scraping). Short-term medical therapy will help relieve pruritus and will allow evaluation of the scabicide later in the course of treatment. Intensification of pruritus following termination of corticosteroids should not be equated with ineffectual scabicidal activity. A rebound phenomenon may be explained by a hypersensitive state. Remember, scabies is a *curable* disease with an *excellent* prognosis.

FELINE SCABIES

Feline scabies (notoedric mange, head mange) is a rare disease in the US. It is caused by the sarcoptiform mite *Notoedres cati*. The life cycle of this parasite is similar to that of *Sarcoptes scabiei*. *Notoedres* is an obligate parasite with species specificity that transiently infests humans and other animals. Clinical signs of feline scabies are comparable to those of canine scabies, with pruritus the earliest and most prominent feature. The ears and facial region are most affected, with lesions consisting of erythema, papules, crusts, scales, and excoriations. *N. cati* is more easily demonstrated in skin scrapings than *S. scabiei;* therefore, confirmation of the diagnosis is easy.

TREATMENT

Treatment of feline scabies is comparable to the regimen for canine scabies. Two per cent lime sulfur applied to the entire body is an excellent choice for cats. Malathion or weak solutions of approved organophosphates such as phosmet (Para-Mite) would be efficacious but have severe toxicity potentials. Weekly applications should be continued for four to six treatments. This disease is highly contagious; therefore, all animals in the household should be

---

*Dermatologics for Veterinary Medicine, Miami, FL.

†Vet-Kem, Dallas, TX.
‡Hart-Delta Inc., Baton Rouge, LA.
§Carson Chemical Co., New Castle, IN.
‖Editor's Note: Amitraz (Mitoban, Upjohn Co., Kalamazoo, MI) is a new topical miticide said to be highly effective for canine scabies that will be available to veterinarians in 1983.

treated. This is another curable disease with an excellent prognosis.

TICK INFESTATION

Ticks are arachnid parasites that may be classified into two major families utilizing morphologic and biologic characteristics. Ixodid (hard shelled) ticks possess a shield-like scutum; their heads extend anteriorly. Ixodid ticks are the most common ticks found on small animals. They include ticks of the *Rhipicephalus sanguineus*, *Dermacentor*, *Amblyomma*, and *Ixodes scapularis* species. Argasid ticks are soft shelled and lack the shield-like scutum. The head (capitulum) is ventral and cannot be seen on a dorsal view.

Otobius megnini is the argasid tick associated with small animal dermatology. The larval and nymphal stages of *O. megnini* parasitize the host; the nonparasitic adult is found in the environment. Parasitism of the exterior ear canal by the tick with its spiny cuticle has led to the common name "spinous ear tick."

LIFE CYCLE

All ticks are blood-sucking parasites and have four stages in their life cycle: egg, larva (seed tick), nymph, and adult. The larval form has only three pairs of legs and is the first parasitic stage. Most species are three-host ticks. The brown dog tick *R. sanguineus* is of particular concern because it is commonly found in the dog's environment (housing, bedding, carpets, and so on) when it is not feeding on the host. Gravid adult females, engorged with blood, detach from the host and lay eggs in the environment. These eggs hatch into the larval form in about one to four weeks. The larvae parasitize a host and after several days of feeding return to the environment to molt. Nymphs are formed in about one week and once again parasitize a new host. They return to the environment and molt to the adult form in several weeks. Both adult males and females feed on the host, but the female usually does so for a shorter period of time. Ixodid ticks other than those of *R. sanguineus* that are located in vegetated areas during their nonfeeding phase are commonly referred to as "wood ticks." They require more moisture and a blood meal from another host animal to complete the life cycle. The adult form engorges on dogs. The life span of ticks is variable and may be in excess of one year. Ticks may be dormant during colder periods and have been observed feeding on their hosts.

Argasid ticks usually lay hundreds of eggs in several batches and have two or more nymphal stages. Both nymphal and argasid ticks feed. They breed repeatedly and lay their eggs after each meal. In contrast, the ixodid ticks feed only once in each developmental stage. Adult female ixodids die after ovipositing their eggs, whereas adult males usually die after mating.

CLINICAL SIGNS

Clinical signs of tick infestation depend on the number of ticks feeding, the reactivity of the host, and potential secondary disease. Ticks transmit a variety of protozoan, viral, rickettsial, and bacterial disease to both humans and animals. *Dermacentor* species in particular are noted for the neurotoxin in the saliva of engorged females that is responsible for the lower motor neuron disease referred to as tick paralysis. Rocky Mountain spotted fever has been reported in dogs (see page 1202).

Tick bites are irritating and usually show a local inflammatory response. Large nodular reactions with surrounding tissue swelling may be the result of a hypersensitivity reaction. These may terminate in a large granulomatous reaction and may persist for a prolonged period of time after the tick is gone. Ticks may attach almost anywhere on the host but are especially common in the ears, around the neck, and between the toes. Numbers of seed ticks have been observed from skin scrapings obtained between toes of dogs and cats exhibiting pododermatitis. Many dogs will tolerate a moderate infestation with minimal clinical signs. Careful inspection of the skin and skin scrapings should be performed routinely. Identification of the tick is desirable.

TREATMENT

An insecticidal solution appropriate for tick infestations should be applied to the entire body. However, if only a few ticks are present manual extraction may be preferred. Care must be taken to remove the entire head and its mouth parts. Engorged females may be difficult to kill. Repeated whole-body dips are essential in geographic areas where the parasites are endemic and reinfestation is chronic. Organophosphates such as Dermaton II Dip,* Para-Mite,† Ectocide,‡ and Adams Flea-Off Dip§ are effective. Carbamates are weaker cholinesterase inhibitors than the organophosphorus compounds but may also be effective. Flea and tick collars or medallions are usually ineffective. Some powders or sprays may offer residual killing and/or repellent effect. Dogs with severe reaction to tick bites may require concurrent systemic corticosteroid therapy in addition to topical wet compresses and/or mild astringents.

Treating the environment is important when *R. sanguineus* is the infesting tick. Buildings, particularly kennels, should be periodically sprayed with a suitable product. Professional pesticide agencies

---

*Burroughs Wellcome Co., Research Triangle Park, NC.
†Vet-Kem, Dallas, TX.
‡Hart-Delta Inc., Baton Rouge, LA.
§Adams Veterinary Research Labs, Inc., Miami, FL.

will provide this service. The outdoor environment may be more difficult to control. Malathion (Ectocide), dimpylate (Diazinon*) and carbaryl (Sevin Dust†) have been used in areas where tick infestation is high.

CHEYLETIELLOSIS

Cheyletiellosis (cheyletiella dermatitis) is a cutaneous parasitic disease caused by *Cheyletiella* spp. of mites. *C. yasguri* is usually isolated from the dog, *C. parasitovorax* from the rabbit, and *C. blakei* from the cat. Limited host specificity is observed, and transient parasitism of humans can occur. The adults live on the skin surface and do not burrow. The entire life cycle takes place on the host. Eggs deposited at the base of hairs hatch in a few days into larvae characterized by three pairs of legs. The first nymph form is formed in about one week and has four pairs of legs. A second nymph stage is seen following another week of maturation. The adult finally develops within the third week.

Clinical signs classically include moderate to severe seborrhea sicca with pruritus, usually affecting young animals. Dorsal truncal distribution is typical, although generalization may occur. The problem is seen in litters and is highly contagious. Pruritus is not as intense as that observed with scabies. This is especially true in cats. Excoriations, erythema, and a mild papular eruption may be seen. Miliary crusted lesions are more commonly seen in cats and should be considered in the differential diagnosis associated with feline miliary dermatitis. An asymptomatic carrier state has been observed in cats.

Diagnosis is confirmed by finding a mite in skin scrapings obtained from areas of scale. In most cases adults, eggs, and immature forms are easily demonstrated.

The mite may also be seen with the aid of a hand lens by placing scales on a dark background and observing movement, hence the term "walking dandruff." The most characteristic morphologic feature of adult *Cheyletiella* mites is the large palpal hooks on the accessory mouth parts.

TREATMENT

Treatment should be directed at eradicating the mite from the affected animal and any possible in-contact carriers. Although *Cheyletiella* is an obligate parasite, environmental extermination is usually recommended. An antiseborrheic shampoo bath such as Sebbafon‡ should be given prior to application of an acaricidal solution. The mites are susceptible to most routinely used preparations. The ideal dip for cats and young animals is 2 per cent lime sulfur solution. Powders and sprays may not be distributed uniformly to the entire body or may not reach the skin in thick-coated animals. Use of flea shampoos has been advocated by some as the only treatment necessary. All animals should be treated at weekly intervals for six to eight treatments. Kennel or pet store infestations require more intensified efforts, and environmental extermination is included in the protocol.

PEDICULOSIS

Lice are highly host specific wingless insects with dorsoventrally flattened bodies. They spend their entire life cycle in the host. Blood-sucking lice (Anoplura) have relatively narrow heads with piercing mouth parts, whereas biting lice (Mallophaga) have broader heads and mouth parts adapted for biting or chewing. Transmission is usually by direct animal contact, although grooming instruments may act as fomites. The life cycle takes from 14 to 21 days to complete. Ovipositing females attach eggs (nits) to the hair shaft. Eggs hatch into an immature version of the adult and, although several molts take place, only minor morphologic changes occur. The metamorphosis is, therefore, incomplete.

Trichodectes canis is the common biting louse of the dog. It is recognized as an intermediate host for *Dipylidium caninum. Heterodoxus spiniger* is the other biting louse of dogs, and *Linognathus setosus* is the only sucking louse. *Felicola subrostratus* is the biting louse of cats.

Lice-infected animals have a dry, rough, unkempt haircoat with varying amounts of scale, crust, and alopecia. Pruritus is usually of moderate intensity. Young, debilitated dogs may develop an anemia if heavily parasitized with *L. setosus*. Diagnosis is made by careful integumentary examination of the skin. Finding adults and nits is usually easy. Microscopic examination, however, may be necessary for identification.

TREATMENT

Lice are susceptible to most insecticidal agents. All appropriate host animals in the household should be treated. Insecticide baths and/or topical dusts, sprays, or dips should be repeated at least once 10 to 14 days following treatment. Grooming instruments should be hygienically cared for.

SUPPLEMENTAL READING

Fadok, V.: Miscellaneous parasites of the skin (Part I). Comp. Cont. Ed. 2:707, 1980.
Fadok, V.: Miscellaneous parasites of the skin (Part II). Comp. Cont. Ed. 2:782, 1980.
Horwood, R. F., and James, M. T.: *Entomology in Human and Animal Health,* 7th ed. New York: Macmillan Co., 1979.
Muller, G. H., Kirk, R. W., and Scott, D. W.: *Small Animal Dermatology,* 3rd ed. Philadelphia: W. B. Saunders, 1983.

---

*Ciba-Geigy Corp., Summit, NJ.
†Stauffer Chemical Co., Westport, CT.
‡Winthrop Laboratories, New York, NY.

FLEA ALLERGY DERMATITIS

RICHARD E. W. HALLIWELL, M.R.C.V.S.

Gainesville, Florida

HABITAT AND LIFE CYCLE

This laterally compressed insect of the order Siphonaptera is the cause of the most common skin disease of dogs and cats and, arguably, of the most common disease entity of domestic animals.

The different species of the genus *Ctenocephalides* are generally not host specific, which has serious implications when control measures are considered. The most common species to parasitize dogs and cats is apparently *Ctenocephalides felis*. A moist, warm environment is most favorable for a rapid completion of the life cycle, which can be as short as 16 days. Fleas do not thrive in the cold (e.g., in parts of northern US and parts of Canada), in hot and dry climates (e.g., in the desert Southwest), or at high altitudes (e.g., in Colorado). In the South the infestation incidence peaks in spring and fall, but the heavy rains of the summer are prejudicial to survival in the outside environment, and an apparent fall in the infestation incidence may occur.

Most internal environments are favorable for completion of the life cycle, although the low humidity usually associated with heating systems often interrupts the cycle in the winter, controlling infestation. The life cycle has three larval stages and a pupa, which hatches into the adult. Eggs may be laid on or off the host, but the major part of the life cycle, and most of the adult stage, is spent in the environment. It is probably true to say that for every flea on the dog, there are 100 in the environment.

In the South, the sticktight flea, *Echidnophaga gallinacea*, which is a natural parasite of poultry, is becoming more common. The female burrows into the skin, where she lays her eggs. When the larva hatches, the remainder of the life cycle is completed in the environment.

PATHOGENESIS

A blood meal is required by the female, who is the major feeder of the two sexes, before reproduction can occur. During the feeding process the flea intradermally injects saliva, which contains a variety of irritant and pruritogenic substances including proteolytic enzymes and histamine-like substances. Thus, the bite of the flea in a normal, unsensitized

animal is somewhat irritating. However, of greater importance is the potential development of hypersensitivity to the injected allergens.

Early workers studying this phenomenon in guinea pigs defined four stages in the sensitization process (Benjamini et al., 1961). Stage I was a phase of delayed (cell-mediated) hypersensitivity only. In stage II, delayed and immediate (presumably IgE-mediated) hypersensitivity were coexistent. Stage III was marked by immediate hypersensitivity only. The animal then spontaneously desensitized upon further antigenic exposure (stage IV) and was no longer reactive to the bites.

Recent studies at the University of Florida using controlled flea exposure indicate that this orderly sequence probably does not occur in the dog. Flea-naive dogs ordinarily became sensitized after six to ten weeks of intermittent flea exposure. However, not all animals developed a clinically or histologically demonstrable delayed phase before showing immediate hypersensitivity. In animals continually exposed to fleas, onset of allergic skin test reactivity took much longer and in some cases did not develop during the course of the studies (up to ten months). Stage IV, or spontaneous desensitization, has only rarely been observed in animals followed in excess of one year.

The major flea antigen has been identified as haptenic in nature (i.e., a simple chemical), which becomes a complete antigen upon combination with dermal collagen (Michaeli et al., 1966). However, haptens, unless they are large and multivalent, cannot induce degranulation of mast cells. The fact that immediate wheals result in sensitive animals not only upon intradermal injection of antigen but also following exposure to fleas indicates that higher molecular weight substances also must be involved.

The factors that determine whether or not a patient will develop hypersensitivity to flea bites are the subject of intensive investigation. Genetics is likely to be involved, as has been shown to be the case in atopy. In a recent survey conducted at the University of Florida, 76 per cent of patients with atopy were shown to be allergic to fleas. Also of possible relevance is the age at which flea exposure first occurs. Many practitioners agree that the most severe cases of flea allergy dermatitis often involve animals reared in the North and brought to a flea-infested environment later in life. Furthermore, Floridian pound dogs, who are presumably massively exposed to fleas from an early age, have a very low incidence of both clinical flea allergy dermatitis and positive responses to intradermal skin tests with flea antigen. These considerations imply that the age at which exposure first occurs and the extent of that exposure may both be factors that determine whether allergy, tolerance, or immunity results.

CLINICAL SIGNS

The clinical signs of flea allergy dermatitis depend on the degree of sensitivity and the level of flea exposure. In the nonallergic pet, the signs of flea infestation may be minimal. The recognition of its existence is dependent upon the tolerance of the dog to the flea bites and on the acuteness of the owner's observations of the pet's responses. Seborrheic changes may result, but neither a clinically demonstrable eruption nor marked evidence of self-trauma would be expected.

If the pet develops hypersensitivity, a variety of changes may result, either primary or secondary. Classically, a small wheal develops at the site of the flea bite that either resolves or, if the animal has delayed hypersensitivity, develops into a papule, which later crusts over. A variety of other secondary changes may result from self-trauma, which can lead to widespread erythema, crusting, hair loss, seborrhea, and lichenification. The distribution often involves the lower back and posterior thighs, but it may become quite generalized in the severe case, leading to total body involvement. Even the head and feet, which are not areas favored by the flea, may be included in the disease process. Surprisingly, staphylococcal infection secondary to flea allergy dermatitis is rather uncommon. However, some dogs are seen who will predictably develop a staphylococcal folliculitis whenever they have a flea infestation.

DIAGNOSIS

The clinical signs together with the observation of fleas and/or flea dirt may be highly suggestive, but a definitive diagnosis is dependent on the demonstration of a positive intradermal skin test. It should also be emphasized that a positive skin test alone does not justify a diagnosis. It merely indicates that the patient has IgE antibodies against flea antigen on its dermal mast cells. Clinical signs compatible with such a diagnosis together with evidence of flea infestation or a history of recent exposure are required.

Despite recent controversy on the value of intradermal tests with flea antigen, the author remains convinced that a 1:1,000 w/v aqueous solution of antigen extract* is a potent and highly specific antigen for diagnostic purposes. An injection of diluent and a 1:100,000 w/v solution of histamine phosphate† should be used as negative and positive controls. The patient must also be observed for the delayed reaction, which peaks at 24 hours. This reaction, which of course is not urticarial, is more subtle and less readily visualized. It must be remembered that recent use of corticosteroids and antihistamines may interfere with the skin test. The author usually requires that patients be off corticosteroids for one week for every month of continued therapy that has taken place immediately prior to the skin test. However, the use of alternate-day short-acting corticosteroids is far less likely to interfere.

As is always the case in dermatology, care must be taken to rule out other factors that may be relevant to the etiology of the dermatitic process. Although the clinical signs of atopy are somewhat different from those of flea allergy dermatitis, atopy can only be conclusively ruled out by allergy testing. If the clinical suspicion of flea allergy dermatitis is high, it is sufficient to use a limited test of perhaps 15 to 20 of the most common inhalant allergens to exclude the possibility of coexistent atopy.

THERAPY

PRODUCTS FOR FLEA CONTROL ON THE PET

Experiences with conventional pesticides approved for use in veterinary medicine differ widely from one part of the country to another. This results from regional variations in the resistance of the flea population. For example, despite the fact that flea collars still have demonstrable efficacy against laboratory-reared fleas, clinical trials with some popular brands have shown them to be of little or no therapeutic value in the state of Florida (Randell et al., 1980). Other preparations, including dips, sprays, and powders, may have efficacy in some areas but may be quite valueless in others.

All clinicians agree, however, that few products have any residual action. This is particularly true when insecticidal shampoos are used, as the active ingredients are washed off in the rinsing process. Such formulations have little place in any flea control regimen. The application of microencapsulation techniques to topical parasiticides, which gives a delayed release of active ingredient, is awaited with eager anticipation. One such product, Sectrol,‡ which is pyrethrin based, already has been shown to be highly efficacious in environmental flea con-

---

*Flea Extract 1:1000, Greer Laboratories, Lenoir, NC.
†Eli Lilly and Co., Indianapolis, IN.
‡3M Co., St. Paul, MN.

trol, and clinical trials in dogs have shown much promise.

It is beyond the scope of this article to review all available pesticides. Instead, the experiences of the author with some newer products will be given.

Oral cythioate,* at a dosage of 30 mg/9 kg, is helpful in many but not all cases. It does not, of course, kill the flea until it bites, and so environmental control is still essential. The author prefers to ensure a negative heartworm status prior to commencing therapy, although this is not listed as a requirement by the manufacturer. The product is not approved for use in cats, but it appears to be safe and fairly effective when used at half the canine dose.

Fenthion† is a cattle insecticide that is widely used on pets in the South, although it is not currently approved for canine use. The recommended dosage is 0.75 ml/5 kg placed in a line down the skin of the back every two weeks, with a total dose not to exceed 7 ml. This technique appears to be quite safe, although the drug should not be used in young puppies. Occasional severe reactions have been noted in heartworm positive animals, and a blood test should be performed to ensure a negative status prior to commencement of therapy. A smaller dose totaling a maximum of 0.3 ml placed behind the ears has been used safely on adult cats and appears to be highly efficacious. Remarkably good results are achieved with this product even in the absence of adequate environmental control. It has spared the lives of many animals whose owners were considering euthanasia on humanitarian grounds, and normal skin and haircoat have usually been restored.

FLEA REPELLENTS

Although topical preparations such as n,n-diethyl-m-toluamide (Deet), produced for mosquito control in humans, are probably efficacious against fleas, practical and esthetic considerations prevent their routine use.

A number of oral products have been advocated in the past, and some are still marketed. Garlic products have many advocates, but although in high doses they act as excellent owner repellents, the flea is usually unimpressed. Vitamin-containing products have also been used (e.g., Fleatabs‡), and vitamin B (thiamine) has been used in the past as a mosquito repellent in humans. However, controlled studies with the latter have failed to demonstrate its efficacy, and a recent controlled study in dogs showed no demonstrable repellent action against

fleas (Halliwell, 1982). It appears that these types of products can rather easily find their way onto the market, and it often takes considerable time for the regulatory agencies to catch up with them. The recent experiences with a diethanolamine-containing product (Flee§), whose efficacy was not documented in controlled trials and which was associated with severe neurotoxicity in at least 50 instances, should serve as a warning. Until the efficacy of such products has been demonstrated by unbiased, well-planned, and controlled studies, their sale should be regarded as highly unethical, and veterinarians have an obligation to inform their clients to this effect.

PRODUCTS FOR ENVIRONMENTAL CONTROL

Depending on the climatic conditions, both the external and internal environment may be a source for renewed infestation of the pet. Careful attention to the particular circumstances pertaining to each case must be given, and a program should be devised bearing in mind the specifics of the life cycle. Client education is the key to success, and lack of such counseling is the major cause of treatment failure, which leads to frustration and disillusionment for the owner. Much time can be saved by preparing a client handout detailing the life cycle and the various approaches to control of flea infestation, leaving space for insertion of the particular program recommended for this patient.

Products available for environmental flea control have been recently reviewed (Bledsoe et al., 1982). Three approaches are available. Many prefer to "do-it-yourself" with commercially available sprays or foggers, but this may be more expensive and less efficacious than the use of a licensed pest control service. Indeed, some of the most potent (and hazardous) products may be restricted in use to licensed pest control officers. Propetamphos (Safrotin‖) and the refined chloropyrifos (Durisban L.O.**) are two such products. Among agents available to the general public, 50 per cent malathion used at a dilution of 2 oz/gal as a spray is still effective in the South.

Foggers are also widely used and may be quite effective. The recently registered agent methoprene, which prevents maturation of the larva, is a welcome addition to the line of available products, as it has good residual action. It is the active ingredient in a number of products and may be combined with a quick-kill agent (e.g., Siphotrol II)†† to give excellent control.

*Proban, American Cyanamid Co., Princeton, NJ.
†Spotton, Cutter Lab, Inc., Shawnee, KS.
‡Fleatabs, Inc., Bowling Green, OH.

§Environmental Products, Hollywood, FL.
‖Sandoz, E. Hanover, NJ.
**The Dow Chemical Co., Midland, MI.
††Vet-Kem, Dallas, TX.

HYPOSENSITIZATION

Although hyposensitization for atopy is widely practiced, with good results, this approach to the management of flea allergy dermatitis has fewer advocates. Recent double-blind studies with three products using six weekly injections via the intradermal route showed little efficacy (Halliwell, 1981). However, these results do not negate the possibility that prolonged (e.g., 6 to 12 months) therapy might give acceptable results. It is indeed irrational to recommend at least that length of therapy for atopy and to expect that a shorter duration of therapy would be efficacious in flea allergy dermatitis. However, the use of products for a total course of three injections, as is recommended by at least one manufacturer, clearly cannot be supported.

If hyposensitization is attempted, the intradermal route, which is an excellent route for antigenic stimulation, is probably preferable, although severe dermal reactions may occur.

ANTI-INFLAMMATORY THERAPY

Despite the vigor with which other methods are pursued, the necessity for anti-inflammatory therapy often cannot be avoided. However, it is important that this therapy be used in conjunction with other therapy rather than instead of such measures. The owner must be told that the apparent success of this therapy does not mean that the problem has gone away.

There is increasing resistance on the part of dermatologists to use long-acting injectable corticosteroids. Such products induce profound pituitary/adrenal suppression and have far more anti-inflammatory effects at the height of their action than are required to induce remission. The increased incidence of severe iatrogenic Cushing's disease is clearly a reflection of the widespread misuse of such products.

Judicious use of alternate-day short-acting corticosteroid therapy (e.g., prednisone or prednisolone) offers a cheaper and far safer alternative if long-term therapy is required. Management by this technique involves finding the minimal dose that will control the condition on an SID basis and changing over three to four days so that twice that dosage is given at around 9 AM on one day, no therapy is given on the next day, and so on. In other cases, short tapered courses (6 to 14 days) of prednisone or prednisolone may be used while flea control is being effected.

CONCLUSION

Each case of flea allergy dermatitis is different, and each case requires a carefully tailored therapeutic approach using varying combinations of the approaches outlined previously. The veterinarian must take care to assess all factors relevant to the particular patient and design the most appropriate program. Client education is the key to success.

REFERENCES

Benjamini, E., Feingold, B. F., and Kartman, L.: Skin reactivity in guinea pigs sensitized to flea bites: The sequence of reactions. Proc. Soc. Exp. Biol. Med. 108:700, 1961.

Bledsoe, W., Fadok, V. A., and Bledsoe, M. E.: Current therapy and new developments in indoor flea control. J.A.A.H.A. 18:415, 1982.

Halliwell, R. E. W.: Hyposensitization in the treatment of flea-bite hypersensitivity: Results of a double-blind study. J.A.A.H.A. 17:249, 1981.

Halliwell, R. E. W.: Ineffectiveness of thiamine as a flea repellant in dogs. J.A.A.H.A. 18:423, 1982.

Michaeli, D., et al.: In vitro studies on the role of collagen in the induction of hypersensitivity to flea bites. J. Immunol. 97:402, 1966.

Randell, W. F., Bradley, R. E., and Brown, D. L.: Field evaluation of anti-flea collars for initial and residual efficacy on dogs. V.M.S.A.C. 75:606, 1980.

THE PRURITIC DOG

WILLIAM H. MILLER, Jr., V.M.D.
Philadelphia, Pennsylvania

Pruritus is an ill-defined sensation that has been described as an unpleasant or uneasy sense of irritation within the skin that provokes the desire to scratch. Pruritus is a frequent complaint in companion animal medicine. Because of the overlap in the various conditions that can cause itching, the diagnosis of the underlying problem can be difficult.

PRURITUS

Heat, cold, touch, and pain are the four classic cutaneous sensations. Pruritus was thought to be a result of an admixture of these sensations but is now felt to be a unique sensation. Pruritus is an epidermal phenomenon that is the result of stimu-

Table 1.   *Steroid-Responsive Pruritic Diseases of the Dog*

Disease	Level of Pruritus	Response to Steroids	Sites of Predilection
Acute moist dermatitis	Intense	Excellent	Anywhere
Atopy	Moderate to intense	Excellent	Face, ears, feet, axillae, anywhere
Cheyletiella	Mild to intense	Good	Dorsum, rump
Contact allergy/dermatitis	Moderate	Poor to good	Feet, ventrum, perineum
Demodicosis	Moderate to intense	Poor to good	Face, feet, anywhere
Flea allergy/bite dermatitis	Moderate to intense	Good to excellent	Rump, thighs, ventrum
Parasitic infestation			
Hookworm larvae			
Pelodera larvae	Moderate to intense	Poor to good	Face, feet, ventrum, perineum
Chiggers			
Lice	Mild to moderate	Good	Dorsum, rump
Pyoderma	Mild to moderate	Poor to good	Anywhere
Seborrhea complex	Mild to intense	Good	Face, ears, intertriginous areas, anywhere

lation of naked nerve endings of the skin, which are most dense at the dermoepidermal junction. The density and/or sensitivity of these nerve endings and the ability to perceive itch varies in different areas of the body. The pruritic impulses are carried to the spinal cord by slowly conducting unmyelinated C fibers and ascend to the sensory cortex in the ventrolateral spinothalamic tract. Local axonal reflexes as well as central neurologic factors can modulate the pruritic sensation. Skin devoid of epidermis is incapable of experiencing itch but can experience the other four primary sensations.

Pruritus can be produced by mechanical, electrical, thermal, or chemical stimulation of the nerve endings. Clinically, pruritus is a chemical phenomenon. Proteolytic enzymes are the major mediators of pruritus, but other substances such as vasoactive amines can also play an important role. The proteolytic enzymes arise from bacteria, fungi, mast cells, polymorphonuclear leukocytes, and damaged epidermal cells as well as from other sources.

Pruritus typically causes inflammation of the skin, which results in the release of proteolytic enzymes. This potentiates the initial inflammation and pruritus. Clinically, this causes the itch-scratch-itch cycle, in which the pruritus can remain even though the initial pruritogenic stimulus may be gone. Additionally, chronically irritated skin can lose its ability to perceive any sensation other than itch. The itch-scratch-itch cycle coupled with the altered sensibility of the skin can make diagnosis and treatment of the initial disease much more difficult.

CLINICAL EVALUATION

Pruritus, which is manifested by licking, chewing, rubbing, or scratching, is a nonspecific sign of disease. Evaluation of a pruritic dog can be time-consuming and frustrating for both the owner and the veterinarian. Tables 1 and 2 list those diseases in which pruritus is a consistent complaint. One should not view these tables as all-inclusive, since any disease can induce pruritus in an individual dog. Careful consideration of the history and physical findings should allow the formulation of a well-ordered list of differential diagnoses.

HISTORY

The history involves three areas of information and is the most useful diagnostic tool available. A cursory examination of the animal prior to or during the history taking can be useful in directing the line of questioning.

Table 2.   *Steroid-Nonresponsive Pruritic Diseases of the Dog*

Disease	Level of Pruritus	Sites of Predilection
Acral pruritic nodule	Moderate	Distal limbs
Bacterial allergy	Moderate to intense	Feet, ventrum, anywhere
Cutaneous lymphomas	Moderate to intense	Face, anywhere
Drug allergy	Mild to intense	Mucocutaneous junctions, anywhere
Food allergy	Moderate to intense	As in flea allergy or atopy, anywhere
Hormonal hypersensitivity	Intense	Perineum, flanks
Neurodermatitis	Mild to intense	Feet, flank folds, tail
Sarcoptic mange	Intense	Ears, legs, ventrum
Subcorneal pustular dermatosis	Intense	Face, trunk

The first area of the history is the signalment (age, breed, and sex) and general information about the dog and its environment. Here one should assess the animal's temperament through observation and questioning. Bored or very nervous dogs may have begun to itch for no medical reason (acral pruritic nodule, neurodermatitis) or may itch well out of proportion to the severity of the pruritic stimulus. The diet should be evaluated both for adequacy and any recent changes, although food allergies are often associated with foods that have been fed for long periods of time. Along the same line, contact allergies usually are not due to sensitization to a new item in the environment. If a dog develops signs of a contact allergy shortly after a new product is introduced into the environment, an irritant contact dermatitis is most likely.

Since many of the pruritic diseases are associated with external parasites, the probability and source of exposure should be investigated. Infestation usually is the result of direct animal contact but can occur via a contaminated environment. Grooming establishments are point sources of infestation that owners may overlook. Involvement of other dogs and cats can be a helpful diagnostic tool. Most parasites are contagious and, except for *Sarcoptes scabiei*, will cross species lines. One should not exclude the diagnosis of a parasitic disease if other dogs in the household are not involved. An asymptomatic carrier state occurs in all the common external parasitic diseases of the dog, even sarcoptic mange.

The owner should be questioned as to whether any relatives of this dog suffer from a similar skin condition. This line of questioning often is less than rewarding, since many owners know nothing about the relatives of their dog or are unable to obtain a satisfactory answer from the breeder. If one suspects an inherited disease such as atopy or demodicosis, the owner should contact the dog's breeder.

The next area of investigation is the previous medical history, which should include any significant disease, dermatologic or not, that the animal has had or is currently being treated for. If the dog is a regular patient of a veterinary hospital, the medical record should include all of this information. In a group practice, the dog may have seen a different veterinarian for each of its problems, and thus the entire medical record should be reviewed. The development of a problem list is very helpful.

One should review all of the previous dermatologic problems of the dog. Particular attention should be paid to the symptomatology, date of occurrence, and duration of the disease. The previous problems may be unrelated to the dog's present condition but may suggest an underlying disease such as atopy.

Since the skin often reflects internal disease, one should consider all systemic diseases that the animal has had. Recurrent infections, either of the skin or internal organs, suggest an immunodeficiency state, either primary or secondary, which would predispose the dog to recurrent pyodermas. If the animal is being treated for a disease, the therapy and its adequacy should be reviewed carefully. If the systemic disease is being poorly controlled, the skin problem may be secondary to that disease. In this situation, both the skin and the underlying disease must be approached. All drugs that the animal is receiving, including vitamins and dietary supplements, should be reviewed. Drug eruptions or drug allergies are reported infrequently in the dog, but they do occur, probably at a higher frequency than the literature suggests. Any dog can become allergic to any drug, but long-term administration, either constant or episodic; simultaneous systemic and topical application of the same drug; or the use of repositol drugs can increase the likelihood of an allergic reaction.

Finally, the present history concerning the current complaint is investigated. When and where did the itching start? Did the pruritus start suddenly or was it gradual in onset? What area of the body was involved first and how did the disease spread? Are certain areas more itchy than others? How pruritic is the dog? To assess the level of pruritus, one can ask the owner to rate it on a scale from one to ten. Intensely pruritic dogs usually will not sleep through the night nor can they be distracted from their itching. If the dog does not appear to be as itchy as the owner describes, one should ask the client what he thinks the normal level of itching is for a dog. Some owners do not know or are not willing to accept more than an occasional scratch.

One should try to determine whether there were any lesions present before the itching started. Often owners are unable to answer this question, since they examine the skin only after the dog has started to scratch. If one is able to determine that the pruritus came first or is the only abnormality present, the dog is likely to be suffering from an allergic disease. If the owner did notice skin changes before the dog started to scratch, allergic diseases are less likely. If the dog is an intact bitch, one should assess whether the onset of the skin problem coincided with an estral cycle. If this association can be made, the next step is to determine whether or not skin changes preceded the pruritus. Dogs with hormonal hypersensitivities scratch normal skin, whereas dogs with ovarian imbalances develop skin changes prior to or without pruritus.

The animal's response to any therapy, either owner or veterinarian instituted, should be determined. Since most pruritic dogs receive corticosteroids at one point or another, the animal's response to these drugs can be a useful diagnostic clue. Table 2 lists those diseases in which the pruritus usually does not decrease significantly with adequate steroid therapy. If the pruritus did decrease, one should determine whether the skin returned to normal or whether the sores remained. Dogs with pruritic pyodermas often will become less itchy with steroid therapy but the lesions will remain.

After completing the history, one should have a reasonable list of differential diagnoses. The physical examination will further refine that list.

PHYSICAL EXAMINATION

The dog should receive a complete physical examination. The general physical is important, since the skin disease could be the first sign of a systemic problem or could be secondary to, or complicated by, an underlying disease. The entire skin surface should be examined carefully, noting both the nature and pattern or distribution of lesions. External parasites should be shown to the owner. If the dog suffers from a recurrent pruritic pyoderma, the oral cavity, ears, and anal sacs should be checked carefully, as these areas can act as subclinical point sources of infection.

Since pruritus is the presenting complaint, the dog should be examined for signs of self-trauma (salivary staining, broken or matted hairs, or excoriations) to substantiate the owner's complaint and identify areas unnoticed by the owner. A crude estimate of the level of pruritus can be made by scratching an area and watching the dog's response. Dogs with sarcoptic mange usually will show a positive ear test, in which the ipsilateral hind leg starts to scratch when the edge of the pinna is scratched. If the dog responds painfully as the skin is palpated, one should consider the possibility of a drug eruption.

During the examination, one should identify the primary skin lesions and all secondary changes. Since most pruritic dogs traumatize their skin, the primary lesions may be obscured. Chronically pruritic dogs are a more difficult diagnostic challenge, since they often have severe secondary skin diseases, which can mask the underlying disease.

DIAGNOSIS AND DIAGNOSTIC EVALUATION

After the history and physical examination are completed, one should have a well-ordered list of differential diagnoses for the primary condition. Since the evaluation of many pruritic dogs is not straightforward, the owner should be advised of the various possibilities and how each is to be approached. It is imperative that the owner recognize that you are approaching the problem in a logical rather than a haphazard fashion. Many pruritic dogs are presented to many different veterinarians needlessly. Often the correct diagnosis was made early in the course of the disease, but because of poor communications the problem was not resolved.

Every pruritic dog should be examined for external parasites, both grossly and microscopically through the aid of skin scrapings or vacuuming of the haircoat. Since demodicosis can assume many different clinical pictures, multiple deep skin scrapings should always be taken. Since the *Demodex* mite is a normal inhabitant of the dog's skin, one must demonstrate many mites before the diagnosis of demodicosis can be offered. If only one mite is seen, the area should be rescraped. If one suspects one of the other external parasitic diseases, the diagnosis should not be abandoned if the parasite was not found. It often is very difficult to demonstrate mites by skin scrapings. Usually, the frequency of mite identification decreases as the chronicity of the pruritus increases. In this situation, a strong clinical suspicion is sufficient grounds for the institution of a trial course of therapy. The therapy should be as specific as possible, and the animal's response should be evaluated early in the course of treatment. If a dog is being treated for a presumptive case of sarcoptic mange, it should be significantly less pruritic after two parasiticidal dips. If the dog is responding in the expected fashion, the therapy should be completed. If there is minimal response, the diagnosis should be re-evaluated.

Diseases such as food allergy, drug allergy, or contact allergy are difficult, if not impossible, to diagnose via testing. In these situations, the food, drug, or contact agent must be avoided to diagnose and correct the problem. If the dog has a secondary pruritic disease such as a pyoderma, it should be resolved before an evaluation of the underlying disease is undertaken. If both problems are addressed simultaneously and the pruritus stops, then one is uncertain whether the pruritus was due to the pyoderma or the suspected disease. If the secondary problem is resolved first, the animal's basal level of pruritus can be determined. If the level of pruritus decreases with the institution of, for example, a hypoallergenic diet, one is certain that the dog does have a food allergy. Along the same line, it is difficult to evaluate an animal's response to a hypoallergenic diet when the diet is instituted during a change of season. If the dog's pruritus decreases, it could be due to the avoidance of a food or the decrease in the pollen count. In this situation, the dog should be challenged with its original diet to see if the pruritus returns. If it does, the food allergy has been documented. If one suspects a drug allergy, the dog should not be challenged with the drug.

Many different diagnostic tests are available to help confirm the clinical suspicion of the various pruritic diseases. It is imperative that these tests be used to confirm a tentative diagnosis and not to make a diagnosis. More often than not, a skin biopsy taken to make a diagnosis will be of little diagnostic help. If an animal is skin tested for inhalant allergies, any significant reactions must correlate with the history before they can be considered truly significant. A strong reaction to house dust in an animal who itches during the spring only must be viewed as a false positive.

If the dog becomes nonpruritic after a secondary skin disease, usually a pyoderma, is treated, the diagnostic evaluation should not be stopped. In this situation the initial pruritogenic stimulus was transient in nature and could recur. If the history suggests what the initial event might have been, that problem can be approached in an appropriate manner. If the history and physical examination are noncontributory, the owners should be advised to return with their dog at the first sign of itching.

THERAPY

Since pruritus is just a sign of disease, the aim of therapy is to resolve the underlying problem and thus eliminate the pruritogenic stimulus. Usually it is advisable to couple temporary antipruritic therapy with specific therapy for the disease in question. This breaks the vicious itch-scratch-itch cycle and hastens the animal's recovery. When pruritus is a chronic problem, prolonged antipruritic therapy may be necessary to allow the skin to heal completely and lose its altered sensibility.

It is common for pruritic dogs to develop secondary skin diseases, such as seborrhea or pyoderma, which add to the dog's itchiness. If the secondary problem is significant, it should be treated. Ideally, the secondary problem should be resolved before the underlying disease is approached. In this fashion, the animal's basal level of pruritus can be determined and its response to the specific therapy is easier to appreciate and, oftentimes, more complete. In most instances in which the seborrhea is secondary to the pruritus, such as in flea allergy dermatitis, the seborrhea does not require specific treatment. If the therapy for the primary problem can easily incorporate a drug that is beneficial in the treatment of seborrhea, that drug should be used. For example, the treatment of sarcoptic mange requires the application of a parasiticidal agent. In this instance, a bath with an antiseborrheic shampoo prior to the application of the dip is very beneficial but oftentimes not absolutely necessary.

Secondary pyodermas do require treatment. Once a significant pyoderma has developed, it will remain even if the inciting disease is resolved. If the pyoderma is of such a nature that systemic antibiotic therapy is necessary, the dog should not be treated concurrently with a glucocorticoid. Steroids make it much more difficult to evaluate an animal's response to an antibiotic and can prolong the treatment of the pyoderma. If the dog's condition necessitates the concurrent administration of a steroid and an antibiotic, the glucocorticoid should be used for as short a period of time as is necessary and should be discontinued well before the antibiotic is stopped. It is not uncommon to have the pyoderma recur when the steroid and antibiotic are discontinued simultaneously. In this situation, the relapse is not actually a recurrence of the pyoderma but rather an exacerbation of a pre-existing infection that was made subclinical by the glucocorticoid.

When the pruritus is initiated or intensified by psychological factors such as boredom or extreme nervousness, therapy must be directed toward both the skin and the mind. A dog with a chronic acral pruritic nodule either will not respond completely to lesional therapy or will start a new lesion unless his psyche is altered either chemically or through behavior modification. Since behavior modification is a time-consuming process, it is best to start with chemical therapy so that the skin disease can be treated and the itch-scratch-itch cycle broken. Behavior modification is used to prevent a recurrence of the problem.

Many different types of drugs are used to modify a dog's psyche, but drugs that provide sedation are most useful. Although many drugs have a sedative effect, phenobarbitol (0.5 to 1.5 mg/kg/8 hr) and diazepam (Valium, 0.1 to 0.25 mg/kg/8 hr) are the most widely used since their effect is rather dose dependent. In most instances, the dose of the drug is adjusted so that the dog is mildly sedated. Hydroxyzine (Atarax) can be useful in dealing with a very nervous or anxious dog. In humans, this drug is a true antianxiety drug that calms without depressing; it has also proved useful in some dogs. Therapy is instituted at a dosage of 0.1 to 0.25 mg/kg/8 hr and adjusted as necessary. Hydroxyzine has antihistaminic effects and can cause relaxation of skeletal muscles. If these side effects are seen, the dose of the drug should be decreased or the drug should be discontinued.

Progestational compounds such as megestrol acetate (Ovaban, Megace) are useful in behavior modification in the dog. The exact mode of action is uncertain, but megestrol acetate (5 to 15 mg/kg/24 hr) usually calms a dog without depressing it. Because of their potential side effects, progestational compounds should be reserved for animals with severe behavior problems.

Nonspecific antipruritic therapy can be approached either on a topical or a systemic basis. Because of the nature of the dog and its pruritic disease, topical therapy usually is inadequate as the sole means of treatment but is often a useful adjuvant to systemic therapy.

Of all the topical agents reported to have an antipruritic effect, corticosteroids are the most reliable and the most beneficial. As with systemic steroids, the potency of the available products varies greatly. Initially, a potent agent such as betamethasone valerate (Valisone) should be applied to the affected area three to four times daily. Once the affected area is healed, a less potent steroid such as 1 per cent hydrocortisone should be used to keep the lesion in remission. Judicious use of topical steroids can decrease the amount of systemic therapy that an animal needs.

Systemic antipruritic therapy in the dog presently revolves around the use of antihistamines and corticosteroids. Nonsteroidal anti-inflammatory agents and drugs that stabilize the mast cell's membrane and therefore block degranulation are being developed and hold great promise. To date, only one nonsteroidal anti-inflammatory agent, orgotein (Palosein), is licensed for use in the dog. Because of its expense, the effectiveness of orgotein as a systemic antipruritic agent is poorly documented, although it is very effective in the lesional treatment of acral pruritic nodules.

Although histamine is not the major mediator of pruritus, it is a potent pruritogenic compound. It directly stimulates the nerve endings of the skin and, through its vasoactive properties, results in the release of extracellular proteases, which contribute to the pruritic stimulus. Histamine is primarily released from mast cells as they degranulate through various immunologic and nonimmunologic mechanisms.

The classical antihistamines are known as H_1 blockers because they competitively interfere with the action of histamine at its receptor sites (H_1 sites). Additionally, they all have some local anesthetic effect and provide mild to heavy sedation. Recently, a second type of histamine receptor, the H_2 site, has been identified and an H_2 blocker, cimetidine (Tagamet), has been developed. This antihistamine has no antipruritic properties and, when administered alone, could potentiate the pruritus associated with allergic disease. Mast cells have H_2 receptors on their cell surface, which are activated by endogenously released histamine. This process inhibits further mast cell degranulation. Administration of cimetidine alone would interfere with this negative feedback mechanism and potentiate the pruritus. Simultaneous administration of a H_1 blocker and cimetidine is reported to be more effective in controlling pruritus than administration of the H_1 blocker alone. Even with this joint therapy, the pruritus is not totally eliminated. Because of the expense of cimetidine, this joint therapy is not widely used but may be of benefit in those situations in which corticosteroids are contraindicated.

Again, antihistamine therapy usually will not completely eliminate pruritus, but it may decrease the level of pruritus such that the dog is "tolerably itchy." If the remaining level of pruritus is unac-

ceptable, corticosteroids can be added to the therapeutic regimen, provided that they are not contraindicated. If steroids and antihistamines are used simultaneously, it is important to demonstrate that the antihistamines are lowering the minimal effective dose of steroids. If the joint therapy is no more effective than the steroid therapy alone, the antihistamine therapy should be modified or discontinued.

The antihistamines most widely used are trimeprazine (Temaril, 1.0 to 2.0 mg/kg/12 hr), diphenhydramine (Benadryl, 2.0 to 4.0 mg/kg/8 hr), and chlorpheniramine (2 to 12 mg every 8 to 12 hours). Chlorpheniramine can be purchased without a prescription. Cimetidine is administered at a dose of 5 to 10 mg/kg/6 hr.

The most obvious side effect of antihistamine therapy is drowsiness. The dose of the drug should be adjusted so that the dog is mildly sedated. The owner should be advised not to increase the dose if the pruritus escalates. Deaths have been attributed to massive antihistamine overdose.

Glucocorticoids are the most effective drugs available to control pruritus in the dog. Steroids suppress inflammation through various mechanisms and stabilize cell and lysosomal membranes to inhibit the release of pruritogenic agents. The action of these drugs usually stops the pruritus and therefore breaks the itch-scratch-itch cycle. As healing occurs, the skin regains its normal pattern of sensibility. Steroids do not cure any skin disease but rather control the signs of disease. Because of their various clinical and metabolic side effects, steroids should be administered carefully and only for as long as is necessary. Chronic steroid administration should be reserved for those cases in which the underlying disease cannot be cured (i.e., atopy) or when conventional therapy is ineffective in reducing the dog's level of pruritus.

Many different glucocorticoids are available in both oral and injectable form. The selection of drug and route of administration depends on the animal and the condition being treated. Generally speaking, injectable drugs are abused in veterinary medicine. There is little or no place in the management of canine pruritus for injectable drug administration that lasts for one month or longer. Repeated injections of shorter-acting drugs are equally inappropriate. Injectable steroids should be reserved for those cases in which seven to ten days of anti-inflammatory therapy are desired and oral therapy is inappropriate.

Oral medication should be used whenever possible, because the effects of the drug can be more easily controlled. For a short course of therapy, most oral steroids will produce the desired effect with minimal side effects. When therapy is to last for two weeks or more, the short-acting glucocorticoids (prednisolone, prednisone, or methylprednisolone) should be used, since these can be used on an alternate-day basis. The alternate-day steroid regimen was developed to minimize the hypothalamic-pituitary-adrenal (HPA) suppression seen with chronic steroid administration. The HPA axis is suppressed by alternate-day steroid administration, but the suppression is not as marked or of as long a duration as it is with daily or injectable therapy. Although alternate-day steroid administration minimizes HPA suppression, suppression does occur and the dog can develop signs of hyperadrenocorticism. Care should be used whenever a steroid is administered, even on an alternate-day basis.

Before an animal is placed on an alternate-day regimen, daily therapy will be necessary to initiate the healing process. Using prednisolone, the animal should be treated with 0.5 to 1.0 mg/kg/12 hr for five to seven days and then 1.0 mg/kg once every other *morning*. Once the dog is on the alternate-day regimen, the dose is adjusted as needed. If the dog is totally nonpruritic, it is receiving too much medication and the dose should be decreased to the point where the dog is slightly more itchy than it would be if it did not have the underlying disease. Alternatively, if the pruritus is too intense, the dose should be increased slowly. By maintaining the dog at a mild level of pruritus, one can be assured that the animal is receiving the minimal effective dose of the drug. Since the animal's condition will change with time, the effective dose of prednisolone will also change, and the owners should be advised to adjust the dose as is necessary to keep the dog "tolerably itchy." Alternate-day steroid administration can be abused; therefore, it is advisable to keep track of the number of pills dispensed and reexamine the dog whenever the prescription needs to be refilled.

SUPPLEMENTAL READING

Eyre, P.: Pharmacology of antipruritic drugs. *In* Kirk, R. W. (ed.): *Current Veterinary Therapy VII*. Philadelphia: W. B. Saunders, 1980.

Halliwell, R. E. W.: Pathogenesis and treatment of pruritus. J.A.V.M.A. 164:793, 1974.

Ihrke, P. J.: Differential diagnosis of the pruritic dog. Proceedings of the American Animal Hospital Association 47:157, 1980.

Muller, G. H., and Kirk, R. W.: *Small Animal Dermatology II*. Philadelphia: W. B. Saunders, 1976.

Pemberton, P. L.: Feline and canine behavior control: Progestin therapy. *In* Kirk, R. W. (ed.): *Current Veterinary Therapy VII*. Philadelphia: W. B. Saunders, 1980.

Soctt, D. W.: Topical cutaneous medicine, or "Now what should I try?" Proceedings of the American Animal Hospital Association 46:89, 1979.

Scott, D. W.: Systemic glucocorticoid therapy. *In* Kirk, R. W. (ed.): *Current Veterinary Therapy VII*. Philadelphia: W. B. Saunders, 1980.

Van Stee, E. W.: Alternative to corticosteroids in the management of pruritus in dogs. V.M./S.A.C. 76:331, 1981.

THE MANAGEMENT OF CANINE PYODERMAS

PETER J. IHRKE, V.M.D.

Davis, California

Canine pyodermas are among the most common skin diseases seen in small animal practice. However, despite their frequency of occurrence, misdiagnosis and therapeutic mismanagement are commonplace. Much of the fault for this situation rests with the fact that surprisingly little is still known about the etiology and pathogenesis of bacterial infections of the skin in any species, including humans. In addition, despite the rather succinct and exact definition of a pyoderma as a cutaneous pyogenic bacterial infection, the diversity seen within this group of diseases is enormous. The lesions seen with pyodermas may be localized or generalized, superficial or deep, and surface characteristics may vary considerably. Visible frank pustules are not a requisite for a diagnosis of pyoderma, since the identifiable histopathologic lesion may not be obvious to the naked eye. Furthermore, pustules may be extremely transitory in the disease process, possibly owing to the thinness of canine skin. Self-trauma associated with pruritus, crusting, or other secondary changes may obliterate all evidence of an initially readily identifiable pyoderma within just a few hours. Actual pus production may vary from minute amounts associated with inapparent microabscess formation to copious purulent debris draining from devitalized fistulous tracts. Variability is also noted in the isolation of bacteria from pus contingent upon the age of the pustule. In addition to the wide variety of clinical manifestations seen with canine pyodermas, this diagnostic challenge is compounded by the fact that pustules may be seen in association with a number of diseases other than bacterial infections. Demodicosis and ringworm may both present as primary pustular diseases. Furthermore, pustules may be seen in less common diseases such as pemphigus foliaceus and subcorneal pustular dermatosis. Consequently, the presence of pustules alone does not warrant a diagnosis of pyoderma.

CUTANEOUS MICROBIOLOGY

Under ordinary circumstances, the bacterial flora of normal canine skin consists primarily of rather small numbers of coagulase-negative micrococci with occasional diphtheroids and clostridia seen. Pathogenic environmental transients such as *Staphylococcus aureus* and *Proteus* and *Pseudomonas* spp. normally do not take up residence on noninflamed skin. A number of rather poorly understood external or internal host factors may create a surface environment compatible with intense colonization by pathogenic coagulase-positive *S. aureus* organisms. If this ecological shift in resident population occurs, other factors, such as seborrhea, ectoparasitism, poor grooming, endocrine imbalances, or trauma, may precipitate or facilitate the formation of a pyoderma.

It is now generally accepted that coagulase-positive forms of *Staphylococcus aureus* are responsible for the great majority of canine pyodermas. In cases in which only one bacterial strain is isolated from a canine pyoderma, over 99 per cent of the isolates are *S. aureus*. Since *S. aureus* is ubiquitous in mixed bacterial canine skin infections and treatment for *S. aureus* alone will frequently resolve a mixed bacterial pyoderma, it may be assumed that *S. aureus* is the primary pathogen in canine skin. Invasion by *Proteus* or *Pseudomonas* species or other gram negative organisms should be considered secondary to the tissue changes seen as a result of *S. aureus* infection.

GENERAL DIAGNOSTIC PROCEDURES

When bacterial infection is suspected, a simple smear of the pustular contents of the exudate is the simplest, most beneficial, and most cost effective procedure. A pustule may be opened with either a 22-gauge needle or a scalpel blade. The pustular contents are then collected on a cotton swab, and multiple impressions are made on glass slides. A rapid stain such as Diff-Quik* or a Gram stain may be used. The author prefers Diff-Quik, since almost

---

*Harleco, Gibbstown, NJ.

as much information may be gleaned from this procedure as from a Gram stain and it is less messy and time-consuming than a Gram stain. The Gram stain offers little advantage, since the coccal bacteria seen would almost always be gram positive *Staphylococcus aureus* and the rod-shaped bacteria from canine skin will most likely be gram negative *Pseudomonas* or *Proteus* species. In addition to this basic information, a bacterial smear will also give the clinician a rough evaluation of the approximate number, incidence, and, hence, importance of various bacteria seen. Bacterial engulfment by phagocytes also indicates some protective leukocyte function.

Bacterial culture, identification, and antibiotic sensitivity testing are overused in veterinary medicine; the information obtained from bacterial smears is, in many cases, sufficient. Specific situations in which bacterial cultures are indicated will be discussed later.

When a defect is suspected in the host animal's immune response to bacterial infection, there is currently no easy, accurate testing procedure readily available to determine immunocompetence. *In vitro* lymphocyte blastogenesis studies and bacteriocidal assays are available only as research tools. A clinician may obtain certain gross information as to immunocompetence from a complete blood count and a serum electrophoresis. One would expect an absolute neutrophilia in an immunocompetent dog with a moderate to severe pyoderma. The absolute lymphocyte count should be at least 1,000 to 1,500 lymphocytes per cubic milliliter of blood if a reasonable cell-mediated response is to occur. A broad-based elevation in both the beta and gamma range should be seen in the B cell–competent dog with a pyoderma. However, it should be emphasized that none of these readily available parameters are function tests.

CLASSIFICATION OF PYODERMAS

The classification of pyodermas with respect to depth of involvement in the skin is useful clinically since, in general, deeper infections require more vigorous combinations of both systemic and topical therapy (Table 1). Although surface pyodermas frequently respond to topical medications as sole methods of therapy, deeper infections generally require systemic antibiotics. The most rapid therapeutic success is usually achieved through the vigorous use of both systemic antibiotics and topical medications for long periods of time.

SURFACE PYODERMA

"Surface pyoderma" is a convenient term used to group several very superficial erosions or ulcerations

Table 1.   *Classification of Canine Pyoderma*

Surface Pyoderma
    Pyotraumatic dermatitis ("hot spots," acute moist
        dermatitis)
    Intertrigo (skin fold pyoderma)
        Lip fold pyoderma
        Facial fold pyoderma (nasal fold pyoderma)
        Vulvar fold pyoderma
        Tail fold pyoderma (screw-tail pyoderma)
        Obesity fold pyoderma
Superficial Pyoderma
    Impetigo (puppy pyoderma)
    Superficial folliculitis
        Intertriginous folliculitis
        Secondary folliculitis
    Pruritic superficial pyoderma
Deep Pyoderma
    Deep folliculitis and furunculosis
        "Canine acne" (muzzle folliculitis and furunculosis)
        Nasal pyoderma
        Interdigital pyoderma
        Pressure point pyoderma
        Folliculitis and furunculosis
    Cellulitis
        Cellulitis (as an extension of a furunculosis)
        Cellulitis (secondary to demodicosis)
Disease formerly classified as pyoderma
    "Hidradenitis suppurativa"
    Juvenile pyoderma (puppy strangles)

of the skin in which bacterial colonization, if not frank bacterial invasion, may play a significant role. Although pathogenic bacteria such as *S. aureus* may be consistently cultured from the exudative debris, their association is most likely secondary in the disease process. Although smears of the exudate using any rapid staining procedure may have some value in indicating the intensity of bacterial colonization, bacterial culture and sensitivity testing is usually not indicated. General diagnostic and therapeutic recommendations are listed in Table 2.

PYOTRAUMATIC DERMATITIS

Despite the frequency of occurrence of pyotraumatic dermatitis or "hot spots," it remains a poorly understood condition. Clinically, it is recognized that thick-coated, long-haired breeds seem to have a predilection for the development of alopecic, exudative, self-traumatized lesions during the warmer months. In most cases, secondary bacterial colonization is probably a more proper term than bacterial infection, since systemic antibiotics alone do not significantly alter the disease process. An underlying reason for the animal's intense interest in such a localized area should be investigated. Clinically, the lesions appear to be secondary to self-trauma. However, no adequate explanation is available to explain the predisposition to this condition seen in some dogs. Ectoparasites, allergy, otitis externa, and poor grooming may be contributing factors. In the author's experience, flea allergy dermatitis is the most frequent underlying cause.

If possible, any potential predisposing factors should be corrected to prevent recurrence. In addition to gentle cleansing, short-term corticosteroid therapy (both systemic and topical) is usually all that is required therapeutically.

INTERTRIGO

Intertrigo, or skin fold pyoderma, is seen in a number of breeds in conjunction with dependent skin folds that create a moist, dark, warm environment for bacterial growth. The continuous frictional microtrauma associated with these anatomic defects may also contribute to inflammation and bacterial colonization. In these related diseases, chronic bacterial involvement appears much more significant than in pyotraumatic dermatitis. Lip fold pyodermas are seen most commonly in breeds such as cocker and springer spaniels and occasionally in Irish setters. Halitosis is the most common owner complaint. Facial fold pyodermas are usually seen in brachycephalic breeds. Corneal ulceration is a frequent sequela to self-trauma. Vulvar fold pyodermas are seen most commonly in obese older bitches that have been spayed before their first estrus. Boston terriers, English bulldogs, and other breeds with corkscrew tails are most susceptible to tail fold pyodermas.

With the advent of 2.5 per cent benzoyl peroxide shampoos, palliative therapy for lip fold pyodermas has become much more practical. Daily cleansing of the affected intertriginous area followed by maintenance cleansing every two to five days may be effective. Alternatively, cleansing may be used to decrease the inflammation in the area before ablative surgery. Benzoyl peroxide shampoo alone is effective in facial fold pyodermas if no other underlying cause of facial pruritus is present. Generally, diets to reduce obesity and corrective surgery are indicated in vulvar fold pyodermas. Tail fold pyodermas may respond to benzoyl peroxide shampoos followed by antibiotic-corticosteroid ointment application. Surgery may be required in more severe cases.

SUPERFICIAL PYODERMA

A superficial pyoderma is a bacterial infection in which multiple abscesses of extremely variable size are present either just below the stratum corneum or within the ostia of hair follicles. The diagnosis of a superficial pyoderma is often quite difficult, since the pustules may not be visible to the naked eye. In addition, the visible pustular stage of the disease may be quite transitory in the dog. Consequently, a superficial pyoderma should be considered in the differential diagnosis of virtually any pustular, pa-

Table 2.　　Management of Surface Pyodermas*

Disease	Differential Diagnosis	Diagnostic Procedures	Therapy	
			Topical	Systemic
Pyotraumatic dermatitis	None common; consider demodicosis, ringworm, lymphosarcoma if persistent	Look for underlying problems (esp. fleas), if persistent; scrape; biopsy; impression smear; culture	Gentle cleansing; corticosteroid creams	Corticosteroids: prednisolone orally for five to seven days, 1 mg/kg daily
Lip fold pyoderma	None common; demodicosis; candidiasis; early immune-mediated disease	Impression smear; if persistent, scrape and biopsy	2.5% benzoyl peroxide shampoo; ablate anatomic defect	None
Facial fold pyoderma	None common	If persistent, look for underlying pruritic disease, atopy, food allergy, etc.	2.5% benzoyl peroxide shampoo; antibiotic-corticosteroid ointment; surgical ablation	
Vulvar fold pyoderma	None common; early immune-mediated disease	Look for cystitis, vaginitis	Surgical ablation	Weight reduction; estrogens?
Tail fold pyoderma	Other perianal pruritic diseases	Explore folds; examine anal sacks	Surgical ablation	
Obesity fold pyoderma	Acanthosis nigricans	Look for underlying problem (esp. hypothyroidism)	2.5% benzoyl peroxide shampoo; antibiotic-corticosteroid ointments	Weight reduction

*Adapted with permission from Ihrke: Proceedings of the American Animal Hospital Association, 61, 1981.

Table 3. Management of Superficial Pyodermas

Disease	Differential Diagnosis	Diagnostic Procedures	Therapy	
			Topical	Systemic
Impetigo	Localized demodicosis; ringworm	Smear pustule; scraping; fungal culture	2.5% benzoyl peroxide shampoo; povidone iodine or chlorhexidine shampoo; grooming	Short-term antibiotics (seven to ten days) if necessary
Intertriginous folliculitis	Demodicosis; ringworm	Smear pustule; scraping; if persistent, culture, look for underlying problem	2.5% benzoyl peroxide shampoo; povidone iodine or chlorhexidine shampoo; grooming	Antibiotics (at least two weeks)
Secondary folliculitis	Demodicosis; uncomplicated intertriginous folliculitis	Look for underlying cause if recurrent problem: seborrhea, fleas, atopy, food allergy	2.5% benzoyl peroxide shampoo; antiseborrheic shampoo	Long-term antibiotics (four to six weeks); treat underlying disease
Pruritic superficial pyoderma	Demodicosis; ringworm; many other diseases	Look for underlying cause; smear pustule; scrape; culture; biopsy	2.5% benzoyl peroxide shampoo; antiseborrheic shampoo	Long-term antibiotics (four to six weeks); treat underlying disease, staphage Lysate? staph. toxoid?

pular, or crusting eruption with or without concomitant pruritus. In general, superficial pyodermas in the dog are much more of a diagnostic challenge than either surface or deep bacterial skin infections.

If frank pustules are present, smears should be made and stained for microscopic evaluation. If coccal bacteria are found, empirical antibiotic therapy is often sufficient when recurrence has not been a problem. General therapeutic recommendations may be found in Table 3. Any pustular disease that is not responsive to conventional methods of therapy for pyodermas or that exhibits an atypical progression should be biopsied.

IMPETIGO

Impetigo, commonly termed "puppy pyoderma," is a common, relatively benign condition in which subcorneal pustules are present in the groin and axilla. This disease is frequently asymptomatic and may be noted by a clinician as an incidental finding during a routine physical examination. Impetigo is seen most frequently in prepubescent dogs. Pustular smears indicate the bacterial origin of the disease. Generally, the use of antibacterial shampoos containing benzoyl peroxide or chlorhexidine is sufficient therapy. Occasionally, the use of short-term (seven to ten days) empirical systemic antibiotic therapy is necessary.

Considerably less common, a bullous impetigo with pustules up to 1 cm in diameter may be seen in association with Cushing's disease or with no apparent underlying cause. In a small number of cases, a bullous impetigo has been seen where large greenish pustules had pure cultures of *Pseudomonas* species grown from them. Contaminated surgical scrub material has been implicated in pyodermas arising postsurgically.

SUPERFICIAL FOLLICULITIS

Both the diagnosis and management of a superficial folliculitis may be considerably more difficult than those of an impetigo. The range of clinical signs commonly seen is quite diverse. Papules, pustules, or crusting may be seen, and primary lesions frequently may be obliterated by self-trauma. Hair loss may be significant.

A folliculitis rather similar to impetigo may be seen in the intertriginous areas of the groin and axilla, especially in young dogs. This intertriginous folliculitis usually requires more vigorous therapy than the visually similar impetigo seen with "puppy pyoderma." Differentiation can sometimes be made visually if the pustules are obviously follicular in their orientation. More inflammation is commonly seen with a folliculitis. Generally, this disease will

respond to two weeks of proper antibiotic therapy. Recurrence may indicate that the folliculitis is secondary to another disease such as flea infestation, seborrhea, or any other pruritic disease. Although a secondary folliculitis may appear visually identical to an uncomplicated intertriginous folliculitis, therapeutic success will not be achieved until the underlying cause is determined and corrected. After the underlying cause is delineated, generally a longer course of four to six weeks of proper systemic antibiotic therapy is indicated.

PRURITIC SUPERFICIAL PYODERMA

Since definitive information is not currently available with respect to this disease or group of diseases, the author has chosen to group the diseases previously described as bacterial hypersensitivity, staphylococcal allergy, inflammatory pyodermas, and short-haired dog pyodermas under the broad descriptive heading of pruritic superficial pyoderma. All of these syndromes have certain clinical features in common. They appear to be a pruritic sequela to a superficial pyoderma. Evidence for this statement includes the transient presence of pustules visually, the presence of pustules in biopsy sections, and the significant response seen with the initial use of proper systemic antibiotic therapy. Clinically, expanding circular patches of alopecia and erythema can be seen in association with a pustular or papular eruption. A peripheral peeling back of the stratum corneum, termed an epidermal collarette, has been espoused as the hallmark of this disease. The clinician should be cautioned against making a specific diagnosis based on these collarettes, since any localized highly inflammatory process beginning from a point source will produce a similar circular lesion. In addition to peripheral collarettes, active lesions may coalesce and may finally heal with variable hyperpigmentation.

Although the inflammatory lesions just described are seen most frequently in the groin and axillary regions, similar lesions may be seen dorsally. Diffuse moth-eaten alopecia may be especially obvious dorsally in short-coated dogs. Pustules may be seen transiently at any time during the course of this disease. Rapid resolution of the inflammatory lesions and gradual regrowth of hair is seen in conjunction with antibiotic therapy. The mechanism to explain this transient hair loss is unknown. There appear to be major differences between domestic animals and humans with respect to nonscarring transient alopecias seen secondary to pyodermas or other inflammatory processes. Although rapid response may be seen with antibiotic therapy, it is essential to search for an underlying cause, since recurrence is common. Hypothyroidism, seborrhea, atopy, food allergy, flea allergy dermatitis, and many other less common entities have all been recognized as potential underlying causes of recurrent pruritic superficial pyodermas. In addition to proper antibiotic therapy and the attempted determination of an underlying cause, the use of bacterial products such as Staphage Lysate* or Staphoid AB† may be beneficial. Although corticosteroids may transiently decrease the pruritus associated with the condition, they are contraindicated in the long-term control of the underlying bacterial infection.

DEEP PYODERMA

Deep pyodermas are serious bacterial infections of the skin involving structures beneath and beyond the confines of the hair follicles. In all cases, except with the localized muzzle pyoderma termed "canine acne," possible underlying causes should be strongly considered. Immunodeficiency should be considered in deep pyodermas involving large areas of the animal's body. An underlying demodicosis must be ruled out before other potential contributing factors, such as hypothyroidism, Cushing's disease, iatrogenic Cushing's disease, tumor-associated immunosuppression, or idiopathic immunodeficiency, are explored. With the exception of "canine acne," all other deep pyodermas should be evaluated with a bacterial culture and antibiotic sensitivity in addition to a smear. In general, in contrast to superficial pyodermas, deep pyodermas present as therapeutic rather than diagnostic problems. Long-term systemic antibiotic therapy in conjunction with vigorous topical therapy is usually indicated. A lack of response to appropriate therapy indicates the need for a skin biopsy and a renewed search for an underlying problem. An overview of the management of deep pyodermas is presented in Table 4.

CANINE ACNE (MUZZLE FOLLICULITIS AND FURUNCULOSIS)

Muzzle folliculitis/furunculosis is a more proper term for this condition than "canine acne," since the histopathologic changes seen bear little resemblance to true acne in humans. However, the term "canine acne" is quite useful in client management, since owners are reminded of the protracted course of human acne and the lack of availability of immediate miracle cures.

This disease is a chronic inflammatory disorder of the chin and lips of young dogs characterized by a somewhat symmetric deep folliculitis and furunculosis. Short-coated breeds such as Doberman pinschers, Great Danes, and German short-haired

pointers appear over-represented. The disease is largely asymptomatic, and owner concern often greatly exceeds the animal's awareness of the condition. This disease is frequently self-limiting by the onset of puberty. An underlying localized demodicosis must always be ruled out. In most cases, the local use of a 2.5 per cent benzoyl peroxide shampoo daily is sufficient. In exacerbating cases, warm water soaks may be beneficial prior to the use of the benzoyl peroxide shampoos. In the most severe cases, systemic antibiotics may be useful in the prevention of scarring.

NASAL PYODERMA

Nasal pyoderma is a comparatively uncommon disease characterized by a painfully swollen, somewhat symmetric area of involvement on the dorsum of the nose. A severe furunculosis is seen on biopsy, with a surprisingly variable number of organisms demonstrated by special stains. The onset is usually rapid, and the underlying etiology is unknown. The differential diagnosis of this condition has become increasingly important, since many of the immune-mediated diseases that have been recently documented in the dog may closely resemble nasal pyoderma. In addition to immune-mediated diseases such as discoid lupus erythematosus, systemic lupus erythematosus, pemphigus foliaceus, and pemphigus erythematosus, one should consider *Trichophyton mentagrophytes* ringworm, demodicosis, and drug eruptions as other possible differential diagnoses. Skin scrapings, exudate smears, fungal cultures, and bacterial culture and sensitivities should always be performed. A lack of response to gentle soaks and proper antibiotic therapy indicates the need of a biopsy for routine histopathology and immunofluorescence.

It should be emphasized that this is a poorly characterized disease at present, and the lack of response to antibiotics may indicate that the pyoderma is only secondary to an undiagnosed underlying disease entity.

INTERDIGITAL PYODERMA

The inflammatory digital and interdigital diseases in the dog are poorly characterized, confusing, and frustrating clinically. Interdigital pyodermas are one small subgrouping in this disease complex. Few cases, if any, are simple, uncomplicated interdigital pyodermas. Most chronic or recurrent interdigital pyodermas are probably secondary to other diseases. Consequently, an aggressive diagnostic approach is necessary to determine any underlying predisposing factors such as localized demodicosis of the distal extremities, food allergy, foreign bodies

---

*Delmont Laboratories Inc., Swarthmore, PA.

†Jensen-Salsbery, Kansas City, MO.

Table 4. Management of Deep Pyodermas

Disease	Differential Diagnosis	Diagnostic Procedures	Therapy Topical	Therapy Systemic
Canine acne (muzzle folliculitis and furunculosis)	Demodicosis; ringworm	Scraping; fungal culture	Benzoyl peroxide shampoo; warm water soaks; povidone iodine soaks	Systemic antibiotics rarely necessary
Nasal pyoderma	Ringworm (*T. mentagrophytes*); pemphigus foliaceus; pemphigus erythematosus; discoid lupus; demodicosis; "nasal solar dermatitis"	Fungal and bacterial culture; smear; biopsy; fluorescent biopsy	Warm water soaks; 2.5% benzoyl peroxide shampoos; gentle application	Systemic antibiotics based on bacterial culture and sensitivity (four to six+ weeks); time?
Interdigital pyoderma	Demodicosis; other digital and interdigital inflammatory diseases	Bacterial and fungal culture; scrape, look for underlying cause (demodicosis, hypothyroidism, atopy, food allergy); biopsy	Povidone iodine or chlorhexidine soaks twice daily; debridement; clip hair	Systemic antibiotics based on bacterial culture and sensitivity (four to six+ weeks); immunostimulation? (levamisole, staph. toxoid, staphage Lysate)
Pressure point pyoderma	None common	Bacterial and fungal culture; CBC; serum electrophoresis; scrapings; biopsy; look for underlying cause (hypothyroidism, immune deficiency, steroid therapy)	Povidone iodine or chlorhexidine whirlpools initially twice daily; benzoyl shampoos; clip hair	Same as above
Folliculitis and furunculosis	Demodicosis; if localized, kerion ringworm, drug eruption	Same as above	Same as above	Same as above
Cellulitis	Demodicosis; severe immune-mediated disease; drug eruption	Same as above	Same as above	Same as above
Cellulitis secondary to demodicosis	Other deep pyodermas	Scraping; bacterial culture and sensitivity	Initially clip hair; benzoyl peroxide shampoo; povidone iodine or chlorhexidine whirlpool; discontinue above topical therapy when miticidal therapy begins	Systemic antibiotics based on bacterial culture and sensitivity; continue for minimum two weeks beyond cessation of suppuration; do NOT try immunostimulation

such as grass awns, and psychogenically induced foot licking or chewing. All cases require skin scrapings and a bacterial culture and sensitivity. Most cases should be biopsied. Successful therapy requires elucidation of the underlying cause, long-term systemic antibiotic therapy, and vigorous topical therapy, including clipping of the involved areas and daily antibacterial soaks in products containing povidone iodine or chlorhexidine.

PRESSURE POINT PYODERMA

Pressure point pyodermas are severe, deep infections characterized by folliculitis and furunculosis. Common sites of involvement include the lateral stifle areas, elbows, hocks, and lateral digits (crusts and matted hair may conceal the severity of the infection). This disease is usually mature in onset, and German shepherds, Dalmatians, and Great Danes are over-represented in this condition. Hypothyroidism is seen rather commonly as an underlying cause of immunodeficiency in this syndrome. In many other cases, immunoincompetency is either confirmed or strongly suspected. When an underlying cause has not been documented, therapy should include clipping of all involved areas and the use of an antibacterial shampoo and whirlpools with a cleansing agent such as povidone iodine. Systemic antibiotics based on bacterial cultures and sensitivities should be given for protracted periods of time. Immunostimulation with drugs such as levamisole (2 to 10 mg/kg PO every other day) may be a helpful adjunct. One author feels that levamisole (2 mg/kg every other day) is most useful in cases of deep pyoderma when eosinophils are not found on biopsy (Scott, 1979). However, any use of this drug should be cautioned, since side effects may be severe.

FOLLICULITIS AND FURUNCULOSIS (MISCELLANEOUS)

Some cases of folliculitis and furunculosis do not conform to the rather specific distribution patterns discussed previously. An underlying demodicosis should always be suspected in any localized or generalized deep pyoderma. Treatment of idiopathic deep pyodermas with any distribution pattern is similar to the therapy mentioned previously.

CELLULITIS

Cellulitis is a severe, deep pyoderma characterized by a rapidly spreading suppurative infection. The areas of infection are poorly defined and tend to dissect widely along and through tissue planes. Visually, areas of cellulitis are similar to areas of furunculosis, except that devitalization of skin is more marked. Dark color changes may be noted in affected areas, and the skin may have a friable, gelatinous character. Since most cases of canine cellulitis are secondary to generalized demodicosis, multiple skin scrapings are mandatory. In cases of cellulitis seen secondary to demodicosis, clipping, antibacterial shampoos, and whirlpools are indicated as adjunctive therapy. Systemic antibiotics are also indicated. When the skin is healthy enough for mitecidal therapy to begin, all other forms of topical therapy are discontinued. It should be emphasized that immunostimulatory drugs such as levamisole are not efficacious in the treatment of demodicosis. Furthermore, combination therapy with a mitecidal drug such as ronnel and levamisole is extremely hazardous.

Cellulitis in the dog may also be seen in association with immunodeficiency or as a sequela to other pyodermas as a result of corticosteroid therapy or other mismanagement. Therapy is essentially similar to that given for the other severe, deep pyodermas. Regardless of underlying cause, a cellulitis should always be viewed as a serious disease with the potential for becoming life-threatening.

DISEASES FORMERLY CLASSIFIED AS PYODERMA

Traditionally, two rather distinct clinical entities have been considered as unusual, uncommon bacterial infections of the skin. Newer information indicates that bacterial involvement in both of these syndromes is only secondary. Hidradenitis suppurativa and juvenile pyoderma will be briefly discussed here only to emphasize that their former definition as bacterial diseases has probably been incorrect.

HIDRADENITIS SUPPURATIVA

In humans, hidradenitis suppurativa is an uncommon, severe, deep pyoderma involving the apocrine sweat glands and adjacent deep dermal structures. A syndrome that visually resembles this condition has been reported in several different breeds of dogs, with an increased incidence in collies and Shetland sheepdogs. The disease is characterized by erythematous, suppurative, sharply demarcated plaques with serpiginous borders. The groin and axilla are commonly reported sites.

In retrospect, the degree of apocrine sweat gland involvement necessary to make this diagnosis in the dog was probably insufficient. Furthermore, oral involvement had been reported, and apocrine sweat glands are not found in the oral cavity. Consequently, the hidradenitis seen was most likely a secondary phenomenon. Previous descriptions of this disease closely approximate the criteria currently established for bullous pemphigoid, a subepidermal bullous, immune-mediated disease. Therefore, the majority of cases formerly reported as canine hidradenitis suppurativa were probably canine bullous pemphigoid.

JUVENILE PYODERMA

Juvenile pyoderma is the name traditionally given to a vesiculopustular disease with a mucocutaneous predilection usually seen in puppies less than four months of age. A similar-appearing disease has been seen rarely in adult dogs. Characteristic lesions include severe, acute swellings of the lips and eyelids, a highly exudative otitis externa, and variable involvement of other mucocutaneous junctions. Regional lymphadenopathy is significant. Solitary puppies or entire litters may be affected. Although *S. aureus* is frequently isolated from fistulous draining lesions, newer, nondraining lesions usually are bacteriologically sterile. A hypersensitivity phenomenon with secondary bacterial involvement has been hypothesized. Although antibiotics are conventionally prescribed to control or prevent secondary infection, dramatic curative response is usually seen with immunosuppressive dosages (1 to 2 mg/kg prednisolone PO daily) of corticosteroids. Scarring may be minimized by the prompt administration of proper levels of corticosteroids.

ANTIBIOTIC THERAPY

Once the diagnosis of a pyoderma has been confirmed, proper systemic antibiotic therapy should be initiated. The correct choice of an antibiotic may be based on either empirical considerations or a bacterial culture and sensitivity. It is also important to establish an effective dosage and maintain therapy long enough to ensure cure.

ANTIBIOTIC SELECTION

In veterinary medicine, the term "empirical" has been used to imply a less than satisfactory approach to therapy. However, realistically it is totally unnecessary and of questionable cost effectiveness to advocate the routine use of bacterial culture and sensitivity in the management of canine pyodermas. Empirical antibiotic therapy is justified routinely in the management of uncomplicated superficial pyodermas. Empirical therapy may also be used in deep pyodermas while awaiting the results of a bacterial culture.

However, if empirical therapy is to be initiated, a rapid staining of the contents of an intact pustule is recommended. The finding of cocci in appropriate numbers is both supportive of the presumptive diagnosis of a pyoderma and informative as to the likelihood of the bacteria being *S. aureus*.

If the staining of pustular contents or purulent debris from a fistulous tract reveals a mixed infection, a culture should be submitted. Other reasons for performing a bacterial culture include a deep or long-standing infection. A culture and sensitivity should also be performed when appropriate antibiotic therapy has been ineffective.

Other factors may be important in the choice of an antibiotic. For example, erythromycin should not be prescribed for an animal with a propensity for vomiting. Similarly, an oral antibiotic that must be given three times daily is inappropriate for a dog that is home alone for 12 hours a day. Drug cost may also be a significant factor.

In the past, much emphasis has been placed on the selection of a bacteriocidal antibiotic. If immunosuppression or immunodeficiency is either confirmed or suspected, a bacteriocidal drug should be used. However, in dogs without evidence of severe impairment of host defense mechanisms, there is little evidence that bacteriocidal agents are more effective than bacteriostatic drugs.

EMPIRICAL CHOICE

Since *Staphylococcus aureus* is the primary pathogen of canine skin, an antibiotic chosen empirically should have a known spectrum of activity against this organism. Furthermore, the organism should not be inactivated by penicillinase, since most canine cutaneous trains of *S. aureus* elaborate this enzyme.

Narrow spectrum antibiotics that have proved useful in empirical therapy include erythromycin, lincomycin, and oxacillin. Erythromycin has the advantage of being available in an inexpensive generic form. However, the dosage limitations are significant; this drug must be film coated since it is a gastric irritant. Lincomycin is more expensive but has a much smaller incidence of side effects and may be given only twice daily. Theoretically, oxacillin is the empirical antibiotic of choice, but high cost usually prohibits its routine use. Since erythromycin and lincomycin share common resistance patterns, the ineffectiveness of one precludes the use of the other.

Broader spectrum antibiotics useful in the empirical treatment of pyodermas include chloramphenicol, Tribrissen, and Keflex. Table 5 lists recommended dosages for empirical antibiotic therapy. However, because of emerging patterns of resistance, Keflex should be used empirically only in life-threatening, deep bacterial infections. Aminoglycoside antibiotics, such as Gentamycin, are not

Table 5. *Systemic Dosages of Antibiotics Useful in Empirical Therapy of Canine Pyodermas*

Generic Name	Trade Name	Spectrum	Route of Administration	Suggested Daily Dosage
Erythromycin	—	*Staphylococcus aureus*	PO	10 to 15 mg/kg t.i.d.
Lincomycin	Lincocin*	*Staphylococcus aureus*	PO	20 mg/kg b.i.d.
Oxacillin	Prostaphlin†	Primarily *Staphylococcus aureus*	PO	12 to 24 mg/kg t.i.d.
Chloramphenicol	—	*Staphylococcus aureus*, some gram negative organisms	PO	20 to 50 mg/kg t.i.d.
Trimethoprim sulfadiazine	Tribrissen‡	*Staphylococcus aureus*, some gram negative organisms	PO	2.2 mg/kg b.i.d.
Cephalexin	Keflex§	*Staphylococcus aureus*, some gram negative organisms	PO	22 mg/kg b.i.d.

*The Upjohn Company, Kalamazoo, MI.
†Bristol Laboratories, Syracuse, NY.
‡Burroughs Wellcome, Research Triangle Park, NC.
§Eli Lilly and Company, Indianapolis, IN.

Table 6. *Systemic Dosage of Broad Spectrum Antibiotics Useful in Life-Threatening Canine Mixed Bacterial Infections of the Skin*

Generic Name	Trade Name	Route of Administration	Suggested Daily Dosage
Kanamycin	Kantrim*	Subcutaneous	6 to 8 mg/kg t.i.d.
Gentamicin	Gentocin†	Subcutaneous	2 to 3 mg/kg t.i.d.
Tobramycin	Nebcin‡	Subcutaneous	1 mg/kg t.i.d.
Amikacin	Amikin*	Subcutaneous	5 mg/kg t.i.d.

*Bristol Laboratories, Syracuse, NY.
†Schering Corp., Kenilworth, NJ.
‡Eli Lilly and Company, Indianapolis, IN

recommended for empirical treatment of pyodermas owing to their toxicity and expense. An exception would be the rare use of an aminoglycoside in conjunction with a synthetic penicillin such as oxacillin in overwhelming life-threatening infections such as the mixed gram positive and gram negative organism sepsis occasionally seen in conjunction with generalized demodicosis. This therapy should be initiated only after both skin and blood bacterial cultures have been taken. Recommended dosages for these drugs are listed in Table 6.

Statistically, the antibiotics that should not be used empirically owing to a less than 20 per cent chance of success include penicillin, ampicillin, amoxicillin, and the tetracyclines and sulfonamides.

CHOICE BASED ON CULTURE

Some controversy exists with regard to antibiotic sensitivity testing. The newer tube dilution, agar dilution, and Ericsson's quantitative disc techniques report results as the minimum inhibitory concentration (MIC). The advantage of these more sophisticated methods is that they provide the clinician with the antibiotic concentration necessary to inhibit growth at the site of infection. The Kirby-Bauer single disc technique is still the most readily obtainable standard method available to the small animal clinician. This method is considered more accurate for gram positive than gram negative organisms. In most cases, results obtained by the Kirby-Bauer method are sufficient.

Based on the sensitivity results, an antibiotic that in the past has been an effective therapeutic agent in the treatment of pyodermas should be chosen. In addition, the agent should have minimal side effects, a reasonable cost, and, ideally, have a narrow spectrum of activity directed against the pathogen.

Under many circumstances, the same antibiotics that are good empirical choices are also good choices based on culture and sensitivity testing. However, other drugs that are poor empirical choices may be excellent agents if bacterial sensitivity is noted. As an example, ampicillin would be an excellent choice in the treatment of a nonpenicillinase–producing *S. aureus*.

If *S. aureus* has not been isolated as the primary pathogen, reculture should be considered. In mixed infections, if all of the isolates are not sensitive to one antibiotic or if they are sensitive only to an aminoglycoside, the antibiotic most effective against *S. aureus* should be chosen. In many mixed infections, the effective elimination of *S. aureus* alone may be sufficient to cure the pyoderma, since *S. aureus* creates an environment favorable to the continued growth of other microorganisms.

ANTIBIOTIC DOSAGE

Since improper dosage is one of the most common reasons for treatment failure in pyodermas, the establishment of effective therapeutic dosages is extremely important. Although certain drugs do not require critical attention to accurate dosage, antibiotics must be given at specific dosage levels. Therefore, all dogs receiving systemic antibiotics should be weighed. Unfortunately, in a busy clinical setting it is all too easy to form a "big dog, big pill; little dog, little pill" habit. Dosage errors are made most frequently in very small and very large dogs. Overdosage is common in smaller dogs, since appropriate small pills or capsules may be unavailable. Human pediatric antibiotic elixirs are useful in the treatment of miniature breeds. In larger dogs, a dosage may be reduced to ineffective levels in the misguided attempt to save the owner money. Ineffective therapy, the establishment of resistant bacterial strains, and toxicity associated with overdose are common sequelae to improper dosage levels.

DURATION OF ANTIBIOTIC THERAPY

After an adequate dosage of a proper antibiotic has been established, the dog must be maintained on the antibiotic long enough to ensure cure rather than a transient remission. As mentioned previously, the depth of involvement and the chronicity of the infection are criteria for determining proper antibiotic administration duration. In general, any dog placed on systemic antibiotic therapy should be maintained on the drug for a minimum of ten days. Animals with superficial pyodermas require from two to six weeks of therapy and should be maintained on antibiotics for a minimum of five to seven days beyond clinical cure. The time necessary to adequately treat deep pyodermas is highly variable and depends on the underlying cause of the infection. However, it is wise to maintain dogs with deep pyodermas on systemic antibiotics for 7 to 14 days beyond apparent clinical cure. It should be emphasized that the veterinary clinician, not the owner of the dog, should make the decision regarding discontinuation of therapy. Owners anxious to discontinue antibiotics in the face of apparent success are frequently responsible for relapse.

THERAPEUTIC EVALUATION

Certainly the most important criterion for the effectiveness of an antibiotic is the response to therapy. If an animal has not responded to initial therapy within seven days, re-examination is indicated. The clinician should ascertain if the medication is being given correctly, re-evaluate the choice of antibiotics, look for an underlying cause for the pyoderma, and possibly even reconsider the initial diagnosis.

Recurrent bacterial infections are particularly frustrating. Since many bacterial infections formerly considered to be primary in nature are now known to be secondary to other disease processes, a thorough search for underlying causes should be made. Hypothyroidism, seborrhea, immunodeficiency, demodicosis, atopy, and food allergy have all been shown to be significant underlying causes of recurrent pyodermas in the dog.

TOPICAL THERAPY

Topical therapy is an important adjunct in the treatment of canine pyodermas. Antibacterial agents in shampoo bases or as soak or whirlpool concentrates are quite useful either as sole therapy in surface or superficial pyodermas or as adjunctive therapy in the management of deep pyodermas. Shampoos containing 2.5 per cent benzoyl peroxide (Oxydex*) and chlorhexidine (Nolvasan†) have proved especially useful.

A whirlpool is one of the most beneficial pieces of equipment for dermatologic use in a small animal hospital. Warm water soaks, ideally with whirlpool agitation, remove debris and promote drainage in deep pyodermas irrespective of underlying etiology. Currently, the most beneficial agents available for use in whirlpools or soaks are povidone iodine (Betadine‡) and chlorhexidine (Nolvasan). Six to eight ounces or more of a concentrate are adequate in a 20- to 30-gallon tub. Fifteen-minute whirlpools or soaks twice daily as an adjunct to systemic antibiotic therapy will greatly accelerate the healing of deep pyodermas.

Topical antibiotics in cream or ointment bases have very limited applicability in veterinary medicine with the exception of otic preparations. There is no use for these common products in the treatment of pyodermas owing to the surface area involved, the cost, and the animal's desire to lick the drug off its skin.

SUPPLEMENTAL READING

Ihrke, P. J.: Topical therapy—use principles and vehicles: dermatologic therapy (Part I). Comp. Cont. Ed. Sm. Anim. Pract. 2:28, 1980.

Ihrke, P. J.: Topical therapy—specific topical pharmacologic agents: dermatologic therapy (Part II). Comp. Cont. Ed. Sm. Anim. Pract. 2:156, 1980.

Ihrke, P. J.: Antibiotic therapy in canine skin disease: dermatologic therapy (Part III). Comp. Cont. Ed. Sm. Anim. Pract. 2:177, 1980.

Ihrke, P. J.: Canine pyoderma: diagnosis and management. Proceedings of the American Animal Hospital Association, 61, 1981.

Ihrke, P. J., Halliwell, R. E. W., and Deubler, M. J.: Canine pyoderma. In Kirk, R. W. (ed.): *Current Veterinary Therapy VI.* Philadelphia: W. B. Saunders, 1977, pp. 513–519.

Scott, D. W.: Topical cutaneous medicine or, "Now what should I try?" Proceedings of the American Animal Hospital Association, 89, 1979.

Scott, D. W., MacDonald, J. M., and Shultz, R. D.: Staphylococcal hypersensitivity in the dog. J.A.A.H.A. 14:760, 1978.

---

*DVM, South Miami, FL.

†Fort Dodge Laboratories, Fort Dodge, IA.

‡Purdue Frederick Co., Norwalk, CT.

MANAGING CANINE SEBORRHEA

G. A. KUNKLE, D.V.M.
Gainesville, Florida

Several extensive reviews of canine seborrhea have been written in recent years. Although the authors categorize and divide seborrhea differently, all agree that it is a clinical symptom, a cutaneous disorder that results from many etiologies. Thus, the veterinarian who confronts a flaky, smelly, greasy patient should not stop with a diagnosis of seborrhea and a bottle of tar shampoo.

Once the clinical diagnosis of seborrhea has been made, two important factors are necessary for future successful therapeutic management. First, the veterinarian must gain the cooperation and understanding of the client. One best accomplishes this by spending considerable time during the first office visit educating the client as to the many predisposing and precipitating factors involved in seborrhea. The owner should understand that the most successful therapy for seborrhea is that specific treatment that corrects the underlying problem. Once convinced of the importance of exploring all etiologic avenues, the owner will better appreciate the necessity of an exhaustive diagnostic work-up. After an extensive search, if the veterinarian diagnoses idiopathic seborrhea, the owner can understand how the final diagnosis was reached and hopefully will be more willing to accept lifetime therapy and control rather than a "cure."

Second, the veterinarian needs to meet the challenge of defining the etiology of each seborrheic dog with enthusiasm. Many seborrheic dogs and their owners have visited several veterinarians. If the practitioner is optimistic and interested in the pet, he is more likely to succeed with therapeutic management. Although the diagnosis and management may be time-consuming for the veterinarian, it is likewise a time-consuming condition for the owner. For the veterinarian, management of seborrhea can be rewarding. The more cases one manages successfully, the easier one will find the approach to the seborrheic patient.

SEBORRHEA COMPLEX

A wide range of clinical signs come to mind when the term "seborrhea" is mentioned. The clinical picture may range from a mild scaling or dandruff to severe, alopecic, greasy, odoriferous skin. Liter-ally, seborrhea means "flow of sebum or flow of suet." However, the term as it is presently used in veterinary medicine refers to a clinical condition that includes not only qualitative and quantitative changes in sebum production but changes in keratinization. Inflammation and irritation may occur as well. These factors may all interrelate, acting in concert to disturb the normal ecological balance of the integument.

Sebum changes may result in an increased epidermal turnover rate and, thus, altered keratinization or increased flaking. Qualitative and/or quantitative changes in sebum may result in inflammation and pyoderma. Dogs with keratinization abnormalities may develop a surface population of pathogenic bacteria, which can result in inflammation. To complicate factors, chronic inflammation and pruritus (e.g., as associated with inhalant allergy) may result in sebum abnormalities. Most often the dog presenting with seborrhea has varying degrees of all three factors (sebum changes, keratinization abnormalities, and inflammation), making determination of the original alteration of the integument a difficult task.

ETIOLOGY

Endocrine abnormalities may result in alterations in sebum production and keratinization. The stimulation of sebum production is determined by hormones, primarily androgens. Hormonal regulation of the sebaceous gland is related to an intricate hormonal balance system in which estrogens, thyroid, progesterone, and corticosteroids play a role. Androgens and thyroid generally stimulate sebum production. Inversely, estrogens and corticosteroids generally decrease sebum production, but sex hormone differences and the production of adrenal androgens in the female may complicate matters. There is significant hormonal interplay functioning in sebum production as well as significant variability between individuals. Therefore, the same dose of hormone in different dogs may result in radically different effects. Hypothyroidism and excess use of corticosteroids are among the most common causes of canine seborrhea (sicca). Hormonal seborrhea tends to be only mildly pruritic unless complicated by pyoderma.

518

Allergic skin diseases often result in seborrhea. Flea allergy classically results in excessive scaling over the rump. Atopic dogs manifest a wide range of seborrheic symptoms. One atopic dog may develop greasy odoriferous seborrhea around the mouth, eyes, feet, and perineum, whereas another dog of the same breed with the same allergies may develop generalized dry, scaly skin. Allergic seborrheas are moderately to severely pruritic.

Ectoparasitism may result in chronic inflammation and irritation, both of which lead to symptoms of seborrhea. Infestation with fleas or *Cheyletiella*, *Sarcoptes*, and *Demodex* mites should be considered. A careful examination of the skin, in addition to scrapings, should be part of the initial diagnostic plan of every new case of seborrhea. Seborrhea caused by ectoparasites is variably pruritic.

Infectious factors may complicate seborrhea, and, although rare, seborrhea may occur with generalized dermatophytosis. Pyoderma can result in symptoms of seborrhea in a previously normal dog. Likewise, a secondary pyoderma may severely worsen the seborrhea in a mildly seborrheic dog. The excess flaking of the skin is probably due to alterations in keratinization as a result of inflammation.

Environmental and metabolic factors should be considered for their possible contribution to seborrheic signs. Environmental humidity and temperature are important for the normal shedding of keratin and the sloughing of the stratum corneum. Inappropriate levels of dietary fats or improper absorption of nutrients can complicate the seborrhea complex. Although the sebaceous glands are directly controlled by hormones, the diet and the pancreas, liver, and intestine indirectly play a role in the production of normal sebum. A thorough history should help one determine if these factors are involved.

DIAGNOSIS

The majority of seborrheic dogs have an underlying problem, which may be revealed by a step-by-step investigation. One may be more pessimistic in certain breeds, but an exhaustive search is always indicated. A diagnosis of idiopathic seborrhea is the worst alternative, condemning a dog to lifetime therapy.

For help in diagnosing and managing the seborrheic patient, the flow chart in Figure 1 may be beneficial. To better explain its applications, a discussion of the common presentations of seborrhea and their clinical management follows. This is not an attempt to indicate the best approach to every seborrheic patient but rather is a problem-solving approach and explanation that is generally effective for the author.

DOBERMAN PINSCHER

The seborrheic Doberman pinscher often presents as a young adult with excessive flaking and scaling over the trunk, dorsal rump, and lateral thighs. This also may be accompanied by focal alopecia. Brushing the skin gently or rubbing one's fingers along the back results in a "snowstorm of dandruff," which feels waxy when one's fingertips are rubbed together. Frequently the Doberman pinscher has small raised "bumps" along his dorsum where the hair stands erect in small tufts. Occasional dorsal nodules may be noted and erythematous papules are seen on the lateral thighs, but the skin in general is not inflamed. Pruritus is variable but is usually directly proportional to the extent of flaking.

Initially, demodicosis should be ruled out by scrapings taken from areas of hair loss. Next, one should establish if a pyoderma is present. Focal areas of alopecia usually indicate that pustules were present previously. If small standing tufts of hair are present, a careful search will usually reveal a few papules, an occasional crust, and a rare pustule. This is typical of a superficial folliculitis on the dorsum of a short-haired dog. The lesions may be misdiagnosed as urticaria or hives because of their clinical appearance and their often sudden onset. Recognizing this condition as a pyoderma secondary to the seborrhea will significantly aid the future successful management of this condition. This superficial pyoderma should be treated with a three- to six-week course of systemic antibiotics. Erythromycin, lincomycin, or oxacillin is a good choice initially. Animals previously treated with antibiotics should receive therapy as determined by culture and sensitivity.

If these lesions of superficial folliculitis are treated as hives with steroids, the pruritus and inflammation resolve temporarily. But the infection is still present and sebum production is suppressed by the corticosteroids, resulting in further drying of the skin and eventual worsening of the flaking. When the effects of corticosteroids diminish, the condition often returns with a more extensive clinical presentation. Corticosteroids are *not* indicated in this dry, flaky type of seborrhea.

A serious search should be made for the source of this scaly, waxy seborrhea. Hypothyroidism deserves a high index of suspicion in the Doberman pinscher and should always be evaluated. If the animal is hypothyroid, supplementation with levothyroxine sodium is indicated. After 30 to 90 days of thyroid supplementation, post-pill triiodothyronine (T_3) and thyroxine (T_4) levels should be evaluated four to six hours after medication. These values should be in the middle to high normal range for the dog. Other hormonal changes associated with puberty or estrus may also result in symptoms of

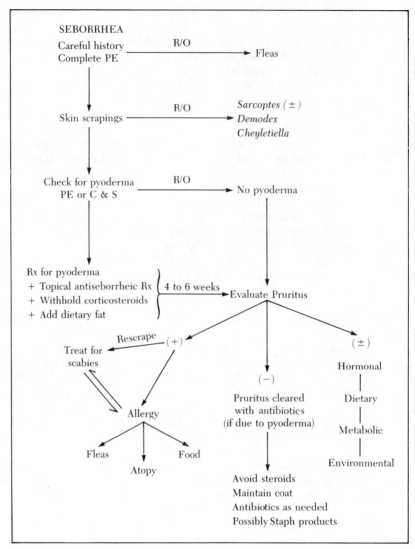

Figure 1. Flow chart for diagnosing canine seborrhea.

seborrhea and pyoderma in the Doberman pinscher.

A thorough history taking is important to help rule out other causes of seborrhea. Many external factors (bathing, dipping, environmental humidity) may contribute to the seborrhea seen in Doberman pinschers. Although Doberman pinschers do not have a high incidence of atopy, flea allergy certainly may occur and may contribute significantly to tail-head and rump seborrhea and pruritus.

Topical therapy is extremely important in the management of the seborrheic Doberman pinscher. The ecologic balance of the skin seems easily altered. Even the drying action of a parasitic dip or flea powder can result in sufficient skin surface changes to allow a superficial pyoderma to develop. Many Doberman pinschers have skin that is acutely sensitive to change, especially to alterations in moisture. Owners should be instructed to conscien-

tiously attempt maintenance of the skin and haircoat as close as possible to normal with various topical products.

For the initial heavy waxing and flaking, a tar shampoo such as Pentrax (Texas Pharm. Co.) seems especially beneficial when used weekly. This shampoo should be massaged gently into the skin for 10 to 15 minutes and rinsed well. Pentrax is an excellent keratolytic shampoo and may also aid in decreasing pruritus. However, in the Doberman pinscher a shampoo with Pentrax should be followed by application of an emollient bath oil and a final water rinse. Alpha Keri Bath Oil (Westwood Pharm. Inc.) or Lubath (Texas Pharm Co.) can be added (1 capful to ½ to 1 gal water) as a final rinse. This serves to rehydrate the skin by trapping water in the superficial layers of the skin. Frequent use of bath oil and water for hydration is essential in the management of the seborrheic Doberman pinscher.

Owners may find it helpful to keep a "plant spritzer" filled with bath oil and water available and spray their dog daily, especially along the dorsal midline and thighs. Several veterinary sprays (e.g., VF Oil Rinse, Neutrogena Corp. and HyLyt, DVM) are currently available for this purpose. On occasion owners may be able to bring initial pustules under control by simply rehydrating the skin in the pustular areas, superseding antibiotic therapy. A newer oil-free product, Humelac (Allerderm), may prove helpful in long-term topical management of the seborrheic Doberman pinscher.

Once the pyoderma is cleared and topical therapy has brought the flaking under control, the frequency of the baths and bath oil/water rinses may be decreased in some cases. Each case requires individual management, but often owners find it necessary to use regular topical therapy.

Occasionally, the skin of Doberman pinschers will not tolerate keratolytic shampoos. Some may become erythematous and pruritic. In these uncommon cases, a mild hypoallergenic shampoo (e.g., Vet Formula, Neutrogena Corp. or Allergroom, Allerderm) may be used.

The addition of dietary fat is often helpful for the seborrheic Doberman pinscher. If the animal is already on a high fat (18 per cent) diet, this would not be indicated. Fat in the form of corn, safflower, peanut, or sunflower oil may be slowly added to the diet until 1 to 2 tablespoons per day are given.

IRISH SETTER

The seborrheic Irish setter usually presents with severe pruritus and extensive alopecia. The neck, trunk, extremities, and even the head may be involved. Although at first glance the Irish setter appears dry and flaky, the skin may feel greasy to the touch, and the owners often complain of a strong "doggy" odor associated with the pruritus. Papules, pustules, and generalized erythema are usually present in addition to excoriations from self-trauma. The ears may have a ceruminous or purulent otitis as well. The generalized pruritus that accompanies seborrhea in the Irish setter may be as severe as that seen with sarcoptic mange.

The history is extremely important in the diagnostic work-up of an Irish setter with chronic dermatitis. Which symptom developed first and how much pruritus is due to an accompanying pyoderma are important details.

Secondary pyoderma frequently occurs in the seborrheic Irish setter and is often very inflammatory. The pyoderma may even extend beyond the superficial layers, and a deep, pruritic furunculosis may occur. The Irish setter can present with such extensive symptoms that the verterinarian may find formulating a diagnostic plan quite difficult. Skin scrapings should be done initially. It is then best to treat the pyoderma with appropriate antibiotics as determined by culture and sensitivity for four to six weeks. Antibacterial and antiseborrheic shampoos may hasten relief, whereas corticosteroids should be withheld. A re-evaluation in one month will allow a much better assessment of the problem.

Once the pyoderma has cleared, the degree of pruritus remaining should be ascertained. If it is minimal, then the severe pruritus was apparently due to the pyoderma, and it is likely that the remaining pyoderma is due to a hormonal or idiopathic seborrhea. As in the Doberman pinscher, hypothyroidism should be considered for the Irish setter. Other hormonal imbalances should also be considered as the source of seborrhea. The previous overuse of corticosteroids is often responsible for the Irish setter's seborrhea. This breed's sebum production seems easily altered with even minimal use of corticosteroids. Although historically Irish setters respond initially to corticosteroid therapy, the rebound effect on sebum production in this breed often results in severe seborrhea and secondary pyoderma.

If the pruritus is still moderate to severe once the pyoderma has resolved, an underlying allergic disease or scabies should be considered. Intradermal allergy testing is indicated at this time. Flea allergy and/or inhalant allergies may be discovered to be the source of the pruritus. A trial course with a hypoallergenic diet may be necessary to rule out food allergy. If the pruritus is severe, the pyoderma gone, and skin scrapings negative, a trial therapy for sarcoptic mange may be indicated. These diagnostic steps should be done independently to define the source of the pruritus.

Unfortunately, in spite of a diligent search, no cause may be found for the pruritus. Idiopathic seborrhea occurs with some frequency in the Irish setter and is often complicated by recurrent pyoderma. Antibiotics are frequently needed in these cases, and they should be given for a minimum of two weeks. Immunization with commercial staphylococcal-derived products (e.g., Staphage Lysate, Delmont Labs or Staphoid AB, Jensen-Salsbery Laboratories) may be useful.

The best topical therapy program for Irish setters varies significantly from dog to dog. Alternating an antibacterial shampoo (e.g., Oxydex, DVM or Sebaffon, Winthrop) with a tar shampoo (e.g., Lytar, DVM or Mycodex Tar & Sulfur, Beecham Labs) every five to seven days usually gives good results. Products containing sulfur, salicylic acid, or selenium disulfide may also benefit Irish setter seborrhea. There is tremendous variability between dogs, and owners should change products until they find a bathing program that repeatedly works on their pet. Again, bath oil and water rinses are usually helpful in maintaining the normal skin hydration.

COCKER SPANIEL

The seborrheic cocker spaniel is usually middle-aged and moderately pruritic. Significant odor reminiscent of rancid fat is associated with cocker spaniel seborrhea. There is usually dorsal wax and grease build-up, often clinging to the base of the hair in clumps. The ears usually have ceruminous otitis, and a similar yellow-brown sebum may be found dorsally between the toes. Large circular plaques with erythema and crusting are often seen on the trunk.

The cocker spaniel presents a unique challenge in the management of seborrhea. Deep scrapings should be done to eliminate demodicosis. Again, any pyoderma should be treated initially. Pyoderma in the cocker spaniel often presents with scaling circular plaques, which are intensely pruritic. Inflammation associated with these plaques varies, depending on the dog. Papules and pustules are rarely found. Surface pyoderma seems to contribute significantly to the pruritus of the cocker spaniel. Animals with abnormal sebum production have increased colonization of the skin by *Staphylococcus aureus*, and this bacteria, in conjunction with an increase in surface fatty acids, causes pruritus and inflammation.

Again, once the pyoderma is successfully treated, the veterinarian should reassess the patient, noting the remaining symptoms. Although cocker spaniels have a decreased incidence of atopy, allergic diseases should be considered. Thyroid status should be assessed as well. The history should be carefully evaluated for any factors that seem to improve or worsen the condition. This is especially important for those cocker spaniels with idiopathic seborrhea; these factors will aid in devising an outline for long-term management.

The cocker spaniel may benefit from a change in diet. The obese patient should be put on a diet. For others, a change from one type of diet to another may be helpful. Again there is tremendous individual variation. A low-fat diet may help some greasy cocker spaniels, but others may be helped by the addition of fat in the diet. Some owners report improvement with zinc or vitamin E supplementation. Vitamin A has proved useful in a few cases, but toxicity can occur, so it should be used with care.

Bathing regimens are not specific for this breed. Oxydex (DVM) seems very useful for this breed as well as those shampoos containing salicylic acid and sulfur (e.g., Sebulex, Westwood Pharm.). Emollient bath oil and water rinses are usually not necessary for common seborrhea of this breed.

Several factors may play a role in the long-term management of seborrhea in the cocker spaniel. The length of the haircoat may affect the seborrhea, depending on individual variation. Some owners find that it is helpful to keep their cockers trimmed closely; the seborrhea seems reduced and bathing is easier. On the other hand, the seborrhea in some cocker spaniels may be exacerbated when they are trimmed. Owners should try both methods and determine which is best for their pet. Environmental humidity and temperature are variables that often contribute significantly to the waxing and waning of symptoms of seborrhea in the cocker spaniel.

The sebum rebound effect occurs in the cocker spaniel after steroid withdrawal. Unfortunately, in spite of frequent antibiotics, extensive bathing, and an intensive search for cause, the idiopathic seborrhea of the cocker spaniel may respond only to corticosteroids. When one finds it necessary to use them for long-term management, short-acting prednisone or prednisolone should be used on alternate days at a minimal dose.

OTHER SEBORRHEIC BREEDS

Virtually any breed can develop symptoms of seborrhea, but some have a higher incidence and the disorder may begin at an early age. Although a breed may be over-represented in the seborrhea complex, closely related family members may not be similarly affected. Springer spaniels and basset hounds manifest a seborrhea somewhat similar to that seen in the cocker spaniel. West Highland white terriers can develop severe seborrheic symptoms, which may be further complicated by a low pruritic threshold. Seborrheic German shepherds exhibit a wide range of symptoms, one of which may be similar to the greasy odor of the seborrheic cocker spaniel. More often, they show a dorsal waxy seborrhea similar to that seen in the seborrheic Doberman pinscher. Middle-aged and geriatric poodles and schnauzers often develop a mixed seborrhea more similar to that seen in the seborrheic Irish setter. Recently, families of severely pruritic seborrheic Labrador retrievers have been recognized.

PRODUCTS FOR THERAPY

Many antiseborrheic shampoos are available today. They may contain one or a combination of the following ingredients: coal tar, salicylic acid, sulfur, selenium disulfide, and benzoyl peroxide. These agents function as keratolytics and keratoplastics. The former act to hydrate, soften, and aid in the peeling of the stratum corneum, whereas the latter aid in normalization of keratinization through unknown mechanisms. The therapeutic effectiveness of various shampoos is different in individual dogs. Some have features such as nonstaining, which should be considered for light-colored haircoats. Ideally, the veterinarian should familiarize himself with the therapeutic properties of four or five shampoos for seborrhea. After attaining knowledge of these through repeated use, new products should be added to the drug list as needed.

Shampoos are most effective when left on the skin for 10 to 15 minutes, followed by thorough rinsing. When a dull haircoat or dry, scaly skin is present, an emollient bath oil (with water) should be used in the final rinse water to provide a light lipid protection for the skin and hair.

A large armamentarium of topical products exists today for use in veterinarian medicine. Several ointments, lotions, and gels (e.g., Keralyt, Westwood or Oxydex Gel, DVM) contain ingredients similar to those in antiseborrheic shampoos. These topical agents have limited application in the dog because of the haircoat, but they may be helpful when applied to alopecia or focal areas of severe crusting. Topical corticosteroids are best avoided for the previously mentioned reasons. After thorough cleansing of the skin, topical corticosteroids in a vanishing cream base may be justified in lieu of systemic corticosteroids. Vitamin A acid (Retin-A, Johnson & Johnson) reduces the cohesiveness of keratinocytes; thus one may find it useful in crusted plaque areas of hyperkeratosis and lichenification. It should be applied in small quantities and massaged in thoroughly. Local irritation can be a problem in some dogs, and, after repeated use, its effectiveness may diminish. Although its cost may prohibit long-term use, its application can be rewarding in the black cocker spaniel with severe seborrhea.

Owners of seborrheic dogs often inquire about the use of nutritional supplements for their pet's skin and haircoat. Because the skin is an actively growing organ, one might expect it to exhibit signs of nutritional imbalance. There are many supplements marketed for "beautiful skin and haircoats." Among their ingredients are fatty acids, amino acids, vitamins, and minerals. In addition to questions regarding the benefit of supplements, there is debate regarding the merits of meat and cereal dog foods. Some dog owners and breeders recommend high protein and high fat and animal protein diets, although many dogs with shiny coats and beautiful skin eat only cereal diets. Again, there is tremendous individual variation.

Dietary fat requirements seem to fluctuate significantly. Major dry dog foods contain 10 to 13 per cent fat, and this may not be optimum for all dogs.

Adding ground beef or canned meat products supplements both the fat and protein intake of dry food. Corn, sunflower, or safflower oil will increase dietary polyunsaturates. Wheat germ oil with added vitamin E is expensive but may benefit some dogs.

High-quality protein may benefit the seborrheic dog. Supplementing a cereal diet with meat, liver, whole milk, and eggs may be advantageous. This is not to say that eating eggs will improve the skin and haircoat of most seborrheics, but a trial diet change certainly has merit. This modification can be from a low fat and protein cereal product to a high animal fat and animal protein product or vice versa. Alternatively, the change can consist of the addition of polyunsaturates, eggs, and liver to the present diet for several weeks. Most prepackaged commercial supplements are expensive and do not have distinct advantages over the previously mentioned additions.

Vitamins and minerals serve numerous roles in the maintenance of normal metabolism. The B vitamins do have profound effects on the skin, but they are readily available in most diets. Vitamin A is being used extensively for many human dermatoses manifested by crusting and scaling. Oral vitamin A supplementation may benefit an occasional case of canine seborrhea, but it should be used cautiously, as toxicity is a potential side effect. Liver provides an excellent dietary source of vitamin A. The usefulness of vitamin E supplementation for the coat is questionable, but as it is relatively safe and inexpensive, a trial course may be attempted. Zinc is a necessary mineral for normal keratinization. True deficiency is uncommon, but a few seborrheic dogs may benefit from its addition to the diet.

In summary, canine seborrhea can be successfully managed in most cases. It requires an astute, motivated clinician willing to search for an underlying etiology. A patient, dedicated owner provides the necessary optimum care for the seborrheic dog.

SUGGESTED READING

Halliwell, R. E. W.: Seborrhea in the dog. Comp. Cont. Ed. 1:227, 1979.
Ihrke, P. J.: Canine seborrheic disease complex. Vet. Clin. North Am. 9:93, 1979.
Kronfeld, D.: Common questions about the nutrition of dogs and cats. Comp. Cont. Ed. 1:33, 1979.
Kunkle, G. A.: Canine seborrhea. Small Anim. Vet. Med. Update 2(6):1, 1979.
Scott, D. W.: Topical cutaneous medicine or, "Now what should I try?" Proceedings of the American Animal Hospital Association, 89, 1979.

ALOPECIA

LLOYD M. REEDY, D.V.M.

Dallas, Texas

Alopecia may be defined as loss or lack of hair. The origin of the term is from the Greek word "alopex" for fox and is believed to refer to the common infestation of that animal with sarcoptic mange mites, resulting in hair loss. Hypotrichosis refers to a partial or complete lack of hair through error of development. The term "pelage" includes the hairs of the body, limbs, and head collectively. Abnormal or excessive hairiness is called hirsutism.

Only mammals, which are also called "trichozoan" (hair mammals) and "Pilfera" (hair bearers), have hair. The major function of hair is thermal insulation. By conserving body heat, warm-blooded animals are relieved of the necessity of absorbing environmental heat. Other functions of hair include protection, camouflage, ornamentation, and communication or tactile sensory perception. The horn of the rhinoceros and the quills of the porcupine are examples of hairs specialized for offense and defense. Mammals that frequently swim increase their buoyancy by trapping air in their fur. As a general rule, where the pelage is thick, the epidermis is thin and uncomplicated.

Hairs consist of compactly cemented keratinized cells produced by follicles, which are epidermal appendages descending into the dermis. These follicles, together with the sebaceous glands that grow from their sides, the apocrine gland, and the arrector pili muscle, form the apopilosebaceous unit. In dogs and cats, hairs are grouped in multiple hair follicles set into the skin at an oblique angle, usually slanted away from the head toward the tips of the appendages. A large primary hair and several secondary hairs share a common opening on the skin surface. Both sebaceous and apocrine glands empty into the hair follicle. The oily film produced by sebaceous glands coats the hair shafts, giving them a glossy sheen. The function of apocrine glands in the dog and cat is unknown but may be related to pheromone communication.

A hair may be divided into the hair shaft, that portion that extends above the skin surface, and the hair root. The hair shaft, viewed in cross section, consists of three parts, the central medulla, the cortex, and the outer cuticle. Hair follicles are richly supplied with vascular and nerve networks. Dog and cat hairs may be divided into three general types: tactile or sinus hair, coarse or guard hair, and fine or secondary hair. One distinctive feature of cat hair is the serrated profile.

Hairs do not grow continuously, since the follicles that produce them have precisely controlled periods of growth and rest, i.e., the hair growth cycle. In many mammals, including humans, follicles grow and rest independently in asynchronous cycles. Anagen is the active growth phase, catagen the transition phase, and telogen the resting phase. When a quiescent follicle grows again, it forms a new hair, which either dislodges the club, or dead hair, or grows alongside it. Each hair follicle has its own growth cycle, which is largely independent of the growth cycle of nearby follicles. Surprisingly little is known about hair growth in dogs and cats, owing to the tedious nature of such investigations as well as the great variety of breeds. One method of determining the anagen:telogen ratio of hairs is to pluck 100 hairs and examine them under the microscope. Anagen hairs have a large moist, glistening and expanded root surrounded by a root sheath. Telogen hairs are club-shaped and keratinized but lack a root sheath. In humans, normal percentages of telogen hairs have been reported to vary from 13 to 22 per cent, with values above 30 per cent considered abnormal. In dogs and cats. normal anagen:telogen ratios have not been studied but would be helpful in evaluating hair loss.

Seasonal shedding is a normal phenomenon in both dogs and cats, especially if unconfined, and is probably related more to the photoperiod than to the environmental temperature. The effects of an artificial environment, such as that produced in most homes with incandescent and fluorescent lighting, on hair growth cycles have not been studied and are unknown. Neutered animals have hair cycles similar to those of intact animals.

Alopecia is a common presenting sign in veterinary dermatology. Normally, except for the nose, footpads, and mucocutaneous junction, the skin of dogs and cats is completely covered with hair. Many external and internal factors can directly or indirectly affect hair follicles to produce hair loss. The four basic distribution patterns of alopecia are focal, multifocal, regional, and generalized. These may be further classified as partial or complete and symmetric or asymmetric.

Alopecia may be divided into two broad etiologic groups, congenital or hereditary and acquired. Examples of acquired or secondary hair loss include losses due to endocrine disorders, bacterial or fungal infections, parasitic infestations, drug or toxin ingestion, nutritional imbalance, stress, neoplasia, physical or chemical injury, and immunologic disorders.

HEREDITARY ALOPECIA

Genetic alopecias are usually irreversible. The pathogenesis involves a genetically controlled faulty growth and development or complete absence of some, many, or all of the hair follicles. Hereditary alopecias may be present at birth (congenital) or may appear during the first several months of life (tardive). Congenital alopecias are not necessarily hereditary.

Feline alopecia universalis is an example of congenital generalized alopecia in the cat. It is an extremely rare condition, but some cat fanciers are trying to produce cats with feline alopecia universalis as a new breed known as "sphinx cats." Microscopically there is a complete absence of primary hairs with sparse lanugo hairs and shorter, abnormal other hairs. The epidermis is thicker than normal. The few hairs present lack a well-formed bulb and can be easily epilated. Sebaceous and apocrine glands are both present but open directly onto the surface of the skin. The dermis is apparently normal.

The Chinese crested dog, the Mexican hairless, and the Chihuahua are examples of canine breeds that have been established by selection for partial alopecia as part of the breed standard. The Chinese crested dog has hair on the top of the head and feet but is almost hairless elsewhere. The Mexican hairless and Chihuahua have varying degrees of hypotrichiasis, with much individual variation. Several cases of congenital alopecia, as well as other ectodermal defects, have been reported in the literature. At times, follicular dysplasias are associated with color coat pattern. Examples include tardive hereditary hypotrichosis in silver miniature poodles, hereditary black hair follicular dysplasia in mongrels, and hereditary partial alopecia associated with blue Dobermans, blue dachshunds, blue whippets, and fawn Irish setters.

ACQUIRED ALOPECIA

ENDOCRINE ALOPECIA

Hair growth requires the normal functioning of several endocrine glands including the thyroid, pituitary, and adrenal. Although bilaterally symmetric alopecia is the common pattern in endocrine-related alopecias, it can occur in nonendocrine conditions.

HYPOTHYROIDISM

Hypothyroidism, a deficiency of effective thyroid hormone, is a common cause of skin and hair abnormalities in the dog. Feline hypothyroidism has not been documented in the literature. The primary hormones secreted by the thyroid gland are thyroxine (T_4) and triiodothyronine (T_3). They exert a profound effect on metabolism as well as on other body functions.

A brief review of the steps in the production and utilization of thyroid hormones will greatly increase the clinician's understanding of the diagnosis and treatment of hypothyroidism. The first step is the concentration of iodine by the thyroid gland. Within the thyroid gland, inorganic iodine reacts with the amino acid tyrosine to form monoiodotyrosine and diiodotyrosine. These are coupled to form triiodothyronine (T_3) and tetraiodothyronine (thyroxine, T_4), which attach to thyroglobulin formed by the glandular cells. Their release from the thyroid gland follows the linkage break between thyroid hormone and thyroglobulin, which remains in the thyroid gland and is not normally found in the circulation. The release of thyroid hormone is controlled by thyroid-stimulating hormone (TSH) secreted by the anterior pituitary. Thyrotropin-releasing factor (TRF) is secreted by the hypothalamus and controls the synthesis and release of TSH. The relationship between circulating thyroid hormone levels and TRF represents a typical biologic negative feedback. As thyroid hormone levels in the circulation decrease, TRF secretion increases and vice versa. Once free of the thyroid gland, thyroxine binds to thyroxine-binding globulin. Small quantities of free thyroxine (T_4) are released from protein binding, carried to the tissues, and deiodinated to T_3, which is considered to be the active cellular thyroid hormone.

Contrary to previous misconceptions, when Hightower and associates studied induced canine hypothyroidism, the first clinical manifestations were changes in the haircoat and skin (1973). These changes preceded the appearance of systemic signs and began several months after ablative levels of radioactive iodine (I^{131}) were given. Because of increased telogen, hairs failed to regrow when clipped and were easily epilated. This resulted in frictional alopecia at points of physical contact. The skin was thickened, hyperpigmented, and seborrheic with characteristic scaling, oiliness, and odor. This does not imply that all seborrheic cases are hypothyroid. Although it must be considered in the differential diagnosis of seborrhea, other factors that alter the keratinization process may be involved in this complex disease.

Systemic changes related to the lowered metabolic rate then followed and included lethargy, obesity despite a clearly reduced appetite, hypersensitivity to cold, anemia, diarrhea, anestrus, and loss of libido in males. Other symptoms were arthralgia and myalgia, especially when cold. Hypothyroidism can affect host immune responses, with a decreased resistance to skin infections. For this reason, recurrent canine pyoderma may be secondary to hypothyroidism.

Histopathology of canine hypothyroid skin is not specifically diagnostic and does not always distinguish hypothyroidism from other alopecic skin diseases. The epidermis is usually thin, with degenerative changes in the collagen fibers of the dermis and hair follicles. The thyroid gland may show leukocytic infiltration and fibrosis followed by follicular collapse and atrophy of thyroid tissue. A TSH deficiency is suggested in those animals with positive clinical and laboratory findings of hypothyroidism without characteristic thyroid gland lesions.

The most common cause of canine hypothyroidism is idiopathic atrophy of the thyroid gland. The etiology of this atrophy is not fully understood but may be related to immune-mediated mechanisms. Autoimmune lymphocytic thyroiditis has been reported in the dog, but the incidence is unknown.

DIAGNOSIS

One reason for the confusion in the diagnosis of canine hypothyroidism is the constant change in laboratory tests. Another problem is that most tests were developed for use in humans, and canine thyroid hormone levels are much lower. Serum cholesterol assessment, protein-bound iodine evaluation, thyroid biopsy, thyroidal radioiodine uptake, thyroid scanning, and serum T_3 and T_4 values by radioimmunoassay (RIA) are examples of the numerous procedures recommended for the diagnosis of canine thyroid dysfunction. Each has drawbacks against routine use in a small animal practice.

Probably the most commonly used test in suspected hypothyroidism is RIA measurement of serum T_3 and T_4 values. The principal problem with this test is that it measures total thyroid hormone as opposed to free thyroid hormone. Normal (euthyroid) dogs may, on any given day, have thyroid hormone levels that approach or overlap established hypothyroid hormone levels. Normal as well as hypothyroid T_3 and T_4 values will vary between laboratories using the same test. For this reason, each laboratory must establish its own normal values for the dog. The ideal test would be the measurement of free thyroid hormone and serum TSH levels, but at present these are not routinely available for veterinary use.

Currently, the author recommends the TSH response test for the diagnosis of canine hypothyroidism. Briefly, a pre-TSH serum T_4 sample is collected, 1 IU TSH*/3 lbs given intramuscularly, and a post-TSH serum T_4 sample taken 8 to 12 hours later. Failure of the second value to be at least twice the first is considered strongly suggestive of hypothyroidism (Hoge, 1974).

THERAPY

Two general categories of thyroid replacement hormone are desiccated or crude animal thyroid preparations and synthetic hormones. In spite of the fact that desiccated thyroid hormones contain both T_3 and T_4 and are cheaper, inconsistencies in formulation and clinical effects as well as shorter shelf life make their use unreliable. Synthetic thyroid hormone products include sodium salts of levothyroxine (T_4), levo-triiodothyronine (T_3), and 4-to-1 mixtures of each. All three synthetic products are capable of returning hypothyroid dogs to the euthyroid state. When compared with doses for humans on a weight basis, dosages required in dogs are quite high. This may be due to the rapid plasma clearance half time of thyroid hormones in dogs. The liver is the most active tissue in concentrating and metabolizing thyroid hormone. Smaller dosages of thyroid hormones two or more times per day may prevent wide fluctuations in plasma concentrations and may be more effective in the treatment of hypothyroidism. Dosages are listed in Table 1.

Response time is variable. The author likes to recheck hypothyroid animals three months after starting supplemental therapy. If there is a satisfactory response, the patient should be continued on medication for life and examined every 6 to 12 months. Most therapeutic failures are due to the owner discontinuing treatment. For unknown reasons, some animals fail to respond upon restarting the thyroid hormone.

The veterinary practitioner will occasionally be presented with an animal with strongly suggestive clinical signs of hypothyroidism but normal or low normal thyroid function tests. Before starting a "therapeutic trial" with supplemental thyroid hormone, it might be wise to consider other differential diagnoses. As a general rule, animals with definitely low thyroid function tests respond better to therapy than those with marginal or "gray area" function tests. The reader is reminded that animals with hyperadrenocorticism as well as other secondary diseases such as demodicosis often have low thyroid values.

Unresponsive animals should be reviewed as to proper dosage and administration, diet, secondary

---

*Sigma Chemical Co., St. Louis, MO.

Table 1. *Recommended Dosages of Thyroid Hormones*

Hormone	Dosage
Desiccated thyroid	20 mg/kg/day
Levothyroxine	0.1 mg/6 kg b.i.d.
Liothyronine (Cytobin, Norden Laboratories)	4.4 mg/kg t.i.d.

problems, and other differential diagnoses. If all are correct, repeat the serum T_4 and T_3 assessments by RIA. Most thyroid-responsive animals will be in the high normal range while on medication. If T_4 and T_3 values are not in this range, dosages of thyroid hormone should be increased.

PITUITARY ALOPECIA

Canine pituitary dwarfism is caused by insufficient growth hormone during the growth phase. It is believed to be associated with cystic Rathke's cleft, resulting in partial or total pituitary insufficiency. This rare disease, which may be due to autosomal recessive inheritance factors, is characterized by smaller body size with normal proportions, retention of a soft, puppy-like haircoat, and eventual bilaterally symmetric alopecia. Usually only one member of a litter is affected.

Canine pituitary dwarfism has been reported more commonly in German shepherds but may occur in other breeds. Other abnormalities include hyperpigmented skin, retention of first dentition, infantile genitalia, and a shrill bark. Both thyroid and adrenal function tests are below normal.

Growth hormone, which is produced by acidophil cells of the anterior pituitary gland, does not act by itself but via growth factors in synergism with thyroid hormones. For this reason, therapy, if undertaken, should consist of parenteral growth hormone as well as oral thyroxine. Regrowth of hair, mostly undercoat, is possible, but an increase in height will not occur, owing to closure of growth plates. Since most owners of these dogs are more concerned about the alopecia than the diminished stature, therapy can be rewarding. However, growth hormone is not commercially available at this time.

Insufficient growth hormone in the mature dog can produce alopecia of the trunk with hyperpigmentation of the skin. Usually the head and legs are spared, but the remaining hairs are dry, lusterless, and easily epilated. Siegel called the condition "pseudo Cushing's" because of the similarity between alopecia and hyperadrenocorticism (1977). The onset is between one and three years of age, with a higher incidence in males than in females. Adult onset insufficient growth hormone alopecia is more common in certain breeds, especially Pomeranians, miniature poodles, chows, and keeshonds. Other than hair and skin abnormalities, the animals are in apparent good health. Thyroid and adrenal function tests are normal. Skin biopsies reveal epidermal hyperkeratosis and melanosis, alopecia, and variable decreases in dermal elastin, but these changes are not completely diagnostic. Regrowth of hair has been reported following parenteral administration of growth hormone on alternate days for ten injections.

HYPERADRENOCORTICISM

Although the first signs of canine hyperadrenocorticism are systemic and classically consist of polyuria, polydipsia, and polyphagia, these may be overlooked by dog owners until dermatologic changes occur some months later. These dermatologic changes include alopecia over the trunk sparing the head and legs, thinning of the skin, and, often, calcinosis cutis. Hyperadrenocorticism should always be included in the differential diagnosis of canine alopecia, especially if accompanied by suggestive systemic signs.

The terms "Cushing's disease" and "Cushing's syndrome" are confusing and should be avoided. Hyperadrenocorticism refers to any condition in which there is increased secretion of glucocorticosteroids by the adrenal glands.

Four factors responsible for the production of hyperadrenocorticism in the dog are anterior pituitary tumor secreting excess adrenocorticotropic hormone (ACTH), functional adrenocortical tumor, abnormality in negative feedback mechanism, and iatrogenesis. A fifth condition, ectopic ACTH syndrome caused by ACTH-like compounds secreted by nonpituitary neoplasms, occurs in humans but has not been reported in dogs.

The majority of canine hyperadrenocorticism cases are caused by hypersecretion of ACTH resulting in bilateral adrenocortical hyperplasia. Such changes can be caused by functional anterior pituitary tumors or by abnormalities in the negative feedback mechanism and are classified as pituitary dependent. Anterior pituitary tumors in the dog are either chromophobic adenomas or adenocarcinoma and are usually slow growing. Abnormalities in the negative feedback mechanism are more common, but the exact mechanism is unknown. A defect in the hypothalamic release of corticotropin-releasing factor (CRF) and ACTH is suspected. In this condition, increasing cortisol levels do not inhibit CRF or ACTH.

Functional adrenocortical tumors are classified as adrenal dependent and are found in less than 5 per cent of animals with hyperadrenocorticism. About half are adenomas and half are adenocarcinomas. They usually are unilateral, with the opposite adrenal gland becoming atrophic. Iatrogenic canine Cushing's syndrome is due to exogenous glucocorticosteroids, which suppress endogenous ACTH secretion, produce atrophy of the zona fasciculata of the adrenal glands, and result in curtailment of endogenous cortisol production. For this reason, despite their signs, these dogs actually have adrenal cortical suppression and may develop glucocorticoid insufficiency when these drugs are discontinued.

CLINICAL SIGNS

Hyperadrenocorticism is rare in dogs younger than five years of age, usually occurring in dogs seven years old or older. Purebred dogs, especially miniature and toy poodles, dachshunds, and Boston terriers, are most commonly affected, although mongrels can develop the disease. Hyperadrenocorticism is rare in cats.

In addition to bilaterally symmetric alopecia, which is more dramatic in long-haired dogs, the remaining hairs are dull, dry, and easily epilated. Because of dermal atrophy, the skin is markedly thin, cool to the touch, and appears to be dehydrated owing to a breakdown of collagen and elastic fibers. Calcinosis cutis occurs in approximately 40 per cent of the cases of hyperadrenocorticism but is not diagnostic since it can be related to nonspecific skin mineralization. Hyperpigmentation is variable and is found also in hypothyroidism and adult onset growth hormone insufficiency. Comedones and keratin plugs are common but not specific for canine hyperadrenocorticism.

Systemic signs are usually present for four to six months before noticeable alopecia develops. In addition to the previously mentioned polydipsia, polyuria, and polyphagia, muscle atrophy and weakness can be quite pronounced. Although the animal appears fat owing to a pendulous abdomen caused by abdominal muscular weakness and an enlarged liver, there is actually a loss of weight. Intact females often are in anestrus and 20 to 30 per cent have an enlarged clitoris, suggesting excessive androgens. Testicular atrophy is found in approximately 30 per cent of the males with hyperadrenocorticism.

LABORATORY TESTS

Although a definitive diagnosis depends on a demonstration of increased secretion of corticosteroids, certain screening tests should be performed first. The most helpful findings are absolute lymphopenia (less than 1000/cm), eosinopenia, and low urine specific gravity. Although absolute lymphopenia may be calculated from a routine CBC, a total eosinophil count is recommended for evaluation of eosinophils. The normal canine total eosinophil count is 300 to 500/cm, but in hyperadrenocorticism it is less than 100/cm and often will be 0. Because of hepatic dysfunction, hypercholesterolemia and elevated serum alkaline phosphatase levels are also found. Mild hyperglycemia is common, and frank diabetes mellitus has been reported. Thyroid function tests are often low. Serum electrolyte values are usually normal.

Histopathology of the skin shows a thin dermis with thickened epidermis due to accumulation of multiple layers of keratin on the surface. These changes are not diagnostic.

A single measurement of plasma cortisol can be misleading. The most commonly used diagnostic test for hyperadrenocorticism is the ACTH response test. A pre-ACTH plasma (not serum) cortisol level is compared with a post-ACTH plasma cortisol level. Normal dogs usually produce a two- to threefold increase, whereas dogs with pituitary-dependent hyperadrenocorticism produce exaggerated responses to ACTH, i.e., often five- to tenfold increases. Animals with adrenal-dependent hyperadrenocorticism will have variable responses to ACTH. Dexamethasone suppression tests help distinguish pituitary-dependent hyperadrenocorticism from adrenal-dependent hyperadrenocorticism as do RIA measurements of ACTH. Since iatrogenic hyperadrenocorticism is associated with atrophy of the adrenal fasciculata, the baseline cortisol level is low and there is no response to ACTH. For complete details on performing and interpreting these tests, the reader is referred to page 863.

THERAPY

The discovery that o,p'-DDD, an analog of DDT, selectively induces necrosis of the adrenal zona fasciculata and zona reticularis is largely responsible for medical management replacing surgery in the treatment of canine hyperadrenocorticism. The veterinarian is cautioned that this is a potentially highly toxic compound and not one to be administered without positive laboratory confirmation and the owner's written consent. The recommended dosage is 50 mg/kg/day, preferably in divided doses, for dogs weighing over 7 kg and 25 mg/kg/day for dogs weighing under 7 kg. The drug is given until the total eosinophil count exceeds 300/cm, the absolute lymphocyte count exceeds 1000/cm, the water consumption returns to normal, or there is no response to ACTH stimulation. The average initial duration of treatment is five to eight days, but some animals require 10 to 21 days. Maintenance therapy is then 50 mg/kg/wk for dogs over 7 kg and less for smaller dogs. The major drawbacks to this drug are the potential toxicity, the possibility of inducing hypoadrenocorticism, and its questionable use in treating pituitary and adrenal tumors. After therapy, some dogs still require supplemental glucocorticosteroids during times of stress. The value of o,p'-DDD in treating canine adrenal tumors is unknown. For this reason, surgical removal is indicated. Since most adrenal tumors are unilateral, the suppressed gland may regain its normal function.

The dosage of corticosteroids in animals with iatrogenic hyperadrenocorticism should be reduced. Dosage once every morning with hydrocortisone for several months may be necessary until the animal's own hypothalamic-pituitary-adrenal axis is functional again.

FELINE ALOPECIA

Feline endocrine alopecia has been reported to occur primarily in castrated domestic short-haired cats. A posterior pattern is most common, especially the ventral abdomen and inguinal and perineal areas. When plucked hairs are examined under the microscope, increased telogen:anagen ratios are found. Feline endocrine alopecia is often confused with psychogenic alopecia, which is more common. In psychogenic alopecia, the hairs are not shed but are broken from excessive grooming with the cat's rasp-like tongue. The secretive grooming habits of some cats make this distinction difficult.

The etiology of feline endocrine alopecia is unclear, but an imbalance of sex hormones is suspected. Before attempting supplemental sex hormone therapy, it is wise to rule out other causes such as dermatomycosis, acariasis, flea bite hypersensitivity, and food and inhalant allergies. The mechanism of action of progesterone compounds such as megestrol acetate in this disease is unknown. Side effects are common, and it is not currently licensed for use in cats.

OTHER CAUSES OF ALOPECIA

Alopecia can occur in association with Sertoli cell tumors, male feminizing syndrome, and ovarian imbalances. Both Sertoli cell tumors and male feminizing syndrome may produce gynecomastia, depressed libido, absence of sperm, and sexual attraction to other male dogs. The etiology is unclear, but excessive estrogens are suspected and neutering is recommended.

Telogen effluvium is the premature precipitation of anagen follicles into telogen, a process which may be regarded as the common response of hair follicles to different types of stress. It can occur following parturition, fever, surgical shock, or other traumatic episodes. Usually no treatment is necessary, and the prognosis for regrowth of hair is good.

Of the drugs and chemicals that may induce alopecia, thallium, heparin, coumarins, antimitotic agents, vitamin A, bismuth, and possibly other heavy metals are probably the best known. Thallium disturbs keratinization by interfering with cystine metabolism. Antimitotic drugs, such as cyclophosphamide and methotrexate, inhibit cell multiplication in anagen hair follicles. Excessive vitamin A (hypervitaminosis A) can also produce desquamation and pruritus. Drug reactions and idiosyncrasies should be considered in unexplained alopecias.

Nutrition-related alopecias are rare. Deficiencies in vitamins A and B-12, zinc, fatty acids, and iron have been reported but are poorly documented. Most commercial dog and cat foods are adequately supplemented and well-balanced for normal pets. Dietary supplementation with extra vitamins, fatty acids, and trace minerals is usually not helpful in treating alopecia.

Patchy alopecia may occur in dermatomycosis, superficial bacterial infections, demodicosis, seborrheic dermatitis, allergic contact dermatitis, and alopecia areata. If the etiology can be determined, appropriate therapy is usually curative. Alopecia areata is a disease of unknown etiology characterized by single or multiple hairless areas with slight erythema and tenderness. Later the alopecic areas become smooth and depressed, indicating atrophic changes. Histopathology is suggestive but usually not diagnostic. It may be a form of an autoimmune disease.

Alopecia can be secondary to trauma and other systemic diseases. Flea bite hypersensitivity, sarcoptic mange, and canine atopic dermatitis often result in secondary alopecia owing to the trauma of pruritus. Neoplasia and autoimmune disease can also result in alopecia.

REFERENCES AND SUPPLEMENTAL READING

Anderson, R.K.: Canine hypothyroidism. Comp. Cont. Ed. 1:103, 1979.
Conroy, J.D.: The etiology and pathogenesis of alopecia. Comp. Cont. Ed. 1:806, 1979.
Fitzpatrick, T.B.: *Dermatology in General Medicine.* New York: McGraw-Hill, 1971.
Hightower, D., et al.: Replacement therapy for induced hypothyroidism in dogs. J.A.V.M.A. 163:979, 1973.
Hoge, W. R.: Response to thyrotropin as a diagnostic aid for canine hypothyroidism. J. Am. Anim. Hosp. Assn. 10:167, 1974.
Lorenz, M.D.: Canine hyperadrenocorticism: diagnosis and treatment. Comp. Cont. Ed. 1:315, 1979.
Muller, G.H., and Kirk, R.W.: *Small Animal Dermatology,* 2nd ed. Philadelphia: W.B. Saunders, 1976.
Parker, W.M., and Scott, D.W.: Growth hormone responsive alopecias in the mature dog: a discussion of 13 cases. J.A.A.H.A. 16:824, 1980.
Siegel, E.T. *Endocrine Diseases of the Dog.* Philadelphia: Lea & Febiger, 1977.

Section

7

OPHTHALMOLOGIC DISEASES

CHARLES L. MARTIN, D.V.M.
Consulting Editor

OCULAR EMERGENCIES

THOMAS J. KERN, D.V.M.

Ithaca, N.Y.

Competent primary care for veterinary ocular emergency patients should be prompt, appropriate, and based on an accurate assessment of clinical signs. Presenting complaints may be generally categorized under four headings according to clients' descriptions: red eyes, swollen eyes, cloudy eyes, and sudden vision loss in "normal" eyes with dilated pupils.

RED EYES

The most common causes of red eyes—glaucoma, hyphema, uveitis, and keratoconjunctivitis—must be distinguished from one another.

ACUTE GLAUCOMA

The hallmarks of acute congestive glaucomatous crises include marked deep episcleral vascular injection, mydriasis, variable corneal edema, and vision loss. Diagnosis is confirmed by tonometric readings well above the normal range (15 to 30 mm Hg). History may suggest a sudden onset of signs or acute exacerbation of intermittent or low-grade signs. Gonioscopic evaluation of iridocorneal angle pathology, although desirable, is frequently inhibited by secondary corneal epithelial and stromal edema.

PRIMARY GLAUCOMA

Immediate therapy with hyperosmotic agents is necessary to prevent permanent blindness. Rapid intraocular pressure (IOP) reduction may be accomplished with intravenous mannitol (2 gm/kg of 15 per cent Mannitol, Abbott) or oral glycerin (2 gm/kg, Osmoglyn, Alcon) therapy, which reduces vitreous volume via dehydration and decreases aqueous humor production.

Following this treatment, aqueous outflow improvement should be attempted using two drops of 2 per cent pilocarpine in the eye hourly for four to six hours. The degree of pupillary constriction does not necessarily correlate with angle outflow relief; each effect is mediated by separate mechanisms. Acetazolamide (50 mg/kg IV; Diamox, Lederle) may be given following the previously mentioned ther-

apy to further decrease aqueous humor production. Oral therapy with dichlorphenamide (2 to 4 mg/kg b.i.d. to t.i.d.; Daranide, Merck, Sharp and Dohme), a carbonic anhydrase inhibitor diuretic, should be added to initiate subsequent IOP control. Oral or intravenous rehydration of the patient must be carefully titrated, as intraocular pressure is monitored as frequently as every half hour for the first few hours following treatment. Rapid rehydration may reverse the benefit derived from initial hyperosmotic therapy if aqueous production and outflow have not been effectively modified by pilocarpine and diuretics.

At the earliest convenience during or following IOP control, complete intraocular evaluation must be performed to rule out lens luxation and/or uveitis as precipitating causes of the pressure rise. Surgical filtering procedures or cyclocryotherapy is indicated shortly following initial medical therapy (1) in breeds with historically intractable primary glaucoma, e.g., cocker spaniels, basset hounds, beagles, and Siberian huskies, or (2) when initial medical treatment is ineffective in lowering IOP. Removal of an anteriorly luxated lens is indicated when this is the cause of glaucoma.

HYPHEMA

Appearance of blood in the anterior chamber is a significant clinical sign for which a cause must be sought. Traumatic iris and ciliary body injury, generalized hemostatic defects, intraocular neoplasms, and uveitis may all cause hyphema. Careful historical review combined with physical examination and indicated laboratory profiles (e.g., hemogram and coagulogram) should be employed to pinpoint a specific etiology and formulate a prognosis.

Treatment objectives include control of uveitis (if present), IOP control, enhancement of hemorrhage resolution, and prevention of further bleeding. To these ends, topical 1 per cent atropine drops for cycloplegia and pupillary dilatation to effect, usually two to four times daily, are recommended for uveitis. IOP should be monitored daily and carbonic anhydrase diuretic treatment instituted if secondary glaucoma ensues. Topical corticosteroids may be judiciously used to control signs of intraocular inflammation, although they may delay clot resolution. Some clinicians prefer topical 2 per cent

531

pilocarpine therapy to atropinization. The suggested advantage is increased iris surface area to facilitate fibrinolysis and erythrocyte removal. Activity restriction by sedation or kennel confinement may reduce the risk of rebleeding. Disadvantages include uveitis exacerbation and sequestration of a small pupil with fibrin.

UVEITIS

Causes of acute uveitis include those of exogenous (acute keratitis, trauma) and endogenous origin (immune-mediated, neoplastic, idiopathic). Diagnostic clinical signs include diffuse conjunctival hyperemia, limbal ciliary vascular injection, miosis, iridal swelling, aqueous flare or hypopyon, corneal edema due to endothelial dysfunction, and decreased IOP. Pending investigation of etiology, mydriatic-cycloplegic therapy (1 per cent atropine or 10 per cent phenylephrine-methylscopolamine; Murocoll, Muro) should be instituted to effect. If improvement is not noted within 12 to 48 hours, topical corticosteroids may be added to the treatment regimen, albeit with consideration of a possible septic origin of the uveitis. Subconjunctival and systemic corticosteroid therapy should be reserved until diagnostic evaluation has ruled out infectious agents. Antibiotic use is discretionary.

KERATOCONJUNCTIVITIS

Acutely red eyes exhibiting diffuse capillary hyperemia of the conjunctiva and significant conjunctival swelling (chemosis) with normal pupils, anterior chambers, and IOPs indicate keratoconjunctivitis until proved otherwise. Diagnostic plans should include a Schirmer tear test if ocular discharge is mucoid or mucopurulent; a swab reserved for bacterial culture; conjunctival cytologic examination; nictitans evaluations; and fluorescein dye staining of the cornea.

Suspected acute bacterial conjunctivitis is best treated initially with broad spectrum triple antibiotic (bacitracin-polymyxin B-neomycin; Neosporin, Burroughs-Wellcome) drops or ointments; the incidence of antibiotic resistance to these drugs by primary bacterial isolates is low owing to their infrequent systemic use.

Suspected feline herpetic keratoconjunctivitis may be treated topically with antiviral drugs (idoxuridine ointment [Stoxil, Smith, Kline, and French] four times daily or drops every two hours; vidarabine drops [Vira-A, Parke-Davis] every two hours) as well as antibiotics to cover frequent bacterial superinfections.

Epithelial and stromal corneal ulceration produces reflex conjunctival hyperemia. Etiologic diagnosis followed by antibiotic therapy is indicated. The presence of a foreign body should be ruled out.

Dry eye syndromes, both primary secretory deficiencies and those secondary to conjunctival inflammation, are frequently overlooked as causes or complications of both acute and chronic keratoconjunctivitis. In animals with low Schirmer tear test values, tear replacement must be added to therapy for other problems such as corneal erosion or bacterial conjunctivitis, and this must be continued indefinitely or until tear test values improve.

SWOLLEN EYES

BLEPHARITIS/BLEPHAREDEMA

Treatment of lid swelling is specified by the suspected problems or proven origin. Only three thin tissue layers—skin, orbicularis muscle, and conjunctiva—comprise the eyelid. Clinically detectable eyelid inflammation or swelling necessarily originates within one of these layers but readily involves the other two by local extension.

Sequelae of acute traumatic contusion may be minimized by prompt cold pack application within the first few hours after injury. Topical DMSO gel (Domoso, Diamond) application improves removal of inflammatory fluid transudates.

Acute bacterial infections of meibomian glands and eyelid sebaceous glands present as discrete nodular swellings or, if extensive, diffuse eyelid thickening; occasionally, subconjunctival or subepidermal abscesses develop. Frequent topical broad spectrum antibiotic ointment use followed by warm compresses usually hastens recovery. Stubborn or recurrent infections should be pursued with bacterial culture. Ophthalmia neonatorum or infectious blepharoconjunctivitis of kittens and puppies prior to eyelid opening must be attended to promptly and correctly to prevent or minimize blinding corneal damage. Eyelid margins should be either gently separated manually or carefully incised to establish drainage of purulent discharge and provide medication access. Attentive nursing care is required to remove all ocular discharge prior to frequent broad spectrum antibiotic ointment instillation. Healing of associated secondary keratitis and uveitis must be monitored. If the bacterial infection is under control, healing of the separated lid margins usually occurs without functional impairment.

Angioneurotic eyelid edema may follow venomous insect stings or bites as a local reaction or may be part of a systemic reaction. Usually more dramatic in appearance than actually serious, this reaction may be inhibited by parenteral corticosteroid therapy (e.g., 0.1 to 0.5. mg/lb prednisone SID) and cold compress application. Recurrent episodes of such swelling in older animals may be caused by a periocular mast cell neoplasm.

CHEMOSIS

Marked conjunctival swelling occurs when the conjunctival vasculature's permeability to intravascular fluids is increased. The vasoactive chemical mediators of inflammation govern the appearance and resolution of such swelling. Hence, severe conjunctival inflammations due to almost any cause appear clinically similar.

The most frequent cause of feline chemosis is incipient upper respiratory agent infection, including viruses (herpesvirus, calicivirus), chlamydia, and mycoplasma. Conjunctival cytology may confirm infection with one of the two last-named agents if characteristic epithelial cell inclusions are noted. Topical and systemic broad spectrum antibiotic therapy (e.g., tetracycline) is indicated. A thorough ocular examination should rule out corneal and intraocular involvement. Topical antiviral therapy (see Keratoconjunctivitis) may be added.

Chemical keratoconjunctivitis resulting from accidental instillation of household chemicals, pesticide sprays, and powders may produce dramatic chemosis. Prompt vigorous irrigation of the external eye with eyewash is the first priority. Topical antibiotic instillation is always indicated; topical corticosteroids initially are helpful but must not be continued if corneal ulceration is present or if alkali was the offending chemical agent. Conscientious follow-up examination is required to avoid iatrogenic corticosteroid-related complications.

Blunt external eye injury may implant a foreign body within the eyelids or conjunctiva, which may be concealed by chemosis. As an aid to diagnosis as well as a nonspecific treatment, use of topical hyperosmotic ointments to effect (40 per cent glucose ointment, Smith, Miller, and Patch; 5 per cent sodium chloride ointment, Muro 128, Muro) is usually indicated. Within minutes to hours, chemosis will decrease enough to allow thorough external ocular examination (and foreign body identification) and to make the patient more comfortable. As conjunctival inflammation resolves, however, hyperosmotic ointments should be discontinued, as they are irritating to the normal conjunctiva.

ORBITAL CELLULITIS

Hallmarks of acute orbital inflammation are rapid onset of exophthalmos, nictitans prolapse, and pain elicitation on extension or flexion of the temporomandibular joint. Variable clinical signs include chemosis, strabismus, restricted ocular motility, and exposure keratoconjunctivitis.

Prior to therapeutic intervention, the clinician should review the potential origins and sequelae of orbital cellulitis. Primary orbital soft tissue inflammation may arise as zygomatic sialoadenitis, lacrimal adenitis, foreign body migration and/or penetration with sepsis (introduced through the oropharynx, conjunctival sac, or eyelids), eosinophilic temporalis myositis, or periodontal abscess. Secondary orbital extension of chronic bacterial or mycotic paranasal sinus infections may produce apparently acute clinical signs. Traumatic injury to the orbital bones and soft tissues (e.g., gunshot wounds) may result in secondary inflammation. Orbital neoplasms seldom produce acute clinical signs unless associated with orbital hemorrhage or tumor necrosis. In the acute episode, diagnostic discrimination between these possible causes is often equivocal despite careful physical examination aided by skull radiography.

Complications of severe untreated or chronic nonresponsive orbital inflammation include optic nerve atrophy, enophthalmos and restricted ocular motility associated with orbital fibrosis and fat atrophy, and exposure keratitis and dry eye syndromes with their sequelae.

Therapy of acute inflammation of presumed bacterial origin should combine broad spectrum systemic antibiotic and hot compress administration. Accessory surgical treatment may include, at the clinician's discretion, peroral drainage of sequestered exudate via incision behind the ipsilateral last upper molar tooth, probing with a blunt instrument, and establishment of a draining tract. This procedure seldom results in immediate drainage of pus but is frequently credited (along with concomitant antibiotic treatment) with marked clinical improvement within 24 hours. This surgery has attendant complications: (1) orbital superinfection with oral bacterial contaminants, and (2) possible damage to optic nerve and large orbital blood vessels during incision. Thus, surgical drainage is best avoided or initially delayed in relatively mild orbital inflammation.

If the above therapy has not resulted in improvement within 24 to 48 hours, the clinician may tentatively assess that nonspecific inflammation is responsible and augment antibiotic treatment with low dose anti-inflammatory systemic corticosteroid administration (e.g., 0.1 mg/lb prednisone SID) for a few days. Resolution of inflammation may be assessed based on degree of remaining exophthalmos and nictitans prolapse and reduction of pain induced during jaw opening.

If signs of orbital cellulitis recur within a few weeks of its apparent improvement, a retained orbital foreign body (e.g., migrating plant material) or a tooth root abscess is the likely cause.

TRAUMATIC PROPTOSIS OF THE GLOBE

The appearance of a proptosed globe instills the pet owner with horror; consequently, nearly all patients with globe proptosis are presented for emergency care.

The pathogenesis of traumatic proptosis involves conformational predisposition and/or forceful blunt trauma applied directly to the orbit and at least indirectly to the eyeball itself. Numerous dog breeds (including but not limited to brachycephalic breeds) and a few cat breeds are characterized by rather large eyeballs situated within small, shallow orbits and tenuously protected by loose, poorly conforming eyelids. In many such individuals, only minimal trauma is required to proptose one or both globes. Animals with normal globe-eyelid-orbit conformation may still sustain proptosis injury, but the traumatic insult responsible is generally major, e.g., automobile accident.

Except for catastrophic globe laceration or rupture, the single most important determinant of vision following injury is extent of the optic nerve damage sustained at impact. If the nerve, with attendant ciliary nerves and blood vessels, is instantly transected, no therapy will prevent blindness. If functional optic nerve damage is not irreversible, intelligent therapy may improve visual outcome.

Formulation of vision prognosis, except in cases in which the optic nerve is visibly transected, is usually inaccurate on initial presentation. Favorable indications are a menace response, direct and consensual pupillary light reflexes originating in the damaged eye, presence of normal retinal vasculature, and short elapsed time between injury and treatment. Unfavorable clinical signs include extensive hyphema, corneal or scleral laceration, obvious retinal detachment, pale fundus vasculature, and marked hypotony. Absolute pupil size is an unreliable indication, as for example, mydriasis may result from oculomotor nerve damage alone or miosis may be a direct traumatic uveitis effect regardless of posterior segment integrity. In general, all proptosed globes of relatively acute presentation without corneoscleral laceration or rupture should be surgically replaced. Even if ultimately blind, such eyes may often be salvaged for cosmetic appearance.

Broadly stated, the objectives of therapy are globe replacement, optic neuritis prevention and treatment, and ocular surface protection. Paracentesis of the globe is *never* indicated.

Minimal hair clipping and surgical preparation are indicated. Under general anesthesia or local anesthetic infiltration, a lateral canthotomy is performed with blunt tipped surgical scissors. This maneuver usually relieves eyelid entrapment at the orbital rim, allowing gently applied pressure on the globe to replace it within the orbit. Frequently, orbital hemorrhage and edema prevent complete replacement, leaving residual exophthalmos. A temporary tarsorrhaphy is performed using 3-0 or 4-0 silk or monofilament nylon horizontal mattress sutures placed through stents in the upper and lower lids of rubber (e.g., short pieces of Penrose drain tubing) or polyethylene tubing. Sutures should pass through the lid skin anterior (external) to the tarsal gland openings on the lid margin to prevent accidental corneal injury when sutures are tightened into place. Two to four snug sutures are sufficient. Near the medial canthus the eyelids should remain slightly separated to allow medication access. The lateral canthotomy may be closed with two suture layers: 4-0 polyglactin (Vicryl, Ethicon) or 4-0 polyglycolic acid (Dexon, Davis and Geck) sutures apposing the deeper subcutaneous layers, and 4-0 silk or nylon horizontal mattress sutures in the skin.

Topical broad spectrum antibiotic and 1 per cent atropine ointments should be administered t.i.d. near the medial canthus to lubricate the cornea and conjunctiva, prevent infection of corneal abrasions, and control traumatic uveitis. Topical corticosteroids are generally contraindicated at presentation owing to their retardation of corneal wound healing.

To treat traumatic optic neuritis, high doses (0.5 to 1.0 mg/lb prednisone SID) of systemic corticosteroids should be given daily for seven days, then tapered and discontinued over the succeeding 14 days. Systemic antibiotic therapy for a similar duration is advisable. The efficacy of such systemically administered medications depends on a functionally intact vascular supply to the orbital optic nerve and posterior segment of the eye.

Seven to ten days following tarsorrhaphy placement, sutures may be removed either all at once or sequentially. The advantage of removing one suture every other day, leaving the most medial and lateral sutures until last, is easier management of residual exophthalmos and lagophthalmos while orbital hemorrhage resolves and eyelid function improves. Lateral or superolateral strabismus due to tearing of medial rectus and/or inferior oblique muscles commonly remains permanently, although over a period of many months globe position may deviate back toward normal. Topical therapy should be modified as assessment of healing keratitis and uveitis is made. In severely exophthalmic animals, bilateral permanent partial tarsorrhaphy should be considered to discourage future proptosis recurrence.

EYELID LACERATIONS

Surgical correction of lid lacerations should be prompt and must restore functional conformation while encouraging healing of tissue in constant motion. In individual animals, loss of up to one-third of the length of the lid margin may be managed without functional impairment. Careful apposition of skin and conjunctival and marginal edges should be the surgeon's goal. The reader is referred to contemporary veterinary ophthalmic surgery texts for details.

CLOUDY EYE

Diagnosis of cloudy eyes presented as emergencies must rule out corneoscleral laceration, descemetocele, uveitis, and glaucoma (previously discussed). In these conditions corneal opacity is mediated via epithelial or endothelial dysfunction, allowing overhydration of the corneal stroma. Corneal endothelium is most responsible for clarity control, and changes in its function create the densest corneal edema.

CORNEAL LACERATION

Full thickness corneal injury results in local endothelial and epithelial damage surrounding the wound. The corneal stroma hydrates, thickens, and may temporarily seal the wound edges, especially if iris prolapse has not occurred. Treatment objectives include sealing the wound, preventing sepsis, and preventing self-mutilation. Under general anesthesia, the conjunctival sac should be thoroughly irrigated with normal saline solution. The prolapsed iris should be excised with electrocautery, the remaining iris separated from the wound edges, and the corneal wound sutured using 6-0 silk, monofilament nylon, polyglactin (Vicryl, Ethicon), or polyglycolic acid polymer (Dexon, Davis and Geck) simple interrupted sutures in a pattern that passes through two-thirds of the stroma. At the surgeon's discretion the corneal wound can then be covered by a conjunctival hood flap.

In the presence of patent corneal wounds, the use of ointments is contraindicated until they are closed. The ointment vehicle, if it penetrates directly into the eye, may induce intractable uveitis.

DESCEMETOCELE

Stromal ulceration deep to Descemet's membrane heralds impending ocular perforation and demands prompt attention. At presentation the cause may not be evident. Corneal ulcers of such severity are best managed surgically with adjunctive medical therapy.

Closure of small (<5 mm diameter) descemetoceles may be accomplished using 6-0 polyglactin (Vicryl, Ethicon) or polyglycolic acid (Dexon, Davis and Geck) simple interrupted or horizontal mattress sutures. Larger defects cannot be closed with sutures.

More frequently useful is a hood or 360° conjunctival flap, which gives immediate coverage of the ulcer, quick adhesion of subconjunctival tissue to the wound, and instant patching of corneal perforations. Contemporary veterinary ophthalmology texts diagram many ways to employ these flaps. Nictitans flaps are poor second choices because they lend little physical support to the weakened cornea, do not adhere to the wound, and prevent daily examination of the eye.

COLLAGENASE-MEDIATED RAPID CORNEAL ULCERATION

These serious corneal ulcers present a gray mucinous appearance; untreated, they quickly deepen and perforate. The corneal stroma liquefies and opacifies as corneal collagen is destroyed by bacterial proteases and/or endogenous corneal collagenase. Peracute inflammatory cellular influx ensues. The ulceration assumes a clear zone as it nears Descemet's membrane. The bacterial organism most often implicated in the evolution of these ulcerations is *Pseudomonas* species, but others may be involved. Unchecked, corneal liquefaction leads to perforation and endophthalmitis within hours.

The most critical diagnostic step is recognition of the progressive nature of the ulcer. Corneal scrapings taken from the ulcer periphery may show neutrophils and gram negative bacilli suggestive of *Pseudomonas* infection. A culture swab taken from the ulcer periphery should be incubated in thioglycollate enrichment broth overnight, then placed onto conventional growth media for bacterial identification and antibiotic sensitivity assessment.

Medical therapy, however, must be started immediately. Topical ophthalmic gentamycin (Garamycin, Schering) or tobramycin (Tobrex, Alcon) solution should be administered at least hourly until signs of stromal liquefaction abate, which may be within hours or not for several days. At that point, frequency of instillation may be reduced. One per cent atropine ophthalmic drops should be used to effect to maintain pupil dilatation and control secondary uveitis. To irreversibly inactivate destructive collagenase enzyme activity, topical acetylcysteine drops (Mucomyst, Mead-Johnson) diluted to 10 per cent concentration should be instilled every one to two hours until corneal liquefaction ceases to progress. Because topical therapy affects only the anterior segment of the eyes, compatible systemic antibiotic treatment (e.g., gentamycin or ampicillin at conventional dosages) should be instituted to protect the eye's posterior segment. Neither drug penetrates the eye well under normal circumstances but both do so during intraocular inflammation. Experimental data suggest that subconjunctival gentamycin injection probably is not medically superior to hourly topical administration when the cornea is ulcerated, but it is recommended when intensive topical therapy cannot be maintained.

Conjunctival flap placement is contraindicated in the face of acute corneal infection but may be considered useful to support deep stromal defects once infection is eliminated.

Topical antibiotic therapy should be modified based on bacterial sensitivity results and clinical response. It should be continued until epithelial regeneration is complete. Corticosteroid use is contraindicated while infection persists but may become useful to minimize later corneal neovascularization and scarring.

If intraocular perforation through an infected corneal wound occurs, the prognosis for vision and retention of the globe is poor. Corneal infection therapy notwithstanding, such eyes may be best managed by enucleation.

SUDDEN VISION LOSS WITH DILATED PUPILS

OPTIC NEURITIS

Emergency presentation of animals suddenly blind with dilated, unresponsive pupils bilaterally should suggest to the clinician acute retinal and/or optic nerve dysfunction. If the fundus background appears normal, implication of the optic nerve as the problem is reasonable, even when the optic disc appears normal. At times the only fundus pathology may be a swollen optic disc with overlying retinal hemorrhages and detachment of the surrounding retina.

The causes of optic neuritis are poorly defined, although canine distemper virus and other neoplastic and inflammatory neurologic disorders (e.g., reticulosis) have been documented. In the absence of localizing neurologic or physical examination findings, therapy is nonspecific. Prior to therapy, cerebrospinal fluid should be examined for evidence of inflammation, hemorrhage, xanthochromia, and protein, any of which might suggest a specific etiology. The majority of cases must be classified as idiopathic. Systemic corticosteroids are administered orally (0.5 to 1.0 mg/lb prednisone SID). Retrobulbar injection of repositol corticosteroid (methylprednisolone acetate [Depo-Medrol, Upjohn] or betamethasone valerate [Betavet Soluspan,

Schering]) may be performed, but its local anti-inflammatory effect would be expected to benefit only inflammation of the orbital portion of the optic nerves. The hazards of retrobulbar injection should be reviewed before using this technique. Adjunctive systemic antibiotic therapy may be indicated at the clinician's discretion.

Oral corticosteroids may be continued at initial levels for up to 14 days. If vision and pupillary light reflexes improve, prognosis is guarded and continuation of therapy indefinitely on an alternate-morning regimen is recommended. If no improvement is noted within two to three weeks, corticosteroid dosage should be reduced, then discontinued, as vision prognosis is poor.

PRESUMED TOXIC RETINOPATHY

Many dogs presenting with signs of optic neuritis have been examined and treated unsuccessfully, only to find on post-mortem ocular examination irreversible degeneration of the outer retinal layers, specifically the rod and cone photoreceptors, and normal optic nerves. No clinical fundus pathology had been detected. The etiologies of such retinal degeneration have been presumed to involve some type of intoxication, though proof has yet to be forthcoming.

This assessment should be borne in mind for dogs and cats that remain blind despite appropriate optic neuritis therapy. Unless the clinician has access to clinical electroretinography, the diagnostic differentiation of optic neuritis from retinotoxicity must be one of exclusion.

SUPPLEMENTAL READING

Bistner, S. I., Aguirre, G., and Batik, B.: *Atlas of Veterinary Ophthalmic Surgery.* Philadelphia: W. B. Saunders Co., 1977.
Slatter, D.: *Fundamentals of Veterinary Ophthalmology.* Philadelphia: W. B. Saunders Co., 1981.
Winston, S. M.: Ocular emergencies. Vet. Clin. North Am. 11:59, 1981.
Wyman, M.: Ocular emergencies. *In* Kirk, R. W. (ed.): *Current Veterinary Therapy VII.* Philadelphia: W. B. Saunders Co., 1980, pp. 542–546.

DISEASES OF THE EYELID

ROBERT J. MUNGER, D.V.M.
Knoxville, Tennessee

The eyelid of domestic animals basically consists of a layer of skin and orbicularis oculi muscle, a layer of tarsoconjunctiva, and glandular elements associated with the conjunctiva, marginal tissues, and eyelid cilia. Because the tarsal plate is very poorly developed in domestic animals as compared with humans and primates, most of the support and shape of the lid is contributed by the lid margin. The eyelids function to protect the eye, to spread the tear film over the eye, and to facilitate drainage of the tears from the conjunctival sac via the lacrimal punctae. Therefore, prompt diagnosis and correction of eyelid defects and diseases can be extremely important to the continued health of the eye. Extensive descriptions of surgical procedures are beyond the scope of this discussion. Recently published textbooks on veterinary ophthalmology and ophthalmic plastic surgery as well as several survey articles contain excellent discussions of eyelid surgeries and are listed in the Supplemental Reading section.

STRUCTURAL AND FUNCTIONAL DEFECTS OF THE EYELIDS

COLOBOMAS

Colobomas of the lids are congenital defects that may range from a small notch in the lid margin to complete absence of the lid. Small colobomas may interfere little with normal lid and tear function, but large defects can result in significant corneal exposure with severe keratitis. Severe exposure can result in perforating corneal ulcers. Artificial tears as well as ocular protectants and lubricants (Lacrilube or Duratears)* should be administered as needed to minimize corneal exposure and drying until the defect can be corrected surgically. With large defects (greater than one-third of the lid), closure may require the use of advancement flaps, bridge flaps, or cross-lid flaps from the opposite lid.

SIZE OF THE PALPEBRAL FISSURE

Congenital abnormalities in the size of the palpebral fissure occur occasionally and are more common in dogs than in other species. Abnormally small palpebral fissures (blepharophimosis, micropalpebral fissure) may occur concurrent with microphthalmia or other ocular anomalies. This defect occurs in chows, Kerry blue terriers, collies, Shetland sheepdogs, and bull terriers. Correction, when desired, is accomplished with a lateral canthoplasty to lengthen the palpebral fissure. The most common technique is von Ammon's lateral canthoplasty in which the temporal conjunctiva is undermined and sutured to the skin edges of the lateral canthotomy incision. Care must be exercised to avoid tension on the conjunctiva, which would result in a shallow and unsightly conjunctival sac (Fox, 1976; Bistner et al., 1977).

Abnormally large palpebral fissures (euryblepharon, macropalpebral fissures) are most commonly observed in brachycephalic dogs with exophthalmos and in St. Bernards and Newfoundlands with associated entropion and/or ectropion. These defects may result in corneal exposure with subsequent drying and irritation from periocular hair. The brachycephalic breeds experience a greater risk for ocular proptosis. Partial, temporary relief may be gained through the use of artificial tears and ocular lubricants. Correction is achieved by shortening the palpebral fissure by a lateral or medial tarsorrhaphy (Fox, 1976; Jenson, 1979). Eye position, lid conformation, and facial features must be considered when choosing between a lateral or medial approach to achieve the best postoperative appearance. In patients with associated lid defects (ectropion, entropion, and so on), multiple surgeries may be required to achieve optimal function and cosmetic improvement.

ANKYLOBLEPHARON AND SYMBLEPHARON

A physiologic, congenital ankyloblepharon (adhesion or fusion of the upper and lower lids along their margins) occurs in dogs and cats and persists for the first 10 to 15 days of life. Premature opening of the eyelids may require treatment with protective ointments and/or temporary tarsorrhaphies until maturation of the cornea and adnexal structures is complete and normal tear function is established (usually complete by 16 days of age).

Delayed opening of the eyelids is more commonly encountered than premature opening. When eyelid opening is delayed, infectious keratoconjunctivitis (neonatal ophthalmia) may develop behind the

---

*Lacrilube, Allergan Pharmaceuticals, Irvine, CA.
Duratears, Alcon Laboratories, Fort Worth, TX.

closed lids, causing the lids to appear distended or swollen. Purulent exudate may be noted at the medial canthus. The infection is usually caused by staphylococci in puppies, although *E. coli* and other bacteria have been incriminated. Neonatal keratoconjunctivitis in kittens is most commonly associated with upper respiratory infections caused by *Chlamydia psittaci* or *Herpes felis*. To minimize damage to the cornea and globe, the lids should be bluntly separated and the exudates irrigated from the conjunctival sac. Separation of the lids can usually be accomplished by carefully inserting one blade of a blunt scissors behind the lids at the lateral canthus and advancing them medially so that no cutting action is used and the normal lid margins are preserved. Cultures of the conjunctival sac with antibiotic sensitivities should be obtained. Broad spectrum topical antibiotic ophthalmic ointments should be instilled in the eyes four to six times daily, and the antibiotic should be changed if indicated by bacterial antibiotic sensitivity. Warm compresses and repeated irrigation of purulent debris from the conjunctival sac are beneficial. Systemic antibiotics are indicated with severe infections, especially when systemic or intraocular infection is suspected. Kittens with systemic *Herpes felis* infections require extensive supportive care and may die regardless of therapy.

Symblepharon is an adhesion of one or both lids to the eyeball and is classified as anterior, not involving the fornix; posterior, involving only the fornix; or complete, involving the entire surface between the lid and the eyeball. Such adhesions may be congenital, as seen in Siamese cats, or acquired as a sequela of trauma, severe conjunctivitis, or keratoconjunctivitis (e.g., neonatal ophthalmitis). When the adhesions are small, simple resection followed by frequent administration of topical ophthalmic antibiotic-corticosteroid ointments may be sufficient. When adhesions are extensive, surgical reconstruction of the conjunctival sac is necessary. Rotating or advancement flaps of bulbar conjunctiva or free grafts of nasal or buccal mucosa can be used to prevent readhesion of the bulbar and palpebral surfaces.

Lagophthalmos

Lagophthalmos is an incomplete closure of the eyelids and occurs most commonly with exophthalmos in brachycephalic breeds. It also occurs with facial nerve paralysis. Failure to achieve complete closure of the lids when blinking (except possibly during forced closure) is noted during the ocular exam, and the owner may have noticed that the dog sleeps with the lids partially opened. Persistent or repeated central corneal ulceration often occurs as a result of exposure and drying of the central cornea. The ulcers may rapidly progress to perforation in severe cases. Treatment consists of medial or lateral permanent tarsorrhaphy to reduce the palpebral fissure by one-third and to decrease corneal exposure. Supportive care consists of the administration of ocular lubricants and artificial tears.

Dermoids

Dermoids, choristomas of skin and dermal appendages, occasionally involve the eyelids as well as the conjunctiva and/or cornea. In some cases, especially when the aberrant tissue is located at or near the lateral canthus, the dermoid may cause little or no irritation and is mainly a cosmetic problem. In other cases the hairs growing from the tumor cause significant ocular irritation. Treatment is by excision of the abnormal tissue and reconstruction of the lids. The lesion may recur with incomplete excision. As with colobomas, dermoids involving large portions of the eyelid may require extensive reconstructive blepharoplasty.

Eyelash abnormalities

Numerous cilia are normally present on the upper lids of most domestic animals. The lower lids of most carnivores lack cilia, and in species in which they are present on the lower lids they are usually shorter and finer than those of the upper eyelids. Most eyelash abnormalities are congenital, but they may occasionally develop secondary to trauma or chronic blepharitis. Dogs are more frequently affected than any other species, and clinical signs are those of extraocular irritation (blepharospasm, epiphora, conjunctival hyperemia). Corneal vascularization and pigmentation with or without corneal ulceration may be present. The three types of eyelash abnormalities are trichiasis, distichiasis, and ectopic cilia.

Trichiasis occurs when hairs arising from normal sites contact the cornea or conjunctiva. This most commonly occurs in conjunction with one or more of the following: entropion, blepharospasm, dermoids, cicatricial defects, and prominent or excessive nasal folds in brachycephalic breeds. Temporary relief can be achieved with ocular lubricants or ointments that reduce ocular irritation from the cilia. In dogs with prominent nasal folds, petrolatum or moustache wax may be used to "wax" down the hairs and prevent contact with the eye. The underlying abnormality should be surgically corrected as soon as possible. A permanent, medial tarsorrhaphy may be performed as an alternative to excising excessive nasal folds in exophthalmic, brachycephalic breeds.

Distichiasis occurs when lashes or cilia originate from abnormally located follicles in the lid margin. The cilia arise from the area of the ducts of the meibomian glands. They may be singular or multiple and involve one or more lids. The condition is thought to be hereditary. Distichiasis occurs most commonly in dogs, with the following breeds most often affected: American cocker spaniel, golden retriever, Shih-Tzu, toy and miniature poodle, Shetland sheepdog, boxer, Bedlington terrier, and Yorkshire terrier. Animals require no treatment as long as they are asymptomatic, such as when the lashes are fine and tend to float on the tear film without causing irritation. When a patient is symptomatic, the frequent use of ocular lubricants and/or plucking the lashes will provide temporary relief. Electroepilation, lid splitting, partial tarsal plate excision, and transconjunctival resection of the lash follicles have been recommended for the treatment of distichiasis. Electroepilation is effective if there are few lashes, but it is tedious and may cause excessive scarring when lashes are numerous. Regrowth of epilated lashes may occur if electrolysis does not completely destroy the follicle. Lid splitting and other procedures designed to resect the lash follicles require surgical precision and high magnification. Distichiasis forceps facilitate surgery by clamping the lid margin, thereby allowing accurate sharp dissection while controlling hemorrhage. All of these procedures except transconjunctival resection weaken the lid margin and result in a certain degree of scarring. Lashes will regrow from any follicles that are missed or incompletely resected, and subsequent procedures contribute further to scarring and deformity of the lid margins.

A simpler procedure requiring less technical skill and no specialized instruments involves a modification of the Hotz-Celsus procedure for entropion. An initial incision is made on the anterior lid surface 1 to 2 mm from the lid margin. A second incision is made 2 mm farther from the margin parallel to the first incision. The intervening strip of skin is excised and the incision closed with simple interrupted sutures of 5-0 and 6-0 silk. Postoperatively, an Elizabethan collar is used to prevent self-mutilation, and an antibiotic-corticosteroid ophthalmic ointment is applied to the eyes three times daily. The sutures are removed in seven days. This creates a slight eversion of the lid margin, thus rolling the offending lashes away from the globe. Since the incisions are close to the lid margin, the eversion does not create significant ectropion. Occasionally, the procedure must be repeated if the degree of eversion is not sufficient to resolve the problem. An added advantage to this procedure is the preservation of the lid margin, which ensures normal shape and support for the eyelid.

Ectopic cilia are cilia that arise from the meibomian glands and emerge through the palpebral conjunctiva. One or more cilia may be present, and detection requires careful examination using a bright light source and magnification. Ectopic cilia usually produce intense irritation and paracentral corneal ulcers corresponding to the position of the cilia. Treatment is by en bloc resection of the cilia with the surrounding conjunctiva and the involved meibomian gland. The conjunctiva is allowed to heal by second intention, and postoperative care consists of topical antibiotic-corticosteroid ophthalmic ointment application three to four times daily for seven to ten days.

ENTROPION

Entropion is an inward rolling of the lid margin and may be congenital or acquired. It is further classified as primary or secondary. Primary entropion is usually bilateral and is frequently hereditary. In the dog it is encountered most often in chows, Chinese Shar-peis, Labrador retrievers, golden retrievers, Chesapeake Bay retrievers, Irish setters, Doberman pinschers, St. Bernards, Great Danes, and English bulldogs. Although much less common in the cat, it does occur in Persians. Secondary entropion is usually unilateral and may occur with scarring of the lids after trauma or with severe blepharospasm (i.e., spastic entropion). Entropion, especially involving the upper lids, is usually more severe in breeds with excessive facial skin folds (chows, Chinese Shar-peis, and bloodhounds), since the weight and proximity of the folds to the eye contribute to the inward rolling of the lids.

Entropion causes signs ranging from mild epiphora to severe blepharospasm with corneal vascularization, edema, pigmentation, and ulceration. Affected animals will often paw or rub the eyes and may exhibit purulent conjunctivitis and photophobia. Severe corneal granulation tissue may develop in chronic cases.

When determining the extent of lid involvement prior to surgical correction of entropion, it is important to eliminate blepharospasm associated with pain and ocular irritation by applying an appropriate topical local anesthetic to the eye. Blepharospasm increases the degree of entropion and leads to an exaggerated assessment of the anatomic defect. Inevitably, this would result in overcorrection of the entropion. Local anesthetics should only be used diagnostically and never for the treatment of pain or ocular irritation, since they are damaging to the corneal epithelium. Spastic entropion is treated by correcting the inciting cause of the ocular irritation. Although this cause may be removed, irritation from secondary trichiasis may persist, and it is often necessary to perform a temporary tarsorrhaphy to hold the lids in normal position until all signs of irritation have subsided. Correction of entropion of the upper and lower lids without involvement of the medial or lateral canthi is best accomplished by a modified Hotz-Celsus procedure or a Y-V blepharoplasty (Bistner et al., 1977; Gelatt, 1981). The latter is particularly beneficial when correcting cicatricial entropion. When the medial aspect of the upper and lower lids is involved in exophthalmic breeds, a permanent medial tarsorrhaphy will simultaneously resolve the entropion and narrow the palpebral fissure. Entropion involving the lateral canthus may be corrected with a lateral canthoplasty either alone or in combination with a modified Hotz-Celsus procedure. When lateral canthal entropion accompanies euryblepharon, a permanent, lateral tarsorrhaphy may be employed in combination with the previously mentioned procedures.

Postponing surgery is often desired in very young and/or debilitated patients. There are two immediate advantages when this can be done without risk of corneal ulceration (and possible perforation) or extensive corneal vascularization, pigmentation, and scarring. First, increased age and improved condition of the patient reduce the anesthetic risk. Second, the surgeon will be better able to assess the degree of lid correction required. Extensive changes in the facial features, head size, and head shape occur during maturation. In debilitated animals, dehydration and loss of body fat enhance enophthalmos, thus accentuating the degree of entropion. With mild entropion causing little or no corneal irritation, surgery may be delayed with little risk as long as the animal is observed daily. Topical ocular lubricants will decrease corneal irritation. With severe entropion prompt correction is more crucial, but a temporary tarsorrhaphy using local anesthesia will hold the lids in normal position and allow temporary postponement (one to three weeks). During that period antibiotic ointments should be applied four times daily through the lid margins at the medial or lateral canthus. This technique has been used successfully in three- to four-week old chows and Chinese Shar-peis. In a few cases the entropion was improved or resolved when the tarsorrhaphy sutures were removed.

ECTROPION

Ectropion is an outward rolling or drooping of the lid. It may arise as a primary familial defect or secondary to trauma and scarring of the lid. Ectropion occurs commonly in the hound breeds and is considered a breed characteristic in basset hounds and bloodhounds. St. Bernards and spaniels are also commonly affected. Ocular irritation with ectropion is related to corneal and conjunctival exposure and the accumulation of debris in the lower conjunctival sac. This results in chronic conjunctivitis, which can lead to decreased tear production and secondary corneal disease.

Primary ectropion with only mild conjunctivitis may be managed conservatively by regular flushing of debris from the conjunctival sacs with a sterile collyrium and by administration of topical antibiotic-corticosteroid ophthalmic ointments as needed to control periodic conjunctivitis. In cases of severe conjunctival exposure, surgical correction is indicated. The modified Kuhnt-Szymanowski procedure is a simple and effective method for correction of primary ectropion, whereas the correction of cicatricial ectropion requires a V-Y blepharoplasty (Bistner et al., 1977). In the St. Bernard and other giant breeds such as the Great Pyrenees and Newfoundlands, the central lid may be ectropic while the lateral and occasionally the medial portions are entropic. In such cases correction may require more extensive blepharoplastic procedures. Lateral canthoplasty, alone or in combination with a modified Hotz-Celsus procedure or a permanent lateral tarsorrhaphy, may be required. Multiple surgical procedures may be necessary to achieve the desired cosmetic results, and the surgeon should avoid trying to accomplish too much at one time.

INFLAMMATIONS OF THE EYELIDS

Blepharitis is a general term describing any inflammation of the eyelids. It may be classified pathologically as deep or superficial; focal or diffuse; acute, subacute, or chronic; and granulomatous or nongranulomatous. Blepharitis may be caused by bacteria, fungi, parasites, trauma, toxic substances, or immune-mediated mechanisms. The signs of blepharitis include epiphora, blepharospasm, hyperemia, swelling, ulceration, serous to purulent exudation, alopecia, scaling, encrustations, and pruritus. Conjunctivitis or keratoconjunctivitis may be present. Skin scrapings, exfoliative cytology, biopsy, and fungal and bacterial cultures with sensitivities are valuable diagnostic procedures.

HORDEOLUM

A hordeolum is an acute, purulent infection of an eyelash follicle (external hordeolum or stye) or of the meibomian glands (internal hordeolum). A painful, reddened, localized swelling is visible on one or both sides of the lid. *Staphylococcus aureus* is most frequently the causative agent. Treatment by application of warm compresses to the site will promote localization and exteriorization of the abscess. The site may then be surgically drained. Topical ophthalmic antibiotic ointments applied to the lid and conjunctival sac are beneficial, and systemic antibiotics are indicated in severe cases. Expression of the contents of these abscesses is contraindicated, as it may result in spread of the infection into surrounding tissues.

CHALAZION

A chalazion is a localized, painless swelling of a meibomian gland resulting from blockage of the duct with inspissated glandular secretions. Rupture of the gland results in spread of the glandular secretions into adjacent tissues and the formation of a lipid granuloma. The swelling is usually yellow in color and is best seen on the conjunctival side of the lid. Incision and curettage of the lesion through the conjunctival surface is curative and is facilitated by general anesthesia and eversion of the lid with a chalazion clamp. A topical antibiotic-corticosteroid ophthalmic preparation should be administered three times daily for seven to ten days postoperatively.

BACTERIAL BLEPHARITIS

Bacterial infections of the eyelids are usually due to staphylococci or streptococci. Infection may be primary or secondary to conjunctivitis, dacryocystitis, generalized seborrhea, or systemic pyodermas. A purulent exudate is generally present, and the lid margins may be depigmented, hyperemic, and swollen. Eversion of the affected lid usually reveals abscessed meibomian glands. Acute infections can often be treated effectively by draining such abscesses, applying warm compresses to the lids, and applying topical broad spectrum antibiotic ophthalmic ointments four times daily. Systemic antibiotics should be given in severe cases.

Chronic nonresponsive cases may occur with staphylococcal hypersensitivity, immune deficiencies, and/or debilitating diseases. Pyogranulomas may develop in such cases. Cultures obtained from the lid margin and conjunctival sac allow identification of the offending organism and specific selection of appropriate antibiotics. Treatment requires systemic antibiotics as well as application of topical antibiotics and warm compresses. Intralesional antibiotic injections should be used if pyogranulomas are present. Autogenous staphylococcal vaccines have proved beneficial in some cases. The effect of these vaccines may be related to hyposensitization or to nonspecific stimulation of T cell–mediated immunity. Topical and systemic corticosteroids may also be beneficial when used in conjunction with antibiotics.

MYCOTIC BLEPHARITIS

Blepharodermatomycosis is usually associated with generalized *Microsporum* and *Trichophyton* skin infections. Fungal culture of skin scrapings is usually diagnostic. Alopecia, scaling, and hyperemia of the lids are generally present. Topical treatment of the lids with miconazole nitrate (Conofite)* and oral griseofulvin (Grifungal, Fulvicin)† at a dose of

50 to 110 mg/kg daily for six weeks is usually curative.

PARASITIC BLEPHARITIS

Demodex canis is a common cause of canine parasitic blepharitis, whereas *Notoedres cati* is often the causative agent in feline parasitic blepharitis. Both may involve only the lids or may occur as part of a generalized process. Generalized sarcoptic mange could also involve the lids. Alopecia and hyperemia with scaling or moist edema are characteristic clinical signs, and animals with sarcoptic or notoedric mange usually exhibit marked pruritus. Diagnosis is confirmed by examination of skin scrapings. Isofluorphate (Floropryl 0.025 per cent)‡ or neostigmine ointment may be massaged into the lids once or twice daily for the treatment of lid lesions due to demodectic or notoedric mange. A 2 per cent sulfur ointment is the treatment of choice for lid lesions due to sarcoptic mange and may be used in cats with notoedric mange. Appropriate parasiticidal therapy should be used for generalized cases. Corticosteroids are contraindicated in demodicosis but are useful in relieving pruritus associated with sarcoptic and notoedric mange. Topical and systemic antibiotics are indicated when secondary bacterial infections are present.

IMMUNE-MEDIATED BLEPHARITIS

Atopic dermatitis (allergic inhalant dermatitis) is an IgE-mediated, immediate type hypersensitivity that usually develops in dogs between one to three years of age. Pruritus with paw licking and face rubbing, generalized erythema, and rust-colored staining of white hair may be present. Epiphora, moist ulcerative blepharitis, and conjunctivitis are also seen, and when pruritus is severe, self-mutilation may occur. Occasionally rhinitis and sneezing are noted. A seasonal occurrence is noted initially, but the problem tends to become constant as the dog ages. Diagnosis is based on history, clinical findings, and results of intradermal allergy testing. Treatment by the elimination of the offending allergen, when possible, is best. Hyposensitization also provides effective long-term control in some cases. Systemic corticosteroids and topical antibiotic-corticosteroid ointments may be used judiciously to control pruritus and secondary infection.

Allergic contact dermatitis is a delayed hypersensitivity (type IV). The inflammation occurs after sensitization by repeated contact with an allergen. It is rarely limited to the periocular region unless sensitivity is associated with a topical ophthalmic preparation. Neomycin is the most common drug incriminated in allergic contact blepharitis, but

---

*Conofite cream 2%, Pitman-Moore Inc., Washington's Crossing, NJ.

†Grifungal, Pitman-Moore; Fulvicin, Schering Corp., Kenilworth, NJ.

---

‡Floropryl, Merck, Sharp and Dohme, West Point, PA.

other drugs, drug carriers, and preservatives may be involved. Pruritus, depigmentation, erythema, alopecia, and excoriations of the lids (especially the lower lids and medial canthi) are common. A seasonal occurrence may be noted with plant hypersensitivities. Diagnosis is based on an accurate history and clinical signs and may be confirmed by elimination and provocative exposure testing and possibly by intradermal skin tests for inhalant allergens. Withdrawal of the offending drug or allergen is curative. Topical corticosteroids may be used, and topical and systemic antibiotics are indicated for secondary infections.

Pemphigus and bullous pemphigoid are the most common autoimmune skin diseases that affect the eyelids of small animals. Eyelid lesions may also be present in animals with discoid or systemic lupus erythematosus. Characteristic lid lesions may be encrusted, exudative, and/or ulcerative with alopecia and erythema. Although history, distribution of lesions, and histologic findings in biopsies of active lesions are suggestive of autoimmune disease, demonstration of autoantibodies in biopsy tissue by immunofluorescence is required for a definitive diagnosis. Therapy with systemic corticosteroids and cytotoxic immunosuppressive agents is effective in many cases. Chrysotherapy with aurothioglucose (Solganal)* was reported to be beneficial, although the exact mechanism of action is unknown (Halliwell, 1981). These therapies may have drastic side effects and should be used only after familiarization with the drugs. Supportive care consists of avoidance of direct sunlight and topical and systemic antibiotics when secondary infection is present.

IDIOPATHIC BLEPHARITIS

Medial canthal blepharitis is a chronic ulcerative blepharitis of dogs involving the inferior medial canthus. It is usually bilateral and occurs in a variety of breeds. An immune-mediated etiopathogenesis has been hypothesized. A similar problem may develop in eyes treated with epinephrine (1 to 2 per cent) ophthalmic drops for the medical management of glaucoma and may be a manifestation of a contact allergic response. Logically, the medial canthus would be involved since tears containing the drug primarily drain from the conjunctival sac via the inferior lacrimal puncta and canaliculus. Biopsy of the lesion reveals an infiltration of lymphocytes and plasma cells. Suspect drugs should be discontinued and antibiotics and corticosteroids applied to the lesion.

Marked depigmentation of the eyelids may occur in association with solar dermatitis. It has been hypothesized that the disease results from a primary hypersensitivity to sunlight and/or autoimmunity

induced by damage to dermal tissues from ultraviolet radiation. Recent studies indicate that many cases of "nasal solar dermatitis" are actually discoid lupus erythematosus (Walton et al., 1981). Treatment consists of protection of affected areas from sunlight and systemic administration of prednisolone at an initial dose of 0.5 mg/kg. The steroid dosage is gradually decreased as the lesions heal. Oral administration of vitamin E (*dl*-α-tocopherol acetate) at a dose of 400 IU twice daily has been used successfully in lieu of systemic corticosteroids for the treatment of discoid lupus erythematosus. Sun screens, marking the lesions with black felt marking pens, and tattooing have been advocated to protect the affected areas from sunlight. Long-term oral administration of para-aminobenzoic acid (PABA) will increase skin pigmentation. The dosage is 2 gm q.i.d. in dogs weighing more than 50 pounds, 2 gm t.i.d. in dogs weighing from 20 to 50 pounds, and 1 gm t.i.d. in dogs weighing less than 20 pounds. In humans, nausea and vomiting, pruritus, drug rash, and drug fever may occur with large doses of PABA. These manifestations subside following withdrawal of the drug. Human patients have received doses as high as 12 to 18 grams daily for as long as a decade without toxic effects. Gastrointestinal upset may be minimized by administration of the drug with food.

EYELID NEOPLASMS

A wide variety of eyelid neoplasms have been reported, especially in older dogs and cats. Sebaceous adenomas, melanomas, and papillomas are most frequently encountered in the dog. Squamous cell carcinomas predominate in cats. Adenomas, melanomas, and papillomas are usually benign, firm, slow growing, and well-delineated. Papillomas occur in dogs of all ages and may be sessile or pedunculated. In young dogs with viral oral papillomatosis, the papillomatous growths may also develop on the eyelids. These tumors usually develop rapidly over several months and then spontaneously regress. Squamous cell carcinomas are malignant, exhibiting local invasion and destruction with frequent ulceration and thickening of the lids. They are associated with actinic radiation, occur most commonly in white cats, and frequently involve the pinnae and nose as well as the eyelids. Adenocarcinomas may initially mimic adenomas but grow more rapidly and are more invasive and destructive. Basal cell carcinomas occur in both dogs and cats and are usually ulcerated, firm, and nodular. They are locally invasive but rarely metastasize. Fibromas, fibrosarcomas, hemangiomas, hemangiosarcomas, histiocytomas, mast cell tumors, neurofibromas, and neurofibrosarcomas have also been reported on the eyelids.

---

*Solganal, Schering Corp., Kenilworth, NJ

As a general rule, eyelid tumors should be removed as early as possible. Papillomas are a possible exception as long as they remain small and cause no ocular irritation. Early resection of tumors increases the likelihood of complete resection, thus decreasing the probability of recurrence. One-fourth to one-third of the lid may be removed by simple "V" or pentagonal full thickness resection. The resulting defect can be simply closed in two layers (tarsoconjunctiva and skin-orbicularis oculi muscle) while maintaining excellent eyelid function and appearance. Excision of larger lid tumors (involving > one-third of the lid) will require reconstructive blepharoplasty. Whenever possible, the surgeon should preserve or reconstruct the upper lid and margin, which is more important to the eye in blinking than the lower lid.

Cryosurgery provides an alternate method for treating selected lid tumors in small animals. It may be performed with local anesthesia under sedation in patients considered high risks for general anesthesia. Treatment of large tumors will usually preserve enough connective tissue matrix so that reconstructive blepharoplasty is not required. Occasionally the tumor regrows, and the procedure must be repeated. Swelling and necrosis of the frozen tissue occur during the first two weeks after freezing, and some depigmentation and scarring of the involved lid tissues will occur. Caution must be exercised, since overzealous freezing can result in extensive sloughing of perilesional tissue.

Radiofrequency-induced hyperthermia therapy provides another possible alternative in the treatment of lid tumors. This technique involves the destruction of tumor tissues by hyperthermia and has yielded favorable results in cattle with ocular squamous cell carcinomas. However, it must be more extensively evaluated for different tumor types and for use in small animals.

Although the incidence of metastasis with primary eyelid tumors is low, their management should not be approached lightly. A thorough physical examination and clinical work-up is necessary to ensure the primary nature of the tumor and the absence of metastasis. Thoracic radiographs are especially important for tumors exhibiting tissue destruction and rapid growth. Adjunctive chemotherapy and immunotherapy should be considered with aggressive tumors, especially when they are recurrent.

SUPPLEMENTAL READING

Barrie, K. P., and Gelatt, K. N.: Diseases of the eyelids (Part I). Comp. Cont. Ed. Pract. Vet. 1:405, 1979.

Bistner, S. I., Aguirre, G., and Batik, G.: Atlas of Veterinary Ophthalmic Surgery. Philadelphia: W. B. Saunders Co., 1977.

Fox, S. A.: Ophthalmic Plastic Surgery, 5th ed. New York: Grune & Stratton, 1976.

Gelatt, K. N. (ed.): Veterinary Ophthalmology. Philadelphia: Lea & Febiger, 1981.

Halliwell, R. E. W.: Skin diseases associated with autoimmunity. Part I. The bullous autoimmune skin diseases. Comp. Cont. Ed. Pract. Vet. 2:911, 1980.

Halliwell, R. E. W.: Skin diseases associated with autoimmunity. Part II. The nonbullous autoimmune skin diseases. Comp. Cont. Ed. Pract. Vet. 3:156, 1981.

Jenson, H. E.: Canthus closure. Comp. Cont. Ed. Pract. Vet. 1:735, 1979.

Krehbiel, J. D., and Langham, R. F.: Eyelid neoplasms of dogs. Am. J. Vet. Res. 36:115, 1975.

Lavach, J. D., and Gelatt, K. N.: Diseases of the eyelids (Part II). Comp. Cont. Ed. Pract., Vet. 1:485, 1979.

Muller, G. H., and Kirk, R. W.: Small Animal Dermatology. Philadelphia: W. B. Saunders Co., 1976.

Munger, R. J., and Gourley, I. M.: Cross lid flap for repair of large upper eyelid defects. J.A.V.M.A. 178:45, 1981.

Northway, R. B.: Chronic solar dermatitis of the dog. Sm. An. Clin. 5:141, 1961.

Slatter, D. H.: Fundamentals of Veterinary Ophthalmology. Philadelphia: W. B. Saunders Co., 1981.

Walton, D. K., et al.: Canine discoid lupus erythematosus. J. Am. Anim. Hosp. Assoc. 17:851, 1981.

DISEASES OF THE CONJUNCTIVA

PAULE BLOUIN, D.M.V.

St. Hyacinthe, Canada

Conjunctival diseases are probably the most frequent ocular problems encountered by the small animal practitioner. They range from mild, self-limiting conditions to chronic diseases that at best can be controlled and are a source of frustration for both the animal owner and the veterinarian.

The conjunctiva consists of a mucous membrane that lines the inner aspect of the superior and inferior eyelids, both surfaces of the nictitating membrane, and the anterior portion of the sclera. It is firmly attached to the globe at the limbus, where its epithelium becomes continuous with that of the cornea. The conjunctiva and third eyelid play a critical role in protection of the eye and production of the tear film (Blogg, 1980; Helper, 1981; Slatter, 1981). They can be involved in a number of different pathologic processes, with inflammation being the most common.

DIFFERENTIATION BETWEEN PRIMARY AND SECONDARY CONJUNCTIVAL DISEASES

Numerous cases of ocular diseases present with signs of conjunctival involvement. The veterinarian must be able to diagnose the problem accurately to give an appropriate prognosis and establish prompt, effective treatment. This calls for a complete, thorough ocular and systemic examination. This cannot be overemphasized since, in many instances, a diagnosis of conjunctivitis is established in the face of a potentially serious intraocular, corneal, lacrimal, orbital, or eyelid problem. One has to remember that signs of conjunctival irritation are the rule rather than the exception in such cases and that unless the primary problem is correctly identified, symptomatic treatment will only mask the evolution of the disease, often leading to permanent and serious complications.

The basic rule to remember when diagnosing a primary conjunctival disease is that all other ocular and adnexal structures should be normal. A detailed examination is thus necessary to rule out other entities. For example, lid problems such as distichiasis, ectopic cilia, entropion, ectropion, and blepharitis will cause variable degrees of conjunctivitis, which will improve with symptomatic treatment but will only recur once the medication is stopped. Similarly, a deficiency in tear production can be diagnosed in its early stages only if a Schirmer tear test is done. Since the test must be performed before any solution is applied to the eye if it is to be valid, the potential diagnosis of keratoconjunctivitis sicca has to be constantly kept in mind. Another disease frequently misdiagnosed as conjunctivitis is dacryocystitis, which can be identified only after an attempt is made to irrigate the nasolacrimal system. One must always look for conjunctival foreign bodies and parasites, and the detection of corneal erosions should be pursued by means of a fluorescein test.

Problems occur when two conditions are present simultaneously. It then becomes a challenge to determine whether there is a cause-and-effect relationship. For example, in the case of a five-year-old St. Bernard with ectropion and a conjunctivitis of sudden onset, it is unlikely that surgical correction of the lid problem will cure the disease, since the animal has been able to live with the ectropion for years with minimal or no symptoms. Another cause for the conjunctivitis should be sought, keeping in mind that the abnormal position of the eyelid may well predispose the animal to another disease

or may increase its severity. The same rationale of diagnosis applies to an eight-year-old cocker spaniel with distichiasis and conjunctivitis of recent onset. Critical judgment has to be used to determine the best therapeutic approach.

Tear deficiencies are often even more complex to interpret, as they can be either the cause or the result of a chronic conjunctivitis. In both cases, lacrimal secretion has to be stimulated or artificially replaced if symptomatic relief is to be expected.

Intraocular diseases such as anterior uveitis and glaucoma also must be ruled out. Particular attention should be paid to vision, corneal transparency, abnormal contents of the anterior chamber, iris color and texture, pupil size and shape, and intraocular tension as evaluated by Schiotz or digital tonometry. These findings must all be normal before making a diagnosis of conjunctivitis. The type of vascular congestion seen is also helpful in differentiating between extraocular and intraocular disease. Conjunctival hyperemia is usually diffuse and more obvious in the palpebral area, whereas episcleral congestion is manifested by large, dark vessels that are most prominent near the limbus and remain stationary when the conjunctiva is moved (Helper, 1981). Conjunctival edema is much less obvious in the presence of intraocular disease.

GENERAL APPROACH TO DIAGNOSIS AND EXAMINATION

A logical, systematic approach should be routinely used to investigate ocular problems. A thorough history can first be taken with particular attention paid to duration of symptoms, possibility of trauma, signs of pain, changes in vision, the type of environment where the animal is kept, and the presence or absence of symptoms relating to other body systems. Vision can then be tested for each eye before proceeding with the examination. The quantity and character of ocular discharge should be evaluated before gently cleaning the excess with a dry gauze pad. A Schirmer tear test is then performed and samples for bacterial cultures taken with a moist, sterile cotton swab. The need for submitting these samples to the laboratory can be determined at the end of the examination, since topical anesthesia is often required later and will interfere with the growth of organisms.

A thorough examination of all adnexal and ocular structures follows. This should be done in a darkened room with a bright source of diffuse light such as that provided by the Finhoff transilluminator and halogen light bulb (Welch Allyn). Magnification is also helpful. Topical anesthesia (0.5 per cent proparacaine HCl, Ophthetic, Allergan) is of benefit in making the animal more tractable. The examination should include a fluorescein stain, examination of the bulbar aspect of the nictitating membrane, and flushing of the nasolacrimal ducts. Inexpensive lacrimal cannulas can be made from hypodermic needles of varying sizes by a thorough filing of the sharp tip. The end is then slightly bent, and the needle is autoclaved after each use. These needles can also be used to irrigate the conjunctival fornices to flush out foreign material or prepare the eye for surgery.

Conjunctival scrapings stained by the Gram and Giemsa methods are extremely helpful in determining the type of inflammatory reaction and the etiologic agent (Slatter, 1981). They are collected from the upper palpebral conjunctiva with a heat-sterilized platinum spatula after topical anesthesia. Their interpretation requires patience and some practice. If canine distemper is suspected, a Shorr's stain will demonstrate the cytoplasmic inclusion bodies. Lastly, a general physical examination is indicated to rule out the presence of a systemic disease or a separate nidus of infection such as skin, ear, and anal sac problems.

CONJUNCTIVAL INJURIES

These are usually divided into hemorrhages, lacerations, and foreign bodies. Subconjunctival hemorrhages can be extensive and most frightening to the owner. They require no treatment, since the blood will resorb within a matter of days. The possibility of a systemic bleeding disorder has to be considered, particularly when the problem is bilateral or when a clear-cut history of trauma cannot be obtained. Traumatic cases should be evaluated thoroughly, since they can be accompanied by other ocular lesions that require prompt treatment, such as corneal injuries, traumatic iridocyclitis, or lens displacement.

Similarly, conjunctival lacerations can be indicative of a more serious problem. They will heal without surgical intervention unless they are extensive, in which case, the defect can be repaired with 5–0 or 6–0 absorbable suture material. Care should be taken to bury the knots or trim the suture ends short to prevent corneal irritation.

One should always suspect and thoroughly search for conjunctival foreign bodies, particularly in a case of acute, unilateral conjunctivitis. They can be minute and are often trapped between folds of swollen conjunctiva, in the fornices, and between the third eyelid and the globe. Once located, they are usually easily removed with thumb forceps after topical anesthesia or by abundant flushing with a sterile irrigating solution.

CHEMOSIS

Chemosis is the term used to describe edema of the conjunctiva. A certain degree of chemosis is present with any type of conjunctivitis and is manifested by excessive folding of the conjunctiva, along with other signs of inflammation. The edema can reach extreme proportions owing to the loose attachment of the bulbar conjunctiva to the underlying episcleral tissues. The conjunctiva can balloon out between the eyelids and prevent their proper closure, leading to exposure keratitis. The exposed conjunctiva can become desiccated and necrotic. This degree of chemosis is usually associated with head trauma, allergic reactions (IgE-mediated response to insect bites, food, drugs, or vaccination), and occasionally acute orbital inflammation. The underlying problem should be appropriately treated, taking care to prevent drying out of the conjunctiva and cornea. Topical steroids are best avoided when a thorough corneal evaluation is impeded by the redundant conjunctiva. Any antibiotic ophthalmic ointment can be liberally applied to the eye. The use of a 5 per cent sodium chloride ointment (Adsorbonac, Burton and Parsons) can also be helpful in decreasing the edema. Lastly, cold wet compresses often provide rapid symptomatic relief.

CONJUNCTIVITIS

Conjunctivitis in small animals ranges from a mild, innocuous disease to long-standing involvement, which can be difficult to control.

CLASSIFICATION

Conjunctivitis can be classified according to cause (primary or secondary, bacterial, viral, and so on), duration (acute or chronic), and the type of ocular discharge present (serous, mucoid, purulent). The term *conjunctivitis* is also often linked to another word to describe conditions in which adjacent ocular structures are simultaneously involved, for example, blepharoconjunctivitis and keratoconjunctivitis. Although a classification based on etiology is logical to provide a rationale for treatment, it is not always possible to establish a definite cause. Other modes of classification can thus be extremely helpful, as they are descriptive and give a good assessment of the type of disease present.

SIGNS

Signs of conjunctivitis vary from almost nonexistent to quite severe. They depend mainly on the intensity of the inflammatory reaction, with etiology, chronicity, and individual variations being other factors to consider. Some type of ocular discharge is almost always present. It can range from serous to purulent, the most common type being mucopurulent. The amount of secretion varies from case to case. It can be misleading to guess the cause based on the type of ocular discharge, since bacterial superinfections may mask the signs of the original disease.

Discomfort is another variable symptom of the disease. It can be virtually nonexistent, but it is often manifested by attempts to rub the eye and narrowing of the palpebral fissure. Severe ocular pain is not a usual component of conjunctivitis. If present, another cause should be carefully investigated, particularly the presence of corneal erosions, iridocyclitis, and glaucoma.

Conjunctival hyperemia is a constant finding in conjunctivitis, but the degree of vasodilatation varies with each case. Chemosis is usually present and occasionally becomes the major clinical sign. The formation of lymphoid follicles is often noted in chronic cases. They appear as small, circular, raised, semitransparent nodules, which are most frequently seen on either face of the nictitating membrane or in the lower conjunctival fornix. They are most easily detected in pigmented areas of the conjunctiva, since the dark background provides a good contrast for their visualization. Although their presence in small numbers is considered normal, excessive follicle formation has been termed *follicular conjunctivitis*, a controversial condition that will be discussed in more detail later.

ETIOLOGY

Ocular irritation by dust, soap, foreign bodies, and anomalies of lid or eyelash position is likely to be the most frequent precipitating factor for the onset of conjunctivitis in dogs. Since the normal bacterial flora of the canine conjunctiva is varied, superinfection by potential pathogens can readily occur once the defense mechanisms of the eye are compromised. This statement is supported by microbiological studies that determined that staphylococci were by far the most common bacteria isolated from both normal and diseased canine eyes (Gaskin, 1980). Bacterial conjunctivitis is thus common in dogs, either as a primary problem or as a sequela to other inciting causes.

Canine viral conjunctivitis has mainly been associated with infection by adenovirus types 1 and 2 and the distemper virus. Signs of systemic disease usually accompany the onset of conjunctivitis and are helpful in establishing a presumptive diagnosis. The problem in canine distemper is compounded by the frequent simultaneous presence of decreased lacrimal secretion and secondary bacterial infection. Although treatment of the systemic disease is of primary importance, the eyes must be monitored carefully to prevent serious complications.

The incidence of bacterial conjunctivitis appears to be lower in cats than in dogs. This is possibly related to the lower incidence of normal bacterial flora in feline eyes than in canine eyes (Gaskin, 1980). The most common cause of feline conjunctivitis is an infection by one of the numerous agents capable of causing upper respiratory infections, such as feline rhinotracheitis, calicivirus and reovirus, chlamydia, and mycoplasma. Furthermore, infection by any of these pathogens is often complicated by the presence of one of the others, with mycoplasma being recognized as a secondary invader that can become active in stressed animals. Although it can be helpful to try to determine the specific etiology of conjunctivitis by the various clinical signs present, one must remember that each agent can cause a disease that can range from mild to purulent conjunctivitis. Respiratory signs may be present or absent too. The only way to establish a definitive diagnosis is to identify the various organisms by culture, a procedure not routinely done by the veterinary practitioner. Conjunctival scrapings fixed for five to ten minutes in acetone-free 95 per cent methanol and stained with Giemsa may confirm the presence of mycoplasma or chlamydia. The presence or absence of a viral infection cannot be conclusively determined by conjunctival scrapings. In the event of a possible chlamydial infection, the owner should be warned that the infection may be transmitted to humans. Owners should wash their hands thoroughly after handling the animal and keep the cat from sleeping on the owner's bed.

Allergic conjunctivitis can occur in small animals, but one should avoid the tendency to make such a diagnosis unless other causes have been ruled out. Local hypersensitivity reactions to any of the components present in topical ophthalmic preparations can develop in dogs and cats. This possibility should be considered when the animal becomes markedly symptomatic shortly after application of the medication. The animal will show signs of increased pain and itching and a worsening of chemosis and hyperemia. Removal of the offending agent is mandatory for successful treatment. Most other cases of allergic conjunctivitis are associated with atopy and are accompanied by dermatitis, rhinitis, blepharitis, and occasionally keratitis.

Other less common causes of conjunctivitis include toxic agents such as acid and alkali, parasites *(Thelazia californiensis)*, and mycotic infections. A specific etiologic agent has not been convincingly shown for follicular conjunctivitis yet. Excessive follicle formation can occur with any type of chronic conjunctivitis. Furthermore, previous hypotheses of canine herpes virus involvement have been contradicted recently by Jackson and Corstvet (1980). The situation is further confused by histologic studies of presumed lymphoid follicles, which showed the presence of glandular tissue rather than inflammatory cells. Further research is needed to solve this controversy.

THERAPEUTIC APPROACH: GENERAL PRINCIPLES

The majority of cases of conjunctivitis can be successfully treated with topical medication alone. Ointments are usually preferred to solutions, since they reach comparable drug levels in ocular tissues with less frequent application. The temperament of the animal also has to be considered, since some owners find it almost impossible to apply ointment to their animal's eyes. Good hygiene is essential for successful treatment. It is necessary to clean the eye thoroughly before each treatment, since conjunctival secretions will interfere with the effectiveness of topical drugs. This is best accomplished by using lukewarm, wet compresses followed by irrigation with a balanced salt solution (Eye-stream, Alcon) or boiled water. Self-mutilation due to pruritus can be avoided by bandaging the dewclaws or, in severe cases, by the use of an Elizabethan collar.

TREATMENT OF CANINE CONJUNCTIVITIS

The first and most important part of treatment of canine conjunctivitis is removal of the offending agent, whenever possible. The administration of antibiotics is required, and the choice of medication depends on many factors. Ideally, bacterial culture and sensitivity tests dictate the most logical therapeutic approach, but in practice these are ordered only in refractory or chronic cases. Even then, culture results can be difficult to interpret because of the presence of potential pathogens such as *Staphylococcus aureus* in the normal conjunctival flora (Gaskin, 1980). In unilateral cases, it can be very useful to culture both eyes to compare the results and select the proper antibiotic. If culture results are unavailable, Gram stains of conjunctival scrapings can help to quickly determine the type of infection present. Bacteria identified by this method are usually significant pathogens, since organisms that are part of the normal flora are seldom numerous enough to be detected in scrapings. As a rule, an antibiotic or a combination of drugs that are broad spectrum, bacteriocidal, and to which there is a low incidence of bacterial resistance is the treatment of choice. The combination of neomycin, bacitracin, and polymyxin B (Neosporin, Burroughs Wellcome) is a good first choice, since it fills these criteria and is relatively inexpensive. Reserve the use of chloramphenicol (Chloroptic, Allergan) and gentamicin (Garamycin, Schering) for refractory cases when a sensitivity is available. Routine use of these agents is likely to promote the emergence of resistant bacteria. The frequency of administration varies with the severity of the case but should be at least every eight hours for effective treatment. The duration of treatment is also variable. Uncomplicated cases should be treated for five to ten days and then re-evaluated. If there is no improvement, the diagnosis and treatment should be reassessed.

The use of systemic antibiotics is reserved for cases in which the animal is intractable or there is an extraocular focus of infection. Chronic infections with *Staphylococcus aureus* can be difficult to control and can lead to complications such as keratitis and decreased tear production. A bacterial sensitivity test is mandatory in such cases, and a combination of topical and systemic antibiotics is usually required to handle the problem initially. Long-term topical medication application is often necessary to prevent recurrences, and in such cases the goal is control rather than cure. Regular follow-ups are necessary and should include close monitoring of tear secretion.

Topical corticosteroids should not be routinely used, as they will interfere with normal ocular defense mechanisms. They are helpful in cases in which pruritus is a problem, however, since they will make the animal more comfortable and will limit the extent of self-mutilation. They are also of great value in chronic cases, particularly those associated with staphylococcal infections; toxic and allergic components appear to play a part in such infections, and they may help to prevent the development of keratoconjunctivitis sicca secondary to conjunctival scarring. Corneal ulceration is obviously a strong contraindication to the use of topical steroids. Animals on long-term treatment with such drugs should be monitored carefully. Owners should be advised to immediately discontinue the medication and have the dog examined promptly if signs of increased pain or discharge present. The choice of the type of steroid depends on the degree of inflammation, but in general preparations with weak steroids such as hydrocortisone are preferred. Exceptions include the presence of large numbers of follicles, which respond only to potent steroids such as dexamethasone. The use of copper sulfate crystals for cauterization is potentially dangerous and unnecessarily traumatic and should be replaced by mechanical abrasion with a gauze sponge.

TREATMENT OF FELINE CONJUNCTIVITIS

Once the possibility of entropion, foreign bodies, or nasolacrimal obstruction is excluded, cases of feline conjunctivitis can be assumed to be associated with one of the agents causing respiratory infections unless proved otherwise. This is due to the high incidence of such infections in the feline population, their degree of contagiousness, the low levels of immunity they induce, the sparse normal bacterial flora of feline conjunctiva, and the low incidence of other precipitating factors such as eyelid anomalies. Since there are no effective antiviral drugs for the treatment of conjunctivitis and since dual infections involving mycoplasma and chlamydia readily occur, the treatment of choice is the topical application of tetracyclines (Terramycin, Pfizer). Chloramphenicol (Chloroptic, Allergan) is also effective, but I prefer to reserve it for proven bacterial infections. Treatment should be administered to both eyes (even in unilateral cases) every eight hours and continued for one week after remission of symptoms. Oral tetracycline (Panmycin, Upjohn, 5 to 16 mg/kg repeated every eight hours for seven to ten days) is reserved for those cases with overt systemic involvement, for cats with recurrent disease, and for breeding queens when they are not pregnant, since carriers of chlamydia will often transmit the infection to their newborns, causing ophthalmia neonatorum. Affected animals should be isolated.

The use of topical steroids is contraindicated in infections with feline rhinotracheitis virus, as it will prolong the course of the disease and lead to serious complications. Particular attention should be paid to fluorescein staining of the cornea in the diagnostic work-up, since early herpetic ulcers are almost impossible to detect by other means. Should they occur, topical antiviral agents are indicated. Vidarabine (Vira-A, Parke-Davis) is preferred to idoxuridine (Stoxil, Smith, Kline and French), since it appears to cause much less irritation.

DISEASES OF THE NICTITATING MEMBRANE

PROTRUSION

Abnormal protrusion of the third eyelid can occur with any condition producing ocular pain. The problem is self-limiting once the primary cause has been corrected. Diseases resulting in changes in the volume of the retrobulbar orbital content can also cause the third eyelid to become elevated. Examples include marked cachexia, dehydration, and retrobulbar masses such as tumors and inflammatory infiltrates. One of the manifestations of Horner's syndrome is a protrusion of the nictitans, and attempts should be made to locate the level of the neurologic defect and establish a cause for it. Topical epinephryl borate (Epinal 1 per cent, Alcon) can provide symptomatic relief but has no curative effect. In cats, bilateral protrusion of the third eyelid can occur without ocular lesions. A history of diarrhea can sometimes be obtained. The disease is thought to be related to a generalized defect of the sympathetic nervous system with a postulated viral etiology. The presence of intestinal parasites and infection with the feline leukemia virus should be ruled out. In many cases, the condition is self-limiting, with a return to normal within a matter of weeks.

Lastly, an excessive protrusion of the nictitans is occasionally seen in dolichocephalic dogs with deep orbits and enophthalmic eyes. This is often unac-ceptable to the owner for cosmetic reasons, and in extreme cases vision can be affected. Recommended treatments have included retrobulbar injection of silicone beads to move the globe forward and resection of the free edge of the nictitating membrane. A better alternative would be shortening of the nictitans without altering its free edge as described by Peruccio (1981).

PROLAPSE OF THE NICTITANS GLAND

This condition, commonly called "cherry eye," occurs in young dogs of many small breeds. It is thought to be hereditary and is related to a defective formation of fibrous attachments to the base of the gland (Helper, 1981). Although benign, the defect is unsightly and often results in conjunctival irritation. Standard operating procedure consists of excision of the protruding portion of the gland. Such treatment appears to predispose the animal to keratoconjunctivitis sicca in later life, and the alternative suggested by Blogg (1979) is reported to give excellent results without removal of any lacrimal tissue. This method consists of incising the conjunctiva over the protruding gland and dissecting inferomedially to anchor the gland to the epibulbar tissues with suture material.

EVERSION OF THE CARTILAGE OF THE THIRD EYELID

This is considered to be a genetic condition occurring mainly in large breeds and is thought to result from either a weakness of the vertical portion of the cartilage or a differential growth rate between the tissues of the anterior and posterior surfaces of the nictitating membrane. Surgical correction of this defect has been well-described and involves excision of the abnormal portion of the cartilage after incision of the conjunctiva covering its bulbar aspect. The technique described by Peruccio (1981) should also be useful when the defect is extensive and associated with marked protrusion of the membrane.

PLASMOCYTIC INFILTRATION OF THE THIRD EYELID

This chronic inflammatory bilateral disease mainly affects adult German shepherd dogs and is thought to be a localized form of an autoimmune disorder. The condition can be observed alone or in association with chronic superficial keratitis ("pannus") and/or ulceration of the medial canthus. Affected dogs show hyperemia, nodular thickenings, and depigmentation of the nictitans, with the lesions being most pronounced along the free edge of the membrane. The disease is accompanied by a mucoid or mucopurulent discharge and in some cases can induce much pruritus. Topical steroids are the only known effective form of control. They must be used for extensive periods, as the problem cannot be cured. Frequent application (every four to six hours) of the more potent steroids (dexamethasone, prednisolone acetate) is necessary to induce remission of the symptoms. The dosage is then gradually decreased over a period of months to eventually reach the lowest frequency effective in preventing recurrences. This can vary from twice a day to once every 48 hours.

REMOVAL OF THE NICTITATING MEMBRANE

It should be emphasized that the only indication for complete removal of the third eyelid is extensive neoplastic involvement. Animals on which this surgery has been performed are predisposed to chronic conjunctivitis, inflammation or ulceration of the medial portion of the cornea, and keratoconjunctivitis sicca. Replacement of the nictitans by means of an oral mucosal graft should be helpful in management of the first two problems (Kuhns, 1977).

REFERENCES

Blogg, J. R.: Surgical replacement of prolapsed gland of the third eyelid ("cherry eye")—a new technique. Aust. Vet. Pract. 9:75, 1979.

Blogg, J. R.: *The Eye in Veterinary Practice—Volume I: Extraocular Disease.* Philadelphia: W. B. Saunders Co., 1980, pp. 338–373.

Gaskin, J. M.: Microbiology of the canine and feline eye. Vet. Clin. North Am. 10:303, 1980.

Helper, L. C.: The canine nictitating membrane and conjunctiva. *In* Gelatt, K. N. (ed.): *Textbook of Veterinary Ophthalmology.* Philadelphia: Lea & Febiger, 1981, pp. 330–342.

Jackson, J. A., and Corstvet, R. E.: Study of nictitating membranes and genitalia of dogs with reference to lymphofollicular hyperplasia and its cause. Am. J. Vet. Res. 41:1814, 1980.

Kuhns, E. L.: Oral mucosal grafts for membrana nictitans replacement. Mod. Vet. Pract. 58:768, 1977.

Martin, C. L.: Conjunctivitis: differential diagnosis and treatment. Vet. Clin. North Am. 3:367, 1973.

Peruccio, C.: Surgical correction of prominent third eyelid in the dog. Calif. Vet. 35:24, 1981.

Slatter, D. H.: *Fundamentals of Veterinary Ophthalmology.* Philadelphia: W. B. Saunders Co., 1981, pp. 275–322.

DISEASES OF THE LACRIMAL APPARATUS

RENEE L. KASWAN, D.V.M.,
and CHARLES L. MARTIN, D.V.M.

Athens, Georgia

The lacrimal apparatus is conveniently divided into secretory and excretory components. Common disorders of the lacrimal system include keratoconjunctivitis sicca due to secretory deficiency and epiphora due to blockage of the lacrimal drainage system. Reflex tearing can also be caused by ocular irritation, which is reviewed adequately elsewhere.

TEAR GLAND ANATOMY AND FUNCTION

The main lacrimal gland and nictitating membrane gland are mixed, mucoserous, compound tubuloacinar glands with parasympathetic innervation. The nictitans gland lies on the inner surface of the nictitating membrane. The lacrimal gland is flattened and lies in a fold of periorbita beneath the orbital ligament. Approximately 70 per cent of tear secretion is produced by the main lacrimal gland and 30 per cent by the nictitating membrane gland, although either gland alone can supply adequate tears in a normal eye (Gillette, 1981). Mucus is also produced by conjunctival goblet cells. Accessory lacrimal glands comparable to the glands of Krause and Wolfring have not been demonstrated in the dog.

The lacrimal glands secrete a slightly alkaline, protein-poor serous fluid with a small component of mucin. The tears lubricate the corneal surface, providing a smooth, regular surface that enhances the optical properties of the cornea. Tears also mechanically cleanse the conjunctival sac and function in the nourishment of the cornea and conjunctiva. Lysozyme and secretory immunoglobulin in tears provide some antibacterial protection.

Although the tear film consists mainly of water, it is not a homogeneous solution. Three layers coat the cornea. The inner layer is hydrophilic mucin, a mixture of glycoproteins, that makes the naturally hydrophobic epithelium wettable. The second and most voluminous layer is aqueous. The thin outer layer of lipids secreted by the meibomian glands in the lid margins increases surface tension and retards evaporation.

KERATOCONJUNCTIVITIS SICCA (KCS)

Commonly called "dry eye," KCS can be defined as progressive inflammatory changes of the cornea and conjunctiva caused by a lack of adequate tear secretion. Increased lid friction and increased tear osmolarity have been specifically implicated in causing pathology. A deficiency of the precorneal tear film is commonly encountered in small animal practice. In a survey of 14 veterinary colleges, approximately 0.24 per cent of the general hospital populations had KCS (Table 1). Occasionally a mucous deficiency is suspected, particularly when lid defects cause inadequate spreading of the tear film. More commonly, a decrease in the aqueous portion of the tears occurs. With loss of the nutritive and protective functions of the tears, a spectrum of acute and chronic keratoconjunctival lesions evolves.

Approximately 70 per cent of KCS occurs bilaterally, although the early presentation is usually asymmetrical. There is no apparent sex predisposition, but the incidence is higher in older dogs (seven to nine years at onset). The English bulldog, cocker spaniel, and dachshund are predisposed to KCS, often with concurrent generalized seborrhea. The West Highland white terrier and miniature schnauzer have a high incidence of KCS independent of skin disease. Lagophthalmos occurs in exophthalmic breeds, causing KCS lesions to be more pronounced. Even when Schirmer tear test (STT) values are only slightly reduced with ineffective blinking, dry spots and exposure keratitis develop easily with lagophthalmos. Additionally, in the pug and Pekingese, melanocyte activity is particularly intense and severe pigmentary keratitis is common. See Table 1 for a list of incidence of KCS in specific canine breeds.

ETIOLOGY

The cause of KCS in the dog is usually unknown. Congenital alacrima occurs occasionally as an extreme xerosis, is usually unilateral, and is most commonly seen in small breeds. Unilateral neurologic xerosis is seen with some cases of facial nerve palsy or peripheral denervation of the parasympathetic lacrimal nerve. Interestingly, aqueous secretory cells in the lacrimal glands require cholinergic innervation, whereas mucous-secreting cells are autonomous.

Atropine, phenazopyridine (Azo Gantrisin), dapsone (Avlosulfon), sulfadiazine, and salicylazosulfapyridine (Azulfidine) can cause transient KCS, which usually is reversed with discontinuation of therapy. However, it sometimes is permanent.

Distemper virus can cause acute lacrimal adenitis. KCS due to distemper usually resolves spontaneously if the animal recovers systemically. Obstruction of the lacrimal ductules due to chemosis or conjunctival cicatrization can cause transient or permanent sicca. Vitamin A deficiency is an unlikely cause of canine KCS.

Hyperadrenocorticoidism, hypothyroidism, diabetes mellitus, demodectic mange, and systemic lupus erythematosus have been empirically associated with canine sicca. Dryness of the nasal and oral mucous membranes occurs in 10 to 30 per cent of KCS cases. Xerostomia is a contraindication to parotid duct transposition because it indicates parotid salivary gland dysfunction.

In a series of 49 nictitating membrane glands or main lacrimal glands dissected from dogs with KCS, no infectious agent was demonstrated by light or electron microscopy (Kaswan, 1982). The most common lesion was multifocal mononuclear cell infiltration with varying degrees of fibrosis. In some sections, acute inflammation, fatty infiltrates, atrophy, and ductal dilatation were predominant lesions. Serum electrophoresis showed elevated beta$_2$ or gammaglobulins in 90 per cent of KCS cases. Investigation is continuing to support a hypothesis of immune-mediated etiology in the dog, similar to KCS and Sjögren's syndrome in humans. To date, two cases of canine Sjögren's syndrome have been definitely documented. When KCS is recognized to occur concurrently with autoimmune hemolytic anemia, SLE, hypothyroidism, rheumatoid arthri-

Table 1. *Canine Breeds with Highest Risk for KCS**

Breed	No. of Dogs	Relative Risk†
English bulldog	187	20.1
West Highland white terrier	104	18.4
Lhasa apso	135	16.6
Pug	46	7.9
Cocker spaniel	276	6.8
Pekingese	91	6.3
Yorkshire terrier	50	5.3
Shih-Tzu	16	4.0
Miniature schnauzer	110	3.9
Boston terrier	43	3.9
Dachshund	64	1.5
Chihuahua	34	1.3
All breeds	1156	1.0
Mixed	317	.82
German shepherd	65	.57
Doberman pinscher	11	.15

*Data from the American Veterinary Data Program, NYSCVM.

†The estimate of relative risk is the ratio of the rate of disease among the exposed group to that of the general population.

tis, or chronic active hepatitis, a complete immunologic evaluation is warranted.

CLINICAL SIGNS

A large proportion of animals with KCS do not appear to have dry eyes. Initially, corneal dryness is painful; it causes blepharospasms, spastic entropion, conjunctival hyperemia, and chemosis. Multifocal punctate or central corneal ulceration, corneal desiccation, and malacia may occur and, if left untreated, may progress to perforation and iris prolapse. In chronic KCS, the cornea develops a dull irregular appearance with neovascularization and superficial haze. The corneal epithelium becomes hypertrophic. Pigment is deposited in patches or can become so dense that the cornea loses all transparency and blindness ensues. Mucin produced by conjunctival goblet cells is not dispersed by an aqueous phase and therefore accumulates in varying degrees as tenacious "ropey" filaments or may resemble mucopurulent blepharoconjunctivitis. Cultured, this exudate often contains staphylococci, or streptococci.

Keratoconjunctivitis sicca ranks high among the most commonly misdiagnosed ophthalmic diseases. Bacterial conjunctivitis, allergic conjunctivitis, and recurrent idiopathic corneal ulcers are common mistaken diagnoses made in cases of KCS. Misdiagnosed cases that are treated frequently with any topical ophthalmic preparation usually show transient improvement, falsely reinforcing the clinician's confidence in his original diagnosis. Virtually all topical medications wet the eye and add lubrication and therefore aid the dry eye condition. A high degree of suspicion should be held for any chronic conjunctivitis, keratitis, or corneal ulceration.

DIAGNOSIS

Even though the cornea may not appear dry, a Schirmer tear test (STT) should be performed as a routine part of the anterior segment ophthalmic examination. A diagnosis of KCS is made when decreased STT values occur with mucopurulent keratoconjunctivitis, corneal inflammation, ulceration, or pigment deposition. Normal dogs wet between 16 to 24 mm/min. KCS cases typically wet less than 10 mm/min, with the majority of cases wetting less than 5 mm/min on repeated trials. Atropinization can cause transient dryness for two to six days postoperatively. Fear-induced sympathetic stimulation also leads to sporadic low STT values, particularly in cats.

TREATMENT OF KCS

Medical therapy of KCS should be attempted for one to two months to evaluate whether it is a transient or permanent deficiency. If the pet is an indoor pet, particularly a "lap" dog, frequent administration of eye drops may be acceptable. Generally, medical therapy of KCS fails to control the progression of lesions owing to the client's inability or reluctance to treat the eyes as often as necessary.

To replace the wetting action of the natural tears, artificial tear preparations are recommended to be used as often as possible. Solutions are used every two to four hours, or minimally q.i.d. Ophthalmic ointments (Lacrilube, Allergan; Duratears, Alcon) are used at night or when frequent administration is impossible. Artificial tear solutions vary in pH, osmolarity, and individual tolerance. Methylcellulose or polyvinyl alcohol is a desirable ingredient to increase surface tension and retard evaporation. Polyvinyl pyrrolidine (PVP) increases the ability of the solution to adhere to the hydrophobic cornea and therefore gives a longer tear break-up time. Adapt (Alcon) and Absorbatears (Alcon) contain both desired characteristics of decreased evaporation and increased wetting. Slow release hydroxypropylcellulose ophthalmic inserts (Lacrisert, Merck, Sharp and Dohme) can be used once or twice daily. Artificial tears are the mainstay of the long-term KCS medical maintenance program.

Pilocarpine is used for its acetylcholine-like action in stimulating residual lacrimal gland secretions. For an average 25-lb dog, one to two drops of 2 per cent pilocarpine placed on a dog food treat every 12 hours is recommended initially. Maximum effect should be seen in 45 to 60 minutes. If no improvement in the STT occurs, the dose can be increased by increments of one drop at a time. If hypersalivation, vomiting, or diarrhea occurs, the medication should be stopped until symptoms abate and then reinstituted at a lower dosage. Bradycardia is a possible side effect, especially in predisposed dogs. Topical dilute (0.25 to 1.0 per cent) solutions of pilocarpine may be preferred in these cases. Pilocarpine appears to be most useful in dogs with marginal tear secretion; responsiveness decreases with disease progression.

Conjunctival overgrowth with commensal bacteria can be treated with topical antibiotics when necessary. If no active corneal ulceration is present, corneal neovascularization or conjunctivitis may be improved with short-term (7 to 14 days) use of topical corticosteroids b.i.d. to q.i.d. A fluorescein dye uptake test is mandatory prior to corticosteroid usage, because many animals with KCS have recurrent ulcerations. To break up tenacious discharge in cases of excessive mucous accumulations, 5 per cent acetylcysteine (half strength Mucomyst, Mead Johnson) can be used as often as every two hours. Acetylcysteine has a short shelf life (four days after opening) and requires refrigeration. Combination preparations of this topical agent can be used effectively if care is taken to use only those ingredients necessary for each individual patient.

Recently, Bromhexidine, a systemic mucolytic agent, has been shown to be safe and effective in decreasing the tenacity of ocular mucus in KCS in humans.

When trial medical therapy is unsuccessful, parotid duct transposition (PDT) is recommended. The basal salivation rate and patency of the parotid duct should be evaluated prior to anesthesia. Many dogs with xerophthalmia have concurrent xerostomia. In general, PDT done by a practiced surgeon is 90 per cent successful.

PREVENTION

Dogs whose nictitating membrane glands (NMG) have been removed for correction of third eyelid gland protrusion have an increased incidence of KCS. In normal dogs, surgical removal of either the NMG or the main lacrimal gland does not cause KCS, as either gland alone can produce sufficient tears. However, individuals who have marginal tear gland function can be decompensated by NMG removal. Therefore, NMG excision is contraindicated in breeds known to be predisposed to KCS.

An alternative to NMG excision is illustrated in Figure 1. The third eyelid is retracted forward. A conjunctival incision is made along the ventral palpebral fornix. Using 4-0 synthetic absorbable suture on a semicircular needle, a single mattress suture is placed horizontally deep into the incision anchored to the fibrous tissue of the orbital rim and exited through the same conjunctival incision. This suture is then passed through the bulbar surface of the third eyelid, around the widest diameter of the gland but not through the palpebral conjunctival surface of the third eyelid; the suture is tightened down tautly. A portion of the free edge of the conjunctival incision is sutured to the distal bulbar surface of the third eyelid with 6–0 chromic catgut to isolate the buried suture from the cornea and to prevent corneal ulceration by the large suture ends.

NASOLACRIMAL DRAINAGE SYSTEM

Tears pool ventrally within the recess of the conjunctival sac in the medial canthus, forming a lacrimal lake. Drainage proceeds into the lacrimal canaliculi through the lacrimal puncta. The lower punctum is normally situated about 5 mm from the medial canthus and within the palpebral conjunctiva, 1 to 2 mm bulbar to the mucocutaneous

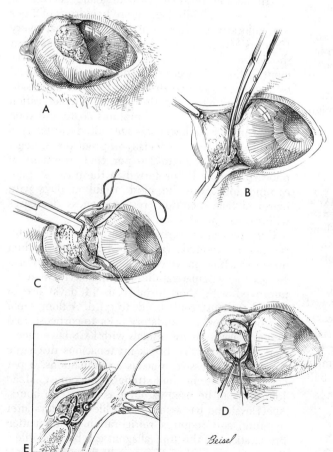

Figure 1.   Replacement of a hypertrophied third eyelid gland. A. Appearance of protrusion preoperatively. B. A conjunctival incision is made along the ventral palpebral fornix. C. Using 4–0 synthetic absorbable suture, a simple single suture is placed, taking a horizontal bite deep into the conjunctival incision and including a portion of the fibrous orbital rim. (Placement of this suture is cumbersome, but inclusion of this fibrous anchor is essential to a secure replacement of the gland.) This suture is then placed through the body of the nictitans gland. D. As the suture is tightened the gland recedes into the ventral fornix. E. A cross-sectional view of the final appearance shows the position of the 6–0 gut sutures used to close the conjunctival surfaces over the 4–0 suture, guarding the cornea from the larger suture ends.

Beisel

margin. The dorsal punctum is similarly situated about 5 to 8 mm from the medial canthus in the dorsal lid. The canaliculi converge in a vestigial lacrimal sac encased within the lacrimal bone. The nasolacrimal duct carries the tears from the lacrimal sac to the anterior end of the nasal vestibule. Tear flow is facilitated by peristalsis and capillary action. Imperfections may occur in the nasolacrimal duct and may result in drainage posteriorly into the nasopharynx or oral cavity. These variations are particularly common in cats and brachiocephalic dogs.

EPIPHORA

Epiphora refers to an abnormal flow of tears down the face. Constant epiphora causes the hair and skin around the medial canthus to be stained brown and occasionally causes a medial canthus moist dermatitis. Once reflex tearing, or hypersecretion, has been ruled out, obstructions of the lacrimal drainage system should be considered in the differential diagnosis of epiphora. See Table 2 for a list of common causes of epiphora.

ABSENCE OF THE LOWER PUNCTUM

Congenital imperforate and microlacrimal puncta occur mainly in golden retrievers, cocker spaniels, Bedlington terriers, and poodles. Reported breed incidence is probably influenced by coat color, as hair staining is much less apparent on dark haircoats. Under illumination and magnification, if the lower punctum is inapparent as either a dimple or pigmented spot, diagnosis is made by cannulation of the upper punctum with a lacrimal cannula. Subsequent lavage frequently tents the area of the lower punctum. Treatment consists of incising the ballooned area, followed by topical antibiotic and steroid administration for three days to prevent infection or adhesions of the newly established orifice.

MALALIGNMENT OF THE VENTRAL PUNCTUM

The ventral punctum may be improperly positioned in its relation to the lacrimal lake so that tears are not readily drawn into the ventral canaliculi. This occurs physiologically in tight-lid breeds such as poodles in which the lacrimal lake is narrowed and the puncta may be held both too tautly and anterior to the pooled tears. Exophthalmic brachiocephalic breeds often have an obscure relative puncta position. Injuries to the ventral lid margin often disturb the normal apposition of the punctum to the lid fissure. Flushing of the nasolacrimal duct does not mimic the physiologic mechanism of tear absorption by the punctum and is

Table 2.   *Causes of Epiphora*

Ventromedial entropion
Distichia, trichiasis
Aberrant dermis or cilia acting as a wick
Prominent nasal folds
Prominence of the eye with a shallow lacrimal lake
Absence, obstruction, or misalignment of the ventral punctum and/or canaliculi
Dacryocystitis
Corneal irritation or pain
Intraocular pain, i.e., uveitis, glaucoma

therefore not adequate to rule out this problem. Fluorescein stain passage from the cornea to the nares occurs via natural drainage and is a more representative test. One source of confusion is that a negative fluorescein test results when the distal nasolacrimal duct orifice is not located in the anterior nasal vestibule. For a quantitative test of tear drainage, a radioactive isotope can be placed in the palpebral fissure and its passage followed with sequential nuclear imaging.

Re-establishing the normal anatomic relationship of the drainage passages is ideal but is often a difficult goal. Conjunctivorhinostomy or conjunctivoralostomy (Gelatt and Gwin, 1981) can create a new tear drainage tract into the nose or mouth, respectively. Transection of the medial canthal ligament (Covitz, 1980) can improve some palpebral conformations. Alternatively, palliative therapy of tear staining can be achieved with long-term oral tetracycline administration (50 mg/dog/day). Tetracycline does not decrease tear flow, but more likely binds the chromatic proteins, which cause staining on lightly pigmented haircoats. Reduction of tear secretion by excision of the nictitans gland is a poor approach because it can precipitate keratoconjunctivitis sicca in a susceptible animal.

DACRYOCYSTITIS

Dacryocystitis, inflammation of the lacrimal canaliculi, lacrimal sac, and nasolacrimal duct, is a relatively uncommon cause of epiphora. Mechanical obstruction by a foreign body, invasive growth, or injury causes stasis of tear drainage, which predisposes to bacterial infection. Conjunctivitis rarely extends to the nasolacrimal duct unless a relative obstruction exists. The presenting signs are usually epiphora and conjunctivitis. Occasionally an abscess of the nasolacrimal duct can rupture just nasal to and below the medial canthus. Diagnosis is usually made while flushing the nasolacrimal duct. Forceful flushing under anesthesia may be necessary to dislodge inspissated pus or a foreign body. Exudates from the procedure should be saved for bacterial culture and sensitivity testing. If the duct is stubbornly resistant to flushing, dacryocystorhinography with viscid radiopaque solutions such as 40 per cent iodized poppy seed oil is advised to demonstrate the nature of the obstruction.

After re-establishing patency, long-term topical antibiotics are used as determined by sensitivity testing. If the blockage recurs, an indwelling nasolacrimal catheter is made from a blunted 2-0 monofilament suture inserted into the upper lacrimal punctum through the nasolacrimal duct, exiting the nostril, and secured on both ends. This remains in place for three weeks with concurrent broad spectrum antibiotic-corticosteroid application.

REFERENCES AND SUPPLEMENTAL READING

Aguirre, G. D., Rubin, L. F., and Harvey, C. E.: Keratoconjunctivitis sicca in dogs. J.A.V.M.A. 161:158, 1971.
Blogg, J. R.: Surgical replacement of a prolapsed gland of the third eyelid. Aust. Vet. Pract. 9:75, 1979.
Covitz, D.: Diseases of the lacrimal apparatus. *In* Kirk, R. W. (ed.): *Veterinary Therapy VII.* Philadelphia: W. B. Saunders Co., 1980.
Gelatt, K. N., and Gwin, R. M.: Canine lacrimal and nasolacrimal systems. *In* Gelatt, K. N. (ed.): *Veterinary Ophthalmology.* Philadelphia, Lea & Febiger, 1981.
Kaswan, R. L., Martin, C. L., and Chapman, W. L.: Keratoconjunctivitis sicca: histopathologic study of the nictitating membrane and lacrimal glands from 28 canine cases. Am. J. Vet. Res. in press, 1983.
Murphy, J. M., Severin, G. A., and Lavach, J. D.: Nasolacrimal catheterization for treating chronic dacryocystitis. V.M./S.A.C. 72:883, 1977.

DISEASES OF THE CORNEA AND SCLERA

KERRY L. KETRING, D.V.M.

Cincinnati, Ohio

Recent textbooks have covered the embryology, anatomy, and physiology of the cornea and sclera in detail. Emphasis will be placed on the recognition of corneal and scleral diseases and the differentiation of primary diseases from diseases involving aqueous dynamics of the adnexa, anterior uvea, and lacrimal apparatus, any of which frequently have corneal involvement as their most obvious sign.

There are several primary corneal diseases, but the majority of cases presented to the practitioner include secondary corneal involvement. In these cases, response to therapy will be poor or temporary unless the primary disease is determined. Failure to identify the primary etiology may lead to loss of vision, unnecessary pain, and even loss of the eye.

SIGNS OF CORNEAL DISEASE

Signs of corneal disease include a change in transparency, pain, hyperemia of the conjunctiva, and/or discharge. Decreased vision may also be associated with corneal diseases. Many of these signs may be found in both primary and secondary corneal disease. However, they also occur in other ocular diseases that have no remarkable corneal involvement.

A change in corneal transparency is the most obvious sign of corneal disease. This change may be due to neovascularization, edema, cellular infiltration of inflammatory or neoplastic cells, pigmentation, calcium and lipid deposits, and scar formation. Large branching or dichotomous vessels are usually found in the superficial corneal layers and indicate chronic irritation. This may be seen in primary corneal disease or corneal involvement in chronic conjunctivitis, adnexal diseases, or exposure keratitis. Smaller straight vessels extending 360° from the limbus can be seen in diseases of the deeper layers of the cornea but usually indicate intraocular disease such as anterior uveitis. These vessels may appear with an acute onset.

Corneal edema may be focal or diffuse. The cornea will have a hazy-blue discoloration. If it is associated with ulceration and damage to the epithelium, the cornea will be thickened and elevated in the area of irritation. Focal corneal edema without epithelial disease may be due to endothelial irritation from an anterior lens luxation. This is usually found in the axial or inferior cornea.

Acute onset of generalized corneal edema is caused by severe damage to the endothelial layer of the cornea with resultant water accumulation between the collagen lamellae of the stroma. This may be associated with anterior uveitis or glaucoma. Deep limbal neovascularization is often also present. The edema may be so extensive as to prevent visualization of intraocular structures.

Digital tonometry may be an excellent diagnostic aid. Decreased intraocular pressure (IOP) associated with anterior uveitis and marked increases in IOP associated with glaucoma can be determined digitally. Corneal edema in these cases is usually transient and will clear if the primary disease is brought under control.

Fluid may accumulate and form vesicles or bullae between layers of the epithelium. The vesicles may rupture, causing acute ulceration and pain. Bullae formation is usually associated with superficial corneal disease or long-standing primary endothelial disease. Primary corneal edema may be focal or diffuse. Its treatment will be discussed under corneal dystrophies.

Pain may be manifested by squinting, blepharospasms, enophthalmia, prolapsed nictitans, and increased lacrimation. With the possible exception of blepharospasms, these signs may not always be indicative of pain, and careful evaluation is needed. The anterior third of the cornea is richly supplied with unmyelinated fibers from the trigeminal nerve. Superficial ulcers involving the epithelial layer and superficial stroma elicit severe ocular pain. Deep stromal ulcers and descemetoceles, which are below the level of innervation, cause little or no pain.

Pain associated with corneal ulceration can be quickly eliminated by the application of topical anesthetics. Use local anesthetics only after fluorescein staining and only as a diagnostic test or an aid to examination. Ocular pain associated with anterior uveitis or glaucoma is not relieved by the application of topical anesthetics. Ocular pain in the absence of corneal ulceration usually indicates additional involvement of the eye, since neovascularization, edema, and cellular infiltrates by themselves or in combination seldom cause pain.

Hyperemia of the conjunctiva and ocular discharge are nonspecific signs of ocular disease. These will be discussed only as they relate to specific disease syndromes.

Blindness is not a common sign of corneal disease. If a tapetal reflex can be seen through a dilated pupil, the cornea is not the cause of total blindness. Corneal disease may cause decreased vision but seldom causes blindness. However, determining degrees of vision in animals is difficult.

KERATITIS

Keratitis is inflammation of the cornea. The inflammatory response may include edema, neovascularization, and the deposit of inflammatory cells, pigment, cholesterol, or calcium. Keratitis is a nonspecific reaction of the cornea to irritation and does not imply a specific etiology. The conditions discussed under this heading are, therefore, secondary corneal diseases. Keratitis will be classified as superficial ulcerative, deep ulcerative, and nonulcerative.

SUPERFICIAL ULCERATIVE KERATITIS

Superficial ulcerative keratitis is indicated by a positive fluorescein dye test and varying degrees of inflammation, depending on the etiology and duration of the ulcer. The ulcer involves only the epithelium and superficial stroma.

Fluorescein is a water-soluble dye that stains the cornea stroma a bright green only if the epithelial layer, which is hydrophobic, is removed. Descemet's membrane does not stain and will appear as either a clear membrane or a black area surrounded by the green staining stroma. Abrasions of the epithelium or removal of only several layers of epithelium will elicit pain, but the fluorescein dye tests will be negative.

Excluding primary corneal ulceration or dystrophies, most cases of superficial corneal ulcers are caused by adnexal diseases, such as entropion, aberrant cilia, decreased tear production, exposure keratitis, and trauma. External trauma is most frequently incriminated by the owner as the cause of ulcerations but is far less common than the others.

Primary bacterial, viral, or fungal involvement is even more rare as a cause of superficial ulceration. Thus, it is not usually necessary to do bacterial culture and sensitivity tests on superficial ulcerations at the initial examination. There is no need to change topical medications after three or four days, because epithelialization is not complete. Slow healing is more likely owing to failure to identify the cause of the ulcer than to resistant bacteria.

If decreased tearing is even a remote possibility, a Schirmer tear test should be done prior to the application of fluorescein dye or a topical anesthetic. Tearing rate should be 15 to 27 mm/min. A rate of 10 mm/min, although not significantly lower, could be the cause of recurring ulceration.

Superficial ulcers are quite painful, but, if possible, fluorescein staining should be done prior to topically anesthetizing the eye. Topical anesthetics disrupt the tear film, and repeated applications may cause false positive stain retention, especially if the eye is examined with a Woods lamp. The location and shape of the corneal ulcer can be clues to etiology. Axial corneal ulcers are usually associated with lagophthalmus and exposure problems commonly found in the exophthalmic and brachiocephalic breeds. A corneal ulcer located nasally may indicate a foreign body under the nictitating membrane. A vertical ulcer near the limbus is often due to ectopic cilia penetrating the palpebral conjunctiva or a foreign body buried in the palpebral conjunctiva. Dogs with ectopic cilia have a characteristic head jerk at the height of the blink as the cilia comes in contact with the cornea. Corneal ulcers located in the temporal and inferior quadrants of the cornea are frequently associated with temporal and inferior entropion. After the shape and location of the ulcer have been noted, the adnexa should be closely examined with the aid of topical anesthesia and magnification.

Associated superficial neovascularization may aid in finding the cause of ulceration. Since these vessels denote chronicity, the ulcer could not have been caused by presumed recent trauma. The eye should be closely examined for a source of chronic irritation such as mild entropion or partial sicca.

After the cause of the superficial ulcer is corrected, epithelialization should be rapid and uncomplicated. Within a maximum of 48 to 72 hours, even a large superficial ulcer will re-epithelialize. If spastic entropion is present, it may be necessary to do a temporary tarsorrhaphy or third eyelid flap until epithelialization is complete. Bacterial contamination is a possible complication, so broad spectrum antibiotics should be applied frequently. Ointments are applied three to four times daily and solutions four to six times daily. It has been shown that ointments retard healing more than solutions, but the significance of this on a clinical level is questionable. If the only problem is a superficial ulcer, there is no rational need for systemic medication.

Anterior uveitis is frequently associated with traumatic superficial ulceration. If present, this should be treated with systemic corticosteroids and topical cycloplegics such as 1 per cent atropine sulfate to effect (dilation of the pupil and decreased ciliary spasms as manifested by blepharospasms). Topical corticosteroids are contraindicated in superficial corneal ulcerations, since they retard the initial phase of re-epithelialization, but should be used systemically if anterior uveitis is present.

If corneal neovascularization and/or edema persists after epithelialization, topical steroids may be used to clear the cornea and reduce scar formation.

DEEP ULCERATIVE KERATITIS

The same causes for superficial ulcers are important here too. Animals with deep stromal ulcers frequently have a history of recurring superficial ulcers. If the owner is unable to document this in the history, examination of the cornea will most likely reveal pigmentation and superficial neovascularization, both of which denote chronicity.

Stromal ulcers and descemetoceles in the brachiocephalic and exophthalmic breeds deserve special emphasis. Owners and many veterinarians believe these are caused by trauma to the eye. The ulcers are usually located in the axial or central cornea and are caused initially by lagophthalmus, which leads to drying of the central cornea. Treatment and the prevention of recurrence include reducing the palpebral fissure by means of a permanent lateral tarsorrhaphy.

Bacteria may play an important role in deep corneal ulcers. Protease enzymes released from bacteria, most notably *Pseudomonas*, cause destruction of the corneal stroma with possible perforation.

Collagenase enzymes, released from necrotic epithelial cells, fibroblasts, and polymorphonuclear leukocytes, cause rapid destruction of the stroma. The end result may be a descemetocele or a white "mushy" cornea that appears to be liquefied. This corneal liquefaction is known as keratomalacia.

After the etiology of the deep corneal ulcer has been determined, collect material from the edge of the ulcer for bacterial culture and sensitivity tests. Avoid topical anesthetics at this time, since they may interfere with culture results. Use tranquilization and careful restraint to avoid rupturing the descemetocele. Initial treatment consists of topical antibiotic solutions that are effective against *Pseudomonas*, such as gentamicin, tobramycin (Tobrex), or polymyxin. I prefer a solution at this stage of treatment because of the ease of administration. Maintain an effective concentration by using drops every one to two hours.

An anticollagenase drug should also be applied initially every one to two hours. The drug of choice is acetylcysteine, which is available in 10 and 20 per cent solutions (Mucomyst). Since high concentrations may be irritating, I prefer to mix 10 cc of the 10 per cent solution with 10 cc of artificial tears. This combination must be refrigerated to avoid deterioration. Since cold drops applied to the eye may be irritating, a day's supply may be kept at room temperature in a separate dropper bottle.

Determine whether anterior uveitis is present. Since the external pressure caused by tonometry may rupture the cornea with a deep ulcer, other signs of anterior uveitis, such as miosis and aqueous flare, may help make the diagnosis. If these cannot be adequately evaluated, the author prefers to treat for anterior uveitis until the eye can be re-evaluated. Apply topical atropine solution two to three times daily. The frequency is based on the desired response. Overtreatment with atropine must be avoided, since it may result in decreased tear production. If the anterior uveitis is severe, a combination of a cycloplegic and a mydriatic may be preferred. A 10 per cent phenylephrine and 0.1 per cent scopolamine ophthalmic solution (Murocoll #2) can be applied every four hours until the desired effect is reached.

Systemic corticosteroids may be necessary in the treatment of severe anterior uveitis. Topical corticosteroids are contraindicated, since they delay epithelialization and augment the activity of collagenase. Antiprostaglandins (aspirin) may also be beneficial in controlling anterior uveitis without interfering with healing of the corneal ulcer.

Show the owner how to restrain the animal for medication without putting excessive pressure on the globe or neck. At least 10 to 15 minutes should lapse between application of different drops. Otherwise, one drug may be diluted below its effective concentration. Intensive therapy is continued until response is noted by decreased corneal necrosis and associated inflammation (i.e., anterior uveitis) and healing of the ulcer.

A descemetocele may be flat and may appear as a clear circle in the bottom of a deep ulcer. Descemet's membrane and endothelium may be forced anterior through the stroma and epithelium to form a bubble above the surface of the cornea.

A descemetocele is an ophthalmic emergency, and medical management alone is not sufficient. A thin conjunctival flap may be sutured directly to the cornea adjacent to the descemetocele, preventing rupture and loss of ocular contents. A corneal-scleral transposition is a better procedure, since the deficit is quickly filled by normal cornea, reducing axial scarring. However, it is a more difficult procedure to perform.

A temporary tarsorrhaphy or third eyelid flap may be an aid to therapy in superficial or stromal ulcer but is not sufficient in the case of a descemetocele. If the ulcer is not down to Descemet's membrane and if lagophthalmus or sicca is not a consideration, the author prefers medical treatment alone for at least the first 24 to 48 hours.

Following epithelialization of the deep ulcer, use a topical corticosteroid to reduce the vascularization. A corneal scar will result from the disorganization of the collagen fibers making up the stroma. In deep stromal ulcers, a depression or crater may remain after epithelialization is complete. This results from a thinning of the stromal layer. In a fluorescein test the dye may have to be flushed from the crater to differentiate it from an ulcer. Although this results in an abnormal curvature or astigmatism, it is not a functional problem for animals.

NONULCERATIVE KERATITIS (INTERSTITIAL KERATITIS, PIGMENTARY KERATITIS, PANNUS)

This is a nonspecific reaction of the cornea to chronic or acute irritation. Various terms have been used to describe keratitis based on the most remarkable inflammatory component present. These terms are descriptive and should not be considered primary corneal diseases but rather signs of an ocular or adnexal disease.

Interstitial keratitis is frequently an acute keratitis with severe corneal edema and deep limbal vascularization. The classic example is the "blue eye" reaction associated with hepatitis. The severe edema is secondary to endotheliitis and anterior uveitis. Treatment must be aimed at the primary disease.

Pigmentary keratitis is the term used to describe corneal inflammation in which pigmentation is the most remarkable and sometimes the only obvious abnormality. In some cases, blood vessels are obscured by the pigment. The source of pigmentation is debatable. Superficial pigment may arise from the basal layer of epithelial cells. Epithelial and stromal pigment may originate from limbal melanoblasts, which migrate into the cornea with and without associated neovascularization. Endothelial pigmentation is due to iris pigment deposited on the endothelium either after sloughing from the iris during severe iritis or as a result of anterior synechia (adhesion of the iris and cornea). Hyphema (blood in the anterior chamber) may produce a reddish-brown appearance of the cornea. This pigment is due to disintegration of red blood cells and deposition of hemosiderin and lipofuscin in the cornea. The prognosis for clearing this pigment is poor, but treatment is indicated for the anterior uveitis or glaucoma that may exist.

Classic examples of pigmentary keratitis are found in pugs and other exophthalmic breeds. The pigmentation located on the nasal aspect of the cornea is due to medial entropion, whereas horizontal and linear pigmentation is due to lagophthalmus. In cases of complete corneal pigmentation, lagophthalmus is also usually involved.

The primary abnormality must be corrected to arrest the progression of pigmentation. Surgical removal of the pigment is not indicated unless the animal is functionally blind. In severe cases, topical corticosteroids may reduce the density of pigmentation. Once the source of chronic irritation is removed, epithelial pigmentation may decrease in time owing to the natural turnover of the epithelial layers. There is little turnover of the stroma, and deep pigmentation normally persists.

Pannus is superficial vascularization of the cornea with granulation tissue. This term is usually reserved for cases of nonulcerative keratitis in which the vascular involvement and inflammatory cell infiltration are the most remarkable findings. This is a nonspecific reaction and should not be confused with the specific disease termed *degenerative pannus*. The superficial vessels denote chronicity. It is not uncommon to have elevated masses of granulation tissue composed of vessels and inflammatory cells. One of the most common causes of pannus is vascular healing of superficial and stromal ulcers.

Topical corticosteroids are indicated in all cases of nonulcerative keratitis to reduce the inflammatory response. They should be used only after the primary defect has been corrected. Ophthalmic antibiotic ointments or drops containing dexamethasone (Maxitrol) or prednisolone acetate (Blephamide, 1 per cent Pred Forte, AK-Tate) are preferred because of their superior anti-inflammatory effect and their ability to penetrate the cornea. Use ointments at least four times daily and solutions or suspensions six times daily. Reduce the frequency of application as the desired response is achieved.

Discontinue medication when there are no longer signs of active inflammation.

To know when to discontinue treatment, it is important to know what may persist in the cornea after active inflammation. Vessels will persist. These ghost vessels stop carrying blood but can always be seen, especially with biomicroscopy. Pigmentation may persist. Calcium or lipid products, which may be deposited in the cornea during active inflammation, will not be removed with topical steroid treatment.

Corneal scars are classified by the depth of corneal involvement and density. With increased density, a corneal scar is termed a *nebula*, a *macula*, or a *leukoma*. Once formed, scars are not reduced by corticosteroids.

These noninflammatory changes, often referred to as keratopathies, are not painful and, if vision is functional, are not treated surgically.

MYCOTIC KERATITIS

Although common in horses, mycotic keratitis is rare in the dog and cat. *Rhinosporidium* has been incriminated as the causative agent in a keratopathy seen in both cats and dogs in the southeastern United States. The affected animal is presented with unilateral or bilateral circular areas of corneal haze. The lesions are present at varying depths in the cornea. The overlying epithelium is intact, and the lesion does not elicit an inflammatory response. The eye is not painful and vision is normal. The condition appears to be self-limiting but does not totally regress. No treatment is indicated.

Many species of fungi have the potential to invade the cornea. The two most common species incriminated in the dog and cat are *Aspergillus* spp. and *Candida albicans*. Although trauma associated with plant material can initiate the infection, the two cases treated by the author had initial corneal ulcers, which were treated for four to six weeks with various topical antibiotics and corticosteroids. *Aspergillus* and *Curvularia* spp. were identified in these cases. In a third case, *Dichotomophthora* was isolated from a corneal ulcer of one week's duration. In addition to stromal ulcers and keratomalacia, animals in both cases had a severe anterior uveitis with aqueous flare, hypopyon, and flocculent material on the anterior lens capsule. A diagnosis was based on the identification of mycelia on cytology. The samples were taken from a thick tenacious material found in the center of the stromal ulcer.

In cases of presumed or cytologically confirmed fungal keratitis, culture and sensitivity tests should be submitted using both Sabouraud medium without inhibitors and blood agar medium.

In addition to the treatment listed previously for a stromal ulcer (including systemic corticosteroids), specific antifungal drugs should be used topically every one to two hours for the first 24 to 48 hours. The most readily available broad spectrum drug is miconazole. This is available as a 10 per cent preparation for IV injection (Monistat IV), which is used topically undiluted. Other nonophthalmic drugs can be used topically if the culture and sensitivity tests indicate that they are the drug of choice; these include amphotericin B, nystatin, and flucytosine. One topical ophthalmic preparation, pimaricin (Natacyn) has a broad spectrum but is not readily available and is quite expensive.

Topical medication alone has been effective in treating cases of mycotic keratitis. The treatment period is prolonged, and if frequent administration cannot be done by the owner, the animal should be hospitalized. After epithelialization, topical corticosteroids can be used in conjunction with antifungal therapy to reduce pannus formation. To date, no corneal recurrence has been noted in the treated cases. One animal has had two episodes of anterior uveitis, both of which responded to topical corticosteroids and atropine.

Candida infection may be seen as an epithelium covered with gray-white plaque. This plaque should be removed by keratectomy and then treated as described previously.

CONGENITAL CORNEAL DISEASE

Microcornea (small cornea) and megalocornea (enlarged cornea) in otherwise normal eyes are rare in animals. Microcornea is usually associated with a congenitally small globe, microphthalmia, which is found in Great Danes, schnauzers, collies, and Australian shepherds. Megalocornea is extremely rare but may be associated with congenital glaucoma and buphthalmia.

Congenital corneal dermoids may be found in any breed but are most frequently reported in the large breeds. This tissue mass, which resembles skin, may be found on the lids or palpebral conjunctiva or, more frequently, on the temporal corneal-scleral junction. Most dermoids contain hairs, which are irritating. As the animal matures, the island of skin grows. These islands should be removed by lamellar keratectomy and sclerectomy. If removed early, scar formation is minimal. The ulcer formed from surgery should be treated as described previously.

Persistent pupillary membrane (PPM) is a cause of congenital corneal opacities. Although all breeds may be affected, the incidence appears to be higher in the basenji, collie, and chow. This incidence may only reflect the popularity of a breed in a given geographic area.

The cornea is involved when these pigmented strands are attached to the corneal endothelium, resulting in a scar or pigmentation. The PPM may have regressed by the time of examination, leaving only the endothelial scar. In severe cases, corneal edema may result from extensive endothelial cell damage. Treatment is seldom indicated, since vision is impaired only in severe cases. We have used topical hyperosmotics to control corneal edema that was progressing to a conical cornea in a severe case in a chow. Although the mode of inheritance has not been established, PPMs may be inherited in the breeds mentioned.

A symblepharon is an abnormal adhesion of the conjunctiva. The adhesion may be to the cornea and may result in a continuation of conjunctival vessels and pigment onto the cornea. This is most frequently caused by infections prior to lid opening in cases of ophthalmia neonatorum. In cats, this is caused by a herpesvirus and in dogs by *Staphylococcus*. It usually does not impair vision, and specific treatment is not indicated.

DEGENERATIVE PANNUS (Überreiter's Syndrome, Chronic Superficial Keratitis)

The exact etiology of this disease is unknown but is believed to be a cell-mediated immune reaction to a yet unidentified corneal protein. It is most frequently seen in German shepherds and German shepherd crosses but has also been reported in dachshunds, corgis, and greyhounds. It is a bilateral disease that starts first in the temporal cornea. The vascular infiltration and associated inflammatory cells (primarily plasma cells and lymphocytes) will progress to involve the entire cornea without treatment. As the disease becomes chronic, corneal pigmentation and fibrovascular changes may become extensive, and lipid deposits may develop. Uncontrolled, vision impairment or blindness results. The temporal conjunctiva usually presents with inflammation and pigmentation.

The free margin of the nictitans may be irregular and eroded and may have focal areas of depigmentation. In some cases, the nictitans is severely hyperemic, friable, thickened, and significantly prolapsed. In this condition, the term *plasmoma* or *plasma cell conjunctivitis* has been used to describe the nictitans, since the predominant cell type is the plasma cell.

Therapy. Although there is no cure for the disease, it can be controlled in most cases. Topical corticosteroid ointments containing dexamethasone or prednisolone acetate applied six times daily will reduce the vascular component of the inflammatory response. After several weeks of rigorous treatment, the frequency of application may be reduced to once or twice daily to prevent recurrence. The frequency of treatment, both initially and for control, varies with individual cases. The complications

of glaucoma, herpes infection, and cataracts seen with long-term topical steroid therapy in humans are not a concern in the dog.

No surgical treatment is indicated in degenerative pannus, as all procedures offer only temporary improvement. The most common cause of failure in medical management is the lack of owner cooperation in treatment. The most difficult component of the disease to control is involvement of the nictitans. It may be necessary to use systemic anti-inflammatory drugs or beta-ray therapy if the nictitans is severely involved.

IDIOPATHIC KERATITIS

This disease may simply be a variant of degenerative pannus, but its clinical appearance, history, and response to therapy differ slightly. This condition has been seen in the poodle, dachshund, spitz, and Siberian husky. Pigmentation and superficial neovascularization without extensive granulation tissue are the most significant findings. It is a bilateral disease, with the pigmentation covering the entire cornea in a swirling pattern. The disease has a chronic course and does not start just in the temporal limbus but at 360° of the limbal area. Treatment consists of topical steroid application as in degenerative pannus. Although the response is not as rewarding, the progression of pigmentation can normally be controlled with continual treatment. Prior to making the diagnosis, all sources of chronic irritation should be evaluated, especially a *partial keratoconjunctivitis sicca*.

PUNCTATE ULCERATIVE KERATITIS

Punctate ulcerative keratitis is a disease of unknown etiology. Although a viral cause has been proposed (mainly DNA viruses), there is no evidence to confirm this etiology.

It is a bilateral disease with an increased incidence in American cocker spaniels, dachshunds, and Shetland sheepdogs. The animal usually has a history of acute pain manifested by squinting, a prolapsed nictitans, and increased lacrimation. The conjunctiva is severely hyperemic. A diffuse corneal neovascularization and pigmentation indicate a chronicity prior to the acute pain. Multiple focal pinhead white opacities are present in the superficial cornea. When stained with fluorescein dye, some, but not all, of the opacities retain dye.

In spite of the superficial ulcers, the treatment of choice is topical corticosteroids. Prednisolone acetate suspension (AK-Tate, 1 per cent Pred Forte) is used initially every four hours. The animal should be rechecked in 48 to 72 hours, and the response to therapy is usually significant. The signs of pain will have subsided, hyperemia will be reduced, and most ulcers will have re-epithelialized. With continual treatment, the neovascularization will be reduced. As improvement is noted, the frequency of medication can be reduced and corticosteroid ointment can be used twice daily in place of the drops. Continual treatment is needed to prevent recurrence.

INDOLENT ULCER (Boxer Ulcer, Refractory Ulcer, Superficial Corneal Erosion, Dendritic Ulcer, Basement Membrane Dystrophy)

Originally described in the boxer, this disease has been seen in the American cocker spaniel, Boston terrier, dachshund, poodle, Welsh corgi, West Highland terrier, wire-haired fox terrier, golden retriever, and mixed breeds. The exact etiology is unknown, but a degeneration or lack of regeneration of the basement membrane of the epithelial layer is suspected. Hemidesmosomes, which anchor the basement membrane to the basal layer of epithelial cells, may also be defective.

Indolent ulcers are usually found in middle-aged to old individuals and are usually unilateral. Although the owners may give a history of trauma, the significance of trauma in the genesis of this disease is questionable. It is important to differentiate an indolent ulcer from other superficial ulcers because of the difference in treatment and prognosis.

An uncomplicated indolent ulcer will present initially with few if any subjective signs of pain, unlike a traumatic superficial ulcer. The dog with an indolent ulcer may show only a mild increase in lacrimation and prolapsed nictitans. When the ulcer is stained with fluorescein dye, a border of lighter staining can be seen around the darker staining ulcer. After a topical anesthetic is applied to the cornea, this lighter staining border can be easily stripped off the cornea with a cotton swab.

The superficial ulcer differs from an indolent ulcer in its lack of a redundant border and its rapid epithelialization (within 24 to 48 hours) or neovascularization. Indolent ulcers do not evoke a vascular response until very late in the course of the disease and usually only after inadequate treatment. If the source of chronic irritation or trauma is not removed, a superficial ulcer may extend into the stroma or to Descemet's membrane. An indolent ulcer, even after as long as six weeks duration, does not extend into the stroma.

Once the diagnosis of an indolent ulcer is correctly made, the owner should be told that the treatment and recovery periods may be prolonged and that recurrence in the same or opposite eye is possible. It is important to assure the owner that this disease will not result in loss of the eye or loss of vision.

Therapy. For an uncomplicated indolent ulcer, initial treatment consists of mechanical and chemical debridement of the redundant border under topical anesthesia. Enough pressure is applied to the cornea with a dry cotton swab to slightly indent the cornea and rub off the redundant epithelium. Frequently, the original ulcer will be enlarged tenfold. All epithelium that can be removed is abnormal. After this, the new border is lightly touched with a swab containing 7 per cent iodine solution as a cautery agent and rinsed with a collyrium.

Since this is not a bacterial ulcer and there is little tendency for these ulcers to penetrate, topical antibiotics are not indicated. Following debridement of the ulcer, a collar should be placed on the dog to prevent rubbing of the eye, since the newly formed epithelium can be easily removed.

If there is an associated anterior uveitis, it should be treated with topical 1 per cent atropine ointment b.i.d. and systemic corticosteroids. If corneal edema is severe, topical hyperosmotic agents (Muro 128) may be useful in reducing the edema, allowing normal epithelialization.

Initial treatment should be re-evaluated in 72 hours. If the size of the ulcer has reduced significantly, no further debridement should be performed. The eye should be re-evaluated in another 72 hours. Debridement is repeated only if the ulcer stops reducing in size. For several weeks following complete re-epithelialization, the epithelium can be easily stripped off by trauma. In refractory cases, it may be necessary to debride the ulcer as previously described and then do a third eyelid flap or temporary tarsorrhaphy. A conjunctival flap is not indicated.

In chronic cases in which neovascularization has become significant, debridement and a temporary tarsorrhaphy may be the best initial treatment. Following epithelialization, topical corticosteroids may be used to reduce corneal edema and vascularization.

FELINE HERPETIC KERATITIS

The herpesvirus, in addition to causing feline rhinotracheitis, causes three ocular disease syndromes in cats: ophthalmia neonatorum in the newborn; bilateral keratoconjunctivitis in the young cat associated with active rhinotracheitis; and unilateral or bilateral keratoconjunctivitis without associated systemic disease in adult cats. The disease found in adult cats will be discussed in this section, but the treatment applies to any cat with ocular involvement with herpesvirus.

The most common form of feline herpes keratitis is presented with a serous to seromucoid discharge, blepharospasms, conjunctival hyperemia, superficial neovascularization, minimal corneal edema, and superficial corneal ulcers. Unstained, these ulcers have a ground glass appearance; they may be multiple small linear lines, or they may have a branching or dendritic pattern. In early cases, the cat may present with severe blepharospasm, swollen hyperemic conjunctiva, and superficial ulcers without additional corneal involvement. The ulcers may be very small, less than 0.5 × 3 mm, and, if located nasally or inferiorly, may be difficult to observe.

In chronic cases, dendritic ulcers may coalesce and form larger superficial ulcers, termed *geographic ulcers*. In severe cases, the corneal stroma may become involved, resulting in severe edema, deep limbal neovascularization, and stromal ulcers.

A clinical diagnosis can be confidently made based on the finding of superficial linear or dendritic ulcers. A compatible history and a large geographic ulcer with associated corneal neovascularization completes the clinical diagnostic picture. If the only involvement is the conjunctiva, it is difficult to make a clinical diagnosis. Conjunctival scrapings may be indicative of herpes infection if a large number of lymphocytes are present. There will be few polymorphonuclear leukocytes unless a bacterial component is also present. Intranuclear inclusion bodies, although possible, are seldom identified in the conjunctival epithelial cells.

A few laboratories are able to do indirect fluorescent antibody tests on conjunctival scrapings. A positive test will identify the viral antigen in epithelial cells. The viral particle is not found in all epithelial cells, so if few cells are submitted a false negative test may result. Also, the viral particles may not be present at all stages of the disease, also resulting in a false negative test. The preparation of a conjunctival scraping for indirect fluorescent antibody testing may vary between laboratories, and one should follow the advice of the laboratory.

Therapy. Response to therapy may be the most practical diagnostic test. If a case of conjunctivitis worsens when topical corticosteroids are used, this may indicate herpes infection. Three solutions are now available with specific antiherpetic activity: idoxuridine (Herplex, Stoxil), vidarabine or adenosine arabinoside (Vira-A), and trifluridine (Viroptic). Idoxuridine is usually the first choice because it is the most readily available and most economical. Initially, one drop is used every 2 hours for the first 24 hours, then every 4 to 6 hours. If the diagnosis is correct, improvement should be noted within 24 to 48 hours. On rare occasions, a cat may be sensitive to idoxuridine, resulting in increased discharge and subjective signs of pain, or the virus may be refractive to idoxuridine, and a change in antiviral solution may be necessary.

Epithelialization should be complete within seven days. Treatment should be continued at least seven to ten days after healing is complete. If a mucopurulent discharge is present initially, a broad spectrum antibiotic such as chloramphenicol should be applied concurrently with the antiviral drug. If corneal neovascularization is still present after two weeks of treatment, a topical corticosteroid can be applied, but an antiviral drug should be continued for an additional week.

The recurrence rate of herpes keratitis is high, and the client should be so advised. In cases of recurrent attacks, the cat may be immunodepressed owing to feline leukemia complex, and this should be evaluated.

EOSINOPHILIC KERATITIS

Eosinophilic keratitis has currently been found only in the adult cat, with no breed predisposition. It may be unilateral or bilateral. The etiology is unknown, and cases examined to date have had no cutaneous lesions of the eosinophilic granuloma complex. A peripheral eosinophilia has been found in some cases but is not a consistent finding. Eosinophilic keratitis is characterized by superficial neovascularization and infiltration of inflammatory cells, beginning at the temporal limbus. The cornea may have a white appearance axially, at the leading edge of the vascularization, and fluorescein dye may be retained. In advanced cases the cornea is extremely thickened and may have an irregular curvature. A characteristic finding in severe cases is superficial white plaques, which can be flushed from the corneal surface with a collyrium or easily removed with a cotton swab. The entire cornea may be involved, resulting in blindness. There may be an associated conjunctivitis and a seromucoid discharge in advanced cases.

A presumptive diagnosis may be made based on the clinical appearance, especially the superficial white plaques and response to therapy. The cytology of conjunctival or corneal scrappings or biopsies is characterized by eosinophils and plasma cells.

Therapy. Although improvement with topical or systemic corticosteroid therapy will occur, the treatment of choice is megestrol acetate (Ovaban). Initially, 5 mg megestrol acetate is given daily until a response is noted, usually in seven to ten days. The entire cornea can be cleared, leaving only residual ghost vessels. Once the cornea is cleared, maintenance therapy will vary but is usually 2.5 to 1.25 mg every three to four days.

The contraindications and side effects of megestrol acetate should be kept in mind. Once controlled, the use of topical corticosteroids may allow further reduction of the total dose of megestrol acetate.

CORNEAL SEQUESTRATION (Corneal Mummification, Cornea Nigrum, Focal Degeneration, Isolated Black Lesions)

This disease is unique to the cat. Although all breeds are susceptible, the incidence is greater in

Persians and Siamese. The etiology is unknown but is believed to be the result of chronic corneal irritation. The exophthalmia found in the Persian may be the source of chronic irritation, since most lesions in this breed are found in the axial cornea. It has also been proposed that herpes keratitis may be the source of chronic irritation.

The condition is usually a unilateral, black or brown axial discoloration on the cornea. The discoloration may be diffuse and may involve the epithelium and stroma, with minimal elevation above the surface of the cornea. It may also form a black, well-defined superficial plaque that extends above the surface of the cornea. In many cases, one edge of the plaque may be free of the cornea and can be elevated with a small spatula. The cat may show varying degrees of blepharospasm, conjunctivitis, corneal edema, and neovascularization. The black plaque, which histologically is desiccated, and degenerated stroma will not stain with fluorescein dye. The cornea adjacent to the sequestrum may be ulcerated, and on close examination with biomicroscopy it can be determined that there is no normal epithelium over the sequestrum. In all cases, the globe and adnexa should be examined closely for a possible source of chronic irritation such as herpes keratitis or entropion and appropriate therapy instituted.

Therapy. If the cat is free of subjective signs of pain, i.e., increased lacrimation and blepharospasm, no treatment may be needed initially, since the sequestrum may slough spontaneously after a period of time. If the eye has no corneal ulcerations yet is painful, topical steroids may control the associated inflammation and reduce the pain. A third eyelid flap may reduce the pain, and, when taken down in several weeks, the sequestrum may have sloughed.

A lamellar keratectomy may be performed to remove the sequestrum, but often there is a core that extends deep into the stroma that cannot be excised. Care should be taken not to perforate the cornea. If excision is incomplete, rapid return of the sequestrum is possible. Following the keratectomy, a third eyelid flap or temporary tarsorrhaphy should be sutured in place and topical antibiotic therapy instituted for 7 to 14 days. If epithelialization is complete after this period of time, topical corticosteroids may be used to treat the keratitis.

If the sequestrum returns but the cat is comfortable, repeated keratectomies are not indicated.

CORNEAL DYSTROPHY AND DEGENERATION

These two terms are often interchanged and used incorrectly. Corneal dystrophies are usually bilaterally symmetric, axial, noninflammatory, nonprogressive or slowly progressive, not associated with systemic disease, frequently found in young animals, and possibly inherited. A corneal degeneration usually follows inflammation. It is often unilateral (if bilateral, it is asymmetric), may be associated with systemic disease or aging, and may be more progressive. Although in some cases the differentiation between dystrophy and degeneration is not easily made, it may be important to make the distinction. If the condition is inherited, the individual and related animals should not be bred. Most corneal dystrophies require no treatment and are neither blinding nor painful. A corneal degeneration, which is caused by or associated with a systemic disease such as hypothyroidism, would be an indication for systemic therapy.

Different corneal layers are involved in various dystrophies and degenerations in different breeds. The layer of involvement may be difficult to determine without biomicroscopy.

Histologically, most epithelial and stromal corneal dystrophies are composed of some form of lipid; neutral fats, cholesterol, cholesterol esters, and phospholipids have all been identified. These deposits may be intracellular or extracellular. There is no consistent relationship of hypercholesteremia or hyperlipemia and lipid corneal dystrophies. This is especially so in cases of true dystrophies, i.e., bilateral corneal opacities without associated corneal neovascularization.

Specific breeds, which will be discussed, have a high incidence of corneal dystrophy. Additional breeds in which corneal dystrophy has been seen include beagle, Boston terrier, boxer, Samoyed, American cocker spaniel, akita, bichon frise, collie, Irish setter, miniature pinscher, Afghan, miniature schnauzer, poodle, pug, Shetland sheepdog, and springer spaniel. In most of these cases, the dystrophic area consists of a round to oval axial or paraxial white opacity. The white opacity is formed by a multitude of white lines or dots in the subepithelial corneal stroma, resulting in a ground glass appearance. In other cases, these white opacities may form arches or concentric rings. They are not painful or blinding, and treatment is not indicated.

SIBERIAN HUSKY CORNEAL DYSTROPHY

A high incidence of bilateral, most often symmetric corneal dystrophy has been identified in the Siberian husky. The incidence of lesions increases with age, but it has been observed in dogs as young as six months old. There is no sex predilection. Lesions can best be detected by retroillumination, directing a focal beam of light through a dilated pupil and observing the reflected light through the cornea. Lesions usually consist of a hazy gray doughnut-shaped axial opacity with a clear center. With biomicroscopy, the typical lesion can be localized deep in the stroma as fine crystals. But in other cases, a hazy opacity is present in the subepithelial and mid stroma. In some cases, both areas are involved. The dystrophy is slowly progressive but seldom results in any visual impairment.

Histochemically, the opacities consist of neutral fats, phospholipids, and cholesterol. Although the mode of inheritance has not been identified, the high incidence in related individuals suggests that the disease is inherited. Not only should affected animals be removed from the breeding program, but all related animals should be used with caution until the exact mode of inheritance has been defined.

CORNEAL DYSTROPHY IN THE AIREDALE

This bilaterally symmetric disease presents as a milky appearance of the axial cornea. The dogs are presented as early as nine months of age, and the opacity gets denser but does not extend grossly to the limbus as the animal ages. By three to four years of age, affected individuals evidence visual impairment. The opacity extends from the subepithelial stroma to as deep as three-fourths of the stromal thickness. Various lipids have been identified by histochemical studies. Lamellar keratectomies have not been therapeutically successful, although full thickness corneal transplant may improve vision. Inheritance has been suggested to be by a sex-linked recessive pattern.

ENDOTHELIAL CORNEAL DYSTROPHY

Although best known as a disease of Boston terriers, Chihuahuas, and dachshunds, a similar disease has been seen in the basset hound, English springer spaniel, West Highland terrier, wire-haired fox terrier, and one domestic cat. Previously undiagnosed anterior uveitis and endotheliitis may have been the causes of endothelial cell death and subsequent corneal edema in some sporadic cases. The endothelium is responsible for maintaining the cornea in a state of controlled hydration. When this layer is not functioning properly, water from the aqueous enters the cornea, increasing the interlamellar spaces. Late in the course of the disease, the epithelium is involved with increased intercellular and intracellular water. Bullae or water-filled clefts form in the epithelial layer. These bullae may rupture, resulting in superficial corneal erosion and pain. Late in the course of the disease the total thickness of the cornea is greatly increased, especially in the axial cornea, resulting in a conical-shaped cornea termed *keratoconus*. At this stage, the axial cornea is further irritated by lagophthalmus. This results in further corneal ulceration. Early in the course of the disease the cornea is free of neovascularization, whereas late in the disease limbal neovascularization and cellular infiltrates contribute to the overall opacity of the cornea.

Affected dogs are usually presented by five years of age. If presented early in the course of the disease, the individual may have only a unilateral focal area of corneal "blueing," usually in the temporal region. The animal may show no conjunctival irritation or subjective signs of pain. The disease will progress as previously described to a complete bilateral corneal edema. In more advanced cases, glaucoma should be considered as a differential, since the Boston terrier and other breeds listed have a high incidence of glaucoma. Also, in advanced cases with ruptured bullae, the animal is presented with conjunctival injection, blepharospasm, and epiphora. Vision may be impaired in advanced cases but seldom progresses to total blindness.

Treatment is palliative at best. Hypertonic sodium chloride ointment (Muro 128) should be used four to six times daily to control the epithelial edema and prevent bullae formation. If there are no corneal ulcers, topical corticosteroids should be used two to four times daily to prevent or control neovascularization. The corticosteroids also seem to help control the corneal edema.

Treatment must be continued throughout life. If the animal is presented with severe keratoconus, a temporary tarsorrhaphy may be needed to protect the cornea while medical management is instituted. Full thickness corneal transplants have been used to improve vision, but they are not routinely successful.

CORNEAL DYSTROPHY IN THE MANX CAT

A bilateral corneal dystrophy, which is believed to be inherited as an autosomal recessive trait, has been described in the Manx cat. Affected cats have been examined at four months of age with a bilateral "haziness" of the axial cornea. The disease progresses to a severe corneal edema and epithelial bullae formation. Unlike the corneal dystrophy in the Boston terrier, the endothelium and deep stroma are not affected. Treatment is not rewarding but should be instituted as described for the Boston terriers.

LIPID CORNEAL DEGENERATION

This may be a unilateral or an asymmetric bilateral disease. The axial or limbal cornea may be involved. The lipid deposits are usually found in the subepithelial or midstromal cornea. The deposits may be so extensive that they are elevated above the normal corneal curvature. Superficial and stromal neovascularization is present. Lipid may be deposited in the cornea after neovascularization if the animal has a hyperlipemia.

Primary lipid deposits in the cornea may stimulate neovascularization, so the often unanswered question is which came first, neovascularization or lipid deposition. In addition to the lipid deposits and neovascularization, the animal may have a mild conjunctivitis.

The globe and adnexa should be closely examined for a source of chronic irritation. The dog should be evaluated for hypercholesteremia or hyperlipemia. A significant number of these cases are hypothyroid and will have systemic signs of the disease.

Treatment is aimed at the hypothyroidism, if present. Topical corticosteroids can be used to control the neovascularization. However, neither treatment regimen will reduce the existing lipid deposits. If vision is reduced, a lamellar keratectomy can be used to remove the lipid deposits after the primary disease is treated.

CORNEAL NEOPLASMS

Primary corneal tumors are rare in the dog and cat. The majority of tumors arise from the limbus or extend into the cornea from the conjunctiva, sclera, and anterior uvea. In all cases of presumed corneal neoplasms, a thorough ocular examination, including indirect ophthalmoscopy, biomicroscopy, and gonioscopy, is indicated. A complete physical examination is also warranted including thoracic radiographs. Viral papillomas, epitheliomas, and squamous cell carcinomas have been successfully removed by lamellar keratectomies. Melanomas originating from the sclera shelf and extending into the cornea have been removed by a corneoscleral resection with transplantation of donor scleral or corneal tissue. Hemangiosarcomas, fibrosarcomas, adenocarcinomas, and melanomas due to extension from uveal tissue are best treated by enucleation.

Lymphosarcoma may involve the cornea and associated sclera and conjunctiva. Affected animals usually have bilateral lesions and intraocular involvement may be present. This form of lymphosarcoma frequently is concurrent with skin lesions. The prognosis is guarded.

FIBROUS HISTIOCYTOMA

This condition is frequently seen in young adult collies and has been termed *pseudotumor, fibrous histiocytoma, histiocytoma, ocular nodular fasciitis,* and *proliferative keratoconjunctivitis.* Part of the confusion arises from trying to fit a disease found in the dog into the nomenclature used for a similar disease in humans. Regardless of the name, the disease in collies presents as a unilateral or bilateral disease. Pink- to flesh-colored, smooth tissue masses are usually found at the limbus. The masses cause little inflammation or pain, with only edema at the corneal edge of the mass. The free margin at the nictitans is also frequently involved with a similar

fleshy swelling. Some cases also have multiple masses on the upper and lower lids, nares, and lips. Histologically, all lesions are similar. They are highly cellular, with varying combinations of lymphocytes, plasma cells, immature fibroblasts, histiocytes, and perivascular polymorphonuclear leukocytes. No neoplastic cells have been identified; therefore, the mass resembles a hyperplasia more than a true tumor.

Isolated limbal lesions may be removed by a lamellar keratectomy and sclerectomy, but the recurrence rate is high. The lesions are sensitive to systemic corticosteroids, but therapy may have to be maintained at a low level indefinitely to control recurrence. In cases in which systemic corticosteroids were not tolerated by the animal or did not give the desired response, azathioprine (Imuran) has been effective in causing regression and preventing recurrence. Initially, the drug is given at a dosage of 2 mg/kg once daily for five to seven days, discontinued for two days, and then repeated. Since azathioprine is a potent bone marrow depressant, complete blood counts should be taken prior to and periodically during its administration. After all lesions have regressed, the previous dosage, given only every three to four days, has been effective in preventing recurrence. To date, no side effects have been noted from the use of azathioprine. Once the limbal mass regresses, an arch of stromal lipid deposits frequently remains.

Isolated masses, similar in appearance, have been

Table 1. *Drugs Used For The Treatment Of Corneal And Scleral Diseases*

Drug	Manufacturer
Antibiotics	
.3% Tobrex	Alcon
Corticosteroids	
Maxidex	Alcon
1% Pred Forte	Allergan
AK-Tate 1%	Akorn
Antibiotic-Corticosteroids Combination	
Maxitrol	Alcon
Blephamide	Allergan
Antiviral	
Viroptic 1%	Burroughs Wellcome
Vira-A, 3%	Parke-Davis
Herplex	Allergan
Stoxil	Smith, Kline and French
Antifungal	
Monistat IV	Ortho
Natacyn	Alcon
Mydriatic and Cycloplegic	
Murocoll-2	Muro
Anticollagenase	
Mucomyst 10 and 20%	Mead Johnson
Miscellaneous	
Ovaban	Schering
Imuran 50 mg	Burroughs Wellcome
Hyperosmotic	
Muro 128	Muro

reported in many breeds of dogs and one cat. These isolated lesions are probably best treated with surgical removal, resorting to medical management only if they recur. All tissues removed should be examined histologically.

DISEASES OF THE SCLERA

Diseases of the sclera are rare in the dog and cat. The sclera may be involved with neoplasms of the cornea or from extension from the uveal tissue.

Episcleritis is an inflammatory disease of unknown etiology most frequently seen in the American cocker spaniel and poodle. It consists of a focal limbal swelling or a diffuse scleral involvement. The overlying conjunctiva is inflamed, and vessels extend into the corneal stroma with resulting limbal edema. Various degrees of pain will be manifested. The condition must be distinguished from extension of intraocular tumors and tumors of the cornea previously described.

Most cases of episcleritis are responsive to topical or systemic corticosteroids. Azathioprine has also been used successfully to control this condition. The recurrence rate is high, and continual or periodic treatment may be needed for control.

SUPPLEMENTAL READING

Bistner, S. I., Aguirre, G., and Batik, G.: *Atlas of Veterinary Ophthalmic Surgery*. Philadelphia: W. B. Saunders Co., 1977.
Blogg, R. J.: *The Eye in Veterinary Practice*. Philadelphia: W. B. Saunders Co., 1980.
Gelatt, K. N.: *Textbook of Veterinary Ophthalmology*. Philadelphia: Lea & Febiger, 1981.
Jones, D. B., O'Day, D. M., and Foster, C. S.: Diagnosis and management of ocular fungal infection. American Academy of Ophthalmology Instruction Course 98, 1980.
Slatter, D. H.: *Fundamentals of Veterinary Ophthalmology*. Philadelphia: W. B. Saunders Co., 1981.

ALTERED OCULAR FLUID DYNAMICS: GLAUCOMA AND HYPOTONY

WILLIAM ARDENE VESTRE, D.V.M.

West Lafayette, Indiana

Altered ocular fluid dynamics may result in increased intraocular pressure (glaucoma) or decreased intraocular pressure (hypotony). These may be transient stages in the course of the disease process, or they may be the end result of altered ocular anatomy and physiology. In many cases one may progress to the other, and the evaluation of this transition must not be bypassed by the clinician. Secondary damage to the nervous structures of the eye occurs rapidly with glaucoma, and early diagnosis and therapy are essential. The clinician must understand both clinical and pathophysiologic aspects to effectively treat and offer a prognosis for glaucoma. An understanding of the mechanisms involved is essential. Because of the threat to vision, the high incidence of the disease, and the availability of therapy the bulk of this article will deal with the glaucoma process.

AQUEOUS HUMOR DYNAMICS

For effective clinical management of glaucoma or hypotony, an understanding of aqueous humor dynamics is essential. Aqueous fills the anterior and posterior chambers of the eye and is responsible for nutrition of the avascular structures of the eye, i.e., the lens, central cornea, and trabecular meshwork.

The aqueous humor is produced by the ciliary body epithelial cells. The ciliary body is composed of fenestrated capillaries embedded in a loose connective tissue stroma. The stroma is lined by a double layer of epithelial cells—outer pigmented (from the retinal pigment epithelium) and inner nonpigmented (from the neural retina). The nonpigmented ciliary epithelium is primarily responsible for the secretion of aqueous humor. Aqueous is produced by a combination of active secretions (Na^+ transport to the posterior chamber dependent on ATP-supplied energy), diffusion, and ultrafiltration. The sodium transport also results in a shift in osmolality across the ciliary epithelium. This increased osmolality is also enhanced by the active transport of chloride (Cl^-) and bicarbonate (HCO_3^-) ions. Carbonic anhydrase is present in high levels in the ciliary epithelium. Oxidative metabolism of glucose is predominantly localized in the nonpigmented epithelium and provides 75 per cent of the ATP required. It is now estimated that diffusion and ultrafiltration contribute about 30 to 50 per cent of aqueous production. Aqueous formation is about 1 to 2 μL/min in the dog and 10 to 20 μL/min in the cat.

The aqueous is secreted and diffuses into the posterior chamber, then flows over the anterior surface of the lens, through the pupil, and into the anterior chamber.

The chemical composition of the posterior aqueous differs from that of the anterior aqueous, since constituents are removed or added during aqueous passage through the eye. There is an appreciable exchange of constituents of the aqueous between anterior aqueous and the iris vessels. Most of the aqueous leaves the anterior chamber by bulk flow through the trabecular meshwork, but some is removed by iris vessel absorption and uveoscleral flow.

The iridocorneal angle is formed where the corneoscleral and uveal tracts of the eye unite. Histologically, it begins where Descemet's membrane ends and terminates at the iris root where the anterior border layer of the iris begins. The innermost structures of the drainage angle are the pectinate ligaments. These originate from the base of the iris, traverse the drainage angle, and insert in the posterior surface of the peripheral cornea. There are at least two rows of ligaments, with the inner row the largest and most heavily pigmented. The ligaments are occasionally tent-like from their origin, and interconnections between ligaments are common. The pectinate ligaments insert at the end of Descemet's membrane in a pigmented band. Behind the pectinate ligaments is a white to blue-gray zone, which is a loose collagenous meshwork that actually arises from the ciliary body and is termed the *ciliary trabecular meshwork*. This trabecular meshwork is the filtering area of the drainage angle. Aqueous is drained through the trabecular meshwork via small sacculated vessels to the plexus venous sclerae (circle of Hovius), which is on the external half of the sclera and is composed of three to four large, interwoven, circumferential veins. The plexus venous sclerae communicates with vortex veins, anterior ciliary veins, and choroidal vessels to transfer aqueous to the general circulation.

GLAUCOMA

Glaucoma is defined quite simply as an increase in intraocular pressure beyond that which is compatible with the normal health and function of the intraocular structures. In the dog and cat this is usually considered to be any pressure greater than 30 mm Hg.

Glaucoma is one of the leading causes of blindness in the middle-aged dog, with an estimated incidence of 0.5 per cent. The disease does present in the cat as well but much less frequently than in the dog.

Glaucoma is one of the most challenging disease processes in veterinary ophthalmology not only for the general practitioner but for the specialist as well. It is often misdiagnosed or ignored in the early stages, and often the definitive diagnosis is made only after irreversible changes have occurred.

CLINICAL SIGNS OF GLAUCOMA

The signs in early glaucoma are often subtle and can be quite variable, depending on the extent of pressure elevation. The clinical signs can be divided into those of acute versus chronic glaucoma, although the clinician must remember that there can be a great deal of overlap and blending of signs as the disease progresses.

ACUTE GLAUCOMA

Acute glaucoma will often be quite painful as evidenced by blepharospasm, an elevated membrana nictitans, epiphora, and photophobia. The conjunctiva is often inflamed, although this can be mild with moderate pressure elevations. The episcleral vessels will be congested if there is a relatively large pressure increase. The cornea becomes edematous owing to a decrease in function of endothelial cells and imbibition of fluid into the corneal stroma. The pupil is dilated and nonresponsive to light as the pupillary constrictor is paralyzed. Visual acuity is decreased early in the course of glaucoma, although this is often not detected by the client even if bilateral disease is present. The retinal vascularity is decreased, and cupping of the optic disc may be detected ophthalmoscopically. This may not be present if the disease is caught early, but it is an important prognostic sign.

CHRONIC GLAUCOMA

Long-standing increases in intraocular pressure lead to irreversible damage. This will present with various combinations and degrees of change in ocular structure and function. A gradual enlargement of the globe or buphthalmos occurs, although this can be rapid in young animals. This generally indicates irreversible loss of vision and a long-standing increase in intraocular pressure. The buphthalmos is not reversible even if the pressure is reduced. Episcleral congestion and occasionally an extreme enlargement of these vessels are common in chronic glaucoma. The veins may remain dilated even after the pressure is controlled. The conjunctival vessels are usually engorged to a much lesser degree. Episcleral engorgement is believed to be due to increased flow via the anastomosing episcleral veins as ciliary flow to the vortex veins is decreased. The corneal edema present in acute cases remains, and striae (white endothelial stretch marks) (striate keratopathy) occur as linear ruptures form in Descemet's membrane. Corneal neovascularization and pigmentation follow in extreme cases. The pupil dilation remains and is often more pronounced than in early glaucoma. In some cases of advanced glaucoma the iris stroma becomes atrophic and assumes a lacy appearance. The lens often becomes cataractous and may luxate owing to zonular rupture as the eye enlarges. Retinal and optic nerve atrophy with cupping of the optic disc and retinal vascular attenuation are usually present in chronic glaucoma. This begins with ganglion cell degeneration but progresses to total retinal degeneration indistinguishable from advanced retinal atrophy from other causes. The end-stage eye usually is not painful unless corneal ulcerations are present owing to exposure keratitis from lagophthalmos. Even these cases may not be painful owing to decreased sensation from nervous tissue destruction. Some cases of long duration have ciliary atrophy and decreased intraocular pressure, however the globe will remain enlarged.

DIAGNOSIS OF GLAUCOMA

The presenting signs and history, e.g., breed predisposition (Table 1), should lead to a high index of suspicion. Recurring episodes of "reddened" or "blue" eyes and indications of ocular pain in the susceptible breeds should alert the clinician. The measurement of intraocular pressure (IOP) is the most important diagnostic test. Because of the dif-

ficulty in diagnosing glaucoma in its early stages, quantitative measurement of IOP is a necessity. Three forms of tonometry are used in veterinary medicine.

Digital tonometry involves placing the index fingers against the globe over the upper eyelid; one finger is pressed against the globe, using the other to estimate pressure. This gives a very crude estimation of IOP and is not recommended.

Indentation tonometry involves the use of a Schiotz tonometer. This is used to measure the indentation of the cornea produced by a plunger of known weight and diameter as the plunger protrudes through the concave footplate. The amount of indentation of the cornea depends primarily on IOP, although scleral rigidity, corneal curvature, and the presence of corneal edema do affect the final reading.

The observed tonometer reading equals 0.05 mm of indentation per unit. The reading is then converted to pressure from calibration tables. To perform Schiotz tonometry, the cornea is anesthetized with topical anesthesia and the animal is held in a sitting position. The head is elevated, the eyelids retracted and the footplate placed as near the central cornea as possible. The unit is allowed to rest on the cornea. Excess pressure on the instrument or the globe must be avoided. The procedure is done three times and an average taken. Additional weights are placed on the instrument if the scale readings are low (less than 3 units). Because of species differences in corneal curvature, ocular rigidity, and tissue characteristics, an underestimation of actual IOP is usually obtained in the dog. However, the range of 3 to 7 units with a 5.5-gm weight is considered normal regardless of the conversion table used.

Applanation tonometry involves the application of a flat disc to the cornea that applanates or flattens a small area on the corneal surface. Either the force

Table 1. Breed Predisposition to Primary Glaucoma

Breed	Classification
American cocker spaniel	Primary closed angle (narrow angle)
Basset hound	Open to narrow; mesodermal dysgenesis (congenital)
Beagle	Open ($\downarrow$ outflow)
Bedlington terrier	Narrow to closed angle
Brittany spaniel	Narrow to closed angle
Dachshund	Narrow to closed angle
Dalmatian	Narrow to closed angle
English cocker spaniel	Open angle
English springer spaniel	Narrow to closed angle
Fox terriers (smooth and wire-haired)	Narrow to closed angle
Malamute	Narrow to closed angle
Norwegian elkhound	Narrow to closed angle
Samoyed	Narrow to closed angle
Sealyham terrier	Narrow to closed angle
Siberian husky	Narrow to closed angle
Toy and miniature poodle	Open angle
Toy terrier	Narrow to closed angle

necessary to flatten a constant area or the area flattened by a constant force can be measured. This type of tonometry is more accurate than the other two forms. It is quick and accurate and requires minimal restraint and positioning. Its cost, however, prohibits use in general practice. For general small animal practice the Schiotz tonometer remains the instrument of choice.

Gonioscopy is the visualization of the drainage angle. Direct observation of the iridocorneal angle is not possible because of the overlying opaque corneoscleral limbus. The difficulty of internal reflection of light is overcome by allowing light to strike the air interface at less of an oblique angle. This is accomplished by placing on the cornea a lens with a curvature different than that of the cornea. In direct gonioscopy the observer looks across the pupil to the opposite angle region. In indirect gonioscopy mirrors are positioned in the lens and the angle observed indirectly.

Numerous lenses are available, but the smaller ones are best suited to veterinary ophthalmology. A good light source is necessary to illuminate the angle. The angle can be examined with a focal light source and magnifying loupe, an indirect ophthalmoscope, a special gonioscope, a portable slit lamp, or a direct ophthalmoscope. I prefer the direct ophthalmoscope, as it provides magnification (14 ×) and is an excellent light source.

Almost all animals can be evaluated with just topical anesthetics on the cornea. General sedation is rarely needed.

All lenses require a fluid between the cornea and lens. A commercial high viscosity methyl cellulose solution is preferred. All quadrants of both eyes must be examined. Gonioscopic evaluation of the iridocorneal angle is essential in the classification of glaucoma and for selection of the most rational therapy.

The structures normally seen and evaluated on gonioscopy are the following:

1. *Peripheral one-half to one-third of the iris.* There is normally a sinuous pulsating vessel (arterial ring of Purtscher).

2. *Pectinate ligaments.* The pigmentation will usually correlate somewhat with haircoat and iris coloration. The length of the strands denotes in general the width of the angle. The variables are pigmentation, length, branching, and stoutness of fibers.

3. *Deep pigmented band.* The insertion of the pectinate ligaments at the end of Descemet's membrane.

4. *Uveal trabecular meshwork.* A gray-white zone visible between and behind the pectinate ligaments (through the spaces of Fontana).

5. *Superficial pigmented band.* More variable in width (and presence) than the deep pigmented band. This is from the normal pigmentation on the internal surface of the scleral shelf, which emerges externally at the limbus. It appears lighter because of the intervening cornea.

Direct or indirect ophthalmoscopy is used to evaluate the retina and optic disc for damage due to the increased pressure. The early changes are cupping and atrophy of the optic disc, which can be followed by retinal degeneration. Indirect ophthalmoscopy is usually superior to direct ophthalmoscopy because of better depth perception and better penetration of the cloudy cornea.

Tonography is the determination of the degree of resistance associated with the flow of aqueous humor from the eye. Tonography requires sedation and placement of an electronic Schiotz tonometer on the corneal surface for two to four minutes. The change in pressure over this period is measured and the facility of outflow calculated. This is usually available only at specialty practices or university centers.

Provocative tests have been used for some time in humans to detect patients with early glaucoma. These tests include water administration, mydriatic testing, dark room testing, and corticosteroid provocation. At present none of these are routinely done in animals, but mydriatic provocation may be useful in the future.

CLASSIFICATION OF GLAUCOMA

Glaucomas can be classified by mechanism of action and by stage of disease.

CLASSIFICATION BY MECHANISM OF ACTION

Classification by mechanism of action is superior to classification by stage of disease because understanding the mechanism is essential for therapy and is necessary in comparative ophthalmic research. The following classification of human glaucoma is adapted from Becker and Shaffers' *Diagnosis and Therapy of the Glaucomas.* The appropriate mechanism has been identified in animals in most forms, and others are being found as better diagnostic methods are used and more clinicians are looking. This classification is based on the state of the drainage angle and includes primary and secondary forms of glaucoma. Primary glaucoma indicates no other ocular abnormality, whereas secondary glaucoma indicates a structure other than the outflow pathway initiated the disease process.

CLOSED-ANGLE GLAUCOMA

With Pupillary Block. This glaucoma occurs typically in hyperopic, narrow-angled eyes, which usually have small anterior segments and shallow anterior chambers. Tension elevation tends to occur abruptly, causing typical symptoms and ocular pain. There may be marked fluctuations in intraocular pressure. A combination of circumstances leads to an acute attack: a pupillary resistance to the forward flow of aqueous humor at the site of iris contact with the anterior lens capsule, a laxity of the peripheral iris, and a possible contribution of vascular factors. The resulting forward displacement of the peripheral iris toward the trabecular meshwork can lead to complete or partial closure of the angle. Iridectomy usually bypasses the pupillary block and normalizes the outflow if the trabecular meshwork has not been damaged and peripheral anterior synechias have not formed.

PRIMARY CLOSED-ANGLE GLAUCOMA. This occurs, for example, in the American cocker spaniel.

SECONDARY CLOSED-ANGLE GLAUCOMA. This can result from a number of causes:

1. Swollen lens—acute unilateral closed-angle glaucoma associated with a rapidly intumescent lens. This occurs most in cocker spaniels and poodles.

2. Posterior synechia to lens—an iris bombé following severe uveitis.

3. Lens subluxation into either the anterior chamber or vitreous humor—more common in terrier breeds.

4. Posterior synechias to vitreous humor in aphakic eyes—a postoperative complication of cataract extraction or luxation of the lens.

5. Malignant glaucoma—as vitreous is displaced forward it blocks the pupil; aqueous goes behind the vitreous and pushes vitreous farther forward.

Without Pupillary Block. In this type of glaucoma the trabecular meshwork is covered by the iris root, but a pupillary block is not responsible for holding the iris against the meshwork.

PRIMARY PLATEAU IRIS. In this type of primary closed-angle glaucoma there is an insignificant amount of pupillary block. The angle is mechanically blocked by the last roll of the iris if the pupil is dilated. Iridectomy is not curative, for it only bypasses the pupillary block.

SECONDARY CLOSED-ANGLE GLAUCOMA. Peripheral anterior synechias are caused by the iris' becoming permanently attached and blocking the trabecular meshwork. In the absence of pupillary block, a chronic form of glaucoma results from a number of causes:

1. Previous pupillary block, which leads to peripheral anterior synechia and angle closure.

2. Flat anterior chamber, which can be seen with lens intumescence.

3. Tumors or cysts, such as uveal melanomas.

4. Inflammation with a severely swollen iris.

5. Neovascular glaucoma (rubeosis iridis); this is more frequent in cats than in dogs.

6. Essential iris atrophy, which is most common in toy poodles.

OPEN-ANGLE GLAUCOMA

With Decreased Facility of Aqueous Outflow. In open-angle glaucoma the iris is not in apposition to the trabecular meshwork. The decreased facility of outflow is caused by interference with aqueous flow through the outflow passages to the venous system. Symptoms are usually negligible until extensive ocular damage has occurred.

PRIMARY OPEN-ANGLE GLAUCOMA

1. Chronic simple glaucoma, such as that seen in cocker spaniels and beagles.

2. Open-angle glaucoma with low tension.

SECONDARY OPEN-ANGLE GLAUCOMA

1. Corticosteroid induced; this has not been established in the dog.

2. Secondary to inflammation, e.g., secondary to uveitis of any cause.

3. Lens-induced or phakoanaphylactic glaucoma occurs as lens material leaks through the capsule and macrophages, blocking the drainage angle.

4. Traumatic.

5. Alpha-chymotrypsin induced.

6. Associated with tumors, most frequently lymphosarcoma in dogs.

7. Secondary to epithelial ingrowths; postoperatively, conjunctival growth can occur through the limbal incision.

8. Neovascular glaucoma (rubeosis iridis) due to severe iritis.

9. Secondary to epidemic dropsy.

10. Secondary to retrobulbar pressure.

Open-angle glaucoma associated with congenital ocular abnormalities or intraocular disease not at the drainage angle is relatively rare in dogs and cats.

With Normal Outflow Facility. This group of cases demonstrates increased intraocular pressure resulting in vision defects. However, at all times the eyes have open angles and normal facilities of outflow.

HYPERSECRETION GLAUCOMA. This form is not documented in animals.

GLAUCOMA WITH INCREASED EPISCLERAL VENOUS PRESSURE. This is not completely documented in animals.

COMBINED MECHANISMS

This category includes various combinations of closed- and open-angle glaucoma.

CONGENITAL GLAUCOMA

Although the primary glaucomas are, at least in part, genetically determined, this category refers only to those cases in which anomalies of the anterior segment are present at birth. The glaucoma may be present at birth or may appear in the first four decades of life. In animals the primary form is mesodermal dysgenesis of bassets and cocker spaniels in which embryonic mesodermal tissue lines and obstructs the drainage angle. This can be easily evaluated gonioscopically.

CLASSIFICATION BY STAGE OF DISEASE

Classification by stage of disease process is valuable in deciding on therapy and offering a prognosis to the owner. This is a personal preference for classifying the disease and deciding on a course of action. This classification is much more practical for the average small animal practice than attempting to classify by mechanism of action.

The four classes used are (A) enlarged blind eye; (B) blind but not enlarged eye; (C) recent attack of congestive glaucoma; and (D) very early attack of glaucoma. Treatment is greatly influenced by the stage of the disease at the time of presentation.

Class A. No therapy will improve the eye. If the pressure is still elevated and the eye painful or if an exposure keratitis is beginning, the options are cyclocryosurgery, an intraocular prosthesis, or, lastly, enucleation. If the pressure is decreased owing to ciliary atrophy and the animal is comfortable it may be best to do nothing.

Class B. The pressure will almost always be elevated and the eye painful, so either cyclocryosurgery, an intraocular prosthesis, or medical therapy should be performed.

Classes C and D. Intense and early medical therapy is required to get the pressure down and save vision. Once the cause (mechanism) is established, a long-term medical and/or surgical treatment regimen can be started.

MEDICAL MANAGEMENT OF GLAUCOMA

Medical therapy must be started as soon as the diagnosis of glaucoma is made, as even a few hours of highly elevated pressure can cause irreversible damage. Medical treatment is directed at opening the drainage angle with miotics and decreasing aqueous production. Numerous drugs are readily available (Table 2). The emergency medical treatment regimen includes combinations of the following drugs.

Mannitol. As initial therapy, 1 to 3 gm/kg IV of a 20 or 25 per cent solution is given. Water must be withheld for the first few hours after administration. This will decrease the pressure by removing fluid, and the low pressure will make the miotics more effective. By shrinking the vitreous, mannitol also helps to pull the iris back and open the drainage angle. Oral glycerol has been recommended as an adjunct to medical therapy but does not seem as effective as mannitol on a one-time basis. Mannitol

administration can be repeated two to four times in the first 48 hours, but the animal must be monitored for signs of dehydration.

Cholinergic Stimulation

DIRECT CHOLINERGICS. The two most commonly used direct cholinergics are pilocarpine and carbachol. Pilocarpine 1, 2, or 4 per cent is given topically every hour until the pupil constricts and then three times a day. This direct-acting stimulant increases the facility of outflow and decreases the amount of aqueous production slightly. Carbachol has a similar mechanism of action to pilocarpine but is less frequently used in animals.

INDIRECT CHOLINERGICS. These are organophosphates, which cause irreversible blockage of the cholinesterases. These are more powerful and longer acting than the direct-acting drugs. The two commonly used are demecarium bromide (Humorsol) and echothiophate (Phospholine Iodide).

Carbonic Anhydrase Inhibitors. These act to decrease aqueous humor production by creating a local acidosis. The effect may be up to 30 to 40 per cent of aqueous production and usually lasts about

Table 2. Drugs and Dosages for Medical Management of Glaucoma

Osmotic Diuretics
Mannitol—20 to 25%, 1 to 2 gm/kg IV, single dose (Mannitol Injection USP, Invenex)
Glycerin—50 to 75%, 1 to 2 gm/kg oral, s.i.d. to b.i.d. (Glycerol, Cooper Vision)
Urea—30%, 1 to 2 gm/kg IV, single dose (Ureaphil, Abbott)

Carbonic Anhydrase Inhibitors
Acetazolamide—10 mg/kg oral, b.i.d. to t.i.d.; 5 to 10 mg/kg IV, single dose (Diamox, Lederle)
Dichlorphenamide—2–5 mg/kg, oral divided b.i.d. to t.i.d. (Daranide, Merck, Sharp and Dohme; Oratrol, Alcon)
Methazolamide—5 to 10 mg/kg b.i.d. to t.i.d. oral (Neptazane, Lederle)
Ethoxzolamide—5 to 7.5 mg/kg b.i.d. to t.i.d. oral (Cardrase, Upjohn)

Cholinergics
Pilocarpine—1 to 4%, 1 drop t.i.d. to b.i.d. (Isopto Carpine, Alcon)
Echothiophate—0.06 to 0.12%, 1 drop s.i.d. to b.i.d. (Phospholine Iodide, Ayerst)
Demecarium bromide—0.125 to 0.25%, 1 drop s.i.d. to b.i.d. (Humorsol, Merck, Sharp and Dohme)
Carbachol—0.75 to 3.0%, 1 drop t.i.d. to q.i.d. (Carbachol, Alcon)

Sympathomimetics
Epinephrine—0.5% to 2.0%, 1 drop b.i.d. to t.i.d. (Epitrate, Ayerst)

Autonomic Blocking Agents
Beta-blocking
Timolol—0.25 to 0.5%, 1 drop b.i.d. (Timoptic, Merck, Sharp and Dohme)
Alpha-blocking
Thymoxamine—0.5%, still investigational and not currently available for routine use

Combination Drugs
Pilocarpine plus epinephrine—2 to 4% pilocarpine and 1% epinephrine, 1 drop t.i.d. to q.i.d. (E-Carpine 2, Alcon)

eight hours when given orally. Intravenous acetazolamide is available for management of acute cases (50 mg/kg administered one time). Acetazolamide 20 mg/kg divided orally three times a day or dichlorphenamide 2 to 5 mg/kg orally three times a day is used. The individual dose may need adjustment to balance the pressure reduction with the side effects of vomition, panting, and weakness.

Sympathomimetics. Epinephrine 1 or 2 per cent applied topically one to three times daily decreases production and increases the outflow of aqueous humor.

Combination Drugs. Pilocarpine plus epinephrine (P_2E_1) seems to be very effective in the dog. Pupil size stays small to moderate, and the facility of outflow is increased.

Autonomic Blocking Agents. These include the beta antagonists, e.g., timolol maleate (Timoptic) and atenolol, and the alpha antagonists, e.g., thymoxamine.

The owners must be counselled that life-long therapy is required and frequent re-evaluation of these animals is necessary.

For acute attacks on sighted eyes I use topical pilocarpine, 2 to 4 per cent hourly, mannitol as the osmotic diuretic (single dose), and acetazolamide as the carbonic anhydrase inhibitor (intravenous initially and oral for maintenance). This is often changed to organophosphates (Humorsol), carbonic anhydrase diuretics (Daranide), and epinephrine as the situation becomes chronic.

SURGICAL MANAGEMENT OF GLAUCOMA

Long-term control of glaucoma is not often achieved medically in animals, so the owner should be counselled that surgical procedures may be necessary. Indeed, many owners are unwilling or unable to medicate frequently enough to control the pressure and may desire surgery in the early stages of the disease. If possible, the pressure should be brought to a normal range by medical management before surgery is attempted.

Surgical therapies are divided into those that decrease production and those that increase the outflow of aqueous.

METHODS TO DECREASE PRODUCTION OF AQUEOUS

Cyclocryosurgery. This is selective destruction of the ciliary body by freezing. It has been used in humans, monkeys, and rabbits and now is widely used in dogs and cats. The cryoprobe is held at $-70°C$ to $-80°C$ and is placed 5 mm behind the limbus. The area is frozen for one-half to three minutes. This is done at four to eight locations on the globe either equally spaced or in a quadrant or

hemisphere on the superior globe. The procedure is rapid and noninvasive and thus is repeatable as necessary. Side effects include conjunctivitis (marked postoperatively), uveitis, and retinal detachments. It is very effective clinically but is still experimental to some degree.

There are several specific cryosurgery units available. In general, a nitrous oxide unit with a 4-mm or less diameter tip should be used. Postoperative therapy should include a topical antibiotic/steroid ointment three times a day for one week. The pressure should be carefully monitored postoperatively, as many cases have a transient pressure rise, which will further damage the retina and optic nerve. After the pressure is controlled with cyclocryosurgery, I recommend re-evaluation at two to three weeks and then every three months. If the pressure begins to rise, low dose medical therapy can be added, or the cyclocryosurgery may be repeated with no adverse effects. If the cryosurgery is too extensive, a phthisical eye may result. This is very rare in my experience. A chronic hypotonic globe with no evidence of pain or irritation has developed in many cases. Cyclocryosurgery is also effective in decreasing the pain of glaucoma, although controlled studies in animals have not been completed.

Cyclodiathermy. Heat cautery is very damaging and results in a large percentage of phthisical eyes and can no longer be recommended.

METHODS TO INCREASE AQUEOUS OUTFLOW

Cyclodialysis. An aqueous outflow channel is created by separating the ciliary body from its scleral attachment, thus making the anterior chamber confluent with the suprachoroidal space. Problems usually arise with hemorrhage and rapid closure of the fistula.

Iridencleisis. A filtering wick is created by bringing a strip of iris through a scleral opening, hoping that as the iris atrophies or scars a draining tract will be left. Often the fistula will close a few months postoperatively.

Scheie Technique. A piece of sclera is removed by cautery with the hope of keeping the tract open longer because of the tissue destruction. This is often combined with iridencleisis.

Corneoscleral Trephination and Iridectomy. A small surgical bypass of the angle is made by making a corneoscleral (limbal) opening to the subconjunctival space. The peripheral iridectomy prevents occlusion by the iris and also any chance of pupillary block.

Numerous combinations of these methods are available.

Because of the low overall success rates reported by most authors with the various filtering procedures, I am currently recommending cyclocryosurgery on all eyes in which the pressure is not easily controlled medically. In cases of secondary glaucoma the initiating cause must be treated before the glaucoma can be adequately controlled either surgically or medically.

For blind, painful, enlarged eyes and in glaucomas due to aseptic uveitis, which may not respond to cyclocryotherapy, an intraocular prosthesis is recommended. These should not be implanted in infected or tumorous globes.

The globe is eviscerated and a silicone ball implanted via a scleral incision. The sclera is closed with interrupted absorbable sutures and the conjunctiva with continuous absorbable suture. Standard intraocular techniques and equipment are required. The postoperative appearance of the eye depends on the preoperative status of the cornea. After two to three weeks no further therapy is required and the globe is essentially maintenance free. Enlarged eyes will conform to a standard size ball in two to three months. The results are cosmetically very acceptable, and this option should be offered as an alternative to enucleation for intractable glaucoma.

HYPOTONY

Persistent hypotony or abnormally low intraocular pressure can be an end result of ciliary body destruction secondary to long-standing glaucoma. It may be due to uveal tract inflammation, or it may be secondary to surgical procedures on the globe. For hypotony secondary to uveal inflammation, the underlying causes need to be evaluated and treated. Primary ocular hypotension does not seem to be a clinical problem in dogs and cats, although it is well-documented in humans. Chronic hypotony secondary to cyclocryosurgery is not associated with discomfort and does not appear to necessitate treatment. If the hypotony progresses and a phthisical globe is eminent, an intraocular prosthesis is recommended.

REFERENCES AND SUPPLEMENTAL READING

Bedford, P. G.: The surgical treatment of canine glaucoma. J. Small Anim. Prac. 18:713, 1977.
Brightman, A. H., Magrane, W. G., Huff, R. W., and Helper, L. C.: Intraocular prosthesis in the dog. J.A.A.H.A. 13:481, 1977.
Brightman, A. H., Vestre, W. A., Helper, L. C., and Jones, J. E.: Cryosurgery for the treatment of canine glaucoma. J.A.A.H.A. 18:319, 1982.
Gelatt, K. N.: The canine glaucomas. In Gelatt, K. N. (ed.): Textbook of Veterinary Ophthalmology. Philadelphia: Lea & Febiger, 1981, pp. 390–435.
Gwin, R. M.: Pharmacologic agents that reduce intraocular pressure. In Gelatt, K. N. (ed.): Textbook of Veterinary Ophthalmology. Philadelphia: Lea & Febiger, 1981, pp. 181–205.
Kolker, A. E., and Hetherington, J.: Becker and Shaffer's Diagnosis and Therapy of the Glaucomas, 4th ed. St. Louis: C. V. Mosby, 1976.

DISEASES OF THE LENS

KATHLEEN P. BARRIE, D.V.M.

Tampa, Florida

The lens, a biconvex transparent organ positioned behind the iris and pupil and in front of the vitreous, transmits and focuses light on the retina. Although it is one of the simplest structures in the body, dysfunction is common and often leads to blindness. Knowledge of the anatomy, physiology, biochemistry, and pathology of the lens can assist the clinician who must diagnose and treat diseases of the lens.

ANATOMY AND PHYSIOLOGY

The lens resides in the fossa hyaloidea suspended by the zonular ligaments. Anteriorly, the iris contacts the lens except in maximum mydriasis. Posteriorly, the anterior vitreous forms a concave depression, the fossa hyaloidea (patellar fossa). The hyaloid membrane in the dog firmly attaches to the posterior lens capsule, making intracapsular lens extraction almost impossible without anterior vitreous displacement.

The volume of the dog and cat lens is approximately 0.5 ml. The canine lens diameter is 9 to 11.5 mm, and the diameter of the feline lens is 12 to 13 mm; the anteroposterior length is 7 and 8 mm, respectively.

The anatomy of the lens is not complex. The lens is surrounded by a capsule, which is the basement membrane of the lens epithelium. In the dog, the anterior capsule is 50 μ thick, although thickness varies with age and disease. The capsule is impermeable to large molecules but permits passage of water, electrolytes, and smaller molecules. The capsule isolates the lens proteins, thus keeping them immunologically foreign to the body.

Immediately beneath the anterior lens capsule is a single layer of epithelium. The cuboidal cells of this layer gradually elongate at the equator to form the lens bow and new lens fibers. The new fibers extend from the equator to the anterior and posterior poles. Because the lens is not a sphere, these fibers do not meet at the same point, thus forming suture lines in the shape of a Y. In the anterior cortex, the Y suture is upright; in the posterior cortex the Y suture is inverted. Lens fibers, formed throughout life, gradually increase the size of the cortex and compress the nucleus. This condition leads to a dense central nucleus, referred to clinically as nuclear sclerosis.

The lens is suspended in the posterior chamber by the ciliary zonules (ligaments). The zonules arise from the ciliary body and fuse with the lens capsule at the equator. Accommodation occurs when the ciliary muscles contract, relaxing the zonular pressure and allowing the lens to become spherical. Accommodation is minimal in most domestic animals, although it is more developed in the dog and cat.

The lens capsule has no direct association with the vascular and lymphatic systems. The energy requirements of the lens are low; the prime energy source is glucose from anaerobic glycolysis. The aqueous humor provides glucose, which diffuses across the epithelium of the lens capsule. Glucose is broken down by four pathways in the epithelium: (1) Embden-Meyerhof pathway, (2) hexose-monophosphate shunt, (3) citric acid cycle, and (4) sorbital pathway.

The lens is 65 per cent water and 35 per cent protein. The protein content of the lens is higher than that of any other organ. Lens proteins are classified as soluble (crystallin, 85 per cent) and insoluble (albuminoid, 15 per cent). The insoluble proteins increase with age. Transparency of the lens is dependent on a normal physiologic and biochemical environment.

CLINICAL EXAMINATION

The lens is best examined after mydriasis. Our choice is 1.0 per cent tropicamide (Mydriacyl), which results in full mydriasis in 15 to 20 minutes. The lens is examined with direct illumination, transillumination, retroillumination, and an oblique beam utilizing either the direct ophthalmoscope, pen light, or slit-lamp biomicroscope. The lens is divided clinically into regions: anterior lens capsule, anterior cortex, nucleus, posterior cortex, and posterior capsule. It can also be divided into axial (polar) and equatorial areas. The center of rotation of the dog's eye is the posterior nucleus; therefore, lesions in front of the nucleus move with the eye and those behind the nucleus move in an opposite direction (Fig. 1).

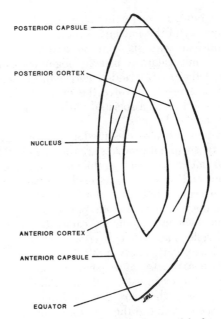

Figure 1. Biomicroscopic anatomy of the lens.

CATARACTS

A cataract is a focal or diffuse opacity within the lens and its capsule. Cataracts are classified by anatomic location, age of onset, degree of maturation, morphology, and cause. Cataracts may be hereditary or nonhereditary.

Cataracts classified by age are congenital, developmental (juvenile), and senile. Congenital cataracts are present at birth but are not necessarily inherited. It is important to get a complete medical history to attempt to determine inheritance. Depending on the anatomic site, congenital cataracts can be progressive or stationary and may even regress with time. Congenital cataracts are usually nuclear or capsular, with the latter often associated with other ocular anomalies such as persistent pupillary membranes, persistent hyaloid, persistent hyperplastic primary vitreous, and multiple ocular anomalies. Persistent pupillary membranes are inherited in the basenji. The persistent strands can attach to the anterior lens capsule, producing a focal cataract. Surgical treatment is not usually necessary because the cataract is rarely progressive. If vision is impaired, 1 per cent atropine two to three times weekly to dilate the pupil may be helpful.

Developmental cataracts may occur in dogs between one and five years of age. Heredity has been proposed in many breeds. Other causes of cataracts at this age may be diabetes mellitus, inflammation, trauma, and toxins and other agents. Cataract formation usually involves the cortex first, then the nucleus. Cataracts are usually progressive. Surgery is indicated in the functionally blind animal.

Senile cataracts generally occur in animals over five years of age. Nuclear sclerosis is not a true cataract but a normal aging change with increased translucency of the nucleus. Vision is not impaired with nuclear sclerosis, and no treatment is indicated. Senile cataracts usually begin with opacification at the equator and/or cortex of the lens and usually progress to involve the entire lens. Senile cataracts are often associated with systemic, toxic, and traumatic diseases.

Cataracts are also classified by their degree of maturity. Incipient cataracts are the earliest changes and do not cause visual problems. They consist of vacuoles and/or water clefts in the equator or subcapsular region. Rate of progression is variable. As the cataract matures, more portions of the lens become involved. Immature cataracts still permit tapetal reflection, although vision can be impaired at this stage, particularly if miosis is present.

Mature cataracts cause complete loss of vision and prohibit examination of the fundus. In the mature stage, the lens can become swollen or intumescent owing to the imbibition of fluid. Lens proteins may escape through the capsule, producing an immune-mediated anterior uveitis. Glaucoma may develop owing to either intumescence decreasing the angle width or lens-induced iridocyclitis embarrassing the iridocorneal angle. In the latter case inflammatory cells and large lens proteins obstruct the aqueous outflow channels. Treatment is surgical excision of the cataract.

Hypermature cataracts contain liquefied lens material, which may leak through the lens capsule and reduce the lens volume. In some hypermature lenses the nucleus remains hard and gravitates ventrally within the liquefied cortex. This is a Morgagnian cataract. Vision can be restored spontaneously in animals with hypermature and Morgagnian cataracts because of the resorption of the cortex. Mydriatics (1 per cent atropine) to maintain dilation may permit partial vision; intraocular pressure should be monitored periodically. Resorption of the lens sufficient to restore vision is more common in young animals (less than four years of age).

Cataracts can also be classified according to location of the opacity within the lens and its capsule (Fig. 2).

ETIOLOGY OF CATARACTS

INHERITED

Inherited cataracts occur in many breeds of dogs and may also be associated with other ocular anomalies. Both dominant and recessive inheritance patterns have been proposed for these cataracts. Breeds with suspected autosomal dominant inheritance include the beagle, German shepherd, golden retriever, pointer, Chesapeake Bay retriever, and Labrador retriever. Breeds with suspected autosomal recessive inheritance include the Afghan hound, American cocker spaniel, Boston terrier, poodle, miniature schnauzer, Old English sheepdog, Staffordshire bull terrier, Welsh springer spaniel, and West Highland white terrier (Table 1).

In some breeds, retinal diseases are concurrent with cataracts. The most common breeds with retinal degeneration and cataracts are the miniature and toy poodle, Labrador retriever, and Old English sheepdog. Inherited cataracts in the cat have not been reported.

METABOLIC

Diabetes mellitus is the most common metabolic disorder producing cataracts in the dog. The cat also develops cataracts from diabetes but not as rapidly as the dog. Glucose, the source of energy for the lens, is transported to the lens by active transport from the aqueous humor. In diabetes, the glucose concentration is greatly increased and overwhelms the hexokinase pathway. The excess glucose is then metabolized via the sorbital pathway to form a nondiffusible alcohol (sorbitol); this changes the osmotic state, causing more water to enter the lens and leading to swelling and disruption of lens fibers. Early stages of the disease are evident as vacuoles at the equator. If the serum glucose level remains elevated, there is rapid progression of the cataract.

Nutritional excesses or deficiencies may also produce cataracts. Experimentally high sugar diets have produced cataracts. Diets deficient in certain amino acids have been reported to produce cataracts in young wolves. Wolves fed commercially prepared canine milk replacers developed posterior sutural cataracts. In another experiment, young puppies were given milk replacer from two days of age until death (five to eight weeks); 50 per cent developed some degree of lens opacity, although the opacities were mild and decreased with time.

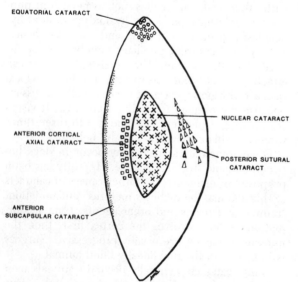

Figure 2. Classification of cataracts by location.

Table 1. *Hereditary Cataracts in the Dog*

Breed	Mode of Inheritance	Age of Onset	Clinical Characteristics
Afghan hound	Autosomal recessive (suspected)	4 mos to 2 yrs	Equatorial cataract with progression
American cocker spaniel	Autosomal recessive (suspected)	Developmental	Anterior and posterior cortical with progression
Beagle	Dominant (suspected)	Congenital	Diffuse and progressive and associated with other ocular anomalies
Boston terrier	Autosomal recessive	8 weeks to adult	Sutural opacities with progression by 1 year of age
Chesapeake Bay retriever	?	Developmental	Nuclear and cortical; progression is variable
English cocker spaniel	?	Congenital	Anterior capsular
German shepherd	Dominant	Congenital	Nuclear; nonprogressive
Golden retriever	Dominant with incomplete penetrance	Developmental	Posterior sutural, triangular; slow progression
Labrador retriever	Dominant	Congenital	Posterior cortical with progression
Miniature poodle	Autosomal recessive	2 to 5 yrs	Diffuse cortical with progression
Miniature schnauzer	Autosomal recessive	Congenital	Nuclear, posterior cortical with progression
Old English sheepdog	Autosomal recessive (suspected)	Developmental	Nuclear, cortical with progression
Siberian husky	?	Developmental	Posterior cortical, may progress
Standard poodle	Autosomal recessive (suspected)	Developmental	Equatorial, cortical with progression

INFLAMMATION

Any inflammatory disease that produces anterior uveitis can lead to cataract formation. Interruption of normal aqueous humor dynamics can disrupt the normal metabolism of the lens, leading to cataracts. Anterior uveitis can result in posterior synechiae with alterations in the lens capsule. In the dog, leptospirosis, hepatitis, systemic mycoses, geotrichosis, toxoplasmosis, leishmaniasis, and primary septicemia can contribute to secondary cataract formation. Feline infectious peritonitis, leukemia virus, toxoplasmosis, and systemic mycoses may produce anterior uveitis with secondary cataracts in the cat.

Severe blunt trauma or penetrating injury to the globe can cause a dislocation of the lens or a tear in the lens capsule, which may result in cataract formation. Lens proteins leaking into the anterior chamber may produce a lens-induced uveitis. Intensive medical therapy with topical mydriatrics (1 per cent atropine) and antibiotic/corticosteroid preparations four times daily are indicated. Surgical removal of the entire lens and medical therapy are indicated in some cases of traumatic dislocation.

A number of toxic substances have been reported to produce cataracts in dogs including dinitrophenol, diazoxide, and radiation.

TREATMENT OF CATARACTS

MEDICAL

Medical treatment for the resolution of cataracts has included vitamins, selenium and vitamin E, sulfadiazine, and, most recently, orgotein (Palosein, Diagnostic Data), gamete factor, and aspirin. None have proved significantly successful.

Medical therapy is indicated in lens-induced uveitis, including topical mydriatics (1 per cent atropine) for pupil dilation and topical corticosteroids two to three times daily. Mydriatics alone may be used in cases of immature or hypermature cataracts to facilitate vision.

SURGICAL

Surgical removal of the lens by phacofragmentation or standard extracapsular extraction methods is the only effective therapy for cataracts at this time.

Phacofragmentation/phacoemulsification consists of the use of high-frequency vibrations to fragment or emulsify the cataract. A well-controlled irrigation-aspiration system, combined with ultrasonic mechanical phacofragmentation, allows removal of the lens while maintaining intraocular pressure. The advantages of this technique include the small limbal or corneal incision required for the probe and the reduction of surgery time, inflammation, and postoperative complications. The major limitation of phacofragmentation is the initial cost of the equipment. In addition, because the lens becomes more dense with age, it may be difficult to fragment old lenses. The extended time and excessive manipulation necessary to remove a hard lens may injure the corneal endothelium and result in chronic bullous keratopathy.

There are three traditional methods of removing a cataractous lens: (1) discission and aspiration, (2) extracapsular extraction, and (3) intracapsular extraction. Discission and aspiration are used infrequently; this method is limited to very young animals with a soft lens. It often results in some lens material remaining in the eye, producing postoperative lens-induced uveitis. Extracapsular extraction (anterior lens capsule, cortex, and nucleus are removed) is the most commonly used procedure in small animals. The major advantage of this technique is the reduced likelihood of vitreous prolapse. The main disadvantage is the release of lens proteins into the anterior chamber, which may increase the intensity of the postoperative anterior uveitis. In addition, the posterior lens capsule may become opaque. Intracapsular extraction is difficult in animals with lenses *in situ;* the zonular fibers tightly adhere to the equator of the lens capsule and are not adequately affected by alpha-chymotrypsin–induced enzymatic zonulolysis as in humans. The anterior hyaloid membrane adheres tightly to the posterior lens capsule, so extraction frequently results in vitreous prolapse.

Many surgical complications are associated with cataract extraction in the dog and cat. Most can be avoided or handled at the time of surgery by a careful surgeon. Surgery should be performed by experienced veterinary ophthalmologists and the postoperative problems managed appropriately.

Selection of the Surgical Candidate

Careful selection of patients for lens extraction is essential for a high success rate. Animals functionally blind from cataracts or those with acute anterior lens luxation and secondary glaucoma are considered prime candidates. Complete ophthalmologic and general physical examinations are imperative. Prior to surgery, CBC and clinical chemistries (BUN, SGPT, glucose) should be performed. Abnormal pupillary light reflexes, although highly variable, may suggest concurrent retinal disease. The pupils should dilate rapidly and completely with 1.0 per cent tropicamide (Mydriacyl, Alcon). If mydriasis is slow and incomplete, a subclinical lens-induced anterior uveitis may be present. Tonometry may also help detect the presence of ocular hypotony suggestive of subclinical anterior uveitis. Any evidence of an anterior uveitis should dictate a delay of cataract extraction until after successful medical treatment.

Fundic examination is often impossible because of advanced lens opacity, but by using maximum dilation a small portion of the fundus occasionally can be observed with indirect ophthalmoscopy. A history of night blindness may indicate retinal degeneration. Fifty to eighty per cent of toy and miniature poodles with cataracts may have progressive retinal degeneration. If possible, electroretinography (ERG) should be performed preoperatively on all potential surgical canine cases, particularly if the ocular fundus cannot be evaluated.

The presence of external ocular diseases, such as keratoconjunctivitis sicca or advanced corneal degeneration, is also a limiting factor for cataract surgery candidates.

Other important considerations are the owner's desire for the surgery and the animal's temperament. The animal must tolerate topical and oral medications several times daily. If it is extremely excitable and cannot be handled by the owner, the animal is a poor candidate. In addition, the owner must be prepared to treat the pet often and must be willing to return for re-examinations. The surgery is expensive; it requires both a financial and an emotional commitment.

Postoperative Complications

Proper postoperative management of the cataract patient is as important as the surgery itself. Initially, the animal must be kept quiet to prevent trauma to the eye. The canine eye reacts more violently to intraocular surgery than does the human eye. The intensity of the anterior uveitis varies with each animal. Immediately after surgery the pupil may become miotic. Mydriatics are necessary to maintain reasonable pupil size. If mydriatic therapy is not successful, the pinpoint pupil can become adhered to the posterior lens capsule or anterior hyaloid membrane and prevent vision. Uncontrolled anterior uveitis can devastate the eye. Complications can vary from posterior synechia, fibropupillary membranes, and anterior peripheral synechia to phthisis bulbi. Secondary glaucoma often can be the end result of acute and chronic uveitis when inflammatory debris and adhesions close the drainage angle.

Other postoperative problems include corneal ulceration due to exposure from lagophthalmos. Persistent corneal edema can result from surgical trauma to the corneal endothelium. Retinal detachment may result from a tear in the retina at the time of surgery. Careful examination during the postoperative period allows detection of a retinal tear while it can still be treated. Retinal detachments rarely occur several months postoperatively.

DISPLACED LENS

Displacement of the lens is relatively common in dogs and is infrequent in cats. Subluxation refers to the partial rupture of zonules, resulting in the lens being displaced but remaining within the patellar fossa. Luxation refers to the complete displacement of the lens from the patellar fossa and loss of all zonular attachments. The lens can be displaced forward into the anterior chamber or posterior into the vitreous.

Lens displacement can be hereditary, trauma induced, or secondary to other ocular diseases (e.g., glaucoma, intraocular tumors). Certain breeds of dogs are predisposed to lens luxations including the wire-haired fox terrier, smooth-coated fox terrier, Sealyham terrier, Jack Russell terrier, Manchester terrier, Norwegian elkhound, and basset hound. The etiopathogenesis is not clearly understood, although inflammatory cells have been demonstrated engulfing defective zonules, possibly indicating an immune-mediated phenomenon.

The clinical signs of lens luxation are iridodonesis, aphakic crescent, change in depth of the anterior chamber, central corneal edema, and frequently glaucoma. If there is an increase in IOP, there may be extensive corneal edema, blepharospasm, epiphora, and blindness.

Management of a displaced lens is dependent on concurrent ocular disease. In subluxation without other complications, conservative treatment is recommended, depending on the cause. The owner must be informed of possible progression of the ocular disease and the resultant clinical signs. In lens luxation, the decision to treat surgically is also dependent on the location of the lens. In acute anterior lens luxation, the lens should be removed immediately. If the lens is tilted anteriorly, producing a pupillary block glaucoma, the block may be relieved medically by cautiously dilating the pupil with 10 per cent phenylephrine (Neo-Synephrine, Winthrop), allowing restoration of the communication between the anterior and posterior chambers. Use of long-acting miotics such as 0.03 per cent echothiopate iodide (Phospholine Iodide), can be used to maintain the lens posterior to the iris although this may be dangerous. If the lens becomes entrapped in the pupil, it would be difficult to relieve the pupillary block. Also, if surgery is necessary there is an increased chance of hemorrhage and inflammation. An alternative is a sympathomimetic mydriatic (10 per cent phenylephrine) to dilate the pupil. If the pupillary block cannot be relieved medically, lens extraction is necessary.

Posterior lens luxations without concurrent ocular disease should be examined periodically. If the posterior lens luxation induces ocular inflammation or glaucoma, removal should be considered. Removal is a difficult procedure, usually resulting in vitreous loss. The close proximity of the retina to the luxated lens necessitates meticulous surgical technique.

SUPPLEMENTAL READING

Barnett, K. C.: Hereditary cataract in the dog. J. Small Anim. Prac. 19:109, 1978.
Barnett, K. C.: Hereditary cataract in the Welsh springer spaniel. J. Small Anim. Prac. 21:621, 1980.
Barrie, K. P., et al.: Posterior lenticonus, microphthalmia, congenital cataracts and retinal folds in an Old English sheepdog. J.A.A.H.A. 15:715, 1979.
Bistner, S. I., Aquirre, G., and Batik, G. Atlas of Veterinary Ophthalmic Surgery. Philadelphia: W. B. Saunders Co., 1977.
Gwin, R. M., and Gelatt, K. N.: The lens. In Gelatt, K. N. (ed.): Veterinary Ophthalmology. Philadelphia: Lea & Febiger, 1981.
Martin, C. L.: Cataract production in experimentally orphaned puppies fed a commercial replacement for bitch's milk. Proceedings of the 10th Annual Meeting, Am. Coll. Vet. Ophthalmol. 241–253, 1979.
Narfstrom, K.: Cataract in the West Highland white terrier. J. Small Anim. Prac. 22:467, 1981.
Playter, R. F.: The development and maturation of a cataract. J.A.A.H.A. 13:317, 1977.
Rathbun, W. B.: Biochemistry of the lens and cataractogenesis: Current concepts. Vet. Clin. North Am.: Small Anim. Prac. 10:377, 1980.
Vainisi, S. J., et al.: Nutritional cataracts in timber wolves. J.A.V.M.A. 11:1175, 1981.

DISEASES OF THE ORBIT

DANIEL M. BETTS, D.V.M.

Ames, Iowa

ANATOMIC CONSIDERATIONS

The orbit is a conical cavity that contains the eyeball and the ocular adnexae. The orbital margin forms the base of the cone, and the apex is directed caudally toward the optic foramen. The medial wall and part of the roof are osseous. The remainder of the roof and lateral wall are formed by the large temporalis muscle that extends from the top of the cranium to surround and insert on the coronoid process of the mandible. The floor of the orbit is formed by the pterygoid muscles, which originate from the bony skull medially and extend laterally to insert on the medial side of the mandible.

The contents of the orbit are totally enclosed in a conical fibrous membrane—the periorbita—with the apex attached to the orbital wall around the optic foramen and the base around the orbital rim and the orbital ligament. Medially and dorsally where bone forms the wall of the orbit, the periorbita and the periosteum are one and the same. The periorbita is a tough fibrous sheet dorsally, laterally, and ventrally where it separates the eye and adnexae from the muscles that form the limits of the orbit.

Within the periorbita are numerous smooth muscle fibers which normally exert some degree of tone that acts to squeeze the eyeball forward in the orbit and causes the normal prominence of the globe. These smooth muscle fibers are innervated by sympathetic nerve fibers. The orbital septum is a sheet of connective tissue that extends from the periorbita and the orbital rim to the tarsi of the lids. It is the anterior limit of the orbit.

Smooth muscle fibers derived from periorbita insert in the upper and lower eyelids and help maintain their retracted position when the palpebral fissure is open. At the base of the cartilage of the third eyelid other smooth muscle fibers also insert and help to maintain it in a retracted position. Innervation of these smooth muscles is also by the sympathetic fibers from the cranial cervical ganglion. Sympathetic denervation causes a sinking of the globe (enophthalmos), protrusion of the third eyelid, and drooping of the upper eyelid (ptosis). These signs, together with miosis, constitute Horner's syndrome.

The zygomatic salivary gland covers the lateral two-thirds of the floor of the orbit just behind the orbital margin and lies against the inner surface of the zygomatic arch. It is outside the periorbita. The lacrimal gland is within the periobita dorsolaterally, adjacent to the medial surface of the orbital ligament.

The eyeball is attached to the posterior of the orbit by the four rectus muscles, which originate around the opening of the optic foramen and insert on the globe anterior to the equator. The retractor bulbi muscle originates at the orbital fissure, penetrates the rectus muscle cone, and then fans out and divides to insert at the equator of the globe. The superior oblique muscle originates at the optic foramen, passes around a trochlea (pulley) in the dorsomedial orbital wall, and inserts on the globe under the dorsal rectus muscle. The inferior oblique muscle originates on the medial orbital wall, passes ventral to the ventral oblique muscle, and fans out to attach to the posterior lateral portion of the globe. Check ligaments are thin bands of tissue joining the anterior portions of the rectus muscles with the periorbita to prevent overaction of these muscles.

A dense connective tissue membrane, Tenon's capsule, surrounds the eyeball from the limbus to the optic nerve. It divides to permit the passage of the extraocular muscles and optic nerve and numerous blood vessels. It is continuous with the dura of the optic nerve and also forms a covering for the rectus muscles and an intermuscular membrane.

Three prominent openings at the apex of the orbital cone permit the passage of the major vessels and nerves of the orbit into the cranium or alar canal. The optic foramen contains the optic nerve and internal ophthalmic artery. The optic chiasm is immediately behind it. The orbital fissure transmits the oculomotor (III), trochlear (IV), and abducens (VI) nerves; the ophthalmic branch of the trigeminal nerve (V); and the orbital vein. The maxillary artery and the maxillary branch of the trigeminal nerve (V) enter the orbit via the round foramen but traverse anteriorly on the floor of the orbit outside the periorbita.

The external ophthalmic artery branches from the maxillary artery at the posterior of the orbit, enters the periorbita, and anastomoses with the much smaller internal ophthalmic artery. They give rise to the long and short posterior ciliary arteries to the eyeball. The maxillary artery branches several times within the orbit and becomes the infraorbital artery as it exits the orbit anteriorly via the infraorbital canal.

Venous drainage from the eye and adnexae passes forward into the facial vein, medial with the veins of the nose, downward with the deep facial vein or veins of the pterygoid fossa or backward via the orbital plexus and into the intracranial cavernous sinus. None of these veins has effective valves, so blood will flow in the direction of least resistance. These arteries and veins are utilized in contrast radiography of the orbit.

Fat fills the spaces within and around the muscle cone, and there is extensive fat ventral and lateral to the periorbita. The fat cushions the orbital contents, contributes to the prominence of the globe, and permits rotation and retraction because it is easily deformed. Orbital or systemic disease that diminishes this fat body may markedly affect the position of the globe.

Demands for increased accommodation within the orbit by edematous fluid, blood, exudates, or neoplastic growth or any encroachment from swellings around it will be met largely by pushing forward the anterior structures, distending soft tissues ventrally to protrude on the roof of the mouth behind the last upper molar tooth or laterally to protrude above the zygomatic arch. In a fully distended palpebral fissure, the globe is a plug in the orbit, and increased intraorbital pressure results in circulatory strangulation and further outpouring of edematous fluid from venous compression, so that the process augments itself.

Four surgical spaces occur in the orbit that control (or determine) the spread of infiltrations and limit the degree of relief from exploratory measures confined to one compartment. (1) The subperiosteal space (potential) is between the bone and the periorbita. (2) The peripheral surgical space is between the periorbita, the muscle cone, and the intermuscular membrane. (3) The central surgical space is within the muscle cone. (4) The episcleral space occurs between Tenon's capsule and the globe. These are rigid constraints, and decompression can be obtained only when the appropriate compartment is breached.

The shape of the head affects the shape and proportions of the orbit, but the size of the dog or its head has little relation to the size of the orbit. A large-headed dog with a large globe may not have a proportionally larger orbit. Space-occupying lesions, including tumors, hemorrhage, exudates, and edema, have little room to accumulate, and working area in the event of surgical exploration does not increase as the dog grows.

The orbit can be the meeting place of surrounding pathologic disturbances involving the sinuses, cranium, bones of the face, lids, and lacrimal apparatus and is a point of spreading that can be rapid and dramatic. The orbital lesion frequently is a menace not only to vision but also to life, more severe than generally encountered in ocular disease.

CLINICAL SIGNS OF ORBITAL DISEASE

Orbital disease is nearly always associated with an abnormal position of the eyeball and pressure on normal orbital contents. Exophthalmos may be created by orbital inflammation or abscess; tumor; edema; hemorrhage; zygomatic gland mucocele, inflammation, or tumor; swollen temporal muscles; orbital vascular anomalies; or extension of lesions from the sinuses, nasal cavity, oral cavity, or teeth. A prominent anterior position of the eyeballs has also been associated with dirofilariasis. The size and position of space-occupying lesions affect the direction of displacement of the eyeball; this is useful in locating the offending mass and selecting a route for surgical exploration. Exophthalmos often results in exposure keratitis and secondary corneal ulceration. Any space-occupying lesion within the orbit may also cause the membrana nictitans to protrude. Strabismus may be caused by rupture of one or more of the extraocular muscles or damage to cranial nerves III, IV, or VI, which innervate them. Orbital disease frequently is accompanied by chemosis, and this may be exacerbated by compression of the orbital veins and diminished posterior venous drainage. Congestion of conjunctival vessels, lid edema, and erythema may be marked, and ischemic degenerative changes may follow. Exophthalmos must be differentiated from apparent exophthalmos associated with shallow orbits (in brachycephaly and hydrocephalus), euryblepharon, glaucoma, and facial paralysis.

Enophthalmos results from loss of tone in the smooth muscle of the periorbita (as in loss of sympathetic innervation or rupture of the membrane). It also is seen in chronic orbital inflammation and debilitation when retrobulbar fat is lost. The globe may be withdrawn deep in the orbit owing to pain on the cornea or intraocular pain. It may also occur with phthisis bulbi following intraocular inflammation. Whatever the cause, the lacrimal lake may be enlarged, interfering with tear drainage and producing a chronic conjunctivitis. The action of the coronoid process in the movement of the mandible will enhance the enophthalmos when the jaws are

opened. Inflammatory disease involving the posterior orbit may be associated with intense pain upon opening the jaw as the coronoid process impinges on the retrobulbar tissues. The pain may make the animal reluctant to eat or drink and may cause it to vigorously resist examination of the mouth.

Ocular discharges may be associated with the conjunctiva or may be traced to periocular draining tracts. Because exudates drain and proliferative tissue grows in the direction of least resistance, a swelling or draining tract is commonly found posterior to the last upper molar tooth.

The temporal aspect of the orbit may be distended with advanced neoplasia and may be confused with eosinophilic myositis. Temporomandibular joint disease could also cause similar swelling and pain on attempting to open the mouth.

Loss of sensation on the cornea is associated with damage to the ophthalmic branch of the trigeminal nerve, and blindness with dilated pupils may be due to compression of the optic nerve or optic neuritis.

If orbital inflammation extends to the lacrimal gland, keratoconjunctivitis sicca may be a sequela that remains after the orbital problem is resolved. Bruits may be palpated or auscultated temporally or through the globe in the rare orbital arteriovenous fistula.

On fundus examination, chorioretinal degeneration, retinal hemorrhage, and possible edema of the optic disc may be observed as a result of direct extension or from retrobulbar pressure on the globe and optic nerve.

DIAGNOSTIC APPROACH

Some orbital diseases and their causes are immediately evident upon inspection, but when they are not, an orderly progression for examination of the orbit and globe is essential. Beyond visual inspection, digital palpation of the orbital rim, zygomatic arch, and soft tissues of the lateral side of the orbit should be undertaken. Open the mouth to determine if there is associated pain and inspect for a swelling or draining tract posterior to the last upper molar tooth. Also inspect the adjacent hard and soft palates, teeth, and pharynx. A general anesthetic may be required before the animal will tolerate this.

Samples of tissues or exudates for cytologic examination or culture may be collected by aspiration from the retrobulbar space. An 18-gauge, 1½-inch needle on a 12-ml syringe is inserted posterior and dorsal to the angle formed by the orbital ligament and the zygomatic arch. The plunger is withdrawn slowly until considerable vacuum is drawn. The plunger is then released slowly so that the collected fluid or tissue will not be lost from the needle. The needle should not be repositioned while great vacuum is being applied. Rather, the vacuum should be released and the needle withdrawn, redirected, and reinserted if another sampling site is desired so that the risk of trauma to one of the several vessels or nerves is minimized. If a sinus tract is noted, it should be explored with a blunt probe.

Systematic examination of the eyeball, including ophthalmoscopy, for signs of neurologic or vascular disturbances is warranted. Radiographic examination of the orbit may be utilized to demonstrate congenital bony malformations, erosion or hyperostosis of bone and fractures, regional or diffuse inflammation, vascular abnormalities, foreign bodies, and neoplasms. Plain films of the ventrodorsal, lateral, and frontal views should be taken. Oblique views are occasionally of value. A metal ring (Fleiringa ring*) should be placed in the conjunctival fornix to delineate the eyeball position.

Several contrast radiographic techniques may be utilized to outline orbital lesions. General anesthesia is required.

Orbital venography (Oliver, 1969) is the easiest and safest contrast radiographic technique to perform. Three to seven milliliters of 50 per cent sodium diatrizoate (Hypaque, Winthrop Labs) are injected into the angularis oculi vein. By occluding the jugular veins at the time of injection, the contrast medium will be carried through the orbital venous system to the cerebral and vertebral venous sinuses. Lesions within the orbit cause displacement, compression, or collapse of the ophthalmic veins or orbital plexus.

Orbital arteriography (Tice, 1975) using the infraorbital artery is more difficult but has some advantages. Although the artery is readily identified, it is easiest to cannulate if the skin is incised over the infraorbital foramen and the artery is isolated by blunt dissection. Both arterial and venous outlines are obtained when 5 to 8 ml of 50 per cent sodium diatrizoate are injected immediately before and at the time of the x-ray exposure. No contrast medium is injected into the intracranial vasculature, and the ventral orbital arteries are outlined.

Pneumorbitography may be accomplished by injecting 5 to 15 ml of air slowly into the bulbar subconjunctival space to give a negative contrast to a radiolucent mass within the orbital cone. A sub-Tenon's capsule injection of air may outline a lesion on or around the posterior of the globe.

Positive contrast orbitography (Munger and Ackerman, 1978) is used to outline lesions as radiolucent areas or filling defects. The most productive technique in the dog is to inject 2 to 3 ml of metrizamide† by Barth's method into the orbit from beneath the zygomatic arch.

---

*Storz Instrument Co., St. Louis, MO.

†Nyegaard & Co., A/S Oslo, Norway. Available through Accurate Chemical and Scientific Corp., Westbury, NY.

Optic thecography (LeCouteur et al., 1982) is an innovative technique for indirect imaging of the optic nerve. Metrizamide is injected into the cerebrospinal fluid space via the foramen magnum. Then, by carefully lowering the dog's head, the contrast medium will gravitate forward and fill the subarachnoid space around both optic nerves. (This method is not without hazard.—Ed.) A filling defect or a deviation of the nerve indicates a space-occupying lesion. The opposite orbit is a control or normal to compare with the side with the lesion.

Ultrasonography, tomography, radioisotope scanning, and thermography are more sophisticated diagnostic techniques used in human ophthalmology for localizing and identifying orbital lesions but are rarely available for veterinary use except in research or experimental facilities.

ORBITAL CELLULITIS AND ABSCESS

An inflammatory process within the orbit may cause a variety of the signs previously discussed, but it is most important to remember that although not all inflammations are septic, they should be considered to be so.

Cellulitis may orginate within the orbit or may extend into it from adjacent tissue. The stimulus for inflammation may be carried into the orbit by hematogenous or lymphatic circulation or may penetrate through the skin, conjunctiva, or roof of the mouth. Its spread may be limited by the periorbita, the muscle cone, and the intermuscular septa or Tenon's capsule. Orbital cellulitis is a diffuse inflammation accompanied generally by pain, pyrexia, and anorexia. An abscess is more localized with more pain and pyrexia and is likely to be accompanied by a history that suggests an onset more acute than it actually was. The etiology is poorly understood but is generally assumed to be bacterial in origin.

Orbital cellulitis and retrobulbar abscess are treated similarly, beginning with establishing ventral drainage. Under general anesthesia a small incision is made in the mucous membrane behind the last upper molar tooth and a hemostat is inserted and opened to dissect a tract into the retrobulbar area. A sharp instrument should never be used. A purulent exudate may erupt if a pocket of pus under pressure is encountered. In many cases only a serosanguinous discharge seeps out. This may be a diffuse cellulitis, or there may be a pocket of exudate in another tissue plane that was not entered. The hemostat may be carefully redirected to other areas, but extensive trauma should be avoided. The orbit is irrigated with a neomycin-polymyxin B solution (Polymycin, Osborn Labs). A broad spectrum antibiotic is administered systemically for five to seven days, and hot packs are applied over the orbit two or three times daily for a few days until the swelling recedes. The cornea and protruding edematous conjunctiva must be protected with frequent applications of an antibiotic ointment. Alternatively, the lids may be sutured together with a horizontal mattress pattern with 4–0 nylon or other nonabsorbable material.

If an abscess pocket is encountered and drained, the signs will diminish rapidly, but cellulitis is apt to resolve slowly over several days. Persistent or recurring clinical signs should make one suspicious of a foreign body or a bone or neoplastic disorder. Radiographs and retrobulbar aspiration for culture and cytology are indicated.

TRAUMATIC PROPTOSIS OF THE GLOBE

This emergency condition is most commonly seen in brachycephalic dogs and occasionally in cats. It usually is the result of a fight or having been hit by a car. Chemosis develops quickly, preventing lid closure, and the cornea becomes dry. Retrobulbar hemorrhage and edema also contribute to the problem. Frequently the medial rectus muscle is torn from its insertion on the globe, resulting in a lateral exotropia.

A recent proptosis in a brachycephalic dog may be replaced after cleaning and lubricating the eye with an antibiotic ointment. If the globe is intact but cannot be replaced easily, anesthetize the patient and locate the lid margins with a muscle hook or other blunt probe. Pull them anteriorly and place three or four simple interrupted sutures of 4–0 nylon in the lids across the palpebral fissure. Then place a Bard-Parker scalpel handle between the eye and the sutures. Pull all the suture ends anteriorly simultaneously—slowly—and gently press the globe back into the orbit. Remove the scalpel handle and tie the sutures. The eye may not return to its original position in the orbit until retrobulbar hemorrhage and edema have resolved.

Inject 10 mg of triamcinolone (Kenalog, Squibb) into the postorbital tissue by directing a 1-inch needle through the skin in the middle of the upper eyelid between the orbital rim and the globe. A topical antibiotic ointment is applied between the lid margins, several times a day, and cold packs are applied to the eye for the first 24 hours. These are changed to hot packs for the following two to three days. A systemic broad spectrum antibiotic such as ampicillin (10 to 20 mg/kg every 6 to 12 hours) is administered. Topical 1 per cent atropine is used to minimize synechia formation, because uveitis frequently occurs. Systemic steroids may be valuable in treating uveitis, but caution should be exercised with topical steroids owing to the frequent corneal trauma.

Leave the lid sutures in place for two to three weeks. If the animal is unable to close its lids over the cornea completely after the sutures are removed, replace the sutures for two or three more weeks or do a tarsorrhaphy.

Nearly all traumatic strabismus improves for several weeks following the injury. If it remains grossly malpositioned, surgical correction may be attempted.

Frequently there is evidence of intraocular injury and damage to the optic nerve or other nerves. Hyphema is an unfavorable sign. A pinpoint pupil is a favorable sign, and a dilated pupil (sympathetic innervation intact) carries a guarded prognosis. A normal-sized pupil occurs when both sympathetic and parasympathetic nerve supplies have been severed. The optic nerve is irreversibly damaged in these cases.

If the globe is ruptured or hanging loosely from the orbit it should be removed.

EOSINOPHILIC MYOSITIS

Symmetric swelling of the masseter, temporal, and pterygoid muscles with associated exophthalmos, protruding nictitans, eyelid edema, and pain on opening the jaws occurs in Weimaraners and German shepherds. The signs of eosinophilic myositis are similar to those of orbital cellulitis. Attacks last 10 to 21 days and commonly recur. The etiology of eosinophilic myositis is unknown, but a characteristic lesion can be found on muscle biopsy specimens. A peripheral eosinophilia is not consistently noted. An immunosuppressive dose of prednisone (2 mg/kg) is given for 10 to 14 days and then halved at weekly intervals for another two to three weeks. After recovery, muscle and orbital fat atrophy occurs and enophthalmos follows.

RETROBULBAR OPTIC NEURITIS

Retrobulbar optic neuritis has been reported with canine distemper, toxoplasmosis, rhinotonsillitis, blastomycosis, reticulosis, sinusitis, cellulitis, hemorrhage, and neoplasia. Any orbital inflammation, degeneration, or ischemic crisis may predispose to the condition. It is characterized by dilated, fixed pupils with a normal fundus. Systemic steroids at immunosuppressive levels (prednisone 2 mg/kg) for three to four days and halved each week for another two to three weeks may result in reduction of clinical signs, but the prognosis is generally poor for eventual recovery of sight.

ZYGOMATIC MUCOCELE

A leakage of saliva from this gland or the duct, with inflammation and granulation following, is supposed to be uncommon, but zygomatic mucocele may be frequently misdiagnosed. It resembles orbital cellulitis, but there is no systemic febrile response or pain. A mass protrudes under the conjunctiva in the inferior temporal fornix. Aspiration of the substance in the sac yields a yellow, tenacious, honey-like fluid. A zygomatic sialogram will delineate the extent of the sialocele. The only effective treatment is dissection and removal of the mass by orbitotomy.

REFERENCES AND SUPPLEMENTAL READING

LeCouteur, R. A., Scogliotti, R. H., Beck, K. A., Gehrmann, J. E., and Holliday, T. A.: Indirect imaging of the canine optic nerve using metrizamide (optic thecography). Submitted for publication Am. J. Vet. Res., 1983.

Munger, R. J., and Ackerman, N.: Retrobulbar injections in the dog. A comparison of three techniques. J. Am. Anim. Hosp. Assoc. 14:490, 1978.

Oliver, J. E.: Cranial sinus venography in the dog. J. Am. Vet. Rad. Soc. 10:70, 1969.

Ticer, J. W.: *Radiographic Techniques in Small Animal Practice*. Philadelphia: W. B. Saunders Co., 1975.

INTRAOCULAR INFLAMMATION

STEPHEN BISTNER, D.V.M.
and DONALD SHAW, D.V.M.

St. Paul, Minnesota

Intraocular inflammation refers to all inflammatory and potentially inflammatory diseases of the inner layers of the eye and includes uveitis, chorioretinitis, and endophthalmitis. Inflammation can be defined as the interaction between a stimulus and a host, invariably resulting in some degree of structural change within the host. Inflammatory responses within the eye can be divided into two general categories: neuronal and non-neuronal. Neuronal inflammation is mediated by axonal reflexes in the cornea. Branches of the ophthalmic nerve (a branch of the trigeminal nerve) can be stimulated by trauma, and impulses are carried to the iris and ciliary body, producing vasodilation, increased vascular permeability, edema, and increased protein levels and cell numbers in the aqueous fluid. These types of reactions are seen with corneal epithelial abrasions, corneal foreign bodies, and contusions of the eye. Infections of the cornea also lead to secondary neuronal inflammation. These types of inflammation are usually short-lived and do not seriously threaten vision.

Non-neuronal ocular inflammation is usually more severe and can result in severe alteration of ocular structure and visual loss. Non-neuronal inflammatory responses are related to anaphylactoid reactions, acute and chronic infections, deposition of immune complexes and binding of complement, and the development of chronic granulomatous processes (O'Connor, 1981).

In classifying intraocular inflammation for prognostic and treatment purposes, the following scheme based on the degree of structural alteration will be used (Arronson and Elliot, 1972):

1. No inflammation, intact ocular structure
2. Active inflammation, no structural alteration
3. Active inflammation, minimal structural alteration
4. Inactive inflammation, minimal structural alteration
5. Active inflammation, marked structural alteration
6. Inactive inflammation, marked structural alteration

In evaluating the patient with intraocular inflammation it is important to: (1) evaluate the extent of intraocular structural change to establish a prognosis and determine what changes can be reversed or altered by treatment; (2) take a history and perform a general assessment of the patient; (3) perform a general physical examination; and (4) establish a general diagnostic work-up looking for specific etiology.

Use the following outline of pathologic ocular structural alterations to evaluate the extent of ocular damage:

1. Active anterior segment inflammation—no structural alteration
   a. deep ciliary vascular injection
   b. aqueous flare, hyphema, or hypopyon
   c. keratitic precipitates
   d. neovascularization
   e. iris edema
2. Active anterior segment inflammation—mild structural change
   a. pigmentary keratitic precipitates
   b. lens precipitates
3. Active anterior segment inflammation—moderate change

a. anterior synechiae
b. posterior synechiae
c. iris atrophy
d. reversible glaucoma
e. early lens opacities

4. Active anterior segment inflammation—severe change
   a. irreversible glaucoma
   b. persistent corneal opacity (edema)
   c. cataract
   d. hypotony
   e. pupillary block

5. Active inflammation posterior segment—no structural alteration
   a. cells and protein in vitreous chamber
   b. hemorrhages in vitreous and retina
   c. edema of the retina
   d. retinal and retinal perivascular exudate formation

6. Active inflammation posterior segment—structural alteration
   a. vitreous veils, bands, cyclytic membranes
   b. retinal detachments
   c. vitreous syneresis
   d. choroidal vascular atrophy
   e. increased pigment cell hypertrophy of pigment epithelium and choroid
   f. atrophy of the pigment epithelium and choroid
   g. cataract formation
   h. lens luxation

An inflammatory stimulus is any agent that can initiate or perpetuate an inflammatory response. Stimuli can be divided into toxic and immune agents. Toxic agents may be necrotizing (i.e., destroying parenchymal and interstitial tissue of the host) or non-necrotizing. Sources of toxins may be exogenous, e.g., changes in the biochemical environment, cellular breakdown secondary to inflammatory, or degenerative or neoplastic diseases.

Non-necrotizing toxic agents indirectly alter structural integrity through intermediate pathways that will activate inflammatory cells, e.g., gamma globulin binders such as plant material, catgut, complement binders such as microbial endotoxins, and antigenic activators of mitogenic pathways.

INFLAMMATIONS OF THE UVEAL TRACT

"Uveitis is defined as that group of diseases, either of endogenous or exogenous origin, involving the inner coats of the eye. No attempt is made to precisely distinguish the uveal tract as the principal source of intraocular inflammation. Uveitis is once again a composite of clinical diseases in which the inflammatory response is the predominant cause of altered ocular function and attenuated structure" (Arronson and Elliot, 1972).

Attempting to organize and categorize the etiology of uveitis is a frustrating task. In the past, categorization was based on descriptive terminology (clinical morphology and clinical history) and histologic examination of inflamed, enucleated eyes. The following classification was developed for uveitis.

I. Infective uveitis
   A. Exogenous infection
   B. Endogenous infection
II. Hypersensitivity uveitis
III. Toxic uveitis
IV. Traumatic uveitis
V. Uveitis associated with noninfective systemic diseases
VI. Uveitis of unknown etiology

Based on this schema, it would appear that most cases of uveitis could be classified easily. Unfortunately, this is not true. Most cases of uveitis fall into the endogenous category with an unknown etiology.

Exogenous Infection—Exogenous Inflammation. These inflammations, caused by the introduction of organisms through an infected perforating wound or a perforated corneal or scleral ulcer, are usually of great significance. The inflammation can be confined to the anterior ocular segment only. It can spread to the vitreous cavity to involve the vitreous and associated retina (endophthalmitis). Or the toxin and inflammatory cells can diffuse through all the ocular tunics (panophthalmitis). This acute inflammation of the globe can result in severe scarring, the loss of all sight, and eventual phthisis bulbi.

Exogenous Infection—Postoperative Exogenous Infection. This may follow intraocular surgery. In spite of the environment in which most of our domestic animals live, there is surprisingly little exogenous postoperative infection.

Endogenous Infection. Bacteria or their by-products infect the eye via the blood stream from some source elsewhere in the body. The role of this mechanism in producing uveitis is not clear. However, this type of uveitis does occur and is associated with the bacteria and their toxic by-products. Classically, many cases of uveitis are associated with tuberculosis and the spread of tubercle bacilli from other areas of the body into the eye.

Recent studies in dogs indicate that *Brucella canis* can produce endogenous uveitis.

Less is known about the role of viral infections in the etiology of uveitis; however, several viruses have been firmly associated with ocular disease. In small animals, spontaneously occurring viral-induced uveitis has been associated with adenovirus-1 infection of canine hepatitis, canine herpesvirus, feline panleukopenia virus, and feline infectious peritonitis virus.

Hypersensitivity Uveitis. It has been demonstrated, utilizing rabbits, that the eye is not an immunologically competent organ by itself. The immunologic sequence of events that can take place in the uveal tract is similar to that which takes place in a regional lymph node under antigenic stimulation. Immunologically competent cells enter the eye from regional lymph nodes. These immunologically competent cells persist in the uveal tract and can be reactivated by antigen to provide the basis for immunologic memory. Mast cells, plasma cells, lymphocytes, and phagocytes are found in the interstitial tissue of the uveal tract. Many melanocytes and fibroblasts occupy the choroidal stroma.

The eye constitutes a type of immunologic microcosm in which various immune mechanisms can operate as they do elsewhere in the body (Arronson and Elliot, 1972). The body reacts to antigenic stimuli by inflammation. If the hypersensitivity reaction occurs in a highly sensitive location, such as the uveal tract, a violent inflammatory reaction with all of its ramifications can result.

The uveal tract is able to support all types of immunogenic inflammatory reactions including the active formation of antibody and anaphylactic and Arthus types of antibody-mediated hypersensitivity inflammations. These lesions often present so similar a clinical picture that their pathogenetic differentiation is difficult. Each appears as a nonspecific, nongranulomatous uveitis. The several inflammations can only be differentiated microscopically, and then only at certain periods during their development.

Lens proteins normally contained within the lens capsule appear to act as foreign proteins when freed (phacoanaphylaxis or phacolytic uveitis). Uveitis also has been produced by the injection of homologous uveal and retinal tissue into experimental animals.

ROLE OF PROSTAGLANDINS IN OCULAR INFLAMMATION

The prostaglandins are a family of naturally occurring, humoral agents characterized by a unique, oxygenated, low molecular weight, fatty acid structure. Prostaglandins are formed by nearly all cells from membrane-located stores of polyunsaturated acids found as phospholipids. Prostaglandins are potent biologic mediators that can cause profound effects at extremely low concentrations, making them among the most important and potent of the naturally occurring substances. It is now established that prostaglandins are locally active in tissues but are rapidly inactivated by specific enzymes located close to their site of formation.

The role of prostaglandins in pathologic and physiologic events must be considered in light of the following general points. First, prostaglandins are released when cell membrane integrity is altered or damaged. Second, most available evidence supports the concept that cells do not store prostaglandins; therefore, all prostaglandin levels depend on new synthesis. Third, most studied cells have microsomal enzymes that can synthesize prostaglandins from precursor molecules. Aspirin-like drugs, such as salicylates and indomethacin, inhibit the synthesis and release of prostaglandins.

The prostaglandins E_2 and $F_{2\alpha}$ have been shown to be actively involved in ocular inflammation and uveitis. The ocular reactions to intraocular or systemic prostaglandins are vasodilation, miosis, and increases in aqueous humor protein level and IOP.

The hyperemia, edema, and cellular and proteinaceous exudation that develop in intraocular inflammatory disease represent a reaction of the tissue to physical, chemical, bacterial, and immunologic insult. The tissue reactions are usually nonspecific in the sense that the clinical appearance is not pathognomonic of one particular cause.

APPROACH TO THE PATIENT WITH INTRAOCULAR INFLAMMATORY DISEASE

Once an active intraocular inflammatory disease is recognized, an etiology should be established if possible. Consider those diagnoses in which we can establish a possible definitive relationshp with intraocular inflammation:

Infectious Uveitis With Exogenous Infection. Is there evidence of a traumatic penetrating wound to the globe, a deep or perforated corneal ulcer, or previous intraocular surgery?

Infectious Uveitis With Endogenous Infection. A careful, systematic physical examination is important. Note associated systemic signs in the history as well as in physical examination. Some areas often overlooked in physical examination but important in endogenous intraocular inflammation are the ears, teeth, heart (bacterial endocarditis), liver (abdominal palpation), bladder (cystitis), prostate, and anal glands. Evaluate all peripheral lymph nodes. When history or physical signs indicate possible systemic disease, screen a blood sample for CBC and microfilaria and obtain a blood chemistry profile. Obtain chest radiographs, especially in those geographic areas where the systemic mycoses are prevalent.

In severe panuveitis, diagnostic paracentesis of aqueous, vitreous, or subretinal fluid may be helpful for cytology as well as for culture on blood agar, thioglycollate media, and Sabouraud agar.

ENDOGENOUS DISEASE THAT CAN RESULT IN INTRAOCULAR INFLAMMATION

The systemic mycoses cryptococcosis, blastomycosis, coccidioidomycosis, and histoplasmosis may all produce intraocular inflammation. The systemic mycoses produce a granulomatous chorioretinitis and uveitis. In most instances, infection is the result of inhalation of spores (or other infectious elements) from fungal colonies growing in nature. Inhalation of the infectious agent results in a primary pulmonary focus from which dissemination may occur. All available evidence indicates that both humans and animals contract these diseases through common exposure to sources in the environment. Resistance to fungal infections appears to be more dependent on cellular immunity than on humoral immunity. Animals that are debilitated, immunodeficient, or immunosuppressed are thought to be more likely to develop clinical disease with any of these agents. Therefore, a search for underlying immunosuppressive factors is indicated. Consider malignancies, particularly lymphosarcoma and other hematologic malignancies; drug therapy, especially corticosteroid and cancer chemotherapy; dysproteinemias; debilitation; and so on. Affected cats should be examined for feline leukemia virus, which suppresses cell-mediated immunity.

When a systemic mycotic infection is suspected, obtain aspirates of intraocular fluid for cytology. Vitreous aspirates are obtained, with the animal under general anesthesia, using a short, beveled, 20-gauge needle. Pass the needle through the pars plana area of the globe approximately 8 mm behind the limbus. The passage of the needle can be visualized with an ophthalmoscope through the dilated pupil.

Toxoplasmosis can produce intraocular inflammation as well as systemic disease. The ocular lesions in dogs involve the retina (chorioretinitis), the extraocular muscles, and the anterior uveal tract. Severe systemic infection may not be present. Cats usually have ocular toxoplasmosis associated with severe systemic disease. It is characterized by high fever, pneumonia, anorexia, neurologic signs, vomiting and diarrhea. Chorioretinitis and granulomatous panuveitis are the ocular manifestations.

There are two basic ways to confirm the diagnosis of toxoplasmosis: serologic examination and fecal examination. The serologic tests are the IFA test, the indirect hemagglutination test, and the complement fixation test.* Cats can develop antibody to *Toxoplasma gondii* in low titers, and up to 60 per cent of cats in the United States have been found to have low level titers to *T. gondii*. Active infections may be indicated by titers greater than 1:256.

Fecal examination involves looking for nonsporulated *Toxoplasma* oocysts, which are 10 to 12 μ in diameter; this is about one-fourth the size of *Isospora felis* oocysts and one-sixth to one-eighth the size of *Toxocara* oocysts.

Cats with uveitis should have a careful general physical examination. Some 25 per cent of cats with uveitis may have feline infectious peritonitis or may be positive for feline leukemia.

FELINE INFECTIOUS PERITONITIS (FIP)

This multisystemic disease of the cat is caused by a coronavirus. Clinical signs of FIP are referable to a multisystemic, immune-mediated vasculitis and an Arthus-like reaction involving viral antigen, antibody, and complement. A severe, granulomatous uveitis is but another manifestation of this generalized immune-mediated inflammatory reaction. Ocular lesions can be observed in both the "wet" and "dry" form of FIP, although there is a greater prevalence for eye changes in the dry form. Ocular lesions are characterized by an intense necrotizing and pyogranulomatous inflammation. There are large keratitic precipitates that form on the corneal endothelium, intense flare, many cells, and rapid synechia formation. Exudative retinal detachments may occur when a panuveitis develops. If optic neuritis is present, it leads to rapid visual loss.

Confirming the diagnosis of FIP depends on clinical signs, clinical pathology evaluation, and antibody titers from serologic studies such as IFA or ELISA. These tests, however, are not specific for FIP because cats are subject to a coronavirus enteritis that produces antibody titers that cross-react with FIP. Antibody titers in the range of 1:25 to 1:1600 by IFA test are almost always associated with FIP, usually the noneffusive type. Titers ranging from 1:400 to 1:1600 may be seen in cats with effusive FIP. Antibody titer results should always be evaluated with clinical findings and clinicopathologic studies.

FELINE LEUKEMIA

Feline leukemia and related diseases are caused by a C-type oncornavirus. Ocular abnormalities are often associated with feline leukemia virus (FeLV). Uveitis and infiltration of the uveal tract with immature lymphoblastic cells may be seen in feline lymphosarcoma. The entire uveal tract may become greatly thickened and the iris very misshapen, and an intense flare and cellular deposit develop in the anterior chamber. FeLV may alter an animal's immune response and may lead to secondary infections that may produce intraocular inflammation, e.g., systemic mycoses.

Confirmation of FeLV is based on detection of FeLV antigens in platelets and leukocytes on blood smears using IFA and ELISA tests and the detection of feline oncovirus-associated cell membrane antigen (FOCMA). These tests are evaluated along with clinical signs, radiographs, CBC, cytology, and biopsy in diagnosis.

Infectious canine hepatitis is caused by canine

---

*An enzyme-linked immunosorbent assay (ELISA) is being developed.

adenovirus type-1 (CAV-1), one of the two presently recognized canine adenoviruses. Immunologically mediated uveitis can be seen in both the naturally occurring disease and in animals vaccinated with modified live virus (MLV) adenovirus-1. This form of uveitis is associated with viral antigen-antibody immune complex formation and the development of an Arthus-like inflammatory reaction in the anterior uveal tract. Inflammation and cellular inflammatory enzymes destroy corneal endothelial cells, leading to severe corneal edema (the "blue eye" of canine hepatitis). Fortunately, the development of an adenovirus type-2 vaccine has obviated the uveitis associated with MLV adenovirus type-1. The uveitis associated with adenovirus type-1 should be treated with the same regimen as that used with most other forms of intraocular inflammation, i.e., reducing intraocular inflammation to prevent secondary sequelae.

LEISHMANIASIS

Leishmaniasis (kala-azar) is an endemic disease affecting both humans and animals in southern Europe, Africa, Asia, and South America. The dog, as well as the fox and the jackal, is an important reservoir host of this infection. The intermediate host is the sandfly (*Phlebotomus*). The disease has been reported only four times in dogs in the United States, and in each case the dog has been brought to the US from Greece.

The causative organism is *Leishmania donovani*. Clinical signs associated with visceral leishmaniasis are anorexia, vomiting, diarrhea, epistasis, ataxia, conjunctivitis, keratitis, and anterior uveitis.

Pathologically, the hallmark of the disease is a massive proliferation of reticuloendothelial cells with distention, disruption, and eventual replacement of normal structures. Organisms have been identified within the cytoplasm of reticuloendothelial cells and monocytes of the bone marrow. They are approximately 2 μ in diameter and are differentiated from *Toxoplasma* and *Histoplasma* by the presence of an intracytoplasmic kinetoplast.

In one case of a six-year-old female mixed breed dog, the presenting signs were bilateral blepharitis and endophthalmitis. In this case, *L. donovani* was cultured from the conjunctiva, eyelid, anterior chamber, and vitreous body.

Ocular manifestations of visceral leishmaniasis in humans are rare, but reports tend to indicate that ocular manifestations are common in animals. Keratitis and conjunctivitis are the predominant signs in animals, but inflammation of the sclera, anterior uveal tract, extraocular muscles, and eyelids is also seen.

Brucella canis can produce a bacteremia. Organisms have been isolated from the aqueous fluid in dogs with intraocular inflammation.

TRAUMATIC UVEITIS

Any form of ocular trauma can result in uveitis. The two most frequent forms of trauma are penetration of the anterior ocular segment with a foreign body and concussive trauma to the eye following a blow, for example, resulting from an automobile accident or from being hit by a blunt object. The presence of a highly vascular uveal tract and uveal blood vessels without a well-developed tunica muscularis predisposes animals to uveal bleeding. Increases in aqueous protein levels are readily produced, with even minor trauma. Following a penetrating injury to the anterior ocular segment (such as by a thorn or a claw from a cat), a plasmoid aqueous humor characterized by increased protein level and cell numbers develops rapidly. The iris becomes miotic, edematous, and vascularized. There is pain, blepharospasm, and photophobia. The globe is usually hypotensive. Intensive treatment to bring the ocular inflammation under control usually quickly resolves the uveitis.

LENS-INDUCED UVEITIS

This form of uveitis may go unrecognized in many small animals, particularly dogs. Embryologically, the lens develops a capsule that surrounds it early in its course of development. Thus, lens proteins are effectively walled off from the rest of the body. These proteins can stimulate a hypersensitivity reaction if released from the confines of the lens capsule. In the dog, lens-induced uveitis is seen most frequently either during development of cataracts with lens resorption or following traumatic injury to the lens capsule and release of lens proteins.

In animals that are developing cataracts, re-examination every three months is recommended to evaluate the possible development of phacolytic uveitis or intumescence (swelling) of the lens leading to secondary glaucoma. Phacolytic uveitis is characterized by the following signs: (1) presence of developing cataract, (2) red eye, (3) miotic pupil (when dilation is attempted with an indirect-reacting mydriatic i.e., tropicamide 1 per cent, the pupil does not dilate as rapidly or as fully as the normal eye), (4) presence of aqueous flare, and (5) mild blepharospasm and photophobia. If left untreated, this type of uveitis can worsen. Early cases of phacolytic uveitis associated with developing cataracts respond well to topical corticosteroids, such as prednisolone acetate 1 per cent drops, and a cycloplegic drug, such as 1 per cent atropine.

Uveitis associated with a ruptured lens capsule and the release of lens protein can produce a more severe uveitis, which is very difficult to control. In these cases, there is an intense uveitis with a secondary increase in IOP. The anterior chamber contains a large amount of protein, and the lens may be subluxated into the anterior chamber or moved forward, forcing the iris diaphragm forward and narrowing the anterior drainage angle. The treatment of choice in this form of uveitis is surgical removal of the lens and anti-inflammatory drug therapy.

THERAPEUTIC PRINCIPLES IN TREATING UVEITIS

Treatment in uveitis should reduce inflammation and its serious sequelae and preserve ocular tissue to maintain normal physiologic function.

First, investigate the initiating source of the inflammation and the qualitative and quantitative aspects of the inflammatory stimulus. How does the agent in question produce disease? What pathways does the agent follow in invading other tissues? How does the agent respond to treatment?

The overriding principle in the treatment of uveitis is removal of the stimulating agent from the eye. This may be possible for nonreplicating agents but is extremely difficult for replicating agents. The role of replicating, infective agents is less understood in the eye than in generalized systemic disease. Replicating agents, in general, are involved with the acute stage of a systemic disease, whereas most cases of uveitis are of a chronic nature. Even in acute uveitis, it has been difficult to incriminate replicating agents, and antibiotics are of questionable value in most cases.

ROLE OF CORTICOSTEROIDS

The eye is capable of responding immunologically just like other areas of the body, and many of these immunologic reactions take place in uveal inflammation. Thus, a regimen of nonspecific therapy has been developed to interfere with the defensive mechanisms of the host and prevent further, more extensive damage to ocular tissues. In general, the adrenocorticosteroids have been the agents of choice. The exact role of these agents in suppressing ocular inflammation has not been completely defined, and their effects seem to include lysosomal stabilization, reduction in number of lymphoid elements, and reduction in antibody production, thereby limiting immunologic reactions.

Corticosteroids are delivered to the eye via three major routes: topical, subconjunctival, and systemic. The topical steroid of choice is prednisolone acetate 1 per cent drops, used at least six to seven times a day. The acetate vehicle provides greater penetration of the drug through the intact epithelium and stroma so that a greater concentration of drug is delivered to the anterior ocular segment.

Corticosteroids can also be given subconjunctivally. The highest available concentration of drug should be used to minimize the volume administered. The corticosteroids used most frequently for subconjunctival injection are methylprednisolone acetate (40 mg/ml; 10 mg average subconjunctival injection), triamcinolone (40 mg/ml; 10 mg average subconjunctival injection), and betamethasone (6 mg/ml; 3 to 6 mg average subconjunctival injection).

In very severe cases of uveitis, the use of systemic steroids is also indicated. Prednisone can be given orally at a dose of 1.5 to 3.5 mg/kg/day.

In acute uveitis, steroids are usually given in high dosages for seven to ten days. If the acute inflammatory reaction is subsiding at that time, steroid dosage can be reduced and an alternate-day regimen of therapy begun.

MYDRIATIC-CYCLOPLEGICS

The use of a mydriatic-cycloplegic agent is also extremely important. Atropine 1 to 4 per cent drops or ointment can be used. In severe uveitis, the use of this indirect-acting agent can be supplemented with a direct-acting agent, such as 10 per cent phenylephrine drops, to achieve maximal pupillary dilatation. In animals, the prolonged use of phenylephrine can lead to topical irritation.

ANTIPROSTAGLANDINS

The role that prostaglandins play in ocular inflammation has been reviewed. The use of antiprostaglandin agents to decrease inflammation is gaining wide acceptance. It has been found that aspirin and indomethacin can prevent the disruption of the blood–aqueous humor barrier that develops in association with prostaglandin release. These substances inhibit the enzyme that catalyzes the production of prostaglandin from its fatty acid precursors. Caution must be used because of the systemic side effects, gastritis, gastrointestinal bleeding, and vomiting. The dose of aspirin in the dog is 25 mg/kg every eight hours and in the cat 12 mg/kg every 24 to 48 hours.

COMPLICATING SEQUELAE

The major clinical problem in the treatment of uveitis is that the ocular inflammatory response may not be controlled until too late in the course of the disease. This leads to sequelae such as anterior synechia formation, cataracts, secondary glaucomas, and buphthalmic and phthisical globes. Effective management of uveitis must involve vigorous attempts to preserve ocular structures and the physiologic integrity of the eye.

In reviewing cases of uveal inflammation, the

following major difficulties have contributed to inflammatory sequelae:

1. Failure to recognize the early clinical signs of uveitis (red eyes, tearing, photophobia, blepharospasm, cells and flare in anterior chamber).

2. Failure to effectively ameliorate the inflammatory process, with the resultant development of chronic sequelae and severe visual loss. Failure to use adequately high levels of corticosteroids to suppress inflammation. Additionally, too rapid withdrawal of corticosteroids, allowing intraocular inflammation to recur. Steroids should be tapered off slowly and the patient observed carefully for recurrence of inflammation.

3. Failure to recognize evidence of chronic ocular change that is irreversible and that results in permanent *structural alteration*. These types of changes can include:

    a. Persistent endothelial damage with permanent corneal edema and deep interstitial keratitis.

    b. Persistent protein leakage into the aqueous fluid because of structurally altered vasculature in the anterior ocular segment.

    c. Anterior or posterior synechia formation.

    d. Secondary glaucoma associated with broad-based anterior synechia and closure of the anterior drainage angle.

    e. Secondary cataract formation.

    f. Exudative retinal detachments.

    g. Optic neuritis and atrophy.

It is important to emphasize that once severe intraocular inflammation takes place and ocular structural damage develops, medical therapy is of no benefit in reversing that damage. Therefore, control of scar tissue formation and active inflammation must be accomplished by the vigorous use of high levels of anti-inflammatory agents.

ENDOPHTHALMITIS

Endophthalmitis refers to severe inflammation of the ocular tunic and its associated cavity. The inflammation in endophthalmitis is appreciably greater than that seen in uveitis, and often an infectious agent is associated with this reaction. In veterinary medicine, endophthalmitis is usually associated with penetrating intraocular wounds, postsurgical infections, and ruptured corneal wounds with secondary infections.

Signs of endophthalmitis are more severe than are signs of uveitis and include extreme pain, very deep scleral vascular engorgement, corneal edema with large numbers of cells and large amounts of protein in the anterior chamber, and a large amount of vitreous exudate.

APPROACH TO THE TREATMENT OF THE PATIENT WITH ENDOPHTHALMITIS

If severe structural damage is not evident and the cornea has not been ruptured (with intraocular tissue loss) one can attempt to treat the eye.

Aspirate the anterior chamber and/or vitreous chamber for culture and cytologic examination. This requires either a short-acting anesthetic or deep sedation of the patient. Experience has indicated that endophthalmitis in animals produces a very plasmoid aqueous and although small gauge needles (25 or 26 gauge) are less traumatic, they frequently become plugged with fibrin. We therefore use a 20-gauge needle and enter the anterior chamber at the limbus. The bevel of the needle should be up and the globe stabilized with a single tooth forceps, grasping the conjunctival-episcleral tissue at the limbus. A 1-cc tuberculin syringe is used, and 0.2 ml of fluid is withdrawn. Material is immediately inoculated into blood agar, thioglycollate broth, and Sabouraud agar. Slides are prepared for Gram and Giemsa staining. The same technique may be used for vitreous aspiration. Enter the vitreous cavity at the pars plana. Because culture results can take 24 hours, initial evaluation based on cytologic examination is extremely important. Evidence of large numbers of polymorphonuclear leukocytes and bacteria (gram negative or positive) is a good indication of an active infection, and treatment should begin immediately.

The rapid determination of glucose content in the vitreous cavity may be an aid in distinguishing infectious from noninfectious endophthalmitis. The technique can be accomplished by using a Dextrostix and applying material obtained from a vitreous tap. In bacterial infections, the organisms utilize glucose in the vitreous and sugar is reduced to absent. In noninfectious endophthalmitis, the vitreous sugar content is normal, usually greater than 10 mg per cent (Wong, 1981).

Routine treatment of endophthalmitis has produced poor results because of inadequate penetration of antibiotics into the eye, especially the vitreous cavity. Newer forms of treatment, although radical, have produced better results. Antibiotics and inflammatory agents are placed into the aqueous and vitreous cavity in appropriate dosage levels. Additionally, in vitreal disease, a vitrectomy may be performed. This technique requires specialized equipment to grind up and aspirate the vitreous body. Although vitrectomy is not within the realm of the nonspecialist, intracameral injections may be performed in an attempt to save infected globes.

Initial therapy for endophthalmitis can include any of the following: intraocular injection of gentamicin 350 to 500 μg or cephaloridine (Loridine) 250 μg; subconjunctival injection of gentamicin 25 mg and cephaloridine 1 mg or methicillin 100 mg or triamcinolone 20 mg (Kenalog 40 mg/cc); topical application of gentamicin ophthalmic ointment; and systemic administration of cephaloridine IV in appropriate dosage.

Intraocular aspiration should be repeated at 48 hours, and, if bacteria are still evident (and are cultured), the intraocular antibiotic regimen should be repeated.

The clinician should be aware that infections associated with endophthalmitis can spread via the optic nerve and the meninges surrounding the nerve. This may result in meningitis. It is important to either vigorously treat the endophthalmitis or enucleate the diseased globe. If treatment of endophthalmitis is not successful, the globe must be enucleated.

Preparation of Gentamicin for Intraocular Injection (Intraocular gentamicin, 500 μg)
1. Withdraw 0.1 ml (5 mg) from the vial containing 50 mg/ml gentamicin and add 1 ml nonbacteriostatic saline.
2. One milliliter contains 5 mg gentamicin, and 0.1 ml contains 0.5 mg or 500 μg.

3. Inject 0.1 ml containing 500 μg gentamicin.

Preparation of Cephaloridine for Intraocular Injection
1. Reconstitute powder with 10 ml sterile sodium chloride (1,000 mg in 10 ml).
2. Add 0.1 ml (10 mg) of suspension to 3.9 ml nonbacteriostatic saline; 10 mg in 4 ml contains 1 mg cephaloridine in 0.4 ml.
3. Inject 0.1 ml containing 0.25 mg cephaloridine.

REFERENCES AND SUPPLEMENTAL READING

Arronson, S., and Elliot, J.: *Ocular Inflammation*. St. Louis: C. V. Mosby, 1972.
Bistner, S. I., Shaw, D., and Riis, R. C.: Diseases of the uveal tract. Parts 1, 2, and 3. Comp. Cont. Ed. Prac. Vet. 1:868, 899, 1979; 2:46, 1980.
Forster, R. K.: Endophthalmitis. *In* Duane, T. (ed.): *Clinical Ophthalmology*. Vol. 4. New York: Harper and Row, 1981.
O'Connor, G. R.: The inflammatory response. *In* Susan, A., Gery, I., and Nussenblatt, R. B. (eds.): Immunology of the Eye. Workshop III. Special supplement to Immunology Abstracts, 225, 1981.
Wong, R.: Endophthalmitis. An exhibit at American Academy of Ophthalmology Meeting, Atlanta, Georgia, 1981.

OCULAR TUMORS OF THE DOG AND CAT

GREGORY M. ACLAND, B.V.Sc.
Philadelphia, Pennsylvania

and STEPHEN GROSS, V.M.D.
New York, New York

Ocular tumors are often potentially blinding and in many cases carry significant risk to the animal's life. Their true incidence may be greater than is suggested by the infrequency with which they are seen clinically. Ocular neoplasia may be the unsuspected cause in ocular diseases such as chronic inflammation or glaucoma. As a general principle, ocular tumors are more likely to be malignant in cats than in dogs.

In assessing these tumors, one must determine whether the tumor is primary, without metastases; or if it has metastasized or is itself a metastatic tumor. This determination must be based on accurate histologic identification of the tumor.

Predictions of ocular tumor behavior are unfortunately based on relatively small numbers of cases, with little long-term follow-up data. Extrapolations are sometimes possible from knowledge of the behavior of comparable tumors in humans, but the validity of these extrapolations is uncertain. Therefore, a cautious approach is advisable in the management of these tumors. As far as is possible, all tumors should be submitted for histopathologic identification, and all patients should have routine follow-up examinations for at least one year after surgical or alternative therapy.

EYELID TUMORS

Tumors of the canine eyelid are significantly different from those of the feline eyelid (Table 1). The former are usually small, firm, discrete, and benign; whereas the latter are more likely to be malignant.

There is considerable overlap in the clinical ap-

Table 1. *Eyelid Tumors*

Canine
    Sebaceous gland adenoma/adenocarcinoma
    Papilloma
    Melanoma
    Histiocytoma
    Mastocytoma
    Basal cell carcinoma
    Squamous cell carcinoma
    Fibroma/fibrosarcoma

Feline
    Squamous cell carcinoma
    Basal cell carcinoma
    Fibroma/fibrosarcoma
    Neurofibroma/neurofibrosarcoma
    Adenoma/adenosarcoma

pearance and behavior of canine eyelid tumors. Some may also have histologic features characteristic of more than one tumor type. Those tumors may be referred to as adnexomas. The risk of metastasis is low in most adnexomas, even those identified histologically as malignant.

The typical and most common of the canine tumors is the sebaceous gland adenoma. This tumor arises from the meibomian glands and is a gray to black mass found at the lid margin. This tumor appears most commonly in dogs eight years of age or older. Secondary low-grade inflammation of the surrounding tissues and superficial ulceration of the tumor are not uncommon. This tumor must be distinguished from chalazia (non-neoplastic, chronic lipogranulomas of the meibomian glands). If the tumor is large and especially if centrally located, it may impinge upon and irritate the cornea. Epiphora, keratitis, and sometimes corneal ulceration may result.

The most commonly encountered tumor of the feline eyelid is the squamous cell carcinoma. This malignant, invasive tumor characteristically affects white cats with nonpigmented eyelid margins. Solar ultraviolet radiation is believed to contribute to the development of this tumor. The tumor is frequently irregular in thickness and ulcerated and grows rapidly. The bulbar and third eyelid conjunctiva may be involved. The risk of metastasis is significant.

Small, slowly growing, discrete tumors may need no treatment beyond observation. However, they should be removed if rapid growth or corneal irritation occurs. Many of these tumors can be removed by a full thickness lid resection, accomplished by taking a margin of surrounding healthy tissue and closing the lid wound by simple sutures. Care must be taken when a mass is excised from the medial region of the lid to identify and preserve the lacrimal puncta and duct. *All tumors removed should be submitted for histopathologic examination* to identify the tumor and determine whether it has been completely excised.

Larger and/or more aggressive tumors, particularly infiltrative ones with indistinct margins, may require wide surgical excision and plastic surgical repair of the lids. Plastic repair is usually necessary if more than one-third of the lid margin is removed. If total surgical excision is not possible, alternative therapies are necessary. Nonetheless, partial surgical excision is advised to obtain biopsy tissue.

Radiation therapy has proved useful in the management of tumors such as squamous cell carcinomas in cats and large animals. The following methods have been used: x-irradiation (2,500 to 5000 rads in divided dosage over 10 to 14 days); gamma-irradiation (radon, gold-198, cobalt-60, or cesium-137 needles; 5000 rads); and beta-irradiation (strontium-90 application).

Cryotherapy may also be useful. Many tumors can be destroyed readily by this technique, and the eyelid does not appear to be harmed by freezing (except from depigmentation). The use of thermocouples to ensure adequate freezing of a sufficient margin around the tumor is recommended for reliable, consistent results.

A variety of other therapies have been found useful in the treatment of lid tumors of other animals and humans. So far, however, they have had limited application in canine or feline lid tumors. These techniques include radiofrequency hyperthermia and immunotherapy (e.g., tumor vaccine, BCG vaccine). Under appropriate circumstances these methods may be worthy of consideration.

THIRD EYELID, CONJUNCTIVAL, AND PERILIMBAL TUMORS

Tumors of the gland of the third eyelid are occasionally seen. The gland lies below and just posterior to the globe when the third eyelid is in its normal position. Thus, a large mass may grow unobserved until it prolapses anterior to the globe. Its appearance may be dramatic, and the tumor may entirely obscure the eye. These tumors are usually adenocarcinomas, and complete excision of the third eyelid is indicated. These tumors need to be differentiated from benign prolapse of the gland of the third eyelid ("cherry eye").

Epibulbar melanomas arising from the limbus (most commonly in the dorsolateral quadrant) occur in dogs. They can be invasive and tend to dissect into the corneal stroma. In our experience they are most common in dogs over five years of age, but their presence in younger dogs has been reported. Successful excision of these tumors can salvage the eye. Removal often necessitates corneoscleral grafting to repair the surgical defect. This should be attempted only by a surgeon experienced in this technique. Epibulbar melanomas are usually benign and appear to have a very low metastatic potential.

There is a group of tumors that occurs in the perilimbal region, and occasionally in adjacent tissues, of the canine eye. These appear to form a spectrum of distinctly non-neoplastic to distinctly neoplastic growths. They arise from episcleral tissue, most commonly in the dorsolateral quadrant, as white, cream, yellow, or pinkish to red masses. There is often considerable inflammation of surrounding tissues, and cholesterol crystals may deposit in the cornea secondary to this inflammation. Histologically they are composed of varying proportions of histiocytic and fibroblastic cells and acellular fibrous tissue. Depending on the histologic appearance, these tumors may be diagnosed as nodular episcleritis, fibrous histiocytomas, nodular fasciitis, proliferative keratoconjunctivitis (seen characteristically in collies), or histiocytomas. Distinction of these entities on clinical grounds is unreliable. The majority of lesions will regress, often completely and permanently, following subconjunctival injection (20 mg methylprednisolone) and topical application (1 per cent prednisolone) of corticosteroids. Large masses may require surgical excision, which may be curative. Any tissue resected should be submitted for histologic examination. If the tumor is persistent or recurrent, local radiation therapy may be advisable.

Other tumors occurring in the conjunctival and adjacent tissues include adenomas, viral papillomas, hemangiomas, and squamous cell carcinomas. These are usually amenable to local excision.

ORBITAL TUMORS

The vast majority of orbital tumors in the dog and cat (Table 2) are malignant, and prognosis is guarded. The clinical signs are those of a space-occupying orbital mass and may include exophthalmos or occasionally enophthalmos, deviation of the globe, protrusion of the third eyelid, and resistance of the globe to retropulsion. Affected animals are typically eight years of age or older and show a relatively slow progression of signs. There may be asymmetry of the bones surrounding the orbit and those overlying the nasal passages. Tumors are usually unilateral and do not cause pain when the mouth is opened. It has been the authors' experience that the majority of orbital tumors in both the dog and cat arise from adjacent structures and invade the orbit secondarily. Thus, a thorough examination of the skull, including the mouth, is essential in the assessment of a suspected space-occupying orbital mass.

Diseases characterized by non-neoplastic space-occupying orbital lesions (e.g., orbital abscessation, orbital cellulitis, myositis of the masticatory muscles and zygomatic adenitis) are primarily found in younger animals (usually less than five years old)

Table 2. *Orbital Tumors*

Canine
  Adenocarcinoma
    Nasal
    Lacrimal, salivary, sinus, or ductal
    Metastatic mammary, thyroid, renal, or pancreatic
  Multilobular osteochondroma of skull
  Primary or metastatic sarcoma
  Fibrosarcoma, rhabdomyosarcoma, neurogenic sarcoma, angiosarcoma, osteosarcoma, anaplastic sarcoma
  Lymphosarcoma
  Meningioma
  Malignant melanoma
  Squamous cell carcinoma

Feline
  Sarcomas
    Lymphosarcoma
    Ocular melanoma
    Osteosarcoma (primary)
    Rhabdomyosarcoma (primary)
    Undifferentiated (primary)
  Carcinoma
    Ocular squamous cell carcinoma
    Metastatic, e.g., pulmonary, mammary

and usually cause pain when the mouth is opened.

Foreign bodies migrating through the oral mucosa and apical inflammation of the carnassial tooth have been incriminated in orbital inflammatory disease. Thus, a thorough examination of the mouth should be undertaken, under anesthesia if necessary, whenever a space-occupying orbital lesion is suspected. Particular attention should be paid to the carnassial tooth and the area of mucosa just behind the last molar. Warmth and erythema of the lids and an elevated white cell count are also indicative of inflammatory orbital disease.

Myositis of the masticatory muscles (including the masseter, temporal, and pterygoid muscles) is usually bilateral and also painful. German shepherds and retrievers appear predisposed. Circulatory eosinophilia, elevated serum creatinine phosphokinase levels, and results of muscle biopsy may help confirm the diagnosis.

Canine and feline orbits lack a bony floor, thus orbital tumors are frequently large before they are noticed. Advanced tumors can cause defective pupillary function and blindness, as nerves are either directly infiltrated or damaged by compression or stretching. Fundus examination may reveal congested tortuous vessels or indentation of the globe.

Because of the likelihood of malignancy, thoracic, abdominal, and skull radiographs should be taken early in the clinical assessment of a suspected orbital neoplasm. Positive or negative contrast orbitography, tomography, and orbital angiography may provide valuable information as to tumor size location and character when survey radiographs are inconclusive. Osteolytic lesions of the zygomatic or vomer bones indicate malignancy and a poor prognosis.

Nasal carcinomas that erode through the medial orbital wall may present as orbital tumors without showing nasal signs. High quality occlusal radiographs of the nose may show disruption of the vomer bone and/or loss of fine turbinate structure.

Orbital exploration (Harvey, 1977) is valuable for both removal of discrete masses and biopsy of nonresectible masses. Owners should be advised that the eye may have to be removed during this procedure. Tissue may be obtained by curettage of nasal and paranasal sinuses when these are also involved. Needle biopsy of the orbit can also be attempted, either through the oral mucosa behind the last molar or percutaneously through a point immediately posterior to the middle of the lateral orbital ligament.

If complete surgical removal of a tumor is not possible, as is often the case, chemotherapy and/or radiation therapy can significantly improve the animal's condition. Such therapy requires specialist supervision.

INTRAOCULAR TUMORS

Although relatively rare, intraocular neoplasia may be the cause of chronic or recurrent ocular disease. Thus the clinician should be alert for an intraocular tumor in any undiagnosed ocular disease. This is particularly true in cases of persistent ocular inflammation or glaucoma (Table 3).

Sometimes the presence of an intraocular tumor is evident on examination, and in early cases there may be little reactionary ocular disease. However, in many cases the secondary effects of the tumor are its most prominent feature and may even mask its presence.

An ophthalmic examination, including direct and indirect ophthalmoscopy and slit-lamp biomicroscopy, will reveal most tumors. However, accessory diagnostic aids may be useful or necessary at times.

Ultrasonography is an extremely useful technique and is essential when ocular media are not clear.

Fluorescence angiography may also be useful in documenting tumor size and vascularity, helping to differentiate tumors from hematomas.

Other techniques developed for ophthalmic oncology in humans, such as radioactive phosphorus uptake and tumor enzymology and immunology, have not yet found significant clinical application in veterinary ophthalmology.

Non-neoplastic ocular conditions sometimes appear similar to intraocular neoplasia. Iridal or ciliary body cysts can resemble melanomas. They usually are translucent to light reflected from the fundus and are easily distinguished by ultrasonography. Any intraocular inflammation, particularly if chronic and/or exudative, should suggest the possibility of neoplasia. Inflammatory and neoplastic processes can sometimes be differentiated by cytology of ocular fluids.

Primary and secondary intraocular tumors may present with similar clinical signs, so differentiation may be difficult. A thorough systemic examination, including thoracoabdominal radiography, is advisable in all cases of suspected intraocular neoplasia.

PRIMARY TUMORS

DOG

The most frequently seen intraocular tumor in the dog is the uveal melanoma (Table 4). In young dogs this tumor is usually a discrete dark nodule, growing slowly in the iris. It is benign histologically, causes little reactive ocular disease, and has a very low metastatic potential.

In older dogs uveal melanomas tend to be larger and may grow into the iris, ciliary body, and occasionally the choroid. Secondary inflammation and intraocular hemorrhage occur. These tumors are more malignant histologically and may have a greater metastatic potential. Whether the tumors in young and old dogs represent different stages of the same type of neoplasm is unknown. That conclusion does appear reasonable, however.

Not all canine uveal melanomas fit the previously mentioned description. Some are nonpigmented, and their diagnosis as melanoma is not obvious. Rarely the tumor may be primary to the choroid, and occasionally it may be secondary to a melanoma elsewhere.

Nonpigmented epithelioid tumors, either adenomas or adenocarcinomas, usually arise in the ciliary body. They are usually discrete nodular or pedunculated masses that may displace the iris and/or the lens. Their color varies from glistening white to cream, tan, pink, or gray and may occasionally be quite dark, largely reflecting varying degrees of vascularity. The risks of intraocular hemorrhage, secondary glaucoma, and metastasis with these tumors are significant.

Table 3. Clinical Signs of Intraocular Neoplasia

Altered color, size, shape, texture, thickness, or mobility of iris
Ocular inflammation
    Conjunctival hyperemia
    Keratitis
    Uveitis
        Anterior
        Posterior
Glaucoma
Blindness
Intraocular hemorrhage
Retinal detachment
Lens luxation and/or opacification (cataract)
Neoplastic disease in other organs

Table 4. Intraocular Tumors

Canine
Primary
- Melanomas
  - Iris and/or ciliary body
  - Choroid (rare)
- Adenomas/adenocarcinomas
  - Ciliary body
- Glioneurogenic tumors
  - Medulloepithelioma
  - Teratoid medulloepitheliomas
  - Astrocytomas
  - Others
- Hemangiomas
- Others

Secondary
- Metastatic to the eye
  - Lymphosarcomas
  - Adenocarcinomas (esp. mammary)
  - Dermal melanoma
  - Hemangiosarcoma
  - Meningioma
  - Rhabdomyosarcoma
  - Canine venereal tumors
  - Neurogenic sarcoma
- Invasive to the eye
  - Meningioma

Feline
Primary
- Melanomas
  - Iris and/or ciliary body
- Adenosarcoma
- Medulloepithelioma

Secondary
- Lymphosarcoma
- Adenocarcinoma

Other primary intraocular tumors (Table 4) are less common in the dog and can only be differentiated by histopathology.

CAT

As in the dog, most primary intraocular tumors in the cat are melanomas (Table 4). Their behavior is far more aggressive, however.

Two forms of melanoma occur. The more frequent is a discrete nodular tumor that appears to be the counterpart of the canine uveal tumor. The risk of metastasis seems much greater in the cat than in the dog. When metastasis occurs it is frequently within one year of diagnosis. The second form of melanoma is a less discrete tumor that diffusely invades the uvea, iridocorneal angle, and aqueous drainage pathway. Glaucoma ensues. This tumor also has significant metastatic potential, although even after enucleation a number of years may elapse before metastatic disease becomes apparent.

Other primary intraocular tumors in the cat (Table 4) are similar to their canine counterpart but appear less frequently.

SECONDARY TUMORS

Lymphosarcomas are the most commonly reported secondary intraocular tumors in both the dog and cat. These may appear as discrete tumors but are commonly infiltrative and may be associated with a considerable degree of intraocular inflammation, exudation, and hemorrhage. They may be bilateral. In the cat they are usually associated with the feline lymphosarcoma leukemia virus. Whenever such a tumor is suspected in a cat (e.g., in any chronic or exudative uveitis), both immunofluorescent viral antigen assay (e.g., FELEUK) and FOCMA tests should be performed. The immunofluorescent test may be negative in cats with these tumors.

Adenocarcinomas are the second most frequently reported secondary tumors, more common in the dog than in the cat. They tend to be more discrete than lymphosarcomas and are less likely to be bilateral. They may grow rapidly, and intraocular hemorrhage may occur.

Many other tumors may metastasize to the eye (Table 3) but are less commonly seen. A thorough ophthalmic exam should be included in any case of systemic neoplasia.

THERAPY OF INTRAOCULAR TUMORS

Three main alternatives exist

Leave the Tumor Alone. This may well be the best option under certain circumstances, for example, if the tumor is small and discrete and is causing no secondary effects, such as a small "benign" iridal melanoma in a young dog. In such a case the tumor should be re-examined at regular intervals of not more than six months and preferably photographed to document any future change.

If the tumor is metastatic to the eye or has already metastasized systemically, it also should be left alone. In such a case the ocular tumor may be secondary in importance to the systemic disease. However, even when the animal has a limited life expectancy, removal of an intractably painful, glaucomatous, or phthisical eye may be advisable.

Local Excision. Discrete tumors such as small iridal melanomas or ciliary body adenomas may be amenable to local surgical excision (e.g., iridocyclectomy). Such surgery should be attempted only by an experienced ophthalmic surgeon.

The beneficial probability of saving a visual eye needs to be weighed in each case against the possibilities of incomplete removal and enhanced metastatic risk. A wide margin of normal tissue must be removed with the tumor and manipulation of the tumor kept to a minimum.

Enucleation or Exenteration. In many cases

these may be the only real options available. *All blind eyes suspected or known to harbor a tumor should be removed.* Current controversy over the relationship in humans between enucleation and metastasis strongly suggests that a healthy margin of extraocular tissue (including optic nerve) be removed with the eye. Manipulation of the eye should be *absolutely* minimal until it is severed from its blood supply. *Do not tug on the eye.* Details of surgical techniques may be found in standard texts.

Alternative therapies, including xenon and argon laser photocoagulation, cobalt plaque radiotherapy, chemotherapy, and cryotherapy, have found application in humans and experimental animals but so far have not found significant clinical application to intraocular tumors in the dog or cat.

SUPPLEMENTAL READING

Acland, G. M.: Intraocular tumors in dogs and cats. Comp. Cont. Ed. 1:558, 1979.
Barron, C. N.: The comparative pathology of neoplasms of the eyelids and conjunctiva with special reference to those of epithelial origin. Acta Derm. Venereol. 41(Suppl. 51):1, 1962.
Bistner, S. I., Aguirre, G. D., and Batik, G.: *Atlas of Veterinary Ophthalmic Surgery.* Philadelphia: W. B. Saunders, 1977.
Gross, S., Harvey, C. E., and Aguirre, G. D.: Orbital tumors in dogs. Manuscript in preparation. Am. Coll. Vet. Ophthal. A.G.M./Conf., 1981.
Harvey, C. E.: Exploration of the orbit. *In* Bistner, S. I., Aguirre, G. D., and Batik, G. (eds.): *Atlas of Veterinary Ophthalmic Surgery.* Philadelphia: W. B. Saunders, 1977, pp. 258–260.
Krehbiehl, J. D., and Langham, R. F.: Eyelid neoplasms of dogs. Am. J. Vet. Res. 36:115, 1975.
Martin, C. L.: Canine epibulbar melanomas and their management. J. Am. Anim. Hosp. Assoc. 17:83, 1981.
Williams, L., Gelatt, K. N., and Gwin, R. M.: Ophthalmic neoplasms in the cat. J. Am. Anim. Hosp. Assoc. 17:999, 1981.

Section

8

DISEASES OF CAGED BIRDS AND EXOTIC PETS

MURRAY E. FOWLER, D.V.M.

Consulting Editor

Additional Pertinent Information found in Current Veterinary
Therapy VII:

Holzworth, Jean, D.V.M.: Control of Feline Infectious Diseases in Catteries and Adoption Shelters, p. 1270.

McDonald, Scott E., D.V.M.: Respiratory Diseases in Psittacine Birds, p. 697.

EPIDERMAL SHEDDING PROBLEMS IN REPTILES

FREDRIC L. FRYE, D.V.M.

Davis, California

Difficulties associated with epidermal shedding or molting usually are encountered only in snakes and lizards. The ancient tuatara, *Sphenodon punctatus*, the crocodilia (alligators, crocodiles, caimans, and gharials or gavials), and most of the chelonians (turtles, terrapins, and tortoises) rarely exhibit conditions related to inhibited or abnormal epidermal renewal.

The process of periodic ecdysis of the keratinized epidermal layers entails a complex series of events mediated and/or initiated by growth, the overall state of nutrition, reproductive activity, endocrine function (especially related to the thyroid gland), humidity, ambient temperature, and environmental abrasion.

Neonatal snakes and lizards shed the outermost layers of keratinized epidermis within a few days or weeks of their birth or hatching. In at least two instances, hatching snakes were observed to be molting while still confined within their egg shells (Cliburn, 1976). As they grow, the outer epidermal layer is shed during the most rapid phase of growth at intervals from every few weeks to three or more times annually. Older, fully mature animals may shed once or twice yearly. Many female oviparous snakes quite predictably exhibit ecdysis a week to ten days prior to ovoposition (Wagner, 1982).

Transcutaneous water loss in snakes has been shown to be greatest immediately after completion of skin shedding (Groves and Altimari, 1977). Interestingly, a water economy study of a genetically scaleless snake tended to cast doubt on the role of scales in preventing water loss in snakes (Licht and Bennett, 1972). Another investigation demonstrated that the permeability barrier to cutaneous water loss in the reptilian (ophidian) epidermis consisted of neutral and polar lipids, particularly in the *mesos layer* of the shed skin (Roberts and Lillywhite, 1980).

Aquatic and semiaquatic turtles shed the senescent epidermis covering their extremities in a piecemeal fashion; they also shed one or more of the laminated keratinized carapacial and plastral shields from time to time (Frye, 1981). Each time one of these plate-like shields is lost, a growth ring is added to the newly exposed carapacial shield beneath. The number of growth rings is *not* synchronous with the passage of time; one *cannot* reliably estimate the age of a turtle or tortoise by counting the number of growth rings in its shields.

The tuatara, the crocodilians, and most lizards shed their old epidermis in small shreds rather than in one whole cast. By contrast, when snakes molt, their outgrown and/or worn epidermal covering

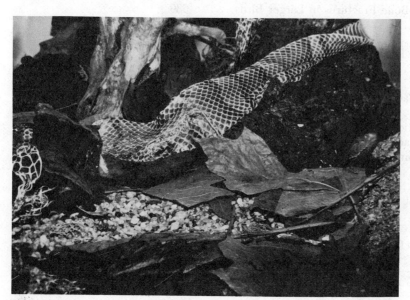

Figure 1. Inverted epidermal skin cast from a snake. Note the branches in the cage, which offer the animal sufficient abrasive surfaces upon which to rub its labial and rostral areas to initiate the shedding process.

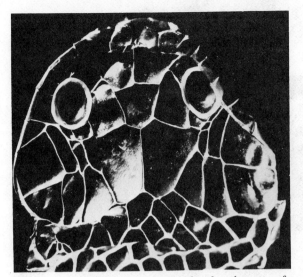

Figure 2. A closer view of the head and neck region of a shed snake skin. Note the attached spectacle shields, which covered the serpent's corneas.

comes away as an intact, inverted tube that faithfully reproduces each scale and textured nuance, including the spectacle shields covering the corneas (Figs. 1 and 2).

The normal process of ophidian ecdysis takes about a week or so to be completed, although the underlying metabolic events are more or less one continuous process throughout the snake's life (Cliburn, 1976; Chiu and Lynn, 1971; Frye, 1981; Jacobson, 1977; Madderson, 1964; 1965; Mays and Nickerson, 1968; Munro, 1952; Semlitsch, 1978). Approximately a week or two prior to skin shedding, a snake usually refuses to feed and its eye color becomes progressively dull, finally assuming an opaque or milky blue hue. The skin also loses its luster. Within a few days, this corneal and integumentary dullness diminishes, but the clarity of the spectacle shields remains less than normal. Soon the snake begins to rub its upper and lower labial surfaces and rostrum on abrasive objects such as logs, branches, or stones within its environment to loosen the old skin from its underlying, freshly exposed skin surface. The old epidermis on the head is pulled inside out, in a stocking-like fashion, as the snake literally crawls out of its shed skin. Some snakes will eat their freshly molted skin (Groves and Altimari, 1977). The author witnessed this behavior in the diminutive desert night lizard, *Xantusia vigilis*.

The predisposing factors of overall malnutrition, dehydration, excessively low environmental humidity, hypothermia, debilitating metabolic or infectious disease, parasitism, thyroidal dysfunction, trauma, and lack of suitable cage "furniture" to provide an abrasive surface contribute to either total lack of shedding or impaired shedding (dysecdysis).

In the case of snakes, dysecdysis may assume the form of one or more retained spectacle shields over the cornea (Fig. 3). Additionally, patches of old epidermis may remain attached to portions of the skin (Fig. 4). Both of these conditions create favored sites for ectoparasitism by the common snake mite, *Ophionyssus natricis*, as well as the nymphal stages of trombiculid grain mites. Rarely, a small ring of retained epidermis may tighten around a snake's tail or a lizard's digit (Fig. 5) (Frye, 1981), causing ischemic necrosis distal to the constriction.

Under inadequate husbandry practices that result in filth, abnormal moisture, and overcrowding, these retained portions of epidermis may predispose the underlying tissues to infection and invasion by a plethora of fungal, bacterial, protozoan, and metazoan pathogens.

Clearly, most instances of dysecdysis in snakes can be prevented by close attention to sound captive housing, husbandry, and feeding practices.

TREATMENT

Treatment of retained epidermal tags or shreds as well as spectacle shields in the uncomplicated case is relatively simple. A 30-minute bath in tepid water often is enough to soften the retained tissue sufficiently to allow it to be rubbed gently away. The depth of the water bath should not be so deep as to endanger drowning the specimen. Another method of softening the retained epidermis is to select a confined area, such as a styrofoam box or picnic chest, in which the snake or lizard can be sandwiched between layers of moistened clean toweling (Frye, 1981). As the snake or lizard crawls among the layers of toweling, its epidermis is loosened and wiped away without additional aid.

Once loosened with warm water, retained spectacle shields usually can be lifted away with a curved fine-pattern forceps by grasping one edge of the shield at the corneal-scleral-cutaneous junction. Exquisite care must be taken when operating the forceps and applying traction; grasping the underlying spectacle or even the cornea along with the softened shield may result in avulsion of the spectacle and/or cornea and destruction of the entire eye.

The small rings of retained epidermis acting as mini tourniquets around tails and digits also can be removed after soaking the animal in warm water. Animals that are too large to conveniently place in warm water baths can be treated with warm water sprays from hand-held bottles or hose nozzles. Larger snakes or lizards are then covered with clean, moist toweling or burlap bagging material. Both fabrics provide sufficient abrasiveness to help remove portions of retained skin as the creature crawls through the layers. A small volume of contact

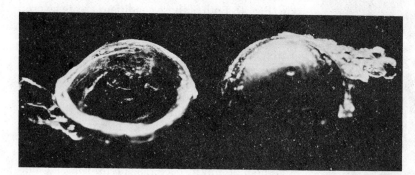

Figure 3. Two multiple-layered spectacle shields or caps from a large snake.

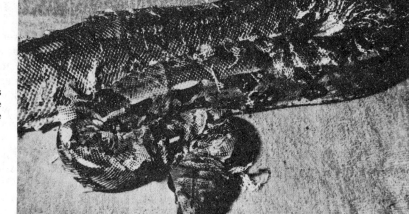

Figure 4. An example of dysecdysis in a captive boa constrictor. Note the shreds of old epidermis adhering to the underlying skin surface.

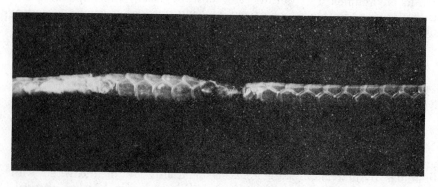

Figure 5. A circumferential lesion on the tail of a snake. This lesion was the result of a retained ring of epidermis, which acted as a tourniquet and produced ischemic necrosis distal to the constriction.

lens wetting solution, liquid household detergent, or similar wetting agent will help in quickly penetrating and moistening the epidermis.

REFERENCES AND SUPPLEMENTAL READING

Chiu, K. W., and Lynn, W. G.: Further observations on the role of the thyroid in skin shedding in the shovel-nosed snake, *Chionactis occipitalis*. Gen. Comp. Endocrinol. 17:508, 1971.

Cliburn, J. W.: Observations of ecdysis in the black pine snake, *Pituophis melanoleucus lodingi* (Reptilia, Serpentes, Colubridae). J. Herpetol. 10:299, 1976.

Frye, F. L.: *Biomedical and Surgical Aspects of Captive Reptile Husbandry*. Edwardsville, KS: Veterinary Medicine Publishing Co., 1981, pp. 187–189.

Groves, J. D., and Altimari, W.: Keratophagy in the slender vine snake, *Uromacer oxyrhynchus*. Herpetol. Rev. 8:124, 1977.

Jacobson, E. R.: Histology, endocrinology and husbandry of ecdysis in snakes (a review). V. M./S. A. C. 72:275, 1977.

Licht, P., and Bennett, A. F.: A scaleless snake: tests of the role of reptilian scales in water loss and heat transfer. Copeia 1972:702, 1972.

Madderson, P. F. A.: The skin of lizards and snakes. Br. J. Herpetol. 3:151, 1964.

Madderson, P. F. A.: Histological changes in the epidermis of snakes during the sloughing cycle. J. Zool. 146:98, 1965.

Mays, C. E., and Nickerson, M. A.: Notes on shedding in the sea snake, *Laticauda semifasciata* (Reinwardt), in captivity. Copeia 1968:619, 1968.

Munro, D. F.: Variation in rates of shedding by young snakes. Herpetologica 8:37, 1952.

Roberts, J. B., and Lillywhite, H. B.: Lipid barrier to water exchange in reptile epidermis. Science 207:1077, 1980.

Semlitsch, R. D.: The influence of temperature on ecdysis in snakes (genus *Natrix*) (Reptilia, Serpentes, Colubridae). J. Herpetol. 13:212, 1978.

Wagner, E.: Unpublished data, 1982.

Zucker, A.: Cutaneous water loss in relation to skin shedding in squamates. Am. Zool. 15:803, 1975.

PARASITIC DISEASES OF REPTILES

ELLIOTT R. JACOBSON, D.V.M.

Gainesville, Florida

Parasitic diseases involving both endoparasites and ectoparasites are commonly encountered in captive reptiles (Marcus, 1981). Although parasitic epizootics are relatively uncommon, *Entamoeba invadens* is responsible for considerable mortality in collections of tortoises, lizards, and particularly snakes. Many parasitic diseases, including cryptosporidiosis and spirorchiasis, are insidious in their expression and often go unrecognized until dramatic changes appear. A few parasites, such as the common snake mite, *Ophionyssus natricis*, may act as either a primary pathogen or a vector for a bacterial pathogen, *Aeromonas hydrophila*.

Although the ideal parasitic relationship is one in which the host is not killed, this optimum state may shift precipitously at any time in favor of the parasite. Unfortunately, many reptile parasites are resistant to chemotherapy. Additionally, a safe drug in species A may not be safe for species B. Thus, extrapolation from species to species may not be simple. Basic knowledge about the life cycle of the parasite will at least often be of value in reducing transmission both intraspecifically and interspecifically.

The following is a review of the commonly encountered endoparasites and ectoparasites of captive reptiles. The object is to enable the clinician to recognize these parasites and, when possible, treat infected animals and reduce transmission to noninfected animals.

AMOEBIASIS

To date, the most significant sarcodine pathogenic for reptiles is *Entamoeba invadens*. This protozoan has been responsible for considerable mortality in collections of lizards and snakes (Donaldson et al., 1975). Although crocodilians and turtles have been considered inapparent carriers of this protozoan, an epizootic involving *Entamoeba invadens* in a group of red-footed tortoises (*Geochelone carbonaria*) has been identified.

As is true of many systemic diseases in captive reptiles, a reptile with an active amoebic infection may show nonspecific signs. Absolutely no clinical signs have been noted in some reptiles up to 24 hours prior to the death of the animal. Snakes that are initially active and that have a good appetite become lethargic, lose weight, dehydrate, and often pass watery, mucoid, and often bloody stools prior to death. Epizootic clinical signs noticed in the red-footed tortoise were severe depression, listlessness, watery diarrhea, dehydration, and lingering death.

The mucoid and bloody diarrhea is generally correlated with the shedding of trophozoites. Trophozoites can be observed in wet preparations or in fecal smears stained by the Wright-Giemsa method. Trophozoites range in size from 16 to 19 μm. Leukocytes, epithelial cells, cellular debris, bacteria, and starch grains may be ingested and may be seen within the cytoplasm of trophozoites.

The diagnosis of amoebiasis may be aided by culturing stools from suspect animals. Techniques for the axenic culturing of *E. invadens* are available using agar plates (Diamond et al., 1978).

Gross necropsy findings in snakes often include extensive gastrointestinal inflammation with ulceration and hemorrhage. The colon appears to be the most severely involved organ, with extreme ulceration and necrosis. In most cases the liver is swollen and mottled throughout with focal to diffuse areas of necrosis. In red-footed tortoises the major lesions included a thickened, edematous duodenum in which the mucosa was necrotic. The common bile duct and gallbladder appeared necrotic, and the liver had multifocal to diffuse areas of necrosis.

The infective stage for the transmission of *E. invadens* is the cyst. Trophozoites are most likely not infective, since they readily desiccate upon release from the host. Cysts that are ingested by snakes develop in the gastrointestinal tract into trophozoites, which divide and become invasive. Encystment is dependent upon the availability of polysaccharides in the lumen of the intestinal tract and, therefore, is favored in turtles on high carbohydrate diets. This may explain the carrier state in these animals. Other factors appear to be involved in the crocodilian carrier state. In any case, mixed exhibits or housing of snakes with crocodilians and/or turtles should be discouraged.

E. invadens is not considered a normal snake parasite in the wild. The recently imported or collected snake is often housed under unsanitary conditions that would expose it to other reptiles that may have active infections. Snakes may become infected under these conditions, with clinical signs of disease seen weeks or months later. It is often this recently acquired snake by the private collector that may become a nidus of infection for an entire colony.

The drugs used for the prevention and control of reptilian amoebiasis have been extrapolated from the human literature. Several drugs have been used successfully, including diloxanide furoate (Furamide) at 0.5 gm/kg body weight orally as a single dose, emitine hydrochloride intramuscularly or subcutaneously at 0.5 mg/kg body weight as a single daily dose for ten days, and paromomycin (Humatin) at 33 to 110 mg/kg body weight given as a single daily dose orally for up to four weeks.

Two drugs that appear safe and effective for use in snakes are dimetridazole (Emtryl) and metronidazole (Flagyl). Flagyl is administered orally as a single dose at 275 mg/kg body weight; this dosage is repeated in two weeks. Administration can be achieved in solution either via a stomach tube or injected into a mouse offered to the snake. Red-footed tortoises suffering from *E. invadens* infection were treated by soaking food in an Emtryl solution of 5 ml per 3.7 liters of water with 5.5 liters of solution per 18.5 liters of food.

In experimental infections it was found that *E. invadens* was unable to result in an active infection when snakes were maintained at high temperatures (above 33°C). Thus, elevating the ambient temperature of a collection may be one way to control an epizootic.

In almost all cases of amoebiasis there is concomitant bacterial infection, with gram negative microorganisms most commonly isolated. Treatment should include the use of broad spectrum antibiotics such as chloramphenicol (Chloromycetin) (50 mg/kg body weight divided b.i.d. for two weeks) or gentamicin (2.2 to 4.4 mg/kg body weight as a single dose every 72 hours for five treatments).

Preventive and control measures should include a vigorous sanitation schedule. Cage to cage contamination should be reduced. Sick animals should be quarantined, and cages should be disinfected with a 3 per cent sodium hypochlorite solution. Recently acquired animals should also be quarantined and stool samples screened for shedding of cysts or trophozoites.

CRYPTOSPORIDIOSIS

Coccidia of the genus *Cryptosporidium* are considered mild pathogens that may infect turkeys, mice, calves, rhesus monkeys, and humans. *Cryptosporidium* associated with hypertrophic gastritis has been reported in zoologic collections of snakes (Brownstein et al., 1977). The author has also seen several cases in individual animals kept in zoologic and private collections. One recently field-collected corn snake was found to have typical signs and lesions.

Persistent post-prandial regurgitation, generally within three days following feeding, is a consistent clinical sign. Although adult snakes appear to be more commonly involved, the field-collected corn snake previously mentioned was a juvenile. The stomach is generally palpably firm and may result in mid body enlargement. Contrast radiography using barium sulfate confirms the stomach involvement. Oocysts and trophozoites may be demonstrated in PAS-stained fecal smears or smears stained by the Jenner-Giemsa method. Oocysts measure 2.6 to 6.0 μm, depending on the staining technique used. Trophozoites measure 1.8×1.2 μm.

Cryptosporidium can also be demonstrated by staining smears of the mucus covering regurgitated mice. Smears of stomach biopsy specimens can be stained by the Wright-Giemsa method and examined for microorganisms. Stomach biopsy specimens should be submitted for histopathology.

Gross pathology includes an increase in the diameter of the stomach with edema and thickening of the gastric mucosa. An abnormal amount of mucus may be adherent to thickened longitudinal rugal folds. Focal necrosis of the mucosa has been described.

The life cycle of reptilian *Cryptosporidium* is unknown. Attempts to establish an active infection in mice using reptile material have been unsuccessful. As in guinea pigs, reptilian cryptosporidiosis may involve a direct life cycle. Thus, isolation of suspect animals and reduction of cage to cage contamination should be a part of the control program.

There is no safe chemotherapeutic agent known to be effective against *Cryptosporidium*. Sulfadimethoxine (Bactrovet) at a single daily dose of 5 mg/kg body weight for five days was unsuccessful in eliminating an infection in a corn snake. Animals suspected of being infected should be isolated and their cages disinfected with a 3 per cent sodium hypochlorite solution. Adult snakes infected with this organism may represent an indefinite source of infection for other snakes.

HEMOGREGARINOSIS

The hemogregarines include the genera *Haemogregarina*, *Hepatozoon*, *Karyolysus*, *Schellackia*, and *Lainsonia*. These comprise the most common group of intracellular sporozoan hemoparasites found in reptiles, infecting all species except marine turtles. All are transmitted by arthropod or annelid vectors.

Hemogregarines are generally diagnosed by examination of a stained peripheral blood smear. The parasites, either single or paired, may be observed within the cytoplasm of both red and white blood cells. Red cells are often distorted by the presence of these parasites, with the nucleus displaced and cells showing both anisocytosis and poikilocytosis.

Although heavy parasitemias of hemogregarines may be seen in both clinicially healthy and ill snakes, it is difficult to relate any significance to the presence of these parasites. There is no experimental work to prove pathogenicity.

There is no information available on chemotherapeutic agents effective against hemogregarines. Possibly some of the antimalarial drugs may prove effective. In any case, since there is no documentation of pathogenicity, treatment would more than likely be an academic pursuit. Since transmission is dependent upon a suitable invertebrate vector, normal control measures for limiting transmission would include arthropod and leech eradication.

TREMATODIASIS

Numerous species of monogenetic and digenetic trematodes are known to infect reptiles. Although most species appear to be clinically insignificant, a definite disease relationship has been identified with several species. The more important pathogens will be discussed.

The family Spirorchidae includes a group of flukes that as adults inhabit the circulatory system of their host. Turtles are the most common reptilian host. Adult parasites are often found within the ventricular chamber or the lumen of the great vessels. Although the adult parasites may cause focal endothelial hyperplasia, no clinical signs have been attributed to these lesions. Major problems result from eggs released by adults into the circulatory system, which ultimately become trapped within terminal arterioles in visceral organs and in peripheral structures such as the limbs and dermal bone of the shell. Eggs collecting at these sites often elicit a granulomatous inflammatory response. Infected turtles may be submitted with pitted ulcerations of the carapace and plastron. These lesions result from an ischemic necrosis. Turtles may also be presented with edematous limbs resulting from vascular obstruction. Granulomatous pneumonia results from eggs trapped within vessels in the lungs; secondary bacterial infection is a common sequela. These turtles may exhibit flotation abnormalities.

Spirorchid trematode eggs ultimately pierce the gastrointestinal mucosa and are released in the feces. Diagnosis of a spirorchid infection is based on demonstration of eggs in the feces or tissues. Eggs of *Spirorchis elegans* measure approximately 100×75 μm and are thin shelled and amber to red in color. *Laeredius laeraedi*, which infect the green turtle, *Chelonia mydas*, produce eggs measuring 43×34 μm.

There is no chemotherapeutic agent known to be effective against reptilian spirorchid infections. The life cycle of the fluke involves a snail as an intermediate host so that infections in captivity are usually self-limiting. Turtles maintained in outdoor enclosures under natural conditions may become infected. Control under such conditions would entail defining and eliminating the intermediate host.

These trematodes represent a group of flukes that include the genera *Dasymetra*, *Lechriorchis*, *Zeugorchis*, *Ochestosoma*, and *Stomatrema*. Adults are commonly seen within the oral cavity of a wide variety of snakes. No lesions are associated with the flukes at this site. Adult flukes may also be found within the esophagus, trachea, and lung/air sac. Adult parasites within the lung attach to the epithelial lining, resulting in focal ulcerating lesions. Secondary bacterial pneumonia is associated with renifer lung infections.

Renifer infections are generally identified upon routine examination of the oral cavity. Eggs are shed within the lung and oral cavity and are ultimately eliminated in the feces. Eggs are yellow-orange in color, measure approximately 40 × 25 μm, and have a pale polar cap. Eggs can be seen on examination of a direct fecal smear or sediment. Lung washings taken from snakes presented with pneumonic problems should be examined for characteristic eggs.

No safe chemotherapeutic agent has been reported for renifer infections. Tetrachlorethylene at a dose of 0.2 ml/kg body weight administered orally was found effective when given to common water snakes *(Natrix sipedon)* (Nelson, 1950). The hepatotoxic effects of this compound limit its use in all identified infections. Adult flukes within the oral cavity can be manually removed.

The intermediate hosts for these parasites are generally amphibians. Thus, captive reptiles that require amphibians as food items generally maintain a continual infection.

STYPHYLODORA

Adult flukes in this genus have been found within renal tubules and ureters of several genera of harmless and poisonous snakes. With few exceptions, the infections are subclinical. In one case report a boa constrictor *(Constrictor constrictor)* was anorexic for approximately six months prior to its death. At necropsy, multifocal firm nodules may be seen throughout the kidneys. Pathologic changes associated with these parasites include renal tubular dilatation, intraluminal tubular debris build-up, and chronic interstitial nephritis. Diagnosis is dependent upon examining a direct smear of urine or urine sediment for eggs. With hematoxylin and eosin stain the eggs have a bright yellow eggshell and a faint polar cap. Eggs measure approximately 40 × 18 μm. There is no chemotherapeutic agent known to be effective against *Styphylodora.*

CESTODIASIS

Tapeworms are known to infect all major groups of reptiles except crocodilians. Although reptiles are generally definitive hosts, with adult tapeworms located in the gastrointestinal tract, several species act as intermediate hosts. All reptilian tapeworms of clinical significance can be grouped into three orders: Pseudophyllidea, Mesocestoididea, and Proteocephalidea.

The pseudophyllidean tapeworms include the genera *Bothridium, Bothriocephalus,* and *Spirometra.* Reptiles (particularly pythons) serve as definitive hosts for *Bothridium* and *Bothriocephalus,* which are generally found as adults in the intestine. Although most infections are subclinical, infection with *Bothridium* sp. in two green tree pythons was

associated with mild chronic enteritis (Toft and Schmidt, 1975). With heavy tapeworm infestations the small intestine may become packed with a bolus of parasites, mechanically obstructing the bowel.

Diagnosis of pseudophyllidean infection is dependent upon finding the adult parasites in the feces. Morphology of eggs varies with the species, being either operculated or nonoperculated and either unembryonated or containing a ciliated larva.

Lizards and snakes serve as intermediate hosts for *Mesocestoides* and *Spirometra,* respectively, with carnivorous mammals acting as definitive hosts. Most infections are subclinical. *Mesocestoides* larvae are often found in the liver, where mechanical damage to hepatocytes may occur. At necropsy multifocal small nodules may be seen throughout the liver and other visceral organs.

Snakes may serve as intermediate hosts for *Spirometra,* with plerocercoids (sparganna) being found in the subcutis or visceral structures; damage is generally mechanical. Snakes may be presented with subcutaneous swellings or nodules. Surgical excision will demonstrate the larval forms. Human infection following the ingestion of raw snake meat has been reported.

The most significant genus of the order Proteocephalidea is *Ophiotaenia.* It is the most common tapeworm found in North American snakes. Frogs act as intermediate hosts for larval forms, and snakes become infected after ingesting infected frogs. Infections in snakes are usually subclinical. Diagnosis is based upon a demonstration of adult tapeworms in feces or an examination of fecal sediments or direct fecal smears for eggs containing oncospheres. Eggs of *Ophiotaenia* measure approximately 50 × 40 μm.

There are no drugs known to be effective against extraintestinal larval pseudophyllideans. For adult tapeworms within the intestine the drugs of choice include niclosamide (Yomesan) administered orally at 150 to 300 mg/kg body weight as a single dose, bunamidine (Scolaban) administered orally at 50 mg/kg body weight as a single dose, and mebendazole (Telmin) in a single oral dose of 20 to 25 mg/ kg body weight repeated in two weeks. No information is available on the use of injectable agents such as praziquantel (Droncit) in reptiles.

NEMATODIASIS

All groups of reptiles are susceptible to infection by a wide variety of nematodes. Almost any system may be involved, with specific adult nematodes found at specific sites. Although there may be rather demonstrable gross lesions at necropsy, infections are often subclinical. Diagnosis is dependent upon recognizing characteristic ova within the feces.

ASCARIDS

Ascarid nematodes have been identified in all major groups of reptiles except the tuatara, *Sphenodon punctatus*. A majority of the species have been described from experience with crocodilians and snakes. *Ophidascaris* is the largest genus, containing several dozen species; it is found only in snakes.

Carnivorous reptiles become infected by eating a suitable intermediate host. Ascarids infecting herbivorous reptiles most likely have a direct life cycle. Infection by ascarids may result in significant lesions as they migrate as larval forms through visceral structures. In snakes and crocodilians adult ascarids often embed through the mucosa into the submucosa of the caudal esophagus and stomach, with several parasites embedding at one site. At these locations a tremendous granulomatous inflammatory response may develop. Secondary bacterial infections with bacteremia have been seen. Snakes are often subclinical, but post-prandial regurgitation may occur. Adult parasites may be identified in regurgitated food or in the feces. Diagnosis is often made based on examination of a fecal flotation specimen for characteristic eggs that have thick shells, typical of mammalian ascarids, that measure 80 to 100 × 60 to 80 μm. A direct examination of the esophagus and stomach can be achieved with a flexible fiberscope.

Mebendazole (Telmin) at 20 to 25 mg/kg body weight and thiabendazole (Omnizole) at 50 mg/kg body weight administered as a single oral dose and repeated in two weeks are the drugs of choice. When severe granulomatous lesions have been identified or suspected, the animal should be additionally treated with a broad spectrum antibiotic.

STRONGYLES

Reptiles are subject to infection by numerous species of strongyles. The spirurid nematode *Physaloptera* is a common gastric parasite of lizards inhabiting the southwestern U.S. *Kalicephalus* is a hookworm that infects numerous species of snakes and may be found anywhere in the alimentary tract. These are generally small parasites that may be overlooked on post-mortem examination.

Although most infections with *Kalicephalus* are subclinical, anorexia, debility, lethargy, and death have been reported in snakes with heavy infections. Inflammatory gastrointestinal lesions with hemorrhage, erosions, and ulcerations may be associated with the presence of these parasites.

Demonstration of eggs in a fecal flotation specimen or adults in feces is diagnostic. Eggs are thin walled, measure 70 to 100 × 40 to 50 μm, and may be seen in either the morula or larvated stage. Lungworm eggs are also larvated and, other than being slightly smaller, are indistinguishable from *Kalicephalus* eggs.

Kalicephalus has a direct life cycle, with infection following either oral ingestion or percutaneous penetration. Unsanitary conditions with fecal build-up in a cage promote a sustained infection. Good sanitation with the administration of thiabendazole at 50 mg/kg body weight and mebendazole at 20 to 25 mg/kg body weight as a single dose repeated in two weeks should eliminate the infection. *Physaloptera* has an indirect life cycle involving insects, so that total elimination in insectivorous lizards may be impossible.

LUNGWORMS

Members of the genus *Rhabdias* are the lungworms of snakes and lizards. Most free-ranging snakes in the southeastern U.S. have substantial lungworm burdens. Adult female *Rhabdias* organisms in the lung are parthenogenetic, producing embryonated eggs that are expelled up the trachea, swallowed, and eliminated in the stool. Eggs hatch in the stool and free-living rhabditiform larvae produce infective filariform larvae that enter a suitable reptile via either the oral or percutaneous route. Larvae ultimately migrate to the lungs, where they mature.

Although most infections with *Rhabdias* are subclinical, they may result in severe respiratory disease, especially in conjunction with bacterial microorganisms. Clinical signs include gaping of the mouth with extended glottis and exudate accumulating around the glottal opening. Ante-mortem diagnosis is based on a demonstration of embryonated eggs measuring approximately 60 × 35 μm either in the feces, in exudate around the nares and glottis, or in lung washings. Lung washings can be easily taken via a polyethylene cannula inserted down the trachea into the lung field.

The drug of choice for the treatment of snakes with lungworm infections is levamisole hydrochloride (Tramisol) administered intraperitoneally at 10 mg/kg body weight as a single dose repeated in two weeks. Although most colubrid snakes are responsive to therapy with this drug, the author has not been able to eliminate lungworm infections in the genus *Bitis* (African vipers). Since *Pseudomonas* and *Proteus* spp. are commonly cultured from lungs of snakes infected with lungworms, therapy should include the administration of a broad spectrum antibiotic.

FILARIDS

All major groups of reptiles are susceptible to infection with filarid nematodes. Although most infections go undetected, there is one report of pathology associated with infection in an aberrant host. *Macdonaldius oschei,* normally infecting boid, colubrid, and viperid snakes from western Mexico, caused extensive dermal lesions in several Southeast Asian pythons in a German zoo (Frank, 1964). The parasites are normally found in the posterior vena cava and renal veins. The mesenteric arteries of the pythons were occluded, and dermal lesions resulted from occlusion of capillaries by microfilariae.

Diagnosis of filarid infections is dependent upon demonstration of microfilariae in the blood or adults in the veins at necropsy. Chemotherapy for reptilian filarid infections has not been reported. Adult *M. oschei* can be killed by maintaining snakes at an ambient temperature of 35 to 37°C for 24 to 48 hours. Since this temperature range is near the critical thermal maximum for some species of snakes, the ambient temperature and snake must be monitored closely.

OTHER NEMATODES

Reptiles are subject to a wide variety of nematode infections not discussed previously. Snakes and lizards may suffer from capillariasis, which is often subclinical. Adult parasites may be found in the intestinal tract or within hepatic bile ducts, where mechanical damage to the liver often occurs. The eggs measure 65 × 35 μm and are typical capillaria eggs, i.e., they are double operculated. Oral thiabendazole at 100 mg/kg body weight as a single dose repeated in two weeks is the treatment of choice.

Oxyurid nematodes commonly infect turtles, lizards, and several species of snakes. In most species these parasites act as saprophytes within the colon, although a fatal impaction in a Fiji Island iguana (*Brachylophus fasciatus*) has been reported (Kane et al., 1976). The eggs are typical oxyurid eggs, being elongated with a flattened side and measuring 130 × 40 μm. Infected animals may be treated with thiabendazole at 50 mg/kg body weight orally as a single dose repeated in two weeks.

ACANTHOCEPHALINIASIS

A number of thorny-headed worms have been demonstrated in reptiles. Aquatic turtles commonly have acanthocephalans within the small intestine, with infections almost invariably being subclinical. Pathology includes ulceration of the intestinal mucosa with a focal inflammatory response. Although snakes are mostly parasitized by larval acanthocephalans, a king cobra was found to have a heavy

infection of the intestinal tract with mature *Sphaerechinorhynchus serpenticola;* several parasites were also found attached to the capsule of the liver. Mature eggs are multi-enveloped and oval, containing an acanthor larva with rostellar hooklets. In most cases acanthocephalans have an indirect life cycle with invertebrate intermediate hosts. Therefore, infection should be self-limiting in captive collections. There is no safe chemotherapeutic agent effective against acanthocephalan infections.

PENTASTOMIASIS

Pentastomes, which used to be categorized with the arthropods, are presently considered a separate phylum of parasites. The adults are worm-like in appearance with pseudosegmentations resulting from superficial cuticular rings. Except for *Linguatula* in domestic mammals and *Reighardia sternae* in gulls, adult pentastomes are found in adult crocodilians (*Sebakia*), lizards (*Rallietiella*), and snakes (*Rallietiella, Kiricephalus, Porocephalus, Armillifer*). Mammals generally serve as intermediate hosts for these parasites.

Adult pentastomes are usually found within the respiratory system of their reptilian hosts, including trachea, lungs, and air sacs. Sexually mature pentastomes have also been found in the coelomic cavity and subcutis. Subcutaneous swellings may be seen in heavy infections, and there are several reports of parasites exiting through ulcerations in the skin upon capture and handling of field-collected snakes. Similarly, adults inhabiting the respiratory system may exit via the glottis and then through the mouth and nares. Larval forms generally migrate to visceral and subcutaneous sites in the intermediate host. Humans may serve as the intermediate host for the genera *Armillifer* and *Rallietiella*. Infected reptiles must be considered a source for human infection.

Most cases of pentastomiasis in the natural host go undetected. Although in most cases there is little in the way of pathology, in some instances adult parasites in the lung will result in focal epithelial necrosis with hemorrhage and an inflammatory response. Secondary bacterial infection adds to the problem. Adult parasites such as *Armillifer* are huge (up to 5 cm) and may physically obstruct the trachea, resulting in suffocation. Snakes may be presented with clinical signs of open-mouth gaping with an extended glottis.

Ante-mortem diagnosis is dependent upon a demonstration of larval or adult forms in subcutaneous swellings or within the respiratory system. With large snake species a rigid fiberscope inserted into the trachea of an anesthetized snake allows visualization of a limited portion of the respiratory system. Pentastomid eggs are often surrounded by a capsule and are large in size, measuring 130 μm in diameter. Larvae containing hooklets may be visualized within the egg. Eggs may be found upon examination of lung washings or fecal smears.

Unfortunately, there are no chemotherapeutic agents effective against pentastomes. Larvae and adults, where possible, may be removed surgically or manually. Since infection is dependent upon ingestion of an infected intermediate host, most infections are self-limiting in captivity, although autoinfection is possible in several species.

ACARIASIS

Numerous species of mites and ticks are known to infest reptiles. The best studied of these is the snake mite, *Ophionyssus natricis*. Although infestations in the wild are rare, burdens in captivity may be enormous. Adults may be located under scales anywhere on the body. Eggs are deposited off the snake in the cage with the entire life cycle requiring 10 to 32 days. With females laying 60 to 80 eggs, a snake may go from a light to heavy burden within one month.

The snake mite causes disease both by feeding upon the host with resulting anemia and by mechanically transmitting the bacterial agent *Aeromonas hydrophila*, which is responsible for pneumonia and septicemia in snakes (Camin, 1948); mortality rates may approach 100 per cent. Not all infestations are associated with the transmission of this organism; therefore, the septicemic state should be first identified before treating an infested individual or colony with broad spectrum antibiotics.

Diagnosis is dependent upon identification of the mite on the host, crawling about in the cage, or within the water bowl. Mites range up to 1.5 mm in length and may be found by brushing the snake over a clean sheet of white paper. The conjunctiva may be edematous, and mites commonly infest the space between the periocular scales and spectacle.

One of the earliest methods used to treat an infected snake was to cover the animal with olive oil, which essentially suffocated the mites. Snakes have also been treated with topical silica gel powder (Dri-Die 67), which desiccates the mite. Dichlorovinyl dimethylphosphate (DDVP) pest strips (Vapona) are quite effective in eliminating mites. One must be cautious in using these strips, since the active ingredient is potentially toxic to reptiles. The strip can be suspended either outside the cage or within the cage for up to four days. The cage should always be well ventilated, water bowls should be removed, and the reptile should not be able to come in direct contact with the strip. A small 2.5-cm square can be placed within a perforated plastic film container and suspended within the cage.

Additional species of mites that the clinician may encounter are lung mites (*Entonyssus* and *Ophiopneumicola*) and chiggers (*Eutrombicula*), both of which are generally innocuous.

Several genera of ticks, including *Amblyomma*, *Aponomma*, and *Ornithodoros*, are known to infest reptiles. Some of these are rather species specific, whereas others are rather indiscriminate in their host preference. Ticks may be found under scales of snakes and attached to periocular sites in lizards and skin and scutes of terrestrial turtles. Heavy burdens could potentially result in anemia, but more importantly these parasites are vectors of blood parasites such as *Macdonaldius oschei*. An outbreak of Q fever (rickettsial infection involving *Coxiella burnetti*) was diagnosed in several workers handling recently imported ball pythons (*Python regius*) that were infested with ticks. Most ticks can be manually removed; DDVP-impregnated strips can be used in a manner similar to that described for mites.

MYIASIS

Infestation with larval forms of sarcophagid flies is not uncommon in wild tortoises and is occasionally seen in crocodilians. Captive animals maintained in outdoor enclosures may be similarly infected. Larvae may be deposited at sites of skin lesions, such as those produced by feeding ticks. Turtles may be presented with either focal or diffuse subcutaneous swellings involving the entire body. Blow holes through the skin are usually seen. The larvae migrate through the subcutaneous tissues, resulting in craters and fistulous tracts. The recommended treatment is surgical removal. Turtles are anesthetized with ketamine hydrochloride at 50 mg/kg body weight administered intramuscularly. The skin should be prepared with an organic iodine solution. Following removal of the larvae, the fistulous tracts should be flushed with a dilute organic iodine solution. The use of a broad spectrum antibiotic is recommended in severe cases.

GENERAL COMMENTS CONCERNING FECAL EXAMINATION

Fecal examination should include examination of a direct smear, sediment, and flotation specimen. It is important to realize that parasite eggs present within food items such as birds, rodents, and rabbits, which are commonly fed to carnivorous reptiles, will be seen within the feces of the reptile. Thus, the picture may become quite confusing and the clinician must be aware of the parasite burdens of the food items to arrive at an accurate diagnosis. Additionally, rodent mites, lice, and their eggs are also commonly encountered.

RECOMMENDATIONS FOR PRESERVING AND SUBMITTING HELMINTHS*

Trematodes and cestodes should be placed in a dish containing tap water, which is placed in a refrigerator overnight to allow the parasites to relax. They should then be placed in a solution (AFA) consisting of 8.5 parts 85 per cent ethanol, 1 part commercial formalin, and 0.5 part glacial acetic acid. Nematodes should be dipped in concentrated glacial acetic acid or hot 70 per cent ethanol for fixation. They are then transferred to a mixture of 9 parts 70 per cent ethanol and 1 part glycerin. They may be stored indefinitely in this solution. It is important to preserve the holdfast organ of spiny-headed worms intact. The parasite should be carefully pulled free or dissected from the host tissue and handled in the same manner as that for cestodes and trematodes. All material presented to a parasitologist should have complete data including host

*Recommendations of Dr. Ellis Greiner, College of Veterinary Medicine, University of Florida, Gainesville, FL.

species, host organ or tissue, collection locality, date of collection, and collector. Many new reptile parasites are yet to be identified and named.

REFERENCES AND SUPPLEMENTAL READING

Brownstein, D. G., Standberg, J. D., Montali, R. J., Bush, M., and Fortner, J.: *Cryptosporidium* in snakes with hypertrophic gastritis. Vet. Pathol. 14:606, 1977.

Camin, J. H.: Mite transmission of a hemorrhagic septicemia in snakes. J. Parasitol. 34:345, 1948.

Diamond, L. S., Harlow, D. R., and Cunnick, C. C.: A new medium for the axenic cultivation of *Entamoeba histolytica* and other *Entamoeba*. Trans. R. Soc. Trop. Med. Hyg. 72:431, 1978.

Donaldson, M., Heyneman, D., Dempster, M. S., and Garcia, L.: Epizootic of fatal amebiasis among exhibited snakes: epidemiologic, pathologic, and chemotherapeutic considerations. Am. J. Vet. Res. 36:807, 1975.

Frank, W.: Die pathogenen Wirkungen von *Macdonaldius oschei* Chaubaud et Frank 1961 (Filaroidea, Onchocercidae) bei verschiedenen Arten von Schlangen (Reptilia, Ophidia). Z. Parasitenk. 24:249, 1964.

Kane, K. K., Corwin, R. M., and Boever, W. J.: Impaction due to oxyurid infection in a Fiji Island iguana. V. M./S. A. C. 71:183, 1976.

Marcus. L. C.: *Veterinary Biology and Medicine of Captive Amphibians and Reptiles*. Philadelphia: Lea & Febiger, 1981.

Nelson, D. J.: Treatment for helminthiasis in ophidia. Herpetologica 6:57, 1950.

Toft, J. D. II, and Schmidt, R. E.: Pseudophyllidean tapeworms in green tree pythons (*Chondropython viridis*). J. Zoo Anim. Med. 6:25, 1975.

DISINFECTANT AND INSECTICIDE USAGE AROUND BIRDS AND REPTILES

MURRAY E. FOWLER, D.V.M.

Davis, California

DISINFECTANTS

Information exists concerning the safety and efficacy of disinfectants used around cage birds and reptiles, but little research has been carried out to establish toxic levels, contraindications, or usage regimens. Some information can be extrapolated from the poultry industry relative to safe disinfectants and insecticides for birds. However, the small size of some cage birds (25 gm for a canary) places them in a higher risk category.

Veterinarians should advise clients requesting information on disinfectants that none should be used indiscriminately. Thorough cleaning with a soap or detergent will usually control microorganisms unless there has been a specific disease outbreak.

Most disinfectants are inactivated in the presence of organic material. A disinfectant solution should be left on a surface for 15 to 30 minutes, after which the surface should be thoroughly rinsed.

The major sources of trouble for bird and reptile owners occur when errors of dilution have been made and when the cage has been insufficiently rinsed before animals are allowed access to the area. Ingestion of the disinfectant by birds may result from preening habits. All of the commercially available disinfectants may be used to sanitize bird or reptile cages if rinsing is thorough before the animal enters the area.

TREATMENT

Before describing the proper use of individual disinfectants, a protocol for management of suspected disinfectant poisoning will be suggested.

Remove the disinfectant from the animal's body or limb surfaces with copious quantities of tap water. If ingestion is suspected, a mild laxative should be given to hasten evacuation of the digestive tract. In birds, the crop can be washed with water by insertion of a large intragastric tube, but if there is a possibility of caustic esophagitis, caution should be used with mechanical intervention.

After removal of the disinfectant, follow-up care will depend on the severity of the lesion. Application of ointments or lotions may suffice, or bandages may be indicated. Systemic poisoning must be treated symptomatically, as no specific antidotes are available. The cage and its paraphernalia must be rinsed to remove residual disinfectant.

SPECIFIC COMPOUNDS (Table 1) (Fowler, 1978; Small, 1974)

PHENOL COMPOUNDS

Phenols, creosol, and biphenols have been used around poultry without major poisoning problems. The phenols are generally potent disinfectants and can be used safely around birds.

Sodium-O-phenylphenol (OPP) is one of the newer effective and safe phenolics. OPP is an ingredient in many household (Lysol*) and industrial disinfectant solutions (One Stroke Environ†). OPP

is effective against most bacteria including mycobacteria, fungi, and lipophilic viruses. The US Department of Agriculture utilizes OPP in official disinfection programs.

Concern has been expressed regarding the use of phenolics around reptiles. One author states, "Phenolics are considered highly toxic to herpetofauna and should be avoided" (Marcus, 1981). OPP may be corrosive to tissues. Signs of poisoning include dermal hyperemia and ulceration. In snakes, absorption or ingestion of OPP causes convulsions.

Pine oil is a phenolic compound obtained from the destructive distillation of pine and other woods and is a common ingredient in household disinfectants and deodorizers (e.g., Hexol,‡ Pine-sol§). Pine oil may be used for sanitizing perches, feeders, waterers, and cages. It is generally safe for use around birds and reptiles, but accidental contact may cause irritation to exposed body surfaces. It is unlikely that systemic signs will be produced.

Pentachlorophenols (PCP) pose a special problem. They are potent fungicides, herbicides, and bacteriocides that are often used as wood preservatives. In one case, a home had to be vacated by its human occupants because of the volatile PCP fumes that emanated from the naturalistic wood used in the home's construction (Fowler, 1978). Birds in such a home would also be at risk.

An interesting case of poisoning in canaries resulted from the use of pentachlorophenol–impregnated binder twine for nest material (Dorrestein and Zeller, 1979). The eggs of breeding canaries declined in hatchability. There was retardation of growth and feathering and a high neonatal mortality in the first week. All chicks died before three months.

---

*Lehn and Fink Consumer Products, Montvale, NJ.
†Vestal Laboratories, St. Louis, MO.

‡Hexol Inc., San Francisco, CA.
§American Cyanamid, Princeton, NJ.

Table 1.   *Characteristics of Disinfectants Used for Birds and Reptiles**

Disinfectant	Bacteriocidal	Virucidal	Fungicidal	Sporocidal	Algaecidal	Mycobacteriocidal	Inactivated in Organic Material	Inactivated by Hard Water	Stability in Solution
Cationic detergents	±	±	−	−	−	−	+	−	+
Phenolics	+ +	+	+	−	?	+	−	−	+
Quaternary NH₄ compounds	+ +	±	±	−	?	−	+ +	−	+
Chlorine compounds	+ +	+	+	±	+	−	+ +	−	±
Chlorhexidine (Nolvasan)	±	+ +	−	−	?	+	+	−	+
Iodophors (tamed iodine)	+ +	+	+	±	?	+	±	−	+
Lye (NaOH)	+	+ +	+	+	+	±	−	±	+
Quicklime	+	+	+	±	±	±	+	−	−
Formalin	+	+	+	+	?	±	+	−	+

*Reprinted with permission from Fowler: *Zoo and Wild Animal Medicine.* Philadelphia: W. B. Saunders, 1978.

QUATERNARY AMMONIUM COMPOUNDS (QUATS)

This is a large class of disinfectants. These compounds are commonly used for a variety of sanitizing purposes. Household quat concentrates are quite dilute. Industrial quats may be highly concentrated and present a significant risk if the user is unaware of the difference between the two. The toxicity of one quat cannot be compared with that of another. A change in formulation may change the toxicity.

Quats are corrosive irritants to epithelial surfaces. Clinical signs and lesions are similar whether the exposure is dermal or by ingestion. In turkey poults, signs include reluctance to drink, cries of discontent, restlessness, persistent swallowing, continual spitting, foamy ocular discharge, head shaking, scratching of eyes and mouth with toe, incessant coughing and chirping, ataxia, convulsions, and death. High concentrations cause respiratory paralysis. Lesions include diphtheritic caseous ulcers at the base of the tongue, diphtheritic membranes in the mouth, thickened mucosa of upper GI tract (pseudomembrane), and erosion at the proventricular orifice.

CHLORINE

Chlorine is effective against a broad range of microorganisms, primarily the vegetative forms of bacteria, viruses, fungi, and algae. Chlorine does not readily destroy spores. Many available forms meet a variety of needs. Chlorine is a deodorizer. It is not affected by water hardness, and it is inexpensive. Colored fabrics may be bleached and the fabric may deteriorate if too high a concentration is used. It is inactivated by organic matter and the presence of ammonia or ammonia compounds and decomposes in the presence of light.

The signs of chlorine intoxication include local skin burns and bleaching of the skin. Chlorine is corrosive in high concentrations. Common lesions include conjunctivitis and keratitis if it is splashed on the animal. If ingested, stomatitis and various degrees of gastroenteritis are produced. Severe burning may result in strictures of the esophagus. Birds that walk in chlorine solutions may suffer footpad burns. Snakes will suffer burns of the ventral scales.

To treat, wash the chlorine from the damaged surface, although it is likely that by the time signs or lesions are noted the chlorine will have dissipated. Nonetheless, the affected area should be cleaned thoroughly and protective ointments or lotions applied. The feet of birds may require bandaging.

CHLORHEXIDINE (NOLVASAN-S*)

Chlorhexidine is an excellent virucide but is less effective against bacteria, especially gram positive bacteria and *Pseudomonas* sp. If used properly, no toxic hazard to birds or reptiles is known. Even concentrated solutions cause only mild irritation to conjunctiva or oral mucosa.

IODINE

Although inorganic iodine solutions have been used traditionally as antiseptics in medicine, it is only since the advent of organic iodine (iodophors) that iodine has become a practical, effective disinfectant. An iodophor is a combination of iodine and a solubilizing agent or carrier, which allows slow release of free iodine when diluted with water.

Iodophor soaps are safe to use as surgical scrubs for birds and reptiles. Dilute solutions (one part iodophor to four parts water) are the most effective and least toxic of solutions used to irrigate wounds and incised abscesses.

Iodophors are effective in both hard and soft water and in a wide pH range. They are noncorrosive, stable in solution, effective in both cold and warm water, and have broad bacteriocidal and fungicidal actions. Disadvantages include expense and initial staining (which washes out).

INSECTICIDES

Numerous insecticide formulations are used on domestic animals. Many have been applied to birds and reptiles, sometimes with disastrous results. There are two major concerns: the toxicity of the insecticide itself, and, perhaps even more importantly, the effect on the bird or reptile of the inert ingredients of the vehicle. No experimental trials have been carried out to determine safe inert carriers.

There are three types of formulations in common use: dusting powders, aerosols, and solutions or suspensions used in dips or sprays.

DUSTING POWDERS

In general, a dusting powder is the best insecticide formulation for use on birds, since a powder is more apt to penetrate the feathers and reach the skin, particularly if manual fluffing of the feathers accompanies application. Sprays and aerosols are

---

*Fort Dodge Laboratories, Fort Dodge, IA.

likely to stay on the surface of the feathers unless the bird is literally soaked with the solution.

It is difficult to ascertain the composition of the inert ingredients in dusting powders. The manufacturer is not legally required to disclose this information, yet such information may be of vital importance to the veterinarian applying the powder to a bird or reptile.

Numerous compounds have been used as the vehicle for active ingredients (boric acid powder, barium sulfate, magnesium stearate, zinc stearate, calcium carbonate, chalk, talc, and cornstarch). The compounds most likely to be used in preparations on animals are talcs, cornstarch, and chalk ($CaCO_3$) (Hoover, 1975).

Probably none of these substances would have deleterious effects on the skin or gastrointestinal epithelium if ingested, although inhalation of the dust may be of some concern. Dusts applied to the feathers of birds may be inhaled during vigorous preening. Carbaryl and malathion dusts are used as inhalation therapy against the respiratory mite *Sternostoma tracheocolum* in canaries and budgerigars.

Medical grade talc (magnesium silicate) may be highly purified. It is quite inert in this form. However, commercial grades may be contaminated with Temolete, one of the asbestos fibers. Asbestos fibers are known to produce pulmonary interstitial fibrosis and calcification and fibrosis of the pleura in humans (Menzel and McClellan, 1980).

Cornstarch has not been reported to cause pulmonary fibrosis but has caused granulomatosis and peritonitis in humans when used on surgical gloves and must be considered an irritant.

SPRAYS

Most insecticides are not water soluble. Thus, in sprays and aerosols the insecticide is dissolved in petroleum distillate plus an emulsifying agent. Petroleum distillate refers to any one of the many fractions (petroleum ether to lubricating oils) obtained from the distillation of crude oil. The more volatile fractions include petroleum ether (benzin, benzine, petroleum benzin) and the closely related petroleum naphtha.

The more likely components of insecticide formulations include kerosene and the more highly purified kerosene, Deobase.

All petroleum distillate fractions are capable of producing skin irritation and, more rarely, photosensitization in humans. Dermal toxicity in birds and reptiles is unknown, but caution should be used in applying these substances to the delicate skin of birds. Ingestion of these compounds is not a major concern, but inhalation is dangerous. Whereas the active ingredient may be minimally toxic, the solvent used may be highly inflammatory to the mucosa of the respiratory tract.

Clinical signs of toxicity may include central nervous system depression and pneumonitis, if aspirated. The high volatile substances may replace oxygen in the lung and may cause anoxic cardiac arrest and/or brain damage.

AEROSOLS

Aerosols are a standard form of topical drug application. The active ingredient (insecticide) plus petroleum distillates and a propellant are sealed in a can (Hoover, 1975; Menzel and McClellan, 1980).

There are a number of fluorinated, chlorinated hydrocarbons that are used as propellants in aerosol preparations. These are marketed under trade names such as Freon, Genetron, Rabon, and Isotron. Freon 12 is the most common propellant used in insect bombs and is usually considered nontoxic; however, high vapor pressure may cause lung irritation, confusion, tremors, and coma in humans. Nothing is known of its effects on birds or reptiles.

Unfortunately, aerosols have been abused by thrill-seeking individuals. The propellant is separated from the active ingredient by tipping the can upside down and releasing the gas into a plastic bag or balloon. Rapid death has occurred from such abuse, probably caused by laryngeal spasm or edema, oxygen displacement, or sensitization of the myocardium to catecholamines. Ventricular fibrillation may ensue.

Another hazard to be reckoned with is the disposal of aerosol cans; heating the can may release highly toxic gases such as chlorine, hydrochloric acid, fluorine, hydrofluoric acid, and phosgene.

SPECIFIC INSECTICIDES

Table 2 lists insecticides recommended for use in and around poultry. These recommendations may be used as a starting point for cage bird formulations, but direct extrapolation is not wise without some testing.

ORGANIC PHOSPHATES

The organic phosphate malathion (Cythion*) and the carbamate carbaryl (Sevin†) are the most commonly used insecticides for cage birds. They are safe when used as directed (Frye, 1981; Feldman and Kruchkenberg, 1975; Marcus, 1981).

---

*American Cyanamid, Princeton, NJ.

†Union Carbide, Nutley, NJ.

Table 2. *Insecticides Recommended for Application In and Around Poultry**

Insecticide	Concentration (%)	Form
Coumaphos (Co-ral, Chemagro, Kansas City, MO)	0.25	Spray
	0.5	Dust
Malathion (Cythion, American Cyanamid, Princeton, NJ)	1.0	Spray
	4.0	Dust
Carbaryl (Sevin, Union Carbide, Nutley, NJ)	0.5	Spray
	5.0	Dust
Stirofos (Rabon, Shell Chemical Co., Atlanta, GA)	0.5	Spray
	1.0†	Spray
Malathion†	3.0	Paint
Nicotine SO₄†	40.0	Paint

*Data from Capizzi et al.: *Pacific Northwest Insect Control Handbook.* Corvallis, OR: OSU Bookstore, 1981.

†Insecticides found in roost paints.

Dichlorvos (DDVP, Vapona*) is a commonly used organic phosphate that is the active ingredient in no-pest strips and cat and dog flea collars.

The client often asks, "Is it safe to put a no-pest strip in a room with a bird in it?" The answer is a qualified "yes." One must ascertain the size of the room and the bird and the general air circulation. Newly opened no-pest strips are quite pungent, and more insecticide is volatilized. Large birds may chew and swallow segments of a no-pest strip if they can reach them.

Mass casualties of canaries (*Serinus canarius*) and zebra finches (*Taeniopygia guttata*) occurred in a closed room aviary in which DDVP-impregnated no-pest strips were used (Leuthgen and Lucas, 1971). Experimental work showed that canaries were more susceptible than budgerigars (*Melopsittacus undulatus*) or weaver birds (*Textor albirostus*). It was also shown that a higher room temperature caused more risk of toxicity.

No-pest strips are used routinely in some reptile collections (Frye, 1981). A small 2- to 5-cm square of the plastic strip is suspended above the cage or laid on a wire screen on the cage (Frye, 1981). Some collection managers are vehemently opposed to their use and cite numerous suspected cases in which snakes and lizards may have died from the effects of DDVP.

Some species are apparently more suspectible than others. Alternatively, size may be a factor. In one instance, anole lizards (*Anolis carolinensis*) were thought to be paralyzed by fumes from a 3-inch strip of a flea collar. Signs abated with removal of the strip (Marcus, 1981).

Pet bird and snake owners may purchase insecticide preparations from pet shops. Of six products randomly taken from a shelf in a pet store, three contained pyrethrins, one rotenone, one paradichlo-robenzene, and the other a mixture of thymol, betanaphthol, naphthalene, and petroleum hydrocarbons.

PYRETHRINS

Pyrethrins are a class of natural insecticides produced by the composite plant Pyrethrum (*Chrysanthemum cinerariaefolium*) (Casida, 1973).

Pyrethrins are usually combined with chemical synergists, such as piperonyl butoxide, to enhance insecticidal activity. Pyrethrins are characterized by rapid knockdown and lethal action on a wide range of insects and nonvertebrate species. There are no residual effects, and the insecticide must contact the parasite. Pyrethrins have negligible toxicity in warm-blooded vertebrates (mammals and birds).

Laboratory studies in birds have shown that mallard ducks (*Anas platyrhynchos*) and coturnix quails (*Coturnix coturnix*) survived oral doses of 10,000 mg/kg pyrethrins.

Studies in reptiles are lacking, but minimal effects would be expected. Contrary to scare statements promulgated by pet store personnel, this author has not found any reports of poisoning in reptiles by pyrethrins.

ROTENONE

Rotenone is an insecticidal chemical obtained from the leguminous plant *Derris eliptica.* Other names include derris powder and cube root. A 0.75 per cent powder is sold in pet stores to control lice.

Rotenone has minimal toxicity for mammals. Fish are highly susceptible. Rotenone has been used as a fish kill agent to rid streams and ponds of unwanted fish. Little is known about the effects of rotenone on reptiles and birds.

Rotenone-containing products are used to treat *Knemidokoptes* (scaly face mite) infestations in birds. Although dermal application is safe, ingestion from too liberal an application may be a hazard.

Older acaricides are still in use and are recommended by veterinarians with stocks on hand. A 10.12 per cent rotenone solution (Canex†) in an oil base is effective. The oil aids in suffocating the mites and penetrating the burrows. Too liberal an application can be hazardous. It would be best to hospitalize the bird and apply this daily for five days.

A common lay preparation for use against *knemidokoptes* mites contains thymol 0.55 per cent, betanaphthol 0.45 per cent, and petroleum hydrocarbon 32.0 per cent (Scalex‡). Thymol is a coal tar phenolic disinfectant that is rarely used. B-naphthol

---

*Shell Chemical Co., Atlanta, GA.

†Pitman-Moore, Washington Crossing, NJ.

‡Arlix Co., Los Angeles, CA.

is an antiseptic anthelmintic, and naphthalene is an ingredient of moth balls. Some aviculturists swear by this product. It is probably safe, but there are more effective products.

OTHER ACARICIDES

Benzyl benzoate and benzene hexachloride (BHC) (Mulzyl)* are both effective insecticides. BHC is a chlorinated hydrocarbon. Again, this product should be applied sparingly and only in a hospital situation.

PARADICHLOROBENZENE

This chemical is the active ingredient of "bird protectors" that are hung on or near a bird cage. This agent has been used as an insect repellant and is one ingredient of clothing moth fumigants. The effect is probably negligible. Toxic hazard is minimal; even consumption by a large psittacine would not be likely to lead to poisoning. Vapors have caused irritation to the skin, throat, and eyes in humans.

NICOTINE

An aqueous solution containing 40 per cent alkaloidal nicotine sulfate (Black Leaf 40†) is available commercially as an insecticide. Older clients who have experience with poultry may remember the use of this insecticide for the control of the red mite, *Dermanyssus gallinae*. It was used as a paint on roosts and is quite effective. It can also be used as a spray.

The problem is that small birds are more likely

---

*Pitman-Moore, Washington Crossing, NJ.
†Black Leaf Products, Elgin, IL.

to be poisoned by nicotine than larger species. Another source of nicotine poisoning in cage birds is the ingestion of tobacco. If cigarettes and cigar butts are accessible, some birds will ingest lethal quantities. Nicotine should not be recommended for use in any aviary or terrarium.

Nicotine is first a stimulant and then a depressant to all autonomic ganglia and the central nervous system. The signs exhibited vary with the stage at which the animal is seen. In the bird one may see excitement and rapid breathing, or depression, incoordination, slow respiration, and paralysis. Death may occur within minutes after signs appear. There is no satisfactory treatment.

REFERENCES AND SUPPLEMENTAL READING

Bahl, A. K., and Pomeroy, B. S.: Acute toxicity in poults associated with carbaryl insecticide. Avian Dis. 22:526, 1978.
Capizzi, J., Fisher, G., Homan, H., Baird, C., Retan, A., and Antonelli, A.: *Pacific Northwest Insect Control Handbook*. Corvallis, OR: OSU Bookstore, 1981, pp. 238–240.
Casida, J. E. (ed.): *Pyrethrum—The Natural Insecticide*. New York: Academic Press, 1973.
Dorrestein, G. M., and Zelle, R.: [Pentachorophenol poisoning in nestling canaries.] Pentachorophenol intoxicatie bij nestjongen van kanaries (*Serinus canarius*). Tijdschr. Diergeneeskd. 104:268, 1979.
Feldman, B. F., and Kruchkenberg, S. A.: Clinical toxicities of domestic and wild cage birds. Vet. Clin. North Am. 5:653, 1975.
Fowler, M. E.: Sanitation and disinfection. *In* Fowler, M. E. (ed.): *Zoo and Wild Animal Medicine*. Philadelphia: W. B. Saunders, 1978, pp. 21–30.
Frye, F. L.: *Biomedical and Surgical Aspects of Captive Reptile Husbandry*. Edwardsville, KS: Veterinary Medicine Publishing, 1981.
Hoover, J. E. (ed.): *Remington's Pharmaceutical Sciences*, 6th ed. Easton, PA: Mack Publishing Co., 1975, pp. 712, 1267, 1644–1664.
Leuthgen, W., and Lucas, H.: [Poisoning of cage birds by DDVP used for the treatment of ectoparasites.] Vergiftungen von Ziervoegln durch DDVP bei der Ektoparasiten—und Schaedlings—bekaempfung. Verhandlungsbericht des. 13th Int. Symposiums ueber die Erkraukungen der Zootier, Berlin, Akademie, 1971, pp. 191–194.
Marcus, L. C.: *Veterinary Biology and Medicine of Captive Amphibians and Reptiles*. Philadelphia: Lea & Febiger, 1981, pp. 62, 196–198.
Menzel, D. B., and McClellan, R. O.: Toxic responses of the respiratory system. *In* Doull, J., Klaassen, C. D., and Amdur, M. O. (eds.): *Toxicology*, 2nd ed. New York: Macmillan, 1980, pp. 246–274.
Small, J. D.: *Disinfectants, Their Chemistry, Use and Evaluation*. Publication 74–5. Joliet, IL: American Association for Laboratory Animal Science, 1974.

ASPERGILLOSIS

PATRICK T. REDIG, D.V.M.

St. Paul, Minnesota

The diagnosis and treatment of aspergillosis in avian species remains one of the most difficult and frequently encountered problems of the avian practitioner. In working with wild raptors, it is the most frequently encountered nontraumatically induced

medical problem. The onset of the disease is insidious and generally progresses to an advanced state before overt clinical signs are exhibited by the bird. Indeed, unless a bird is subjected to regular exercise, such as that which a hunting falcon receives, the early stages of respiratory system involvement may pass unnoticed. Little experimental work dealing with definitive ante-mortem diagnostic techniques or therapeutic regimens has been reported in the literature. The approach to diagnosis and therapy presented herein is based on experience derived from encounters with this disease in birds of prey, domestic turkeys, a variety of waterfowl, and a few psittacines. The literature on pathogenesis, diagnosis, and treatment in a variety of avian and mammalian species may be reviewed by consulting references in the supplemental reading list.

PATHOGENESIS

Both acute and chronic forms of aspergillosis are encountered. Since the pathogenesis for each form is different, recognition of the particular syndrome is important for determining the proper treatment approach, the likelihood of success, and advice to the owner as to the cause and means of prevention. The acute form occurs as the result of the inhalation of an overwhelming number of spores by an otherwise healthy bird. Clinical signs are variable and rapid in onset. They include sudden loss of appetite, polydypsia, polyuria, polypnea, and dyspnea, in that order. The course usually runs less than one week and culminates in death. Treatment is ineffective.

The definitive diagnosis is made post mortem, at which time one finds the lungs studded with thousands of miliary granulomas. An owner should be advised that the bird had received an overwhelming exposure to a point source of spores. Prevention of future exposure to other birds can be accomplished by maintaining a clean environment. Several cases of this form of aspergillosis have been encountered in trained raptors; the birds probably encountered spores stirred up in grass and leaf litter while struggling with their quarry.

The chronic form of aspergillosis is the classic form. It appears that stress-induced immunosuppression renders a host susceptible to "background" numbers of *Aspergillus fumigatus* organisms. The posterior thoracic and abdominal air sacs are the usual sites of primary colonization. A second important site of primary colonization is the bifurcation of the trachea. After four days of unfettered growth at either of these sites, the colony sporulates and spores may be spread throughout the respiratory system. The extent of colonization at this point depends on the status of the intrapulmonary defense mechanisms, which may have changed since the first exposure. As more spores are infused into the system, a struggle ensues between the spores attempting to germinate and the macrophages attempting to contain and destroy them. The rapidity of progression and the severity of the disease depend on the balance of this interplay. The ultimate

respiratory distress that is seen terminally is associated with inflammation of the air sacs and blockage of airways within the lungs. Systemic effects, caused perhaps by elaboration of toxins from the colonizing organisms, may be seen much earlier and include slight depression, vomiting, polydypsia, and polyuria. These toxins may also contribute to persistent immunosuppression.

When the trachea or syrinx is a site of colonization, there is a progressive change and, ultimately, a loss of voice. If the lungs and air sacs are well defended, the disease may not progress beyond a lesion in the trachea. As the lesion grows and occludes a bronchus, severe dyspnea develops. This form is not usually accompanied by other systemic effects.

DIAGNOSIS

The goals of diagnosis are to differentiate aspergillosis from other causes of chronic respiratory diseases and, more importantly, to localize the site of the lesions within the respiratory system. For these purposes, a hematologic screen, tracheal culture, endoscopic examination of the trachea, and exploratory surgery provide the most effective tools. Hematologically, one finds an elevated total white count, neutrophilia, and lymphopenia. Cultures taken from deep within the trachea by means of a small nasopharyngeal swab will often yield an abundance of *A. fumigatus* growth on a Sabouraud's dextrose agar culture plate. The probability of recovering this organism from the trachea of an afflicted bird is much greater than background contaminant recovery rates and hence may be regarded as a useful diagnostic tool. Examination of the trachea with an arthroscope can be easily accomplished under general anesthesia (ketamine 8 mg/kg and Xylazine 2 mg/kg). In many birds examination can be extended past the tracheal bifurcation into the bronchi. When an arthroscope is unavailable or when the neck of the bird is too long, examination has been accomplished by direct incision of the trachea just above the bifurcation.

Exploratory abdominal surgery (celiotomy) via a ventral midline incision extending from the sternum to the pubic bones has been well tolerated by various hawks, eagles, ducks, and parrots and provides a direct means for assessing the severity of the disease and allows initial treatment by direct removal of caseous lesions from the air sacs. Whether incised air sacs repair themselves is not yet properly evaluated; however, no long-term negative effects have been noted in birds subjected to this procedure including several trained falcons, which were subsequently returned to the field for hunting. The celiotomy offers a good opportunity to rule out other problems and permits ready access to visceral organs for biopsy purposes. Other procedures such as radiology have been much less effective in establishing a definitive diagnosis.

THERAPY

The goals of therapy are to (1) locate and remove the primary site of infection, (2) inhibit the growth of invasive mycelia, and (3) enhance immune function of the host. Lesions located in the trachea and bronchi have been removed by direct surgical intervention through a longitudinal cut in the trachea just above the bifurcation. The success of this procedure varies with the extent of damage done to the wall of the trachea. When there is extensive involvement of the syringeal membranes such that removal of the lesion would leave a defect, one might remove that part of the lesion obstructing the lumen and lightly cauterize what is left to kill the organisms. The latter has not been attempted. Lesions encountered in the air sacs can be removed most easily with an appropriately sized curette or other instrument as indicated by their size, location, and consistency. Air sacs filled with liquid exudate should be emptied via aspiration. Following removal of the lesions, the body cavity can be flushed with 20 cc of sterile water containing 5 mg of amphotericin B,* which is then taken up by gentle aspiration or swabbing with gauze sponges. The abdominal incision can be closed by a row of 3-0 gut continuous sutures in the muscular layer followed by a similar row in the skin.

Postoperative medical care is directed toward the second and third treatment objectives. The duration of treatment is determined largely by the response of the host. The following protocol is recommended:

1. Amphotericin B intravenously at 1.5 mg/kg three times a day.

2. Amphotericin B intratracheally (transglottis) at 1 mg/kg two times a day (in practice, amphotericin B is diluted to a volume of 2 to 3 cc with sterile water to enhance distribution).

3. 5-Fluorocytosine† orally at 100 to 120 mg/kg three or four times a day.

4. Rifampicin‡ orally at 30 mg/kg two to three times a day.

All of those procedures have been undertaken simultaneously. Although the amphotericin B doses are very high when compared with those given to mammals, pharmacodynamic determinations of this drug in birds have revealed a T½ of about three hours and no evidence of nephrotoxicity. One occasionally

encounters transitory ataxia immediately following the intravenous injection of amphotericin B. Lastly, immunostimulation is attempted by the intramuscular administration of levamisole§ at 2 mg/kg at four- to six-day intervals. That such immunoenhancement actually plays an effective role in the treatment has yet to be clinically or experimentally established.

Supportive care in the form of force feeding, nutritive supplementation, and fluid therapy is provided depending on the needs and condition of the patient. Obviously the treatment protocol itself is rigorous and one must weigh the stress of additional handling against the benefits to be gained. When a patient has abundant fat reserves, one need simply supply fluids subcutaneously for the first few days of treatment. The course of treatment may run four to six weeks, with frequency of manipulation tapering off toward the end. Patients undergoing treatment should be kept hospitalized.

Prevention of the disease involves the usual sanitation procedures and reduction of stress, which is felt to render the bird susceptible. However, one must emphasize the subtle nature of stresses that have been noted to accompany the development of the disease. Among trained raptors, long-distance transportation to field meets in personal vehicles under nearly ideal conditions, changes in ownership or housing conditions, and forced inactivity during adolescence have been followed by the development of aspergillosis. Eider ducks imported as unhatched eggs and reared under good housing and feeding conditions have developed an undefined maladaptation syndrome (although outwardly appearing contented) that has been accompanied by aspergillosis. Certain species are more likely to contract aspergillosis, and certain individuals of even so-called more resistant species have temperaments that seem to render them more easily stressed than other members of their species. For those individuals and those species subjected to management alterations that are likely to be stressful, the oral administration of 5-fluorocytosine at 100 mg/kg b.i.d. is recommended during the period of adaptation, usually 10 to 14 days.

SUPPLEMENTAL READING

Redig, P. T.: The diagnosis and treatment of aspergillosis in birds. Ph.D. Thesis, Department of Veterinary Biology, College of Veterinary Medicine, St. Paul, MN, 1980.

Redig, P. T.: Aspergillosis in raptors. *In* Cooper, J. E. (ed.): *Recent Advances in the Study of Raptor Diseases.* Keighly, West Yorkshire: Chiron Publications Ltd., 1981.

---

*Fungizone, E. R. Squibb & Sons, Inc., Princeton, NJ.

†Ancobon, Roche Laboratories, Nutley, NJ.

‡Rifadin, Dow Chemical, Indianapolis, IN.

§Levasole, Pitman-Moore, Inc., Washington Crossing, NJ.

BUMBLEFOOT IN RAPTORS

BARBARA ANN SAWYER, D.V.M.*

Merced, California

Bumblefoot, or pododermatitis, is seen primarily in large cage birds, waterfowl, and penguins. It is an entity of clinical importance in captive raptors. This debilitating disease can range from small bruises on the footpads to corns to extensive proliferative lesions involving the joints and bones of the foot. It is more common in falcons than in hawks and is seldom seen in owls.

ETIOLOGY

Staphylococcus aureus is the bacteria isolated in pure culture from 80 to 90 per cent of the cases, although other organisms such as *Pseudomonas*, *Proteus*, *Streptococcus*, and coliforms can be grown in mixed or pure culture (Halliwell, 1979). However, the disease is more than just a bacterial infection; a number of other factors contribute to the development of the lesions. If the disease has been chronic, there may be mycotic involvement with *Candida albicans* or *Aspergillus* as well (Halliwell, 1978).

PATHOGENESIS

The pathogenesis of the disease involves chronic trauma or constant pressure to the foot coupled with secondary bacterial infection. Normally the raptor foot is protected by stratified squamous epithelium covered with keratin. There are papillae on the plantar surface to aid in grasping prey. Constant pressure on the epithelium leads to thinning of the stratified layers, weakening this protective barrier. Once the initial break in the epithelium has been established and the bacteria have entered, cellulitis is seen. Often a fibrous connective tissue capsule will encapsulate the abscess. This may rupture, allowing infection to spread to tendon sheaths and ligaments. If the bacteria reach the synovial sheaths, pyogenic arthritis, osteomyelitis, and septicemia can result.

Wounds on the feet of birds are not as resistant to infection as wounds elsewhere on the body, owing in part to the lower body temperature and/or the relatively poor blood supply of the foot

(Cooper, 1978). The foot is more apt to be contaminated with feces and dirt than any other part of the body. Although *Staphylococcus* is uncommon in raptor feces, it is found on the epithelial surfaces of the feet and body.

It is felt that the development of the bird's immune system may dictate the progression of the lesions (Halliwell, 1979). If the immune system is functional, the infection can be eliminated by the body at the initial stage. A bird whose immune system is not as complete may "wall off" the bacterial invasion by encapsulation, but with repeated or continued trauma breaks in the connective tissue capsule will appear, allowing the bacteria to spread into the tissues. As the infection spreads around the tendons, ligaments, and nerves, the capsule spreads as well in an attempt to contain the problem.

PREDISPOSING FACTORS

There are many predisposing factors to bumblefoot. Overweight birds that are not active (as is seen more in captive birds that are perched than in wild or free-flying raptors) are more prone to trauma of the epithelium because of the constant pressure on the footpads. Heavy-bodied birds with small weight-bearing surfaces such as the gyrfalcon or peregrine falcon have similar problems.

Vitamin A is vital for epithelial development and integrity. Diets deficient in vitamin A can lead to epithelial damage and corn development. Normally, epidermal layers are replaced regularly, similar to feathers through a molt. This does not occur with vitamin A deficiency. Birds can store vitamin A for several months, so this deficiency does not appear immediately but is seen in birds in prolonged captivity without proper nutrition.

Unsanitary cage conditions, resulting in fecal contamination of perches, will allow coliforms and other bacteria to secondarily infect the original foot lesions.

Talons that are too long can puncture or irritate the pad while the bird is perching, especially on perches of inadequate diameter, contributing to self-inflicted trauma. Any trauma or injury to the foot can allow bacteria to enter, although foreign objects in the foot are not a common cause of trauma. Poor perch design or utilization will also predispose the foot to epithelial damage.

---

*It is with great sadness that we report the death of Dr. Sawyer in the fall of 1982.

CLINICAL SIGNS

Clinical signs of the disease vary according to the stage of infection. A swollen metatarsal pad with or without a small ulcerative lesion (corn) is seen early. This may spread to involve an entire digit as well. The bird may favor one leg, and the foot may be swollen, warm, and painful on palpation. There may be scabs on the plantar surface with purulent or, more often, caseous exudate beneath. More severe lesions can inhibit weight bearing and can cause gross deformity of the foot. Radiographs are helpful to assess the extent of the damage and aid in evaluation of potential osteomyelitis.

DIAGNOSIS

The diagnosis is based on clinical signs and culture of the exudate. The lesions of bumblefoot are fairly distinctive. Avian pox can affect the epithelial surfaces of the foot but can be distinguished from bumblefoot by the proliferative and noninvasive nature of the pox lesions. Pox is not limited to the foot and often has concomitant oral or facial lesions. Pox lesions may, however, become secondarily infected with *Staphylococcus*.

TREATMENT

Treatment of bumblefoot must be prompt and vigorous to ensure the best results. Treatment of chronic lesions can be very discouraging. Depending on the stage of the lesions, therapy will vary in intensity and duration. Early treatment with appropriate antibiotics is important, as chemotherapy is less successful once encapsulation has started, and this can occur as early as three to five days after initial tissue damage (Cooper, 1978). The foot should be scrubbed with soap and water, rinsed with betadine, and dried. A small (23- to 25-gauge) needle is inserted to aspirate the exudate. Culture and sensitivity testing should be done on each case. Parenteral as well as topical antibiotics are most efficacious when combined with padded dressings on the foot.

Depending on the sensitivity testing, a number of antibiotics can be used, including gentamicin (4 mg/kg b.i.d. IM), chloramphenicol (4 to 50 mg/kg t.i.d. PO or 6 to 10 mg/kg b.i.d. IM), and ampicillin (25 to 50 mg/kg t.i.d. PO or 6 to 10 mg/kg b.i.d. IM) (Halliwell, 1978). Antibiotics are often combined with topical steroid and dimethyl sulfoxide (DMSO) therapy. A combination of DMSO (240 ml), dexamethasone (4 mg), and appropriate antibiotics can be applied topically for two to three weeks (Redig, 1979). It is important to wash the foot well each time before applying the mixture so that the lesion is not contaminated. An enzyme preparation such as Granulex* is also effective as a topical agent to remove necrotic debris. The foot should be soaked daily in betadine if the lesions are early and mild. The foot should be padded with cotton and gauze and kept wrapped, with the dressing changed daily. With any treatment, swelling should decrease within five days. If there is no response, therapy needs to be re-evaluated.

Supplemental vitamin A is also given in the form of a whole-animal diet, raw liver, egg yolk, day-old chicks, or cod liver oil, as raptors need preformed vitamin A, which is not present in an all-meat diet.

Radiation and cryotherapy may be considered as adjuncts to medical treatment.

Because of the relationship of the immune system to the progression of the lesions, immunotherapy has been tried in conjunction with vaccination against the *Staphylococcus* organism. Autogenous vaccines have been found to be of more benefit than commercial vaccines. The toxins of *Staphylococcus* are necrotoxins and are responsible for most of the tissue damage.

Encouraging success with a combination of an antibiotic, an immunomodulator, and a *Staphylococcus* vaccination has recently been reported from the Boston zoo. Minocycline, a tetracycline that is actively transported into the *Staphylococcus* organism, was used in those birds that were sensitive to tetracycline at a dosage of 5 mg/kg b.i.d. orally (sprinkled on food). Levamisole (Levasole†), 3 mg/kg every fifth day for five treatments orally or subcutaneously, was used to optimize the cell-mediated immune response. *Staphylococcus* toxoid was given intramuscularly one day following the levamisole treatment, using doses for humans suggested by the manufacturer (Satterfield and O'Rourke, 1981). This combination has shown encouraging clinical efficacy in early cases, but more work needs to be done to complete its evaluation.

In conjunction with medical treatment, perches need to be well padded. When encapsulation has occurred, systemic antibiotics are ineffective owing to impaired circulation and irreversible tissue damage. The prognosis is guarded in these cases. Surgery is a last resort because of the extensive involvement of the foot and the poor healing of the epithelium. If the lesion is localized and osteomyelitis has not spread, amputation of a digit may be helpful as long as the back toe is not removed. The raptor cannot perch or hunt well without the rear toe.

For surgery the bird is anesthetized (the author prefers ketamine at a dosage of 15 to 25 mg/kg IM). Radiographs should be taken prior to surgery to assess bone involvement. Surgery must be done in a sterile environment or more contamination and spread of the infection will result.

---

*Dow B. Hickam Inc., Houston, TX.

†Pitman-Moore, Washington Crossing, NJ.

The lesions are opened, and all infected and necrotic tissue is removed. The enzyme trypsin can be used to facilitate removal of all necrotic tissue (Cooper, 1978). The wound is flushed with an antibiotic solution. The integrity of the ligaments and nerves should be maintained to minimize the damage. Skin should be closed with mattress sutures of nonabsorbable material.

The wound should be wrapped and padded. The administration of oral antibiotics and vitamin A is continued postsurgically. Good nursing care is important to keep the foot clean and the bird in good weight with a minimum of stress.

If the whole foot is involved and osteomyelitis is present, the bird may need to be euthanized. Amputation of the entire foot is not a viable option in most birds, because the remaining foot will develop severe bumblefoot lesions fairly soon, having to constantly support the total weight of the bird. Pioneering work on the use of prosthetic devices for amputated legs has been done on bald eagles at one rehabilitation center (Crawford, 1972), but this is not a practical solution for the majority of cases.

PREVENTION

The best treatment for bumblefoot is prevention. Many of the contributing factors can be eliminated or alleviated.

Birds should be fed diets that are nutritionally sound and balanced for all vitamins, especially A. This means feeding either a whole-animal diet or a balanced preformed food (such as Zupreem*) or using proper supplements to supply at least 1,500 to 2,000 IU of vitamin A weekly.

Whenever possible, stress should be kept to a minimum for captive birds. Environment and the behavior of the bird should be matched to minimize potential problems; e.g., nervous birds, such as accipiters and white-tailed kites, should not be kept in open mews.

Minimize trauma to the feet by having perches

---

*Hills Division, Riviana Foods, Inc., Topeka, KS.

of uneven thickness and varying surfaces. Free-flying aviaries are best because the birds can move at will and can select a variety of perching surfaces. Perches should be of adequate diameter for the size of the bird; too small a perch may allow the back talon to damage the metatarsal pad. If necessary, the back talon may be clipped with a nail trimmer. Smooth dowels are not advisable as perches, as the foot needs some abrasiveness to stimulate normal sloughing of epithelium, which in turn helps maintain epithelial integrity. Natural wood perches have worked best in our flight cage.

If a bird must be tethered, a ring perch is better for the feet than a block perch, especially for falcons. Fecal contamination on a block perch can aggravate existing problems. Sisal rope is often used on the ring perches. The size of the rope varies with the bird (e.g., ½-inch rope for eagles, ⅜-inch for hawks, ¼-inch for kestrels) (Garcelon and Bogue, 1977). Astroturf has been used as well, although there have been a few instances in which it has irritated the feet. Concrete is a poor substrate for feet for prolonged contact, especially for heavier birds. All perches and cages should be kept clean to decrease bacterial build-up and contamination.

Feet of all birds should be checked at least twice a week to find early lesions. Bumblefoot is a complex entity, but with proper management and prompt detection and treatment of early lesions it can be controlled and eliminated.

REFERENCES AND SUPPLEMENTAL READING

Cooper, J. E.: *Veterinary Aspects of Captive Birds of Prey.* Gloucestershire, England: Standfast Press, 1978.

Crawford, W.: Raptor research meeting, Davis, California, 1979.

Garcelon, D., and Bogue, G.: *Raptor Care and Rehabilitation.* Walnut Creek, CA: Wildlife Rehabilitation Council (c/o Alexander Lindsay Jr. Museum), 1977.

Halliwell, W. H.: Raptors (Falconiformes and Strigiformes). *In* Fowler, M. E. (ed.): *Zoo and Wild Animal Medicine.* Philadelphia: W. B. Saunders, 1978, pp. 221–290.

Halliwell, W. H.: Diseases of birds of prey. Vet. Clin. North Am. 9:541, 1979.

Redig, P. T.: Infectious diseases. *In* Cooper, J. E., and Eley, J. T. (eds.): *First Aid and Care of Wild Birds.* Devon, England: David and Charles, 1979.

Satterfield, W. C., and O'Rourke, K. I.: Staphylococcal bumblefoot: vaccination and immunomodulation in the early treatment and management. J. Zoo Anim. Med. 12:95, 1981.

ACUTE HEMORRHAGIC SYNDROME OF BIRDS

CHUCK GALVIN, D.V.M.

Novato, California

Occasionally the veterinarian is presented with an Amazon parrot with a very sudden onset of a severe intravascular hemolytic crisis. Although the etiology has yet to be determined, the onset, course, and response to therapy in 20 such cases that I have treated over a ten-year period are very similar. A definite syndrome appears to exist. This syndrome may occur in other types of birds, but so far I have only seen it in various species of Amazon parrots.

SIGNS AND STAGES OF DISEASE

The first sign of the disease is usually a very sudden onset of watery, red-orange urine, which the bird owner and sometimes the veterinarian incorrectly assume is bloody diarrhea. The hemoglobin mixes with the urate component of the droppings and imparts a color and consistency similar to that of tomato soup rather than a port wine color, as is seen in mammals with hemoglobinuria. In some cases, the sudden onset of clear, colorless, watery urine is the first sign, followed within a few hours to a day by the red-orange urine. The parrot is usually only mildly depressed at this stage but usually becomes more severely depressed over the next 12 hours.

Regurgitation usually becomes a prominent sign simultaneous with the onset of hemoglobinuria. It is possible that the hemolysis itself causes the nausea and regurgitation. As the depression progresses, anorexia usually occurs.

Although 19 out of 20 birds I have personally treated have responded well to therapy, veterinarians have described similar cases in which the patient died two to four days following the onset of signs. It is my feeling that this is not a self-limiting syndrome and that most cases could be expected to progress to the point of death if not treated early, vigorously, and correctly. Based on the extremely rapid rate of hemolysis in some individuals with this syndrome, I feel that death could occur within 24 hours of the onset of signs. Thus, a guarded prognosis should be given to the client initially.

In none of the cases did a detailed history suggest the cause. A gross and microscopic post-mortem examination on the patient that died and post-

mortem examinations on other patients that died from this syndrome described to me by other veterinarians did not reveal the cause. Mild, nonspecific microscopic liver changes were common. Some cases occurred in multiple bird households, and in some cases another bird was in the same cage. The other birds did not develop the syndrome.

DIFFERENTIAL DIAGNOSIS

The idiopathic hemolytic crisis should be differentiated from hematuria and bloody diarrhea caused by such things as urinary and gastrointestinal infections, gastrointestinal parasites, cloacal hemorrhage, and some cases of egg binding with large wet droppings (sometimes with blood). It should also be differentiated from hemorrhagic syndromes due to clotting defects, such as from vitamin K deficiency, warfarin poisoning, platelet deficiency, liver diseases, and some cases of septicemia with suspected disseminated intravascular coagulation. The differentiation is simple in that red blood cells are not found with hemolysis, in contrast to the hemorrhagic syndromes mentioned previously.

Of course, it should also be differentiated from other causes of hemolytic anemia similar to those that might occur in mammals: (1) red blood cell parasites, e.g., *Plasmodium, Haemoproteus,* and avian *Piroplasma* (note: gross hemoglobinuria would be uncommon with red cell parasites of birds); (2) severe bacterial or viral disease, uncommon as a cause of intravascular hemolysis; (3) some poisons, such as lead, copper, and other poisons; (4) drug reactions; and (5) immune-mediated diseases.

It should be noted that the most common disease to mimic the idiopathic hemolytic syndrome is acute lead toxicity. In some practices with a large number of birds, parrots presented with "tomato soup" urine almost always have lead poisoning. I personally have seen more cases of the idiopathic syndrome. Lead poisoning can present in a variety of ways, ranging from only mild depression to violent seizures, behavioral abnormalities, neurologic abnormalities, and sometimes coma. Watery urine and upward tilting of the head are common. Seizures and neurologic abnormalities are not part of the idiopathic syndrome. However, a bird dying from any cause may at times show a central nervous system disturbance, including seizures, just prior to death. It should be noted that some birds with acute lead toxicity will present with signs indistinguishable from those seen with the idiopathic syndrome. In lead toxicity, a severe intravascular hemolytic crisis may be the major sign without any neurologic abnormalities. Neurologic abnormalities, including seizures, may occur later in the course of the disease or may not appear at all.

LABORATORY EVALUATION

The two most important laboratory tests are the hematocrit and the radiograph. The hematocrit tube shows hemolyzed plasma and usually an anemia. The best way to monitor therapy in addition to observing the patient and its droppings is to compare daily hematocrit tubes, looking for levels of anemia and degrees of hemolysis in plasma. After the second day of therapy, the plasma is often less hemolyzed and is sometimes clear of any evidence of hemolysis, but the hematocrit is usually lower than the day before. From this point, if response to therapy occurs, the hematocrit either declines at a slower rate, stabilizes, or starts to climb. One patient with an extremely rapid rate of hemolysis dropped from a hematocrit of 52 to one of 16 within eight hours. The following day, with therapy, the hematocrit dropped to 11. It then stabilized and started to climb the following day. This patient was seen on the first day of the disease. It would have died if the owner had waited until the second day.

The radiograph is helpful in demonstrating the presence of radiopaque substances in the gizzard or other parts of the gastrointestinal tract that may represent lead. One cannot always eliminate the possibility of lead poisoning based on negative radiographic findings, although in most cases of lead poisoning the lead shows up radiographically. For example, one case of lead poisoning occurred when a parrot was given gravel from the bottom of a fish tank as grit. There were lead weights on the bottom of the fish tank, and sufficient lead went into solution to contaminate the gravel given to the bird. This lead did not show up radiographically, of course. Birds that I have seen with the idiopathic syndrome were radiographically normal. I suggest that a severely depressed avian patient not be sedated or anesthetized to be radiographed. Exact positioning is not essential for evaluating the presence or absence of radiodense objects within the digestive tract.

Elevations in white blood cell counts are common but are not present in all cases. Elevations may be presence in SGOT, LDH, and/or uric acid levels. They may be in normal ranges in other cases. As the patient improves, the hematologic and chemical values return to normal.

If lead poisoning remains a possibility but radiographs are inconclusive or negative, a blood-lead determination would be helpful. Some laboratories are equipped to perform blood-lead determinations on a single standard capillary tube of heparinized blood. Normal ranges may vary slightly from lab to lab. A guideline to aid in interpreting results would be the following: (1) under 10 ppm: negative for lead poisoning; (2) 10 to 20 ppm: highly suspect; and (3) over 20 ppm: diagnostic of lead poisoning.

Some birds with chronic lead poisoning with acute exacerbations will have a large percentage of very young-looking red cells. They are less elliptical, with darker-staining cytoplasm and less tightly packed nuclear chromatin than mature red cells. Not all birds show this blood picture, but I have had a number of cases of lead poisoning in which I knew that lead poisoning was a likely possibility as soon as I glanced at the blood picture.

THERAPY

The very first bird with idiopathic hemolytic syndrome that I treated ten years ago with "shotgun therapy" and general supportive care responded favorably and made a complete recovery. My second case responded in a similarly favorable manner to the same treatment program. I have been reluctant to treat subsequent cases in any different manner. Out of 20 cases to date that I have personally treated, only one patient died. That patient was presented on the third day following the onset of signs and was presented in a state of severe depression and was barely able to stand. All others were presented for therapy usually less than 24 hours and none more than 36 hours following the onset of signs noted by the owner.

The treatment program consisted of the following: (1) antibiotics: chloramphenicol (Chloromycetin* 100 mg/ml) at a dosage of 0.00035 ml/gm body weight IM b.i.d.; (2) corticosteroids: dexamethasone 2 per cent solution (Azium injectable 2 per cent† at a dosage of 0.0011 ml/gm body weight given once daily for two days; (3) multiple vitamins: e.g., Injecom 100 plus B Complex‡ at a dose of 0.01 ml/ 100 gm body weight daily for one week, then twice weekly if still hospitalized; (4) fluid therapy to combat fluid loss and shock from regurgitation, watery urine, and rapidly plunging hematocrit: lactated Ringer's solution or half-strength saline and dextrose at a dosage of 0.09 ml/gm body weight divided b.i.d. subcutaneously; (5) a warm environment (85 to 90°F) with minimal stress.

Nineteen out of twenty patients responded to this therapy and were discharged after three to seven

---

*Parke-Davis, Detroit, MI.
†Schering Corp., Kenilworth, NJ.
‡Hoffman-La Roche Inc., Nutley, NJ.

days. Home treatment consisted of Chloromycetin given orally at the same dosage given by injection in the hospital. Multiple vitamins were also given for administration in the drinking water. Home treatment was continued for one week, and the patient was then rechecked. If follow-up examination was favorable, antibiotics were discontinued and vitamins were continued indefinitely.

Of the 19 cases reponding to therapy, I am aware of only one recurrence with episodes of hemolysis months later.

Patients presented with acute intravascular hemolysis due to lead poisoning are treated the same way as those with the idiopathic syndrome. In addition, chelation therapy is given, using CaEDTA (calcium disodium versenate*). An attempt is also made to rid the gastrointestinal tract of lead. If frequent seizures are present, they are controlled with diazepam (Valium†) at a dosage of 0.0005 to 0.001 mg/gm given IM two to three times daily as needed. It should be noted that two birds with acute hemolysis that was not discovered to be lead toxicity until the following day were treated as for the idiopathic syndrome without CaEDTA and were markedly improved and showed no hemolysis in the plasma 12 hours after therapy. Chelation therapy was begun at this time. The dosages and durations of treatment suggested in the literature for CaEDTA are varied. I give an undiluted dosage of 0.11 mg/gm body weight divided twice daily intramuscularly for up to five days. If lead poisoning is a possibility in a specific case, I suggest starting chelation therapy prior to laboratory confirmation. So far, I have not observed signs of renal toxicity. Whether longer therapy would result in toxicity, I do not know.

If lead still remained in the digestive tract after five days but the patient was not showing signs of

hemolysis or central nervous system abnormalities, I would stop the CaEDTA for five days, continue efforts to eliminate lead from the digestive tract, and give another five-day course if lead remains. If small particles of lead are present in the gizzard, these tend to remain, as do pieces of grit. To encourage their passage from the gizzard, I tube feed a mixture of peanut butter and corn oil. This often, but not always, successfully empties the gizzard of lead particles within a few days or sometimes longer. Cathartics can also be given and have been reported to be helpful in moving the lead particles through the digestive tract.

Magnesium sulfate (epsom salts), for example, may be given at a dosage of 0.5 to 1.0 gm/kg to precipitate lead and act as a saline purgative. Asymptomatic patients with lead still in the digestive tract can be treated at home with a 5 per cent solution of magnesium sulfate in the drinking water; it is hoped that the lead will pass out of the digestive tract over a period of days or weeks. Periodic follow-up radiographs will indicate whether the lead has gone. Unusual cases in which large amounts of lead are present and are not expected to pass may require surgical removal from the gizzard. This has been performed successfully but should be considered high risk surgery and should not be undertaken unless absolutely necessary. Surgical removal of pieces of lead from the crop is much less risky and would be indicated before they move further down the digestive tract.

CONCLUSION

It is hoped that in the future we will learn more about the pathogenesis of the idiopathic hemolytic syndrome of birds and will be able to make more scientific statements and suggestions. It is also hoped that the clinical impressions and empirical approaches presented here will help the practitioner recognize and deal with this syndrome.

*Riker Laboratories, Inc., Northridge, CA.
†Hoffman-La Roche Inc., Nutley, NJ.

AVIAN TRICHOMONIASIS

SANDRA EMANUELSON, D.V.M.

Walnut Creek, California

Trichomoniasis is an infectious disease whose primary host is the domestic pigeon (*Columba livia*). It is caused by the protozoa *Trichomonas gallinae* (also known as *T. columbae*). Trichomoniasis is called "canker" in pigeons, chickens, and turkeys and "frounce" in raptors.

T. gallinae is present in an asymptomatic form in approximately 80 to 100 per cent of domestic pigeons. It causes disease in nestlings two to five weeks of age and in weak or debilitated adult birds. The disease occurs in raptors that feed on pigeons either in the wild or in captivity. *T. gallinarum* causes lower digestive tract disease in turkeys and domestic fowl. Infections of *T. gallinae* and/or *T. gallinarum* in chickens and turkeys can occur naturally or from the ingestion of contaminated feed or water. Many strains of *T. gallinae* vary in virulence from non-disease–producing strains to severely virulent strains. There are many nonpathogenic *Trichomonas* organisms.

SYMPTOMS

Affected birds often lose weight through reluctance to feed. Other symptoms that may be seen are diarrhea, a sour crop (atonic crop distended with fluid), gasping while flying, and drooling of a green-yellow fluid. Sick birds may merely have fluffed feathers. Diseased birds are the very young (two to five weeks of age) and those that are stressed by other disease, poor nutrition, unsanitary conditions, racing, or breeding.

Healthy individual birds are frequently carriers and do not exhibit any signs of disease. The incubation time for *T. gallinae* is 4 to 14 days. Young birds may die within one to a few days after developing the disease. Older birds may die after two to three weeks of illness.

TRANSMISSION

The organism does not encyst and can remain alive in tap or distilled water for two to five days at 5 to 10°C. At 21°C it survives for one day. The organism dies immediately in a dry environment.

Adult-to-adult transmission occurs primarily from affected or carrier birds picking up seeds and then dropping them. Susceptible birds feeding in the same area may then ingest the infected seeds. Adult-to-offspring transmission occurs when the organism is transferred in the crop milk given to the young by adult pigeons or doves. One case involving a cockatiel was the result of an owner hand feeding a fledgling dove and cockatiel at the same time. Contaminated feeding apparatus has transmitted the disease among songbirds raised by rehabilitators. Sinusitis symptoms were produced without visible lesions. Yellow caseous lesions described hereafter were found on opening the sinuses.

GROSS LESIONS

Lesions are most frequently found in the oral and pharyngeal areas. They range in size from 1 mm to approximately 1 cm, are yellowish in color, elevated, and can be peeled off the mucosa with little or no bleeding. They are thought to originate from tiny excoriations in the mucous membrane and,

therefore, can occur in aberrant sites such as the tip of the tongue.

Diseases that can be confused with trichomoniasis are avian pox, hypovitaminosis A, avian tuberculosis, bacterial diseases such as salmonellosis, and fungal diseases such as candidiasis. Secondary bacterial infection may be present as well as the primary trichomoniasis. The systemic form exhibits well-defined yellow nodules in the liver. More unusual forms involve the navel or cloaca of nestlings, in whom there are yellow crusty or nodular lesions.

DIAGNOSIS

The organism can be demonstrated microscopically by swabbing the lesion and placing the smear on a warm slide with a small amount of saline. The organism is a flagellated protozoan that is pear shaped to rounded. It measures approximately 6.2 to 18.9 μm $\times$ 2.3 to 8.5 μm. It has four free anterior flagella and a fifth that trails posteriorly. There is an undulating membrane along approximately two-thirds of its length and an axostyle that extends along and beyond the long axis of the body. In some media, various cytoplasmic bodies can be seen. Its characteristic spiral movements differentiate *T. gallinae* from other flagellates that may be commensal organisms unrelated to the lesions.

TREATMENT AND CONTROL IN THE FLOCK

Pigeon breeders can greatly minimize the risk of disease by maintaining a well-fed, minimally stressed flock. Equally important is maintenance of proper sanitary conditions in the loft. This should include a clean, nonporous, dry floor; feeders and waterers that provide ample, good quality food; and provisions for avoiding cross contamination. Routine treatment three to four times a year, especially prior to the breeding season and following the racing season, will keep the number of organisms low.

The safest, most commonly used drug in the flock is Emtryl* (1,2-dimethyl-5-nitro-1H-imidazole). The dosage rate is 50 mg of active ingredient/kg body weight or 1 pouch (36.4 gm)/200 liters water (0.02 per cent) for five days. The drug is available in livestock stores that sell feed to pigeon breeders. Treatment may be inhibited by the lack of patient acceptance of the treated water. Individual treat-

---

*Emtryl (Salsbury Laboratories, Charles City, IA) is difficult to obtain through veterinary suppliers. It is usually available from poultry supply outlets.

Dimetridazole is also known as RP 8595, Emtrymix, and Histostat 50. It is available in 182-gm pouches (36.4 gm active ingredient).

ment is preferred whenever possible. Other drugs used for treatment and control of trichomoniasis are Enheptin* and copper sulfate. Enheptin is given at the rate of one 5-mg capsule per pigeon weighing 350 to 550 gm daily for seven days; or 1 gm/liter of water for six days; or up to 40 mg/kg/day for six days. Medicated water is somewhat unpalatable. Enheptin will kill the organisms in an infected or carrier bird. Copper sulfate has been used in the past at the rate of 100 mg/100 cc water for 20 days. Copper sulfate can, however, cause liver damage. Enheptin is not considered as safe as Emtryl.

TREATMENT AND CONTROL IN THE INDIVIDUAL

There are several facets of the treatment of individual birds. The safest drug currently used is Emtryl,† at the rate of 50 mg active ingredient/kg body weight daily for five days. An easy formula to use in dosing Emtryl is 1 cc of Emtryl powder per 10 cc water. Give 0.5 cc of the solution per 100 gm body weight PO daily for five days. A 250- to 300-gm pigeon would receive 1.5 cc of the solution once daily for five days. A 100- to 120-gm dove would receive approximately 0.50 cc once daily for five days. If a bird has difficulty swallowing, divide the dose into two to three smaller doses or give by gavage.

As with any sick bird, warmth should be provided to a level at which the bird is no longer fluffed. If the bird is not eating it should be force fed. If it has not eaten for two to three days, it should be treated very gently and given 20 to 25 per cent glucose solution at the rate of 0.5 to 1.0 cc/30 gm body weight in small birds and 0.25 to 0.50 cc/30 gm body weight in larger birds (i.e., about 4 to 6 cc per adult pigeon, 2 to 4 cc per adult dove). The glucose feeding should be repeated two to four times a day (when the crop empties) for the first one-half to one and one-half days. Then a mixture of force-feeding formula can be added to the glucose

solution over the next day or so until the bird is receiving straight force-feeding formula two times a day by gavage with either a red rubber catheter‡ or rodent feeding needle.§ Force feeding formulae may vary. One that works well for a variety of species of birds and reptiles consists of the following:

> 1 jar Gerber baby food egg yolks (4 oz)
> 1½ tsp cooking oil
> ¼ cup Sustagen‖ vanilla
> 20 grains (1200 mg) calcium gluconate or calcium lactate
> 1 tsp Superpreen** or other avian vitamin

Grind the calcium to a *very fine* powder and add egg yolk and Sustagen. Mix well. Add enough water so that the mixture will *very* easily pass through a feeding tube. Freeze in 3- to 60-cc syringes to be thawed and used as needed. Mixture will thicken upon freezing.

Even birds that are severely affected with trichomoniasis can survive if handled carefully. Those with organ involvement can survive too, if the disease has not progressed to involve large areas of the liver.

SUPPLEMENTAL READING

Galvin, C.: *Avian Drugs and Dosages.* Walnut Creek, CA: Wildlife Rehabilitation Council (c/o Alexander Lindsay Jr. Museum), 1973.

Hill, J.: Trichomoniasis in cockatiel nestlings. Proceedings of the Western States Pathological Conference, Palo Alto, CA, 1981.

Hofstad, M. S., et al.: *Diseases of Poultry,* 7th ed. Ames, IA: Iowa University State Press, 1978, pp. 841–843.

Honingberg, B. M.: Trichomonads of veterinary importance. In Kreir, J. P.: *Parasitic Protozoa, 2.* New York: Academic Press, 1978, pp. 276–424.

Kocan, R. M., and Herman, C. M.: Trichomoniasis. In Davis, J. W., et al. (eds.): *Infectious and Parasitic Diseases of Wild Birds.* Ames, IA: Iowa University State Press, 1971, pp. 282–289.

Petrak, M. L. (ed.): *Diseases of Cage and Aviary Birds,* 2nd ed. Philadelphia: Lea & Febiger, pp. 538–539.

Schrag, L.: *Healthy Pigeons.* West Germany: Verlag Ludwig Schober, 1978, pp. 99–115.

Theis, J.: Personal communication, 1982.

---

*American Cyanamid, Princeton, NJ.
†Salsbury Laboratories, Charles City, IA.

‡Sovereign red rubber feeding tubes, Sherwood Medical Industries, Inc., St. Louis, MO.
§Rodent feeding tubes, Corners Ltd., Kalamazoo, MI.
‖Sustagen, Meade Johnson Nutritional Division, Evansville, IN.
**Superpreen, RHB Laboratories, Santa Ana, CA.

HYPOVITAMINOSIS A IN PSITTACINES

CLYDE PITTS, D.V.M.

Studio City, California

Fat–soluble vitamin A was first postulated to exist in 1915 and was first produced synthetically in 1939. Since that time extensive research has established requirements for humans and other animal species. Since the body is incapable of producing vitamin A, all higher animals must ingest animal products containing the vitamin or plant-produced carotenes that can be converted to vitamin A. The liver acts as the primary storage depot, and liver excesses compensate for temporary deficiencies.

Many studies have investigated vitamin A's role in growth, health, and disease. Classically, hypovitaminosis A produces lesions of the respiratory, alimentary, and genitourinary tracts and the external ocular tissues. In humans, vitamin A deficiency results in "night blindness" owing to lowered levels of rhodopsin, a phenomenon of lesser significance in lower animals. Research results indicate that certain disease states may markedly increase minimum body requirements of this vitamin.

A review of the current literature reveals many references of a general nature to hypovitaminosis A in caged birds. Detailed studies have been confined to the human species, domestic and research species, and domestic fowl. Little work has been done with exotics. In fact, I found no reports of a definitive nature on vitamin A requirements or deficiency responses in any of the over 300 psittacine species known worldwide. Therefore, much of the material in this article is extrapolated to the psittacine from research on the domestic fowl.

DIAGNOSIS

GROSS DIAGNOSIS

Cases involving hypovitaminosis A are seen frequently in our practice, and insufficiencies of varying degrees are treated even more commonly. A dietary history revealing inadequate carotene or vitamin A intake should alert one to possible deficiency states, even in birds that appear normal. Deficient diets are unfortunately all too common in psittacines because the majority of seeds fed these birds contain little or no carotene.

Most clinical cases involving decreased vitamin A levels present with respiratory complaints, but many exhibit only the "sick bird syndrome" of generalized unthriftiness and lethargy. Observable symptoms generally arise from the upper respiratory area and may include sneezing, wheezing, nasal discharge, and crusted or plugged nares. Ocular lesions, if present, include: xerophthalmia, conjunctival inflammation and swelling, and ocular discharge. Oral membranes can appear dryer or "stickier" than normal. Plate-like swellings—pinpoint to large and confluent—may be visible on any area of the oral cavity but are generally palatine and commonly grouped around the choana. If advanced, these lesions may contain white to greyish, dry caseation. A culture of this material can reveal any of several bacterial agents, most commonly coliforms, *Klebsiella,* or *Staphylococcus.*

We see oral abscesses most commonly in the Amazon parrot group. In smaller psittacines, nasal and ocular discharge is the rule. Unfortunately, many lesions appear similar to those produced in infectious states uncomplicated by lack of vitamin A.

Since respiratory disorders are among the most common problems seen in psittacines, differential considerations should include (in decreasing order of frequency in our practice) infectious agents (bacterial, fungal, or viral; not uncommonly multiple or mixed); inhalant irritations (paint fumes, aerosol sprays, smoke, household cleaners, and so on); respiratory distress secondary to organic dysfunction (hepatic, renal, cardiac, and so on); foreign bodies (most commonly seeds and husks); parasitism; and neoplasia.

HISTOPATHOLOGY

RESEARCH ON FOWL

Studies of vitamin A–deficient domestic chicks indicate that the earliest lesions involve a change in the mucous protective blanket overlying the epithelial membranes. There is an increase in mucous membrane viscosity, reducing the flow rate of the blanket. This change reduces epithelial resistance to invasion by pathogens.

In the early stages of vitamin A deficiency few histopathologic changes were observed in the chicks. Nasal and oral tissues appeared predominantly normal. Subsequent histopathologic changes

622

included reduction in number and height of both ciliated and mucous acinar cells, followed by increased keratinization of mucous membranes and degeneration and atrophy of mucosal glands. Thus, vitamin A deficiency not only allows more frequent or serious infectious penetration across mucous membrane barriers, but also prevents normal cellular regeneration of damaged tissues.

Additionally, it is important to note that in studies conducted on chicks deficient in vitamin A but uncomplicated by infection, these chicks showed minimal histopathologic changes, even under malnourished and growth-stunted conditions. Thus it is apparent that histopathologic changes are mainly due to the combined effects of vitamin A deficiency and damage to cellular structures, generally by microorganism invasion.

Other research findings of a histopathologic nature in vitamin A–deficient fowl include marked depletion of lymphoid and plasma cell populations in the cell–mediated immune system; increased plasma uric acid levels owing to reduced kidney clearance; increased severity of gastrointestinal parasitism; and increased incidence and severity of candidiasis.

CLINICAL PROCEDURES

In suspected cases of hypovitaminosis A, a punch biopsy of an affected oral area may confirm the diagnosis. This is most feasibly performed on those birds with oral abscesses large enough to warrant lancing and curettage. However, this procedure is not without risk, especially in debilitated patients. The oral cavity of psittacines is highly vascular and hemostasis must be maintained. Oral ulcerations produced by surgical manipulations may induce temporary anorexia in a patient that can ill afford it. If possible, tissue sections should be read by a pathologist familiar with avian tissue. In any case, advise the pathologist of your suspicions.

An assay of liver tissue for vitamin A content is a fairly reliable (but by no means infallible) determination of deficiency states. In studies on many species, including domestic fowl, birds with induced avitaminosis A often assayed as depleted in liver stores while exhibiting no symptoms of deficiency. In most cases a sizeable piece of liver tissue must be submitted to those labs capable of performing this test, thus limiting the value of the test on living birds. However, the assay may be useful as a tool in determining unexplained deaths of valuable birds.

THERAPY

Precise therapy recommendations are difficult to offer because the pet birds we are dealing with are highly dissimilar with regard to geographic region, normal diet, size, and metabolic functions. A young, 30-gm parakeet is likely to convert carotene to vitamin A at a much different rate than an aged 1-kg macaw. In addition, chronic disorders (especially of liver and digestion) necessitate higher levels of vitamin A for these birds. For these reasons the following support therapy recommendations are general in nature and must be tailored to each individual case.

VITAMIN A THERAPY

Since ill or debilitated patients may not efficiently convert carotene to a useable form, oral or parenteral vitamin A supplementation is necessary for initial therapy. Therapeutic doses of vitamin A at 5 to 50 IU/gm body weight should be used daily for approximately two to four weeks. A maintenance dose of 0.25 to 1 IU/gm body weight should be continued on a daily basis if no dietary corrections are possible or two to three times weekly as a supplement if the bird is eating adequately.

Supplementation may be in injectable or oral form. The oral route is by far the most practical for long-term administration. However, additions to water or seed are, at best, a calculated guess with regard to final ingested dose. Furthermore, a bird may fail to drink or eat adequately owing to the presence of the additive, hence contributing dehydration or caloric deprivation to the initial problems. Therefore, when adding any material to water or food, watch closely for reduction in food or water intake. If possible, begin with a small quantity and gradually increase the dosage during the prescribed time period.

There are many oral preparations containing vitamin A. A sampling follows.

Vitamin A only
  Aquasol-A (aqueous)
  USV Labs (Tuckahoe, NY)
  1 drop = approximately 1,600 IU

  Vitamin A capsules (oil)—25,000 IU
  1 drop = approx. 3000 IU

Multiple-vitamin preparations
  Cod liver oil (with A and D)
  1 drop = approx. 125 IU

  Avitron
  Lambert Kay (Cranbury, NJ)
  1 drop = approx. 50 IU

  Poly-Vi-Sol
  Mead Johnson (Evansville, IN)
  1 drop = approx. 40 IU

  Abdec
  Parke-Davis (Detroit, MI)
  1 drop = approx. 260 IU

Note: Many human multiple vitamins deliver vitamin A in useable form but may not deliver vitamin D in the D_3 form necessary for use by birds.

There are two basic forms of injectable vitamin A.

Lipo Aqueous Vitamin Complex
10,000 IU vit. A/cc; also 1000 IU vit. D/cc and small amounts of vit. B. complex

Vitamin A palmitate in sesame oil
100,000 IU vitamin A/cc

Note: the aqueous injectable is less irritating than the oil product but does contain other vitamin additives (not necessarily undesirable).

There are two notes of caution in using vitamin A compounds. First, these products can lose efficacy with prolonged exposure to sunlight, excessive heat, age, or rancidity. Second, significant overdosing with vitamin A for long periods of time can lead to hypervitaminosis A toxicosis.

DIETARY THERAPY

Dietary therapy includes not only the addition of foodstuffs high in carotene or vitamin A (Table 1), but also dietary changes to eliminate other nutrient imbalances. Factual information on the diets of free-living psittacines is lacking, and that which is known is often difficult to duplicate. Consequently, seeds have been widely used as a substitute diet since they are readily available, relatively inexpensive, nonperishable, and, most importantly, are well liked by the birds.

When seeds are used as a dietary base, supplements should include additional high-quality protein in the form of small bits of cooked egg, meat, cottage cheese, and so on. Calcium:phosphorus balances should also be corrected (most seeds have a Ca:P ratio of 1:5 or more) using oyster shell, eggshell, mineral blocks, or bits of cheddar or Limburger cheese. Green leafy vegetables, yellow vegetables, or tiny bits of cooked liver supply A vitamins and other nutrients. A broad spectrum of mixed fruits and vegetables will supply important nutrients as well as fiber to the diet.

Dietary changes should initially involve only small quantities of supplemental food to avoid major changes in elimination. Most diet-induced "diarrhea" (which often worries owners) is in reality a transitory increase in the urine component of the droppings.

Close observation will determine which supplements added to the diet are actually eaten by the bird. Anorexic and badly debilitated birds should be tube fed as needed.

THERAPY OF COEXISTENT DISEASE STATES

Just as a deficiency of vitamin A can aggravate infectious states, certain disorders can deplete the body's supply of vitamin A. Especially notable are liver and intestinal disorders, which may prevent conversion and absorption of vitamin A compounds or reduce body storage levels. In these cases therapy is aimed at those disease states that cause or compound the problem and will depend on causative agents.

WARMTH

Application of heat is a very important therapeutic device. It is a valuable aid, and often a necessity, in treating the vast majority of illnesses in the psittacine family. Ill birds benefit from temperatures of 80 to 90°F, maintained 24 hours per day. An open container of water outside the cage will maintain humidity. Warmth should be maintained for a period extending beyond recovery and should be withdrawn gradually.

A light bulb, although commonly recommended, is a poor source of heat. When positioned near enough to the cage to produce adequate warmth it can cause glare and can interefere with vital rest or sleep. A heating pad is a preferred means of providing warmth. Placed outside and beneath the cage, it will radiate enough heat for all except very large cages. Blankets or towels covering the top and three sides of the cage will effectively trap the heat within.

STRESS REDUCTION

Rest and quiet are important for any ill bird, but they are imperative for a nervous or frightened avian. Many of the vitamin-deficient birds presented to us have been recently acquired by the owner. Most are newly purchased from pet shops, quarantine stations, or, all too commonly, smugglers. Many of these birds are malnourished and have been stressed by numerous moves, temperature changes, overcrowding, and/or a variety of handlers. House these birds in an out-of-the-way corner. Limit noise and activity around the bird. Stop, or at least minimize, handling or training

Table 1.   *Foodstuffs High in Vitamin A*

Food Item	IU/100 gm
Beet greens	6,000
Carrots	11,000
Dandelion greens	14,000
Spinach	8,000
Sweet potatoes	9,000
Turnip greens	7,500
Butter	3,300
Beef liver	45,000
Dried red peppers*	77,000
Egg yolks	3,000

*Included in most parrot mixes; excellent source of vitamin A if the bird will eat them.

procedures. Allow adequate hours of darkness or dim light for sleep.

If the bird has cage mates, be watchful for aggression toward the ill animal. Often the hindrance of rest by an overattentive "friend" can be deleterious. Separate the birds unless they are close companions. Placing cages side by side often eliminates separation trauma.

PREVENTION

If the old adage "an ounce of prevention is worth a pound of cure" were applied to the psittacine, it would read ". . . is worth ten pounds of cure." Psittacines in general are quite resistant to disease but once affected are often difficult to cure. Prevention is truly the most important form of avian therapy.

By far the majority of vitamin–A deficiency cases in psittacines are caused by inadequate diets. Accordingly, prevention should be aimed at the consumption of fresh foodstuffs in addition to seed. Most psittacines habituate readily to a seed-only diet, and many are reluctant to try new products. Force or tube feeding is impractical on a long-term basis. For many of these birds patience and persistence are necessary when adjusting their diet. Covering the seed with supplemental products will force the bird to handle and even taste new foods. Long-term daily use of these foodstuffs may allow an apprehensive bird to become familiar with the new products. In healthy birds, limiting hours of seed consumption to two or three hours morning and afternoon or moderately reducing the quantity of daily seeds may stimulate new food interests through mild hunger. However, a total withholding of seed in favor of "better" foods may result in weakness or even starvation. In very tame birds, hand feeding may be possible.

A multiple vitamin supplement alone is not sufficient to compensate for the lack of other needed nutrients but is a good adjunct to the dietary program and is a necessity in those birds refusing dietary supplements.

It is likely that excessive gravel ingestion interferes with digestion and assimilation of many products, including carotenes. This is a common problem in some caged birds, notably budgerigars.

One unexplained quandary in psittacine nutrition is the fact that many birds consume an exclusive diet of seeds and yet exhibit no signs of vitamin A deficiency. It is possible that these birds have very low vitamin A requirements or highly efficient liver recycling processes. Also, some seeds might contain very small amounts of carotene products. It may also be that many of these birds are chronically A insufficient, appearing normal as long as they are free of stress.

SUMMARY

The effects of hypovitaminosis A in psittacines are variable and complex because most cases do not indicate a "pure" vitamin A deficiency. As in humans, the majority of vitamin A–deficient diets are also lacking in other vitamins, proteins, or minerals. Therefore, therapy must be aimed at the overall improvement of nutrition.

Vitamin A's primary understood activity is to ensure the integrity of the epithelial defense barrier, especially the lining tissue of the mucous membranes. Often the clinical signs observable in deficiencies are those of infections. Therapy should therefore be aimed at controlling infection in addition to correcting faulty diets and replacing vitamin A. Prevention primarily involves dietary education of bird owners.

SUPPLEMENTAL READING

Altman, P. L., and Dittmer, D. S.: *Metabolism.* Bethesda, MD: Federation of American Societies for Experimental Biology, 1968, pp. 10–46.

Altman, R. B.: Respiratory diseases of caged birds. Vet. Clin. North Am. 9:527, 1979.

Arnall, L.: Diseases of the respiratory system. In Petrak, M. E. (ed.): *Diseases of Cage and Aviary Birds.* Philadelphia: Lea & Febiger, 1969, pp. 263–89.

Arnall, L., and Keymer, I. F.: *Bird Diseases.* Neptune City, NJ: T.F.H. Publications, 1975, pp. 71–83, 331–45.

Bang, B. G., and Bang, F. B.: Experimentally induced changes in nasal mucous secretory systems and their effect on virus infection in chickens. J. Exp. Med. 130:105, 1969.

Bang, B. G., Bang, F. B., and Foard, M. A.: Lymphocyte depression induced in chickens on diets deficient in vitamin A and other components. Am. J. Pathol. 68:147, 1972.

Bang, F. B., and Bang, B. G.: Defense mechanisms against viruses in the upper respiratory tract. Ann. Otol. Rhinol. Laryngol. 79:489, 1970.

Bang, F. B., Bang, B. G., and Foard, M.: Acute Newcastle viral infection of the upper respiratory tract of the chicken. Am. J. Pathol. 78:417, 1975.

Fisher, H.: The nutrition of birds. In Farner, D. S., and King, J. R. (eds.): *Avian Biology—Volume II.* New York: Academic Press, 1972, pp. 431–72.

Gendron, A. P., and Howard, E. B.: *Pathology of Pet Birds—Training and Study Aids,* Vol. X. Downey, Cal. Comparative Medicine and Veterinary Services, County of Los Angeles, 1980.

Herrick, J. B.: The influence of vitamin A on disease status. V.M./S.A.C. 67:906, 1972.

Newberne, P. M.: The influence of nutrition in response to infectious disease. Adv. Vet. Sci. Comp. Med. 17:265, 1973.

Scott, M. L., and Norris, L. C.: Vitamins and vitamin deficiencies. In Biester, H. E., and Schwarte, L. H. (eds.): *Diseases of Poultry,* 5th ed. Ames, IA: Iowa State University Press, 1965, pp. 181–219.

Tollefson, C. I.: Nutrition. In Petrak, M. E. (ed.): *Diseases of Cage and Aviary Birds.* Philadelphia: Lea & Febiger, 1969, pp. 143–65.

Ullrey, D. E.: Biological availability of fat-soluble vitamins: vitamin A and carotene. J. Anim. Sci. 35:648, 1972.

Vitamin A, 1st ed. New York: Chas. Pfizer & Co., Inc., 1963.

Wallach, J. D.: The mechanics of nutrition for exotic pets. Vet. Clin. North Am. 9:405, 1979.

SCALY FACE IN BUDGERIGARS

MARY E. MAINSTER, D.V.M.

San Antonio, Texas

Scaly face in budgerigars is a very common problem for both the individual bird owner and the breeder. The condition is caused by a minute arthropod, *Knemidokoptes pilae*, that attacks the nonfeathered parts of the bird, resulting in scaly, warty, or scabby excrescences around the beak, cere, eyelids, legs, and vent and on the keel (Fig. 1).

The condition seems to be more prevalent in spring and summer. It is most often seen in fledgling budgerigars; therefore these birds should be closely examined. All birds with unusual beaks should be suspect. Any encrustations on the legs or irritation around the vent should be checked. Skin scrapings are usually diagnostic.

The most common form of transmission is thought to be direct from parent to nestling during feeding. Transmission can also be indirect when a bird rubs its face against the perch, cuttlebone, or nest box. A third possibility is that seed may become contaminated. Wild birds may contaminate seed when scavenging. Alternatively, seed may be accidentally contaminated if it is improperly stored, as, for example, when uncovered food is kept too close to the cage of an infected bird. This could occur in the aviary or the pet store or at home.

The disease usually does not involve the entire flock but only a percentage of the birds. Hence, there is thought to be some predisposing factor that creates an imbalance in the host-parasite relationship, resulting in clinical signs. This factor could be nutritional stress, change of location, overcrowding, or a subtle psychological stress we do not yet understand. Sanitation and husbandry practices should be evaluated as well. Some birds exposed to mites as nestlings develop lesions later in life, whereas other birds exposed at the same time never have a problem. Pruritus is not necessarily a feature of this disease.

Early recognition will shorten the duration of treatment and decrease the possibility of beak deformity. A fine, white, crusty coating or film at the margins of the cere may be the first sign seen by the owner. In others, a beige-colored deposit is noted below the beak; around the eyes or vent; and on the eyelids, scaly parts of the feet, and/or the legs. In advance cases a guarded prognosis should be given.

Knemidokoptes pilae spends its entire life cycle on the host. It burrows into the skin and feather follicles, where it feeds on connective tissue. Its many burrowing tunnels give infected tissue its characteristic honeycomb appearance, which can be seen with a hand lens. It often burrows into the germinal layer of the upper beak, causing distorted growth. This can result in malocclusion and various types of beak deformities. Later, these may cause a problem in feeding. Some beak anomalies may be correctable by beak trimming and/or a change in diet. Others may result in the bird being unable to feed at all and could result in the bird starving to death. Ankylosis of the hock and other joints can occur as hyperkeratotic crusts overgrow the affected joints, making it difficult for the bird to move or feed. Toes may become necrotic and may slough off, making it impossible for the bird to perch.

The major goals of therapy are to soften crusts with emollients and kill the mites with a topical acaricidal lotion or oil. Early diagnosis allows for effective treatment. Advanced cases carry a grave prognosis.

There are two drugs used for the specific treatment of scaly mite in birds: crotamiton and rotenone

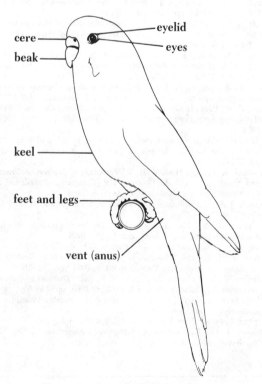

Figure 1. Sites of scaly mite invasion.

plus O-phenyl phenol. Crotamiton (Eurax*) is thought to be the safer treatment and is normally applied to the lesions every three days for two weeks and then once weekly until the lesions are healed. Rotenone plus O-phenyl phenol (Goodwinol Ointment†) is usually applied once weekly until healing occurs. *With either drug extreme care must be practiced so that the bird does not ingest any medication.* Other drugs used are mesulphen, mineral oil, olive oil, and p-chlorosym-m-xylenol plus terpineol. Drugs that are potentially toxic and should *not* be used are benzyl benzoate, coumaphos, and lindane. Commercial products available are Scalex and Avi-scale. These can be harmful or fatal if not used properly. Dusting powders do not affect scaly mite.

In advanced cases one can use light mineral oil or olive oil for the first three to five applications. This breaks down the encrustations and reduces the amount of acaricidal ointment needed. Antibiotic ointments can be used around the eyes to protect the corneas. One should instruct the owner to hold the beak closed to prevent ingestion of any medication. The medication should be applied directly to the area around the face with an applicator stick, using a rotary motion to break down the crusty materials. Apply medication to the legs by massaging in well with the fingertips. Remove all excess ointment to prevent ingestion or matting down of the feathers. Rub the ointment away from the feathers, not toward them. Tolerance to treatment among birds can vary greatly and in some cases any treatment may cause death.

The mite can be readily transmitted, and infected birds should be isolated. Reinfestation is always a possibility. Therefore the treatment of asymptomatic in-contact birds is warranted. In an aviary situation the house should be thoroughly cleaned, especially the roosts, and sprayed as recommended for chicken mites. It is best to do this during the non-nesting season if possible. With a caged pet, the bird or birds should be removed from the cage on the third day of treatment. In both cases all cage enrichment materials (toys, nest boxes, seed sprays, cuttle bones, and so on) that cannot be sterilized should be discarded. The cage, wooden perches, and dishes should be sprayed with a commercial dog and cat flea spray. Allow 15 minutes for the spray to penetrate all areas. Then wash the cage and all the items thoroughly with a mild household detergent. Rinse well. If possible, allow to dry in the sun. Return the treated bird to the treated cage. A temporary holding area for birds during this procedure can be made by placing the birds in a strong paper bag. Make some small air holes and secure the top with staples or paper clips. A diluted

form of Avi-scale may be used to treat for mite eggs.

Ointments should be applied only to unfeathered areas of the body. Any topical administration of ointment should be done sparingly or the bird while preening may distribute the ointment all over its body, which may result in matting of the feathers. If this happens the bird can no longer elevate its feathers and it loses its capacity for thermoregulation. The bird will then lose body heat at an accelerated rate. This can result in a respiratory problem or even death.

In severe cases, absorption of the topical acaricidal medication can be deadly.

Some practitioners advise using a vitamin A ointment to treat denuded areas. Others believe that a vitamin A deficiency may contribute to the problem and recommend adding vitamin A to the diet. This can be done by mixing a powdered vitamin supplement in the food or using pulverized dog food in a 50/50 mixture with seed.

Histopathologic examination of affected tissues shows marked papillomatous proliferation of the skin with cystic degeneration of the feather follicles, focal hyperkeratosis, and parakeratosis in both passeriformes and psittaceformes. In budgerigars lesions usually involve the cere. Other regions of the face and feet are frequently affected. In canaries and passerines leg lesions are common. Rarely, one finds involvement of the wing tips.

Causative agents in various species of birds are as follows:

Knemidokoptes pilae—budgerigars, canaries, psittacines

Proknemidokoptes jansseni—love birds, psittacines

Knemidokoptes philomelae — passeriformes

Knemidokoptes jamacicesis—passeriformes

Knemidokoptes fossor—evening grosbeak, goldfinches, sparrows, red-winged blackbirds, grackles, cowbirds, chickadees, flycatchers, nightingales, munia, thrushes, other passeriformes

Knemidokoptes mutans—poultry

Knemidokoptes gallinae—chickens, pigeons, and pheasants

Melopsithacus undulatus—kakarikis, lovebirds, cockatiels, parrots, goldfinches

Kakarikis can have mites over the entire body. Treatment consists of nebulizing the birds with a solution of ortho-malathion 50 insect spray diluted in 20 ml saline. The birds should be treated for 15 minutes weekly for one month. Routine treatment should also be carried out.

Convalescent birds can be aided by maintaining good sanitation and husbandry practices. Eliminate all possible stress situations. Supply good nutrition and trim the beak and toenails.

Prevention depends on maintaining good nutrition and good sanitation, and husbandry practices.

*Geigy Pharmaceuticals, Ardsley, NY.
†Goodwinol Products, Huntington Station, NY.

All newly purchased birds should be prophylactically treated with Avi-scale per package directions and kept isolated for 30 days (Kray, 1981).

SUPPLEMENTAL READING

Altman, R. B.: Parasitic diseases of caged birds. *In* Kirk, R. (ed.): *Current Veterinary Therapy VI*. Philadelphia: W. B. Saunders, 1977, pp. 683–684.

Altman, R. B.: Perching birds, parrots, cockatoos, and macaws (psittacines and passerines). *In* Fowler, M. E. (ed.): *Zoo and Wild Animal Medicine*. Philadelphia: W. B. Saunders, 1978, pp. 375–377.

Arnall, L., and Keymer, I. F.: *Bird Diseases*. Neptune City, NJ: TFH Publications, Inc., 1975, pp. 164–165, 168, 340–350.

Ensley, P.: Caged bird medicine and husbandry. Vet. Clin. North Am. 9:517, 1979.

Kray, R. A.: Scaly face—scaly face and leg dermatitis revisited. Bird World, Oct–Nov.: 20, 1981.

Loomis, E. C.: External parasites. *In* Hofsted, M. S. (ed.): *Diseases of Poultry*, 7th ed. Ames, IA: Iowa State University Press, 1978, p. 695.

Olsen, D. E., Dolphin, R. E.: Parasitism in the companion bird. V.M./S.A.C. 73:640, 1978.

Saunders, E. B.: Olive oil treatment of *Cnemidocoptes* mange in parakeets. V.M./S.A.C. 7:248, 1976.

Steiner, C. V., Jr.: *Caged Bird Medicine—Selected Topics*. Ames, IA: Iowa State University Press, 1981, pp. 36, 62, 92.

Woerpel, R. W., and Rosskopf, W. J.: Avian therapeutics. Mod. Vet. Pract. 62:947, 1981.

VISCEROTROPIC VELOGENIC NEWCASTLE DISEASE IN PET BIRDS

SUSAN L. CLUBB, D.V.M.

Miami, Florida

Newcastle disease (ND) is a highly contagious viral disease affecting most species of birds. Four major pathotypes have been described in domestic poultry, with varying degrees of pathogenicity and organ specificity. Viscerotropic velogenic Newcastle disease (VVND) is the most virulent form, producing high mortality in chickens, psittacines, and other species.

Imported pet birds, especially psittacines, are often incriminated as the source of virus leading to outbreaks of VVND in poultry. VVND is endemic in many countries and has been eradicated from poultry flocks in the US at great expense. The fear of re-entry of VVND into domestic poultry flocks resulted in the establishment of an avian quarantine program in 1974. All avian species must undergo a 30-day quarantine period and must be free of VVND prior to release from quarantine.

VVND was first recognized in Java in 1926. Psittacine birds were incriminated in the spread of the disease to Europe and South America between the years 1926 and 1942. VVND was first reported in the US is 1944. An epornitic of a very virulent strain reached all continents between the years 1968 and 1972. Owing to a successful eradication program in the US and the intensive vaccination in other countries, VVND was not a significant problem in most countries by 1976.

VVND was isolated from 12 of 483 (2.48 per cent) commercial shipments of imported birds in 1981. Shipments from Mexico, Central America, and Southeast Asia are most commonly affected. However, it has been reported in almost every country from which exotic birds are exported. VVND appears to have a seasonal incidence in Mexico and Central America corresponding to the rainy season (from March to June). Poultry flocks in these countries are vaccinated annually at this time.

ETIOLOGY AND PROPERTIES OF THE VIRUS

The etiologic agent of ND is a paramyxovirus, an RNA virus 120 to 300 nm in size. The virus is protected by a lipid envelope. The virus is unstable at high temperatures and is rapidly inactivated at a pH of 3.0 or by lipid solvents or UV light. Warm temperatures and sunlight facilitate the destruction of the virus by chemicals, and it is protected by suspension in proteinaceous material (feces or tissues). Freezing temperatures suspend the inactivation of the virus by chemicals. For proper disinfection all objects must be physically cleaned and supplemental heat must be provided in winter. Phenolic compounds are recommended for disinfection.

EPIDEMIOLOGY AND CLINICAL SIGNS

Aerosols are the primary means of spread of ND virus (NDV) within a closely confined susceptible flock of chickens. Approximately two days after exposure to the virus, an infected bird begins to liberate virus from its respiratory tract and continues to do so for several days. Coughing or sneezing is not required for production of the aerosols. Other means of transmission, which may be more important in pet birds, include direct contact with infected birds and contamination of food and water supplies. Humans are the primary vehicle for spread of the virus from one poultry premise to another by way of contaminated clothing, shoes, and other fomites. Spread of virus between exotic bird facilities is primarily by the movement of birds incubating the virus between facilities.

VVND can be a peracute disease in chickens, resulting in high mortality. The incubation period is 2 to 15 days, with an average of 5 to 6 days. Clinical signs include acute depression, anorexia, conjunctivitis, marked dyspnea, and diarrhea. The head may become edematous and paralysis may be present, but other neurologic signs are rare unless the course of the disease is protracted. Death usually occurs within one to three days after the onset of clinical signs. Post-mortem lesions include ecchymotic hemorrhages with occasional necrosis throughout the digestive tract, especially the small intestine, proventriculus, and sometimes the ventriculus. Tracheal hemorrhages and peritracheal edema may be present.

VVND is an extremly variable disease in exotic birds. The incubation period in psittacines is 3 to 16 days. In some cases the only signs are acute death and high flock mortality, with no response to antibiotics. This is especially true of young birds, which are more severely affected than mature birds. Severity of the disease also varies with the virulence of the virus, the species involved, and the viral dosage. Older or more resistant birds may initially show anorexia and depression. Bright yellow or bloody diarrhea may be present, and coughing, sneezing, and dyspnea may occur. In some birds the course of the disease is protracted. In these birds, neurologic signs are seen including ataxia, incoordination, torticollis, hyperexcitability, opisthotonus, head tremors, and unilateral or bilateral wing and leg paralysis. Neurologic signs may persist in birds that recover from active infection.

Post-mortem lesions in exotic birds are also extremely variable. The most consistently observed lesions include petechial hemorrhages on serosal surfaces of the intestines, proventriculus, pericardium and air sacs and petechiae in the tracheal lumen. Air sac inflammation, hepatomegaly, and splenomegaly may be found as well. The lungs, proventriculus, and trachea may be congested. Petechiae may be found on the mucosal surface of the proventriculus and under the lining of the ventriculus. Visceral lesions of VVND commonly observed in chickens are rarely seen in exotic birds. No truly pathognomonic lesions or signs have been recognized. The overall pattern of clinical signs and gross post-mortem lesions are more significant than signs observed in individual birds.

Infection, with or without disease, has been induced in many species of exotic birds experimentally. Amazon parrots (*Amazona* sp.) have been documented as shedding virus for over one year following recovery. Mynahs, conures, and budgerigars have also been shown to shed virus for a prolonged period of time. Shedding of virus may be intermittent and may be stress induced.

SPECIES SUSCEPTIBILITY

Species susceptibility to VVND is variable among psittacines and nonpsittacines. Cockatoos and cockatiels are highly susceptible, and infection often results in high morbidity, high mortality, and acute deaths. Amazon parrots and conures are very susceptible to the disease but usually linger longer than cockatoos, therefore showing a higher incidence of neurologic signs. Morbidity and mortality are usually high in Amazon parrots; however, mortality is lower in conures. Macaws, parakeets, lories, and African parrots are usually less susceptible; neurologic signs are uncommon and many birds recover completely from the disease. VVND has also been reported in birds of prey and many softbilled birds. Canaries and finches are relatively resistant to the disease, usually exhibiting only transient infection with low morbidity and mortality.

Severity of the disease will also vary in the species to which it has become adapted. Some strains show increased virulence for psittacines but cause a milder syndrome in chickens. Some strains increase or decrease in virulence with each passage through birds. Clinical signs may be more severe at high ambient temperatures.

DIAGNOSTIC PROCEDURES

Diagnosis must be based on the isolation of the virus by a USDA-approved laboratory. Virus may be isolated from cloacal or pharyngeal swabs of live birds. Samples of brain, lung, colon, spleen, and trachea should be submitted from dead birds. Swabs and tissues should be placed in brain heart infusion broth, frozen, and shipped to the lab on dry ice. NDV is isolated in the allantoic chamber of embryonated chicken eggs. Hemagglutination and hemagglutination inhibition tests are performed on eggs that die within five days of inoculation. If both tests are positive the virus is inoculated into specific pathogen-free chickens for pathotyping. The local USDA offices should be contacted for the designated laboratory that processes swabs in your state. Although most samples are processed by the National Animal Disease Center in Ames, Iowa, some state labs have also been approved for NDV isolation.

VACCINATION

Vaccination has made the control of VVND possible in poultry. Some of the available vaccines have been used safely in pet birds. However, federal regulations strictly prohibit the vaccination of exotic birds intended for import. The use of vaccines would produce an immune flock, thereby masking the presence of asymptomatic carriers. In quarantines of large numbers of birds, testing of each individual bird is impossible. However, the shedding of virus in a closely confined population would result in the rapid spread of infection and the easy detection of the virus.

MANAGEMENT OF SUSPECTED CASES

VVND is a disease that must be reported immediately to the local office of the USDA. The policy of the USDA for birds in commercial trade is that once a bird is exposed it is considered infected and must be given up for diagnostic evaluation. The USDA will pay indemnity on all birds they destroy. In the case of isolated pet birds, breeding collections, and zoo birds, arrangements may sometimes be made for isolation and testing of suspect birds. Federal regulations for the handling of suspect birds change rapidly; contact any local USDA office for the most up-to-date regulations.

EXTERNAL FIXATION TO REPAIR LONG BONE FRACTURES IN LARGER BIRDS

MITCHELL BUSH, D.V.M.

Washington, D.C.

The repair of extremity fractures in small companion birds has been well described in previous editions. These fractures are usually not severe and heal satisfactorily with cage rest and/or coaptation splinting. Also, the post-repair function of the injured extremity is not usually critical owing to the limited opportunity or demands for flight in these birds.

When repairing fractures of long bones of larger birds (500 gm and up) that are free living (e.g., raptors) or zoologic specimens, the return to near-normal function is a major concern. In free-living species destined for rehabilitation and release, the functional repair of a fractured wing is mandatory. Likewise, in a zoologic environment, the return to normal flight is desirable. Even more important is the return to normal courtship and breeding activity, which would be inhibited by a wing or leg with limited function.

Preoperative patient care is critical to the successful outcome of a fracture repair in a bird.

Initially, the patient is usually stressed owing to the trauma and is a poor candidate for extensive manipulation or surgery until it has stabilized. The patient should be handled only to evaluate the fracture by palpation and to provide temporary stabilization via splinting and/or bandaging to minimize further damage to the fracture and surrounding tissue. If bleeding is present, it is controlled by a pressure bandage or vessel ligation. If indicated, an antibiotic and/or corticosteroid can be administered at this time. Wild birds with fractures that may be several days old may be hypoglycemic when admitted and should receive intravenous and/or oral glucose solutions to meet their immediate metabolic needs. The bird should be placed in a warm, dark environment for several hours until it has time to stabilize. Once stabilized, a more detailed examination including radiographs is conducted to help assess the fracture so a repair method can be determined and implemented.

The basic principles of fracture repair are the

same whether the patient is a mammal or bird. Following repair, there should be rigid fixation of an anatomically aligned fracture in good apposition with the absence of infection. This allows early return to function by minimizing joint stiffness and muscle atrophy and contractures. The avian fracture presents unique problems not seen in mammalian fractures. First, avian bone is brittle owing to a higher calcium content and tends to shatter and crack when broken, causing comminuted fractures. The extent of the splintering cannot always be visualized by regular radiographs. Second, birds have pneumatized bones with larger intramedullary spaces, which complicate adequate stabilization with intramedullary (IM) pins.

External fixation was determined to be an acceptable method of repair of avian fractures following a study that radiographically and histologically evaluated the healing of avian bones. The basic mechanism for repair was found to be similar in both birds and mammals. The study found that avian fractures heal rapidly, in about three weeks in a well-aligned stable fracture, by forming a large endosteal callous. The endosteal callous is much larger than the resultant periosteal callous unless the fracture is unstable. Delayed healing can result from two factors: a nonstable fracture and/or a repair

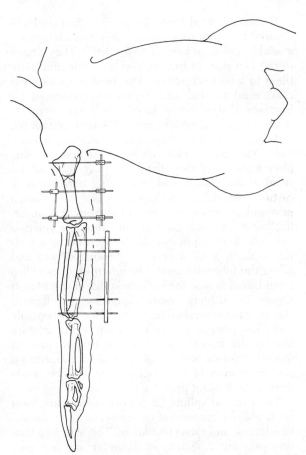

Figure 2. Applying the half-pin external splint to the ulna and combination half- and full-pin external splint to the humerus.

technique that disrupts the endosteal callous (i.e., IM pin).

The technique for applying the external splint (either half-pin or full-pin) is simple. With the full-pin external splint, the fixation pins penetrate perpendicularly through the bone and the skin on both sides of the fracture (as seen on the tibiotarsus in Figure 1). The external support rods are then attached to the fixation pins both medially and laterally to the fracture. This provides the most rigid fixation but creates a heavier splint and in lighter birds may be too heavy for the affected limb and may impair post-surgical ambulation. For the half-pin external splint, the fixation pins penetrate the skin and both cortices but do not emerge through the skin on the opposite side; thus the external support rod is attached to the fixation pins on one side of the fracture only (as seen in the femur in Figure 1 and ulna in Figure 2). In some fractures, a combination of the two splints is needed when it is not possible for all fixation pins to exit through the skin on the opposite side. This occurs, for example, on the medial aspect of the proximal end of the humerus (see Fig. 2) and on the medial aspect of the femur in selected distally occurring fractures.

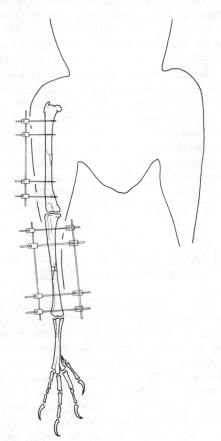

Figure 1. Applying the full-pin external splint to the tibiotarsus and the half-pin external splint to the femur.

The exteriorized fixation pins are connected and secured by various techniques. Fixation clamps are available commercially in two sizes.* They attach to the two sizes of fixation pins available and unite them to a connecting bar. The smaller fixation pin (2.03 mm) is used almost exclusively, except for fractures that occur in larger birds (i.e., cranes, storks, eagles), in which case a 3.0–mm fixation pin and larger fixation clamp and connecting bar are used. The fixation pins can be connected by using fiber glass† or polyurethane‡ casting material instead of the clamps and connecting bar. Strips of casting material are wrapped around the fixation pins and, when cured, form a lightweight connecting bar to stabilize the pins and thus the fracture site. The fixation pin can also be secured by inserting a plastic tube over the exteriorized pins and filling the tube with an acrylic mixture§ to establish a rigid fixation (see the half-pin splint of the ulna in Figure 2). Although more expensive, the fixation clamps have several advantages. They are reusable and allow compression or extension to the fracture site by the forces applied to the fixation pins. A major advantage is that adjustments in compression and angulation of the fracture site can be made during the healing period if necessary.

The external splints for fracture repair are most applicable for fractures of the humerus, ulna, femur, tibiotarsus, and tarsometatarsus. The standard fixation pins are 2.03 mm in diameter and are very sharp. They fit the commercially available clamps. Using a hand drill, these pins are placed through the cortex, taking care to prevent further splintering. The pins should be placed perpendicular to the axis of the bone, using many rotations while penetrating the cortex and keeping the pin in a single axis. The perpendicular placement of the fixation pins in birds, which differs from techniques described in mammals, is preferred because of the ease of alignment and compression of the fracture segments. If the fixation pin is not going to exit through the skin and is going to be placed in half-pin fashion, the opposite cortical surface is engaged but not completely penetrated.

Ideally, two fixation pins are placed on each side of the fracture. This provides the most rigid fixation. Some fractures preclude the placement of a second pin, although satisfactory stabilization can usually be obtained, as seen in the humeral fracture in Figure 2. The entrance point and expected exit point of the fixation pins on the skin are surgically prepared by carefully plucking the feathers, cleansing the area with surgical soap, and rinsing it with an organic iodine preparation.

*KE Clamps, Kirschner Scientific Division, Hazelton Laboratories, Seattle, WA.
†Lightcast II, Orthopedic Products, Surgical Products Div., 3M, St. Paul, MN
‡Cutter cast, Haver-Lockhart Labs, Shawnee Mission, KS.
§Technovit, Dr. Jorgensen Labs, Loveland, CO.

Ideally, the fracture site is not surgically invaded during the repair to minimize further disruption to the vascular supply and possible wound contamination. The first two fixation pins are placed farthest away (proximally and distally) from the fracture site. The fracture is reduced and the connecting bar is attached by means of fixation clamps applied to these two pins. The two remaining pins are placed adjacent to the fracture site, along the line of the connecting bar, so that reduction and stabilization of the fracture can be properly maintained. If it is impossible to align the fixation pins with one connecting bar, additional bars can be used. The disadvantage of this method is the additional weight. The exposed sharp metal edges and fixation clamps must be padded, especially on the medial aspect, to prevent self-trauma by the bird.

Although immediate postoperative use of the fractured area is desirable, there are situations in which some support through coaptation splinting is initially required until the bird regains strength and can adapt to the weight of the splint. If the fracture was compounded, a systemic broad spectrum antibiotic is indicated in the postoperative period.

External fixation can be used in combination with other fixation methods such as IM pins to prevent rotation at the fracture site, but one of the advantages of external fixation is that there is no further disruption at the fracture site and no metal to interfere with the endosteal callous. If an IM pin is needed for alignment of the fracture prior to application of the fixation pins, removal of the IM pin within the first postoperative week after alignment and fixation are secured would be indicated to prevent further disruption of the endosteal callous.

The external splint can be used to reduce and stabilize simple fractures and can also be used to provide stabilization and preserve length to a comminuted fracture without surgical intervention and disruption of the fracture site. Another use of the external splint is to maintain length of a fractured bone in the event a bone graft is indicated.

EXTERNAL SPLINT PLACEMENT FOR LONG BONE FRACTURES

Humerus. Most humeral fractures have to be repaired using a half-pin splint with connecting bars placed on the dorsal/lateral aspect of the humerus. In some situations, a partial full-pin splint can be used in fractures that are most distal (see Fig. 2).

Radius and/or Ulna. In larger birds, the external splints can usually be applied to the ulna when an unstable fracture occurs. These splints can either be full- or half-pin splints (see Fig. 2), depending on the stability required and the weight factor of the splint.

Femur. External fixation of a fractured femur is

usually limited to half-pin splints with the connecting rod on the lateral aspect of the leg (see Fig. 1). These fractures are the most common type employing the combination of an IM pin and a half-pin splint.

Tibiotarsus. Fractures of the tibiotarsus can be repaired using full-pin splints on the lateral and medial aspects of the leg (see Fig. 1).

Tarsometatarsus. These fractures can be repaired using a full-pin splint on the lateral and medial aspects of the leg.

DISCUSSION

The use of external splints for fixation of avian fractures has several distinct advantages as follows:
1. Minimal specialized equipment is needed,
2. The technique for application is not difficult,
3. The surgery and anesthesia time are short,
4. Rigid fixation is possible,
5. Early return to function is maximized,
6. Postoperative care is minimal, and
7. Adjustments in tension and alignment during healing are possible.

The disadvantages of an external splint are as follows:
1. The weight of the device, and
2. The protuberance of the fixation pins and connecting rod from the surface of the skin.

The use of external splints is not the answer to the repair of all avian fractures, but when used on appropriate cases in larger birds by a surgeon who understands the principles and techniques involved, it is a useful technique and provides good results, especially in the all-too-common, severely comminuted fracture.

This type of fixation also aids early return to function of a bird with a fractured humerus. The external splint allows movement of the wing and maintains bone length, thereby preventing muscle and tendon contracture, which can render a bird flightless. These splints also minimize external or periosteal callous formation and promote an internal callous. This is beneficial because a large periosteal callous can affect muscle activity and can hinder return to normal flight.

AVIAN POX IN CAGED BIRDS

SUZANNE KENNEDY-STOSKOPF, D.V.M.

Baltimore, Maryland

Avian pox, also known as avian diphtheria and contagious epithelioma, is caused by the *Avipoxvirus* genus and appears to affect all avian species. Reported strains of the virus include fowl poxvirus, canarypox, pigeonpox, juncopox, quailpox, sparrowpox, starlingpox, turkeypox, and parakeetpox. Although all strains are related antigenically and a few are pathogenic for only one host species, the majority appear to be able to infect several host species. Natural infections occur sporadically in wild bird populations, which act as a reservoir for the disease. Mosquitoes act as mechanical vectors and can transmit the virus for as long as one month after an infected meal. Consequently, birds housed in outdoor facilities or facilities with open-window ventilation are subject to outbreaks. There is evidence indicating that latent infections can be activated by stress.

CLINICAL COURSE

Under natural conditions the incubation period for avian pox is usually four to ten days. The disease occurs in two forms, cutaneous and diphtheritic, and may present as separate entities or together. The cutaneous form involves the development of wart-like nodules on the unfeathered portions of the body. The legs, feet, base of the beak, and periorbital skin are most commonly involved. Cutaneous lesions may appear on feathered portions of the body with canarypox. The course of the lesions varies with the species of bird infected and the virulence of the virus. In general, by two weeks after the appearance of the first nodules the lesions have progressed through the papular and vesicular stages and have coalesced, turning a dark brown or grey color, with inflammation present at the base. Scab formation then occurs, which may last one to two weeks or longer in the case of wild birds. If the scabs are removed early, a moist seropurulent exudate is seen covering a hemorrhagic and granulating surface.

In the diphtheritic form of the disease, white, opaque, slightly raised nodules develop on the mucous membranes of the oral cavity, crop, esophagus, trachea, and sinuses. These lesions coalesce rapidly to form a cheesy, yellowish pseudomembrane. When removed, it leaves a hemorrhagic, eroded surface. Lesions may be restricted to the oral cavity, crop, and esophagus, causing anorexia, or may involve only the trachea and sinuses, causing dyspnea. In some cases all mucosal surfaces may be affected at once. Secondary bacterial and fungal infections exacerbate these lesions. Prognosis is usually poor with the diphtheritic form of the disease.

Canaries may develop a fatal septicemia with canarypox. Mortalities often approach 100 per cent. Initially, the owner will notice the bird rubbing its eyes on the perches and scratching at its beak. Lacrimation is present, followed by the appearance of yellowish proliferative lesions on the eyelids. During the course of the next few days, the lesions rapidly progress to the classic cutaneous and diphtheritic lesions previously described. Birds become anorexic when respiratory signs appear, and diarrhea often develops. The course of the disease lasts three to ten days. With particularly virulent strains, acute respiratory distress and death may occur without the appearance of cutaneous lesions. At necropsy, liver necrosis and fibrinous pneumonitis may be observed. The spread of the disease is usually slow, except in crowded aviaries where there is evidence of aerosol transmission. Normally, the virus must enter through a break in the skin or mucosa.

DIAGNOSIS

An accurate diagnosis is essential, since many other diseases that are treatable may resemble avian pox. A quick, presumptive diagnosis can be made in the practitioner's office by making a smear of a pox lesion, staining it by the Wright method, and looking for elementary (Borrel) bodies. These spherical structures stain light pink and measure approximately 0.25 μm in diameter. They may be arranged in short chains or in diplococcal forms resembling bacteria. Thousands of these elementary bodies form the intracytoplasmic eosinophilic inclusions (Bollinger's bodies) seen on histologic preparations of lesions. The presence of inclusions confirms the diagnosis. Biopsies of lesions should be submitted to a pathologist in 10 per cent buffered neutral formalin.

If further verification is necessary, specimens may be submitted for viral isolation to an appropriate diagnostic laboratory. Preferred samples include newly formed vesicles and diphtheritic membranes. If possible, specimens should be submitted fresh at room temperature but may be frozen at −20° C. Identification of the strain of avian pox is not routinely performed. Serologic techniques are available, but there is considerable cross reactivity between strains.

DIFFERENTIAL DIAGNOSIS

The differential diagnosis for the cutaneous form of the disease includes pantothenic acid deficiency, bumblefoot, and *Knemidokoptes* infestations (scaly leg and beak) of parakeets and canaries. The last-named can be easily checked by scraping the skin and looking for the offending mites. Depending on the clinical signs and the species affected, there are several differential diagnoses for the diphtheritic form of avian pox. The lesions seen in vitamin A deficiency, candidiasis, and trichomoniasis can mimic the oral and esophageal lesions of avian pox. A preliminary diagnosis of *Candida* infestation can be made by an unstained wet smear of a lesion or one stained with Gram stain to demonstrate the presence of budding yeast cells and hyphae. A definitive diagnosis, however, must be made with cultures incubated on Sabouraud's agar at 37°C and room temperature. Growth must be heavy to confirm a diagnosis.

Trichomonas gallinae affects pigeons, raptors, canaries, and other species of passerines. The flagellated protozoan can easily be recognized on fresh smears. Laryngotracheitis and *Syngamus trachea* (gapeworm) can cause severe dyspnea and can be confused with the tracheal form of avian pox. Only chickens and pheasants are susceptible to laryngotracheitis, which is caused by a herpesvirus and produces intranuclear inclusion bodies. Virtually all species of birds may be affected by *Syngamus*, the presence of which can be diagnosed by the characteristic double-operculated eggs present in the droppings or occasionally in the mucus, which accumulates in the trachea and is either coughed up or gently swabbed out of the trachea of a lightly anesthetized bird. A diagnosis of a vitamin deficiency is usually based on a history of poor nutrition and exclusion of infectious etiologies.

TREATMENT

Treatment is purely supportive. Birds with clinical signs should be isolated. Cutaneous lesions may be treated with an antiseptic or topical antibiotic to prevent secondary infections. A solution of 1 to 3 per cent Mercurochrome in 70 per cent alcohol to which a trace of acetone has been added is applied once or twice daily in managing cutaneous lesions of canarypox (Petrak, 1982). Birds with particularly severe lesions around the beak may be unable to eat and will have to be tube fed until the lesions resolve. Likewise, birds with severe periorbital lesions may temporarily lose their vision due to blepharal swelling and may require tube feeding. As stated earlier, prognosis is poor with the diphtheritic form of the disease unless the lesions are mild. Careful tube feeding will be necessary to maintain the patient until it feels like eating on its own. Birds that recover from either form of the disease are resistant to reinfection with that strain of the virus but not necessarily to other strains.

CONTROL AND PREVENTION

In the face of a large outbreak of avian pox in open facilities, consideration should be given to wild birds as a possible source of infection. Equally important is the prevalence of mosquitoes and their proper control. All new birds should be strictly quarantined, preferably in mosquito-proof enclosures, for at least two weeks before being introduced into an established collection to avoid possible introduction of avian pox or other infectious diseases. After an outbreak, the facilities should be thoroughly disinfected, since the poxvirus is fairly resistant to most environmental influences. Poxvirus is most readily destroyed by oxidizing disinfectants such as hypochlorites and potassium permanganate. Formaldehyde at a concentration of 0.2 per cent destroys infectivity in 24 hours at room temperature.

Although vaccines have been used for chickens, turkeys, pheasants, and pigeons, the use of any attenuated live virus preparation is strongly discouraged. Vaccination in the face of an outbreak is not effective, since it takes about four weeks to develop immunity and immunity is not permanent. Owing to the number of strains of poxviruses and their rather haphazard cross reactivity and consequent cross protection, introduction of an attenuated strain of live virus into a facility may afford no protection or, worse, may introduce a new strain of virus pathogenic for the vaccinated birds. Thus, emphasis for elimination of the virus should be placed on isolation, disinfection, and vector control.

REFERENCES AND SUPPLEMENTAL READING

Cunningham, C. H.: Avian pox. In Hofstad, M. S. (ed.): *Diseases of Poultry*, 6th ed. Ames, IA: Iowa State University Press, 1972.
Karstad, L.: Pox. In Davis, J. W., Anderson, R. C., Karstad, L., and Trainer, D. O. (eds.): *Infectious and Parasitic Diseases of Wild Birds.* Ames, IA: Iowa State University Press, 1971.
Petrak, M. L. (ed.): *Diseases of Cage and Aviary Birds*, 2nd ed. Philadelphia: Lea & Febiger, 1982.

GOUT

KAY G. MEHREN, D.V.M.
West Hill, Ontario

Gout, a relatively common metabolic disorder of birds, is characterized by the abnormal deposition of insoluble crystals of uric acid and related waste substances in various areas of the body. It occurs most frequently in gallinaceous birds, budgerigars, and waterfowl; less frequently in large psittacines and raptors; and rarely in pigeons and canaries (Arnall and Keymer, 1975).

The etiology of gout is uncertain. Although gout is often associated with renal disease, gout lesions may occur without associated renal lesions, and vice versa (Petrak, 1969; Steiner and Davis, 1981).

Two forms of gout—visceral and articular—may occur separately or in combination. Clinical signs vary depending on the distribution of urate deposits. The literature indicates that opinions on relative frequency of occurrence of articular and visceral gout and types of birds affected vary considerably, depending on each author's experience.

ARTICULAR GOUT

Viscid to pasty masses of urate accumulate within joints and along tendon sheaths, usually peripher-

ally in the legs and/or wings. Early signs might include nonspecific restlessness and frequent shifting of weight from foot to foot. As the disease progresses, the bird may become lame or unsteady on its feet; cage birds may also have difficulty perching, preferring instead to sit on the cage floor (Petrak, 1969; Steiner and Davis, 1981). Sometimes the affected bird will be unable to fly, and one or both wings may droop (Petrak, 1969). Characteristic urate tophi may develop as small, pale, firm swellings adjacent to joints. Soft, fluctuant swellings may fill tendon sheaths, especially those proximal to the hock and the base of the foot.

VISCERAL GOUT

Dry, chalky urates form a "frost" on the serous membranes, most frequently on the epicardium, pericardium, the surface of the liver, and on the air sacs (Arnall and Keymer, 1975; Petrak, 1969). Deposits may also occur in the interstitial connective tissue of the liver and kidneys and may fill the excretory ducts of the kidneys (Petrak, 1969). Clinical signs of visceral gout are insidious and difficult to detect. They may include poor appetite, changes in temperament, lethargy, variable stool consistency, emaciation, or sudden death with little or no indication of illness (Arnall and Keymer, 1975; Fowler, 1978; Petrak, 1969; Steiner and Davis, 1981).

CLINICAL DIAGNOSIS

Clinical diagnosis poses problems. Early articular gout may resemble an acute, infective arthritis, and gout tophi may be mistaken for abscesses (Arnall and Keymer, 1975). Radiographs are not useful in visualizing gout deposits. If gout tophi are present, one may be incised to aid diagnosis; the contents will be opaque, chalk-white to beige, and range in consistency from creamy to powdery. Microscopically, the contents are composed of needle-shaped or amorphous crystals. The presence of uric acid can be confirmed by the murexide test (Petrak, 1969; Steiner and Davis, 1981).

An elevated uric acid level in the blood plasma occurs in gout and may aid in making a diagnosis. Normal blood uric acid levels are stated as 1.2 to 8 mg/100 ml (average 4.5 mg/100 ml) but vary owing to species differences and physiological factors including reproductive state, amount and kinds of food, and state of health (Petrak, 1969).

Suggested predisposing factors are important to consider in attempting to establish therapy and prevention of gout. They include factors that increase levels of uric acid presented to the kidneys for excretion (e.g., high-protein diet or overeating; or inactivity: decreased blood circulation and decreased water intake) and factors that impair renal function (e.g., exposure to cold and dampness; vitamin A deficiency; poor nutrition: high carbohydrate–low protein diet with inadequate vitamin-mineral supplementation; and infectious disease or intoxication) (Arnall and Keymer, 1975; Petrak, 1969; Steiner and Davis, 1981).

GOALS OF THERAPY

Gout in birds is considered incurable. Treatment may influence the bird's general condition but cannot mobilize previous deposits of urate crystals. Therapy is directed toward improving the affected bird's comfort and prolonging its life (by months) and involves dietary and environmental management, administration of systemic drugs to reduce uric acid levels, and possible curettage of local lesions (Steiner and Davis, 1981).

SPECIFIC THERAPY

When gout is diagnosed, euthanasia is indicated. In the case of pet birds or valuable birds, an effort at treatment may be desirable. The owner should be advised that the treatment is not a cure and that daily medication as well as changes in diet and management will be required for the remainder of the bird's life.

Allopurinol (Zyloprim*) reduces the amount of uric acid being formed by the liver and kidneys, thereby reducing crystalization and deposition of uric acid crystals. It has no effect on previously formed urate deposits (Steiner and Davis, 1981). Zyloprim may be administered at the rate of 10 to 15 mg/kg daily for the rest of the bird's life. One 100-mg Zyloprim tablet crushed and added to 5 ml of water makes a stock solution of 20 mg/ml. One drop of stock solution daily would be an adequate dosage for a budgerigar. The medication may be offered on a treat food to avoid the stress of daily handling.

Acetylsalicylic acid (aspirin) may provide some analgesia; 0.3 gm (5 gr) of aspirin dissolved in 240 ml of water may be used as the sole source of drinking water or may be given by eyedropper.

Local treatment of urate tophi by surgical curettage followed by cautery with 1 per cent AgNO₃ has been suggested by some authors (Petrak, 1969; Steiner and Davis, 1981). However, it must be pointed out that these wounds heal poorly and that deposition of urates will continue in other parts of the body.

ANCILLARY TREATMENT

Nonstressful management and improved diet are probably the most important factors in treating (and preventing) gout.

The bird should be kept at a fairly constant warm temperature, away from drafts. Perches should be smooth and broad and should be placed at low levels. Food and water dishes should be placed within easy reach (Petrak, 1969; Steiner and Davis, 1981).

An effort should be made to evaluate and balance the bird's diet. If the present diet is high protein, offer cereals and low-protein seed mixtures and vegetables supplemented with vitamin A; avoid concentrates (especially those of animal origin) (Arnall and Keymer, 1975; Petrak, 1969; Steiner and Davis, 1981). If the bird is on a low-protein diet,

---

*Burroughs Wellcome Co., Research Triangle Park, NC.

add cooked eggs, grubs, and insects (Arnall and Keymer, 1975; Steiner and Davis, 1981). Vitamin and mineral supplementation should be offered.

If the bird is able, it may benefit from daily flying exercise. Muscular activity stimulates blood circulation and also increases thirst; this may increase the dispersal and excretion of urates (Arnall and Keymer, 1975).

REFERENCES

Arnall, L., and Keymer, I. F.: *Bird Diseases.* Neptune City, NJ: T. F. H. Publications, 1975.
Fowler, M. E. (ed.): *Zoo and Wild Animal Medicine.* Philadelphia: W. B. Saunders, 1978.
Petrak, M. L.: *Disease of Cage and Aviary Birds.* Philadelphia: Lea & Febiger, 1969.
Steiner, C. V., and Davis, R. B.: *Caged Bird Medicine, Selected Topics.* Ames, IA: Iowa State University Press, 1981.

SALMONELLOSIS AND OTHER BACTERIAL ENTERITIDES IN BIRDS

JANE E. MEIER, D.V.M.

San Diego, California

Diarrhea is a common problem in captive birds. One major cause is bacterial enteritis, and mortality rates can approach 100 per cent in some outbreaks. Along with bacterial enteritis, the differential diagnosis of diarrhea should include parasitic infections, viral diarrheas, dietary problems, and renal disease. Renal disease is included because initially it can be difficult to tell which portion of a bird's droppings—urates or feces—is abnormal.

Differentiating bacterial enteritides requires bacteriologic culturing of feces or necropsy specimens, since clinical signs and necropsy results are similar with different causative organisms. Typical necropsy findings include hemorrhagic thickened intestinal walls; fibrinonecrotic exudate on the intestinal mucosa; and increased fluid in the intestinal lumen. Abscesses may be present in the liver, heart, and/or spleen.

Many different microorganisms can cause avian enteritis. Some are opportunists, whereas others are primary pathogens. *Salmonella* can cause disease in mammals, birds, and reptiles. In domestic fowl, salmonellosis is classified according to causative organism: fowl typhoid, *S. gallinarum*; pullorum disease, *S. pullorum*; and paratyphoid, *Salmonella* sp. In cage birds the syndromes are indistinct and all are considered together as salmonellosis.

Avian colibacillosis is caused by pathogenic strains of *Escherichia coli,* and *Pasteurella* sp. can cause fowl cholera. *Arizona* sp., *Clostridium colinum* (quail disease), *Streptococcus* sp., *Staphylococcus* sp., *Erysipelothrix* sp., and *Mycobacterium* sp. can also produce avian enteritis. Occasionally other organisms are isolated from birds with enteritis. The disease produced by these organisms may include organ systems other than the gastrointestinal tract. However, the primary presenting sign is generally diarrhea.

Treatment of bacterial enteritis in captive birds is similar whatever the causative organism. It is based on the clinical signs, physical examination, and antibiotic sensitivities. Treatment involves supportive care to reduce the effects of damage to the intestinal wall (i.e., diarrhea, dehydration, electrolyte imbalance) and antibiotic therapy to help the bird's immune system overcome the bacterial infection.

Control and prevention of bacterial enteritides are based on good husbandry and sanitation practices and vector control.

BACTERIAL ENTERITIDES

SALMONELLOSIS

Salmonellosis is caused by any one of over 1,500 serotypes of *Salmonella*. All serotypes are pathogenic, but there is some variation in severity depending on the age and susceptibility of the birds, the size of the inoculum, and the virulence of the serotype. Young birds are usually more severely affected. Adult birds may have only minimal signs, whereas mortality rates in young birds can be over 90 per cent.

Salmonellosis can cause several different syndromes in birds. Peracute disease is characterized by sudden death. Birds are normally of good weight and often do not have signs of diarrhea. Anorexia and depression may not be obvious. Necropsy results indicate an overwhelming septicemia.

In acute disease, birds become ill within a few days to two weeks after exposure. The course of the disease is generally rapid. Over a period of several days, the birds become depressed and have a watery green, yellow, gray, or bloody diarrhea. The vent and vent feathers become matted with fecal material. Other signs include huddling, fluffed feathers, incoordination, shivering, decreased appetite, vomiting, weight loss, increased respiratory rate, increased or decreased thirst, and severe dehydration. As the disease progresses, birds can exhibit an inability to stand or perch, tremors, blindness, convulsions, and death.

Newly hatched birds with acute salmonellosis are small and weak, have diarrhea, and tend to fade during the first few days of life. Infected eggs have low hatchability.

Birds with chronic salmonellosis are often "poor doers." Diarrhea may be present intermittently, although not all birds have diarrhea. Septic arthritis and localized abscesses can occur with chronic salmonellosis.

Inapparent *Salmonella* carriers appear clinically normal but shed the organism in their feces. They can harbor the bacteria in their oviducts as well as lay infected eggs. These birds may only shed *Salmonella* intermittently. Birds that survive an outbreak of salmonellosis may or may not become carriers. Some birds are inapparent carriers without ever having clinical signs. As in mammals, eliminating the state can be extremely difficult. Birds with any form of salmonellosis can pose a risk to other birds, pets, and caretakers, and sanitary precautions should be taken. Carrier birds are especially dangerous because the problem may be unrecognized.

COLIBACILLOSIS

Considerable variation exists in the pathogenicity of *Escherichia coli* in different bird species. *E. coli* is a normal enteric inhabitant of insectivorous and carnivorous species. Even though *E. coli* is not thought to be normal gut flora in granivorous and fructivorous species, especially psittacines, it has been recovered from clinically normal captive birds. When *E. coli* is isolated from birds not normally hosting the organism, it should be considered a potential pathogen. The decision to treat a bird with

E. coli must be based on clinical signs, pathology, and history of the particular bird or aviary.

E. coli tends to be an opportunist, and colibacillosis is seen most often in stressed, weakened, or young birds. Signs vary when different organ systems are affected. In avian enteritis, the organism breaches the integrity of the gut mucosa, causing septicemia and peritonitis. Birds with this form of colibacillosis have severe diarrhea and die suddenly. Signs are similar to those seen with peracute and acute salmonellosis.

E. coli can also produce purulent pericarditis, hepatic abscesses, granulomas, salpingitis with egg retention, pneumonia especially associated with aspergillosis, chronic air sacculitis, and septic arthritis. It has been connected with bumblefoot infections.

PASTEURELLOSIS

Pasteurellosis, fowl cholera or hemorrhagic septicemia, usually refers to disease caused by *Pasteurella septica*, *P. avium*, or *P. multocida*. Mortality rates may be greater than 90 per cent. In the peracute form, there may be multiple rapid deaths with few clinical signs. Birds may die while singing, eating, preening, or flying.

In acute pasteurellosis, signs appear three to ten days after inoculation. Birds become depressed, fluffed, and uncoordinated. Severe bloody or watery diarrhea develops with concurrent weight loss and dehydration. There may be an increased respiratory rate with sneezing and nasal discharge. Feathers around the face and vent may be matted. Birds with chronic pasteurellosis fail to thrive and are thin and inactive and may have septic arthritis. These birds may become carriers, shedding the organism in feces or nasal exudate.

In addition to enteritis, there may be splenic enlargement with pinpoint necrotic foci in the spleen, heart, and liver. Petechial hemorrhages may be present in the lungs, air sacs, and kidneys.

CLINICAL PATHOLOGY

Microbiology is necessary to differentiate bacterial enteritides. Cultures of feces and necropsy specimens should be done whenever possible to make a definite diagnosis. Antibiotic sensitivities help determine the drug of choice for treatment. In avian enteritis, antibiotic therapy is generally begun prior to obtaining culture and sensitivity results. Therapy is then adjusted according to the bird's response and the laboratory findings.

Hemograms and serum electrolytes may be useful in gauging the severity of the enteritis, determining the degree of electrolyte imbalance and dehydration, and managing the patient.

In diarrhea, feces contain excessive amounts of water, sodium, potassium, chloride, and bicarbonate. The consequences include metabolic acidosis, dehydration, electrolyte imbalances, impaired renal function, and shock. Only birds of adequate size and stable clinical state are bled. Severely ill birds can die from the stress of handling. Samples are taken from the brachial vein with a 26-gauge needle with or without a syringe. The blood is drawn into a syringe or can be allowed to run directly into a heparinized capillary tube. The same technique is used with a toe clip. Normal values for psittacines should be in the following ranges: total protein 2.5 to 4.9 gm/dl; packed cell volume 38 to 50 per cent; serum calcium 8.2 to 10.4 mg/dl; serum chloride 104 to 120 mEq/liter; serum potassium 2.2 to 4.2 mEq/liter; serum sodium 144 to 160 mEq/liter. Total white cell counts have not been consistent enough to be diagnostic in avian enteritis.

TREATMENT

SUPPORTIVE CARE

Sick birds tend to become hypothermic. The ambient temperature should be kept at approximately 85°F, and drafts should be avoided. Incubators, heat lamps, and space heaters can be used to provide extra heat, and a high/low thermometer is helpful in regulating the temperature.

The object of fluid therapy in avian enteritis is to replace fluid and electrolyte losses due to diarrhea, meet maintenance requirements, and provide caloric support. Fluids should be given as needed. Daily weighing and hematologic assessment are helpful in making these calculations. Fluids may be given orally, subcutaneously, or intravenously. All fluids should be warmed before administration.

Caution should be used when giving oral fluids to birds with enteritis. Oral fluids should not be given to severely hypothermic birds. In severely hypothermic individuals, gut peristalsis and metabolism absorption are impaired, and giving fluids or food *per os* can cause bloat and may encourage bacterial proliferation. If strongly hypertonic, they can produce an osmotic diarrhea. Several oral electrolyte solutions are well tolerated (e.g., Lytren*). They may be given at a dosage of 0.03 to 0.05 ml/gm body weight up to four times daily by feeding tube. When birds are started back on solids, bland foods or tube formulas are recommended. Lactated Ringer's solution and 5 per cent dextrose 1:1 are excellent for rehydration and maintenance of birds with enteritis.

Maintenance requirements of 0.05 to 0.125 ml/gm body weight/day may be given subcutaneously or intravenously. Deficit requirements due to dehydration should be added to this. Administration of intravenous fluids can be quite stressful to birds, and hematomas may result. However, it is the most rapid means of meeting fluid needs. Fluids should be given over a 10- to 15-minute period in the brachial or medial tarsal vein.

An energy source, often 5 per cent dextrose, should be supplied because hypoglycemia may be serious enough to cause incoordination and convulsions. Birds are often anorectic, and even if they continue to eat, digestion and absorption are disrupted. Potassium supplementation may also be necessary either orally or parenterally.

Kaopectate may be given orally at 0.005 ml/gm body weight three to four times daily to help reduce the severity of the diarrhea. Vitamin supplementation, especially the water-soluble vitamins, should be given orally or parenterally. Several preparations are available for birds. Follow the manufacturer's recommended doses. Vitamin B complex can also be given. *Lactobacillus acidophilus* may be used in the recuperative stages of treatment to help reestablish gut flora. A 250-mg tablet may be crushed into the food for several days.

ANTIBIOTIC THERAPY

Antibiotic sensitivities are the best way to determine the drug of choice in avian bacterial enteritis. This is not always practical, so a broad spectrum antibiotic should be selected. Treatment may be prolonged and may be repeated when dealing with chronic infections or birds that have become carriers, especially with salmonellosis. Bacteriologic cultures are necessary when attempting to eliminate inapparent carriers. Organisms are shed intermittently, so birds are not usually considered free of the organism until they have had three consecutive weekly negative fecal cultures. Treatment is continued until negative cultures are obtained. This generally takes from three to eight weeks. Many anti-

Table 1. *Normal Body Weights of Representative Avian Species*

Bird	Body Weight (gm)
Finch	6–12
Canary	18–40
Budgerigar	30–60
Lovebird	55–75
Cockatiel	75–125
Parakeet	125–175
Small parrot	350–400
Large parrot	500–600
Macaw	700–1500

*Mead Johnson Nutritional Division, Evansville, IN.

Table 2.   *Antibiotics and Other Drugs Commonly Used in Birds With Bacterial Enteritis*

Drug	Dosage (gm body weight)	Manufacturer
Antibiotics		
Ampicillin (Polycillin-N)	0.1 mg/gm IM b.i.d. or t.i.d.	Bristol Laboratories, Syracuse, NY
Ampicillin (Polycillin)	0.1 mg/gm PO b.i.d. or t.i.d.	Bristol Laboratories, Syracuse, NY
Chloramphenicol palmitate (Chloromycetin palmitate)	0.05 mg/gm PO t.i.d. or q.i.d.	Teuco, Morris Plains, NJ
Chloramphenicol (Tevcocin)	0.01 to 0.03 mg/gm IM b.i.d. to q.i.d.	International Multifoods, Minneapolis, MN
Gentamicin Sulfate (Gentavet)	0.005 mg/gm IM SID	Burns-Biotec, Omaha, NE
Oxytetracycline HCl (Liquamycin 100)	0.01 to 0.03 mg/gm IM SID	Pfizer Inc., New York, NY
Tetracycline (Panmycin)	0.01 to 0.03 mg/gm PO b.i.d.	Upjohn Co., Kalamazoo, MI
Trimethoprim 8 mg/ml/ sulfamethoxazole 40 mg/ml (Septra)	0.005 mg trimethoprim/gm PO b.i.d.	Burroughs Wellcome Co., Research Triangle Park, NC
Fluids		
Lactated Ringer's injection	As needed IV, SQ	Abbott Laboratories, North Chicago, IL
5% dextrose injection	As needed IV, SQ	McGaw Laboratories, Irvine, CA
Oral electrolyte solution (Lytren)	As needed PO	Mead Johnson, Evansville, IN
Vitamins		
Baby vitamins (Abdec)	0.01 mg/gm PO SID	Parke-Davis, Detroit, MI
Vitamin-mineral powder (Vionate)	Follow manufacturer's directions	E. R. Squibb, Princeton, NJ
Others		
Kaopectate	0.005 ml/gm PO t.i.d. or q.i.d.	Upjohn Co., Kalamazoo, MI
Lactobacillus acidophilus (Acidophilus)	250 mg on feed SID	Kovac Labs, Oceanside, CA

biotics tend to prolong the carrier state in salmonellosis; however, initial results with trimethoprim and sulfamethoxazole (Septra*) have been encouraging.

In peracute or acute bacterial enteritis, antibiotic therapy is generally given for 5 to 14 days. Antibiotics may be administered in the food or water; however, sick birds do not always eat or drink normally. Oral or intramuscular administration may be more suitable early in the course of the disease. Table 1 provides average weights of some common cage birds, and Table 2 provides commonly used antibiotics and their dosages. All exposed birds in an aviary should be treated, not just those with clinical signs.

CONTROL

Control of bacterial enteritis in an aviary can be difficult because of the high incidence of carriers in free-ranging birds, rodents, flies, and so on. Sources of infection include contact with a newly acquired inapparent carrier bird or a human carrier, contamination of food at the manufacturer; or contamination of the food, food preparation equipment, or environment where the birds are housed. Some organisms, notably *Salmonella*, can survive for long periods in the environment. *Salmonella* can survive for over four months in stagnant water and even longer in soil. Bacterial enteritides are more likely

*Burroughs Wellcome Co., Research Triangle Park, NC.

to spread through an aviary if there is overcrowding, improper food storage, stale food/water, and poor sanitation.

Prevention depends on good sanitation and hygiene practices. Food and water dishes should be cleaned regularly in detergent and water hotter than 140°F. Cages, perches, and so on should be routinely disinfected with chlorine bleach or another germicidal solution and rinsed with water. Feed only good quality foodstuffs, and store them properly to avoid contamination. Cages and aviaries should be vermin proofed as much as possible. New birds should be isolated from other birds for at least several weeks, and in some cases fecal culturing is recommended.

SUPPLEMENTAL READING

Arnall, L., and Keymer, I. F.: *Bird Diseases.* Neptune City, NJ: T. F. H. Publications, Inc., 1975.
Bowman, T. A., and Jacobson, E. R.: Cloacal flora of clinically normal captive psittacine birds. J. Zoo Anim. Med. 11:81, 1980.
Fowler, M. E. (ed.): *Zoo and Wild Animal Medicine.* Philadelphia: W. B. Saunders, 1978.
Graham, C. L., and Graham, D. L.: Occurrence of *Escherichia coli* in feces of psittacine birds. Avian Dis. 22:717, 1978.
Hofstad, M. S., et al.: *Diseases of Poultry,* 6th ed. Ames, IA: Iowa State University Press, 1972.
Jones, D. M., and Nisbet, D. J.: The gram negative bacterial flora of the avian gut. Avian Pathol. 9:33, 1980.
Kirk, R. W. (ed.): *Current Veterinary Therapy VII.* Philadelphia: W. B. Saunders, 1980.
Tizard, I. R., Fish, N. A., and Harmeson, J.: Salmonella bird vectors. Can. Vet. J. 20:143, 1979.
Whitford, H. W., and Jones, L. P.: Bacterial pathogens from exotic birds. Proceedings of the 21st Annual Meeting of the American Association of Veterinary Laboratory Diagnosticians. 243, 1978.

PARASITIC DISEASES OF CAGE BIRDS

PHILIP ENSLEY, D.V.M.

San Diego, California

Veterinarians diagnose and treat parasitism in cage birds that are kept by the single- or multiple-bird owner, the serious aviculturalist, and zoos. Therapy for a single isolated parrot in a client's home differs from a management program in a large outdoor aviary or zoo collection exposed to transient or feral birds and other vectors. Each situation requires therapy tailored for each bird or group of birds.

Cures for some parasitisms evade the clinician. As comprehension of avian parasites improves, new anthelmintics will become available. The author will briefly describe current therapy for the more common parasitisms a practitioner will encounter.

INTERNAL PARASITISM

Healthy-appearing birds may harbor internal parasites. Clinical evaluation of all birds, healthy or ill, should include a fecal examination for protozoans and ova of adult worms (Table 1).

Internal parasitism, if found, may not be the major malady of a sick bird; therefore, in treating the parasitism, the clinician must not overlook other disease. Owing to the diversity of avian species and their parasites, medication of a bird or group of birds may not eliminate the parasite. After treatment, a follow-up fecal examination will aid in evaluating the effectiveness of treatment.

GUIDELINES FOR TREATMENT OF INTERNAL PARASITISM (Table 2)

1. Accurate gram scales are critical in weighing birds to determine drug dosages.

2. Large birds, 400 gm and over, should be fasted up to four hours prior to and after treatment.

3. Clients should be advised about reactions to drugs such as parenteral levamisole hydrochloride.

4. Follow-up fecal examination several days following treatment is essential to evaluate effectiveness of medication.

5. Stress should be kept to a minimum if the medication is given daily for several days.

NEMATODES

ASCARIS

Ascaris sp. are the most common parasites encountered by the clinician. They are generally found in the intestine. In small numbers they cause no obvious problems; however, in large numbers they cause weight loss and poor condition and, in severe cases, mechanical obstruction and death. The life cycle of the parasite is direct, with infection occurring after ingestion of infective eggs. Diagnosis is made by identification of ova (Fig. 1) on fecal flotation. Treatment using either piperazine, thiabendazole, or levamisole hydrochloride (oral or injectable) is relatively effective; however, fenbendazole is becoming more widely used.

CAPILLARIA

Capillaria sp. occur in a variety of sites in the gastrointestinal tract such as the crop, esophagus, and intestine and in the oral cavity in some cases. They are important because they cause tissue damage by burrowing into the mucosa. In significant numbers, this activity causes debilitation of infected birds. Diagnosis is made by identifying bipolar eggs (Fig. 2) on fecal flotation or by wet mount preparation of swabs of oral and crop secretions. Like ascarids, *Capillaria* sp. have a direct life cycle. Treatment of this burrowing worm with thiabendazole, piperazine, or levamisole can be difficult, and five to seven days of oral fenbendazole therapy may be more effective.

HETERAKIS

Heterakis sp. is a common parasite of fowl. The life cycle is direct; however, earthworms ingest the eggs of this nematode and can act as a transport host. This nematode is more commonly found in the cecum and colon and can cause injury to the cecal wall, resulting in digestive disturbances. This parasite acts as a carrier for *Histomonas melegridis*, which causes enterohepatitis (blackhead) in poultry and pea fowl.

The author wishes to thank Gerry Cosgrove, M.D., and Tom Olson for the photographs in this article.

641

Table 1. Summary of Common Parasites Found in Cage Birds

Parasite	Location in Bird	Diagnosis	Therapy*	Control
Nematodes				
Capillaria (threadworm)	Oropharynx, crop, esophagus, small intestine	Fecal flotation: bipolar eggs; oral and crop secretion: bipolar eggs	Fenbendazole	Cage sanitation, periodic worming
Ascaridia (roundworm)	Gizzard	Fecal flotation: eggs	Piperazine, fenbendazole, thiabendazole, levamisole (oral or injectable)	Cage sanitation, periodic worming
Heterakis	Cecum, colon	Fecal flotation: Ascarid-like eggs	Same as *Ascaridia*	Remove earthworms (transport host), cage sanitation
Acuaria	Proventriculus, gizzard	Necropsy lesions	None	Isolate from invertebrate intermediate hosts (insects and crustaceans)
Syngamus (gapeworm)	Trachea	Tracheal exam, necropsy, fecal flotation: bipolar eggs	Thiabendazole	Remove invertebrate intermediate hosts and earthworm transport hosts
Filarids	Adults: muscle; microfilariae: blood	Blood smears: microfilariae	Levamisole (oral) is microfilaricidal; adulticidal activity is not known	Eliminate biting insect vectors
Cestodes				
(Tapeworm)	Small intestine	Proglottids or eggs in fecal smears	Niclosamide	Cage sanitation
Protozoa				
Giardia	Small intestine	Cysts or trophozoites in fecal smears	Dimetridazole	Cage sanitation
Trichomonas	Oral cavity, small intestine	Smears of secretions or feces	2-Amino-5-nitrothiazole, metronidazole, dimetridazole	Cage sanitation, clean water and food sources
Coccidia	Intestine, cecum	Fecal flotation: oocysts	Sulfamethazine (or comparable agent)	Cage and litter sanitation, reduce crowding of birds
Blood Vascular Protozoa				
Plasmodium (avian malaria)	Blood, spleen, liver	Blood smears, intraerythrocytic schizonts and gametocytes	Chloroquine phosphate, quinacrine hydrochloride	Insect vector control
Haemoproteus	Blood	Blood smears, gametocytes in RBCs	Chloroquine phosphate, quinacrine hydrochloride	Insect vector control
Leucocytozoon	Blood	Blood smears, gametocytes in RBCs and WBCs, schizonts in tissues of internal organs	Cloroquine phosphate, quinacrine hydrochloride	Insect vector control
Ectoparasites				
Cnemidocoptes (scaly leg or scaly face mite)	In skin around beak, cere, eyelids, legs, and feet	Skin scrapings of honeycomb-like lesions	Crotamiton or rotenone ointment	Treat affected birds and maintain mite-free stock
Lice, ticks, fleas, feather mites	Skin, feathers	Gross and microscopic identification of parasite	Carbaryl powder	Treat affected birds and maintain cage sanitation

*Refer to Table 2 for dosage.

Table 2. *Therapeutic Recommendations*

Drug	Manufacturer	Dosage and Method of Administration
Chloroquine phosphate (Aralen)	Winthrop Labs, New York, NY	Per os: 25 mg/kg in divided doses (see text)
Quinacrine hydrochloride (Atabrine)	Winthrop Labs, New York, NY	Per os: 50 mg/kg SID for seven days 0.25 mg/gm (small birds) SID for seven days
2-Amino-5-nitrothiazole (Enheptin)	American Cyanamid, Princeton, NJ	Per os: 40 mg/kg SID for seven days Drinking water: 0.03 to 0.015 per cent for 7 to 14 days
Dimetridazole (Emtryl)	Salsbury Laboratories, Charles City, IA	Per os: for Giardia 1.5 mg/30 gm every 12 hr for three doses (see text) Drinking water: for *Trichomonas* 0.02 to 0.04 per cent for five days
Crotamiton (Eurax)	Geigy Pharmaceuticals, Ardsley, NY	Topical: to affected areas weekly for four wk
Fenbendazole (Panacur)	American Hoechst Corp., Somerville, NJ	Per os: for ascarids 10 to 50 mg/kg (repeat in two wk); for *Capillaria* 10 to 50 mg/kg SID for five days
Metronidazole (Flagyl)	Searle and Co., San Juan, PR	Per os: for trichomonads 50 to 500 mg/kg SID for five days
Rotenone (Goodwinol)	Goodwinol Products, Huntington Station, NY	Topical: to affected areas weekly for four wk (toxic reaction if ingested)
Levamisole hydrochloride (Levasole 1.8%)	Pitman-Moore, Inc., Washington Crossing, NJ	IM: 20 mg/kg (repeat in two wk)
Tramisol	Cyanamid Agricultural de Puerto Rico, Inc., Manati, PR	Per os: 15 mg/kg (repeat in two wk)
Piperazine (Pipzine or comparable product)	Affiliated Labs, Horsham, PA	Per os: 100 to 500 mg/kg (repeat in two wk)
Carbaryl (Sevin 5%)	Union Carbide Corp., Salinas, CA	Topical: lightly dust body and limbs
Sulfamethazine (Sulmet)	American Cyanamid, Princeton, NJ	Drinking water: 0.1 to 0.2 per cent for five days
Thiabendazole (Mintezol or comparable product)	Merck & Co., Inc., Rahway, NJ	Per os: for Ascarids 250 to 500 mg/kg (repeat in two wk); for gapeworms 100 mg/kg SID for seven to ten days
Niclosamide (Yomesan)	Bayvet Division of Cutter Laboratories Inc., Shawnee Mission, KS	Per os: 150 to 250 mg/kg

Identification of ascarid-like eggs (Fig. 3) on fecal flotation may indicate the presence of *Heterakis* infection. Treatment is the same as that for ascariasis.

ACUARIA

This genus of nematodes attaches to the mucosal surface of the proventriculus, causing a reactive process resembling a tumor-like growth. The digestive tract cannot function, and an infected bird loses condition and starves to death. Young growing birds are more often affected by this nematode. Diagnosis is generally made at necropsy. The life cycle of this parasite is indirect; intermediate host insects or crustaceans are necessary for transmission. Prevention of this parasitism by isolation of young growing birds from intermediate hosts may offer the best solution.

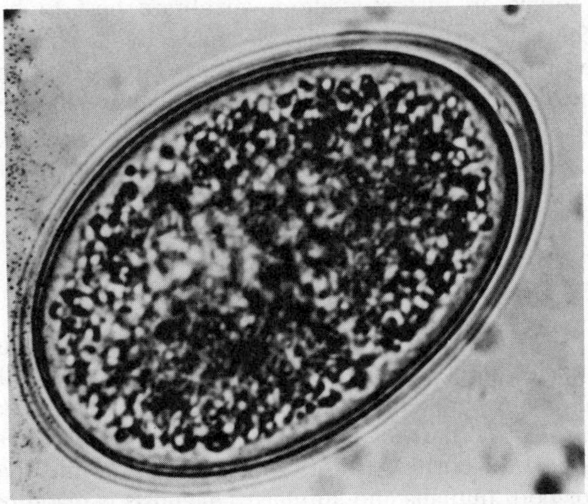

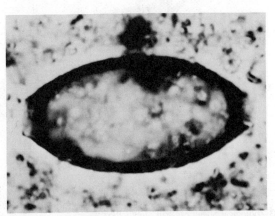

Figure 1. Ascarid ova. © Zoological Society of San Diego 1982.

Figure 2. *Capillaria* ova. © Zoological Society of San Diego 1982.

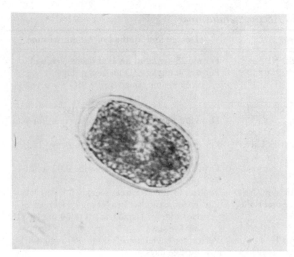

Figure 3.   Heterakid ova. © Zoological Society of San Diego 1982.

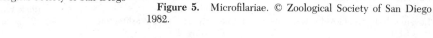

Figure 5.   Microfilariae. © Zoological Society of San Diego 1982.

SYNGAMUS

The adult worms of *Syngamus* sp. (gapeworms) are found in the trachea of a variety of bird orders, although more frequently they are associated with galliforms and passeriforms. The female worms with males attached (Fig. 4) cause damage, irritation, and partial obstruction of the trachea. Birds with heavy infection exhibit dyspnea and debilitation. The life cycle is direct; however, earthworms and other invertebrate hosts can act as intermediate hosts. Diagnosis is made by observing nematodes in the trachea or at necropsy. Biopolar eggs may be found on fecal flotation. Daily treatment with thiabendazole for seven to ten days is recommended.

FILARIA

Microfilariae (Fig. 5) are occasionally found in peripheral blood smears of avian species and probably do not cause illness. The adult nematodes are sometimes located in facial planes and are not considered pathogenic. However, adult filarial nematodiasis has been documented in the cardiovascular system of a few avian species (Ensley, 1978). Levamisole hydrochloride given orally for up to four days may provide microfilaricidal activity; however, adulticidal activity is not known.

CESTODES

Tapeworms are found in the small intestine of avian species. There are few reports of these worms causing serious damage. They are sometimes found at necropsy in birds that have died from other causes. Some have a direct life cycle, whereas others require an intermediate invertebrate host to become infective. Diagnosis is made by identifying proglottids or eggs (Fig. 6) in feces. Treatment with niclosamide has been shown to be effective in most species of birds.

PROTOZOA

GIARDIA

Giardia sp. have been documented in wild avian species and, more recently, as a pathogen in adult and baby parakeets (Panigrahy et al., 1981). Affected birds have diarrhea and a high mortality. Giardiasis is a water-borne disease, with cysts being infective for both humans and animals. Diagnosis is made by

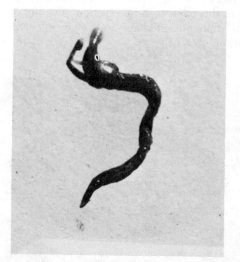

Figure 4.   Female gapeworm with smaller male attached. © Zoological Society of San Diego 1982.

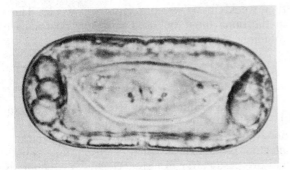

Figure 6. Tapeworm ova. © Zoological Society of San Diego 1982.

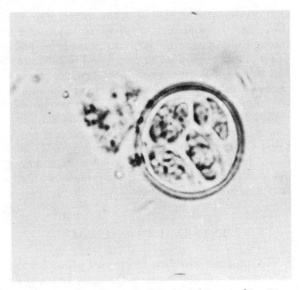

Figure 8. *Coccidia* oocyst. © Zoological Society of San Diego 1982.

identifying cysts or trophozoites (Fig. 7) in fecal smears. Metronidazole is the treatment of choice in human giardiasis. Investigations of different treatment protocols with dimetridazole in parakeets indicate that the most effective treatment is three oral doses at the rate of 1.5 mg/30 gm of body weight every 12 hours (Scholtens et al., 1982).

TRICHOMONAS

Of the several species of *Trichomonas* found in a wide variety of birds, *T. gallinae* is considered to be the only pathogen. Virulent strains of this protozoa cause caseous oral lesions in pigeons, doves, and raptors. Systemic invasion of trichomonads to the liver, lungs, and other organs may also occur. Less virulent strains are associated with mild inflammation of the mouth, crop, and esophagus. It is not uncommon to find trichomonads in fecal smears of clinically healthy birds. Diagnosis is made by microscopic examination of swabs of lesions.

Transmission of this protozoan occurs through contaminated food and water sources. Favorable response to medications such as 2-amino-5-nitrothiazole, dimetridazole, or metronidazole may depend on the severity of the lesion or debilitation of the bird under treatment. Use of these medications may be indicated as supportive care for birds with digestive disturbances in which trichomonads are found in fecal smears.

COCCIDIA

Coccidia sp. cause protozoal intestinal disease more commonly in poultry. Coccidiosis is diagnosed in a wide variety of wild and captive birds. It causes enteritis, diarrhea, and debilitation, particularly in growing birds in overcrowded enclosures. Transmission occurs through contaminated litter and soil. Diagnosis is made by identifying oocysts (Fig. 8) on fecal flotation. (Oocyst morphology may vary considerably between species of *Coccidia*.) Treatment may not be satisfactory. Medication of water with sulfamethazine or comparable agents is recommended. Prevention by reduced crowding and improved cage sanitation is more beneficial.

BLOOD VASCULAR PROTOZOANS (AVIAN MALARIA)

PLASMODIUM, HAEMOPROTEUS, AND LEUCOCYTOZOON

Blood vascular protozoans are occasionally found by the practitioner. Their clinical significance, when found in more commonly kept pet birds, is not as

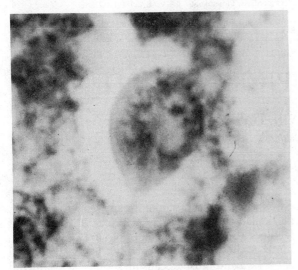

Figure 7. *Giardia* trophozoite. © Zoological Society of San Diego 1982.

well documented as that of avian species found in the wild. Transmission of avian malarias occurs through biting insects. Diagnosis is made by identification of the parasite in peripheral blood smears and histopathology. When pathogenicity is suspected, treatment with quinacrine hydrochloride or chloroquine phosphate has been tried with variable results. In one case involving a *Plasmodium* infection in gyrfalcons, clinical improvement was noted using chloroquine phosphate, 25 mg/kg in divided doses. Initially, 10 mg/kg was given orally, followed in 6 and 12 hours by 5 mg/kg, and 5 mg/kg 24 hours later as a final dose (Kingston et al., 1976).

EXTERNAL PARASITISM

The most common form of external parasitism the practitioner will encounter is the scaly leg or scaly face mite in parakeets. Canary breeders will frequently find a tracheal mite in their birds. The majority of lice, ticks, fleas, and feather mite cases will be found in large aviaries or in wild species brought to veterinarians while undergoing rehabilitation.

KNEMIDOKOPTES

Scaly leg or scaly face mites are commonly found in parakeets. The mite burrows into the skin around the beak, cere, eyelids, legs, and feet and occasionally around the cloaca and wing tips. Diagnosis is made by observing the honeycomb appearance of the skin where the mite has tunnelled or by finding the mite on microscopic examination of skin scrapings from the affected areas.

Treatment consists of topical application of crotamiton or rotenone ointment on a biweekly and then weekly basis for up to four to six weeks. These medications must be used sparingly, particularly rotenone, as it is highly toxic if ingested.

STERNOSTOMA

Little clinical information exists about therapy for the tracheal mite *S. tracheocolum* seen most frequently in canaries and some finches. Typically, affected birds exhibit wheezy respiratory sounds and tire easily after exercise. Diagnosis is generally made by identifying the mite in the trachea at necropsy. Convincing successful treatment against this mite has not yet been developed.

LICE, TICKS, FLEAS, AND FEATHER MITES

These ectoparasites are most frequently found in large aviaries and wild birds. They are most often found while physically restraining a bird. Identification of these parasites is made by microscopic evaluation of the parasite's morphology. Treatment is all cases is topical application of carbaryl powder along the bird's neck and back and under the wings and legs. When these parasites are found in an aviary, all nest boxes must be cleaned and the premises fumigated.

REFERENCES

Ensley, P. K.: Levamisole hydrochloride for treatment of *Paronchocerca ciconarum* microfilariae in a marabou stork. J.A.V.M.A. 173:1246, 1978.
Kingston, N., Kemple, J. D., Burnham, W., Stabler, R. M., and McGhee, R. B.: Malaria in a captivity-produced F_1 Gyrfalcon and in two F_2 peregrine falcons. J. Wildl. Dis. 12:562, 1976.
Panigrahy, B., Craig, T. M., and Glass, S. E.: Intestinal parasitism in budgerigars. J.A.V.M.A. 179:573, 1981.
Scholtens, R. G., New, J. C., and Johnson, S.: The nature and treatment of giardiasis in parakeets. J.A.V.M.A. 180:170, 1982.

THE FEATHER PICKING BIRD

CHUCK GALVIN, D.V.M.

Novato, California

Feather picking or chewing is a very common problem among pet birds, particularly the psittacines. It is a frustrating problem from the pet owner's standpoint and can also be a frustrating and challenging management problem for the veterinarian. In most cases the consequences of feather picking are mostly esthetic problems. However, chronic feather replacement can weaken the bird, particularly if nutrition is marginal. Birds without feathers also are more susceptible to chilling. Some birds go beyond pulling or chewing feathers and chew skin and muscle, causing serious, self-inflicted damage. In addition, blood loss from broken or chewed pin feathers can be significant.

CAUSES OF FEATHER PICKING

A bird is a social animal and needs environmental stimulation to maintain normal mental balance. It is normal for a bird to preen its feathers and remove the keratin sheath that surrounds a newly formed feather. This normal preening can become exaggerated, however, with the bird chewing or pulling out feathers. The usual causes, in decreasing order of importance, are considered to be the following: (1) boredom or nervousness, similar to fingernail biting in humans; (2) emotional disturbance; (3) lack of privacy; (4) endocrine or dietary imbalance; and (5) feather mites. Feather mites are rarely a cause of feather picking, although they are commonly assumed to be the cause by bird owners and pet shop employees. It should be noted that there are many feather picking birds that are properly fed, have many toys to play with, receive much attention, and appear to have a good relationship with their owner.

DIAGNOSIS

The diagnosis is easy. The pet bird owner has usually already made the diagnosis and is seeking a solution. However, clients occasionally do not realize that their bird is a feather picker. They do not realize that the preening activity is exaggerated, or in some cases the bird only plucks its feathers when the owner is not around. The clue is the feather loss; typical feather loss in a feather picker appears only in areas where the bird's beak can reach. The beak can reach everywhere except the head; therefore, typical areas of picking include the breast, legs, tail, back, wings, and so on. Another clue, of course, is the presence of many feathers in the cage. It is possible for feather loss to be present on the head as well if the bird scratches at its head or rubs its head on objects or if the bird is being plucked by another bird. Also, there are usually pin feathers present. Some birds pull out the pin feathers so that none are visible. If there is a question as to whether there is feather follicle activity, put an Elizabethan collar on the bird and recheck the bird in two weeks to look for pin feathers. The bare skin of feather pickers may show just the gray down feathers.

Some birds, instead of being feather pluckers, are feather chewers and mutilate and fray the feathers instead of pulling them out. These birds take longer to improve because the chewed feathers have to be molted out, in contrast to the plucked feathers, which start to grow right away. Some birds squawk when they pull out a feather. In some cases this is the primary complaint, an unexplained squawking out during the night when the bird is unobserved. The owner may not associate the squawking with a feather being pulled. In most cases the skin itself appears normal, but in some cases the bird may pick at the skin and cause open sores, which are slow to heal. The featherless areas are easily bruised; therefore, examination should be gentle but firm.

THERAPY

The treatment of feather picking in cage birds is often difficult and sometimes discouraging. Once the bird has established the habit, it can be hard to break. In my practice, I have a success rate of approximately 70 per cent. The following suggestions have helped a number of my feather picking patients. In some cases, just trying one of the suggestions cured the problem. In a minority of cases, all the suggestions were tried with no success and the bird remained a feather picker. Some birds responded initially but reverted back to plucking later on.

Make sure that nutrition is adequate (i.e., regular seed mixtures, treats and condition foods, vitamins and minerals, table foods, and miscellaneous supplements). It takes a lot of protein, calcium, and energy to replace pulled out feathers. Feather picking can be corrected in some birds by adjusting the diet and supplying nutritional supplements. In most cases, however, improving the diet by itself does not alleviate the problem. Ask the client what the bird is fed and what it actually eats.

Suggest that the owner give the bird a lot of direct attention. Play with it, talk to it, hand feed it, take it from room to room, and so on. Some clients may be reluctant or unable to give the pet bird more of their time; others are quite willing. It may be helpful to have all the family members present when suggestions are discussed.

Some birds respond to environmental sounds, such as music, radio, television, records, and so on. Suggest that the owner leave a radio or television on when no one is home.

Toys can be helpful. They must be safe and kept clean and must not overcrowd the cage. Examples include swings, bells, mirrors, balls, chains (heavy enough so that the bird cannot hang itself), and balls of paper. Chewing toys, e.g., rawhide bones, pieces of wood, alfalfa cubes, or other novelties, may also be helpful. Entire avian "playgrounds" can be made. Soft fabrics, strings, and yarn should be avoided, since the bird can injure itself by getting its claws or neck caught in the frayed fabrics or string. Or the bird can ingest the string, resulting in an intestinal obstruction. The sturdiness of the toys, of course, varies with the size of the bird. Larger birds can easily destroy plastic toys. There are wide selections of "keet toys" in pet shops. Not all birds play with toys; some are afraid of them.

Try moving the cage to another area of the house (away from drafts). Perhaps the bird would like to look out the window during the warm part of the day. (Do not allow the bird access to lead-based paint on windowsills.) Move the cage away from the window when it gets cold and allow access to a shaded area if it gets too warm. Perhaps the bird would be happier in a room where there is more family activity. Birds do not like to be left alone. They appear to want to feel that they are part of the activity. In fact, some birds will only pick their feathers when their owners are away.

The cage should be of an adequate size to allow the bird room for physical activity. If the cage is small, suggest a larger cage. A flight cage might be helpful. Some avian practitioners advocate providing a place for the bird to hide and "get away from it all." A dark box that attaches to the bird's cage so that the bird can retreat into it at leisure would be sufficient. It should be easily accessible for cleaning.

Make sure the bird gets 8 to 12 hours of sleep in a dark area. Some birds can sleep whether a light is on or not, whereas a light can result in lack of sleep, nervousness, and feather pulling in other birds.

Remove the feathers that fall to the bottom of the cage. Some feel that if the bird has the opportunity to play with its plucked feathers the feather plucking habit can be aggravated.

Some chronic feather pickers may cut down on the practice following baths. Frequent sprays with lukewarm water or baths may alleviate the picking habit if it is caught before it becomes a firmly entrenched habit. Not all birds like to bathe. Some learn to like it in time. Many appreciate a fine spray. They can be sprayed several times daily. Some birds like to bathe in their water cup or in wet greens. Some bird owners take their parrots into the shower with them. Some birds prefer to bathe under a running faucet (carefully regulate the temperature). After a bird has bathed, make sure that it is thoroughly dry before nightfall and that it is not subjected to drafts. Bathing is best done outside of the cage so that perches, seed, and grit do not get wet. Once learned, a bath can become an enjoyable part of a bird's daily routine.

Try using a branch of a tree as a perch. Do not use a softwood perch that a parrot can destroy immediately. There are many reasonable hardwoods, such as apple, pear, peach, plum, cherry, willow, maple, eucalyptus, nut, madrone, and manzanita, to mention a few, that are readily available. The bird can pick at the bark and also exercise its feet. Do not overcrowd the cage with branches.

If the bird is tame, give it an opportunity to fly around the room. The owner should be present to watch so that the bird does not get into trouble. The bird should be kept away from open flames, boiling pots, hot running water, electric mixers, toasters, fans, dishwashers, uncovered light bulbs, opened doors or windows, uncovered windows, poisonous plants, and so.

Avoid stressful situations, e.g., other pets that threaten the bird, humans who tease the bird, and so on. Feather picking may sometimes be a reaction to stress.

Suggest feeding the bird so that it has to work harder at eating. For example, add small pebbles (big enough so that they cannot be swallowed) in the food cups so that the bird has to move the pebbles around to get at the seeds. If the bird has to hunt for the food it might pick at its feathers less.

Sometimes a change in the photo period helps, i.e., alternating short and long days every two weeks. The short day should consist of 8 hours of light and 16 hours of dark (such as in a closet). The long days should be reversed, i.e., 8 hours of dark and 16 hours of light. Encouraging results are sometimes obtained within two months.

Try playing a record or tape of bird sounds. If this is unsuccessful, suggest that the owner acquire a companion bird. If there already is a companion bird, try separating them and observe any favorable behavior change. I do not encourage obtaining another bird unless the client really wants a second bird. Some clients who obtain a second bird end up with two feather pickers. The first bird can teach the second bird to pick.

Tranquilizers may be helpful. Often, but not always, the dose required to stop the picking would sedate the bird outwardly and thus would be undesirable. The dosage varies, and trial and error is needed to determine the correct dosage. Start low and increase the dose until either feather picking ceases or obvious sedation occurs. Examples of drugs that may be tried include diazepam (injectable Valium,* 5 mg/ml) given in drinking water at a starting dose of 2 drops/oz of drinking water; and phenobarbital oral suspension, given by direct oral administration at a starting dose of 0.003 mg/gm body weight two times daily.

Rarely, birds will start to pull their feathers because of mites, which cause itching. These birds may be scratching as well as picking. Red mites are tiny gray bugs that do not usually live on the birds during the day. Rather, they live in tiny crevices of the perches and cage or aviary. They usually come out at night and feast on the blood of the birds and then return to their holes in the morning. They often look red because of the blood they have engorged. The birds are often agitated by their presence. If their presence is suspected, suggest that the client cover the cage with a piece of white cloth at night and check it the following morning for tiny red specks. These mites are uncommon in individual pet birds.

---

*Roche Labs, Nutley, NJ.

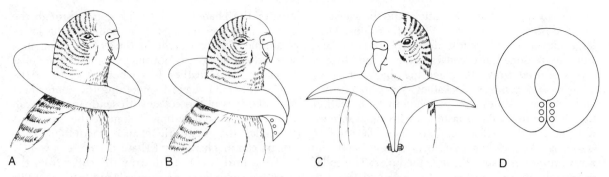

Figure 1. Elizabethan collar. *A*, For budgerigar. *B*, For large parrot, side view; (*C*) front view. Note that the screws are placed on the posterior surface. *D*, Pattern for Elizabethan collar before it is attached with screws and bent posteriorly.

Thyroid hormone can decrease or stop feather picking in a small percentage of pickers. I use levothyroxine sodium (Synthroid* 0.1-mg tablets) at a dosage of ¼ tablet crushed and dissolved per oz of drinking water.

The use of progestational drugs can be helpful in a small percentage of cases. One such drug is medroxyprogesterone acetate (Depo/Provera† 100 mg/ml injectable suspension) given at a dosage of 0.07 mg/gm body weight as a single intramuscular injection. Side effects can include quietness, increased appetite, polydypsia, and polyuria. Another progestational drug that is beneficial in a small number of cases is megestrol acetate (Ovaban‡ 5-mg tablets) at a dosage of ¼ tablet (for a 400- to 600-gm parrot) crushed and placed in a small amount of food such as a banana. This dosage is given once daily for seven to ten days and then once or twice weekly.

Some clinicians feel that corticosteroids are helpful. I have used steroids on a limited number of birds without benefit. They may help relieve the rare case of self-inflicted skin irritation.

Negative reinforcement can be useful in some cases. Such tactics as squirting the bird with a water gun, scolding it verbally, making loud noises, scolding it with a fly swatter, and so on are helpful at times. Birds appear to realize that they are displeasing their owners.

The use of a restraint collar may stop the feather picking. Nothing less than physically inhibiting the bird from chewing itself or pulling its feathers is necessary in many birds. Keeping the collar on long enough for the feathers to grow back (two to three months) may stop feather pulling even after its removal. Other birds may start pulling feathers as soon as the collar is removed and need to wear the collar continuously. Some birds only pull their feathers during certain times of the year or during their molt or at certain times of the day (e.g., when the owner is at work). They may only have to wear collars during these times. With a collar on, the

feather sheath remains on the feather and does not allow the feather to open up. In such cases, owners can work these sheaths off or temporarily remove the collar and let the bird do it. In other birds the general activity of the bird seems to get the sheath off without the help of the beak.

A variety of mechanical devices may be used to inhibit birds from picking feathers. The most commonly used are the Elizabethan collar (Fig. 1) and the tubular collar (Fig. 2) and combinations thereof. Many experienced avian practitioners choose a collar as a last resort when other conservative attempts have failed. I used to take that approach. At present, I use the collar as an initial approach while instituting environmental changes. I feel that my results are quicker and better.

SUGGESTIONS FOR MAKING AND APPLYING ELIZABETHAN COLLARS

The proper use of the Elizabethan collar requires experience and patience. Application can be frustrating and time consuming. The goal is to fit a collar so that it is tolerated, not destroyed by the bird, does not injure the bird mechanically or psychologically, and keeps the bird from reaching the picked areas of the body. The collar should also be neat and attractive in appearance. These goals can be achieved in over 90 per cent of patients that I fit with collars.

The larger the bird's beak, the greater its ability

*Flint Laboratories, Deerfield, IL.
†Upjohn Co., Kalamazoo, MI.
‡Schering Corp., Kenilworth, NJ.

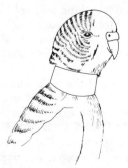

Figure 2. Tube collar.

to destroy the collar. Cockatiels and budgerigars rarely destroy collars, even soft leather ones. Most large parrots could rapidly destroy leather collars. For this reason, I use collars made of four to five layers of used x-ray film glued together with spray adhesive for conures, cockatoos, Amazon parrots, and macaws. Holes are punched with a leather punch, and the collar is fastened with small screws, nuts, and washers. The holes are placed face to face (see Fig. 1D) rather than overlapping, and the screws are then placed through the holes. The collar is then bent backward (see Fig. 1B and C). The bird is unable to loosen the screws with its beak because they are on the posterior surface of the collar. I also feel that the bending backwards of the collar makes the bird more able to tolerate the collar, as the bird can see behind it better. Three to four screws are used to fasten the collar. They should be close enough together to prevent the bird's beak from reaching between the screw holes from the anterior surface of the collar and loosening the screws. The screws should be tightened well so that the bird's movements do not loosen them.

In small birds such as budgerigars and cockatiels in which removal of the collar by the bird is not usually a problem, I do not bend the collar backward (see Fig. 1A). A piece of clear tape is placed on the posterior surface to keep the cut edges of the collar together. If staples are used, do not place the loops of the staples on the posterior surface of the collar where the bird's nails may become caught. If x-ray film is used on these smaller birds, one to two layers are usually sufficient. Tube collars can also be made of x-ray film padded with tape and then secured with tape in a tubular fashion around the neck (see Fig. 2).

The size of the Elizabethan collar varies, of course, with the size of the bird. The following are average diameters of patterns that I use for Elizabethan collars for commonly seen psittacine birds (specific birds may require larger or smaller collars depending on variations in size within a species, tolerance to the collar, and dexterity in getting around the collar): budgerigar, 6 cm; small cockatiel, 9 cm; large cockatiel, half-moon conure, 11 cm; 200- to 400-gm Amazon parrot, rose-breasted cockatoo, severe macaw, 17 cm; 400- to 500-gm Amazon parrot, 20 cm; 500- to 600-gm Amazon parrot, 23 cm; military macaw, blue and gold macaw, scarlet macaw, large Moluccan cockatoo, 33 cm; green-winged macaw, hyacinth macaw, 40 cm (note: 14 × 17-inch x-ray film is large enough for this size collar).

The center hole of the collar should allow you to freely move the collar without it touching the neck. On an Amazon parrot's collar, for example, there should be about ¼ inch or more between the collar and the skin of the neck. The larger the hole, the less the chance of mechanical irritation but the greater the chance of the beak going through the center hole and damaging the collar or the lower mandible getting caught in the collar. Even in a well-fitted collar, it is not uncommon for the collar to cause some feather loss where it rubs on the neck feathers. I suggest smoothing the center hole and all edges of the collar with sandpaper to minimize mechanical irritation. The more the bird fights the collar, the greater the chance of irritation. Tube collars can mechanically irritate the neck as well.

If the bird is able to destroy the collar from the neck hole or if the bird still pulls out feathers on its neck anterior to the collar, a small tube collar may be placed below the Elizabethan collar to push the Elizabethan collar closer to the head so that the beak cannot reach it.

If your practice sees a significant number of birds, I suggest making up collars of various sizes ahead of time and having them ready for future feather pickers. In addition to the increased efficiency of storing preassembled collars, if you bend the collar and insert the screws before the glue sets completely, the layers are bonded together better and the collar is fixed in the bent shape for easier application to the feather picker later.

The adjustment period following placement of a collar varies from immediate acceptance (rare), to a few hours, to few days, to total inacceptance (rare). The initial adjustment period can be violent, with the bird acting as if it has lost its balance. It may flap wildly about the cage, hold its head down, vocalize, lie on its back or side with its feet on the back of the collar, and so on. Some are so violent that injury may result unless the collar is removed. In such cases, I usually put on a smaller collar and let the bird get used to that before going to a larger collar. The smaller collar may not prevent the bird from reaching its feathers to pick but may accustom the bird to having something around its neck. In some cases the bigger collar can be applied the following day. In other cases I wait a few weeks. I routinely hospitalize birds for placement of collars. I explain the adjustment period to the client, but I do not feel that it is good for them to observe this initial adjustment behavior. Furthermore, time is needed for the veterinarian to evaluate whether the collar meets all of the desired criteria mentioned previously. Hospitalization allows this time. The patient usually goes home the next day, but sometimes it will take several days and several adjustments before an acceptable collar is created.

Upon admission, the patient is usually given a few hours to adjust to the hospitalization before a collar is applied. Some birds will not eat in the hospital, and some birds will not eat with a collar on. The first few hours of hospitalization without a collar on helps the clinician evaluate this aspect. Some birds will not eat with the collar on in the hospital but will eat with it on at home. If the budgerigar does not eat after 24 hours at home or if the Amazon parrot does not eat after a few days at home, the collar should be removed and a smaller collar applied later after appetite has returned to normal. The client is instructed to observe the bird closely for loss of appetite and signs of irritation from the collar or loosening of the screws and to notify the hospital if problems arise. Problems are uncommon with properly applied collars. Another aspect of adjustment involves the bird's ability to climb around its cage with the collar on. At first the feet bump the collar as the bird climbs. Most birds learn to adjust after a few days. If the hospital bird housing areas do not have bars, this aspect of adjustment will have to begin at home, and the client should be informed of this.

THE CLIENT HANDOUT

The time allotted for an office visit for a client with a feather picker can be quite extensive. To save time and make it easier on the client, a handout is suggested. The client should read the handout before the veterinarian even walks into the examination room. I encourage the client to use the handout as a guide for his own imagination. After reading the handout, many clients come up with their own ideas for their particular bird. Even if the suggestions turn out not to be helpful, clients develop a more favorable, pleasurable, and mutually rewarding relationship with their pet bird after trying various suggestions.

THE WORK-UP SHEET

A mimeographed work-up sheet may help the veterinarian collect his observations concerning a particular case. The sheet should include the following:

1. Presenting complaint?
2. Duration of complaint?
3. Has the bird been a feather picker before?
4. Is the feather picking seasonal?
5. Does the bird pick all day long or just when owner is away, etc.?
6. Any attempted treatments? What? Results?
7. Duration of ownership?
8. Any environmental changes concurrent with the start of feather picking, e.g., a move, new family, change in diet, other new pet, etc.?
9. Is the bird apparently healthy in other respects? Is it listless? Does it talk less, eat less, squawk less, etc.?
10. Does the bird actually eat the food provided? Source of minerals, grit, vitamins?
11. Does the bird receive a lot of direct attention?

12. Does the bird appear to listen to radio or television or outside birds?
13. Any other birds in the house? If so, do they have a feather picking problem?
14. What toys does the bird have and how does it react to them?
15. Is there a mirror accessible to the bird?
16. Where is the cage located? Has the location been changed recently? Is there a lot of family activity in this location?
17. Does the owner see the bird pulling its feathers?
18. If there is another bird in the same cage, could that bird be pulling this bird's feathers?
19. Is the cage an adequate size?
20. How much sleep does the bird get? Is the cage covered at night?
21. Are fallen feathers removed from the cage?
22. At what rate is the bird pulling out its feathers and what areas does it pick at most? Diagram areas of feather loss.
23. Does the bird bathe or get sprayed?
24. What types of perches are used?
25. When was the bird's last molt? What is this bird's usual molting pattern?
26. Has the owner seen mites, fleas, lice, etc., on the bird or in the cage?
27. How tame is the bird?
28. Are the wings clipped?
29. Does the bird get out of the cage?
30. Does the bird scratch as well as pick at its feathers?
31. Does the bird lay eggs or rear young?
32. Any change in environmental temperature?
33. Assessment of the owner's attitude about the problem; i.e., how much effort will the owner put forth and how upset will he be if all attempts fail?

IF THERAPY IS UNSUCCESSFUL

If you run out of things to try and are still not getting results, the client will have to learn to live with a feather picking bird. There are worse problems that could afflict the bird. Most feather pickers can remain in good health if properly cared for and kept out of drafts. In some unsuccessful cases when clients are told that it is okay that their bird is a feather picker and that they should not feel guilty, they accept the habit and it does not bother them as much.

SUPPLEMENTAL READING

Lafeber, T. J.: Feather disorders of common caged birds. *In* Kirk, R. W. (ed.): *Current Veterinary Therapy* V. Philadelphia: W. B. Saunders, 1974.

RHINOTRACHEITIS IN NONDOMESTIC CATS

WILLIAM J. BOEVER, D.V.M.

St. Louis, Missouri

Feline viral rhinotracheitis is the most common and most serious disease of the exotic feline respiratory system. Feline calicivirus is also a common respiratory disease of cats but is much less serious. It often occurs concurrently with feline viral rhinotracheitis.

Feline viral rhinotracheitis virus has a tropism for the upper respiratory tract and conjunctiva, whereas calicivirus more commonly infects the oral mucosa and lungs.

Feline viral rhinotracheitis, a herpesvirus with worldwide distribution, has been reported in numerous nondomestic cats including cheetahs, clouded leopards, jaguars, Asiatic and African leopards, mountain lions, and fishing cats. It is suspected that all felines have the potential susceptibility to feline viral rhinotracheitis.

VIRAL CHARACTERISTICS

Feline viral rhinotracheitis virus produces a characteristic cytopathic effect in feline tissue cultures and forms acidophylic intranuclear inclusion bodies in infected cultured cells as well as in cells of the respiratory tract. The virus is fragile and survives less than 18 hours outside the host.

ROUTE OF INFECTION AND TRANSMISSION

The route of infection is by means of infectious aerosols entering through either the nasal, oral, or conjunctival membranes. The virus reproduces rapidly in the epithelial cells of the upper respiratory tract and the conjunctiva, resulting in the characteristic lesions and symptoms. During the course of the infection, large amounts of highly infectious virus are shed in the oropharyngeal, ocular, and nasal secretions for a period of one to three weeks. It has been reported that carrier cats may shed the virus intermittently for at least one year.

CLINICAL SYNDROME

The clinical syndrome as presented in exotic cats is similar to that seen in domestic cats; however, not all symptoms are always present. Depression is sometimes present, although this is often difficult to judge in the nondomestic cat. Serous to mucopurulent conjunctival or nasal discharge is almost always present. The temperature elevation that results in the domestic cat is difficult to assess in the exotic cat because of the temperature variability caused by restraint. Anorexia and dehydration are of grave significance, since they can often lead to emaciation and death in the exotic cat. Secondary bacterial invaders often complicate the disease, adding to its severity. In one case of five clouded leopards, there were minimal ocular lesions with severe ulceration of the nasal and oral mucous membranes. In a separate case involving six cheetahs, ulcerative keratitis and corneal opacities were the most significant lesions, with only mild upper respiratory symptomatology.

Feline viral rhinotracheitis has been responsible for abortions in domestic cats, and the same syndrome has been reported in clouded leopards with feline viral rhinotracheitis.

The duration of the clinical illness is usually only 7 to 21 days; however, when anorexia and severe dehydration occur in the exotic cats, causing general debility, it is often life-threatening. The nondomestic cats seem to take longer to recover from the disease, and severely affected animals often die; however, in my experience, those that recover do not usually have chronic sequelae, as do their domestic counterparts.

The morbidity may reach 100 per cent in susceptible cats, and the mortality is usually higher than 25 per cent in nondomestic cats because of the difficulty in administering supportive care.

DIAGNOSIS

A leukocytosis is usually present throughout the course of the disease, and intranuclear inclusion bodies may be present in the tissues of cats that die from feline viral rhinotracheitis. The herpesvirus responsible for feline viral rhinotracheitis can be isolated from the tissues of infected cats or from swabbings from the ocular, nasal, or oropharyngeal mucosa. These are best demonstrated in the early stages of the disease. Virus-neutralizing antibody can be detected in the serum of cats during the convalescent stage.

THERAPY

The goal of therapy is to offer supportive care during the acute and convalescent stages of infection by preventing dehydration, starvation, and secondary invasion. The aim is to bring the cat through the disease with minimal long-term sequelae.

There are no drugs available to counteract feline viral rhinotracheitis; however, treatment should be tailored to combat the specific symptoms presented. Antibiotics should be used to control secondary bacterial infections. The choice of antibiotics should be determined from cultures and sensitivities obtained from smears of the nasal and ocular discharges. Intramuscular drugs are almost always preferred with nondomestic cats because of the difficulty of oral administration. Physically administering a drug to a nondomestic feline on a regular basis is usually impossible, and mixing the medication in the food makes the food less attractive to a cat that is potentially anorexic.

The nursing care that is so essential is the most difficult part of the treatment process. Affected cats should be kept clean and warm, and the discharge from the eyes and nose should be removed frequently. The ulcerated lesions in the nose may be flushed with povidone iodine (Betadine) solution. Antihistamines and mucolytic agents may be useful in maintaining clear airways. The eyes, if severely involved, will require subconjunctival injection with antibiotics as well as daily (preferably four times a day) administration of antibiotics, steroids, atropine, or other eye medications, depending on how the lesions are progressing and whether or not ulcerations of the cornea are present.

The animal must continue to eat. This more than any other sign will determine the outcome. Eating should first be encouraged by giving the regular diet. Once the animal stops consuming that diet, start changing to more appealing diets, stronger flavored foods or freshly killed rats or guinea pigs. If the cat refuses to eat completely, force feeding with a stomach tube is required and a pharyngostomy may be indicated, especially in the highly fractious individual. If dehydration is evident, subcutaneous or intravenous fluid administration is also indicated.

It is very difficult to maintain good supportive care in the nondomestic cat. An aggressive approach is necessary. If the cat is small, very young, or gentle, nursing care can be carried out by catching the animal daily and restraining it by physical means; however, this is not the case with all nondomestics. If chemical immobilization is required to administer supportive care, then total treatment can only be carried out every other day. If the cat has to be chemically immobilized so that fluids can be administered or stomach tubes can be passed, some compromises have to be made. Ideally, daily or twice daily treatment is desired; however, chemical immobilization on a daily basis is counterproductive. A more aggressive approach is to chemically immobilize the cat, attach a pharyngostomy tube, and pass an IV catheter; then place the cat in a squeeze cage for daily administration of fluids and food during the course of the disease.

The treatment for feline viral rhinotracheitis is essentially the same for exotic and domestic cats. The trick is to devise ingenious methods to administer and carry out the treatment.

Little is known about chronically affected nondomestic cats. Most of the long-term problems are a result of secondary invasion: recurrent rhinitis, conjunctivitis, corneal scarring, and so on.

Over 80 per cent of recovered domestic cats are said to remain viral carriers, which have recurrent problems. Work has not been done to determine if this is true in nondomestic cats as well. In my experience the incidence of recurrent problems in recovered individuals is low. This may be due to a lower number of exotic cats recovering from the disease.

CONTROL AND PREVENTION

The ideal approach to control and prevention is vaccination. There are numerous vaccines against feline viral rhinotracheitis on the market for domestic cats. Some are modified live vaccines; others are killed vaccines. Some are for intramuscular use; others are to be given by the intranasal or intraocular route. All are recommended for use in healthy, unexposed domestic cats, and annual or six-month boosters are recommended.

Recent evidence, however, indicates that there should be some concern about using modified live virus vaccines for feline viral rhinotracheitis in exotic cats. The vaccine sometimes causes mild symptoms in domestic cats, and there is reason to believe that these symptoms can become quite severe in nondomestic felines.

The killed intramuscular feline viral rhinotracheitis vaccine would appear to be the safest. The cats should be vaccinated annually unless there is a high incidence of feline viral rhinotracheitis in the area, in which case six-month boosters would be advisable.

Exotic cats develop antibody titers against feline viral rhinotracheitis just as domestic cats do. Whether they have protection and immunity has not been determined, although one would suspect that immunity is established if antibody titers are obtained. It has long been a practice in nondomestic animal medicine to establish antibody titers by vaccinating the larger exotic cats with twice the domestic cat dose. Recent evidence indicates that this is no longer necessary. Single doses should be used on all cats.

Young cats should be vaccinated at 9 weeks of age and then every two to four weeks until 16 weeks of age. Adult cats being vaccinated for the first time should receive two doses of vaccine three to four weeks apart.

SUPPLEMENTAL READING

Boever, W. J., McDonald, S., and Solorzano, R. F.: Feline viral rhinotracheitis in a colony of clouded leopards. V.M./S.A.C. 72:1859, 1977.
Bush, M., Povey, R. C., and Koonse, H.: Antibody response to an inactivated vaccine for rhinotracheitis, caliciviral disease and panleukopenia in nondomestic felids. J.A.V.M.A. 179:1203, 1981.
Gaskell, R., and Wardley, R. C.: Feline viral respiratory disease: a review with particular reference to its epizootiology and control. J. Small Anim. Pract. 19:1, 1977.
Kahn, D. E., and Hoover, E. A.: Infectious respiratory diseases of cats. Vet. Clin. North Am. 6:399, 1976.

RABBIT GASTROINTESTINAL DISORDERS

DALE L. BROOKS, D.V.M.
Davis, California

Gastrointestinal problems with primary signs of anorexia and diarrhea are the major causes of significant losses in rabbits. The etiology of GI disorders is often multifactorial and may include malocclusion of the jaw, tooth abscesses, osteomyelitis of the jaw, gastric hairballs, enteropathogenic bacteria, and coccidiosis. The stresses of transportation, restraint, weather changes, feed changes, competition for or restricted access to food and water, parturition, lactation, weaning, old age, uterine adenocarcinoma, pasteurellosis, ectoparasites, pain, husbandry practices, and other poorly understood factors may predispose rabbits to anorexia and diarrhea.

TEETH

Anorexia and drooling, which sometimes causes a wet dewlap with a moist bacterial dermatitis, may be controlled by clipping the overgrown incisor teeth every six to eight weeks using a dog nail trimmer. These malocclusions may also affect the molar teeth (and are difficult to correct), resulting in a chronic wasting with eventual death. Since malocclusion of the rabbit's jaw is genetically inherited, breeding stock passing this trait should be culled. Molar teeth with caries not uncommonly develop fistulas, resulting in osteomyelitis of the jaw. Careful palpation will reveal bony irregularities of the jaw, which may progress to skin abscesses. Radiographs easily provide a positive diagnosis. Early removal of the affected tooth may be helpful, but the osteomyelitis responds poorly to therapy and the prognosis is guarded.

HAIRBALLS

The gastric hairball of the cat is similar to that of the rabbit; however, the rabbit cannot vomit. Cat laxatives preparations* are occasionally successful in eliminating the rabbit's gastric hairball. Identification of a gastric trichobezoar obstruction is difficult, and rabbits may die within three to four weeks of starvation. Animals with a partial obstruction may live for several months, showing increased cachexia. Abdominal palpation is frequently inconclusive and may traumatize the very friable liver and stomach. Both plain and contrast radiography are not diagnostic, since hairballs and fasted rabbits show similar findings of delayed emptying and filling defects in the gastric lumen. Definitive diagnosis requires an exploratory gastrotomy. Operative management includes correcting fluid, electrolyte, vitamin, and caloric imbalances. Broad spectrum antibiotics are administered to decrease commonly occurring secondary *Pasteurella* infections or infection secondary to the gastrotomy. Often a true trichobezoar is not found, so it is important to carefully empty all the ingesta from the stomach. Small multiple hairballs, a less discrete aggregate of hair, or only a plug of hair occluding the narrow pyloric lumen may be present. Postoperative administration of fluids, vitamins, antibiotics, and *per os* live *Lactobacillus* culture is critical to successful surgery and resolution of anorexia.

---

*Kit-Tonne Laxative, Haver-Lockhart, Bayvet Div., Cutter Labs, Shawnee, KS.

BACTERIAL DIARRHEA

The enteropathy complex of rabbits is poorly defined and difficult to manage. The known etiologies include enteropathogenic *E. coli*, *Clostridium perfringens* type E, *Bacillus piliformis* (Tyzzer's disease), *Yersinia pseudotuberculosis*, *Salmonella typhimurium*, and yeast overgrowths of the intestinal flora. The enteropathy complex is called hemorrhagic and nonhemorrhagic diarrhea, typhlitis, impaction, and bloat. The term most commonly used is *mucoid enteritis* (mucoid enteropathy). Mortality ranges from 5 to 90 per cent. Bacterial diarrheic deaths occur in the following age groups: seven- to ten-day-old suckling rabbits, four- to eight-week-old late suckling to weanling rabbits, mature does a few days pre and post partum, and recently stressed young and mature adults.

Dead seven- to ten-day-old suckling rabbits frequently have fully distended stomachs containing a large firm milk curd. Baby rabbits need only nurse once for three to five minutes every 24 hours. Often orphaned neonates are fed too frequently, causing distention of the stomach and an increased tendency for aspiration pneumonia. Frequently, there are no clinical signs other than hypothermia with body temperatures one to two degrees below normal (101°F average) and an ileus. Gross necropsy findings vary from no lesions to a mildly hyperemic small intestine and an occasional hemorrhagic typhlitis. A cold nest box is a significant predisposing factor, depending on environmental temperature and quantity of fur in the nest made by the doe. Once affected, the entire litter is usually lost within 24 hours. The doe of affected sucklings frequently remains healthy. These baby rabbits may not have the normal antimicrobial "milk oil" that maintains an essentially sterile gut during the first two to three weeks of life prior to eating solid foods. *Clostridium perfringens* type E toxins and some enterotoxic *E. coli* are the primary isolates in these early deaths and in older rabbits with diarrhea. Other than the preventive measures of adding fur that has been saved from a clean weaned nest box and heating the environment, there is no treatment.

The second age group with diarrhea is the four- to eight-week-old late suckling to weanling rabbits. These rabbits are usually growing well, appear healthy, and are fed pelleted rations *ad libitum*. There is no set pattern to the diarrhea outbreak. Diarrhea affects two to three rabbits per litter or, at times, the entire litter, with a sporadic cage incidence throughout the rabbitry. The does are usually healthy, and the disease does not appear to be contagious. The course and signs of diarrhea are variable, lasting from a few hours to one week. Very few rabbits recover, and an ileus is often present 12 to 72 hours before death. The stomachs are frequently fully distended, with ingesta varying in consistency from a semiliquid to a solidly packed, wet alfalfa meal food ball. The intestine is fluid and gas filled with variable amounts of clear gelatinous mucin with and without paintbrush-like hemorrhages in the subserosa of the cecum. These hemorrhages may extend to the distal ileum and proximal colon. Petechial hemorrhages are occasionally seen in the gastric mucosa. The small intestine may be hyperemic, although generally there are no signs of inflammation. The cecum, in about 25 per cent of cases, contains a semisolid to dry impacted mass of ingesta. The commonly reported mucin-filled colon is present in only 30 per cent of the necropsies.

Tyzzer's disease is called acute bacillary typhlitis owing to the increased hemorrhage and pathology in this area. The liver may show multi-focal pinpoint areas of necrosis, and similar changes may be seen in the myocardium. *Bacillus piliformis* will not grow on ordinary laboratory media, and positive diagnosis is based on histologic demonstration of the filamentous clumps of organisms by periodic acid–Schiff, Giemsa, or Wartin-Starry stain. Paratyphoid is much less commonly reported, and diagnosis is based on positive cultures. *Yersina pseudotuberculosis* is also uncommon and is caused by ingestion of feeds contaminated by the feces of birds and rodents. Diagnosis is confirmed by finding gross, whitish-yellow caseous nodules in the gut mucosal wall and abdominal organs. Smears and cultures from these lesions are diagnostic. The feeding of "greens" obtained from the grocery may be the source of diarrhea, since the discarded outer leaves are more apt to be contaminated by feces, insecticides, and fertilizers.

The third age group of rabbits in which diarrhea is seen consists of mature does a few days pre or post partum. The fourth group comprises weanling and mature animals recently stressed by restraint procedures, injection, sampling techniques, changes in environment, and dietary intake. Signs and known etiologies of anorexia and diarrhea for these groups are similar to those for the four- to eight-week-old group.

The predisposition of rabbits to the enteritis complex has become more widespread with the common practice of *ad libitum* feeding of pelleted rations. Caged rabbits tend to overeat, producing a semidry compact food mass in the stomach that is poorly penetrated by antimicrobial gastric acids. This condition forms a suitable environment for growth and toxin production by enterotoxic bacteria. It is during the critical transition from the relatively sparse gastrointestinal flora of the suckling (controlled by the antimicrobial "milk oil") with a stomach pH of 5 to 6 to the established flora of the weanling–young adult with a stomach pH of 1 to 2 that most diarrheas occur. The incidence of diarrhea may be reduced by limiting the intake of pelleted feeds, increasing the crude fiber content of the pellets to 16 to 25 per cent, and supplementing the diet with whole grains and good quality hays. The resulting gastric food mass is of larger particle size and greater porosity. This allows for a thorough penetration of the food mass by gastric acids, thus a more rapidly lowering pH to inhibit populations of potentially infective organisms.

Complete control of anorexia and diarrhea is difficult, but at times a careful history and correction of any modifications of the normal rabbitry routine may be sufficient to restore the situation to normal. Often just the supplementation of a high quality hay for five to ten days will stop an outbreak, especially when a new batch of pellets has been fed. Most stress-induced anorexia and diarrhea of the rabbit respond to supportive therapy and dietary supplementation of the pelleted ration within five to seven days. The addition of calf manna* may quickly stimulate the rabbit's appetite and may curtail diarrhea.

Non-responsive rabbits require more aggressive measures. Correction of the dehydration and electrolyte balance is essential through administration of lactated Ringer's solution at a dose of 20 ml/kg subcutaneously twice daily for three to five days. Corticosteroids, such as dexamethasone, 0.5 mg/kg, will enhance stress tolerance. Since sick rabbits do not practice their normal coprophagy, a multi-B vitamin supplement at a dose of 0.5 to 1 ml is often useful. Systemic broad spectrum antibiotics are administered to the rabbit at cat dosages for three to five days.

An imbalance in the rabbit's gastrointestinal flora may be the cause of diarrhea, the result of diarrhea, or the result of antibiotic therapy. A slurry of Nutrical,† live *Lactobacillus* culture,‡ and 50 per cent dextrose is given via stomach tube at an initial dose not to exceed 30 ml. This mixture or plain yogurt is continued for up to ten days at a dose of 6 ml twice daily inserted in the rabbit's cheekspace with a disposable syringe. The use of a live *Lactobacillus* culture decreases the number of enteric *E. coli* and may have prophylactic benefit in preventing an overgrowth of enterotoxic bacteria. It also is a good nutritive supplement.

The anorexia-diarrhea therapy described previously may benefit individual cases, but it is not practical for large numbers of rabbits. Strict husbandry practices of effective hygiene, group segregation of rabbits by size, and careful observation to supply adequate rations for economic production without overeating must be instituted. The daily intake of pelleted ration may need to be limited to 4 to 8 oz per rabbit. Changing the crude fiber content of the pellets up to 16 to 25 per cent and/or adding a hay supplement may be beneficial.

The drinking water may be supplemented with a calf scours vitamin-electrolyte preparation.§ Most treatments are nonspecific and are aimed at reducing the number of enteric organisms. The rabbits' drinking water may be medicated with chlorotetracycline‖ or dimetridazole. Chlortetracycline reduces aerobic enteric organisms when given at a dosage of 0.25 per cent in the drinking water. Dimetridazole (Emtryl**) reduces enteric clostridial organisms when given at a dosage of 0.025 per cent (45 gm/190 l or 50 gal) of the drinking water. The dispensing of some drinking water preparations is greatly facilitated by using a poultry drug proportionater in rabbitries with automatic watering systems. A word of caution: rabbits may be further dehydrated by not drinking unpalatable medicated water.

Sulfaquinoxaline- and tetracycline-medicated rabbit pellets are both available commercially. Some rabbitries routinely use medicated feeds for three to seven days each month or during the critical three- to eight-week-old age period as a "sometimes successful" method of controlling diarrhea losses. Since the enteric bacterial synthesis of the B group of vitamins is reduced by these antimicrobial drugs, the rabbit needs a vitamin B supplement. The rabbit's medication schedule must comply with specific drug withdrawal rules (ranging from 5 to 30 days post treatment) for slaughter animals; however, most veterinary products do not have specific FDA clearance for use in the rabbit. The complex etiology of the anorexia-diarrhea syndrome is still poorly defined, and many of the suggested courses of therapy are of little value in the rabbit.

YEASTS

A wet mount and flotation technique examination of the feces or intestinal contents may be useful aids in the diagnosis of rabbit diarrhea. The yeast *Saccharomyces guttulatus* is found in small numbers in healthy rabbits. The cells are about 15 to 18 μ long with parallel sides and may be confused with coccidial oocysts. Little is known of its pathogenicity, and it may be the predominant finding in a anorexic-diarrheic rabbit, especially after a course of antibiotic therapy. Nystatin, which is readily available in some canine ear medications (Panalog††), given at a dose of 3 to 5 ml *per os* for several days, greatly reduces the numbers of this

---

*Carnation Milling Div., Kansas City, MO.
†Evsco Pharmaceutical Corp., Damon Co., Buena, NJ.
‡Bio-Max 10, CHR-Hansen Labs Inc., Milwaukee, WI.

§Ellradd-4000, Haver-Lockhart, Bayvet Div., Cutter Labs. Shawnee, KS.
‖Polyotic Solution Powder, American Cyanamid, Princeton, NJ.
**Salsbury Laboratories, Charles City, IA.
††E. R. Squibb & Sons, Inc., Princeton, NJ.

yeast. Live *Lactobacillus* cultures or a slurry of parasite-free fresh feces from a normal rabbit is essential to help re-establish the affected rabbit's appetite and gut flora.

COCCIDIOSIS

Coccidiosis is a very common finding in rabbits and is usually caused by a subclinical, opportunistic parasite. Owing to the prevalence of coccidiosis, its overall role in rabbit disease is difficult to assess. It is possible to have fatal coccidiosis without fecal shedding of oocysts and to have oocysts in the feces without the rabbit showing any clinical signs. Theoretically, strict hygiene, J-shaped feeders, automatic lixit valve waterers, and suspended wire-floored cages should adequately reduce fecal contamination. However, coccidiosis is rarely eliminated in practice. Many suckling rabbits are infected during the first three weeks of life inside the nest box, which is soiled by an asymptomatic carrier doe. Selection of does that maintain a clean nest box, thorough sanitization of nest boxes between litters, and regular cleaning of feces stuck to the cage wire surfaces, followed by application of a 10 per cent solution of household ammonia, are effective preventive measures. Coccidial oocysts are not infective when first passed in the feces and, depending on environmental temperature and humidity, take several days to sporulate (spores are the infective state ingested by the rabbit). Coccidiosis is best controlled by routine thorough sanitization one to two times per week, culling of dirty nest-box does, and periodic anticoccidial therapy. The dams of rabbits who show spotted livers (hepatic coccidiosis) at butchering should be culled. Drug therapy is not very effective in eliminating either intestinal or hepatic coccidiosis, but along with sanitization will reduce infectivity to subclinical levels. This will improve the rabbits' feed utilization, weight gain, and resistance to other diseases.

Sulfaquinoxaline* at a dose of 3.5 gm powder or 180 ml of a 20 per cent stock solution mixed in 4 liters of the rabbit's drinking water produces an approximate 0.1 per cent drug concentration. The rabbits are administered this medicated water for 14 to 21 days. After no medicated water for the next five to ten days, this therapy schedule should be repeated. Commercial rabbit pellets† are available with 0.025 per cent sulfaquinoxaline. This medicated ration may be fed for the stressful period of 3 to 8 weeks of age or up to 12 weeks of age. Some problem rabbitries routinely use medicated feed or water 3 to 14 days each month. Sulfaquinoxaline is one of the few rabbit medications approved by the Federal Food and Drug Administration. Treated animals should not be butchered for ten days post treatment. To date, the newer anticoccidial drugs have not been very palatable to the rabbit.

SUPPLEMENTAL READING

Cheeke, R. R., Patton, N. M., and Templeton, G. S.: Rabbit production. Oregon State Univ. Rabbit Res. Center, 1982.
Harkness, J. E., and Wagner, J. E.: *The Biology and Medicine of Rabbits and Rodents*. Philadelphia: Lea & Febiger, 1977.
Hime, J., and O'Donoghue, P. N.: *Handbook of Disease of Laboratory Animals*. London: Heinemann, 1979.
Weisbroth, S. H., Flatt, R. E., and Kraus, A. L.: *The Biology of the Laboratory Rabbit*. New York: Academic Press, 1974.
Williams, C. S. F.: *Practical Guide to Laboratory Animals*. St. Louis: C. V. Mosby, 1976.

*SQ 20% Solution, Merck Chem. Div., Rahway, NJ.
†RabbitAde, Carnation Co., Milling Div., Kansas City, MO.

TOTAL PARENTERAL NUTRITION IN EXOTIC ANIMALS

LYNDSAY G. PHILLIPS, Jr., D.V.M.

Omaha, Nebraska

We are sometimes presented with an animal in a cachectic state or with a disease condition that develops into a progressive, catabolic, nutritional condition. These cases prove difficult to manage with conservative methods; many animals fail to recover. Total parenteral nutrition (TPN), or parenteral hyperalimentation, in which all nutritional needs are provided intravenously, is an optional therapy available to any practitioner willing to devote the effort to attempt it. The major disadvantages of TPN include expense, time (the patient requires almost constant monitoring), and the risk of sepsis. However, there are situations (Table 1) in which the disadvantages are far outweighed by the animal's value.

Exotic, or nondomestic, pets are presented in

Table 1. *Indications for Total Parenteral Nutrition*

Severe malnourishment, catabolism
Inability to support nutritional needs enterally
Severe enteric losses
     Intractable diarrhea, ileus from any cause
     Gastrointestinal disease or trauma
Acute renal failure
Acute pancreatitis
Pre- and post-gastrointestinal surgery

depleted states most often because of chronic situations such as severe stress, poor management, improper nutrition, infection, or trauma. These result from the owners' lack of knowledge or inability to provide for the special needs of this type of animal.

The goal of TPN is to convert an animal in a negative nitrogen balance or severe catabolic state, starving and approaching death, to a stable condition of positive nitrogen balance, allowing time for resolution of the condition preventing enteral nutrition, producing a balanced metabolic state, and returning the animal to normal nutritional intake. This is accomplished by providing all of the patient's nutritional and caloric needs with continuous intravenous administration of a composite solution that provides essential calories, proteins, water and electrolytes, vitamins, and trace elements. Adequate levels of carbohydrates and lipids are provided to meet maintenance caloric needs, prevent loss of body protein, and provide energy. Nitrogen sources are added to produce an anabolic state.

CALORIC SOURCES

Glucose is the body's primary energy source; however, it cannot be the sole source of the patient's total caloric requirement in TPN. Used alone in levels sufficiently concentrated to supply maintenance caloric requirements, the glucose solution must be hypertonic (six times the osmolality of plasma). This solution will produce a severe lactic acidosis, hyperglycemia, glycosuria, and diuresis and must be infused into a large central vein, which will cause phlebitis and thrombosis in peripheral vessels. To avoid these complications, 10 per cent dextrose is used as a caloric source in total parenteral hyperalimentation mixtures. It is present in most of the commercial amino acid solutions designed for TPN. In patients exhibiting hyperglycemia using standard 10 per cent dextrose in the TPN solution, the addition of insulin is indicated to maximize glucose utilization and minimize hyperglycemia. It should be added to the parenteral nutrition solution so as to allow continuous administration rather than intermittently as in intramus-

cular injection. Starting levels in humans are 6 to 10 units of regular insulin added per 250 gm of glucose given (Grant, 1980). Other carbohydrate sources, such as fructose, sorbitol, and xylitol (in a ratio of 2:1:1), have been used in hyperglycemic patients with elevated insulin levels (Strombeck, 1979). These sugars are metabolized independently of insulin activity and glucose metabolism, are protein sparing, and are metabolized in the liver (limiting their use to patients with normal liver function). This mixture also reduces the chance of metabolic acidosis by limiting the production of lactic acid.

Lipid emulsion solutions (Intralipid* 10%, 20%; Liposyn†) are available that can provide up to 75 per cent of the animal's daily caloric needs when infused at a rate of 6 gm/kg/day (Strombeck, 1979). When used as the major source of calories in conjunction with glucose and amino acid administration, a positive nitrogen balance can be achieved. It can be infused into peripheral veins, as it exerts little osmolar pressure. The lipid solution is mixed with other infused fluids by allowing it to flow into the administration tubing as close as possible to the IV catheter. Peripheral administration allows easier catheter placement and reduces the risk of sepsis seen with large central venous catheterization. As the lipids become the major source of calories, the potential for hyperglycemia, seen with infusion of hypertonic glucose solutions, decreases.

With short-term therapy, no fatty acid deficiency is seen; however, this deficiency may occur during long-term therapy. Supplying linoleic acid in adequate levels (0.1 gm/kg/day) can prevent most fatty acid deficiencies. In the initial stage of therapy, the infusion of lipid should be cyclic to monitor the serum for clearance of lipemia. Serum Intralipid levels greater than 100 to 150 mg/dl indicate the need for a reduction in the volume of lipids infused to prevent overloading the patient with fats (represented clinically by hyperlipemia, fever, lethargy, hepatic damage, and coagulation disorders) (Kerner and Sunshine, 1979).

PROTEIN SOURCES

Formerly, the source of protein for TPN was limited to protein hydrolysates. These solutions, composed of large and small peptides, varied in their amino acid levels, were high in ammonia (resulting in azotemia, hyperaminoaciduria, hyperaminoacidemia, and hepatic encephalopathies in patients with liver disease), and could potentially cause hypersensitivity reactions owing to their an-

---

*Cutter Animal Health Laboratory, Shawnee, KS.
†Abbott Labs, North Chicago, IL.

tigenicity. Many of the peptides were unavailable for metabolism, as they were removed from the circulation by the reticuloendothelial and urinary systems.

Presently, nitrogen is provided using free, crystalline amino acids of various concentrations (Freeamine II;* Travasol, Travenol;† Aminosyn‡). Use of crystalline amino acids, rather than protein hydrolysates, allows for more efficient nitrogen use by decreasing the amount of protein required to achieve positive nitrogen balance (with simultaneous carbohydrate administration). With glucose in the infusate, nitrogen is spared as an energy source and is saved for building body tissue. These solutions more closely approach normal serum amino acid levels and can be individually formulated as needed by adding specific amino acids.

Measuring serum ammonia levels is necessary during TPN to prevent hyperammonemia. In neonates and seriously ill, malnourished adults, the addition of arginine, ornithine, and/or aspartic acid can alleviate hyperammonemia by working within the Kreb's cycle to convert ammonia to urea. Cessation of amino acid infusion is required if serum ammonia levels rise and cannot be controlled. It should be noted that administration of amino acid solutions containing hydrochloride salts may result in hyperchloremic acidosis; however, providing the acetate salts of the amino acids will prevent this pH imbalance.

ELECTROLYTE SOURCES

Amino acid and glucose solutions administered alone quickly lead to metabolic derangement, as tissue synthesis in the anabolic state consumes not only protein and calories but also electrolytes for intracellular incorporation. The water provided in the TPN solution usually meets the fluid requirements; more often, the animal receives fluid overloads during the attempt to supply sufficient nutrients. Supplying sufficient calories for anabolism in fluid volumes the animal can handle necessitates the use of hypertonic solutions.

The serum levels of potassium, calcium/phosphorus, sodium, chloride, and magnesium have to be monitored throughout TPN therapy to guard against ionic imbalances. Acid-base homeostasis is monitored by measuring bicarbonate levels in the serum.

In determining the electrolytes needed to restore the serum to normal levels during the first 24 hours of treatment, consider the cause that prompted use of parenteral hyperalimentation. With subsequent electrolyte therapy, additional amounts of intracellular electrolytes are required to meet the needs for reconstruction of lean body mass.

Potassium requirements increase greatly with TPN (usually double) to meet the intracellular requirements of tissue synthesis and the constant urinary excretion rate. Hypertonic glucose and insulin accelerate intracellular utilization of potassium. In dogs, 3 mEq potassium is utilized for each gram of nitrogen replaced in the body. Malnourished adults should be started at a rate of 1.2 to 1.5 mEq/kg/day (Grant, 1980). Neonates should be started at a rate of 2 to 3 mEq/kg/day (Kerner and Sunshine, 1979) and adjusted according to body needs as indicated by serum levels. Supplying potassium in the form of potassium phosphate and potassium chloride will reduce the potential for hyperchloremic acidosis.

Phosphate is another intracellular ion that the body requires. For each kilogram of lean body tissue replaced during TPN, administer phosphate levels of 80 mEq. With low serum phosphate levels the patient may develop weakness, seizures, anemia, neurologic disorders, and possibly death. Extracellular stores need to be replaced in ill animals and maintained at normal serum levels to prevent resorption of phosphate from the skeletal system. Minimally, 2 mM/kg/day should be administered in the infusate. This can be increased up to a maximum of 40 mEq/liter (Kerner and Sunshine, 1979), Strombeck, 1978). Calcium should be included to prevent hypocalcemia.

Most TPN solutions provide sufficient sodium to meet body needs; however, with hyperglycemia and glycosuria, diuresis occurs, resulting in an excess sodium loss that must be corrected during fluid administration. Care must be taken to decrease sodium levels administered to patients with renal failure or heart disease.

Magnesium is efficiently conserved by the body but is lost to some degree with catabolism and to a greater extent with starvation combined with high gastrointestinal and renal losses. The addition of magnesium sulfate at the rate of 4 to 8 mEq/liter of infusate (0.25 to 0.5 mEq/kg/day) will alleviate hypomagnesemia (Grant, 1980).

The chloride level should be adjusted to equal the level of sodium to prevent hyperchloremic acidosis. This is most efficiently achieved by using nonchloride salts as sources of sodium and potassium.

In most animals requiring TPN, therapy is short enough that stores of trace elements are not depleted. However, with long-term therapy or in the neonate, blood and bone changes can manifest as zinc and copper deficiencies. In these cases, after seven days of treatment, zinc sulfate should be added at a rate of 40 mEq/kg/day and copper sulfate at a rate of 30 mEq/kg/day (Kerner and Sunshine, 1979).

---

*American McGaw, Irvine, CA.
†Cutter Animal Health Laboratory, Shawnee, KS.
‡Abbott Labs, North Chicago, IL.

VITAMINS

Vitamin therapy is indicated in the debilitated patient. Care should be taken to avoid indiscriminate administration of vitamins, however. Both the B and C complexes can be given intravenously daily; however, the fat-soluble vitamins should be supplemented by giving 1 ml of M.V.I. (Multi-Vitamin Infusate*) once weekly in the infusate. Folic acid, vitamin B_{12}, and vitamin K should be given weekly as intramuscular injections, since these vitamins are oxidized if placed in the glucose–amino acid IV solutions.

Homeostasis of serum acid-base levels is mandatory. Maintaining proper pH is aided by adding sodium, potassium, calcium, and magnesium as acetate, lactate, phosphate, and sulfate salts, respectively. Bicarbonate should not be added to the TPN solution, as this will result in precipitation of calcium and magnesium in the infusate.

METHOD OF ADMINISTRATION

Total nutritional therapy normally is a continuous process. When lipid emulsions are added as the main caloric source, the osmolality of the solutions is decreased; therefore, they may be administered through a peripheral vessel, with much less risk of phlebitis and thrombosis. If hypertonic glucose solutions (greater than 10 per cent) are used, they must be administered into a large central vein. This increases the risk of sepsis. With this in mind, calculations of dosages of protein, glucose, and lipid solutions should be made for a 24-hour period. Table 2 provides an example of a TPN solution formula.

Alternatively, parenteral hyperalimentation can be given on a cyclic basis. Provide the lipids and amino acids during 10- to 12-hour periods only, and administered glucose and electrolytes continuously. Another method of parenteral hyperalimentation is to withhold glucose eight to ten hours each day and

*U.S. Vitamin and Pharmaceutical Corp., Tuckahoe, NY.

Table 2. *Daily Dietary Composition—*
*Total Parenteral Nutrition**†*

Nutrient	Source	Vol (ml)	Gm	Cal (Kcal)
Fats	Intralipid 10%	350	35	325
Carbohydrates	Dextrose 10%	100	10	41
Proteins (and electrolytes)	Travasol 8.5%	100	8.5	35
Total		550		401

*For a 10-kg adult dog.
†Data from Strombeck: *Small Animal Gastroenterology.* Davis, CA: Stonegate Publishing, 1979.

use only a 3 per cent amino acid or a 3 per cent amino acid with lipid emulsion during that period. This produces a more normal postabsorptive state so that (1) serum insulin levels (stimulated by glucose infusion) will fall as well as serum glucose levels; (2) infused amino acids may be utilized for visceral synthesis rather than being forced into muscle compartments; and (3) lipogenesis will be reduced, aiding in prevention of fatty, enlarged livers due to glycogen storage and allowing calories to be available for use in metabolic processes. TPN fluids can be given using conventional intravenous administration sets, microdrip administrations sets, or burette-type precision infusion sets (Soluset†) by gravity flow. However, for ease and accuracy of administration and to maintain catheter patency, positive pressure intravenous administration should be utilized with an IV infusion pump (IMED Volumetric Infusion Pump‡).

Whenever a TPN solution must be stopped, 5 per cent dextrose infusion should be continued to avoid sudden hypoglycemia due to the high endogenous insulin secretion stimulated by the composite solutions.

As previously mentioned, careful monitoring of the patient is essential during parenteral hyperalimentation. Serum potassium, phosphate, sodium, and chloride levels; BUN; and ammonia, acid/base, and urine glucose values should be determined daily until they remain stable and then at least twice weekly. Complete blood counts are important, as they signal anemia or sepsis. Hydration status, body temperature, body weight, and vital signs should be checked frequently to monitor patient status and the possibility of sepsis. Complete, constant, aseptic catheter care is as important as biochemical tests. Dressings should be replaced frequently and should be kept clean. The TPN system and catheter should not be used for administration products other than hyperalimentation solutions.

COMPLICATIONS

A variety of factors may require solution adjustment or catheter removal. Hyper- or hypoglycemia, acidosis or alkalosis, hydration upset, electrolyte imbalances, and hyperammonemia can be corrected by adjusting the composition of the TPN solution. Sepsis must be treated with antibiotics but may also require removal of the catheter to eliminate the source of contamination. Some patients develop increased levels of serum enzymes and signs of cholestasis, but these usually subside with discontinuation of TPN therapy. Parenteral hyperalimen-

†Abbott Labs, North Chicago, IL.
‡IMED Corp., San Diego, CA.

tation can be attempted again once complications have been resolved.

WITHDRAWAL FROM THERAPY

With patient improvement, i.e., weight gain, stabilization of the starved patient, correction of gastrointestinal problems, stabilization of serum BUN levels in acute renal failure, or return of the ability to take sufficient enteral nutrition, steps should be taken to remove TPN therapy. Begin limited oral intake and reduce intravenous therapy. As patient intake achieves half of the caloric and fluid needs, the volume of infusion should be reduced by one-third to one-half. If the patient tolerates this and can take three-fourths of daily main-tainance calories orally, administer 5 per cent dextrose at a low flow rate overnight and remove the catheter the following morning.

REFERENCES AND SUPPLEMENTAL READING

Advances in parenteral nutrition. Proceedings of the International Symposium of Intensive Therapy, Bermuda, May, 1977.
Berry, W. R., Press, H., and Hirztz, R. M.: Hyperalimentation: a review. Milit. Med. 144:(1), November, 1979.
Fisher, J. F. (ed.): *Total Parenteral Nutrition*. Boston: Little, Brown and Co., 1976.
Grant, J. P.: *Handbook of Total Parenteral Nutrition*. Philadelphia: W. B. Saunders, 1980.
Kerner, J. A., and Sunshine, P.: *Parenteral Alimentation*, Seminars in Perinatology, Vol. III (4), October, 1979.
Strombeck, D. R.: Parenteral hyperalimentation. *In Small Animal Gastroenterology*. Davis, CA: Stonegate Publishing, 1979, pp. 540–545.
Total parenteral alimentation. Proceedings of the International Symposium of Intensive Therapy, Rome, 1975.

SKIN DISORDERS OF NONDOMESTIC CARNIVORES

THAD E. THORSON, D.V.M.

Long Beach, California

The order Carnivora, which has 7 families and over 200 species, contains animals that are found in diverse ecological zones and niches. These animals are distributed from the Arctic tundra to the tropical forest and may be aquatic, terrestrial, arboreal, or fossorial in habitat.

The skin acts as a barrier, protecting the body from physical, chemical, or microbiologic injury. It also provides temperature regulation; sensory perception; storage of fats, electrolytes, and other materials as well as a myriad of other functions.

Animals inhabiting the areas of lower temperature zones have a denser coat of primary and secondary hairs and a thinner skin than animals of warmer climes. The success of many of these predators is largely dependent on protective coloration. The color of the haircoat may vary in intensity owing to natural selectivity. Thus, the haircoat of an animal found in the desert will be a shade lighter than that of an animal of the same color found in the forest. Some carnivores, such as the Arctic fox and the weasel, actually have seasonal molts; the color of the haircoat changes from natural to white in the winter.

DISEASE ENTITIES

PARASITIC DISEASES

SARCOPTIC MANGE

This has been reported in, among other animals, ferrets, foxes, wolves, fishers, coyotes, ocelots, and some of the procyonids. The lesions usually appear on the head and neck initially and then spread to the legs and belly. They can, however, appear almost anywhere. The first visible change is an increase in scale formation, followed by erythema and pustules. Intense pruritus is present. Thickening of the skin ensues with scab formation. Hairs break off or fall out. Severe skin changes can cause blindness, breathing difficulty, dehydration, exhaustion, and death. In foxes the disease is likely to appear first on the metatarsal, metacarpal, and elbow joints and ischial protuberances.

Treatment consists of dipping the animal (those in the Canidae and possibly the Hyaenidae and

Ursidae families) weekly for five weeks in Paramite* at the canine dose on the label. Dip all other animals weekly at one-half the feline dose and watch for toxicity. Atropine counteracts the action of the drug. Use Ectoral† only on canines, bears, and hyenas. Lime/sulfur‡ or Lym-Dyp§ can be used weekly for five weeks on all other species at the recommended dose.

NOTOEDRIC MANGE

Depilation, scruffiness, and scabs occur with this parasitism, particularly around the head. Damaged ears and crusts on the head and tail have been reported in bobcats. The treatment for notoedric mange is the same as that described for sarcoptic mange.

PSOROPTIC MANGE

This skin disease produces scabbiness, depilation, and crusty lesions and is found in polecats, genets, and dogs. The treatment for psoroptic mange is the same as that described for sarcoptic mange.

CHEYLETIELLOSIS

The clinical signs are a mild dermatitis or sometimes a hairless skin. Utilization of a flea powder that is safe for cats is usually sufficient treatment.

DEMODECTIC MANGE

Demodicosis is an infestation with *Demodex* thought to be linked with immunodeficiency, primarily of the Canidae. The lesions may be localized or generalized. Local lesions are erythematous lesions with partial alopecia. They are usually found on the face and forelegs. Generalized lesions begin as localized lesions but quickly worsen. Numerous lesions are found on the head, legs, and trunk. The generalized form is highly pruritic and usually is secondarily infected with *Staphylococcus aureus*.

The immunodeficiency is frequently caused by some other disease process, which the history and basic laboratory tests would reveal. Improper nutrition, particularly in a growing animal, parasitism, hypothyroidism, and a chronic bacterial infection frequently underlie the skin manifestation. The immunodeficiency could be hereditary, but this is not likely in nondomestic carnivores.

Treatment consists of determining the cause of the immunodeficiency and correcting it, in addition to attempting to eliminate the mite. Ectoral‖ and Dermaton‖ are two insecticidal dips that may be used at weekly intervals on the canids at dog dilutions. Goodwinol Ointment** can be used for localized topical treatment of lesions. Mitaban probably will be the drug of choice in the future but is not thoroughly tested in exotics as yet.

Demodex cati infestation has been diagnosed in snow leopard cubs and treated successfully with lime/sulfur dips. Lime/sulfur is not a specific drug for *Demodex*. A correction of the immunodeficiency probably occurred concurrently.

OTODECTIC MANGE

This skin disorder occurs in the fox, raccoon, and ferret. The mites may occlude the auditory meatus. The condition may be complicated by secondary infection. Treatment for otodectic mange in nondomestic carnivores is the same as that in domestic carnivores.

FLEA AND LICE INFESTATION

These conditions may be treated with the same products for nondomestic carnivores as those used for fleas in domestic cats.

MYIASIS

The adult form of many dypteric flies lays eggs on the warm skin of debilitated and weakened animals with draining wounds. The larvae are very destructive, producing punched-out, round holes in the skin. The larvae may be found under the skin and in the tissue. Frequent locations are the nose, eyes, mouth, arms, and genitalia and adjacent to infected wounds.

CUTEREBRA INFESTATION

The larval form of *Cuterebra* is a large, ¾-inch grub found singly or in pairs in large subcutaneous pockets. The larvae require air; therefore, the cystic structure has an air opening in the skin. It is found in young members of the Canidae and Felidae families in July, August, and September.

---

*Vet-Kem, Dallas, TX.
†Pitman-Moore, Inc., Washington Crossing, NJ.
‡L. A. City Chemical, South Gates, CA.
§D.V.M. Co., Miami, FL.

‖Burroughs Wellcome Co., Research Triangle Park, NC.
**Goodwinol Products, Huntington Station, NY.

FUNGAL DISEASES

DERMATOMYCOSIS

This condition is diagnosed by fungal culture. *Microsporum* and *Trichophyton* are the most common genera found. All carnivores are susceptible to dermatomycosis, but the disease is most commonly seen in the Canidae and Felidae families.

The lesions are most commonly found on the head and lateral surfaces of the limbs and feet. The gross appearance is usually scaly encrustations of epithelial debris and loss of hair. The hair is brittle and is broken off near the skin surface. Lesions are frequently, but not necessarily, circular. Sometimes large portions of the body are affected. The lesions may be secondarily infected by bacteria.

Treatment consists of griseofulvin administration daily for at least six weeks. If administration is difficult, megadoses may be administered weekly at 20 ml/kg. The dosages should be adjusted according to the response noted. If feasible, weekly dipping with an iodine-based shampoo is beneficial as well as topical application of Conofite.*

BACTERIAL DISEASES

Usually skin infections are caused by *Staphylococcus aureus* and are secondary to some underlying cause. The infection may be localized or generalized.

GENERALIZED SKIN INFECTIONS

The generalized infection is usually secondary to some systemic condition such as allergy, hypothyroidism, diabetes, or nutritional or congenital disease.

LOCALIZED SKIN INFECTIONS

Localized infection occurs when obesity or congenital faults, with their concurrent folds of tissue, produce anatomically susceptible areas such as the vulvar folds, lip folds, and so on. Moisture, erythema, and alopecia are found in the folds of the tissue. Localized skin infections respond to long-term antibiotic therapy and drying agents. The underlying cause should be corrected as rapidly as possible. Surgical correction is sometimes necessary.

Trauma, with its resultant secondary infection, can be produced by behavioral problems such as excessive pacing. The footpads become raw, in-

fected, and chronically thickened. Improper caging with improper drainage plus rough cage surfaces can also produce various foot lesions. Elbow calluses can be produced with concomitant secondary infections if the animal lies on hard surfaces. Treatment, therefore, is aimed at eliminating these hard surfaces; the surface of the cage can be made smooth, or Fuller's earth can be used in the area the animal is likely to occupy.

PRIMARY BACTERIAL, VIRAL, AND INTERNAL FUNGAL DISEASES

Various systemic infectious diseases may elicit dermatologic changes in carnivores. These diseases are rare but should be considered.

Anthrax has been reported in large cats fed infected meat.

Tuberculosis (*Mycobacterium bovis*) has been discovered in Siberian tigers, mink, and otters fed infected meat. Depigmentation of the nares plus systemic signs were noticed.

Oral papillomatosis, which is found in members of the Canidae family, has been reported in cougars. The warts are found on the head, lips, gums, and buccal mucosa. Surgical removal by electric cautery or cryosurgery is recommended. An autogenous vaccine may be successful in refractive cases.

Coccidiomycosis, which has been reported in coyotes, is a respiratory infection that may become generalized. It is characterized by fungating and ulcerated lesions in the skin.

Actinomycosis (*Actinomycosis bovis*) produces soft tissue abscesses in wild Canidae members.

NONSPECIFIC DISEASES

Telogen effluvium is caused by stress such as that from fever, shock, pregnancy, malnutrition, lactation, and severe debilitating illness. This condition may be localized or generalized. It can be aggravated by mechanical factors that pull out loose club hairs. Any systemic disease may produce this condition, but hepatitis, nephritis, and pancreatitis are the most common.

NUTRITIONAL DISEASES

The nutritional factors influencing the skin are complex. When deficiencies are produced in laboratory animals, they often result in cutaneous disorders. Generally speaking, malnutrition causes the skin to be dry, inelastic, and scaly. In this condition it has a greater susceptibility to infection, hemorrhage, and pigment disturbances. Certain problems that arise in the maintenance of captive carnivores should be particularly noted.

---

*Pitman-Moore Co., Washington Crossing, NJ.

ZINC DEFICIENCY

In an effort to prevent metabolic bone disease, an abundance of calcium, which inhibits the absorption of zinc and manganese, is sometimes fed. This deficiency produces parakeratosis and alopecia, primarily at the mucocutaneous junctions of the mouth, anus, inner surface of the ear, scrotum, and feet. There is also a slippage of the fur. Treatment consists of zinc methionine,* 15 mg/20 lb daily.

THIAMINE DEFICIENCY

When fish containing thiaminase are fed, the resultant lack of thiamine may produce a dry, unkempt coat.

IODINE DEFICIENCY

Hypothyroidism results from an iodine deficiency, producing a nonpruritic, bilateral alopecia. The lesions are not necessarily symmetric. They may become secondarily infected.

COPPER DEFICIENCY

A lack of this mineral produces a very pale coat.

HEREDITARY DISORDERS

In certain species of carnivores the number of individuals in captivity are few. Line or inbreeding (which elicits hereditary disease factors) may be necessary to preserve the species. Consequently, congenital or hereditary disorders are likely to become more prevalent.

Certain carnivora have had anaphylactic reactions to immunologic products. Atopic dermatitis and other allergic disorders may be present also. The likelihood of this disease, which has hereditary tendencies, to persist in a feral state is slight but must be recognized as a possibility. Atopic disease in the wild state would bring about an early demise of the animal.

ALLERGIC DISEASES AND TREATMENT

Atopy is a hereditary clinical hypersensitivity that is accompanied, in Canidae, by pruritus, scratching, face rubbing, and sneezing. In Felidae, a miliary dermatitis occurs, with miliary pustules, hemorrhagic crusts, partial alopecia, and pruritus. Flea

bite dermatitis in nondomestic carnivores exhibits symptoms similar to those of the domestic dog and cat. The fox exhibits both the atopic and miliary signs found in the dog and cat.

The previously mentioned conditions may be controlled by avoidance of the allergen or by medical or biologic treatment. The specific allergens may be determined by intradermal testing, history, or exclusion and provocative exposure. Biologic treatment has not been attempted in exotic carnivores but might be of benefit. Medical treatment consists of the judicious use of systemic corticosteroids, which give relief from pruritus. The types of drugs and dosages must be selected to suit the individual patient. It is reasonable to maintain the animal on oral therapeutic levels of short-acting corticosteroids over long periods of time. The dose should be as low as possible to just control the symptoms and should be given every other or every third day. Extreme care should be taken to eliminate the possibility of any viral, bacterial, microbiologic, or parasitic infection, because systemic corticosteroids are immunosuppressive. In my practice, allergic diseases have been refractory to antihistamines.

Food allergy dermatitis is a disease that is easy to test for but is frequently overlooked. Food allergy may be due to either an immediate or a delayed hypersensitivity. Food allergy dermatitis may or may not produce pruritus, alopecia, erythema, lichenification, crusts, and excoriations in any location on the body. It frequently causes otitis externa with no other symptoms or conditions.

An animal cannot become sensitized to any food unless it has been fed that food. Therefore, if the problem is a food allergy, giving a new food for a period of two weeks will cause the symptoms to abate dramatically. Once the diagnosis is confirmed, a new diet that is economically feasible and nutritionally sound must be started. This may be expanded by adding one new food substance to the diet for a period of two weeks. If no symptoms develop, another new food may be added and so on until the diet is nutritionally sound.

CONTACT DERMATITIS

Contact dermatitis is an inflammatory skin reaction caused by contact with an offending substance. There are two types. *Primary irritant contact dermatitis* causes an acute inflammation without an allergic response. Substances such as soap, detergents, insecticidal sprays, or strong acids and alkalies are potential primary irritating agents.

Allergic contact dermatitis is a delayed hypersensitivity that follows repeated exposure to a specific allergen. Flea collars (producing neck lesions), plastic or rubber feeding dishes (producing muzzle

---

*Zinpro, Chaska, MN.

lesions), and dyes in carpets (producing generalized lesions) are frequent causative agents.

The signs produced are intensive pruritus and self-trauma. The areas most affected are those usually in contact with the offending substance. Thus, the abdomen, chest, axillae, flanks, interdigital space, and perianal region are the most susceptible areas.

Treatment consists of determining the offending substance and removing it. Corticosteroids may be utilized systemically and topically until the offending substance is ascertained and removed, but they may not be completely effective.

CUTANEOUS ENDOCRINOLOGY

The absence of pruritus, a chronic course, a bilateral symmetric alopecia, and hyperpigmentation are common characteristics of endocrine skin disorders. However, secondary bacterial infection may produce pruritus, and hypothyroidism is frequently not bilaterally symmetric.

Hypothyroidism is a state of decreased thyroid hormone that results in alopecia; a thin, dry haircoat; and dry, brittle hair that epilates easily. The coat is coarse and sparse. The skin is dry, slightly scaly, and sometimes hyperpigmented. Secondary seborrhea and ceruminous otitis may be associated with systemic signs such as lethargy, weight gain, anestrus, and decreased libido.

Hypothyroidism may be primary or secondary. The primary type, which is most common in captive carnivores, is due to dietary lack of iodine. This condition is frequently seen in bears. The secondary type results from pituitary insufficiency, which results in a decreased thyroid-stimulation hormone (TSH) output.

Primary hypothyroidism responds nicely to the addition of iodine to the diet. Iodized salt may be used in small carnivores. The simple addition of salt-water fish to the diet of bears may be adequate therapy.

The pituitary insufficiency that results in secondary hypothyroidism should be determined by testing the T_3 and T_4 levels. The normal values for exotic carnivores are not known but possibly may be extrapolated from those of domestic dogs. A TSH stimulation test should be recommended if at all feasible.

If the T_4 level is low, L-thyroxine at a dose of 0.2 mg/10 kg is administered b.i.d. orally for one month. T_4 blood levels are then rechecked. If the T_4 is normal and a good clinical response occurs, maintain the dose indefinitely and recheck every six months. If the T_4 level is too high, adjust the dosage.

If the T_3 level is low, L-thyroxine should be given at the same dose as that for low T_4 levels and the blood rechecked in 30 days. If the T_3 level is normal, follow through as if treating for a T_4 deficiency. If the T_3 level remains low, use Cytobin* as directed on the label for dogs in addition to L-thyroxine, and recheck the T_3 level in 30 days.

OVARIAN IMBALANCE

There are two types of cutaneous syndromes associated with this endocrine disorder. Ovarian imbalance type I is characterized by alopecia, hyperpigmentation, and lichenification of the perigenital, perianal, and axillary areas. Pseudocyesis is a common finding in the history. Cystic ovaries are often found when the animal is spayed. The surgery frequently corrects the condition. This condition is seen most frequently in ocelots and margays.

Animals with ovarian imbalance type II present with a normal skin and coat until the animal is spayed. The imbalance is then characterized by a complete alopecia of the perineum, ears, ventral neck, chest, and abdomen. The skin is soft, thin, and pliable. Replacement therapy with small doses of diethylstilbestrol usually results in a return of normal haircoat. This is seen most commonly in spayed raccoons.

Diabetes mellitus produces atrophy and ulceration of the skin. Diagnosis is by blood and urine tests. Owing to the fact that the animal's blood glucose level rises with excitement, determining the correct dose of insulin is extremely difficult. Treat the animal as you would a domestic dog and use the lack of glucose in the urine when the animal is not excited to judge the correct dose of insulin. Some hyperglycemias can be almost completely corrected by diet.

SUPPLEMENTAL READING

Davis, J. W., and Anderson, R. C. (eds.): *Parasitic Diseases of Wild Mammals.* Ames, IA: Iowa State University Press, 1971.

Davis, J. W., Karstad, L. H., and Trainer, D. O. (eds.): *Infectious Diseases of Wild Mammals.* Ames, IA: Iowa State University Press, 1970.

Fowler, M. D. (ed.): *Zoo and Wild Animal Medicine.* Philadelphia: W. B. Saunders, 1978.

Hamilton, W. J. (ed.): *American Mammals.* York, PA: Maple Press Co., 1939.

Kirk, R. W. (ed.): *Current Veterinary Therapy VII.* Philadelphia, W. B. Saunders, 1980.

Muller, G. H., and Kirk, R. W. (eds.): *Small Animal Dermatology.* Philadelphia: W. B. Saunders, 1976.

---

*Norden Laboratories Inc., Lincoln, NE.

DIAGNOSIS AND MANAGEMENT OF SALMONELLOSIS AND SHIGELLOSIS IN NONHUMAN PRIMATES

GEORGE V. KOLLIAS, JR., D.V.M.

Gainesville, Florida

Physical signs referrable to gastrointestinal disease in nonhuman primates represent one of the most common reasons for clinical presentation. The etiology of these problems may be multifactorial and often includes a nutritional, infectious, or psychogenic basis. Bacterial infections resulting in enteritis or enterocolitis comprise approximately 30 per cent of these cases. The rate of recovery of enteric pathogens is comparable to the reported isolation of bacterial pathogens in 20 to 40 per cent of human cases of diarrheal disease (Gardner and Povine, 1975; McClure, 1980).

ETIOLOGY

The most commonly isolated bacterial agents associated with diarrheal disease in nonhuman primates include *Shigella* spp., *Salmonella* spp., enteropathogenic serotypes of *Escherichia coli*, *Yersinia enterocolitica*, *Yersinia pseudotuberculosis*, and, more recently, *Campylobacter fetus* subsp. *jejuni* (McClure, 1980; Tribe and Frank, 1980). The majority of these agents have been incriminated as causes of diarrheal and systemic disease in humans. The use of protective clothing, including disposable surgical gowns, surgical masks, and gloves, should be considered when handling clinically ill as well as apparently healthy nonhuman primates. The remainder of this discussion will be centered around *Shigella* and *Salmonella* spp. owing to their documented zoonotic potential and relatively high incidence rate in nonhuman primates and man (Fiennes, 1967).

Shigella and *Salmonella* spp. have been isolated from most species of nonhuman primates, including great and lesser apes, and various species of New and Old World monkeys, including prosimians.

Reports of carrier rates of *Shigella* spp. for clinically normal colony animals range from 5 to 6 per cent (McClure, 1980). These organisms are frequently isolated from recently imported nonhuman primates as well as from animals that have been in captivity for prolonged periods of time. *Shigella flexneri*, including serotypes 1, 2, 3, 4, and 6, is most frequently isolated; other less frequently encountered species include *Shigella sonnei*, *S. boydii*, *S. dysenteriae*, and *S. schmitzii*.

Isolates of *Salmonella* spp. from nonhuman primates include *S. anatum*, *S. derby*, *S. stanley*, *S. oranienburg*, *S. miami*, and *S. typhimurium*. The most frequently isolated species associated with gastrointestinal disease in nonhuman primates is *Salmonella typhimurium* ser. *enteritidis*. Geographic variation of isolates frequently occurs.

TRANSMISSION

Many species of insects, birds, mammals, and reptiles have been shown to harbor a variety of *Salmonella* species, which can potentially be transmitted to humans and nonhuman primates. In addition, certain animal products may be a source of transmission. It is thought by some investigators that humans are the actual reservoir for *Shigella* spp. and that nonhuman primates may become initially infected by contact through contaminated food or water prior to importation. Nonclinically affected carrier animals may also act as a continual source of infection with *Salmonella* and *Shigella* spp. The direct fecal/oral route is the commonest mode of transmission with both of these agents, although fomites may act as an indirect means by which infection can occur. Thorough sanitation of contaminated areas is essential to eliminate the organisms in the environment. Ingestion of food or fecal material present on cage or enclosure floors is a common means of reinfection.

CLINICAL FINDINGS

SIGNS

The clinical manifestations of shigellosis and salmonellosis are similar and can vary with the age of the animal affected and the virulence of the particular variant of bacteria. Carrier animals generally show no clinical manifestations of infection. Individual animals may exhibit mild to severe clinical signs when stresses, such as changes in husbandry practices or concurrent disease, exist and may contribute to the induction of changes in the intestinal microflora. Mild to moderate signs include partial anorexia and soft to semifluid stool developing gradually over a 24- to 48-hour period. Severe signs are abrupt in onset and include anorexia and refusal to drink, depression, tenesmus, fluid or hemorrhagic diarrhea, fever of 40 to 41°C, vomiting, and prostration. Clinical manifestations in infant and juvenile animals are generally much more severe than those in adults and can be characterized by fever and projectile fluid diarrhea variably containing blood and mucus. Rapid dehydration can ultimately proceed to death unless intensively managed. Blood in the stool appears to be a less consistent finding with all forms of enteric *Salmonella* infections than with *Shigella* infections.

Extraintestinal *Shigella* infections have been reported in both humans and nonhuman primates (McClure, 1980). In nonhuman primates, specifically macaques, gingivitis and periodontitis have been associated with *Shigella flexneri* isolates from the oral cavity.

LABORATORY FINDINGS

The white blood cell count is generally elevated, often with a marked shift to the left in moderate to severe infections. Toxic neutrophilia and a predominance of band forms in the differential smear may be an important diagnostic clue. Fibrinogen levels are often elevated (800 to 1200 gm/dl). Methylene blue–stained rectal swab smears examined for the presence of leukocytes are of diagnostic value in differentiating non-toxin–producing bacterial enteric infections from other etiologic agents. Enteric diseases due to toxin-producing agents such as *Vibrio cholerae*, certain noninvasive *E. coli*, *Staphylococcus aureus* (food poisoning), *Clostridium perfringes*, and *C. botulinum* are not characterized by inflammation of the bowel; therefore, leukocytes are not usually found in the stool. In addition, gastroenteritis due to presumed viral etiologies is not associated with inflammatory cells in the stool.

The staining procedure involves placing a small fleck of mucus (stool if no mucus is present) on a clean glass slide and mixing thoroughly with two drops of methylene blue stain. A coverslip is applied to the slide. A period of two to three minutes is necessary for good nuclear staining. The slide is examined first under low power to note the presence of cells and then under high dry power to perform a differential white blood cell count. In one experimental study in humans, the presence of fecal leukocytes was more reliable in establishing infection than was a bacterial culture of the stool (Nelson and Haltalin, 1971). The differential white cell count in stool specimens is of diagnostic interest. Stools of animals with shigellosis and invasive *E. coli* infection are characterized by large numbers of WBCs (greater than 50 per high-power field), more than 80 per cent of which are polymorphonuclear leukocytes, often band forms. In salmonellosis, the total count tends to be lower, with a greater proportion, approximately 25 per cent, being mononuclear cells. Individuals with inflammatory bowel disease due to noninfectious causes (regional enteritis, ulcerative colitis) often have many eosinophils among the fecal leukocytes, as demonstrated by Wright's stain.

Stool cultures are usually positive with salmonellosis and shigellosis, but owing to the fragile nature of the organism results may be negative if the stool specimen is improperly collected, transported, or inoculated. Following isolation on selective media for the Enterobacteriaceae, members of the group are differentiated on the basis of their antigenic characteristics. Serotyping is an important epidemiologic tool in determining sources and distributions of infections. *Salmonella* spp. are grouped on the basis of O and H antigens, with several hundred serotypes known. Using polyvalent O antisera, a laboratory can determine the group of *Salmonella* in question. Species typing and speciation on the basis of H antigens must be performed in a reference laboratory. *Shigella* organisms are grouped using biochemical characteristics and O antigenic relationships as mentioned previously. *Shigella flexneri*, the most common isolate, contains a number of serotypes. Chronic subclinical carriers appear to intermittently shed organisms in their stool; therefore, serial collection of samples for culture may be necessary to isolate the agent. Rarely, *Shigella* and *Salmonella* spp. may coexist in the same animal.

PATHOLOGIC FINDINGS

Lesions associated with *Shigella* and *Salmonella* spp. are often limited to the jejunum, ileum, colon, and, rarely, the stomach. Grossly, the lumen of the colon is often filled with semiliquid fecal material mixed with blood and mucus. Petechial hemorrhages are often present on the serosa of the colon. The mesenteric lymph nodes may be swollen, edematous, or hemorrhagic. In severe cases, necrosis of the colonic mucosa is present, and the intestinal wall may appear gangrenous. The spleen may be enlarged and soft, with prominent subcapsular petechial hemorrhages. Extraintestinal *Shigella* infections have resulted in swollen, hyperemic gums that contain scattered yellowish-white foci of necrosis. Gingival biopsies show prominent submucosal infiltration of mononuclear inflammatory cells, with scattered areas of polymorphonuclear leukocyte accumulation. Although rare, extraintestinal localization with *Salmonella* spp. can result in pyogenic infections in almost any anatomic site.

Histologic examination reveals some differences between *Shigella* and *Salmonella* infections. Experimentally infected animals frequently exhibit involvement of the ileum with salmonellosis and infrequent involvement in shigellosis. Crypt abscesses, described as numerous, and lymphoid abscesses frequently appear in experimental shigellosis, whereas they are infrequent in salmonellosis. Mucosal ulceration is not present in salmonellosis but occurs in some individuals with shigellosis. Organisms are numerous and easily seen in Giemsa-stained gut sections of animals infected with *Shigella* but are less easily demonstrated in sections of gut from *Salmonella*-infected monkeys (Carlton and Hunt, 1978).

TREATMENT

SPECIFIC MEASURES

Antimicrobial agents should not be given for mild enteritis or enterocolitis caused by *Salmonella* or *Shigella* spp., since treatment is ineffective and prolongs the carrier state. Exceptions to this rule include animals with impaired cellular immunity, concurrent systemic disease, and infants less than one year of age, who appear to be at risk of developing systemic effects of *Salmonella* or *Shigella* infections. Antimicrobial therapy is indicated in individuals with moderate to severe infections exhibiting fever, leukocytosis, and blood and/or mucus in the stool. Although antimicrobial sensitivity patterns vary between facilities, chloramphenicol (50 to 100 mg/kg daily divided q.i.d., PO or IM) or ampicillin (200 mg/kg daily divided t.i.d., PO or SQ) is the drug of choice for treating enteric *Salmonella* and *Shigella* infections in adults and infants. Chloramphenicol palmitate, although well tolerated, is not recommended because of irregular absorption of this lipase-dependent compound. A suspension of the crystalline form from the capsule is preferred when the drug is administered orally (Yeager and Kempe, 1980). Treatment is generally continued for five to seven days. Trimethoprim-sulfamethoxazole appears to be effective in areas where resistant strains are prevalent. The recommended dosage is 8 to 10 mg/kg of trimethoprim and 40 to 50 mg/kg sulfamethoxazole or sulfadiazine daily divided b.i.d. PO or SQ for five to seven days (SQ for trimethoprim/sulfadiazine only). One report concludes that the carrier state of *Shigella* infection was eliminated in a colony of macaques utilizing

trimethoprim-sulfamethoxazole (Pucak et al., 1977). Essentially all strains of *Salmonella* and *Shigella* have shown sensitivity to gentamicin and kanamycin, but these agents should only be considered in special clinical situations.

GENERAL MEASURES

Vigorous fluid therapy based on serum electrolytes, packed cell volume, total solids, and blood gas studies is imperative in the management of nonhuman primates with severe diarrhea, especially infants. An infant or juvenile may become severely dehydrated and semicomatose within six to eight hours of abrupt onset with salmonellosis or shigellosis. Immediate rehydration is critical (see Fluid Therapy, page 28). Accessible sites for venoclysis include the antecubital, saphenous, femoral, and jugular veins. In severely dehydrated animals a cutdown procedure and cannulation of the femoral vein may be necessary. Fluids may be given subcutaneously in mild to moderate cases. After initial rehydration with parenteral fluids, clear liquids may be required orally for two to three days, followed by glucose-containing preparations such as grape juice, apple juice, liquid Jello-O, ginger ale, or Gatorade. In addition, oral potassium supplementation (Kaon Elixir*) as indicated by serum determination enhances recovery. In very young animals daily caloric maintenance is critical. Supplementation with strained vegetable, egg, and fruit baby foods or complete dietary preparations such as Portagen† is indicated. A mild form of chronic malabsorption syndrome may supervene and may require prolonged dietary control.

Antispasmotics, such as diphenoxylate (Lomotil Liquid‡), 0.1 to 0.4 mg/kg divided t.i.d., are indicated when tenesmus is severe or unrelenting after initiating fluid therapy. Overdose with diphenoxylate, as evidenced by depression or respiratory embarrassment, can be treated with 0.02 mg/kg naloxone IV. Administration of whole blood, B-complex vitamin injections, and iron supplementation are indicated with severe blood loss.

If toxicity is marked, a short course of corticosteroids may be indicated when antibiotics are begun. Prednisone, 1 mg/kg/day orally, during the first four days of antibiotic therapy results in marked improvement (McIntosh et al., 1980).

COMPLICATIONS

Dehydration, acidosis, and shock occur in infancy. In some cases, a chronic diarrhea results,

*Warren-Teed, North Chicago, IL.
†Mead Johnson Nutritional Division, Evansville, IN.
‡G. D. Searle & Co., Chicago, IL.

characterized by mucoid stools and chronic debilitation. In older animals gastrointestinal hemorrhage and perforation may occur acutely or with chronic, severe infection. The clinical signs of serious hemorrhage are those of acute blood loss, including the appearance of gross blood in the stools and evidence of shock. Intestinal perforation generally occurs at the terminal ileum or the proximal segment of the colon. The clinical manifestations include pain, tenderness, and rigidity in the lower right abdominal quadrant. A radiographic finding of free air in the peritoneal cavity is diagnostic. Bacterial pneumonia, meningitis, septic arthritis, and osteomyelitis are uncommon complications if specific treatment is given promptly in severe cases.

Protozoal and metazoan parasite infections may coexist with bacterial enteritis or enterocolitis in nonhuman primates. When this occurs, as determined by wet mount smears of rectal swabs or fecal flotation, specific therapy for these agents must also be considered. As an example, overgrowth of symbiotic flagellates, such as *Trichomonas* spp., commonly occurs with bacterial enteric infections and in some cases produces manifestations of invasive disease. Treatment with metronidazole (Flagyl*), 35 to 40 mg/kg divided t.i.d. PO (infants and adults) for five days, in addition to specific antibacterial therapy, often reduces recovery time.

PROGNOSIS AND PREVENTION

The prognosis is generally good when immediate attention is directed toward specific and general supportive therapy. Infant mortality is high if therapy is not initiated rapidly.

Prevention is directed toward avoiding contact between normal animals and human or animal carriers. Chronic carriers are common and are difficult to eliminate in some instances.

Carrier animals should be isolated from other nonhuman primates in situations such as breeding facilities, zoos, and research colonies. In addition, contaminated environments, foods, and fomites should be properly sterilized or eliminated.

REFERENCES AND SUPPLEMENTAL READING

Carlton, W. W., and Hunt, R. D.: Bacterial diseases. *In* Benirschke, K., Garner, F. M., and Jones, T. C. (eds.): *Pathology of Laboratory Animals.* New York: Springer Verlag, 1978.

Fiennes, R.: *Zoonoses of Primates.* Ithaca, NY: Cornell University Press, 1967.

Gardner, P., and Povine, H. T.: *Manual of Acute Bacterial Infections—Early Diagnosis and Treatment.* Boston: Little, Brown and Company, 1975.

McClure, H. M.: Bacterial diseases of non-human primates. *In* Montali, R. J., and Migaki, G. (eds.): *The Comparative Pathology of Zoo Animals.* Washington, D.C.: Smithsonian Institution Press, 1980.

McIntosh, K., Lauer, B. A., and Eller, J. J.: Infections—bacterial and spirochetal. *In* Kempe, H. C., Silver, H. K., and O'Brien, D. (eds.): *Current Pediatric Diagnosis and Treatment.* Los Altos, CA: Lange Medical Publications, 1980.

Nelson, J. D., and Haltalin, K. C.: Accuracy of diagnosis of bacterial diarrheal disease by clinical features. J. Pediatr. 83:519, 1971.

Pucak, G. J., Orcutt, R. P., Judge, R. J., and Rendon, F.: Elimination of the *Shigella* carrier state in rhesus monkeys (*Macaca mulatta*) by trimethoprim-sulfamethoxazole. J. Med. Primatol. 6:127, 1977.

Roy, C. C., and Silverman, A.: The gastrointestinal tract. *In* Kempe, H. C., Silver, H. K., and O'Brien, D. (eds.): *Current Pediatric Diagnosis and Treatment.* Los Altos, CA: Lange Medical Publications, 1980.

Tribe, G. W., and Frank, A.: *Campylobacter* in monkeys. Vet. Rec. 106:365, 1980.

Yeager, S., and Kempe, H. C.: Anti-infective chemotherapeutic agents and antibiotic drugs. *In* Kempe, H. C., Silver, H. K., and O'Brien, D. (eds.): *Current Pediatric Diagnosis and Treatment.* Los Altos, CA: Lange Medical Publications, 1980.

*G. D. Searle & Co., Chicago, IL.

RABBIT PASTEURELLOSIS

J. DERRELL CLARK, D.V.M.

Athens, Georgia

Pasteurella multocida is normally carried as a commensal in the upper respiratory tract of many domestic and wild animals including cattle, sheep, swine, dogs, cats, rabbits, rats, and birds. Many strains of *P. multocida* have very low pathogenicity and do not produce disease in healthy animals that are well cared for. Frequently disease only occurs when certain predisposing factors give the bacteria the opportunity to multiply uncontrollably and overwhelm the physiologic and immunologic defenses of the respiratory tract. During these episodes, clones of virulent bacteria increase. These virulent strains of bacteria can be more easily transmitted and are pathogenic for other animals of the same species. However, they rarely are pathogenic for other host species. Diseases caused by *P. multocida* include fowl cholera, pneumonia and shipping fever in cattle and sheep, swine pasteurellosis, and several clinical entities in rabbits.

Pasteurellosis is a frequently occurring, highly

contagious, and complex disease of domestic rabbits. It causes important clinical problems in pet rabbits and is responsible for severe economic losses in research and commercial colonies. A number of clinical forms occur including snuffles, enzootic pneumonia, septicemia, otitis media, conjunctivitis, pyometra, orchitis, abscesses, and mastitis. *P. multocida* is considered to be the primary etiologic agent. The bacteria are presumed to be spread by direct contact with infected rabbits and contaminated fomites and through the air. Conditions creating stress in animals are thought to contribute to the development of overt disease. Common predisposing factors include shipping, chilling, unfavorable weather, poor management, pregnancy, concurrent disease, and experimentation. Diagnosis of pasteurellosis is based on clinical signs, isolation of the causative organism from affected tissues, and pathologic findings.

P. multocida is a prevalent infection in clinically normal rabbits and may be isolated from the nares, conjunctiva, lungs, and middle ear. It is enzootic in many colonies unless specific measures are taken to prevent it. Results of several surveys indicate that approximately 40 to 80 per cent of conventionally raised adult rabbits harbor *P. multocida* in their respiratory tracts. Prevalence rates in immature rabbits are lower. It is believed that natural transmission from mother to offspring takes place via the respiratory tract within a few days to a few weeks after birth. Apparently, as rabbits age, the opportunities for exposure to *P. multocida* are increased, and consequently the prevalence rate increases. There is also variation in the number of infected animals in different colonies.

STAGES OF DISEASE

Pasteurellosis is characterized by acute, subacute, or chronic disease. Since the organism frequently infects the respiratory tract of apparently normal rabbits, it is not surprising that rhinitis, pneumonia, and otitis media are common forms of the disease. From the respiratory tract, the bacteria may invade other systems of the body to produce disease.

A chronic form of the disease, snuffles, is one of the most commonly observed diseases in domestic rabbits maintained for pets, research, or food consumption. Snuffles is a rhinitis and paranasal sinusitis characterized by a serous, mucoid, or mucopurulent nasal discharge; sneezing and coughing; respiratory distress; and stained and matted fur on the inner aspect of the forepaws caused by rubbing exudate from the nose.

Bronchopneumonia caused by *P. multocida* is also enzootic in rabbits. Clinical signs, if observed, include anorexia, depression, labored breathing, and fever. Sudden deaths in rabbits with no previous clinical signs are common. Mortality rates up to 50 per cent have been reported. Frequently, rabbits that appear to be clinically normal have gross pneumonic lesions when examined post mortem.

Otitis media is another manifestation of pasteurellosis in rabbits. Torticollis is the primary clinical sign in this condition. This may range from a slightly tilted head to a rotation approaching 180°. When examined at necropsy, approximately one-third of adult rabbits may have suppurative exudate in one or both middle ears. *P. multocida* can be isolated from many of these lesions. However, the incidence of clinical torticollis is much lower than the occurrence of otitis media observed at post-mortem examination.

Septicemia caused by *P. multocida* may occur following other forms of pasteurellosis, or it may be the initial manifestation of the disease. Clinical signs are rarely observed. Usually affected rabbits are found dead.

Other forms of pasteurellosis include conjunctivitis, subcutaneous abscesses, lung abscesses, metritis, and orchitis.

GOALS OF THERAPY

Goals of treatment in rabbit pasteurellosis are twofold. Specific chemotherapeutic measures are primarily supportive because it is nearly impossible to eliminate the bacteria from infected animals. Second, since predisposing factors are important in initiating disease, correction of management deficiencies will contribute to the reduction of signs and mortality and to the effectiveness of specific chemotherapy.

SPECIFIC THERAPY

Antibacterial chemotherapy has been used extensively in the treatment of rabbit pasteurellosis with varying success. Sensitivity testing may be advantageous, since strains of *P. multocida* vary in susceptibility to chemotherapeutic agents, and R factor–mediated antibiotic resistance has been found in pasteurellosis from some animals. *In vitro*, *P. multocida* isolated from rabbits is generally sensitive to a number of antimicrobial agents including several commonly used antibiotics such as penicillin, oxytetracycline, erythromycin, chloramphenicol, ampicillin, gentamicin, and kanamycin; nitrofurans; and some sulfonamides. It may be resistant to streptomycin and some sulfonamides.

Most clinicians agree that therapy with antimicrobial agents is relatively unrewarding and results are inconsistent. In general, the more advanced the disease, the less effective the treatment. Rabbits may show remission of the clinical signs during the treatment period. However, *P. multocida* can continue to be recovered from the respiratory tract, and clinical relapses are common after therapy is discontinued.

For treatment of snuffles and enzootic pneumonia, penicillin and tetracyclines have been used both parenterally and orally. The following drugs and dosage regimens have been used:

Individual treatment

1. Procaine penicillin G—60,000 IU/kg body weight, IM, once daily for ten days
2. Oxytetracycline—5 mg/kg body weight, IM, twice daily for ten days
3. Tetracycline—50 to 100 mg/kg body weight, PO, daily in divided doses for ten days

Group treatment

1. Sulfaquinoxaline—0.025 per cent in water or feed
2. Oxytetracycline—55 to 100 mg/kg body weight in water (0.055 to 0.1 per cent)
3. Sulfamethazine or sulfamerazine—100 mg/kg body weight in water (0.1 per cent)

Systemic treatment of otitis media is usually unrewarding. However, tympanocentesis in conjunction with systemic antibiotic administration and antibiotic flush into the ear canal may relieve the clinical signs of torticollis.

Subcutaneous abscesses may be incised, drained, flushed with antiseptics, and treated with topical and systemic antibiotics. Conjunctivitis can be treated with ophthalmic ointments containing antibiotics.

COMPLICATIONS

Several antibiotics, including penicillin and ampicillin, have been associated with diarrhea, colitis, and death in domestic rabbits. Diarrhea usually is first observed several days after the beginning of antibiotic treatment. Clinicians should recognize that antibiotic therapy of rabbits could result in fatal colitis. Rabbits being treated with antibiotics should be closely monitored; if diarrhea occurs, antibiotic therapy should be stopped and appropriate supportive therapy begun immediately.

PREVENTION

In controlling pasteurellosis, specific preventive measures for individual pets or small groups of conventionally housed rabbits are not totally effective. The risk of disease is reduced in one or a few pet rabbits maintained in a household or on prem-

ises apart from other rabbits. Since predisposing factors are often responsible for lowering resistance and contributing to overt disease, management procedures should eliminate as much stress as possible. Poor management practices, substandard husbandry, inadequate ventilation, other environmental deficiencies, and overcrowding should be corrected. Newly acquired rabbits should be quarantined, and ill animals should be isolated. Good husbandry, care, and facilities will reduce the incidence of pasteurellosis but will not eliminate the infection or disease.

For long-term maintenance of *P. multocida*–free rabbits, the most effective method of preventing the infection involves caesarian delivery and hand rearing of animals. If maintained in specific pathogen-free conditions, these animals can be used as breeding stock to establish colonies free of pasteurellosis. A method that is less definitive but has been used successfully by some producers involves the selection of breeding stock free of clinical signs and free of *P. multocida* as determined by negative bacterial examination. Maintenance of these animals in clean facilities and constant elimination of infected or diseased animals may result in *Pasteurella*-free animals or at least animals with a minimal incidence of infection.

In the past, there have been several attempts to produce a *P. multocida* bacterin that could be used in the control of pasteurellosis. The effectiveness of experimental bacterins in protecting against pasteurellosis has been variable. None are commercially available, but research is continuing in an effort to develop an effective bacterin.

SUPPLEMENTAL READING

Chengappa, M. M., Myers, R. C., and Carter, G. R.: A streptomycin dependent live *Pasteurella multocida* vaccine for the prevention of rabbit pasteurellosis. Lab. Anim. Sci. 30:515, 1980.
Flatt, R. E.: Bacterial diseases. *In* Weisbroth, S. H., Flatt, R. E., and Kraus, A. L. (eds.): *The Biology of the Laboratory Rabbit*. New York: Academic Press, 1974, pp. 194–205.
Flatt, R. E., Deyoung, D. W., and Hogle, R. M.: Suppurative otitis media in the rabbit: prevalence, pathology, and microbiology. Lab. Anim. Sci. 27:343, 1977.
Flatt, R. E., and Dungworth, D. L.: Enzootic pneumonia in rabbits: naturally occurring lesions in lungs of apparently healthy young rabbits. Am. J. Vet. Res. 32:621, 1971.
Harkness, J. E., and Wagner, J. E.: *The Biology and Medicine of Rabbits and Rodents*. Philadelphia: Lea & Febiger, 1977, pp. 102–104.
Jaslow, B. W., Ringler, D. H., Rush, H. G., et al.: Pasteurella-associated rhinitis of rabbits: efficacy of penicillin therapy. Lab. Anim. Sci. 31:382, 1981.
Lu, Y.-S., Ringler, D. H., and Park, J. S.: Characterization of *Pasteurella multocida* isolates from the nares of healthy rabbits and rabbits with pneumonia. Lab. Anim. Sci. 28:691, 1978.
Rehg, J. E., and Lu, Y.-S.: *Clostridium difficile* colitis in a rabbit following antibiotic therapy for pasteurellosis. J.A.V.M.A. 179:1296, 1981.

EAR MITES IN LAGOMORPHS, RODENTS, MUSTELIDS, AND NONDOMESTIC CARNIVORES

MICHAEL K. STOSKOPF, D.V.M.

Baltimore, Maryland

Many practitioners are called upon to treat the occasional pet rabbit, rat, hamster, or ferret. Even fractious animals such as fox and mink are kept as household pets, although most encounters with these animals come through clients with fur-farming operations. Many of these animals are presented for ear problems. This is probably due to the readily observable nature of an animals' reaction to ear disease. Crusts and scabs in the ears, intense scratching resulting in trauma, head shaking, head tilting, circling, torticollis, and convulsions are all easily recognized by owners as abnormal even when the animal is observed from a distance. Ear mite infestations of the canal and pinna are commonly associated with these signs. The alert practitioner should be aware of the importance of ear mites as a major cause of ear disease.

Synonyms for infestations of mites in the ears include ear canker, ear mange, auricular mange, parasitic otitis, otoacariasis, otodectic mange, and aural acariasis. Many infestations are completely asymptomatic and are detected only through ear examination during a routine work-up. This is particularly true in young animals. Classical signs of symptomatic ear mite infestation include intense pruritus and crusty earwax build-up, which may range in color from light yellow in rabbits to dark brown–black in foxes. Infected ears may also show inflammation, edema, and hyperemia. The disease is normally bilateral and may be accompanied by gross trauma as a result of the extreme pruritus.

Several species of mites are known to affect the ears of animals, but for most practical purposes they can be divided into two groups. The classical ear mites of the family Psoroptidae are surface-dwelling mites that do not burrow into the skin. They feed either on serum and tissue fluids obtained by puncturing the skin or on debris in the ear. Their entire life cycle is maintained on the host and takes three to four weeks to complete. *Psoroptes cuniculi*, the most common ear mite of rabbits, falls into this group as well as *Otodectes cynotis*, the major ear mite affecting fox, mink, ferrets, and other carnivores and mustelids. *Otodectes cynotis* is not host specific, and human ear infections caused by this organism are reported.

The second major group of mites affecting ears are those of the family Sarcoptidae. These are burrowing mites and are more frequently found elsewhere on the body but can infest the ears. The most common ear mites of rats and hamsters are members of this family in the genus *Notoedres*. Rabbits can be infested with *Notoedres*, but this is relatively rare. Foxes suffer from the same *Notoedres* mite that affects domestic cats and dogs, but, as would be expected in a domestic carnivore, lesions are more commonly seen on the top of the head, under the throat, and on the elbows. Foxes and other carnivores are also susceptible to major zoonotic species of this mite family, the *Sarcoptes scabiei*. This mite has a more generalized pattern of infestation but may affect the ears only. In general, the burrowing mites are less specific in location, cause greater skin reactions and thickening, and have greater zoonotic potential. They complete their life cycle on the host, are passed primarily by direct contact, and are not host specific.

As in demodectic mange, there is evidence that a defect in the host's immune response system allows the exacerbation of ear mite infestation to a recognizable level. Allergen testing with mite extracts has shown that most animals have been exposed to ear mites at some time during their life. It has also been shown that an allergic mechanism may be involved in the development of disease. This may be related to atopy seen in humans exposed to various pollens.

DIAGNOSIS

Diagnostic methods for ear mite infestations are essentially the same in all species. The small animal clinician should have little trouble diagnosing a case in even the most unusual of patients. For true ear mites, a complete otoscopic examination of both ear canals can provide a positive diagnosis when mites are visualized moving over the caked wax in the ears. These mites are usually white and are readily seen with minimal magnification. General anesthesia or strong sedation may be required to complete this examination in animals that defy restraint. Erythema, irritation, and ceruminous build-up are strong indications of mite infestation even if mites

672

are not visualized. Samples of wax from the patient's ears should be tested for the presence of mites. White mites can often be seen by placing a small amount of earwax on carbon paper and observing for movement as the wax is slowly heated by a strong light. A more reliable technique involves microscopic examination of ear debris for mites or ova after clearing with 10 per cent potassium hydroxide or after dissolving the wax with chlorallactophenol. Chlorallactophenol is made by mixing equal parts of 85 per cent lactic acid, phenol, and chloral hydrate.

Infestations of the Sarcoptidae mites can be diagnosed in the same way as those of Psoroptidae mites. Males and some larval forms do not burrow and may be found moving over the ear debris. Burrowing forms may be discovered by careful examination of dewaxed debris, looking for mites that use the caked wax as a protective environment. If burrowing mites are suspected because of thick skin and intense pruritus and they are not demonstrated by examining ear debris, a skin scraping of a thickened area is often successful.

Major differentials to be excluded during diagnosis include otitis interna, otitis media, or otitis externa due to bacterial, fungal, or yeast infections. Foreign bodies in the ear, pediculosis, and traumatic otitis must also be ruled out. The routine blood parameters, including total and differential leukocyte count, will not be affected by a simple ear mite infestation. Alterations in these parameters should lead the clinician to investigate complex etiologies.

THERAPY

All diagnosed cases of ear mites should be treated. The initial step in any case of ear mites is to gently clean the ears with light mineral oil to remove the build-up of cerumen and debris that serves as the protective matrix and food source for the parasites. Light or moderate infestations of nonburrowing mites will respond to mineral oil therapy alone. Weekly cleaning with light mineral oil for five weeks is adequate to cure many cases. More severely affected animals with extensive crusting, hyperemia, and inflammation of the ears will respond better if the weekly cleansing of the ears is followed by administration of an oil-based ointment containing a steroid, an antibacterial agent, and an acaricidal drug. A combination of thiabendazole, dexamethasone, and neomycin sulfate in an oil base (Tresaderm*) is very successful. Infestations of burrowing mites also respond well to this mixture or to rotenone 0.25 per cent in mineral oil (Canex†).

Animals with severe infestations should be treated for mites on the rest of the body to prevent continual reinfection. Areas of primary concern are the tip of the tail, which often contacts the ears in the sleeping posture, the feet, and the rest of the head. Pyrethrin powders are usually the best choice for this treatment. Shampoos and dips are often unable to adequately penetrate the thick pelage of fur-bearing animals such as fox and mink. All animals in direct contact with the patient should be treated to avoid reinfection through this route.

COMPLICATIONS

The major complications of ear mite infestation have already been listed as bacterial, fungal, and yeast infections as well as aural trauma. Pyogenic otitis and severely inflamed cases of ear mites should be cultured and tested for antibiotic sensitivities. Concomitant topical antibacterial or antifungal therapy may be indicated.

Ear trauma is a frequent complication. Relief of pruritus with corticosteroids may be enough to prevent self-mutilation, but more difficult cases may require Elizabethan collars, protective mitts, or bandage helmets to prevent the patient from destroying its ears. If these are unsuccessful, an aural hematoma is a likely result of self-inflicted trauma. Simple repeated aspiration of a hematoma may be adequate to prevent permanent deformity in small lesions, particularly in small-eared predators. Rabbits and large-eared animals, however, are prone to large hematomas, which often require pressure bandaging. This can be accomplished by packing the inside of the pinna, but not the canal, with gauze sponges. Support the back of the ear with discarded x-ray film and tape to apply pressure on the ear. The x-ray film is not always necessary. Aspiration is only effective if the hematoma is fresh. This is rarely the case. When presented with a partially organized hematoma, take measures to prevent further trauma, apply a pressure wrap, and wait approximately ten days for the hematoma to completely organize. This will reduce hemorrhage during surgery. With the animal under anesthesia, clip and prep both sides of the ear. Make an S-shaped incision over the hematoma on the concave surface of the ear and remove the clot. Suture using through-and-through dexon horizontal mattress sutures tied on the convex surface of the ear, leaving a 4- to 5-mm gap in your incision. These sutures appose the skin to the cartilage for proper scarring. A pressure bandage on the ear aids healing.

PREVENTION

Prevention is based on several factors. The life cycle of both families of mites is completed on the host, alleviating the need to treat the environment. Ear mites are primarily transmitted by direct con-

---

*Merck Sharpe & Dohme, Rahway, NJ.

†Pitman-Moore Co., Washington Crossing, NJ.

tact, and inapparent infections are common. This emphasizes the need to examine and treat all animals in contact with an identified case. Active examination for ear mites during quarantine periods can prevent severe problems for colony or farm situations. There is some evidence that some mites can be mechanically transmitted by flies. Severe fly problems may contribute to spread when direct contact is not likely. Many, if not all, ear mites have at least some zoonotic potential. Human contact with active cases should be appropriately monitored, particularly when young children are involved.

SUPPLEMENTAL READING

Flynn, R. J.: *Parasites of Laboratory Animals*. Ames, IA: Iowa State University Press, 1973.

Harrison, G., and Fowler, M. E.: Rabbits, hares, and pika. *In* Fowler, M. E. (ed.): *Zoo and Wild Animal Medicine*. Philadelphia: W. B. Saunders, 1978.

Krull, W. H.: *Notes in Veterinary Parasitology*. Lawrence, KS: University Press of Kansas, 1969.

Ott, R. L.: Ears. *In* Archibald, J. (ed.): *Canine Surgery*. Santa Barbara, CA: American Veterinary Publications, 1974.

Van de Heyning, J.: Otitis externa in man caused by the mite *Otodectes cynotis*. Laryngoscope 87:1938, 1977.

Weisbroth, S. H., Powell, M. D., Roth, L., and Scher, S.: Immunopathology of naturally occurring otodectic otoacariasis in the domestic cat. J.A.V.M.A. 165:1088, 1979.

Section
9

NEUROLOGIC AND NEUROMUSCULAR DISORDERS

ALEXANDER DE LaHUNTA, D.V.M.
Consulting Editor

Additional Pertinent Information found in Current Veterinary Therapy VII:

Barrett, Ralph E., D.V.M.: Canine Hepatic Encephalopathy, p. 822.
Barrett, Ralph E., D.V.M.: Canine Polyarthritis, p. 795.
Barsanti, Jeanne A., D.V.M.: Botulism, Tick Paralysis, and Acute Poly-radiculoneuritis (Coonhound Paralysis), p. 773.

Duncan, E.D., B.V.M.S., and Griffiths, I.R., B.V.M.S.: Inflammatory Muscle Disease in the Dog, p. 779.
Gannon, James R., B.V.Sc.: Exertional Rhabdomyolysis (Myoglobinuria) in the Racing Greyhound, p. 783.
Olsson, Sten-Erik, V.M.D.: Canine Hip Dysplasia, p. 802.
Olsson, Sten-Erik, V.M.D.: Osteochondrosis in the Dog, p. 809.

CEREBROSPINAL FLUID
EVALUATION

CHERYL L. CHRISMAN, D.V.M.

Gainesville, Florida

When an animal is presented with a potential neurologic problem, a history analysis, physical and neurologic examinations, and initial clinicopathologic tests are performed. The information collected from these evaluations is assessed to determine the probability of neurologic disease, the location of lesions within the nervous system, the severity of involvement, and the most likely mechanisms of disease. A differential diagnosis list is formulated and an initial diagnostic plan outlined to aid in the selection of the appropriate diagnosis.

Cerebrospinal fluid (CSF) collection and analysis is often part of the initial diagnostic plan. For lesions affecting the spinal cord or nerve roots, the diagnostic plan often includes electromyography (EMG), CSF analysis, plain vertebral column radiography, and possibly myelography. Electroencephalography (EEG), CSF analysis, and plain radiography of the skull often constitute the initial diagnostic plan for lesions affecting the brain stem, cerebellum, or cerebrum. CSF analysis is another objective piece of information to be used in the overall evaluation of the problem, regardless of the location of the lesion.

The mechanisms of disease that most frequently produce the greatest alterations in CSF include inflammatory, traumatic, vascular, degenerative, and neoplastic disorders. Except for some nonspecific EEG and EMG abnormalities, CSF alterations may be the only abnormal diagnostic aid associated with inflammatory disorders of the brain and spinal cord. In these cases, CSF analysis is necessary to make the diagnosis.

Normal CSF does not preclude the possibility of one of the mechanisms of disease that usually alters CSF, but those diseases that usually do not should be carefully considered. Those mechanisms of disease that rarely alter the CSF are congenital, metabolic, toxic, nutritional, and idiopathic disorders.

The CSF analysis is a very valuable diagnostic aid when interpreted in relation to the initial information collected, the differential diagnosis, and the results of other diagnostic aids. Past frustrations that some practitioners may have had with CSF analysis as a meaningful diagnostic tool may be partly due to improper analysis techniques. These yield inaccurate results and make interpreting the results

difficult. This discussion will emphasize analysis techniques and interpretation of results.

The techniques, indications, and contraindications for the collection of CSF are well described elsewhere (Averill, 1977; De Lahunta, 1977; Kay et al., 1974; Spano and Hoerlein, 1978; Wilson, 1980). With a little practice and care, CSF may be easily collected with minimal risk to the animal. Most routine analysis techniques may be performed on 1 to 2 ml of fluid.

CSF ANALYSIS TECHNIQUES AND RESULTS

Much of the equipment necessary to evaluate CSF is already in the veterinary hospital clinicopathology laboratory and includes a refractometer, urinary reagent strips, a hemocytometer, microscope slides, test tubes, and coverslips. Other equipment may be adapted, and solutions may be purchased at a low cost. The analysis techniques are simple and can be easily performed by a technical assistant (Coles, 1971; Kay et al., 1974; Mayhew and Beal, 1980; Spano and Hoerlein, 1978).

All parameters of the CSF except the determination of protein content must be evaluated within 30 minutes from the time of collection to obtain accurate results. Therefore, the analysis must be performed in the individual veterinary hospital and not in a commercial laboratory. The parameters routinely evaluated and normal values are found in Table 1.

PRESSURE

As CSF is collected from the cerebellomedullary cistern with the animal in lateral recumbency, the pressure may be measured with a spinal fluid manometer.* Compression of the jugular veins by extreme neck flexion during collection may falsely elevate CSF pressure. If CSF pressure is elevated by a disease process, only 1 ml of fluid of the contents in the manometer should be removed,

---

*Pharmaseal Laboratories, Glendale, CA.

676

Table 1. *Cerebrospinal Fluid Parameters and Normal Values*

Parameter	Normal Values
Pressure (cerebellomedullary cistern)	<100 mm (cats) <170 mm (dogs)
Color	Transparent
Clarity	Clear
Refractive index	1.3347 to 1.3350
Urinary reagent strips	pH 8 ± 1 Glucose: trace to + Protein: trace to 30 Blood: negative
Total cell count	<8 WBC, no RBC
Cell type	Small lymphocytes, few monocytes
Spectrophotometer protein determination	10 to 25 mg/dl
Pandy's test	No turbulence
Nonne-Apelt or Ross-Jones test	No ring formation

because excessive removal of CSF may produce a low pressure area at the cistern. The brain can shift caudally into the low pressure region, producing herniation of the cerebellar vermis through the foramen magnum, compression of vital centers in the medulla oblongata, and death. CSF collection is contraindicated in known cases of cranial trauma owing to this potential for herniation and compression.

Anything that can produce cerebral edema will produce elevated CSF pressure. The most common cause of elevated CSF pressure is neoplasia of the cerebrum, cerebellum, or brain stem. Other causes are status epilepticus, severe metabolic and toxic disturbances, abscesses, and meningitis.

Abnormally low CSF pressure is most frequently due to an improper collection technique but may be seen with noncommunicating obstructive hydrocephalus and severe dehydration.

COLOR AND CLARITY

A tube of CSF and a tube of distilled water are compared against a white background and should appear the same, i.e., colorless. The tubes are then placed against a background with black printed words; the words should be equally legible through each, as both fluids should be clear.

Pink or red CSF is most commonly due to contamination of the CSF sample with blood during the collection procedure. If contaminated with fresh blood, the sample may be centrifuged. The red blood cells will collect in the bottom of the tube, clearing the fluid in the supernate. If the supernate does not clear but remains pink or red, recent hemorrhage within the nervous system is likely. After 24 to 48 hours, hemorrhage in the CSF appears xanthochromic or yellow. Hemorrhage

within the nervous system may be associated with trauma, vascular disorders, and infections. Xanthochromic CSF is occasionally associated with severely elevated protein content or systemic icterus.

Increased turbidity and an opaque CSF are often due to an extreme increase in cell numbers or protein content. Mild to moderate elevations in either parameter rarely alter CSF clarity. The presence of bacterial or mycotic organisms in the CSF may also contribute to the turbidity.

REFRACTIVE INDEX

CSF may be placed in the chamber of a standard refractometer* used for urinalysis, the refraction read, and a refractive index calculated. A refraction between 17 and 20 with a refractive index between 1.3347 and 1.3350 is normal. The refractive index increases when either cell numbers or protein content is greatly increased.

URINARY REAGENT STRIPS

CSF may be dropped on urinary reagent strips† used during urinalysis and an estimate of pH, glucose, protein, and blood values obtained. Normal values are listed in Table 1. The pH may be reduced in severe acidosis. The glucose level may be elevated with diabetes mellitus. Protein elevations between 30 and 100 mg/dl (as determined by a spectrophotometer method) may not be detected, but increases greater than 100 mg/dl usually alter the reagent strip. Blood contamination or hemorrhage will be detected. The urinary reagent strips are a quick and easy screening test for CSF.

TOTAL CELL COUNT

The number of cells in the CSF is one of the important parameters and must be performed within 30 minutes of collection to ensure accuracy. After that time cells degenerate and numbers are unreliable.

A standard dual-chambered hemocytometer‡ used to count red and white blood cells in the peripheral blood may be used to count cells in CSF. One chamber is filled with gently mixed CSF alone. The other chamber is filled with a mixture of CSF and a diluting fluid composed of 0.2 gm of crystal or methyl violet dissolved in 10 ml of glacial acetic acid brought to a volume of 100 ml with distilled water. In a 1:10 white blood cell (WBC) diluting

---

*Goldberg Refractometer, American Optical, Buffalo, NY.
†Hemacombistix, Ames Company, Elkhart, IN.
‡Neubauer Hemocytometer, Fisher Scientific Company, Fairlawn, NJ.

pipette, the diluting fluid is drawn to the 1 mark. CSF is then drawn to the 11 mark and the two fluids gently mixed. The first few drops of the mixture are discarded and the hemocytometer chamber is filled. The diluting fluid lyses red blood cells (RBCs) and stains the nuclei of WBCs. The filled chambers are allowed to settle for two minutes before the cells are counted.

All cells on each side in five of the 1-mm² areas are counted. On the undiluted side the number is multiplied by two and represents the combined number of RBCs and WBCs per microliter of fluid. On the diluted side the number is multiplied by 2.2 and represents the number of WBCs per microliter only. The number of RBCs is determined by subtracting the number of WBCs from the combined number.

Normal CSF has no RBCs and eight or fewer WBCs. An increase in RBCs is usually due to contamination with peripheral blood during collection. The significance of an elevated WBC count in a contaminated sample is difficult to interpret. There is no accurate way to estimate how many WBCs are present owing to contamination and how many are due to an actual disease process in the nervous system, since WBCs marginate in blood vessels. The CSF may be contaminated with larger numbers of WBCs than is considered reasonable for the number of RBCs. If the CSF sample is significantly contaminated with peripheral blood, it is best to wait and re-evaluate the CSF in a week.

Elevated WBC counts unassociated with contamination indicate inflammation and are commonly associated with viral, protozoal, bacterial, and fungal infections and immune-mediated disorders. On rare occasions intervertebral disc herniation and brain or spinal cord neoplasia may produce a slight elevation of WBCs in CSF, but usually cell counts are normal in these conditions.

DIFFERENTIAL CELL COUNT

If the number of WBCs in the CSF is elevated, it is important to determine the type of cells to characterize the inflammatory process.

A direct smear of CSF on a slide is inadequate, as cell numbers are low. A method of concentrating the cells is needed; two techniques that are readily adaptable to a private veterinary hospital are outlined.

For the first technique, a sedimentation chamber and a standard glass microscope slide are needed (Mayhew and Beal, 1980). A sedimentation chamber can be fashioned from a glass test tube cut to form a double, open-ended cylinder. The smooth end of the glass cylinder is dipped in melted paraffin wax and placed on a warm slide. A thin ring of wax seals the cylinder to the slide, leaving a circle of clear glass on the bottom of the chamber. Shortly after collection, approximately 0.25 to 0.50 ml of CSF is placed in the chamber and allowed to sit undisturbed for 25 minutes. The cells settle to the bottom of the chamber onto the glass slide. If the CSF sits longer than 25 minutes, cell distortion results, making interpretation difficult. At the appropriate time, the supernate is gently aspirated and the cylinder removed by breaking the paraffin ring. A small bleb of CSF remains on the glass slide within the paraffin ring. The slide is then dried and sprayed with a cell fixative.* The paraffin ring is removed with a razor blade and the slide stained with a commercial white blood cell stain.† After staining, a coverslip is applied with a mounting medium.‡ A differential cell count and morphologic study may then be performed.

In a second technique for CSF cell collection, CSF is passed through a millipore filter (Mayhew and Beal, 1980; Roszel, 1972; Vandervelde and Spano, 1977). Ten drops to 1 ml of CSF are mixed with 2 ml of 40 per cent ethanol. Once mixed with the ethanol, the cells are preserved and will not degenerate if immediate examination is impossible. A Swinny-type hypodermic adapter§ contains a 13-mm diameter millipore filter.‖ The CSF-ethanol mixture is placed in a syringe attached to the adapter and gently passed through the millipore filter. The pores of the filter measure 5μ, which is smaller than most cells; therefore all cells within a CSF sample are collected.

The membrane filter containing the cells is then lifted from the adapter with forceps and immediately immersed in 95 per cent ethanol for two minutes. The filter is then placed sequentially in distilled water for 30 seconds, Harris' hematoxylin stain for 10 to 15 seconds, distilled water for 30 seconds, and then back into 95 per cent ethanol for 30 seconds. Finally, the filter is placed in absolute alcohol and xylene for one minute each. Following the xylene soak, the membrane should be transparent and can be placed on a standard glass microscope slide. A few drops of mounting media and a coverslip may then be applied.

Although the membrane filtration technique does require the purchase of special equipment, it does collect approximately ten times more cells than the sedimentation technique and with less distortion. Tumor cells and fungi, which may be found in small numbers within the CSF, are more likely to be collected and visualized with the membrane filtration technique. The examiner must adjust to viewing the cells at several angles in the filter, because

---

*Profixx, Scientific Products, McGraw Park, IL.

†Wright Stain Solution, Fisher Scientific Company, Fairlawn, NJ.

‡Permount, Fisher Scientific Company, Fairlawn, NJ.

§Gelman Instrument Company, Ann Arbor, MI.

‖Millipore Corporation, Bedford, MA.

they are not flattened as in the sedimentation technique. Both techniques concentrate cells onto a small area of the slide and facilitate rapid microscopic examination.

The cell population of normal CSF is comprised primarily of mononuclear cells, mainly lymphocytes and some monocytes. Differentiating between lymphocytes and monocytes may be difficult owing to the wide range in size. Monocytes generally have a greater abundance of cytoplasm than lymphocytes. Neutrophils and eosinophils are rarely seen in CSF, and their presence should be considered abnormal.

A CSF cytology composed of mainly increased numbers of mononuclear cells is most often associated with viral infections but can be seen in immune-mediated and other inflammatory disorders in which no agent can be isolated. Occasionally a small percentage of neutrophils will be seen, but lymphocytes, monocytes, and macrophages (phagocytic monocytes) predominate.

A CSF cytology composed of mainly increased numbers of neutrophils is most compatible with a bacterial infection. A Gram stain applied to a cell sedimentation slide may show the organisms.

A mixed population of mononuclear cells and neutrophils may be seen in fungal and protozoal infections. *Cryptococcus* organisms may be visualized after an India ink stain is applied to a cell sedimentation slide. Fungal organisms may be seen in the membrane filter.

On rare occasions the membrane filter may trap large, irregularly shaped cells that 'are clumped together, which might be identified as tumor cells. Tumor cells are not likely to be identified on sedimentation slides.

CULTURE

If the WBC count is elevated and a bacterial or fungal infection is suspected, the CSF should be cultured for the organism. Since the number of organisms may be low, at least 0.25 to 0.50 ml should be cultured. An antibiotic sensitivity may be performed on bacterial cultures. If a viral infection is suspected, CSF may be sent to a special laboratory for virus isolation attempts.

PROTEIN DETERMINATION

Along with cell number and type determinations, the evaluation of protein content of the CSF is most important. Unlike cytology studies, the protein content does not have to be tested immediately. The CSF may be frozen and then thawed when analysis is convenient.

If the veterinary hospital clinicopathology laboratory has a standard laboratory spectrophotometer,* a simple quantitative determination of protein content can be made using a turbidimetric procedure with CSF and trichloroacetic acid. Details of the technique are described elsewhere (Mayhew and Beal, 1980). Normal values using this technique in our laboratory are found in Table 1. Normal values should be established for each individual laboratory.

If a spectrophotometer is not available, CSF may be sent to a commercial laboratory. Techniques that measure small quantities of protein in fluids must be used, as normal CSF usually contains less than 25 mg/dl. Normal ranges must be established for each individual laboratory.

There are several qualitative tests of protein content that may be used to screen the CSF while waiting for results from the commercial laboratory. Urinary reagent strips may detect large increases in protein content but may miss mild but significant increases.

Pandy's test is another qualitative protein test. Pandy's solution is made by mixing 10 mg of carbolic acid crystals in 100 ml of distilled water. A few drops of CSF and 1 ml of Pandy's solution are mixed in a test tube and then shaken thoroughly. A positive Pandy's test is seen with increased turbidity of the CSF and is proportional to the globulin content.

The Nonne-Apelt or Ross-Jones test is another quick qualitative test for protein content. One milliliter of saturated ammonium sulfate is pipetted into a small test tube. CSF is carefully overlaid onto this and allowed to sit for three minutes. If the CSF contains increased amounts of globulin, a white to grayish ring will form at the interface of the CSF and ammonium sulfate.

CSF protein content increases with diseases that alter the blood-brain and blood-CSF barriers, block cerebrospinal fluid absorption, or increase gamma globulin synthesis in the nervous system. When serum gamma globulin is greatly elevated, there may be some diffusion into the CSF. Severe metabolic and toxic disorders may elevate CSF protein, but the mechanisms are not well understood (Eliasson et al., 1978).

CSF protein content may be elevated with inflammations. On occasion there may be only an elevation of protein content, with no increase in number of cells. If the inflammation is focal and does not contact any CSF spaces, the CSF may be normal.

Traumatic and vascular disorders produce elevated CSF protein levels owing to vascular leakage. Xanthochromic CSF, along with the elevated protein content, may further support traumatic and vascular disease. Widespread spinal cord degeneration or focal spinal cord compression, as seen with

---

*Bausch and Lomb Spectronic 70, Fisher Scientific Company, Fairlawn, NJ.

intervertebral disc protrusions and herniations, also produces increased CSF protein content.

Many primary and metastatic neoplasms of the nervous system produce an elevated CSF protein content. Neoplasia of the cerebrum, cerebellum, and brain stem may also produce elevated CSF pressure along with the elevation of CSF protein content.

CSF protein content may be mildly elevated in severe or chronic metabolic disorders such as anoxia, hypoxia, hypoglycemia, acidosis, and hyperthermia, especially when cerebrocortical or cerebellar necrosis has occurred.

MISCELLANEOUS TESTS ON CSF

If CSF protein content is elevated, a protein electrophoresis may be obtained to determine the type of protein present.

Immunoelectrophoresis of CSF may be performed to determine the specific types of immunoglobulins if globulins are elevated in the CSF.

CSF may be analyzed for the enzymes creatine phosphokinase (CPK), lactic dehydrogenase (LDH), and glutamic oxalic transaminase (GOT). The levels of these enzymes may be elevated in severe necrosis and may be a guide to prognosis for certain disorders.

A complete chemistry profile may be obtained on CSF evaluated in an automated unit that analyzes serum. The accuracy and usefulness of this information for diagnosis of specific disorders needs to be determined.

Canine distemper fluorescent antibody tests may be performed on CSF cell preparations by some special laboratories. Canine distemper virus titers of CSF may be obtained by other special laboratories and may aid in the diagnosis of infection by this organism.

CSF pH and osmolality may be determined when nervous system acidosis or hyperosmolar or hyposmolar syndromes are suspected.

INTERPRETATION OF THE RESULTS

Once an accurate analysis of the CSF is obtained, the results must be added to the other information collected so that meaningful interpretation can be made. An elevated CSF protein content may be associated with many different diseases. However, if an older dog is demented and convulsing and has elevated CSF pressure and protein content with no increase in cell number, cerebral neoplasia is a likely diagnosis. If a cat is paralyzed in all four limbs and has an extradural mass compressing the spinal cord, the CSF protein content often increases. The

Table 2. *Diseases and Associated Cerebrospinal Fluid Changes*

Disorder	Pressure	Appearance	Cell Count	Primary Cell Type	Protein
Congenital and familial disorders					
Hydrocephalus (congenital)	N	Clear	N	N	N
Hydrocephalus (post-natal)	N	Turbid	↑	Neutrophils	↑
Globoid leukodystrophy	N	Turbid	↑	Globoid cells, macrophages	↑
Inflammations					
Canine distemper virus	N or ↑	Clear or turbid	N or ↑	Mononuclear	N or ↑
Feline infectious peritonitis	N or ↑	Clear or turbid	N or ↑	Mononuclear	N or ↑
Cryptococcosis	N or viscous	Turbid, xanthochromic	↑	Neutrophils, mononuclear, and eosinophils	↑
Toxoplasmosis	N or ↑	Xanthochromic	↑	Neutrophils and mononuclear	↑
Bacterial	N or ↑	Turbid	↑	Neutrophils	↑
Granulomatous meningoencephalitis	N	Clear or turbid	↑	Mononuclear	↑
Trauma					
Fracture or spinal hemorrhage	N	Xanthochromic	N	N	↑
Intervertebral disc protrusion	N	Clear, xanthochromic	N or ↑	Mononuclear	↑
Vascular disorders					
Fibrocartilaginous infarct	N	Clear	N	N	↑
Degenerative disorders					
Degenerative myelopathy	N	Clear	N	N	↑ (lumbar)
Neoplasia					
Cerebral	↑ or N	Clear	N	N	↑
Spinal cord	N	Clear	N	N	↑

N = Normal.
↑ = increased.

interpretation of the results is the most difficult part of CSF evaluation and is a skill that comes only with experience.

Table 2 outlines common CSF alterations that may be associated with certain disease processes. These alterations do not always occur, but when they do this table may serve as a guide to interpretation when used in conjunction with the other information collected supporting the diagnosis.

REFERENCES AND SUPPLEMENTAL READING

Averill, D. R., Jr.: Examination of cerebrospinal fluid. In Kirk, R. W. (ed.): Current Veterinary Therapy VI. Philadelphia: W. B. Saunders, 1977.

Coles, E. H.: Cerebrospinal fluid. In Kaneko, J. J., and Cornelius, C. E. (eds.): Clinical Biochemistry of Domestic Animals, Vol. 2, 2nd ed., New York: Academic Press, 1971.

De Lahunta, A.: Cerebrospinal fluid and hydrocephalus. In Veterinary Neuroanatomy and Clinical Neurology. Philadelphia: W. B. Saunders, 1977.

Eliasson, S. G., Prensky, A. L., and Hardin, W. B. (eds.): Pathophysiology of the cerebrospinal fluid. In Neurological Pathophysiology, 2nd ed. New York: Oxford University Press, 1978.

Kay, W. J., Israel, E., and Prata, R. G.: Cerebrospinal fluid. Vet. Clin. North Am. 4:419, 1974.

Mayhew, I. G., and Beal, C. R.: Techniques of analysis of cerebrospinal fluid. Vet. Clin. North Am. 10:155, 1980.

Roszel, J. F.: Membrane filtration of canine and feline cerebrospinal fluid for cytologic evaluation. J.A.V.M.A. 160:720, 1972.

Spano, J. S., and Hoerlein, B. F.: Laboratory examinations. In Hoerlein, B. F. (ed.): Canine Neurology, Diagnosis and Treatment. Philadelphia: W. B. Saunders, 1978.

Vandervelde, M., and Spano, J. S.: Cerebrospinal fluid cytology in canine neurological diseases. Am. J. Vet. Res. 38:1827, 1977.

Wilson, J. W.: Cerebrospinal fluid analysis. In Kirk, R. W. (ed.): Current Veterinary Therapy VII. Philadelphia: W. B. Saunders, 1980.

CANINE MYOSITIS

GEORGE C. FARNBACH, V.M.D.

Philadelphia, Pennsylvania

Idiopathic inflammatory muscle disease (myositis) has been recognized and variously described in the dog for almost half a century. The first reported cases of this condition reflected the most dramatic and easily recognizable aspects of the disease process, i.e., acutely swollen muscles of mastication, trismus, and peripheral eosinophilia (Whitney, 1970). In our experience, this form of myositis is rare. A more frequent but less dramatic form of myositis, which has a subtle onset and produces a profound trismus not associated with peripheral eosinophilia, has also been known for a long time (Whitney, 1957).

The first of these two conditions was called eosinophilic myositis, whereas the second has various labels but is most often referred to as atrophic myositis. Because of the apparent similarities between atrophic myositis and eosinophilic myositis in the chronic phase, considerable debate has arisen regarding the relationship of these two conditions. This debate has been further muddled by the inclusion of a few cases of noninflammatory degeneration of the masticatory musculature (Whitney, 1970).

Before considering this debate, it is important to take note of the fact that canine myositis is not limited to the masticatory musculature. In an early report of the eosinophilic form of myositis, inflammatory involvement included muscles of the forearms, neck, and esophagus (Harding and Owen, 1956); in one case, lesions were limited to the hind quarters (Whitney, 1955). Since these early reports, additional cases with truncal weakness (Scott and de Lahunta, 1974) and other distributions of muscle inflammation with and without evidence of masticatory involvement have been reported.

Averill (1977) has used the term polymyositis (PM) for these cases. This term seems appropriate, since many muscles are involved in the inflammatory process. These more recent findings indicate that in the dog, as in humans (Bohan and Peter, 1975), inflammatory muscle disease represents a spectrum of clinical signs, possibly with common pathogenetic mechanisms.

In reviewing cases of polymyositis presented at the Veterinary Hospital of the University of Pennsylvania (VHUP) over the past three years, a variety of presenting signs have been seen. The majority of cases have been presented because of trismus and wasting of the masticatory muscles, but a significant number of animals have been presented for other signs related to their myositis. Many of the dogs had additional signs that were also seen in dogs presented for reasons other than trismus. The variety of physical and clinical findings in dogs with polymyositis is presented in Table 1.

The most frequent finding is wasting of the masticatory musculature, but this is not unique in most dogs, nor is it always accompanied by trismus (one dog). Approximately one-third of the dogs with polymyositis were presented for reasons not directly

Table 1. *Physical Findings Seen with Canine Polymyositis*

Wasting or swelling of masticatory muscles with trismus
Gait abnormalities
Dysphagia
Profound weakness

related to this atrophy or trismus. Indications in animals presented for reasons other than masticatory muscle involvement were gait abnormalities, dysphagia, and acute, profound weakness. In these animals masticatory involvement could often, but not always, be demonstrated by wasting and some degree of trismus.

The facts that evidence for more general muscle involvement can often be found in connection with masticatory signs and that masticatory signs can be seen with generalized myositis strongly support the concept that canine myositis can produce a broad spectrum of clinical signs, any of which may or may not be present in a single case.

The high incidence of multiple muscle involvement suggests that the term *polymyositis* would best serve nosologic interests, even in those cases in which masticatory involvement is most dramatic.

Such a classification would allow us to concentrate more on the disease process than on the variety of signs, which can be randomly selected from the spectrum of possibilities produced by the disease.

PATHOGENESIS AND ETIOLOGY

The unifying feature of all the possible indications of myositis is the histopathologic finding of intramuscular inflammation. Figure 1A shows some of the characteristic findings. Patchy areas of individual myofibers have virtually been replaced by inflammatory cells, whereas surrounding myofibers appear essentially normal. This section is from a mildly affected muscle. In more severely affected muscle sections similar inflammatory cells can often be seen involving almost every muscle fiber.

Figure 1B is a transverse section of human muscle from a patient with polymyositis. Similarities between the histopathology of human and canine polymyositis can be appreciated; however, differences also exist. In humans the types of cells involved in the inflammatory infiltrate are predominantly those associated with cell-mediated immunity, i.e., mononuclear cells, which are chiefly

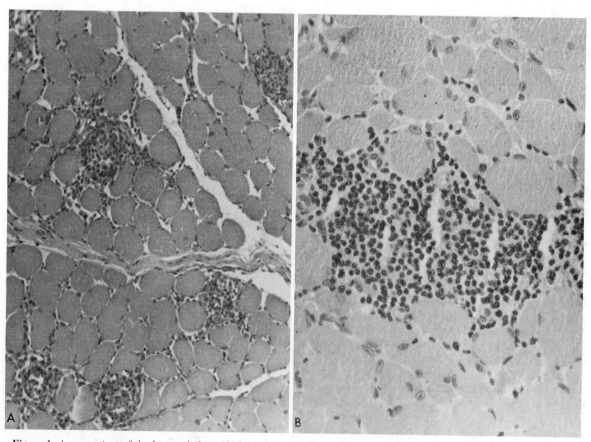

Figure 1. A comparison of the histopathology of canine (A) and human (B) polymyositis. Both diseases show a marked cellular replacement of individual muscle fibers in cross section.

ymphocytes (Bohan and Peter, 1975). Eosinophils are seen sometimes, however, and a few cases of human polymyositis with marked eosinophilia have been reported (Schumacher, 1976). In the dog the inflammatory infiltrate often includes cells identified with both the humoral (plasma cells, macrophages, and polymorphonuclear cells) and the cellular (lymphocytes) aspects of the immune system.

Historically, the degree of eosinophilia has been a crucial point in the distinction between the *eosinophilic* and *atrophic* forms of canine polymyositis. This was of particular clinical importance, since the atrophic form of the disease carried a somewhat more favorable prognosis than the eosinophilic form. The advent of steroid therapy in the treatment of polymyositis (Moon and Wood, 1954) has made eosinophilia a clinically moot point, however. Since the role of the eosinophil in the immune system remains relatively obscure and the numbers of circulating and peripheral eosinophils in the dog seem to vary, the importance of this aspect in the pathogenesis of polymyositis is questionable.

Very little is known of the etiology of either canine or human polymyositis. There is, however, some suggestive evidence concerning the pathogenesis of these diseases. First, the histopathology strongly incriminates the immune system, since the hallmark of the microscopic lesion is an inflammatory process directly involving muscle fibers. Second, the disease is frequently seen in connection with immune system diseases in both humans (Bohan and Peter, 1975) and dogs (Lewis, 1977). The responsiveness of the disease to immunosuppressive therapy in both human and canine species supports the notion that the pathogenesis is immune mediated. Finally, there is preliminary but persuasive laboratory evidence from the evaluation of delayed hypersensitivity mechanisms in humans indicating that the polymyositis includes an altered responsiveness of cell-mediated immunity (Bohan and Peter, 1975). What induces these alterations, however, remains unclear.

DIAGNOSIS

In arriving at a diagnosis of canine polymyositis, considerations should be made in at least four main cagetories. These are (1) history and presentation, (2) serum enzyme determinations, (3) electromyography (if available), and (4) muscle biopsy. Frequently, positive findings in all these areas are found and a comfortable diagnosis is made. However, it is not uncommon to find normal results in some areas and positive results in others. In these cases the diagnosis may be somewhat less clear, but if results indicative of myositis are found in three of the four areas the diagnosis should be considered positive.

HISTORY AND PRESENTATION

In our experience, polymyositis has no breed, age, or sex predilection. This is contrary to some reports (Roberts et al., 1975; Whitney, 1955), but we have seen the disease in both small and large breeds and in brachycephalic dogs. In any event, when an animal is presented with a history and signs suggestive of myositis this possibility should not be ignored, regardless of breed.

Myositis can be seen in an acute, subacute, or chronic form. Both the acute and subacute forms may manifest fever and marked lymph node swelling. In the acute form affected muscles are swollen and usually painful. In the subacute form marked bilateral atrophy of relatively sudden onset is noted. When the masticatory musculature is involved in these cases, a complete trismus with or without pain is usually found.

In the chronic form, the animal usually suffers a slow, subtle wasting and/or debilitation. Generally no episode of transient fever or illness can be recalled by the owner. In some instances the owner, in fact, may not be aware of the problem, and it is first observed by the veterinarian on physical examination associated with a routine vaccination visit. In other cases the owner may be concerned about slowly appearing bumps, which are, in fact, bony protuberances (occipital crest, scapular spines) that are being uncovered by the gradually receding muscle mass. Although we have divided the presentations here into three categories, in reality they represent a continuous spectrum, and only rarely does a case represent a single dimension.

The muscles most often recognized as affected by the disease process are the muscles of mastication. These animals almost invariably have a decreased range of motion in the jaw and may have a complete trismus. One of the hallmarks of the distribution of the disease is bilateral wasting of the masticatory musculature and trismus. The veterinarian should have a high index of suspicion for polymyositis when presented with an animal with these signs. However, since disuse also can produce wasting and since disuse of the temporomandibular joint can be produced by either a painful joint or a painful palate, other criteria must also be considered.

After the masticatory muscles, the muscles of the neck, shoulders, and forearms are those most often found to be involved. Here again a perfectly bilateral wasting without underlying evidence of either skeletal or neurologic disorder is highly suggestive of polymyositis. Other signs include truncal and pelvic limb weakness with or without obvious wasting. In these cases the animal's gait often appears painful, with short, choppy limb action and frequent tremors while either standing or rising. Occasionally animals are seen with voice changes, dysphagia, coughing, and megaesophagus.

Clinical criteria, physical findings, and historic evidence prompt a possible diagnosis of polymyositis. Supporting evidence can be obtained by specific muscle enzyme determinations. In our experience, serum CPK (creatine phosphokinase) is the most informative of these determinations. Interpretation of results, however, must be made with some caution, since serum CPK can be elevated for a variety of reasons.

In our laboratory normal values for CPK are less than 100 IU/l. In severe myositis cases the serum levels may approach 1000 IU/l, and in milder cases the values are almost never less than 200 IU/l. In neurogenic myopathy serum CPK may be greater than 100 IU/l but generally does not exceed 200 IU/l.

Trauma, surgery, intramuscular injections, electromyography, and a variety of less common myopathies may also cause extreme elevations of serum CPK levels. Consequently, serum CPK determinations should be made prior to other diagnostic or treatment procedures. In humans (Bohan and Peter, 1975) and dogs (Kornegay et al., 1980), normal serum CPK determinations have been reported in many of the histologically confirmed cases. (Our experience does not confirm this, however.)

The most reliable positive evidence for confirming a diagnosis of polymyositis lies in the histopathology of the muscle biopsy specimen. Negative results from these studies do not rule out myositis, however, since the biopsy technique is not trouble-free. In dogs with polymyositis there is frequently a very patchy distribution of inflammatory foci in affected muscles. This introduces the problem of sampling error in choosing a necessarily small site for biopsy. Biopsy of masticatory musculature in severely affected animals is also frequently fruitless because of the paucity of muscle fibers.

The variety of presentations and physical findings associated with canine PM is paralleled by a variety of possible abnormalities found on EMG studies. These changes run from complete electrical silence to bizarre pseudomyotonic discharges in affected muscles (Table 2). Essentially similar findings are reported in humans (Bohan and Peter, 1975). The pathogenesis of this electrical activity is unclear. Careful survey by needle EMG frequently reveals a much broader distribution of involvement of muscle in the disease process than can be appreciated on physical examination. This survey technique can be useful in selecting muscle for biopsy. Because of

the marked bilateral symmetry of the disease, one side of the animal can be studied with the EMG and the other side used for biopsy, thus avoiding needle artifacts in the histopathology.

Other diagnostic work that should be considered in canine PM includes antinuclear antibody (ANA) titers and thoracic radiographs if clinically indicated. In approximately one-fourth of our cases of PM in which ANA titers were done, significant elevations (> 1:80) were found. This finding supports the concept of an immunopathologic basis for the disease and is an indication for very careful control and monitoring of the disease process in these animals, since the higher titer is probably indicative of more severe immunopathology. Thoracic radiographs are indicated in animals with dysphagia and/or post-prandial regurgitation, since the disease may also effect esophageal musculature and may produce hyomotility or megaesophagus.

TREATMENT AND PROGNOSIS

The use of corticosteroid therapy to control the inflammatory muscle destruction seen with canine PM was introduced in 1954 (Moon and Wood, 1954) and has provided much benefit to animals with all forms of the disease. Recent literature suggests the use of immunosuppressive levels of steroids (1.0 mg of prednisolone/kg divided three times daily) until remission occurs and then tapering off the drug over a short period (Averill, 1977). In some instances physical force has been recommended to correct chronic trismus.

Our experience does not support these recommendations. We have found that recurrence of the disease process is fairly general and that the single disease episode is a rare occurrence. Recurrence appears to be much more frequent in those animals tapered off steroids over a short period of time.

Our approach to treatment in the dog is similar to that taken in human PM, wherein the immediate goal is restoration of muscle function followed by control of the disease by long-term, low-dose, alternate-day steroid therapy. Initial treatment consists of immunosuppressive levels of either prednisolone or prednisone (available in larger pill sizes) on a daily basis.

In those animals with acute presentations—regardless of the presence or absence of eosinophils—the response is usually dramatic, with clinical remission beginning in one or two days and return of CPK levels to normal within one week. In these cases, dose reduction can begin immediately; the daily dosage is halved and given once every other day (resulting in effectively reducing weekly intake by a factor of four). This new dose level is maintained for at least two to four weeks, and then serum CPK levels and motor function are re-eval-

Table 2.   *Electromyographic Changes Seen with Canine Polymyositis*

Fibrillations
Positive sharp waves
Pseudomyotonic discharges
Electrical silence

uated. If these factors remain normal the dose can again be reduced by half.

This process should be repeated at increasingly longer intervals until a very low corticosteroid dose is attained (2.5 to 5 mg every other day). At this point, the low dose is maintained for at least two months before complete withdrawal is attempted. Once this is obtained, the animal should be monitored closely for return of clinical signs and/or CPK elevations. If at any point clinical signs reappear or CPK levels begin to elevate, the last dose should be used again. Further reductions are probably contraindicated.

In more chronic cases initial reversal of clinical signs may be less dramatic, particularly in those with long-term progressive trismus. The principles of treatment and control remain the same in chronic cases as in acute cases, but dose reductions are made in smaller steps. After two weeks of high-dose therapy, the animals are re-evaluated in terms of jaw opening and serum CPK levels. By this time CPK levels are invariably normal and jaw opening is improved, although by no means normal. At this point the corticosteroid dose should be halved by switching to alternate-day therapy. The complete dose given once every other day seems to be most effective, and occasionally clients note a difference between dose days and no-dose days. As long as continued improvement—although slow—is noted, this dose level is continued until near norml function is restored. Then dose tapering and maintenance, as in acute cases, can be attempted.

Using this treatment and control regimen, we have not found that prying of jaws or other surgical intervention is necessary. Figure 2 shows the long-term progress of an illustrative case of chronic polymyositis with trismus in an eight-year-old mal-

amute in terms of prescribed steroid levels, serum CPK levels, and jaw opening. Prior to this animal's presentation at the VHUP, an attempt had been made to pry the mouth open, the result of which was two broken premolars and no improvement in mouth opening. Euthanasia was declined by the owner.

At the time of presentation at the VHUP, the serum CPK level was 877 IU/l. There was extreme wasting of the masticatory musculature with mild wasting of epaxial musculature as far caudal as the mid thoracic spine. Two weeks of prednisolone therapy (25 mg b.i.d.) resulted in a decrease in serum CPK activity to 129 IU/l and an approximate doubling of jaw excursion. At this point alternate-day therapy was begun at 50 mg prednisolone every other day. On the next and subsequent visits, serum CPK values remained below 70 IU/l. Jaw mobility continued to improve, and muscle mass returned to normal everywhere except over the head, where slow but incomplete improvement in muscle mass occurred. The animal has continued to require 5 to 10 mg prednisolone every other day for the last three years.

In human PM, high levels of steroids are used until signs of iatrogenic Cushing's disease are produced or until control is obtained. If signs of Cushing's disease develop before control is achieved, other nonsteroidal immunusuppressive drugs (such as Azothioprine) are used. In the treatment of more than ten animals over two or more years, we have not seen one animal fail to respond to nontoxic levels of chronic steroid therapy.

Clearly, a dosage of prednisolone that controls the disease and has minimal side effects must be achieved. We are currently treating and monitoring a number of dogs with PM with time courses

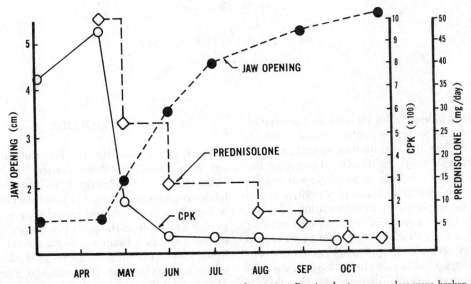

Figure 2. The course of steroid therapy and control of canine polymyositis. Previously, two premolars were broken in an attempt to pry the mouth open. Prompt improvement is noted in serum enzyme levels and jaw opening after steroid therapy.

essentially parallel to this case and have found no complications at the dose rate of 5 mg prednisolone every other day. The disease has recurred in two animals in which steroids were briefly discontinued.

On the basis of these cases we have begun to conclude that the prognosis for canine PM is relatively favorable under certain conditions. The first of these conditions is that treatment must be approached with the philosophy of *control* rather than *cure*, since the disease appears to be an ongoing process with frequent remissions. Second, the owner must participate in the process of monitoring the animal's condition. This includes a daily check on the animal's status, which is very effective in the early detection of loss of control or remission and therapeutic complications if they occur. In those cases with involvement of the muscles of the esophagus and deglutition, the prognosis is far less favorable, since a constant risk of inhalation pneumonia exists throughout the long recovery period.

CONCLUSION

Polymyositis is probably the most frequently recognized muscle disease in the dog. The etiology is unknown, but several bits of clinical and histopathologic evidence suggest an immunopathologic basis. Polymyositis produces a spectrum of clinical signs ranging from wasting and trismus to painful gait abnormalities and generalized weakness. A diagnosis of PM is based on history and signs, serum enzyme determinations, electromyography, and histopathology. The disease is generally controllable through the use of adrenocorticosteroids, and prognosis need not be as guarded as has been previously reported.

REFERENCES AND SUPPLEMENTAL READING

Averill, D. A.: Polymyositis in the dog. *In* Kirk, R. W. (ed.): *Current Veterinary Therapy VI.* Philadelphia: W. B. Saunders, 1977, pp. 822–825.

Bohan, A. B., and Peter, A. B.: Polymyositis and dermatomyositis. N. Engl. J. Med. 292:344, 1975.

Harding, H. P., and Owen, L. N.: Eosinophilic myositis in the dog. J. Comp. Pathol. 66:109, 1956.

Kornegay, J. N., Gorgacz, E. J., et al.: Polymyositis in dogs. J.A.V.M.A. 176:431, 1980.

Lewis, R. M.: Canine systemic lupus erythematosus. *In* Kirk, R. W. (ed.): *Current Veterinary Therapy VI.* Philadelphia: W. B. Saunders, 1977, pp. 463–465.

Moon, C., and Wood, A. C.: Eosinophilic myositis in a dog. J.A.V.M.A. 125:312, 1954.

Roberts, K. E., Hanson, P., and Zaslow, I. M.: Masticator myopathy in the dog. V.M./S.A.C. 70:840, 1975.

Schumacher, H. R.: A scleroderma-like syndrome with fasciitis, myositis, and eosinophilia. Ann. Intern. Med. 84:49, 1976.

Scott, D. W., and de Lahunta, A.: Eosinophilic polymositis in a dog. Cornell Vet. 64:47, 1974.

Whitney, J. C.: Eosinophilic myositis in dogs. Vet. Rec. 67:1140, 1955.

Whitney, J. C.: Atrophic myositis in a dog: the differentiation of this disease from eosinophilic myositis. Vet. Rec. 69:130, 1957.

Whitney, J. C.: A case of cranial myodegeneration (atrophic myositis) in a dog. J. Small Anim. Pract. 11:735, 1970.

MYOTONIA IN THE DOG

I. D. DUNCAN, B.V.M.S.,

Madison, Wisconsin

and I. R. GRIFFITHS, B.V.M.S.

Glasgow, Scotland

Myotonia is a disorder of skeletal muscle characterized clinically by active contraction of a muscle that persists after the cessation of voluntary effort or stimulation (Walton, 1974). The underlying defect is thought to originate in an abnormal muscle membrane that discharges trains of repetitive action potentials in response to depolarization (Bryant, 1974). In humans, myotonia is found in a number of different muscle diseases, the most important of which are myotonia dystrophica and myotonia congenita. Myotonia has been found in association with several different muscle diseases in the dog, a number of which appear to be breed specific.

ETIOLOGY

Much of the investigation into the pathophysiology of myotonia has been carried out in the myotonic goat and in chemically induced myotonia in laboratory animals (Bryant, 1974; Kwiecinski, 1981). A low–membrane chloride conductance is thought to play a key role in the pathophysiology of myotonia in the goat, in human myotonia congenita, and in human myotonia congenita seen after administration of the carboxylic acids (Furman and Barchi, 1978). This is related to accumulation of potassium in the t-tubular system, which leads to progressive post-excitation depolarization of the muscle membrane. 20,25-Diazacholesterol, a cholesterol lowering agent, has also been used to induce myotonia in experimental animals following the discovery that chronic administration of the drug could produce myotonia. However, in this form of myotonia and in myotonic dystrophy it appears unlikely that reductions in sarcolemmal conductance are involved in the pathophysiology (Furman and Barchi, 1981). It can therefore be suggested that the pathophysiology of myotonia is multifactorial.

MYOTONIA IN THE CHOW CHOW

Myotonia has been reported in chow chows in four countries: the United Kingdom (Griffiths and Duncan, 1973), Holland (Wentink et al., 1972), Australia (Farrow and Malik, 1981), and New Zealand (Jones et al., 1978). It therefore seems likely that myotonia is more widespread in the chow than in any other breed. To date there is no unequivocal evidence that the disease is inherited in this breed, but the evidence appears strong. (1) In the report of Wentink and colleagues (1972), affected dogs were found in two successive litters bred from the same parents. (2) In the report of Jones and associates (1978), members of the same litter were found to be affected. (3) Farrow and Malik (1981) reported a few related chows with myotonia. The first two were littermates (male and female) in a litter of three. The third pup was fathered by the same sire as the first two pups, and a daughter of this same sire produced the fourth affected pup. The authors described the suspect sire as being very muscular and stiff, although he was not examined electromyographically. (4) In our experience of four chows with the disorder (two male, two female), all have come from litters produced by normal parents, and each has been the only member of the litter to be affected. This combined evidence strongly suggests that the disease is inherited, perhaps as an autosomal recessive trait.

CLINICAL SIGNS

In all instances the clinical signs appear as early as two to three months of age, but whether myotonia is present at birth is not known. The signs are first noted when the animal attempts to rise. Marked abduction or splaying of the forelimbs often occurs, and after struggling to rise the dog walks with a stiff gait and arched back. Farrow and Malik (1981) suggested that this initial splaying of the forelimbs was the result of transient pectoral muscle weakness. They noted that such a phenomenon can be seen in humans with myotonia congenita. There is marked inability to flex the stifle joints, and the dog may move with a "bunny-hop gait" and may be unable to climb stairs. In all reported cases this stiffness lessens with exercise but worsens with cold weather. If the dog is suddenly rotated onto its side or back, the resultant hyperextension of the limbs will persist for up to a minute and will prevent the dog from righting itself. On palpation of skeletal muscles (proximal and distal muscles in the fore- and hind limbs and the masticatory muscles), marked hypertrophy can be detected. This can perhaps be felt best in the proximal muscles of the fore- and hind limbs, where individual muscles can easily be palpated as a result of their hypertrophy. All voluntary muscles can be hypertrophied including the tongue and external anal sphincter (Farrow and Malik, 1981).

An additional clinical test can be of significant value in diagnosing the disease. Percussion of a muscle with a blunt instrument results in a furrow that will persist for up to 30 to 45 seconds (myotonic dimple) (Fig. 1). Either a proximal fore- or hind

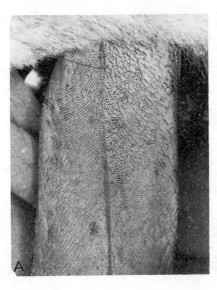
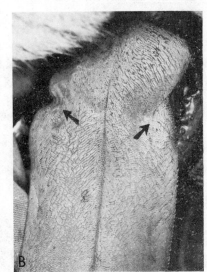

Figure 1. *A*, Tongue of a myotonic chow prior to percussion. *B*, After percussion with a blunt instrument a furrow forms (arrows) and persists for 30 to 45 seconds.

limb muscle can be percussed with the animal lying on its side, although the hair has to be clipped over the muscle to visualize the dimple. If the dog is anesthetized, percussion of the tongue often reveals a very obvious myotonic dimple.

Care should be taken when anesthetizing animals suspected of having myotonia, because stenosis of the laryngeal glottis can result in difficulties in intubation. In two dogs, stenosis of the glottis was thought to be responsible for the moderate dyspnea from which the dog was suffering. Dysphagia may be present, especially at the start of the meal. Muscle tone as judged by passive flexion of the joints is not increased. In some cases, patellar luxation and secondary arthritis may be found, possibly as an initial result of the continued contraction of the hind limb extensor muscles. Abnormalities of other organs aside from the muscular system have not been reported. Measurement of serum creatine phosphokinase (CPK) should be carried out, as in some cases this may be raised and may indicate myopathic damage. Serum cholesterol should be checked, as one dog in the Australian series showed a hypocholesterolemia (Farrow and Malik, 1981).

ELECTROMYOGRAPHY (EMG)

An unequivocal diagnosis of myotonia in the chow can be made on EMG examination, although the clinical signs, breed, and presence of a myotonic dimple should indicate the diagnosis. The insertion of a concentric needle electrode into almost any muscle in the resting or anesthetized dog will induce high-frequency discharges that can be heard on the EMG loudspeaker. These sounds, which have been likened to noise produced by a dive bomber, are the result of waxing and waning of the amplitude and frequency of the discharges. Currently, the analogy between these sounds and a motorbike revving up might be more appropriate. Insertion of the needle and needle movement will elicit these discharges, but following this activity spontaneous discharges also occur (Fig. 2). Percussion of the muscle while the needle is in place will also induce myotonic discharges. In general, these discharges have a frequency of 100 to 200/sec and last for one-half to one second. They persist after both depolarizing and nondepolarizing muscle relaxants are given, thus proving that the activity arises in the muscle. The reaction to succinylcholine is somewhat unusual in that, instead of the normal fasciculations that occur shortly after the drug is given, opisthotonos, tonic spasm of all the limbs, and apnea as a result of fixation of the thorax are found (Griffiths and Duncan, 1973; Jones et al., 1978). This has also been noted in human patients with myotonia and in the myotonic goat (Bryant, 1974). To date there have been insufficient reports of EMG results of voluntary activity, but in one case the interference pattern was normal (Griffiths and Duncan, 1973). Nerve conduction velocities are within normal range. Repetitive nerve stimulation

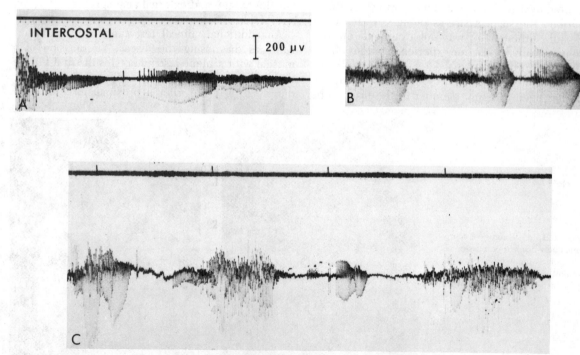

Figure 2. Typical myotonic discharges. *A*, Intercostal muscle. Note the increase and decrease in both frequency and amplitude of the high-frequency potentials. *B*, Lateral triceps. *C*, Biceps femoris. In *B* and *C* time marker = 1 second.

can result in decrement of the compound–evoked muscle action potential, and this may be related to the transient muscle weakness seen at the start of exercise (Farrow and Malik, 1981).

PATHOLOGY

Although muscle biopsy is not an essential part of the investigation of this disease, it can provide some useful information. To date there has been some variance (Duncan et al., 1975; Wentink et al., 1972; Jones et al., 1978) in the description of the pathologic changes found, and in our recent cases there have been differences among individual chows. In two of our cases the only abnormality noted in the proximal muscle biopsies from the fore- and hind limbs was pronounced hypertrophy, probably of both type I and II muscle fibers. In the remaining cases there was a marked variation in muscle fiber size in biopsies from the same muscle, with both hypertrophic and atrophic fibers (Duncan et al., 1975; Jones et al., 1978). The incidence of other myopathic changes in our cases and in those of Jones and associates (1978) is variable. These changes include muscle fiber degeneration and regeneration, hyaline fibers, split fibers, internal nuclei, and increased connective tissue. These changes have led us to suggest that these cases may represent a true muscular dystrophy (Walton, 1974); i.e., there is evidence of a primary inherited progressive degenerative myopathy. However, there is no evidence of those changes regarded as hallmarks of human myotonia dystrophica, i.e., ringed fibers and sarcoplasmic masses. Interestingly, however, it appears probable that some groups of muscle (e.g., the ventral neck muscles) may be more severely "myopathic" than limb muscles (Duncan et al., 1975). This may be analogous to many of the human dystrophies in which the predilection for various groups of muscles to be more severely affected has given rise to many of their appellations, e.g., facioscapulohumeral dystrophy. Very recent observations following autopsy of an older chow have shown profuse myopathic features, mainly internal nuclei, in certain muscles (Griffiths and Duncan, 1982). Further documentation of the muscle pathology in the chow is required.

TREATMENT

Attempts at treating myotonia are aimed at stabilizing the muscle fiber membrane using such compounds as procainamide and phenytoin. The mode of action of these compounds is to block dynamic sodium-conduction channels (Bryant, 1974). The latter drug has been used by us with little success. Farrow and Malik (1981) reported in some detail on the use of procainamide, quinidine, and phenytoin. Oral administration of the first two drugs proved beneficial in lessening the initial weakness and concomitant stiffness. The success of these drugs in the canine disease may be limited in the long term if dystrophic muscle changes become significant. Currently, however, it appears that muscle hypertrophy may predominate, and therefore some treatment may be feasible. Once the diagnosis has been established, the owner should be advised that treatment is still experimental and that while there may be no progression of signs, improvement may be unlikely. The owner should also be advised to avoid exposing the animal to cold weather. Because of the possible inherited nature of this condition, affected dogs and their parents should not be used for breeding.

In summary, myotonia in the chow has some similarities to human myotonia congenita (Thomsen's disease): very early onset, clinical signs, muscle hypertrophy, and significant lack of involvement of other organs. It is unlike human myotonia dystrophica, in which alopecia, cataracts, gonadal hypoplasia, and endocrine and immunoglobulin abnormalities are found. Unequivocal evidence of a familial nature requires further breeding trials, and, although similarities between it and its human counterparts remain interesting, caution should be exercised in further extrapolation. Indeed, Farrow and Malik (1981) suggest that because there may be evidence of mild myopathic process in affected chows, the canine disease is not identical to either of the human conditions and that a better term for the chow disorder is hereditary myotonia.

SEX-LINKED MYOPATHY IN IRISH TERRIERS

Five male puppies from one litter were found to have difficulty in walking associated with stiffness and weakness from eight weeks of age onward (Wentink et al., 1972). Dysphagia was present in all cases, and there was lumbar kyphosis and muscle atrophy. A myotonic dimple was not elicitable on percussion. Myopathic changes were prominent in the skeletal muscles examined and consisted of degeneration, regeneration, calcification, and some inflammatory cell infiltration. Prolonged high-frequency discharges that decreased in frequency were found on EMG examination. These are unlike the discharges seen in the myotonic chow, which are short in duration and increase and decrease in both amplitude and frequency.

AUTOSOMAL RECESSIVE MYOPATHY ASSOCIATED WITH MYOTONIA AND A DEFICIENCY OF TYPE II MUSCLE FIBERS IN LABRADOR RETRIEVERS

This disease was described in five retrievers from three separate litters and was first seen at the age of six months or less (Kramer et al., 1976). A further study has shown that the disease is inherited as an autosomal recessive trait (Kramer et al., 1981). The dogs were stiff, walked with a hopping gait, and had abnormal head and neck posture. Muscle atrophy was noticeable. Unlike the condition seen in the chow and human cases of myotonia congenita, exercise increased the weakness and cold weather also exacerbated the signs. There was no note of the presence of a myotonic dimple. Serum CPK levels were lower than normal, unlike the values found in the chow (Griffiths and Duncan, 1973; Jones et al., 1978). Discharges found on EMG examination were classified as myotonic. Muscle biopsy showed a variation in fiber size, and an increase in connective tissue and histochemistry demonstrated a decrease in the number of type II fibers. There was no apparent progression of clinical signs with age.

MYOPATHY IN ASSOCIATION WITH CUSHING'S DISEASE

The clinical signs of muscle weakness and atrophy in the majority of dogs with hyperadrenocorticism are well known. Muscle weakness often results in excess abduction of the elbows, and a pendulous abdomen and generalized muscle atrophy, often most noted in the temporal muscles, can be seen. Iatrogenic Cushing's disease can result from the protracted overdosage of steroids, and animals with this condition can present with a myopathy. In both spontaneous and iatrogenic Cushing's disease a few animals may present with limb rigidity and a stiff gait (Duncan et al., 1977; Greene et al., 1979). In these cases there is hyperextension of all four limbs, especially the hind limbs, and flexion of the limb may be impossible even under general anesthesia. A myotonic dimple can be found on percussion of the muscles, which are often hypertrophic.

EMG of dogs with Cushing's disease either with muscle weakness and atrophy or stiffness revealed the presence of high-frequency discharges, mainly in the proximal muscles (Duncan et al., 1977; Greene et al., 1979). These discharges were mainly pseudomyotonic (Fig. 3); i.e., they did not wax and wane. They were often stimulated by needle insertion and started and stopped abruptly after periods of up to 30 seconds. After careful searching, however, spontaneous myotonic discharges were also found (Duncan et al., 1977). Pseudomyotonic discharges can be found in many primary disorders of muscle and can also be found in neurogenic atrophy. Use of the term "pseudomyotonic" should perhaps be discontinued in favor of the more accurate term, "bizarre high-frequency discharge" (Eisen and Karpati, 1971). The origin of these high-frequency discharges is not known, but the association between them and the abnormal calcium metabolism found in canine Cushing's disease has been suggested. Muscle biopsy from affected cases shows

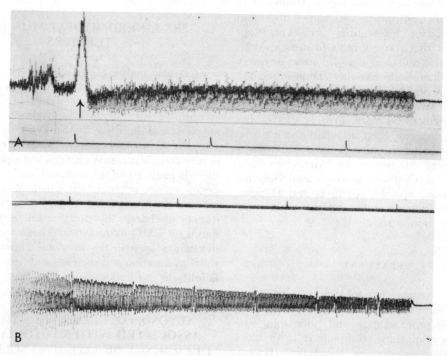

Figure 3. Typical bizarre high-frequency discharge (pseudomyotonia). *A*, Needle movement (arrow) has triggered this discharge, which does not vary in frequency or amplitude and which terminates abruptly. *B*, In this high-frequency discharge (pseudomyotonia) there is a slight variation in frequency and amplitude. In *A* and *B* time marker = 1 second.

atrophy, some fiber necrosis and regeneration, and an increase in fat and connective tissue. Skeletal muscle calcification can occasionally be seen. Treatment of Cushing's disease using adrenocorticolytic drugs can occasionally result in resolution of the weakness and muscle atrophy (Greene et al., 1979), but in most instances, although polydipsia and polyuria may be reduced, the weakness remains and myotonic discharges can still be found.

CONCLUSIONS

Single cases of myotonia in a variety of breeds have also been reported (West Highland terrier, Griffiths and Duncan, 1973; Labrador retriever, Duncan and Griffiths, 1982; Samoyed, Cardinet and Holliday, 1979). More cases will be seen in the future, and genetic analysis, careful EMG examination, and muscle biopsy will help determine whether there is a range of myotonic syndromes in the dog as in humans.

REFERENCES AND SUPPLEMENTARY READING

Bryant, S. H.: The electrophysiology of myotonia, with a review of congenital myotonia in goats. In Desmedt, J. E. (ed.): New Development in Electromyography and Clinical Neurophysiology, Vol. 1. Basel; Karger, 1974, p. 420.

Cardinet, G. H., and Holliday, T. A.: Neuromuscular diseases of domestic animals: a summary of muscle biopsies from 159 cases. Ann. N. Y. Acad. Sci. 26:290, 1979.
Duncan, I. D., Griffiths, I. R., and McQueen, A.: A myopathy associated with myotonia in the dog. Acta Neuropathol. 31:297, 1975.
Duncan, I. D., Griffiths, I. R., and Nash, A. S.: Myotonia in canine Cushing's disease. Vet. Rec. 100:30, 1977.
Eisen, A. A., and Karpati, G.: Spontaneous electrical activity in muscle description of two patients with motor neuron disease. J. Neurol. Sci. 12:121, 1971.
Farrow, B. R. H., and Malik, R.: Hereditary myotonia in the Chow Chow. J. Small Anim. Pract. 22:451, 1981.
Furman, R. E., and Barchi, R. L.: The pathophysiology of myotonia produced by aromatic carboxylic acids. Ann. Neurol. 4:357, 1978.
Furman, R. E., and Barchi, R. L.: 20,25 Diazacholesterol myotonia: an electrophysiological study. Ann. Neurol. 10:251, 1981.
Greene, C. E., Lorenz, M. D., Munnell, J. Jr., Prase, K. W., White, L. A., and Bowen, J. M.: Myopathy associated with hyperadrenocorticism in the dog. J.A.V.M.A. 174:1310,1979.
Griffiths, I. R., and Duncan, I. D.: Myotonia in the dog: A report of four cases. Vet. Rec. 93:184, 1973.
Griffiths, I. R., and Duncan, I. D.: Unpublished data, 1982.
Jones, B. R., Anderson, L. J., Barnes, G. R. G., Johnstone, A. C., and Juby, W. D.: Myotonia in related chow chow dogs. N. Z. Vet. J. 25:217, 1978.
Kramer, J. W., Hegreberg, G. A., Braun, G. M., Meyers, K., and Ott, R. L.: A muscle disorder of Labrador retrievers characterized by deficiency of type II muscle fibers. J.A.V.M.A. 169:817, 1976.
Kramer, J. W., Hegreberg, G. A., and Hamilton, M. J.: Inheritance of a neuromuscular disorder of Labrador retriever dogs. J.A.V.M.A. 179:380, 1981.
Kwiecinski, H.: Myotonia induced by chemical agents. C.R.C. Crit. Rev. Toxicol. 8:279, 1981.
Walton, J. N.: Disorders of Voluntary Muscle, 3rd ed. New York; Longman, 1974.
Wentink, G. H., van der Line-Sipman, J. S., Keijer, A. E. F. H., Kamphuisen, H. A. C., van Vorstenbosch, C. J. A. H. V., Hartman, W., and Kendriks, H. J.: Myopathy with a possible recessive x-linked inheritance in a litter of Irish terriers. Vet. Pathol. 9:328, 1972.
Wentink, G. H., Hartman, D., and Koeman, J. P.: Three cases of myotonia in a family of chows. Tijdschr. Diergeneeskd. 99:729, 1974.

TICK PARALYSIS IN AUSTRALIA

JAN E. ILKIW, B.V.Sc.

Sydney, Australia

Tick paralysis in Australia is a disease produced by *Ixodes holocyclus*. Other species, *I. cornuatus* and *I. hirsti*, have been reported in association with cases of tick paralysis.

Ixodes holocyclus is a three-host tick that engorges and then falls off the host between each successive stage of the life cycle. The disease usually follows infestation with adult female ticks but may follow infestation with nymphs or larvae.

Cases of tick paralysis are restricted to the coastal areas of eastern Australia, especially in bush and scrub country.

CLINICAL SIGNS

Severe disease with death is reported in all species: humans (principally infants), foals, calves, pigs, sheep, and poultry, but it is most common in the dog and cat. In contrast, death is rarely observed in native fauna. In the dog one tick is sufficient to cause paralysis with progression to death, but not all adult female ticks are capable of causing the disease. Clinical signs are usually observed six to seven days after attachment of the tick, and even with mass infestation signs do not appear before the fourth day.

In the dog the signs are those of a rapidly ascending, flaccid motor paralysis. Altered voice, cough, and dysphagia may be early signs, but the first consistent sign is a slight incoordination of the hindquarters. Whether the ticks are removed at this stage or not, the incoordination becomes more marked and soon the dog is unable to stand. Respiration is slow and embarrassed, and violent retching occurs in some animals. The disease progresses to the forelimbs until the dog lies in lateral recumbency; the pupils are usually dilated and unresponsive to light, and the dog makes feeble convulsive movements usually associated with respiration. In contrast to the severity of the motor disturbance, other signs are slight. The afferent sensory pathways are usually not affected; consciousness is not lost, and the animal is aware of activity in its immediate surroundings.

In the cat the signs are similar to those seen in dogs, but vomiting is uncommon.

PATHOGENESIS OF THE DISEASE

Studies by Cooper (1976) indicated that the paralysis is produced by an abnormality in the mechanism that couples nerve terminal depolarization and acetylcholine release. No abnormality in nerve conduction was found, but the release of acetylcholine in response to nerve stimulation was depressed owing to a reduction in quantal content rather than quantal size. This effect was found to be markedly temperature dependent, in that lowering the temperature resulted in a reduction of the effect.

Studies of the cardiovascular and respiratory effects of *Ixodes holocyclus* in the dog (Ilkiw, 1979) have shown that both these systems also are involved. There is a progressive fall in respiratory rate with no change in tidal volume. This contrasts with other diseases that cause neuromuscular paralysis in which respiration is rapid and shallow. In tick paralysis this is probably the result of central respiratory depression. The "grunting" type of respiration characteristic of a dog with tick paralysis is due to closure of the vocal cords during expiration. No abnormalities in blood-gas or acid-base status are found until quite late in the disease. Just prior to death, moderate hypoxemia with acute ventilatory failure and a mild metabolic acidosis are present. Abnormalities in the electrocardiogram (sinus tachycardia, ventricular tachycardia, sinus arrest, and sinus bradycardia) frequently are found. The sinus bradycardia observed terminally is due to increased vagal tone. Within the cardiovascular system there is an increase in peripheral vascular resistance, leading to a significant elevation in mean arterial pressure. The elevation in pulmonary arterial pressure despite a fall in cardiac output indicates an increase in pulmonary vascular resistance. These changes appear to be due to central sympathetic stimulation.

IMMUNITY

It is possible to produce immunity to tick paralysis by allowing ticks to engorge for short periods of time. After two to three months the dog can tolerate a number of ticks to full engorgement. The serum from such dogs was found to be beneficial in the treatment of tick paralysis and is now commerically available.

TREATMENT

Treatment of animals with tick paralysis falls into three categories.

REMOVAL OF THE TICK OR TICKS

Once the diagnosis has been made, a thorough search by palpation should be made. In small animals the favorite sites for attachment are on the head and neck, especially in the ears or under the collar; behind the elbows; and between the scapulae. Although one tick may be found, the search should be a complete one, because other ticks will prevent recovery, even with treatment.

Ticks are best removed with tweezers or fingernails, taking care not to squeeze the body of the tick, because further toxin may be expressed into the animal. If the animal is showing signs of the disease, removal of the tick is not enough, as the disease may progress for 48 more hours.

NEUTRALIZATION OF THE TOXIN

Hyperimmune serum should then be injected slowly intravenously. The dose administered depends on the severity of the clinical signs and the size of the animal, but as a guide a dose rate of 0.5 ml/kg body weight may be used. In the cat care should be taken to avoid reactions to the serum. Hyperimmune dog serum may be administered intravenously to cats after an antihistamine, or it may be given intraperitoneally.

It appears that hyperimmune serum is totally effective in those animals with a straightforward ascending paralysis (Allan and Pursell, 1971). However, some deaths can be expected if the animal is showing signs of vomiting, laryngeal paralysis, sialosis, and pulmonary edema.

SUPPORTIVE TREATMENT

Good nursing care is vitally important in animals with tick paralysis. Dogs should be watched carefully for changes in respiratory and heart rates and nursed through crisis periods. After retching or vomiting the pharynx should be swabbed clean, and if the animal is in lateral recumbency it should be turned every four to six hours to prevent the development of hypostatic pneumonia.

Stress of any type, such as excitement, fear, or heat, has an adverse effect on the course of the disease. Quiet cage rest with minimal interference should be provided in a cool environment. All water and food should be withheld until the patient is mobile and has been free from vomiting for 12 to 24 hours. Water can then be given in small amounts, and if no vomiting occurs food can be given.

Although symptomatic treatment of tick paralysis with various drugs is common, some of these drugs can have deleterious effects. Atropine sulfate, which is administered to dry up salivary and bronchial secretions, should not be given if the animal is in an advanced stage of the disease or if bradycardia is present. Intravenous fluid replacement is generally not required unless recovery is prolonged. If fluids are administered, they should be given very slowly, with careful monitoring of the patient for signs of pulmonary congestion.

Recent work (Ilkiw, 1979) has demonstrated that phenoxybenzamine hydrochloride (Dibenyline*), an α-adrenergic blocking drug, is beneficial when used in conjunction with hyperimmune serum in the treatment of dogs presented in advanced stages of the disease. It should be administered at a dose rate of 1 mg/kg body weight, diluted in at least 20 ml of normal saline, and given slowly intravenously over a period of at least 20 minutes. Care must be taken not to overload the circulation if the drug is administered in a large volume of diluent. To aid removal of fluid from the lungs, a diuretic may be given.

Many practitioners are now using the phenothiazine tranquilizer acetylpromazine maleate (Acepromazine†) for its α-adrenergic blocking and sedative properties. It is administered slowly intravenously at a dose of 0.05 to 0.1 mg/kg body weight.

If respiratory arrest is imminent or if excessive secretions in the trachea are impairing respiration, tracheostomy may be performed. This allows suction of fluid from the trachea and intermittent positive pressure ventilation (IPPV) to be initiated. Constant cleaning of the tracheotomy tube is important to prevent respiratory obstruction. Postural drainage may also be advantageous.

After recovery, a convalescent period of up to two weeks with restricted exercise and avoidance of high temperatures should be advised to prevent death from cardiac complications.

PREVENTION

Bathing with the organophosphate coumaphos 50 g/liter (Asuntol‡) according to the manufacturer's instructions has been shown to prevent attachment of *Ixodes holocyclus* for one week.

Daily examination of the animal is also a very effective means of protection, because the disease cannot be produced from attachment of the tick in less than four days.

Collars impregnated with the organophosphate propoxur are reported by Bayer Australia Ltd. to be up to 95 per cent effective in the control of *Ixodes holocyclus* for four weeks.

REFERENCES AND SUPPLEMENTAL READING

Allan, G. S., and Pursell, R. T.: Pulmonary involvement and other sequelae of tick poisoning. Aust. Vet. Pract. 1:39, 1971.
Cooper, B. J.: Studies on the pathogenesis of tick paralysis. Ph.D. Thesis, University of Sydney, Sydney, Australia, 1976.
Ilkiw, J. E.: A study of the effects in the dog of *Ixodes holocyclus*. Ph.D. Thesis, University of Sydney, Sydney, Australia, 1979.

---

*Smith Kline & French Laboratories, Philadelphia, PA.
†Arnolds of Reading, Pty. Ltd., Baronia, Victoria, Australia.

‡Bayer Australia Ltd., Botany N.S.W., Australia.

LARYNGEAL PARALYSIS IN HYPOTHYROID DOGS

H. J. HARVEY, D.V.M.,
Ithaca, New York

N. L. IRBY, D.V.M.,
Philadelphia, Pennsylvania

and B. J. WATROUS, D.V.M.
Corvallis, Oregon

Laryngeal paralysis has been described as a cause of respiratory obstruction in dogs. It is usually a disease of older, large breed dogs, although congenital laryngeal paralysis occurs in sled dogs and in the Bouvier des Flandres breed.

Clinical findings depend on the severity of airway obstruction. Early clinical signs include coughing, hoarseness, change in voice, repeated throat clearing, and slight to moderate decrease in exercise tolerance. In later stages of the disease affected dogs may experience inspiratory dyspnea severe enough to cause cyanosis and collapse. Clinical signs are frequently minimal until the animal is stressed by excitement, exertion, or hot, humid weather.

Confirmation of the diagnosis is made by visualizing the glottis. However, because visualization requires anesthesia or heavy sedation, caution should be used in dogs in severe respiratory distress. Most dogs presented as upper respiratory emergencies benefit from the immediate administration of corticosteroids and tranquilizers and placement in a quiet, oxygen-rich environment. Emergency tracheotomy is necessary in a few instances. Once the respiratory status of the animal permits, a light plane of anesthesia or tranquilization is used to allow visualization of the glottis. Anesthesia must be light enough to avoid obliterating the action of the arytenoid cartilages and vocal cords.

Normally, the diameter of the glottis is increased during inspiration by active bilateral abduction of the arytenoid cartilages and vocal cords. In dogs with laryngeal paralysis, these structures move passively and ineffectively, if they move at all. In some cases, one or both vocal cords appear to be fixed in a median position. Usually there is secondary edema of the laryngeal mucosa and hyperemia of the pharynx and tonsils.

Radiography yields information of value in selected cases. Although lateral radiographs of the larynx are unremarkable in most cases, the examination rules out other causes of upper airway obstruction, such as foreign bodies, tracheal collapse, hypoplastic trachea, and edema or distortion of the larynx secondary to trauma or other causes. Laryngeal edema is seen as a loss of detail of the laryngeal cartilages and the normally air-filled lateral ventricles. Fluoroscopic examination of laryngeal function in a dorsoventral view may allow visualization of the arytenoid cartilages. The failure of symmetric retraction of these structures during inspiration supports the diagnosis of paralysis.

The thoracic radiographic signs of upper airway obstruction when present are subtle and often overlooked. The morphologic changes are related to the physiologic effects of Müller's maneuver, which consists of inspiration against a closed glottis. The resulting decrease in intrathoracic pressure causes an inward pull of the intercostal muscles, which creates a scalloped appearance of the parietal surface of the lung. In addition, the pulmonary vasculature dilates, increasing vessel caliber and blood flow. The intrathoracic trachea dilates, whereas the cervical trachea tends to narrow. Pulmonary edema is rare but may be encountered secondary to a decrease in interstitial pressure.

Laryngeal paralysis should be differentiated from the laryngeal collapse that occurs in brachiocephalic breeds. The latter condition is secondary to increased supraglottic pressure resulting from the effects of the brachiocephalic airway syndrome (stenotic nares, elongated soft palate, everted lateral ventricles, and, occasionally, hypoplastic trachea). In laryngeal collapse, the arytenoid cartilages and aryepiglottic folds are flaccid and tend to collapse medially and ventrally during inspiration.

Surgery is the best method of treating laryngeal paralysis, although mildly affected dogs respond to short-term corticosteroid therapy and avoidance of stress. Two types of surgical correction have been

694

described: partial laryngectomy via oral or ventral laryngotomy approach, and arytenoid lateralization, similar to the "roarer's" operation in horses. We prefer partial laryngectomy and vocal cordectomy through the oral approach because of its simplicity, effectiveness, and lack of complications. In mildly affected dogs, we have occasionally limited surgery to bilateral vocal cordectomy with good results. Otherwise, partial laryngectomy (arytenoidectomy, aryepiglottic fold excision, and vocal cordectomy) is performed. Partial laryngectomy is performed on one side of the glottis only. Bilateral arytenoidectomy is not done because webs of scar tissue may form across the glottis as healing progresses. Aspiration pneumonia is also more common with bilateral surgery, since the diameter of the glottis can be made too large for effective closure by the epiglottis during swallowing.

Prior to definitive surgery, a tracheotomy tube is placed. Laryngeal cup forceps or uterine biopsy forceps are used to excise the medial portion of the arytenoid cartilage and aryepiglottic fold on the side most severely affected. Unilateral removal of the vocal cord is also performed. The usually mild hemorrhage is controlled by direct pressure. The tracheotomy tube can usually be removed within 24 hours. Corticosteroids are continued for two or three days postoperatively.

LARYNGEAL PARALYSIS AND HYPOTHYROIDISM

The cause of laryngeal paralysis in dogs is not known. Mechanical injury to the left recurrent laryngeal or vagus nerves, pressure on the nerves by neoplasms, neoplastic infiltration of the nerves, and enlarged thyroid glands have been mentioned as contributing factors. Laryngeal paralysis in a cat was attributed to infiltration of the vagus nerve by lymphosarcoma. Congenital laryngeal paralysis occurs in sled dogs and in the Bouvier des Flandres breed (Venker-van Haagen, 1980).

O'Brien and coworkers (1973) have described neurogenic atrophy of the laryngeal musculature in seven large breed dogs with laryngeal paralysis. Biopsies were obtained as part of therapeutic surgical procedures (unilateral partial laryngectomy and vocal cordectomy). Histologic changes included diffuse inflammatory infiltrate of the lamina propria and hyperplasia of surface epithelium. Muscular changes seen were small fibers, scattered among normal fibers, that were strongly eosinophilic with pyknotic nuclei. Necrotic myofibers were also seen with an increase in perimysial connective tissue, interpreted as consistent with long-standing neurogenic atrophy. Neurologic tissue seen in several biopsies showed vacuolization, beading of myelin, loss of axons, and perineural fibrosis. Two patients

exhibited hind limb weakness. One of these animals was necropsied and showed evidence of a central degenerative neurologic disease. Wallerian degeneration and fibrosis were also found in sciatic and recurrent laryngeal nerve sections of this animal.

Laryngeal paralysis in the horse has been associated with a peripheral neuropathy. The changes in the larynx were typical of a chronic degenerative neuropathy progressing to the final stages of neurogenic atrophy: muscle fiber atrophy, fatty invasion in the perimysium and endomysium, and fibrosis of nerve bundles. The early muscular changes observed in subclinical cases were fiber-type grouping, fiber size variation, angulation of fibers, and fiber atrophy. Also seen were increased amounts of connective tissue. Nerve changes observed in two horses were described as a distally progressive loss of myelinated nerve fibers. Duncan and associates (1974) stated that "the length of the recurrent laryngeal nerves and the distally progressive loss of myelinated fibers suggests that a dying-back phenomenon is taking place," perhaps related to decreased axoplasmic flow in longer fibers.

We are currently investigating the hypothesis that laryngeal paralysis in dogs is related to hypothyroidism. We have detected hypothyroidism in nine of the ten dogs with laryngeal paralysis that have been tested for thyroid function. These cases are summarized in Table 1. Although the relationship between hypothyroidism and laryngeal paralysis in dogs is speculative, other neuropathies and myopathies in hypothyroid humans and dogs have been previously diagnosed. In humans the laryngeal dysfunction associated with hypothyroidism is thought to be caused by myxedematous changes in the larynx itself. However, diffuse polyneuropathy is often a feature of human hypothyroidism. The polyneuropathy is characterized histologically as segmental demyelination and remyelination with aggregates of glycogen granules, abnormal mitochondria, and lipid droplets in Schwann cell cytoplasm. Conduction velocities are decreased. Clinical signs consist of numbness of the feet and hands, unsteady gait, fatigue, and constipation. Treatment with thyroid hormone reverses both the histologic and clinical abnormalities of the neuropathy.

Myopathies associated with hypothyroidism in humans have been discussed by McKerna and colleagues (1980). Syndromes they observed included (1) muscle weakness with muscular hypertrophy; (2) muscular hypertrophy with proximal muscle weakness, bradykinesia, post-exercise stiffness, decreased tendon responses, and pseudomyotoma; (3) atrophic myopathy (rarely); and (4) myasthenic syndrome with poor response to edrophonium. Their patients were assessed before and during thyroid replacement treatment by serial muscle biopsies. Characteristic muscular changes included type II fiber atrophy and increased central nuclear counts,

Table 1.   Nine Dogs with Laryngeal Paralysis and Hypothyroidism

Case No.	Breed	Sex	Age	Other Clinical Findings	Thyroid Hormone				Treatment	Follow-up
					T_4 ($\mu g/dl$)*		T_3 (ng/dl)†			
					Base	Post-TSH	Base	Post-TSH		
1	Irish setter	F/S	11	None	1.40	2.39	1.2	1.78	Bilateral vocal cordectomy; thyroid hormone	Normal
2	Old English sheepdog	M	9	Diabetes mellitus, proprioceptive deficits of hindlimbs	0.0	0.64	NOT DONE		Bilateral vocal cordectomy; thyroid hormone	Normal
3	Brittany spaniel	M	13	Megaesophagus	1.40	2.68	NOT DONE		Bilateral vocal cordectomy	Improved
4	Mix	M	10	Alopecia	0.83	1.99	0.68	1.18	Bilateral vocal cordectomy; thyroid hormone	Normal
5	Irish setter	M	14	Cardiomyopathy	1.8	3.56	NOT DONE		For heart disease	Cardiac function improved
6	Labrador retriever	F/S	10	Dysphagia, megaesophagus, hiatal hernia, hindlimb weakness, muscle atrophy	0.0	0.97	0.21	0.68	Bilateral vocal cordectomy; thyroid hormone	Improved to nearly normal for all abnormalities
7	Labrador retriever	F/S	12	Laryngeal paralysis, mild occasional dysphagia	1.2		NOT DONE		None	Unchanged
8	German wire-haired pointer	F/S	12	Fibrosarcoma of left humerus	0.43	2.52	0.60	1.18	Limb amputation; vocal cordectomy; thyroid hormone	Breathing improved
9	Irish setter	M	9	Megaesophagus	3.30	4.58	1.75	2.56	Unilateral vocal cordectomy; partial laryngectomy	Breathing improved
10	Old English sheepdog	M	10	Eighth cranial nerve deficit	0.29	1.70	0.83	1.47	Thyroid hormone only	Pending

*Normal values: base: 2.5–3.0; post-TSH: 3.0–6.0.
†Normal values: base: 1.0–2.0; post-TSH: 2.0–4.0.

which returned to normal with treatment. These changes were believed to relate to altered glycogen storage and mitochondrial metabolism.

Hypothyroid myopathy in dogs has been described as a type II muscle fiber atrophy. However, the dogs described were not clinically abnormal and there was no histologic pathology associated with peripheral nerves.

The results of thyroid hormone supplementation given to dogs with laryngeal paralysis are provocative. Each dog in our clinic that received exogenous thyroid hormone became asymptomatic or showed improvement for the laryngeal disease even when minimal surgery was performed. In addition, several of the dogs with laryngeal paralysis diagnosed in our clinic had concurrent abnormalities, including symptomatic megaesophagus in two dogs, air in the esophagus not diagnosed as megaesophagus in four dogs, neurologic abnormalities (proprioceptive deficits, hypermetria) of the rear limbs in two dogs, and muscle atrophy of the shoulders, neck and head in one dog. These conditions also showed marked improvement after thyroid hormone administration.

These findings are only the most superficial evidence that laryngeal paralysis, as well as other neuromuscular disease, may be related to hypothyroidism. We are currently designing studies to more thoroughly investigate this relationship.

REFERENCES AND SUPPLEMENTAL READING

Braund, K. G., Dillon, A. R., August, J. R., and Ganjam, V. K.: Hypothyroid myopathy in two dogs. Vet. Pathol. 18:589, 1981.

Duncan, I. D., et al.: The pathology of equine laryngeal hemiplegia. Acta Neuropathol. 27:337, 1974.

Harvey, C. E., and Venker-van Haagen, A. J.: Surgical management of pharyngeal and laryngeal airway obstruction in the dog. Vet. Clin. North Am. 5:515, 1975.

Kurdjaver, T.: Neurologic complications of thyroid dysfunction. Adv. Neurol. 19:619, 1978.

McKerna, R. O., et al.: Hypothyroid myopathy. A clinical and pathological study. J. Pathol. 132:35, 1980.

O'Brien, J. A., Harvey, C. E., Kelly, A. M., and Tucker, J. A.: Neurogenic atrophy of the laryngeal muscles of the dog. J. Small Anim. Pract. 14:521, 1973.

Schaer, M., Zaki, F., Harvey, H. J., and O'Reilly, W. J.: Laryngeal hemiplegia due to lymphosarcoma involvement of the vagus nerve in a cat. J.A.V.M.A. 174:513, 1979.

Venker-van Haagen, A. J.: Laryngeal paralysis in young Bouviers. In Kirk, R. W. (ed.): Current Veterinary Therapy VII. Philadelphia: W. B. Saunders, 1980, pp. 290–292.

EPISODIC WEAKNESS

BRIAN R. H. FARROW, B.V.Sc.

Sydney, Australia

Episodic weakness may be a manifestation of a variety of different diseases and presents an interesting diagnostic problem for the clinician. Weakness interspersed with periods of apparent normality can result from neuromuscular, cardiovascular, or metabolic disease. Diseases that may produce weakness of an episodic nature are indicated in Table 1, together with pertinent diagnostic aids and appropriate therapy.

NEUROMUSCULAR DISEASES

MYASTHENIA GRAVIS

Myasthenia gravis (MG) is a neuromuscular disorder manifested by weakness and fatigability of muscles. The weakness is alleviated by rest or the administration of anticholinesterase drugs. After variable amounts of exercise, weakness in the appendicular muscles is evident. Affected animals become fatigued, shorten their stride, and lie down and refuse to move. After a short period of rest they are able to walk again before the weakness returns. Drooping of facial features reflects facial muscle weakness in some cases. Sialosis, regurgitation of food, and megaesophagus in a high percentage of cases are manifestations of pharyngeal and esophageal striated muscle weakness. The response in MG to the administration of anticholinesterase drugs is diagnostic. Edrophonium chloride (Tensilon*), a short-acting anticholinesterase drug, or neostigmine methylsulfate (Prostigmin*), a longer-acting drug, may be used for diagnostic testing.

Following IV administration of edrophonium chloride (total dose 0.5 to 5.0 mg, depending on size), there is obvious clinical improvement within 10 to 30 seconds and then a return of weakness within five minutes. Neostigmine methylsulfate is given by intramuscular injection (0.05 mg/kg), fol-

---

*Roche Laboratories, Nutley, NJ.

Table 1. *Episodic Weakness*

Disease	Diagnostic Aids	Treatment
Neuromuscular		
Myasthenia gravis	Anticholinesterase response Electromyographic studies	Prostigmine Pyridostigmine
Polymyopathy	Enzymology: SGOT ↑ , CPK ↑ Muscle biopsy	Specific therapy where indicated Glucocorticosteroids
Cardiovascular		

Arrhythmias	ECG	Antiarrhythmic agents
		    (ventricular)
		        Lidocaine
		        Quinidine
		        Procainamide
		Cardiac glycosides
		    (supraventricular)

Conduction blocks	ECG	Depends on degree and course (see elsewhere in text).
Congestive heart failure	Radiography	Cardiac glycosides Diuretics
Heartworm disease	Microfilariae in blood Radiography	Treat CHF if necessary Caparsolate
Metabolic		
Hypoglycemia	Fasting blood glucose	Surgery (pancreatic neoplasia) Diazoxide
Adrenal insufficiency	Na ↓ , K ↑ ECG Plasma cortisol ↓ ACTH response	Fludrocortisone acetate Glucocorticosteroids, when necessary
Other disturbances	Electrolyte determinations	Appropriate fluid therapy Specific treatment as indicated

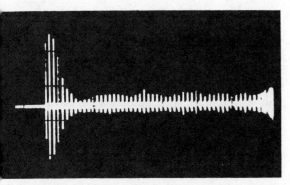

Figure 1. Electromyographic recording of evoked motor unit potentials from a dog with myasthenia gravis. The potentials were recorded from the palmar interosseous muscles during repetitive supramaximal stimulation of the ulnar nerve at a rate of 30 per second. Note the significant and progressive decrease in successive responses in the early phase of stimulation.

owed by clinical improvement in 15 to 30 minutes that lasts for some hours. Undesirable muscarinic effects such as vomiting or defecation should be prevented by prior administration of atropine. Care should be taken with anticholinesterase test dosing, since the possibility of a cholinergic crisis (i.e., excessive muscle depolarization and weakness) exists with dosage of nonmyasthenic individuals or overdosage. Facilities for resuscitation should be readily accessible should the need arise. The use of electrodiagnostic testing, when available, enables demonstration of characteristic decremental responses to repetitive nerve stimulation. Repetitive supramaximal stimuli are applied to a peripheral nerve (e.g., the ulnar nerve), and the induced action potentials are observed in an appropriate muscle (e.g., the interosseus muscles). In normal animals successive stimuli produce action potentials of the same magnitude, whereas in myasthenic individuals successive stimuli produce action potentials of decreasing magnitude (Fig. 1).

The basic defect in MG is a reduction of available acetylcholine receptors at neuromuscular junctions, which in the majority of adult onset cases is the result of an antibody-mediated autoimmune attack directed against the postsynaptic neuromuscular junction. The decreased number of available receptors reduces the probability of interactions between acetylcholine and receptor molecules.

Therapy in MG is based on symptomatic control by the use of anticholinesterases. Although therapy does nothing to repair the basic deficiency in receptors, it does delay the degradation of acetylcholine released by the nerve and allows it to interact with more receptors, thereby improving neuromuscular transmission and the animal's strength. Neostigmine bromide (Prostigmin*) and pyridostigmine bromide (Mestinon*) are the anticholinesterase drugs generally used for oral administration in MG. Pyridostigmine bromide is also available as a sustained-release tablet,* making less frequent administration

possible. There is marked variability in dosage requirements, and it is necessary to individualize the dose for each case. Suggested starting doses are indicated in Table 2. Glucocorticosteroid therapy, directed against the autoimmune mechanisms involved in the pathogenesis of the disease in adults, may also be indicated as an adjunct to anticholinesterase therapy in certain individuals.

Although the association between thymic disorders and MG is not as well documented in dogs as it is in humans, thymoma has been reported in some dogs with MG. For this reason the cranial mediastinum of dogs with MG should be evaluated radiographically. The etiologic connection between thymic abnormalities and MG remains the subject of speculation.

MG in dogs is often of a transitory nature, with spontaneous remissions occurring after some weeks. During this time appropriate anticholinesterase medication is necessary to provide adequate muscular strength and minimize the risk of aspiration pneumonia. In many cases the need for therapy diminishes with time, and treatment may be discontinued after several weeks when strength returns to normal.

MG has been reported as a congenital problem in Jack Russell terriers, in which a decrease in acetylcholine receptor numbers is present at birth that is not associated with antireceptor antibodies. It has also been observed in puppies of other breeds, in which the onset of the disease is some weeks after birth. Slightly different mechanisms may be involved in the pathogenesis of the neuromuscular disorder in these cases, but the approach to therapy is the same. The disease has also been recorded in cats.

POLYMYOPATHY

The weakness that accompanies various myopathies can be difficult to distinguish clinically from MG. The disability in dogs with myopathic weakness tends to be progressive but may vary in intensity and is generally made worse by exercise. Pain may be present on palpation of muscle groups but is frequently absent.

In addition to weakness, muscle trembling may be apparent following minimal exercise. Diagnosis is aided by demonstration of elevated levels of serum enzymes of muscle origin, particularly crea-

Table 2. *Anticholinesterase Therapy in Myasthenia Gravis*

Drug	Dosage*
Neostigmine bromide†	0.5 mg/kg per os
Pyridostigmine bromide‡	2.0 mg/kg per os

*Dosages of both drugs to be administered as required.
†Prostigmin, Roche Laboratories, Nutley, NJ.
‡Mestinon, Roche Laboratories, Nutley, NJ.

*Roche Laboratories, Nutley, NJ.

tine phosphokinase (CPK), although these may be normal at the time of sampling. Confirmation of the diagnosis is by demonstration of histologic changes in muscle biopsies. Electromyographic detection of increased insertional activity, trains of high-frequency discharges that start and stop suddenly, and motor unit action potentials that are reduced in amplitude and duration are all suggestive of myopathy. Some specific infectious agents, such as *Toxoplasma gondii* and *Leptospira icterohaemorrhagiae*, may produce a polymyositis, but in most cases of polymyositis the etiology is obscure. The nature of the inflammatory infiltrate in many cases suggests that immune mechanisms may be involved. When biopsies fail to implicate an infectious agent, vigorous use of glucocorticosteroid therapy generally produces a favorable response. Other acquired and congenital myopathies of a noninflammatory nature have also been observed in dogs but have not been well documented to date. However, the diagnosis should be considered in young animals presented because of weakness.

CARDIOVASCULAR DISEASES

The initial physical examination of the animal presented for episodic weakness could reveal the presence of congestive heart failure (CHF) and other cardiovascular abnormalities, if present. Careful auscultation of the chest will detect the presence of valvular abnormalities. Arrhythmias may also be detected at this time, although the arrhythmias may not always be present or detectable at the time of the examination. Electrocardiographic examination is necessary to define the arrhythmias and conduction disturbances more precisely to select the appropriate therapy. This aspect of therapy is discussed in detail elsewhere in the text (see Section 4, Cardiovascular Diseases).

Dogs with heartworm disease are occasionally presented with a history of episodic weakness and no other signs of CHF. In these cases physical examination may be unrewarding, and the diagnosis depends on demonstration of microfilariae in the peripheral circulation together with characteristic changes on thoracic radiography. A detailed discussion of diagnosis and treatment of heartworm disease may be found elsewhere in the text.

METABOLIC DISEASES

HYPOGLYCEMIA

Hypoglycemia is probably the most frequently encountered metabolic change that results in weakness of an episodic nature. This may result from increased utilization of glucose, as in hyperinsulin-ism, or from interference with normal glucose availability, as in the glycogen storage diseases, adrenal insufficiency, hepatic insufficiency, and starvation.

Blood glucose determination should be part of the initial laboratory investigation of animals presented with episodic weakness in which examination fails to implicate neuromuscular or cardiovascular disease. It is important to remember that blood glucose levels may be normal at the time of presentation or at a single sampling in cases in which the weakness is in fact of hypoglycemic origin. It is therefore necessary in some cases to repeat blood glucose determinations after withholding food for 12 to 24 hours before hypoglycemia can be excluded as a possible cause.

The clinical signs of hypoglycemia vary in severity from mild weakness and behavioral changes to grand mal seizure episodes. Which particular clinical picture dominates is not so much a manifestation of the degree of hypoglycemia as of the rapidity with which the blood glucose level is lowered. Some animals can adapt to changes in blood glucose that occur slowly over a long period and so display neurologic signs infrequently. Others, in which hypoglycemia occurs precipitously, manifest severe signs.

Once established, the precise cause of hypoglycemia should be investigated. Young puppies may develop transient hypoglycemia as a result of starvation or gastrointestinal disease that interferes with glucose uptake. A persistent or recurrent hypoglycemia occurs in young puppies, particularly of the toy breeds, that have inherited abnormalities in carbohydrate metabolism. These diseases (glycogen storage diseases) are not well defined in the dog.

Hyperinsulinism. The commonest cause of maturity-onset hypoglycemia is hyperinsulinism from a functional pancreatic beta-cell neoplasm. In cases in which hypoglycemia is established as the cause of neurologic dysfunction in a mature dog that is free of significant liver disease, exploratory laparotomy and a search for a pancreatic tumor are warranted. It should be remembered that these tumors are frequently small and may be difficult to find. It should also be remembered that in dogs these tumors tend to be malignant, metastasizing to portal lymph nodes and the liver early in the course of disease. Where facilities allow, establishment of the diagnosis by demonstration of inappropriately high insulin levels in desirable. This should be performed in conjunction with blood glucose estimations. Provocative testing utilizing intravenous tolbutamide is rarely necessary to establish the diagnosis in the clinical situation.

The treatment of choice is surgical removal of the tumor. However, because of the highly metastatic behavior of this tumor in dogs, surgery may not be successful. In these cases symptomatic relief can frequently be attained by the use of oral diazoxide

(10 mg/kg initially, increasing as required up to 40 mg/kg) daily), a nondiuretic thiazide with hyperglycemic effects. Streptozotocin, an antibiotic and cytotoxic agent derived from *Streptomyces achromogenes*, is known to have cytotoxic effects against both normal and neoplastic pancreatic beta cells and has been used for the treatment of metastatic insulinomas in people. The drug has not been adequately evaluated in the dog; however, it is very expensive and has a fairly narrow margin of safety, with toxic effects predominantly on the renal tubules. Therefore, further work is necessary to evaluate the role, if any, of steptozotocin in the management of metastatic pancreatic beta-cell neoplasia in the dog.

ADRENOCORTICAL INSUFFICIENCY

The fluctuating and often severe electrolyte disturbances and changes in blood pressure that result from adrenocortical insufficiency are responsible for the episodic weakness associated with this disease. A history of gastrointestinal disturbances is frequently present in these cases. On physical examination bradycardia may be present. Flattened P waves and tall peaked T waves on the electrocardiogram reflect the hyperkalemia that may be present at the time of examination. Hematologic examination often reveals eosinophilia and lymphocytosis, and plasma electrolyte determinations may show hyperkalemia and hyponatremia. However, the laboratory features traditionally ascribed to hypoadrenocorticism often are absent at the time of examination, particularly in mild cases, and in cases in which the index of suspicion is high, confirmation of the diagnosis should be sought by direct assay of plasma cortisol levels before and after administration of ACTH. Animals with adrenocortical insufficiency should receive specific hormone replacement therapy consisting of 9α-fluorohydrocortisone, together with glucocorticosteroid supplementation at times of stress. The detailed management of these animals and those that may be presented in a more critical state is dealt with in Section 11 (Endocrine and Metabolic Disorders).

OTHER METABOLIC CAUSES

Other electrolyte disturbances secondary to such events as severe vomiting or diarrhea or diabetic ketoacidosis may also produce weakness. These disorders are less likely to be episodic in their manifestations. Therapy should be directed at correction of the electrolyte disturbances and treatment of the fundamental disorder.

SUPPLEMENTAL READING

Capen, C. C., Belshaw, B. E., and Martin, S. C.: Endocrine disorders. *In* Ettinger, S. J. (ed.): *Textbook of Veterinary Internal Medicine.* Philadelphia: W. B. Saunders, 1975, pp. 1351–1452.

Drachman, D. B.: Myasthenia gravis. N. Engl. J. Med. 298:136, 186, 1978.

Ettinger, S. J., and Suter, P. F.: *Canine Cardiology.* Philadelphia: W. B. Saunders, 1970.

Garlepp, M., Farrow, B. R. H., Kay, P., and Dawkins, R. L.: Antibodies to the acetylcholine receptor in myasthenic dogs. Immunology 37:807, 1979.

Grob, D. (ed.): Myasthenia gravis: pathophysiology and management. Ann. N.Y. Acad. Sci., 377:1, 1981.

SCOTTY CRAMP

K. M. MEYERS, Ph.D.,
Pullman, Washington

and R. M. CLEMMONS, D.V.M.
Gainesville, Florida

The Scottish terrier breed of dogs is affected by an inherited neurologic disorder with a recessive mode of transmission that is characterized by transient episodes of muscular hypertonicity resulting in postural abnormalities and locomotion difficulties that can be induced by excitement or exercise. The condition was first described by Klavenbeck and associates in 1942 and is commonly known as "Scotch cramp" or "Scotty cramp."

CLINICAL SIGNS (Meyers et al., 1969; 1971)

Dogs appear normal at rest, and locomotion is normal under most conditions of light or moderate exercise. However, with continued exercise, excitement, or fear, clinical signs may be seen. The initial sign may be a slight abduction ("winging") of the forelimbs, whereas in others an arching of the lumbar spine or overflexing of the rear limbs while walking is the initial sign. If the dog is running, the initial sign may be a sudden "catapulting" of the rear limbs into the air. From this point the dog's ability to move may progressively decrease. A goose-stepping gait is observed, and, when the dog is walking briskly, a pronounced rotation of the hind quarters is seen. When an exciting stimulus is continued in the severely affected dog, the dog assumes a pillar-like stance and locomotor activity becomes impossible. If the dog falls over it may curl into a ball, respiration may momentarily cease, and facial musculature may show signs of involvement. Once the stimulus is removed, the clinical signs progressively decrease and then disappear. The dog does not lose consciousness and does not appear to be experiencing pain.

Individual variations in severity of involvement are common and exhibit a complete spectrum that appears to have a normal distribution. A few dogs are mildly affected; locomotor activity is only slightly altered and then only under special circumstances. A few dogs are severely affected and are nearly incapacitated after short exercise periods. In the majority of affected dogs the most severe clinical sign is an arching of the back coupled with a goose-step gait. Several factors alter the clinical severity of Scotty cramp and may explain the individual variations in severity; the most prominent are the

environment, the physiologic state of the dog, psychological factors, and genetic differences.

The intelligence and spirit of the dog do not appear altered. The dog's general health is not affected, and its life span is not shortened. An increased incidence of post-natal mortality has not been reported. Scotty cramp can be observed in puppies as young as six to eight weeks of age if they are heavily exercised while excited. If the puppy has matured normally the clinical signs are usually seen within five minutes of excited exercise. The condition does not increase in severity unless other factors in the dog's environment or its health status are altered.

FACTORS MODIFYING THE CLINICAL SIGNS OF SCOTTY CRAMP

The elicitation of an episode of Scotty cramp is highly dependent upon factors that modify the behavior of the dog. By identifying those situations in which an episode will predictably be elicited, an owner may reduce the incidence of episodes by not exposing the dog to the stimulus or, if this is not possible, by behaviorally training the dog to accept the stimulus. Potent inducers of an episode are events that make the dog excited such as feeding or the anticipation of going for a walk. Fear may also be a potent inducer. It is common to find dogs with Scotty cramp exhibiting signs when confronted with stairs. In one case, the veterinarian sedated the dog and, through repetitive exposure to stairs, was able to eliminate them as an initiator of cramp. Furthermore, in new and unusual situations where the dog may be uneasy it is often difficult to elicit clinical signs. For example, it is hard to induce the clinical signs of Scotty cramp in the veterinarian's office.

Dogs may suppress the elicitation of clinical signs by modifying their activity. Young puppies often exercise freely until severe clinical signs become evident. Thereafter, they may stop exercising or may modify the intensity of exercise when they feel the beginning of clinical signs. It is, therefore, not uncommon to find clinical signs more prevalent in younger dogs. The owner may think that the adult

702

dog, showing fewer clinical signs, has outgrown the disease.

The environment of the dog may also influence the expression of the disease. Most, if not all, stressful conditions have the potential to modify the clinical signs of Scotty cramp. This means that dogs with Scotty cramp raised in a quiet home may exhibit fewer clinical signs than dogs raised with other dogs or placed in a more intense environment. Thus, the dog may again appear to grow out of the disorder when taken from the kennel to a home environment at a young age.

If the health of the dog with Scotty cramp deteriorates, the clinical signs become more severe; in fact, Scotty cramp is an excellent barometer of the health of the dog. The increase in clinical signs can be marked. When presented with a mature dog that suddenly exhibits clinical signs of Scotty cramp, it must be realized that the dog was born with Scotty cramp, that the owner did not recognize the dog as having Scotty cramp, and that some other event is increasing the severity of clinical signs. The owner and veterinarian should direct their efforts toward defining these other events. We have had reports of dogs in which the clinical signs of Scotty cramp suddenly increased owing to a viral or bacterial infection, liver disease, or kidney dysfunction. With the correction of the secondary problem and cessation of treatment, the severity of clinical signs of Scotty cramp dissipated and the animal returned to the predisease state.

PATHOPHYSIOLOGY (Meyers et al., 1971; 1973; 1974; Peters and Meyers, 1977; 1980; Clemmons et al., 1980)

Clinical laboratory findings were normal, and pathologic examination of dogs with Scotty cramp did not reveal any abnormalities. In these studies, special emphasis was placed on the muscles and the central nervous system (CNS). Physiologic studies demonstrated that the defect resides in the CNS and appears to be in those neuronal systems that control or moderate muscle contraction. At the beginning of exercise the electrical activity of the muscle is normal. However, as exercise continues the electrical activity of a given muscle first increases in intensity and then becomes more prolonged, until finally, in severely affected dogs, the muscles do not relax but remain contracted. Since the clinical signs are due to alteration in control of normal muscle activity, Scotty cramp is not analogous to a muscle cramp, and pain would not be obligatory. The name Scotty cramp, therefore, describes the clinical signs and not the pathology of the disease.

The clinical signs of Scotty cramp coupled with the physiologic observations and the absence of observable pathologic signs suggest that Scotty cramp might result from a progressive depletion or accumulation of a compound within the CNS. Meyers and coworkers (1973) examined the possibility that the clinical signs resulted from an anomaly within a neurotransmitter system in the CNS and found that the clinical signs of Scotty cramp are closely related to the functional status of serotonergic neurons. Administration of agents that decrease serotonin function, such as inhibitors of enzymes that are responsible for serotonin synthesis, serotonin receptor blockers, or inhibitors of prostaglandin synthesis, markedly increases the severity of clinical signs and shortens the exercise time required to elicit the clinical signs. Aspirin, indomethacin and phenylbutazone, penicillin G, and flumixin meglumine are examples of drugs that reduce prostaglandin formation and increase the severity of Scotty cramp. The increased severity with aspirin and penicillin G occurred at the recommended therapeutic dosage. However, the effect is not permanent and clinical signs return to previous levels following withdrawal of medication.

Agents that enhance serotonergic function, such as precursors of serotonin and inhibitors of enzymes that are responsible for serotonin catabolism, provide substantial improvement in Scotty cramp behavior.

GENETIC BASIS OF SCOTTY CRAMP

Based on pedigree analysis, a genetic basis with a recessive mode of transmission has been suggested for Scotty cramp. This theory is supported by the fact that only the Scottish terrier breed has been shown to exhibit the disorder and successive matings of affected males to affected females at Washington State University have resulted in more than 30 offspring, all affected with Scotty cramp. Outcross mating to nonaffected dogs produced only normal offspring. Not all dogs were affected to the same extent, and there was not a good correlation between the severity of affection of the offspring and that of the parents. This is apparently due to the transmission of other genetic information, which may influence or modify the expression of a defective gene. This difference in genetic make-up may be one reason why some Scottish terriers become incapacitated.

DIAGNOSIS

There is no laboratory test for the diagnosis of Scotty cramp. Diagnosis is made on the observation of clinical signs. There may be a question as to whether a dog with tonic epileptic seizures has severe Scotty cramp or epilepsy. If the dog with

Scotty cramp is affected severely enough to produce signs of tonic immobility, then the less severe signs of arching of the back and a goose-step gait are very easily and repetitively induced with only mild exercise and excitement. Because of this, the dog can be diagnosed as having Scotty cramp. Since the diagnosis of Scotty cramp is based on the observation of clinical signs and since it may be difficult to induce the signs, the clinical and family history are highly significant.

To induce the clinical signs we recommend excited exercise. If this is not effective, methysergide (Sanserf*) treatment may be used. Methysergide blocks serotonin receptors and markedly increases the severity of clinical signs so that clinical signs are quick and easily observed. We suggest administering 0.3 mg/kg of methysergide orally and then exercising the dog two hours later. If clinical signs are not observed, another 0.3 mg/kg is given and the dog retested two hours later. The action of methysergide dissipates within eight hours.

If prompt remission of signs is desirable, the dog can be treated with diazepam (Valium†). Some transient nausea and gastrointestinal irritation may be seen with methysergide, but other side effects are not obvious. The gastrointestinal irritation may be exacerbated by the presence of an existing problem; therefore, the dog should be free of gastrointestinal parasites prior to initiating methysergide treatment. We have used methysergide on dogs as young as 8 weeks of age without incident. We are not aware of an affected dog that failed to exhibit observable clinical signs with exercise following methysergide treatment. Likewise, we are not aware of an unaffected dog that exhibited clinical signs of Scotty cramp following methysergide treatment.

TREATMENT

Several options are available when treating the dog with Scotty cramp. Often behavioral modification or environmental change may be sufficient. If

---

these are unsatisfactory, either diazepam or vitamin E may be employed. Diazepam, at a dosage from 0.5 to 1.5 mg/kg, reduces the clinical signs of Scotty cramp in an acute episode and, if given chronically, prevents the expression of clinical signs up to eight hours after treatment. Diazepam has several central nervous system actions including skeletal muscle relaxation. This action occurs at low diazepam concentrations, and, in most dogs, it is possible to titrate the dose so that the clinical signs of Scotty cramp are suppressed without significant alteration in the psychological state of the dog. Diazepam is very beneficial when administered prior to exposing the dog to a situation in which clinical signs are known or are likely to be expressed.

Vitamin E (125 IU/kg/day) is also effective in suppressing the clinical signs of Scotty cramp. Vitamin E does not reduce the severity of an episode but reduces the likelihood that an episode will occur. Lower doses (70 IU/kg/day) were also found to be effective, but platelet aggregation was enhanced with lower doses, and dogs receiving 70 IU/kg/day of vitamin E for long periods of time may be at risk for thromboembolic complications. Aggregation of platelets from dogs treated with 120 IU/kg/day was not enhanced. In severe cases of Scotty cramp, maintaining the dog on vitamin E and, when needed, diazepam may effectively control the condition.

REFERENCES AND SUPPLEMENTAL READING

Clemmons, R. G., Peters, R. I., and Meyers, K. M.: Scotty cramp: A review of cause, characteristics, diagnosis and treatment. Comp. Cont. Ed. Pract. Vet. 5:395, 1980.

Klavenbeck, A. S., et al.: Een aavalsgewijs optrendende stoornes in de regulatie van de spiertonus: Waargenomen bij Schotsche Terriers. Tijdschr. Diergeneesk. 69:14, 1942.

Meyers, K. M., and Schaub, R. G.: The relationship of serotonin to a motor disorder of Scottish Terrier dogs. Life Sci. 14:1895, 1974.

Meyers, K. M., et al.: Hyperkinetic episodes in Scottish Terrier dogs. J.A.V.M.A. 155:129, 1969.

Meyers, K. M., et al.: The genetic basis of a kinetic disorder of Scottish Terrier dogs. J. Hered. 61:189, 1970.

Meyers, K. M., et al.: Muscular hypertonicity: Episodes in Scottish Terrier dogs. Arch. Neurol. 25:61, 1971.

Meyers, K. M., et al.: Serotonin involvement in a motor disorder of Scottish Terrier dogs. Life Sci. 13:1261, 1973.

Peters, R. I., and Meyers, K. M.: Precursor regulation of serotonergic neuronal function in Scottish Terrier dogs. J. Neurochem. 29:753, 1977.

Peters, R. I., and Meyers, K. M.: Serotonergic-catecholaminergic antagonism and locomotor control. Exper. Neurol. 69:22, 1980.

---

*Sandoz Pharmaceuticals, East Hanover, NJ.
†Hoffman-LaRoche, Nutley, NJ.

TETANUS

CRAIG E. GREENE, D.V.M.
Athens, Georgia

Tetanus is caused by the action of a potent neurotoxin that is formed in the body during the vegetative growth of *Clostridium tetani*. It develops when resistant spores from the environment are introduced into wounds or penetrating injuries. The spores vegetate as a response to decreased oxygenation at the site of injury. The presence of a foreign body, tissue necrosis, other microorganisms, and abscessation contribute to the development of tetanus. The incidence of the disease in dogs and cats is relatively low compared with that of other domesticated animals.

Many experimental studies have been performed on dogs, cats, and other laboratory animals to determine the mechanism by which toxin enters and affects the central nervous system. Toxin enters the axons of the nearest motor nerves, presumably at the end-plate, and migrates by retrograde axonal transport to the neuronal cell body within the spinal cord (regional tetanus). Spread of toxin within the nervous system occurs in an ascending fashion bilaterally in the spinal cord until the brain is reached. Alternatively, hematogenously liberated toxin is thought to localize preferentially in the neuromuscular endings of motor nerves throughout the body (generalized tetanus). From here it may ascend by retrograde axonal transport into many areas of the nervous system, causing generalized signs initially.

The clinical signs of tetanus intoxication can be explained by the known pathophysiologic effects of tetanus toxin. Evidence has accumulated for its action on the spinal cord, brain, neuromuscular junctions, and sympathetic nervous system. In the spinal cord and brain stem tetanus toxin appears to interfere with inhibitory synapses on cranial nerve and motor neurons.

Death from tetanus is usually associated with respiratory difficulty. Respiratory distress may be caused by rigidity of respiratory musculature, reflex spasms of the larynx, increased secretions in upper airways, prolonged hypoventilation during seizures, and central arrest of breathing from medullary intoxication.

Clinical signs of tetanus usually occur within five to ten days of wounding, although intervals of up to three weeks have been reported. The onset, progression, and severity of signs are frequently controlled by the distance of the wound from the brain. Wounds near the head are associated with more rapid onset and generalization of signs as compared with injuries of distant extremities.

Localized tetanus is more common in dogs and cats as compared with humans because of relatively increased resistance of these animals to intoxication. This process may extend over a variable interval to involve the entire central nervous system. Affected animals walk with a stiff gait and a generally outstretched tail. They have difficulty standing or lying down in comfortable positions because of their extreme rigidity. Rectal temperature is usually increased as a result of excessive muscular activity.

Postural reactions requiring minimal motor function such as proprioception are usually normal despite the presence of stiffness. Protrusion of the third eyelid and enophthalmos result in retraction of the globe from extraocular motor nuclei involvement. The ears are held erect, the lips are drawn back (risus sardonicus), and the forehead is wrinkled as a result of facial muscle spasms. Trismus (lockjaw) is caused by contraction of masticatory muscles. Increased salivation, heart rate, respiratory rate, laryngeal spasm, and dysphagia can occur from involvement of parasympathetic cranial nerve nuclei.

Reflex muscle spasms occur in animals with generalized tetanus or intracranial involvement. Animals become apprehensive and react strongly to tactile or auditory stimulation. Generalized muscular contraction is characterized by sudden tonic contracture of all muscles and opisthotonus. The interval between such tonic spasms may decrease until the animal reaches a convulsive state. Dogs and cats are usually conscious until they develop severe convulsions. They frequently have a desire to eat but may have trouble in prehending or swallowing solid food. Reflex muscle spasms are painful, and dogs may vocalize during such episodes. Dysuria and urinary retention, constipation, and gaseous distention are commonly a result of persistent anal and urinary sphincter contractions. Death is usually caused by respiratory arrest, which culminates the progression of clinical signs.

DIAGNOSIS

The history of a recent wound and the clinical signs are the primary means of making a diagnosis of tetanus. Hematologic abnormalities, including a leukocytosis with a neutrophilia and left shift, are a result of wounds that may be present. They resolve when appropriate therapy is used. Blood chemical values are unaffected with the exception of muscle enzyme elevations, which may be present. These changes are usually mild or inconsistent. The cerebrospinal fluid is normal.

Electromyographic findings of tetanus are characteristic. Nerve conduction velocities are normal. There is, however, a lack of the usually observed electrical silence following insertion of the needle or tapping of muscles or tendons.

Isolation of *C. tetani* from wounds can be a difficult and frequently unrewarding procedure. The organisms are usually present in such wounds in very low concentrations. Gram-stained smears may demonstrate the organism, but the morphology is not different from that of other anaerobic bacteria. Culture should be performed under strict anaerobic conditions at 37°C for 12 days.

THERAPY

Therapy for tetanus is costly and time-consuming in severely affected animals. Owners must be advised of the possible complications and lengthy hospitalization. Untreated cases are frequently fatal. Fortunately, however, the disease is often localized or mild in dogs and cats as compared with other animals because of their innate resistance to the toxin.

The immediate concern in treating tetanus in most species is to administer antitoxin as soon as a diagnosis is made. Less concern is usually needed in mildly affected dogs and cats. Timing and the route of therapy are extremely important in determining the effectiveness of antitoxin. Given parenterally, it only neutralizes toxin that is still unbound to the CNS.

Intravenous administration of antitoxin is superior to the intramuscular or subcutaneous route in producing a rapid and marked increase of circulating antitoxin. Unfortunately, the use of intravenous antitoxin is associated with a higher incidence of anaphylaxis, requiring appropriate precautions during administration. A single dosage of 100 to 500 U/kg is recommended for dogs and cats; larger animals should receive a proportionally lower dosage rate based on body weight. Total dosages greater than 20,000 U will probably not be more effective; they also increase the antigenic mass and are costly. An initial test dose (0.1 to 0.2 ml) of antitoxin should be administered subcutaneously 15 to 30 minutes prior to the intravenous dosage, and the animal should be observed for allergic reactions. Glucocorticoids and antihistamines can be administered prior to the intravenous dose, which is given slowly over five to ten minutes. Repeated administration is not recommended, as it increases the risk of anaphylactic reactions and a therapeutic blood level of antitoxin persists in dogs for 14 days following injection (Mason, 1964).

Local intramuscular injection of small dosages of antitoxin (1000 U) around and proximal to the wound site has been shown to be beneficial in experimental studies on local tetanus. Intracisternal or intracerebral injection of antitoxin in laboratory animals has been shown to be beneficial in treating tetanus under experimental conditions. Intracisternal injections of one-tenth of the intravenous dosage of antitoxin may reduce the mortality in dogs with mild or moderate tetanus compared with animals receiving intravenous or lumbar intrathecal injections. In severe cases intracisternal injections may prolong the life of animals but may not alter the mortality rate. Toxin that has penetrated into the CNS may be partially neutralized if antitoxin also reaches the CNS by direct injection. Appropriate clinical trials have not been performed to establish the superiority of this route of therapy. Furthermore, the antitoxin, being of equine origin, has potential toxicity in the subarachnoid space. It should be reserved for severely affected animals.

Local and parenteral antibiotic therapy should be instituted to kill any vegetative *C. tetani* organisms present in the wound. Penicillin is the drug of choice at a dosage of 10 to 15 × 10³ U/kg given every 12 hours. It may be injected intramuscularly in close proximity to the wound site. Effects of penicillin on the vegetative organisms may vary, and tetracycline has been recommended as an alternative choice (66 mg/kg given every eight hours). The prognosis for recovery does not always improve when the organism is eliminated because of the already impending intoxication. Antibiotic therapy should be continued until clinical signs improve, because the degree and site of infection cannot always be determined.

Various drugs alone or in combination have been used to control the reflex spasms and convulsions seen with tetanus. Phenothiazines appear to be highly effective in controlling the hyperexcitable state when used either alone or in combination with barbiturates. Chlorpromazine is the drug of choice at a dosage of 2 mg/kg given every 12 hours, although acetylpromazine or methotrimeprazine can be substituted.

Barbiturates can be used most successfully to control grand mal convulsions that may occur. Pentobarbital (3 to 5 mg/kg IM) may have to be given every two to three hours, but the actual dose should be titered to the clinical signs of the patient. Oral or injectable phenobarbital can be given for longer duration of action.

Benzimidazole derivatives such as diazepam (2 to 20 mg every two to eight hours as needed) can be substituted for barbiturates in controlling seizures.

Methocarbamol is a frequently recommended but less commonly used centrally acting muscle relaxant. It has a relatively short duration of action, as does diazepam. Narcotics should never be given in tetanus therapy because they depress the respiratory centers and may cause increased excitability of the CNS. Parasympatholytic drugs such as atropine should also be avoided.

Supportive measures are imperative in the successful management of tetanus in dogs and cats. Constant nursing may be required in severely affected animals. They should be placed in a dark, quiet environment with a minimum amount of stimulation. All therapeutic measures should be carried out at the same time each day so that a minimal amount of handling and stimulation occurs.

Surgery may be required if tissue necrosis or abscessation is extensive. General anesthesia is usually required to debride wounds and remove necrotic tissue. Antitoxin should be administered prior to surgery because of the potential release of toxin in the circulation during tissue manipulation. Hydrogen peroxide may be beneficial in flushing the wound because it increases oxygen tension, inhibiting obligate anaerobes. Foreign bodies should not be overlooked in wounds or abscesses.

Soft, comfortable bedding is required because tetanus causes incapacitation and animals frequently develop decubital ulcers. Animals should be encouraged to eat and drink on their own. They frequently have difficulty in prehending and swallowing solid foods. They can usually obtain blended foods or fluids by sucking through clenched teeth. A stomach tube may be passed if they are reluctant to eat, but it is frequently stressful for conscious animals and esophageal spasm may restrict passage. The hematocrit, plasma protein, and body weight should be evaluated daily to determine if an adequate fluid balance is being maintained. Balanced polyionic isotonic fluids should be given parenterally to meet any deficits. Parenteral alimentation requires continual intravenous fluid administration and considerable expense.

Complications in dogs and cats with tetanus are numerous. Fractures of the long bones, spine, or skull may result from trauma incurred during sudden muscular spasms or convulsions. Other problems can include sepsis from intravenous catheterization and aspiration pneumonia from difficult swallowing. Tracheostomy may be required if obstructive respiration develops from laryngeal spasm. Urinary and fecal retention occur as a result of hypertonic anal and urethral sphincters. Repeated urinary catheterization may be needed with dysuria or reflex dyssynergia may occur. Simethicone, gastric intubation, and enemas may be required to relieve gas or obstipation.

Glucocorticoid therapy has never been proved to be beneficial in tetanus and should be avoided. Hyperbaric oxygenation has been tried on humans and on one dog with tetanus in an attempt to inactivate *C. tetani*. There is little proof of benefit of such procedures. Neuromuscular blocking agents have been used in human tetanus in an attempt to control convulsions or to paralyze patients completely while placing them on artificial respirators. Such therapy is impractical in veterinary medicine because of the intensive monitoring required.

Most dogs and cats have a self-limiting course of tetanus intoxication with rapid and appropriate therapy. Improvement is usually noticeable by one week after therapy is instituted, and complete but gradual recovery has taken as long as two to three weeks.

Active immunoprophylaxis with tetanus toxoid is not recommended for tetanus in dogs and cats as it is in more susceptible species such as humans and horses. Routine tetanus boosters or post-exposure prophylaxis is not required. Appropriate care of infected wounds and rational antibiotic use should minimize its occurrence.

REFERENCES AND SUPPLEMENTAL READING

Killingsworth, C., Chiapella, A., Veralli, P., and deLahunta, A.: Feline tetanus. J. Am. Anim. Hosp. Assoc. 13:209, 1977.
Mason, J. H.: Tetanus in the dog and cat: a review with comments. J. S. Afr. Vet. Assoc. 35:209, 1964.
Stogdale, L.: Canine tetanus. J. S. Afr. Vet. Assoc. 47:299, 1976.

CERVICAL AND THORACOLUMBAR DISC DISEASE IN THE DOG

RAYMOND G. PRATA, D.V.M.

New York, New York

Numerous medical and surgical procedures have been advocated for the treatment of neck pain, back pain, paresis, or plegia in the dog resulting from extruded disc material attenuating the spinal cord and/or nerve roots. The management of such injuries has long been the subject of debate concerning the preservation or restoration of neurologic function. Although it is generally agreed that surgical decompression of the paretic or plegic dog is the treatment of choice, the decompressive procedure itself and the philosophy regarding its use are subjects of great controversy among veterinary surgeons. Likewise, the understanding and medical or surgical management of pain are variable.

Spinal cord injury must be discussed as a cause and effect relationship. The causes are numerous, and the effects are varied and often devastating. The ability to differentially diagnose, prognosticate, and appropriately manage all forms of spinal cord injury resulting from extruded disc herniation is directly related to the surgeon's knowledge of basic principles of neurology, neurophysiology, neuroradiology, neurosurgery, and neuropathology.

Of major concern in the management and prognosis of space-occupying lesions such as discs is the pathophysiologic response of the spinal cord. The pathologic process associated with acute spinal cord injury has been shown to be directly related to the degree of force transmitted to the spinal cord. Physiologic studies have demonstrated chemical, neuronal, and blood flow alterations in the wounded spinal cord, resulting in various degrees of pathology and neurologic deficits. Since traumatic lesions (with or without persistent mechanical compression) are produced by an inherent and variable destructive spinal cord process; bone removal procedures (laminectomy, hemilaminectomy, ventral cervical decompression) alone cannot be expected to resolve the neurologic deficits in the severely injured dog.

The age-old question of when to operate and with what prognosis will always be subject to controversy. The appropriate surgical treatment for some spinal cord injuries can be determined by the type of injury. For example, spinal cord injuries associated with mechanical extra-axial compression lend themselves to surgical decompression. The mass attenuating the spinal cord, however, must be removed to afford a decompressive procedure. This principle has long been respected in the treatment of spinal cord injuries in humans. Laminectomy, hemilaminectomy, or ventral cervical decompression procedures alone without mass removal may be compared to "making a hole in the roof of a house to let the water out of the basement" or, as another surgeon put it, "attempting to remove the patient from his lesion." All decompressive procedures are purely bone removal techniques, which provide access to the spinal canal. Decompression of attenuated spinal cord and/or nerve root is achieved only following mass removal (disc).

From a purely mechanical point of view, it seems reasonable to remove demonstrable mechanical neural obstruction. However, the logic approaches reality only when partial neural loss and extra-axial compression coexist.

The objectives in the management of spinal cord trauma with cord and/or nerve root entrapment associated with extruded fragments of disc include (1) establishing the onset, course, and severity of spinal cord injury or radicular (nerve root) signs; (2) establishing the neurologic localization; (3) predicting the reversibility or irreversibility of the lesion; and (4) affording the appropriate medical and/or surgical treatment. The cause of pain, a frequent accompaniment to disc extrusion, must also be considered to effectively manage and achieve relief of signs.

NEUROLOGIC CONSIDERATIONS

The neurologic examination remains a most important aspect in the diagnosis, localization, and prognosis of spinal cord and/or nerve root dysfunction. The motor, proprioceptive, and sensory components of the examination must be simultaneously approached and assimilated.

The historic development of neurologic disease, an often neglected clinical approach, is most important in documenting the onset and course of the

708

disease as well as enabling the clinician to establish the differential diagnoses. Acute injuries resulting in tetraplegia or paraplegia (complete motor and sensory loss) generally hold a more guarded prognosis when compared with more gradual onsets of motor and sensory disturbances. An extruded disc fragment must be viewed as a mass of variable size, expelled from a given interspace with variable velocity and striking the spinal cord with variable force. The resultant neurologic deficits are related to the pathophysiologic insult sustained from the initial impact as well as the persistent space-occupying lesion attenuating the cord and/or nerve roots.

Critical serial neurologic examinations complement the historic evaluation in conclusively establishing the state of plegia or the degree of paresis. Likewise, they permit confirmation and localization of neck or back pain with or without presenting motor or proprioceptive deficits.

In cases of intervertebral disc disease, neck or back pain may be discogenic or radicular (nerve root) in origin. Discogenic pain is associated with desiccation of the nucleus pulposus with concomitant degenerative pathology of the annulus fibrosis without extrusion of disc material into the spinal canal. Pain originates from the inflammatory changes of the pain-sensitive structures of the dorsal longitudinal ligament and superficial layers of the dorsal annulus, which have been shown to be innervated by the sinuvertebral nerve (a branch of the dorsal root). The diagnosis of discogenic pain in humans is confirmed by a negative myelogram, a positive discogram demonstrating tearing of the annulus, and elicitation of pain upon performing discography of the pathologic disc.

In the author's experience, neck or back pain associated with degenerative disc disease, with little exception, is caused by the dorsolateral extrusion of disc material and subsequent entrapment of a nerve root, which is defined as radicular pain. This has been consistently documented with cervical or lumbar myelography and confirmed surgically. Ischemia of the nerve root, as a direct result of root entrapment, has been postulated as the pathophysiologic mechanism of radicular pain. Neck or back pain may be minimal or nonexistent in some dogs with varying degrees of tetraparesis or paraparesis. In these cases, disc material has extruded ventrally and on the midline, not attenuating existing nerve roots.

The elicitation of back pain, by application of digital pressure on the spine at the site of disc extrusion, is a reliable method of establishing the localization of disease. This hyperpathic level is accurate within two to three interspaces. The accuracy of localizing the level of cervical disease by digital manipulation is not as consistently valuable as that with thoracolumbar disease. However, elicitation of hyperpathia upon digital manipulation of the ventral tubercles of the cervical vertebra may provide for a high, middle, or low cervical level of localization.

The hyperpathic level, as with each individual neurologic component of the examination, is only valuable in localizing the lesion when all the components of the examination support a focal spinal cord dysfunction.

Disc extrusions attenuating nerve roots result in radicular pain and associated referred pain and/or spasm of the muscles innervated. When nerve roots, contributing to the innervation of an extremity, are attenuated, a "root signature" may be historically described and/or clinically observed. A root signature is defined as referred pain radiating down the front or rear limb associated with nerve root entrapment (C_{4-8}, T_{1-2}, L_{4-7}, S_1) resulting in lameness or elevation of the limb. Awareness of this sign is of great importance to the clinician, as many dogs with cervical or lumbar discs are initially treated for obscure lameness. A root signature will not be observed at the C_{2-3} disc interspace (C_3 root) or at the T_{3-4} to L_{3-4} disc interspaces. It must be emphasized that a root signature may not be observed despite entrapment of a root that innervates an extremity.

When examining a nonambulatory dog, it is extremely helpful to ascertain if a root signature had been historically present prior to paresis or plegia. Accurate localization is enhanced with this information.

Motor deficits ranging from paresis to plegia are frequent sequelae to disc extrusion in the dog. Although most frequently associated with thoracolumbar disc extrusion, paresis and plegia are not uncommonly associated with cervical disc extrusions. The resultant paresis or plegia is classified as upper motor neuron (UMN) or lower motor neuron (LMN) by means of the neurologic examination and demonstration of altered reflexes in the extremities. LMN signs are those of hyporeflexia, areflexia, hypotonia, atonia, and a rapid onset of atrophy (within five to seven days). UMN signs are those of hyperreflexia, hypertonia, and crossed extensor reflexes. The crossed extensor reflex, most often elicited with UMN disease, is purely localizing and affords no basis for prognostication. Flaccidity is the hallmark of LMN disease, as spasticity is that of UMN disease.

The term *spinal shock* has often been used to describe an acute spinal cord injury and reflects upon the areflexic state despite an UMN level of localization. Flaccid paralysis has also been used in the same manner. Although acute spinal cord wounding may produce this neurologic picture, it often does not occur, as previously reported, or is extremely transient (6 to 12 hours). Such cases, with confirmed focal UMN pathology, are most often complete (sensorimotor paralysis), with associated focal hemorrhagic necrosis of the spinal cord at the extruded disc level. Flaccid paralysis denotes localization to the cervical or lumbar enlargements and must be reserved for this condition.

The reflex alterations are strictly a means of localizing pathology to the UMN segments (C_{1-6}, $T_{3-}L_3$) versus the LMN segments (C_7-T_2, L_{4-7}, S_{1-3}). These reflexes provide the clinician with no prognostic information in and of themselves. However, depending on the degree of injury sustained, it is our experience that LMN disorders do hold a less favorable prognosis. It must be emphasized that many disc extrusions at the LMN and cauda equina levels may be surgically corrected with rewarding results in animals with incomplete lesions.

The motor examination also permits categorization of the degree of reported paresis, which ultimately aids in prognostication. We have concluded in previous reports that ambulatory paraparetics respond more favorably to surgery than nonambulatory paraparetics with voluntary movement, who, in turn, respond more favorably than nonambulatory paraparetics without voluntary movement. Likewise, we have demonstrated the importance of correlating the historic onset of motor signs (acute versus chronic progressive) with the degree of motor deficits exhibited and subsequent recovery rates. A dog with an acute onset of nonambulatory paraparesis (zero to four hours) with preservation of moderate voluntary movement responds more slowly to surgical treatment than a dog attaining the same level of motor weakness progressively over a 48-hour period or longer. Likewise, the restoration of more normal ambulatory capabilities was more favorable in the progressively deteriorating groups. The duration of compression has also been shown to affect the dog's recuperation; those with prolonged compression recovered more slowly. It must be stressed that surgical decompressive procedures should not be limited to those dogs presenting within a specific time frame, after which surgery is denied. Of importance are preservation of sensation and a knowledge, when available, of the onset (acute or progressive) of the paresis. Rewarding results are not infrequently attained.

Cervical disc extrusion not uncommonly presents with moderate to severe tetraparesis. Tetraplegia (sensorimotor paralysis) is extremely rare. Despite rather severe nonambulatory disturbances, ventral cervical decompression is extremely rewarding when compared with comparable thoracolumbar motor deficits. Again, of major importance is the historic information, when available, regarding onset (acute versus progressive). Acute disc extrusions of the cervical spine at the C_{2-5} levels may result in profound motor deficits of an UMN nature, most demonstrable in the forelimbs with relative sparing of rear limbs. These dogs are nonambulatory. This is referred to as a "central cord" phenomenon and

is a reflection of the front limb motor fibers lying more medial within the spinal cord motor pathways than the rear limb fibers. The acute injury results in central cord edema and/or hemorrhage affecting the forelimb fibers to a greater degree than the more laterally placed rear limb fibers. The sensory status is most often fully preserved. Surgical decompression and mass removal may be rewarding, but the prognosis must be guarded based on potential permanent central cord dysfunction. In general, surgical management of pain and paresis (mild or profound) related to cervical disc extrusion is much more gratifying than thoracolumbar disc extrusions. Nonlocalizing loss of conscious proprioception (CP) reflects dorsal column dysfunction and neurologic dysfunction of either the UMN or LMN segments and is of minimal prognostic value to the clinician.

Establishing the integrity of the sensory system is of major importance in determining the ultimate prognosis. Because of its subjectivity, documentation of the sensory status necessitates numerous critically performed examinations. It is imperative that an appropriate response to noxious stimuli applied to the digits be elicited, including barking, whining, or an attempt to bite the examiner. Pure withdrawal, in and of itself, is not appropriate, as it may reflect a reflex withdrawal only. An anesthetic state bespeaks a severe, complete lesion and holds an extremely guarded prognosis regardless of the type or time interval of management. Profound sensory disturbances, when associated with a progressive state of deterioration, hold a more favorable prognosis than those presented with an acute injury. Acute spinal cord injuries with moderate to severe hypesthesia respond more favorably when surgically treated within the first 48 hours. However, dogs with progressive disease, presented with profound sensory disturbances, may respond favorably to surgery even after days or weeks have elapsed. As a rule, we advocate surgery, despite the time frame from onset to time of presentation, provided an appropriate response to noxious stimuli is established.

PATHOPHYSIOLOGIC CONSIDERATIONS

Pathophysiologic as well as pathomechanical aspects of spinal cord dysfunction must be examined to ensure appropriate management. Ultimately, the prognosis of reversible versus irreversible disease is foremost in one's mind. Four factors must be considered following spinal cord injury: (1) mechanical pressure on and distortion of the spinal cord; (2) the intrinsic chemical, neural, and blood flow alterations within the spinal cord, (3) the onset (acute versus progressive) of spinal cord attenuation; and (4) the duration of attenuation.

Current research on spinal cord injury has demonstrated that a blow of 400 G/cm or more to the spinal cord of dogs results in immediate permanent plegia. Complete spinal cord dissolution progresses over 24 to 48 hours. This is related to an inherent autodestructive process in the cord rather than to actual, immediate physical disruption. The pathophysiologic basis for the autodestructive process has been shown to be associated with the post-traumatic toxic release of certain vasoactive substances such as norepinephrine, serotonin, and dopamine within the spinal cord. The toxic concentration of catecholamines has been shown to have a profound effect on the microvasculature of the spinal cord. Vasospasm, decreased blood flow, and the development of endothelial gaps and ruptures in the walls of small vessels within the cord result in perivascular accumulation of red cells, which in themselves are toxic to neural substance. Decreased perfusion, hypoxia, and a self-perpetuating hemorrhagic necrosis result in a spinal cord that is composed mainly of an amorphous necrotic tissue (myelomalacia) and aggregated red blood cells with only a small rim of identifiable white matter 24 to 48 hours after the injury (400 G/cm). Surgical decompressive procedures are ineffective in the management of such devastation.

Hematomyelia, in effect, is the end result of acute spinal cord injury associated with an impact of 400 G/cm force or greater. Hematomyelia, in the strictest sense of the definition, refers to a nonextending, expansile, limited saccular mass of blood in the spinal cord and must be distinguished from the extended bleeding and hemorrhagic necrosis associated with some rare cases of peracute spinal cord injuries. In veterinary medicine, the term *hematomyelia* has been inappropriately used to describe the ascending and descending progressive, devastating hemorrhagic necrosis that results in complete dissolution of the spinal cord. This pathologic process is most frequently associated with peracute explosive extrusions of thoracolumbar discs resulting in instantaneous plegia. This condition is uncommon. The cause is unknown but is likely to be related to the massive autodestructive process previously described. Serial neurologic examinations are required to ascertain the presence of ascending-descending disease. Surgical intervention and/or present-day medical therapy is not rewarding.

Impact injuries of less magnitude produce transient spinal cord dysfunction with varying resultant deficits. The autodestructive process and progressive hemorrhagic necrosis are not initiated. When present, hemorrhage within the gray matter is variable but does not spread extensively into the white matter. The transient deficits are related to reversible tissue ischemia, hypoxia, and edema, which subsequently result in varying degrees of demyelination of intact axons.

Disc extrusions deliver forces of varying intensity to the spinal cord, mechanically distort it, and produce neuronal dysfunction related to microvascular disturbances. If the force is sufficient, autodestruction and permanent paralysis ensue. However, disc extrusion must be examined in light of its mass effect attenuating the spinal cord as well as its effect on the microvasculature. It has been shown that progressive attenuation of the spinal cord experimentally and clinically holds a much more favorable prognosis than acute injuries. Mass lesions of gradual onset produce demyelination by direct pressure and/or vascular deprivation. Restoration of function by decompressive procedures is dependent on degrees of degeneration and, more importantly, axonal integrity.

The duration of compression is also important in establishing the restoration of function but must also be assessed in light of the acute or slow progressive onset of dysfunction. Acute space-occupying lesions are more devastating and may require earlier decompression than chronic progressive forms of spinal cord dysfunction.

The progressive neurologic signs associated with progressive mechanical deformation and ischemia are related to a demyelination process. Those fibers that are most heavily myelinated show the earliest dysfunction. Therefore, the signs of progressive neurologic deterioration of the spinal cord in order of presentation are (1) proprioceptive and joint position sense loss (spinal ataxia), (2) motor dysfunction (reflex alterations, ambulation, voluntary movement), and (3) sensory disturbances. The neurologic recovery rate occurs in reverse. In our experience, months are usually required for restoration of appropriate joint position sense. In many instances, mild to moderate deficits are permanent.

MEDICAL MANAGEMENT

Medical management must address and provide for symptomatic treatment of pain, paresis, and sphincter dysfunction. Although there are limitations, numerous drugs have substantial value in the management of intervertebral disc disease.

NECK AND BACK PAIN

Neck and back pain, invariably associated with extruded fragments of disc attenuating nerve roots (radicular pain), most favorably benefit from a combination of corticosteroids and muscle relaxants. Corticosteroids reduce the inflammatory process about the nerve root and the resultant ischemia of the root, which produces pain. Dexamethasone

(Azium* 0.25 to 0.5 mg t.i.d.; total dose) or prednisone† (5 to 10 mg t.i.d.; total dose) tapered over seven to ten days is recommended. There is no justification for higher dosages despite the size of the dog. Methocarbamol (Robaxin‡ 10 mg/lb t.i.d.) provides relief of the myalgia associated with nerve root entrapment. It is our experience, however, that diazepam (Valium§) administered at a dosage of 2 to 5 mg t.i.d. (total dose) provides more complete relief of the associated muscle spasms. The dosage may vary in individual patients to avoid excessive sedation. We do not encourage cage confinement nor do we advocate full activity for the ensuing two to three weeks. Increased recurrences or treatment failures have not been documented. Likewise, we do not support the philosophy of providing the dog with incomplete therapeutic relief of pain for the sake of beneficial self-limiting pain. Radicular pain is devastating and should be dispelled in the most efficacious therapeutic mode available.

Hospitalization and specific diagnostic protocols leading to surgery are discussed upon recurrence of neck or back pain or in the event that medical therapy fails. Approximately 30 per cent of our surgically treated cervical and thoracolumbar cases presented with prior episodes of pain and/or mild paresis. The recurrence rate of the overall population, although not statistically evaluated, is approximately 10 per cent.

At our institution, motor and sensory deficits are categorized as follows: (1) ambulatory paresis, (2) nonambulatory paresis with voluntary movement, (3) nonambulatory paresis without voluntary movement, and (4) plegia. The preservation of sensation, as subjectively assessed, is preserved in the paretic states.

MYELOPATHY

Medical management of myelopathy in the dog is presently practically limited to the use of corticosteroids. Corticosteroids maintain vascular integrity following injury, protect cellular membranes during hypoperfusion states, and support lysozymes. They also depress catecholamine metabolism and accumulation and have remarkable stabilization properties of white matter. Steroids have a definite influence on recovery from moderate spinal cord injuries (< 300 G/cm), whereas severe injuries fare poorly. The most effective steroid dosage has not yet been determined; however, it is felt by some that massive dosages are more beneficial (as high as 10 gm prednisolone [Solu-Delta Cor-

tef‖]/day and tapered). Mannitol (2 gm/kg) has been used to treat spinal cord injury. Additional studies, however, are needed to assess the efficacy of mannitol in functional recovery following spinal cord trauma. We believe, purely on a clinical level, that the use of steroids with mannitol does not afford better results than the use of steroids alone.

MILD PARESIS

The mildly paretic dog (with ataxia, CP deficits, no reflex changes) is managed conservatively on steroids and Robaxin or Valium. The steroid administration varies with the size of each patient and is tapered over seven to ten days. The steroid dosage range used is 1 to 5 mg t.i.d. (total dose) and slowly tapered. We do not routinely advocate massive steroid administration schedules and find extremely rewarding results at these low levels. These dogs are treated as outpatients with client instruction to minimize activity and report every two days. Reexamination is conducted in two weeks. Clients are advised of potential further extrusion and more profound deficits. This is of particular concern for thoracolumbar discs but is rarely a complicating feature with cervical discs. The incidence of recurrence following such regimentation has not been accurately determined; however, we have established an overall 20 to 25 per cent recurrence rate. A nonresponsive course or subsequent relapse signifies the need for surgical considerations.

MODERATE TO SEVERE PARESIS

Dogs with moderate to severe paresis are hospitalized and placed on corticosteroids at dosages ranging from 5 to 20 mg of dexamethasone t.i.d. (total dose). The cortisone is tapered over seven to ten days. A complete diagnostic work-up is performed inclusive of spinal radiographs under general anesthesia. Myelography is selectively performed, followed by a decompressive, mass removal procedure.

Gastrointestinal hemorrhage, acute ulceration, and perforation may be initiated by the administration of steroids, especially when massive dosages are administered. We rarely encounter this pathophysiologic process at the given steroid regimentation. Tagamet** may be administered for gastric ulceration; however, it is ineffective in the management of associated hemorrhagic enteritis. In the latter instances, steroids should be immediately discontinued. Kaopectate and/or other coating agents should be given as appropriate.

The catecholamine theory of severe spinal cord injury with subsequent neurovascular alterations

---

*Schering Corp., Kenilworth, NJ.
†Danbury Pharmacal, Inc., Danbury, CT.
‡A. H. Robins Co., Richmond, VA.
§Hoffman-LaRoche Inc., Nutley, NJ.

‖The Upjohn Co., Kalamazoo, MI.
**Smith Kline & French, Philadelphia, PA

and hemorrhagic necrosis has led to alternate means of treatment aimed at arresting this devastating process. Numerous anticatecholamine drugs (alpha-methyltyrosine, reserpine, phenoxybenzamine) have been administered with encouraging results. Antifibrinolytic therapy with aminocaproic acid also has been used with some success. These treatments are experimental, and further investigation must be conducted prior to their routine administration. At present, these forms of therapy are rewarding in experiments, but only if administered prior to or immediately after the spinal cord has been wounded. Naloxone is under investigation for its blocking effect on endogenous endorphins, which when released at the time of spinal cord injury result in systemic hypotension and subsequent decreased cord perfusion. Beneficial results have been described. Thyrotropin-releasing hormone is also under investigation for its similar action on reducing systemic hypotension following spinal cord injury. Thyrotropin has an added advantage over naloxone in not blocking the analgesic action of endorphins and thus exacerbating post-trauma pain.

Urinary bladder management is of crucial importance to the overall successful management of the spinally injured dog. Urinary tract infection and ascending renal disease are not infrequent sequelae in poorly managed cases. Intermittent catheterization three times daily is most effective in the male dog, whereas bladder expression is most practical in the female dog. However, when faced with incomplete evacuation in the female, placement of a Foley catheter is advised. These catheters must not remain in place longer than 48 hours. These permanent catheters are a frequent cause of cystitis from mechanical abrasion of the bladder wall and associated ascending infection. Appropriate antibiotics must be administered concomitant with corticosteroids and muscle relaxants.

NEURORADIOLOGY

Neuroradiographic procedures, following serial neurologic examinations, provide accurate means for localizing the level of pathology. Spinal radiographs must be taken under general anesthesia to provide for high quality films and accurate interpretation. In many instances, correlation of the neurologic and radiographic level is confirmed without myelography. However, myelography is indicated when a discrepancy between the neurologic and neuroradiographic level occurs, when survey films produce no visible lesion, or when more than one lesion is suspected on spinal films. It is our experience that all cervical disc cases should be myelographed to establish the most appropriate surgical approach (ventral decompression, laminectomy, hemilaminectomy) to provide for complete mass removal with minimal cord manipulation.

Multiple disc extrusions of the cervical or thoracolumbar spine, as demonstrated by myelography, are extremely rare. We have reported one case in the thoracolumbar spine and none in the cervical spine. This statement refers specifically to acute disc extrusions and not to chronic disc disease (spondylosis), which may deflect the dye column at multiple levels.

NEUROSURGICAL CONSIDERATIONS

Surgical considerations are reserved for those dogs with recurrent neck or back pain, recurrent paresis preceded by a favorable steroid response, progressive paresis despite steroid therapy, or moderate to severe acute paresis with preservation of sensation of the limbs. We do not impose any time restrictions on surgical correction.

Thoracolumbar discs, following neurologic localization and identification by neuroradiology, are surgically treated by laminectomy or hemilaminectomy. Our surgical technique consists of laminectomy carried out over two vertebral bodies combined with bilateral facetectomy and foramenotomy at the site of disc extrusion. Variable amounts of pedicle (lateral wall) are removed bilaterally to facilitate visualization and complete removal of the disc. Manipulation of the dural tube and spinal cord should be avoided at all times. Double-action pediatric laminectomy rongeurs or a Hall air drill* is used. Hemostasis, of critical importance, is achieved with bipolar cautery,† thrombin-soaked absorbable gelatin sponges,‡ and bone wax.§

Unless the neurologic examination lateralizes the weakness to the right or left side of the body or unless myelography is performed in each case, hemilaminectomy will fail to expose the disc approximately half of the time. We have found no statistical difference in the percentage of right versus left extrusions. Decompression is achieved only following complete mass removal and is not achieved by simply removing bone. We frequently use a hemilaminectomy approach but only when accurate localization and lateralization have been established.

Laminectomy over two vertebral bodies has been discouraged because of the unsightly cosmetic defect and the potential laminectomy scar formation. We have eliminated the defect by spanning the laminectomy site with a 20- or 22-gauge orthopedic wire. A loop of wire is placed around the rostral and caudal spinous processes and moderately tightened. The thoracolumbar muscles and fascia are

---

*Amsco Hall Surgical Division, Santa Barbara, CA.
†Martin Elektrom, 72 Tuttlinger, Germany.
‡The Upjohn Co., Kalamazoo, MI.
§Ethicon Inc., Somerville, NJ.

sutured in a simple interrupted pattern over the wire with 3-0 or 2-0 nylon.

A laminectomy scar was reported in only 2 of 187 of our laminectomized dogs. The probable reason is that, although variable amounts of pedicle were removed, the dural tube was not left completely exposed. Also, direct contact of muscle tissue on the dural tube was precluded by the use of the spanning wire. Lastly, and very importantly, the laminectomy defect was covered with adipose tissue (free fat graft) resected from the incision site. This has been clearly shown to reduce scar formation. Gelfoam has been shown, however, to substantially increase scar formation and therefore should not be used.

Cervical disc extrusions may be surgically treated using laminectomy, hemilaminectomy, or ventral decompressive procedures. However, the gratifying results associated with ventral decompressive procedures far outweigh any advantages of the dorsal approaches.

The ventral approach, using a Hall air drill to remove disc and adjacent vertebral end-plates, provides direct access to the ventral aspect of the spinal canal, wherein lie the extruded fragments of disc. Technical experience enables the surgeon to avoid the venous sinuses and establish complete mass removal with no manipulation of the spinal cord. Should hemorrhage from the venous sinuses occur, direct application of Gelfoam to the sinuses establishes hemostasis.

Laminectomy or hemilaminectomy of the cervical spine should be reserved for those rare instances in which disc extrusion occurs totally lateral within the canal or when disc extrudes into the intervertebral foramen, causing pure root entrapment. The use of a laminectomy or hemilaminectomy approach, with the exception of the aforementioned, often results in excessive cord manipulation to achieve full decompression. The result is a worsened neurologic state, which is most often permanent.

Myelography, when dealing with cervical disc disease, is of extreme importance and provides the surgeon with valuable information dictating the surgical approach. Oblique radiographs are valuable in identifying intraforaminal disc extrusions.

We have not yet documented evidence to support a rationale for the use of fenestration in the definitive or prophylactic treatment of disc disease.

The signs of pain and/or paresis are, with rare exceptions, associated with solitary extrusion and subsequent attenuation of neural structures. Definitive treatment is established consistently only by removal of the mass entrapping the cord and/or root. Recurrence at other levels, subsequent to surgery, is extremely rare in both cervical and thoracolumbar spinal levels.

SUPPLEMENTAL READING

Albin, M. S., White, R. J., Locke, G. S., et al.: Localized spinal cord hypothermia: Anesthetic effects and application to spinal cord injury. Anesthesiol. Analg. 46:8, 1967.

Brown, N. O., Helphrey, M. L., and Prata, R. G.: Thoracolumbar disc disease in the dog: A retrospective analysis of 187 cases. J. Am. Anim. Hosp. Assoc. 13:665, 1977.

Cloward, R. B.: Treatment of lesions of the cervical spine by the anterior surgical approach. *In* Austin, G. (ed.): *The Spinal Cord: Basic Aspects and Surgical Considerations*, 2nd ed. Springfield, IL: Charles C Thomas, 1972, pp. 392, 403–405, 429.

Doppman, J. L.: Angiographic changes following acute spinal cord compression: an experimental study in monkeys. Br. J. Radiol. 49:398, 1976.

Doppman, J. L., and Girtow, M.: Angiographic study of the effect of laminectomy in the presence of acute anterior epidural masses. J. Neurosurg. 45:195, 1976.

Gage, E. D.: Incidence of clinical disc disease in the dog. J. Am. Anim. Hosp. Assoc. 11:135, 1975.

Gill, G. G., Sakovich, L., and Thompson, E.: Pedicle fat grafts for prevention of small scar formation after laminectomy: An experimental study in dogs. Spine 4:176, 1979.

Gooding, M. R., Wilson, C. B., and Hoff, J. T.: Experimental cervical myelopathy: Effect of ischemia and compression of the canine cervical spinal cord. J. Neurosurg. 43:9, 1975.

Henry, W. G.: Dorsal decompressive laminectomy in the treatment of thoracolumbar disc disease. J. Am. Anim. Hosp. Assoc. 11:627, 1975.

Hoerlein, B. F.: Intervertebral disc protrusions in the dog. No. 1: incidence and pathological lesions. Am. J. Vet. Res. 14:260, 1953.

Hukuda, S., and Wilson, C. B.: Experimental cervical myelopathy: Effects of compression and ischemia on the canine cervical cord. J. Neurosurg. 49:412, 1978.

Keller, J. T., Dunster, S. B., McWorter, J. M., et al.: The fate of autogenous grafts to the spinal dura: An experimental study. J. Neurosurg. 49:412, 1978.

Knecht, C. D.: The effect of delay hemilaminectomy in the treatment of intervertebral disc protrusion in dogs. J.A.A.H.A. 6:71, 1970.

Langenshiold, A., and Kiviluoto, O.: Prevention of epidural scar formation after operations on the lumbar spine by means of free fat transplants: A preliminary report. Clin. Orthop. 115:92, 1976.

LaRocca, H., and Macnab, I.: The laminectomy membrane: Studies in its evolution, characteristics, effects, and prophylaxis in dogs. J. Bone Joint Surg. 56-B:545, 1974.

Minckler, J.: Surgical pathology of the spinal cord. *In* Austin, G. (ed.): *The Spinal Cord: Basic Aspects and Surgical Considerations*, 2nd ed. Springfield, IL: Charles C Thomas, 1972, p. 220.

Nelson, E., et al.: Spinal cord injury: Role of vascular damage in the pathogenesis of central hemorrhagic necrosis. Arch. Neurol. 34:332, 1977.

Osterholm, J. L.: The pathophysiological response to spinal cord injury. J. Neurosurg. 40:5, 1974.

Parker, A. J., Park, R. D., and Stowater, J. L.: Reduction of trauma-induced edema of spinal cord in dogs given mannitol. Am. J. Vet. Res. 34:1355, 1973.

Prata, R. G.: Diagnosis of spinal cord tumors in the dog. Vet. Clin. North Am. 7:165, 1977.

Prata, R. G., and Stoll, S. G.: Ventral decompression and fusion for the treatment of cervical disk disease in the dog. J. Am. Anim. Hosp. Assoc. 9:462, 1973.

Prata, R. G., Stoll, S. G., and Zaki, F. A.: Spinal cord compression caused by osteocartilaginous exostoses of the spine in two dogs. J.A.V.M.A. 166:371, 1975.

Rawe, S. E., et al.: Norepinephrine levels in experimental spinal cord trauma. Part I: Biochemical study of hemorrhagic necrosis. J. Neurosurg. 46:342, 1977.

Rawe, S. E., et al.: Norepinephrine levels in experimental spinal cord trauma. Part II: Histopathologic study of hemorrhagic necrosis. J. Neurosurg. 46:350, 1977.

Reed, J. E., Allen, W. E. III, and Dohrmann, G. J.: Effect of mannitol on traumatized spinal cord. Spine 4:391, 1979.

Sandler, A. N., et al.: Review of effect of spinal cord trauma on vessels and blood flow in the spinal cord. J. Neurosurg. 45:638, 1976.

Seim, H., and Prata, R. G.: Ventral decompression for the treatment of cervical disk disease in the dog: A review of 54 cases. J. Am. Anim. Hosp. Assoc. 18:233, 1982.

Swaim, S. F., and Vandevelde, M.: Clinical and histological evaluation of bilateral hemilaminectomy and deep dorsal laminectomy for extensive spinal cord decompression in the dog. J.A.V.M.A. 170:407, 1977.

Tarlov, I. M.: *Spinal Cord Compression: Mechanical Paralysis and Treatment.* Springfield, IL: Charles C Thomas, 1957.

Tator, C. H., and Deeke, L.: Value of normothermic perfusion, hypothermic perfusion, and durotomy in the treatment of experimental acute spinal cord trauma. J. Neurosurg. 39:52, 1973.

Trotter, E. J.: Canine intervertebral disc disease. *In* Kirk, R. W. (ed.): *Current Veterinary Therapy VI.* Philadelphia: W. B. Saunders, 1977.

Wagner, R. E., Jr., et al.: The development of intramedullary cavitation following spinal cord injury: An experimental pathologic study. Paraplegia 14:245, 1977.

CONSIDERATIONS FOR MEDICAL TREATMENT OF SPINAL CORD INJURY

C. D. KNECHT, V.M.D.

Auburn, Alabama

Trauma to the vertebral column is not uncommon as a result of automobile accidents and gunshot wounds. The extent of injury to the spinal cord is often greater than might be expected when considering the protective musculoskeletal structure of the vertebrae and epaxial musculature. Fracture or luxation of the vertebrae or penetration wounds from missiles may cause compression, laceration, or contusion of the spinal cord. Severe neurologic deficit resulting from spinal cord trauma is perhaps the most common indication for euthanasia in veterinary practice following trauma. Nevertheless, care is essential in localizing and confirming the lesion in the central nervous system before this irrevocable step is taken.

Trauma may produce a number of signs that resemble spinal cord injury. Pelvic fractures mimic paraparesis; cranial contusion and shock may appear as tetraplegia. The effects of trauma are rarely static. Signs may progress, as in continued spinal instability and increasing compression, or regress, as in recovery from concussion. Spinal shock, defined as the absence of all spinal reflexes following trauma, lasts only minutes in the dog and cat and is generally absent by the time of presentation at the veterinary clinic. Because the severity and signs of neurologic damage may change (worsen) following trauma, conservative treatment should begin as soon as possible.

The goals of therapy are multiple. The first goal in the treatment of trauma is to preserve the animal's life by the prevention and treatment of shock, support of respiration, and control of hemorrhage. In the event of real or suspected trauma to the spinal cord, simultaneous treatment must be given to prevent increased damage to the cord, which might result from vertebral instability. Such treatment should begin as soon after the traumatic episode as possible. Treatment at a primary care facility is directed to lessening the secondary hemodynamic effects on the spinal cord. This treatment may be medical or surgical, depending on the severity of signs. As the need for surgical treatment is deliberated, medical therapy should be combined with continued temporary immobilization of the injured site.

Treatment should be given by the owner at the time of trauma. It is the veterinarian's responsibility to advise the owner not only to bring the injured animal to the hospital but *how* to do so. Just as hemorrhage can be reduced with a pressure bandage and apparent fractures can be immobilized by a rolled magazine or bath towel securely taped to the limb, further cord damage from fractured or luxated vertebrae can be prevented. The paretic animal should be handled with minimal movement of the back or neck. A gauze muzzle may be applied for the safety of the owner and the animal slid onto a pallet (wood or window screen) or a blanket by two people (Fig. 1). The animal should be restrained on the pallet manually or with straps.

Physical, neurologic, and radiographic examinations at the veterinary hospital should be completed with similar restraint. A vertebral body splint may be necessary. Following proper immobilization, emergency therapy for shock and hemorrhage may be administered without delay. The physical and neurologic findings should be recorded at the earliest convenience, noting the date and time of the observations. Comparisons with the findings at the time of entrance may alter subsequent therapy.

Neurologic examination is the keystone to locali-

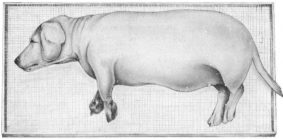

Figure 1. A window screen pallet. (Reproduced with permission from Knecht et al.: *Fundamental Techniques in Veterinary Surgery*, 2nd ed. Philadelphia: W. B. Saunders, 1981.)

zation, reducing the manipulation for and cost of radiographic examination, treatment, and prognosis. Not all neurologic reflexes need to be tested. Flexor and myotatic reflexes can be elicited without excess manipulation and will define normal peripheral nerves and lumbosacral and brachial plexuses. Absence of voluntary motion and tone is common caudal to the site of spinal cord trauma and may lessen the need for postural or attitudinal reaction testing. If the clinician is in doubt and the animal's vertebrae are adequately stabilized, placing and extensor postural thrust reactions may be used to demonstrate an upper motor neuron lesion cranial to the deficit. Induction of the panniculus reflex with a safety pin will frequently localize the thoracolumbar lesion between T_2 and L_4. Malalignment of spinous processes may be apparent with careful palpation. The cranial nerves should be examined and the level of consciousness determined before sedation.

In spinal cord trauma, the prognosis is better if the animal is in pain or is paretic and not paralyzed. Animals with Schiff-Sherrington reaction, that is, extensor rigidity of the forelimbs and flaccidity of the rear limbs, have a poor prognosis. In evaluating the Schiff-Sherrington reaction, one should recall that the closer the lesion is to T_2, the less severe it need be to cause the reaction. In addition, dogs with paraplegia and severe pain may extend the forelimbs, mimicking the reaction. When placed in sternal recumbency, these dogs will usually demonstrate the ability to flex the forelimbs.

The crossed-extensor reflex is normal in the upright position. When observed in the lateral position, it signals upper motor neuron disease and may be used as an indication of the severity of the lesion. The crossed-extensor reflex is a rapid extension of the contralateral limb when flexion is induced. If it does not occur simultaneously with flexion or if it only occurs when the leg beneath the dog is flexed, one should suspect a partial righting reaction and not a crossed-extensor reaction. Examination for deep pain will usually validate the crossed-extensor reflex and is the best prognostic neurologic test.

The digital nerves are pressed vigorously with the examiner's thumb nail and the dog observed for cognition in the form of vocal efforts or attempts to move away or bite. Limb flexion is only a reflex and does not indicate cognition. If the dog does not respond, a hemostat may be used to squeeze the nail or digit. The absence of a pain response is a grave prognostic sign.

Radiographic examination is valuable to confirm the diagnosis and indicates the need for surgical decompression of bony fragments and the method of surgical repair. Radiographic appearance is less reliable for prognosis than neurologic signs because, in the conventional radiographic views, damage to the spinal cord frequently differs from that indicated by malaligned vertebral fragments.

Many drugs have been used singly or in combination for the treatment of trauma to the spinal cord and most of these in combination with decompressive surgery. Few controlled studies have demonstrated the efficacy of individual drugs, and a recent study indicates minimal benefits resulting from any single medicament.

Naloxone did cause improvement following trauma, but more trials are needed. The author continues to use adrenocorticosteroids and immobilization of the injured area with or without surgery. Dexamethasone (2 mg/kg) is given intramuscularly on first examination and is repeated at the time of surgery at 1 mg/kg if the surgery is delayed more than four hours. If surgical decompression is not indicated, the vertebrae should be immobilized with a vertebral cast or splint for no less than three weeks. Only the initial intramuscular dose of dexamethasone is administered if surgery is not done.

The indications for surgery in trauma to the spinal cord are (1) progression from paresis to paralysis, (2) worsening paresis, (3) vertebral fracture that cannot be stabilized by a cast, as might occur in a fracture at L_6, (4) paralysis caudal to the lesion and the presence of deep pain sensation, and (5) paralysis without deep pain sensation if the owner requires confirmation that the spinal cord is irreparably damaged. Surgery should not be delayed more than a few hours. The surgical procedure should include decompression of the spinal cord by laminectomy or hemilaminectomy, decompression of the spinal cord by durotomy, and internal fixation of the vertebral fracture/luxation.

Ancillary treatment is important. Stabilization of the vertebrae by splint or cast for at least three weeks or internal fixation and accessory external splintage for at least seven days is mandatory (Fig. 2). The external fixation device should be kept dry and scrupulously clean. The edges should be well padded and powdered to prevent irritation to the skin. Splints further reduce the ability of the animal to right itself. They also inhibit evaluation of emptying and expression of the urinary bladder. Until

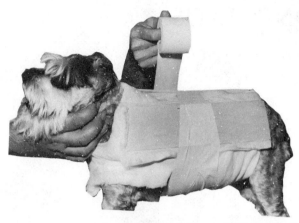

Figure 2. A vertebral splint using basswood. (Reproduced with permission from Knecht et al.: *Fundamental Techniques in Veterinary Surgery*, 2nd ed. Philadelphia: W. B. Saunders, 1981.)

the animal can right itself, it should be propped in a sternal position with towels or rolled from side to side frequently. A whole body sling, appropriately adjusted to the size of the animal, is used for four to six hours daily and all limbs moved through a full range of motion 10 to 20 times at least three times daily. If the urinary bladder cannot be manually expressed and the dog is not micturating when placed in a vertical position, the bladder must be emptied at least three times daily with a urinary catheter or by paracentesis. If the animal is recumbent, an indwelling urinary catheter is placed and attached to a closed collection system. Prophylactic broad spectrum antibiotics should be administered until the animal is continent. Naturally, adequate fluid and nutritional intake is assured.

The complications of medical therapy are related to inadequate immobilization and corticosteroid therapy. Inadequate immobilization results in a worsening of clinical signs. Evaluation of the neurologic status should be recorded every hour for the first six hours, every three or four hours for the next 24 hours, and twice daily thereafter. A worsening neurologic status is an indication for surgical intervention. Gastric hemorrhage and ulceration may result from adrenocorticosteroid therapy and the stress of trauma or surgery. The complication is less likely to occur if steroid therapy is not continued for more than 24 hours.

Other complications are associated with splintage and can be prevented by adequate splint care. Prevention of urinary tract complications has been discussed. Decubital ulcers are prevented by scrupulous cleanliness, clean and well-padded bedding, and frequent repositioning.

Convalescence from spinal trauma may be slow. Some voluntary limb flexion should occur within one week and urinary control and attempts at ambulation within one to three weeks. The sling is useful to encourage supporting motions. As soon as the animal attempts support, it should be assisted with straps or towels under the abdomen and encouraged to exercise on grass or other nontraumatizing surfaces. If not walking when the splint is removed in three weeks, the animal is given whirlpool baths or is placed in shoulder-high warm water baths for 15 to 20 minutes twice daily. Animals are generally discharged to home care as soon as they are continent and making partial walking movements.

Medical therapy in the form of corticosteroids, proper immobilization of the vertebrae, and dedicated physical therapy and care of urinary tract function is indicated for paretic dogs and those requiring surgery because of more severe lesions. Future studies will hopefully reveal more specific therapy, but as of this writing surgical decompression is the most definitive treatment.

SUPPLEMENTAL READING

Griffiths, I. R.: Spinal cord blood flow in dogs. J. Neurol. Neurosurg. Psych. 36:34, 1973.

Hoerlein, B. F.: Personal communication, 1981.

Mendenhall, H. V., Litwak, P., and Yturraspe, D. J.: Aggressive pharmacologic and surgical treatment of spinal cord injuries in dogs and cats. J.A.V.M.A. 168:1026, 1976.

Osterholm, J. L.: The pathophysiological response to spinal cord injury. J. Neurosurg. 40:5, 1974.

Osterholm, J. L., and Mathews, G. J.: Altered norepinephrine metabolism following experimental spinal cord injury. J. Neurosurg. 36:395, 1972.

DISKOSPONDYLITIS

JOE N. KORNEGAY, D.V.M.

Raleigh, North Carolina

Diskospondylitis is intervertebral disk infection concurrent with vertebral osteomyelitis of contiguous vertebrae. First reported in humans as early as 1887 and in dogs in the 1960s, diskospondylitis has been diagnosed in 56 dogs evaluated at the University of Georgia Veterinary Medical Teaching Hospital (GVMTH) since 1976. The clinical features and treatment of these 56 dogs are the basis of this article.

CASE SIGNALMENT AND CLINICAL FEATURES

Diskospondylitis primarily affects large dogs (Fig. 1), and males outnumber females by approximately 2 to 1. Affected dogs evaluated at the GVMTH usually are middle aged (Fig. 2). German shepherds and Great Danes appear to be affected disproportionately.

Clinical signs include hyperesthesia, paresis/paralysis, stilted gait, depression, weight loss, and pyrexia (Table 1). Both neurologic dysfunction and evidence of systemic disease are usually seen, but each can occur separately.

The mid thoracic spine, C_{6-7}, and L_7-S_1 are the most common sites involved (Fig. 3). Multiple disk space involvement occasionally is seen and usually occurs at adjacent disk spaces, suggesting local spread of infection. The thoracic spine is predisposed to multiple adjacent disk space involvement.

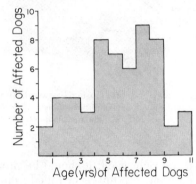

Figure 2. Age (yrs) of dogs with diskospondylitis evaluated at the GVMTH.

ETIOLOGY AND PATHOGENESIS

Causes of diskospondylitis in dogs include foreign body migration and fungal and bacterial infection. *Staphylococcus aureus* is the most common organism associated with diskospondylitis in dogs. It is frequently isolated by culture of either blood, urine, or bone. *Brucella canis* and *Streptococcus* sp. are occasionally cultured from affected dogs. Other bacteria are viewed as contaminants unless isolated on multiple cultures of blood or bone.

In humans, diskospondylitis generally occurs secondary to hematogenous dissemination of bacteria from infections elsewhere in the body. Humans commonly have concurrent urinary tract infections that may serve as the primary site of infection. Concurrent bacteremia and urinary tract infection also are seen occasionally in dogs with diskospondylitis. However, a direct cause-and-effect relationship has not been established in most of these cases.

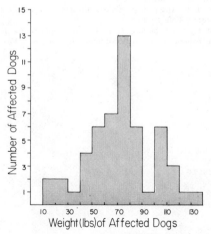

Figure 1. Weight (lbs) of dogs with diskospondylitis evaluated at the GVMTH.

Table 1. *Clinical Signs Seen in Dogs with Diskospondylitis**

Clinical Sign	Number of Affected Dogs
Hyperesthesia	42
Paresis/paralysis	26
Pyrexia	18
Stilted gait	16
Depression	15
Weight loss	14
Anorexia	10
Lameness	7
Abdominal pain	4

*Evaluated at GVMTH.

718

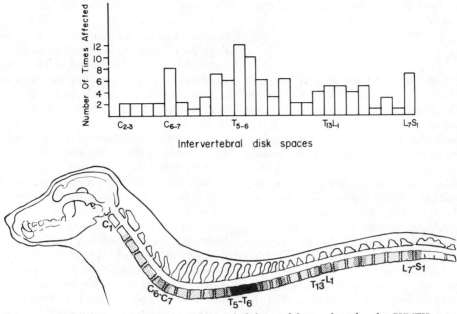

Figure 3. Distribution of lesions in dogs with diskospondylitis evaluated at the GVMTH.

Other potential primary sites of infection identified in affected dogs include bacterial endocarditis, dermal abscessation, and orchitis due to *B. canis*.

Diskospondylitis can occur secondary to disk surgery in humans and has been diagnosed in three dogs subsequent to disk fenestration at the GVMTH. Although one of these dogs was a dachshund, the rarity of diskospondylitis in this breed suggests that neither disk disease nor disk surgery significantly predisposes dogs to its occurrence.

Although trauma has been reported as a possible predisposing factor in dogs with diskospondylitis, a history of trauma is rarely present in affected dogs evaluated at the GVMTH. However, the prevalence of diskospondylitis in large male dogs suggests that stresses placed on the spine due to increased size and activity may play a role.

DIAGNOSIS

RADIOLOGY

Diagnosis of diskospondylitis is made principally by evaluation of radiographs in which varying degrees of vertebral lysis, sclerosis, and spondylosis are seen (Fig. 4). Radiographic changes may not occur until four to six weeks after the onset of infection; thus, dogs may have clinical signs of diskospondylitis and may be radiographically normal. Serologic evaluation for *B. canis* and cultures of blood and urine indirectly identify the causative organism in such cases, allowing for initiation of antibiotic therapy before radiographic confirmation is possible.

Diskospondylitis should not be confused with spondylosis deformans, a common, usually benign, vertebral lesion often present in older large dogs. Although spondylosis and sclerosis are features of both spondylosis deformans and diskospondylitis, vertebral lysis is seen only in diskospondylitis. Vertebral tumors also cause bone lysis but do not affect adjacent vertebrae.

CLINICOPATHOLOGY

Consistent blood chemistry abnormalities are not present in dogs with diskospondylitis. Leukocytosis is present infrequently. Pyuria, bacteriuria, or both

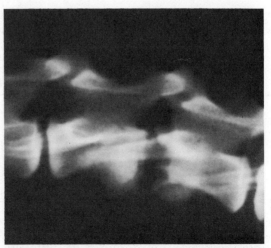

Figure 4. Radiographic demonstration of diskospondylitis. Note the vertebral lysis, sclerosis, and spondylosis.

are present in about 50 per cent of cases. Cerebrospinal fluid analysis is usually normal.

MICROBIOLOGY

Bacterial cultures of blood are positive in about 75 per cent of dogs with diskospondylitis evaluated at the GVMTH. *Staphylococcus aureus* is the most common organism identified. *B. canis* and *Streptococcus* sp. are isolated occasionally. Other bacteria are considered to be contaminants unless isolated on multiple cultures.

Cultures of bone are done if treatment includes vertebral curettage. When cultures of bone are obtained at the GVMTH, bacteria usually are cultured with antibiotic sensitivities similar, if not identical, to those from blood. For this reason, bacteria identified on blood cultures are regarded as the causative organisms.

Urine cultures are positive in only about 25 per cent of dogs with diskospondylitis evaluated at the GVMTH. Urinary organisms other than *S. aureus* are not considered the cause of the vertebral lesion unless also cultured from either blood or bone.

The tube agglutination test for *B. canis* is positive in about 10 per cent of dogs with diskospondylitis evaluated at the GVMTH. Titers from 1:250 to 1:500 are indicative of bacteremia; titers between 1:50 and 1:100 suggest exposure with possible bacteremia; a titer of 1:25 may occur owing to cross agglutination with another organism.

Brucella canis usually is isolated from cultures of blood in seropositive dogs. Cultures of bone have been obtained from only three affected dogs at the GVMTH, and results were positive in one dog. Three other cases have been reported in which *B. canis* was isolated from bone of dogs with diskospondylitis.

TREATMENT

Various regimens have been used to treat dogs with diskospondylitis. A combination of spinal cord decompression, spinal column immobilization, and systemic antibiotic therapy resulted in clinical resolution of diskospondylitis in 28 of 30 dogs. Other dogs have been managed successfully with curettage, drainage, and irrigation of the vertebral lesion. Antibiotic therapy alone has also been used.

Criteria utilized in selecting a therapeutic regimen at the GVMTH include (1) degree of neurologic dysfunction, (2) results of *B. canis* titer and blood cultures, (3) multiplicity of lesions, and (4) surgical accessibility of the lesion site.

Dogs with little or no neurologic dysfunction are treated with antibiotics alone. The antibiotic selection is based on serology results or blood cultures. If cultures and serology are negative, the causative organism is assumed to be *S. aureus* and the antibiotic is chosen accordingly (Table 2). Dogs that fail to improve clinically within five days of the onset of antibiotic therapy are reassessed. Those with solitary, readily accessible lesions are operated on, at which time the lesion is curetted and cultured. Dogs with multiple widely spaced lesions or lesions that are not readily accessible are treated with a different antibiotic.

Dogs with moderate to marked neurologic dysfunction usually have spinal cord compression due to either fibrosis or exostosis. A myelograph is done to determine the extent and location of the compression. Surgery is performed to remove the offending bone or fibrous tissue. Either a hemilaminectomy or dorsal laminectomy can be used. A dorsal laminectomy provides better exposure but also entails removal of the dorsal spinous processes, which are needed if spinal stabilization is required. Hemilaminectomies are usually done at the GVMTH in affected dogs requiring decompressive surgery. Stability is assessed at surgery, and vertebral immobilization is accomplished using plates on the dorsal spinous processes if needed. The lesion is curetted, and necrotic bone and disk material are removed. Antibiotic therapy is instituted on the basis of cultures of affected bone and is continued for at least four to six weeks after surgery.

Table 2.   *Results of Antibiotic Sensitivities of Bacteria Isolated from Blood or Bone from Dogs with Diskospondylitis**

| | | Antibiotic and *In Vitro* Sensitivity (percentage) | | | | | | | | | | | | |
Bacterium	No. of Isolates	Ampicillin	Cephalothin	Chloramphenicol	Cloxacillin	Erythromycin	Gentamicin	Lincomycin	Penicillin	Streptomycin	Sulfadimethoxine	Tetracycline	Trimethoprim	Triple sulfa
S. aureus	30	27	97	83	93	77	83	46	20	60	11	57	65	10
B. canis	5	100	60	100	20	100	100	20	100	100	0	100	40	0
β-hemolytic streptococcus	2	100	100	100	100	100	0	100	100	0	0	100	100	0

*Evaluated at GVMTH.

Table 3. *Antibiotics and Dosages Recommended for Treatment of Diskospondylitis in Dogs*

Bacterium	Antibiotic and Dosage
S. aureus*	Cephradine† 20 mg/kg t.i.d. PO for 4 to 6 weeks Cloxacillin 10 mg/kg q.i.d. PO for 4 to 6 weeks
B. canis	Tetracycline hydrochloride‡ 20 mg/kg t.i.d. PO for 3 weeks Streptomycin 20 mg/kg b.i.d. IM for 5 days at onset of tetracycline regimen Skip 3 weeks and repeat this regimen
β-hemolytic streptococcus*	Ampicillin 20 mg/kg t.i.d. PO for 4 to 6 weeks Penicillin 40 mg/kg q.i.d. PO for 4 to 6 weeks

*Dogs with acutely progressive clinical signs should be treated parenterally for five days and then orally for at least four to six weeks.

†A number of cephalosporins are available. Cephradine (Velosef) is used because of its availability and low cost. Cephalexin (Keflex) also has been used.

‡Minocycline hydrochloride also has been used and may be more efficacious. However, it also is more expensive.

Parenteral antibiotic therapy generally is recommended when treating vertebral osteomyelitis in humans. Dogs with acutely progressive clinical signs due to diskospondylitis also are treated parenterally while hospitalized at the GVMTH. However, after five days parenteral antibiotic therapy is generally replaced by oral antibiotic therapy. This is continued for at least four to six weeks. The importance of administration at the prescribed full dosage must be emphasized to the owner.

Table 2 lists results of antibiotic sensitivities of bacteria isolated from either blood or bone from dogs with diskospondylitis evaluated at the GVMTH. Table 3 lists antibiotics and the dosages used to treat affected dogs. The preferred antibiotic is listed first. Bacteriocidal antibiotics such as the cephalosporins and semisynthetic penicillinase-resistant penicillins are preferred in treating S. aureus infections. Less expensive antibiotics such as chloramphenicol and trimethoprim do not appear to be as effective. Penicillin and ampicillin usually are clinically ineffective. A staged-treatment regimen using tetracycline and streptomycin is used to treat diskospondylitis due to B. canis at the GVMTH (see Table 3). Intact dogs with brucellosis also are neutered. Streptococcus sp. infection is treated with a bacteriocidal antibiotic selected on the basis of blood or bone culture and sensitivity tests. Ampicillin and penicillin usually are effective.

Affected dogs are evaluated clinically and radiographically at two-week intervals during treatment. Dogs with evidence of clinical or radiographic deterioration are either operated on or placed on a different antibiotic regimen. Blood cultures are repeated at this time and in all dogs two weeks after cessation of antibiotic therapy.

PROGNOSIS

Dogs with little or no neurologic dysfunction usually respond to antibiotic therapy alone or to antibiotics used in combination with vertebral curettage. Occasionally, however, dogs deteriorate despite treatment, so owners should be informed of this possibility. The prognosis for dogs with marked neurologic dysfunction is guarded.

Recurrence rarely is a problem in dogs with S. aureus infection but is common in dogs with B. canis infection. Owners should be advised that it is difficult to eliminate B. canis from the infected animal and cautioned as to the potential need for repeated treatment. However, all dogs with diskospondylitis due to B. canis evaluated at the GVMTH have either been cured or kept relatively free of clinical signs with periodic treatment.

Diskospondylitis due to B. canis does not progress as rapidly as that due to S. aureus and rarely necessitates spinal cord decompression or spinal immobilization. In contrast, lesions resulting from S. aureus often progress rapidly and are likely to require extensive therapy.

PUBLIC HEALTH SIGNIFICANCE

Human infections with B. canis are rare but do occur. They are usually mild and respond to tetracycline therapy. Owners should be advised of this rare potential public health risk.

SUPPLEMENTAL READING

Kornegay, J. N.: Canine diskospondylitis. Comp. Cont. Ed. Pract. Vet. 1:930, 1979.
Kornegay, J. N., and Barber, D. L.: Diskospondylitis in dogs. J.A.V.M.A. 177:337, 1980.

MICTURITION DISORDERS IN CATS WITH SACROCAUDAL VERTEBRAL LESIONS

N. SYDNEY MOISE, D.V.M.,

and JAMES A. FLANDERS, D.V.M.,
Ithaca, New York

Cats sustaining damage to the sacrum and caudal vertebrae often have nerve damage that results in disorders of micturition. Radiography may reveal a fracture or dislocation between the second and third sacral vertebrae, the third sacral and first caudal vertebrae, or the first few caudal vertebrae. The location of the skeletal lesion does not correspond to the degree or type of neurologic damage. The nerve damage may vary from stretching to transection of the nerves. The prognosis for recovery of nerve function depends on the extent of damage.

The nerve roots that are present in the sacrocaudal spinal canal give rise to the pelvic, pudendal, and caudal nerves. In the cat, the spinal cord segments containing the cell bodies of the sacral nerves (pelvic and pudendal) are located at the L_5–L_6 interspace or at the level of L_6. The caudal segments containing the cell bodies of the caudal nerves are located in the conus medullaris over L_6 and L_7. Although the spinal cord terminates cranial to the sacrum in the cat, sacrocaudal skeletal damage may be associated with sacral segment damage as well as with damage to the cauda equina.

PELVIC, PUDENDAL, AND CAUDAL NERVE FUNCTION

The pelvic nerve is a part of the parasympathetic nervous system. It is most commonly composed of branches from the second and third sacral nerves, but in many cats the first sacral nerve also contributes parasympathetic fibers. The pelvic nerve provides innervation to the caudal colon and rectum, the detrusor muscle of the bladder, and the smooth muscles of the genitalia.

The pudendal nerve is composed of branches from spinal nerves S_1, S_2, and S_3. It is a somatic motor nerve supplying the striated anal and external urethral sphincters and muscles of the genitalia. It also provides somatic sensation to the perineal area and external genitalia via its peripheral branches (perineal nerve, dorsal nerve of penis, nerve of clitoris).

The caudal nerves provide sensory and motor innervation to the tail.

If an injury destroys the pelvic, pudendal, and caudal nerves, the cat will have a flaccid, noncontracting bladder; atonic anal and urethral sphincters; a flaccid, analgesic tail; and an analgesic anus and perineum.

If the sacral segments or all of the nerve roots of the pelvic nerve are damaged secondary to sacrocaudal trauma, serious deficiencies in defecation and urination develop. The pelvic nerve increases the resting tone of the colon and rectum and aids in fecal propulsion during defecation. Cats with pelvic nerve damage cannot effectively defecate, and large amounts of feces accumulate in the colon if not managed properly.

Perhaps the most serious complication produced by pelvic nerve damage is the loss of the ability to contract the detrusor muscle of the bladder. In addition to the motor paralysis, cats with pelvic nerve destruction lose sensation to the bladder and cannot reflexly contract the bladder even when excessive urine volumes accumulate. The bladder lacks tone, and urine leaks from the urethra when the volume becomes excessive. The great bladder distention does not cause discomfort to the cat, since the information from the bladder stretch receptors can no longer reach the brain.

Complete damage to the pudendal nerve results in a flaccid anal sphincter and a defective external urethral sphincter. Voluntary control of defecation is lost, and affected cats are unaware of any involuntary fecal loss. The sensation of the anal sphincter, perineal skin, and genitalia is lost. Although loss of external urethral sphincter innervation occurs with a pudendal nerve lesion, if normal internal urethral sphincter and bladder neck muscle layer arrangement is present, urinary continence is maintained. In the normal cat, urine is retained in the bladder at the level of the internal urethral sphincter. The sympathetic nervous system plays a role in the tone of this sphincter (see CVT VII, pages 1122–1127). Also, the detrusor muscles are arranged in a specific manner at the bladder neck, which provides for an anatomic closing of the vesicourethral junction when the bladder is distended.

The external urethral sphincter is located caudal to the internal urethral sphincter, just distal to the prostate in the male cat and at mid urethra in the female. The striated sphincter allows for voluntary control. If the bladder is greatly distended with urine, sufficient intravesicular pressure can be generated during contraction to overcome the internal urethral sphincter. Voluntary control of the external sphincter may interrupt the urine stream by contracting or may allow it to pass by relaxing. Additionally, if urine does leak into the urethra in the absence of detrusor contraction, the external urethral sphincter provides for reflex contraction to prevent urine passage. Therefore, urine is retained in the bladder primarily before reaching the external urethral sphincter, and loss of pudendal nerve function alone causes loss of voluntary urethral control but usually does not cause urinary incontinence.

Damage to the caudal nerves secondary to sacrocaudal trauma results in a flaccid, analgesic tail. Occasionally in chronic cases, sufficient muscle atrophy and fibrosis occur to cause partial elevation of the tail base.

PHYSICAL EXAMINATION

In addition to a thorough physical examination, a complete neurologic examination should be done on cats sustaining sacrocaudal trauma. Specific attention should be paid to pain sensation, muscle tone, and reflexes in the perineal area. These cats resist the manipulation involved in a neurologic examination because of pain. Patience and careful observation are therefore necessary for accurate interpretation of neurologic findings.

The most obvious physical abnormality associated with sacrocaudal trauma is a flaccid, analgesic tail. Damage to the caudal nerves as they pass through the sacral spinal canal deprives the tail of normal tonus and voluntary movement. Sensation is tested by pinching the skin of the tail with mosquito forceps. Usually the entire length of the tail is analgesic; however, some cats may have sensation near the tailhead. Accurate delineation of the area of analgesia is important in determining the amount of nerve damage. It also provides a basis upon

which reinnervation can be assessed. In addition to the nerve damage, circulation of the tail may be interrupted in some cats, resulting in vascular necrosis of the tail.

The tone of the anal sphincter is evaluated by direct observation and by spreading the anus open with mosquito forceps. A normal cat will resist insertion of lubricated forceps in the anus and will contract the anal sphincter tightly in response. Damage to the pudendal nerve causes a loss of anal tone, which may vary from a dilated anus to an anus that appears closed but does not reflexly contract.

The status of the pelvic nerve is evaluated by observing the cat urinate and checking the amount of residual urine. A normal cat should have less than 2 ml of residual urine after micturition. If there is doubt about pelvic nerve function, a cystometrogram (CMG) can be made. A CMG is a record of intracystic pressure changes that occur as the bladder volume is increased. A reflex detrusor contraction that occurs when the threshold urine volume is reached indicates intact pelvic nerve reflex.

CLASSIFICATIONS OF MICTURITION DISORDERS

Based on neurologic examination, cats with sacrocaudal lesions are divided into four groups. Although individual variations exist, common features are present within each group (Table 1).

GROUP 1

Group 1 cats have flaccid, analgesic tails. Anal tone, perineal reflex, bulbourethral reflex, and perineal pain sensation are normal. Micturition and defecation are normal. These cats do not have damage to the nerves of micturition, although the caudal nerves are injured. The prognosis for a normal life in these cats is excellent.

GROUP 2

Group 2 cats have flaccid, analgesic tails. Anal tone, perineal reflex, bulbourethral reflex, and perineal pain sensation are normal. Although these cats posture and strain to urinate, they are unable to void urine. Attempts to manually express urine from the bladder are not successful. Steady pressure

Table 1. *Classifications of Micturition Disorders in Cats with Sacrocaudal Vertebral Lesions*

Group	Detrusor Reflex	Perineal Pain Sensation	Perineal/Bulbo- urethral Reflexes	Urethral Tone
1	Present	Present	Present	Normal
2	Absent	Present	Present	Increased
3	Absent	Absent	Absent	Increased
4	Absent	Absent	Absent	Decreased

applied to the bladder cannot overcome the urethral resistance. After one to two weeks these cats begin to urinate and then continue to make a complete recovery.

In Group 2 cats normal anal tone, perineal pain perception, and segmental spinal reflexes indicate functional pudendal nerves. The cats posture to urinate, and this observation also supports normal pudendal nerve innervation. The lack of urination seen in these cats is due to an inadequate detrusor contraction coupled with inadequate urethral relaxation. This disorder of micturition is termed detrusor-sphincter dyssynergia. Because the detrusor muscle does not adequately contract, the muscle layers in the bladder neck do not funnel to form an orifice for urine passage. Also, the poor bladder contraction does not increase the intravesicular pressure enough to overcome urethral resistance. Impaired pelvic nerve function accounts for the poor detrusor reflex. The increased urethral resistance is also due to impaired pelvic nerve function. Afferent pelvic nerve impulses stimulate external urethral sphincter relaxation via inhibitory interneurons. These interneurons, once stimulated, synapse on the cell bodies of the pudendal nerves, causing pudendal nerve inhibition and external urethral sphincter relaxation. If this normal inhibitory process is interrupted, external urethral sphincter spasticity results. Part of the efferent pudendal nerve must be intact for this skeletal muscle spasticity to occur. Another reason for the increased urethral resistance is excess internal urethral sphincter tone. The smooth muscle of the internal urethral sphincter has alpha-adrenergic receptors that, during the voiding stage of micturition, are inhibited and thereby cause the internal urethral sphincter to relax. It is believed that the efferent pelvic nerve plays a role in the inhibition of these receptors. Therefore, poor pelvic nerve function may allow excess sympathetic tone of the alpha-adrenergic receptors.

Group 2 cats usually return to normal micturition function within one to two weeks after injury, indicating a stretching or contusion of the pelvic nerve or its branches.

GROUP 3

Group 3 cats have flaccid, analgesic tails. Anal tone is depressed, but the anus is not widely dilated and open. Pain perception around the anus and perineal area is absent. Perineal and bulbourethral reflexes are depressed or absent. In most of the male cats spastic twitching of the penis occurs when pressure is applied to the bladder. Manual expression of urine from the bladder is not possible. For one to four weeks after injury the cats do not seem aware of a distended bladder. The cats do not attempt to urinate. After this time the cats begin to

posture and strain to urinate, but urine is not voided. Four to eight weeks after injury most cats are able to void small amounts of urine and manual expression is easier. Anal tone improves in a few cats, but sensation usually does not return. Most of these cats have residual urine volumes of 20 to 50 ml after urinating.

Group 3 cats have damage to the pelvic, caudal, and pudendal nerves. The pudendal nerve is more severely damaged in group 3 cats than in group 2 cats, but the innervation of the striated sphincter remains intact and produces excessive urethral resistance. Post-mortem examination of these cats reveals partial destruction of the sacral segments or cauda equina. Some nerve branches from the sacral segments are left intact. The explanation for the detrusor-sphincter dyssynergia described for group 2 cats is applicable for group 3 cats.

Prognosis for complete recovery of group 3 cats is poor. A few cats will make a complete recovery, most will recover to a satisfactory state with minimal residual urine volumes after urination, and others will improve minimally with large residual urine volumes after urination.

GROUP 4

Group 4 cats have flaccid, analgesic tails. Anal tone is poor and the anus is usually dilated. Pain perception of the anus and perineal area is absent. Perineal and bulbourethral reflexes are usually absent. Urinary incontinence is present, and the cats' bladders are easily expressed with abdominal pressure. Urethral tone is depressed. Most of the cats do not posture to urinate. Only an occasional cat in this group will recover after four to six weeks.

Group 4 cats have complete interruption of the pelvic, pudendal, and caudal nerves. The cats' bladders are easy to express because complete pudendal nerve damage produces an atonic, striated external sphincter. The detrusor contractions are ineffectual because pelvic nerve function is lost. Urine loss is mainly due to overflow incontinence, although such an autonomous bladder does have weak intrinsic contractions, which produce voiding of small amounts of urine. Post-mortem examination of group 4 cats reveals either complete destruction of the sacral segments or complete severance of the cauda equina. If a group 4 cat recovers, complete yet temporary interruption of sacral nerve function has occurred.

Prognosis for group 4 cats is poor. Most cats never regain bladder function.

THERAPY

The most important aspect of treatment for cats with sacrocaudal vertebral lesions is supportive care. In cats with neurologic dysfunction of the bladder and urethra it is important to keep the bladder empty. If urine retention is excessive, infection and stretching of the tight junctions can occur. Overdistention and infection for prolonged periods can cause irreversible fibrosis of the bladder wall. In group 2 and 3 cats it is necessary to catheterize the bladder. Intermittent catheterizations are preferred to a permanent indwelling catheter, which necessitates hospitalization of the cats for prolonged periods of time. Owners may be encouraged to treat group 2 cats at home because hospitalization will usually be from 7 to 14 days. Group 3 cats require prolonged hospitalization of 30 to 60 days, which few clients will be able to afford. Cats in group 4 usually do not need catheterization, because the bladder is easily expressed. This should be done three times daily, and owners can learn to manage these cats at home.

Of the cats requiring catheterization, most adapt well to the procedure. Catheterization is done twice daily employing sterile technique. The 3.5 French soft polyvinyl feline urinary catheters* are preferred. After catheterization, the urine is aspirated from the bladder with a 60-ml syringe attached to the catheter. The urine sediment should be examined weekly for evidence of cystitis. Ideally, antibiotics should only be used when bacterial infection is documented; however, we do recommend therapy with amoxicillin (Amoxi-Tabs†), 15 to 25 mg/kg twice daily until normal urinary tract function returns. If bacteriuria is present, antibiotic therapy should be based on antibiotic sensitivity testing or, better yet, minimum inhibitory concentration of antibiotics to the specific bacterial organism.

Certain drugs have been advocated for treating disorders of micturition. Treatment of detrusor-sphincter dyssynergia includes the combined use of parasympathomimetic drugs to enhance detrusor contraction and alpha-adrenergic blockers or skeletal muscle relaxants to decrease the urethral tone. The most common drug used for parasympathetic stimulation is bethanechol (Urecholine‡), 2.5 to 5.0 mg orally two to three times daily. This drug can enhance a detrusor contraction, but it cannot initiate a contraction. Bethanechol is often effective in group 2 cats but not in group 3 and 4 cats. At higher dosages, bethanechol may cause diarrhea, vomiting, salivation, and anorexia.

Phenoxybenzamine (Dibenzyline§) is an alpha-adrenergic blocker and is used at a starting dose of 0.25 mg/kg orally three times daily. The dose is gradually increased to 0.5 mg/kg orally three times daily. This drug is used to decrease the internal urethral sphincter tone. Hypotension can be produced with higher dosages of phenoxybenzamine. Aminopropazine (Jenatone||), 2.0 to 3.5 mg/kg orally, is advocated as a smooth muscle relaxant. This drug theoretically acts on the internal urethral sphincter. Unfortunately, the results of therapy with phenoxybenzamine and aminopropazine are disappointing. The skeletal muscle relaxant dantrolene (Dantrium**) has a predilection for spastic skeletal muscles. This drug has been of some value in cats with excessive urethral tone. A starting dose of 0.5 mg/kg orally twice daily is used and then is gradually increased to 2.0 mg/kg orally twice daily. In humans this drug causes elevations of liver enzyme levels. We have not identified any problems to date with dantrolene use in the cat; however, caution should be exercised. Other skeletal muscle relaxants, such as methocarbamol (Robaxin††) and diazepam (Valium‡‡), have been used with minimal success in cats with detrusor-sphincter dyssynergia.

Constipation in cats with sacrocaudal vertebral lesions is usually controlled with a diet of canned cat food, one teaspoon of a laxative (e.g., Metamucil§§), and three tablespoons of bran cereal. If this mixture is moistened with warm water, most cats eat it readily. If the stools are kept light and bulky, the peristaltic waves of the transverse colon can move the feces through the descending colon and out the rectum. Enemas may be needed in some cats.

Taylor (1981) advocates dorsal decompression of the sacrum and amputation of the tail for the treatment of sacrocaudal vertebral injuries in cats. We provide supportive care without surgical intervention. Controlled studies are needed to define the best therapy. Amputation of the tail does ease management and prevent avascular necrosis of the tail and may prevent a pendulum action on an injured cauda equina.

COMPLICATIONS

Complications encountered in cats with micturition disorders caused by sacrocaudal vertebral lesions include cystitis, hydronephrosis, ascending pyelonephritis, perineal scalding, and avascular necrosis of the tail. We have had two cats return three and twenty months after injury with compromised renal function. The renal disease is caused by an ascending infection originating from residual infected urine in the bladder. The residual urine is present because of incomplete bladder contraction and emptying. This major complication is of concern

---

*Sovereign sterile disposable feeding tube and urethral catheter, Sherwood Medical Industries, St. Louis, MO.
†Beecham Laboratories, Bristol, TN.
‡Merck Sharp and Dohme, West Point, PA.
§Smith Kline & French, Philadelphia, PA.

||Jensen-Salsbery Laboratories, Kansas City, MO.
**Norwich-Eaton Pharmaceuticals, Norwich, NY.
††A. H. Robins Co., Richmond, VA.
‡‡Hoffman-La Roche Laboratories, Nutley, NJ.
§§Searle Consumer Products, Chicago, IL.

in treating these cats. Perhaps bladder contraction can be enhanced in these partially recovered cats with bethanechol.

SUPPLEMENTAL READING

Bradley, W. E., and Teague, C. T.: Electrophysiology of pelvic and pudendal nerves in the cat. Exper. Neurol. 35:378, 1972.
Bradley, W. E., and Timm, G. W.: Physiology of micturition. Vet. Clin. North Am. 3:487, 1974.
Hackler R. H., Broecker, B. H., Klein, F. A., and Brady, S. M.: A clinical experience with dantrolene sodium for external urinary sphincter hypertonicity in spinal cord injured patients. J. Urol. 124:78, 1980.
Khanna, O. P.: Disorders of micturition, neuropharmacologic basis and results of drug therapy. Urology VIII:316, 1976.
McGuire, E. J., and Brady, S.: Detrusor-sphincter dyssynergia. J. Neurol. 121:774, 1979.
Moreau, P. M.: Neurogenic disorders of micturition in the dog and cat. Comp. Cont. Ed. 4:12, 1982.
Oliver, J. E., and Young, W. O.: Air cystometry in dogs under xylazine-induced restraint. Am. J. Vet. Res. 34:1433, 1973.
Tanagho, E. A., and Smith, D. R.: The anatomy and function of the bladder neck. Br. J. Urol. 38:54, 1966.
Taylor, R. A.: Treatment of the sacrum and sacrococcygeal region. Vet. Surg. 10:119, 1981.

DISEASES OF THE VESTIBULAR SYSTEM

STEPHEN SIMPSON, D.V.M.
Auburn, Alabama

The vestibular system in mammals is a complex neuronal arrangement deeply involved with other nervous system components. Specially derived receptor mechanisms provide sensory information about gravity and changes in linear and angular motion. Peripheral nerves conduct the sensory information, and several neuronal structures within the central nervous system (CNS) integrate the sensory information.

Disorders of the vestibular system are not uncommon and are frequently confusing to the veterinary practitioner. An elementary understanding of normal anatomic relationships and physiologic functions is necessary to determine the etiology of the vestibular disease and provide an accurate prognosis and proper treatment.

NORMAL ANATOMIC AND PHYSIOLOGIC RELATIONSHIPS

The peripheral structures consist of the inner ear (membranous labyrinth) and the vestibular portion of the eighth cranial nerve. The central components are the four vestibular nuclei, the descending spinal cord tracts, and the ascending brain stem tracts. These components are present bilaterally.

PERIPHERAL COMPONENTS

The membranous labyrinth is a delicate structure buried in a bony labyrinth in the petrosal bone. It is fluid filled (endolymph) and consists of two compartments: the vestibular and cochlear compartments. The membranous labyrinth is surrounded by a fluid (perilymph) that communicates with the cerebrospinal fluid (CSF) through the perilymphatic duct. The perilymphatic space ends blindly at the cochlear window in the middle ear.

The membranous labyrinth of the vestibular compartment consists of five parts: the utricle, saccule, and three semicircular ducts (Fig. 1). Each part contains a region of specialized receptor structures, which are innervated by the sensory endings of the eighth cranial nerve.

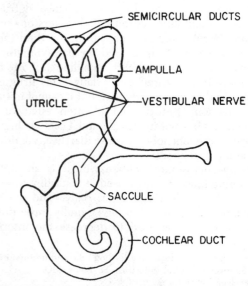

Figure 1. Membranous labyrinth demonstrating the relationship between the vestibular and cochlear components.

The vestibular system is bilaterally symmetric. The utricle and saccule are primarily responsible for detecting the direction of gravity relative to head position. In addition, the utricle is responsible for detection of alteration in linear movement (acceleration or deceleration). The semicircular ducts are oriented approximately 90° from one another so that each set can perceive changes in angular movement about any axis.

Because of the bilateral configuration of the semicircular ducts, when one side is stimulated the other side is inhibited, maintaining a perception of motion. Once the velocity of motion is constant the vestibular organs are no longer stimulated and the perception of motion is absent.

The eighth cranial nerve (vestibulocochlear) enters the brain stem in the ventrolateral portion of the medulla immediately caudal to the emergence site of the trigeminal nerve (CN V). It is intimate with the facial nerve. Peripherally, the vestibulocochlear nerve enters the internal acoustic meatus with the facial nerve. The vestibulocochlear nerve continues into the petrosal bone to the respective sensory organs in the membranous labyrinth. The facial nerve continues and turns laterally and ventrally to proceed through the caudal portion of the middle ear and exits through the facial canal caudal to the external auditory meatus (Getty, 1979).

Additionally, nerves enter the osseous bulla from the caudomedial aspect. These nerves are some of the fibers of the glossopharyngeal nerves (CN IX) that innervate salivary glands and the fibers of the sympathetic nervous system. The sympathetic fibers course with the internal carotid artery blood supply to the head. These fibers provide sympathetic supply to the head and eye (Blauch and Strafuss, 1973).

CENTRAL COMPONENTS

The peripheral vestibular nerves enter the brain stem to supply the vestibular information to the central portion of the system. There are four major vestibular nuclei. They lie in the dorsolateral and lateral walls of the fourth ventricle in the rostral medulla and pons. The individual function of each nucleus provides different efferent components to the system, but they will be considered as one. The peripheral vestibular nerve also projects into the rostral portion of the cerebellum.

The vestibular nuclei have three major efferent projection pathways that are of clinical significance. The vestibulospinal tract arises from the vestibular nuclei and descends the brain stem and spinal cord in the ventral funiculus.

The descending medial longitudinal fasciculus (MLF) descends the brain stem and spinal cord. It is also a bilateral system and descends in the ventral funniculus near the midline. It descends to rostral thoracic levels (de Lahunta, 1977).

The ascending MLF arises from the vestibular nuclei. This is a complex arrangement of neurons that ascend the brain stem mostly near the midline to influence the nuclei of the extraocular muscles.

NORMAL PHYSIOLOGIC FUNCTION

The peripheral end-organs are specially adapted to perceive changes in motion, direction, and gravity and to transduce the information into nerve impulses. The eighth cranial nerve conducts those impulses to the vestibular nuclei and cerebellum. The impulses from one peripheral vestibular system provide the tone to the vestibular nuclei to maintain adequate ipsilateral antigravity muscle tone to prevent falling toward that side. The two systems working together provide complete antigravity maintenance.

The vestibulospinal tracts descend to all four limbs (de Lahunta, 1977). They provide the major extensor facilitation to the trunk and limbs. The descending MLF descends the spinal cord only to rostral thoracic levels. It provides the major antigravity tone to the head and neck and some to the front limbs. The ascending MLF influences the nuclei of extraocular muscles. This system helps to provide conjugate gaze (both eyes looking at the same object), especially when the head or full visual field is in motion. It is this system that is responsible for nystagmus.

ABNORMAL VESTIBULAR FUNCTION

CLINICAL SIGNS

The clinical signs associated with vestibular disease are related to the absence of normal antigravity tone in the two descending spinal cord systems and the presence of abnormal nystagmus findings.

Animals with unilateral vestibular disease will fall toward the side of the lesion. There will be a curvature of the trunk with the concavity on the side of the lesion. These findings are largely due to absence of normal vestibulospinal tone.

Head tilts and leaning toward the side of the lesion are also common findings. The head tilt is the most common sign associated with vestibular disease. It is caused by lack of antigravity tone to the ipsilateral descending MLF. The support muscles of the head lose antigravity strength, thereby causing that side of the head to fall toward the side of the lesion.

Nystagmus is usually associated with vestibular disease. Nystagmus is a rhythmic oscillation of the eyes. It usually has a fast and a slow phase. It is described according to the direction of the fast phase.

Table 1. *Observation of Nystagmus*

Spontaneous nystagmus
    Resting nystagmus
    Positional nystagmus
Induced nystagmus
    Vestibular (physiologic) nystagmus
    Post-rotatory nystagmus

Table 2. *Neurologic Signs of Peripheral or Central Vestibular Disease*

Sign	Central Disease	Peripheral Disease
Head tilt	Present	Present
Falling, rolling	Present	Present
Nystagmus		
Horizontal	Present	Present
Rotary	Present	Present
Vertical	Present	Absent
With change in position	Yes	No
Cranial nerve lesions	V, VI, VII	VII
Horner's syndrome	No	Yes
Gait dysfunction	Severe ataxia, ipsilateral hemiparesis	Mild ataxia
Cerebellar signs	Possible	Not possible

The types of nystagmus are described in Table 1. Resting nystagmus is the observation of nystagmus when the animal is allowed to hold its head in the normal position. Positional nystagmus is nystagmus produced when the animal's head is placed in an unusual position, e.g., upside down or extended. Any form of spontaneous nystagmus is abnormal.

Induced nystagmus means that some mechanism is employed to determine whether nystagmus can be induced. The failure to observe symmetric induced nystagmus is abnormal. Vestibular nystagmus occurs when the animal's head is gently turned from side to side (or up and down). The nystagmus induced should be in the same direction as the head movement. This form of testing has been called tonic eye reflexes and the oculocephalic reflex elsewhere. The author prefers the term *vestibular nystagmus*.

Post-rotatory nystagmus occurs after fast rotation of the patient. During rotation the unobserved patient will develop nystagmus in the direction of the movement. After an abrupt halt of the rotation, the patient is observed. The nystagmus induced is described by direction, velocity, and number of movements. The nystagmus should be in the direction opposite that of the rotation. When the nystagmus has stopped, the same procedure should be performed in the other direction. The induced nystagmus should be equal in either direction.

The absence of induced nystagmus suggests an abnormality in the vestibular system or ascending MLF. Asymmetric induced nystagmus suggests an abnormal vestibular system with normal ascending MLF.

Central vestibular signs are often worse for longer periods of time. Spontaneous nystagmus may be in any direction: horizontal, rotary, or vertical. In addition, nystagmus of central origin may exhibit changes in direction from time to time or with changes in head position. With lesions of central vestibular structures there is usually involvement of other central structures. Other cranial nerves commonly affected are the trigeminal (CN V), abducent (CN VI), and facial (CN VII). In addition, other ipsilateral upper motor neuron pathways are affected, causing an ipsilateral hemiparesis or lateralizing tetraparesis (Table 2).

Occasionally, a patient is observed to exhibit vestibular signs (head tilt, nystagmus) suggestive of a lesion on one side but with gait and postural reaction abnormalities suggestive of a lesion on the other side. These signs are termed the paradoxical vestibular syndrome (de Lahunta, 1977). They are suggestive of a lesion in the cerebellar peduncles on the side opposite the head tilt and, hence, are paradoxical.

Peripheral vestibular signs may be quite similar. Vertical nystagmus does not occur with peripheral lesions. Changes in nystagmus direction are usually not seen with peripheral vestibular disease. Motor disabilities may be difficult to evaluate because of the severe disorientation. If motor capabilities indicate that postural reactions are intact and that a paresis does not exist, motor signs are related to vestibular incoordination and vertigo (see Table 2).

Paravestibular syndromes exist with both central and peripheral lesions. A central lesion, as stated previously, can produce lesions in other cranial nerves. Middle ear lesions can produce profound vestibular signs by producing pressure or inflammation of the inner ear. In addition, involvement of the facial (CN VII) nerve and sympathetic supply to the eye (Horner's syndrome) is commonly seen as these nerves course through the middle ear. Not as easily detectable is paralysis of the parasympathetic supply to the sublingual and maxillary salivary glands and the lacrimal gland.

Bilateral vestibular signs are somewhat different and warrant separate description. In acute disease there is a rather dramatic tendency to maintain the head and neck in a flexed position (the animal apparently is unable to raise the head adequately to look upward). Nystagmus may or may not be present. If present, it suggests an asymmetric lesion. In a more chronic or congenital bilateral lesion, patients will exhibit a mildly ataxic gait that may be described as loose and clumsy. The head will make wider than expected excursions when the animal moves it from side to side. Also, the patient's trunk will usually sway in the direction of head movement.

DISORDERS OF THE VESTIBULAR SYSTEM

CONGENITAL DISORDERS

Congenital vestibular disease should be suspected in any purebred animal that exhibits vestibular signs at an early age. The clinical signs usually are observable by three months of age and often by the time the animal begins to ambulate.

Vestibular signs of head tilt and mild ataxia with an acute onset have been reported in related German shepherds and Siamese cats (de Lahunta, 1977). The disease first appears at three to four weeks of age, and slow improvement is noted until recovery or compensation by four months of age.

Burmese cats have been reported to have vestibular signs soon after birth (de Lahunta, 1977). Signs exhibited include rolling, often continuous, and a head tilt.

Other animals have been seen with vestibular lesions of a congenital nature. This author has observed part of a litter of Doberman pinschers affected with symmetrically bilateral vestibular signs. The onset was apparently insidious, and the age of onset was unknown. Another group of Doberman pinschers was reported with acute vestibular signs at 12 weeks of age (Chrisman, 1980). Signs consisted of a head tilt and mild ataxia. Occasionally cerebellar dysfunction was also noted.

The author has observed two young Shetland sheepdogs with vestibular signs. The first dog was observed at three months of age, whose vestibular signs had been progressive for several weeks. The disorder was apparently bilateral, and other CNS abnormalities were noted. This dog had congenital CNS deficits including hydrocephalus with severe dilation of the fourth ventricle. The second Shetland sheepdog was presented at three days of age. It continually rolled in one direction and was unable to right itself to suckle. Post-mortem examination revealed hydrocephalus and agenesis of the corpus callosum. No direct cause of vestibular signs was found.

A congenital, bilateral, vestibular anomaly has been reported in beagles (de Lahunta, 1977). They exhibited wide excursions of the head and ataxia from the beginning of ambulation. The dogs were also deaf.

A unilateral, congenital, vestibular syndrome was reported in a litter of seven English cocker spaniels (Bedford, 1979). Two puppies had died post partum. The remaining five puppies were noted to be small and unstable. They had a tendency to roll, and suckling was made difficult by their inability to remain sternal. Three puppies developed normal posture by four weeks of age. The other two puppies were affected to different degrees. One was destroyed, and the other slowly improved but was left with a residual head tilt. There was no spontaneous nystagmus nor could vestibular nystagmus be elicited. At 11 months of age there was a persistent head tilt and enophthalmus.

Occasionally an oscillatory nystagmus, equal in both directions, can be observed in young animals. This is most common in Siamese and Siamese cross cats. No other vestibular signs are observed. Lesions have been localized to the visual system (Guillery et al., 1974).

INFLAMMATORY DISEASE

Extension of otitis media to otitis interna is the most common cause of inflammatory vestibular disease (Chrisman, 1980). This is not necessarily the most common cause of all vestibular syndromes. Otitis media occurs most commonly by extension from otitis externa (redundant ear breeds) and extension from the pharynx via the auditory tube.

Cocker spaniels and other breeds with redundant ears commonly have continual otitis externa. Extension of this condition into an otitis media is common, especially if the tympanic membrane erodes or ruptures. A chronic or acute otitis media may then develop. Signs may develop rapidly, and the patient may present with head tilt, nystagmus, and falling. The signs may develop so slowly that the patient may not exhibit obvious signs. Often otitis externa may be diagnosed, topical therapy applied, or the ear canals cleaned, only to have the dog return a few days later exhibiting acute vestibular signs and/or deafness. The clinician should suspect a ruptured tympanic membrane.

Otitis media or externa can produce so much pain that the dog holds its head tilted because of discomfort rather than because of abnormal vestibular function. Physical palpation elicits pain, whereas other signs of vestibular disease (nystagmus, ataxia) may be absent. Otitis media can also cause dysfunction in the facial nerve (CN VII) and in sympathetic fibers in the middle ear. The dog will exhibit a drooped upper lip (CN VII), inability to close the eyelids (CN VII), a lowered ear (CN VII), and miotic pupil, ptosis, and enophthalmos (sympathetic fibers).

Observation of the eardrum is absolutely necessary in cases of otitis media–interna. Frequently anesthesia is required for adequate observation of the tympanic membrane. An unobstructed view of the tympanic membrane should normally allow limited visualization into the tympanic bulla. The eardrum is normally translucent, and the manubrium of the malleus can be observed. In addition to direct observation, the functional integrity of the eardrum should be tested. This is best performed with a diagnostic head otoscope* and a bulb syringe at-

---

*Welch Allyn Diagnostic Otoscope No. 20160, Welch Allyn, Skaneateles Falls, NY.

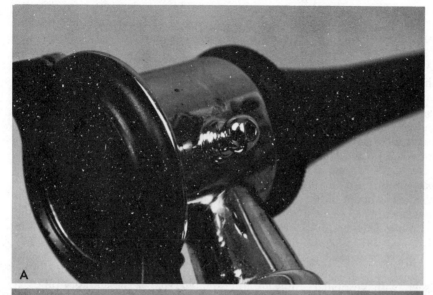

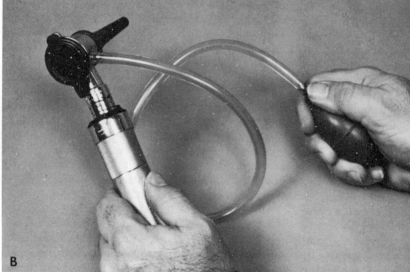

Figure 2. *A*, Otoscope exhibiting the connecting port on the side of the chamber. *B*, Otoscope with the tubing set up to examine the functional integrity of the tympanic membrane.

tached to the vent port on the right side of the otoscope (Fig. 2). By this method positive and negative pressure can be applied to the eardrum and its movement can be observed. Normally the eardrum has two portions, a tense portion ventrally (pars tensa) comprising more than half of the membrane and a flaccid portion dorsally (pars flaccida). The malleus is attached to the tense portion.

Radiography of the bulla may reveal a fluid-filled osseous bulla or a sclerotic bone around the bulla. A fluid-filled bulla is usually observed by direct examination of the ear.

Fluid or caseous material within the middle ear is inflammatory debris from an otitis media. If the eardrum is intact, a myringotomy may be needed to relieve pressure and pain and obtain cytology and culture material. Chronic, recurrent otitis may

require a bulla osteotomy to allow continual drainage.

In the author's experience, corrective surgery (myringotomy or bulla osteotomy) is of little benefit if bulla sclerosis but no otoscopic abnormality is found. The sclerosis suggests previous otitis media but not current disease. Prolonged antibiotic therapy may help, but drainage appears to have little benefit.

If central vestibular disease has resulted from extension of otitis media–interna, a CSF tap should be performed to determine CSF pressure, cytology, and culture.

Primary central vestibular inflammatory disease is usually the result of multifocal or diffuse CNS disease. Canine distemper in the dog and feline infectious peritonitis in the cat are the most common etiologic agents causing central vestibular inflammatory disease. History and physical findings usually suggest these diseases. A more chronic inflammatory disease of dogs may produce profound central vestibular signs. This is also a multifocal process, and other neurologic signs may be detected. The diagnosis at necropsy is a granulomatous encephalomyelitis or reticulosis of the central nervous system.

Membranous labyrinths of people made deaf by viral infections show cochlear, saccular, and macular degeneration (Davis et al., 1975). In addition, hamsters have been found to develop active viral labyrinthitis following experimental inoculations of certain viruses (Davis et al., 1975). Research is needed to elucidate causes of idiopathic acute vestibular diseases, including acute viral infections of the membranous labyrinth.

NUTRITIONAL VESTIBULAR DISEASE

Feline thiamine deficiency is the major disease in this category. It is reported to be a periventricular polioencephalomalacia, causing hemorrhagic necrosis of periventricular brain stem nuclei including the vestibular nucleus (de Lahunta, 1977). The earliest clinical signs of thiamine deficiency include ventroflexion of the head and neck and ataxia. Other signs include dilated and poorly responsive pupils, dementia, seizures, and blindness. Response to intramuscular injections of 1 to 2 mg of thiamine is rapid.

TRAUMATIC VESTIBULAR DISEASE

Severe blunt trauma to the head of a dog or cat is a common cause of acute vestibular disease. With peripheral nerve trauma, the animal will usually present with severe signs of head tilt, nystagmus, rolling, and circling. Serial neurologic evaluation should be performed to detect any change suggestive of intracranial hemorrhage or cerebral edema. Dexamethasone (2 mg/kg IV) may be beneficial in preventing cerebral edema.

CSF collection should not be attempted in acute head trauma, because of the potential of brain herniation.

Signs similar to those seen with severe blunt trauma may be observed with brain stem contusion or hemorrhage. These dogs usually have a more severe curvature to their body, to the point of having their head bent under their tail. Significant improvement within 72 hours is a favorable prognostic sign and suggests more peripheral than central involvement. Postural reactions should not be evaluated until improvement is seen.

TOXIC VESTIBULAR DISEASE

Toxic vestibular abnormalities are rare. The most likely disease is vestibular degeneration due to administration of an aminoglycoside antibiotic. Cats are more susceptible than dogs. Serial evaluations of vestibular and hearing function should be performed when these drugs are used. Damage is usually irreversible, although compensation may occur (Chrisman, 1980).

NEOPLASTIC VESTIBULAR DISEASE

Neoplastic conditions of the peripheral vestibular region are rarely reported, partly because histopathology of the inner ear is difficult to evaluate. Neither primary nor metastatic neoplasms are reported with significant frequency.

Invasion of peripheral vestibular structures by adjacent neoplasms has been reported infrequently (Chrisman, 1980). Primary bone tumors of the skull or mandible could invade vestibular structures. Tonsilar sarcomas or pharyngeal adenomas could invade skull tissue and cause peripheral vestibular signs.

Primary CNS tumors are the most common neoplastic cause of vestibular disease. Meningiomas of the caudal fossa may affect vestibular or cranial nerves or nuclei.

A six-year-old Doberman pinscher developed right unilateral temporal muscle atrophy, which progressed for more than two years and involved other muscles of mastication. The animal exhibited a mild right head tilt, ataxia, and, eventually, laryngeal esophageal paresis. The animal was euthanized. A flattened meningioma was attached to the floor of the skull, compressing the brain stem from right to left. The right trigeminal nerve was absent, and the rootlets of the right glossopharyngeal nerve were diminished. The tumor extended bilaterally from the level of the rostral pons to the middle medulla but was more massive on the right.

Gliomas infrequently occur in the brain stem. They are more frequent in other regions of the CNS. Signs are usually progressive for weeks to months and are dependent on location of the tumor. Most animals with gliomas are more than five years old.

The common tumor involving the vestibular system is the choroid plexus papilloma of the fourth ventricle. Animals usually present with a head tilt, ataxia, hemiparesis, and nystagmus. The head tilt may be opposite the side of the lesion, creating a paradoxical vestibular syndrome (de Lahunta, 1977). They have not been successfully removed, are fairly rapidly growing, and are both invasive and compressive in nature; the prognosis, therefore, is poor.

They may respond transiently to moderate levels of steroids. This fact may be of diagnostic significance.

IDIOPATHIC VESTIBULAR DISORDER

The most common disease in this category is the idiopathic feline vestibular syndrome. Its pathogenesis is unknown. Adult cats are usually affected with an acute bilateral peripheral vestibular disease. Owners report a normal cat that a few hours later is found twisted, rolling, and crying. On presentation, they have a severe head tilt and are rolling and falling to the same side. They have horizontal or rotary nystagmus to the opposite side. The nystagmus usually disappears within two or three days, but a positional nystagmus may be detectable. Several days may pass before the cat can remain in a stable sternal position. A crouching walk is slowly attempted, and eventually the cat becomes reasonably normal. The entire disease process takes two or three weeks. A residual head tilt may persist.

The disease occurs seasonally, with the higher incidence in the summer and early fall. In warmer climates it may occur year round. Some regions of the United States appear to have a much reduced incidence.

No laboratory test assists in the diagnosis of idiopathic feline vestibular syndrome. All findings are normal. Diagnosis is made by ruling out other causes and observing a fairly rapid recovery. No therapy appears to shorten the course of the disease. Diazepam (2 mg IM three or four times a day) may relax the cat enough to prevent self-injury.

An idiopathic geriatric vestibular syndrome occurs in dogs. The disease occurs in older dogs as an acute, peripheral vestibular disease. It is commonly diagnosed as a "stroke" but without confirmation. No pathology has been found. A peripheral vestibular disease is suspected. Animals improve rapidly and are often normal within one to two weeks. Because these animals are old and the signs are fairly severe, they are often euthanized before they have a chance to improve (Chrisman, 1980).

Both the feline and geriatric vestibular syndromes behave as if they are either vascular or inflammatory in nature. The feline disease may be of an allergic nature since it is seasonal and does not occur everywhere. A seasonal infectious disease cannot be overlooked as a cause of vestibular syndromes. An inflammatory process could produce severe vasospasm or the disease could result from hypoxia or direct labyrinthitis.

REFERENCES AND SUPPLEMENTAL READING

Bedford, B. G. C.: Congenital vestibular disease in the English cocker spaniel. Vet. Rec. 105:530, 1979.
Blauch, B., and Strafuss, A. C.: Ganglia of the middle ear. Am. J. Vet. Res. 34:685, 1973.
Chrisman, C. L.: Vestibular diseases. Vet. Clin. North Am. 10:103, 1980.
Davis, L. E., Shurin, S., and Johnson, R. T.: Experimental Viral Labyrinthitis. Nature 254:329, 1975.
de Lahunta, A. (ed.): Vestibular system—special proprioception. In Veterinary Neuroanatomy and Clinical Neurology. Philadelphia: W. B. Saunders, 1977, p. 221.
Getty, R.: The ear. In Evans, H. E., and Christensen, G. C. (eds.): Miller's Anatomy of the Dog, 2nd ed. Philadelphia: W. B. Saunders, 1979.
Guillery, R. W., Casagrande, V. A., and Oberdorfer, M. D.: Congenitally abnormal vision in Siamese cats. Nature 252:195, 1974.

PRIMARY RETICULOSIS OF THE CENTRAL NERVOUS SYSTEM IN DOGS

(Granulomatous Meningoencephalitis)

MARK E. RUSSO, V.M.D.

Kingston, Massachusetts

The term *reticulosis* is frequently used to designate proliferation of elements of the reticuloendothelial system. Although this type of cellular reaction can occur throughout the body in several diseases, primary reticulosis limited to the central nervous system is thought to be a specific entity. It is a progressive disease of unknown etiology seen most frequently in dogs.

Primary reticulosis of the canine central nervous system is characterized histologically by a proliferation and accumulation of mesenchymal cells around the blood vessels of the nervous system. These reactive cells fill the Virchow-Robin space of the vessels and invade the surrounding parenchyma. Cytologic evaluation reveals a large number of macrophages (histiocytes), with a varying admixture of lymphocytes and plasma cells.

Three patterns of cell accumulation are recognized. In some dogs, lesions are diffusely scattered throughout the brain and spinal cord and appear as isolated areas of microscopically apparent perivascular cuffs and local infiltrations. The heaviest concentration of these lesions is usually seen in the brain stem. This pattern has sometimes been referred to as *disseminated reticulosis*.

In other dogs, a different pattern called *focal reticulosis* is seen. In this condition, adjacent and localized cellular lesions coalesce to form a large, macroscopically apparent tumor-like mass, which destroys or replaces pre-existing nervous tissue. These isolated masses occur singly and are usually unilateral. They are found most often in the brain stem or forebrain and are infrequently found in the spinal cord. Occasionally the mass lesion of focal reticulosis and the scattered lesions of disseminated reticulosis are observed in the same animal.

. A third pattern is called *ocular reticulosis*. In this type, the typical cellular accumulations are found in the uveal tract or optic nerves. Ocular lesions may occur alone but are more often associated with reticulosis of the brain and/or spinal cord.

The current discussion of reticulosis is marked by profound confusion, much of which arises from a lack of understanding of the etiopathogenesis of the disease. Debate is often reduced to a matter of semantics. Based on the relative number of cell types and their degree of differentiation, some pathologists make a distinction between inflammatory and neoplastic reticulosis. However, intermediate forms are common and distinctions are not clearly defined. Some investigators believe that reticulosis represents a single disease entity manifesting itself as a continuous spectrum of cellular response ranging from inflammatory to neoplastic.

Similar debate over terminology has occurred in relation to a disease reported in the veterinary literature under the name "granulomatous meningoencephalomyelitis." The histopathology and clinical signs of this disease are so similar to those of disseminated reticulosis that they are considered by some to be variants of the same disease.

The morphology of reticulosis resembles several forms of encephalitis of known etiology. Reticulosis is differentiated from these by the absence of microscopically demonstrable organisms, a somewhat different distribution of lesions, and a lack of systemic involvement. Because of the similar morphology, there has been considerable speculation that reticulosis is caused by an infectious agent. The possibility that reticulosis is a variant of distemper encephalomyelitis is often mentioned. Alternatively, the morphologic changes may represent the response of the nervous system to a yet unknown virus, or they could be the result of an altered or deranged immune response.

These etiologic questions remain unresolved. Consequently, the question remains whether the various forms of reticulosis represent a single disease entity or whether reticulosis is several diseases of various causes linked by their common ability to incite a characteristic cellular response. Despite all these problems, the disease is an acknowledged clinical entity. The problem for the clinician is to recognize that the disease exists and to diagnose and treat it.

INCIDENCE

Although reticulosis is considered to be infrequent in occurrence, this may be the result of a low index of suspicion for the diagnosis as well as the difficulty in making an antemortem diagnosis. Reticulosis may represent up to 25 per cent of the primary central nervous system neoplasms diagnosed post mortem. Although the disease can occur in any breed, some clinicians believe it is more common in miniature poodles and other small breeds. Peak age incidence is two to six years, but up to 30 per cent of the cases occur in dogs two years old or younger. There is no clear-cut sex predilection.

CLINICAL SIGNS AND COURSE

The onset, clinical signs, and course of the disease appear to differ for the various forms of reticulosis. Each form is therefore considered separately. Although the clinical manifestations can vary considerably, the following represent reasonable generalizations.

FOCAL RETICULOSIS

Dogs with focal reticulosis generally are seen after a subtle onset of signs. The most frequent presenting complaints include incoordination, falling, depression, head tilt, circling, blindness, and seizures. Abnormalities found on neurologic examination are generally suggestive of a focal, unilateral lesion. Even in those cases in which the mass lesion of focal reticulosis coexists with disseminated reticulosis, the signs can usually be explained by dysfunction caused by the mass lesion alone.

As would be expected, the clinical signs vary according to the location of the lesion. Focal reticulosis of the forebrain most often manifests itself as abnormalities of the visual and motor systems. Seizure disorders and behavioral changes are also common. The most frequent signs of a brain stem mass are related to dysfunction of the vestibular system, motor system, and cranial nerves. Generally, focal reticulosis of the spinal cord causes signs of motor dysfunction and pain. Lesions in any of these locations produce signs that progress steadily and slowly over a period of weeks or months.

DISSEMINATED RETICULOSIS

Dogs with disseminated reticulosis often have a short history that suggests a rapidly evolving intracranial disease. Owner complaints at presentation are similar to those of dogs with focal reticulosis, but the clinical signs usually start abruptly and progress rapidly. As befits the multifocal distribution of the lesions, neurologic examination almost always reveals abnormalities indicating dysfunction of two or more areas of the nervous system. Signs of brain stem disturbance are the most frequent. Some dogs have intermittent fever. The course is often fulminant, with progressive deterioration occurring over a few days.

OCULAR RETICULOSIS

Blindness is the usual presenting complaint in dogs with ocular reticulosis. The visual deficit can be due to retinal detachment secondary to uveal invasion or cellular infiltration of the optic nerves. In the latter case, signs are usually typical of optic neuritis (i.e., sudden loss of vision associated with dilated pupils that are unresponsive to light). If the optic nerve is affected within or immediately behind the globe, ophthalmoscopic examination may reveal a swollen optic disc. The signs of ocular reticulosis may occur alone or in concert with signs of brain involvement.

ANCILLARY DIAGNOSTIC AIDS

The majority of dogs show changes of the cerebrospinal fluid. Sometimes only a moderate increase in protein is seen. More often, one sees increases in both protein and cell counts. When cell counts are increased, cytologic evaluation is useful. The cells are usually an admixture of lymphocytes and undifferentiated cells of the mononuclear phagocytic system. The latter are sometimes referred to as reticulum cells. This cytologic pattern is highly suggestive of reticulosis.

Routine hematology, serum biochemistries, and urinalysis are normal. Other diagnostic aids may facilitate the localization of the lesion and may help in ruling out other neurologic diseases. Electroencephalographic changes are sometimes noted. These changes are nonspecific but may be of localizing value. Skull radiographs are normal. In cases of focal reticulosis of the spinal cord, myelography may be useful in demonstrating the intramedullary lesion. Although limited in use, cerebral angiography, radioisotope brain scans, and computerized axial tomography have been helpful in localizing the intracranial mass lesion of focal reticulosis. Brain biopsy, although rarely performed, can demonstrate typical histopathologic lesions.

DIAGNOSIS

One of the first steps in making a neurologic diagnosis is to localize the lesion on the basis of clinical signs. Deciding whether one is confronted with a unifocal or multifocal central nervous system disorder allows the clinician to limit the etiologic differential diagnosis list to those diseases that cause the corresponding distribution of lesions. Reticulosis may manifest itself with unifocal signs in focal reticulosis or with multifocal signs in disseminated reticulosis.

Focal reticulosis must be differentiated from other space-occupying masses that cause similar focal, slowly progressive signs. These include neoplasms and focal inflammatory lesions (i.e., abscesses and granulomas). The rapid progression of multifocal signs seen in disseminated reticulosis resembles that seen in other multifocal neurologic disorders and, in particular, infectious diseases. It must be differentiated from the encephalomyelitides caused by viruses (distemper), protozoa (toxoplasmosis), fungi (cryptococcosis), and bacteria.

Antemortem differentiation of reticulosis from these other diseases can be difficult. It requires typical cytologic findings in cerebrospinal fluid. When these are not present, a firm diagnosis may not be possible.

In summary, although reticulosis is not a common disease, it must be considered in the differential diagnosis of a wide variety of neurologic disturbances. It should be considered in any progressive neurologic syndrome. Special attention should be given to this diagnosis in young or middle-aged dogs. It should be especially considered when retinal or optic nerve disease is associated with progressive neurologic deficits. Typical cerebrospinal fluid findings or observation of response to therapy strongly supports the diagnosis. Final diagnosis requires corroboration by history, clinical signs, course, and cerebrospinal fluid examination.

PROGNOSIS AND TREATMENT

Since the underlying cause of the cellular proliferation seen in reticulosis is unknown, specific therapy is not available. Consequently, the long-term prognosis is poor. In almost all cases, the disease is progressive and irreversible. However, the progression of signs often can be temporarily halted or reversed. Many animals with ocular and focal reticulosis respond dramatically to the use of corticosteroids.

No definite dosage has been established; however, oral administration of prednisone at the rate of 1 to 2 mg/kg/day is frequently effective. Response is often dramatic and rapid, with marked improvement seen within several days. After stabilization or elimination of signs, attempts to gradually reduce dosage to a lower maintenance dose are made. If possible, long-term maintenance with alternate-day corticosteroid dosage is used. Too rapid a reduction of the dose may result in acute exacerbation of clinical signs. Cessation of treatment almost always causes prompt deterioration. In cases with seizure disorders, anticonvulsant drugs are used as well.

Survival times for dogs on corticosteroid therapy vary. Animals with focal reticulosis and/or ocular reticulosis can be sustained for several months with corticosteroids before signs progress. In general,

results of such therapy in a limited number of cases of disseminated reticulosis have been variable and disappointing, with most animals deteriorating over a period of days or weeks.

Other forms of therapy, including chemotherapy, immunotherapy, and radiation therapy, have not been adequately evaluated. Theoretically, they might be helpful. More frequent antemortem diagnosis is necessary to allow further evaluation of these types of therapy.

SUPPLEMENTAL READING

Braund, K. G., Vandevelde, M., et al.: Granulomatous meningoencephalomyelitis in six dogs. J.A.V.M.A. 172:1195, 1978.
Fankhauser, R., Fatzer, R., et al.: Reticulosis of the central nervous system of dogs. Adv. Vet. Sci. Comp. Med. 16:35, 1972.
Fischer, C. A., and Liu, S. K.: Neuro-ophthalmologic manifestations of primary reticulosis of the central nervous system in a dog. J.A.V.M.A. 158:1240, 1971.
Roszel, J. F.: Membrane filtration of canine and feline cerebrospinal fluid for cytologic evaluations. J.A.V.M.A. 160:720, 1972.
Russo, M. E.: Primary reticulosis of the central nervous system in dogs. J.A.V.M.A. 174:492, 1979.
Vandevelde, M.: Primary reticulosis of the central nervous system. Vet. Clin. North Am. 10:57, 1980.

MENINGITIS

CRAIG E. GREENE, D.V.M.

Athens, Georgia

Meningitis is inflammation of the tissue coverings of the brain and spinal cord. It may result secondarily from inflammatory processes within the nervous system or from primary infection of meningeal or ependymal tissue. Primary meningitis, which will be the basis of this discussion, is usually caused by non-neurotropic bacteria and fungi. *Pasteurella, Staphylococcus, Streptococcus,* and systemic fungal pathogens are the most frequent offending organisms in dogs and cats. Meningeal inflammation can also be caused by viruses, immunologic disease, hemorrhage, and neoplasia, but it is less common and will not be discussed. Organisms causing meningitis usually enter the subarachnoid space hematogenously from extracranial foci of infection. Retrograde spread up emissary venous sinuses is also possible. Local spread can occur from structures adjacent to the central nervous system (CNS). Defense mechanisms in the body are relatively effective in restricting the spread of infection into the CNS but do little to control the spread of infection

once it has already entered the CNS or cerebrospinal fluid (CSF).

Complications such as CNS edema and increased intracranial pressure can result from CNS infections. Communicating hydrocephalus may develop from decreased CSF absorption by arachnoid villi of the venous sinuses. Obstruction of CSF flow patterns may cause noncommunicating hydrocephalus. CSF collection in animals with suspected meningitis should be attempted with extreme caution and should be avoided if papilledema is present.

CLINICAL SIGNS

The clinical syndrome associated with meningeal inflammation depends on the anatomic location and severity of infection. Hyperesthesia is usually prominent and occurs early owing to dense innervation of meningeal tissue. Neurologic deficits, when present, are mild and occur later because of secondary involvement of the CNS. Hyperesthesia is a predominant clinical sign observed with polyarthritis, polymyositis, polyneuritis, discospondylitis, and intervertebral disc disease. These diseases can usually be differentiated from meningitis by historical, physical, and neurologic examinations. Laboratory testing is usually helpful.

Hyperesthesia from meningitis is manifest by difficulty or reluctance to walk, "board-like" stance, and resistance to passive manipulation or traction of the head, neck, and limbs. Stretching of the animal's limbs causes traction on nerve roots and the meninges and is usually associated with obvious discomfort.

Cranial or spinal nerves are commonly diseased with meningeal inflammation as they leave the brain stem or spinal cord and enter the subarachnoid space. Clinical signs associated with cranial nerve involvement usually include blindness (II), anisocoria (II, III), facial hyperesthesia (V), facial paralysis (VII), and nystagmus and head tilt (VIII). Dense focal cranial nerve deficits with associated postural reaction deficits and upper motor neuron (UMN) signs in the limbs usually indicate an intracranial abscess or inflammation with adjacent brain stem involvement. Lower motor neuron (LMN) signs in one or more limbs indicate spinal cord or nerve root involvement at a particular segment.

Seizures with meningitis may be caused by excessively high fever, hypoglycemia, forebrain edema, or inflammation. Progression of signs to coma, opisthotonus, and pupillary dilation or constriction usually indicates severe cerebral hypoxia or tentorial herniation.

Shock, hypotension, coagulopathy, heart murmur, and multisystemic clinical signs in the presence of the previously mentioned neurologic signs suggest that an underlying bacteremia is the cause of the meningitis.

Extraneural signs caused by meningitis include vomiting and nausea, presumably resulting from increased intracranial pressure or direct stimulation of the vomiting center. Pyrexia is usually caused by muscular rigidity and the effects of endogenous pyrogens derived from the inflammatory process. Bradycardia and slowed respiration are caused by increased intracranial pressure. Multisystemic signs are frequently present with deep mycotic infections.

DIAGNOSIS

Meningitis should be suspected on the basis of historic and physical examination findings. Hematologic and biochemical parameters of peripheral blood are not affected by meningeal or CNS inflammation. CSF examination is the only way to confirm a diagnosis of meningitis. Collection and analysis of CSF have been described elsewhere. CSF should be examined grossly immediately following collection. Turbidity is only present with cell concentrations greater than 500/dl. CNS or CSF inflammation cannot be eliminated from consideration on the basis of clear CSF.

Further cytologic and chemical analyses are essential to determine the degree and type of inflammatory process. Marked increases in cell numbers (>1000/dl) are common with bacterial or fungal meningitis. Neutrophils predominate in acute bacterial infection, and a predominance of lymphocytes is more characteristic of viral infections. Chronic bacterial or fungal infections are usually characterized by a mixed population. A predominance of lymphocytes may be noted following antibiotic therapy or with abscess formation.

Increased protein concentration (>100 mg/dl) is typical of primary or extensive meningeal inflammation. The blood-CSF (B-CSF) barrier is normally impermeable to globulin and slightly permeable to albumin. Protein concentration of CSF increases in infection as a result of increased permeability of the B-CSF barrier and increased production of globulin from local immune responses.

Glucose concentration in CSF is normally 60 to 70 per cent of simultaneous blood concentration. A decreased blood glucose level (hypoglycorrhachia) is thought to be specific for bacterial meningitis, differentiating it from fungal and viral infection. Hypoglycorrhachia has not been a consistent finding in canine or feline bacterial meningoencephalitis.

CSF pressure (normally <180 mm CSF) is frequently elevated with meningeal inflammation to greater than 220 to 300 mm CSF. This may be subjectively detected by rapid efflux of CSF from the needle after penetration of the subarachnoid space during collection. More accurate pressure measurements require a manometer.

Microorganisms are best identified on Gram-stained smears of the sediment from centrifuged CSF. Cryptococcal organisms are best identified by adding a drop of India ink to a wet mount preparation. Other fungi can be found with routine staining for cytology.

Bacterial or fungal culture of CSF should only be performed when increased protein and neutrophil counts are present. Routine culture is expensive and unrewarding. Positive cultures obtained in the absence of pleocytosis usually indicate contamination during collection or the presence of bacteremia. False negative cultures are more common and result from failure to use transport media or appropriate culture media or failure to culture anaerobically. Anaerobic culture is a worthwhile consideration when focal neurologic signs in conjunction with CSF analysis suggest an abscess.

Electroencephalography is frequently abnormal but nonspecifically altered in meningoencephalitis.

Depressed electrical voltage and abnormal spiking have been described. Serologic examination of CSF may reveal increased titers to infectious agents. Titers in the CSF may represent nonspecific leakage of globulin in the CSF during inflammatory processes. Neurotropic viruses usually cause immunospecific increases in CSF globulin that are more diagnostic. Serial or duplicate titers demonstrate changes between acute and convalescent measurements.

Specific antibacterial therapy should be instituted in many circumstances on the basis of CSF findings prior to the results of culture and sensitivity. Therapy should also be continued when clinical improvement is found, even if culture results are negative.

THERAPY

Meningitis should be treated as expeditiously as possible, which usually involves immediate hospitalization. Animals are usually depressed, dehydrated, anorectic, or semicomatose. General nursing care may involve force feeding or parenteral fluid therapy.

Body temperature should be monitored closely in animals with meningitis. Hyperthermia commonly results from increased neuromuscular activity from an irritative process. Fever may occur as a direct effect of the infectious process on hypothalamic thermoregulation. Cold-water baths or other means of lowering body temperature may be required if body temperature fails to respond to antibiotic therapy alone or becomes dangerously elevated.

Convulsions occur as the result of inflammation, causing edema and irritation of forebrain structures. Status epilepticus is initially treated with intravenous diazepam or intermediate-acting barbiturates such as pentobarbital. Animals should be switched to oral anticonvulsants as soon as possible. Anticonvulsants should be administered for one to two months after clinical improvement occurs and the dosage slowly reduced thereafter. Administration may have to be continued indefinitely if seizures recur during the interval.

Antibiotics are the most important agents used in treating bacterial meningitis. Therapy usually begins prior to the return of culture and sensitivity results. Antibiotics are administered immediately after the CSF is collected with the understanding that appropriate changes will be made. The initial choice of antibiotics should be based on the type of organisms suspected as judged by the history, clinical findings, Gram staining of CSF, and the knowledge of antibiotic pharmacodynamics within the CSF and CNS. Antibiotics with high lipid solubility, low ionization, and low protein binding penetrate the blood-brain (BB) and B-CSF barriers most ef-

fectively. To ensure the highest concentration possible, intravenous therapy is most desirable with any antibiotic used. Other forms of parenteral therapy should only be considered as a second choice when cost or difficulty precludes intravenous administration.

The choice of appropriate antibiotic therapy is also difficult in meningitis because *in vivo* response does not always correlate with *in vitro* testing. Many animals with meningitis respond to antibacterial therapy when organisms cannot be cultured or in contrast to sensitivity testing. Bacteriocidal antibiotics should be used whenever possible to ensure complete destruction of the organisms within the relatively immunodeficient subarachnoid space. Therapy should continue for a minimum of three to four weeks once a good response is obtained.

Penicillin and its derivatives are extremely effective in treating bacterial meningitis despite their ionized state and relatively poor passage through the BB and B-CSF barriers. Penetration is increased with meningeal inflammation. As inflammation subsides, the concentration of the penicillins may decrease to the point at which they are no longer effective. For this reason, large and preferably intravenous dosages should be administered for long periods despite clinical improvement. Penicillin is primarily reserved for gram positive infections, and oxacillin can be used when infections involve resistant staphylococci. Ampicillin and carbenicillin, whose penetration of the BB and B-CSF barriers is equal to that of penicillin, are used to treat gram negative and anaerobic infections, respectively.

Chloramphenicol is the only antibiotic that reaches higher concentrations in the brain as compared with serum. Its concentration in CSF in the absence of inflammation is relatively higher than that of most other antibiotics. Intravenous therapy is desirable but not essential because of the high concentration attained. Chloramphenicol is a second choice of therapy under most circumstances after penicillin derivatives. Its use in treating gram negative infections is associated with failures and relapses presumably because it is bacteriostatic at even the highest dosages.

Aminoglycosides are extremely ionic and diffuse poorly into the CNS or CSF in the presence of inflammation. High-dosage gentamicin therapy (2.2 mg/kg at eight-hour intervals) has been recommended, but its use potentiates the development of renal toxicity.

Cephalosporins as a class have relatively poor penetration into the brain and CSF tissue. Only relatively ineffective and toxic, cephaloridine has been shown to reach adequate concentrations in the presence of inflammation. Intrathecal therapy is a possible alternative. Cephacetrile (Celospor) penetrates the CSF in an amount sufficient to eradicate most encountered pathogens. These drugs frequently fail in the clinical setting despite their experimental success.

Other antibiotics, such as tetracycline and erythromycin, have limited penetration in the CSF. They are rarely used because they are bacteriostatic, have a narrow spectrum of activity, and are frequently toxic at the doses employed.

Metronidazole has been used to treat meningitis caused by anaerobic pathogens. It is effective because it is bacteriocidal and diffuses into all tissues, including the CNS, in high concentrations. Leukopenia is a transient side effect that occurs following its administration.

Gram positive infections are treated first with intravenous penicillin. Penicillinase-resistant organisms are treated with a resistant penicillin derivative or chloramphenicol. Cephalosporins should be used only as a last resort. Gram negative infections are treated with intravenous ampicillin, since they are usually susceptible to it. Aminoglycosides can be used in addition. Chloramphenicol can be substituted if these fail. Anaerobic infections should respond to penicillin, chloramphenicol, or metronidazole.

Treatment of infection of the CNS or CSF by mycotic agents most frequently involves amphotericin B. Intravenous therapy is primarily and most practically used, although intrathecal therapy has been recommended. Flucytosine and amphotericin B have been used to treat cryptococcosis. Together these greatly reduce the rate of relapse and increase efficacy of therapy. These drugs have been combined alone and with rifampin to treat histoplasmosis and aspergillosis. The use of ketoconazole has not been thoroughly evaluated.

Combinations of antimicrobial agents may be beneficial and have been most frequently recommended in the treatment of fungal meningitis or encephalitis. Problems have arisen with routine and indiscriminate use of antibacterial agents. Cidal and static agents should not be combined. One justified combination is the use of two bacteriocidal agents such as penicillin and an aminoglycoside. Aminoglycosides should never be used as the sole therapeutic agents in the therapy of meningitis because of their limited efficacy.

Intrathecal therapy has been advocated in treating bacterial or fungal meningitis. In general, it should never be considered unless intravenous antimicrobial therapy has failed. A major disadvantage to the use of this therapy in animals is the multiple anesthetic episodes that must be performed at frequent intervals. Intrathecal gentamicin therapy has been recommended for treating meningitis. The rationale for such therapy has never been established.

Glucocorticoids have been advocated for routine use in the therapy of meningitis in an attempt to minimize the inflammatory process. Their use has been associated with increased morbidity, mortality, and relapses. They may minimize meningeal inflammation, but they compromise an already impaired host defense mechanism. Edema or swelling of the CNS from bacterial or fungal infection is better controlled with osmotic agents than with glucocorticoids. Unfortunately, these cannot be administered over the long run. Intravenous fluid therapy for symptomatic management of cases must be used with caution if cerebral edema is present.

Neurologic deficits or permanent sequelae may be present following successful therapy of meningitis. Abscess formation may result from localization of a more disseminated infection and may be managed by combining antimicrobial therapy and surgical drainage. The latter requires extensive training in neurosurgery.

Frequent monitoring of meningeal infections has shown that culture, gram stain, and CSF glucose level should be normal within 48 hours after successful therapy. CSF protein level and cytology may lag behind for several days to weeks as the inflammatory process subsides. Repeated evaluation of the CSF is difficult in animals that require anesthesia. It may be used if intrathecal administration of antibiotics is being performed. The inability to frequently obtain CSF means that clinical signs are primarily used to evaluate therapy. Evaluation should continue for at least three to four weeks following improvement. Some neurologic signs are permanent as a result of injury caused by the inflammatory process.

SUPPLEMENTAL READING

Bullmore, C. C., and Sevedge, J. P.: Canine meningoencephalitis. J. Am. Anim. Hosp. Assoc. 14:387, 1978.
Kornegay, J. N., Lorenz, M. D., and Zenoble, R. D.: Bacterial meningoencephalitis in two dogs. J.A.V.M.A. 173:1334, 1978.

HEAD TRAUMA AND NERVOUS SYSTEM INJURY

WILLIAM R. FENNER, D.V.M.

Columbus, Ohio

Traumatic injuries involving the head are common in dogs and cats. They are often severe and are frequently frustrating to manage. In a recent review it was found that about 20 per cent of all traumatic injuries in the dog and approximately 35 per cent in the cat involved the head. Of the total number of injuries, 10 per cent were severe and 10 per cent life-threatening (Kolata et al., 1974). The bony skull and spinal fluid afford the central nervous system (CNS) considerable protection from injury. For this reason, trauma that causes CNS injury is usually major and clearly identifiable, either historically or on physical examination.

Head injuries may cause neurologic signs by damaging the peripheral nervous system (PNS), the CNS, or both. Although the signs of PNS injury are often permanent, they are rarely life-threatening. CNS injury often is life-threatening but causes fewer long-term deficits. The diagnostic approach to both types of injury is the same but the therapeutic approach differs.

GOALS OF THERAPY

The principal goals of therapy in head injury are to reduce tissue swelling, decrease intracranial pressure, and maintain vascular perfusion and thus oxygenation. Achieving these goals serves to preserve the greatest amount of functional tissue. Regardless of therapy, a certain amount of neural tissue will be irreparably injured at the time of trauma. The clinician cannot reverse this initial damage but can attempt to prevent its progression (Averill, 1981; Cooper, 1979).

To improve the survival rate in head trauma as well as the quality of survival, the clinician must rapidly classify the location, extent, and severity of the injury. This allows the prompt establishment of appropriate therapy.

PATIENT APPROACH

The history of trauma to the nervous system (NS) usually indicates an acute injury. The signs usually reach their maximum severity within hours of the accident, and, if the injury is not fatal, they are followed by a period of stabilization and resolution.

The first step in evaluating the patient is to diagnose and correct life-threatening non-neural injuries. Shock, with its associated hypotension, can cause CNS hypoxia and brain edema. CNS hypoxia may be potentiated by severe pneumothorax or traumatic cardiac arrhythmia if these injuries are not fatal in themselves. When instituting fluid therapy for shock, be aware that the blood-brain barrier will not be intact in the patient with CNS disease. In this situation, the massive volumes of fluid required for treatment of shock may aggravate cerebral swelling and attendant neurologic signs. After ensuring an airway, stabilizing cardiac output, and controlling any life-threatening hemorrhage, the neurologic evaluation should begin.

The neurologic history should include not only the trauma but other major concurrent metabolic or neurologic disease as well. A patient with pre-existing neurologic disease such as epilepsy may display abnormalities not related to the head injury. Animals with severe metabolic diseases such as diabetes will be more difficult to treat if their underlying disease is not recognized.

The neurologic examination should be rapid and complete, with emphasis on the level of consciousness, pupil size and symmetry, eye movements, and spinal reflexes. The injury should be localized and classified as either CNS or PNS and diffuse or focal.

CLASSIFICATION OF INJURY

The neurologic examination is the first step in differentiating a CNS injury from a PNS injury. The CNS above the foramen magnum consists of three parts: the cerebrum, cerebellum, and brain stem. Each of these parts serves some separate or unique function, and each has some function in association with other parts of the CNS (Fig. 1). Thus, an injury to any portion of the CNS can cause varying degrees of loss of coordination (ataxia) or weakness (paresis) in one or more limbs. In addition, an injury to either the cerebrum or brain stem can cause increased tone and abnormal (increased) reflexes in the limbs. These reflex changes reflect the loss of upper motor neuron (UMN) influence over the limbs.

The changes in the unique (localizing) function in

739

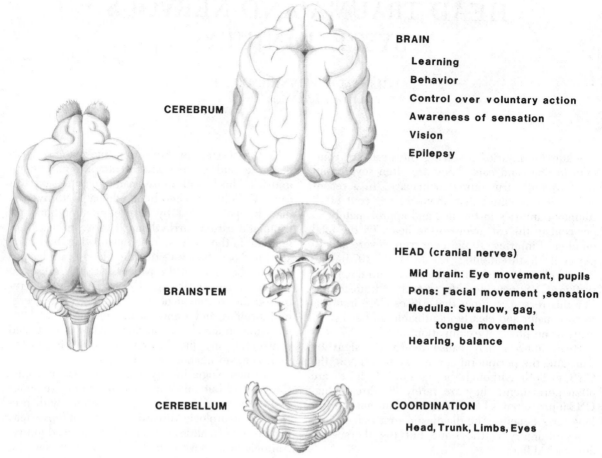

CEREBRUM

BRAINSTEM

CEREBELLUM

BRAIN

   Learning

   Behavior

   Control over voluntary action

   Awareness of sensation

   Vision

   Epilepsy

HEAD (cranial nerves)

   Mid brain: Eye movement, pupils

   Pons: Facial movement ,sensation

   Medulla: Swallow, gag,

            tongue movement

   Hearing, balance

COORDINATION

   Head, Trunk, Limbs, Eyes

Figure 1. Summary of functions associated with major anatomic levels. (Adapted from Daube: *Medical Neurosciences.* Boston: Little, Brown and Co., 1978.)

combination with the reflex changes allow the clinician to decide which portion of the CNS is affected. The cerebral functions are those of intellect and vision. The unique signs of cerebral disease include epilepsy and visual, behavioral, and mental changes. Brain stem function can be thought of as controlling the "head" and vegetative body functions. Dysfunction of the brain stem will be seen as paralysis of cranial nerves, loss of balance, loss of consciousness, and cardiac and respiratory abnormalities. The cerebellum serves to coordinate motor movements. Cerebellar injury may cause ataxia of the head and body.

In contrast to CNS injury, which causes limb signs and evidence of brain dysfunction, PNS injuries usually cause signs limited to the areas innervated by the damaged cranial nerve. An exception to this is the vestibular nerve (CN VIII), which is responsible for maintaining balance. Damage to this nerve may cause ataxia, circling, falling, and disorientation. Injury to the peripheral portion of the eighth cranial nerve is common and is often mistaken for injury to the CNS. The facts that other cranial nerves are not involved, that limb reflexes are normal, and that consciousness is preserved all suggest peripheral nerve injury. A review of the neurologic examination can be found in textbooks of veterinary neurology (de Lahunta, 1977; Hoerlein, 1980; Palmer, 1977).

TREATMENT OF PNS INJURIES

After localizing the injury, therapy can be instituted. In injuries of the PNS that do not involve the vestibular nerve, treatment is usually not required. A careful examination should be performed for skull fractures that may have entrapped or severed a peripheral nerve. If these are found, surgical correction of the fracture may result in return of function to the injured nerve. There may be a concomitant loss of lacrimation in animals with facial paralysis. Tear production should be evaluated by a Schirmer tear test. If lacrimation is inadequate, the cornea should be moistened at frequent intervals with artificial tears.

Animals with peripheral vestibular disease may injure themselves further because their disorientation causes them to roll and thrash about violently. These animals may require mild sedation or light restraint to prevent additional injury. If physical restraint is used, body temperature should be monitored frequently, because these animals may become hyperthermic while struggling to free themselves.

Vestibular disorders usually appear worse than they actually are, and the tendency is to overtreat a benign PNS injury rather than perform a critical neurologic examination. Even with total destruction of the inner ear, signs begin to resolve in less than two weeks with or without treatment (Baloh and Honrubia, 1980). An otoscopic examination should be performed to detect hemotympanum.

In summary, peripheral nerve injuries are usually complete (total loss of function of the involved nerve); they rarely require treatment; and, with the exception of vestibular injuries, they rarely cause signs beyond focal loss of function.

EVALUATION OF CNS INJURIES

When evaluating a patient with CNS injury, several steps should be taken rapidly. First, palpate for skull fractures. If skull fractures are present and fragments are depressed into the cranial vault, they may compound the injury. Depressed fractures should be elevated as soon as the animal's condition is stable. Second, a record should be made of the animal's level of consciousness, pupil size and symmetry, pupillary responsiveness, and the presence or absence of physiologic nystagmus (doll's eye maneuver). These tests aid in differentiating animals with cerebral and brain stem injury. Brain stem injury carries a grave prognosis. An animal with such an injury is more likely to have permanent sequelae and least likely to be responsive to therapy.

The level of consciousness may be abnormal in one of two ways (Fig. 2). The animal may have an abnormal content of consciousness; i.e., it appears to be awake but does not respond properly to its environment. In this case, cerebral injury should be suspected. If the animal has an abnormal level of consciousness such as stupor or coma, either generalized cerebral injury or brain stem injury should be suspected. A change in the level of consciousness during the observation period is more significant than the level at any one time. In humans, 50 per cent of head injury patients with coma die. If coma persists beyond six hours, mortality increases. The anatomic site of the lesion causing coma is also important, because 85 to 95 per cent of humans with coma and signs related to brain stem injury will die (Plum and Posner, 1980). My experience with dogs supports the observation in humans that cerebral injuries respond more favorably than brain stem injuries.

Abnormal pupil size may be seen with either cerebral or brain stem injury. The animal with cerebral injury will have abnormally small pupils that are responsive to light and will still display physiologic nystagmus (Fig. 3). The animal with brain stem injury may have abnormally large or abnormally small pupils. If the injury is in the mid brain, the pupils will be abnormally large and nonresponsive to light and physiologic nystagmus will be absent. If the injury is in the pons, the pupils will be abnormally small (pinpoint) and poorly responsive or nonresponsive to light and physiologic nystagmus will be absent. Recent reports indicate that certain cerebellar injuries also may cause abnormal pupil size. The animals with cerebral or brain stem injury and abnormal pupil size that I have seen have also had an abnormal level of consciousness. This would not be expected with cerebellar injury. Therefore, if the animal has abnormal pupil size, normal consciousness, and normal physiologic nystagmus, cerebellar injury (or a peripheral nerve injury) should be suspected.

When evaluating animals with abnormal pupil size, remember that ocular injury may be responsible. Careful examination of the globe should reveal the injury. Animals may also suffer injury to the optic nerve. If both optic nerves are involved, the pupils will be abnormally large and nonresponsive

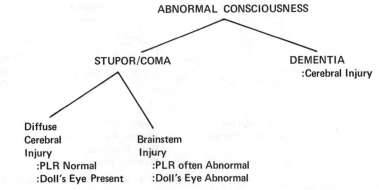

Figure 2. Two ways in which the level of consciousness may be abnormal.

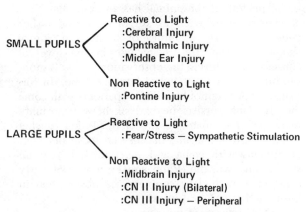

Figure 3. Abnormal pupil size.

opisthotonus of cerebellar disease. Decerebrate posturing is more commonly episodic than constant and is induced by noxious stimuli. It is a poor prognostic sign in an otherwise stable patient.

Examination of the spinal reflexes helps to confirm the presence of a lesion involving the CNS and may show that the animal has spinal as well as intracranial injury. This combination of injuries is rare in my experience, but when it does occur the spinal injury is often overlooked, whereas the intracranial injury is treated. Later, when the patient remains nonambulatory following apparent improvement of the head injury, a complete neurologic examination is performed and the second lesion is localized.

to light, but normal physiologic nystagmus should be present.

Record the animal's posture and response to external stimuli. Animals with lesions of the rostral brain stem (mid brain) may have spasms of decerebrate posturing, which look very similar to the opisthotonic posture of cerebellar injury. The presence of coma or stupor serves to identify the behavior as decerebrate posturing, as opposed to the

THERAPY OF INTRACRANIAL INJURY

After having localized the animal's injury to the cerebrum, brain stem, or cerebellum, therapy should be instituted (Fig. 4).

When treating injuries of the CNS, an attempt is made to decrease the size of any intracranial masses and the metabolic needs of the CNS and to provide oxygen and glucose for the metabolic needs that remain.

As a rule, I hospitalize and observe for at least 24 hours any traumatized animal with either historic

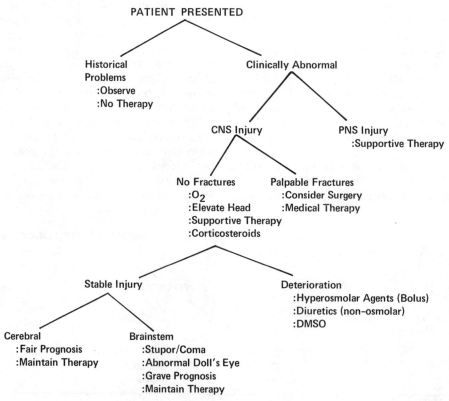

Figure 4. Therapy for intracranial injury.

or clinical evidence of neurologic dysfunction. The first line of treatment in intracranial injury is corticosteroids. Although there is no standard dosage for corticosteroids in head trauma, I use a dosage of 0.2 mg dexamethasone/kg of body weight given as a bolus, followed by the same amount on a daily basis in two or three divided doses. This dosage is lower than those recommended by others, and dosages as high as 2.0 mg/kg of body weight three times per day have been suggested (Kirk and Bistner, 1975). I use the lower dosage in the absence of shock. If the animal is in shock, a dosage of 2.0 mg/kg of body weight is given as the initial bolus.

The animal is then placed in 40 per cent oxygen with its head elevated and is observed and evaluated. If necessary, the animal is carefully restrained to prevent further self-injury; sedative drugs are avoided. Supportive fluid therapy is provided if warranted by the animal's clinical condition. The head is elevated to improve venous drainage, thereby decreasing the size of the vascular component of intracranial contents. The enriched oxygen atmosphere is used because hypoxia potentiates CNS edema.

Hypercarbia causes vasodilatation and a decrease in cerebral perfusion pressure, which increases edema and intracranial pressure. A decrease in consciousness often causes decreased ventilation. Although maintenance of airways is often difficult in small animals, the high oxygen atmosphere may help prevent hypercarbia.

Although steroids have not been clearly demonstrated to be beneficial experimentally, they are routinely used because of the clinical impression that they are efficacious. Large volumes of fluids are not administered to the animal with head trauma unless shock is present. Fluids are given judiciously to prevent extravasation of excess fluid across an already damaged blood-brain barrier, which may worsen cerebral edema.

Although the use of hyperosmolar agents has been advocated, I rarely use them except in animals that are *in extremis* or in those that display rapid deterioration. The animal with intracranial injury may have an altered blood-brain barrier, and hyperosmolar agents can leak across this barrier into the damaged neural parenchyma. Fluid will follow the hyperosmolar agent into the central nervous system rather than being removed from it into the vascular compartment. In addition, there is evidence that hyperosmolar agents are effective only in acute states and should only be used once rather than on a repeated basis (Fishman, 1980; Sklar, 1979).

If the animal has seizures, I administer diazepam (Valium) intravenously at 0.25 to 0.50 mg/kg of body weight as needed. If diazepam is ineffective, I use phenobarbital to effect. I attempt oral maintenance therapy with phenytoin (Dilantin) 30 mg/kg t.i.d. in animals weighing less than 10 kg. In animals over 10 kg, I use phenobarbital (1 to 2 mg/kg b.i.d.) for oral therapy. Although phenytoin is less sedative than barbiturates, its short half-life and poor absorption necessitate dosage that is cost prohibitive in animals over 10 kg.

At this point, initial therapy is complete. The patient is re-evaluated on an hourly basis. If the animal shows deterioration despite therapy, hyperosmolar agents may be used. Mannitol is given once only at a dosage of 2 gm/kg body weight. Other drugs that may be tried are acetazolamide (Diamox) and furosemide (Lasix). Although they act by different mechanisms, both are believed to decrease the production of cerebrospinal fluid and may lower intracranial pressure. Lowering intracranial pressure would facilitate resolution of edema. The use of dimethyl sulfoxide (DMSO) intravenously in conjunction with corticosteroids has been advocated. I have not had personal experience with this drug.

Signs of deterioration include a decline in the level of consciousness, development of bradycardia, loss of physiologic nystagmus, and loss of pupillary responsiveness to light. An animal that is recumbent owing to cerebral or brain stem injury may develop ataxia and other signs of cerebellar disease as it improves and begins to walk. This is an unmasking of a previous injury and not a sign of deterioration.

In my experience, exploratory craniotomies in animals with head trauma are rarely required. If there is no objective surgical lesion (e.g., fracture), surgery is not indicated.

The objectives of treatment of intracranial injury are alleviation of brain edema and prevention of deterioration. A certain amount of irreversible injury that is present cannot be treated and may result in sequelae.

The sequelae of head trauma include neurogenic pulmonary edema, permanent neurologic deficits, epilepsy, and internal hydrocephalus. Permanent neurologic deficits may be central or peripheral in nature. Peripheral nerve injuries are usually focal and are rarely debilitating. Sequelae to central nervous system injuries include marked personality changes, visual deficits, circling, weakness in one or more limbs, and other deficits that may make the animal an unacceptable pet. On the initial neurologic examination it is impossible to determine whether an animal will have residual sequelae. The animal with brain stem injury is more likely to have permanent deficits than the animal with cerebral injury. Animals with cerebellar injury are likely to recover completely.

The onset of epilepsy may be at the time of head trauma or may be delayed for hours, days, or weeks. I feel that in most cases post-traumatic epilepsy begins within one week of injury. Delayed post-traumatic epilepsy is relatively easy to manage and does not usually require special therapy. Hydrocephalus as a sequela to head trauma is a reported phenomenon that I have rarely seen. It is reported to cause a rapidly progressive decline in the level of consciousness days or weeks after the animal appears to have recovered from head injury. The prognosis in these animals is considered to be grave.

In summary, the treatment of head trauma consists of preventing further injury and administering corticosteroids, enriched oxygen mixtures, and supportive care. The prognosis is largely determined by the site of injury. Animals with peripheral nervous system injuries tend to have good prognoses. Animals with CNS injuries can be divided into three categories. Animals with cerebellar injuries have a good prognosis, those with cerebral injury have a guarded to fair prognosis, and those with brain stem injuries have a grave prognosis.

REFERENCES AND SUPPLEMENTAL READING

Averill, D. R.: Brain injury. *In* Bojrab, M. (ed.): *Pathophysiology in Small Animal Surgery*. Philadelphia: Lea & Febiger, 1981.

Baloh, R. W., and Honrubia, V.: *Clinical Neurophysiology of the Vestibular System, Contemporary Neurology Series*, Vol. 18. Philadelphia: F. A. Davis, 1980.
Cooper, P. R.: The treatment of head injury. *In* Rosenberg, R. (ed.): *The Treatment of Neurological Diseases*. New York: Spectrum Publications, 1979.
de Lahunta, A.: *Veterinary Neuroanatomy and Clinical Neurology*. Philadelphia: W. B. Saunders, 1977.
Fenner, W. R.: Seizures and head trauma. Vet. Clin. North Am. 11:31, 1981.
Fishman, R. A.: *Cerebrospinal Fluid in Diseases of the Nervous System*. Philadelphia: W. B. Saunders, 1980.
Hoerlein, B. F.: *Canine Neurology*, 3rd ed. Philadelphia: W. B. Saunders, 1978.
Kirk, R. W., and Bistner, S.: *Handbook of Veterinary Procedures and Emergency Treatment*, 2nd ed. Philadelphia: W. B. Saunders, 1975.
Kolata, R. J., Kraut, N. H., and Johnston, D. L.: Patterns of trauma in urban dogs and cats: A study of 1000 cases. J.A.V.M.A. 164:499, 1974.
Palmer, A. C.: *Introduction to Animal Neurology*. London: Blackwell Scientific Publications, 1977.
Plum, F., and Posner, J. B.: *The Diagnosis of Stupor and Coma*, 3rd ed., *Contemporary Neurology Series*, Vol. 19. Philadelphia: F. A. Davis, 1980.
Sklar, F. H.: Treatment of increased intracranial pressure. *In* Rosenberg, R. (ed.): *The Treatment of Neurological Diseases*. New York: Spectrum Publications, 1979.

STORAGE DISEASES

BRIAN R. H. FARROW, B.V.Sc.

Sydney, Australia

The storage diseases are a relatively rare group of diseases that result from deficiency of specific intracellular enzymes contained within membrane-bound structures in cells known as lysosomes. These enzymes are responsible for the normal degradation of proteins, polysaccharides, and lipids. When a particular enzyme deficiency exists, that enzyme's substrate accumulates within cells, and this ultimately interferes with function. The tissue distribution of the undegradable substrate determines the organs most affected and the clinical signs.

Certain characteristic features of the storage diseases, summarized here, are adapted from Blakemore (1974).

1. Animals are normal at birth.
2. Affected animals may fail to grow as rapidly as their littermates.
3. There is usually a recessive mode of inheritance, with only certain members of a litter likely to be affected.
4. There often is a history of inbreeding, clinical signs being expressed in the homozygous recessive individual.

5. Specific deficiencies of single enzymes are known to occur in certain breeds.
6. Young animals are presented with signs of multifocal neurologic disease which is progressive in nature and ultimately fatal.
7. Systems other than the nervous system may be involved.

In humans, more than 30 of these inborn errors of metabolism are known to occur, and in domestic animals a smaller but increasing number have been described. The diseases are named after the main substance stored, the enzyme that is deficient, or the person who first described the syndrome. Examples of storage diseases in dogs and cats are given in Table 1. Most of the inherited lysosomal storage diseases are accompanied by severe neurologic disease. In the case of the glycogen storage diseases, although there are neuronal lesions and neurologic disturbances, the main clinical sign is weakness.

Diagnosis in suspected cases can be confirmed by enzymatic analysis of peripheral blood leukocytes or tissues such as skin, which can be biopsied, cell cultured, and subsequently analyzed. Laboratories

Table 1. *Examples of Storage Diseases in the Dog and Cat*

Disease	Breeds Affected	Selected Reference
Glycogenoses		
α-Glucosidase deficiency (Pompe's disease)	Dog	Mostafa, 1970
α-Glucosidase deficiency	Cat (DSH)*	Sandstrom et al., 1969
Mucopolysaccharidoses		
α-L-iduronidase deficiency (mucopolysaccharidosis I: Hurler's syndrome)	Cat (DSH)	Haskins et al., 1979
Arylsulfatase B deficiency (mucopolysaccharidosis VI; Maroteaux-Lamy syndrome)	Cat (Siamese)	Langweiler et al., 1978
Sphingolipidoses		
β-Galactocerebrosidase deficiency (Krabbe's disease)	Dog (Cairn terrier, WHW,† beagle, miniature poodle) Cat (DSH)	Fletcher et al., 1971
β-Glucocerebrosidase deficiency (Gaucher's disease)	Dog (Australian silkie terrier)	Farrow et al., 1982
Hexosaminidase deficiency (GM$_2$ gangliosidosis; Tay-Sachs disease)	Dog (German short-haired pointer) Cat (DSH)	Karbe, 1973
β-Galactosidase deficiency (GM$_1$ gangliosidosis, type I)	Cat (DSH)	Blakemore, 1972
Partial β-galactosidase deficiency	Cat (Siamese)	Baker et al., 1971
Sphingomyelinase deficiency (Niemann-Pick disease)	Cat (DSH), Siamese	Wenger et al., 1980

*Domestic short-haired cat.
†West Highland white terrier.

with facilities for lysosomal enzyme assay should be consulted regarding particular specimen requirements. Diagnosis can also be confirmed by histologic examination of appropriate biopsy or necropsy material in which the stored substrate may cause characteristic ultrastructural changes. Biochemical identification of the stored material enables specific diagnosis.

INHERITANCE

Most of the diseases due to deficiency of a lysosomal enzyme are inherited as autosomal recessive traits. Heterozygotes, having one normal and one defective gene, are clinically normal, although their specific lysosomal enzyme level is intermediate between homozygous recessive and homozygous normal individuals. It is therefore possible, using lysosomal enzyme assays, to detect the heterozygote carrier animals and manage breeding programs accordingly. Peripheral blood leukocyte enzyme assay of puppies may also be used to detect homozygous recessive individuals that will subsequently develop the disease.

TREATMENT

Treatment for the lysosomal storage diseases is not available at present. In veterinary medicine attention should be directed toward detection and elimination from the breeding population of carrier animals. Current emphasis in research on storage diseases is directed toward enzyme replacement therapy. The rationale for this is based on the assumption that exogenously administered enzyme can enter lysosomes through a process of endocytosis and function in the degradation of accumulated substrate. Although this approach is promising, problems with enzyme uptake and inactivation have prevented successful application of it. The use of lipid vesicles (liposomes) to protect and stabilize replacement enzymes and enhance uptake and subcellular distribution holds some promise for the treatment of humans with these disorders. It may also be possible to replace or add genetic material to affected individuals so that they gain the capability to produce active enzyme. The naturally occurring storage diseases of animals provide valuable models in which new approaches to therapy may be studied.

REFERENCES AND SUPPLEMENTAL READING

Baker, H. J., Lindsey, J. R., McKhann, G. M., and Farrel, D. F.: Neuronal GM₁ gangliosidosis in a Siamese cat with beta-galactosidase deficiency. Science 174:838, 1971.

Blakemore, W. F.: GM₁ gangliosidosis in the cat. J. Comp. Pathol. 82:179, 1972.

Blakemore, W. F.: Lysosomal storage diseases. *In* Grunsell, C. S. G., and Hill, F. W. G. (eds.): *Veterinary Annual*, 15th issue. Bristol, England: Wright-Scientechnica, 1974, p. 242.

Farrow, B. R. H., Hartley, W. J., Pollard, A. C., Desnick, R. J., Grabowski, G., and Fabro, D.: Gaucher disease in the dog. *In Gaucher Disease: A Century of Delineation and Research*. New York: Alan R. Liss, Inc., 1982.

Fletcher, T. F., Lee, D. G., and Hammer, R. F.: Ultrastructural features of globoid-cell leukodystrophy in the dog. Am. J. Vet. Res. 32:177, 1971.

Haskins, M. E., Jezyk, P. F., Desnick, R. J., McDonough, S. K., and Patterson, D. F.: Mucopolysaccharidosis in a domestic short-haired cat. A disease distinct from that seen in the Siamese cat. J.A.V.M.A. 175:384, 1979.

Karbe, E.: Animal model of human disease: GM$_2$-gangliosidoses (amaurotic idiocies) types I, II, and III. Animal model: canine GM$_2$ gangliosidosis. Am. J. Pathol. 71:151, 1973.

Kolodny, E. H.: Lysosomal storage diseases. N. Engl. J. Med. 294:1217, 1976.

Langweiler, M., Haskins, M. E., and Jezyk, P. F.: Mucopolysaccharidosis in a litter of cats. J. Am. Anim. Hosp. Assoc. 14:748, 1978.

Mostafa, I. R.: A case of glycogenic cardiomegaly in the dog. Acta Vet. Scand. 11:197, 1970.

Reynolds, G. D., Baker, H. J., and Reynolds, R. H.: Enzyme replacement using liposome carriers in feline GM$_1$ gangliosidosis fibroblasts. Nature 275:754, 1978.

Sandstrom, B., Westman, J., and Ockerman, P. A.: Glycogenesis of the central nervous system in the cat. Acta Neuropathol. (Berl.) 14:194, 1969.

Wenger, D. A., Sattler, M., Kudoh, T., Snyder, S. P., and Kingston, R. S.: Niemann-Pick disease: a genetic model in Siamese cats. Science 208:1471, 1980.

ANTICONVULSANT DRUG THERAPY IN COMPANION ANIMALS

SUSAN E. BUNCH, D.V.M.

Raleigh, North Carolina

INTRODUCTION

INCIDENCE OF SEIZURE DISORDERS

The seizure disorder is a common clinical problem requiring chronic medical management in small animals. Published epidemiologic reports in humans indicate an incidence of 0.5 to 1.0 per cent. The only comparable veterinary data available were collected in one study that showed that seizure disorders comprised 1 per cent of all canine illnesses diagnosed at a veterinary tecahing hospital. A retrospective evaluation of canine and feline hospital records over a six-year period at the New York State College of Veterinary Medicine (NYSCVM) revealed an incidence of 2.3 per cent of all sick dogs examined and 1 per cent of all sick cats examined, suggesting that seizures are more common in dogs than in cats.

DEFINITIONS OF SEIZURES AND SEIZURE PHASES

Seizures are the clinical manifestation of a paroxysmal cerebral disorder. They may represent a systemic illness that causes central nervous system (CNS) dysfunction or a primary intracranial disease. In either case, the fundamental event is a disturbance in the excitability of the CNS that results in a focus of excessive neuronal discharge. It is important to note that even normal nervous tissue can be made hyperexcitable under appropriate conditions.

If the stimulus is sufficient, the seizure threshold is exceeded, and normal inhibitory mechanisms fail; this abnormal discharge is allowed to spread, resulting in a seizure. When seizures become recurrent and are associated with nonprogressive intracranial disease that may be inherited or acquired, the term *epilepsy* may be used.

The two basic categories of seizures are focal, or partial, and generalized. *Focal seizures* are caused by a localized area of neuronal dysfunction that results in clinical signs compatible with the area of involvement in the brain and are usually acquired. The prototype of focal seizures in humans is the scar left by trauma to the head that remains as an irritable focus. Examples in the dog include psychomotor seizures characterized by marked changes in behavior or hallucinations ("fly biting"). Frequently, seizures may begin as partial seizures and develop into generalized seizures by a process termed *secondary generalization*.

Generalized seizures begin abruptly, are distinguished by the absence of localizing signs, and are usually accompanied by interruptions in consciousness. Generalized seizures may be classified by the presence of violent muscular activity, *grand mal seizures*, or the absence of such activity, *petit mal seizures*. Most seizure disorders seen in small animals are of the grand mal type. Although many petit mal seizures probably occur in small animals, documentation has been difficult because the more common focal motor seizure is frequently misinterpreted as a petit mal seizure.

The mechanisms involved in the initiation, spread, and termination of a seizure discharge are not clearly understood, although considerable advancements in the comprehension of these events have been made in recent years. Currently under investigation is the role of neurotransmitter metabolism, the contribution of CNS inhibitory substances such as gamma aminobutyric acid, and changes in neuronal cell membrane physiology. The importance of these studies lies not only in clarification of the pathogenesis of seizures but also in the pharmacology of the therapeutic agents selected to control them.

The actual seizure (ictus) is preceded by an aural or *preictal phase* commonly characterized by behavioral changes and autonomic signs that may last minutes to days. The next phase, the *seizure* itself, usually lasts one to two minutes unless *status epilepticus* is developing. Finally, the *postictal phase* may be very short, with immediate return to normalcy, or may last for hours, during which behavioral changes, disorientation, and temporary blindness are typical. The description and duration of the seizure phases may be useful in localizing the excitable focus, especially in partial seizure disorders. However, they do not provide information as to the exact cause or severity of the seizure disorder nor do they influence the choice of therapy.

CAUSES OF SEIZURES

The causes of seizures have been addressed in previous publications and will not be considered in depth here. Intracranial causes include various infections (canine distemper, feline infectious peritonitis, blastomycosis, toxoplasmosis, cryptococcosis), head trauma, developmental abnormalities (hydrocephalus, lissencephaly), lysosomal storage diseases, neoplasia (primary or metastatic), inflammatory conditions (parasitic migration, reticulosis), vascular impairment (feline ischemic encephalopathy), genetic predisposition (German shepherd, beagle, Belgian shepherd, Irish setter, keeshond, poodle, and Saint Bernard breeds suspected), and idiopathic epilepsy. Systemic illnesses that may have central nervous system sequelae include hypocalcemia, hypoglycemia, cardiopulmonary insufficiency, thiamine deficiency, intoxication (lead, strychnine, organophosphates), uremia, hepatic failure, hyperlipidemia, polycythemia, and heat stroke.

DIAGNOSIS

The diagnostic approach to a patient presented for evaluation of a seizure disorder consists of a careful analysis of the history of the patient, a physical examination, a neurologic examination, clinical laboratory analyses, and radiography.

History. The attending veterinarian must rely on the owner's description to differentiate seizures from other episodic syndromes such as syncope, cataplexy, myasthenia gravis, or polymyositis. Once it has been established that a seizure actually occurred, specific attention is given to elements of the history that would contribute to the differential diagnosis. The age of the patient is valuable, since inherited or congenital seizures usually begin at less than three years of age. Geriatric patients with seizures beginning late in life, especially with localizing neurologic signs, are most likely to have a space-occupying lesion in the CNS. Since certain breeds are predisposed to particular CNS diseases, breeding information is useful also. Background history should include vaccinations received, illnesses unrelated to the current complaint of seizures such as difficult delivery as a puppy or head trauma, evidence of infectious disease, and information regarding other animals at home and littermates and parents and their state of health. Information about environmental conditions is essential in determining whether there has been exposure to toxins or contagious agents endemic to specific geographic locations. A detailed account of all phases of the seizure is needed to classify the seizure as focal or generalized and to determine what conditions, if any, might be considered provocative. For example, cats with thiamine deficiency may seize with handling. Equally important is knowledge of the interictal period. Patients genetically predisposed to seizures appear healthy between episodes, whereas those with structural lesions of the CNS are likely to have clinical signs of illness between seizures.

Physical Examination. A careful physical examination may reveal the presence of systemic infection, cardiac irregularities, respiratory inadequacy, external trauma, or perhaps tumors. Although seizures can accompany advanced renal or hepatic disease, it is unlikely that they will be the sole presenting clinical sign. Eye examination is also important, since fundic lesions are often associated with various systemic and intracranial disorders.

Neurologic Examination. A complete neurologic examination is only valid if performed during the interictal period. Evaluate all aspects of the nervous system including spinal reflexes, postural reactions, and cranial nerves. If interictal neurologic signs are present, then there is structural brain disease. Single mass lesions such as a tumor or infarct produce specific localizing signs. Metabolic diseases may produce diffuse cerebral signs or no interictal signs. Abnormal findings in more than one part of the nervous system suggest multifocal involvement. A normal interictal neurologic examination supports a tentative diagnosis of *idiopathic epilepsy* or an episodic metabolic illness such as hypoglycemia. Regardless of the cause of seizures, serial neurologic examinations are invaluable in assessing the course of illness.

Clinical Laboratory Evaluation. Ideally, baseline laboratory data should be obtained for all seizure patients before therapy is instituted, not only for diagnostic purposes but to supply a reference point should problems develop in the future. Clinical laboratory evaluation should include a hemogram, to determine whether *lead intoxication* (large numbers of nucleated red blood cells, basophilic stippling) or *systemic infection* (leukocytosis or leukopenia, depending on the offending organism) is present; a chemistry profile to assess *liver and kidney function;* urinalysis; and, in selected cases, a 30-minute BSP per cent retention test and a plasma ammonia concentration determination.

Whole blood obtained after at least a 12-hour fast and preserved in sodium fluoride is preferred for accurate determination of glucose concentration. *Hypocalcemia* of sufficient magnitude to cause seizures is usually detectable by routine serum analysis. The persistence of conspicuous *lipemia* in a serum sample harvested more than eight hours post prandially signifies altered lipid metabolism and may be related to metabolic diseases such as diabetes mellitus or may be without an identifiable cause. Idiopathic hyperlipidemia is occasionally associated with seizures in both humans and dogs. *Elevated serum proteins*, especially in the globulin fraction, are frequently seen with feline infectious peritonitis.

Evaluate cerebrospinal fluid (CSF) when empirical anticonvulsant therapy has not been successful; when abnormalities are detected in the neurologic examination; or when neoplasia, meningeal infection, encephalitis, or other intracranial disease is suspected. A complete evaluation of the CSF includes measurement of opening pressure and protein and cytologic examination. Perform these additional analyses when indicated: (1) culture and sensitivity when there are more than 5 WBC/high power field or if the predominant cell is the polymorphonuclear cell, (2) CSF creatine phosphokinase activity—this is of prognostic value; higher values (>1 sigma units/ml) are associated with poor prognoses, (3) antibody titers to canine distemper, feline infectious peritonitis, and toxoplasmosis, which may indicate active infection, and (4) a strong, positive reaction to the Pandy's test indicates elevated CSF protein, mostly of the globulin fraction.

Radiography. Radiographs of the skull are generally only helpful in cases of head trauma or intracranial neoplasia. Fractures or superficial tumors that may be treated surgically are rarely identified. However, most patients with seizure disorders have normal survey radiographs of the skull. Contrast procedures using a positive or negative medium may outline the dilated ventricles of hydrocephalus. Angiography may reveal abnormal vascular patterns in neoplasms, hematomas, and infarctions but is not used routinely. Survey thoracic radiographs may occasionally disclose evidence of primary or metastatic neoplasia that may be related to CNS neoplasia.

For selected cases and usually only at referral institutions where specialized equipment is available, electroencephalography and scintigraphy may confirm a working diagnosis. Each procedure is relatively safe and noninvasive.

This introduction represents only a summary of the information available on seizure disorders in companion animals. Thorough reports of the pathophysiology, description, and diagnosis of seizures have been published previously, and readers are encouraged to consult the references listed at the end of this article.

CHRONIC MEDICAL THERAPY OF SEIZURE DISORDERS

INDICATIONS FOR THERAPY

If specifically treatable intra- or extracranial diseases have been ruled out during the diagnostic evaluation, one must assume that a nonprogressive seizure disorder exists. The remaining discussion will pertain only to canine and feline patients with a seizure disorder of this type.

The many factors influencing the decision to begin therapy can be placed in two groups: patient factors and client factors. Patient factors are as follows.

Seizure Frequency. It is not necessary to begin continued anticonvulsant therapy in a young patient that has experienced only one seizure. Rather, establish that a pattern of repetitive seizures exists before making a long-term commitment to therapy. Patients with seizures that occur more than once monthly or patients that have clusters of seizures are candidates for extended therapy.

Character of the Various Seizure Phases. If the seizures are particularly objectionable, such as psychomotor seizures during which the patient becomes vicious, or if the pre- and postictal phases are characterized by intolerable changes in excretory habits, then control of the episodes must be attempted.

Perhaps more important than the patient factors are the client factors. Be sure to inform the owner of all the ramifications of seizure disorders and continued anticonvulsant therapy. Frequently, owners interpret anticonvulsant therapy as curative. The definition of successful management of most veterinary patients is a reduction in the severity, frequency, and, possibly, duration of seizures. Although a majority of patients will improve with drug therapy, 20 to 30 per cent will never be controlled despite intensive medical treatment. Each patient must be treated individually, and many medication changes may be required to reach optimal control. If high dosages of drugs are required, the risk of developing drug-induced complications increases and must be weighed against the benefits of therapy. Explain to the client that once therapy has begun, the prescribed dosage schedule must be followed *exactly*, usually for the life of the patient. Be sure the client understands that the drugs most commonly used must be given two to four times every day, regardless of the inconvenience. Moreover, the cost of the drugs can be considerable. Polydipsia, polyuria, and sometimes polyphagia and weight gain are expected side effects of all the commonly used anticonvulsant drugs. With barbiturate derivatives, personality changes are common. These considerations must be made clear to the owner before initiating therapy so that maximal owner compliance can be achieved.

PRIMARY ANTICONVULSANT DRUGS

In keeping with the goal of anticonvulsant therapy, the perfect drug should control seizures without toxic effects. Many drugs are available to treat the large variety of seizure disorders that occur in humans. Because a vast majority of seizures seen in companion animals are of the generalized, grand mal type, the drugs found efficacious for these seizures in humans are the most commonly used anticonvulsant drugs in animals. The recommended dose ranges for dogs and cats and the desirable serum concentrations for humans are listed in Table 1.

PHENOBARBITAL

Phenobarbital (Luminal*) was the first barbiturate derivative approved for anticonvulsant use in humans. It has been found effective for generalized grand mal seizures as well as simple partial seizures. It acts by raising the threshold of electrical excitability and shortening the duration of afterdischarges in the motor cortex. Thus, the overall effect is to suppress the spontaneous electrical discharges and, to a limited extent, prevent their spread to other areas of the brain. It is interesting to note that phenobarbital is the most effective of the primary anticonvulsants in delaying the progressive intensification of seizure activity known as "kindling." Experimental evidence suggests that repeated application of certain drugs or an electrical stimulus to the cerebral cortex induces changes in excitability that facilitate the development of recurrent seizures. This implies that the probability of establishing repetitive seizures increases with each episode. It is not known with certainty whether "kindling" occurs in spontaneous seizure disorders; however, human patients seem to be more effectively controlled when anticonvulsant therapy is started early.

Biotransformation of phenobarbital to inactive metabolites that are excreted in the urine takes place in the microsomal enzyme fraction of the liver. The elimination half-life has been found to be 36 to 46 hours in the dog; data are not available for the cat. With continued oral administration of phenobarbital, effective steady-state serum and tissue concen-

*Winthrop Laboratories, New York, NY.

Table 1. *Drugs, Dosages (Animal), and Therapeutic Serum Concentrations (Human) of Anticonvulsant Drugs*

Drug	Dose Range Dog	Dose Range Cat	Therapeutic Serum Concentration (μg/ml)
Phenobarbital	1–6 mg/kg/day divided b.i.d. or t.i.d.	1–3 mg/kg/day divided b.i.d. or t.i.d.	10–30
Primidone*	10–25 mg/kg b.i.d.	—	10–30 (phenobarbital metabolite)
Phenytoin†	50–80 mg/kg t.i.d.	2–3 mg/kg/day; 20 mg/kg/week	10–20
Carbamazepine‡	4–8 mg/kg b.i.d.	—	5–10
Valproic acid‡	75–200 mg/kg t.i.d.	—	50–100
Diazepam	5–15 mg t.i.d.	2.5–5.0 mg t.i.d.	—

*Not approved for use in cats.
†Not approved or recommended for use in cats (see page 750).
‡Not approved for use in dogs or cats.

trations are achieved only after seven days. As a result, there is a lag period during which there is limited anticonvulsant efficacy. To expedite therapeutic effect, the recommended dosages of 1 to 6 mg/kg/day for the dog and 1 to 3 mg/kg/day for the cat divided b.i.d. or t.i.d. may be doubled for the first four days. Unfortunately, the anticipated side effects of sedation, ataxia, polydipsia, and polyuria may be especially marked during the loading period, making this practice undesirable. These side effects generally diminish with time even with continued administration.

Despite the long-standing availability of phenobarbital, little is known about its metabolism. Although it is a controlled substance, it is a safe, inexpensive, effective anticonvulsant for the dog and is *the* drug of choice in cats. I do not feel that the drug classification of phenobarbital should discourage its use as the first drug chosen for a seizure control regimen.

PRIMIDONE

Primidone (Mylepsin*) is a desoxybarbiturate that is metabolized by the microsomal enzyme fraction of the liver to phenobarbital and phenylethylmalonamide (PEMA). All three components have inherent anticonvulsant activity and contribute to the efficacy of the drug. With repeated dosing, the phenobarbital fraction accumulates and the remaining fractions do not. It is likely that phenobarbital is responsible for most of the anticonvulsant activity of primidone. Like phenobarbital, primidone generally causes polydipsia, polyuria, and polyphagia and may cause personality changes in certain patients.

Primidone is approved for use only in the dog. It is not a controlled substance but is five to ten times more expensive than phenobarbital at beginning recommended dosages (10 mg/kg b.i.d.). When primidone is administered in doses less than 50 mg/kg/day, three to four weeks must elapse before serum concentrations of the phenobarbital metabolite reach the therapeutic range established for human patients (see Table 1). Nevertheless, clinical improvement generally occurs well before the end of this period.

PHENYTOIN

Of the three primary anticonvulsant drugs traditionally used in veterinary medicine, phenytoin (Dilantin†) has received the most attention recently

*Fort Dodge Laboratories, Fort Dodge, IA.
†Parke-Davis, Morris Plains, NJ.

because of several interesting experimental studies. In humans, phenytoin is degraded to parahydroxy metabolites and has a half-life of 22 hours. In contrast, in dogs phenytoin is rapidly transformed to primarily a metahydroxy metabolite and has a half-life of four hours. The biotransformational reactions take place in the microsomal enzyme fraction of the liver in both species. However, phenytoin stimulates its own degradation in the dog, a process that occurs in humans only at high dosages. It is possible that the metahydroxylation step in dogs occurs more rapidly than the parahydroxylation step in humans, which may also contribute to the difference in phenytoin half-life in the two species. Since brain concentrations of phenytoin are directly related to serum levels, phenytoin is of questionable efficacy as an anticonvulsant because serum levels cannot be maintained. To achieve and sustain effective blood levels of phenytoin in the dog based on human therapeutic ranges, 60 to 100 mg/kg t.i.d. must be given. Unfortunately, studies to determine the dose and serum level of phenytoin necessary to protect against chemically or electrically induced seizures have not been done in the dog. Cardiac arrhythmias caused by digitalis intoxication in dogs can be suppressed with phenytoin at a serum concentration of 10 μg/ml. Whether a similar serum concentration would be effective in anticonvulsant therapy is not known. Only one study in dogs has been reported correlating successful therapy using 6.6 to 11 mg/kg t.i.d. with serum concentrations of 1.5 to 3.0 μg/ml.

Phenytoin acts by stabilizing neuronal membranes and subduing the spread of electrical activity from the seizure focus. There is a negligible effect on the focus itself. Although phenytoin has been in use for years, many clinicians consider it inadequate. Not until recently, however, were there experimental data to support these observations. Some individuals improve with phenytoin therapy, perhaps because of individual variation in biotransformation of the drug. However, I cannot recommend it as an effective anticonvulsant drug because of its short half-life and the unreasonable dosages required.

Pharmacokinetic studies of phenytoin in cats have revealed a plasma half-life that varies from 41.5 hours in kittens to 24 to 108 hours in adult cats. Signs of toxicity developed with low daily doses of phenytoin and were associated with high plasma concentrations. Because of these findings, phenytoin is considered unsuitable as an anticonvulsant drug for cats unless it is given at 2 to 3 mg/kg/day or 20 mg/kg/week and suspended as soon as sedation, ataxia, or anorexia is noticed.

MISCELLANEOUS PRIMARY ANTICONVULSANT DRUGS

PARAMETHADIONE

The main indication for use of paramethadione (Paradione*) in humans is petit mal seizures. The drug has also been found effective against experimentally induced seizures in dogs. For this reason, a pilot study was designed in 1975 using canine seizure patients uncontrolled with conventional therapy and seizure patients not receiving drugs. Sixty five per cent of the previously uncontrolled patients improved, and the response in the new patients was similar to that achieved with traditional anticonvulsants (70 per cent improvement). Paramethadione has not been stringently studied in dogs and cannot be recommended until more information is available.

CARBAMAZEPINE

Although carbamazepine (Tegretol†) is the first drug of choice for trigeminal neuralgia in humans, it has been found to be as effective as phenytoin in the treatment of grand mal seizures and psychomotor seizures. Both the parent drug and its main metabolite, carbamazepine-10,11-epoxide, have potent anticonvulsant activity. The half-life of the drug decreases from 35 hours to 10 to 20 hours with repetitive administration. The recommended starting dosage is 100 to 200 mg b.i.d., but because there is marked tendency for the drug to stimulate its own degradation, the dosage must be increased to maintain optimum serum concentrations (see Table 1). The most common side effects are bone marrow depression and, occasionally, hepatitis. There is no sedation with carbamazepine as there frequently is with phenobarbital and phenytoin in humans.

Recently, carbamazepine has been evaluated in dogs as both a liquid and a tablet. The liquid was absorbed rapidly, but serum concentrations were variable and declined rapidly (half-life of one to two hours). As in humans, dogs transform the parent drug to the epoxide metabolite, but serum levels of both compounds decrease considerably with repeated administration. Because of these characteristics, carbamazepine has not been found to be suitable for extended anticonvulsant therapy in dogs.

Carbamazepine has not been evaluated in cats.

---

*Abbott Laboratories, North Chicago, IL.
†Geigy Pharmaceuticals, Ardsley, NY.

VALPROIC ACID

Over the past few years since its approval in 1978, valproic acid (VPA) (Depakene*) has shown considerable promise in the treatment of various types of epilepsy in humans. Pharamacologic characteristics of the drug in dogs are different from those in humans. The average half-life in dogs is 2.8 hours, and it does not change with prolonged treatment, in contrast to phenytoin. In addition to VPA, two metabolites found in the plasma of dogs have anticonvulsant activity. Moreover, there is less protein binding of VPA in dogs than in humans, which allows greater concentrations of the free, active drug to enter the CNS. These two factors suggest that lower dosages, and thus lower serum levels, might be sufficient to control seizures in dogs. However, because of its short half-life, VPA must be given either at very high dosages or very frequently to maintain a steady serum concentration.

In a recent clinical study of 57 canine seizure patients, VPA (30 to 40 mg/kg/day) was added to the existing therapy of phenytoin and phenobarbital or primidone or was given alone or in combination with phenobarbital. The most improvement was observed in dogs treated with a combination of VPA and phenobarbital. Serum concentrations were not evaluated, so conclusions about adequacy of the dosage cannot be made. On the basis of the canine pharmacology of VPA and using the accepted human therapeutic serum ranges (see Table 1), the estimated dosage of VPA alone needed to achieve effective levels is 220 mg/kg t.i.d. If the increased serum level of phenobarbital in the presence of VPA observed in humans occurs in dogs, then the improvement observed in the dogs treated at the lower dosage of VPA in the clinical study may be a result of this effect.

A distinct advantage of VPA as an anticonvulsant drug is that the half-life does not decrease with chronic administration. However, until more experimental work with VPA has been done in dogs, we can only speculate on the dosage, serum therapeutic ranges, efficacy, and long-term side effects.

The clinical usefulness of VPA in cats has not been investigated.

COMBINATIONS OF DRUGS

It is preferable to begin therapy with one drug, usually phenobarbital or primidone, and wait for three seizure cycles before assessing the effectiveness of the treatment. If there has been no improvement, increase the dosage and wait. If there still is no improvement, consider adding other drugs. Always begin at the lower end of the dose range, then increase the dose when necessary. Some patients cannot be controlled with one drug, and some respond to one drug and not another, even if they are of the same class of drugs and are given in adequate dosages.

The use of combination preparations such as Dilantin with phenobarbital or Mebroin* (60 mg phenytoin plus 90 mg mephobarbital per tablet) is not advisable. Separate preparations allow you to treat each patient more accurately.

If you need to change therapy and wish to withdraw a drug completely, DO NOT make sudden changes. This is especially important when using the barbiturate derivatives, which cause habituation. When these drugs are stopped abruptly, seizures may become more severe and more difficult to control or may progress to *status epilepticus*. To be safe, reduce the dosage by 30 per cent every seven days. This rule of thumb also applies to patients whose dosages you are reducing to the minimum maintenance level after a period of satisfactory control, usually six months to one year.

SUMMARY

The two drugs that remain effective for seizures in dogs are phenobarbital and primidone. Recent experimental studies of phenytoin in both dogs and cats have shown it to be unsatisfactory for various pharmacologic reasons. The limited information available on newer drugs, such as carbamazepine and valproic acid, is an insufficient basis on which to make recommendations. Phenobarbital remains the drug of choice for seizure disorders of cats. Single agents are preferable, but combinations of drugs may be necessary.

SECONDARY OR ADJUNCT ANTICONVULSANT DRUGS

DIAZEPAM

If the preictal phase is long enough and clearly demarcated, you can use diazepam (Valium†) during that time in both dogs and cats to reduce the severity of the coming seizure. The usual starting dose is 2.5 to 15 mg t.i.d. As a primary anticonvulsant, diazepam has not been useful because of expense, controlled drug classification, and short half-life. Its primary indication is in the treatment of *status epilepticus*, which will be discussed later.

---

*Winthrop Laboratories, New York, NY.
†Roche Laboratories, Nutley, NJ.

COMPLICATIONS OF CHRONIC THERAPY

Much has been learned about the many adverse effects of chronic anticonvulsant therapy in humans in recent years. The factors that influence the development of these problems are duration of therapy; use of multiple drugs, perhaps at high dosages; and failure to recognize subtle evidence of toxicity.

Similar complications may occur in animals since the same anticonvulsant drugs are used in their treatment as in human therapy. However, animals seem to be remarkably resistant to most of the toxic effects seen in humans. For this reason, only the complications that have been reported or that I have seen will be discussed. No adverse effects were recognized in the few cats that underwent long-term anticonvulsant therapy examined at the NYSCVM, so the following discussion pertains only to dogs.

ENZYME INDUCTION

Phenobarbital, primidone, and phenytoin belong to the group of compounds capable of altering the activity of the metabolizing enzymes located in the smooth endoplasmic reticulum of the liver. The biotransformation of both endogenous and exogenous compounds can be accelerated by this process of *enzyme induction*. Substances given concurrently with anticonvulsants will be metabolized more rapidly, resulting in lower serum concentrations of the parent drug. Some drugs, including phenytoin and carbamazepine, given chronically will stimulate their own degradation as well. In addition, endogenous compounds such as cortisol are affected, leading to stimulation of ACTH and adrenal hypertrophy. Enzyme induction has been implicated in the pathogenesis of such drug-induced complications as folate deficiency and metabolic bone disease in humans.

Membrane-bound enzymes other than drug-metabolizing enzymes can also be induced by the anticonvulsant drugs. The best example is alkaline phosphatase (AP) of hepatic origin. Elevated serum AP activity not related to hepatic injury can be expected within one month of initiating anticonvulsant therapy. Because the AP isoenzyme induced by the anticonvulsants is the same as that associated with hepatic injury, it is difficult to distinguish the benign drug-induced effect from a more serious hepatotoxic reaction without the benefit of other tests of liver function.

When more than one anticonvulsant drug is used, drug interactions can be expected. Concurrent administration of phenytoin and a barbiturate derivative in humans results in lower serum concentrations of phenytoin and higher concentrations of phenobarbital than when either is administered alone. This does not appear to be of clinical significance. Similar studies have not been done in dogs, but the successful use of phenytoin/bariturate combinations is probably attributable to the barbiturate contribution in most cases. In addition, as mentioned before, the metabolism of phenytoin is too rapid to be of long-term benefit, especially in the presence of a barbiturate.

The activity of drug-metabolizing enzymes can be inhibited by certain compounds. For example, administration of chloramphenicol in addition to phenytoin or phenobarbital results in accumulation of the anticonvulsant drug and clinical signs of toxicity (sedation, ataxia, prolonged anesthesia).

FOLATE DEFICIENCY

Megaloblastic anemia caused by folate deficiency is seen in 0.15 to 0.75 per cent of human seizure patients. It is most commonly associated with the administration of phenytoin and can occur at any time after initiation of therapy. Folate concentrations are classically subnormal in the serum, RBCs, and CSF. The condition can be reversed with folic acid supplementation, using 1 to 2 mg/day. I have observed megaloblastic anemia, leukopenia, and thrombocytopenia in dogs given phenytoin experimentally. Because seizures may be aggravated in some human patients given folic acid for megaloblastic anemia, folic acid must be used cautiously.

GINGIVAL HYPERPLASIA

The most common chronic toxic effect of phenytoin therapy in humans is gingival hyperplasia, occurring in as many as 50 per cent of treated patients. Periodontal disease or other diseases caused by poor oral hygiene aggravate the gingival hyperplasia. The hyperplasia will regress within six months if phenytoin is discontinued and secondary infection is controlled. Gingival hyperplasia was reported in a dog receiving 100 mg b.i.d. of phenytoin for three years. I have not recognized this complication caused by phenytoin in dogs.

HEPATOTOXICITY

Liver disease caused by anticonvulsant drug therapy in humans is most commonly associated with phenytoin. Phenytoin hepatotoxicity has been determined to be an idiosyncratic hypersensitivity reaction resulting in lesions varying from mild cholestatic hepatitis to massive hepatic necrosis. In a published review of 23 human cases, 17 (74 per cent) developed signs of hepatotoxicity within six weeks of starting therapy and nine (39 per cent) subsequently died.

Published reports of hepatic injury associated with anticonvulsant therapy in dogs are rare. Reports of single cases of toxic reactions caused by primidone and phenytoin suggest that these are idiosyncratic drug reactions. Cirrhosis of the liver was diagnosed at the NYSCVM in five dogs that received primidone alone or in combination with other anticonvulsant drugs for two to three years. Increased activities of AP, alanine aminotransferase (ALT), and BSP retention may be observed in as many as 50 per cent of seizure patients receiving anticonvulsant therapy. This may represent a tolerable degree of hepatic injury. However, *severe* hepatic disease occurs much less frequently.

Hepatic function should be evaluated before and every six months after starting anticonvulsant therapy. Increased serum gamma glutamyl transferase activity (GGT) (>2 to 4 IU/L), bile acid retention (>10 μmol/L), and BSP retention (>5 per cent at 30 minutes) suggest hepatic dysfunction. When this occurs, the anticonvulsant drug dosages should be reduced to the minimum needed to control seizures. In the presence of liver disease, the metabolism of the primary anticonvulsants is delayed and toxicity could result if dosages are not decreased. More importantly, the drugs may be the cause of the liver disease.

ACUTE MEDICAL THERAPY—STATUS EPILEPTICUS

Repeated seizures within a short period of time and without recovery constitute *status epilepticus*. The neuronal damage, hyperthermia, acidosis, and possible cardiac arrhythmias that occur during *status epilepticus* may cause death unless the seizures are stopped. Thus, *status epilepticus* is a true medical emergency.

The following diagnostic and therapeutic approach is recommended.

1. If there is not too much muscular activity, place an indwelling intravenous catheter, not only to administer medications but to draw blood samples for laboratory analysis. *If possible*, collect a blood sample for determination of glucose and calcium concentrations.

2. To stop the seizures, give diazepam, 5 to 20 mg intravenously depending on the size of the patient. Slow test boluses of glucose and calcium gluconate may be given first to determine whether hypoglycemia or hypocalcemia is causative. If not and if one bolus of diazepam is inadequate, repeat the diazepam every ten minutes for three doses.

3. If diazepam is not sufficient, give pentobarbital slowly to effect. The onset of action of pentobarbital is faster than that of phenobarbital, although phenobarbital has more anticonvulsant activity.

4. Ensure a patent airway, using an endotracheal tube if necessary. Regulate body temperature, acid-

base balance, electrolyte status, fluid balance, and cardiovascular integrity.

5. Once the seizures are controlled, the remaining diagnostic tests may be pursued. Remember not to make definitive judgments about neurologic status until the patient is fully recovered, which may be days.

6. During recovery, phenobarbital may be given intramuscularly in low doses (0.5 mg/kg t.i.d.) to provide anticonvulsant effects. When the patient is able to swallow, switch to oral phenobarbital at the usual recommended dosages.

7. Occasional seizure activity during recovery is acceptable. Do not attempt to stop it completely, because oversedation may be dangerous.

SUMMARY OF RECOMMENDATIONS

For chronic therapy of both canine and feline seizure patients, the following recommendations are given.

1. Start with phenobarbital at the low end of the recommended dose range. Wait for three seizure cycles before determining the efficacy of your regimen. You can increase the dose of phenobarbital to the high end of the suggested range before deciding that it is ineffective.

2. If phenobarbital is considered ineffective, add primidone (dogs only) at the low end of the dose range. You can increase it if necessary.

3. Consider adding phenytoin only if phenobarbital and primidone have not been effective. Other unapproved drugs may be tried only with the informed consent of the owner.

4. Recheck your patient every six months, evaluating the drug regimen, the seizure history, hematology, and, especially, liver function. After a period of *satisfactory* control, usually six months to one year, you may attempt to gradually reduce the amount of drugs given.

5. Maximal seizure control has been improved in human patients through the use of established serum concentrations of anticonvulsant drugs (see Table 1). Although this information is not available for dogs and cats, cautious reference to human values combined with clinical assessment may be useful. The serum sample for such analysis should be collected immediately before a scheduled dose.

6. Because most seizures in cats seen at the NYSCVM have been caused by organic diseases, there is little information available on prognosis and side effects of long-term therapy in cats with nonprogressive seizure disorders.

7. Euthanasia must remain as an option for owners who choose not to start or continue a lifelong commitment to a dog with seizures.

SUPPLEMENTAL READING

Holliday, T. A.: Seizure disorders. Vet. Clin. North Am. 10:3, 1980.

Kay, W. J.: Epilepsy in cats. J.A.A.H.A. 11:77, 1975.

Loscher, W.: Plasma levels of valproic acid and its metabolites during continued treatment in dogs. J. Vet. Pharmacol. Therap. 4:111, 1981.

Oliver, J. E.: Seizure disorders in companion animals. Comp. Cont. Ed. 2:77, 1980.

Prichard, J. W.: Phenobarbital: Introduction. *In*, Glaser, G. H., Penry, J. K., and Woodbury, D. M. (eds.): *Antiepileptic Drugs: Mechanisms of Action.* New York: Raven Press, 1980, pp. 473–491.

Roye, D. B., Serrano, E. E., Hammer, R. H., and Wilder, B. J.: Plasma kinetics of diphenylhydantoin in dogs and cats. Am. J. Vet. Res. 34:947, 1973.

Russo, M. E.: The pathophysiology of epilepsy. Cornell Vet. 71:221, 1981.

Shepherd, D. E., and de Lahunta, A.: Central nervous system disease in the cat. Comp. Cont. Ed. 2:306, 1980.

Woodbury, D. M., Penry, J. K., and Schmidt, R. P. (eds.): *Antiepileptic Drugs.* New York: Raven Press, 1972.

Yeary, R. A.: Serum concentrations of primidone and its metabolites, phenylethylmalonamide and phenobarbital, in the dog. Am. J. Vet. Res. 41:1643, 1980.

DIAGNOSIS AND TREATMENT OF NARCOLEPSY IN ANIMALS

THEODORE L. BAKER, Ph.D.,
Stanford, California

MERRILL M. MITLER, Ph.D.,
Stony Brook, New York

ARTHUR S. FOUTZ, Ph.D.,
CNRS, France

and WILLIAM C. DEMENT, M.D., Ph.D.
Stanford, California

The first International Symposium on Narcolepsy (La Grande Motte, France, 1975) made the following conclusion:

Narcolepsy refers to a syndrome of unknown origin that is characterized by abnormal sleep tendencies including excessive daytime sleepiness and often disturbed nocturnal sleep and pathological manifestations of REM sleep. The REM sleep abnormalities include sleep onset REM periods and the dissociated REM sleep inhibitory processes; cataplexy and sleep paralysis and hypnagogic hallucinations are the major symptoms of the disease.

Thus, narcolepsy is a well-defined neurologic disorder that can be evaluated by clinical polysomnographic techniques. Current estimates suggest that as many as 250,000 Americans suffer from narcolepsy. The most problematic symptoms in humans are excessive daytime somnolence (EDS) and cataplexy. EDS is manifested as abrupt, irresistible "sleep attacks" and as continuous sleepiness that waxes and wanes throughout the day. Cataplectic attacks are sudden episodes of flaccid paralysis, usually associated in humans with laughter or other affective behaviors. Symptoms range from mild to extremely disabling. Treatment of human patients is tailored to individual needs and typically involves the use of central nervous system stimulants to control somnolence (e.g., amphetamine-type compounds and methylphenidate) and tricyclic antidepressants to control REM sleep–related symptoms such as cataplexy (e.g., protriptyline and imipramine).

Knecht and colleagues in 1973 and Mitler and colleagues in 1974 independently reported a syndrome in the dog that resembles human nacrolepsy. These discoveries prompted a research group at Stanford University to begin acquisition of narcoleptic animals for research into ontogenetic, pharmacologic, physiologic, electrographic, and hereditary issues associated with this canine disorder.

Since 1974, over 100 narcoleptic dogs have been studied in the Stanford Canine Narcolepsy Research Project. More than 18 purebred and mixed-breed dogs have been diagnosed as having the disease including the poodle, Doberman pinscher, dachshund, beagle, wire-haired griffon, Saint Bernard, cocker spaniel, Welsh corgi, Labrador retriever, Irish setter, and cockapoo. At present, the Stanford Canine Narcolepsy Colony is composed of over 30 affected animals, including a stable breeding population used for genetic studies.

In collaboration with Dr. T. A. Holliday and other colleagues at the University of California at Davis School of Veterinary Medicine, the Stanford group has also studied several ponies and a miniature horse with a syndrome clinically identical to that affecting dogs. Collectively these data suggest that narcolepsy in animals is far more prevalent than could have been predicted from a review of the veterinary literature. Furthermore, records suggest that animals affected with narcolepsy, like human patients, are frequently misdiagnosed during their initial clinical encounters.

CLINICAL SIGNS

The clearest clinical sign of narcolepsy in canines and equines is cataplexy. Cataplectic episodes frequently are precipitated by play or the pursuit of desired goals such as food, water, or sex. Cataplexy can also occur in what appears to be a spontaneous fashion. Age at onset of first cataplexy symptoms

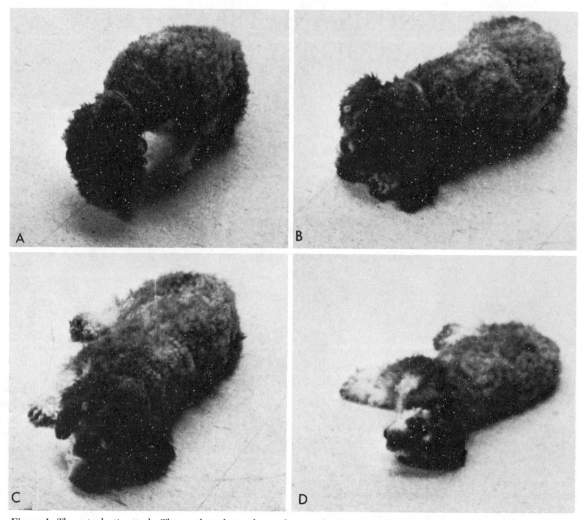

Figure 1. The cataplectic attack. These selected time-lapse photographs (from a series shot during an interval of approximately 2500 msec) show the development of a cataplectic episode in an adult female miniature poodle. The attack begins with hind limb flaccidity *(A)* that spreads to the forelimbs *(B)* and neck *(C)*. In *D*, the dog has regained some head and neck control and has managed to look at the photographer.

varies from a few weeks to several years. Cataplectic attacks are characterized by: (1) rapid onset and termination; (2) partial to complete flaccid paralysis, which may involve all skeletal musculature or may be localized to the front or hind quarters (Fig. 1); (3) variable duration (ranging from a few seconds to more than 20 minutes); (4) no impairment of vegetative function; and (5) simultaneous occurrence of REM sleep–like phasic events such as rapid eye movements, twitches of distal musculature, weak vocalizations, and facial grimaces. A "cataplectic fugue-state" may occur at the beginning or end of a complete cataplectic attack, during which the patient is unable to move but seems to be aware of the surroundings and may be able to perform limited motor activities such as chewing, tail wagging, and visual tracking.

Cataplectic episodes are reversible in nature. Petting the patient or making loud, startling noises can terminate an attack and reinstitute normal locomotor behavior. In some cases attack frequency is less than one per day, but other animals may experience hundreds of paralytic episodes daily. Frequently the client may report that the patient has "bad days and good days." This may be related to changes in routine such as a bath, automobile ride, or visit to the veterinary clinic. In general, intimidating or novel situations decrease the frequency of attacks.

Electroencephalographic evidence in dogs suggests that narcoleptic canines also have symptoms of excessive somnolence. Narcoleptic dogs, when given multiple opportunities to sleep interspersed with longer periods of wakefulness—such as 30 minutes of enforced wakefulness alternated with 30 minutes of *ad libitum* sleep—differ from control dogs with respect to the rapidity with which they fall asleep. Futhermore, once sleep begins narcoeptic animals show an increased tendency to have REM sleep shortly after sleep onset. This observation is consistent with analogous observations in human narcoleptic patients.

FAMILY HISTORY

The client may disclose that the patient's littermates, parents, or other less closely related relatives had shown similar cataplectic behavior. The evidence for a hereditary component to canine narcolepsy is strong for Doberman pinschers and Labrador retrievers. The Stanford colony has successfully produced 61 viable affected offspring in 11 litters (eight litters Doberman-Doberman cross, two litters Doberman-Labrador cross; one litter Labrador-Labrador cross). When both parents are narcoleptic, all pups in the litter are affected. These direct breeding experiments, coupled with evidence derived from the extremely positive family history in the dogs' pedigrees, suggest that transmission occurs via the same autosomal recessive gene in the Doberman and Labrador breeds (Baker et al., 1982).

Breedings in affected poodles and beagles have yielded three litters of each breed, but none of the offspring to date have developed symptoms. This finding suggests that there may be both genetic and nongenetic etiologies in canine narcolepsy. Other observations support this hypothesis. Narcoleptic Dobermans and Labradors invariably display the first symptoms between one and four months of age. In these apparently genetically transmitted cases, cataplexy symptoms are severe early in life but are ameliorated to varying degrees in adulthood. In the 16 assorted breeds for which no positive family history has been established, age of onset varies from ten weeks to seven years with no consistent pattern within any given breed. When precise observations were possible it was noted that the disease developed quite abruptly and symptoms usually stabilized within a week. Afterward, little change in severity of symptoms was observed throughout the patient's life.

These findings suggest that there may be several forms of canine narcolepsy with different etiologies: (1) an inheritable form involving a single-allele recessive mechanism; (2) a noninheritable type that may be related to neurologic accidents during fetal or pubescent development; and (3) more complex patterns of inheritance, such as multiple genes or incomplete penetrance, which could account for the negative genetic findings in some dog breeds.

Although the severity of symptoms, age of onset, and genetic mechanisms differ considerably in the various canine breeds, the clinical picture is otherwise remarkably similar. In all dogs, the cataplectic attacks appear identical to an observer, they are elicited by similar appetitive behaviors, and they respond in the same fashion to drug interventions.

CLINICAL TESTING

The clinician may elect to do clinical tests to confirm the presumptive diagnosis of narcolepsy. Assessment of excessive somnolence presents unique technical problems in canine patients, since this requires long-term electrographic recordings of freely moving animals. The situation is complicated by the fact that normal dogs spend over 50 per cent of their lives asleep and have extremely fragmented sleep-waking cycles. Therefore, it would be extremely difficult to demonstrate pathologic levels of sleepiness in the usual clinical setting.

Assessment of cataplexy involves more straightforward procedures. Tests should be aimed at distinguishing cataplexy from epileptic phenomena and from other flaccid, reversible paralytic disorders such as myasthenia and hypokalemia. In such diagnostic tests the clinician must be certain that any changes in the frequency or duration of paralytic episodes are due to experimental factors that can be controlled and not due to changes in environment or the stress of drug administration.

It is important to determine whether any ancillary epileptiform behavior is present during suspected paralytic episodes. During cataplexy there is no fecal or urinary incontinence; there is no excessive salivation; and there is no tonic rigidity of musculature. In addition, animals suspected of having narcolepsy should not show significant improvement with anticonvulsants such as phenytoin or phenobarbital. To rule out myasthenia, the condition of suspected animals should not worsen with repetitive electrical stimulation of the limb or improve with anticholinesterases given in sufficient doses to produce peripheral effects.

Pharmacologic provocative testing is often used by the Stanford research group to assist in establishing a diagnosis of narcolepsy in canines and equines. Anticholinesterase compounds that cross the blood-brain barrier dramatically increase both frequency and duration of cataplectic attacks in narcoleptic patients but have no effect on normal animals. For example, physostigmine salicylate given IV in a single dose ranging from 0.025 to 0.10 mg/kg, in combination with an appropriate behavioral test, consistently induces cataplectic attacks in susceptible patients. This procedure may be useful for screening a mildly affected patient that may otherwise exhibit only subtle or infrequent cataplectic episodes and shows no spontaneous symptoms in the clinic. The actual protocol for behavioral testing can vary, depending on the pattern of clinical signs presented by the patient. Several minutes of controlled observation during play with other animals might suffice for certain patients. For others, quantifying attacks during the eating of a specified amount of food may be useful.

TREATMENT

Few data are available on long-term treatment regimens for narcolepsy in animals. In narcoleptic humans pharmacologic interventions are divided into two groups: therapy to control excessive somnolence and therapy to control cataplexy.

In treating animals, the control of excessive somnolence may not be a high clinical priority. Of greater concern to the client may be cataplectic episodes. In some cases it may be possible to satisfy the client by explaining that cataplexy is not, in and of itself, a life-threatening problem to the patient and instructing the client to avoid placing the patient in situations in which cataplexy could become a dangerous liability (e.g., hunting and roaming in dangerous terrain). Clients may express concern because cataplectic attacks often occur during eating and drinking. At Stanford, behavioral testing usually involves presentation of food pieces, but episodes of upper airway obstruction have never been observed during eating; swallowing and cough reflexes appear to be intact during cataplexy. Finally, patients that present with severe cataplexy during the first few months of life may experience a substantial amelioration of symptoms as adults, in a manner analogous to the Stanford Doberman and Labrador populations.

Client education may be supplemented with therapeutic trials of stimulants such as methylphenidate. Available data on these drugs in dogs can only confirm short-term efficacy. The use of methylphenidate to control cataplexy in humans is not thought to be of permanent effectiveness. There are no long-term data available for antidepressant compounds or stimulating compounds in the treatment of narcoplepsy in animals.

One treatment that is strongly contraindicated in narcolepsy is the use of inhibitors of the enzyme monoamine oxidase (MAOI), despite their high anticataplectic potency. MAOI drugs such as pargyline and phenelzine have been discontinued in humans because they have dangerous cardiovascular side effects when the diet contains tyramine. Furthermore, studies at Stanford suggest that narcoleptic canines may be much more susceptible to harmful side effects of MAOI compounds than normal animals.

SELECTING PROPER DOSE LEVELS

The optimum dose levels for drugs that control cataplexy are not readily definable. For humans the physician titrates anticataplectic and stimulant drugs to individual needs. The veterinary practitioner who chooses to treat narcolepsy must use an analogous titration procedure.

A reasonable beginning range for the anticataplectic compound imipramine is 0.5 to 1.0 mg/kg t.i.d. The only route of administration tested to date has been IV, but forms suitable for oral administration are available in various milligram levels. The practitioner should be aware of an important side effect in human males, impotency, which is thought to be related to the anticholinergic properties of imipramine.

A reasonable beginning range for methylphenidate is 0.25 mg/kg IV. For oral administration, appropriate divisions and multiples of 5-mg tablets may be tried. Methylphenidate has short-term anticataplectic properties and does not cause impotency; low doses are sometimes used to minimize cataplexy and facilitate natural breeding in the Stanford canine colony.

As a final point about dose level, the practitioner should not attempt to eliminate cataplexy completely, because the required dose levels may run dangerously high. Rather, some acceptable reduction in frequency and duration of cataplexy should be sought. A favorable treatment strategy is to instruct the client to administer anticataplectic medication intermittently only as the need arises. In this way, the canine patient could receive short-term benefit during an occasional trip away from home, for example, while minimizing the risk of developing tolerance to medications.

TREATMENT RATIONALE

The efficacy of imipramine in controlling cataplexy may derive from one or both of the following actions: (1) blockade of serotonin uptake, thus potentiating serotonergic mechanisms. Serotonin-containing neurons are thought by some theorists to control the REM sleep mechanisms and to sequester REM sleep episodes within relatively long periods of sleep; and (2) anticholinergic properties of the tricyclic antidepressant compounds, which may suppress the REM inhibitory processes.

Available evidence supports both of these hypotheses. Using gas chromatography–mass spectrometry, Faull and colleagues (1982) at Stanford developed data suggesting that narcoleptic poodles have a decreased concentration and a decreased turnover of serotonin. Additionally, they show a decreased turnover of norepinephrine and a decreased concentration of dopamine. Studies in progress at Stanford conducted by Mefford and coworkers (in press), using a more sensitive technique of regional neurochemical analysis, indicate that in Dobermans many brain regions have decreased turnover and/or utilization of dopamine.

These findings are consistent with pharmacologic

tudies directed by Foutz and associates (1982) that
how that several drugs that potentiate monoamine
ystems ameliorate cataplexy symptoms. Drugs such
s atropine and scopolamine that inhibit cholinergic
ystems also reduce cataplexy. Thus, it has become
ncreasingly clear that distinct neurochemical ab-
ormalities underlie the canine narcolepsy syn-
lrome. In some breeds these neurochemical prob-
ems are probably genetically determined, whereas
n other breeds analogous neurochemical aberra-
ions may be the consequence of neuropa-
hology later in life.

Finally, it should be noted that narcolepsy in all
nimals studied to date is an incurable neurologic
lisorder. In humans chemotherapies are useful in
controlling symptoms but are eventually only pallia-
ive. Thus, in severely affected animal patients that
present clinical management problems it may be
better to discuss the possibility of donating the
nimal for research purposes* rather than have the
client administer the various drug regimens and
manage the necessary periodic drug withdrawal
programs when tolerance develops to therapeutic
agents.

---

*Further information may be obtained from the Director,
Narcoleptic Dog Colony, Stanford University, (415) 497-9391,
497-9380, or 497-6601.

REFERENCES AND SUPPLEMENTARY READING

Babcock, D. A., Narver, E. L., Dement, W. C., and Mitler, M. M.: The
effects of imipramine chlorimipramine, and fluoxetine on cataplexy in
dogs. Pharmacol. Biochem. Behav. 5:599, 1976.

Baker, T. L., Foutz, A. S., McNerny, V., Mitler, M. M., and Dement,
W. C.: Canine model of narcolepsy: genetic and developmental deter-
minants. Exper. Neurol. 75:729, 1982.
Delashaw, J. B., Jr., Foutz, A., Guillemenault, C., and Dement, W. C.:
Cholinergic mechanisms and cataplexy in dogs. Exper. Neurol. 66:745,
1979.
Faull, K. F., Barchas, J. D., Foutz, A. S., Dement, W. C., and Holman,
R. B.: Monoamine metabolic concentrations in cerebrospinal fluid of
normal and narcoleptic dogs. Brain Res. 242:137, 1982.
Foutz, A. S., Delashaw, J. B., Jr., Guilleminault, C., and Dement, W.
C.: Monoaminergic mechanisms and experimental cataplexy. Ann.
Neurol. 10:369, 1982.
Foutz, A. S., Mitler, M. M., Cavalli-Sforza, L. L., and Dement, W. C.:
Genetic factors in canine narcolepsy. Sleep 1:413, 1979.
Foutz, A. S., Mitler, M. M., and Dement, W. C.: Narcolepsy. Vet. Clin.
North Am. 10:65, 1980.
Knecht, C. D., Oliver, J. E., Redding, R., Selcer, R., and Johnson, G.:
Narcolepsy in a dog and a cat. J.A.V.M.A. 162:1052, 1973.
Lucas, E. A., Foutz, A. S., Dement, W. C., and Mitler, M. M.: Sleep
cycle organization in narcoleptic and normal dogs. Physiol. Behav.
23:737, 1979.
Mefford, I. N., Baker, T. L., Boehme, R., Foutz, A. S., Ciaranello, R.,
Barchas, J. D., and Dement, W. C.: Narcolepsy: biogenic amine deficits
in an animal model. Science (in press).
Mitler, M. M.: Toward an animal model of canine narcolepsy-cataplexy.
In Guilleminault, C., Dement, W. C., and Passouant, P. (eds.):
Narcolepsy. Vol. 3 of Advances in Sleep Research. New York: Spectrum
Publications, 1976, pp. 387–410.
Mitler, M. M., Boysen, B. G., Campbell, L., and Dement, W. C.:
Narcolepsy-cataplexy in a female dog. Exper. Neurol. 45:332, 1974.
Mitler, M. M., and Dement, W. C.: Sleep studies on canine narcolepsy:
Pattern and cycle comparisons between affected and normal dogs.
Electroencephalogr. Clin. Neurophysiol. 43:691, 1977.
Mitler, M. M., and Dement, W. C.: Canine narcolepsy. *In* Andrews, E.,
Ward, B., and Altman, N. (eds.): *Spontaneous Animal Models of Human
Disease.* Vol. 2. New York: Academic Press, 1979, pp. 165–170.
Mitler, M. M., Soave, O., and Dement, W. C.: Narcolepsy in seven
dogs. J.A.V.M.A. 168:1036, 1976.

Section
10

GASTROINTESTINAL DISORDERS

DONALD R. STROMBECK, D.V.M.
Consulting Editor

DISORDERS OF GASTRIC RETENTION

DAVID C. TWEDT, D.V.M.

Fort Collins, Colorado

The retention of gastric contents results from either obstructive lesions associated with the antral or pyloric region or functional motility disorders. Intrinsic, extrinsic, or obturative lesions of the pylorus have been incriminated as the predominant cause of delayed gastric emptying. However, recent evidence suggests that gastric motility disorders may also be an important cause of gastric retention. Although physiologic concepts have been rapidly evolving, practical methods for the study and diagnosis of gastric motility problems in the dog and cat are yet to be developed. Currently, the diagnosis of motility disorders is made when gastric retention occurs in the absence of an outflow obstructive lesion.

NORMAL GASTRIC MOTILITY

The control and regulation of gastric emptying is a complex and controversial mechanism. Simplistically, the stomach can be divided into two distinct motor regions, each with a specific function. The proximal region includes the fundus, cardia, and body, which controls emptying of liquids. The proximal stomach acts as a reservoir, expanding to accommodate food. The passage of liquids from the stomach occurs when sustained or tonal contractions of this region press liquid contents into the pylorus for passage into the duodenum.

The distal stomach is composed of the antrum and pylorus, both of which act as a gastric grinder. This region allows liquids to empty and acts to retain solids in the stomach for further grinding. This is accomplished by antral peristalsis. Antral peristaltic waves press the solids forward against the pylorus. Unable to pass in a forward direction, the solids are ground together by an advancing peristaltic wave and are then retropelled backward to the more proximal stomach, only to be thrust forward again by the next peristaltic wave. This propulsion, grinding, and retropulsion occurs over and over again until solids are broken into particles of about 1 mm, which are passed through the pylorus.

Large, nondigestible particles (> 2 mm) are retained by the stomach during the digestive period. These particles are emptied during fasting by strong contractions known as special interdigestive "housekeeper" contractions.

The pylorus is the distalmost portion of the stomach. It is a muscular thickening continuous with the muscle layers of the antrum. Normally, the pyloric sphincter is open, closing only as an antral contraction reaches the pylorus. Controversy exists as to whether the pylorus has an actual sphincter function with a zone of increased pressure. The pylorus is important in limiting the emptying of solids but not liquids and in the prevention of the reflux of duodenal contents.

There is no normal rate of gastric emptying. Gastric emptying is regulated by dietary composition and by hormonal and neurologic influences. Liquids empty faster than solids. Diets comprised of carbohydrates empty faster than those comprised of protein; fats leave the stomach last.

DISORDERS OF MOTILITY

GASTRIC STASIS

Many factors reduce the motility of the stomach and result in retention of gastric contents (Fig. 1). When gastric retention persists, signs similar to those of an outflow obstruction occur, manifested predominantly by vomiting. The inhibition of gastric motility is generally mediated through the sympathetic nervous system. Acute stress, trauma, or psychogenic causes reduce the rate of gastric emptying. This clinical condition has been observed in animals without primary organic gastric disease. Once the precipitating cause is corrected, the signs abate. Primary gastric lesions also alter normal gastric motility. Gastric stasis can result from such conditions as gastritis, gastric ulcers, or serosal inflammation (peritonitis). Infiltrative lesions such as those seen with granulomatous or neoplastic disease impair normal gastric contractions and cause prolonged retention of gastric contents.

Hypokalemia as well as certain drugs have a direct effect on gastric motility. Anticholinergic agents commonly used for controlling vomiting markedly decrease gastric motility. The prolonged use of these drugs results in severe gastric atony with gastric retention. It is not unusual for overuse of

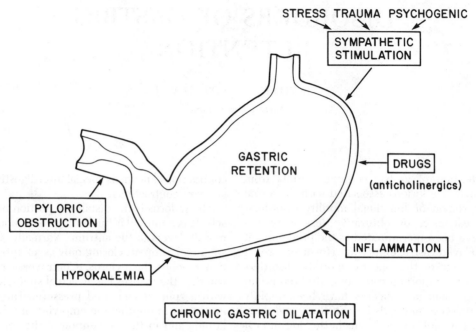

Figure 1. Factors reducing gastric motility, thereby leading to gastric retention.

these agents to cause an iatrogenic gastric emptying disorder accompanied by persistent vomiting.

Dogs with chronic gastric dilatation and/or volvulus typically have large hypomotile stomachs. It has been suggested that gastric stasis with chronic gastric retention is one predisposing factor in this syndrome. Chronic pyloric obstructions also result in gastric distention and hypomotility. Gastric stasis has been described in humans following certain viral gastrointestinal infections. A similar syndrome may occur in animals. Persistent vomiting owing to gastric atony has been observed in some dogs several days following recovery from parvovirus infections.

The occurrence of chronic trichobezoar formation in certain animals is probably due to a motility abnormality. It is interesting to speculate that the abnormal retention of nondigestible substances such as hair is due to an absence of the normal interdigestive "housekeeper" contractions.

Pylorospasm

A syndrome of pylorospasm has been described in which contraction of the pyloric musculature results in persistent closure of the pyloric canal and an outflow obstruction. This is a radiographic diagnosis commonly made when delayed gastric emptying occurs with failure of the barium to fill the pyloric canal. True pylorospasm has not been adequately documented in small animals. It is a well-established fact that both the gastric antrum and pylorus function as a single muscle unit and that gastric evacuation is controlled through gastric peristalsis rather than through pyloric closure. The previously described condition is probably the result of abnormal gastric motility rather than a true pylorospasm.

GASTRIC OUTLET OBSTRUCTIONS

Obstruction of pyloric emptying may result from either extrinsic, intrinsic, or obturative lesions. Extrinsic pyloric lesions are uncommon but can result from such things as hepatic or pancreatic abscesses, inflammatory lesions, and neoplasia. More common are intrinsic lesions of the pylorus that result from either hypertrophy of the circular muscle fibers or infiltrative neoplastic or granulomatous lesions. Adenocarcinoma is the most common type of gastric neoplasia found in the dog, arising most frequently as an infiltrative lesion in the pyloric and antral regions, obstructing normal gastric emptying. Foreign bodies, gastric or duodenal ulcers, antral polyps, or gastric mucosal hypertrophy can result in obturative pyloric lesions.

Pyloric Stenosis

Stenosis of the pylorus can result from hypertrophy of the circular muscle fibers reducing the luminal diameter of the pyloric canal. Two rather distinct clinical syndromes occur with pyloric stenosis. The first is *congenital pyloric stenosis*, which is most often encountered in brachycephalic dogs, especially the Boston terrier and boxer. An increased incidence also has been reported in Siamese eats. The signs of pyloric outflow obstruction usually begin at a young age and progressively increase in severity. The second type, *acquired pyloric stenosis*, occurs in middle-aged to older dogs with no breed or sex predilection.

The etiology of pyloric stenosis is unknown. It may result from excessive secretion of gastrointestinal hormones. The hormone gastrin has a potent trophic effect on gastric smooth muscle. Gastrin injections given to pregnant bitches caused 28 per cent of the pups to be born with pyloric stenosis. The circular muscle is hypertrophied as in spontaneous disease. Pyloric stenosis may also be associated with a neurogenic dysfunction. In these cases, the overall number of myenteric ganglion cells and nerve fiber tracts is reduced in the pyloric region. Pyloric stenosis with antral dilatation and muscular hypertrophy can be produced by selective destruction of the intramural ganglia of the pylorus.

Obstruction of gastric outflow results in gastric distention, which then becomes a stimulus for gastrin secretion. Gastrin stimulates hydrochloric acid secretion and causes mucosal hypertrophy, which may explain the antral ulcers and the redundant mucosal folds observed in some cases of pyloric stenosis.

CLINICAL FINDINGS

The primary sign of gastric retention is postprandial vomiting with accompanying gastric distention. Vomiting from gastric retention is frequently projectile, occurring abruptly without the warning of increased salivation and retching. The vomitus may be thrown for a considerable distance. Since vomiting may occur at varying intervals following eating, the character of the vomitus may range from undigested to partially digested food. The vomitus may also contain swallowed salivary and gastric secretions but is rarely bile stained.

Most animals with congenital pyloric stenosis appear healthy, although they are usually thin and stunted in stature. These animals begin vomiting shortly after weaning, and the frequency of vomiting increases with age. Chronic and persistent vomiting from any cause may be associated with dehydration and electrolyte loss. Anorexia and abdominal discomfort may also accompany conditions resulting from gastric emptying disorders.

DIAGNOSIS

A tentative diagnosis of a gastric emptying disorder can be made based on the history. Normally, the stomach is empty six to eight hours following a meal. Vomiting of an undigested meal when the stomach should be empty is diagnostic of abnormal gastric retention. An observation of the act of emesis may be helpful if the vomiting is projectile in nature.

Laboratory assessment is often noncontributory. Animals that vomit infrequently generally do not demonstrate dehydration, electrolyte loss, or acid-base abnormalities. When vomiting becomes severe, electrolyte and acid-base imbalances occur. Profuse vomiting from a gastric outflow obstruction may result in a net loss of hydrogen ions, resulting in hypochloremia, hypokalemia, and a metabolic alkalosis. A *paradoxical aciduria* is observed in some dogs with a metabolic alkalosis occurring from vomiting owing to a pyloric outflow obstruction. Paradoxical loss of acid in the urine in conjunction with a metabolic alkalosis results from two mechanisms: chloride depletion with contraction of the extracellular volume, and severe hypokalemia. Renal conservation of bicarbonate occurs in the proximal tubules in response to hypochloremia. Sodium is normally reabsorbed in the proximal nephron with the anion chloride; when chloride levels are reduced another anion, bicarbonate, must be reabsorbed to maintain electrical neutrality. With severe hypokalemia, sodium reabsorption in the distal nephron exchanges only with hydrogen ions to conserve potassium. The result of the two mechanisms is a net loss of the acid in the urine.

Radiography affords the most definitive method of diagnosing gastric retention. Gastric distention with food and/or air long after ingesta should be in the intestine is diagnostic of gastric retention. Contrast radiography is required to outline the luminal surface and assess the rate of gastric emptying. The term *gastric emptying time* is that time required for the stomach to begin to empty, not the time for the stomach to completely empty. Less than 30 minutes is reported to be a normal gastric emptying time; however, barium is normally retained for only 5 to 15 minutes. The presence of barium within the stomach for more than 12 to 24 hours is abnormal and should be considered a sign of gastric retention.

Radiologic evaluation based on the time of disappearance of a barium solution is, at best, only a crude index of the rate of emptying. Excitement, stress, certain drugs, and manual restraint may all delay gastric emptying. Another reason for inaccuracy is the unphysiologic composition of barium. Since the proximal stomach regulates emptying of liquids and the distal stomach regulates emptying of solids, a liquid barium medium may empty normally, whereas a barium-mixed meal may empty abnormally. In suspected cases of gastric retention, a barium meal is required when a routine barium study fails to demonstrate delayed emptying. Retention of portions of a barium meal for 12 to 24 hours is diagnostic of gastric retention.

The radiographic features of a pyloric stenosis include a delay in gastric emptying, distention of the stomach, and failure of the contrast to fill the pyloric canal. Frequently, stenosis resulting from hypertrophy of the muscle results in a radiographic pyloric "beak" sign. The barium contrast appears as a beak-like projection entering the pyloric canal. In addition to pyloric stenosis, other lesions resulting in outflow obstruction may be identified in the pyloric or antral region.

Fluoroscopy with contrast material is useful for assessing gastric motility. A loss of normal antral contractions is observed with motility disorders. A hypermotile stomach is often observed in cases of pyloric stenosis, but when the obstruction is prolonged, hypomotility ensues.

Endoscopic examination of the stomach is not useful for detection of motility disorders. Pyloric stenosis from hypertrophic circular musculature is often appreciated by a grossly thickened and closed pyloric sphincter. Frequently, antral ulcers are observed as they occur secondary to pyloric outflow lesions. Foreign bodies, ulcers, neoplasms, inflammation, or obturative lesions may be observed and biopsies taken for diagnosis.

In cases of gastric retention due to a suspected outflow obstructive lesion, exploratory surgery becomes a valuable diagnostic procedure. During surgery, extrinsic lesions can be observed and the stomach palpated for infiltrative intrinsic lesions or pyloric hypertrophy. A simple gastrotomy is often required to examine the stomach for obturative lesions.

TREATMENT

GASTRIC STASIS

Motility disorders of the stomach have received little attention in veterinary medicine. Therapy has generally been directed toward controlling the symptoms by the use of central-acting antiemetics or anticholinergics. When chronic vomiting occurs with delayed gastric emptying and there is no evidence of organic disease, a gastric motility disorder should be considered. When true gastric stasis occurs, surgery will do little to correct the problem; these animals must be managed medically.

Signs of gastric stasis result following a meal owing to ineffective stimulation of gastric evacuation. The first line of therapy should be dietary management. It is known that liquids empty faster than solids and carbohydrates empty faster than proteins, whereas fats are the last to leave the stomach. With these general principles, a diet should be formulated as a low-fat, low osmolar solution. Frequent small feedings of a liquid carbohydrate–rich diet are best suited for this purpose.

Recently, drug therapy has been beneficial in some cases. Spasmolytic drugs such as atropine or propantheline bromide are reported to be effective in relieving the symptoms of pylorospasm. Since true pylorospasm probably does not exist but rather is gastric stasis, anticholinergic drugs should not be used. Although they may mask vomiting, they will actually promote further gastric stasis. Drugs that stimulate gastric motility may be effective as well. Parasympathomimetic agents such as bethanechol (Urecholine) may be used with meals.

Recent investigation suggests that metoclopramide (Reglan) may be beneficial in cases of gastric stasis. This drug increases the tone and amplitude of gastric contractions and relaxes the pyloric sphincter, resulting in accelerated gastric emptying. It has been used by the author at a dose of 0.5 to 1.0 mg/kg body weight orally. It is given one-half hour before meals three to four times a day. No serious side effects have been observed at this dose. Metoclopramide also has a central-acting antiemetic effect when used at a dose of 0.1 to 0.2 mg/kg once or twice a day either orally or parenterally.

GASTRIC OUTFLOW OBSTRUCTIONS

Profuse vomiting from a gastric outflow obstruction may result in serious fluid, electrolyte, and acid-base abnormalities. Immediate parenteral fluid therapy should be instituted to replace these deficits. The fluid of choice for vomiting animals should contain adequate chloride and potassium concentrations. Ideally, pH and bicarbonate levels should be known before selecting the type of fluid. Without knowledge of specific acid-base or electrolyte levels and with the knowledge that many vomiting animals with pyloric obstructions are alkalotic, a nonbuffered, polyionic extracellular replacement fluid such as Ringer's solution should be used. This solution contains high levels of chloride (156 mEq/L), supplies potassium (4 mEq/L), and will adequately expand volume, rehydrate, and replace the usual electrolyte deficits. In some conditions, critical potassium depletion may exist and will require additional potassium supplementation. A rate of 20 to 60 mEq of potassium chloride can be added to each liter of maintenance fluids following the usual precautions for potassium administration.

An alternative fluid that is unbuffered and isotonic is normal saline (0.9 per cent NaCl). This solution lacks potassium, an electrolyte usually depleted with vomiting. Potassium chloride should be routinely added to the fluids at the rate of 20 to 60 mEq/L, depending on the severity of the hypokalemia. Buffered solutions such as lactated Ringer's solution should be avoided.

Lesions obstructing gastric outflow are treated surgically. Pyloric stenosis caused by intrinsic hypertrophy of the pylorus is managed successfully with a pyloromyotomy or pyloroplasty. With either technique, an incision is made longitudinally along the pylorus and extended well onto the antrum as well as the duodenum to alleviate the area of hypertrophied muscle. Should redundant gastric mucosa appear to block the pylorus, a pyloroplasty should be done. With this technique, the pyloromyotomy incision is carried through the mucosa, and the longitudinal incision is closed transversely. Because neoplasia cannot be ruled out, a biopsy of the hypertrophied muscle area should always be done. Surgery on the pylorus only slightly increases the emptying rate of solids but greatly accelerates the emptying rate of liquids. A liquid diet should be instituted following surgery for pyloric stenosis, with a gradual return to a normal diet. The prognosis for animals with pyloric stenosis caused by muscular hypertrophy is very good.

Obturative lesions due to neoplasia, ulceration, or mucosal hypertrophy must be carefully evaluated. It is usually necessary to excise the affected area, which often requires elaborate surgical techniques such as gastrojejunostomy. Gastric neoplasia commonly metastasizes to the regional lymph nodes, and surgical excision of these nodes is indicated for therapeutic and prognostic reasons. These surgical techniques are not without complication, and the prognosis varies with the type of lesion and its amenability to surgery.

SUPPLEMENTAL READING

Archibald, J. A., Cawley, A. J., and Reed, J. H.: Surgical technique for correcting pyloric stenosis. Mod. Vet. Pract. 41:28, 1960.

Cooke, A. R.: Control of gastric emptying and motility. Gastroenterology 68:804, 1975.

Dodge, J. A.: Production of duodenal ulcers and hypertrophic pyloric stenosis by administration of pentagastrin to pregnant and newborn dogs. Nature 225:284, 1970.

Douglas, S. W., Hall, L. W., and Walker, R. G.: The surgical relief of gastric lesions in the dog: Report of seven cases. Vet. Rec. 86:743, 1970.

Dumler, F.: Primary metabolic alkalosis. Am. Fam. Physician 23:193, 1981.

Hunt, J. N., and Stubbs, D. F.: The volume and energy content of meals as determinants of gastric emptying. J. Physiol. 245:209, 1975.

Malagelda, J. R.: Physiologic basis and clinical significance of gastric emptying disorders. Dig. Dis. Sci. 24:657, 1979.

Strombeck, D. R.: Chronic gastritis, gastric retention and gastric neoplasms. In Strombeck, D. R. (ed.): Small Animal Gastroenterology. Davis, CA: Stonegate Publishing, 1979, p. 110.

Twaddle, A. A.: Pyloric stenosis in three cats and its correction by pyloroplasty. N. Z. Vet. J. 18:15, 1970.

Wingfield, W. E.: Small animal gastric disease. In Anderson, N. V. (ed.): Veterinary Gastroenterology. Philadelphia: Lea & Febiger, 1980, p. 433.

GASTRIC ULCERS

DAVID C. TWEDT,   D.V.M.

Fort Collins, Colorado

Gastric ulcers are more frequently diagnosed today in the dog and cat than in previous years. This is due to both an increased professional awareness and a pursuit of a definitive diagnosis through radiology, endoscopy, and necropsy.

Gastric ulcers are simply defects in the gastric mucosa that result from a variety of factors. The location, morphologic characteristics, and clinical manifestations vary with the underlying pathogenesis. Acute lesions are often observed as multiple superficial erosions, whereas chronic lesions are usually single circumscribed mucosal defects that extend through the muscularis mucosae and have a firm, raised margin. Gastric ulcers are also usually peptic in that they develop through the presence of gastric acid and pepsin. The location of most "peptic ulcers" is between the gastric body and the proximal duodenum. This area, i.e., the antrum, pylorus, and proximal duodenum, is most sensitive to the effects of acid.

ETIOPATHOGENESIS

The normal stomach has the ability to resist damage during digestion from both the abrasive action of foodstuffs and the generated hydrochloric acid and the proteolytic enzyme pepsin. The unique ability of the stomach to withstand damage is referred to as the *gastric mucosal barrier*. This barrier consists of two parts: the mucous layer lining the surface of the epithelial cells, and the mucosal cells comprising the epithelial membrane. Damage to the barrier allows a "back-diffusion" of luminal acid into the mucosa. This back-diffusion of luminal acid is essential in the pathogenesis of peptic gastric ulceration (Fig. 1). Also of importance in maintaining a normal gastric mucosa is adequate gastric blood flow. Normally there is always a small back-diffusion of acid into the mucosa. This leakage occurs at a very slow rate, and the acid is removed by the gastric microcirculation. Alterations in gastric

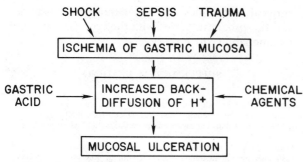

Figure 1. The back-diffusion of luminal acid into the gastric mucosa is essential for ulceration. The pathogenesis includes conditions causing mucosal ischemia, agents altering the mucosal surface, and factors increasing acid production.

blood flow allow this back-diffusion of acid to damage the gastric wall. Gastric ischemia is generally accepted as a cause of gastric ulceration.

The topical action of certain endogenous or exogenous agents can alter the gastric mucosal barrier, leading to increased mucosal permeability and gastric ulceration. Those agents incriminated in acute or chronic gastritis may also produce gastric ulcers. Other factors that affect mucosal resistance include conditions that increase gastric acid production and those that alter the acid-base balance or nutritional status. Table 1 lists the causes of gastric ulcers in small animals.

DRUGS

Drugs that are commonly ulcerogenic include aspirin, indomethacin, flunixin (Banamine), and phenylbutazone (Table 2). The mechanism of ulcerogenesis of many drugs is not completely understood. Most act by altering the gastric mucosal barrier and not by stimulating increased acid production. The best studied ulcerogenic drug used in small animals is aspirin. Gastric ulcers due to aspirin are directly related to the dose and duration of

Table 1. *Causes of Gastric Ulcers in Small Animals*

Drugs
Stress factors
    Shock
    Trauma
    Severe illness
    Environmental stress
Gastric ischemia
Bile reflux
Neurologic disease
Metabolic disease
    Renal failure
    Liver disease
    Adrenocortical insufficiency
    Gastric outflow obstruction
Gastric hyperacidity
    Systemic mastocytosis
    Gastrinoma

Table 2. *Ulcerogenic Agents*

Aspirin
Indomethacin
Phenylbutazone
Flunixin
Bile salts
Pancreatic juice
Hypertonic solutions
Alcohols
Certain heavy metals
Acetazolamide
Urea

administration. Buffered aspirin also causes gastric lesions, whereas enteric-coated aspirin produces fewer gastric lesions but has inconsistent drug absorption. Corticosteroids also play an important role in the etiology of gastric ulcers. Alone they do not directly alter the permeability of the gastric mucosa but significantly enhance the ulcerogenic effect of other factors. Corticosteroids decrease mucosal cell turnover and mucous production and increase gastrin levels, thus enhancing gastric acid output. Hypertonic agents, corrosive agents, and heavy metals such as lead also cause gastric lesions.

STRESS

Acute erosion of the gastric mucosa may occur secondary to such factors as shock, trauma, hypotension, neurologic disease, and severe illness. Lesions resulting from these conditions are referred to as "stress ulcers." The lesions usually occur as multiple superficial erosions located in the body region of the stomach but occasionally can result in a large penetrating ulcer. Although stress ulceration is infrequently recognized clinically, it is not uncommon to detect gastric mucosal erosions on necropsies of animals with the previously mentioned conditions. When there is evidence of clinical disease, the mortality may be quite significant.

GASTRIC ISCHEMIA

Ischemia is proposed as one mechanism in the formation of stress ulcers. Mucosal ischemia occurs when the normal gastric microcirculation is altered by conditions such as hypotension, shock, and sepsis, which result in a mucosal energy deficit. This is particularly severe in the body of the stomach, in which there can be a profound decrease in gastric aerobic metabolism and rapid cellular death. Focal ischemic necrosis then undergoes acid-peptic digestion and ulcer formation.

BILE ACID REFLUX

Bile acids are ulcerogenic and work synergistically with acid and ischemia to destroy the mucosal barrier. The prevalence of bile reflux in small animals is unknown, but its importance has been emphasized in studies of experimental hemorrhagic shock in dogs. Dogs in hemorrhagic shock that had their pylorus surgically occluded, preventing duodenal reflux of bile, had a significantly lower incidence of gastric ulceration than control animals.

NEUROENDOCRINE MECHANISMS

Animals enduring conditions of environmental or physical stress have increased blood levels of catecholamines and cortisol. Although the precise mechanism of stress-related ulcers is obscure, the endogenous release of corticosteroids, vasoactive catecholamines, and serotonin is postulated to have an ulcerogenic effect. Gastric mucosal ischemia occurs as a result of sympathetically mediated vasoconstriction of the vascular bed promoting vascular stasis. The combination of hormonal and neural influences during certain stress episodes can lead to the formation of discrete multiple erosions characteristic of the stress ulcer syndrome (Fig. 2).

NEUROLOGIC DISEASE

The relationship of neurologic disease and gastric lesions has long been observed in humans and more recently in some dogs with spinal cord lesions. Dogs with spinal cord lesions undergoing surgery and receiving corticosteroids may develop diffuse hemorrhagic gastritis or a deep or perforating gastric ulcer. The course of the disease is often acute and fulminant, with a high mortality.

Gastric ulcers associated with spinal cord lesions are believed to arise from the previously described stress-related factors and through an imbalance in the sympathetic and parasympathetic nervous innervation to the stomach. When a loss of sympathetic influences occurs, there is a paralytic vasodilation and vagotonia in the vessels of the gastric wall, which in turn result in mucosal ischemia. Parasympathetic overdrive further stimulates an increase in gastric acid and enzyme secretion. The formation of gastric ulcers is then potentiated by endogenous administration of corticosteroids (Fig. 3). It appears that the clinical incidence of gastric lesions is greatest in dogs receiving very high levels of corticosteroids.

METABOLIC DISEASE

Gastric ulcers frequently occur secondary to certain metabolic diseases. Renal failure results in the accumulation of uremic toxins that damage the gastric mucosa and vessels of the gastric wall. Renal failure also results in elevated serum gastrin levels owing to reduced renal clearance of gastrin. Increased gastrin levels stimulate gastric acid production, which contributes to uremic ulcer formation. Gastric ulcers occur with liver failure, although the exact mechanism is not completely understood. Damage occurs at least in part from reduced mucosal blood flow, elevated serum gastrin and histamine levels, and a loss of the normal mucous barrier. Gastric ulcers have been observed in some animals suffering from conditions causing chronic gastric retention and in animals with chronic adrenocortical insufficiency.

GASTRIC HYPERACIDITY

Few clinical syndromes have been documented to cause an increase in gastric acid production with peptic ulcer formation. Acid secretion by the parietal cells of the stomach is mediated through vagal

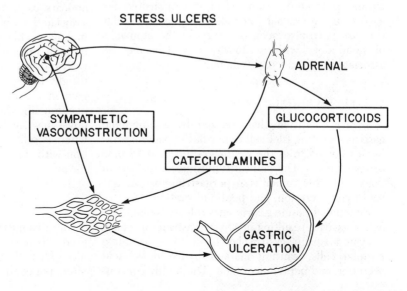

Figure 2. Stress ulcers occur through a combination of hormonal and neural influences, causing gastric ischemia, and the ulcerogenic effect of endogenous glucocorticoids.

STRESS ULCERS

ADRENAL

SYMPATHETIC VASOCONSTRICTION

GLUCOCORTICOIDS

CATECHOLAMINES

GASTRIC ULCERATION

GASTRIC LESIONS AND CNS TRAUMA

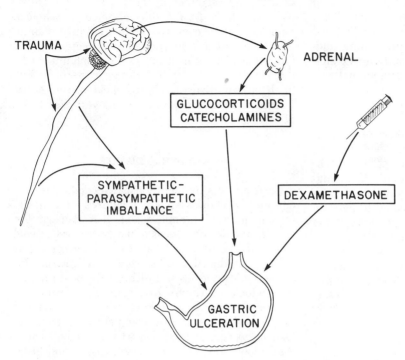

Figure 3. The proposed mechanism of gastric ulceration occurring with neurologic disease.

stimulation and gastrin and histamine secretion. Experimental studies in which high levels of histamine or gastrin are injected in dogs result in gastric hyperacidity and peptic ulcer formation in the gastric antrum or proximal duodenum. Clinical gastric hyperacidity occurs in association with gastrin-secreting tumors and systemic mast cell neoplasia.

SYSTEMIC MASTOCYTOSIS

Peptic ulcers frequently occur as a complication of systemic mast cell neoplasia. Histamine produced by the mast cells is released and mediates abnormal parietal cell hydrochloric acid production. The histamine–generated luminal acid is responsible for gastric or duodenal ulceration. Small vascular thrombi have also been observed in the stomachs of some dogs with mastocytosis, which may be associated with mucosal ischemia.

GASTRIN-SECRETING TUMOR

A rare condition characterized by a functional gastrin-secreting islet cell tumor of the pancreas has been referred to as the *Zollinger-Ellison syndrome* or *gastrinoma*. The clinical syndrome described in dogs with this tumor is hypergastrinemia, gastric acid hypersecretion, and peptic ulceration.

Functional canine gastrinomas release biologically active gastrin, resulting in a hypergastrinemic state. Elevated serum gastrin levels in turn stimulate parietal cells, causing marked hydrochloric acid secretion and peptic ulceration. The highly concen-

trated acid secretions may also cause esophagitis from gastric acid reflux or diarrhea from the acid's damage to bile salts, pancreatic enzymes, and the intestine.

CLINICAL FINDINGS

Vomiting is the most frequent clinical sign of gastric disease, and the presence of blood in the vomitus generally signifies gastric ulceration. Fresh blood may be present as small, red flecks or as large blood clots. Blood that has remained in the stomach for some time soon becomes partially digested and appears as brown "coffee grounds." Other signs associated with gastric ulcers include anemia and melena, or black tarry stools that occur with gastric or high intestinal bleeding. Less specific signs of gastric disease include nausea, a variable appetite, weight loss, and polydipsia. Animals with gastric pain may exhibit a position of relief or a "praying position" in which the rear legs are elevated. Some dogs may be asymptomatic with gastric ulcers, whereas others are encountered following perforation with signs of peritonitis.

DIAGNOSIS

The diagnosis of gastric ulcers should be considered when the clinical situations that potentiate ulcer formation exist. The physical examination is often noncontributory, but abdominal pain is the most frequent finding. The stomach's location prevents direct palpation, but abdominal splinting should cause the clinician to include gastric ulceration in the differential diagnosis. The animal suspected of having gastric ulcers should be carefully examined for cutaneous mast cell tumors. A fine needle aspirate of suspected skin tumors followed by cytologic examination easily confirms mast cell neoplasia.

There are few biochemical and hematologic alterations consistently associated with gastric ulceration. A regenerative anemia is often associated with an acute peptic ulcer. Chronic gastrointestinal blood loss eventually results in an iron deficiency anemia with microcytic hypochromic red blood cell indices. Biochemical profiles and urinalyses should be run to exclude metabolic disease from the differential diagnosis.

Gastric ulcers may be demonstrated by contrast radiology. Large chronic ulcers appear as a collection of contrast material that extends beyond the confines of the gut wall. Gastric ulcers will not be observed if the barium fails to collect in the ulcer or if the radiographic positions used do not show the ulcer in profile. Superficial stress erosions cannot be seen with a barium contrast examination.

Endoscopy affords the best objective evidence of gastric ulcers. With acute ulcers, the mucosal lesions may be bleeding and may have an inflammatory appearance around their periphery, with no evidence of fibrin in the ulcer crater. Chronic ulcers show little inflammatory response around the ulcer crater. Early stress ulcers appear as small punctate submucosal hemorrhages. Later, small, well-delineated punctate erosions can be identified along the crests of the rugae of the proximal stomach. These lesions are usually only a few millimeters in size.

Exploratory surgery and gastrotomy are diagnostic tools useful in documenting suspected gastric ulcers. Since gastric ulcers can occur in association with malignant neoplasia, histopathology should be performed on all animals with gastric ulceration. All surgical cases should include careful examination of the pancreas for small gastrin-secreting tumors.

When the cause of chronic gastric ulceration cannot be determined, plasma gastrin levels are assessed to rule out a gastrin-secreting tumor. Standard radioimmunoassay (RIA) techniques used for human determinations are also used for canine measurements. In our laboratory normal fasting gastrin levels in the dog range from 20 to 70 pg/ml. Most animals with gastrinomas have marked elevations in gastrin levels, which are diagnostic, but some may require specific provocative testing using calcium or secretin. It must be noted that fasting hypergastrinemias may occur with some types of gastritis, chronic gastric retention, hepatic disease, and renal failure.

TREATMENT

The treatment of gastric ulcers begins with a determination of the etiology, proceeding to correction of the cause. Once gastric ulcers are recognized, measures must be taken to prevent further damage to the gastric mucosa and promote healing. The secretion of hydrochloric acid perpetuates mucosal lesions. Specific treatment is largely empirical and is directed toward decreasing hydrogen ion and peptic activity or increasing the ability of the gut to deal with or resist the effects of these agents. Two common pharmacologic drugs used in the management of gastric ulcerations are antacids and H_2–receptor blocking agents. When gastric ulceration results in severe hemorrhage or acute perforation, immediate measures must be taken to correct these life-threatening problems.

ANTACIDS

Antacids are used in the treatment of gastric ulcers to neutralize gastric acid and inactivate pepsin. Antacids reduce the total amount of available hydrogen ions and irreversibly inactivate pepsin, if the gastric contents can be brought above a pH of 6. Antacids also diminish peptic activity as the pH is raised above the optimal range for proteolysis.

Antacids must be given frequently, as infrequent antacid administration may result in a rebound hypersecretion of acid. This results because an acid pH in the antrum inhibits the release of gastrin; antacid neutralization of gastric contents impedes this inhibition. Gastrin release then continues and results in a greater quantity of acid secretion. This rebound effect occurs when antacids are given only a few times a day. The rate of gastric emptying is also a factor in antacid effectiveness. Continued gastric emptying means that infrequent doses are less likely to provide a sustained buffering action. Antacids must be given every two to four hours for adequate buffering.

Many available preparations consist of mixtures of magnesium, aluminum, and calcium salts. No antacid, however, is free of hazard. Sodium bicarbonate may produce sodium overload and systemic alkalosis. Magnesium preparations may lead to diarrhea and are hazardous to animals with renal failure. Calcium salts may cause hypercalcemia or renal impairment. Aluminum hydroxide may lead to phosphate depletion.

H_2 RECEPTOR ANTAGONISTS

Histamine analogs such as cimetidine are effective in reducing gastric acid production in the dog and cat by blocking the histamine receptor of the parietal cells. The therapeutic role of cimetidine in gastric disease is evolving, but clinical indications for its use in animals still needs to be described. This drug has been shown to be useful in the treatment of some types of gastritis and gastric or duodenal ulcers. It may also be helpful in the prevention and treatment of acute gastric hemorrhage, gastrinomas, and gastric ulcers from mast cell tumors. Many dogs with uremic gastritis and ulcers appear to respond favorably to cimetidine therapy. A suggested dose of cimetidine (Tagamet) for dogs is 5 mg/kg three to four times a day. No toxicities have been observed at this dose level.

ANTICHOLINERGIC DRUGS

These drugs reduce gastric motility and spasms, both of which stimulate vomiting and pain with gastric ulcers. In addition to blocking parasympathetic stimulation of the smooth muscles of the gastric wall, they also block vagal–stimulated gastric acid secretion but do not block histamine or gastrin–stimulated acid secretion. Anticholinergic drugs have the disadvantage of reducing gastric emptying. This results in gastric distention, which promotes further gastric acid secretion. For these reasons they *should be avoided* in the management of gastric ulcers.

OTHER TREATMENTS

Drugs such as prostaglandin compounds have been effective experimentally in reducing gastric acid secretion in the dog. They may be generally available in the future. Carbenoxolone, a drug that protects the gastric mucosa, and drugs with antipepsin activity may also prove clinically useful in the management of gastric ulcers.

EMERGENCY TREATMENT

Severe gastric hemorrhage should be treated as an emergency condition with whole blood and fluids to replace losses. Attempts then are directed toward controlling bleeding through gastric lavage and local vasoconstriction. This is best accomplished with intragastric lavage with ice water. Norepinephrine may be added to the ice water solution at the rate of 8 mg/500 ml to aid in controlling hemorrhage through vasoconstriction. This potent alpha-adrenergic agent acts locally but is also absorbed systemically. However, it is almost completely destroyed in one passage through the normal liver. The lavage should be instilled in the stomach, left for 5 to 30 minutes, and then removed to assess for continued gastric bleeding. The lavage is repeated until gastric bleeding ceases.

SURGERY

Occasionally surgical therapy is required for gastric ulceration. A partial gastrectomy is generally required for removal of a chronic ulcer. This technique, in conjunction with a pyloromyotomy and vagotomy, has been used successfully in dogs with gastric ulcers. With continued gastric bleeding or with peritonitis secondary to ulcer perforation, immediate surgery is mandatory.

SUPPLEMENTAL READING

Ader, P.: Penetrating gastric ulceration in a dog. J.A.V.M.A. 175:710, 1979.

Cheville, N. F.: Uremic gastropathy in the dog. Vet. Pathol. 16:29, 1979.

Happé, R. P., van der Gaag, I., Lamers, C. B., van Toorenburg, J. Rehfeld, J. F., and Larsson, L. I.: Zollinger-Ellison syndrome in three dogs. Vet. Pathol. 17:177, 1980.

Howard, E. B., Sawa, T. R., Nielsen, S. W., and Kenyond, A. J. Mastocytoma and gastroduodenal ulceration. Path. Vet. 6:146, 1969.

Kuo, Y. J., and Shanbour, L. L.: Mechanism of action of aspirin on canine gastric mucosa. Am. J. Physiol. 230:762, 1976.

Moody, F. G., and Cheung, L. Y.: Stress ulcers: Their pathogenesis, diagnosis, and treatment. Surg. Clin. North Am. 56:1469, 1976.

Morrissey, J. F., and Barreras, R. F.: Antacid therapy. N. Engl. J. Med. 290:550, 1974.

Murray, M., Robinson, P. B., McKearing, F. J., and Sauder, I. M. Peptic ulceration in the dog: A clinico-pathological study. Vet. Rec. 91:441, 1972.

Skillman, J. J., and Slen, W.: Gastric mucosal barrier. Surg. Ann. 4:213, 1972.

Straus, E., Johnson, G. F., and Yalow, R. S.: Canine Zollinger-Ellison syndrome. Gastroenterology 72:380, 1977.

Strombeck, D. R.: Chronic gastritis, gastric retention and gastric neoplasms. *In* Strombeck, D. R. (ed.): *Small Animal Gastroenterology.* Davis, CA: Stonegate Publishing, 1979, p. 110.

Toombs, J. P., Caywood, D. D., Lipowitz, A. J., and Stevens, J. R. Colonic perforation following neurosurgical procedures and corticosteroid therapy in four dogs. J.A.V.M.A. 177:68, 1980.

Wingfield, W. E.: Small animal gastric disease. *In* Anderson, N. V. (ed. *Veterinary Gastroenterology.* Philadelphia: Lea & Febiger, 1980, p. 433.

APUDOMAS

MICHAEL D. WILLARD, D.V.M.,
Mississippi State, Mississippi

and WILLIAM D. SCHALL, D.V.M.
East Lansing, Michigan

APUD is an acronym for Amine, Precursor, Uptake, and Decarboxylation. These four terms describe certain characteristics of cells that, according to the hypotheses of Pearse (1969) and Friesen (1982) but contrary to the hypothesis of Roth and coworkers (1982), originate from the embryonic neural crest and function to secrete polypeptide hormones throughout the body. In humans, tumors derived from such cells are collectively termed *APUDomas*. Neoplasia of the APUD system is most often detected because of paraneoplastic effects due to uncontrolled hormone production (Fig. 1).

The most frequently diagnosed APUDoma of dogs and humans is insulinoma, a functional beta-cell tumor of the pancreas that results in hypoglycemia. The diagnosis and treatment of this well known APUDoma is discussed in detail elsewhere.

The overproduction of gastrin due to neoplasia is termed *gastrinoma* or *Zollinger-Ellison syndrome* and has been a recognized syndrome in humans for over 25 years. In humans the causative APUDoma is usually a non-beta-cell tumor of the pancreas, although neoplasia of the stomach, intestine, and spleen has also been implicated. Excessive production of gastrin causes hyperplasia of gastric parietal cells and increased gastric acid secretion. This hyperacidity usually causes ulcers of the stomach or duodenum, although the jejunum or esophagus may be affected. Pain, melena, hematemesis, and vomiting may be secondary to peptic ulceration. The release of large amounts of acid into the intestinal tract is thought to be responsible for the diarrhea seen in over 30 per cent of humans with Zollinger-Ellison syndrome. Resultant diarrhea may be due to inactivation of pancreatic lipase secondary to a low duodenal pH, interference with micelle formation in the duodenum, or alterations of the intestinal mucosa.

Diagnosis of gastrinomas in humans is based on history, physical examination, and adjunctive laboratory tests. Radiographic findings of atypical ulcers, thickened gastric mucosal folds, and fluid in the stomach and upper small intestine may suggest the syndrome, but the actual tumors are usually too small to be detected radiographically (< 5 mm in diameter). An inappropriately increased basal or stimulated circulating gastrin concentration is the most diagnostic finding. Gastrinomas may be associated with greater than to near-normal basal serum gastrin concentrations. Extremely increased concentrations (i.e., more than 1000 pg/ml) are considered diagnostic; however, other disorders such as antral G-cell hyperplasia, atrophic gastritis, short bowel syndrome, hyperthyroidism, retained gastric antrum, and renal insufficiency may have mild to moderate increases in basal circulating gastrin levels. If the diagnosis is in question, the response of the serum gastrin concentration to stimuli such as oral protein intake or the administration of secretion may be tested. Intravenous secretin normally causes no change or a slight decrease in serum gastrin concentration. Gastrinomas paradoxically respond with an increased output of gastrin instead of the expected decrease.

Recently six dogs have been reported with data consistent with those of gastrinoma (Drazner, 1981; Happé et al., 1980; Jones et al., 1976; Straus et al., 1977). Five dogs were over six years of age, and there was no obvious sex or breed predilection. All dogs presented with weight loss. Vomiting or diarrhea was seen in five of the six dogs. Each dog had a pancreatic tumor, all but one having metastasized to regional lymph nodes or liver. Other physical findings included inflamed distal esophageal mucosa, hypertrophied gastric mucosa, and pyloric or duodenal ulceration found during endoscopy or at necropsy. Serum albumin concentration was often decreased, whereas serum alkaline phosphatase activity was usually increased. Fasting blood gastrin concentrations, when measured, ranged from three to ten times above the upper limit of normal. One dog had an increase in circulating gastrin concentration in response to both calcium and secretin (Straus et al., 1977).

In dogs with evidence of gastric, duodenal, and/or esophageal ulcers, gastrinoma should be ruled out. Fasting serum gastrin determinations can be used as a screening test in these patients. Serum gastrin concentration in dogs can be determined at The Clinical Endocrinology Laboratory at Michigan

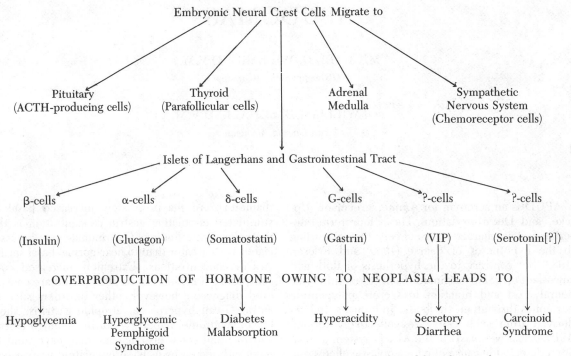

Figure 1. Paraneoplastic effects that may occur owing to neoplasia of cells derived from the neural crest.

State University.* The current protocol requires 0.5 cc serum obtained before and 15, 30, 45, and 60 minutes after feeding one-half can of meat dog food plus one-half can of beef broth.

Gastrinomas are usually malignant in humans and dogs but tend to grow slowly. Control of acid secretion, the principal cause of morbidity and mortality, is currently the therapeutic goal rather than control of the neoplasm.

One dog transiently responded to cimetidine therapy (regained 4 of 7 kg body weight originally lost) for less than two months (Drazner, 1981), and surgical resection of pancreatic neoplasia did palliate one dog for four and one-half months (Happé et al., 1980). Treatment in humans principally consists of resection of the tumor, total gastric resection (to remove the site of acid production), and/or treatment with cimetidine and vagotomy (to block acid production). Cimetidine, an H_2 blocker, offers control of gastric secretion with little risk of iatrogenic disease. Total gastric resection has the disadvantage of significant morbidity and mortality but is sometimes required if the hyperacidity is resistant to cimetidine or if poor patient compliance occurs with cimetidine therapy. Therapy with streptozotocin is reserved for human patients with large tumor burdens.

Some human patients treated with cimetidine alone have been controlled for at least 30 months.

Aggressive surgical resection of the tumor plus cimetidine therapy has produced mean human survival rates in excess of seven years. Perhaps a similar approach should be used in veterinary medicine.

Vasoactive intestinal polypeptide (VIP) is another hormone that, when overproduced in humans, has been associated with dramatic gastrointestinal signs (Verner-Morrison syndrome, pancreatic cholera, WDHA syndrome [watery diarrhea, hypokalemia, achlorhydria], or VIPoma). Although recognized in humans for ten years, this syndrome has not yet been documented in veterinary medicine. In humans, pancreatic tumors are the most common cause of increased plasma VIP concentrations, although pancreatic islet cell hyperplasia, ganglioneuroblastomas, and bronchiogenic carcinomas have also been implicated. Patients with excessive plasma VIP concentrations due to VIP-producing tumors usually have "torrential" pancreatic secretion and increased intestinal secretion, resulting in watery diarrhea with potassium loss sufficient to result in hypokalemia. Steatorrhea occurs, and significant weight loss is commonly seen but rarely marked. In suspected cases a trial of corticosteroids is begun. Such therapy will often produce symptomatic relief. If improvement occurs, abdominal surgery is performed to search for a pancreatic neoplasm, which, if found, is resected. If a neoplasm is not found, 75 per cent pancreatectomy may be performed for possible islet cell hyperplasia or undetected pancreatic neoplasia.

In veterinary patients suspected of having VIPomas, plasma should be saved and portions of

*Ray Nachreiner, Clinical Endocrinology Laboratory, Veterinary Clinical Center, Michigan State University, East Lansing, MI 48824.

suspected VIPoma tissue should be frozen at $-20°C$ for VIP extraction and immunohistochemical characterization after clinical response to prednisolone therapy is assessed.

Syndromes resulting from APUDomas in animals may not be identical to those in humans, but those that have been documented are associated with similar clinical signs. The purpose of this article is to alert veterinarians to the potential occurrence of APUDomas in animals. Finally, it is important to recognize that the pluripotential of APUD cells, regardless of origin, can result in the production of unexpected hormones, two or more hormones simultaneously, or different hormones sequentially. The interested reader is directed to the recent review of Friesen (1982).

REFERENCES AND SUPPLEMENTAL READING

Barraclough, M. A., and Bloom, S. R.: Vipoma of the pancreas. Arch. Intern. Med. 139:467, 1979.

Bloom, S. R., and Gardner, J. D.: The VIP controversy. Dig. Dis. 23:370, 1978.

Bloom, S. R., Polak, J. M., and Wellbourn, R. B.: Pancreatic apudomas. World J. Surg. 3:587, 1979.

Bonfils, S., Mignon, M., and Gratton, J.: Cimetidine treatment of acute and chronic Zollinger-Ellison syndrome. World J. Surg. 3:597, 1979.

Broor, S. L., Soergel, K. H., Garancis, J. C., and Wilson, S. D.: Case report. Hormone-producing pancreatic islet cell carcinoma: Changing clinical presentations. Am. J. Med. Sci. 278:229, 1979.

Drazner, F. H.: Canine gastrinoma: A condition analogous to the Zollinger-Ellison syndrome in man. Cal. Vet. 11:6, 1981.

Friesen, S. R.: Tumors of the endocrine pancreas. N. Engl. J. Med. 306:580, 1982.

Happé, R. P., van der Gaag, I., Lamers, C. B., van Toorenburg, J., Rehfeld, J. F., and Larsson, L. I.: Zollinger-Ellison syndrome in three dogs. Vet. Path. 17:177, 1980.

Johnston, J. A., Fabri, P. J., and Lott, J. A.: Serum gastrin in Zollinger-Ellison syndrome: Identification of localized disease. Clin. Chem. 26:867, 1980.

Jones, B. R., Nicholls, M. R., and Badman, R.: Peptic ulceration in a dog associated with an islet cell carcinoma of the pancreas and an elevated plasma gastrin level. J. Small Anim. Pract. 17:593, 1976.

Long, R. G., Bryant, M. G., Yuille, P. M., Polak, J. M., and Bloom, S. R.: Mixed pancreatic apudoma with symptoms of excess vasoactive intestinal polypeptide and insulin: Improvement of diarrhea with metaclopramide. Gut 22:505, 1981.

Marshall, J. B., and Settles, R. H.: Zollinger-Ellison syndrome. A clinical update. Postgrad. Med. 68:28, 1980.

McCarthy, D. M.: The place of surgery in the Zollinger-Ellison syndrome. N. Engl. J. Med. 302:1344, 1980.

Pearse, A. G. E.: The cytochemistry and ultrastructure of polypeptide hormone-producing cells of the APUD series and the embryonic, physiologic and pathologic implications of the concept. J. Histochem. Cytochem. 17:303, 1969.

Roth, J., LeRoith, D., Shiloach, J., et al.: The evolutionary origins of hormones, neurotransmitters, and other extracellular chemical messengers. N. Engl. J. Med. 306:523, 1982.

Said, S. I., and Faloona, G. R.: Elevated plasma and tissue levels of vasoactive intestinal polypeptide in the watery-diarrhea syndrome due to pancreatic, bronchogenic and other tumors. N. Engl. J. Med. 293:155, 1975.

Straus, E., Johnson, G. F., Yalow, R. S.: Canine Zollinger-Ellison syndrome. Gastroenterology 72:380, 1977.

Wyke, R. J., Hill, G. L., and Axon, A. T. R.: A review of the Zollinger-Ellison syndrome—with particular reference to a patient treated with cimetidine. Postgrad. Med. J. 55:716, 1979.

Zollinger, R. M., Ellison, E. C., Fabri, P. J., Johnson, J., Sparks, J., and Carey, L. C.: Primary peptic ulcerations of the jejunum associated with islet cell tumors. Twenty-five-year appraisal. Ann. Surg. 192:422, 1980.

MECHANISMS OF DIARRHEAL DISEASE

FREDERICK H. DRAZNER, D.V.M.

Des Plaines, Illinois

Profuse and relentless diarrhea is a characteristic sign of many enteropathies. Many of these diseases have similar clinical consequences (e.g., fluid/electrolyte imbalance, malnutrition, metabolic acidosis, shock, death, and impaired somatic development). Although the clinical symptomatology of these diseases may be identical, the pathogenetic mechanisms producing the diarrhea may be quite varied. To properly diagnose and manage affected patients it is essential that the clinician understand these various mechanisms.

GENERAL CONSIDERATIONS

Diarrhea may be defined as a marked variation of the bowel movement with increases in one or all of the following parameters: frequency, fluid content, and volume. A 20-kg dog has approximately 2,700 ml of fluid entering the alimentary canal daily. Of this volume, approximately 95 per cent is absorbed, leaving only a small amount to be excreted in the feces. Because most fluid is absorbed in the small intestine, diseases in this segment of the alimentary canal are characterized by voluminous diarrhea as well as failure to maintain nutritional homeostasis. Disease that is confined to the large bowel (ceeum, colon, and rectum), on the other hand, has little effect on body condition and is usually associated with smaller volumes of fecal material passed more frequently (Table 1).

CLASSIFICATION OF DIARRHEA ACCORDING TO PATHOGENESIS (Table 2)

Most medical problems involve multiple mechanisms that cause diarrhea, hence they may be found in more than one place in this classification.

OSMOTIC (MALABSORPTIVE) DIARRHEA

Increased fecal excretion of osmotically active particles augments fecal water excretion because these particles hold water. Some of the unabsorbed osmotically active substances (monosaccharides and fatty acids) are fermented by the colonic flora (producing volatile substances, low weight organic acids), which further increases the number of osmotically active particles excreted. In addition, unabsorbed fatty acids are hydroxylated by the colonic flora (especially ricinoleic acid) to produce chemicals that reduce colonic salt and water absorption (the so-called castor oil effect). The end result is a watery, voluminous diarrhea, often laden with fat and starch droplets. Examples of conditions that may produce an osmotic diarrhea include dietary overload, pancreatic exocrine insufficiency, bile-salt deficiency, and small intestinal mucosal disease.

Pancreatic exocrine insufficiency, either congenital or acquired, produces a classic voluminous fatty diarrhea (steatorrhea). The inability of the pancreas to deliver adequate quantities of lipase and amylase to the intestinal lumen results in inadequate digestion of fats and starches. With certain clinical entities inactivation of intraluminal pancreatic enzyme activity results in a malabsorptive diarrhea. Patients with pyloroplasties may deliver such large amounts of gastric acid to the duodenum and jejunum that the pH of duodenal contents remains low enough

to destroy lipase and amylase activity. A functional gastrin-secreting non-beta islet cell tumor (gastrinoma or Zollinger-Ellison syndrome in humans) can produce the same results by stimulating gastric secretion of excess acid, which enters the duodenum in large amounts.

Bile acid deficiency (due to extrahepatic biliary obstruction; intrahepatic disease; chronic ileitis, which impairs the recycling of bile acids; or stagnant intestinal bowel loops, which result in deconjugation of bile acids) can produce a watery osmotic diarrhea. Bile acids emulsify neutral fats (triglycerides), enhance the enzymatic activity of pancreatic lipase and phospholipase A, and participate in micelle formation. Formation of micelles (a conglomeration of fatty acids, bile acids, and beta monoglycerides) enhances the absorption of long–chained fatty acids by the intestinal mucosa, where they are esterified, converted to chylomicrons, and removed by the intestinal lymphatics.

Duodenal mucosal disease may result in inadequate release of hormones necessary for normal assimilation of nutrients. Reductions in cholecystokinin (CCK) and secretin release result in impaired secretion of pancreatic digestive enzymes and bicarbonate. The inability to secrete enterokinase prevents the intraluminal activation of trypsin, which in turn activates the remainder of the proteolytic enzymes as well as phospholipase A. Deficient production and release of duodenal enterogastrone prevents the orderly regulation of gastric emptying, thereby overwhelming the duodenal lumen with gastric acid and inactivating pancreatic enzymes.

Small intestinal mucosal diseases result in the loss of brush border disaccharidases (lactase, maltase, and sucrase) and proteases, impairing the digestion of disaccharides (especially lactose) and peptides. Examples of such diseases include giardiasis, coccidiosis, canine coronavirus (CCV), and possibly canine rotavirus (CRV). In these conditions the intestinal villi are shortened, blunted, and fused. Thus the surface area necessary for proper absorption is markedly reduced. Canine parvovirus (CPV) destroys the villous crypt precursor cells, leading to necrosis, sloughing, and collapse of the crypt-villus unit.

Intramural diseases of the small intestine produce

Table 1. *Localizing Characteristics of Small Intestine versus Large Bowel Diarrhea*

	Small Intestine	Large Bowel
Character of stool	Watery; may see fat droplets, undigested food, or melena	Loose, mucoid; often with fresh blood (hematochezia)
Volume of stool	Increased	Normal to increased
Frequency of defecation	Normal to increased	Always increased
Effect on nutritional status	Important; may see fluid electrolyte imbalances, weight loss, poor hair coat, anorexia, hypoproteinemia, etc.	Of little importance; little or no weight loss
Secondary signs	Abdominal distention (ascites), polydipsia, vomition, pallor of mucus membranes	Tenesmus, abdominal pain, anal pruritus

Table 2. *Mechanisms by Which Diarrhea Occurs*

I. Osmotic Diarrheas
   A. Dietary overload
   B. Maldigestion
      1. Pancreatic exocrine insufficiency
         a. Juvenile pancreatic hypoplasia
         b. Chronic pancreatitis
         c. Pancreatic ductal obstruction—adenocarcinoma
      2. Deactivation of pancreatic enzymes
         a. Post pyloroplasty
         b. Canine gastrinoma (Zollinger-Ellison–like syndrome)
      3. Bile deficiency
         a. Post parenchymal disease—cirrhosis, bile duct carcinoma
         b. Post-hepatic obstruction
            (1) Cholelithiasis
            (2) Pancreatitis causing stenosis of bile duct
            (3) Pancreatic adenocarcinoma with regional metastases
         c. Regional ileitis—loss of recycling of bile acids through enterohepatic circulation
         d. Drug induced (neomycin, calcium carbonate)
   C. Malabsorption
      1. Duodenal mucosal disease (duodenitis, neoplasia, gluten enteropathy, parasitism)
         a. Inhibition of secretion of enterokinase
         b. Inhibition of CCK and secretin release
         c. Inhibition of release of enterogastrone
      2. Jejunal and ileal mucosal disease
         a. Loss of disaccharidases and peptidases from brush border
         b. Loss of absorptive mechanisms via active transport
         c. Inability to transport lipids across mucous membrane
      3. Jejunal and ileac intramural disease
         a. Lymphoma
         b. Lymphangiectasis
         c. Mastocytosis
         d. Lymphocytic plasmacytic enteritis
         e. Gluten enteropathy
         f. Regional enteritis
         g. Eosinophilic enteritis
         h. Amyloidosis
II. Secretory Diarrheas
   A. Secretory agent or toxin
      1. Bacterial enterotoxins
      2. Methylxanthines (theophylline)
      3. Prostaglandins
      4. Dihydroxy bile acids (owing to bacterial action)
      5. Vasoactive intestinal peptide (VIP—proved in humans)
      6. Glucagon
      7. Secretin
      8. Calcitonin (medullary carcinoma of the thyroid gland)
   B. Mucosal injury
      1. Viruses
         a. Feline panleukopenia
         b. CPV
         c. Canine distemper
      2. Bacteria
         a. Salmonellosis
         b. Invasive *E. coli*
      3. Inflammatory bowel disease
         a. Ulcerative enterocolitis
         b. Regional enteritis
      4. Antibiotics (pseudomembranous enterocolitis)
         a. Clindamycin
         b. Lincomycin
         c. Ampicillin
         d. Chloramphenicol
   C. Neoplasms with hormone production—canine gastrinoma
III. Increased Intestinal Permeability
   A. Increased intestinal capillary hydrostatic pressure (right-sided CHF)
   B. Disorders of intestinal lymphatics
   C. Inflammatory exudation
      1. Intact mucosa
      2. Ulcerative mucosa
IV. Disorders of Motility
   A. Increased transit rate
      1. Flaccid alimentary canal with peristaltic rush (any type of osmotic, secretory, or hyperpermeability mechanism)
      2. Spastic diarrhea (hyperperistaltic diarrhea)
   B. Decreased transit rate (stagnant bowel loops)

an osmotic, watery diarrhea by physically impairing the absorption of particulate material of inflammatory cells (lymphocytic-plasmacytic enteritis, regional enteritis, eosinophilic enteritis, or gluten enteropathy) or neoplastic cells (intestinal lymphoma), producing a marked thickening of the lamina propria and thus a physical barrier against absorption.

From the previous discussion of osmotic diarrhea it is apparent that, left unchecked, such diseases will produce chronic deteriorations of nutritional hemostasis known as *maldigestion* (pancreatic exocrine insufficiency, bile acid deficiency, and disaccharidase deficiency) and *malabsorption* (small intestinal mucosal disease). For convenience, malassimilation syndrome is used to describe both entities. Besides having a voluminous, watery diarrhea, patients with a malassimilation syndrome may exhibit signs of secondary polysystemic involvement, including a roughened seborrheic-like haircoat, marked weight loss, listlessness, anemia, coagulation problems, bone pain, tetany, and so on (Tables 3 and 4).

SECRETORY DIARRHEA

Abnormal amounts of extracellular fluid enter the gut lumen with a secretory diarrhea. This can be due to increased capillary hydrostatic pressure within the lamina propria due to inflammation and mucosal injury or to a response to stimulated active ion secretion. The latter mechanism is best illustrated by examining the pathogenesis of enterotoxic colibacillosis *(E. coli)*. In this disease the intestinal villi are not damaged; they retain their absorptive functions. The *E. coli* enterotoxin, via the chemical mediator cyclic adenosine monophosphate (cyclic AMP), stimulates the intestinal crypt cells to secrete massive quantities of sodium, chloride, and bicarbonate ions, resulting in a marked efflux of water into the lumen. Secretory diarrheas differ from osmotic diarrheas in that they continue during fasting because the diarrhea results from a mechanism not dependent on chyme in the lumen. Since osmotic diarrhea results from the malabsorption of ingested solutes, fasting causes the diarrhea to cease.

INCREASED PERMEABILITY

In the normal intestinal tract the total fluxes of fluid leaving the lumen exceed those entering the lumen, and this results in absorption. The amount of fluid secreted into the alimentary canal of a 20-kg dog is considerable (approximately 2,700 ml), so

Table 3.   Etiology of Maldigestion and Malabsorption (Malassimilation)

I. Maldigestion
   A. Pancreatic exocrine insufficiency
      1. Congenital
      2. Acquired—relapsing chronic pancreatitis
   B. Inactivation of pancreatic enzymes
      1. Pyloroplasty
      2. Canine gastrinoma
      3. Mastocytosis
      4. Chronic uremia with inadequate excretion of gastrin
   C. Bile acid deficiency
      1. Intrahepatic biliary obstruction (advanced cirrhosis)
      2. Extrahepatic biliary obstruction
         a. Cholelithiasis
         b. Biliary flukes in cats (*Eurythrema* sp., *Opisthorcis felineus*)
         c. Relapsing pancreatitis
         d. Pancreatic carcinoma
      3. Chronic ileal disease
         a. Regional ileitis
         b. Lymphoma
      4. Stagnant bowel loop syndrome
      5. Drug induced (sequestration of bile salts)
         a. Neomycin
         b. Calcium carbonate
   D. Brush border enzyme deficiency
      1. Disaccharidase deficiency
      2. Protease deficiency
II. Malabsorption
   A. Villous atrophy and derangement and infiltration of lamina propria
      1. Lymphocytic-plasmacytic enteritis
      2. Eosinophilic enteritis
      3. Gluten enteropathy
      4. Histoplasmosis
      5. Amyloidosis
      6. Sarcoma
   B. Lymphangiectasia

Table 4. *Pathophysiologic Correlations of Clinical Signs Seen in Malassimilation Disorders*

Clinical Sign	Pathophysiologic Correlation
Weight loss, poor nutritional state	Inadequate absorption of proteins, fats, and carbohydrates—negative caloric intake
Diarrhea (bulky, voluminous, and fatty)	Dihydroxylation of fatty acids and bile acids—decreased colonic absorption of sodium and water; carbohydrate malabsorption—osmotically active particles; absorptive capacity of colon is far exceeded
Weakness, listlessness	Depletion of electrolytes (K^+ and Mg^{++}); anemia
Petechiations and ecchymoses	Malabsorption of vitamin K (fat-soluble vitamin)—hypoprothrombinemia
Integumentary changes (seborrhea, eczema, alopecia)	Impaired absorption of vitamin A
Anemia	Impaired absorption of iron, folate, vitamin B_{12}
Tetany	Vitamin D, calcium, and magnesium malabsorption
Bone pain	Vitamin D and calcium malabsorption—osteomalacia
Nocturia, polyuria	Hyposthenuria owing to hypokalemia
Edema	Malabsorption of amino acids—hypoproteinemia

that the amount that must be absorbed is approximately twice the normal blood volume. When permeability of the mucosa is increased by inflammation or increased interstitial fluid pressure, the flux of fluid entering the intestine increases. When this flux exceeds the amount leaving the lumen, diarrhea ensues.

With increased permeability, the loss of large molecules into the gut (such as proteins) can be accelerated. In contrast to glomerular disease, enteropathies characterized by increased mucosal permeability are commonly associated with leakage of large as well as small molecular weight proteins (i.e., globulins, molecular weights ranging from 200,000 to 1,000,000 daltons; and albumin, molecular weight approximately 65,000 daltons). The loss of excess plasma proteins into the intestinal lumen has been termed protein-losing enteropathy (PLE) and may be due to various causes (Table 5). Besides the chronic diarrhea, listlessness, and emaciation, patients with severe PLE may present with pitting edema, ascites, or hydrothorax due to hypoalbuminemia.

It is obvious that many clinical entities (e.g., lymphoma, intestinal lymphangiectasia, histoplasmosis, lymphocytic-plasmacytic enteritis) that result in a malabsorption syndrome with steatorrhea may also produce PLE.

MOBILITY DERANGEMENT

In general, small animal clinicians show a poor understanding of intestinal motility changes with diarrhea as evidenced by the widespread use of anticholinergic agents in the treatment of diarrhea in dogs and cats. To gain a therapeutic advantage in the management of motility disorders, it is important to first review the normal physiology of motility in the small intestine and large bowel.

The smooth muscle within the alimentary canal performs two basic functions: (1) it slows the passage of chyme via the random contractions of circular smooth muscles (rhythmic segmentation) to allow proper digestion and absorption, and (2) it continuously moves chyme in an aboral direction (peristalsis). Rhythmic segmentation offers resistance within the alimentary canal against the continuous propulsive movements of the peristaltic waves. It also allows complete mixture of chyme with the digestive enzymes and promotes contact of this mixture with the absorptive surfaces of the intestine. Rhythmic segmentation is greatly enhanced by the action of acetylcholine released by vagus nerve fibers, especially in the post-prandial state. Peristalsis, on the other hand, is not only influenced by vagal nerve activity but also by various endocrines including 5-hydroxytryptamine (serotonin),

Table 5. *Disorders That May Result in PLE*

I. Cardiac (increased capillary hydrostatic pressure due to right-sided CHF)
   A. Tricuspid insufficiency
   B. Idiopathic congestive cardiomyopathy
   C. Ventricular septal defect
   D. Constrictive pericarditis
II. Gastric (exudation of massive quantities of protein)
   A. Gastric ulceration
   B. Giant cell hypertrophy of basenji dogs (analogous to Menetrier's disease in humans)
   C. Gastric carcinoma
III. Intestinal
   A. Mucosal ulceration with exudation of proteins
     1. Acute infectious enteritis
       a. CPV
       b. Salmonellosis
     2. Chronic foreign body
     3. Intestinal carcinoma
     4. Parasitic enteritis
     5. Hemorrhagic gastroenteritis (HGE)
     6. Regional enteritis
   B. Inflammatory exudation with intact mucosa
     1. Lymphocytic-plasmacytic enteritis
     2. Histoplasmosis
     3. Gluten enteropathy
     4. Eosinophilic enteritis
   C. Derangement of intestinal lymphatics
     1. Intestinal lymphangiectasia
     2. Intestinal lymphoma

cholecystokinin (CCK), gastrin, motilin, and prostaglandins.

It is evident that the administration of anticholinergic agents in an animal with normal intestinal function would inhibit rhythmic segmentation activity, thus converting the alimentary canal into a flaccid tube. This state offers little or no resistance to the driving forces of peristalsis, and thus the chyme is propelled long distances by relatively weak peristaltic waves. The vast majority of patients seen in small animal practice with diarrhea have a "hypomotile" bowel that offers little resistance to the rapid movement of contents passing through it. The use of anticholinergic agents in such situations is thus irrational and contraindicated, for it would further inhibit any remaining rhythmic segmentation activity without affecting peristalsis.

Augmented motility can be the basis for some cases of diarrhea. As stated previously, peristalsis is unaffected by vagal activity but appears to be influenced by gut hormones. Some diarrheas appear to result from the release of abnormal amounts of prostaglandins. Since treatment with an inhibitor of prostaglandin synthetase (sulfasalazine) results in remission and since prostaglandins also stimulate secretion of fluids, it is not possible to determine which effect is more important. Gastrin participates in normal gastrointestinal motility. Human patients with gastrinoma (Zollinger-Ellison syndrome) exhibit spasms and hyperperistalsis owing to the effect of marked hypergastrinemia on the gastrointestinal tract. Exercise increases colonic motor activity and propulsive movements in normal dogs. Exercise will worsen diarrhea due to any cause but may make diarrhea reappear in a dog in which inactivity had allowed the dog to recover from a previous bout of diarrhea. Emotion is believed by many to play an important role in the motor function of the colon in a number of chronic bowel diseases in humans. This has not been supported by research on humans with these problems. Treatment with tranquilizers and antispasmotics is ineffective in their management.

Diseases that are characterized by diarrhea as a result of a markedly diminished transit time are those associated with a stagnant bowel loop (intussusception, foreign body, infiltrative neoplasia, and acute necrotizing pancreatitis with localized peritonitis and fibrinous adhesions to bowel serosal surfaces). Stagnation of bowel loops allows for bacterial overgrowth and dehydroxylation of fatty acids and bile acids, resulting in the inhibition of colonic reabsorption of water.

DIAGNOSTIC APPROACH

PHYSICAL EXAMINATION

The cornerstones of any good diagnostic work-up are a detailed and accurate history and a meticulous physical examination. The pet owner should be questioned thoroughly regarding the number of stools per day; the relative volume of fecal material passed daily; and the color, character, and consistency of the feces. As stated previously (see Table 1), patients with small intestinal disease will have a voluminous, watery diarrhea, whereas those with pure colonic disease may pass scant volumes of stool rather frequently. Blackish, tarry stools are indicative of intraluminal bleeding in the cranial portion of the alimentary canal, whereas bright red blood often mixed with mucus is characteristic of large bowel pathology. Vomition often accompanies small intestinal disease. Questions regarding the patient's appetite and diet are helpful. As a rule of thumb, patients with pancreatic exocrine insufficiency (except owing to pancreatic adenocarcinoma) usually have voracious appetites but are unable to maintain normal body weight. In contrast, patients with malassimilation due to intestinal mucosal or intraluminal disease rarely have a good appetite. The type of food that is fed is important when considering the possibility of food hypersensitivity (gluten enteropathy; eosinophilic gastroenteritis, especially in dogs that are fed horsemeat).

Questions regarding the patient's immediate environment may be helpful when considering enteritis due to heavy metal or organophosphorus intoxication. The pet owner should be asked about the patient's geographic (traveling) history, because some diseases are endemic to certain regions of the United States (e.g., giardiasis in the Rocky Mountain area, histoplasmosis in the Ohio and Mississippi River Valleys). If the patient has not been previously seen by the clinician, important points to note include vaccination history (feline panleukopenia, canine distemper, CPV, and so on), any medications that the patient is being given (theophylline, neomycin, cardiac glycosides), and past pertinent medical history (relapsing pancreatitis, surgery for pyloric stenosis, atopic dermatitis, and so on).

Close physical inspection of the patient may either be quite helpful or unrevealing. The patient should be initially assessed to appreciate any weight loss or cachexia. The haircoat should be inspected for dullness or seborrhea. If the sclera and mucous membranes are jaundiced, this may indicate a cholestatic process with bile acid deficiency. Pallor of the mucous membranes is indicative of anemia and may be the result of malabsorption of iron, vitamin B_{12}, or folate or may be due to prolonged gastrointestinal bleeding. Petechiations of mucous membranes or integument may indicate hypoprothrombinemia due to malabsorption of vitamin K. The heart and lungs should be carefully auscultated for any murmurs (right-sided congestive heart failure causing increased intestinal mucosa permeability), muffled heart sounds (constrictive pericarditis), or pleural friction rubs (hydrothorax due to hypoproteinemia). Generalized lymphadenopathy may be an early indication of intestinal lymphoma or histoplasmosis. Palpation of the abdomen may reveal ascites (PLE) or bone pain (osteomalacia due to malabsorption of vitamin D and calcium). Finally, digital palpation of the rectum is helpful in detecting blood, mucus, strictures, intraluminal masses, or deep ulcerations.

LABORATORY EVALUATION (Table 6)

The simplest and most useful screening test in the evaluation of diarrhea is a complete qualitative fecal analysis. The stool should be examined grossly for consistency and presence of fat droplets, undigested muscle fibers, mucus, and blood. The color

of the feces should be noted. Normally the color of the stool is dark brown owing to bacterial conversion of conjugated bilirubin into stercobilin. Grey or acholic feces is a rare occurrence and is due to complete biliary obstruction; thus, the patient should exhibit marked jaundice. Light-colored feces (usually a shade of mustard) may be due to a variety of causes: reduction of bacterial flora by intestinal antibiotics, milk proteins, and rapid transit of fecal material with little time for bacterial conversion of bilirubin to stercobilin.

Microscopic examination of feces should include (1) a direct smear and flotation inspection for parasites and/or ova, (2) Sudan III stain for neutral fats (and fatty acids), (3) Lugol's iodine stain for starch granules, (4) Wright's stain to document inflamma-

Table 6. *Tests Useful in the Diagnosis of Malassimilation or PLE*

Test	Normal Value	Comment
Stool Analyses		
Parasites/ova	Negative	Chronic giardiasis is often difficult to document and most often produces an osmotic diarrhea
Fecal fat (neutral and fatty acids)	0 to 3 droplets/hpf*	Reliable screening test; may not be sensitive enough to document minimal steatorrhea
Starch	0 to 4 droplets/hpf	Helpful in detecting alpha-amylase deficiency due to pancreatic exocrine insufficiency
Trypsin	Positive	Helpful in detecting pancreatic protease deficiency; subject to false positive and false negative results (use the gel test instead of x-ray film test)
Occult blood	Negative	Helpful in detecting melena due to GI neoplasia or inflammatory bowel disease; subject to false positive results
24-hour fecal fat quantitation	< 0.2 gm/kg/24 hr	Valuable test to document steatorrhea; may be technically cumbersome
Bacterial culture	Negative for *Salmonella, Shigella, Campylobacter jejuni*, hemolytic *E. coli, Candida albicans*	May be helpful in immunosuppressed patient or in patient that has received oral antibiotics (positive yield is quite low)
Pancreatic Function Test		
Oral PABA test	60 to 75 per cent excretion of PABA in urine	Dogs with urinary PABA excretion < 16 per cent require pancreatic replacement
Absorption Tests		
Fat absorption	Plasma turbidity (lipemia) within two to three hours	A good inexpensive and simple test for determining malassimilation of fat; may be repeated with pancreatic enzyme powder added
D-xylose	> 50 mg/dl (blood level)	A valuable test to help document intestinal malabsorption; may get falsely lowered values owing to gastric emptying or intestinal bacterial overgrowth
Oral glucose tolerance test (OGTT)	Peak level 160 mg/dl in 60 min; return to fasting level in 180 min	Less reliable than oral D-xylose absorption; however, is easier and less expensive to run; may detect prediabetic state in patients with pancreatic maldigestion
Hemogram		
CBC	————————	Leukopenia (severe) often accompanies CPV; leukocytosis with a left shift may be seen in bacterial enteritis; eosinophilia may accompany parasitism or allergy; anemia (normochromic/normocytic) may be seen in patients with chronic melena
Prothrombin time	8 to 12 sec	Frequently prolonged owing to malabsorption of vitamin K
Biochemical Tests		
Serum protein (total)	5.4 to 7.2 gm/dl	Markedly decreased in PLE; losses in both albumin and globulin fractions
Serum calcium	9.0 to 12.0 mg/dl	Frequently decreased owing to malabsorption
Serum cholesterol	130 to 250 mg/dl	Frequently decreased owing to steatorrhea

*hpf = high power field.

tory cells (neutrophils and eosinophils), and (5) Gram's stain to identify microorganisms, especially *Staphylococcus aureus* and *Candida albicans*, which may represent a superinfection as a result of prolonged antibiotic usage.

Sudan III saturated in 95 per cent ethyl alcohol will demonstrate neutral fats as orange-red droplets. More than four droplets per high power field is abnormal and suggests a deficiency of pancreatic lipase or phospholipase A. Intestinal mucosal disease causing malabsorption may be suspected by identifying split fats (fatty acids) in the feces. In this instance there is adequate pancreatic lipolytic enzymatic activity. However, there is a defect in mucosal transport of the fatty acids. The clinician or technician may identify fatty acids by heating a mixture of the fecal smear with 4 drops of 36 per cent acetic acid. The fatty acid soaps are thus transformed into free fatty acids, which are fat soluble. Staining this suspension again with Sudan III will reveal many orange-red droplets.

Alpha-amylase deficiency may be suspected by Lugol's iodine stain, in which unsplit starch appears as blue-black granules.

There is no uniform agreement among small animal internists regarding the value of fecal cultures, which only identify aerobic members of the fecal flora. Since most diarrheas result in, or are the result of, a rapid bowel transit time, causing an overall decrease in bacterial populations, and since greater than 99 per cent of the total bacterial population is comprised of anaerobic bacteria (*Clostridium, Bacteroides, Fusobacterium, Peptostreptococcus*, and so on), a quantitation of fecal bacterial numbers is not done. The author considers the following to be indications for stool culture: (1) if a potential public health problem exists, especially if there is a young child in the household (*Salmonella* sp., *Shigella* sp., or *Campylobacter jejuni*), (2) if many neutrophils are seen on the Wright's stain of the feces and the patient is febrile and has a circulating leukocytosis, or (3) if there is a possibility of overgrowth of *Staphylococcus aureus* or *Candida albicans* because of antibiotic therapy.

After completing the microscopic examination, the stool should be evaluated biochemically. A good screening test for pancreatic protease activity is the trypsin gelatin liquifaction test. Trypsin activity is documented if the gelatin in a tube is liquified by a fecal homogenate. False negative reactions can occur when normal trypsin activity in the small intestine is destroyed in the colon or feces by bacteria. This can occur with abnormally long retention of feces in the colon or with analysis of feces that were not recently passed. False positive findings may result from bacteria liquifying the gelatin instead of the trypsin.

Melena may be detected by tests employing benzidine or orthotoluidine chemicals, which oxi-

dize the feces, producing a color change. One drawback of these tests (Hema-Chek Fecal Occult Blood Test*) is that a diet containing red meat may give a false positive reaction. It is best to withhold red meat for 72 hours prior to testing.

Determination of the quality of fecal fat excreted in 24 hours is the most reliable method of documenting steatorrhea. The author uses C/D† as a constant diet (one can has 8.3 per cent fat or approximately 37 gm fat/can) for 72 hours before a 24-hour collection is performed. A 1979 study by Burrows and associates revealed that dogs with either pancreatic maldigestion or intestinal malabsorption excrete more than 1.0 gm/kg/24 hr of fat, whereas dogs with normal assimilation ability excrete less than 0.2 gm/kg/24 hr.

A simple yet helpful screening test for fat absorption ability is the oral administration of corn oil (Lipomul‡) at the dosage of 3 ml/kg. Plasma samples using CaEDTA are collected at one, two, and three hours post feeding and are centrifuged. The failure of plasma turbidity to appear is indicative of either pancreatic maldigestion or intestinal malabsorption. The test may be repeated after giving desiccated pancreatic enzyme powder (Viokase§) mixed with the corn oil and 1½ tsp of baking soda (to alkalinize the suspension for maximal lipase activity). Allow the mixture to stand at room temperature for 30 minutes before feeding. The appearance of plasma turbidity (lipemia) in the second test is highly suggestive of pancreatic exocrine insufficiency and maldigestion.

Testing the ability of the patient to absorb monosaccharides may yield valuable information regarding the capabilities of small intestinal absorption. The oral glucose tolerance test (OGTT) is simple to perform and is relatively inexpensive. Glucose, a hexose monosaccharide, requires no digestion by pancreatic or brush border enzymatic activity and is transported intact across the brush border of the epithelial cells. A 20 per cent solution of glucose is given orally at a rate of 2 gm/kg, and plasma glucose levels are measured every 30 minutes for 180 minutes. Patients with normal intestinal absorptive functions reach maximal blood glucose levels between 30 and 60 minutes and rarely exceed 160 mg/ dl. The return to levels comparable to those of the fasting glucose state should be achieved within 180 minutes. Patients with intestinal malabsorption have a "flattened curve," with blood glucose levels rarely exceeding 115 mg/dl. Patients with pancreatic exocrine insufficiency and maldigestion will have a normal OGTT curve but may exhibit prolonged hyperglycemia, indicating previous relapsing pan-

---

*Ames Division, Miles Laboratories, Inc., Elkhart, IN.
†Hills Division, Rivinia Foods, Inc., Topeka, KS.
‡Upjohn Co., Kalamazoo, MI.
§A. H. Robbins Co., Richmond, VA.

creatitis with some degree of islet cell destruction and a prediabetic state.

A more sensitive but technically more difficult and more expensive monosaccharide absorption test employs D-xylose as the sugar source. D-xylose is a pentose monosaccharide that is not metabolized by animals but is passively absorbed through the intestinal mucosa and into the portal circulation. The patient is fasted for at least 12 hours prior to administration of D-xylose (500 mg/kg in a 10 per cent solution via stomach tube). Blood samples for determination of D-xylose serum levels are taken every half hour for three hours. Within 60 minutes, normal animals will have reached a maximal serum level of D-xylose (> 45 mg/dl). Patients with intestinal malabsorption will have a "flattened" C-xylose curve with blood levels substantially less than 45 mg/dl. The major advantage of D-xylose assessment over OGTT is that blood levels of D-xylose are not affected by insulin or glucagon. Both the D-xylose test and OGTT may yield false negative results owing to delayed gastric emptying or impaired intestinal circulation. Dogs with lymphangiectasis and some forms of small intestinal mucosa disease will have abnormally depressed D-xylose absorption test results.

Evaluation of pancreatic protease activity may be achieved by the paraaminobenzoic acid (PABA) test. In this test, a synthetic peptide comprised of *n*-benzoyl-*l*-tyrosine and PABA is given by stomach tube at a dosage of 16.7 mg/kg (0.25 ml) after a 28-hour fast. The ingested synthetic peptide stimulates the release of pancreatic chymotrypsin, which cleaves the compound and allows the freed PABA to be absorbed into the systemic circulation and excreted in the urine. The rates of digestion and absorption of PABA are determined by measuring PABA levels in blood or urine. Dogs that have urine PABA excretion levels of less than 16 per cent in six hours or blood levels less than 125 μg/dl require pancreatic enzyme replacement. Spurious results may occur in patients with renal failure (because the clearance of plasma PABA into the glomerular filtrate would be impaired) and in those receiving sulfonamides or other antibiotics or furosemide.

A complete blood count (CBC) may yield valuable supplemental information regarding the etiology of the diarrhea. Leukocytosis with a left shift may be found in patients with enteropathogenic bacterial infection (*E. coli*, *Salmonella*, and *Shigella* sp.). Profound leukopenia is a common finding in canine parvovirus (CPV) enteritis. A relative and absolute eosinophilia may accompany intestinal parasitism or allergic gastroenteritis. A microcytic, hypochromic anemia may be seen in patients with chronic ancylostomiasis with chronic blood loss or intestinal malabsorption in which there is insufficient iron absorption.

A urinalysis is an important supplemental tool for all patients that present with hypoproteinemia that may be associated with pitting limb edema and/or ascites. The absence of proteinuria excludes a nephrotic syndrome as a cause of the hypoproteinemia. In patients with biliary obstruction causing steatorrhea, relatively acholic feces and a jaundice urinalysis reveal bilirubinuria and no urobilinogen in the urine.

Serum biochemical surveys may yield valuable information in the evaluation of a patient with suspected intestinal malabsorption. The abnormalities may include moderate to marked hypocholesterolemia, a blood glucose in the low-normal range, and mild hypocalcemia. Patients suspected of having a protein-losing enteropathy (PLE) can have hypoproteinemia (total protein < 4.0 gm/dl, albumin < 1.5 mg/dl, and globulins 2.5 mg/dl). Fractionation of the serum proteins via serum protein electrophoresis will show a uniform reduction in both the albumin and globulin migratory regions. Thus, a patient presenting with pitting leg edema that reveals no proteinuria, a marked reduction of both serum albumin and globulins, normal liver function tests (BSP retention, ammonia tolerance test, and serum bile acid levels), and a normal cardiovascular examination (ECG and thoracic and abdominal radiographs) is a prime candidate for a diagnosis of PLE.

A prolonged prothrombin time (> 13 sec) may be seen (but very seldom) in patients with intestinal malabsorption or bile acid deficiency causing a defect in absorption of fat–soluble vitamin K.

Abdominal radiography, either plain films or barium contrast studies, seldom yields specific diagnostic information. Exceptions include regional enterocolitis in which roughened mucosal borders ("paint-brush borders") and narrowing ("stringing") of various bowel segments occur, stagnant bowel loop syndrome (gas ileus with air/fluid levels), infiltrative neoplasia (lymphoma or leiomyosarcoma), and various strictures of the bowel segments.

Proctoscopy with biopsy of the colon is essential in the evaluation of unexplained diarrhea. A definitive diagnosis of colonic disease is possible only with a colon biopsy. This procedure can be done in most dogs without any sedation. The gastrointestinal anatomy of dogs and cats does not readily lend itself to endoscopic examination of the small intestine and pancreatic/bile ducts. Biopsy of the small intestine utilizing Oregon or Quinton biopsy instruments is not highly successful except in larger dogs. Ultimately, if the small intestine appears to be the region in question, an exploratory celiotomy with full-thickness biopsies is indicated. Patients with PLE heal very slowly and often inadequately, possibly resulting in dehiscence and/or evisceration.

THERAPEUTIC PRINCIPLES (Table 7)

Re-establishment and maintenance of fluid and electrolyte balance is the foremost consideration in the supportive care of the patient with diarrheal

Table 7.   *Treatment of Specific Diarrheal Diseases*

Condition	Treatment	Comment
Parasitic		
Giardiasis	Metronidazole (Flagyl, Searle Laboratories) 60 mg/kg SID for five days	*Giardia* organisms may be difficult to demonstrate; may treat with flagyl to achieve a therapeutic diagnosis
Coccidiosis	Sulfadimethoxine (Bactrovet, Pitman-Moore) 25 mg/kg SID for ten days	Treatment is highly effective in eradicating organisms
Inflammatory		
Eosinophilic enterocolitis	Prednisone 0.50 mg/kg/day, then taper dosage	Can manage with controlled diet if eosinophilia disappears after feeding for ten days; sulfasalazine can cause keratitis sicca
Ulcerative colitis	Sulfasalazine (Azulfidine, Pharmacia Inc.) 20 mg/kg t.i.d. Prednisone 0.50 mg/kg/day for six days, then taper dosage	
Lymphocytic-plasmacytic enteritis	Prednisone (see above dose schedule) Tylan powder with vitamins (Elanco Co.) ½ to 1 tsp mixed with food	Good response may be achieved with long-term Tylan powder therapy
Gluten enteropathy	Dietary: boiled rice, dry cottage cheese, and boiled chicken	Prednisone may be used in refractory cases
Post-Inflammatory		
Pancreatic exocrine insufficiency	Pancreatin (Viokase, A.H. Robbins Co.; Pancrease capsules, Johnson & Johnson)	Same treatment applies for juvenile pancreatic atrophy; refractory conditions may improve after adding Tagamet (Smith Kline & French)
Intestinal lymphangiectasia	MCT or Portagen (Mead Johnson Co.) as nutritional source along with R/D or I/D (Hills Pet Food Co.)	Refractory cases in humans have temporarily responded to prednisone
Neoplastic		
Intestinal lymphoma	C.O.M.P. (Cytoxan, Mead Johnson; Oncovin, Lilly; Methotrexate, Lederle; prednisone)	Prognosis is grave; patients usually are too debilitated to undergo chemotherapy

disease. Patients with profuse diarrhea will often be markedly dehydrated (5 to 8 per cent of body weight) and depleted of sodium, potassium, and bicarbonate ions. Hypokalemia is clinically manifested as muscular weakness and may complicate diarrhea by intensifying intestinal hypomotility, resulting in a paralytic ileus with subsequent bacterial overgrowth. Copious loss of bicarbonate will result in metabolic acidosis. In the ideal situation, measurement of serum sodium, potassium, chloride, and plasma bicarbonate is carried out to assist the clinician in selecting the proper replacement fluid. If such measurement is not possible or if the patient requires intravenous fluid therapy before the results are available, it is wise to select a balanced, polyionic alkalinizing solution such as Ringer's lactate or Multisol-R.*

Patients with severe PLE are markedly depleted of plasma proteins, especially albumin. Attempts to replenish lost proteins by infusion of intravenous plasma or albumin may be unsuccessful.

The use of antibiotics in patients with diarrheal disease is controversial and often unnecessary. The rationale for their usage is that the diarrhea is the result of or is complicated by pathogenic bacteria in the gut. Except for patients with salmonellosis, shigellosis, *Campylobacter jejuni* infection, and stagnant bowel loop syndromes with bacterial overgrowth, the widespread use of antibiotics is usually unnecessary. Antibiotics such as tetracycline, ampicillin, and neomycin may actually cause diarrhea in patients with previously normal bowel movement. Macrolide antibiotics such as lincomycin (Lincocin†) and clindamycin (Cleocin†) have been implicated in a lethal form of hemorrhagic pseudomembranous enterocolitis in humans.

One sound indication for the use of prophylactic antibiotics is in patients with hemorrhagic diarrhea, especially if leukopenia (often owing to CPV) is present. The presence of occult or fresh blood in the stool indicates a loss of the intestinal mucosal barrier and the potential for bacterial invasion and septicemia. Rational administration of antibiotics is based on the knowledge that the anaerobes outnumber aerobes (especially in the colon) by one-thousandfold. Thus, any antibiotic regimen should include an agent that is effective against these organisms (*Clostridia, Bacteroides, Fusiformis, Peptostreptococcus,* and so on). In addition, the agents should be administered parenterally, preferably intravenously. A combination that is relatively inexpensive and effectively covers the patient against coliform and anaerobic invasion is kanamycin (Kantrim‡) at a rate of 5 mg/kg intravenously b.i.d. and potassium penicillin-G at a rate of 20,000 U/kg

---

*Abbott Laboratories, North Chicago, IL.

†Upjohn Co., Kalamazoo, MI.
‡Bristol Laboratories, Syracuse, NY.

intravenously q6h. If nephrotoxicity is a problem and an aminoglycoside antibiotic (such as kanamycin) is contraindicated, this combination may be replaced by intravenous chloramphenicol at a rate of 20 to 30 mg/kg q6h.

Motility modifiers can be used as adjunct symptomatic therapy for diarrhea. Since diarrheal disease usually is associated with a loss of normal motility, anticholinergics, which further reduce motility (rhythmic segmentation), should not be used. Their usage can contribute to paralytic ileus and bacterial overgrowth. The only indication for the use of anticholinergic agents is diarrhea accompanied by intestinal spasms, which occurs infrequently. Symptomatic relief of the majority of diarrheal conditions may be achieved by the use of opiate derivatives, which increase rhythmic segmentation and slow the rate of transit through the intestines. Effective agents include paregoric, diphenoxylate and atropine (Lomotil*), and loperamide (Imodium†).

Agents that contain bismuth salicylate may be effective in treating secretory diarrhea due to prostaglandin stimulation of cyclic AMP. The bismuth salicylate in these agents (Corrective Mixture,‡ Pepto Bismol§) blocks prostaglandin release. Although widely used, agents that contain kaolin and pectin have never been shown to be effective in the symptomatic treatment of diarrhea in carefully controlled clinical trials.

One agent that has been shown to be effective in some cases of pediatric enterocolitis is cholestyramine (Questran‖), which binds hydroxylated acids, which impair colonic water absorption.

Nutritional management of the patient with diarrheal disease is important yet difficult. Patients recovering from acute diarrheal disease should be given a bland, easily digested, low-lactose diet. This may include boiled rice mixed with dry cottage cheese and boiled chicken added for flavor, or prescription diets such as I/D.** Since it takes

*Searle & Co., San Juan, PR.
†Ortho Pharmaceutical Corp., Raritan, N.J.
‡Beecham Laboratories, Bristol, IN.
§Norwich-Eaton Pharmaceuticals, Norwich, N.Y.
‖Mead Johnson, Evansville, IN.
**Hills Division, Rivinia Foods, Inc., Topeka, KS.

approximately 10 to 14 days to re-establish proper brush border disaccharidase levels, milk products, which are high in lactose, should be avoided. Patients that have been found to have intestinal lipid malabsorption may exhibit marked alleviation of symptoms with the use of powdered food supplements that contain medium-chain triglycerides (MCTs). When digested, these lipids release fatty acids that can be readily absorbed and transported through the portal circulation rather than the lymphatics. This is especially useful in treating lymphangiectasia. Available products include MCT‖ and Portagen.‖ Parenteral supplementation with vitamins (A, D, E, and K) is often beneficial in treating secondary deficiencies due to steatorrhea.

SUMMARY

Although diarrhea is a common clinical sign, it is often a frustrating problem to treat successfully. Understanding the basic pathophysiologic mechanisms of diarrheal disease will enable the clinician to form a relevant diagnostic plan and a rational therapeutic approach.

REFERENCES AND SUPPLEMENTAL READING

Burrows, C. F., Merritt, A. M., and Chiapella, A. M.: Determination of fecal fat and trypsin output in the evaluation of chronic canine diarrhea. J.A.V.M.A. 174:62, 1979.

Drazner, F. H.: Current concepts of gastroenterology. Paper presented at the Symposium on Small Animal Diseases, Mexico City, November, 1980.

Drazner, F. H.: The diseases of the pancreas—a pathophysiologic approach. American Animal Hospital Association Scientific Proceedings, 105, South Bend, Indiana, 1981.

Greenberger, N. J.: *Gastrointestinal Disorders—A Pathophysiologic Approach.* Chicago: Year Book Medical Publishers, 1981, pp. 117–174.

Lorenz, M. D.: Canine malabsorption syndromes. Comp. Cont. Ed. 2:885, 1980.

Moon, H. W.: Mechanisms in the pathogenesis of diarrhea: A review. J.A.V.M.A. 172:443, 1978.

Moreau, P. W.: Canine viral enteritis. Comp. Cont. Ed. 2:540, 1980.

Sherding, R. G.: Canine large bowel diarrhea. Comp. Cont. Ed. 2:279, 1979.

Strombeck, D. R.: *Small Animal Gastroenterology.* Davis, CA: Stonegate Publishing, 1979, pp. 172–290.

Tams, T. R., and Twedt, D. C.: Canine protein-losing gastroenterology syndrome. Comp. Cont. Ed. 3:105, 1981.

THE TREATMENT OF DIARRHEA

COLIN F. BURROWS, B.V.M.S.

Gainesville, Florida

Diarrhea, defined as the passage of loose or liquid feces at an increased frequency, is one of the most common complaints in veterinary medicine. There are no reliable data for the overall incidence of diarrhea in the dog and cat, but in one study gastrointestinal disease ranked second only to skin disease as a reason for consultation with a veterinarian.

Even though diarrhea is defined as the passage of loose or liquid feces, there is such a wide variation in both the character and consistency of normal canine and feline feces, as well as in the frequency of defecation, that the normal feces and patterns of defecation for the individual patient should always be utilized for comparison when evaluating an animal presented for treatment of diarrhea.

Diet appears to be the major influence on fecal consistency, since dogs fed dry food have bulkier, softer feces that weigh approximately twice as much as the feces of animals fed canned food. However, the frequency of defecation is also important, since the more frequently an animal defecates, the less time is available for colonic water absorption and the softer the feces will appear. The canine colon is usually completely evacuated at defecation, and it is perfectly normal for the terminal portion of the feces to appear soft or semiformed, especially if the animal is fed dry dog food. Clients frequently present animals for treatment of this spurious "diarrhea," a situation in which a detailed history and effective client education would be of much greater benefit than ineffectual attempts at treatment.

The fact that an animal has diarrhea does not always indicate primary gastrointestinal disease, an important clinical consideration, since treatment should always be directed at correction of the underlying disorder. Nevertheless, treatment of diarrhea, at least on a symptomatic basis, may be essential while diagnosis of the underlying disorder is pursued.

GASTROINTESTINAL PHYSIOLOGY

The gastrointestinal tract and its accessory organs, the liver and pancreas, should be thought of as a tightly integrated system for the provision and conservation of water, nutrients, and essential ions. Such a system is subject to disruption in a number of ways, but the end result is usually manifested as vomiting and/or diarrhea.

It is important to realize that diarrhea is a sign, not a specific disease process, and as such it reflects a disruption of normal intestinal salt and water transport. For this reason, an understanding of intestinal salt and water transport is essential for both diagnosis and logical treatment of the various manifestations of diarrhea.

INTESTINAL SALT AND WATER TRANSPORT

Large volumes of isotonic fluid enter the lumen of the proximal bowel every day; most is reabsorbed, and only a fraction is actually excreted in the feces. This fluid comes partly from the diet but mainly from the endogenous secretions of the upper intestinal tract. The daily volume of fluid exchanged greatly exceeds that of the extracellular fluid volume and explains why dehydration can occur so rapidly if this fluid is lost in acute diarrhea.

There are no reliable data for the exact volumes of fluid exchanged across the gastrointestinal tract of the dog or cat, but, depending to some extent on the environment and diet, a 20-kg dog will consume about 500 ml of water per day, to which must be added an estimated 3 liters of gastric, pancreatic, and intestinal secretions. This represents a total daily volume of 3 to 3.5 liters presented to the small intestine. Most of this fluid (about 80 per cent) is absorbed in the small intestine and the remainder in the colon, with only about 2 per cent excreted in the feces.

FUNCTIONAL ANATOMY

The functional units of the small intestine are the villi. These structures account for a tenfold amplification of the absorptive surface area of the bowel, whereas microvilli on the surface of each epithelial cell are responsible for a further twentyfold amplification of the surface area. Intestinal epithelial cells perform a number of specialized functions including digestion, secretion, absorption, and the synthesis of a variety of hormones. These cells, formed by division in the crypts of the villi, have a very rapid turnover rate. After division they migrate up the villus, reaching the tip in three to five days, maturing as they do so and changing their primary func-

784

ion from secretion to surface digestion and absorp-ion. When they reach the tip of the villus the cells ire shed into the bowel lumen, where they are ligested and their constituents reabsorbed. This apid cell turnover is the major reason why most icute diseases of the small intestine are self-limiting. Normal mucosal integrity and function are usually estored in two to three days, providing the inciting ause is eliminated and the initial insult is not ufficiently severe to damage the crypts.

Diseases that decrease the surface area of the gut educe water and electrolyte absorption and cause liarrhea. Since absorption and secretion are contin-ous processes in the small intestine, with absorp-ion normally just exceeding secretion, small in-reases in secretion or decreases in absorption result n large volumes of fluid being presented to the olon. This frequently overwhelms the absorptive apacity of the colon and results in diarrhea. Diar-hea also occurs in colitis, both as a result of lisruption of the normal absorptive function of the olon and from stimulation of colonic secretion. The lifference between small bowel diarrhea (increased luid load to the colon) and large bowel diarrhea lecreased absorption and/or increased secretion) is eflected in the history and signs of specific diarrheal liseases. Differentiation is very important for diag-osis, prognosis, and therapy (Burrows, 1982).

PATHOPHYSIOLOGY OF DIARRHEA

Diarrhea can occur in three ways: (1) increased smotic solute load, (2) abnormal electrolyte and rater transport (increased secretion or exudation), nd (3) altered intestinal motility. More than one of iese mechanisms is usually involved in an individ-al patient (Phillips, 1972; Binder, 1979).

SMOTIC DIARRHEA

Causes of *acute* osmotic diarrhea include inges-on of poorly absorbed osmotically active sub-ances, ingestion of a very large meal, or an abrupt nange in diet, all of which can overwhelm normal igestive and absorptive processes. Malabsorption f nutrients as a result of either pancreatic exocrine isufficiency or diffuse small intestinal mucosal dis-ase causes *chronic* osmotic diarrhea. Osmotically :tive compounds induce water influx into the je-num, with the severity depending on the ability the ileum and colon to compensate by absorbing :cess fluid. Osmotic diarrhea results predomi-ntly in fluid loss rather than electrolyte depletion hillips, 1972).

CRETORY AND EXUDATIVE DIARRHEA

Passive secretion is a result of increased mucosal rmeability associated with inflammation or dam-

age to the intestinal mucosa; inflammatory bowel diseases are the most common cause. Active elec-trolyte secretion can result from the presence of toxin-producing bacteria, hydroxyfatty acids, and bile acids. Although the major alteration in water and electrolyte transport in diarrhea is probably hypersecretion, inhibition of absorption through a decrease in surface area may also play a role (Binder, 1979).

MOTILITY ABNORMALITIES IN DIARRHEA

The contribution of intestinal motility disorders to diarrhea is still poorly understood. A variety of mechanisms have been proposed, but their relation-ship to disorders of secretion and absorption re-mains to be elucidated. Although a few specific disease entities have been associated with either an increase in motility or abnormal motor patterns, most authorities now agree that intestinal contractile activity is decreased, in the majority of intestinal diseases.

ACUTE VERSUS CHRONIC DIARRHEA

Diarrhea in the dog and cat can be conveniently divided into two categories: acute and chronic. Each mandates a different diagnostic and therapeutic approach. Acute diarrhea is more common and usually self-limiting, even if mucosal damage is severe, since the rapid intestinal epithelial cell turnover quickly restores normal intestinal function. Treatment of acute diarrhea usually need be only supportive and symptomatic, since most animals that die from diarrhea do so not as a result of the inciting cause but from the loss of electrolytes and water, with subsequent dehydration, acidosis, and shock. Treatment of chronic diarrhea is an entirely different matter, since it is rarely self-limiting. It is essential to establish an accurate diagnosis and prescribe appropriate and specific therapy for effec-tive treatment.

THE APPROACH TO TREATMENT

The management of diarrhea can be divided into three basic categories: supportive, symptomatic, and specific.

Supportive treatment consists of replacing fluid and electrolyte losses and, in acute disturbances, resting the intestinal tract by restricting food intake for 24 to 48 hours. Dietary restriction allows resto-ration of intestinal epithelial integrity without the added complication of ongoing fluid loss from os-motic diarrhea and the possibility of intestinal irri-tation from ingested foodstuffs.

Symptomatic treatment involves the use of drugs such as motility modifiers and absorbents. These neither alter the underlying pathophysiology nor correct electrolyte or fluid losses but may reduce the number of bowel movements and improve fecal consistency. This type of treatment frequently placates the client, but there is no evidence that these agents actually benefit the patient. If prescribed at all, these compounds should be restricted to the treatment of acute diarrheal disease. Together with supportive care they are usually sufficient to allow restoration of normal gut function.

Specific therapy is aimed at treating the underlying condition and blocking cellular mechanisms of fluid and electrolyte loss. It is most appropriate in the treatment of chronic diarrhea and includes dietary modification, administration of antimicrobials and anthelmintics, replacement of pancreatic enzymes, discontinuation of diarrhea-causing drugs, and, on rare occasions, administration of corticosteroids. Specific treatment of any underlying metabolic disorder also falls into this category.

TREATMENT CATEGORIES

There are seven broad symptomatic or specific treatment categories for diarrheal disease. These are (1) dietary modification or manipulation, (2) antimicrobials, (3) motility modifiers, (4) gastrointestinal protectants, (5) anthelmintics, (6) pancreatic enzyme replacement, and (7) corticosteroids. The appropriate use of anthelmintics, pancreatic enzyme replacement therapy, and corticosteroids is discussed elsewhere in this text (page 797).

DIETARY MODIFICATION

Restriction or manipulation of individual dietary constituents is the single most important treatment of both acute and chronic diarrhea; it is also the least understood and the most neglected.

DIET AND ACUTE DIARRHEA

Placing the intestinal tract in a state of physiologic rest is perhaps the single most important aspect of the treatment of acute diarrhea. It is not possible to reduce the function of many of the internal organs to expedite the return of normal function, but this can be done with the gastrointestinal tract and its accessory organs, the liver and pancreas, by completely restricting the oral intake of food. After 24 to 48 hours of dietary restriction, with the duration depending on the severity of signs, the patient may be gradually reintroduced to food. This reintroduction should be comprised of small quantities of bland, easily digested, low-fat foods, such as boiled chicken or hamburger mixed with boiled rice in a ratio of approximately 1:4. Provision of the total daily caloric requirement is not important, and the food should be offered in small quantities four to six times a day to avoid rapid delivery into the small intestine and exacerbation of diarrhea. If this regimen is accepted by the patient without exacerbation of signs, the original diet can gradually be reintroduced over a two- to three-day period. Water is usually not contraindicated; the volume offered depends on the fluid requirements of the patient and whether or not it is vomiting.

DIET AND CHRONIC DIARRHEA

Dietary modification is also an important part of the treatment of chronic diarrhea. Indeed, it is frequently possible to control diarrhea of small intestinal origin by dietary means alone. The principles of diet formulation for a dog with chronic diarrhea have been described in detail (Strombeck 1979). An ideal diet should (1) require minimal digestion, (2) be low in fat, (3) contain no lactose, (4) be nonallergenic, (5) be designed so that it can be fed frequently in small quantities, and (6) be acceptable to the patient.

The requirement of minimal digestion is thought to reduce the digestive workload placed on the gut particularly when the normal digestive process may be reduced by disease.

A diet low in fat is usually essential, even though fat is a valuable source of calories and an important component of the normal carnivore diet. This is because unabsorbed fatty acids can be hydroxylated by intestinal bacteria to substances that stimulate colonic water secretion and exacerbate diarrhea and fluid loss.

Intestinal disease frequently results in destruction or reduction of mucosal brush border enzymes; for this reason milk or other substances containing lactose should be avoided. Failure to digest lactose results in bacterial degradation of the sugar to volatile fatty acids which can cause osmotic diarrhea.

Although there is no conclusive evidence that dietary allergy or sensitivity causes chronic diarrhea in the dog or cat, clinical experience and anecdotal reports suggest that it may occasionally be a causative factor. For these reasons, especially when food allergy is suspected, an attempt should be made to feed a nonallergenic diet. Admittedly this is difficult in the dog or cat, but can best be achieved by feeding meat, such as lamb or mutton, to which the animal has not been previously exposed.

The basis of a diet that fulfills many of the previously mentioned criteria and provides nutritional homeostasis, at least on a short-term basis, is four parts boiled rice or potatoes and one part cottage cheese, lean meat, or eggs. Vitamin supplements should be added as necessary. Commercial low-fat diets such as ID,* RD,† and Cycle 3‡ are reasonable alternatives for clients who do not wish to prepare meals. The daily nutritional requirement should be calculated and fed in three or four small meals rather than one large one. Low-fat or home-prepared diets are especially useful in diseases associated with disordered fat digestion or absorption; their use makes no sense in diarrhea caused by diseases of the large bowel. If a low-fat diet controls the diarrhea, a gradual return to a normal diet can be attempted. The long-range goal of dietary therapy is the eventual return of the patient to its original diet.

Medium-chain triglycerides (coconut oil, Portagen,§ or MCT oil§) fed at a rate of about 1 tbs/400 gm canned food provide an additional source of calories in dogs suffering from lymphangiectasia. Medium-chain triglycerides (< 14 carbon chain length) are more rapidly hydrolyzed, and are not dependent on bile salts for emulsification. They are carried via the portal system and are not dependent on chylomicron synthesis or lymphatic transport. They therefore bypass the lymphatics and prevent exacerbation of lymphatic disease.

Dogs and cats are occasionally presented with a history of an inability to tolerate commercial diets; the history in these animals is usually characterized by a combination of one or more of the following: vomiting, flatulence, borborygmus, and diarrhea. A specific diagnosis in these apparently hypersensitive animals is frequently elusive, but so-called pure foods such as Eukanuba‖ are sometimes beneficial in dogs, whereas semimoist foods such as Tender Vittles** may be useful as an adjunct to the control of diarrhea in cats.

The addition of an indigestible bulk-forming agent in the form of dietary fiber can be useful in the treatment of both diarrhea and constipation. This apparent paradox is best explained by the water-retaining properties of most intestinal bulk-producing agents and the effect of increased fecal bulk on colonic motility. Fiber slows the speed of intestinal transit in diarrhea and increases it in constipation. Most bulking agents consist of either a purified component of dietary fiber, such as cellulose, or a natural preparation such as bran. Over-the-counter preparations such as Siblin†† or Metamucil‡‡ are sometimes quite effective as an adjunct to the symptomatic control of chronic diarrhea; however, bran is cheaper and just as effective. One cup of coarse bran mixed with the diet is usually adequate to correct diarrhea in a 35-kg dog. Contrary to general belief, increasing fecal bulk decreases canine colonic motility and is therefore most useful in the treatment of functional diarrheas, some of which may be associated with a disturbance of colonic smooth muscle function.

ANTIMICROBIALS

ANTIBIOTICS IN ACUTE DIARRHEA

Antibiotics have long been part of the standard treatment of both acute and chronic diarrhea in the dog and cat, and yet there is still no evidence for either bacterial infection as a major cause of diarrhea or the efficacy of antibiotics in its treatment. Most of the combination drugs marketed for the treatment of diarrhea contain nonabsorbable sulfonamides or antibiotics combined with motility modifiers, adsorbents, or intestinal protectives. These compounds are of no proven value in the treatment of either acute or chronic diarrhea in the dog and cat and are best avoided. Most animals with acute diarrhea will recover without them, and, with a few exceptions detailed hereafter, animals with chronic diarrhea fail to permanently respond to this type of treatment. There is, in fact, absolutely *no indication* for the *routine use* of oral antimicrobials in the treatment of acute diarrhea in the dog and cat. The only specific indication for their use is in salmonellosis and other invasive bacterial infections, which are extremely rare.

As a general principle, antibiotics should only be used in those patients in which damage to the intestinal mucosal barrier is suspected (evidenced by acute hemorrhagic diarrhea) and in those that have a leucocytosis or fever ascribed to the diarrheal disease. Mucosal damage is thought to allow penetration of the intestinal wall by bacteria, with their subsequent release into the systemic circulation. Although unproved, this might occur following severe acute enterocolitis, intussusception, parvovirus infection, and hemorrhagic gastroenteritis. In all cases *parenteral* antibiotic therapy is probably more appropriate.

Antimicrobials are routinely used by many clinicians to treat animals that are presented with any form of acute enterocolitis, but their use is simply not warranted in patients in which the barrier is intact. In fact, they are potentially harmful in that they disturb the distribution of normal flora and may prolong the return of normal intestinal function and homeostasis.

ANTIBIOTICS IN CHRONIC DIARRHEA

There are some exceptions to the preceding general principles that apply to the treatment of diarrhea associated with colitis, to overgrowth of bac-

---

*Intestinal Diet, Hills Pet Products, Topeka, KS.
†Reducing Diet, Hills Pet Products, Topeka, KS.
‡Cycle 3, General Foods Corporation, White Plains, NY.
§Mead Johnson, Evansville, IN.
‖Iams Food Company, Lewisburg, OH.
**Ralston Purina, St. Louis, MI.
††Parke-Davis, Morris Plains, NJ.
‡‡Searle Pharmaceuticals, Chicago, IL.

teria in the small intestine, and perhaps to some of the chronic inflammatory diseases of the small intestine. Sulfasalazine is the drug of choice for the treatment of colitis, and although many antibiotics have been used in chronic small intestinal disease, tylosin and metronidazole are perhaps the most effective.

Sulfasalazine. Sulfasalazine (Azulfidine*) is the drug of choice for the treatment of idiopathic chronic canine colitis. This drug, a combination of sulfapyridine and 5-amino-salicylate, was initially developed for the treatment of rheumatoid arthritis in humans. Although of no proven efficacy against this disease, it has been shown to be useful in the treatment and prophylaxis of ulcerative colitis in humans and in the treatment of idiopathic chronic colitis in the dog and cat. Cleavage of the azo bond, the initial step in sulfasalazine metabolism, occurs in the colon and is attributed exclusively to the action of intestinal bacteria. The drug is split into sulfapyridine, which is absorbed and excreted in the urine, and 5-amino-salicylate, which is excreted in the feces. Rectal infusion of the separate ingredients into human patients suffering from ulcerative colitis has recently shown that 5-amino-salicylate is the probable therapeutic ingredient.

The mechanism of action of sulfasalazine is unclear. Several mechanisms have been proposed, but current evidence suggests that it most likely acts through an effect on prostaglandins in the colonic epithelial cell.

The dose is 50 mg/kg/day divided into three or four equal doses, and treatment for at least 21 to 28 days is generally necessary. Side effects of sulfasalazine in the dog are rare but include allergic dermatitis, nausea and vomiting, and cholestatic jaundice. Keratoconjunctivitis sicca (KCS) has been observed in dogs treated for a long period of time. KCS also occurs rapidly in some dogs if there has been prior exposure to any sulfonamide. Sulfasalazine should be used with caution in the cat, since signs of salicylate toxicity may be exhibited at doses recommended for the dog.

Tylosin. Tylosin (Tylan-plus-Vitamins†) is reportedly effective in the treatment of a wide spectrum of canine inflammatory bowel diseases. The drug is now supplied only as a vitamin-powder mix, and dosage for the dog is thus imprecise. A dose range of 11 to 200 mg/kg/day (½ to 1 teaspoonful of mix twice daily) has been reported to be effective. The drug appears to be useful in the control of chronic inflammatory diseases of the small intestine and in those diseases in which bacterial overgrowth is suspected. This author uses a dose of approximately 40 mg/kg of tylosin powder twice daily.

Metronidazole. Metronidazole (Flagyl‡) is another antibacterial drug that has occasionally proved useful in the treatment of both colitis and chronic diarrhea of unknown etiology in the dog and cat. In addition to its antiprotozoal action, metronidazole suppresses cell-mediated immune reactions and has been used in the treatment of granulomatous enterocolitis in humans. The drug has also been shown to have a protective effect against experimental colitis. Metronidazole is effective against anaerobic bacteria and has proved useful in the treatment of anaerobic infections. This is relevant, since it has been postulated that the predominantly anaerobic intestinal flora may be a source of antigens participating in immunologic reactions of possible significance in inflammatory bowel disease. It is quite possible that in many dogs a favorable response may be due to elimination of undiagnosed protozoal infections. Dosage is 30 mg/kg body weight once a day for five days, but treatment for longer periods is not contraindicated and may sometimes be necessary.

Other antibiotics have been used in the treatment of chronic diarrhea associated with bacterial overgrowth in the small intestine. Tetracycline, chloramphenicol, and ampicillin appear to be effective, but it must be emphasized that these compounds are not indicated in the *routine* treatment of chronic diarrheal disease.

MOTILITY MODIFIERS

A widespread but probably fallacious belief is that the bowel is hypermotile in most diarrheal disease. The role of disordered motility in the pathogenesis of most types of diarrhea still remains to be clarified, but current evidence suggests decreased rather than increased motility. There are, therefore, few specific indications for motility modifiers in the treatment of diarrhea. These compounds have been used as symptomatic treatment for acute diarrhea in the belief that they reduce the number of bowel movements and improve fecal consistency, but there is no evidence that they actually benefit the patient. They may be contraindicated in many diarrheal diseases in that they impair elimination of the inciting cause. They are, however, of some apparent benefit in the symptomatic control of chronic functional diarrhea.

There are three basic classes of drugs that modify intestinal motility: narcotic analgesics, anticholinergics (antispasmodics), and combinations of central nervous system depressants and anticholinergics.

NARCOTIC ANALGESICS

Narcotic analgesics are the drugs of choice for the symptomatic treatment of diarrhea. Of these, opiates have been the most widely used, since they purportedly cause an increase in the strength of rhythmic segmentation and thus inhibit aborad pro-

*Pharmacia Laboratories, Piscataway, NJ.
†Elanco Products, Indianapolis, IN.
‡Searle and Co., San Juan, PR.

pulsive activity (peristalsis). Other possible beneficial effects of these drugs are the analgesia they produce and their enhancement of fluid and electrolyte transport. The drugs most commonly used as antidiarrheals are paregoric and tincture of opium. Paregoric is given at the rate of 0.05 to 0.06 mg/kg of body weight two to three times a day. Tincture of opium is given at one-fourth that dose. Codeine and meperidine have the same effect on the bowel and can also be used. Codeine is a particularly effective antidiarrheal drug at a dose of 0.25 to 0.50 mg/kg three to four times daily.

Diphenoxylate is a synthetic compound that is similar to the opiates in structure and function. This drug is purported to act directly on intestinal smooth muscle to stimulate rhythmic segmentation. This feature is an important consideration in the use of the commercial preparation, in which diphenoxylate is combined with atropine and marketed as a preparation called Lomotil.* Atropine has a pharmacologic effect opposite that of diphenoxylate, but the combination is effective, since diphenoxylate acts directly on smooth muscle whereas the anticholinergic acts one step before the muscle in the ganglionic synapses of the intrinsic nerves. In humans, atropine is added to diphenoxylate to prevent overdosage, allowing it to be distributed with less stringent narcotic controls. The dose is 0.05 to 0.1 mg/kg body weight three to four times a day. A similar drug is loperamide (Imodium†), perhaps the most potent of the currently available antidiarrheal drugs. Unfortunately, this drug is only available in 2-mg capsules, which are too large for small dogs. The approximate dose is 1 capsule/25 kg body weight four times daily.

ANTICHOLINERGICS

Atropine, tincture of belladonna, propantheline (Pro-Banthine*), isopropamide, and numerous other anticholinergic products are often used in the treatment of diarrhea, but no controlled studies on their efficacy are available. Recent evidence suggests that anticholinergics enhance electrolyte and water absorption, and it is possible that this action is more important in the control of diarrhea than their effect on motility. A decrease in gastrointestinal motility and tone usually occurs only with doses sufficient to cause unpleasant side effects. However, there is no doubt that inflammatory diseases of the distal colon and rectum can cause tenesmus, which can be relieved by antispasmodic therapy. These drugs are also of occasional use in the treatment of problems that may have a nervous or psychologic basis.

Drugs classified as antispasmodics can be grouped as (1) belladonna alkaloids such as atropine; (2) anticholinergics such as propantheline (Pro-Banthine*), isopropamide, and antihistamines; and (3) direct-acting smooth muscle relaxants such as dicyclomine (Bentyl‡). These agents are effective when excessive intestinal contractile activity occurs either as a result of acute enteritis caused by an invasive organism or following many of the chronic inflammatory bowel diseases, since in both these conditions the pathologic process frequently extends to the muscle layers.

Contraindications to the use of antispasmodics include those diseases that result in a paralytic ileus, in which they delay the return of normal intestinal motility; those that result in gastric atony and gastric outlet obstruction; and any diarrheal disease associated with an infectious agent in which antispasmodics may delay elimination of the organism and prolong the intestinal disease.

THE COMBINATION OF CNS DEPRESSANTS AND ANTISPASMODICS

There are a number of products that combine a central nervous system depressant with an antispasmodic to form compounds that are possibly effective in the treatment of psychomotor disturbances of the gastrointestinal tract. Definitive evidence is lacking for the existence of this type of disease in small animal medicine, but extensive clinical experience has indicated that these compounds have definite therapeutic benefit in a variety of gastrointestinal diseases. Darbazine§ (isopropamide and prochlorperazine) probably falls into this category, even though prochlorperazine is more commonly prescribed for its antiemetic effects. Librax‖, a combination of chlordiazepoxide and clidinium, is another useful preparation in the treatment of diarrhea resulting from psychomotor disturbances of the canine gastrointestinal tract. Of these, the most common is a chronic diarrheal disease of colonic origin, which is apparently stress associated and in which no inflammatory component can be identified.

PROTECTANTS AND ADSORBENTS

These are a group of inert insoluble compounds that are purported to coat "irritated" gastrointestinal mucosa and adsorb or bind "noxious" agents. Some of these products have been used in the treatment of diarrhea since ancient times, but well-controlled clinical trials of their effectiveness are still lacking.

---

*Searle and Co., San Juan, PR.
†Ortho Pharmaceuticals, Raritan, NJ.

‡Merrell-National Laboratories, Cincinnati, OH.
§Norden Laboratories, Lincoln, NE.
‖ Roche Laboratories, Inc., Nutley, NJ.

Most widely used are compounds containing various combinations of kaolin and pectin.

Pectin is a polyuronic polymer consisting of purified carbohydrate extracted from citrus fruit or apple pumice. Up to 90 per cent of this drug is decomposed in the gastrointestinal tract, but it does increase the thickness of the unstirred layer and decreases the absorption of several substances. The effect of pectin in diarrhea is still unknown.

Kaolin is a widely used antidiarrheal and a native hydrated aluminum silicate with an unproved ability to absorb large numbers of bacteria and toxins such as those of *E. coli* and *Clostridium welchii*. Kaopectate* is a popular proprietary product that contains 25 per cent kaolin and 1 per cent pectin. Its effectiveness is not proved. In one study of diarrhea in South American children, feces appeared to be more formed with this product, but there was no decrease in the frequency of defecation or in fecal weight or water content. Recent studies have also shown fecal sodium output to be increased by Kaopectate in diarrheal disease. In addition to its questionable efficacy, the absorption of digoxin and lincomycin may be impaired if given concurrently with Kaopectate. The use of this compound is probably no longer acceptable in veterinary practice.

Pepto-Bismol† is a similar compound but appears to be a more effective antidiarrheal in that it contains bismuth subsalicylate, which may inhibit the action of prostaglandins and thereby inhibit secretion. The manufacturer also claims that Pepto-Bismol binds toxins that aggravate diarrhea, that it "turns off" cyclic AMP, and that it may increase epithelial cell absorption. It is probably the antidiarrheal drug of choice in the symptomatic treatment of most acute diarrheas. The dose is about 1 ml/kg divided into six to eight equal daily doses. The drug tastes unpleasant, but some of the resistance to administration may be overcome, especially in the cat, by keeping the drug in the refrigerator and administering it when cold.

Parepectolin† and Donnagel-PG‡ are over-the-counter preparations that contain opiates as well as kaolin and pectin. These drugs are useful in the symptomatic treatment of simple diarrhea; the opiates are the probable active ingredients. Corrective

Mixture§ is another effective liquid antidiarrheal that contains both subsalicylate and paregoric.

CONCLUSION

Diarrhea is a very frequent complaint in small animal practice and can be either acute or chronic. Differentiation is important, since each type mandates a different therapeutic approach. Acute diarrhea is usually self-limiting and in most instances requires only supportive and symptomatic therapy. Relief of the clinical signs and restoration of normal fecal consistency can usually be achieved by restriction of food intake for 24 to 48 hours, restoration and maintenance of fluid balance, treatment with a liquid antidiarrheal such as Pepto-Bismol, and, in exceptional circumstances, the use of drugs that modify intestinal motility.

The approach to the treatment of chronic diarrhea is quite different; the nature of the disease processes necessitates a specific diagnosis for appropriate treatment. Treatment usually includes a combination of dietary modification and selected antimicrobials, or pancreatic enzyme replacement. In some instances corticosteroids, CNS depressants, or drugs that modify intestinal motility may also be indicated.

REFERENCES AND SUPPLEMENTAL READING

Binder, H. J. (ed.): Net fluid and electrolyte secretion: The pathophysiologic basis for diarrhea. *In Mechanisms of Intestinal Secretion.* New York: Alan R. Liss Inc., 1979, p. 1.

Burrows, C. F.: Diarrhea and constipation. *In* Ettinger, S. J. (ed.): *A Textbook of Veterinary Internal Medicine.* Philadelphia: W. B. Saunders, 1982, p. 56.

Greenberger, N. J., Arvanitakin, C., and Hurwitz, A.: *Drug Treatment of Gastrointestinal Disorders,* Vol. 3. New York: Churchill Livingstone, 1978.

Longe, R. L., and Ansel, H. L.: Antidiarrheal and other gastrointestinal products. *In Handbook of Nonprescription Drugs,* 5th ed. Washington, D. C.: American Pharmaceutical Association, 1979, pp. 25–36.

Netchvolodoff, C. V., and Hargrove, M. D.: Recent advances in treatment of diarrhea. Arch. Intern. Med. 139:813, 1979.

Phillips, S. F.: Diarrhea: A current view of the pathophysiology. Gastroenterology 63:495, 1972.

Pietrosko, R. G.: Pharmacotherapy of diarrhea. Am. J. Hosp. Pharm. 36:757, 1979.

Strombeck, D. R.: *Small Animal Gastroenterology.* Davis, CA: Stonegate Publishing, 1979.

---

*The Upjohn Company, Kalamazoo, MI.
†Norwich Pharmaceuticals, Norwich, NY.
‡A. H. Robins, Richmond, VA.

---

§Beecham Labs, Bristol, TN.

FELINE EOSINOPHILIC ENTERITIS

RONDA PROUTY MOORE, D.V.M.

Boston, Massachusetts

Gastrointestinal disease in the cat is a common problem; however, a specific diagnosis is seldom made. Feline eosinophilic enteritis (FEE) is an uncommon disease characterized by segmental or diffuse thickening of the bowel caused by eosinophilic infiltration or effacement of the bowel wall. A tentative diagnosis can be rendered from the history, physical exam, and hemogram and is confirmed by histopathologic examination of the intestine.

HISTORY

Cats with eosinophilic enteritis are middle aged or older (range 3 to 11 years, median 8 years). They are domestic cats with long or short hair and may be of either sex. At Angell Memorial Animal Hospital (AMAH), FEE has not been found in Siamese, Burmese, Abyssinian, or Himalayan breeds.

Vomiting is a frequent complaint associated with these cats. It is usually an early sign, although it may not occur at all. In one cat, vomiting did not occur until six months after a peripheral eosinophilia was detected. The vomitus has no distinctive gross characteristics, and a consistent relationship between vomiting and eating has not been observed.

Diarrhea occurred in 75 per cent of the cases diagnosed at AMAH. Almost one-half of these cats also had hematochezia, melena, and eosinophilic infiltration of the colon. Mucus in the stool was found in only two cats, both of which also had blood in the stool.

Anorexia and weight loss are presenting signs in most cats with FEE. Often weight loss is insidious and is not apparent to the owner until late in the disease course.

PHYSICAL EXAMINATION

The most consistent and characteristic physical finding is a uniformly diffuse or segmental thickening of the intestinal tract found on abdominal palpation. The loops of bowel are nonpainful, firm, and rigid, "like a hose." The intestine can be easily palpated throughout its length. The colon as well as the small intestine may be abnormal. Ruffled, matted haircoat, moderate to severe weight loss, and dehydration are frequent physical findings. Hepatosplenomegaly and enlarged mesenteric lymph nodes may be detected. Blood or mucus is sometimes found on rectal examination or adhering to the end of the thermometer.

LABORATORY FINDINGS

The packed cell volume is usually normal or slightly elevated if the cat is dehydrated. Occasionally a mild anemia is found. The total white blood cell count is often greater than 25,000 cells/mm^3; the range is 12,000 to 100,000/mm^3. Total eosinophil counts are consistently elevated (greater than 1500 cells/mm^3) and may be as high as 44,000 cells/mm^3. Occasionally immature band-type eosinophils are observed in the peripheral blood smear. Bone marrow aspirates and impressions have been characterized by massive infiltration of eosinophils in more than 90 per cent of cases examined at AMAH.

RADIOGRAPHS

Radiographs are not diagnostic of FEE, but radiographic evidence of pulmonary metastasis assists the clinician in differentiating neoplasia from eosinophilic enteritis. Abdominal radiographs may demonstrate enlarged mesenteric lymph nodes, a thickened or fluid-filled bowel, obstructive ileus, hepatomegaly, or a radiopaque intestinal foreign body. Without radiographs, careful palpation alone should disclose the size, consistency, shape, and location of an abdominal mass or the presence of thick, rigid loops of intestine. Radiographic contrast studies of the gastrointestinal tract markedly increase hospitalization costs and contribute little toward a specific diagnosis of FEE.

DIFFERENTIAL DIAGNOSIS

In most cats acute episodes of *vomiting* will subside when food is withheld for a day or two. The

Table 1. A Guide to the Differential Diagnosis of Feline Gastrointestinal Disease

	FEE	GIFB	GIN	PEI	FH	PLKP
History						
Vomiting	+	+	+	−	±	+
Diarrhea	+	+	+	+	+	+
Weight loss	+	±	+	+	+	±
Anorexia	+	+	+	−	−	+
↑ appetite	−	−	−	+	+	−
PE						
↑ Intestinal diameter	+	+	+	−	−	±
Melena or hematochezia	±	±	±	−	−	±
CBC						
Eosinophilia	+	−	−	−	−	−
↓ WBC	−	−	−	−	−	+

Notes: FEE = feline eosinophilic enteritis.
GIFB = gastrointestinal foreign body (or intussusception).
GIN = gastrointestinal neoplasia.
PEI = pancreatic exocrine insufficiency.
FH = feline hyperthyroidism.
PLKP = feline panleukopenia.

cat that continues to vomit or lose weight warrants a careful examination (Table 1). FEE as well as a number of other diseases must be considered. Age, vaccination status, and presence of fever are important, especially in ruling out panleukopenia. A good history is helpful but is not always reliable when considering an intestinal foreign body. Intussusception and gastric or intestinal neoplasms such as lymphoma, adenocarcinoma, or mast cell tumors should be considered. Pancreatitis occurs in the cat but is rarely diagnosed, partly because of its poor correlation with hyperamylasemia. Hepatobiliary disease is common but is usually associated with icterus. Extragastrointestinal causes of vomiting, such as kidney disease, vestibular disease, and lead poisoning, should not be overlooked.

The specific cause of *diarrhea* in adult cats is often elusive. Even in adult cats the *acute* onset of severe bloody or mucoid diarrhea may indicate panleukopenia. The stool of a cat with FEE may be indistinguishable from that of a cat with panleukopenia, but the course of diarrhea in a cat with FEE, unlike that in a cat with panleukopenia, is always chronic. A hemogram is most helpful in distinguishing these two diseases.

Chronic diarrhea and weight loss are characteristic of feline hyperthyroidism and feline pancreatic exocrine insufficiency. These two important cat diseases must also be distinguished from FEE. Elevated serum thyroxine (T_4) or triiodothyronine (T_3) levels are consistent findings in hyperthyroidism (Holzworth et al., 1980). Feline pancreatic exocrine insufficiency is usually diagnosed on the basis of steatorrhea, negative fecal protease, favorable response to clinical trials using pancreatic extract, and exclusion of other causes of diarrhea. Cats with pancreatic exocrine insufficiency and hyperthyroidism often have a voracious appetite, whereas a diminished appetite is more characteristic of FEE.

Intestinal neoplasia, especially malignant lymphoma, may be difficult to differentiate from FEE. Biopsy of the small intestine will provide the diagnosis but is not without risk to the patient. The bowel of cats with FEE heals with difficulty, and stricture formation at the biopsy site has occurred in at least one cat. Most cats with FEE with bloody stools also have eosinophilic infiltration of the colon. Since nearly one-half of the cats have bloody stools, a colon biopsy may render a specific diagnosis. In addition, biopsy by colonoscopy is less invasive and less costly than biopsy of the small intestine.

A hemogram is more helpful than any other noninvasive procedure in differentiating FEE from other causes of chronic vomiting or diarrhea. With the exception of one cat, a peripheral eosinophilia was found in all cases of FEE. Melena, vomiting, and a peripheral eosinophilia may coexist with mast cell tumors, but the thickened intestine characteristic of FEE is not found with these tumors.

CLINICAL MANAGEMENT

A presumptive diagnosis of FEE can be made and therapy initiated on the basis of characteristic clinical signs, physical findings, and a peripheral eosinophilia. Supportive therapy and steroid therapy such as prednisone or prednisolone at a dose of 1.0 to 2.0 mg/kg/day have been the usual course of treatment.* Initially, notable improvement in appetite and activity is seen. Episodes of vomiting diminish in frequency and may cease altogether. Stools may return to normal consistency and color. This "well-being" is short-lived, and by the third or fourth week of treatment the original signs recur and may be more severe than on initial presentation. One cat was treated at different times with busulfan (Myleran†), and vincristine (Oncovin‡). There was no response to these drugs.

*Editor's Note: A better response may be achieved with 2 mg/lb, a dose well tolerated in cats.
†Burroughs Wellcome Co., Research Triangle Park, NC.
‡Eli Lilly and Co., Indianapolis, IN.

Because of the poor response to treatment, most cats are euthanatized within a month of diagnosis. One cat that was presented initially for upper respiratory signs did not begin to vomit or have diarrhea until six months after a peripheral eosinophilia was detected. The cat was treated for four months with prednisone and improved considerably before signs recurred. Unfortunately, this is the longest survival time of a cat with confirmed FEE. Two other cats were not euthanatized. One was untreated and died within a week, and the other died within eight weeks of diagnosis while on steroid therapy.

PATHOLOGY

Hendrick (1981) described the lesions of FEE and suggested that it is a component of a hypereosinophilic syndrome comparable to a similar syndrome in humans. In her review of six cases at AMAH, all six cats had an eosinophilic infiltrate of the small intestine. Since that time, we have autopsied a cat with involvement of the colon and other organs but not the small intestine. The stomach is affected infrequently. A circumferential band of fibrosis in the lamina propria of the small intestine was described by Hendrick in three of six cats. We have observed this same lesion in subsequent cases of FEE. Presumably the fibrosis and the eosinophilic transmural infiltrate cause a malabsorption syndrome and an osmotic diarrhea. In some cats a segmental transmural infiltrate almost completely occludes the intestinal lumen. At this time, correlation between the severity of clinical signs and the extent of segmental or diffuse involvement of the intestine cannot be made.

As in the hypereosinophilic syndrome of humans,

involvement of organs other than the gastrointestinal tract is common. Frequently, mesenteric lymph nodes and occasionally peripheral nodes are affected. An eosinophilic infiltrate is sometimes found in the spleen, liver, kidney, pancreas, heart, and adrenal gland. The bone marrow is hypercellular, and mature as well as immature eosinophils may be present. In some cases, immature forms of eosinophils predominate (Hendrick, 1981). Because there is no universal agreement on the normal maturation sequence of the feline eosinophil, the criteria used to distinguish eosinophilic leukemia from disseminated eosinophilic disease are highly controversial. It is difficult, therefore, to determine if these cats have a deranged proliferation of eosinophils. In FEE, regardless of the presence of disseminated eosinophilic disease or leukemia, it appears that the disease is invariably fatal.

SUMMARY

The clinical signs of FEE are vomiting, diarrhea, anorexia, and weight loss. A tentative diagnosis is based on history, a dramatically thickened small bowel, and a peripheral eosinophilia. The diagnosis is confirmed by microscopic examination of the intestine. The prognosis is grave, and most cats survive only a few months with or without treatment.

REFERENCES

Hendrick, M.: A spectrum of hypereosinophilic syndromes exemplified by six cats with eosinophilic enteritis. Vet. Pathol. 18:188, 1981.
Holzworth, J., Theran, P., Carpenter, J. L., Harpster, N. K., and Todoroff, R. J.: Hyperthyroidism in the cat: Ten cases. J.A.V.M.A. 176:345, 1980.

THE USE OF ANTIMICROBIAL DRUGS IN THE TREATMENT OF DISEASES OF THE GASTROINTESTINAL TRACT

DWIGHT C. HIRSH, D.V.M.,

and L. REED ENOS, Pharm.D.

Davis, California

Many diarrheal diseases are treated with antimicrobial agents. For treatment purposes these diseases are in two categories. The first category encompasses those conditions in which the etiology is unknown. Antimicrobial therapy for such conditions is irrational. The second category encompasses those conditions in which a specific microbial etiology is suspected or known. There is no evidence that antimicrobial therapy is of value in treating these diseases as long as the infectious agent is confined to the gastrointestinal tract. With this in mind, it is obvious that the efficacy of antimicrobial agents in the treatment of these diseases is marginal at best. Traditionally these drugs have been used with little expectation of any success, but the deleterious effects of such therapy on the patient and the environment have gone unrecognized. In addition to the intrinsic toxicity of these antimicrobial agents, it is now apparent that the effects of these drugs on microbial populations are more far-reaching and potentially more dangerous than was first thought.

Rational or irrational use of an antimicrobial agent results in changes in the normal flora throughout the body. These changes can have such deleterious effects that it is imperative that some thought be given prior to prescribing such drugs.

The normal flora acts as a primary host defense barrier. As such, it is vital to the host that such a barrier remain intact. This barrier results from the optimal relationship between microbes and the host. This relationship is part of the complex ecosystem of the body. Microbes do not distribute themselves in a random, haphazard manner throughout the ecosystem; each microbe exists in a niche especially suited for it. If a new microbe can successfully compete against the existing niche dweller, then the newcomer will occupy the niche.

To produce disease, most, if not all, bacterial pathogens must first attach or interact with a target cell. Following this interaction, the microbe, depending on its genetic make-up, will produce disease by a variety of means, e.g., toxin production, invasion, and so on. If, however, the target cell is in a niche occupied by another group of microbes, then the pathogen must successfully compete against these niche dwellers to gain access to the target cell. Most bacterial pathogens cannot do this without help.

One way to disrupt the ecosystem and thereby help the pathogen successfully compete with the niche dweller is through the use of antimicrobial agents. There is no more efficient method of producing such an effect. For example, it takes one million times more *Salmonella* to produce disease in an untreated animal than in an animal pretreated with an antimicrobial agent. The difference between these animals is the presence (or absence) of an intact normal flora. It is our opinion that the risk is unwarranted in view of the limited efficacy of antimicrobial agents in disease of the gastrointestinal tract.

In addition to allowing a potential pathogen access to target cells, antimicrobial agents shift the microbial flora from a normal, well-studied, and well-characterized flora to one that is largely unknown. If the aim is to cover or protect a compromised site located near a microbial ecosystem, prediction of the infecting microorganism will become impossible when infection occurs.

The complex ecosystem of the body forms a barrier to microorganisms that are in the environment of the animal. These include bacteria living in the water, soil, and fecal matter from other animals. These microorganisms belong to a variety of bacterial families but share one common trait: they are all very resistant to antimicrobial agents. Disruption of the normal flora, especially the obligatory anaerobic bacteria, results in proliferation of resistant strains of gram negative enteric bacteria (e.g., *E. coli*) (Table 1) and colonization of the oral cavity and gastrointestinal tract with environmental microorganisms (e.g., *Pseudomonas*). If the animal is compromised or becomes compromised, the com-

Table 1. *Incidence of Tetracycline-Resistant Coliforms in the Rectum of Healthy, Non-Medicated Dogs (n = 94)**

Incidence of Resistant Coliforms (%)	No. of Animals (%)
80 to 100	65 (69)
20 to 80	19 (20)
< 20	10 (11)

*Modified from Hirsh, Ling, and Ruby: Antimicrob. Agents Chemother. 17:313, 1980.

Note: Approximately 50 per cent of the tetracycline-resistant strains studied were also resistant to other agents. Eighteen per cent were resistant to kanamycin (Km), neomycin (Nm), streptomycin (Sm), sulfonamides (Su), and tetracycline (Tc). Eighteen per cent were resistant to ampicillin (Ap) and chloramphenicol (Cm) in addition to those agents previously mentioned. Thirteen per cent were resistant to *all* agents previously mentioned *plus* cephalothin (Cp).

Table 2. *Effect of Certain Antimicrobial Agents on Colonization Resistance**

Drug	Effect
Doxycycline	None
Cephradine	None
Trimethoprim-sulfa	None
Polymyxin B	None
Nystatin	None
Amoxicillin	Some
Cephalexin	Some
Ampicillin	Great
Cloxacillin	Great
Tetracycline	Great

*Modified from Van der Waaij and Verhoef: *New Criteria for Antimicrobial Therapy: Maintenance of Digestive Tract Colonization Resistance.* Amsterdam: Excerpta Medica, 1979.

Table 3. *Effect of Polymyxin B–Neomycin* on the Concentration of Gram Negative Enteric Bacteria in the Feces of the Dog†*

No. of Bacteria/gm Feces	Days of Treatment
10^7	1
10^6	3
10^3	5
10^2	7
< 10	9

*Polymyxin B is given at 20 mg/kg body weight orally, neomycin at 200 mg/kg body weight, divided in two doses, orally.

†Modified from Heidt *In* Van der Waaij and Verhoef: *New Criteria for Antimicrobial Therapy: Maintenance of Digestive Tract Colonization Resistance.* Amsterdam: Excerpta Medica, 1979.

promised site will almost always be infected with those microorganisms that have proliferated in the oral cavity and gastrointestinal tract or colonized from without. This is due to the large numbers of these microorganisms now in or on the mucosal surfaces of the animal.

In the severely compromised host, it is imperative that antimicrobics, if they must be used, be used with some thought to the effects they might have on the anaerobic flora. Not to do so is to put the patient at unnecessary risk. Table 2 lists some commonly used antimicrobials and their effects on colonization resistance and proliferation of gram negative enteric bacteria. In high-risk patients (e.g., granulocytopenic animals) in which the presence of gram negative bacteria may pose a problem, selective decontamination of the oral cavity and the gastrointestinal tract might be indicated. Selective decontamination is the use of antimicrobial agents that leave the anaerobic flora intact yet suppress the gram negative bacteria. Such selective decontamination is used with great success to treat at-risk humans. Antimicrobics such as trimethoprim-sulfa alone or in combination with neomycin and polymyxin-B have been used (Table 3). If fungal overgrowth occurs, nystatin is added to the regimen.

Aside from the more immediate changes in the microenvironment of the animal, more far-reaching changes are presently occurring in our environment that are directly related to antimicrobial usage: vast pools of resistance genes are being created. This phenomenon is of such a serious nature that every antimicrobial agent must be used only in a rational and responsible fashion. These resistance genes are literally moving throughout the microbial populations of the world. The genes move via plasmids, which are self-transmitting, nonessential, autonomous units of DNA. The plasmids usually contain more than one resistance gene. Selection of plasmid-containing bacteria by one drug results in resistance to a number of antimicrobial agents. It now seems certain that the resistance genes found in previously sensitive strains of *Hemophilus influenzae* (the leading cause of meningitis in children), *H. pleuropneumoniae* (in swine), *Neisseria gonorrhoeae*, *Pasteurella multocida* (in poultry and cattle), and *P. haemolytica* (in cattle) arose from this environmental pool. Each time an antimicrobial agent is used, the environmental pool grows larger. As the pool of resistance genes becomes larger, more and more previously sensitive strains become resistant, and bacterial infections become refractory to treatment.

REFERENCES AND SUPPLEMENTAL READING

Hirsh, D. C., Ling, G. V., and Ruby, A. L.: Incidence of R plasmids in fecal flora of healthy household dogs. Antimicrob. Agents Chemother. 17:313, 1980.

Van der Waaij, D., and Verhoef, J.: *New Criteria for Antimicrobial Therapy: Maintenance of Digestive Tract Colonization Resistance.* Amsterdam: Excerpta Medica, 1979.

GIARDIASIS

ROGER P. PITTS, D.V.M.

Madison, Wisconsin

Giardiasis is a diarrheal disease that affects humans and many animal species. Surveys have shown it to be the most common intestinal parasite of humans in the United States and the world. Giardiasis has been observed in dogs and cats throughout the United States. In a number of studies, identification of *Giardia* sp. in diarrhetic feces of companion animals has ranged from 6 to 33 per cent.

Giardia sp. primarily affect the duodenum and upper jejunum. Many mechanisms have been proposed as causing giardiasis. Most likely the pathogenesis is multifactorial. Physical obstruction of mucosal surfaces may result in malabsorption. Microvillus damage caused by the sucking disc may also prevent nutrient absorption. Bile salt deconjugation caused by the organism can result in maldigestion of dietary fat and steatorrhea.

Immunologic disease may play a role in individual susceptibility to *Giardia* in humans. Hypogammaglobulinemia, lack of intestinal IgA, and deficiency of gut IgG have been found in humans with giardiasis. Studies to confirm this in companion animals are lacking.

Transmission of *Giardia* is via oral ingestion of the infective cyst from feces or contaminated food or water. Epidemics have been identified in humans and are linked to ingestion of the cysts from contaminated municipal water supplies where filtration and sedimentation procedures were inadequate to kill the organism. Outbreaks have also resulted from consumption of stream water that was contaminated by feces of beaver, elk, and other animals.

CLINICAL SIGNS

Clinical signs of giardiasis vary considerably. Large volumes of a watery, tan-colored, "cow-pie" like stool are often observed with steatorrhea. Although primarily a small bowel parasitism, giardiasis may mimic large bowel disease by the presence of mucus, tenesmus, flatulence, or rectal prolapse. Steatorrhea is a common clinical finding. A frequent historical finding is weight loss, despite a good appetite and an adequate diet. Intermittent bouts of diarrhea are often reported. Subclinical giardiasis is common, but nonetheless important, owing to the potential transmission to other animals.

Giardia sp. are often present in addition to other endoparasites, and thus diarrhea following treatment for nematode infestation indicates the need for careful examination for the organism.

The observation has been made that many subclinical bitches harboring *Giardia* may "break" with diarrhea at the time of whelping. Although this diarrhea may be attributed to stress, the clinician should be aware of the danger of *Giardia* to the puppies and should undertake identification of the parasite and proper treatment.

DIAGNOSIS

Diagnosis of giardiasis can pose a challenge to the veterinarian. Direct saline smears or smears stained with iodine may reveal the trophozoite form. The trophozoite is motile, pyriform in shape, dorsally convex, and ventrally flattened and has a ventral sucker for attachment to the intestinal mucosa. Rapid deterioration of the trophozoite in feces necessitates examination soon after the sample is obtained.

The encysted form, more commonly found in feces, is oval or ellipsoid in shape and contains two to four nuclei, giving it the appearance of a face. Its small size (12 μm) requires examination under oil immersion and helps distinguish it from *Coccidia* organisms, which are usually twice as large. Fecal flotation, with or without iodine, will often reveal the cysts.

Encystation and fecal passage of *Giardia* is often intermittent, so multiple fecal examinations may be required to reveal the parasite. Duodenal aspiration is useful for detection of the parasite and can be done during exploratory laparotomy or endoscopy. Studies by the author have shown that in only four of ten dogs in which *Giardia* organisms were found on duodenal aspiration were the organisms found on a single fecal flotation specimen.

Immunologic assays have been developed in humans for the detection of *Giardia* infection. Precipitin and indirect immunofluorescence testing show a systemic response to the disease. These tests have not been adopted for use in animals.

TREATMENT

Treatment of giardiasis usually is successful. Metronidazole (Flagyl*) given at a dosage of 65 mg/kg s.i.d. for five days or quinicrine (Atabrine†) at a dosage of 9 mg/kg s.i.d. for six days usually results in clinical remission. Clinical trials in humans have

---

*Searle Laboratories, Chicago, IL.
†Winthrop Laboratories, New York, NY.

796

shown that a single large dose of metronidazole is more effective in clearing the organism, but similar studies in animals are lacking. It is the feeling of the author that, when giardiasis is strongly suspected but not demonstrated on fecal examination, therapy that results in the disappearance of clinical signs may be diagnostic. Reinfection is common, and requires retreatment, a possibility that should be explained to the client.

PUBLIC HEALTH SIGNIFICANCE

Although *Giardia* have been classified into separate species depending on the host infected, it is now agreed that all species are morphologically similar. Cross infectivity does occur between animal species and humans. Because of the danger of transmission of giardiasis from humans to pets and vice versa, identification of this pathogen in domestic pets and proper treatment must be goals of the practicing veterinarian.

SUPPLEMENTAL READING

Barlough, J. E.: Canine giardiasis, a review. J. Small Anim. Pract. 20:613, 1979.
Brightman, A. H., and Slonka, G. F.: A review of five clinical cases of giardiasis in cats. J.A.A.H.A. 12:492, 1976.
Davies, R. B., and Hibler, C. P.: Animal reservoirs and cross species transmission of *Giardia*. In *Waterborne Transmission of Giardiasis*: Proceedings of a Symposium at Cincinnati, Ohio, Sept. 18–20, 1978. Washington, DC: US Environmental Protection Agency, 1978, pp. 104–126.
Williams, J. F., and Zajac, A.: *Diagnosis of Gastrointestinal Parasitism in Dogs and Cats*. St. Louis: Ralston Purina Co., 1980, pp. 31–32.

GASTROINTESTINAL PARASITISM

EDWARD L. ROBERSON, D.V.M.,

and LARRY M. CORNELIUS, D.V.M.

Athens, Georgia

PREVALENCE OF HELMINTH INFECTIONS IN DOGS

Despite many years of attention to parasitic infections of small animals, the prevalence of ascarids, hookworms, whipworms, and tapeworms is still quite high and widespread. Table 1 presents prevalences of these parasites in pound dogs (all ages) from five different locations in the U.S. Overall, more than 50 per cent of these dogs were infected with ascarids, hookworms, whipworms, or a combination of these.

A further study in Georgia (Table 2) compares the prevalences of canine helminths in pups (less than six months old) and adult dogs obtained from pounds. Ascarids (*Toxocara canis*) were much more prevalent among pups (74 per cent) than among dogs more than six months old (13 per cent); whipworms (*Trichuris vulpis*) were more prevalent among older dogs (62 per cent as compared with 15 per cent in pups); and hookworms (*Ancylostoma caninum*) were equally prevalent in both age groups (82 to 85 per cent).

The Georgia study also surveyed owned dogs seen as patients at the University of Georgia Veterinary Teaching Hospital. Table 2 suggests that routine and therapeutic deworming of owned animals (and perhaps an increased level of nutrition and improved living conditions) substantially reduces the overall prevalence of ascarids, hookworms, and whipworms.

HOOKWORMS

MEANS OF INFECTION AND CLINICAL SIGNS

Infections of the more common hookworms of dogs (*Ancylostoma caninum* and *Uncinaria stenocephala*) and cats (*Ancylostoma tubaeforme*) may be obtained by the ingestion of food and water contaminated with infective L_3 larvae or by penetration of the skin by these larvae. Another evidently important means of infection documented for *A. caninum* is the passage of L_3 larvae to pups via the bitch's milk. In this transmammary route infective larvae that the pregnant bitch has picked up orally or by skin penetration accumulate in her mammary glands and subsequently pass via the milk to her nursing pups, especially during the first weeks of nursing.

Hookworm larvae obtained orally (via the bitch's milk or contaminated water or food) are confined to development in the digestive tract, especially in young animals. Larvae of *A. caninum*, when ingested orally, enter the gastric glands of the stomach or glands of Lieberkühn in the small intestine, where they develop for a few days and subsequently return to the gut lumen to molt to the fourth stage,

Table 1. *Incidence of Parasitic Infections at Necropsy of Dogs from Five States**

Infection†	Georgia	Ohio	North Carolina	Texas	Calif.	Total
No. Dogs Sampled	177	1128	868	737	188	3098
Ascarids % Infected	51	51	40	58	93	52
Hookworms % Infected	81	51	87	82	46	70
Whipworms % Infected	55	72	62	10	27	51
Tapeworms % Infected	NR‡	19	44	17	9	26§

*Modified from Hass, Collins, and Flick: Canine Pract., 2:42, 1975.
†Ascarids: *Toxocara* and *Toxascaris*.
 Hookworms: *Ancylostoma* and *Uncinaria*.
 Whipworms: *Trichuris*.
 Tapeworms: *Taenia* and *Dipylidium*.
‡NR = not recorded by investigator.
§Based on 2,921 dogs; the prevalence of tapeworms was not recorded by the Georgia investigators.

then to the fifth stage, after which they mature to the adult stage. Hookworm eggs may be seen in the host's feces as early as 15 to 18 days after the initial oral infection.

The blood letting by hookworms will have begun with the fourth-stage larvae (i.e., about eight days following the initial infection, several days before eggs are passed). The fourth-stage larvae, young immature adults (fifth stage), and adult worms feed by pulling a plug of mucosa into the large buccal cavity. The digestion of this plug occurs within approximately 30 minutes, resulting in disruption of the vasculature and loss of blood into the surrounding tissue. After ingesting as many as two or three mucosal plugs, the worms move to another site, leaving the first site bleeding. This graze-type feeding results in numerous punctiform hemorrhages of the small intestinal mucosa.

A. caninum is the most pathogenic hookworm for dogs, and *A. tubaeforme* is most pathogenic for cats. The pathogenicity of *A. braziliense* and *Unicinaria* is 50 to 100 times less than that of *A. caninum*. Maximum blood loss is seen 10 to 25 days after infection. Pups with 66 to 132 worms (*A. caninum*)/kg of body weight will show approximately a 45 per cent decrease in hematocrit value; 165 worms/kg is considered the LD_{50} in young pups.

The loss of blood into the lumen of the canine digestive tract gives a tarry appearance to the feces, which may become foul smelling and completely fluid. Such pups quickly develop pale mucous membranes and demonstrate signs of weakness and ema-

Table 2. *Prevalence of Nematodes in Pound Versus Owned Dogs in North Georgia**

	Percent of Dogs Infected			
	Pound Dogs		Owned Dogs	
Organism	Pups	Adults	Pups	Adults
Toxocara canis	74	13	39	6
Ancylostoma caninum	85	82	37	37
Uncinaria stenocephala	12	28	1	1
Trichuris vulpis	15	62	10	23
Toxascaris leonina	0	0	1	<1
Capillaria spp.	0	<1	0	<1
Physaloptera spp.	<1	0	0	0
Spirocera lupi	0	<1	0	0
No parasites	6	6	43	50

*Data obtained by D. E. Burgess and T. M. Burke, Athens, GA.

ciation. Older dogs may develop regenerative microcytic hypochromic anemia as a result of iron deficiency caused by chronic blood loss.

TREATMENT

In young pups and kittens and in older animals that are clinically anemic and listless from hookworm infection it is necessary to eliminate the parasites as quickly as possible. Anthelmintics requiring a single dose (rather than five daily doses) are most satisfactory for these animals. These include dichlorvos (Task or Task Tabs), pyrantel pamoate (Nemex-2), and disophenol (D.N.P.) (Table 3). Dichlorvos seems to bring about the most immediate expulsion of worms (within eight hours or so), whereas disophenol given subcutaneously requires 24 hours or more to effect expulsion. Dichlorvos is contraindicated if severe diarrhea accompanies the clinical anemia and listlessness; in these cases pyrantel pamoate or disophenol is preferred. Percutaneously acquired larval stages in the lungs at the time of treatment are not affected by any of these drugs. Many of these larvae will cycle to the intestine and mature within two weeks. Thus, retreatment should be given two weeks after the initial treatment. To determine if subsequent treatments are needed, feces should be rechecked for eggs at two-week intervals until previously ill young animals are about four months of age.

Necessary supportive therapy depends on the severity of the anemia. When the packed cell volume is 15 per cent or lower, whole blood probably should be administered, at a rate of about 10 to 15 ml/lb (22 to 33 ml/kg). This is especially important if the animal's clinical condition seems to be deteriorating. The intravenous route is preferred, but injection into the femoral bone marrow cavity through the trocanteric fossa is simple in pups and kittens and should be used whenever intravenous injection is too difficult. Intraperitoneal transfusion can be done, but results are less satisfactory. Other supportive measures include keeping the animal warm and quiet, with no undue stress. It is critical that handling of severely anemic animals be gentle during blood transfusion. Excessive struggling can result in the patient's death. Hematinic drugs are generally unnecessary in animals consuming a proper diet; however, nursing pups or kittens probably should receive iron supplementation.

In the case of a bitch that lost pups in a previous litter owing to transmammary passage of hookworms, it should be assumed that she will also pass heavy hookworm infections to her subsequent litters when the pups are nursing. Further losses can be prevented by treating these litters weekly during the five- to six-week nursing period, starting one week after birth. This regimen will eliminate hookworms acquired via the milk before they cause extensive damage to the gut. As a suspension, pyrantel pamoate is the drug of choice for this use; it is relatively easy to administer by syringe and has a wide margin of safety for young pups.

In less critical hookworm infections, in which immediate expulsion of worms is not essential, or in routine dewormings, a single treatment with dichlorvos, toluene (Vermiplex), or thenium closylate (Canopar) or a three-day treatment with mebendazole (Telmintic) gives relatively equal hookworm expulsion. Some concern currently exists about the routine use of certain of these drugs because of occasional drug-related deaths; i.e., with mebendazole and with thenium closylate (especially collie and Airedale breeds).

Experimentally, fenbendazole at 50 mg/kg body weight for three days has expelled hookworms satisfactorily (see Table 3). The feces of pups so treated were normal and formed following a three-day treatment with fenbendazole, as compared with the dysenteric stools of untreated infected littermates.

Two older compounds that have little merit in treating hookworms today are *n*-butyl chloride and tetrachloroethylene. The former is only 60 per cent effective for hookworms, and the latter, although 90 per cent effective, has numerous disadvantages (hepatotoxicity and contraindication in debilitated or tapeworm-positive animals) that newer synthetic anthelmintics have overcome.

ASCARIDS

MEANS OF INFECTION AND CLINICAL SIGNS

Two species of ascarids, *Toxocara canis* and *Toxascaris leonina*, infect dogs. Cats are infected by a feline strain of *Toxascaris leonina* and their own species of *Toxocara*, *T. cati*. These three ascarids differ in the extent of larval migration in the host and, thus, in the degree of larval pathogenicity. Larvae of *Toxocara canis* migrate most extensively, i.e., liver-lung migration or somatic tissue migration. Larvae of *Toxocara cati* are confined predominately to a liver-lung migration; somatic migration of this ascarid is fairly insignificant. Larvae of *Toxascaris leonina* are confined to gut mucosal invasion and do not migrate through hepatic, pulmonary, or somatic tissues. Thus the pathogenesis of *Toxascaris* is considerably less than that of either species of *Toxocara*, and treatment for the gut-dwelling *Toxascaris* is less complicated than that for *Toxocara*, since none of the currently available anthelmintics significantly reduce the number of extraintestinal larvae of *Toxocara*.

The greatest larval damage occurs to the liver and lungs. Following ingestion of infective eggs of *Toxocara canis* and release of the larvae in the stomach and small intestine of pups (especially pups

Table 3. Anthelmintics for Dogs and Cats

Drugs	Efficacy*					Dosage	Comments
	Hookworms	Ascarids	Whipworms	Tapeworms	Strongyloides		
D.N.P. (disophenol) (American Cyanamid)	95%	—	—	—	—	10 mg/kg SC	36 mg/kg is fatal. Do not administer to overheated animals or those with respiratory problems. Can be used on nursing young.
Tetrachlorethylene (Several manufacturers)	90%	—	—	—	—	0.22 ml/kg after 12-hr fast	Hepatotoxic. Contraindicated in sick, debilitated, or tapeworm-positive animals.
Canopar (thenium closylate) (Burroughs Wellcome)	89%	±	—	—	—	1 tablet (500 mg) for dogs over 10 lb (5 kg), regardless of weight; ¼ tablet (125 mg) b.i.d. (q 12 hr) for 5- and 10-lb (2.5- to 5-kg) dogs	Some emesis. Cannot use in nursing pups or those less than 5 lb (2.5 kg). Occasional deaths (collies and airedales).
Piperazine (many manufacturers)	—	52–100%	—	—	—	45–65 mg base/kg orally; maximum of 250 mg for pups under 2.5 kg and for cats and kittens	No contraindications except long-standing renal or liver disease.
Caricide (diethylcarbamazine) (American Cyanamid)	—	80%	—	—	—	6.6 mg/kg/day orally as a preventive	Substantial adult ascarid burden is eliminated when DEC is given as a heart-worm preventive. Contraindicated if microfilariae present.
Styrid-Caricide (DEC + styrylpyridinium chloride) (American Cyanamid)	80%	80%	—	—	—	6.6 mg DEC and 5.5 mg Styryl. Cl./kg/day orally	Used as a heartworm preventive and as an aid in control of ascarids and hookworms.
Whipcide (phthalofyne) (Pitman-Moore)	—	—	90%	—	—	200 mg/kg orally after 24-hr fast; 250 mg/kg IV, no fasting	Side effects. Foul odor of by-products.
Milibis-V (glycobiarsol) (Winthrop)	—	—	90%	—	—	220 mg/kg daily × 5 days	Developed for treatment of amebiasis. ½ dose × 10 days recommended for debilitated dogs.

Drug						Dosage	Remarks
Thiabendazole (Merck Sharp & Dohme)	±	±	—	—	—	95%	55 mg/kg daily × 3 days orally	Some emesis. Repeat treatment monthly if needed.
Nemex-2 (pyrantel pamoate) (Pfizer)	95%	95%	±	—	—	18 mg/kg in tablet or suspension (Nemex-2, Strongid-T, Imathal)	Used in dogs of all ages, including nursing pups. No contraindications.
n-Butyl chloride (Several manufacturers)	60%	90%	—	—	—	1 ml (618 mg)/kg after 12-hr fast	Cathartic recommended.
Task (dichlorvos) (Shell)	95%	95%	90%	—	—	Dog: 27–33 mg/kg; Puppy & cat: 11 mg/kg	Contraindications include heartworm disease and liver or kidney damage. Do not use in conjunction with other cholinesterase inhibitors. Split dosage b.i.d. for debilitated animals.
Styquin (butamisole HCl) (American Cyanimide)	92%	—	99%	—	—	2.4 mg/kg SC	A fourfold overdose is lethal; do not use simultaneously with Scolaban or in heartworm-positive or debilitated dogs.
Telmintic (mebendazole) (Pitman-Moore)	95%	95%	95%	85% T† / 0% D	—	22 mg/kg in food daily × 3 days (nematodes) or 5 days (*Taenia*)	Approved for dogs; experimental in cats. Evidence suggests occasional drug-induced acute hepatic necrosis in dogs.
Vermiplex (toluene and dichlorophene) (Pitman-Moore)	82%	90%	—	72% T / 85% D	—	Size capsule as directed by manufacturer	Incoordination, emesis, toxicity in excess.
Scolaban (bunamidine HCl) (Burroughs Wellcome)	—	—	—	100% T / 56–90% D / 86–100% E	—	25–50 mg/kg on empty stomach; feed lightly in 3 hr	Occasional idiosyncratic reaction. Do not use simultaneously with Styquin.
Yomesan (niclosamide) (Chemagro)	—	—	—	80% T / 18–56% D	—	100–157 mg/kg orally	Heavy mucus interferes with elimination of scolex.

Table continued on following page

Table 3. *Anthelmintics for Dogs and Cats (Continued)*

Drugs	Efficacy*							Dosage	Comments
	Hook-worms	Ascarids	Whip-worms	Tape-worms	Strongy-loides				
Nemural (arecoline-acetarsol) (Winthrop)	—	—	—	50% T, D >75% E	—			4–6 mg/kg orally after light feeding	Severe vomiting and diarrhea may occur and may be difficult to control.
Droncit (praziquantel) (Haver Lockhart)	—	—	—	100% T, D, E				Dog: 5 mg/kg, single oral, SC, or IM dose Cat: 11 mg total (1–3 lbs) 22 mg total (3–11 lbs) 33 mg total (>11 lbs)	10 mg/kg required for *Echinococcus* juveniles. Effective against tapeworm larvae in many intermediate hosts. No effect on nematodes.
Fenbendazole (experimental) (American Hoechst)	98%	99%	100%	88–100% T 0% D				50 mg/kg/day × 3 consecutive days	Suspension or granules (added to moist food). Single dose, even at 150 mg/kg, is not effective in dogs or cats. Current FDA approval only in horses (Panacur).

*Percentages in "Tapeworms" column refer to % of dogs cleared of infection; all others refer to % of nematodes expelled.
†T = *Taenia* sp.; D = *Dipylidium caninum*; E = *Echinococcus* sp.

less than five weeks old), the larvae enter the hepatic portal system, migrate through the liver for several days, and are carried in the blood via the heart to the lungs, where additional migration and disruption of tissue occur until they enter the respiratory tree, from which they are coughed up, swallowed, and returned to the gut. Almost all *Toxocara* larvae take this route in very young pups (less than five weeks old) and eventually mature as adult worms in the gut. Assuming that there is a continuous source of infective eggs, as the pup grows older fewer larvae will enter the respiratory passage that returns them to the gut; instead, more and more larvae in the lung will burrow through the pulmonary vein and will be distributed with oxygenated blood to somatic tissues, where they will remain without further development, perhaps for the life of the animal. Practically all larvae infecting three-month-old pups will become somatically located.

For male dogs there is no release from the continually growing burden of somatic ascarid larvae. In females, however, pregnancy and subsequent lactation afford a chance for the bitch to reduce her somatic numbers—at the expense of the pups. Transplacental (prenatal) migration of the bitch's larvae begins following day 42 of pregnancy. These larvae will enter the liver and lung of the fetus and await the birth of the pup before passing to the gut. Extremely heavy prenatal infections may cause stillbirths. A bitch with a moderate somatic infection of ascarids, if prevented from further ingestion of eggs, will require three or four pregnancies to pass all of her larval burden to her pups. Following birth, the number of *Toxocara* larvae that pass to nursing pups via the milk is insignificant. The lactogenic root is the important root in cats; prenatal infections of *T. cati* do not occur.

In heavy prenatal and transmammary infections the pulmonary phase may be lethal for pups within a few days of birth. Generally, however, pups do not succumb immediately but clinically become unthrifty, demonstrate evidence of respiratory distress and a dull haircoat, develop a distended abdomen primarily as a result of the physical presence of numerous large worms (potbellied appearance), and experience varying degrees of digestive disturbance (colic, vomiting, diarrhea, or alternating diarrhea and constipation). Only very rarely do adult worms wander into and block the bile or pancreatic ducts. Somewhat more frequently, however, wandering larval stages enter the central nervous system, resulting in meningitis-like signs.

TREATMENT

Treatment of young pups or kittens for heavy ascarid burdens (especially *Toxocara*) involves repeated dosing (perhaps three or four treatments at two-week intervals beginning at two weeks of age). Repeated treatments are necessary because none of the currently available drugs have any significant effect against larvae (stages L_2 and L_3) that may be present in the liver or lungs at the time medication is administered. Following treatment, some of these larvae will complete their migration, returning to the digestive tract and continuing development through a fourth larval stage and immature adulthood to become adult worms. Another treatment will be necessary to expel these intestinal stages. While kittens (and, to some degree, pups) are nursing, transmammary infections are continuously occurring and add to the necessity for repeated treatments. Multiple treatments generally are not needed for older animals infected with *Toxocara*.

A wide variety of anthelmintics are available for treating ascarid infections: piperazine, *n*-butyl chloride, dichlorvos, methylbenzene (toluene), mebendazole, and pyrantel pamoate (see Table 3). All are substantially effective, and the selection of one drug over another is not necessary when routinely treating healthy pups, eight weeks of age or older, that are taking solid food (mebendazole is administered in the food). Nursing pups, however, especially those clinically ill from heavy ascarid infections, seem to tolerate the relatively new pyrantel pamoate (Nemex-2) best. This compound is supplied in suspension form, is caramel flavored, and is often easier to administer orally by syringe to nursing pups of small breeds than are tablet and capsule formulations of the other anthelmintics. Nemex-2 also has excellent activity against hookworms.

Supportive treatment for toxocariasis consists primarily of good nursing care. For nursing pups or kittens, it is beneficial to provide warm, dry housing and to be certain that the bitch or queen is lactating properly. Older animals should be provided with a palatable, balanced diet.

In light of the ubiquity of prenatal and transmammary infections of ascarids and hookworms, an anthelmintic that is effective against somatic stages in the bitch, thus preventing infection of her pups, clearly is needed. Such a drug most likely would require daily long-term administration. Preliminary success along these lines has been obtained in Germany and the United States with fenbendazole, an anthelmintic that currently is approved in the United States only for use in horses (Panacur). Greater than 90 per cent reduction in prenatal transmission of *T. canis* and lactogenic transmission of *A. caninum* from bitch to pups can be expected when Panacur is administered once daily to the bitch from the fortieth day of pregnancy until two weeks after parturition. The dosage is 50 mg/kg/day. This is approximately 37 days of drug administration and would be economically prohibitive except in special cases of valuable dogs that have had previous heavily infected litters or in colonies of dogs where total elimination of ascarid and hookworm infections is desired.

WHIPWORMS

MEANS OF INFECTION AND CLINICAL SIGNS

Whipworm (*Trichuris vulpis*) infections of dogs occur by direct ingestion of eggs containing the infective stage. The hatched larva burrows into the upper small intestine for approximately one week (without consequent pathology), emerges, and subsequently moves to the cecum to develop to adulthood.

Although the morbidity associated with whipworm infection has been suggested in the past to be relatively low, more recent clinical observation has indicated that the opposite is true. At the University of Georgia Veterinary Teaching Hospital whipworms are one of the most common causes of chronic mucoid bloody diarrhea (large bowel diarrhea). Whipworm ova are frequently absent in the feces in such cases, making diagnosis difficult. By using a flexible fiberoptic endoscope we have been able to visualize whipworms in the cecum of dogs with large bowel diarrhea when fecal flotation tests were repeatedly negative. It is suggested that, whenever a cause for chronic large bowel diarrhea cannot be established by routine diagnostic methods, whipworm treatment should be given before resorting to more elaborate diagnostic procedures.

Cats are not infected by the canine species of whipworm. A few reports of feline infection with *Trichuris campanula* have been made in the U.S., South America, Cuba, and the Bahamas.

TREATMENT

Five anthelmintics that give satisfactory activity against canine whipworms are now available. The activity of two of these—phthalofyne (Whipcide) and glycobiarsol (Milibis V)—is strictly against whipworms, whereas the others—butamisole HCl (Styquin), dichlorvos (Task), and mebendazole (Telmintic)—also are effective against ascarids and/or hookworms (see Table 3). Three of these have the advantage of requiring only a single dose; glycobiarsol requires five and mebendazole three daily doses. However, dichlorvos is contraindicated in heartworm-positive dogs, and both dichlorvos and phthalofyne are contraindicated in dogs that have chronic nephritis, hepatitis, pancreatitis, or cardiac insufficiencies. Intravenous phthalofyne is seldom used now because of the occurrence of vomiting, ataxia, and drowsiness in approximately 40 per cent of dogs treated in this manner. Another disadvantage of intravenous phthalofyne is accidental perivascular leakage, which causes cellulitis and subsequent necrosis. Side effects occur less frequently in dogs given phthalofyne orally; ataxia and drowsiness

seldom occur but vomition is fairly common. These disadvantages of phthalofyne favor the routine use of dichlorvos for treating whipworm infections in areas in which heartworms are not endemic.

Fenbendazole (Panacur for horses) has given highly satisfactory activity for canine whipworms at a daily dose of 50 mg/kg for three days. The granulated formulation can be added to canned food, or the suspension formulation can be administered by syringe directly into the dog's mouth. Either is acceptably palatable.

The degree of success of dichlorvos (and perhaps of the other drugs) seems to be inversely proportional to the whipworm burden. In dogs harboring fewer than 100 worms, greater than 90 per cent expulsion can be expected. When the burden exceeds 100 worms, the efficacy of dichlorvos is reduced, and retreatment within one to two weeks is necessary.

In general, the expulsion of whipworms from a treated dog requires a longer period of time (usually 72 hours) than the expulsion of ascarids or hookworms (less than 48 hours). Thus, collection of feces for a post-treatment evaluation of whipworm eggs should not be made within 72 hours of treatment. Submission of a fecal sample one week after treatment is the routine policy of practitioners and is preferred. In obstinate cases, a second regimen of medication can be given in one to two weeks. Such animals should be checked routinely at three-month intervals for the establishment of additional patent infections.

In cases in which clients are adept and conscientious about treating their dogs, the five-day regimen of either glycobiarsol or mebendazole may be handled by the client. No fasting is required with either drug. If there is difficulty in administering the rather large glycobiarsol tablets, they can be crushed and added to the food. Mebendazole is prepared as a powder for addition to the food. It is advantageous to use moist food when either drug is added; this allows the drug to stick to it and results in consumption of the entire dose. Again, mebendazole has previously been preferred over glycobiarsol because of its slightly greater activity against whipworms and its broader anthelmintic range (ascarids, hookworms, and *Taenia* but not *Dipylidium* tapeworms). Recent reports of mebendazole-induced hepatotoxicity, however, have encouraged many practitioners to use fenbendazole instead of mebendazole for treatment of whipworm infections.

Supportive therapy generally is unnecessary in whipworm-infected dogs.

TAPEWORMS

MEANS OF INFECTION AND DIAGNOSIS

Tapeworms that commonly infect dogs include *Dipylidium caninum* and *Taenia pisiformis*. Those commonly infecting cats are *D. caninum* and *T. taeniaeformis*. Cats and dogs acquire *Dipylidium* infections by ingesting fleas or biting lice that carry the infective cysticercoid. Dogs become infected with *T. pisiformis* and cats with *T. taeniaeformis* by ingestion of infective cysticerci from rabbit and rat or mouse tissues, respectively.

Gravid (egg-filled) proglottids detach from these tapeworms and pass with the feces. The proglottid may be seen crawling on or near freshly passed feces or on the perineum of the dog. In dry weather they desiccate and shrink quickly and thus may go undetected. The proglottid may be identified by teasing it open with forceps in a couple of drops of water on a glass slide, placing a coverslip over it, and examining it under a compound microscope for packets containing several to 20 eggs (*Dipylidium*) or for single eggs with a dark, thick, striated wall (*Taenia*). A dried proglottid should be allowed to rehydrate for 15 minutes or more before attempting to tease it open. Identification of the tapeworm is needed to advise clients on appropriate preventive measures and to treat the infection effectively (*Dipylidium* is not eliminated by some drugs that expel *Taenia*).

Although still uncommon, infections of *Spirometra mansonoides* are being seen with increasing frequency in the southeastern U.S. These tapeworms do not shed proglottids. Fluke-like operculated eggs (slightly larger than those of *D. caninum*) are passed in the feces and are recovered easily by salt flotation procedures that are used routinely to detect nematode eggs. The intermediate hosts of this tapeworm include water copepods (first host) and amphibians or reptiles (second host), on which dogs or cats occasionally feed.

Each of these tapeworm infections is of negligible pathologic importance. In our laboratory, Burke has recovered over 8000 *Dipylidium* scolices from a single three-month-old pup that had normal stool consistency and appetite. However, clients are esthetically offended by seeing crawling proglottids issuing from their pets and demand that something be done to stop it.

TREATMENT

Until marketing of praziquantel (Droncit) in early 1981, there was no anticestodal drug that had particularly good activity against *Dipylidium caninum*. Praziquantel has 100 per cent activity for this obstinate tapeworm and for *Taenia* and *Echinococcus* infections in dogs (see Table 3). Nematodes are not affected. Oral, subcutaneous, or intramuscular administration provides a choice of easy and safe routes for treating dogs. The single therapeutic dose is 5 mg/kg; dogs, however, tolerate prolonged daily doses of 60 mg/kg without toxicosis or changes in hematologic or clinicochemical parameters. FDA approval has been obtained for use of this drug against tapeworms in cats.

Bunamidine hydrochloride (Scolaban) has variable activity against *Dipylidium caninum*. At the recommended dose of 25 to 50 mg/kg of body weight in dogs or cats, 56 to 90 per cent of *Dipylidium*-infected animals and 100 per cent of *Taenia*-infected animals can be expected to be cleared. *Echinococcus* also is expelled by this drug. Fewer than one of every ten animals will vomit following dosing with tablets. The enteric-coated tablets should not be crushed for administration in suspension, since the drug is irritating to the oral mucosa and oral absorption is more liable to result in toxic manifestations (emesis and diarrhea).

Bunamidine hydrochloride can be administered to females during all stages of pregnancy and during lactation without ill effects to the bitch or her pups. Reduced spermatogenesis has been found in male dogs but not in male cats 4 to 28 days following administration of twice the current recommended dosage, i.e., 2×25 to 50 mg/kg.

One rare complication of the use of bunamidine hydrochloride is the occasional sudden death of an apparently healthy dog. This idiosyncratic reaction occurs most often in large, heavily exercised, working-type dogs that have developed ventricular fibrillation and died upon sudden exertion within a 24-hour period following treatment. There is evidence that in these cases the drug had sensitized the heart musculature to epinephrine, the level of which at the time of sudden exercise increased in the blood and may have triggered fibrillation of the cardiac muscle. The occurrence of sudden death appears to be dose-related in view of the greater frequency of deaths in Australia (1 of 3000 dogs treated at a dose of 44 mg/kg) than in the U.S. (1 of an estimated 600,000 dogs treated at a dose of 25 mg/kg). In Canada and the United Kingdom, where even lower doses are used, no drug-related deaths have been reported.

Niclosamide (Yomesan) has been used widely by veterinary practitioners for tapeworm infections. Whereas this compound clears approximately 80 per cent of dogs harboring *Taenia* infections, less than 50 per cent of dogs with *Dipylidium* infections will be cleared. The drug does destrobilate (remove the body of) the tapeworm, but the remaining intact scolex will regenerate another body and shed gravid proglottids three to four weeks after treatment. Thus, the client returns again complaining about the "crawly things" on his pet. Similarly, mebendazole in five daily treatments or fenbendazole (Panacur) in three daily treatments is about 85 per cent effective for taeniad tapeworms but has no activity against *Dipylidium*.

Vermiplex and Anaplex (commercial combinations of toluene and dichlorophene) are frequently used to treat ascarids and hookworms simultaneously (toluene) and to "aid in the control of" tapeworms (dichlorophene) (see Table 3). These drugs are used primarily in young dogs and cats during the ascarid-positive months. Studies suggest that he efficacy of these drugs for *Taenia* and for *Dipylidium* is 72 and 85 per cent, respectively, but these figures may be high, since no reported search was made following treatment for destrobilated scolices that may have remained attached to the intestinal mucosa.

Arecoline-acetarsol (Nemural), an old purging compound used in both dogs and cats, is still used by some practitioners to treat *Taenia* and *Dipylidium* infections. This drug narcotizes the tapeworm for two to three hours, during which it must be expelled; otherwise, reattachment occurs. The purgative action of arecoline, however, usually brings about catharsis within the desired three hours.

It is difficult to assess the efficacy of Nemural for tapeworms in the absence of any recent experimental investigations. This fact, plus occasionally adverse reactions (vomition, salivation, discomfort, restlessness, ataxia, and labored breathing); restrictions against its use in pups less than three months old and cats less than one year old; and contraindications in animals having febrile conditions, intestinal disturbances, or severe cardiac or circulatory disturbances have greatly limited use of the drug today.

The currently used synthetic anticestodals (Droncit, Scolaban, Yomesan, Telmintic, and Vermiplex) kill the tapeworm so that it becomes completely or partially digested before being voided in feces. Detection of voided worms by examination of the feces is therefore not possible. Arecoline-acetarsol, on the other hand, simply narcotizes worms so that they remain alive and can be detected in the feces. The occurrence of some worms in the feces, however, gives no indication of how many tapeworms still remain attached in the gut.

PROTOZOAN INFECTIONS

FLAGELLATES

Giardia sp. and *Pentatrichomonas* sp. are found in approximately 10 per cent of dogs and only occasionally in cats. The clinical significance of either of these protozoans is disputed. They may be seen in perfectly normal feces (saline smear), yet they are far more likely to be detected in soft or loose feces, especially in young dogs. It has been suggested that they may be nonpathogenic opportunists, frequently present in the small intestine in low numbers but multiplying to large populations when the gut environment is favorable (for example, in mucoid enteritis). The fact that direct treatment of these organisms favors re-establishment of normal bowel function suggests that these flagellates are primary pathogens. In humans, *Giardia*-induced diarrhea may occur without evidence of either cysts or trophozoites in the feces. In these cases duodenal aspirates are needed to demonstrate the parasite. The incidence of similar findings in dogs and cats is unknown, but if giardiasis is strongly suspected in a patient with negative fecal findings, it may be prudent to treat for *Giardia*. It is not known with certainty whether or not the canine and feline species of *Giardia* and trichomonads are infective for humans. Current information on *Giardia*, however, suggests that this parasite is not so host specific as previously thought. Suspected *Giardia* transmissions have occurred from nonhuman primates and beavers to humans, from beavers to dogs, and from humans to dogs. These cases compel veterinarians to advise clients to handle all *Giardia* infections as if they are of public health significance (see page 796).

Details of diagnostic morphology and procedures other than the direct saline smear can be obtained from the 6th edition of *Current Veterinary Therapy*.

Infections of either *Giardia* or *Pentatrichomonas* respond rather dramatically to treatment with a human trichomonad drug, metronidazole (Flagyl). The drug is given orally at the rate of 25 mg/kg every 12 hours for five days for *Giardia* and at the rate of 66 mg/kg/day for five days for *Pentatrichomonas*. Treatment with glycobiarsol (Milibis), using the whipworm regimen, is also suggested to be effective for trichomonads, but its use is not well documented. *Giardia* infections alternately can be treated with quinacrine (Atabrine) orally at 50 to 100 mg every 12 hours for three days, with rest for three days; then the regimen is repeated.

COCCIDIA

Traditionally, the coccidia of dogs and cats have been reviewed as consisting of but a few species of *Cystoisospora*. Closely controlled experimental work in the past eight years, however, has uncovered several other genera—at least 13 feline species and 13 canine species of coccidia (Table 4). Future investigations very likely will discover more. Furthermore, it is now known that, unlike the monoxenous (single-host) infections of *Eimeria* in ruminants and birds, feline and canine coccidian infections can involve an intermediate host. Cat-to-cat or dog-to-dog infections of the species of coccidia listed in Table 4 can occur by direct ingestion of sporulated oocysts. Additionally, certain other animals (listed as intermediate hosts in the table) may become infected by ingesting oocysts or sporocysts from the cat or dog. The coccidian stages in intermediate hosts become located as asexually multiplying cystic forms in extraintestinal tissues (muscles, endothelium, brain, connective tissues, and others) that are infective for felids or canids that prey on

Table 4. *Coccidia of Cats and Dogs**

Organism	Average Size† (μm)	Intermediate Host
Coccidia of Cats		
Cystoisospora felis	40 × 30	Mammals
Cystoisospora rivolta	25 × 20	Mammals
Besnoitia besnoiti	15 × 13	Cattle
Besnoitia wallacei	17 × 12	Mouse
Besnoitia darlingi	12 × 12	Opossum
Toxoplasma gondii	12 × 10	Mammals, birds
Hammondia hammondi	12 × 11	Mouse
Sarcocystis hirsuta	12 × 8	Ox
Sarcocystis tenella	12 × 8	Sheep
Sarcocystis porcifelis	13 × 8	Pig
Sarcocystis muris	10 × 8	Mouse
Sarcocystis leporum	10 × 13	Cottontail
Sarcocystis sp.	11 × 8	White-tailed deer
Coccidia of Dogs		
Cystoisospora canis	38 × 30	Mammals
Cystoisospora ohioensis	23 × 19	Mammals
Cystoisospora neorivolta	11 × 13	Mammals
Cystoisospora burrowsi	20 × 17	Mammals
Hammondia heydorni	11 × 12	Ox
Sarcocystis cruzi	16 × 11	Ox
Sarcocystis capracanis	—	Goat
Sarcocystis ovicanis	15 × 10	Sheep
Sarcocystis miescheriana	13 × 10	Pig
Sarcocystis bertrami	15 × 10	Horse
Sarcocystis fayeri	12 × 8	Horse
Sarcocystis hemionilatrantis	14 × 9	Mule deer
Sarcocystis odocoileocanis	11 × 15	White-tailed deer

*Prepared by A. K. Prestwood, Athens, GA.
†Sporocyst of *Sarcocystis*; oocysts of other genera.

animal tissues. The intermediate hosts do not produce oocysts.

Relative to pathogenicity, it is usually the intermediate hosts rather than the dog or cat (definitive host) that are adversely affected. Dalmaney disease of cattle, for example, represents the clinical manifestations of damage to bovine vascular endothelium caused by multiplying coccidial stages, the infection having been obtained by cattle ingesting infective sporocysts shed in the feces of dogs. More information about the effect of these coccidia on cattle and other intermediate hosts can be obtained from references listed in the supplemental reading section.

Clinical coccidiosis in dogs or cats apparently is caused only by certain species of *Cystoisospora* and by *Toxoplasma gondii* (toxoplasmosis). The cat is the only definitive host for *T. gondii*, i.e., the only host in which oocysts are produced in the intestine and shed in the feces. Following accidental ingestion of *T. gondii* oocysts, pathogenic extraintestinal infections can develop in virtually all mammals, including dogs and the cat itself. Most of these are subclinical infections, but occasionally a severely pathogenic case is seen, especially in immunologically naive pups and kittens or in immunologically deprived older animals. A detailed discussion of toxoplasmosis may be found elsewhere in this text.

Little is known about clinical coccidiosis due to infections of *Cystoisospora* in dogs and cats. The pathogenicity of the intestinal stages of this coccidium is only now beginning to be evaluated experimentally. For example, recent work by Dubey (1978) gives evidence that *C. ohioensis* can cause clinical disease in newborn pups—diarrhea resulting from inflammation of the intestinal cysts, with necrosis and massive desquamation of the tips of villi and contents of the lamina propria, especially in the lower part of the small intestine. Only 5 of 21 newborn pups given large numbers of oocysts, however, developed clinical illness, and none of 26 weaned pups, similarly infected, became ill despite apparent infections as judged by the shedding of oocysts from four days to two weeks after initial exposure. Subsequent re-exposure did not produce apparent reinfection.

Until experimental studies are performed with other species of *Cystoisospora* in dogs and cats, it seems safe to assume that intestinal coccidiosis in general is a self-limiting disease. Apparently most pups and kittens acquire low-level infections soon after birth and rapidly become immune to clinical disease. Clinical disease may result if massive numbers of oocysts are ingested by nonimmune animals. Overcrowding, poor sanitation, and inadequate disease control are conditions that may favor clinical coccidiosis. In clinical cases peak numbers of oocysts are shed within the first week following exposure. Shedding of oocysts continues only for about two weeks in weaned pups but may last as long as five weeks in nursing pups, suggesting a delay in acquisition of immunity in younger pups.

DIAGNOSTIC PROCEDURES

Although a saturated solution of $NaNO_3$ used for routine fecal flotations will recover the larger size oocyst of *Cystoisospora*, all coccidian oocysts (especially *Toxoplasma* and *Sarcocystis*) are best recovered by using Sheather's sugar centrifugal flotation technique. Sheather's sugar solution is prepared by mixing 500 gm of regular table sugar with 320 ml of distilled water; add to this 6.5 gm of phenol crystals that have been melted in a hot-water bath (avoid excessive inhalation of fumes).

The procedure for using the Sheather's technique is as follows:

1. Soften feces with tap water to a fluid consistency.
2. Pass the aqueous fecal suspension through a tea strainer or two layers of gauze (to remove excessive debris).
3. Thoroughly mix one part of the strained fecal suspension with two parts of Sheather's sugar solution. Pour into a 15-ml centrifuge tube and add sufficient sugar solution to form a meniscus at the top of the tube. Place a circular overslip on top. (If an air bubble appears under the coverslip, add more sugar solution to the tube and put the coverslip on again.) Balance with a tube of exactly equal weight on the opposite side. Centrifuge at 1500 rpm for 10 minutes.
4. Remove coverslip (twist slightly and lift straight up) and place on a microscope slide. Examine with a $20\times$ or $42\times$ objective (since the eyepiece is $10\times$, the total magnification will be 200 to 420 times actual size).

This technique is especially beneficial in recovering oocysts of *Toxoplasma* and sporocysts of *Sarcocystis*. It also reveals most nematode eggs and protozoan cysts as *Giardia*. Fluke eggs are not demonstrated well nor are tapeworm eggs or nematode larvae.

Differential diagnosis of coccidian infections (whether clinical or subclinical) deserves some attention in light of the specific need to identify oocysts of *T. gondii* in cats and the need to separate the potentially pathogenic *Cystoisospora* from other nonpathogenic coccidia of dogs or cats. Such a separation is fairly easily accomplished on the basis of differences in size of oocysts (see Table 4), provided that the compound microscope is equipped with a calibrated ocular micrometer. The largest oocysts (more than $20 \times 17\mu$) shed by either

dogs or cats are all species of *Cystoisospora*. The other genera of coccidia have smaller oocysts that are relatively similar in size. Morphologic features can be used to separate *Sarcocystis* from the other genera. The oocysts of all of the species of *Sarcocystis* undergo sporulation and rupture before being shed in the feces; thus, small "sporocysts" each containing four minute sporozoites are recovered by flotation of fresh feces. The small, similar-appearing oocysts of *Besnoitia*, *Hammondia*, and *Toxoplasma* are passed unsporulated (as are *Cystoisospora*) and require two days or more for the protoplasmic mass to develop into two sporocysts each containing four sporozoites (all within a single oocyst). Isolation of these three types of oocysts from feces, inoculation of the oocyst into mice, and histosectioning of the mouse brain to check for *Toxoplasma cysts* are procedures that are handled more readily by a diagnostic laboratory. Feces containing unknown oocysts should be fixed in 2 per cent potassium dichromate for shipping to a laboratory.

TREATMENT

Several drugs are used as coccidiostatic agents, including intestinal sulfas, sulfadimethoxine, and nitrofurazone. These drugs are probably indicated only in animals showing clinical signs of coccidiosis (see previous discussion). Dosage is according to manufacturers' recommendations for 14 to 21 days. Spiramycin (Rhode-Pulene) and amprolium (Corid) are drugs reported to be coccidiocidal. We have not used these drugs in dogs or cats with coccidiosis.

Supportive care is important, especially in puppies and kittens. Parenteral fluid therapy with lactated Ringer's solution should be given according to estimations of dehydration. Intestinal protectants such as Kaopectate are helpful when administered in adequate amounts (3 to 5 ml/kg every six to eight hours). Other measures, such as whole blood transfusion (22 to 33 ml/kg) and the use of blankets or heating pads, may be required in anemic, hypothermic animals. Prolonged use of enteric antibiotics or potent parasympatholytic agents should be avoided because they alter the normal intestinal microflora and cause ileus, thereby favoring multiplication of enteric pathogens and the subsequent production and absorption of their toxins.

PREVENTIVE AND CONTROL MEASURES FOR HELMINTH AND PROTOZOAN PARASITES

All gastrointestinal parasites shed some stage (egg, oocyst, or other stage) in feces, which after an appropriate incubation period can directly reinfect logs or cats or, with certain parasites, intermediate hosts. It is at this point that attempts to break the organism's life cycle can be particularly beneficial. There is no better preventive measure than simple removal of the feces on a regular basis, preferably daily. Parasite eggs are trapped in the fecal mass until it becomes disseminated by rain or tracking. Dogs isolated individually on concrete-floored runs that are hosed down with water daily usually do not track their feces and seldom increase their existing parasite burden. Over a period of one year, even in the absence of anthelmintic treatment, dogs under these ideal conditions probably will lose more GI parasites by natural expulsion of aged worms than they will gain. Housing several dogs in the same run makes thorough removal of feces more difficult but all the more important. Dissemination of the feces (and thus of parasite eggs) by tracking is much more likely to occur. Even so, approximately six days are required for freshly passed hookworm eggs to develop, hatch, and reach the infective larval stage; almost two weeks are needed for ascarid eggs to become infective; and only two days are required for coccidian oocysts to sporulate to the infective stage. Tapeworm eggs are immediately infective for their respective intermediate hosts. Once these stages are spread in cracks and corners of the run, they are not so easily flushed away by water spray. Ascarid eggs have a sticky coat that allows them to adhere easily even to smooth surfaces like glass and especially to rough surfaces like concrete or soil. Thus, every effort should be made to remove the fecal mass while it is intact.

Most clinical cases of whipworm infection seem to occur in dogs confined to a small yard pen, where defecation continuously seeds the ground with eggs and allows for reinfection of the dog, especially if food is eaten from the ground. This often occurs with hunting-type dogs and is much more likely to occur in clay soil than in sandy soil. Perhaps the physical rain washing of whipworm eggs deep into the less compact sand prevents access to the eggs, whereas eggs in clay soil remain nearer the surface. The reverse is true of hookworm infective larvae, which seem to infect dogs more readily from sandy soil. It must be remembered, however, that whipworm eggs are not motile, whereas hatched hookworm larvae can migrate deeper in sandy soil when the surface is dry and return to the surface when moisture is available.

Direct sunlight is an excellent all-round means of reducing the level of infective stages of parasites on premises (concrete or ground). Hatched hookworm larvae are more susceptible to dessication than are the intact eggs of ascarids and whipworms; nevertheless, burdens of ascarids or whipworms are generally lower in dogs housed in bright sunlight than in dogs housed in shaded areas. Of course, in geographic areas of uncomfortably high temperatures, some shading may be a necessity.

If heavy hookworm infections are not being controlled by anthelmintics in dogs confined to yard plots where daily removal of feces may not be practical, reduction of the number of larvae contaminating the premises can be accomplished chemically. Sodium borate, sold in grocery stores for washing clothes, can be sprinkled dry over concrete or dirt areas (10 lb/100 sq ft) and wet by sprinkler. Hookworm larvae are effectively killed by this method. The effect on unhatched hookworm eggs or eggs of ascarids or whipworms is questionable. Repeated applications at one- to two-month intervals are recommended during the spring and summer months. Grass is killed but no adverse effects to dogs' feet have been reported. A commercial spray (VIP Hookworm Spray Concentrate) is available for use in a power sprayer for yards and kennels. It can be used at two-week intervals and does not kill grass, as sodium borate does. Tests indicate a good level of reduction in infective hookworm larvae. However, the residual activity evidently lasts but a few days, and intact fecal material is not penetrated by the compound.

Low-level use of diethylcarbamazine (Caricide, Dirocide, Cypip, Filarabits) has tremendous preventive benefit not only for heartworm but also for ascarid infections. Tablet or syrup formulations are available for daily oral administrations, either directly in the mouth or in the food (6.6 mg/kg BW/day). A powdered formulation (Cypip) for administration in the food requires a daily dosage of 2.75 mg of base/kg BW.

Although it is known that diethylcarbamazine prevents heartworm infection by destroying the infective third-stage larvae, which are transmitted by mosquitoes, it is not known with certainty which stages of ascarids are adversely affected by the drug. We do know that patent ascarid infections in the gut are usually prevented. Apparently, there is no effect against somatic stages of ascarid larvae in the extraintestinal tissues.

The addition of styrylpyridinium chloride to diethylcarbamazine (Styrid-Caricide) provides a compound that is effective in "preventing the establishment of patent hookworm infections." Again, somatic hookworm larvae seem to be unaffected. Daily use of Styrid-Caricide is recommended in pups from the time of weaning until approximately six months of age, when the most critical hookworm period is past. Thereafter, diethylcarbamazine alone may be used for the continued prevention of heartworms. Use of these compounds has the effect of lowering the overall environmental contamination with parasite eggs and therefore reducing the chance of overwhelming infections being contracted by other dogs.

Control of tapeworms depends not only on the

effectiveness of the anthelmintic used but also on the availability of reinfections from appropriate intermediate hosts. To control *Dipylidium* in either dogs or cats, fleas and, less frequently, chewing lice must be controlled. The consistent use of flea collars, although not completely effective in eliminating fleas, does much to reduce the total population and thus restricts the opportunity of reinfection with *Dipylidium*. Similarly, *Taenia* infections do not occur if dogs do not eat wild cottontail rabbits and cats do not eat wild rodents. Prevention of these carnivorous habits of outdoor animals is hardly feasible, but clients should at least be told how their animals continue to be reinfected with these tapeworms.

REFERENCES AND SUPPLEMENTAL READING

Dubey, J. P.: A review of *Sarcocystis* of domestic animals and of other coccidia of cats and dogs. J.A.V.M.A., 169:1061, 1976.
Dubey, J. P.: Pathogenicity of *Isospora ohioensis* infection in dogs. J.A.V.M.A., 173:192, 1978.
Hass, D. K., Collins, J. A., and Flick, S. C.: Canine parasitism. Canine Pract. 2:42, 1975.
Polzin, D. J., Stowe, C. M., O'Leary, T. P., et al.: Acute hepatic necrosis associated with the administration of mebendazole to dogs. J.A.V.M.A. 179:1013, 1981.
Roberson, E. L.: Antinematodal drugs; anticestodal and antitrematodal drugs. *In* Booth, N. H., and McDonald, L. E. (eds.): *Veterinary Pharmacology and Therapeutics*. Ames, IA: Iowa State University Press, 1982, pp. 803–873.

ACUTE PANCREATITIS

DONALD R. STROMBECK, D.V.M.,

and BERNARD F. FELDMAN, D.V.M.

Davis, California

Despite new information, the identification and management of acute pancreatitis have not improved appreciably in the six years since the disease was a topic in *Current Veterinary Therapy VI*.

The etiopathogenesis of acute pancreatitis includes nutrition, drugs, and pancreatic ischemia. Acute pancreatitis can be induced experimentally when dogs are fed a diet containing 70 per cent fat. In contrast, animals fed a nutritionally balanced diet with proper exercise rarely develop the disease. Pancreatitis has also been associated with the administration of glucocorticoids, sulfamethizole, salicylazosulfapyridine, chlorpromazine, and isoniazid. Pancreatic ischemia may result from hypovolemic shock, production of fat emboli during hyperlipemia, obstruction of pancreatic ducts by parasite migration, and spasms of the ducts due to duodenal inflammatory problems. Other proposed etiologies include chronic renal disease, hypercalcemia, immune-mediated disease, and trauma.

CLINICAL FINDINGS

Pancreatitis occurs more frequently in obese, middle-aged dogs. Clinical signs are inconsistent and may include vomiting, pain, anorexia, depression, fever, diarrhea, abdominal distention, dehydration, shock, cardiac arrhythmias, and respiratory distress. Based on frequency in experimental dogs, anorexia, depression, dehydration, generalized abdominal pain, and vomiting occurred in more than 90 per cent of the animals; diarrhea in 54 per cent; fever greater than 39.2°C (102.5°F) in 46 per cent; and cardiac arrhythmias in 23 per cent.

LABORATORY FINDINGS

Laboratory findings may include leukocytosis or a degenerative left shift on a hemogram. Changes in blood chemistries can include hyperglycemia, fasting hyperlipidemia, and increases in serum activities of alanine aminotransferase and alkaline phosphatase. The best means of diagnosing pancreatitis is thought to be by finding serum lipase activity increased above the normal range or by finding serum amylase activity increased to levels three to four times normal.

A recent retrospective study compared serum activities of amylase and lipase in a large group of dogs suspected of having pancreatitis. These clinical pathologic data were correlated with pathology findings in 90 of the dogs. The results of this study showed that there was no correlation between serum amylase and lipase activities until lipase activity was greater than 800 U/L. It was concluded that information on serum amylase activity is of little value in identifying pancreatitis and that use of this test as a diagnostic tool will suggest pancreatitis in many cases in which the disease does not exist. Pathology results indicated that dogs with serum lipase activities less than 500 U/L seldom had pancreatitis, whereas approximately 75 per cent of those with activities greater than 500 U/L did have pancreatitis. Thus, it was also concluded that, although high serum lipase activity findings are useful in identifying pancreatitis, they are not pathognomonic for the disease.

DIAGNOSIS

A diagnosis of pancreatitis cannot be made on any single finding. The diagnosis is based on information gained from clinical signs, hemograms, blood chemical analyses, and radiographs. More so than in many other diseases, the diagnosis is made probabilistically. With all clinical evidence consistent with pancreatitis and a very high lipase value (the single best test to identify the problem), the probability for pancreatitis is only 75 per cent.

TREATMENT

The treatment of a patient with acute pancreatitis should be based on the following therapeutic goals: (1) restoration and maintenance of normal fluid volume, thus preventing hypovolemic shock; (2) minimization of secretion by the pancreas; and (3) control or prevention of secondary infection. Management of pancreatitis, however, has been largely empirical with no information from controlled studies to support any single treatment. Accepted routine management has included giving nothing by mouth; giving anticholinergics to reduce pancreatic secretion; and supportive use of antibiotics, corticosteroids, and fluids.

Complete restriction of oral feeding is essential to gain remission. Restricting oral intake causes a reduction in pancreatic secretory activity by preventing pancreatic stimulation by gastric distention, the presence of fats and amino acids, or low duodenal pH. Ideally, food should be restricted for at least five days. Water may be given orally for the succeeding several days.

Antibiotics should be used, since acute inflammation of the pancreas can extend to the adjacent loops of both the small and large intestine and the bacterial microflora of the intestinal lumen can invade those tissues and cause infection. Since pancreatitis complicated by peritoneal infection and abscessation is difficult to treat, antibiotics are indicated as prophylaxis. Antibiotic therapy should include a penicillin and an aminoglycoside, both of which are required to manage invasion by the anaerobic and aerobic bacteria found in the intestines.

Fluid therapy is the most essential aspect of treatment for remission of pancreatitis. Studies in dogs with a severe form of experimentally induced hemorrhagic pancreatitis indicated that vigorous fluid therapy enabled animals to survive. In fact, dogs survived when the pancreas was found to be almost totally absent three months after recognition of the acute problem.

Balanced electrolyte solutions such as lactated Ringer's solution are given intravenously and in amounts sufficient to treat hypovolemia and shock. There is a tendency to undertreat with fluids. There is more risk in giving insufficient fluids (losing the patient) than in giving excessive amounts (which might produce pulmonary edema). The only accurate means of determining how much fluid to give is to monitor central venous pressure during administration.

Hypoproteinemia is an invariable complication of the early phase of acute pancreatitis. When this is recognized, fluid therapy can include the intravenous administration of canine plasma or other colloids such as low molecular weight dextran (10 per cent dextran at 5 ml/kg/hr) to decrease viscosity, improve pancreatic microcirculation and peripheral circulation, and impede platelet function, thus preventing thrombus formation.

Anticholinergic therapy has no effect on the clinical course or clinical pathology associated with acute pancreatitis. These drugs not only fail to control vomiting but also reduce gastrointestinal motility, which is already reduced in dogs with acute pancreatitis. Thus, since no benefits can be gained from the use of anticholinergics and if complications can be aggravated by their use, it is recommended that this type of drug be avoided.

Similarly, corticosteroids have not been demonstrated to have significant effects on the course of the disease. A recent study showed that steroid therapy did not reduce inflammation associated with pancreatitis. Moreover, their use can precipitate pancreatitis. Steroid therapy may be useful in managing complications of shock or myocarditis, and their use should be limited to these very specific indications.

A number of other treatments have been suggested for acute pancreatitis. The premise supporting their use in clinical cases is based on results of experimental studies in animals. The suggested treatments have included the use of proteolytic enzyme inhibitors; hormones such as glucagon and insulin to inhibit pancreatic enzyme secretion; and vasopressin, fibrinolysin, or heparin to improve the reduced circulation in the inflamed pancreas. None of these treatments has been shown to be effective in clinical cases. If adequate therapy with fluids and antibiotics is provided, it is doubtful whether any other treatment is necessary.

CONVALESCENCE

Resumption of oral feeding should not begin until clinical signs disappear and serum lipase activity returns to normal. The dog's appetite often returns within three to four days, whereas the lipase activity is not normal until seven to eight days following the initiation of treatment. Relapses are most often associated with premature resumption of feeding. Some dogs can appear to be in complete clinical remission yet still have high serum lipase activity, reflecting chronic pancreatitis. Nutrients offered first on resumption of feeding should be those that stimulate pancreatic enzyme secretion the least. Carbohydrates have this property and are given in a form that requires minimal digestion. Glucose or small polymers of glucose (Polycose*) result in minimal pancreatic secretion (a net effect of glucose solutions stimulating the gastric phase and inhibiting the intestinal phase of pancreatic secretion). With improvement, the carbohydrate source is gradually changed to an easily digested source of starch (such as boiled rice) and a small quantity of protein. Protein should be of high biologic value, such as cooked egg white, cottage cheese, or lean meat, and should be added gradually in amounts not to exceed minimum requirements. With improvement, commercial products can be fed. Serum enzyme activities sometimes increase following a return to commercial foods, although the animal may remain clinically normal. Persistence of high enzyme activity in clinically normal dogs can reflect chronic pancreatitis requiring continuous management with a controlled diet.

Owing to the fact that protein is a more potent stimulator of pancreatic secretion than lipid, a high-protein diet should not be fed. However, since a high level of dietary fat also is an important factor in the development of acute pancreatitis, the animal should be maintained on a minimal level of dietary lipids. If the animal is returned to commercial dog food, it must be remembered that different preparations differ in fat content. Low-fat prescription diets are a satisfactory food source for these patients. If a long-term goal is a fat-free diet, minimum fat requirements can be met by supplementing this diet with triglycerides made up of medium-chain fatty acids (MCT Oil†). Fatty acids containing fewer than nine carbon atoms do not stimulate the pancreas to secrete bicarbonate or enzymes. Fatty acids of greater length and monoglycerides containing these fatty acids are potent stimulators of pancreatic secretion.

_____

*Ross Laboratories, Columbus, OH.
†Mead Johnson Nutritional Division, Evansville, IN.

Patients with acute pancreatitis may need to have some of their nutritional requirements met parenterally before oral feeding can be resumed. The ideal method is total parenteral nutrition, which does not affect pancreatic secretion. Elemental diets may be of limited use in selected cases of pancreatitis. Pancreatic secretion of fluid and enzymes is as great with orally administered elemental diets as it is with conventional diets. Infusion of an elemental diet directly into the duodenum results in persistence of the normal response to secrete enzymes but not the normal response to secrete fluid and bicarbonate. The acid-pH stimulus for secretin release is lacking during this infusion. If, however, an elemental diet with a neutral pH is infused into the jejunum, the pancreas secretes neither enzymes nor fluid and bicarbonate.

PROGNOSIS

Prognosis is dependent upon early recognition and prevention of complicating factors such as shock, peritonitis caused by infection, disseminated intravascular coagulation, acute renal failure, and pulmonary hypoxemia. Proper medical management results in survival in most patients. Some survivors later develop complications that may require surgery. These include pancreatic abscesses, stricture of the bile duct, and stenosis of the duodenum.

Client education must include information on possible deficiencies in pancreatic exocrine and endocrine functions as sequelae to acute pancreatitis. To reduce the risk of their occurrence, the importance of strict dietary restrictions should be discussed. Signs of weight loss, steatorrhea, polyuria, polydipsia, and polyphagia should be used as indicators of possible future pancreatic disease.

SUPPLEMENTAL READING

Attix, E., Strombeck, D. R., Wheeldon, E. B., and Stern, J. S.: Effects of an anticholinergic and a corticosteroid on acute pancreatitis in experimental dogs. Am. J. Vet. Res. 42:1668, 1981.
Feldman, B. F., Attix, E., Strombeck, D. R., and O'Neill, S.: Biochemical and coagulation changes in a canine model of acute necrotizing pancreatitis. Am. J. Vet. Res. 42:805, 1981.
Strombeck, D. R.: *Small Animal Gastroenterology.* Davis, CA: Stonegate Publishing, 1979, pp. 301–331.
Strombeck, D. R,. Farver, T. F., and Kaneko, J. J.: Serum amylase and lipase activities in the diagnosis of pancreatitis in dogs. Am. J. Vet. Res. 42:1966, 1981.

HEPATIC BIOPSY

ROBERT M. HARDY, D.V.M.

St. Paul, Minnesota

Hepatic biopsy is the single most important *diagnostic* test in evaluating the majority of animals with hepatic disease. All other components of the patient's medical evaluation, i.e., history, physical exam, hematology, biochemistry, radiology, and so on, primarily serve a localizing function. The findings of these studies usually indicate that hepatobiliary disease exists and may give some indication as to relative severity or duration of the disease process, but rarely do they establish a definitive diagnosis. In many cases hepatic biopsy serves as the only means of establishing a definitive diagnosis. Veterinarians interested in providing the highest degree of diagnostic accuracy to patients with hepatobiliary disease should develop the skills necessary to consistently obtain hepatic tissue samples. Since hepatic needle biopsy is the fastest, least expensive, safest, and most often utilized technique for obtaining hepatic tissue in veterinary practice, this discussion will relate primarily to needle biopsy rather than to more invasive procedures utilizing laparoscopy, laparotomy, or key-hole techniques.

INDICATIONS (Osborne et al., 1969; 1974; Strombeck, 1979)

I have utilized one primary philosophy in the evaluation of patients with hepatic disease regarding the need for a liver biopsy. If the patient has significant clinical illness such that the owner sought veterinary counsel for the animal, if liver disease is identified as the most likely cause of the patient's illness, and if the cause of the liver disease has not been identified by less invasive techniques, then biopsy is warranted if the patient's condition will tolerate it. The primary indication is to establish a diagnosis of liver disease, preferably an etiologic one, when such a diagnosis is not available by other means.

Many other indications for hepatic biopsy exist. Even though an etiologic diagnosis may not be established, morphologic changes in the animal's liver often give valuable prognostic information and may indicate certain therapies. The relative degree of inflammation and cell necrosis and the presence or absence of fibrosis and/or biliary tract involvement all aid in formulating accurate prognostic and therapeutic plans. Biopsy is also indicated as a direct means of assessing the patient's response to therapy.

Although clinical signs and biochemical profiles usually indicate whether the disease process is resolving, evidence of morphologic improvement or deterioration is only available via biopsy. This evidence may contradict clinical and laboratory findings. Hepatic biopsy may also be utilized when abnormal hepatic enzyme or function tests are found in animals without other evidence of hepatic disease. The need for biopsy in animals with occult hepatic disease is determined by the presence or absence of other major diseases, the magnitude of the enzymatic or functional abnormalities, and whether such abnormalities persist on serial metabolic profiles. The presence of unexplained hepatomegaly is another primary indication for biopsy.

A number of hepatic diseases may be manifested as hepatomegaly in the absence of dramatic biochemical abnormalities. Biopsy is an efficient, easy method for diagnosing the cause of the hepatic enlargement. Occasionally, biopsy may also help in differentiating intrahepatic jaundice from extrahepatic jaundice. In most cases of extrahepatic biliary obstruction, clinical and biochemical parameters are such that exploratory celiotomy is chosen over biopsy to establish the diagnosis as well as institute appropriate therapy. However, when the risk of complications during surgery makes an exploratory less advisable or when the biochemical evaluation of the patient does not clearly indicate intrahepatic versus extrahepatic cholestasis, needle biopsy may be chosen. In humans, hepatic needle biopsy in patients with major bile duct occlusion is contraindicated owing to the risk of puncturing a major bile duct and creating bile peritonitis. Although such a complication is possible in dogs and cats, it rarely occurs following needle biopsy. Furthermore, the diagnosis of extrahepatic obstruction can be made from a biopsy sample, and surgery can then be recommended with certainty.

Hepatic needle biopsy is obviously of greatest value in patients with diffuse hepatic disease in which lesions are randomly distributed throughout the liver. To consistently obtain accurate diagnoses using blind, percutaneous biopsy techniques, lesions must be diffuse in all hepatic lobes. For signs of hepatic failure to be present, 80 per cent or more of the liver's functional mass must be compromised, making the probability of collecting a specimen from an affected area very high. Furthermore, postmortem data indicate that needle biopsy diagnoses

813

correlated well with necropsy results in 80 per cent (Edwards, 1977; Osborne, 1969) of cases. Even when searching for hepatic metastases, positive confirmation is possible in 20 to 75 per cent of cases using needle biopsy alone (Osborne et al., 1974).

Proper handling and evaluation of the biopsy is as important as obtaining the biopsy. Veterinary pathologists experienced in evaluating needle biopsy samples should be utilized whenever possible. Individuals familiar with artifacts induced by needle biopsy as well as with interpreting pathologic changes present in small samples are most likely to provide diagnostically useful information. In addition to the biopsy sample, all physical, radiographic, and laboratory data pertinent to the case should be included. By utilizing information from these multiple sources it is often possible to establish a diagnosis.

CONTRAINDICATIONS (Edwards, 1977; Osborne et al.,1969; 1974; Strombeck, 1979).

Contraindications to hepatic biopsy may be either absolute or relative. Absolute contraindications are situations in which severe injury to the patient would likely result if a biopsy were taken. The most important absolute contraindications include significant coagulation abnormalities, intrahepatic vascular tumors, hepatic cysts or abscesses, and severe anemia. Except for detecting bleeding tendencies and anemia presurgically, other absolute contraindications are unlikely to be identified until after the biopsy is performed. In addition, significant bleeding problems that would preclude hepatic needle biopsy are extremely uncommon.

Relative contraindications are primarily associated with the inexperience of the person performing the biopsy. Nearly every study evaluating the risks of hepatic biopsy confirms that the number of biopsy complications is directly proportional to the inexperience of the surgeon. Another relative contraindication is a patient with extrahepatic jaundice. It has already been mentioned that the risk in biopsying a patient with obstructive jaundice is very low; the value of an accurate diagnosis usually outweighs the minimal risk. One relative contraindication relates to inadequate patient restraint. A major cause of bleeding after liver biopsy is laceration of the liver capsule during the biopsy procedure. Lacerations most often occur when the patient moves unexpectedly while the needle is in the intrahepatic phase of the procedure. Adequate chemical restraint almost always prevents this complication.

PATIENT PREPARATION

Preparing the patient for hepatic needle biopsy is relatively simple. The animal should be fasted 12 to 24 hours preceding the procedure to reduce the possibility of puncturing the stomach. Feeding the animal a fatty meal (5 to 30 ml of Lipomul*) 30 to 60 minutes prior to biopsy may stimulate gallbladder contraction. However, radiographic evaluations during cholangiography, both before and after a fatty meal, indicated no significant change in gallbladder size, so I no longer routinely feed fatty meals prior to biopsy. Some assessment of the animal's clotting ability must be made. Any of the following coagulation tests effectively screens for major coagulation abnormalities: activated clotting time, prothrombin time, partial thromboplastin time, and whole blood clotting time. It is advisable to scan a fresh blood smear to be sure that there are adequate circulating platelets. Routine survey abdominal radiographs prior to biopsy are also valuable. If the liver is nonpalpable, radiographs indicating liver size, shape, and position may lead one to select an alternative biopsy approach.

Chemical restraint is often required for adequate patient immobilization and prevents unpredictable movement of the patient during the biopsy procedure. I routinely utilize 2 per cent sodium thiamylal for patient immobilization during needle biopsy. The patient is clipped and a surgical scrub of the biopsy site is completed before administering the anesthetic. This reduces the anesthesia time. The dose of anesthetic is titrated by monitoring the animal's response to the drug. Give just enough anesthetic so that the patient will lie quietly on its back or side. Rarely is the plane of anesthesia deep enough to require intubation of the animal. This extremely light plane of anesthesia allows three to five minutes of relaxation, which is more than sufficient to perform a needle biopsy. There have been no complications related to anesthetic administration in over 250 biopsies. The animal is usually up and ambulatory within 10 to 30 minutes. Alternative measures include using local anesthetics alone, combinations of Innovar-Vet† (0.04 to 0.09 mg/kg IV) plus atropine, and ketamine hydrochloride at 1 to 2 mg/kg IV (in cats). Animals may also be masked down with inhalant anesthetics.

TECHNIQUES (Edwards, 1977; Feldman and Ettinger, 1976; Osborne et al., 1969; Strombeck, 1979)

Several techniques are available for obtaining hepatic tissue. Selection primarily involves personal preference; the location through which the biopsy is taken, i.e., transabdominal versus transthoracic; and whether a needle or wedge biopsy is taken. Unless large tissue samples are needed, such as for

---

*The Upjohn Co., Kalamazoo, MI.
†Pitman-Moore, Inc., Washington Crossing, NJ.

quantitative determination of toxins, heavy metals, or microsomal enzyme activities, needle core biopsies usually provide sufficient material. Needle core biopsies are also quicker to obtain, less expensive to perform, less risky for the patient, and technically easier than wedge biopsies. They also readily lend themselves to repeat biopsies for prognostic purposes because they are less objectionable to the owner. This discussion will be limited to the blind percutaneous transabdominal needle biopsy technique because I have the most experience with this technique and have found it to be extremely safe, reliable, and easy for neophyte biopsiers to master. Alternative biopsy procedures have been well described elsewhere (Feldman and Ettinger, 1976; 1977; Osborne et al., 1974; Strombeck, 1976).

The animal is prepared as previously described. A small (5 × 5 cm) area over the tip of the xiphoid is clipped and sterilely scrubbed. Light sodium thiamylal anesthesia is administered. The patient is placed either in dorsal recumbency or turned toward its right side at a 45° angle from the midline. If a tilt table is available, the animal's head is raised to a 45° angle to allow the viscera to fall away from the liver. This also tends to drop the liver margins, making them more easily palpable. For dogs with normal liver size, the puncture site is located midway between the *tip* of the xiphoid cartilage and the costal margins on the dog's *left* side. There is a "V" formed by the xiphoid process and the rib cage. It is important to stay adjacent to the tip of the xiphoid and not introduce the needle too anteriorly in the xiphoid notch. If the needle is placed too far cranially, it may enter the thoracic cavity. The skin is incised with a #11 scalpel blade. This gives the biopsy needle access to subcutaneous tissues. Most needles are not designed to puncture the skin.

Several biopsy needles are available. The two most widely used are the Menghini needle* or its recent modification (Jamshidi soft tissue biopsy needle†) and the Tru-Cut disposable biopsy needle.‡ The best needle sizes for obtaining hepatic biopsies are 70 × 1.2 mm for the Menghini, 70 × 1.9 mm for the Jamshidi, and 11.4-cm, 14-gauge for the Tru-Cut. Both the Menghini and Jamshidi needles can be operated with one hand and have a very rapid intrahepatic phase (< 1 sec). The Tru-Cut needle requires the use of both hands and has a slightly longer intrahepatic phase. All three needles consistently obtain high-quality hepatic biopsy material. The Menghini needle is very desirable and is designed for multiple use and repeated autoclaving. Although the Jamshidi and Tru-Cut needles are disposable, they may be washed, gas sterilized, and reused a number of times. If more than one biopsy sample is desired, the needle

should be rinsed in sterile saline between biopsies to remove any blood. Blood drying on or in the needle causes the sides and/or cutting prong to drag as it passes through the skin and hepatic tissue. Details relative to the use of each of these needles have been well described elsewhere (Feldman and Ettinger, 1977; Osborne et al., 1974). In addition, instructions on the use of each needle are included as packaged by the manufacturer.

The biopsy needle should be angled approximately 20° anteriorly and 20 to 30° toward the dog's *left* side, i.e., in a left anterolateral direction. The needle is angled to reduce the risk of puncturing the gallbladder, which lies adjacent and *right* of the xiphoid process. If hepatomegaly is present, any palpable area of liver tissue away from the gallbladder may be biopsied. If a Menghini-type needle is used, it is advanced through the skin and subcutaneous tissues until its tip is just within the peritoneal cavity. The Tru-Cut needle is also advanced until the tip has just entered the abdominal cavity. The normal liver lies very close to the parietal peritoneal surface, and the needle does *not* have to be advanced deep into the peritoneal cavity to obtain hepatic tissue. Do not expect to feel any cutting sensation or resistance to the passage of these needles within the liver. In many cases one can ascertain that liver was obtained only after removing the needle and observing for liver tissue. Always check the biopsy port of the Tru-Cut needle after each attempt to obtain tissues.

Postbiopsy care is minimal. The patient is left in a sternal position to recover. The weight of the liver may help provide some degree of hemostasis to the puncture site. Animals should be kept quiet for 24 to 48 hours to reduce the possibility of traumatizing the biopsy area. There is no need for routine use of prophylactic antibiotics.

Hepatic biopsy samples are often quite friable, so they should be handled with care to avoid unnecessary fragmentation. A small piece of the biopsy tissue may be transferred to a glass slide and impression smears evaluated immediately. Hepatic neoplasia occasionally may be diagnosed cytologically without waiting for fixation and processing of the sample. The biopsy needle may also be cultured if a bacterial hepatitis/cholangitis is suspected. The rest of the sample should be gently transferred to 10 per cent buffered formalin for fixation.

COMPLICATIONS (Edwards, 1977; Feldman and Ettinger, 1976; Osborne et al., 1969; Strombeck, 1979)

The fear of complications associated with any biopsy keeps many individuals from attempting the procedure. Fortunately, significant morbidity and mortality following liver biopsy are low. When

---

*V. Mueller Co., Chicago, IL.
†Kormed, Inc., St. Paul, MN.
‡Travenol Laboratories, Inc. Deerfield, IL.

complications do occur, they are most often related to errors in technique or inexperience of the operator. Published mortality figures vary from 0 to 4.7 per cent, and significant morbidity occurs in 2.7 to 14 per cent of patients.

Significant complications occurring in dogs and cats following hepatic biopsy include hemorrhage, biopsy of adjacent tissues (stomach, spleen, diaphragm, pancreas, kidney, lung), puncture of the gallbladder or a major bile duct leading to bile peritonitis, and transfer of ascitic fluid into the thorax through a puncture hole in the diaphragm. Although hemorrhage is the most important complication, it is a rare event. Cases of hemorrhage have occurred following liver biopsy even though prebiopsy coagulation tests were normal. Significant bleeding is most often associated with laceration of the liver during the biopsy procedure. Attempts to control bleeding should be made initially with transfusions, reserving laparotomy as a salvage procedure. Biopsy of tissues from organs adjacent to the liver occurs with some regularity, but other than embarrassment for the clinician, it causes no demonstrable problems for the patient. Puncture of the gallbladder or a major bile duct may lead to bile peritonitis, which necessitates exploratory surgery to seal the leak, but it usually seals spontaneously. Signs exhibited when bile peritonitis develops include vomiting and abdominal pain. Abdominocentesis confirms the diagnosis. Surgical repair of the rent is usually easy.

RESULTS

The goal of every biopsy is to obtain useful information for the diagnosis, prognosis, or therapy of the patient. Any series of biopsy data reflects the personal bias of the investigator; his inclination to biopsy patients with mild, moderate, or severe liver disease; and the expertise of the individuals interpreting the histopathology. Nonetheless, there is value in looking at the types of diagnoses made by individuals interested in hepatic disease to see what types of diseases are documented. To that end, data from two recently published reports on large numbers of liver biopsies (Edwards, 1977; Feldman and Ettinger, 1977) plus the results of 213 biopsies compiled at the University of Minnesota over a ten-year period have been tabulated (Table 1).

This table shows that certain diagnoses were made much more frequently at certain diagnostic centers than at others; e.g., vacuolated hepatosis, a morphologic alteration induced predominantly by glucocorticoids, was diagnosed at only two of the three hospitals. The same is true of chronic active hepatitis. Toxic hepatitis was a diagnosis made only by the University of Minnesota. Such differences may reflect a multitude of factors including different population bases, investigator interests, and pathologist interpretive variabilities. What is probably most enlightening is an examination of the four most common biopsy diagnoses: vacuolated hepatosis, normal, neoplasia, and lipidosis. These four diag-

Table 1. *Summary of Histologic Diagnoses From 395 Hepatic Biopsies**

Histologic Diagnosis	Berkeley†	UCD‡	UM	Total	Per Cent
Vacuolated hepatosis	0	33	29	62	15.7
Normal	15	14	21	50	12.7
Neoplasia	11	13	26	50	12.7
Lipidosis	14	3	27	44	11.1
Focal hepatitis/necrosis	5	16	6	27	6.8
Cholestasis	8	0	15	23	5.8
Cirrhosis	2	0	20	22	5.6
Chronic active hepatitis	0	16	5	21	5.3
Insufficient tissue/no diagnosis	5	6	10	21	5.3
Toxic hepatitis	0	0	20	20	5.1
Hepatitis	11	0	8	19	4.8
Cholangitis	4	0	9	13	3.3
Hemosiderosis	0	0	6	6	1.5
Passive congestion	0	3	2	5	1.3
Biliary hyperplasia	0	1	3	4	1.0
Extramedullary myelopoiesis	0	2	1	3	0.7
Hepatic atrophy	0	0	3	3	0.7
Histoplasmosis	0	0	1	1	0.3
Microabscesses	0	0	1	1	0.3
Total number of biopsies	75	107	213	395	100

*Taken from 345 dogs and 33 cats at three veterinary referral centers: Berkeley Veterinary Medical Group, Berkeley, CA; University of California, Davis, CA; University of Minnesota, St. Paul, MN.
†Data from Feldman and Ettinger: J.A.A.H.A. 13:17, 1977.
‡Data from Edwards: Calif. Vet. 4:9, 1977.

noses accounted for 52 per cent of the 395 biopsies. Vacuolated hepatosis is usually secondary to either exogenous or endogenous glucocorticoids and nonsteroidal toxic injury. The frequency with which this diagnosis is made reflects both the widespread use of glucocorticoids in the dog and the prevalence of canine hyperadrenocorticism.

The finding of one dog in eight biopsied to be normal histologically is unexpected. Liver biopsies are rarely performed to confirm a normal liver. Obtaining a normal biopsy sample in an animal suspected of having liver disease suggests either that the lesion was missed or that whatever damage is present is not evident at the light microscopic level.

Hepatic neoplasia is one of the most important diagnoses to confirm. Animals with hepatic failure secondary to neoplasia generally have a very poor prognosis, and any attempts at supportive and symptomatic care should only be made with the owner's full knowledge of the prognosis.

Hepatic lipidosis may be induced by a number of causes ranging from toxic to nutritional and metabolic. However, the prognosis for animals with lipidosis is generally guarded to good, except for cats with the idiopathic feline lipidosis syndrome. One comment is necessary regarding the interpretation of hepatic vacuolar change as lipidosis. It is probable that some of the cases diagnosed as lipidosis actually involved steroid-induced vacuolated changes. Only a retrospective evaluation of all these biopsies would allow better clarification of this point.

Improvements in our knowledge concerning many hepatic diseases have occurred primarily because a few individuals were willing to biopsy dogs and cats with hepatic diseases. Hepatic biopsy is the one procedure that may allow a definitive etiologic diagnosis to be made in hepatic diseases. Otherwise "they all look the same." Hepatic biopsy is an easy, rapid, safe, and worthwhile procedure to learn. All it takes is the courage to do the first one.

REFERENCES

Edwards, D. F.: Blind percutaneous liver biopsy: A safe diagnostic procedure. Calif. Vet. 4:9, 1977.
Feldman, E. C., and Ettinger, S. J.: Percutaneous transthoracic liver biopsy in the dog. J.A.V.M.A. 169:805, 1976.
Feldman, E. C., and Ettinger, S. J.: Percutaneous transthoracic liver biopsy in the dog: A review of 75 cases. J.A.A.H.A. 13:17, 1977.
Osborne, C. A., Hardy, R. M., Stevens, J. B., and Perman, V.: Liver biopsy. Vet. Clin. North Am. 4:333, 1974.
Osborne, C. A., Stevens, J. B., and Perman, V.: Needle biopsy of the liver. J.A.V.M.A. 155:1605, 1969.
Strombeck, D. R.: Liver Biopsy. In Strombeck, D. R. (ed.): Small Animal Gastroenterology. Davis, CA: Stonegate Publishing, 1979.

DIETARY THERAPY FOR DOGS WITH CHRONIC HEPATIC INSUFFICIENCY

DONALD R. STROMBECK, D.V.M.,
M. C. SCHAEFFER, M.P.H.,
and Q. R. ROGERS, Ph.D.

Davis, California

Hepatic encephalopathy is an important clinical manifestation of hepatic insufficiency. Early signs of encephalopathy are subtle and include decreased food intake and possibly depression. Pronounced signs of hepatic encephalopathy do not usually appear until the pathology is severe and involves the entire organ.

Successful management is possible if the pathology can be reversed. Portosystemic vascular anastomosis, which can often be corrected by surgery to partially close the shunt, is one of the few problems in which dramatic improvement and lasting remission can be realized. Management is usually not as successful with other forms of hepatic disease, including some cases of chronic active hepatitis, all cases of cirrhosis, and cases of massive necrosis due to toxins, drugs, or infections in which 60 to 90 per cent of hepatic function is lost. Hepatic diseases such as steroid-induced hepatopathy and hepatic lipidosis seldom show signs of hepatic encephalopathy and are usually resolved after successful management of the primary problem. Primary and metastatic cancers of the liver are usually not associated with signs of hepatic encephalopathy.

Management of hepatic encephalopathy is directed toward removing the cause of liver pathology and supporting regeneration of the liver. The causes of hepatic disease that can result in encephalopathy are poorly understood. When chemicals or infectious agents have produced hepatitis, the initiating agent is usually no longer a factor by the time signs of hepatic encephalopathy appear. Since the liver has a remarkable capacity to regenerate, removal of the cause of pathology should result in restoration of normal hepatic structure and function. Regeneration to restore normal function is not always possible because the normal architecture of the liver is irretrievably lost.

Regeneration may also be impaired by a continuation of destructive processes that are unrelated to the original cause of liver damage. Such a perpetuation of liver damage can be produced by toxins originating within the intestines that are not removed by the liver's reticuloendothelial system because of hepatic insufficiency. An example is bacterial endotoxin, which is able to produce disease when it is not removed and is, therefore, degraded. Thus, since one important goal of management of hepatic disease is the arrest of active pathologic processes, it is apparent that the absorption of toxins from the intestine should be minimized.

Control of the colonic environment to minimize the production and absorption of toxins can be partially achieved by daily administration of agents with a laxative effect. The most popular of such agents is lactulose, which is described on page 773. We believe that a better effect could be achieved by feeding a diet that is well digested and absorbed in the small intestine. Such a diet should contain ingredients with nearly 100 per cent digestibility, i.e., resulting in very little residue. This would be advantageous since the growth of bacteria in the colon is supported largely by fermentation of polysaccharides and other foodstuffs that are not digested in the small intestine. The diet should contain sufficient protein to at least meet the minimum requirements for normal dogs. The protein should have high digestibility and a high biologic value so that, when fed, it is nearly completely absorbed in the small intestine and nearly completely used by the dog for synthesis of new protein. Milk protein is highly recommended because not only is it a very high-quality protein, but more importantly, there are suggestions in the literature that dogs with experimentally produced hepatic insufficiency do better when fed milk protein than when fed other kinds of protein.

We have formulated a diet for dogs with experimentally induced hepatic disease and have used it to treat a number of clinic patients with hepatic insufficiency due to portosystemic vascular anastomosis, chronic active hepatitis, hepatic necrosis, or hepatic cirrhosis. When clinic patients were fed the diet, they showed an improvement in appetite and activity and fewer signs of encephalopathy. Exceptions were several dogs with terminal hepatic insufficiency caused by cirrhosis, where death followed within ten days of identifying the basis for the hepatic problem. In a small group of dogs with experimentally induced liver disease, those fed a diet of similar composition were still living more than two years after the induction of chronic active hepatitis. After long-term feeding of this diet, significant regeneration was evident in this model when liver mass was reduced by a toxin to one-third of normal. Such improvement would not be expected with a conventional diet. In fact, improvement in the condition of these dogs did not begin until dogs were switched from a conventional dry diet to this purified diet.

The composition of the diet we prepare for use by our clinic patients with liver disease is as follows:

Ingredient	gm/100 gm dry diet
Casein	9.0
Animal fat	20.0
Sucrose	32.35
Corn starch	32.35
Vitamin mix	1.0
Mineral mix	5.0
Choline chloride	0.3

Because some of the ingredients used are available only to research facilities, we have approximated the formula using ingredients readily available to the client. Two separate recipes for low-protein, low-fiber diets are presented with instructions for preparation. Both contain no meat or meat products, and casein is their principal protein source. Diet 1 provides most micronutrients without requiring extensive supplementation, and, as a dry diet, is fairly resistant to spoilage. Diet 2 requires more supplementation to ensure a balanced diet, but it contains somewhat less ash and crude fiber than Diet 1. This diet is also lower in copper. Hepatic copper levels often increase with hepatic disease, and they sometimes reach levels that further damage the liver. Thus, it is desirable to feed nutrients low in copper content. Because tastes and availability of ingredients vary, one diet may be more palatable or easier to prepare than the other. It is important that the instructions be followed closely and that substitutions of ingredients not be made so that the diet is nutritionally complete.

MIXING DIRECTIONS FOR DIET 1

Mix wheat germ and cold safflower oil in electric mixer if possible. If beef tallow is used, allow to

Diet 1

	Gm (As Is) Per Batch	Oz (As Is) Per Batch	Measurements* (As Is) Per Batch
Instant non-fat dry milk *fortified* with vits. A and D	208	7 3/8	3 C
Blackstrap molasses†	133	4 3/4	2/5 C between 1/3 and 1/2 cup)
Wheat germ, raw ground if possible‡	114	4	1 C and 2 T (1 1/8 C)
Bone meal§	37	1 3/10	1/5 C
Safflower oil	100	3 1/2	1/2 C
Animal fat‖	100	3 1/2	1/2 C
Table salt, *iodized***	10	3/8	1 1/2 t
Cornstarch	403	14 1/5	3 C
Vitamin C (ascorbic acid††)	Provide vitamin C as a supplement at 10 mg/lb BW/day		
Choline‡‡	A dog weighing 33 lb or less should be given 250 mg choline per day; 500 mg per day should be given to larger dogs		

*C = cup, T = tablespoon, t = teaspoon. If possible, ingredients should be weighed rather than measured, since weighing is more accurate.

†Blackstrap molasses is available at most health food stores and in some supermarkets. Blackstrap is the most "crude" form of molasses available and is highest in nutritional quality (i.e., has the highest mineral content).

‡Raw wheat germ is available in bulk in most health food stores. The toasted wheat germ available in supermarkets is not acceptable. Raw wheat germ spoils fairly quickly so it should be bought fresh regularly. If the equipment is available, the wheat germ should be ground into smaller particles, using a coffee mill, mortar and pestle, or blender.

§Bone meal is available at pet care stores. It should be the kind prepared specifically for consumption by animals, i.e., sterilized.

‖Lard or beef tallow may be used. Because the type of fat used is an important component of a diet's palatability, this choice should be tailored to the individual's taste.

**If a lower sodium content is desired, the NaCl level may be reduced. However, if the diet is to be fed over a long period of time, an additional source of iodine, an essential nutrient, must be provided. See discussion following Diet 2.

††See discussion following Diet 2.

‡‡Choline tablets (either choline chloride or choline bitartrate) can be bought at health food stores. Also, see discussion following Diet 2.

come to room temperature before mixing. Add animal fat and mix. Mix salt, bone meal, and cornstarch separately and add to above ingredients. Add dry instant milk and molasses and mix.

COMMENTS

1. Diet will be dark golden brown and slightly granular. It can be fed as is or formed into chunks with hands. A small amount of water can be added at the time of feeding to improve palatability. Water should not be added to the whole batch at once; this would reduce the stability of the ingredients. Garlic or onion powder sprinkled on the food might further improve palatability to some dogs.

2. Diet should be refrigerated or frozen to minimize rancidity and bacterial degradation. Always keep lard, beef tallow, oil, and wheat germ refrigerated.

3. One batch should feed a 33-lb dog for about four days if the dog is already at normal weight. At current prices, it should cost $.60 to $.70 per day to feed a 33-lb dog this diet (with supplements), about 20 per cent more than feeding the most appropriate prescription diet, K/D (Hills Division, Riviana Foods, Inc.).

4. Although lactase deficiency is rare in dogs, lactose intolerance may occasionally be a problem in dogs fed this diet. If diarrhea occurs, the diet

should be fed in smaller amounts for a time, or Diet 2 should be fed instead.

5. Nutritional information on Diet 1 (*by calculation* and not including supplements) is as follows:

Nutrient	gm/100 gm dry weight
Protein	11.1
Fat	21.2
NFE	55.2
Ash	6.9
Crude fiber	0.44
Ca	1.44
P	.82
K	.85
Na	.54*

Calories = 4.6 kcal/gm dry weight

*Can be reduced by reducing NaCl content; if low NaCl content is desired for a long period of time, however, an additional source of iodine, an essential nutrient, must be provided.

MIXING DIRECTIONS FOR DIET 2

Mix the sugar, cornstarch, bone meal, and salt. If beef tallow is used, allow to come to room temperature before mixing. Blend animal fat with the sugar mixture. Mix the cottage cheese and safflower oil and blend in with other ingredients.

COMMENTS

1. Diet must be refrigerated. Garlic or onion powder sprinkled on the diet may increase its palatability for some dogs.

2. If Centrum (Lederle) is not available, an equally "potent" supplement should be used. Most of the vitamins and minerals in this diet are supplied by this supplement, and the amounts of bone meal and salt have been determined assuming this supplement will be used. If another supplement must be substituted, refer to the National Academy of Sciences' *Nutrient Requirements of Dogs* (NRC) when determining nutritional adequacy of the diet plus supplement.

3. One batch of diet (5 lbs) should feed a 33-lb dog for five days. At current prices it should cost $.80 to $.90 per day to feed a 33-lb dog this diet (with supplements), about 45 per cent more than feeding the most appropriate prescription diet, K/D.

4. Nutritional information on Diet 2 (*by calculation* and not including supplements) is as follows:

Nutrient	gm/100 gm dry weight
Protein	10.3
Fat	19.0
NFE	65.5
Ash	4.4
Crude fiber	0.1
Ca	.81
P	.47
K	.56
Na*	.50*

Calories = 4.7 kcal/gm dry weight
           3.2 kcal/gm wet weight

*Can be reduced by reducing NaCl content. If low NaCl content is desired for a long period of time, however, an additional source of iodine, an essential nutrient, must be provided.

Approximate daily maintenance food intakes for adult dogs for each diet are given in Table 1. More will be required by poorly nourished or growing dogs. It may be better to divide total daily food into more than one meal. Diets with supplements are nutritionally adequate, and no other food or supplement should be given.

Although healthy dogs probably have no dietary requirement for ascorbic acid, we have recommended ascorbic acid supplementation for both diets described. Our unpublished studies in dogs with experimentally induced hepatic insufficiency showed that plasma ascorbic acid concentrations decreased early and markedly with acute hepatic necrosis and remained low during ensuing chronic hepatic insufficiency. With hepatic necrosis, the reduction in ascorbate levels was one of the earliest changes seen and the reductions in some cases were to 10 per cent of normal. We found that oral supplementation with ascorbic acid at 25 mg/kg BW/day maintained normal plasma concentrations. We therefore recommend dietary supplementation of ascorbic acid at this level for dogs with hepatic insufficiency.

Neither diet contains adequate choline to meet the nutritional lipotropic needs of a dog. Choline tablets should therefore be provided as previously described. There is no need to administer additional lipotropic agents that include methionine. Administration of commercially prepared lipotropic combinations containing methionine have been shown to precipitate signs of encephalopathy in dogs with hepatic insufficiency.

A low sodium intake may be necessary to manage ascites, which often develops with hepatic insufficiency and which may obviate the need for diuretics. The sodium content of both diets can be minimized by reducing or eliminating the added NaCl. With no added table salt, Diets 1 and 2 contain 0.16 and 0.19 per cent sodium, respectively, or 37 and 47 per cent, respectively, of the amount recommended by the NRC (1974). Without added salt, the diets contain 30 to 35 per cent of the sodium found in most commercial diets and about 75 per cent of the sodium in the most appropriate commercial prescription diet (see hereafter). The diets as such would provide 10 to 12 mg sodium per pound body weight, approximating the level of intake recommended for dogs with signs of congestive heart failure. Note, however, that if either diet without added table salt is fed for a long period of time, an additional source of iodine, an essential nutrient, must be provided periodically.

Table 1. *Approximate Daily Maintenance Food Intake for Adult Dogs*

Body lb	Weight kg	Required for Adult Maintenance (Calories)	Diet 1 gm	oz	Diet 2 gm	oz
10	4.5	410	89	3.2	128	4.5
20	9.1	692	150	5.3	216	7.6
30	13.6	935	203	7.2	292	10.3
35	15.9	1051	228	8.1	328	11.6
45	20.4	1267	275	9.7	396	14.0
55	25.0	1476	321	11.3	461	16.3
80	36.4	1956	425	15.0	611	21.6

Diet 2

	Measurements Per Batch*
Low-fat cottage cheese	2 lb
Animal fat†	½ lb
Safflower oil	¼ C
Sugar	1 lb plus 3 T
Cornstarch	1 lb plus 5 T
Bone meal‡	1 ⅓ oz (a little less than ¼ C)
Salt substitute (KCl) *iodized*§	3 ¼ t
Table salt (NaCl) *iodized*‖	2 t
Vitamin C (ascorbic acid)**	Provided as supplement at 10 mg/lb BW/day
Choline††	Provided as supplement: 33-lb dog or less, 250-mg tablet per day; large dogs, 500 mg per day
Centrum‡‡	High-potency multivitamin and multimineral formula designed for human use; one tablet daily

*C = cup, T = tablespoon, t = teaspoon. If possible, ingredients should be weighed rather than measured, since weighing is more accurate.

†Lard or beef tallow may be used. Because the type of fat used is an important component of a diet's palatability, this choice should be tailored to the individual's taste.

‡Bone meal is available at pet care stores. It should be the kind prepared specifically for consumption by animals, i.e., sterilized.

§Only iodized salt (e.g., that manufactured by Schilling) should be used. This addition is important because the diet would otherwise be very low in K+, and dogs with hepatic insufficiency are often depleted of potassium owing to vomiting, diarrhea, increased renal losses, and reduced food intake. Note that salt substitute (KCl) is not the same as "Lite Salt," which is a combination of NaCl and KCl.

‖If a lower sodium content is desired, the NaCl level may be reduced. However, if the diet is to be fed over a long period of time, an additional source of iodine, an essential nutrient, must be provided. See discussion following Diet 2.

**See discussion following Diet 2.

††Choline tablets (either choline chloride or choline bitartrate) can be bought at health food stores. Also, see discussion following Diet 2.

‡‡Centrum (Lederle) is widely available.

As an alternative to the diets described here, a commercially prepared dog food may be used to achieve good results in some individuals. The current formulation of *dry* K/D Prescription Diet* approximates the composition of these homemade diets. This prescription diet contains, in decreasing order of abundance, ground corn, brewer's rice, dried whole egg, whey, and animal fat. The diet is low in protein (14 per cent) and contains moderate amounts of fat (15 per cent). Like the homemade diets, it contains no meat, which could minimize the occurrence of hepatic encephalopathy, sometimes called "meat intoxication." *Dry* K/D may be less costly to feed than the homemade diets, and its acceptance is such that dogs with hepatic insufficiency may eat it more willingly than the homemade diets. However, dry K/D with egg protein contains more sulfur–containing amino acids than the homemade diets. There is some evidence that

the dietary levels of these amino acids may be involved in the etiology of hepatic encephalopathy. Another possible disadvantage of dry K/D for dogs with hepatic insufficiency is its relatively high crude fiber content, over four times higher than the highest crude fiber content of our homemade diets. Moreover, zein (corn protein) is a relatively poor-quality protein that is less well digested than casein or albumin. Also, the processing involved in commercial food preparation leads to a decrease in digestibility of nutrients. Overall, dry K/D probably has a poorer digestibility than either of the homemade diets. Decreased digestibility would increase the appearance in the large intestine of nutrients for fermentation by the bacterial population, a detriment to animals with hepatic insufficiency.

Dietary therapy should continue indefinitely for dogs with hepatic insufficiency. It is only when liver function tests (such as sulfobromophthalein retention at 30 minutes or an ammonia tolerance test) return to normal that consideration can be given to returning to a conventional type of dog food.

---

*Hills Division, Riviana Foods, Inc., Topeka, KS.

ICTERUS IN CATS

LARRY M. CORNELIUS, D.V.M.,

Athens, Georgia

and ROBERT C. DeNOVO, Jr., D.V.M.

Knoxville, Tennessee

Icterus* is a syndrome characterized by hyperbilirubinemia and deposition of bile pigment in tissues, including the skin and mucous membranes. Icterus is a relatively common problem in cats and is usually a diagnostic and therapeutic challenge. Icterus can result from many diverse causes, and therefore a standard, logical approach is very important if one is to consistently diagnose and manage this problem in cats. The primary objectives of this article will be to (1) summarize diagnostic plans for evaluating icteric cats, (2) describe the most common causes of icterus in cats, and (3) outline symptomatic treatment for this problem.

ASSOCIATED CLINICAL SIGNS

Although bilirubin is potentially cytotoxic, clinical signs attributable to bilirubin toxicity apparently are unusual. In newborn animals (not adults), unconjugated bilirubin can cross the blood-brain barrier, enter neurons, and result in CNS damage termed *kernicterus*. In experimental hyperbilirubinemia in dogs, significantly decreased glomerular filtration rate and renal plasma flow as well as histologic evidence of damage to proximal tubular epithelial cells were observed with plasma bilirubin concentrations of 19.2 and 23.9 mg/dl, respectively (Masumoto and Masuoka, 1980). The clinical significance of this is uncertain.

Signs associated with icterus depend on the cause. In general, clinical signs are more acute and severe when icterus results from hemolysis and/or hepatocellular disease than from obstruction of bile flow. Varying degrees of depression, anorexia, weight loss, and weakness often accompany icterus. Icteric cats seem especially prone to severe anorexia, and efforts to provide calories are extremely important in many cases. Pale mucous membranes usually indicate anemia, which may be the result of hemolysis, blood loss, or reduced erythropoiesis. Vomiting and/or diarrhea may be present. Diarrhea may be characterized by hematochezia and/or melena if gastrointestinal ulcers or clotting or bleeding

disorders accompany hepatocellular disease or biliary obstruction. Complete biliary obstruction is uncommon but may cause clay-colored stools owing to lack of bile pigment. Excessive bilirubin production, as would occur with hemolysis, will cause the feces to appear dark orangish-brown. Urine containing increased amounts of bilirubin will be dark brown, whereas hemoglobin causes urine to be red or port-wine colored. Abdominal pain may accompany icterus caused by acute pancreatitis or peritonitis. Abdominal enlargement may be present with hepatocellular disease (ascites, hepatomegaly) or intra-abdominal neoplasia.

If thrombocytopenia accompanies icterus, petechiae and/or ecchymoses may be observed on mucous membranes and hematuria may be observed. The liver normally synthesizes several clotting factors, and in severe, diffuse hepatocellular disease, this function may be impaired. Biliary obstruction may cause decreased absorption of fat-soluble vitamins A, D, E, and K because bile is needed for emulsification of fat prior to its intestinal absorption. Vitamin K is necessary for hepatic synthesis of the clotting factors of prothrombin. Injection of vitamin K should correct the prolonged prothrombin time associated with biliary obstruction but not that caused by severe hepatocellular disease.

Severe hepatic disease may cause abnormal central nervous system signs (hepatic encephalopathy). Although a variety of signs may be observed, the most common are intermittent depression, stupor or coma, transient apparent blindness, head pressing, circling, and excessive salivation. Ingestion of meat or meat by-products frequently exacerbates these signs.

DIAGNOSTIC PLAN

Initially, efforts should be made to categorize icterus into hemolytic, hepatocellular, or obstructive causes, realizing that combinations of these basic causes frequently occur in clinical disorders. Even so, such categorization will usually help narrow down the list of diagnoses to be considered. History and physical examination may sometimes

---

*In this article, icterus refers to tissue and/or serum jaundice.

suggest one of these categories, but laboratory evaluation is usually necessary (Table 1). By far the most common categories of icterus in cats are hepatocellular and intrahepatic biliary obstruction (partial).

HISTORY

A thorough, orderly history is valuable. It is especially important to know if the cat spends any time outside, whether there are other cats (healthy or ill) in the immediate environment, and if there has been previous illness or injury or medication administration. The course of signs may suggest a particular category of icterus. Signs associated with hemolytic icterus (weakness, exercise intolerance) usually occur suddenly and dramatically, whereas obstructive icterus is generally associated with slowly progressive and insidious signs (decreased appetite, weight loss, and so on). The history with hepatocellular disease is variable.

PHYSICAL EXAMINATION

Physical findings in an icteric cat vary, depending on the cause of the icterus and the severity of the causative disease process (see previous section on Associated Clinical Signs). Subtle icterus is most easily detected by observing the caudal palate and sclera. A thorough ophthalmoscopic examination should be done, since some causes of icterus (e.g., lymphosarcoma, feline infectious peritonitis) may produce ocular lesions.

LABORATORY EVALUATION

Initial laboratory testing in an icteric cat should include a CBC, urinalysis, and a screening serum biochemical profile including serum urea nitrogen (SUN), alanine aminotransferase (formerly SGPT), alkaline phosphatase (SAP), glucose, total protein, albumin, and globulin. We still include van den Bergh's test (total serum bilirubin, conjugated and unconjugated) in our initial data base for icteric cats, although we recognize that it often contributes no more information regarding the pathogenesis of jaundice than other more readily available tests. Unfortunately there are no currently available laboratory tests that reliably distinguish those icteric cats that require surgery from those that need only medical treatment. Expected results of initial laboratory evaluation for each category of icterus are shown in Table 1.

Species differences between cats and dogs for some of these laboratory tests should be emphasized. Normal SAP values in the cat are approximately one-third canine SAP values. Alkaline phosphatase in the cat has a serum half-life of only 6 hours as compared with 72 hours for dogs (Hornbuckle and Allan, 1980). Therefore, even slight increases in SAP in cats are significant and usually indicate biliary stasis. In dogs with partial biliary obstruction, an increase in SAP nearly always precedes the onset of icterus. In our experience, icteric cats with partial biliary obstruction often have normal SAP values. It has been reported that, at the usual clinical doses, neither glucocorticoids nor

Table 1. *Initial Plan for Icterus in Cats**

Diagnosis†		Most Common Findings
Hemolytic	Hx and PE:	Sudden onset of weakness and exercise intolerance; very pale mucous membranes with slight yellow tinge; holosystolic mitral murmur common (anemic)
	Lab:	PCV <15; ↑ reticulocytes and NRBCs if three to four days since onset; WBC variable; slightly ↑ urine bilirubin and urobilinogen; increased total serum bilirubin with >50% unconjugated (three to four days after onset may have >50% conjugated); SGPT normal or ↑ slightly (two to five times normal); rest of data base normal
Hepatocellular	Hx and PE:	Lethargy; anorexia; vomiting; diarrhea; dehydration; mild to marked icterus
	Lab:	PCV normal or ↑; WBC variable; moderately to markedly ↑ urine bilirubin; slightly ↑ urine urobilinogen, increased total serum bilirubin with >50% conjugated; SGPT moderately to markedly ↑ (5 to 50 times normal); SAP mildly to moderately ↑ (two to five times normal); total protein variable, albumin normal or ↓; globulin normal or ↑; SUN normal or ↓; glucose variable
Obstructive	Hx and PE:	Mild to moderate lethargy; variable appetite; occasional vomiting and weight loss; mild to marked icterus (not as ill clinically as with hemolytic or hepatocellular icterus)
	Lab:	PCV normal; WBC variable; moderately to markedly ↑ urine bilirubin; urine urobilinogen variable (may be negative with complete extrahepatic obstruction); increased total serum bilirubin with >50% conjugated (may be >80% conjugated with complete extrahepatic obstruction); SGPT mildly to moderately ↑ (two to ten times normal); SAP moderately to markedly ↑ (5 to 20 times normal); rest of data base variable

*Data base: history (Hx); physical examination (PE); CBC; reticulocyte count; urinalysis; serum urea nitrogen (SUN); serum glutamic pyruvic transaminase (SGPT); serum alkaline phosphatase (SAP); total protein; albumin; globulin; glucose; total, conjugated, and unconjugated serum bilirubin; fecal examination.
†Combinations of these three types of icterus are frequently present in clinical cases.

Table 2. Causes of Icterus in Cats and Associated Findings

Cause	History	Physical Examination	Laboratory Data
Hemolytic*			
1. Hemobartonellosis	Lethargy; weakness; anorexia; often associated with stress such as fighting and abscesses	Fever (103 to 105°F); depression; dehydration; pale mucous membranes; icterus, when present, is mild	Regenerative anemia (unless associated with feline leukemia virus); variable WBC; organisms seen in erythrocytes intermittently; mildly ↑ SGPT (two to five times normal)
2. Drugs a. Acetaminophen b. Methylene blue	Depression; weakness; dyspnea; vomiting; drug administration	Severe depression; pale or cyanotic mucous membranes; icterus, when present, is mild; subnormal body temperature; dyspnea	Hemoglobinemia, stress leukogram†; anemia (too acute for regenerative response); markedly ↑ SGPT (5 to 20 times normal); Heinz bodies in erythrocytes with methylene blue
3. Bacteremia/septicemia	Depression; anorexia; weakness	Subnormal temperature or fever; depression; dehydration; icterus, when present, is mild; sources of infection may be observed (abscess, purulent vaginal discharge, etc.)	Nonregenerative anemia; neutropenia with inappropriate left shift; thrombocytopenia; mildly ↑ SGPT (two to five times normal); mildly to moderately ↑ SAP (two to five times normal); positive blood cultures in some cases
Hepatocellular			
1. Feline leukemia virus–associated diseases (lymphosarcoma, myeloproliferative disorders, lymphoproliferative disorders, immunosuppression with bacterial infection)	Lethargy; anorexia; vomiting; weight loss	Fever; depression; dehydration; icteric mucous membranes; sometimes hepatomegaly	Nonregenerative anemia; neutropenia with inappropriate left shift; neoplastic cells sometimes present in blood; thrombocytopenia; normal to slightly ↑ SGPT (two to three times normal); mildly to markedly ↑ SAP (two to ten times normal); feline leukemia virus positive; neoplastic mass or effusion observed on radiographs; malignant lymphocytes may be observed in the effusion stained with Wright-Giemsa stain
2. Cholangitis/hepatitis/cholangiohepatitis	Intermittent episodes of decreased appetite; lethargy; weight loss; occasional vomiting	Depression; unkempt appearance; icteric mucous membranes; thin (some cats are asymptomatic except for mild, intermittent lethargy and anorexia)	Mild nonregenerative anemia; WBC normal or ↑ (neutrophilia with left shift); mildly to markedly ↑ SGPT (2 to 40 times normal); mildly to moderately ↑ SAP (two to five times normal, may be the only laboratory abnormality in some cases); ↓ albumin; ↑ globulin; ↓ BUN; ↑ plasma ammonia or ↓ ammonia tolerance; ↑ BSP retention
3. Idiopathic hepatic lipidosis	Chronic, total anorexia; lethargy; weight loss	Depression; unkempt appearance; icteric mucous membranes; thin; dehydrated	Mild nonregenerative anemia; WBC normal; mildly to moderately ↑ SGPT (two to ten times normal); moderately to markedly ↑ SAP (5 to 20 times normal); ↓ albumin; ↓ BUN; ↑ plasma ammonia or ↓ ammonia tolerance; ↑ BSP retention time; in some cases, ↑ activated clotting time; ↑ prothrombin time; ↑ partial thromboplastin time; increased thrombin time

4. Feline infectious peritonitis	Chronic lethargy; decreased appetite; weight loss	Depression; dehydration; fever (103 to 105°F), icteric mucous membranes in a few cases; abdominal enlargement (ascites) and dyspnea (pleural effusion) in effusive form; anterior and posterior uveitis in some cases	Mild to moderate nonregenerative anemia; WBC variable; SGPT and SAP normal; ↑ globulin in some cases; ascitic and pleural fluids are modified transudates with high protein (>3.0 gm/dl); FIP titer variable; feline leukemia virus test positive in one-half of cats
5. Bacteremia/endotoxemia	See bacteremia/septicemia under Hemolytic		Hepatocyte secretion of conjugated bilirubin is impaired, resulting in functional cholestasis; mildly to moderately ↑ SAP (two to five times normal); normal or mildly ↑ SGPT (one and one-half to two times normal)
6. Drugs or toxins			
a. Acetaminophen	See acetaminophen under Hemolytic		
7. Neoplasia			
a. Feline leukemia virus–related diseases (lymphosarcoma, reticuloendotheliosis)	See Feline leukemia virus–associated diseases under Hemolytic		
b. Others (primary or metastatic)	Depression; decreased appetite; weight loss; sporadic vomiting and diarrhea	Depression; weight loss; icteric mucosa; palpably enlarged liver; abdominal mass; ascites in a few	Mild to moderate nonregenerative anemia; normal to ↑ WBC with either inflammatory or stress leukogram†; SGPT usually normal to slightly ↑ (one and one-half to two times normal); SAP normal to markedly ↑ (5 to 20 times normal); neoplastic mass, ascites, or hepatomegaly observed radiographically in some; ascites is a nonseptic exudate with moderate protein content (3.0 to 4.5 gm/dl) and a preponderance of nondegenerate neutrophils
Obstructive*			
1. Intrahepatic			
a. Cholangitis/hepatitis/cholangiohepatitis	See cholangitis/hepatitis/cholangiohepatitis under Hepatocellular		
b. Neoplasia (primary or metastatic)	See Neoplasia under Hepatocellular		
2. Extrahepatic			
a. Neoplasm compressing bile duct	See Neoplasia under Hepatocellular		
b. Trauma-ruptured gallbladder or bile duct	History of trauma or opportunity for trauma; depression; anorexia; vomiting	Fever 103 to 104°F; depression; dehydration; icteric mucosa; abdominal pain upon palpation	↑PCV and total solids (dehydration); ↑WBC with neutrophilia and left shift; moderately to markedly ↑SGPT (5 to 40 times normal); normal to slightly ↑SAP (two times normal); abdominal fluid observed radiographically; fluid has a moderate protein level (3.0 to 4.5 gm/dl); nonseptic exudate with a preponderance of nondegenerate neutrophils; bilirubin concentration of fluid is higher than in plasma in acute stage
c. Cholelithiasis	Usually secondary to chronic cholestasis and bile inspissation associated with cholangitis/hepatitis/cholangiohepatitis—see above		

*See Table 1 for general characteristics and associated findings.

†Leukocytosis characterized by mature neutrophilia, lymphopenia, eosinopenia, and monocytosis.

phenobarbital causes increases in SAP in cats as they commonly do in dogs (Hornbuckle and Allan, 1980).

The renal threshold for conjugated bilirubin is apparently higher in cats than in dogs. Therefore, even small amounts of bilirubin in a cat's urine are abnormal (Hardy, 1981).

Transient hyperglycemia (150 to 300 mg/dl) and glucosuria (1+ to 4+) commonly occur in stressed or sick cats (including icteric cats) that are not diabetic. Hypoglycemia (< 70 mg/dl) occasionally occurs with a severely reduced hepatic functional mass in both cats and dogs.

Follow-up diagnostic plans for an icteric cat depend on which diagnoses are suspected after results of initial tests are returned (Table 2). With hemolytic icterus, further detailed history for drug or toxin ingestion is indicated. Careful examination of a blood smear for *Hemobartonella* organisms should be done, and blood cultures should be submitted if septicemia is suspected.

For icterus due to hepatocellular disease, abdominal radiographs may be indicated. Plasma ammonia or the ammonia tolerance test can be used to evaluate liver function. It is often wise to be conservative and repeat serum biochemical analysis to monitor the progress of hepatic disease before proceeding to more expensive and/or invasive diagnostic procedures. If no improvement or an actual deterioration in clinical appearance and/or laboratory data is observed, liver biopsy is indicated. If the liver is palpably enlarged, percutaneous needle biopsy is simple and relatively safe. If the liver is normal in size or small, biopsy via laparoscopy or celiotomy is preferred. All liver biopsy procedures should be preceded by laboratory evaluation of blood coagulation.

Follow-up plans for icterus due to biliary obstruction (partial or complete) are similar to those for hepatocellular disease. It is probably safer to biopsy the liver via laparoscopy or celiotomy than to risk bile peritonitis from puncture of a distended gallbladder or bile duct during blind percutaneous liver biopsy with a needle.

ETIOLOGY OF ICTERUS IN CATS

Table 3 lists the final diagnoses recorded for 80 icteric cats at the University of Georgia Veterinary Teaching Hospital during a nine-year period (1973–81). Only those cases with a histologic (biopsy or necropsy), cytologic, or serologic diagnosis were included in the survey. The histopathologic complex of cholangitis/hepatitis/cholangiohepatitis was the most common cause of icterus in the 80 cats (30 per cent), followed by neoplasia (21.2 per cent), hepatic lipidosis (12.5 per cent), and feline infectious peritonitis (11.2 per cent). Most icteric cats were fairly

young (mean age 3.8 years), and 77.5 per cent either died or were euthanized (see Table 3).

Table 4 illustrates selected laboratory values from cats with icterus due to the most common hepatic disorders in this series of cases. Important points to observe are as follows: (1) SGPT was highest in the cholangitis/hepatitis/cholangiohepatitis complex and lowest (usually normal) in feline infectious peritonitis; (2) SAP was highest in hepatic lipidosis and lowest (usually normal) in feline infectious peritonitis; (3) serum total bilirubin was higher in cholangitis/hepatitis/cholangiohepatitis and hepatic lipidosis than in feline infectious peritonitis and neoplasia.

The causes of cholangitis/hepatitis/cholangiohepatitis and hepatic lipidosis are usually unknown (Kelly et al., 1975; Prasse et al., 1982; Barsanti et al., 1977). Indeed, it is probable that a variety of inciting factors may cause the hepatic lesions seen in these disorders. *E. coli* is sometimes cultured from the bile of cats with cholangiohepatitis, but it is unclear whether this represents a primary pathogen or a secondary invader of the biliary tree from the intestinal tract associated with cholestasis. In any event, treatment with antibiotics seems to be beneficial. The prognosis for cats with cholangiohepatitis is usually guarded to fair (see Table 3), although affected cats may have several exacerbations over a period of months to years and eventually die of hepatic failure. A few cats with hepatic lipidosis have diabetes mellitus, but most have near-normal blood glucose levels and the cause is unknown. The prognosis for cats with idiopathic hepatic lipidosis is poor to grave (see Table 3). Early diagnosis and prolonged (three to four weeks) forced feeding, generally via a pharyngostomy tube, may sometimes allow for recovery.

SYMPTOMATIC THERAPY

Every effort should be made to make a specific diagnosis and treat appropriately. Whenever this is not possible, or while the diagnostic work-up is underway, symptomatic therapy may be indicated. The type of symptomatic treatment used to support a jaundiced cat depends somewhat on the category of icterus suspected, but some measures are common to all types. It is important to allow the cat to rest and avoid stress. Whenever feasible, supportive care given in the home environment with opportunity for fresh air, sunshine, and contact with the owner is preferred.

Ensuring adequate caloric and fluid intake is especially important in sick cats, and the oral route is the only practical means of supplying enough calories. If vomiting is present, it must be controlled so that oral intake can proceed. The cat should be tempted to eat if possible. Otherwise, either force

Table 3. *Final Diagnoses in 80 Icteric Cats**

Disorder	No. (%)	Mean Age (yrs)	Discharge Status			FeLV Status		
			Alive	Dead	Euthanized	Pos.	Neg.	ND†
Cholangitis/hepatitis/ cholangiohepatitis	24(30.0)	5.1	10	9	5	6	10	8
Neoplasia	17(21.2)	3.2	2	2	13	9	4	4
Myeloproliferative	10(12.5)	2.1	2	2	6	6	2	2
Lymphosarcoma	5(6.2)	5.0	0	0	5	2	2	1
Lymphoproliferative	2(2.5)	3.2	0	0	2	1	0	1
Hepatic lipidosis	10(12.5)	5.8	0	8	2	0	9	1
Idiopathic	8(10.0)	5.2	0	6	2	0	8	0
Diabetes mellitus	2(2.5)	8.0	0	2	0	0	1	1
Feline infectious peritonitis	9(11.2)	2.7	1	3	5	2	3	4
Normal liver‡	7(8.8)	2.7	1	4	2	2	2	3
Probable sepsis	6(7.5)	2.8	0	4	2	1	2	3
FeLV positive	1(1.2)	2.0	1	0	0	1	0	0
Hemobartonellosis	6(7.5)	1.5	2	1	3	5	0	1
Miscellaneous	7(8.8)	1.5	2	1	4	3	2	2
FeLV-associated erythroid and myeloid hypoplasia	2(2.5)	1.5	0	1	1	2	0	0
Panleukopenia	1(1.2)	ND	0	0	1	1	0	0
Ruptured gallbladder	1(1.2)	1.0	0	0	1	0	0	1
Heartworms	1(1.2)	ND	0	0	1	0	0	1
Granulocyte maturation arrest	1(1.2)	ND	1	0	0	0	1	0
Erythroid hypoplasia/ granulocyte hyperplasia	1(1.2)	2.0	1	0	0	0	1	0
All icteric cats	80(100)	3.8	18 (22.5%)	28 (35%)	34 (42.5%)	27 (33.7%)	30 (37.5%)	23 (28.7%)

*Data from the University of Georgia Veterinary Teaching Hospital, 1973–81.
†ND = no data.
‡Histologically normal.

Table 4. *Laboratory Data from 80 Cats with Icterus due to Hepatic Disease**

Value	Cholangitis/ Hepatitis/ Cholangiohepatitis	Hepatic Lipidosis	Feline Infectious Peritonitis	Neoplasia†	Normal*
PCV (%)	27.4 ± 7.8‡ (24)	29 ± 10 (10)	21 ± 6 (9)	19.8 ± 9.3 (17)	30–45
WBC (mm³)	13,570 ± 10,193 (24)	15,916 ± 7,483 (10)	7192 ± 6,907 (9)	15,178 ± 19,166 (17)	5,500–19,500
SGPT (mU/ml)	465 ± 668 (24) (276 ± 188)§	219 ± 207 (10)	30 ± 26 (8)	115 ± 165 (17)	1–64
SAP (mU/ml)	79 ± 78.5 (23)	366 ± 271 (10)	6.0 ± 5.3 (8)	85 ± 102 (13)	2.2–37.8
Albumin (gm/dl)	2.9 ± 1.0 (23)	2.5 ± 0.8 (10)	2.3 ± 0.5 (8)	2.6 ± 0.6 (14)	1.9–3.8
Glucose (mg/dl)	143 ± 62 (20)	310 ± 503 (6) (153 ± 78)‖	108 ± 44 (6)	123 ± 32 (14)	53–120
Bilirubin (mg/dl)	11.7 ± 17.6 (20) (8.4 ± 10.0)**	8.4 ± 3.8 (10)	3.3 ± 1.8 (7)	3.3 ± 2.5 (12)	0.15–0.30

*Data from the University of Georgia Veterinary Teaching Hospital, 1973–81.
†Includes lymphosarcoma and myeloproliferative and lymphoproliferative disorders.
‡Mean ± 1 standard deviation.
§Two extremely high values (2,748 and 2,344) were not included.
‖One extremely high value (1,725) was not included.
**One extremely high value (74) was not included.
Note: Numbers in parentheses indicate number of cats.

feeding, stomach-tube feeding, or feeding through a pharyngostomy tube is necessary.

Total caloric intake should be about 80 to 100 kcal/kg/day. It is generally sufficient to use well-balanced, commercial cat foods. These can be mixed into a watery gruel with an electric blender and then administered via pharyngostomy tube. To minimize vomiting and diarrhea, it is best to administer small amounts of gruel (5 to 10 ml/kg) at frequent intervals (six to eight times daily). It may be possible to gradually increase the amount administered at each feeding and reduce the number of daily feedings. Total daily fluid requirements (about 50 to 60 ml/kg) must be supplied orally and/or parenterally. Whenever parenteral fluids are necessary, balanced electrolyte solutions such as Ringer's solution are recommended. Icteric cats with hepatic disease may be hypoglycemic, and 50 per cent glucose solution can be added to the Ringer's in sufficient amounts to yield a final concentration of 10 per cent glucose solution. This hypertonic solution should be given intravenously. Potassium deficit may be present in icteric, anorectic cats. Enough potassium chloride solution should be added to the Ringer's solution to supply a minimum of 1 to 3 mEq of potassium/kg/day, assuming renal function is adequate. Serum potassium should be measured frequently to assess the adequacy of potassium therapy. Once oral administration of cat food gruel is begun, it is not necessary to supply extra glucose or potassium parenterally.

Transfusion of fresh whole blood (about 20 ml/kg intravenously) may be indicated in some debilitated icteric cats. Indications are severe anemia (PCV < 15), hypoalbuminemia (serum albumin < 1.5 gm/dl), and evidence of coagulopathy due to decreased hepatic synthesis of clotting factors. Blood transfusion is especially important if cats with these laboratory abnormalities are to undergo surgery for liver biopsy. Transfusion should be avoided in cats with diseases characterized by ongoing hemolysis unless the anemia is life-threatening. Body weight should be checked frequently to assess the adequacy of total daily caloric and fluid therapy.

Hepatic encephalopathy may be present in icteric cats with severe hepatic disease (see following article for treatment of hepatic encephalopathy). Management of hepatic encephalopathy necessitates several dietary modifications. Reduction of protein intake is essential because bacteria in the distal small intestine and colon metabolize amino acids to potentially toxic nitrogenous wastes such as ammonia. However, some dietary protein is necessary to prevent breakdown of body proteins for energy. For dogs with hepatic encephalopathy, it has been suggested that the minimum daily dietary protein intake should be 1 gm/20 kcal (Strombeck, 1979). Similar information for cats with hepatic encephalopathy is unavailable. Since normal cats have

Table 5. *Nutritive Value of Common Foods*

	Protein (gm)	Calories
Bread (1 slice)	2.0	60
Butter or margarine (1 tsp)	0	50
Cake (poundcake 2″ × 3″ × 5″)	2.1	130
Cheese* (1 cup cottage)	43.0	260
(1 oz Swiss)	7.8	106
(1 oz cream)	2.6	106
Cream (1 oz light)	0	50
Egg (cooked)	7.0	120
Gravy (1 Tbsp)	0	80
Ice cream (1 oz)	1.2	62
Macaroni and cheese (1 cup)	17.8	460
Milk (2 oz white)	2.0	40
Rice* (1 cup cooked)	4.2	200
Spaghetti (1 cup cooked)	7.4	355
Sugar or honey (1 tsp)	0	20
Vegetable shortening (1 Tbsp)	0	120

*The diet for the management of chronic hepatic diseases should be composed mainly of cottage cheese as the primary protein source and boiled rice as the primary carbohydrate/calorie source. Other foodstuffs can be added to improve palatability.

higher dietary protein needs (Morris, 1972) than normal dogs, it is possible that this figure should be increased. The animal should be closely observed for signs of hepatic encephalopathy and dietary protein adjusted as indicated. In general, cats with liver disease should be fed as much of their normal protein requirements as they will tolerate without developing hepatic encephalopathy.

Whenever hepatic encephalopathy develops, the type of protein fed is very important. Meat proteins should be avoided because they worsen signs of hepatic encephalopathy. Cottage cheese provides high biologic value protein and is the best main protein source.

Boiled white rice is an excellent source of carbohydrate because it is well digested and leaves little residue for bacterial fermentation to potentially toxic volatile fatty acids. Basic fat requirements should be supplied. Table 5 lists protein and calorie contents of selected foods that are useful to animals with hepatic failure. If the owner is unwilling to feed a homemade diet, prescription diet Feline K-D* is a reasonable alternative. A sample calculation of dietary requirements of a 5-kg cat with hepatic encephalopathy follows.

Protein: 1 gm protein/20 kcal/day assuming 80 kcal/kg/day = 4 gm protein/kg body wt/day

4 gm protein/kg × 5 kg = 20 gm protein/day

Carbohydrate: 6 gm carbohydrate/kg/day × 5 kg = 30 gm carbohydrate/day

Fat: 4.4 gm fat/kg/day × 5 kg = 22.2 gm fat/day

*Hill's Division, Riviana Foods, Inc., Topeka, KS.

1. 5-kg cat × 80 kcal/kg/day = 400 kcal/day
   a. 20 gm protein/day × 4 kcal/gm
      = 80 kcal from protein
   b. 30 gm carbohydrate/day × 4 kcal/gm
      = 120 kcal from carbohydrate
   c. 22.2 gm fat/day × 9 kcal/gm = 200 kcal from fat
2. 5-kg cat × 50 ml H_2O/kg/day = 250 ml H_2O/day

Both B-complex and fat-soluble vitamins (A, D, E, K) should be given in standard doses by mixing oral vitamin preparations in the blended gruel. The fat-soluble vitamins are especially needed if severe cholestasis is present, as this impairs fat emulsification and decreases fat absorption. We do not recommend lipotrophic compounds (choline and methionine) because their efficacy in hepatic failure is doubtful and because methionine will worsen hepatic encephalopathy.

If antibiotics are used for icteric cats with hepatic disease, those concentrated in bile and effective against enteric organisms are preferred. Gentamicin (2.2 mg/kg every eight hours SC) is best for gram negative bacteria, and ampicillin (22 mg/kg every eight hours PO) is effective against anaerobes and is well concentrated in bile. The following antimicrobial agents may be hepatotoxic and should be avoided or used with caution: chloramphenicol, chlortetracycline, erythromycin, oxytetracycline, neomycin, streptomycin, and sulfonamides.

Icterus due to hepatic disease (especially cholan-giohepatitis) is frequently accompanied by partial biliary obstruction, resulting in severe cholestasis and inspissated bile. In this situation, use of a hydrocholeretic drug may help stimulate bile flow by increasing biliary secretion of thin, watery bile. Decholin* is a hydrocholeretic drug containing dehydrocholic acid, a bile acid. Our usual dosage is 10 to 15 mg/kg every eight hours PO for seven to ten days. Use of hydrocholeretics is contraindicated in cats with total biliary obstruction.

*Dome Laboratories, Westhaven, CT.

REFERENCES AND SUPPLEMENTAL READING

Barsanti, J. A., Jones, B. D., Spano, J. S., and Taylor, H. W.: Prolonged anorexia associated with hepatic lipidosis in 3 cats. Feline Pract. 7:52, 1977.
Hardy, R. M.: Pathophysiology of hepatic disease. Proceedings of 6th Annual Conference in Internal Medicine—Medical Disorders of the Abdomen, Santa Cruz, CA, 1981.
Hornbuckle, W. E., and Allan, G. S.: Feline liver disease. In Kirk, R. W. (ed.): Current Veterinary Therapy VII. Philadelphia: W. B. Saunders, 1980, pp. 891–895.
Kelly, D. F., Baggott, D. G., and Gaskell, C. J.: Jaundice in the cat associated with inflammation of the biliary tract and pancreas. J. Small Anim. Prac. 16:163, 1975.
Masumoto, T., and Masuoka, S.: Kidney function in the severely jaundiced dog. Am. J. Surg. 140:426, 1980.
Morris, M. L., Jr.: Feline Dietetics. Topeka, KS: Mark Morris Associates, 1972.
Prasse, K. W., Mahaffey, E. A., DeNovo, R. C., and Cornelius, L. M.: Chronic lymphocytic cholangitis in 3 cats. Vet. Pathol. 19:99, 1982.
Strombeck, D. R.: Small Animal Gastroenterology. Davis, CA: Stonegate Publishing, 1979.

HEPATIC ENCEPHALOPATHY IN THE DOG

FREDERICK H. DRAZNER, D.V.M.

Des Plaines, Illinois

In the past ten years, the syndrome of hepatic encephalopathy (HE) has been documented on numerous occasions in small animal practice. Hepatic encephalopathy is a complex metabolic disorder manifested by diverse central nervous system (CNS) signs that develop as a result of acute or chronic hepatic insufficiency.

ETIOLOGIC CONSIDERATIONS (Table 1)

Canine HE has thus far been most often documented in young dogs with anomalous connections between the portal vein and the systemic circulation. The congenital anomaly most commonly asso-ciated with HE is the patent ductus venosus, occurring in 50 per cent of all reported cases. The breed most frequently represented thus far is the miniature schnauzer. The ductus venosus is a fetal vessel that bypasses the liver and delivers blood from the umbilical vein into the caudal vena cava. In the dog it normally closes within 60 hours after birth, probably as a response to vasoactive substances such as prostaglandins and to changes in oxygen tension and blood flow and pressure.

The second most common congenital shunt connects the portal vein with the vena cava caudal to the liver. Another shunt frequently reported in the dog allows communication between the portal and azygous veins.

Table 1. *Etiology of Canine HE*

I. Congenital Anomalies
   A. Anatomic
      1. Patent ductus venosus (with or without hypoplastic hepatic portal branches)
      2. Connection of portal vein to vena cava caudal to liver
      3. Connection of portal vein to azygous vein
      4. Connection of portal vein and vena cava with azygous vein
      5. Portal vein atresia with collateral portosystemic shunts
      6. Large central portopostcaval anastomoses
   B. Inborn biochemical errors
      1. Urea cycle deficiency
         a. Arginosuccinate synthetase
         b. Carbamyl phosphate synthetase I
      2. Defect in copper metabolism—hepatolenticular degeneration (Wilson's disease of Bedlington terriers)
II. Acquired Hepatic Diseases
   A. Chronic parenchymal destruction
      1. Cirrhosis
      2. Extensive infiltrative neoplasia (hepatocellular carcinoma, bile duct carcinoma)
   B. Chronic hepatic disease (cirrhosis) associated with portal hypertension and portosystemic shunts
      1. Gastroesophageal collaterals
      2. Mesenteric to renal collaterals
      3. Mesenteric to rectal collaterals
      4. Mesenteric to deep circumflex iliac collaterals
      5. Splenorenal collaterals
   C. Acute fulminant liver failure owing to hepatocellular destruction
      1. Hepatotoxins
         a. Carbon tetrachloride, nitrotoluene
         b. Acetaminophen
         c. Copper, arsenic, mercury
         d. Tannic acid (acorns)
         e. Aflatoxins (molds)
         f. Drugs (testosterone derivatives with C-17 alkyl group, acetaminophen, chlorpromazine, nitrofurantoin, albamycin, tetracycline)
      2. Infectious canine hepatitis
      3. Leptospirosis
      4. Hepatic lipidosis
         a. Diabetes mellitus with ketoacidosis
         b. Iatrogenic hyperadrenocorticism
      5. Circulatory factors (fulminant right-sided congestive heart failure)

Acquired portosystemic shunts have been reported in the dog and have been associated with end-stage liver disease (cirrhosis). In cirrhotic patients with extensive fibroplastic infiltration and loss of the normal architecture of hepatic lobules, there is a marked increased resistance to portal blood flow, resulting in portal hypertension. This impedance to intrahepatic blood flow stimulates the development of venous collaterals, which divert portal blood flow away from the liver, reduce hepatic circulation, and can be expected to worsen hepatic atrophy.

Extensive hepatocellular destruction due to infiltrative neoplasia, inflammatory changes, infections, chemical toxins, and drugs may render the liver ineffective in its ability to detoxify catabolic substances and may ultimately result in HE.

Dogs with congenital inborn errors of metabolism resulting in hepatic urea cycle enzyme deficiency have been seen by the author and have been described in the literature by others. These patients have been found to have HE associated with hyperammonemia without any evidence of hepatocellular destruction or portosystemic shunting.

PATHOPHYSIOLOGY OF HEPATIC ENCEPHALOPATHY

The traditional and probably most important concept regarding the pathogenesis of HE in most patients involves alterations in normal ammonia (NH_3) metabolism. To better understand these alterations it is useful to summarize the origin and fate of NH_3 in the dog.

The gastrointestinal tract is the major source of NH_3 in the body, beginning in the oral cavity where small concentrations of NH_3 are generated by the activity of bacteria on ingested proteins. Gastric juice may contain detectable concentrations of ammonium ions (NH_4^+), which originate from urease-containing bacteria acting on blood urea. The colon is the major source of NH_3 formation in the body because of its large resident population of urease-producing coliform bacteria (*E. coli*, *Proteus* sp.).

Peripheral tissue, especially the skeletal muscle, may be an important source of uptake and metabolism of blood NH_3, with approximately 50 per cent of labeled arterial N-ammonia 13 being metabolized in normal (noncirrhotic) human subjects.

The kidneys have the potential to play an important role in NH_3 metabolism by providing NH_3 for excretion and by being an endogenous source of ammonium ion (NH_4^+). Glutamine removed from plasma by the kidneys is broken down by renal glutaminase to glutamate and NH_3. Hypokalemia increases the rate of production and renal vein concentration of NH_3. With inadequate acidification of urine in the distal tubule, the ammonia secreted into the urine is not completely converted to NH_4^+, and abnormal amounts of NH_3 (which is permeable to phospholipid cell membranes) diffuse back into the circulation. In addition, the azotemia seen with renal failure results in increased NH_3 production because large amounts of urea diffuse across membranes into the colon, where it is hydrolyzed by bacterial ureases.

After its production, NH_3 is transported to the liver via the hepatic portal circulation, where it diffuses into the hepatocytes. Utilizing the complex enzyme system of the Krebs-Henseleit urea cycle, the hepatocytes convert NH_3 into urea. Seventy-five per cent of the urea generated by the liver is excreted by the kidneys, whereas the remaining 25 per cent migrates back into the alimentary canal, where it is again decomposed into NH_3 and returned to the liver.

In patients with severe hepatic insufficiency due to either extensive parenchymal destruction or portosystemic shunting, the liver is unable to clear and convert NH_3 and other toxic substances, and HE ensues.

Hyperammonemia is important in the pathogenesis of HE as shown by the following: (1) Coma may be induced in experimental animals with normal hepatic function by administering massive amounts of NH_4^+ salts. (2) Coma may be induced in cirrhotic patients by feeding excess dietary protein, which causes blood ammonia concentrations to increase. (3) In humans, there seems to be a good correlation between blood ammonia levels and deterioration in mentation.* (4) The symptoms of HE are often ameliorated by feeding reduced dietary protein, which lowers arterial NH_3.

The biochemical mechanism by which hyperammonemia produces encephalopathy is unknown. Studies in human patients whose clinical signs were compatible with HE but whose laboratory studies (fasting blood NH_3 and ammonia tolerance tests) did *not* suggest abnormal NH_3 metabolism prompted the search for other causative metabolic factors in the etiopathogenesis of HE. Several compounds, including short–chain fatty acids (SCFA), mercaptans, and false neurotransmitters, have been detected in abnormally high concentrations from the blood, cerebrospinal fluid (CSF), and cerebral tissue in human HE patients.

Short–chain fatty acids, which are produced in the intestine by the action of gut bacteria, have been shown to be present in abnormally high concentrations in the blood and CSF of human HE patients. Furthermore, large concentrations of SCFA can induce coma when administered to experimental animals. It is thought that SCFAs disrupt normal NH_3 metabolism and act in concert with mercaptans and NH_3 to disrupt cerebral function. It appears that octanoic acid is the SCFA with the most potent coma-producing effects. Some SCFAs are produced from incomplete metabolism of lipids in the liver.

Mercaptans are the deaminated products of intestinal bacterial degradation of sulfur–containing amino acids such as methionine. These products (methanethiol, ethanethiol, and dimethyl sulfide) act synergistically with NH_3 and SCFA to inhibit normal brain activity. Ironically, lipotropic agents that contain methionine are widely used by many small animal clinicians for virtually all hepatopathies regardless of the type or etiology. By its conversion to mercaptans, the methionine administered may produce iatrogenic HE in patients with hepatic insufficiency.

Another important factor in the pathogenesis of HE is the development of abnormal ratios of plasma amino acids, with a marked increase in the concentration of aromatic amino acids (tyrosine, tryptophan, and phenylalanine) and a decrease in the concentration of the branched–chain variety (leucine, isoleucine, and valine). It appears that, with the development of hepatic insufficiency, the body depletes the levels of branched–chain amino acids for use in energy production, whereas the diseased liver has lost its normal capacity to metabolize aromatic amino acids. The ratio of branched–chain amino acids to aromatic amino acids in both humans and dogs with normal hepatic function is in the range of 3:4, whereas individuals with HE have a ratio of only 1:1.5. The high plasma levels of aromatic amino acids are associated with abnormalities in brain neurotransmitters, including decreases in the excitatory neurotransmitter (norepinephrine) and increases in inhibitory neurotransmitters (octopamine, phenylethanolamine, 5-hydroxytryptamine, or serotonin). In addition, false neurotransmitters may be produced in large amounts and may play a role. The resultant CNS signs include somnolence, confusion, obtundation, and coma.

Other suspected cerebral toxins include indoles, skatols (which are produced as a result of bacterial deamination of tryptophan in the alimentary canal), and various peptides. As in the case of NH_3, mercaptans, SCFAs, and aromatic amino acids, the diseased liver is unable to catabolize these substances (or they are shunted around the liver) and they accumulate in the plasma, cross the blood-brain barrier, and exert a toxic effect on the brain.

There are many factors that may precipitate overt coma in patients with impaired liver function. Azotemia (either spontaneous or owing to vigorous diuretic therapy in ascitic patients) results in a markedly increased endogenous production of ammonia as well as a directly suppressive effect on the brain by the toxic products of uremia. Likewise, gastrointestinal hemorrhage (a common occurrence in advanced liver disease, usually due to portal hypertension or coagulopathy) provides a substrate for ammonia formation. Transfusions with stored blood can induce hyperammonemia (blood ammonia concentrations, storage of blood at 4°C: 1 day, 170 $\mu g/dl$; 4 days, 330 $\mu g/dl$; 21 days, 900 $\mu g/dl$. Widespread infection may also increase blood ammonia levels by increasing tissue catabolism. Hypokalemia with metabolic alkalosis (often as a result of intensive thiazide diuretic therapy) may induce hyperammonemia. Metabolic alkalosis leads to an increased transfer of ammonia across the blood-brain barrier.

Hepatic coma may develop as result of constipation, which promotes the excessive production and absorption of ammonia and other nitrogenous substances.

The use of tranquilizers (especially phenothiazine derivatives), sedatives (diazepam [Valium]), anticon-

---

*Editor's note: This is not true in dogs.

vulsants (primidone), and anesthetics may result in HE because of a direct depressant effect on the brain and because of the diminished metabolic clearance of these pharmacologic agents due to hepatocellular insufficiency. Some of these agents (especially the phenothiazine derivatives) are themselves potentially hepatoxic and by causing parenchymal cell damage may induce HE.

An iatrogenic precipitating factor in the development of HE in the dog is the injudicious use of lipotropic agents that contain methionine. The methionine is converted by the intestinal flora into mercaptans, which increase the degree of clinical obtundation in patients with HE.

CLINICAL SIGNS OF HEPATIC ENCEPHALOPATHY

Historically, most patients with HE present with a variety of symptoms, which are paroxysmal in character. Neurologic signs include depression, behavior changes (either withdrawal, aggression, or hysteria), stupor, coma, and seizures. Often these parozysmal CNS signs are more apparent one to three hours post prandial (correlating with the digestion and deamination of dietary protein and generation of high concentrations of NH_3). More specific motor dysfunctions include head pressing; ataxia; pacing; amaurosis; and loose, bidirectional circling. Puppies born with portosystemic shunts are often stunted in their development and sometimes develop ascites and signs of a coagulopathy.

An early clue in identifying a patient with HE may be intolerance to anesthesia or tranquilization, since most of these agents require hepatic catabolism. Other nonspecific signs include vomition, diarrhea, polyuria, polydipsia, and hyposthenuria.

DIAGNOSTIC EVALUATION OF HEPATIC ENCEPHALOPATHY

The hemogram of many canine HE patients often reveals microcytosis and hypochromia of the erythron, which are usually not accompanied by anemia. These patients usually have a normal serum iron concentration and total iron binding capacity (TIBC). Explanations for the microcytosis and hypochromia include interference of heme synthesis by ammonia and erythrocyte oxidation with Heinz body formation owing to changes in lipid and bile salt metabolism.

In the vast majority of the patients (except those with acute fulminant hepatitis), the serum transaminases (SGPT and SGOT) and alkaline phosphatase levels are within normal limits, refuting the likelihood of active hepatocellular necrosis. A nearly constant finding is a reduction of plasma protein concentrations, which can be explained by diminished protein production as a result of hepatic

atrophy. Reduction of the blood urea nitrogen (BUN) is commonly encountered and is due to the inability of the liver to receive or convert intestinal NH_3 into urea.

A nearly constant laboratory finding is the increased retention of sulfobromophthalein (BSP). Dogs with normal hepatocellular function and circulation should retain less than 5 per cent of BSP (injected intravenously) after 30 minutes, whereas dogs with HE will often retain greater than 10 per cent. Because of the widespread use of radioisotope liver scanning procedures in human medicine, the BSP retention test is no longer widely utilized and thus BSP dye may be difficult to acquire from diagnostic suppliers. Alternatively, the measure of serum bile acids via radioimmunoassay (RIA) may be a useful tool in the evaluation of liver function. The normal liver absorbs nearly 99 per cent of the bile acids (cholic and chenodeoxycholic acid) from the portal circulation, with only 1 per cent entering the systemic circulation. Thus, impairment of hepatocellular function and/or portosystemic shunting results in a marked increase in the concentration of serum bile acids in the systemic circulation.

Urinalysis of HE patients often reveals substantial concentrations of ammonium biurate crystals (approximately a 50 per cent incidence). They are less likely to be found in dilute urine. Their presence in the urine is thus a valuable screening aid for the detection of hyperammonemia.

Plain abdominal radiographs may reveal microhepatica, a constant finding in patients with portosystemic shunts and secondary hepatic atrophy. Because these patients are often thin, emaciated, and stunted, the liver may not be well visualized on plain radiography owing to lack of detail from the absence of body fat. Because ascites may be encountered in some HE patients, the liver again may be poorly visualized on abdominal radiographs. Patients with HE due to acute fulminant hepatitis may show hepatomegaly on abdominal radiographs.

Electroencephalography (EEG) employed by the author in 25 HE patients has thus far revealed mainly generalized slow-wave activity with increased amplitude, a pattern seen in most human HE patients (consistent with a metabolic encephalopathy). CSF analysis is consistently normal.

Documentation of HE depends on the demonstration of deranged ammonia metabolism. The vast majority (90 per cent) of HE patients have an elevated fasting blood ammonia level (normal canine NH_3 ranges from 10 to 74 µg/dl), with values ranging from 95 to 750 µg/dl. In those patients with normal fasting blood NH_3 levels, the ammonia tolerance test (100 mg/kg of oral ammonium chloride; take a sample prior to administration and 30 minutes after) will reveal a three- to fourfold increase in blood ammonia levels.

Identification of the etiology of HE may be achieved by selective angiography of the celiac or cranial mesenteric artery, splenic or portal venography, or splenoportography. Of these techniques, portal venography offers the advantages of selectivity, accuracy, and safety (no damage to the spleen). Because portal venography is performed via laparotomy, a liver biopsy may be obtained during the procedure.

PATHOLOGIC LESIONS ASSOCIATED WITH HEPATIC ENCEPHALOPATHY

In patients whose symptomatology indicates congenital portosystemic shunts, the primary liver lesion is atrophy of the hepatocytes. Patients with acquired HE may exhibit cirrhosis or generalized massive hepatocellular necrosis.

Microscopic examination of the brain yields variable pathologic lesions. Patients with acute HE exhibit varying degrees of cerebral edema. In chronic HE due to congenital portosystemic shunts, the cerebral lesions may include hyperplasia of the astrocytes (Alzheimer type II astrocytosis) and vacuolization of the cerebral hemispheres. These lesions are thought to be the result of a glial cell (astrocyte) response to a chronically toxic environment and a derangement of protein synthesis, respectively.

TREATMENT OF HEPATIC ENCEPHALOPATHY

Acute hepatic coma constitutes a medical emergency. The primary goal in the treatment of this phenomenon is the rapid reduction of blood ammonia and related cerebral toxin levels. Therapeutic principles include (1) cessation of protein intake; (2) control of gastrointestinal bleeding; (3) withdrawal of drugs that may elevate blood ammonia, further sedate the patient, or increase circulating mercaptan levels (diuretics, tranquilizers, and methionine, respectively); (4) control of infection; and (5) correction of fluid, electrolyte (especially hypokalemia), and acid-base (especially alkalosis) imbalances.

Specific measures to rapidly lower blood ammonia levels include administering cleansing enemas and nonadsorbable aminoglycoside antibiotics such as neomycin or kanamycin, which are bacteriocidal against urease-producing organisms (*Proteus* sp. and *E. coli*). Neomycin (Neovet*) may be administered via a high retention enema (15 mg/kg q6h). Sorbitol, a simple sugar that acts as an osmotic cathartic, may be combined with oral neomycin. The two drugs appear to act synergistically to lower blood NH_3.

Toxic hepatitis and HE are sometimes treated with prednisolone. There is no scientific evidence for the efficacy of steroid therapy, however. In the past six years, the author has used lactulose (Cephulac†) in the long-term management of chronic HE regardless of etiology. Lactulose is a synthetic disaccharide sugar (4-o-beta-galacto-pyranosyl-D-fructofuranose) that is effective in lowering blood NH_3 levels and improving the EEG pattern and mental status of HE patients. Lactulose suppresses absorption of ammonia from the gut by a combination of the following factors: (1) bacterial degradation of lactulose acidifies colonic contents resulting in more ammonia in the form of NH_4^+ (a relatively nondiffusable cation); (2) lactulose acts as a laxative, thereby cleaning out the colon; (3) lactulose suppresses bacterial urease activity on urea degradation. Recent studies in human patients with acute HE indicate that lactulose may be just as effective as the neomycin-sorbitol combination in lowering blood NH_3 in crisis situations. One may speculate that the combination of neomycin and lactulose may prove to be of greater efficacy in the treatment of acute fulminant hepatic coma than either drug used by itself. One potential objection to such a combination is that the neomycin may alter the bacterial flora in such a manner as to interfere with degradation of lactulose, thus inhibiting the acidification of colonic contents. The average canine dose of lactulose is 1 tbs t.i.d.

Long-term management of HE is dependent upon the establishment of a readily digested diet that contains optimal amounts of protein that do not cause HE. In dogs with HE due to identifiable congenital portosystemic shunts, partial surgical closure is usually the preferred treatment. Closure of acquired portosystemic shunts (as a result of hepatic cirrhosis) is not effective in treating HE. Hepatic portal blood flow increases following partial closure, and the subsequent increase in hormonal hepatotropic factors (namely, insulin and glucagon) reaching the liver supports growth and regeneration of the atrophied liver. The liver can achieve normal size, and blood ammonia levels diminish as the patient's protein tolerance and mental status improve.

There are few new therapeutic measures that could be practical and effective in the management of HE in dogs. Infusions of solutions containing branched–chain amino acids (leucine, valine, and isoleucine) may normalize deranged amino acid ratios and improve the CNS status in refractory HE. The author is currently evaluating the efficacy of levodopa (Larodopa, Roche) in patients with CNS signs. It is thought that levodopa provides the substrate (dopa) for the production of norepinephrine, an excitatory or legitimate neurotransmitter, and inhibits the formation of 5-hydroxytryptamine (serotonin), a false neurotransmitter.

---

*Med-Tech, Inc., Elwood, KS.

†Merrell Dow Pharmaceuticals Inc., Cincinnati, OH.

SUPPLEMENTAL READING

Barrett, R. E., et al.: Four cases of congenital portocaval shunts in the dog. J. Small Anim. Pract. 17:71, 1976.

Conn, H. O., et al.: Comparison of lactulose and neomycin/sorbitol in treatment of chronic portalsystemic encephalopathy: double blind controlled study. Gastroenterology 72:573, 1977.

Gofton, N.: Surgical ligation of congenital portosystemic venous shunts in the dog: a report of three cases. J. Am. Anim. Hosp. Assoc. 14:728, 1978.

Griffiths, G. L., Lumeden, J. H., and Valli, V. E. O.: Hematologic and biochemical changes in dogs with portosystemic shunts. J. Am. Anim. Hosp. Assoc. 17:705, 1981.

Nuchbauer, C. A., and Fischer, J. E.: The failing liver. Surg. Clin. North Am. 61:221, 1981.

Strombeck, D. R., Meyer, D. J., and Friedland, R. A.: Hyperammonemia due to a urea cycle deficiency in two dogs. J.A.V.M.A. 166:1109, 1975.

Strombeck, D. R., Weiser, M. G., and Kaneko, J. J.: Hyperammonemia and hepatic encephalopathy in the dog. J.A.V.M.A. 166:1105, 1975.

COPPER-ASSOCIATED HEPATITIS IN BEDLINGTON TERRIERS

ROBERT M. HARDY, D.V.M.

St. Paul, Minnesota

Bedlington terriers have a unique, genetically predisposed liver disease caused by a marked accumulation of copper within hepatocytes. This disorder was first described in 1975 (Hardy et al., 1975). Although the disease is inherited as an autosomal recessive trait (Johnson et al., 1980), its prevalence within this breed appears to be quite high. Of 144 Bedlingtons screened, 66 per cent had biochemical and/or histologic evidence of hepatic pathology.

HISTORY AND PHYSICAL EXAM

Clinical signs and physical findings associated with Bedlington liver disease are highly variable. Affected dogs generally can be placed in one of three groups. The first group includes young adults of either sex. They have a relatively short, often fulminant clinical course in which the onset of signs frequently follows some stressful event (whelping, showing). The second group has a more chronic course, typical of slowly progressive hepatic disease. The last group is clinically asymptomatic, and evidence for hepatic disease is derived from biochemical evidence of active hepatocellular damage or necrosis, i.e., elevated serum alanine aminotransferase (S-ALT), or biopsy abnormalities.

Animals in the *first group* tend to be young (two to six years of age) and usually have had no apparent illnesses prior to the onset of hepatic failure. In some cases, the association of stress preceding the illness, as observed by breeders, appears to be a valid one. Female Bedlington terriers appear to be particularly susceptible to acute hepatic failure within a few weeks of whelping.

Signs exhibited by the dogs are relatively non-specific. They include depression, lethargy, anorexia, and vomiting, all of acute onset. Jaundice tends to be prominent in the more severely affected dogs, appearing one to two days following the onset of signs. Another physical finding of localizing value is hepatomegaly, although it is not common. Generally, biochemical profiles are necessary to confirm the existence of hepatic failure. A less common but more dramatic physical finding is severe hemolytic anemia. It is characterized by a rapid fall in packed cell volume, severe jaundice, hemoglobinemia, and hemoglobinuria. Serum copper concentrations have been noted to increase dramatically during the hemolytic crisis.

The acute hepatic failure group is characterized by high mortality in spite of massive supportive care. Death may occur within 48 to 72 hours following the onset of signs. Animals surviving an acute attack may remain clinically asymptomatic for years or may suffer recurrent attacks of a similar but less severe nature later in life.

The *second group* of animals is comprised of middle-aged to older dogs. The clinical signs of this group are similar to those of the first group, although less severe. Appropriately, chronic weight loss and ascites may be evident. Previous attacks of acute hepatitis have generally not been observed or recognized. The liver is nonpalpable and will often appear reduced in size radiographically.

The *third group* is asymptomatic, comprised of clinically normal but affected dogs. This group is only detected via abnormal biochemical tests (S-ALT) and/or biopsy evidence characteristic of the disease. This segment of the Bedlington terrier population represents younger dogs that have not experienced an acute crisis or the preclinical stages of the chronic progressive group. Until screening of large numbers of Bedlington terriers for evidence of hepatic disease began, this group went undetected.

PATHOGENESIS

The pathogenesis of this disease is not completely understood but of primary importance is the progressive accumulation of dietary copper within lysosomes of hepatocytes. Copper is known to be hepatotoxic once significant intracellular concentrations develop. In affected Bedlingtons, hepatic copper concentrations may be increased by 8 to 12 weeks of age, or as long as one year may be required for pathologic increases to be detected. Generally, hepatic copper concentrations continue to increase until the dogs reach five to six years of age; after that time, assuming the dog does not die of acute failure, hepatic copper levels tend to slowly decline but never return to normal (Ludwig et al., 1980; Twedt et al., 1979).

Normal hepatic copper concentrations range from 91 to 377 µg/gm on a dry weight basis. From a diagnostic standpoint, dogs are considered to be affected if hepatic copper concentrations exceed 350 µm/gm. Most affected Bedlingtons have hepatic copper concentrations 5 to 50 times normal. Copper accumulates within lysosomes of hepatocytes and gives them a somewhat characteristic histologic picture (Fig. 1). Hepatic copper concentrations above 2000 µg/gm dry weight have been consistently associated with signs of progressive disease both morphologically and functionally (Twedt et al., 1979). Recent evidence suggests that the copper accumulation is secondary to functional impairment of biliary excretion of the metal. It is theorized that dogs remain relatively asymptomatic until the ability of hepatic lysosomes to store copper is exhausted. Once the lysosomal storage capacity is exceeded, copper is released to the cytoplasm of the hepatocytes, where it becomes toxic. When massive numbers of hepatocytes undergo rapid lysis, large quantities of copper are released to the circulation; this phenomenon has been associated with acute hemolytic crisis, a relatively uncommon clinical event.

Initial clinical, biochemical, and histologic findings in the disease strongly resemble an inherited human disorder, Wilson's disease (hepatolenticular degeneration). Although many features of these two disorders are similar, enough differences exist that they are no longer considered identical genetic disorders. Serum copper concentrations are normal in Bedlingtons (except during massive hepatic necrosis) but are very low in humans. Serum copper binding protein, ceruloplasmin, is normal or increased in affected dogs but low in humans. Histologic features also differ between the two species. Nonetheless, the canine disease has served as a valuable biomedical model for copper storage disorders of humans.

DIAGNOSIS

A definitive diagnosis of this disease requires liver biopsy. Occasionally, biopsy and quantitative hepatic copper assays are necessary. Biochemical evidence of hepatocellular inflammation, i.e., elevated S-ALT, is only suggestive of the disease. Conversely, a normal S-ALT does not rule out Bedlington liver disease. Significant numbers of biopsy–confirmed affected dogs have normal S-ALT con-

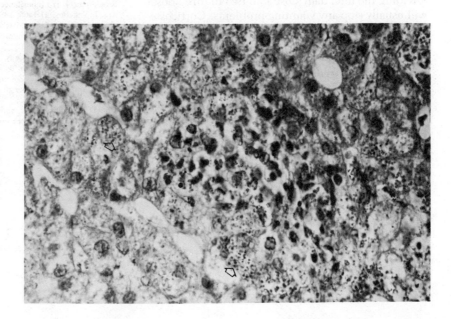

Figure 1. Foci of neutrophils associated with necrotic hepatocytes in a liver biopsy from a Bedlington terrier with copper storage disease. Prominent copper-containing lysosomal granules are present throughout the specimen (arrows) (320×).

centrations. Histologically, these livers vary greatly in terms of lesions observed. Some dogs have no structural injury present, the only pathology being increased copper concentrations as determined histochemically. More severe pathology is indicated by focal hepatitis, which progresses to lesions identical to those described for chronic active hepatitis and which ultimately leads to micro- or macronodular cirrhosis. Hepatocyte cytoplasm contains numerous brownish eosinophilic granules. These lysosomal granules react strongly to three stains used to detect copper (rubeanic, Timm's, and rhodamine). When histochemical determination of hepatic copper content is equivocal, quantitative copper assay is the only way to confirm a diagnosis.

THERAPY

Therapy of this disorder is both specific and symptomatic. This is one of a select group of hepatic diseases for which a specific mode of therapy exists. Drugs thought to have a beneficial effect in this disease include D-penicillamine, glucocorticoids, and ascorbic acid. D-penicillamine (Cupramine) is the only one for which objective data are available to substantiate its efficacy. This drug has been used for years to treat Wilson's disease, and its beneficial effects are thought to be due to its ability to chelate copper within the circulation and promote its elimination in urine. Quantitative hepatic copper concentrations from an affected dog treated for 26 months with D-penicillamine were reduced from 5,298 to 228 μg/gm dry weight (Ludwig et al., 1980). Recommended dosages are 125 to 250 mg/day in adult dogs, given 30 minutes prior to feeding. No toxic side effects except vomiting have been observed in dogs treated for over three years. Dividing the total daily dose into two to three doses will usually stop any vomiting problems. Corticosteroids, because of their lysosomal stabilizing effect, may be useful in this disease, particularly in acute crisis states; 0.5 to 1.0 mg/kg/day may be useful in acute therapy. Ascorbic acid is known to augment copper excretion in urine. Dosages have been empirical, 500 to 1000 mg/day being administered. Other therapy utilized in these patients is supportive and symptomatic.

Attempts to limit dietary copper intake may be undertaken but are difficult. Most commercial dog foods contain from 5 to 10 mg/kg of copper.

In experimental studies in Bedlington terriers, daily copper absorption was on the order of 1 mg (Su et al., 1981). An intake of 1 mg/day is equivalent to what a 70-kg human normally ingests. This extremely high dietary copper appears to reflect the recommendations of the National Research Council (Nutrient requirements of dogs, 1974). It is interesting to note that reported normal hepatic copper concentrations for the dog have progressively increased from 6.8 μg/gm (dry weight) in 1929 to 200 μg/gm in 1981 (Su et al., 1981).

Objective evidence of therapeutic efficacy, i.e., reduction in S-ALT or hepatic copper content, often takes weeks or months of continuous therapy. Clinical improvement, however, is frequently seen much sooner. Patients often gain weight and improve in activity, condition, and alertness in a few weeks. No objective criteria have as yet been established for determining which affected Bedlingtons should receive therapy with D-penicillamine. We routinely initiate therapy in any dog that has had one attack of liver disease and that will tolerate the drug. Therapy is also indicated in asymptomatic dogs with persistently increased S-ALT concentrations of 300 to 400 IU or higher in an attempt to prevent an acute crisis. At this time we recommend treating such dogs for life on the premise that hepatic copper will continue to rise unless therapy is maintained.

REFERENCES AND SUPPLEMENTAL READING

Hardy, R. M., Stevens, J. B., and Stowe, C. M.: Chronic progressive hepatitis in Bedlington terriers associated with elevated liver copper concentrations. Minn. Vet. 15:13, 1975.

Johnson, G. F., Sternlieb, I., Twedt, D. C., Grushoff, P. S., and Scheinberg, I. H.: Inheritance of copper toxicosis in Bedlington terriers. Am. J. Vet. Res. 41:1865, 1980.

Ludwig, J., Owen, C. A., Barham, S. S., McCall, J. T., and Hardy, R. M.: The liver in the inherited copper disease of Bedlington terriers. Lab. Invest. 43:82, 1980.

Nutrient requirements of dogs. Washington, D.C.: National Academy of Sciences, Publication No. 0–309–02315–7, 1974.

Su, L. C., Owen, C. A., Zollman, P E., and Hardy, R. M.: A defect of biliary excretion of copper in copper-laden Bedlington terriers. Am. J. Physiol. 243:G231, 1982.

Twedt, D. C., Sternlieb, I., and Gilbertson, R.: Clinical morphologic and chemical studies on copper toxicosis of Bedlington terriers. J.A.V.M.A. 175:269, 1979.

Section
11

ENDOCRINE AND METABOLIC DISORDERS

JOHN A. MULNIX, D.V.M.

Consulting Editor

DIABETES MELLITUS

DAVID B. CHURCH, B.V.Sc.

Sydney, Australia

UNCOMPLICATED DIABETES MELLITUS

The syndromes collectively known as diabetes mellitus are characterized by an absolute or relative lack of circulating insulin and some form of glucose intolerance. Although the disturbances in protein and lipid catabolism that also accompany this condition are important in producing the clinical signs seen with diabetes mellitus, the abnormalities in carbohydrate metabolism are more readily quantified, allowing more accurate diagnosis of the condition, particularly in its earlier stages or milder forms.

DIAGNOSIS

Often in these less severe forms, the only detectable abnormality is prolonged or excessive postprandial hyperglycemia. As insulin deficiency progresses, the pancreas becomes unable to maintain blood glucose at normal levels, even between meals. The development of fasting hyperglycemia heralds the onset of the major clinical signs (such as polydipsia, polyuria, polyphagia, and weight loss) that traditionally characterize the diabetic syndrome. Because the animals are invariably obese prior to the onset of these signs, the weight loss may not be apparent or obvious at presentation. Although fasting hyperglycemia confirms glucose intolerance in a suspected diabetic (and its presence eliminates the need for any form of dynamic testing), early cases with mild glucose intolerance can easily pass undetected if the fasting plasma glucose level is the sole criterion used to confirm a diagnosis.

In these mild forms, the patient's ability to metabolize a standard glucose load is a simple means of defining this type of abnormality. In the dog, quantitation of the glucose intolerance is most reliably demonstrated by an *intravenous* glucose tolerance test, since a readily calculable index for glucose tolerance—the glucose disappearance coefficient—can be derived (Church, 1980). Any inability to metabolize a glucose load will be demonstrated as a subnormal glucose disappearance coefficient or, more simply, as an abnormally flat plasma glucose versus time curve.

All these diabetic syndromes develop as a consequence of the imbalance between insulin production/release and the hormonal or tissue factors that modify insulin requirements. These two broad categories can be differentiated by measuring the *insulin response* to the intravenous glucose load: the former having diminished or delayed insulin release, the latter normal to excessive release, which may or may not be delayed. Differentiation of these categories is initially important, since most of the diabetic syndromes associated with "peripheral insulin resistance" (i.e., a modified tissue insulin requirement) are almost impossible to treat adequately by insulin administration and require instead correction of the underlying abnormality. The peripheral insulin resistance may be due to a variety of abnormalities acting either singly or in combination. Some of the more commonly recognized "diabetogenic factors" are listed in Table 1.

Even in the presence of a number of these factors, *overt* glucose tolerance (i.e., abnormal fasting blood glucose) is unlikely to develop without some degree of diminished β-cell reserve. Whether this reduction in maximal pancreatic insulin production has been created by the increased demand or whether the increased demand has simply exacerbated an underlying congenital or acquired β-cell defect is still unknown.

Regardless of the actual etiologic sequence, the association between chronic excessive insulin demand and β-cell deficiency means that animals with glucose intolerance due to peripheral insulin resistance will ultimately require some form of exogenous insulin.

ORAL HYPOGLYCEMICS

If there is a measurable insulin response to a glucose challenge, some benefit may be obtained from oral hypoglycemic therapy. A number of these so-called oral hypoglycemics improve glucose tolerance in the dog by increasing the rate and amount of insulin released as well as increasing peripheral

Table 1. *Some of the More Common "Diabetogenic Factors"*

Obesity	Azotemia
Endogenous glucocorticoids	Catecholamines
Exogenous glucocorticoids	Glucagon
Progestogens	Growth hormone
Estrogens	Thyroxine

insulin sensitivity. Among the variety of different compounds commercially available at present (some of which appear ineffective in the dog), glipizide (Glibenese* 0.24 to 0.5 mg/kg b.i.d.) and glibenclamide (Daonil† 0.2 mg/kg daily) are probably the drugs of choice for the dog. Once the animal's insulin reserve has diminished significantly, however, some form of exogenous insulin supplementation is required.

INSULIN THERAPY

Traditionally, treatment regimens employed in uncomplicated cases have involved once daily administration of a prolonged-duration insulin, usually isophane (NPH) or protamine zinc insulin (PZI). The *average* durations of these insulins are approximately 24 and 30 hours, respectively. Their administration is usually combined with twice daily feeding, close to the time of insulin administration and at the expected time of peak insulin activity, around 8 to 12 hours after administration. Unfortunately, although once daily insulin administration is convenient, it seems less than satisfactory in many animals. One problem constantly encountered is the marked variability in the duration of action and time of maximum effect of both NPH and PZI insulin preparations in the dog.

The unpredictability of the time of peak effect for these insulins may be important in preventing satisfactory stabilization. For example, if the insulin's maximum effect occurs four hours before the expected time on one day and four hours after it on the next, maintenance of normoglycemia throughout a 24-hour period will be difficult, particularly as feeding at a fixed time each day may sometimes result in the animal receiving half its daily caloric intake (a substantial hyperglycemic stimulus) *after* the time when the administered insulin was acting maximally.

Furthermore, because the animal's total daily insulin requirement is administered in one bolus, the chance of hypoglycemia is always present. This danger is heightened if the time of peak activity is variable, particularly since rebound hyperglycemia (the Somogyi effect) can make the detection of hypoglycemia difficult. In addition, if the blood glucose concentration at the anticipated time of peak effect is used to assess the adequacy of insulin dosage, an animal may be falsely stabilized at an excessive dose of insulin. This is simply because the insulin's maximum effect is occurring earlier than expected, and the blood glucose level at the time of sampling reflects both the waning insulin effect and the effect of the animal's subsequent hyperglycemic response. Monitoring urine glucose is also of

little use, since the more severe the hypoglycemia the greater the subsequent rebound hyperglycemia owing to the unhampered release of catecholamines, glucocorticoids, glucagon, and growth hormone. The resultant glucosuria created by the rebound effect may be incorrectly interpreted as an indication to further increase the insulin dose. For these reasons, the use of an insulin preparation with a relatively predictable time of peak activity is very important.

In diabetic dogs a relatively predictable peak effect is rapidly attained four to six hours after administration of a highly purified porcine insulin-zinc suspension (IZS-P) (Monotard‡) containing 70 per cent insulin-zinc crystals and 30 per cent insulin-zinc amorphous particles (Church, 1981). This is a traditional lente physicochemical formulation, but with insulin of entirely porcine origin, resulting in an overall duration of approximately 14 hours.

An additional advantage of this preparation is its minimal antigenicity (Schlichtkrull et al., 1975). This is presumably because it lacks impurities, and the amino acid sequences of porcine and canine insulin are identical. Unlike animals that have been treated with other insulin preparations that are not highly purified, no detectable circulating insulin antibodies have been found in dogs treated for up to three years with IZS-P. Because of the generally more rapid absorption of porcine insulin, the shorter duration, and earlier peak activity time, IZS-P generally cannot be used on a once daily basis. However, the potential advantages in diabetic control achieved by utilizing a nonantigenic insulin with an early, relatively predictable peak activity time often outweigh the increased inconvenience of twice daily injections.

In the normal animal the time of major insulin requirement is the post-prandial period, whereas only small amounts are needed during fasting to maintain euglycemia and control lipid and protein metabolism. Although the duration of action of IZS-P is about 14 to 16 hours, much of its "glucose lowering activity" occurs within 6 hours of administration. Therefore, IZS-P administration every 12 hours, with feeding timed to utilize the acute hypoglycemic effect of the insulin to minimize the post-prandial hyperglycemia, should achieve a relatively stable 24-hour plasma glucose profile. Logically most of the hyperglycemic trend should occur during the period when insulin is tending to lower the blood glucose at a maximal rate, not at the time when the blood glucose is lowest.

IZS-P is administered every 12 hours at an initial dose of 0.25 to 0.50 U/kg; the animal is fed one-half its daily caloric requirement one to one and one-half hours later. The adequacy of the insulin dose can then be assessed by measuring the blood glu-

---

*Pfizer Laboratories, New York, NY.
†Hoechst-Roussel Pharmaceuticals Inc., Somerville, NJ.

‡Novo Industri A/S, Copenhagen, Denmark.

cose approximately six hours after insulin administration. This regimen has the additional advantage of a relatively reproducible 12-hour cycle. The morning and evening insulin dosage for the following day can be adjusted according to the blood glucose level of the previous day, and the veterinarian knows that changes in blood glucose after the evening injection should be similar to those after the morning injection.

If circumstances demand a once daily insulin regimen, either NPH, PZI, or a traditional lente preparation may be used, with serial blood samples taken every 2 to 3 hours for the first 12 hours after insulin administration to determine the expected peak activity time in individual patients. Also, with these insulins it would seem preferable to minimize blood glucose fluctuations by feeding the animal during the time that the insulin is producing the most rapid decrease in glucose levels, that time being determined by the results of the initial assessment of the insulin's action in the individual. Because these insulins produce a relatively slow glucose decrement, acute glucose fluctuations can be minimized by feeding the animal's caloric requirement in three or, if possible, four meals during this previously determined period.

Regardless of the type of insulin used or the frequency of administration, the two principal and equally important aims of therapy are to lower the average blood glucose concentration over each 24-hour period and to minimize blood glucose fluctuations. With reasonable care and close monitoring on the part of both owner and veterinarian, a degree of control can be achieved that allows the diabetic dog to lead a relatively normal life.

The cornerstone of long-term diabetic management is *consistency*. Once the animal's insulin dose has been individualized—preferably in the hospital—the ration and the time of feeding should be continued at home. It is imperative that the owner be made fully aware of his obligations and that the food and insulin regimens established be compatible with the normal routine of each household. The type of food given after stabilization must be kept as constant as possible. Usually a commercial canned preparation with small amounts of dry food is preferable, as their caloric content is relatively predictable. Changes in the dog's diet can only be made if the overall caloric content remains unchanged. Within these caloric restrictions, additional supplementation with high-fiber vegetables such as celery, turnips, and cabbage may also be useful, as there is increasing evidence suggesting that certain high-fiber diets may decrease, to some extent, the rate of post-prandial glucose elevation and also the daily insulin requirement (Jenkins et al., 1979; Schwartz and Levine, 1980).

Whatever the diet chosen, the food given should meet the normal maintenance requirements for the patient's ideal body weight, usually 75 to 90 kcal/kg for dogs up to 10 kg and 55 to 57 kcal/kg for dogs up to 30 kg.

Another frequently neglected area of diabetic therapy is the injection site. Areas that are subject to variations in movement and stretching should be avoided. Experiments in humans and rabbits have demonstrated that insulin is more slowly absorbed from sites on the thigh and arm than from sites on the abdomen, and these differences tend to be exacerbated by exercise. For this reason it seems preferable to limit the site of injection to the right and left abdominal walls.

The amount of exercise should also be kept relatively constant, since exercise reduces the insulin requirement. The two main insulin-dependent tissues in the body are muscle and adipose tissue, and the increased blood supply and accelerated intracellular metabolism of glucose seen in exercised muscle can significantly lower the insulin requirements. This is particularly important in working dogs. In general, if exercise is planned to last only a few hours the morning injection should be reduced by about one-third and a small snack offered just prior to performance.

Because female sex steroids, both natural and synthetic, are potent insulin antagonists, intact bitches should be spayed as soon as possible after their diabetes has been stabilized. Indeed, ovariohysterectomy may result in a significant reduction in glucose intolerance, occasionally allowing the animal, at least in the short term, to be managed without exogenous insulin supplementation. The problem is made worse in the breeding bitch, in which the estrogen and progesterone levels present during pregnancy produce marked insulin resistance. This diabetogenic effect is enhanced by a placental insulinase and the markedly increased energy demands placed on the bitch by the developing fetus. In addition, the incidence of dystocia is increased in poorly controlled diabetics because of abnormally large fetuses. The fetal pancreas secretes increased amounts of insulin in response to the elevated amino acids and fat present in the plasma of the poorly controlled diabetic dam (surprisingly, the *fetal* pancreas does not secrete insulin in response to hyperglycemia), and the resultant fetal hyperinsulinemia accelerates growth by a direct somatotrophic effect and also probably by cross reacting with receptors for somatomedins (growth factors structurally related to insulin).

The problem of long-term management and maintenance of adequate insulin dosage in the animal's home environment is difficult. Urine monitoring is widely used as a guide to chronic diabetic control even though numerous factors besides mean blood glucose concentration may alter the urine glucose concentration during the day. This inherent variability, combined with a lack of sensitivity due to the renal threshold for glucose of 180 to 220 mg/dl, minimizes its value. Most well-stabilized diabetic animals have no detectable glucosuria at any time. Urine glucose monitoring in these cases is only of value in allowing early detection of altered control.

A more sensitive method of determining overall diabetic control is the measurement of glycosylated hemoglobin (GHb). This altered hemoglobin accrues after glycosylation (binding of glucose molecules to amino groups) of specific molecular sites on the hemoglobin molecule. Because this modification occurs slowly and nearly irreversibly throughout the life span of the red cell at a rate dependent on the average glucose concentration during that time, its measurement provides an estimate of the mean blood glucose level over the preceding four to six weeks (Gabbay et al., 1979).

Although the early assay methods for measurement of GHb were technically difficult and inconvenient, a recent alternative method for its estimation appears to be less troublesome as well as being non-species-specific (Yue et al., 1982). Wider availability of this method should provide veterinarians with a more accurate means of monitoring diabetic control than either urine glucose monitoring or spot blood glucose samples.

DIABETIC KETOACIDOSIS

Despite the tendency in recent years for early detection of diabetes mellitus, diabetic ketoacidosis (DKA) remains one of the few endocrine emergencies regularly encountered in veterinary practice. Its diagnosis and treatment require a clear understanding of the biochemical genesis and sequelae of ketoacidosis. The three major areas of deranged metabolism seen in DKA (lipolysis, ketogenesis, and glucose homeostasis) are identical to those present in uncomplicated diabetes mellitus; the difference is merely one of severity.

In essence, insulin deficiency produces an increased lipolysis/lipogenesis ratio peripherally as well as accelerated hepatic ketone body and triglyceride synthesis and release. These changes are exacerbated by impaired utilization of ketone bodies and lipid metabolites in insulin-dependent tissues, principally muscle and adipose tissue. The resultant accumulation of ketone bodies in the circulation tends to produce acidosis, since the two principal ketone bodies, β-OH butyrate and acetoacetate, are both acids that are fully dissociated at physiologic pH levels. Every diabetic animal, therefore, has some degree of ketonemia, but it is only when the concentration of ketone bodies reaches high levels (causing ketonuria) that their presence becomes significant and the very different clinical picture of diabetic ketoacidosis arises. These metabolic derangements are described in detail hereafter.

Lipolysis. In the normal animal there is a fine balance between triglyceride (TG) synthesis and lipolysis. The glycerol released as a result of lipolysis within adipocytes, however, cannot be reused for TG synthesis, as its re-esterification with fatty acids (FAs) requires it to be first phosphorylated to α-glycerophosphate, and adipose tissue lacks the appropriate enzyme, glycerokinase. α-Glycerophosphate, however, is an intermediate in glycolysis; thus TG synthesis in adipocytes depends partly on the provision of new α-glycerophosphate from glucose. In addition, lipolysis itself is controlled by a hormone-dependent lipase, which is inhibited by insulin and enhanced by the catabolic hormones.

Thus, insulin deficiency alone will result in increased lipolysis as well as decreased TG synthesis (since insulin is required for glucose's entry into adipocytes), thereby increasing the release of FA into the circulation.

Ketogenesis. The FAs released from adipose tissue are utilized as fuel extrahepatically (although the rate is partly insulin-dependent and hence reduced in insulin deficiency) as well as being assimilated by the liver at a rate that is dependent on their plasma concentration. However, their intracellular metabolism is under hormonal control. In insulin-rich states most of the FAs are converted to TG in the cytosol and excreted as lipoproteins. In insulin-deficient states, on the other hand, and particularly in the presence of hyperglucagonemia, most of the FAs are transported into the mitochondria by the carnitine transport system. Once inside the mitochondria, the FAs are oxidized to acetyl coenzyme A (CoA). The disposal of acetyl CoA depends on the availability of oxaloacetate and the activity of the enzyme citrate synthase, since acetyl CoA can be channelled into the Kreb's cycle. Whatever remains is diverted into the methyl-glutaryl CoA pathway, which is primarily responsible for ketone body synthesis. In insulin-deficient states the carnitine transport system is increased and the synthesis of citrate decreased; consequently, ketogenesis is markedly increased and this trend is exacerbated by an increased volume of substrate owing to accelerated lipolysis.

In hypoinsulinemic states, despite the increased rate of ketogenesis, the supply of FAs may exceed the mitochondrial oxidative capacity. These excess FAs are then esterified with α-glycerophosphate to form triglycerides, which enter the circulation in increased amounts and also accumulate in the liver. Thus there is an overall increase in the level of circulating lipid metabolites owing to increased peripheral lipolysis and accelerated hepatic synthesis of triglycerides and ketone bodies. At the same time, there is a decreased ability of peripheral tissues to use either FAs or ketone bodies.

Hyperglycemia. The two main causes of hyperglycemia are decreased tissue uptake and increased hepatic production. By far the most important insulin-dependent tissues are muscle and adipose tissues. The liver, on the other hand, does not require insulin for glucose uptake but is dependent on insulin for control of glucose metabolism. It is presently believed that insulin controls blood glucose principally through its effects on certain enzymes involved in hepatic glucose metabolism. Insulin stimulates hexokinase/glucokinase, which converts absorbed glucose to glucose-6-phosphate, the first step in its breakdown, thereby *indirectly* promoting intracellular movement of glucose down its concentration gradient. There is further inhibition of glycolysis in diabetic hepatocytes, since conversion of fructose-6-phosphate (F6P) to fructose 1,6-diphosphate (F1,6dP) is also decreased in insulin deficiency.

Impaired glucose breakdown occurs with a simultaneous tendency for increased gluconeogenesis, since the key enzyme that converts oxaloacetate to phosphoenolpyruvate (an early step in gluconeogenesis) is inhibited by insulin. This effect is exacerbated by the continued favoring of conversion of F1,6dP to F6P as well as the stimulation of gluconeogenesis provided by the increased levels of gluconeogenic amino acids accruing from accelerated protein catabolism, another consequence of insulin deficiency.

DIAGNOSIS

Ketoacidosis should be suspected in any animal with a relatively acute history of vomiting, inappetance, lethargy, and weakness, particularly if these abnormalities were preceded by polydipsia and polyuria. Findings on physical examination include dehydration, weakness, depression (sometimes coma), abdominal pain, hepatomegaly, increased minute respiratory volume with a prolonged expiratory phase (Kussmaul's respiration), acetone breath odor, and, occasionally, hypothermia. Whenever ketoacidosis is suspected, a thorough physical examination is obligatory, since it is essential to eliminate possible precipitating factors such as infection, trauma, and acute pancreatitis.

The diagnosis can be confirmed by the demonstration of concurrent ketonemia and hyperglycemia (using Acetest* tablets and Dextrostix*) or ketonuria and glycosuria using urine reagent strips. Although confirmation of ketonemia/ketonuria with hyperglycemia is sufficient reason to initiate therapy, the minimum additional biochemical information required includes complete blood count; plasma sodium, potassium, chloride, and bicarbonate; blood urea nitrogen or creatinine; blood pH (preferably arterial); and urinalysis.

---

*Ames Division, Miles Laboratories, Inc., Elkhart, IN.

FLUID REPLACEMENT

Establishment of a patent airway, by endotracheal intubation if necessary, may be required in obtunded patients, particularly if vomiting is a problem. Introduction of an intravenous line, either cephalic or jugular, is essential; the latter is preferred, as it enables monitoring of central venous pressure (CVP). Measurement of urine output should also be considered, particularly in those animals with marked azotemia.

Animals with diabetic ketoacidosis, because of their obligate diuresis and hyperosmolality, are usually profoundly dehydrated; frequently the dehydration approaches an amount equivalent to 10 to 15 per cent of body weight. Although the total water deficit can be corrected over the first 24 to 48 hours, the circulating blood volume must be rapidly restored, and, provided CVP is not raised excessively, fluids should be administered at a rate of 5 to 15 ml/kg/hour, although this rate maybe higher for the first one to two hours.

Although some free water loss (both extracellular and intracellular) is inevitable in DKA (and is partly responsible for the hyperosmolar state), the use of a relatively isotonic fluid is preferable owing to the potential problem of cerebral edema (see hereafter). The requirements of electrolyte inserts (dictated principally by the animal's potassium and pH status) and later dextrose invariably necessitate the use of an initially hypotonic medium (0.45 per cent NaCl) to maintain near isotonicity of the fluid that is actually administered.

INSULIN THERAPY

Regular or crystalline insulin is always used in the treatment of diabetic ketoacidosis. As equally important as the type of insulin is its route of administration. The conventional insulin regimen has been relatively high-dose (1.1 to 2.2 U/kg) boluses, one-half administered intravenously and the remainder administered intramuscularly. The rationale for high-dose therapy was a fear of insulin resistance due to acidosis and the presence of elevated levels of glucagon, cortisol, and the catecholamines. However, in both humans and the dog there seems to be little evidence to support an effect of ketoacidosis, "insulin resistance," or even previous insulin therapy on the glucose response to insulin. This is particularly true when the insulin is administered as a continuous IV infusion or as hourly IM injections (Goriya et al., 1978; Chastain and Nichols, 1981). Although some clinicians advocate low-dose intramuscular therapy (Chastain and Nichols, 1981), the requirement for hourly injections is cumbersome, and the method is theoretically still subject to variations in response owing to alterations in injection site perfusion, tissue acidity (which may affect insulin solubility and hence its absorption), and the presence of tissue insulinases in certain individuals.

Since the various metabolic disturbances in diabetic ketoacidosis are the result of lack of insulin, it is reasonable to anticipate that metabolic recovery will occur more rapidly and smoothly if insulin is continuously present in effective physiologic amounts and not subject to wide swings in concentration. In addition, both hypoglycemia and hypokalemia are less likely, partly because of the relatively smooth transition but also because their development can be anticipated by extrapolating from the rate of fall of their plasma concentrations and avoided by decreasing the insulin infusion rate. The amount of insulin required should be sufficient to inhibit lipolysis, ketogenesis, and gluconeogenesis; improve extrahepatic utilization of both glucose and ketones; and restore normal transmembrane electrolyte balance. Because too rapid a correction of the hyperglycemia and ketonemia/acidosis may create a number of complications (see hereafter), a graded response is preferable. This may best be achieved by what would be traditionally regarded as a low dose of insulin, i.e., one that produces a circulating peripheral insulin concentration of approximately 50 to 70 μU/ml, which inhibits gluconeogenesis but does not *unduly* enhance extrahepatic glucose utilization. This plasma insulin concentration can be achieved by infusing insulin at a rate of 20 to 30 mU/min/m^2 (about 0.038 to 0.057 U/kg/hr). Although an infusion pump provides the most accurate means of delivering a constant insulin infusion, a pediatric drip set is sufficiently accurate for flow rate regulation.

Because insulin adheres to glass and plastic surfaces, approximately 50 ml of the insulin-containing fluid should be run through the drip set before it is attached to the patient. This then ensures that the animal receives a constant insulin concentration in the administered fluid (Peterson et al., 1976). Furthermore, soluble neutral insulin in phosphate buffer should always be used, since neutral insulin preparations dissolved in acetate buffer tend to crystallize in plastic tubing.

Although peripheral lipolysis, hepatic ketogenesis, and intracellular potassium movement are slightly more sensitive than hepatic gluconeogenesis to insulin's action, all three require only small increments in plasma insulin above fasting levels for their inhibition, certainly much less than is needed for maximal extrahepatic glucose uptake. Despite these varying sensitivities, it is always important to remember that hyperglycemia will be corrected well before the hyperketonemia and acidosis. The relative delay in the correction of the ketonemia and acidosis is primarily due to the even less potent effect of insulin on extrahepatic ketoacid utilization.

The disparity in insulin sensitivity means that insulin therapy must be continued even when the blood glucose concentration has returned to normal. To prevent hypoglycemia and still allow insulin to be infused at a rate that promotes peripheral ketone body utilization, dextrose solution needs to be introduced at a rate of approximately 2 to 3 mg/kg/min once blood glucose concentrations fall to 200 mg/dl. At this stage it is advisable to slow the insulin infusion rate to 15 to 20 mU/min/m^2. The dextrose and insulin should be continued until the animal is accepting food without emesis. The insulin/dextrose infusion is then stopped and subcutaneous insulin administered, as for the uncomplicated diabetic.

Although low-dose intravenous insulin infusion avoids the problems associated with tissue absorption and bolus dosing and produces a slow and predictable decline in plasma glucose, individual variation still exists, necessitating frequent determinations of plasma glucose. Some individual variation is associated with differences in the degree of elevation of the various anti-insulin hormones. Their elevated levels all decrease rapidly with the initiation of insulin therapy alone, although they are more likely to remain elevated when stress factors exist, such as concurrent infections.

ELECTROLYTES

The total body potassium deficit can be profound, particularly if the patient has been vomiting and/or anorectic for some days, even though plasma potassium concentration may be normal or elevated. This apparent paradox is caused by a constant flux of potassium from the intracellular compartment (where normally 95 per cent of total body potassium is located) into the extracellular fluid (ECF), resulting in enormous urinary losses because of impaired renal conservation of electrolytes in the presence of osmotic diuresis. The constant efflux of intracellular potassium is principally due to exchange across cellular membranes of hydrogen ions in the ECF with intracellular cations, mainly potassium.

It is neither possible nor desirable to replace this potassium deficit acutely. There are two distinct aims with potassium replacement. The first is to maintain a normal extracellular potassium concentration during the acute phases of treatment using parenteral supplements. The second is to replace the total, mainly intracellular, deficit using oral supplementation over a period of days or weeks. If insulin and fluids without potassium are given in a ketoacidotic patient, the plasma potassium concentration will fall. This decrease, apart from a mild effect due to some urinary loss and extracellular dilution that occurs with fluid replacement, is primarily dependent on the insulin concentration. The intracellular movement of potassium is enhanced not only by glucose uptake but also through a primary effect of insulin. For this reason plasma potassium concentrations should be determined regularly (at least every five to six hours) throughout the first 12 to 24 hours of insulin therapy. Potassium should be administered in the fluids at a rate not exceeding 0.5 mEq/kg/hr and usually much less than this. It is impossible to determine the exact amount of potassium that is required, but as a guide 20 to 40 mEq of potassium is added to each liter of fluids, and this amount can be adjusted depending on the level and rate of fall of the serum potassium.

Although ketoacidotic diabetics are also phosphorus, magnesium, and calcium depleted, these deficiencies are usually small and self-correcting once insulin and fluid therapies are initiated.

ACIDOSIS

Because of the ketonemia and azotemia, the diabetic with ketosis is always acidotic. The degree of acidosis is best determined by the plasma bicarbonate concentration and pH, although blood CO_2 concentration or the anion gap can provide a reasonable estimate.

Despite the presence of metabolic acidosis, the administration of alkali to animals with diabetic ketoacidosis remains controversial. The problem is balancing the potential ill effects of the acidemia against the problems that may be created by bicarbonate administration. The acidosis leads to hyperventilation, loss of intracellular potassium, peripheral vasodilation and hypotension, negative ionotropism, and, in severe acidemia, CNS and respiratory depression. The use of alkali, however, raises a number of potential problems. By far the most important is the exacerbation, by bicarbonate, of any tendency toward hypokalemia. Bicarbonate does this by lowering the hydrogen ion concentration in the ECF and accelerating the intracellular movement of potassium. Paradoxically, with alkali administration CSF pH may fall because of the disparity in the blood-brain barrier's permeability for CO_2 and bicarbonate, although the importance of this phenomenon may have been overemphasized. Spinal fluid and cisternal pH are not necessarily equivalent, and the problem is relatively easily avoided if the bicarbonate deficit is corrected slowly.

Overzealous administration of alkali may also negate the rightward shifting of the oxyhemoglobin dissociation curve produced by the acidosis, which partially compensates for the leftward shift produced by the decreased erythrocyte 2,3 diphosphoglycerate concentration present in diabetics. Two other hazards that also should be considered are alkalosis and the potential for sodium overload.

It would seem preferable to administer bicarbonate only when the plasma pH is less than 7.0 or in cases of distressing hyperventilation, but very little is needed and certainly its use is not recommended once the pH is greater than 7.1.

COMPLICATIONS

PANCREATITIS

Pancreatitis is the most common complication of diabetic ketoacidosis. Hyperamylasemia (greater than twice the upper limit of normal) is strongly suggestive of acute pancreatitis, although false negatives are not uncommon. Because of the difficulty in ruling out pancreatitis, any ketoacidotic animal should not be offered food until the amylase concentration approaches normal and emesis has ceased. The effectiveness of various medications such as atropine, anti-inflammatories, cimetidine, somatostatin, and antimicrobial agents is highly debatable, and their routine use appears unwarranted.

HYPEROSMOLAR COMA

This is a relatively rare occurrence in the dog and is usually seen in the absence of ketoacidosis. The hyperosmolality produces depression, stupor, and even coma. The animal is frequently a borderline diabetic exposed to some stress, often infection, and the resultant elevation of the hyperglycemic hormones produces sufficient insulin resistance to minimize extrahepatic glucose utilization without negating insulin's inhibition of lipolysis and ketogenesis.

The hyperosmolality is due to the profound hyperglycemia and/or hypernatremia that may result. Plasma osmolality can be measured directly or estimated from the following formula

$$\text{Osmolality} = 2(\text{Na}^+ + \text{K}^+) \times \frac{\text{blood glucose}}{18}$$

when sodium and potassium are expressed in mEq/L and blood glucose in mg/dl.

The treatment of hyperglycemic coma should always begin with a simple infusion of 0.45 per cent saline alone. At the end of the first two hours the blood glucose should be rechecked, as often quite rapid reductions can be achieved without insulin administration.

CEREBRAL EDEMA

This is a compounding problem in the treatment of both ketoacidosis and hyperglycemic coma. The condition is caused by too rapid correction of the metabolic disturbances, thereby creating a significant osmotic gradient between the ECF and the brain. The mechanism remains obscure, although the phenomenon only attains clinical significance when the blood glucose returns too rapidly to levels of less than 250 to 300 mg/dl (Arieff and Kleeman, 1974).

Continuous intravenous insulin administration avoids the vagaries of absorption from tissue depots and overcomes the problem of the short half-life of IV bolus injections, providing a slow and predictable drop in plasma glucose concentration. Although this standardized therapeutic regimen simplifies the management of diabetic ketoacidosis, it must not be allowed to foster a false sense of security. Diabetic ketoacidosis remains one of the few medical emergencies seen in veterinary endocrinology, and the ketoacidotic diabetic animal requires constant care and attention.

REFERENCES AND SUPPLEMENTAL READING

Arieff, A. I., and Kleeman, C. R.: Cerebral edema in diabetic comas. II. Effects of hyperosmolality, hyperglycemia and insulin in diabetic rabbits. J. Clin. Endo. Metab. 38:1057, 1974.

Chastain, C. B., and Nichols, C. E.: Low-dose intramuscular insulin therapy for diabetic ketoacidosis in dogs. J. Am. Vet. Med. Assn. 178:561, 1981.

Church, D. B.: A comparison of intravenous and oral glucose tolerance tests in the dog. Res. Vet. Sci. 29:353, 1980.

Church, D. B.: The blood glucose response to three prolonged duration insulins in canine diabetes mellitus. J. Small Anim. Pract. 22:301, 1981.

Feldman, E. C.: Diabetes mellitus. In Kirk, R. W. (ed): Current Veterinary Therapy VII. Philadelphia: W. B. Saunders Company, 1980.

Gabbay, K. H., Sosenko, H. M., Banuchi, G. A., Mininsohn, M. J., and Fluckiger, R.: Glycosylated hemoglobins: Increased glycosylation of hemoglobin A in diabetic patients. Diabetes 28:337, 1979.

Goriya, Y., Kawamori, R., Shichiri, M., Kikuchi, M., Yamasaki, Y., Shigeta, Y., and Abe, H.: Validation of I.V. small-dose insulin infusion therapy in diabetic ketoacidosis of depancreatized dogs. Acta Diabet. Lat. 15:236, 1978.

Jenkins, D. J. A., Taylor, R. H., Nineham, R., Goff, D. V., Bloom, S. R., Sarson, D., and Alberti, K. G. M. M.: Combined use of guar and acarbase in reduction of postprandial glycaemia. Lancet 2:924, 1979.

Kaneko, J. J., Mattheeuws, D., Rottiers, R. P., and Vermeulen, A.: Glucose tolerance and insulin response in diabetes mellitus of dogs. J. Small Anim. Pract. 19:85, 1978.

Peterson, L., Caldwell, J., and Hoffman, J.: Insulin adsorbance to polyvinylchloride surfaces with implications for constant-infusion therapy. Diabetes 25:72, 1976.

Schlichtkrull, J., Pingel, M., Heding, L. G., Brange, J., and Jorgensen, K. H.: Insulin preparations with prolonged effect. In Hasselblatt, A., and Bruchhausen, B. V. (eds.): Insulin II. Heidelberg, Springer-Verlag, Berlin, 1975.

Schwartz, S. E., and Levine, G. D.: Effects of dietary fibre on intestinal glucose absorption and glucose tolerance in rats. Gastroenterology. 79:833, 1980.

Wood, P. A., and Smith, J. E.: Glycosylated hemoglobin and canine diabetes mellitus. J. Am. Vet. Med. Assn. 176:1267, 1980.

Yue, D. K., McClennan, S., Church, D. B., and Turtle, J. R.: Measurement of glycosylated hemoglobin in man and animals by aminophenylboronic acid affinity chromatography. Submitted for publication, 1982.

CANINE HYPOGLYCEMIA

TIMOTHY A. ALLEN, D.V.M.

Ft. Collins, Colorado

Maintenance of the blood glucose concentration within a relatively narrow range is an essential part of homeostasis. A blood glucose level below the lower limits of normal can result from overutilization or underproduction of glucose or a combination of both. Utilization of glucose depends on the rate of entry into the cell, intracellular metabolism, and excretion. Glucose production is a function of mobilization of glucose from glycogen stores, absorption of ingested carbohydrate, and synthesis of carbohydrate from nonglucose sources, i.e., gluconeogenesis. Therefore, interference with the homeostatic mechanisms that regulate the blood glucose level can take place at different steps of metabolism and in different tissues.

Canine hypoglycemia is a constellation of signs associated with a variety of diseases rather than a specific diagnosis. For the sake of this discussion, hypoglycemia is defined by the presence of clinical signs rather than by a blood glucose concentration below an arbitrary limit. The physical examination and historic findings associated with hypoglycemia are the same regardless of the underlying etiology. The clinical signs commonly observed in hypoglycemic dogs can be attributed to decreased uptake of glucose and decreased utilization of oxygen by the brain. Since glucose enters neuronal tissue principally by diffusion rather than by an insulin-dependent process, the blood glucose concentration reflects the glucose concentration in the neuronal tissue. The neuropathologic lesions associated with severe hypoglycemia closely resemble the lesions associated with hypoxic-ischemic brain injury. Recent case reports in humans indicate that the distribution of neuropathologic lesions with these two syndromes is slightly different; therefore, different mechanisms may be involved.

The neurologic signs commonly observed in the hypoglycemic dog can be either diffuse or focal. These signs include weakness of the rear legs, generalized weakness, focal or diffuse muscle twitching, ataxia, blindness, generalized seizures, and behavioral abnormalities. Behavioral abnormalities include fractious behavior and hysteria or anxiety evidenced by incessant running, barking, and loss of bowel and bladder control. The clinical manifestations of hypoglycemia tend to be episodic in nature regardless of etiology.

The signs that appear in a given animal depend on individual susceptibility and the degree and rate of decline of the blood glucose concentration. When the blood glucose drops rapidly there is a prompt increase in the concentrations of epinephrine, norepinephrine, cortisol, glucagon, and growth hormone. The net effect of this homeostatic response is a stabilization or increase in the blood glucose by an increase in the release of glucose from the liver, inhibiting normal pancreatic insulin release and decreasing peripheral glucose utilization. Some of the clinical signs observed may be due, in part, to the catecholamine excess that results from these counter-regulatory mechanisms, e.g., muscle twitching. When the blood glucose drops slowly the response mechanisms may not be activated, or if hypoglycemia occurs repetitively over a period of time these homeostatic mechanisms may be exhausted. The final result of either process is a severe hypoglycemia that may result in severe, irreversible cerebral damage. The immature nervous system appears to be less susceptible to these permanent changes owing to the ability of newborn pups to increase cerebral lactate utilization, thereby supplementing glucose as the primary energy source. The severity or reversibility of clinical signs cannot be determined with a single blood glucose determination.

Hypoglycemia should be considered in any dog presented in seizure or coma. After a sample has been drawn for blood glucose measurement, a bolus of glucose should be given intravenously. Response to glucose infusion is usually considered diagnostic of hypoglycemia; however, lack of response to a single bolus does not eliminate this possibility. In this emergency setting, the use of semiquantitative reagent strips (Dextrostix) can be valuable. The strips must be stored properly and label instructions followed exactly. Fluoride will inhibit the enzyme system in the strips.

Although hypoglycemia is caused by a variety of clinical syndromes, a precise, meaningful classification scheme based on etiology or pathogenesis is impossible. Classification is also difficult because of the paucity of documented cases in the literature. The following clinical entities should be considered in the differential diagnosis when evaluating a dog with hypoglycemia.

FUNCTIONAL PANCREATIC ISLET CELL TUMORS (INSULINOMAS)

Functional pancreatic islet cell tumors (insulinomas) arise from beta cells in the islets of Langerhans and produce excessive amounts of insulin. Although this is an infrequent tumor type, it is one of the more frequent causes of hypoglycemia in the mature dog. All of the clinical signs associated with this tumor can be attributed to hypoglycemia. Surprisingly, the hypoglycemia in human insulinoma patients has been shown to be due to suppression of glucose production rather than to increased utilization. The majority of canine tumors are adenocarcinomas rather than adenomas. Metastasis is initially limited to the regional lymph nodes. However, eventually more widespread metastasis occurs.

All reported functional islet cell tumors have been in dogs older than three and one-half years of age. The average age at the time of diagnosis is nine years. No sex predilection has been recognized. Boxers, poodles, and terriers seem to be the most commonly affected breeds. This clinical impression has not been documented statistically.

Any of the signs of hypoglycemia previously described can occur. Since these signs are relatively nonspecific, it is important to rule out other potential causes of these signs, e.g., viral encephalitis, brain tumor, hypocalcemia, and so on. The signs tend to be episodic, and with growth of the tumor the frequency and severity of signs increase. Significant compensation is possible because of the typical chronic course. Consequently, it is possible for dogs with severe hypoglycemia to appear clinically normal.

A tentative diagnosis can be based on the demonstration of Whipple's triad. Whipple's triad consists of neurologic signs associated with hypoglycemia, a fasting blood glucose of less than 40 mg/dl, and amelioration of neurologic signs by feeding or glucose administration. This triad establishes that the neurologic signs were due to hypoglycemia. However, it does not reveal the specific etiology of the hypoglycemia.

Definitive diagnosis of an insulinoma requires further testing. The glucagon tolerance test is the provocative test of choice. Other provocative tests include the leucine and tolbutamide tolerance tests. Intravenous administration of glucagon produces rapid glycogenolysis and subsequent hyperglycemia. Glucagon has an early direct effect on insulin release and a later indirect effect that results from the glucagon-induced hyperglycemia. In dogs with functional pancreatic islet cell tumors, the effect of glucagon on insulin release is exaggerated.

The glucagon tolerance test is performed after an overnight fast. An intravenous dose of 0.03 mg/kg glucagon is administered. Blood glucose samples are drawn at 0, 1, 5, 15, 30, 45, 60, 90, and 120 minutes. If the number of samples must be limited, samples at 0, 15, 30, 60, and 120 minutes constitute the minimum acceptable sampling. In dogs with pancreatic islet cell tumors, the glucose concentration does not exceed 135 mg/dl and drops to less than 50 mg/dl by approximately 60 minutes. Since the injection of glucagon can produce a profound hypoglycemia, the dog should be monitored closely during the test. If signs of hypoglycemia develop, intravenous glucose should be administered after obtaining a blood glucose sample.

Serum immunoreactive insulin (IRI) concentrations can also be used to diagnose functional pancreatic islet cell tumors. Many commercial laboratories measure serum IRI; however, results should be interpreted with caution unless the radioimmunoassay is a validated canine assay.

With some insulinomas serum IRI levels may fall in the normal range (8 to 20 μU/ml). To refine the diagnostic specificity of the serum IRI, several computed ratios have been advocated. The most useful ratio is the amended insulin-glucose ratio (AIGR). The AIGR is calculated by using the following equation:

$$\frac{\text{Serum insulin (μU/ml)} \times 100}{\text{Plasma glucose (mg/dl)} - 30}$$

This equation is based on the experimental observation that IRI values drop to 0 when plasma glucose concentrations are less than 30 mg/dl. Reported normal values for this ratio are less than 30 μU/mg glucose. The AIGR appears to be the most specific diagnostic test for functional pancreatic islet cell tumors. The diagnostic specificity of the glucagon tolerance test can be enhanced by drawing a serum IRI sample one minute after the glucagon injection and calculating the AIGR. One rationale for combining the glucagon tolerance test and the AIGR is if preliminary information is desired while awaiting the serum IRI results.

Unfortunately, there are no laboratory tests that reveal whether metastasis has occurred. Exploratory celiotomy is recommended because it is the treatment of choice and because it provides a means of determining prognosis. Exploratory celiotomy should include careful inspection of the liver, mesentery, and regional lymph nodes. Most pancreatic islet cell tumors are grossly visible.

Surgery should be considered palliative. Because of frequent metastasis, complete excision is rarely accomplished. Controlled clinical series comparing treated and untreated dogs are not available; however, it appears that surgery prolongs life.

Several problems can be associated with surgical management. Surgical manipulation can produce an intraoperative hypoglycemic crisis because of sudden insulin release or a postoperative pancreatitis. Although these sequelae are rare, intravenous glucose administration during surgery and close monitoring postoperatively for pancreatitis are warranted. Diabetes mellitus can occur postoperatively. This is usually transient. The presumed mechanism is prolonged increased levels of insulin, which result in feedback inhibition of the normal islet cells.

Medical treatment should be considered if surgery alone is not successful. The available drugs are not antineoplastic agents; however, they do exert a hyperglycemic effect. Diazoxide (Proglycem*) is effective orally at a dose of 10 mg/kg daily. As signs become refractory the dose can be increased to a maximum of 40 mg/kg daily. Unfortunately, eventually signs will recur even at the maximum dose. Propanolol has been shown to have a hyperglycemic effect in humans with functional pancreatic tumors. The value of this drug in dogs with insulinoma has not been demonstrated. Streptozotocin has been reported to be temporarily effective in controlling clinical signs; however, hepatic and nephrotoxicity are significant problems. Glucocorticoids may be temporarily effective in alleviating signs. Frequent high-protein meals are also recommended.

NONPANCREATIC TUMORS

Nonpancreatic islet cell tumors have also been implicated as a cause of hypoglycemia. Several mechanisms have been suggested for the development of hypoglycemia. Hypoglycemia could be due to the elaboration of insulin or other related hormonal factors by the neoplastic tissue. Another possibility is that large, rapidly growing tumors might utilize excessive amounts of glucose. Any tumor that has produced extensive hepatic destruction might potentially cause hypoglycemia, since the liver is the primary organ involved with glucogenesis. It has also been hypothesized that certain tumors might alter metabolic pathways in the liver.

In hypoglycemic humans with nonpancreatic tumors, increased levels of insulin-like growth factor have been demonstrated by means of a radioreceptor assay. Tumor types that have been associated with the reduced blood glucose levels and increased insulin-like growth factor levels include hemangiopericytoma, adrenocortical carcinoma, hepatocellular carcinoma, hepatoma, mesothelioma, and leiomyosarcoma.

Hypoglycemia has been reported in a dog with lymphosarcoma and a dog with a hepatoma. The precise pathogenesis of the hypoglycemia was not established in either case.

HYPOGLYCEMIA-KETONEMIA IN PREGNANT BITCHES

A well-documented and investigated case of hypoglycemia accompanied by ketonemia and ketonuria in a pregnant bitch was reported recently.

---

*Schering Corporation, Kenilworth, NJ.

Clinical signs were alleviated by the parenteral administration of glucose. Permanent remission of signs occurred following delivery of the pups by cesarean section. A variety of metabolic tests were performed following parturition to investigate the pathogenesis of the hypoglycemia. The precise mechanisms of the hypoglycemic episodes were not established, although several potential mechanisms were either directly or indirectly ruled out.

There are several similarities between this case and pregnancy toxemia of ewes. However, because of differences in carbohydrate metabolism in the ruminant it is not completely analogous.

IATROGENIC HYPOGLYCEMIA

The administration of excessively high doses of insulin to diabetic dogs is one of the more common causes of hypoglycemia. In most instances this is due to the failure to adequately control diet and exercise or to properly adjust the dose of insulin based on the daily urine glucose measurement. If the principles of diabetic regulation are reviewed with the client, this is usually a temporary problem. If problems with regulation persist even after correction of management or technical problems, a few unusual situations should be considered.

One possibility is that asymptomatic nocturnal hypoglycemia is activating the compensatory counter-regulatory hormonal mechanisms so that a rebound hyperglycemia occurs (Somogyi phenomenon). Testing of the morning urine reveals a significant glucosuria. If the dose of insulin is increased based on the presence of excessive urine glucose, the problem persists. Objective diagnostic criteria and incidence figures for this syndrome have not been established in the dog. Treatment is aimed at reducing rather than increasing the dose of insulin.

Another possibility that has recently been described in an insulin-dependent diabetic human is the absence of the normal release of counter-regulatory hormones in response to insulin-induced hypoglycemia. The nature and specific location of the lesion responsible for this defect was not identified. This problem has not been documented in the dog.

Drug interactions with insulin are another potential cause of hypoglycemia. Severe hypoglycemia has been reported in a human diabetic patient following high epidural anesthesia. Splanchnic sympathetic outflow is abolished during epidural block of spinal cord segments T_5 to L_1. This results in inhibition of hepatic glycogenolysis and catecholamine release by the adrenal medulla. This is unlikely to cause a problem in a normal dog; however, in an insulin-treated diabetic it might produce hypoglycemia. The infusion of intravenous glucose and reduction in the dose of local anesthetic should prevent the problem.

Hypoglycemia has been reported in humans as an untoward effect of disopyramide (Norpace), a new antiarrhythmic agent with quinidine-like actions. Since this drug is gaining acceptance as a canine antiarrhythmic, awareness of this potential side effect is important.

GLYCOGEN STORAGE DISEASES

The biosynthesis and degradation of glycogen are relatively complex. As a result of both chain elongation and branching, glycogen is a large molecule that resembles a bush in shape. Glycogen is the ready source of free blood glucose for emergencies. If any of the enzymes providing this free glucose are missing, serious metabolic consequences result.

The diseases of glycogen storage result when some defect in the pathways of glycogen synthesis or degradation results in the formation of an abnormal form of glycogen or excess amounts of glycogen. The standard classification of glycogenoses in humans is based on the enzyme whose defect causes the abnormality. Although various clinical parameters may be suggestive, ultimate documentation requires specific assay of the various enzymes on an appropriate biopsy specimen. Since some of these enzymes are quite labile, such specimens must be frozen immediately and assayed without delay. If these precautions are not taken, falsely low values may be obtained.

The only glycogen storage disease that has been documented in dogs is a deficiency of debranching enzyme. In the absence of this enzyme, phosphorylase cannot degrade glycogen beyond a certain point because the branch points cannot be attacked. According to the standard human classification scheme, this is type III or debrancher glycogen storage disease. This syndrome was reported in four young German shepherd dogs. These dogs displayed poor growth, weakness, ascites, and hypoglycemia.

Treatment in humans consists of frequent feedings and, in severely affected patients, surgical portocaval anastomosis. Phenytoin is useful in mildly affected individuals. Phenytoin does not alter levels of debrancher enzyme activity; therefore, a possible inhibitory action on insulin release has been postulated.

Type I glycogen storage disease or von Gierke's disease has frequently been discussed in the veterinary literature; however, no cases have been proven by assaying the specific enzyme, hepatic glucose-6-phosphatase. Humans with this disorder have an enlarged liver and kidneys, growth retardation, severe hypoglycemia, ketoacidosis, and elevated plasma lipids and lactate levels. Severe hepatomegaly and profound hypoglycemia are usually evident in the first few months of life. In man this is the most common form of glycogenosis. The indiscriminate use of this diagnosis in hypoglycemic pups is probably not warranted.

JUVENILE HYPOGLYCEMIA

This form of hypoglycemia is seen most frequently in 6- to 12-week-old puppies of toy or miniature breeds. Clinical signs include weakness, muscle twitching, ataxia, stupor, coma, and seizures. This form of hypoglycemia is frequently associated with an identifiable precipitating cause. Possible predisposing events include anorexia, hypothermia, starvation, gastrointestinal disturbances, and environmental changes. Inappropriate or incomplete development of various metabolic pathways has been suggested as the etiology of this syndrome. A case suggestive of this proposed mechanism has been reported. An 11-week-old Pomeranian was evaluated for hypoglycemia. A fasting blood glucose concentration of 16 mg/dl and abnormally low plasma alanine and pyruvate concentrations were demonstrated. Based on the laboratory results, glycogen storage disease, deficiency of gluconeogenic enzymes, and hyperinsulinemia were excluded. The authors concluded that because of the decreased plasma alanine and pyruvate levels, insufficient substrate was available for glucose production. The pup was maintained by providing a glucose solution *ad libitum* until 18 weeks of age. Beyond this age oral glucose solutions were not required. The dog was still normal at two years of age.

Prompt treatment of juvenile hypoglycemia is important. The intravenous administration of 50 per cent dextrose at the approximate dose of 1 to 2 ml/kg is recommended. This dose can be repeated as needed. Since 50 per cent dextrose is a hyperosmotic solution, it should be diluted with an equal volume of sterile water and infused slowly. In conscious dogs, honey or Karo syrup can be given orally. Dietary recommendations consist of small, frequent meals of high-protein, high-carbohydrate food. Identification and correction of any predisposing factors are essential parts of successful management of juvenile hypoglycemia.

NEONATAL HYPOGLYCEMIA

The neonatal animal is particularly prone to fasting hypoglycemia. There are several reasons for this predilection. The glucose requirements of neonates on a weight basis are two to three times greater than those of the adult. Proportionally, the protein content of the neonatal body is less than that of the adult, so there is less substrate available for gluconeogenesis. It has also been suggested that the normal glucose homeostatic mechanisms are not fully developed at birth and require several days for maturation.

Fortunately, the neonate appears to have unique protective mechanisms to avert irreversible damage. The neonatal heart and brain appear to be able to substitute lactic acid as the fuel for oxidative metabolism during hypoglycemia. Thus the neonate is more prone to hypoglycemia but is protected to a certain extent from its permanent pathologic consequences.

Hypoglycemia is frequently present in premature pups, hypothermic pups, septic pups, and pups suffering from toxic milk syndrome. The management of any sick neonate, regardless of apparent etiology, should include the administration of bitch's milk replacer or glucose and a balanced electrolyte solution by stomach tube.

SEPTIC SHOCK

Severe sepsis with concomitant hypoglycemia has recently been reported in four dogs. This is one of the few reports describing this as a clinical entity; however, there is a wealth of experimental literature detailing this syndrome. Extensive experimental studies have been performed in the dog to clarify the role of endotoxins and sepsis in the development of hypoglycemia. The precise pathogenesis of the hypoglycemia remains controversial, and there is experimental support for several different mechanisms. It has been shown that the endotoxic pancreas elaborates increased levels of insulin. Other investigations have demonstrated increased local utilization of glucose by muscle tissue independent of systemic insulin levels. Increased glucose utilization by bacteria and neutrophils either *in vivo* or artifactually *in vitro* has also been shown. Although the mechanism of the hypoglycemia has not been clarified, it has been established that the severity of hypoglycemia correlates with survival from experimentally induced sepsis.

Recent experiments in dogs have demonstrated enhanced survival from sepsis when antibiotics and glucocorticoids are used concurrently. The intravenous infusion of glucose-containing solutions may further enhance survival of septic patients.

MISCELLANEOUS

Canine Parvoviral Enteritis. In a recent clinical series of 134 dogs hospitalized with signs of parvoviral enteritis, 8.3 per cent had blood glucose concentrations of less than 75 mg/dl. Although hypoglycemia is not a common finding in dogs presenting with parvoviral enteritis, prompt recognition and appropriate therapy with intravenous infusions of glucose are important parts of the overall management of this infection. The mechanism of the hypoglycemia is unknown; however, it does not appear to be sepsis in the majority of cases.

Poisonings. Hypoglycemia is also occasionally associated with accidental poisonings. Mushrooms and other plant toxins such as tropical akee act as hepatotoxins and depress glycogen storage and gluconeogenesis. Certain acetylcholinesterase inhibitors produce hypoglycemia by effecting insulin release from the pancreas. Salicylate intoxication can produce hypoglycemia by increasing glucose utilization.

Hunting-dog Hypoglycemia. Hypoglycemia in hunting dogs has been described. The syndrome reportedly affects very nervous dogs one to two hours after beginning a hunt. Clinical signs include initial disorientation followed by generalized seizures. Recovery is prompt; however, the dog's performance is diminished for the rest of the day. Feeding a high-protein food frequently during the hunt appears to be prophylactic. Pulmonary edema has been associated with this syndrome. Extensive laboratory data substantiating this syndrome have not been published.

Hepatic Disease. Occasionally, dogs with severe liver disease are hypoglycemic. Clinically, it can be difficult to differentiate signs due to hepatic encephalopathy from those due to hypoglycemia.

Inanition. An infrequent cause of hypoglycemia in inanition due to intestinal malassimilation, starvation, neoplasia, or any severe debilitating disease.

Hypoadrenocorticism. A recent article comparing a series of cases of hypoadrenocorticism at one institution with previously reported cases indicates that hypoglycemia is not common in hypoadrenocorticism. Sixteen per cent of the previously reported cases were hypoglycemic, whereas 3 per cent of the cases at the single institution were hypoglycemic. The discrepancy in the frequency of hypoglycemia was attributed to differences in specimen handling, laboratory technique, or the cases themselves.

Primary Renal Glycosuria. Primary renal glycosuria has been mentioned as a cause of hypoglycemia. However, the published cases of proximal and distal renal tubular acidosis do not verify this.

Insulin Autoimmune Hypoglycemia. A small number of human cases have been described in which hypoglycemia has been associated with circulating antibodies to endogenous insulin. These patients have no history of exogenous insulin administration. The postulated mechanism of hypoglycemia is the sudden release of free insulin from a large pool of antibody-bound insulin. The cause of autoantibody production against endogenous insulin is unknown. This problem has not been reported in the dog.

SUPPLEMENTAL READING

Breitschwerdt, E. B., Loar, A. S., Hribernik, T. N., and McGrath, R. K.: Hypoglycemia in four dogs with sepsis. J.A.V.M.A. 178:1072, 1981.
Caywood, D. D., et al.: Pancreatic islet cell adenocarcinoma. Clinical and diagnostic features of 6 cases. J.A.V.M.A. 174:714, 1979.
DeSchepper, J., Van Der Stock, J., and DeRick, A.: Hypercalcemia and hypoglycemia in a case of lymphatic leukemia in the dog. Vet. Rec. 94:602, 1974.
Felig, P.: Disorders of carbohydrate metabolism. In Bondy, P. K., and Rosenberg, L. E. (eds.): Metabolic Control and Disease, 8th ed. Philadelphia: W. B. Saunders, 1980, pp. 364–369.
Jackson, R. F., Bruss, M. L., Growney, P. J., and Seymour, W. G.: Hypoglycemia-ketonemia in a pregnant bitch. J.A.V.M.A. 177:1123, 1980.
Johnson, R. K.: Insulinoma in the dog. Vet. Clin. North Am. 7:629, 1977.
Kahn, C. R.: The riddle of tumor hypoglycaemia revisited. Clin. Endocrinol. Metab. 9:355, 1980.
Strombeck, D. R., Krum, S., Meyer, D., et al.: Hypoglycemia and hypoinsulinemia associated with hepatoma in a dog. J.A.V.M.A. 169:811, 1976.
Strombeck, D. R., Rogers, Q., Freedland, R., et al.: Fasting hypoglycemia in a pup. J.A.V.M.A. 173:299, 1978.
Vannucci, R. C., Nardis, E. E., Vannucci, S. J., and Campbell, P. A.: Cerebral carbohydrate and energy metabolism during hypoglycemia in newborn dogs. Am. J. Physiol. 240:R192, 1981.

DIABETES INSIPIDUS

JOHN A. MULNIX, D.V.M.

Ft. Collins, Colorado

Diabetes insipidus (DI) is the syndrome that results from failure of the neurohypophyseal system to produce or release a quantity of antidiuretic hormone (ADH) sufficient to bring about the normal homeostatic renal conservation of free water. DI may be complete or partial, permanent or temporary, and is usually characterized by the production of large volumes of hypotonic urine. Figure 1 diagrammatically depicts the thirst-ADH-renal axis. Urine production in the dog and cat should not exceed 50 ml/kg of body weight per day, and the upper limit for normal water consumption is approximately 100 ml/kg of body weight per day.

The cause of DI in the majority of the cases is

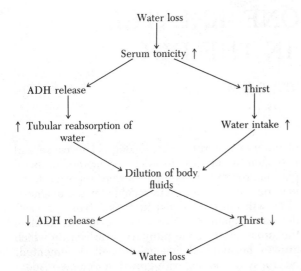

Figure 1. A double negative-feedback system of the thirst-ADH-renal axis to maintain a normal fluid balance in all body fluids (osmolality). (Modified from Oliver and Jamison: Postgrad. Med. 68:120, 1980.)

idiopathic. Other causes include congenital lack of ADH, primary or metastatic tumors, trauma, and vascular disease. DI may also be iatrogenic owing to surgical manipulation.

CLINICAL SIGNS

The main signs of disease are polyuria (PU) and polydipsia (PD), which may be severe with extreme volumes or mild with barely detectable PU/PD. In severe cases, patients may become emaciated owing to reduced intake of food. Vomiting due to stomach overdistension with water may also be observed. In many cases, the owner may note that the PU/PD was of sudden onset. Other signs may be present, depending on the underlying cause of ADH deficiency. These include incoordination, disorientation, convulsions, generalized lymphadenopathy, and others.

DIAGNOSIS

Demonstration of the production of an increased volume of urine that is hyposthenuric is the first step in diagnosis. The specific gravity of the urine is usually 1.001 to 1.005, and the urine osmolality is usually below 300 mOsm/kg (below the normal plasma osmolality). Plasma or serum osmolality is almost always elevated (greater than 320 mOsm/kg in severe cases of DI). In uncomplicated cases of DI, serum biochemical panels and complete blood counts (CBCs) may be within normal limits. When the cause of the DI is lymphosarcoma, the blood chemistry and CBC may reflect abnormalities.

For confirmation of the diagnosis of DI, it is necessary to demonstrate that the patient (1) cannot increase urine concentration during simple water deprivation but (2) can increase urine concentration following exogenous administration of ADH. For specific details on the protocol of testing water metabolism, the reader is referred to articles on the subject (Joles and Mulnix, 1977; Mulnix et al., 1976).

It is important to point out that the patient with severe DI cannot tolerate more than three to four hours maximum of water deprivation. Fluid loss due to iatrogenic water deprivation should not be allowed to exceed more than 5 per cent of total body weight.

TREATMENT

Several drugs are available for replacement of deficient ADH. Long-acting vasopressin tannate in oil (Pitressin Tannate in Oil* 5 pressor units/ml) is the most commonly used preparation in the management of chronic DI in the dog. A dose of 2.5 units given subcutaneously or intramuscularly through a 20-gauge needle will control polyuria for an average of 36 to 72 hours regardless of the size of the dog. Care must be taken to shake the preparation vigorously before injection, since the hormone gradually settles from the vehicle. The drug should not be readministered until some return of PU/PD is evident. This prevents hyponatremia from cumulative water retention (Oliver and Jamison, 1980).

Desmopressin acetate (APDDV†) intranasal drops are supplied in 2.5-ml vials. The product should be stored in the refrigerator. One drop is administered every eight hours intranasally. In patients that will not tolerate intranasal administration, one drop may be administered in the conjunctival sac.

Lypressin (Diapid Nasal Spray‡) does not appear to be suitable for treatment of DI in the dog or cat because of its short duration of action.

---

*Parke-Davis, Morris Plains, NJ.
†Armour Pharmaceutical Co., Tarrytown, NY.
‡Sandoz Pharmaceuticals, East Hanover, NJ.

REFERENCES

Joles, J. A., and Mulnix, J. A.: Polyuria and polydipsia. *In* Kirk, R. W. (ed.): *Current Veterinary Therapy VI*. Philadelphia, W. B. Saunders, 1977, pp. 1050–1054.
Mulnix, J. A., Rijnberk, A., and Hendricks, H. J.: Evaluation of a modified water deprivation test for diagnosis of polyuric disorders in dogs. J.A.V.M.A. 169:1327, 1976.
Oliver, R. E., and Jamison, R. L.: Diabetes insipidus, a physiologic approach to diagnosis. Postgrad. Med. 68:120, 1980.

GROWTH HORMONE–RELATED DERMATOSES IN THE DOG

DANNY W. SCOTT, D.V.M.

Ithaca, New York

Growth hormone–related dermatoses are rare in the dog. Three syndromes have been described: pituitary dwarfism, growth hormone–responsive dermatosis in the mature dog, and acromegaly.

PITUITARY DWARFISM

Canine pituitary dwarfism is usually a hereditary hypopituitarism associated with bilaterally symmetric alopecia and hyperpigmentation and variable thyroidal, adrenocortical, and gonadal abnormalities.

In the German shepherd dog and Carnelian bear dog, pituitary dwarfism is thought to be inherited as a simple autosomal recessive condition. Most affected dogs have a variably sized cyst (cystic Rathke's cleft) in the pituitary gland, resulting in varying degrees of anterior pituitary (adenohypophyseal) insufficiency. However, a few dogs have had either hypoplastic or normal anterior pituitary glands. The clinical signs are related to growth hormone (somatotropin) deficiency, with or without concurrent thyroid, adrenocortical, and gonadal abnormalities.

Canine pituitary dwarfism has been reported in many breeds but predominantly in the German shepherd dog and Carnelian bear dog breeds. No sex predilection is evident.

For the first two to three months of life, the dogs may appear normal. After this time, the dogs fail to grow and the haircoat is notably short, with no development of primary hairs. The puppy coat of secondary hairs, which is soft, woolly, and easily epilated, is retained. Primary hairs are often present only on the face and distal extremities. Bilaterally symmetric alopecia then develops, especially in the wear areas of the neck and caudolateral aspects of the thighs. The alopecic skin is at first normally pigmented, then progresses through increasing degrees of hyperpigmentation. The skin becomes thin, hypotonic, and scaly. Comedones may be numerous. Gonadal status may vary from atrophic testicles and absence of estrus to normal development.

GROWTH HORMONE–RESPONSIVE DERMATOSIS IN THE MATURE DOG (PSEUDO-CUSHING'S SYNDROME)

Growth hormone–responsive dermatosis is a bilaterally symmetric alopecia and hyperpigmentation of otherwise normal mature dogs. The cause and pathogenesis of this disorder are unknown. Basal plasma growth hormone levels were reported to be low, but such levels are unreliable for the diagnosis of growth hormone deficiency. Skin biopsy reveals decreased amounts of dermal elastin, identical to the situation in canine pituitary dwarfism, in which growth hormone deficiency is well documented. Necropsy of one dog with growth hormone–responsive dermatosis demonstrated moderate atrophy of the pituitary gland.

Growth hormone–responsive dermatosis has been recognized predominantly in male dogs of the chow chow, Keeshond, Pomeranian, and miniature poodle breeds. Age of onset is usually one to two years old. The disorder is characterized by bilaterally symmetric alopecia and hyperpigmentation, which occurs mainly on the trunk, neck, pinnae, tail, and caudomedial thighs. Hairs in affected areas are easily epilated. In chronic cases, the skin may be thin, hypotonic, and scaly. Aside from the dermatologic signs, the dogs are otherwise normal.

ACROMEGALY

Canine acromegaly is characterized by inspiratory stridor, thick skin, hypertrichosis, abdominal enlargement, polyuria-polydipsia, and fatigue associated with hypersecretion of growth hormone in the mature animal.

Acromegaly is caused by hypersecretion of growth hormone in the mature animal (after epiphyseal closure). In the dog, acromegaly has been reported in association with injections of anterior pituitary gland extracts, eosinophilic hyperplasia of the anterior pituitary gland, diestrus in the intact cycling bitch, and administration of progestational compounds.

There are no evident breed or age predilections for canine acromegaly. Most cases have occurred in intact female dogs either in diestrus or being treated with progestational compounds. The most common signs noted in canine acromegaly include inspiratory stridor (due to soft tissue increases in the orolingual/oropharyngeal regions), increased body size, abdominal enlargement, polyuria/polydipsia, fatigue, and frequent panting. Cutaneous changes include thickened, myxedematous skin thrown into excessive folds and hypertrichosis. Some dogs have enlarged interdental spaces.

852

DIAGNOSIS OF GROWTH HORMONE–RELATED DERMATOSES

Diagnosis of these disorders is based on history, physical examination, laboratory findings, skin biopsy, and plasma growth hormone level and stimulation tests. Depending on the degree of anterior pituitary insufficiency, dogs with *pituitary dwarfism* may have laboratory findings consistent with hypothyroidism and secondary adrenocortical insufficiency. In addition, radiographic examination of dogs with pituitary dwarfism may reveal failure of the epiphyses of long bones to close, delayed eruption of permanent teeth, and failure of the os penis to completely mineralize by one year of age.

Skin biopsy in dogs with *pituitary dwarfism and growth hormone–responsive dermatosis* reveals changes consistent with endocrinopathy (orthokeratotic hyperkeratosis, follicular keratosis, follicular dilatation, follicular atrophy, telogen hair follicles predominating, sebaceous gland atrophy, epidermal melanosis, and thin dermis). A highly suggestive finding is decreased amount and size of dermal elastin fibers. In dogs with *acromegaly*, skin biopsy reveals increased amounts of collagen and mucin as well as hyperplasia of the epidermis and appendages.

Basal plasma growth hormone levels (by radioimmunoassay) in normal dogs approximate 1.8 to 4.5 µg/ml in most reports. However, basal plasma growth hormone levels are very unreliable for the documentation of growth hormone deficiency. Clonidine (Catapres*), an alpha-adrenergic/antihypertensive drug, has been used to stimulate growth hormone release in the dog and document growth hormone deficiencies. Normal dogs show a marked increase in plasma growth hormone levels within 15 to 30 minutes after the intravenous injection of 10 to 30 µg/kg of clonidine, whereas pituitary dwarfs and hypophysectomized dogs fail to respond. Xylazine (Rompun†) gives similar results when administered intravenously at 100 to 300 µg/kg.

Dogs with *acromegaly* have markedly elevated basal plasma growth hormone levels (11 to 1476 ng/ml), which are not suppressible by an intravenous glucose load (1 gm glucose/kg).

---

*Boehringer Ingelheim Ltd., Ridgefield, CT.

†Bayvet Div., Cutter Laboratories Inc., Shawnee Mission, KS.

TREATMENT OF GROWTH HORMONE–RELATED DERMATOSES

Bovine or porcine growth hormone has been used to treat *pituitary dwarfism and growth hormone–responsive dermatosis.* Five to ten units are administered subcutaneously every other day for 5 to 15 injections. A beneficial response in the skin and haircoat is seen within one to three months. Remission may last from six months to over three years. In dogs with pituitary dwarfism, growth plates close rapidly, and no appreciable increase in stature is achieved.

Repeated injections of bovine and porcine products into dogs could produce hypersensitivity reactions, but such reactions have not been reported. Induction of diabetes mellitus is a known side effect of growth hormone administration in the dog, and two dogs with growth hormone–responsive dermatosis became transiently diabetic after three to five injections of bovine growth hormone. At that time therapy was terminated. Bovine or porcine growth hormone is not presently available commercially.

Dogs with acromegaly associated with diestrus or progestational compound administration have responded well to ovariohysterectomy or cessation of progestogen therapy, respectively.

SUPPLEMENTAL READING

Andresen, E., and Willeberg, P.: Pituitary dwarfism in German Shepherd dogs: additional evidence of simple, autosomal recessive inheritance. Nord. Vet. Med. 28:481, 1976.

Andresen, E., and Willeberg, P.: Pituitary dwarfism in Carnelian bear-dogs: evidence of simple, autosomal recessive inheritance. Hereditas 84:232, 1976.

Eigenmann, J. E.: Diagnosis and treatment of dwarfism in a German Shepherd dog. J. Am. Anim. Hosp. Assoc. 17:798, 1981.

Eigenmann, J. E., and Venker-van Haagen, A. J.: Progestogen-induced and spontaneous canine acromegaly due to reversible growth hormone overproduction: clinical picture and pathogenesis. J. Am. Anim. Hosp. Assoc. 17:813, 1981.

Hampshire, J., and Altszuler, N.: Clonidine or xylazine as provocative tests for growth hormone secretion in the dog. Am. J. Vet. Res. 42:1073, 1981.

Lund-Larsen, T. R., and Grondalen, J.: Ateliotic dwarfism in the German Shepherd dog. Low somatomedin activity associated with apparently normal pituitary function (2 cases) and with pan-adenopituitary dysfunction (1 case). Acta Vet. Scand. 17:298, 1976.

Parker, W. M., and Scott, D. W.: Growth hormone responsive alopecia in the mature dog: a discussion of 13 cases. J. Am. Anim. Hosp. Assoc. 16:824, 1980.

Scott, D. W., Kirk, R. W., Hampshire, J., and Altszuler, N.: Clinicopathological findings in a German Shepherd with pituitary dwarfism. J. Am. Anim. Hosp. Assoc. 14:183, 1978.

Siegel, E. T.: *Endocrine Diseases of the Dog.* Philadelphia: Lea & Febiger, 1977.

GLUCOCORTICOID THERAPY

ROBERT C. ROSENTHAL, D.V.M.,

Urbana, Illinois

and JEFF R. WILCKE, D.V.M.

Blacksburg, Virginia

Adrenal corticosteroids that process glucocorticoid activity, represented by cortisol and corticosterone, influence the metabolic processes of nearly every cell in the body. Glucocorticoids possess an unparalleled range of effects because the cell type affected determines the nature of the response. The structural differences among the glucocorticoids influence the intensity, duration, and subsequent clinical significance of these effects. These effects also vary over a wide range of tissue concentrations.

PHYSIOLOGIC CONTROL OF SECRETION

Glucocorticoids play a critical role in the maintenance of homeostasis. To fulfill this role, concentrations of circulating glucocorticoid must be responsive to the animal's external as well as internal environment. The central nervous system responds to these environments and moderates the anterior pituitary and, ultimately, the adrenal gland by regulating the production of corticotropin-releasing factor (CRF) in the hypothalamus (Fig. 1). CRF secretion is increased in response to stimuli that signal increased glucocorticoid need. Exercise, trauma, and cold are among the stimuli to which the hypothalamus responds. CRF secretion is inhibited by adrenocorticotropic hormone (ACTH) and cortisol.

ACTH, produced by the anterior pituitary, directly mediates the concentration of circulating glucocorticoids produced by the adrenal gland. Its release is stimulated by CRF and inhibited by cortisol (see Fig. 1). Glucocorticoid concentrations are independent of ACTH control when a cortisol-producing tumor that does not require ACTH for its function is present or when exogenous glucocorticoids are administered.

The cortisol secreted by the zona fasciculata of the adrenal cortex represents new synthesis rather than release from storage. ACTH interacts with receptors on the surface of adrenocortical cells to activate adenylate cyclase. Increased levels of cyclic adenosine monophosphate (cAMP) produced by this enzyme appear to cause the phosphorylation (activation) of another enzyme that is rate limiting in the synthesis of corticosteroids.

The secretion rate of glucocorticoid in the dog, represented by a variety of compounds, is physiologically equivalent to 1.0 mg/kg/day of cortisol. For the cat, cow, and horse this secretion rate has not been established, but for purposes of calculating replacement doses it is often assumed to be the same.

Corticosteroids, secreted directly into the blood stream, are transported either as free steroid or bound to plasma protein. Corticosteroids are either specifically bound to corticosteroid-binding globulin (CBG) or nonspecifically to albumin. The equilibrium established between free and protein-bound glucocorticoid is influenced by the structure of the glucocorticoid molecule such that synthetic glucocorticoids are, in general, less avidly bound. Because only free glucocorticoid is active, decreased protein binding increases the relative potency of a particular product. Hypoproteinemia may also cause increases in the free glucocorticoid concentration, necessitating a reduction in dose to achieve an equivalent amount of activity.

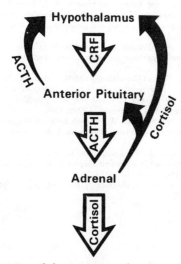

Figure 1. Hypothalamic-pituitary-adrenal axis. Solid black arrows represent negative feedback.

EFFECTS ON INTERMEDIARY METABOLISM

The regulation of intermediary metabolism is of central importance to the actions of the glucocorticoids. The physiologic and pharmacologic effects can, by and large, be related to changes in the metabolism of glucose, proteins, and lipids.

EFFECTS ON GLUCOSE METABOLISM

Administration of a glucocorticoid results in an increase in the concentration of glucose in the blood. An increase in gluconeogenesis, a decrease in new protein synthesis, altered lipid metabolism, and an anti-insulin effect all contribute to this action.

An increase in the synthesis of glucose from noncarbohydrate sources, gluconeogenesis, is the result of an increase in the quantity of necessary precursors. Induction of messenger RNA directly, via new enzyme production, results in an increase in tyrosine transaminase and tryptophan 2,3 dioxygenase. Increased concentrations of these enzymes hasten the catabolism of their amino acid substrates, tyrosine and tryptophan, which can serve as glucose precursors.

Increased gluconeogenic precursors, released from protein and lipid stores, cause a decrease in glucose breakdown via the Embden-Meyerhof pathway. There is concurrently an indirect induction of the enzymes of this pathway that make gluconeogenesis possible.

EFFECTS ON PROTEIN AND LIPID METABOLISM

Peripheral protein synthesis is also decreased, resulting in a relative increase in catabolism as compared with anabolism. This effect is exhibited clinically as muscle atrophy, thinning of the skin, and delayed healing as a result of decreased collagen synthesis.

Lipid metabolism is also affected by the glucocorticoids. Long–chain fatty acid synthesis is inhibited. Glucocorticoids must be present for the mobilization of free fatty acids from fat stores.

ANTI-INSULIN EFFECTS

Glucocorticoids exert an anti-insulin effect by decreasing glucose utilization peripherally and increasing glycogen synthesis in the liver. Although glucocorticoid administration does not, in itself, cause diabetes mellitus, it can unmask an animal's predisposition to the disease. A possible exception would be the appearance of diabetes mellitus sec-

Table 1. *Systemic Effects of Glucocorticoids*

Tissue, Organ, or Function	Effects
Central nervous system	Euphoria and behavioral changes
	Maintenance of alpha rhythm
	Lower seizure threshold
Autonomic nervous system	Required for normal sensitivity of adrenergic receptors
Gastrointestinal tract	Decreased calcium and iron absorption
	Facilitation of fat absorption
	Increased in acid, pepsin, and trypsin secretion
	Structural alteration of mucin
Skeletal muscle	Weakness (excess and deficiency)
	Muscle atrophy (excess)
Skin	Atrophy and thinning (excess)
Hematopoietic system	Involution of lymphoid tissue
	Decrease in peripheral lymphocytes, monocytes, and eosinophils
	Increase in neutrophils, platelets, and RBCs
	Decreased clotting time
	Decreased phagocyte competence
Cardiovascular system	Positive ionotropic effect
	Increased blood pressure owing to increased blood volume
Kidneys	Increased reabsorption of water, sodium, and chloride
	Increased excretion of potassium and calcium
	Increased extracellular fluid volume
Bone	Inhibition of collagen synthesis by fibroblasts
	Acceleration of bone resorption
	Antagonism of vitamin D
Cells	Stabilization of liposomal membranes
	Inhibition of macrophage response to migration-inhibiting factor
	Sensitization of lymphocytes blocked
	Cellular response to inflammatory mediators blocked
	Inhibition of fibroblast proliferation
Reproductive tract	Parturition induced during the latter part of pregnancy in ruminants and horses; effect in dog and cat unknown
	Teratogenesis during early pregnancy

ondary to glucocorticoid-induced pancreatitis. It should be remembered that insulin therapy for regulated diabetics may have to be altered if glucocorticoids are administered.

SYSTEMIC EFFECTS

An outline of the systemic effects of glucocorticoids appears in Table 1. Some of the effects are essential for homeostasis, such as the maintenance of normal alpha rhythm and adrenergic receptor responsiveness. Effects such as stabilization of lysosomal membranes and inhibition of fibroblast proliferation become apparent at supraphysiologic doses and represent desirable pharmacologic effects. Muscle atrophy and thinning of the skin appear only after prolonged glucocorticoid administration or abnormal secretion. The extent of these effects is dependent on the quantity of glucocorticoid administered, the potency of the preparation (related to structure), the time of administration relative to the diurnal cycle, the tissue half-life (also structure related), and the duration of glucocorticoid administration.

GLUCOCORTICOIDS AS DRUGS

STRUCTURE-ACTIVITY RELATIONSHIPS

The carbon skeleton common to all steroid hormones is depicted in Figure 2A. This carbon skeleton imparts to the steroid hormones considerable affinity for proteins, most specifically the steroid receptor found in the cytoplasm of target cells. Protein affinity also leads to the high degree of plasma protein binding associated with steroid hormones. Substitutions on this carbon skeleton produce sex hormones, mineralocorticoids, and glucocorticoids.

Critical to the differential clinical effects of various corticosteroids is the absolute dependence of function on structure. The structure of cortisol (hydrocortisone) is shown in Figure 2B. Certain structural features of hydrocortisone (circled) are essential for glucocorticoid activity. Alterations in the chemical nature or steric configuration of these features abolish this activity. For example, prednisone has an 11-ketol substituted for the 11-hydroxyl radical of prednisolone. Prednisone must be converted to prednisolone by reduction of the 11-ketol in the liver before it is active. *If hepatic function is in doubt, the active drug prednisolone should be administered in preference to the pro-drug prednisone.*

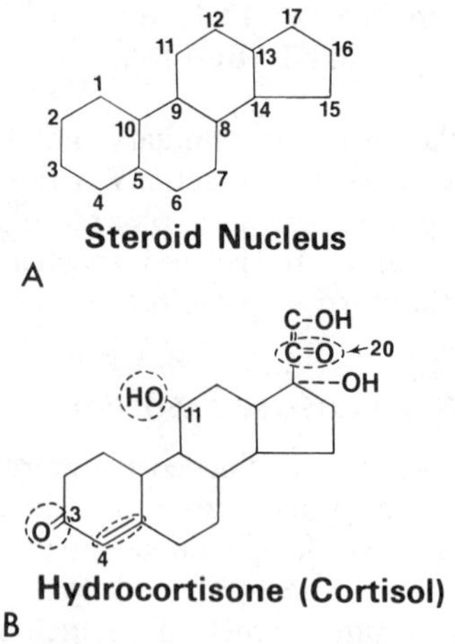

Steroid Nucleus

A

Hydrocortisone (Cortisol)

B

Figure 2. *A*, Steroid nucleus. *B*, Structure of cortisol. Circled structures are essential for glucocorticoid activity.

Synthetic glucocorticoids have been produced to minimize undesirable mineralocorticoid effects and enhance glucocorticoid activity. For example, the addition of 1,2 double bond to the cortisol molecule produces the compound prednisolone with approximately a fourfold increase in glucocorticoid activity. The addition of further substituents to the prednisolone molecule produces dexamethasone (16 methyl, 9 fluoroprednisolone), a compound with markedly enhanced anti-inflammatory activity and negligible mineralocorticoid effect. It is unfortunate that attempts to decrease metabolic effects while maintaining anti-inflammatory potency have been unsuccessful. It would appear that increases in anti-inflammatory properties lead to increases in undesirable hypothalamic-pituitary-adrenal axis suppression.

Modifications of glucocorticoid molecular structure also produce changes in biotransformation, binding to cortisol-binding globulin, and tissue affinity. The net result of these changes is an increase in biologic half-life and subsequent duration of effect of the synthetic glucocorticoids as compared with cortisol. Table 2 lists the common glucocorticoids, their substituents, relative glucocorticoid potencies, and approximate durations of hypothalamic-pituitary-adrenal axis suppression.

ESTERS OF GLUCOCORTICOIDS

Parenteral solutions of glucocorticoids are available as esters that vary in water solubility and hence the rate at which they are absorbed from injection sites. If therapy is to be rational, the clinician must know not only the duration of activity for the particular glucocorticoid base he has chosen but also the absorption and bioavailability characteristics of the ester.

Table 2. *Comparison of Corticosteroid Bases*

Base	Relative Glucocorticoid Potency	Mineralocorticoid Effect	Daily Replacement Equivalent Dose (mg)*	Duration of Hypothalamic-Pituitary-Adrenal Suppression (hr)	Modifications of Hydrocortisone to Produce New Compounds
Short-Acting					
Hydrocortisone	1	+ +	20	12	
Cortisone	0.8	+ +	25	12	11 ketol
Intermediate-Acting					
Prednisone	3.5	+	5	12–36	11 ketol; 1,2% bond
Prednisolone	4.0	+	5	12–36	1,2% bond
Methylprednisolone	5.0	0	4	12–36	6 # methyl; 1,2,% bond
Triamcinolone	5.0	0	4	12–36	9 # fluoro; 16 # hydroxyl; 1,2% bond
Long-Acting					
Paramethasone	10	0	2	> 48	6 # fluoro; 16 # methyl; 1,2% bond
Betamethasone	25	0	0.6	> 48	9 # fluoro; 16 β methyl; 1,2% bond
Dexamethasone	30	0	0.75	> 48	9 # fluoro; 16 # methyl; 1,2% bond

*For 20-kg dog.

Hemisuccinate and phosphate esters are the most water-soluble products available. They should be selected when rapid glucocorticoid effect is desired and whenever the intravenous route of administration is chosen. They are also suitable for intramuscular and subcutaneous injections. Absorption from intramuscular and subcutaneous sites will be complete in 30 to 60 minutes, giving high blood concentrations rapidly. The duration of activity will be that of the glucocorticoid base.

Acetate, diacetate, and tebutate glucocorticoid esters are poorly water soluble. Absorption from these suspensions is slow and sustained, making them suitable for intra-articular or intralesional injection. High concentrations of glucocorticoids will be maintained in these sites for extended periods of time. Given intramuscularly, these esters form depots, maintaining concentrations of glucocorticoid in the serum for 2 to 14 days, depending on the total dose employed and the particular product selected. This method of administration is sometimes employed when sustained glucocorticoid effect is desired and oral administration is inadvisable or impossible. However, the therapist should be aware that such use may cause prolonged suppression of the hypothalamic-pituitary-adrenal axis.

Acetonide esters are also poorly water soluble. In addition, they bind specifically to keratin, leading to their use as topical medications with relatively less systemic absorption and subsequent toxicity. Injected intramuscularly, acetonides also form sustained release depots and should be utilized accordingly.

Preparations of commonly used glucocorticoids are listed in Table 3.

REPLACEMENT GLUCOCORTICOID THERAPY

Primary adrenocortical insufficiency (Addison's disease) results from any disease process that destroys the adrenal cortex. Idiopathic hypoadrenocorticism, thought to be an immune-mediated disease, is the most frequent diagnosis, although granulomatous inflammation, hemorrhagic infarctions, metastatic disease of the adrenal glands, and amyloidosis of the adrenal cortices have been diagnosed in the dog. The adrenolytic drug *o,p'*-DDD (Lysodren), useful in the management of hyperadrenocorticism, may produce iatrogenic primary adrenocortical insufficiency. The clinical signs produced result primarily from aldosterone loss and the ensuing mineral imbalances.

Secondary hypoadrenocorticism occurs with prolonged reduction in the secretion of ACTH. Destructive disease processes of the pituitary or hypothalamus, most often pituitary or central nervous system tumors, may result in such a reduction. More commonly, the hypothalamic-pituitary-adrenal axis suppression that accompanies chronic glucocorticoid administration results in the appearance of hypoadrenocorticism when the glucocorticoids are withdrawn.

The management of primary hypoadrenocorticism requires replacement therapy with mineralocorticoids, which is accomplished in a variety of ways. Patients can be maintained by the subcutaneous implantation of desoxycorticosterone acetate pellets (Percorten) or with monthly injections of desoxycorticosterone pivalate. Daily oral administration of 9-fluorohydrocortisone acetate (Florinef) has been used successfully. The dose of Florinef is adjusted

Table 3. *Available Glucocorticoid Products*

Base	Oral	Intravenous, Rapid Intramuscular	Intralesional, Intra-articular, Depot, Intramuscular	Topical
		Route of Administration		
Betamethasone	Free base	Sodium phosphate	Sodium phosphate + acetate	Free base Benzoate Dipropionate Valerate
Cortisone	Acetate		Acetate	
Dexamethasone	Free base	Sodium phosphate	Acetate	Free base
Fluprednisolone	Free base			
Hydrocortisone	Free base Cypionate	Sodium phosphate Sodium succinate	Acetate	Free base Acetate
Meprednisone	Free base			
Methylprednisolone	Free base	Sodium succinate	Acetate	Acetate
Paramethasone	Acetate			
Prednisolone	Free base	Sodium phosphate Sodium succinate	Acetate Tebutate Sodium phosphate + acetate	Free base Acetate Sodium succinate powder
Prednisone	Free base			
Triamcinolone	Free base Acetonide Diacetate		Acetonide Diacetate Hexacetonide	Free base Acetonide

according to concentrations of serum electrolytes. Although Florinef has some glucocorticoid activity itself, some dogs will require replacement with additional glucocorticoid. This is best accomplished with daily doses of short- to intermediate-acting glucocorticoids. The dosage should be kept as low as possible while still controlling clinical signs.

The treatment of secondary adrenal insufficiency requires the replacement of glucocorticoid activity. The aim of this therapy is to mimic normal adrenal secretion of cortisol. This can be achieved in the dog by administering 0.2 mg/kg of prednisolone each morning. As mineralocorticoid activity is often normal in these dogs, it is usually desirable to administer drugs in which glucocorticoid activity is present and mineralocorticoid activity is minimal. Equivalent doses of prednisone, prednisolone, and other glucocorticoid bases are presented in Table 2.

In addition to daily replacement doses of corticosteroids, additional glucocorticoid must be administered to these dogs any time stress occurs. The daily dose of glucocorticoid should be increased from two to five times until the stressful situation is resolved.

ANTI-INFLAMMATORY AND IMMUNOSUPPRESSIVE THERAPY

Glucocorticoids profoundly affect both immunologic and inflammatory activity in numerous ways. They have nonspecific vascular and tissue effects as well as those more specifically related to their anti-inflammatory and immunosuppressive actions. Important glucocorticoid effects, with regard to inflammatory and immunologic activity, include those on (1) traffic, movement, and circulatory capability of cells; (2) functional capability of cells; and (3) production, secretion, and binding of and response to some humoral factors.

The impact of glucocorticoids on cell movement is very important. Mononuclear and polymorphonuclear cells are affected. Neutrophils are released from bone marrow stores under the influence of glucocorticoids. Their half-life is prolonged and their migration to and accumulation at inflammatory sites is blocked. Glucocorticoids reduce neutrophil adherence to vascular endothelium. These alterations in neutrophil kinetics result in a granulocytosis. The major anti-inflammatory mechanism of glucocorticoids on cellular elements is to prevent neutrophils from reaching the inflammatory site. Eosinophils are redirected out of the peripheral circulation into other body compartments. Lymphocytes are also redirected from the peripheral circulation. It is important to remember, however, that the various subpopulations of lymphocytes are affected to different degrees. T-lymphocytes appear to be more profoundly affected than other lymphocyte populations. T-lymphocytes with IgM receptors may be more affected than those with IgG receptors. The final effects, expressed as functional response, will depend on the relative depletion of both the responding cells and accessory cell populations (helper and suppressor T-lymphocytes) necessary for their activity.

Glucocorticoids affect cell function by modifying

inflammatory and immunologic responses. Glucocorticoids stabilize the lysosomal membranes of neutrophil granules, inhibiting the release of enzymes, which are important in the inflammatory response. The phagocytic and bacteriocidal ability of neutrophils may also be decreased by glucocorticoids *in vitro*, but it is less clear whether this is also true *in vivo* with attainable drug concentrations. Monocyte microbicidal function is impaired at lower drug concentrations. Lymphocyte functions are also profoundly affected. A wide range of lymphocyte functions, including but not limited to, cell activitation, proliferation, differentiation, mediator production and release, response to mediators, antigen recognition, and cytotoxic effector function, is important in inflammatory and immunologic responses. The effects on both effector and mediator lymphocyte populations must again be considered. The final functional lymphocyte capability will be affected by the response of various lymphocyte subpopulations.

Although antibody production does not seem to be suppressed by glucocorticoid administration, there may be a decreased response and antibody effect. Another important humoral effect is the inhibition of macrophage response to lymphocytes that modulate their activity. Glucocorticoid interference with binding to cell receptors affects functions related to humoral factors. Glucocorticoids may also affect prostaglandin production and release.

There are other factors involved in inflammatory and immunologic reactions. It is not always possible to clearly differentiate where one begins and the other ends. The effects of glucocorticoids are seen on both types of reactions (Fig. 3). There are several principles to keep in mind regarding glucocorticoid protection against inflammatory damage.

1. The response is nonspecific relative to the noxious stimulant. Inflammation due to bacterial invasion, immune complex deposition, trauma, snake bite, or other causes will be inhibited by glucocorticoid action.

2. The drug must reach the site of inflammation to be effective, and its effect, in that respect, is local action.

3. The degree of anti-inflammatory response and cellular protection from injury is proportionate to the concentration of glucocorticoids in the involved inflamed tissue.

Because of the overlap of inflammatory and immunologic reactions and their parallel response to glucocorticoids, the specific goal of therapy with these drugs varies depending on the nature and severity of the disease process. This implies that doses and dose intervals should vary depending on the patient's specific needs. Initially an accelerated inflammatory response, as in flea allergy dermatitis, must be inhibited and the deleterious effects checked. Therapy is often initiated at 0.5 to 1.0 mg/ kg of prednisolone or its equivalent every 12 hours for three to five days. Inhibition of the immune system, as required for therapy of pemphigoid diseases, may require twice this amount. Once initiated, glucocorticoid therapy should be modified to achieve the smallest dose necessary to control the

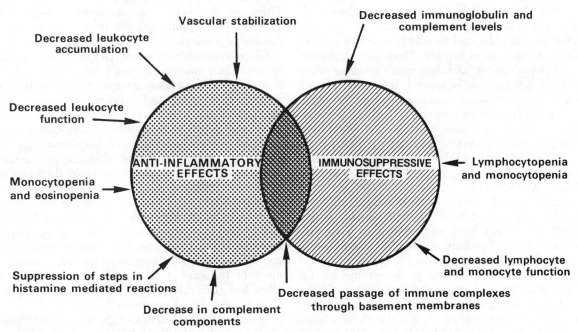

Figure 3. The overlap of anti-inflammatory and immunosuppressive effects of glucocorticoid therapy. (After Fauci et al.: Ann. Intern. Med. 84:304, 1976.)

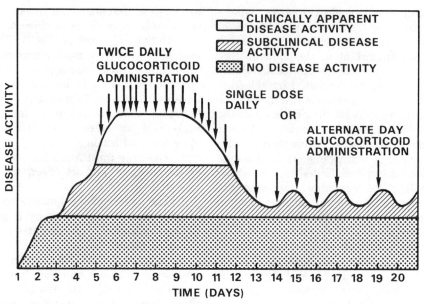

Figure 4. The effect of glucocorticoid administration on the manifestation of disease. (After Fauci et al.: Ann. Intern. Med. 84:304, 1976.)

disease. If the stimulus for the reaction is removed, therapy can be stopped. If the stimulus remains but the response has been controlled, once-a-day therapy may be instituted. It is advisable for patients requiring long-term glucocorticoid administration to utilize alternate-morning therapy to minimize adverse drug effects (Fig. 4).

ANTINEOPLASTIC THERAPY

Most chemotherapeutic agents are selected for their ability to kill cancer cells. Cytotoxic drugs also affect normal cells, and toxicity is usually a limiting factor in this type of therapy. Hormones, however, have the advantage of being much more selective in their actions and, in general, less toxic. Several mechanisms of hormone action relevant to cancer treatment have been proposed. Steroid hormones enter the cell and bind to a specific cytoplasmic receptor protein, forming a complex. "Transformation" ("activation") of this complex allows its translocation across the nuclear membrane, where it binds to DNA. Once bound to DNA, the steroid hormone has effectively altered the transcription of the cell's messenger RNA, resulting in new protein synthesis. It has been suggested that a steroid-induced rise in free fatty acids causes dissolution of the nuclear membrane, leading to cell death.

Corticosteroids are used in cancer therapy for both their primary and secondary effects. Of the corticosteroids, prednisone is most commonly used as a chemotherapeutic agent. It is the glucocorticoid action of these hormones that is important in their antineoplastic effect. Prednisone has been chosen

by oncologists because of its relative freedom from undesirable side effects. It has no specific antitumor properties not found in other glucocorticoids. Because prednisone must be converted to the active form, prednisolone, by the liver, the question arises "Why prednisone rather than prednisolone?" In theory, it is preferable to avoid the use of a prodrug when the active form is available. In practice, the conversion of prednisone to prednisolone is rapid and essentially complete in the normal liver. There are, however, instances in which such conversion may be impaired. On theoretical grounds, the use of prednisolone should be encouraged.

Glucocorticoids may be used for their tumoricidal effects. Their most widespread use in this context is certainly in the chemotherapy of lymphoreticular neoplasms. Prednisone has been used, often with dramatic (if not long-term) results as both a single agent and as part of combination chemotherapeutic protocols for canine and feline lymphosarcoma. It should be remembered that although prednisone alone may cause a marked and rapid decrease in the size of enlarged peripheral lymph nodes, such therapy should not be instituted in the absence of at least a cytologic diagnosis. Glucocorticoid therapy could send a lymphosarcoma into an apparent, although brief, remission. Early single-agent therapy of this type can complicate the later management of the case. Combination chemotherapy is often less successful when it follows an early glucocorticoid-induced remission.

In addition to its use as a single agent, prednisone is often used with other chemotherapeutic agents. The fraction of tumor cells killed by each drug is independent of that killed by the others. Such combination chemotherapies are, therefore, structured to employ drugs that (1) attack the cell cycle at different points and (2) have different toxicities. The place of glucocorticoids in such a scheme is that of a cell cycle nonspecific agent with limited myelosuppressive potential. The single best chemotherapeutic approach to lymphosarcoma is not known. Many protocols result in a remission, but true cure of lymphosarcoma remains elusive. It is, therefore, important to understand the role of glucocorticoids in such therapies. The recognition of the parts played by the various chemotherapeutic agents leads to a more rationale structuring of protocols and, hopefully, to more effective ones. In the search for the "best chemotherapy," protocols undergo frequent revision. The astute clinician should keep abreast of the details of current protocols and chose one that best suits the needs of his patients.

Glucocorticoids are used as primary therapy in neoplasms other than lymphoreticular tumors. As for lymphosarcoma, prednisone has been used as both a single agent and in combination chemotherapy for mast cell tumors. The effect of cortisone on mass cell tumors was first reported in 1952, but a specific mechanism of tumor killing, other than those already alluded to, has not been defined. Although it has been suggested that combination chemotherapy is more efficacious than single-agent therapy, mast cell tumors may follow an unpredictable course, and it is difficult to identify the true best therapy. Single-agent therapy may be as effective as combined modalities and seems to be finding renewed favor. The use of prednisone alone has the advantage of being relatively safe and free of serious side effects.

Long-acting glucocorticoids have also been used in the treatment of mast cell tumors. Triamcinolone acetonide or diacetate (0.25 mg/kg) can be injected intralesionally at weekly intervals until the tumor disappears. It appears that there is a direct effect on the tumor as well as control of localized inflammatory responses. This approach seems best suited to the treatment of localized rather than disseminated disease.

In addition to its use in lymphoreticular neoplasm and mast cell tumors, glucocorticoids may be useful in the treatment of other solid cancers. The effects of glucocorticoids are by no means limited to those on lymphoid cells. As a glucocorticoid, prednisone has widespread effects on carbohydrate metabolism as well as protein and fat synthesis. When given in large doses, powerful suppressant effects on these functions of both normal and neoplastic cells might be expected. These effects would apply to neoplastic tissues that were not necessarily hormone dependent for their growth. However, such a chemotherapeutic strategy is not commonly undertaken. High-dose glucocorticoid therapy of solid tumors, in general, would probably result in a therapeutic index (median toxic dose divided by median effective dose) of 1 or less. This low therapeutic index is an expression of the high relative toxicity of the protocol in question and is unacceptable in the clinical situation. Keeping in mind that it is usually toxicity that limits chemotherapy, it is best to avoid high-dose glucocorticoid therapy for tumors not known to be particularly susceptible to the effects of corticosteroids.

Glucocorticoids have the unique advantage among the chemotherapeutic agents of being able to cross the blood-brain barrier. This opens for consideration the possibility of their use in the treatment of tumors of the central nervous system. The approach seems most reasonable in lymphoreticular neoplasms of the central nervous system. It is generally considered that the important role of glucocorticoids in the therapy of brain tumors is secondary. The reduction of intracranial pressure and the lessening of cerebral edema surrounding brain tumors may relieve symptoms without actually killing tumor cells. The use of glucocorticoids in brain tumors may provide some palliation but cannot be recommended as effective long-term primary therapy.

INTENSIVE SHORT-TERM THERAPY

Glucorticoids in high doses for short periods of time (48 hours or less) have been advocated to reduce the morbidity and mortality that accompany a variety of disease states. In some cases, glucocorticoids are an essential part of emergency therapy; in others their use is considered controversial.

Glucocorticoids are of considerable value in the treatment of shock, which accompanies acute adrenocortical insufficiency. The first objective of therapy is to restore circulating blood volume by administering 0.9 per cent sodium chloride solution. Glucocorticoid therapy then restores vascular sensitivity to norepinephrine from sympathetic nerves, increases blood glucose, and reverses weakness and depression. Hydrocortisone is chosen because it provides glucocorticoid as well as mineralocorticoid activity. When the patient's condition is stable, 0.09 mg/kg desoxycorticosterone is given to provide control of electrolyte homeostasis.

Glucocorticoids are considered to be lifesaving in animals that have suffered inhalation of smoke or noxious gases (sulfur dioxide, nitrogen dioxide) or aspiration of gastric contents. They inhibit the increased pulmonary capillary permeability that follows these insults and often leads to fulminant pulmonary edema.

The use of massive doses of glucocorticoids for therapy of shock other than that associated with hypoadrenocorticism remains controversial. We quote the conclusions of Reichgott and Melmon, who state: "The available data concerning the efficacy of corticosteroids in shock are not as conclusive as the common use of these agents would imply." A protective effect of glucocorticoids has been demonstrated for endotoxemic, hemorrhagic, and cardiogenic shock when massive doses are given prior to or at the time of the shock stimulus. However, these studies do not represent the clinical setting in which an animal is in the advanced stages of shock when presented for treatment.

The utility of glucocorticoids for the reduction of central nervous system edema is also equivocal. As stated previously, most studies support their usefulness in improving the neurologic status of human and animal patients with brain tumors. A decrease in edema by dexamethasone administration following trauma or hemorrhage has been demonstrated by some investigators and refuted by others. The mechanisms by which glucocorticoids may benefit the neurologic patient have not been elucidated. Generally, dosages of dexamethasone in the range of 2 mg/kg every eight hours are recommended.

Although complications of short-term (48 to 72 hours) glucocorticoid therapy are rare, they have been reported in the veterinary medical literature. Toombs and coworkers reported four cases of fatal colonic perforation in dachshunds treated with dexamethasone following neurosurgical procedures (1980). Knecht and associates (1978) noted behavioral changes (aggressive and paranoid behavior, amaurosis, disorientation, and ataxia) in a Doberman pinscher following the accidental ingestion of 250 mg of prednisone and, at a later date, a tube of triamcinolone acetonide ointment. In human patients, glucocorticoid therapy has been associated with pseudotumor cerebri; gastric ulcer; perforation of the colon, cecum, and rectum; as well as pancreatitis and a variety of metabolic disturbances. Until the benefits of acute, high-dose glucocorticoid therapy are better elucidated, it is prudent to consider the potential risks of such therapy. Without demonstrable benefit, benefit/risk ratios cannot be favorable to the patient.

ALTERNATE-DAY GLUCOCORTICOID THERAPY

Any patient receiving glucocorticoid therapy for longer than 14 days is a candidate for alternate-day therapy. The initial therapy for these patients will likely be once or twice daily administration to achieve remission of clinical signs. Once the disease is in remission, a single dose of an intermediate-acting glucocorticoid can be administered on alternate days in a dose equivalent to that being employed over a 48-hour period. For example, a patient receiving 10 mg of prednisolone once a day would be given 20 mg of prednisolone on alternate days.

Glucocorticoids suitable for this method should have a duration of action of 12 to 36 hours. Prednisolone, prednisone, and methylprednisolone are suitable for this method. It can be seen that the hypothalamic-pituitary-adrenal axis will be given a steroid-free rest for a portion of the 48-hour period. This steroid-free interval will allow the axis to maintain some degree of responsiveness to external stimuli. Triamcinolone, considered intermediate in the duration of its effects, has been proved neither satisfactory nor unsatisfactory for this method. Dexamethasone, betamethasone, and paramethasone certainly are not suitable, because single doses of these agents suppress the hypothalamic-pituitary-adrenal axis for 48 hours or longer.

It is often recommended that the daily dose schedule be "tapered" to alternate days. That is, the daily steroid dose is increased prudently on day one, decreased by an equal amount on day two, increased on day three, and so on until the total dose is the same as that given for 48 hours during the initial therapy. This tapering is likely to be essential only for patients already experiencing suppression of the hypothalamic-pituitary-adrenal axis. If the decision to begin alternate-day therapy is made early in the treatment course, tapering is probably unnecessary. It is important to note that exacerbations of the disease need to be treated with high doses of glucocorticoids daily until remission is again evident.

Alternate-day therapy does not *eliminate* undesirable side effects. In a study involving 28 healthy dogs, Chastain and Graham (1979) showed that both daily and alternate-day prednisone therapy resulted in adrenocortical atrophy and hypofunction, but the suppression was less severe and of slower onset when alternate-day treatment was given. Even when alternate-day therapy is optimal, the clinician should be mindful of the potential adverse effects of glucocorticoid therapy (Table 4).

TERMINATION OF GLUCOCORTICOID THERAPY

As stated previously, hypothalamic-pituitary-adrenal axis suppression produced by glucocorticoid therapy is influenced by the chemical nature and dosage of glucocorticoid used, the duration of therapy, and the time of glucocorticoid administration relative to the diurnal cycle. The degree of this suppression will, in part, determine the manner in which glucocorticoid therapy may safely be terminated. In addition, the activity of the underlying disease process will affect the success of such termination.

The hypothalamic-pituitary-adrenal axis recovers in three stages. Initially, plasma concentrations of both ACTH and cortisol will remain low. As the pituitary gland recovers its function, ACTH concentrations rise and cortisol remains low. Finally, the

HYPERADRENOCORTICISM

Table 4. *Clinical Complications of Corticosteroid Therapy*

Endocrine effects	Iatrogenic hyperadrenocorticism
	Adrenal insufficiency following withdrawal
	Unmasking of preclinical diabetes mellitus
CNS effects	Nervousness
	Mood changes
	Pseudotumor cerebri
Ocular effects	Cataracts
Digestive effects	Pancreatitis
	Ulceration
	Hepatopathy
Metabolic effects	Growth retardation
	Hyperglycemia
	Generalized catabolism
Musculoskeletal effects	Osteoporosis
	Myopathy, weakness, wasting
Dermatologic effects	Urticaria
	Calcinosis cutis

adrenal gland begins to function and cortisol concentrations rise. In humans, this process may take 9 to 12 months to be completed, depending on the initial degree of suppression. In the dog, there have been no studies completed to determine the time course for this recovery. Clinical experience suggests that this time is shorter in dogs than in humans.

For patients withdrawn from chronic therapy, it is advisable to taper the dose of glucocorticoid over a period of several months. As mentioned previously, in some cases it may be necessary to change gradually to an alternate-day regimen before attempting to further reduce the dosage and finally eliminate it altogether. Many of these patients require supplemental glucocorticoids to survive stressful situations during the recovery period and certainly need such supplementation if surgery is to be performed.

It is unclear at this time what role ACTH administration may play in the recovery of chronically suppressed patients. It may, in fact, be contraindicated. It should be stated, however, that ACTH will only hasten the recovery of the adrenal gland. The hypothalamus and pituitary will remain unresponsive. For these reasons, we have not used ACTH in the treatment of secondary hypoadrenocorticism.

SUMMARY

Individual patients and diverse disorders respond differently to given doses of glucocorticoid. Therefore, it is impossible to make specific dose recommendations for glucocorticoid therapy. Such therapy is facilitated by an understanding of (1) the physiology of the hypothalamic-pituitary-adrenal axis; (2) the comparative potencies, durations, and adverse effects of the available corticosteroid bases and their esters; and especially (3) the specific goals of the therapy for a wide variety of diseases.

REFERENCES AND SUPPLEMENTAL READING

Azarnoff, D. L. (ed.): *Steroid Therapy*. Philadelphia: W. B. Saunders, 1975.

Chastain, C. B., and Graham, C. L.: Adrenocortical suppression in dogs on daily and alternate-day prednisone administration. Am. J. Vet. Res. 40:936, 1979.

Fauci, A. S.: Mechanisms of the immunosuppressive and antiinflammatory effects of glucocorticosteroids. J. Immunopharmacol. 1:1, 1978.

Fauci, A. S., Dale, D. C., and Balow, J. C.: Corticosteroid therapy: mechanisms of action and clinical considerations. Ann. Intern. Med. 84:304, 1976.

Feldman, E. C., and Owens, J. M.: Fundamentals of physiology of the adrenal cortex. Vet. Clin. North Am. 7:549, 1977.

Knecht, C. D., Henderson, B., and Richardson, R. C.: Central nervous system depression associated with glucocorticoid ingestion in the dog. J.A.V.M.A. 173:91, 1978.

Rosenthal, R. C.: Hormones in cancer therapy. Vet. Clin. North Am. 12:1, 1982.

Toombs, J. P., Caywood, D. D., Lipowitz, A. J., et al.: Colonic perforation following neurosurgical procedures and corticosteroid therapy in four dogs. J.A.V.M.A. 177:68, 1980.

Wilcke, J. R., and Davis, L. E.: Review of glucocorticoid pharmacology. Vet. Clin. North Am. 12:1, 1982.

HYPERADRENOCORTICISM

MARK E. PETERSON, D.V.M.

New York, New York

Spontaneous canine hyperadrenocorticism (Cushing's syndrome) is a disorder that results from excessive cortisol production by the adrenal cortex. The clinical signs of canine Cushing's syndrome include polyuria and polydipsia (approximately 85 per cent of cases), abdominal distention (75 per cent), anestrus (70 per cent), lethargy (70 per cent), hepatomegaly (70 per cent), polyphagia (70 per cent), muscular weakness and atrophy (50 per cent), bilateral symmetric alopecia (40 per cent), testicular atrophy (40 per cent), comedones (35 per cent), and calcinosis cutis (10 per cent). Hematologic testing may show leukocytosis, eosinopenia, lymphopenia, and mild erythrocytosis. Serum biochemical abnormalities may include elevated alkaline phosphatase, alanine aminotransferase, asparate aminotransferase, cholesterol, and glucose concentrations. Several of these clinical signs and abnormal laboratory findings occurring together suggest Cushing's syndrome; however, many dogs with the disorder exhibit only a few of them.

Two separate conditions cause spontaneous canine Cushing's syndrome: in pituitary-dependent Cushing's disease, the pituitary produces excessive adrenocorticotropic hormone (ACTH) and causes bilateral adrenocortical hyperplasia; in hyperadrenocorticism caused by adenoma or carcinoma of the adrenal cortex, excessive cortisol is autonomously secreted. Treatment is different for these two conditions. Specific laboratory tests must be used to definitively diagnose Cushing's syndrome and to differentiate pituitary-dependent Cushing's disease from adrenal tumors.

LABORATORY DIAGNOSIS

PLASMA CORTISOL DETERMINATIONS

Three techniques can be used to measure plasma cortisol concentration: fluorometric assay, competitive protein binding, and radioimmunoassay. Fluorometric assay is less specific and sensitive and tends to give false high values of cortisol concentration. Whatever method is used for measurement, cortisol values may differ significantly from laboratory to laboratory.

Single basal plasma cortisol determinations are not very useful in diagnosis, because values overlap between normal dogs and dogs with Cushing's syndrome. In both normal and cushingoid dogs the adrenal glands secrete cortisol episodically, i.e., in intermittent short bursts throughout the day; in addition, the half-life of cortisol is only about 60 minutes. Stress is another factor that stimulates the adrenal glands to secrete unpredictably. Consequently, the episodic secretion and short half-life of cortisol plus extrinsic factors can cause wide variations in plasma cortisol concentrations, resulting in a pattern of peaks and valleys throughout the day. Peaks of cortisol concentration in a normal dog frequently overlap with valleys in a cushingoid dog, so that a single cortisol determination reveals little about a dog's adrenal function.

ACTH STIMULATION TEST

A useful test for diagnosing Cushing's syndrome is the ACTH stimulation test. Several ACTH preparations are available, and many regimens for ACTH stimulation testing have been described. One method is to collect plasma samples for cortisol determination before and two hours after intramuscular administration of ACTH gel (20 units). With this regimen, a maximum rise in plasma cortisol concentrations occurs two hours after administration of ACTH; cortisol concentrations usually return to basal levels within ten hours after injection.

Post-ACTH cortisol concentrations in normal dogs are at least two to three times higher than basal levels. Results of an ACTH stimulation test are diagnostic for Cushing's syndrome when the post-ACTH cortisol concentration exceeds the upper limit of normal, indicating a greater than normal adrenal response. Approximately 90 per cent of dogs with pituitary-dependent Cushing's disease have an excessive response to ACTH stimulation. Over one-half of dogs with adrenocortical tumors hyperrespond; of these, dogs with adrenal carcinoma tend to hyperrespond more frequently and have higher responses than dogs with adenomas.

The ACTH stimulation test is a valuable screening test for canine Cushing's syndrome because it tests the functional capacity of the adrenal glands to secrete cortisol. The ACTH stimulation test is, however, limited in its usefulness. If Cushing's syndrome is suspected clinically, the diagnosis should not be excluded based on normal ACTH stimulation test results, since many dogs with adrenal tumors respond normally to ACTH stimulation. The test is also limited because it cannot be used to reliably distinguish pituitary-dependent Cushing's disease from that caused by adrenal tumors, since the majority of dogs with pituitary-dependent Cushing's syndrome and approximately one-half of dogs with functional adrenocortical tumors have an exaggerated response.

LOW-DOSE DEXAMETHASONE SUPPRESSION TEST

In normal dogs, pituitary ACTH secretion is regulated by the central nervous system (CNS). Neurotransmitters such as serotonin, dopamine, and norepinephrine direct the hypothalamus to produce corticotropin-releasing factor, which travels to the pars distalis via the hypophyseal portal system and stimulates ACTH secretion. The canine pituitary pars intermedia also secretes ACTH, but unlike the pars distalis it is avascular and is controlled by serotonergic and dopaminergic fibers from the brain. Pituitary ACTH is the major regulator of cortisol secretion. Normally, rising circulating cortisol concentrations decrease secretion of ACTH through CNS and pituitary negative feedback inhibition; as ACTH secretion decreases, cortisol secretion also decreases and physiologic levels of circulating cortisol are maintained. This negative feedback control system of ACTH-cortisol secretion is called the hypothalamic-pituitary-adrenal axis. Potent synthetic analogues of cortisol, such as dexamethasone, also inhibit pituitary ACTH release through negative feedback. In Cushing's syndrome, the pituitary-adrenal axis controlling ACTH and cortisol secretion is abnormally resistant to suppression by dexamethasone.

To perform the low-dose dexamethasone suppression test, we collect a baseline morning plasma sample for cortisol assay, administer dexamethasone (0.015 mg/kg IM), and collect additional plasma samples two, four, six, and eight hours post injection. In a normal dog, this small dose of dexamethasone consistently suppresses cortisol concentrations to less than 1.0 µg/dl for the eight-hour test period.

Figure 1 shows mean low-dose dexamethasone suppression test results from dogs with pituitary-dependent Cushing's disease, dogs with adrenal tumors, and normal dogs; compared with normal dogs, the two groups of cushingoid dogs are resistant to suppression with this dose of dexamethasone. In many of the dogs with pituitary-dependent Cushing's disease, cortisol is suppressed to near-normal

concentrations two and four hours after injection but rises to the presuppression level by the eighth hour, whereas in normal dogs suppression continues throughout the test. The samples drawn six and eight hours after injection are the most important for interpretation of the test.

The low-dose dexamethasone suppression test can be used to confirm Cushing's syndrome, but it cannot reliably differentiate between pituitary-dependent Cushing's disease and adrenal tumors. These two conditions should be distinguished by measurement of plasma ACTH concentrations and high-dose dexamethasone suppression testing.

PLASMA ACTH DETERMINATIONS

Plasma ACTH concentrations determined by radioimmunoassay are useful in determining the cause of Cushing's syndrome. Plasma ACTH concentrations are normal to elevated in dogs with pituitary-dependent Cushing's disease and are low in dogs with adrenocortical tumors. Determination of single basal plasma ACTH concentrations is not useful as a screening test for Cushing's syndrome, because, like cortisol, ACTH is secreted episodically with overlapping values in normal and cushingoid dogs.

The normal to high plasma ACTH concentrations in dogs with pituitary-dependent Cushing's disease indicate secretion of inappropriate and excessive amounts of ACTH by a pituitary tumor and/or defect in the CNS negative feedback mechanism. Low to undetectable concentrations of ACTH in dogs with adrenal tumors reflect normal negative feedback control of pituitary ACTH secretion; high circulating cortisol concentrations suppress ACTH secretion through the negative feedback system to low or undetectable levels.

Difficulty in obtaining plasma ACTH assays may offset their usefulness. Plasma ACTH assays are technically difficult to perform, and many commercial laboratories may be unable to give consistently reliable results. Cost may be prohibitive. Samples must be collected and stored carefully, because plasma ACTH adheres to glass and is unstable in unfrozen plasma. Blood for ACTH assay should be drawn in cold, heparinized, plastic syringes; placed on ice; and spun immediately in plastic tubes in a refrigerated centrifuge. Plasma should then be separated into plastic tubes and kept frozen until assayed.

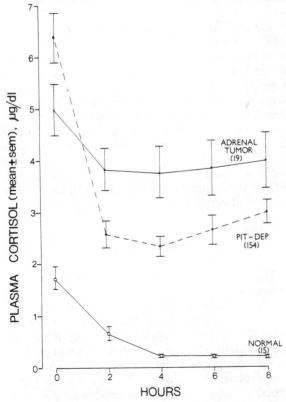

Figure 1. Mean plasma cortisol concentrations during low-dose dexamethasone suppression testing in normal dogs and dogs with pituitary-dependent Cushing's disease and adrenocortical tumors. Plasma cortisol concentrations in both groups of cushingoid dogs are resistant to suppression compared with normal dogs.

HIGH-DOSE DEXAMETHASONE SUPPRESSION TEST

The high-dose dexamethasone suppression test is very useful in determining the cause of canine Cushing's syndrome. The low-dose dexamethasone suppression test, discussed earlier, is a screening test for Cushing's syndrome; the low dose of dexamethasone suppresses ACTH and subsequently cortisol in normal dogs but does not suppress cortisol secretion in dogs with either pituitary-dependent Cushing's or functional adrenal tumors. In dogs with functional adrenal tumors, dexamethasone at any dosage will not suppress cortisol levels, because ACTH secretion has been suppressed by high circulating concentrations of cortisol from the tumor. In pituitary-dependent Cushing's disease, the threshold for glucocorticoid negative feedback of ACTH is higher than normal; ACTH secretion is relatively resistant to glucocorticoid suppression, but high doses of dexamethasone can suppress ACTH secretion in pituitary-dependent Cushing's disease.

To perform the high-dose dexamethasone suppression test, we collect samples for plasma cortisol assay before and two, four, six, and eight hours after administration of dexamethasone (1.0 mg/kg). Figure 2 shows mean high-dose dexamethasone suppression test results in dogs with pituitary-dependent Cushing's disease and adrenal tumors. The high dose of dexamethasone suppresses cortisol in the dogs with pituitary-dependent Cushing's disease; cortisol is not suppressed in the dogs with adrenal tumors, clearly separating them from the

pituitary-dependent group. In our laboratory we have established that suppression of cortisol concentrations below 1.5 µg/dl is diagnostic for pituitary-dependent Cushing's disease, but this value will not necessarily be the same for other laboratories. The six- and eight-hour samples are the most important, because suppression is greatest at these times.

This test reliably distinguishes pituitary-dependent Cushing's disease from adrenal tumors in most cases, but in approximately 10 per cent of dogs with pituitary-dependent Cushing's disease, adequate cortisol suppression does not occur. In most of these dogs adequate cortisol suppression occurs when testing is repeated with a higher dose of dexamethasone, but in a few dogs suppression does not occur even with a dexamethasone dose as high as 2 mg/kg. Dogs in which adequate suppression does not occur invariably have pituitary tumors; however, even if adequate suppression does occur, pituitary adenomas cannot be excluded, since about 80 per cent of all dogs with pituitary-dependent Cushing's disease have tumors arising from either the pars distalis or the pars intermedia, identifiable at necropsy. Most of these tumors are not prognostically ominous because they are small and slow growing and rarely compromise the dog's neurologic function.

Figure 3 shows a flow sheet of diagnostic tests useful in evaluating a dog suspected of having Cushing's syndrome. The screening tests confirm or exclude persistent cortisol overproduction. In approximately 85 per cent of dogs with Cushing's syndrome, both the ACTH stimulation test and the low-dose dexamethasone suppression test are abnormal; in about 15 per cent of dogs, only one of these screening tests will be abnormal. For the dogs in which adequate suppression does not occur even with very high doses of dexamethasone, plasma ACTH determination or surgical exploration of the adrenal glands is diagnostic.

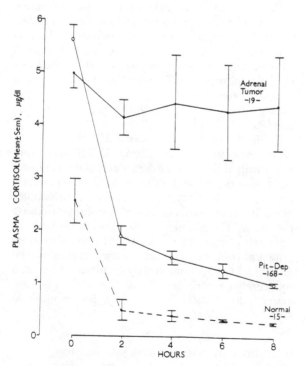

Figure 2. Mean plasma cortisol concentrations determined during high-dose dexamethasone suppression testing in dogs with pituitary-dependent Cushing's disease and adrenocortical tumors. Plasma cortisol is suppressed in the dogs with pituitary-dependent Cushing's; no suppression occurs in dogs with adrenal tumors.

TREATMENT

The cause of Cushing's syndrome determines treatment. Unilateral adrenocortical tumors should be surgically removed. Pituitary-dependent Cushing's disease may be treated surgically with bilateral adrenalectomy or hypophysectomy, or it may be treated medically with *o,p'*-DDD, cyproheptadine, or bromocriptine. Without treatment, canine pituitary-dependent Cushing's disease is usually a progressive disorder with an unfavorable prognosis. In a minority of dogs with very mild, slowly progressive disease, the clinical signs may be intermittent with periods of remission and relapse; observation may be the treatment of choice in these dogs.

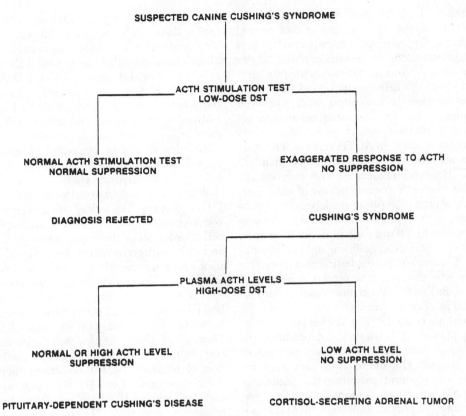

Figure 3. Flow chart for evaluation of suspected canine Cushing's syndrome. DST = dexamethasone suppression test.

ADRENOCORTICAL TUMORS

Adrenocortical tumors should be surgically removed. Using a ventral midline approach, the surgeon can inspect both adrenal glands and search for possible metastasis. With unilateral adrenocortical tumors, the contralateral adrenal gland atrophies and may be difficult to identify. If both adrenals are enlarged, nonsuppressible pituitary-dependent Cushing's disease should be suspected; biopsy of one adrenal gland confirms this diagnosis. After the unilateral adrenal tumor is located, the ventral midline incision can be extended paracostally for better exposure. Because the unaffected adrenal gland is chronically suppressed and atrophied, large doses of glucocorticoids must be given during and immediately after surgery. During surgery 100 to 200 mg hydrocortisone, 25 to 50 mg prednisolone sodium succinate, or 3 to 5 mg dexamethasone should be added to the infusion drip. During the first postoperative day, glucocorticoid supplementation should be continued at five times maintenance dosage using either cortisone acetate (2.5 mg/kg b.i.d.) or prednisone (0.5 mg/kg b.i.d.). The glucocorticoid should be gradually tapered to maintenance dosage (cortisone acetate, 0.5 mg/kg b.i.d., or prednisone, 0.2 mg/kg s.i.d.) over the first postoperative week; the medication can be given orally when tolerated. Glucocorticoids should be continued at maintenance dosage until the remaining adrenal is functioning normally as shown by ACTH stimulation testing; in most dogs glucocorticoids can be discontinued within two months of surgery.

About one-half of adrenal tumors are carcinomas with liver metastasis. These can be treated with o,p'-DDD in dosages as high as 50 to 150 mg/kg daily; however, because of the poor prognosis and very limited success in treatment, euthanasia should be considered. If the owner refuses euthanasia and o,p'-DDD therapy is ineffective, inhibitors of adrenocortical secretion such as aminoglutethimide or metyrapone can be used; although both drugs decrease steroid production, neither destroys tumor cells.

PITUITARY-DEPENDENT CUSHING'S DISEASE

Pituitary-dependent Cushing's disease can be treated with either bilateral adrenalectomy or hypophysectomy; both require a skilled surgeon, intensive monitoring during and after surgery, and lifelong hormone replacement therapy. Surgical techniques and management are described in *Current Veterinary Therapy VII*.

Pituitary-dependent Cushing's disease can also

be managed with drugs that act on either the adrenal glands or the pituitary gland and central nervous system. Cyproheptadine (Periactin*), a serotinin antagonist, produces remission about 50 per cent of the time in human patients with pituitary-dependent Cushing's disease. Increased CNS serotonin concentration is associated with increased pituitary-adrenal function; cyproheptadine may act to block the stimulatory effect of increased CNS serotonin concentration on ACTH release. The drug might also act directly on the pituitary gland to inhibit ACTH secretion because the pars distalis also contains moderate concentrations of serotonin. In our study of dogs with pituitary-dependent Cushing's disease, cyproheptadine was given in dosages ranging from 0.3 to 3.0 mg daily in divided dosages; only 10 per cent of dogs had clinical and biochemical remission. Although cyproheptadine is a very safe drug (major side effects are increased appetite and weight gain), its limited effectiveness makes it useful only for trial in very mild cases.

Bromocriptine (Parlodel†), a dopamine agonist, also lowers plasma ACTH levels and produces remission in some humans with pituitary-dependent Cushing's disease. Dopamine is a precursor for norepinephrine, a neurotransmitter that indirectly inhibits ACTH secretion. Bromocriptine may enhance the norepinephrine inhibition of ACTH secretion; alternately, the drug may directly affect the pituitary to decrease ACTH secretion. In our study of seven dogs with pituitary-dependent Cushing's disease, bromocriptine was given orally in slowly increasing dosages up to 0.1 mg/kg daily in divided doses. Side effects were common and included vomiting, anorexia, depression, and behavior changes; treatment was discontinued after one to two weeks in three of these dogs because of severe side effects. The remaining four dogs were treated for two to seven months. Only one of these dogs had a clinical remission, whereas the remaining three dogs failed to improve clinically.

Cyproheptadine and bromocriptine appear to have limited usefulness in the management of canine pituitary-dependent Cushing's disease. The drugs can induce remission in some dogs, but daily administration to maintain remission, frequent relapse, and serious side effects are problems associated with the administration of these drugs.

The drug used most frequently in the treatment of canine pituitary-dependent Cushing's disease is *o,p'*DDD (Lysodren‡). It decreases cortisol production by selective necrosis and atrophy of the adrenocortical zona fasciculata and zona reticularis. Initial dosage of *o,p'*-DDD is 50 mg/kg daily for ten days; glucocorticoid supplementation with either predni-

sone (0.2 to 0.4 mg/kg daily) or cortisone (1 to 2 mg/kg daily) reduces many side effects associated with acute glucocorticoid withdrawal in the initial phase. In dogs with concomitant diabetes mellitus, a reduced initial dosage of *o,p'*-DDD (25 to 35 mg/kg daily) prevents rapid reduction in daily insulin requirement, which predisposes to hypoglycemia. With adequate instruction most owners can manage this treatment successfully at home.

The dog should be evaluated after the induction period. Most dogs are more active and no longer polydipsic or polyuric. There are many parameters that can be used to assess the effectiveness of *o,p'*-DDD therapy, including measurement of daily water consumption and eosinophil and lymphocyte cell counts. All of these parameters are nonspecific and only indirectly reflect the level of plasma cortisol. A more direct approach to determine the effectiveness of *o,p'*-DDD therapy is to repeat the ACTH stimulation test; if control is adequate, both basal and post-ACTH cortisol concentrations should be within the normal resting range (1 to 4 μg/dl). During *o,p'*-DDD therapy, a decrease in circulating cortisol results in loss of negative feedback inhibition of pituitary ACTH secretion; therefore, episodic secretion of ACTH continues at extremely elevated levels. If adequate adrenocortical tissue remains, elevated ACTH concentrations still cause plasma cortisol concentrations to rise above normal range at frequent intervals throughout the day. In dogs that continue to respond to exogenous ACTH with post-ACTH cortisol concentrations above the normal resting range (4 μg/dl), daily therapy should be continued until a response is seen; this may require as long as 45 days in some dogs.

Once normal cortisol levels are documented by ACTH stimulation testing, *o,p'*-DDD should be continued at maintenance dosages of 50 mg/kg weekly in divided doses. Glucocorticoid supplementation is rarely required during maintenance therapy; however, during periods of stress appropriate dosages of glucocorticoid should be administered. Complete remission of all clinical signs may take from three to five months in some dogs. Dogs on maintenance *o,p'*-DDD therapy commonly have relapses; approximately one-half of those treated have a relapse within the first year. To ensure continued control and prevent serious relapse during *o,p'*-DDD therapy, ACTH stimulation testing should be repeated after three months of maintenance therapy and every six months thereafter. If basal and post-ACTH cortisol concentrations rise above the normal range (4 μg/dl), the *o,p'*-DDD dosage should be increased to 50 mg/kg daily for five days, and the weekly maintenance dosage should be increased by approximately 50 per cent to prevent further relapse.

The most common side effects observed during *o,p'*-DDD therapy include anorexia, vomiting, leth-

---

*Merck Sharp & Dohme Research Laboratories, Rahway, NJ.
†Sandoz Pharmaceuticals, East Hanover, NJ.
‡Bristol Laboratories, Syracuse, NY.

argy, and depression. In most cases these signs result from inadequate concentrations of cortisol and resolve promptly with glucocorticoid supplementation; few, if any, adverse signs result from a direct o,p'-DDD effect. If adverse signs occur during loading or maintenance o,p'-DDD therapy, the drug should be stopped and glucocorticoid supplementation given; if clinical signs persist longer than two to three hours after glucocorticoid therapy, the dog should be re-evaluated to exclude other medical problems. In most cases, low basal and ACTH-stimulated cortisol values (1.0 µg/dl) causing clinical signs increase spontaneously within two weeks; maintenance o,p'-DDD therapy should then be resumed.

SUPPLEMENTAL READING

Peterson, M. E., and Drucker, W. D.: Advances in the diagnosis and treatment of canine Cushing's syndrome. Gaines Vet. Symp. 1981, p. 17.

Peterson, M. E., Gilbertson, S. R., and Drucker, W. D.: Plasma cortisol responses to exogenous ACTH in 22 dogs with hyperadrenocorticism caused by adrenocortical tumor. J.A.V.M.A. 180:542, 1982.

Peterson, M. E., Nesbitt, G. H., and Schaer, M.: Diagnosis and managment of concurrent diabetes mellitus and hyperadrenocorticism in 30 dogs. J.A.V.M.A. 178:66, 1981.

Schechter, R. D., Stabenfeldt, G. H., Gribbe, D. H., and Ling, G. V.: Treatment of Cushing's syndrome in the dog with an adrenocorticolytic agent (o,p'-DDD). J.A.V.M.A. 162:629, 1973.

Scott, D. W.: Hyperadrenocorticism (hyperadrenocorticoidism, hyperadrenocorticalism, Cushing's disease, Cushing's syndrome). Vet. Clin. North Am. 9:3, 1979.

MANAGEMENT OF HYPOTHYROIDISM

ROD ROSYCHUK, D.V.M.

Urbana, Illinois

Hypothyroidism, the disease associated with decreased circulating thyroid hormone concentrations, is the most common endocrinopathy in the dog.

A basic understanding of hypothyroidism, its etiologies, diagnosis, and rational approach to therapy is best preceded by a short review of normal thyroid physiology as it is understood to date.

NORMAL THYROID PHYSIOLOGY

The thyroid is responsible for the production of two physiologically active hormones, thyroxine (also known as L-thyroxine, levothyroxine, or T_4) and triiodothyronine (also known as levothyronine or T_3).

Once released into the blood, more than 99 per cent of both hormones is bound to various plasma proteins (primarily globulins), leaving less than 1 per cent of the "free" hormone available for diffusion into the tissues for binding to various cellular receptor sites. Only this small "free" hormone component is actually physiologically active and responsible for mediating the thyroid effect at the tissue level. The "free" hormone component exists in a reversible equilibrium with plasma protein and tissue receptor–bound pools, which serve as reservoirs to help maintain fluctuating "free" hormone concentrations.

Stimulation of the thyroid to produce both T_4 and T_3 is provided by thyroid-stimulating hormone (TSH) released from the anterior pituitary gland, which is stimulated by thyrotropin-releasing hormone (TRH) from the hypothalamus. The continual maintenance of normal circulating thyroid hormone levels is provided by a sensitive feedback system between the hypothalamus-anterior pituitary and circulating levels of "free" T_3/T_4.

Although all measured serum concentrations of T_4 are produced by the thyroid, the majority of measured T_3 is thought to arise from the conversion (monodeiodination) of T_4 to T_3, which occurs in the peripheral tissues. Although a small quantity of another product of T_4 monodeiodination, reverse T_3, is also produced, it is not likely to be metabolically active.

T_3, with its greater volume of distribution (Rosychuk, 1982) and biologic potency (Table 1), is considered the major physiologically active hormone at the cellular level. Although T_4 is capable of some biologic function, it is thought to primarily serve as a prohormone for T_3 production.

The physiologic and biochemical actions of thyroid hormones have been reviewed elsewhere (Rosychuk, 1982).

Metabolism of T_3 and T_4 is by both deiodination and conjugation (primarily in the liver), with subsequent biliary excretion and fecal loss.

Table 1. *Physiologic and Biochemical Characteristics of Thyroxine (T$_4$) and Triiodothyronine (T$_3$) in the Dog**

	Triiodothyronine (T$_3$)	Thyroxine (T$_4$)
Total serum concentrations	0.75–2.0 ng/ml† (75–200 ng/dl)‡	10–40 ng/ml† (1–4 µg/dl)‡
Serum half-life (hr)	5–6§	Approx. 12§
Comparative biologic potency	4	1

*Modified from Rosychuk: Vet. Clin. North Am. 12:111, 1982.
†Done by radioimmunoassay. A range of normal canine values should be established for each laboratory assaying samples to allow for more accurate interpretation (Nachreiner, 1982).
‡1 µg/100 ml = 10 ng/ml; dl = 100 ml.
§Nachreiner: Personal communication, 1982.

PRIMARY HYPOTHYROIDISM

ETIOLOGIES OF HYPOTHYROIDISM

Hypothyroidism may be produced when circulating T$_3$ and/or T$_4$ concentrations are insufficient to meet physiologic needs.

The vast majority of canine hypothyroidism is of primary origin, wherein the thyroid gland itself is dysfunctional and incapable of maintaining adequate T$_3$ and/or T$_4$ production. In most cases this is histologically represented as atrophy of the follicles with subsequent replacement by adipose tissue. Its cause is unknown. Less commonly, the thyroid may be diffusely infiltrated with lymphocytes, plasma cells, and macrophages, resulting in the destruction of the follicles and, finally, replacement with fibrous connective tissue. Because a significant percentage of these animals may have circulating thyroglobulin autoantibodies, this lymphocytic thyroiditis has been suggested to be immune mediated (Gosselin et al., 1981).

Primary hypothyroidism is rarely associated with obliteration of the thyroid by neoplastic processes. It may be a sequela of surgical thyroidectomy or radioiodine therapy for thyroid neoplasms.

Secondary hypothyroidism is a comparatively uncommon abnormality associated with a lack of normal pituitary production of TSH, which results in eventual thyroid atrophy and decreased T$_3$/T$_4$ production. Congenital abnormalities (cystic Rathke's cleft), neoplasia, or trauma involving the anterior pituitary is the most common cause. Characteristic histologic changes of the thyroid have been reviewed (Belshaw and Rijnberk, 1980).

Tertiary hypothyroidism, associated with the specific lack of hypothalamic TRH production, has not been documented to date in the dog.

The differentiation of primary from secondary hypothyroidism is often not considered important because the replacement hormone regimens for both syndromes are identical. However, documentation of a secondary hypothyroid problem may suggest other potential hormonal/CNS problems that could be prognostically significant (e.g., in the case of neoplasia) or that may suggest potential therapeutic complications (see Complications of Therapy).

Other more uncommon causes of canine hypothyroidism include the following:

1. Apparent sluggish or even absent peripheral conversion of T$_4$ to T$_3$ with subsequently normal serum T$_4$ but low T$_3$ concentrations.

2. Iodine deficiency states. However, owing to the commonplace addition of iodine as iodized salts to both human and animal foods, these have become clinical rarities. The thyroid is characteristically enlarged (goiterous) and histologically hyperplastic. The addition of 1 per cent iodized salt to the diet or the feeding of a good commercial dog food is therapeutic.

3. Congenital thyroid agenesis. Although described, this entity is rare because the clinical problems associated with the disease usually result in early neonatal death.

4. Autoantibodies directed at one or both thyroid hormones, resulting in hormone destruction. Although described, this appears to be a rare problem.

BREED INCIDENCE

Hypothyroidism is noted to occur with a greater frequency in several breeds of dogs including the golden retriever, Doberman pinscher, dachshund, Shetland sheepdog, Irish setter, Pomeranian, miniature schnauzer, cocker spaniel, and airedale (Hilne and Hayes, 1981). Bulldogs, basenjis, Great Danes, poodles, boxers, and beagles have also been noted to have a higher incidence of occurrence than normal (Nesbit et al., 1980). In these higher risk breeds, clinical symptoms are often first noted at two to five years of age, with the giant breeds often manifesting symptoms the earliest. In low-risk and mixed-breed individuals, hypothyroidism tends to be a disease of older age.

Although genetic studies concerning the heritability of hypothyroidism are lacking at present, these suggestive data of a heritable predisposition (breed incidence, early age of onset) would seem to support the recommendation that affected individuals in high-risk breeds not be used for breeding purposes.

PHYSICAL FINDINGS AND RESPONSE TO THERAPY

Abnormalities associated with hypothyroidism that warrant consideration of the diagnosis are discussed hereafter. More thorough discussions of symptoms and pathogenesis have been reviewed elsewhere (Anderson, 1979). Emphasis has been placed on the expected response associated with adequate thyroid hormone supplementation.

Behavioral abnormalities associated with hypothyroidism include mental dullness, lethargy, easy fatigability, and development of an uncommonly good nature. Rarely is irritable behavior seen. Significant increases in mental alertness and activity are usually noted within the first one to two weeks of therapy.

Obesity is often present despite normal or decreased appetite and is worsened by decreased activity. Generally, other signs of hypothyroidism help differentiate this obesity from the obesity seen in the otherwise normal dog. Weight loss following initiation of therapy will often be significant within four to six weeks but must usually be combined with a good dietary/exercise program for the dog to reach its ideal weight.

Thermoregulation abnormalities associated with hypothyroidism include heat seeking, increased tolerance to warm environments, hypothermic rectal temperature, and possible profound hypothermia with heavy sedation or anesthesia. These abnormalities are usually readily reversible with adequate hormone therapy.

Dermatologic symptoms vary widely, depending on breed coat and skin characteristics and duration and severity of disease. Early in the disease the coat is dry and brittle; hairs are easily epilated by normal wear and abrasion. A patchy alopecia appears over points of wear and eventually progresses to a more bilaterally symmetric truncal alopecia sparing the head and limbs. Slow or absent regrowth follows clipping. Short-coated breeds (e.g., boxer, Doberman pinscher) may have a retardation in hair turnover in the cheek and temporal regions, giving a carpet-like appearance. Long-coated breeds (e.g., golden retriever, Irish setter) may develop a fine, "puppy coat"-like pelage.

The skin often becomes dry, variably scaly, thickened, and cool on palpation. Symmetric hyperpigmentation may be present. Comedones appear primarily on the ventral abdomen. In severe cases, skin thickening (dermal mucin or myxedema) produces drooping of facial skin, particularly the eyelids (the dog may have a tragic expression). All forms of seborrhea are possible: seborrhea sicca and oleosa and seborrheic dermatitis. The hypothyroid dog is predisposed to recurrent pyodermas and occasionally bacterial hypersensitivity. Poor wound healing and easy skin bruisability may be noted. Pruritus, if present, is usually secondary to bacterial or seborrheic complications.

Following initiation of therapy, the reactivation of normal cutaneous metabolism may result in the shedding of increased amounts of old hair and keratin, which may give the appearance of a transient worsening of the skin condition. This problem is usually controllable with antiseborrheic shampoos and moisturizers. Hair regrowth should be significant within four to six weeks but may not be complete for five to six months. Hyperpigmentation also tends to resolve slowly over a period of months.

Several weeks of replacement hormone therapy may be required before recurrent pyodermas associated with hypothyroidism are noted to resolve or decrease in severity. Concurrent antibiotic and topical germicidal and antiseborrheic shampoo therapy is usually required initially to clear up and control the bacterial problem while awaiting this effect.

Cardiovascular symptoms are usually seen with more severe hypothyroidism and include bradycardia, a weak apex beat, and decreased amplitudes of QRS complexes in all EKG leads. These changes are generally reversible with therapy.

Cardiac dysrhythmias (PVCs, atrial fibrillation) have also been occasionally noted in hypothyroid large-breed dogs such as the Doberman pinscher and boxer. The clinical course may terminate in sudden death or congestive heart failure. Histologic myocardial changes resemble those seen in the idiopathic cardiomyopathies of large-breed dogs but for the presence of a higher incidence of atherosclerosis in the hypothyroid patients. The potential causal relationship between hypothyroidism and cardiomyopathy awaits further clarification. In the majority of patients to date, adequate thyroid supplementation has not significantly altered the course of the problem. For recommendations regarding therapy, see Complications of Therapy.

Musculoskeletal/neurologic symptoms are usually seen with more severe hypothyroidism and may include weakness, limb stiffness, and dragging or knuckling of feet, possibly owing to a polyneuropathy or myopathy (Braund et al., 1981). These symptoms are usually responsive to therapy.

Unilateral or bilateral peripheral vestibular disorders (head tilt) with or without facial paralysis have occasionally been associated with more severe hypothyroidism, but response to therapy has been generally very poor unless the problem is relatively mild or of short duration.

Reproductive abnormalities in the female associated with hypothyroidism include infertility, prolonged interestral periods, failure to cycle, prolonged estral bleeding, and decreases in intensity and duration of estrous cycles. Male reproductive abnormalities include lack of libido, testicular atrophy, and hypospermatogenesis (in more severe cases). Abnormalities in both the male and female are generally reversible with adequate therapy. Rarely following institution of therapy, a severe exacerbation of endometrial hyperplasia may be noted in the first estral period following a prolonged anestrus.

Although there appears to be a high incidence of hypothyroidism in dogs with keratoconjunctivitis sicca (KCS), hormonal replacement therapy has not improved tear production in the vast majority of patients, suggesting an interesting but unlikely causal relationship. Although a relationship between hypothyroidism and indolent corneal ulcers in the boxer breed has been rumored to occur, poor responses to replacement thyroid hormone therapy make the direct association of problems questionable.

Gastrointestinal symptoms seen in hypothyroid dogs include constipation and mild diarrhea. Both are uncommon and usually are not clinically significant.

Clinicopathologic abnormalities, which are often found with longer-standing, more severe hypothyroidism, include mild to moderate normocytic, normochromic anemia; serum lipid abnormalities, e.g., fasting lipemia; hypercholesterolemia (in about 50 per cent of patients, with values in excess of 500 mg/dl, it is usually well correlated with the diagnosis); and hypertriglyceridemia. All these abnormalities are generally reversible with therapy.

SECONDARY HYPOTHYROIDISM

Generally, the clinical signs of secondary hypothyroidism do not tend to be as severe as those associated with primary hypothyroidism, most likely because the thyroid is capable of some basal production of hormones without input from higher centers. In these cases, symptoms associated with excesses or deficits of other pituitary hormones may be present (e.g., a lack of adrenocorticotropic hormone [ACTH] resulting in hypoadrenocorticism, a lack of antidiuretic hormone [ADH] resulting in diabetes insipidus, or an excess of ACTH resulting in hyperadrenocorticism). Neurologic abnormalities may also contribute to the symptomatology. Response to therapy is usually good but is dependent upon the degree of severity of the associated problems (see also Complications of Therapy).

DIAGNOSIS

When presented with a patient with signs suggestive of hypothyroidism, the clinician must essentially "build" a diagnosis with the use of supportive history, physical findings, clinicopathologic data, and one or more specific laboratory evaluations of thyroid function. If results are equivocal, response to a trial hormone therapy may prove to be the ultimate diagnostic aid. Because they are easy to perform and usually readily available, a CBC, serum cholesterol determination, and EKG should be considered part of the routine work-up.

At present, based on sensitivity, availability, and cost, the screening test routinely recommended to assess the adequacy of thyroid function is the measurement by radioimmunoassay (RIA) of both total serum T_4 and T_3. Hypothyroidism, although usually associated with reductions of both T_4 and T_3, is occasionally noted to occur with only low T_4 or T_3 concentrations. In the majority of cases, measurement of a single resting T_4 or T_3 by RIA is adequate to differentiate between normal and hypothyroid patients. However, some hypothyroid dogs have been noted to have normal resting T_3/T_4 concentrations. These patients may require a TSH challenge or response to trial therapy to confirm the diagnosis.

Important factors to consider before being potentially misled by abnormal resting T_3 and/or T_4 results include the following:

1. The assays must be standardized for use in the dog and cat, which have much lower circulating hormone concentrations than humans.

2. Values should be interpreted using normal ranges established for the laboratory running the test. Comparison to published values from the veterinary literature should not be used for this purpose.

3. Glucocorticoids (either exogenous or endogenous, i.e., cushingoid animals), phenylbutazone, phenytoin, phenobarbital, or *o,p'*-DDD may decrease T_4 and T_3 values into the hypothyroid range (Belshaw and Rijnberk, 1980). Fasting for three to five days or longer or the presence of severe, often terminal, stages of many nonthyroidal illnesses has also been reported to have a similar effect (Belshaw and Rijnberk, 1980). These changes are thought to be brought about by reductions in hormonal binding affinity for plasma proteins or actual reductions in thyroid binding protein concentrations with subsequent decreases in the amount of total bound hormone. In spite of these changes, however, "free" T_3 and T_4 concentrations are maintained and the individual remains euthyroid (normal thyroid status). Because only total T_3 and T_4 (both bound and free hormones) are measured in most veterinary diagnostic laboratories, a reduction of T_3/T_4 values into the hypothyroid range may reflect only bound hormone changes and may, therefore, give a false impression of hypothyroidism. These individuals do not benefit from hormonal supplementation, and values of total serum T_3 and T_4 usually spontaneously return to normal once the disease has

resolved or the drug has been discontinued. This phenomenon has been called the "euthyroid sick" or "low triiodothyronine" syndrome. It must be considered a potential reason for therapeutic failures in dogs diagnosed on the basis of resting T_3/T_4 values when exposed to these extrathyroidal influences.

Because the response of T_4 to TSH stimulation remains normal or at least significantly greater in these animals when compared with those with primary hypothyroidism, a TSH challenge would be indicated to more accurately evaluate thyroid function in such cases (Belshaw and Rijnberk, 1980).

4. The thyroid of a normal animal placed on an exogenous thyroid hormone supplement usually atrophies, resulting in depressed resting hormone levels when the supplement is discontinued. A one-month period following discontinuation of therapy is therefore recommended prior to T_3/T_4 screening to allow for more accurate interpretation of the patient's thyroid while at its fullest functional capacity.

5. Owing to the greater potential for extrathyroidal influences on T_3 concentrations, a T_4 evaluation would be considered preferential to a T_3 evaluation if both were not available to help assess thyroid function.

TSH RESPONSE TEST

The TSH response test is performed by establishing a baseline serum T_4 value and administering 5 IU ($\leq$50 lb body weight) or 10 IU (>50 lb) of bovine TSH intramuscularly or intravenously, with a recheck of T_4 values at 8 to 12 hours (for IM route) or 4 hours (for IV route). Normal results of a TSH response test show at least a two- to threefold increase in total serum T_4 from baseline. Primary hypothyroidism is indicated by a minimal or no

increase in T_4. The "euthyroid sick" syndrome or secondary hypothyroidism is indicated by a subnormal resting T_4 and a normal slope of response (Belshaw and Rijnberk, 1980).

The TSH response test is usually presented to clients as a costly but potentially unambiguous method of determining the thyroid status of the dog. However, at present, because of the reliability of resting T_3/T_4 values as determined by RIA in the majority of cases (80 to 85 per cent?) and our tendency to attempt trial therapy in highly suggestive cases with borderline laboratory data, the TSH response is only routinely used when the patient is suffering from intercurrent illness (e.g., cushingoid) or is receiving an intercurrent drug therapy expected to falsely lower resting total T_3 and/or T_4 values.

TRIAL THERAPY AS A DIAGNOSTIC AID

The ultimate confirmation of the diagnosis of hypothyroidism is usually the clinical observation of improvement following establishment of an adequate thyroid hormone replacement regimen. A trial replacement therapy is therefore performed routinely if clinical signs are strongly suggestive and if (1) the results of resting T_4 and/or T_3 values are borderline; (2) there is some question about the presence of secondary hypothyroidism rather than a "euthyroid sick" situation on the basis of TSH response data; or (3) the owners are unwilling to proceed with diagnostic laboratory testing. T_4 therapy at recommended dosages (Table 2) is instituted for a four- to five-week period. Following this time, a thorough clinical and laboratory examination (T_3/T_4 post-pill test) is performed. If thyroid hormone levels are adequate at this time but no clinical response is noted, the diagnosis of hypothyroidism is eliminated.

Table 2. *Dose Recommendations for Thyroid Hormone Replacement Therapy**

Preparation†	Generic Name	Dog	Cat
Synthetic products L-thyroxine (T_4)	Levothyroxine	20–32 μg/kg‡ once daily (use higher dose per kg for smaller animals) OR 20 μg/kg§ every 12 hr	20 μg/kg§ every 12 or 24 hr
L-triiodothyronine (T_3)	Liothyronine	4.4 μg/kg‖ every 8 hr	Same
L-thyroxine and L-triiodothyronine combined (T_4: T_3)	Liotrix	20 μg/kg T_4, 5 μg/kg T_3 every 12 hr (dosage actually computed on basis of T_4 content of product)**	
Crude hormone products	Desiccated thyroid thyroglobulin	15–20 mg/kg once daily (in higher range may be divided and given every 12 hr)	10–15 mg/kg once daily (in higher range may be divided and given every 12 hr)

*Modified from Rosychuk: Vet. Clin. North Am. 12:111, 1982.
†Approximate biologic dose equivalents: 0.1 mg T_4 = 25 μg T_3 = 1 grain (65 mg) desiccated thyroid/thyroglobulin.
‡20–32 μg/kg = 0.02–0.032 mg/kg or 0.1 mg/7–11 lb.
§20 μg/kg = 0.1 mg/11 lb. See text for rationale.
‖4.4 μg/kg = 2 μg/lb.
** Computed on basis of T_4 content of product. 1 grain equivalent of these products equals 50–60 μg T_4 and 12.5–15 μg T_3 and is equivalent in biologic potency to 1 grain desiccated thyroid.

MISCELLANEOUS DIAGNOSTIC AIDS

Thyroid biopsy, thyroid radioiodine uptake measurement, or the measurement of serum TSH levels may help determine the presence and type of hypothyroidism, but time, cost, and equipment requirements or lack of reliability (TSH) make them prohibitive.

Skin biopsies from hypothyroid patients generally reflect changes associated with nonspecific endocrinopathies, although some alterations may suggest hypothyroidism (Scott, 1982).

TREATMENT

Once a diagnosis of hypothyroidism is established, the following important points concerning the choice and management of replacement hormone therapy regimens should be considered:

1. Because of potential individual variation in degrees of gastrointestinal absorption and rates of catabolism of thyroid hormones, there is no fixed dose of supplementation that satisfies all patients. Only periodic, regular laboratory and clinical examinations determine the maximally effective maintenance dosage regimen for the animal.

2. Hormonal supplementation is generally considered to be required for the life of the hypothyroid patient.

3. Thyroid hormone requirements do seem to vary inversely with size. Large animals require smaller dosages on a per unit weight basis.

4. Following the initiation of therapy, each animal should be re-examined in four to six weeks to evaluate clinical response to therapy. At this time T_3 and T_4 concentrations should again be evaluated at some fixed time (see hereafter) following the daily administration of medication to assess the adequacy of supplementation. This monitoring technique is called post-pill testing. If the post-pill values are well within the normal range but no clinical response is noted, the diagnosis of hypothyroidism should be considered unlikely. Subnormal results suggest possible alterations in dose or product (see hereafter).

5. Routine clinical and laboratory checks of hypothyroid individuals are recommended four to six weeks following each dose or product change. Once a maintenance regimen is established, a clinical re-examination and T_3/T_4 post-pill recheck are recommended every 6 to 12 months. Post-pill data should also be interpreted in light of the fact that drug-induced and "euthyroid sick" reductions in T_3 and T_4 may occur in animals on supplementation, producing a false suggestion of inadequacy of therapy. Clinical response may have to be emphasized heavily in such individuals.

THYROID HORMONE PREPARATIONS AND DOSAGE REGIMENS

Several preparations are available for thyroid hormone therapy. Among the synthetic thyroid hormones, the sodium salts of thyroxine (T_4) and triiodothyronine (T_3) are available either as individual compounds or in T_3:T_4 combinations. They generally offer the advantages of better stability and standardization of potency when compared with the desiccated or crude hormonal products.

Synthetic L-thyroxine sodium (levothyroxine or T_4) is recommended for the routine initiation of therapy in almost all hypothyroid and suspected hypothyroid patients. Following administration, conversion of T_4 to T_3 occurs as it does naturally in the animal, returning low T_4 and T_3 concentrations to normal. This is considered more physiologic than using T_3 or combination T_3:T_4 product therapy, both of which circumvent this mechanism. Generally, a once-a-day dosage of T_4 (see Table 2) is adequate to maintain the euthyroid state in the majority of dogs and is used routinely for initiation of therapy by the author. A range is given to allow for variations in requirement depending on the animal's size. Dogs over 60 lb seldom require more than 0.6 mg of T_4 given once daily as a maintenance regimen. Because of the generally short average half-life of T_4 (see Table 1) in the dog and the somewhat controversial number of animals whose poor hormone absorption/rapid metabolism produces very short T_4 half-lives, administration every 12 hours can be rationalized (see Table 2). However, rather than commit an animal to this more frequent and costly dose of medication for a lifetime, this regimen is recommended for a four- to six-week trial period until clinical and laboratory (post pill) evidence of response has been established. The dose can then be adjusted for once-a-day dosage. Only the reappearance of clinical or laboratory signs of hormone deficiency warrant return to twice-a-day dosage. An initial full replacement dose is usually well tolerated by the animal despite old age and/or severe hypothyroidism.

Post-pill testing is routinely performed at peak post-pill absorption time (four to eight hours post pill for T_4). Values for both T_4 and T_3 should be well within the high normal range at this time to assure adequate duration of effect (ideally 24 hours). This protocol seems to be satisfactory in the majority of cases, although an alternative technique would be to check values at 24 hours post pill (but no later). Expect values to remain within the normal range for this period of time with adequate supplementation. This technique would be specifically indicated if there was a question about the duration of maintenance of adequate T_4, T_3 concentration on a once-a-day regimen.

Low-normal to subnormal values on post-pill testing indicate the need to increase the dose of supplement by 0.1- to 0.2-mg increments. If response is still poor (low T_3, T_4, poor clinical response) following apparently adequate supplementation, the dog may not be routinely getting the pill, may have poor gastrointestinal absorption, or may be directing an antibody at the thyroid hormones. The "euthyroid sick" syndrome should also be considered. A suggestion of poor absorption would warrant trial therapy with a T_3 source, which should have somewhat better absorption potential. High-normal T_4 values with subnormal T_3 values on post-pill testing suggest possible conversion problems, again warranting trial therapy with a T_3 source.

Synthetic L-triiodothyronine (levothyronine or T_3) is a much more potent and faster-acting hormone, with a shorter half-life than T_4 (see Table 1). It should be used only rarely in the management of hypothyroidism. It is primarily indicated when clinical response to a T_4 source is poor because of poor gastrointestinal absorption or in the presence of T_4 to T_3 conversion problems. T_3 is initially administered every eight hours (see Table 2), with testing performed three hours post pill. Values should be in the high-normal range. Persistently low concentrations suggest inconsistent medication, poor absorption, an autoantibody directed at the hormone, or the "euthyroid sick" syndrome. On post-pill examination, T_4 values will be very low in these T_3-treated patients because of the expected negative feedback suppression of thyroid T_4 production.

Because some animals respond well to a dose of 2 µg/lb given only every 12 hours, this dosage reduction can be achieved once adequate response to t.i.d. administration has been documented. When conversion of T_4 to T_3 is suspected to be sluggish but not absent (indicated by high-normal T_4 values but slightly subnormal T_3 values and only a partial clinical response), the addition of T_3 at a dose of 2 µg/lb every 12 hours to the T_4 regimen may prove beneficial.

Combination products (liotrix, 1:4 combinations of T_3:T_4) are seldom used clinically, primarily because of their cost. They may have some rationale with sluggish T_4 to T_3 conversion problems as noted previously. They are generally dosed twice daily to take advantage of the T_3 content of the product (see Table 2).

COMPLICATIONS OF THERAPY

Thyrotoxicosis is an uncommon problem associated with thyroid hormone supplementation, primarily because of the dog's great ability to metabolize and excrete these hormones. Because the biologic potency of T_3 is much greater than that of T_4, one is more likely to see problems when this product is part of the therapeutic regimen. Suggestive clinical signs include polydipsia, polyuria, nervousness, panting, weight loss despite a normal or increased appetite, tachycardia, "forceful heart beats," and an increased pulse pressure. Observation of this symptomatology dictates immediate discontinuation of therapy. Thyrotoxic symptoms usually abate rapidly (although exceptions to this observation have been noted), following which a lower dose of supplementation may be instituted. The development of this problem warrants re-examination of dose, frequency of administration, and product being used.

In hypothyroid patients with concurrent heart problems, the institution of replacement therapy may, through resultant increases in cellular oxygen consumption and general patient activity, threaten to decompensate a potentially borderline congestive heart failure. Institution of therapy at one-half the recommended dose and gradually increasing this to a full replacement regimen over a two- to four-week period is recommended to help circumvent this possibility in such patients. Other potential problems related to treating the patient with cardiovascular disease have been reviewed (Rosychuk, 1982).

Animals with suspected concurrent hypoadrenal problems should have this problem diagnosed and adequately treated prior to the initiation of thyroid supplementation. Thyroid hormone supplementation in a borderline hypoadrenal patient may result in increased metabolism of already borderline adrenal hormone concentrations, potentially exhausting adrenal reserves and precipitating a hypoadrenal crisis.

The institution of therapy with drugs noted to stimulate hepatic microsomal enzyme function (phenobarbital, primidone, diphenylhydantoin) may result in the more rapid metabolism of thyroid hormones in patients on hormone therapy and suggests the need for possible increases in supplementation dosages.

FELINE HYPOTHYROIDISM

Although spontaneous hypothyroidism has been suggested to occur in the cat by many clinicians, well-documented cases are lacking in the veterinary literature. Hypothyroidism in this species is now most commonly noted in cats that have had bilateral thyroidectomies or propylthiouracil therapy for the treatment of feline hyperthyroidism. Suggestive clinical signs have been reviewed (Holzworth et al., 1980; Scott, 1980). Because circulating hormone concentrations and daily thyroid hormone replacement therapy dosages in the cat are noted to be similar to those in the dog, diagnostic and therapeutic plans should be similar (see Table 2).

REFERENCES AND SUPPLEMENTAL READING

Anderson, R. K.: Canine hypothyroidism. Comp. Cont. Ed. 1:103, 1979.

Belshaw, B. E., and Rijnberk, A.: Radioimmunoassay of plasma T_4 and T_3 in the diagnosis of primary hypothyroidism in dogs. J. Am. Anim. Hosp. Assoc. 15:17, 1979.

Belshaw, B. E., and Rijnberk, A.: Hypothyroidism. In Kirk, R. W. (ed.): Current Veterinary Therapy VII. Philadelphia: W. B. Saunders, 1980.

Braund, K. G., Dillon, J. R. A., and Ganjam, V. K.: Hypothyroid myopathy in two dogs. Vet. Pathol. 18:589, 1981.

Fox, L. E., and Nachreiner, R. F.: The pharmakokinetics of T_3 and T_4 in the dog. Proceedings of the 62nd Conference of Research Workers in Animal Diseases. 13, 1981.

Gosselin, S. J., Capen, C. C., and Martin, S. L.: Histologic and ultrastructural evaluation of thyroid lesions associated with hypothyroidism in dogs. Vet. Pathol. 18:299, 1981.

Holzworth, J., Theran, P., Carpenter, J. L., et al.: Hyperthyroidism in the cat: Ten cases. J.A.V.M.A. 176:345, 1980.

Milne, K. L., and Hayes, H. M., Jr.: Epidemiologic features of canine hypothyroidism. Cornell Vet. 71:3, 1981.

Nachreiner, R. F.: Personal communication, 1982.

Nesbitt, G. H., Izzo, J., Perterson, L., et al.: Canine hypothyroidism: A retrospective study of 108 cases. J.A.V.M.A. 177:1117, 1980.

Rosychuk, R. A. W.: Thyroid hormones and antithyroid drugs. Vet. Clin. North Am. 12:111, 1982.

Scott, D. W.: Hormonal and metabolic disorders. J. Am. Anim. Hosp. Assoc. 16:392, 1980.

Scott, D. W.: Histopathologic findings in endocrine skin disorders of the dog. J. Am. Anim. Hosp. Assoc. 18:173, 1982.

HYPOPARATHYROIDISM

GEORGE E. LEES, D.V.M.

College Station, Texas

Hypoparathyroidism is an uncommon metabolic disorder that occurs when parathyroid hormone production is not sufficient to maintain an adequate serum concentration of calcium. Normally, homeostasis of calcium and phosphorus is maintained by the multiple actions and interactions of parathyroid hormone, calcitonin, and vitamin D. These hormones and the responses of their target organs (primarily bone, intestines, and kidneys) normally cause serum calcium and phosphorus to be sustained at relatively uniform levels. Parathyroid insufficiency results in hypocalcemia and hyperphosphatemia. Clinical manifestations of the disorder are primarily the metabolic consequences of hypocalcemia.

When categorized by their causes, instances of hypoparathyroidism form two groups: postoperative and idiopathic. Postoperative parathyroid insufficiency is generally the result of purposeful or inadvertent removal of or damage to parathyroid glands during cervical surgery in the region of the thyroid glands. Animals that have hyperparathyroidism caused by functional parathyroid neoplasms typically will have hypoparathyroidism following tumor excision. This type of parathyroid insufficiency is usually temporary and occurs because the "normal" parathyroid glands are functionally quiescent and become atrophic while the tumor is producing excessive amounts of hormone. Hypoparathyroidism may also occur following thyroid surgery if the parathyroid glands are removed or if their blood supply is compromised. This outcome is particularly likely when bilateral thyroidectomy is performed (e.g., in animals with bilateral thyroid neoplasms). Whether postoperative hypoparathyroidism will be temporary or permanent is determined by the extent to which parathyroid tissue is removed or irreversibly injured. If there is residual parathyroid tissue, it will tend to hypertrophy and restore adequate hormone secretion. Hypoparathyroidism will be permanent, however, if all parathyroid tissue is removed or destroyed.

Idiopathic hypoparathyroidism occurs in dogs. Approximately 20 to 25 cases of the condition have been either described in the veterinary literature or seen by the author. Most affected animals have been of small breeds, particularly miniature poodles and schnauzers, but the condition has been diagnosed in large-breed dogs as well. Dogs are usually two to eight years of age when the diagnosis is established, but idiopathic hypoparathyroidism has been reported in dogs as young as 6 weeks and as old as 12 years of age. Interestingly, most affected dogs are female; only three instances of idiopathic hypoparathyroidism have been reported in male dogs.

The parathyroid glands of dogs with idiopathic hypoparathyroidism typically contain numerous lymphocytes and plasma cells. Glandular parenchyma is destroyed and replaced by connective tissue. Destruction of the glands may be so complete that parathyroid tissue cannot be identified grossly or microscopically. Autoimmune mechanisms are probably responsible for the parathyroiditis. Isoimmune hypoparathyroidism has been experimentally produced in dogs by repeated inoculation of homologous parathyroid tissue.

SIGNS

Neuromuscular irritability, tetany, and seizures caused by hypocalcemia are the predominant signs of hypoparathyroidism in animals. Tetanic muscle spasms, particularly in the facial muscles and forelimbs, may occur spontaneously, but tetany is frequently latent and is revealed only by occurrence of muscle spasms following certain stimuli. In human medicine, for example, unilateral spasm of facial muscles resulting from percussion of the muscles or branches of the ipsilateral facial nerve (Chvostek's sign) and spasm of muscles in an extremity made ischemic by a tourniquet (Trousseau's sign) are crude indicators of latent tetany. Although such discrete phenomena have not been described in animals, it has been observed that handling or excitement may elicit tetany in hypocalcemic dogs. Additionally, generalized major motor (grand mal) seizures have been initiated in hypoparathyroid dogs by similar stimuli.

Neurologic manifestations of hypocalcemia are not limited to tetany and seizures. Although they cannot be documented in animals, numbness or tingling (paresthesias) in the face and distal extremities occur in hypocalcemic humans and probably in animals, too. Restlessness, irritability, confusion, and irrational behavior are other signs that have been associated with hypocalcemia in humans and animals. Electroencephalographic abnormalities may also be demonstrated. These usually disappear following calcium infusion, but chronic hypocalcemia can produce organic brain disease, which might cause the EEG abnormalities to persist despite correction of hypocalcemia.

Gastrointestinal, cardiac, and ocular signs have also been associated with hypocalcemia. Anorexia, nausea, vomiting, and abdominal pain may occur. Electrocardiographic changes may include prolongation of the Q-T interval, and severe tachycardia (>350 beats/min) has been observed during a hypocalcemic crisis in a dog with hypoparathyroidism. A distinctive type of cataract may develop in hypocalcemic patients. Small white punctate to linear opacities may be seen in the anterior and posterior cortical subcapsular region of the lens.

The clinical course of untreated hypoparathyroidism is unpredictable. The condition can develop rapidly and can produce severe hypocalcemia and profound clinical signs in a few hours or days. This pattern is particularly likely for postoperative hypoparathyroidism. Some dogs with idiopathic hypoparathyroidism have had brief clinical courses characterized by mild signs despite severe hypocalcemia and terminated by unexpected death. Other dogs have had protracted clinical courses characterized by intermittent periods of abnormality that have not always included tetany or seizures.

DIAGNOSIS

Usually, a diagnosis of hypoparathyroidism is considered when significant hypocalcemia (<8.5 mg/dl) is discovered during clinical investigation of tetany, seizures, and so on or by routine use of serum biochemical profiles that include a calcium determination. Thus, hypoparathyroidism must be differentiated from other possible causes of hypocalcemia.

Reduced total serum calcium concentration may be associated with hypoalbuminemia due to any cause (e.g., protein-losing enteropathy, nephrotic syndrome, liver disease, and others). This type of hypocalcemia is not usually associated with hyperphosphatemia and does not produce clinical signs. Although total serum calcium concentration is decreased, the reduction is of protein-bound calcium; the level of biologically active unbound calcium remains at or near normal. For recognition of hypocalcemia that merely reflects hypoalbuminemia, it is useful to adjust serum calcium values for serum protein concentration when interpreting test results. In dogs, the formulas for this purpose are as follows: adjusted calcium (mg/dl) = calcium (mg/dl) − albumin (gm/dl) + 3.5, or adjusted calcium (mg/dl) = calcium (mg/dl) − 0.4(total serum protein [gm/dl]) + 3.3.

Hypocalcemia not attributable to hypoalbuminemia has numerous possible causes. These include acute or chronic renal failure, puerperal tetany, acute pancreatitis, malabsorption or excessive intestinal loss of calcium, osteoblastic metastatic bone disease, administration of certain drugs (e.g., diphenylhydantoin), inadequate or ineffective amounts of vitamin D metabolites, hypomagnesemia, hypoparathyroidism, and pseudohypoparathyroidism. Many of these diagnostic possibilities are often suggested or excluded in a hypocalcemic patient by historic data, findings from physical examination, and results of other routine laboratory tests. Once uremia, eclampsia, gastrointestinal disorders including acute pancreatitis, and iatrogenic causes have been excluded, however, accurate diagnosis of disorders causing hypocalcemia becomes more difficult.

Hypoparathyroidism is a reasonable presumptive diagnosis when hypocalcemia and hyperphosphatemia are discovered in an animal with normal renal function. To confirm the diagnosis, however, additional information is needed. Relative or absolute lack of circulating parathyroid hormone is optimum confirmatory evidence of hypoparathyroidism, but parathyroid hormone assays are expensive and not widely available. Furthermore, the validity of assays that have been used to obtain parathyroid hormone values that have thus far been reported in the veterinary clinical literature is uncertain. Suspected hypoparathyroidism may also be confirmed by examination and biopsy of parathyroid glands. Chronic hypocalcemia not caused by hypoparathyroidism should be associated with hypertrophy and hyperplasia of parathyroid tissue. In dogs with hypoparathyroidism, however, parathyroid glands typically are not grossly evident during necropsy or surgical exploration of the neck, and careful microscopic examination of tissue removed from the normal locations of parathyroid glands may reveal a remnant of tissue containing an infiltrate of lymphocytes and plasma cells.

Hypomagnesemia is often associated with hypocalcemia, and serum magnesium concentration should be evaluated in all hypocalcemic patients. Magnesium depletion may cause decreased parathyroid hormone synthesis and action, may enhance net movement of calcium from extracellular fluid to bone, or both. In any event, hypocalcemia usually does not respond to treatment when there is hypomagnesemia that is not corrected as well.

Parathyroid hormone effects on kidneys normally result in increased renal excretion of phosphate and cyclic adenosine monophosphate. Evaluation of these target-organ responses may be used to differentiate hypoparathyroidism from pseudohypoparathyroidism. Clinical manifestations of both conditions are similar, but in pseudohypoparathyroidism it is the target-organ response rather than the hormone itself that is deficient.

TREATMENT

Severe hypocalcemia (<6.0 mg/dl) is a life-threatening medical emergency and should be treated accordingly regardless of the apparent chronicity or mildness of associated clinical signs. The goal of initial therapy is to prevent a fatal episode of hypocalcemic signs during the period that will elapse before an adequate serum calcium concentration can be maintained by administration of vitamin D analogues. Initially, 10 per cent calcium gluconate solution is given intravenously at a dosage of 0.5 to 1.5 ml/kg body weight, up to a maximum total dose of 10 ml. Infusion of calcium should be done slowly over a 15- to 30-minute period and should be carefully monitored by electrocardiography. Occurrence of S-T segment elevation, Q-T interval shortening, or bradycardia requires that calcium infusion cease temporarily, then begin again at a slower rate when the signs of cardiotoxicity have abated. Subsequently, intravenous calcium administration is repeated at six- to eight-hour intervals as needed.

Judicious treatment of hypocalcemia with intravenous calcium administration is more difficult than treatment of hypoglycemia with intravenous glucose, for example, and much greater caution is required. Two factors account for the difference in these clinical situations. First, calcium is cardiotoxic, whereas mild to moderate hyperglycemia produces few or no adverse effects. In fact, a "normal" serum calcium concentration can be cardiotoxic just because it is raised to that level too rapidly. Additionally, whereas resolution of neuro-

logic signs due to hypoglycemia usually is abrupt and virtually complete when glucose is given, signs of hypocalcemia abate more slowly following calcium infusion. In the author's experience, this is particularly true of behavioral aberrations accompanying hypocalcemia in some animals. Resolution of clinical signs, therefore, is an unreliable immediate guide to the adequacy of calcium administration. Some hypocalcemic signs may actually persist when cardiotoxic effects of calcium infusion occur.

Eventual control of hypocalcemia caused by hypoparathyroidism is accomplished by administering appropriate amounts of vitamin D. Although there are several synthetic vitamin D analogues that can be used successfully, the author considers dihydroxytachysterol in oil* to be the best presently available product for treating hypoparathyroidism. In addition to being relatively inexpensive and widely available, formulation of the drug in oil optimizes stability, absorption, and accuracy of dosage for pharmaceutical reasons. Furthermore, onset and offset of drug effects on serum calcium concentration are more rapid for dihydroxytachysterol than for ergocalciferol (vitamin D_2) or for calcifediol (25-hydroxy-vitamin D_3). This means that normocalcemia can be established more rapidly following initiation of therapy and that hypercalcemia will abate more quickly following cessation of therapy in the event of overdosage. Finally, the liquid form of the drug is convenient for appropriate dosage of cats and small dogs. Use of tuberculin syringe for accurate measurement of each dose is advised when the liquid is used.

The daily maintenance dose of dihydroxytachysterol for hypoparathyroid dogs is approximately 0.007 to 0.010 mg/kg body weight. The dose for cats is undetermined but is probably similar. Oral administration of the daily maintenance dose of dihydroxytachysterol to hypoparathyroid animals restores normocalcemia in one to two weeks and produces maximal effects in two to four weeks. Restoration of normocalcemia can be accelerated by using loading doses that are multiples of the daily maintenance dose (i.e., 4-4-2-2-1-1-1- etc.) on the first few days of treatment.

Because the delay before vitamin D therapy will increase serum calcium concentration sufficiently, it is necessary to administer supplemental calcium during the initial phases of treatment. As discussed previously, this is first done by giving calcium gluconate intravenously to combat symptomatic hypocalcemia. As soon as possible, however, oral supplementation of calcium intake should be begun. Calcium carbonate, lactate, and gluconate contain 40, 13, and 9 per cent calcium, respectively. Administration of as much as 1 gm calcium (e.g., 10 to 12 gm calcium gluconate) daily in divided doses may

---

*Hytakerol: 0.125-mg capsules or 0.25 mg/ml liquid.

be needed for the first few days. Oral calcium supplementation, however, must be tapered and stopped as the effects of vitamin D administration develop. Ultimately, regular administration of an optimum amount of vitamin D will sustain normocalcemia without calcium supplementation, the calcium contained in a normal balanced diet being sufficient.

Treatment of hypoparathyroid patients must be individualized. Hospitalization, careful observation, daily determination of serum calcium concentration, and adjustment of therapy as needed are advised during initial phases of treatment. The therapeutic goal is to obtain serum calcium concentrations that are consistently in the low-normal range (i.e., about 9 mg/dl). Once the animal is on maintenance vitamin D therapy and an adequate serum calcium concentration has been obtained, hypercalcemia caused by excessive vitamin D therapy is a greater danger than recurrence of hypocalcemia. This is because the maximum effects of a particular rate of dihydroxytachysterol administration are produced after two to four weeks. Serum calcium concentration should be determined at one- to two-week intervals and the vitamin D dosage adjusted accordingly until the animal's optimum daily dihydroxytachysterol dose is determined.

Development of hypercalcemia may be signaled by the onset of polyuria and polydipsia. If hypercalcemia occurs, calcium supplementation is inappropriate and vitamin D therapy should be temporarily suspended. Additionally, diuresis induced by administration of saline and furosemide together with glucocorticoid therapy may be needed to lower the serum calcium concentration. Although hypercalcemia usually abates in a few days, effects of dihydroxytachysterol on serum calcium values persist for one to three weeks following cessation of its administration, and recurrence of symptomatic hypocalcemia is unlikely. Three to five days after hypercalcemia resolves, vitamin D therapy should be reinstituted using a lower dose.

In patients with hypoparathyroidism that might be transient (i.e., those with postoperative parathyroid insufficiency), care must be taken to detect recovery of parathyroid function if it occurs. In such an instance, continued vitamin D therapy will certainly produce hypercalcemia. Serum calcium concentration should be monitored at weekly intervals during treatment of postoperative hypoparathyroidism. Again, if hypercalcemia develops, dihydroxytachysterol administration must be discontinued, but it should be reinstituted only if a serious hypocalcemic tendency is actually observed (calcium <8.0 mg/dl). When postoperative hypoparathyroidism continues such that therapy is required for more than six to eight weeks, however, it is most likely that the condition is permanent.

Prognosis for carefully managed hypoparathyroidism is excellent. Serum calcium concentration should be checked every three to four months and the dihydroxytachysterol dose adjusted if necessary. In the author's experience, however, animals with hypoparathyroidism have done well for extended periods of time with serum calcium levels adequately maintained by relatively uniform dihydroxytachysterol therapy. This experience differs from that reported by some others who found that serum calcium concentration fluctuated while treatment remained unchanged and that hypercalcemia occurred frequently. The probable explanation for these differences in experience is related to the vitamin D products chosen for use. The key to uniform regulation of serum calcium in hypoparathyroid patients is the use of pharmaceutical products that are appropriately forumlated for optimum stability, absorption, and accuracy of dosage of the vitamin D analogues they contain (Parfitt, 1978).

REFERENCES AND SUPPLEMENTAL READING

Juan, D.: Hypocalcemia: Differential diagnosis and mechanisms. Arch. Intern. Med. 139:1166, 1979.
Kornegay, J. N., Greene, C. E., Martin, C., et al.: Idiopathic hypocalcemia in four dogs. J. Am. Anim. Hosp. Assoc. 16:723, 1980.
Parfitt, A. M.: Adult hypoparathyroidism: Treatment with calcifediol. Arch. Intern. Med. 138:874, 1978.
Sherding, R. G., Meuten, D. J., Chew, D. J., et al.: Primary hypoparathyroidism in the dog. J.A.V.M.A. 176:439, 1980.

PRIMARY HYPERPARATHYROIDISM

DENNIS J. CHEW, D.V.M.,

Columbus, Ohio

and DONALD J. MEUTEN, D.V.M.

College Station, Texas

Primary hyperparathyroidism (HPT) is a disease of older dogs resulting from excessive secretion of parathyroid hormone (PTH) by the parathyroid glands. The normal parathyroid gland decreases its secretion of PTH as ionized serum calcium increases. In primary HPT, this negative feedback inhibition is lost and the parathyroid gland continues to secrete excess PTH. The clinical signs and biochemical alterations in this disease are caused by the exaggerated action of PTH on its target organs (bone, gut, and kidney).

Primary HPT is uncommon. Referral institutions may anticipate about one case per year. When encountered, the underlying lesion is usually a solitary parathyroid adenoma or generalized parathyroid hyperplasia. Rarely, parathyroid gland adenocarcinoma (chief-cell carcinoma) may be found. In humans, primary HPT may develop from long-standing secondary HPT, but this has not been proved in dogs. Recently, primary HPT due to parathyroid gland hyperplasia was identified in two of four puppies from a litter of German shepherd dogs; this lesion was suspected to be familial.

CLINICAL SIGNS

Most of the clinical signs can be attributed to the effects of hypercalcemia (Table 1). Excess PTH promotes increased gastrointestinal absorption of calcium and phosphorus, increased renal tubular reabsorption of calcium, decreased renal tubular reabsorption of phosphorus, and mobilization of both calcium and phosphorus from bone. Hypercalcemia and hypophosphatemia are the net results of these effects. The clinical signs of hypercalcemia are similar regardless of the underlying cause, involving mainly the nervous, gastrointestinal, and urinary systems.

Decreased neuromuscular excitability may result in generalized skeletal muscle weakness and decreased motility of the smooth muscle of the gastrointestinal tract. Depression, stupor, coma, and muscle twitching may occur when serum calcium levels exceed 15 mg/dl. Vomiting, anorexia, and constipation may also result.

Hypercalcemia frequently causes defective urinary concentrating ability, and the owner may present the dog for evaluation of polyuria and polydipsia. The urine is usually hyposthenuric (1.001 to 1.007 SG) or isosthenuric (1.008 to 1.012 SG). In some instances the urine specific gravity may be greater than 1.012. Early in the course of hypercalcemia, normal renal function is maintained (BUN and serum creatinine are normal). As hypercalcemia persists or becomes more severe, progressive functional and structural alterations occur in the kidney, leading to primary renal failure (increased BUN and serum creatinine). (Hypercalcemic nephropathy and associated disorders are discussed in greater detail in *Current Veterinary Therapy VII*, pages 1067 to 1072.) Nephrocalcinosis may occur histologically and occasionally can be observed radiographically. Kidney stones have been seen in dogs with hyperparathyroidism but are rare.

Osteoporosis from excessive PTH secretion may result in bone pain and pathologic fractures. Compression fractures of the vertebrae may cause paresis or paralysis. Fractures that occur after minimal trauma should alert the clinician to the possibility of metabolic bone disease, including that caused by primary HPT. Loose teeth and subsequent pain while eating may be seen as bone around the tooth roots is reabsorbed. Fibrous osteodystrophy may result in maxillary and facial bone enlargement.

HPT should be suspected upon finding hypercalcemia on a routine serum chemistry profile submitted from a dog with vague clinical signs. The search for the cause of hypercalcemia should first eliminate the more likely possibilities (Table 2). Pathologic hypercalcemia is often caused by underlying malignancy. Lymphosarcoma (LSA) is the most common

Table 1. *Categories of Clinical Presentation of Hypercalcemic Patients with HPT*

Asymptomatic—fortuitously discovered
Polyuria/polydipsia—no other systemic signs
Systemically ill—anorexia, vomiting, depression
Renal failure/urinary stones
Bone pain—osteoporosis/fractures
Combinations of the above

Table 2.　*Conditions Associated with Hypercalcemia**

Young growing animal (normal)
Cancer-associated hypercalcemia
　　Lymphosarcoma
　　Apocrine gland adenocarcinoma of the anal sac
　　Other tumors (no bone involvement)
　　Bone tumors
　　　　Primary/metastatic
Hypoadrenocorticism
Primary renal failure
　　Chronic renal failure
　　Acute renal failure (diuretic phase)
Septic osteomyelitis
　　Bacterial/fungal
Hypervitaminosis D
Hemoconcentration (hyperproteinemia)
Primary hyperparathyroidism
Disuse osteoporosis
Severe hypothermia
Laboratory error

*In decreasing order of likelihood.

disease associated with hypercalcemia in the dog and should be suspected as the cause of hypercalcemia until proved otherwise. Estimates of the incidence of hypercalcemia in dogs with LSA vary from 10 to 40 per cent. Many dogs with hypercalcemia caused by LSA will have a radiographically visible mediastinal mass. Apocrine gland adenocarcinoma of the anal sac may also cause hypercalcemia and is usually found in older female dogs. This perirectal tumor may not be obvious externally, as it often remains covered with hair and creates little discomfort for the dog. Consequently, a careful rectal examination is necessary for diagnosis. Lymphosarcoma, apocrine gland adenocarcinoma of the anal sac, and other malignancies are thought to elaborate substances that promote bone dissolution and phosphaturia in the absence of bone metastasis. This creates hypercalcemia and hypophosphatemia indistinguishable from primary HPT (referred to in the past as pseudohyperparathyroidism). The chemical substances elaborated appear to be distinct from PTH.

Bone tumors, either primary or metastatic, rarely cause enough bone dissolution to result in hypercalcemia, often accompanied by hyperphosphatemia. Septic osteomyelitis (bacterial or fungal) also may rarely result in hypercalcemia and hyperphosphatemia owing to direct bone dissolution.

In a recent review of hypercalcemic dogs at The Ohio State University Veterinary Hospital, approximately 10 per cent (6/57) were found to have hypoadrenocorticism. The mechanism for hypercalcemia in hypoadrenocorticism is unknown; it is usually transient and rapidly disappears after appropriate therapy for Addison's disease.

Primary renal failure is occasionally associated with hypercalcemia, but more often serum calcium values are normal or slightly low. In chronic renal disease, long-standing secondary HPT may contribute to the development of hypercalcemia, but other mechanisms have not been adequately evaluated. Occasionally in the diuretic phase of acute renal failure hypercalcemia will develop, possibly as a result of mobilization of calcium from soft tissue where it was deposited during the oliguric phase.

Theoretically, severe hemoconcentration and hyperproteinemia could result in hypercalcemia, because approximately 50 per cent of total serum calcium is protein bound. In a review of 2000 serum biochemical profiles of dogs at The Ohio State University Veterinary Hospital, we were unable to identify any cases in which hypercalcemia could be directly attributed to hyperproteinemia alone. In some cases, hyperproteinemia probably contributed to hypercalcemia, but other disorders involving calcium metabolism were also present.

Hypervitaminosis D may cause hypercalcemia and hyperphosphatemia. Review of the patient history should be undertaken once hypercalcemia is known to be a problem, and specific questions should be asked about dietary supplementation with vitamin D and calcium-containing products. This is particularly important when the animal is owned by a breeder who insists upon feeding special dietary supplements. Overdosage of vitamin D as therapy for hypoparathyroidism may also lead to hypercalcemia. Ingestion of the houseplant day-blooming jessamine (*Cestrus diurnum*) is a potential cause of hypercalcemia, since this plant contains pharmacologic quantities of active vitamin D_3.

Mild hypercalcemia is rarely seen in dogs immobilized owing to extensive neurologic or skeletal injury. Continued bone resorption with decreased bone accretion may be responsible for hypercalcemia. Severe hypothermia has recently been reported as a cause of transient hypercalcemia in a dog, but the mechanism was not addressed.

APPROACH TO THE CLINICAL WORK-UP

The evaluation of an animal with hypercalcemia is presented in Table 3. After hypercalcemia has been documented, a repeat laboratory determination of serum calcium content should be performed to exclude laboratory error. It is important to remember that young growing dogs (less than one year of age) may have serum calcium values considerably higher than those customarily considered normal. Often these dogs will also have increased serum phosphorus and serum alkaline phosphatase values. Uncommonly, severe hyperproteinemia may be associated with hypercalcemia; consequently, the serum calcium and serum protein levels should be evaluated together.

Table 3.   *Sequential Work-Up of Hypercalcemia*

1. Consider age—could hypercalcemia be due
   to normal growth?
2. Consider influence of total protein/albumin on
   serum calcium
3. Repeat serum calcium—verify accuracy/persistence
4. Repeat the history—access to drugs?
   a. Vitamin D
   b. Calcium chloride/gluconate
   c. Day-blooming jessamine (houseplant)
5. Repeat physical examination
   a. Lymph node enlargement?
   b. Abdominal organomegaly?
   c. Rectal/perirectal exam—mass?
   d. Ophthalmoscopic examination—retinal
      infiltrates/hemorrhage?
   e. Any unexplained nodules or growths?
   f. Clip hair and palpate thyroparathyroids—mass?
6. Additional data evaluation
   a. Serum phosphorus
   b. Serum alkaline phosphatase
   c. Urinalysis/BUN/serum creatinine
   d. Chest radiograph
      1. Exclude possibility of mediastinal mass
      2. Exclude metastases
      3. Evaluate bone density
   e. CBC—exclude leukemia
   f. Abdominal radiograph
      1. Rule out nonpalpable organomegaly
      2. Evaluate bone density
      3. Evaluate sublumbar masses
   g. Bone marrow evaluation
      1. Exclude LSA/leukemia
      2. Multiple myeloma
7. Special tests
   a. IPTH
   b. Radioisotope thyroid scan
   c. Bone survey radiography
   d. Bone scan
8. Parathyroid gland exploratory/excision

The diagnostic approach must exclude malignancy as the cause of persistent hypercalcemia, especially lymphosarcoma. The diagnosis of primary HPT is considered only after nonparathyroid malignancy has been excluded. There is no singular laboratory test that is diagnostic for primary HPT. It is prudent to reassess the initial history after hypercalcemia has been documented. Specific questions about the administration of dietary supplements or medications in the form of vitamin D or calcium salts should be asked. Access to the houseplant day-blooming jessamine should be determined.

A careful rectal examination should be performed to rule out apocrine gland adenocarcinoma of the anal sac. It is unlikely that a parathyroid adenoma or parathyroid hyperplasia will be palpated, but palpation is more likely to be successful if the cervical region hair is clipped. All lymph nodes should be examined in an effort to detect subtle lymphadenopathy that may not have initially aroused suspicion. Repeated abdominal palpation to disclose organomegaly (hepatomegaly, splenomeg-

aly, mesenteric or sublumbar lymphadenopathy) should be performed. Ophthalmoscopic evaluation will exclude retinal infiltrates or hemorrhages that may accompany LSA or the systemic mycoses.

Serum phosphorus is usually evaluated simultaneously with serum calcium. Hypophosphatemia due to phosphaturia often accompanies hypercalcemia due to primary HPT but can also occur in malignancies (LSA, apocrine gland adenocarcinoma of the anal sac). Hypophosphatemia is a less consistent feature of primary HPT than is hypercalcemia, and its absence does not exclude the diagnosis. Indeed, renal failure caused by hypercalcemic nephropathy may result in hyperphosphatemia.

Serum alkaline phosphatase (SAP) may be elevated in patients with long-standing primary HPT. Increased SAP of bone origin reflects osteoblastic activity. This may also be seen in other disorders associated with accelerated bone remodeling. Increased SAP in a hypercalcemic animal also may be of liver origin owing to infiltrative lesions (LSA, liver metastasis, mycoses). Elevation of SAP by the prior administration of glucocorticosteroids should also be considered.

Renal function should be evaluated in all dogs with hypercalcemia because of the known deleterious effects of hypercalcemia on renal function. It is sometimes difficult to decide whether hypercalcemia is a cause or an effect of renal failure. Prior to the onset of azotemia (normal BUN/serum creatinine), varying degrees of impaired renal concentrating ability may be caused by hypercalcemia.

Thoracic radiographs should be obtained in all hypercalcemic dogs to exclude the possibility of thymic LSA or metastatic neoplasia. Bone density can be qualitatively evaluated on routine thoracic and abdominal radiographs. Severe osteoporosis may be seen in dogs with HPT because these dogs may survive longer with their disease than those with nonparathyroid malignancies, which cause distant bone dissolution. The vertebrae are often demineralized in long-standing primary HPT, and loss of the lamina dura dentes may be the earliest radiographic abnormality in primary HPT.

A complete blood count (CBC) and bone marrow evaluation should be normal in dogs with primary HPT, whereas they could support a diagnosis of malignancy in dogs with LSA or multiple myeloma.

The determination of immunoreactive PTH (IPTH) is of value in confirming cases of primary HPT when other causes of hypercalcemia cannot be documented. An elevated serum IPTH value from a dog with normal renal function and hypercalcemia virtually assures the diagnosis of primary HPT. Dogs with nonparathyroid-mediated hypercalcemia will have IPTH values that are either low or, in some cases, within normal limits. This is because the parathyroid glands decrease their synthesis and release of PTH as a negative feedback response to the hypercalcemia. Studies in dogs have failed to document elevated IPTH values in animals with hypercalcemia caused by nonparathyroid malignancy. Extremely elevated IPTH values can, however, be found in dogs with severe renal disease. The serum IPTH value should be interpreted in relation to the serum calcium value. A decreased IPTH value is anticipated if the hypercalcemia is due to a nonparathyroid lesion. Elevated serum IPTH values are not appropriate if the serum calcium is elevated.

Standard laboratory determinations of serum IPTH are not yet widely available for dogs. A recent study has suggested measuring canine serum IPTH activity in human commercial laboratories. These procedures use antisera against bovine PTH and predominantly measure C-terminal IPTH. These methods were able to differentiate and accurately identify primary HPT, primary hypoparathyroidism, secondary HPT, and normal dogs. Normal values must be established for the particular laboratory performing this test, as procedural differences may result in different normal serum IPTH values. The current cost of measuring serum IPTH is about $70, and special handling of the blood sample is required. For some assays, the sample must be taken following an overnight fast, allowed to clot for four to five hours at 4°C, centrifuged, and the serum transferred to plastic tubes prior to freezing and delivery to the lab. The expense and special handling required presently limit the widespread use of this test, but its value should be appreciated in selected cases.

Radioisotope scans of the thyroid gland may show abnormalities in the presence of a parathyroid tumor but can be normal if the tumor is very small. Skeletal survey radiographs and bone scans may reveal isolated bone lesions that could account for hypercalcemia.

When all of the more common causes of hypercalcemia have been excluded, exploratory surgery of the neck may be required to diagnose parathyroid gland adenoma or hyperplasia.

TREATMENT OF PRIMARY HYPERPARATHYROIDISM

Initial treatment directed at reducing the deleterious effects of hypercalcemia may be necessary prior to definitive diagnosis and parathyroid gland surgery. The most important considerations are to correct any pre-existing dehydration and maintain normal hydration. Dehydration diminishes renal excretion of calcium, and hemoconcentration increases the relative concentration of all fractions of serum calcium. Enhanced renal excretion of calcium is further accomplished by infusing 0.9 per cent NaCl as the fluid of choice, since it contains no calcium and the large quantity of sodium subsequently filtered by the kidney reduces tubular reabsorption of calcium. Volume expansion will reduce the severity of hypercalcemia but will not usually return serum calcium to normal.

Diuretic therapy may provide additional benefit in lowering serum calcium. Furosemide at 5 mg/kg initially and 5 mg/kg/hr thereafter is effective in lowering serum calcium in experimental dogs. Meticulous attention must be paid to intravenous fluid replacement volume if this technique is to be effective. A maximal decrease in serum calcium of 3 mg/dl can be anticipated. Thiazide diuretics should not be used, since they decrease renal calcium excretion and may increase the severity of hypercalcemia.

Glucocorticosteroids may be useful in the management of hypercalcemia, since they limit bone resorption, decrease intestinal absorption of calcium, and increase renal excretion of calcium. Additionally, direct cytolytic effect on certain neoplasms may be seen. A dramatic response with rapid return of serum calcium to normal often occurs in those dogs whose hypercalcemia is related to LSA. If possible, the use of glucocorticosteroids should be withheld until all diagnostic tissue and serum samples have been obtained. Hypercalcemia caused by primary HPT is usually refractory to the beneficial effects of glucocorticosteroids.

Other therapeutic modalities directed toward lowering serum calcium have not been widely used in veterinary medicine but include phosphate infusions, calcitonin, antiprostaglandins, mithramycin, diphosphonates, EDTA, and dialysis. Of these, the use of calcitonin seems most deserving of future study for the temporary management of hypercalcemia in dogs.

When other causes of hypercalcemia have been excluded, surgical exploration of the cervical region is undertaken and an attempt is made to identify all four parathyroid glands. Particular care in maintaining hemostasis is required to facilitate identification of normal or abnormal parathyroid tissue. The cranial parathyroid glands are more easily visualized, as the caudal glands may be embedded in thyroid tissue. A single adenoma will be obvious in comparison to the remaining atrophic parathyroid glands, which often cannot be identified at surgery. A single adenoma should be completely excised. When all identifiable parathyroid glands are enlarged owing to hyperplasia, subtotal parathyroidectomy with removal of three of the four glands is recommended. In some instances the parathyroid glands will not be obviously hyperplastic, but hyperplasia and hypertrophy may be observed histopathologically. A subtotal parathyroidectomy is recommended in the presence of hypercalcemia and normal-appearing parathyroids at surgery. In the rare event that a parathyroid gland carcinoma is encountered, invasion of adjacent tissue and metastases to regional lymph nodes can be anticipated.

If hypercalcemia persists following parathyroidectomy, an additional parathyroid gland lesion must be suspected. Examples include another adenoma not detected at surgery, functional metastases, and ectopic parathyroid tissue in the mediastinum releasing excessive PTH. It is wise to reconsider all diagnostic possibilities to ensure that they have indeed been excluded prior to thoracotomy and mediastinal exploration for ectopic parathyroid gland tissue.

Since the half-life of intact PTH is short (about 20 minutes), resolution of hypercalcemia may occur within one to two hours following successful parathyroid gland surgery. Symptomatic hypocalcemia may occur within the initial 24 to 48 hours after parathyroid gland surgery and may result in restlessness, tetanic seizures, muscle cramping, or twitching. Severe hypocalcemia may result in cardiopulmonary arrest. The development of postoperative hypocalcemia may be the result of hypofunction of the remaining atrophied parathyroid tissue (decreased PTH secretion) and may also be due to surgically induced damage to the remaining parathyroid tissue or its vascular supply. Postoperative hypocalcemia can also develop in the presence of normal PTH secretion if accelerated bone mineralization takes place ("hungry-bone syndrome"). Symptomatic hypocalcemia is a common finding following parathyroidectomy in animals with severe bone demineralization and may be difficult to control even with parenteral calcium administration. Other causes of hypercalcemia are not often associated with post-treatment symptomatic hypocalcemia, as the severity of bone demineralization in other disorders is not nearly as great. Serum calcium should be monitored after surgery to evaluate the magnitude of hypocalcemia. Patients with severe bone demineralization should be started on an intravenous calcium-containing infusion immediately following surgery prior to the advent of a symptomatic tetany. An infusion rate of 0.5 to 2.0 mg calcium/kg/hr has been suggested as a starting rate, with further adjustments based on serial serum calcium determinations. Symptomatic tetany can be managed with infusions of 10 per cent calcium gluconate, given slowly to effect. Oral calcium and vitamin D supplementation may be necessary to maintain normocalcemia.

The prognosis for primary HPT is usually guarded to poor since end-organ (bone, kidney) damage is often long-standing at the time of definitive diagnosis. Patients with renal failure caused by hypercalcemia and those with severe bone demineralization have the poorest prognosis. Early detection prior to primary renal failure and severe bone demineralization will result in improved success following parathyroid gland surgery.

SUPPLEMENTAL READING

Capen, C. C., and Martin, S. L.: Parathyroid glands and calcium metabolism. *In* Kirk, R. W. (ed.): *Current Veterinary Therapy VI.* Philadelphia: W. B. Saunders, 1977.

Chew, D. J., and Capen, C. C.: Hypercalcemic nephropathy and associated disorders. *In* Kirk, R. W. (ed.): *Current Veterinary Therapy VII.* Philadelphia: W. B. Saunders, 1980.

Chew, D. J., and Meuten, D. J.: Disorders of calcium and phosphorus metabolism. Vet. Clin. North Am. 12:411, 1982.

Feldman, E., and Krutzik, S.: Case reports of parathyroid levels in spontaneous canine parathyroid disorders. J.A.A.H.A. 17:393, 1981.

Finco, D. R., and Rowland, G. N.: Hypercalcemia secondary to chronic renal failure in the dog. A report from cases. J.A.V.M.A. 173:990, 1978.

Legendre, A. M.: Primary hyperparathyroidism. *In* Kirk, R. W. (ed.): *Current Veterinary Therapy VII.* Philadelphia: W. B. Saunders, 1980.

Thomson, K. G., Jones, L. T., et al.: Hereditary primary hyperparathyroidism in German shepherd dogs. Am. J. Pathol., in press.

Section 12

REPRODUCTIVE DISORDERS

DONALD H. LEIN, D.V.M.
Consulting Editor

REPRODUCTIVE PHYSIOLOGY AND ENDOCRINE PATTERNS OF THE BITCH

P. W. CONCANNON, Ph.D.

Ithaca, New York

THE OVARIAN CYCLE: FOLLICULAR AND LUTEAL PHASES

FOLLICULAR PHASE

Bitches ovulate spontaneously following a one– to three–week *follicular phase* during which circulating estradiol levels progressively increase from basal levels of 2 to 10 pg/ml of serum to peak levels of 50 to 120 pg/ml. Concurrent increases in estrone have also been reported. During the follicular phase the elevated estrogen causes increasingly evident external signs of *proestrus:* vaginal discharge of uterine blood; enlargement, edema, and hyperemia of the vulva and perineum; secretion of sex pheromones; and attraction of males. In proestrus the bitch will not permit mounting and intromission. Proestrus often lasts 5 to 10 days but ranges from 2 to 22 days. The transition from proestrus to *estrus* is, by definition, a behavioral one: that is, the bitch stands for the stud. It occurs, in most instances, in association with the events that comprise the culmination of follicle development: a decline in estrogen secretion and serum estrogen levels; a rapid increase in previously initiated follicle luteinization; a corresponding increase in serum progesterone levels; and the preovulatory surge release of luteinizing hormone (LH) from the anterior pituitary. Ovulation occurs about two days after the LH surge. These and other events of the nonpregnant cycle are outlined in Figure 1.

The behavioral change in the transition from proestrus to estrus may occur rapidly (over an 8- to 12-hour period) or slowly (over one to three days). Although it most often occurs synchronously with the preovulatory LH surge, it can occur out of synchrony with the LH surge. The onset of estrus (and the potential first day of mating) may be as early as two to three days before the LH peak or as late as four to five days after the peak. Therefore, the first day of estrus—the first day the bitch stands firmly for the male, shows steady reflex tail deviation, and reflexly presents the vulva to allow intromission—may occur as early as five days before ovulation or as late as two to three days after ovulation.

PREOVULATORY LUTEINIZATION

The endocrine events of late proestrus and early estrus represent the preovulatory transition from the follicular phase to the *luteal phase* of the cycle. Strictly defined, corpora lutea are the histologically transformed progesterone-secreting structures that form from follicles after ovulation, and the luteal phase is a postovulatory period. In the bitch, however, follicles slowly begin to luteinize during proestrus before estrogen secretion is maximal and then undergo a rapid, extensive luteinization during the preovulatory LH surge such that the ovulating follicles have all the characteristics of, and in fact are, rapidly developing corpora lutea. Serum progesterone levels during proestrus rise from 0.4 to 0.6 ng/ml to 0.8 to 1.2 ng/ml at the time of the estrogen peak. Progesterone then increases rapidly throughout the LH surge as estrogen levels decline, reaching 2 to 4 ng/ml at the time of the LH peak and 4 to 10 ng/ml by the time of ovulation two days later.

LUTEAL PHASE

The progesterone level continues to increase throughout the 5 to 10 days during which estrus is usually observed and reaches peak levels of 15 to 80 ng/ml between 15 and 25 days after the LH peak. Corpora lutea continue to secrete progesterone, and serum progesterone levels are maintained above baseline values for two months or more after the LH peak and onset of estrus, although the pattern of secretion and the variability in duration of secretion differ in pregnant and nonpregnant bitches. In nonpregnant bitches progesterone levels slowly decline to reach 1 ng/ml by 55 to 110 days but may not reach basal levels of 0.3 to 0.4 ng/ml until 120 to 150 days after the LH peak. The duration of the luteal phase, and thus of the postestrus or metestrus period of ovarian activity, is not clear-cut and depends on one's point of view. It can be considered to last about two months, as in pregnancy; or two to three months, until mammary development associated with pseudopregnancy subsides; or around 80 days, when mean progesterone

886

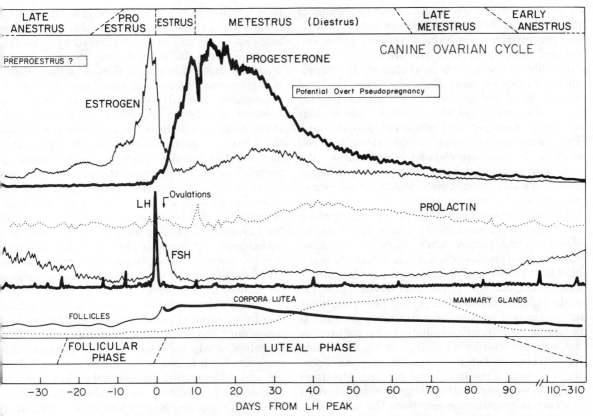

Figure 1. A schematic representation of typical endocrine changes reported or presumed to occur during the nonpregnant canine ovarian cycle and their relation to observable stages and functional phases of the cycle.

levels near 1 ng/ml; or 100 to 160 days, when progesterone levels reach anestrous, basal values; or 120 to 140 days, when the effect of progesterone on the histologically examined endometrium is no longer evident. The transition from a nonpregnant luteal phase (metestrus) to anestrus involves progressive, subtle changes that are variable within and among bitches. Likewise, the transition from anestrus to the subsequent proestrus also probably involves progressive, subtle changes associated with the onset of the next follicular phase.

CYCLE INTERVALS

The interval between one cycle and the next can range from 4 to 13 months and may be consistent or variable within individual bitches. In the author's beagle colony, the shortest and longest intervals consistently recorded for individual bitches have been about four and ten months, respectively. The longest single interval that could be verified by serial progesterone measurement was 13 months. Intervals between subsequent periods of observed estrus longer than 13 months have always included an intervening ovulatory cycle and luteal phase for which external signs were not observed. The mean interval between cycles is seven months. Studies on differences in mean interestrus intervals between breeds have involved too few animals to be mean-

ingful but suggest that it may be only five to six months in German shepherds.

NEW FOLLICULAR PHASE

Regarding the transition from the end of one cycle to the beginning of the next, the possibility that a pre-proestrus phase of follicular activity regularly occurs should be acknowledged. In the author's laboratory each of six "anestrus" bitches ovariohysterectomized between 150 and 180 days following the onset of estrus, although showing no external signs of impending proestrus, exhibited evidence of ovarian follicular activity including gross uterine and oviductal hyperemia, enlarged oviductal fimbria protruding through the bursal slit, and a markedly sanguine endometrium. It is possible, then, that the period of "anestrus" is a physiologic "nonevent," at least following a nonpregnant cycle, and represents the transition from the late luteal phase of one cycle to the early follicular phase of the next cycle.

THE ESTROUS CYCLE: OBSERVABLE STAGES

The canine ovarian cycle can best be understood in terms of the follicular and luteal phases, which in turn are endocrinologically defined in terms of the circulating hormone profiles of estrogen, LH, and progesterone. However, veterinary practitioners and serious breeders are often restricted to externally visible criteria in evaluating the reproductive history or status of a bitch. Hence the need to understand and appreciate the classical stages of the canine cycle and the extent to which their definition, meaning, and usage can and do vary. The stages are *proestrus, estrus, metestrus,* and *anestrus,* the common element being "estrus." Estrus is a behavioral term with an etymological history of gadfly, sting, frenzy, female sexual frenzy, presentation to males, acceptance of a male. *Estrus* lasts about one week and is the period during which the bitch accepts mounting by a male and shows an obvious sexual posture while doing so, including standing firmly with marked extensor activity in the hind legs, raising and presenting the perineum in a lordosis-like manner, and reflexly deviating the tail to the side. In contrast, during the preceding week or so of *proestrus,* the bitch frustrates attempts at mounting or intromission, initially by confronting the male and later by retreating, sitting, or crouching, although in late proestrus she may stand passively without a positive sexual posture. *Metestrus* is the period after estrus during which there is evidence of progesterone secretion. The subsequent *anestrus* is usually described as a period of ovarian quiescence because there is no external evidence of ovarian activity.

PROESTRUS

The first evidence of proestrus may be vulval enlargement or a bloody vaginal discharge, one preceding the other by one to four days; alternatively, the two may occur simultaneously. Some bitches may be so fastidious in licking their genitalia that the bloody discharge is not observed on the vulva although it is present intravaginally. Proestrus is observed an average of five to nine days but in the extreme may be as short as two to three days or as long as three weeks. Vulval tumescence increases throughout proestrus, reaching a maximum in size and turgidity by late proestrus at the time of the estrogen peak. The transition from the passive or confused behavior of late proestrus to the positive, reflex sexual behavior of estrus can be determined by testing the bitch's response daily with a male.

ESTRUS

The onset of estrus often occurs rapidly over an 8- to 32-hour period and within one day of the LH surge. Experiments on ovariectomized bitches administered exogenous sex steroids demonstrated that proestrous behavior is caused by continuous increases in blood levels of estrogen, whereas estrous behavior is triggered by a subsequent fall in estrogen levels and can be facilitated by a simultaneous increase in progesterone. Similar experiments indicated that a rapid decline in the circulating estrogen:progesterone ratio also produces a preovulatory-like LH surge. The onset of estrus, however, may be asynchronous with the LH peak. It can be as early as three, or even five, days before the LH surge, particularly in sexually experienced and sociable bitches. Such an "early estrus" is probably caused by a transient decline in estrogen levels or a rise in progesterone during the follicular phase but prior to a final estrogen peak. The onset of estrus can also be as late as four to five days after the LH surge and two to three days after ovulation, particularly in pubertal bitches, and may indicate a relative insensitivity of behavioral centers to the initial decline in the estrogen:progesterone ratio at the time of the LH peak.

Estrous Abnormalities. The behavioral transition from proestrus to estrus in some instances may not occur, and what appears to be a prolonged proestrus slowly subsides. In some instances this can occur because of a failure in LH release, following which the mature follicles fail to luteinize and ovulate but continue to produce diminishing amounts of estrogen for a period of time without an acute fall in estrogen levels. More often, however, the "prolonged-proestrus, estrus-failure" syndrome occurs in the presence of normal periovulatory endocrine events to which behavioral centers fail to respond. Another type of "false heat" can also occur. A bitch can develop a normal proestrus during follicular development and then, in the absence of an LH surge and/or ovulation, display an apparently normal estrus or intermittent periods of estrous behavior, presumably in response to the declining estrogen levels associated with atresia of the non-ovulating follicles. A false proestrus or false estrus related to ovulation failure is often followed by a normal cycle within three to eight weeks.

Duration of Estrus. Behavioral estrus in a typical cycle lasts 6 to 12 days. It may be abbreviated to two to three days in cycles in which estrus onset is delayed in relation to the LH peak and ovulation. It can also be protracted, with up to three weeks of constant estrous behavior, and in extreme cases may occur intermittently or to a variable degree for even longer periods. In one instance in the author's colony a bitch demonstrated behavioral estrus daily through the fortieth day of pregnancy. Even in normal or typical cycles the end of estrus may not be acute but may involve three to six days of less intense or intermittent receptivity. Vaginal cytology and morphology are better indices of the end of estrus (vaginal estrus) and the beginning of metestrus and can be used to determine the end of the fertile period or to estimate, retrospectively, the time of previous matings in relation to ovulation.

Period of Fertility. Terms such as *in heat* or *in season* represent an unfortunate but unavoidable problem when discussing the condition of a bitch concerning fertility or reproductive status. Although such terms can be useful in detailing much of the reproductive history of a bitch, they are useless when considering the actual events and time course of any individual cycle or breeding attempts, past or present. It is important to make clear to owners that a bitch's normal "heat," or full period of attractiveness to males, bleeding, and vulval swelling, has two distinct parts: a preparatory phase *(proestrus)* of variable length during which she will not allow attempts at copulation, and a receptive period *(estrus)* of variable duration during part of which fertility is maximal. In the author's experience single matings as early as three days before the LH peak (five days before ovulation, six to seven days before ovum maturation) can be fertile, and matings as late as seven to eight days after the LH peak can be fertile, but not routinely. Peak fertility is associated with matings zero to four days after the LH peak. Therefore, because of the variability in the onset of estrus and potential time of first mating, it is advisable to recommend matings as early as possible in estrus, followed by second and third matings at two-day intervals. Such a mating scheme provides an early mating for a bitch that does not *stand* (show estrus) until after ovulation and provides a late

mating for a bitch that starts accepting the male five or more days before she ovulates.

In the absence of a sexually aggressive male or when the bitch has a history of conception failure or abnormal estrous behavior, scheduling of breeding or artificial insemination can be a problem. Nonbehavioral parameters can be used to assess the time of ovulation or to monitor the transition from the follicular phase to the luteal phase. Considering the variability that can be encountered with normal proestrus and estrus, serial assessment of vaginal exfoliate cytology, vaginal morphology, and vulval swelling should be considered when making any breeding recommendations.

Vaginal Smears. The examination of vaginal smears at one- to two-day intervals can confirm the progression of proestrus to the completion of vaginal cornification indicative of follicle maturation or may indicate a failure in such progression. The expected changes in vaginal exfoliate cytology are outlined in Figure 2. A progression of partially cornified cells to 95 to 100 per cent of the smear, with a concomitant loss of leukocytes and nonsuperficial epithelial cells, can be taken as an indication of estrogen secretion and follicle maturation to the point where an LH surge will result in ovulation. However, a distinct, readily discernible change in the smear indicative of the occurrence of the LH surge, ovulation, or preovulatory progesterone secretion has

Figure 2. A schematic summary of temporal relationships among periovulatory endocrine events, behavioral and vulval changes, and changes in vaginal exfoliate cytology associated with proestrous and estrous periods in the bitch.

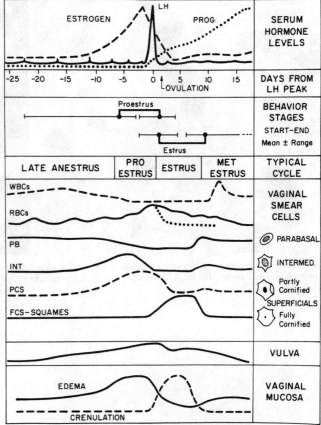

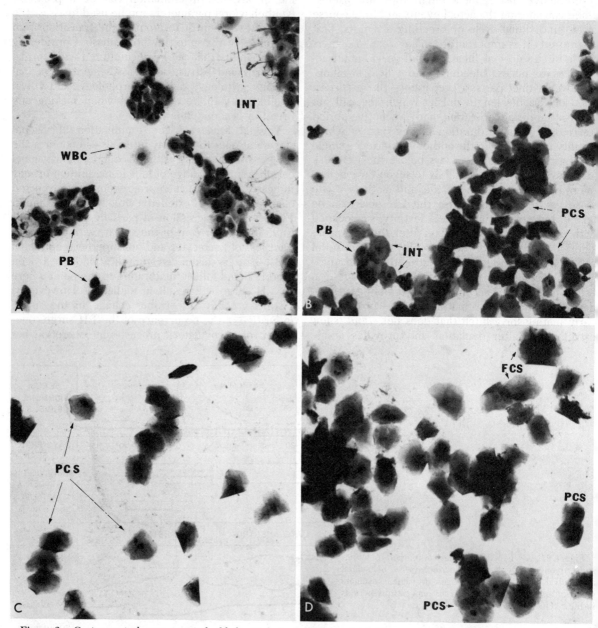

Figure 3. Canine vaginal smears typical of behavioral stages of the cycle and/or specified days before (−) or after (+) the preovulatory LH surge (day 0). *A*, Late anestrus. *B*, Early to mid proestrus (day −6). *C*, Late proestrus (day −1). *D*, Early estrus (day +1).

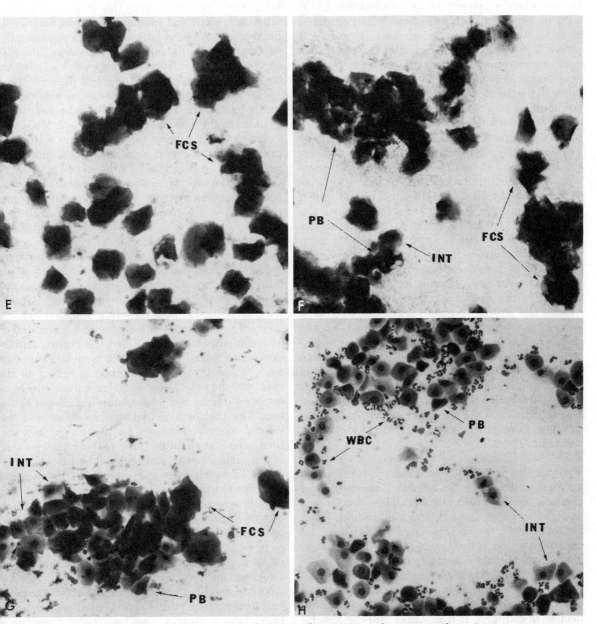

Figure 3. *Continued.* E, Mid estrus (day +4). F, End of estrus (day +7). G, Early metestrus (day +9). H, Distinct metestrus (day +11). PB = parabasal cells; INT = small or large intermediate cells; PCS = partly cornified superficial cells; FCS = fully cornified superficial cells; WBC = white blood cells.

not been found. By three to four days after the LH peak, fully cornified superficial cells almost completely replace the partially cornified cells and dominate the smear from mid to late estrus. Near the time of the LH peak a clearing of the background in the vaginal smear, possibly related to a decrease in mucoprotein content of the vaginal mucus, is seen in some but not all bitches. When observed in serial vaginal smears of individual bitches it is probably indicative of the decline in the estrogen:progesterone ratio near the time of the LH peak and thus is indicative of the beginning of the optimal period to begin breeding. The extent of cornification may not be as reliable an index of the onset of endocrinologic estrus (the occurrence of the estrogen peak) as some reports would suggest. Furthermore, the details of cornification vary with the fixation and staining methods used. For example, with Shorr's trichrome stain or the rapid hematology stain from Harleco (Dif-Quik) fully cornified cells may not have discernible nuclei, but with the Sano-Pollack trichrome staining procedure described by Roszel (1975) nuclear elements remain visible in the cornified cells. The hematology stain mentioned is fast, inexpensive, easy to use, and useful for routine examination of progressive changes in the vaginal smear. A decrease in red blood cells in the vaginal smear, as well as a decrease in the vaginal discharge of blood, usually occurs in early estrus during preovulatory progesterone secretion, but it is by no means a routine occurrence; a delay in breeding in anticipation of its occurrence is not recommended. In many cycles the bloody discharge will continue throughout and beyond estrus and the fertile period. Vaginal smears common to several stages of the cycle are reproduced in Figure 3.

The examination of vaginal smears on a daily or alternate-day basis after full vaginal cornification and/or breeding may be helpful. The abrupt decrease in cornified cells that takes place about seven or eight days after the LH peak can confirm, albeit retrospectively, the occurrence of the LH peak and ovulation as well as the times, relative to ovulation, of attempts at mating or insemination.

The loss of cornification and reappearance of intermediate and parabasal cells appear to occur at a rather precise time after the abrupt preovulatory decline in estrogen. It is probably also the last day that a previously unmated bitch is likely to be fertile. In the author's laboratory this estrus-to-metestrus shift in the vaginal smear is considered to represent the start of metestrus because of its constant temporal relationship to the periovulatory endocrine events and its coincidence with the end of the fertile lifespan of oviductal oocytes. Phemister and colleagues (1973) were the first to emphasize the value of this unique change in the vaginal smear and its timing. They termed the event the "onset of diestrus."

The term *diestrus* has been suggested by several reviewers as a replacement for the long-standing use of *metestrus* in the canine ovarian cycle based on the concept that *diestrus* is more appropriate for indicating the period of luteal activity and more compatable with descriptions for several other species. Such revision of terminology seems unnecessary, however, considering the uniquely long durations of estrus and spontaneous luteal function in the dog. Since *estrus* lasts for some time during the beginning of the luteal phase, *metestrus* (literally the period after estrus) would appear a satisfactory term for the remainder of the luteal phase.

The reappearance of leukocytes in the vaginal smear toward the end of estrus has also been used to indicate the end of the fertile period. However, it may occur at a more variable time in relation to prior endocrine events than does the abrupt reappearance of nonsuperficial epithelial cells. Although the reappearance of leukocytes may be coincident with the metestrus shift in epithelial cells, it may also occur one to two days earlier or two to four days later and in some cases may not be abrupt.

Vaginoscopy. Visualization of gross changes in the vaginal mucosa may also be used to advantage. As estrogen increases during proestrus, the vaginal mucosa becomes progressively more edematous, rounded, puffy, and turgid in appearance. Around the time of the LH peak the white, rounded, smooth mucosal prominences initially become sacculated or folded in appearance, and then the mucosa rapidly develops a wrinkled, peaked, or crenulated appearance. These gross changes probably reflect an abrupt withdrawal of the water retention effects of estrogen during the preovulatory decline in estrogen. The crenated, dehydrated appearance of the vaginal mucosa continues for five to six days and then is lost, at about the time of the metestrus shift in the vaginal smear, and replaced by flaccid vaginal folds. These changes and their value in assessing the reproductive status of normal cycling bitches were first reported by Lindsay (1980). The condition of the vaginal mucosa can be most readily and critically viewed using fiberoptic endoscopy (see page 912). The changes can also be appreciated using a small, light-fitted proctoscope and direct visualization.

Vulval Swelling. The vulva and adjoining perineal area become progressively enlarged and turgid throughout proestrus. Swelling is maintained to a considerable degree throughout proestrus and estrus, but in many bitches there is a distinct softening and decrease in swelling following the LH surge and before ovulation. This softening has also been used as an indicator of the appropriate time for insemination of bitches in which the cycle was induced by exogenous gonadotropins.

METESTRUS

The onset of metestrus varies with the parameter measured and may be described by loss of estrous behavior, vaginal cornification, or vaginal crenulation or reappearance of leukocytes in the vaginal smear. The duration of metestrus likewise varies, depending on the criteria used. It lasts until the effects of the remaining two to three months of luteal progesterone secretion are no longer evident.

ANESTRUS

Representing the transition of one cycle to the next, anestrus is characterized by very low progesterone levels and may last one to six months.

REPRODUCTIVE HORMONES AND ENDOCRINE REGULATION OF THE CYCLE

PITUITARY HORMONES

Those pituitary hormones of interest include the glycoprotein hormones LH and follicle-stimulating hormone (FSH) and the protein hormones prolactin and growth hormone (GH).

LH

LH secretion during the follicular and luteal phases of the cycle has been monitored and reported by several laboratories, but detailed analyses of subtle changes in basal levels or of pulsatile release throughout the cycle have not been reported. However, the general mechanisms regulating LH release in the dog appear similar to those reported for other species, based on results reported to date. A hypothalamic decapeptide, gonadotropin-releasing hormone (GnRH), stimulates release of LH (and FSH) from the pituitary. Exogenous GnRH causes LH release within minutes. LH release is suppressed by ovarian estrogen through a negative feedback inhibition mechanism. LH levels are chronically elevated after ovariectomy and can subsequently be suppressed by estrogen administration. Studies in the author's laboratory demonstrated that continuous increases in estradiol will keep LH at basal levels in ovariectomized bitches and that a subsequent decline in estrogen causes a surge in LH that can be facilitated by a simultaneous increase in progesterone. Thus, in the normal transition from proestrus to estrus, the decline in the estrogen:progesterone ratio that occurs as the follicles reach maturity is probably the trigger for the preovulatory surge release of LH. Similar studies in ovariectomized bitches administered estrogen and progesterone suggested that proestrous and estrous behavior are likewise caused by estrogen stimulation and estrogen withdrawal, respectively, the latter being facilitated by a concomitant rise in progesterone. Pulses of LH release prior to and during proestrus appear to promote and ensure completion of follicle maturation. The preovulatory

surge in LH lasts 24 to 48 hours and causes accelerated follicle enlargement, luteinization, and ovulation. Ovulations occur 36 to 50 hours after the LH surge. LH is luteotropic, and basal LH levels are required for progesterone secretion during the luteal phase of the cycle.

FSH

FSH secretion and regulation have not been extensively studied in the bitch. Reimers and co-workers (1978) have shown that FSH is released simultaneously with LH following GnRH administration and during the preovulatory surge of LH. The preovulatory rise in serum FSH is longer than that of LH because the circulating half-life of FSH is longer. Olson (1980) very recently found that FSH levels are elevated above baseline during anestrus and subsequently depressed during proestrus. Apparently, follicles for the next cycle are recruited by elevated FSH secretion, and once recruited, they selectively regulate FSH secretion by a negative feedback mechanism. FSH inhibition may be caused by elevated estrogen or, as proposed for several other species, elevated serum levels of inhibin, a follicular peptide that selectively inhibits FSH secretion.

PROLACTIN

Prolactin secretion has been studied to a limited extent in the bitch primarily in relation to pregnancy, parturition, and lactation. Besides being a metabolic and lactogenic hormone, prolactin is also part of the pituitary luteotropic requirement along with LH. Prolactin secretion also seems to be inversely proportional to progesterone secretion. Serum prolactin levels surge ante partum as progesterone levels decline. Graf (1978) also found transient rises in prolactin in a few bitches during the early luteal phase at times when progesterone levels transiently decreased.

Both prolactin and thyroid-stimulating hormone (TSH) are released following an injection of the hypothalamic tripeptide thyrotropin-releasing hormone (TRH). Thus, factors that affect endogenous TRH release probably affect prolactin as well as thyrotropin release. Prolactin secretion is normally held to basal rates by a hypothalamic prolactin-release inhibitory factor (PIF), which may be dopamine. Bromoergocryptine, a plant alkaloid derivative, is a dopamine agonist and reduces prolactin secretion in the dog as in other species. Bromoergocryptine administration will reduce the severity of overt pseudopregnancies that can occur during the second or third month of the luteal phase. It thus appears likely that an elevation in prolactin levels at that time may play a major role in the development of overt pseudopregnancy. Such elevation may be variable among bitches to the extent that pseudocyesis is observed among various individuals or breeds. The influence of the photoperiod on prolactin secretion has not been studied in the dog as it has in other species.

GROWTH HORMONE

Growth hormone (GH) is primarily a metabolic hormone, but it is also lactogenic in some species. GH secretion is regulated, at least in part, by the hypothalamic tetradecapeptide somatostatin, an inhibitor of GH secretion, and by GH releasing factor activity found in hypothalamic extracts of dogs as well as other species. In addition, however, GH secretion in the dog can be affected by progesterone secretion during the ovarian cycle as well as by treatment with the contraceptive progestin medroxyprogesterone acetate (MPA). In studies at Cornell, pharmacologic doses of MPA elevated GH levels early in the course of treatment and over a 6- to 18-month period caused acromegaly-like changes, including overgrowth of the skin and alterations in glucose and insulin levels. More recently, Eigenmann and Venker-van Haagen (1981) reported that elevated GH levels and acromegaly-like symptoms may occur with contraceptive doses of MPA in some bitches, and furthermore, that some aged bitches may undergo such changes spontaneously and transiently in response to the progesterone secretion of the luteal phase of the cycle. Such findings may be relevant to understanding the etiology of mammary gland tumors in older bitches. In the Cornell study bitches that developed the most severe mammary neoplasias in response to high doses of MPA only did so following elevations in serum GH levels.

OVARIAN STEROID HORMONE SECRETION

ESTROGEN

During proestrus, follicles increase from 1 to 2 mm to 3 to 4 mm in diameter. The estradiol secreted by proestrus follicles is first evidenced externally by vulval swelling and/or the vaginal discharge of blood originating in the uterus by diapedesis. The pituitary gonadotropin requirement for follicle maturation and estradiol secretion in the dog has not been studied in detail. But, as in several other species, it probably includes FSH, promoting aromatase activity in granulosa cells, and LH, promoting progesterone and, consequently, androgen production, with the androgen serving as aromatase substrate for estradiol synthesis in the granulosa cells. Chakraborty and coworkers (1980) demonstrated that levels of estrone, a weakly estrogenic steroid, are also elevated during proestrus and in general parallel those of estradiol before and after the LH surge. However, estrone appears to be a less reliable indicator of follicular development than is estradiol. Serum estradiol levels reach peak levels (40 to 120 pg/ml) in late proestrus or early estrus, one to two days before the LH peak, and decrease sharply thereafter. The sharp decline in estradiol during and following the LH peak probably reflects an aromatase inhibiting effect of LH on fully matured follicles. In response to the LH surge the follicles rapidly enlarge, bulge from the surface of the ovary, and are about 8 to 10 mm in diameter at ovulation. Wildt and associates have photographically documented the gross appearance of proestrus follicles, ovulation, and luteinization *in situ* (1977).

During proestrus, estradiol promotes vaginal cornification, edema, and elongation; hyperemia and elongation of the uterine horns with a concomitant folding or flexing of the horns along their length; enlargement of the oviduct; and proliferation of the fimbriated end of the oviduct through the bursal slit. Except for minor elevations in mid metestrus, estrogen levels remain near baseline (5 to 15 pg/ml) during the nonpregnant luteal phase. We did find, however, that estrogen levels are increased during the later third of pregnancy (see hereafter) but are not as high as those observed during proestrus.

PROGESTERONE

Progesterone secretion is negligible in late anestrus. At about 40 days prior to the next estrus, serum levels are the same as in ovariectomized bitches, and the 0.2 to 0.5 ng/ml probably represents adrenal progesterone secretion. Administration of ACTH to ovariectomized bitches can cause an elevation of progesterone up to 2 ng/ml. From late anestrus through the onset of proestrus serum progesterone levels remain low; they may fluctuate between 0.4 and 0.8 ng/ml but, in general, tend to increase slightly. This increase, as well as the further increase to 0.6 to 1.0 ng/ml observed during proestrus, is probably due to secretion by developing ovarian follicles. During the second half of proestrus, in fact, follicles undergo partial luteinization prior to the beginning of the LH surge. In late proestrus and concomitant with the beginning of the LH surge, progesterone levels increase sharply, reaching 1 to 3 ng/ml at the time of the LH peak and 2 to 8 ng/ml at the time of ovulation two days later. In frequently collected samples, a pause in the rate of increase is often noted in association with ovulation. Levels then rise toward the maximum concentrations of 15 to 80 ng/ml observed 15 to 25 days after the LH peak. A brief fall in progesterone and rise in prolactin 8 to 12 days after the LH peak was reported in a limited number of bitches. After attainment of peak levels around day 25, progesterone levels slowly decrease over the remainder of the nonpregnant metestrus and fall below 1 ng/ml by days 55 to 90 and reach 0.3 to

0.5 ng/ml by days 100 to 160. Structural regression of the corpora lutea appears to parallel the progesterone profile.

Luteal progesterone secretion is dependent on pituitary LH and prolactin support throughout the luteal phase and ceases following hypophysectomy. Administration of anti-LH serum caused a dramatic decline in progesterone secretion, as did the administration of bromoergocryptine, a dopamine agonist known to reduce prolactin secretion in the bitch. Smith and McDonald (1974) found no significant differences in progesterone levels between overtly pseudopregnant bitches and bitches experiencing a "normal" metestrus. The possibility that the rate of decline in progesterone is a significant factor, with more abrupt declines causing greater elevations in prolactin, could be relevant to the etiology of pseudocyesis. This would perhaps explain the acute onset of pseudopregnancy in some bitches following spaying during metestrus and the often temporary amelioration of the symptoms of pseudopregnancy obtained by short-term treatment with megesterol acetate, a synthetic progestin.

The rapid increase in progesterone that occurs at the start of the preovulatory LH surge concomitant with the fall in estrogen facilitates the completion, if not the start, of the LH surge. This rapid facilitation of estrogen withdrawal at the time of the LH peak may be the basis of the consistent timing of the subsequent loss of vaginal cornification in relation to the LH peak. The continued increase in progesterone during the first part of the luteal phase promotes the growth and development of the uterine mucosa and mammary epithelium, although neither show significant secretory activity until later, during the phase of declining progesterone levels. Rising progesterone levels also cause the uterine horns to elongate and "coil" (actually fold) further such that by day 12 the turns of the horns may be mistaken for early implantation swellings. By days 20 to 25 the enlongated uterine horns no longer appear coiled and have become accommodated by the mesenteries. The endometrium then becomes obviously secretory for one or more months, during which time cystic endometrial hyperplasia may develop and promote a long-lasting mucometra or pyometra. In normal bitches obvious secretory activity slowly subsides as the progesterone levels decline to 1 ng/ml. Complete "repair" of the endometrium to the anestrous state has been reported by Andersen and Simpson (1973) to occur rather consistently between days 120 and 130 of the nonpregnant cycle.

The protracted period of luteal retrogression and decline in serum progesterone, together with the absence of any dramatic or consistent effects of hysterectomy on luteal function, suggest that there is no uterine luteolytic mechanism involved in canine luteolysis. Furthermore, the observations of Ginther indicate that the dog does not possess the intimate relationship between the uterovarian vein and ovarian artery seen in species in which hysterectomy prolongs luteal function and in which the transfer of uterine prostaglandin to the ovarian artery has been proposed as the basis of the uterine luteolytic mechanism (1976). Prostaglandin $F_{2\alpha}$ is luteolytic in the bitch, although relatively large doses must be administered repeatedly for several days to obtain complete luteolysis. The developing corpora lutea are particularly resistant to $PGF_{2\alpha}$, but after day 30 doses of 30 to 50 µg/kg administered two or three times a day will effect a complete luteolysis in nonpregnant bitches.

STEROID MECHANISM OF ACTION AND INTERACTION

In sex steroid target tissues there are specific cytoplasmic and nuclear receptors for both estrogen and progesterone. Each hormone acts on target cells by binding to its specific receptors in the cytoplasm and causing their translocation to the nucleus. Interaction of hormone-receptor complexes with the genome then results in hormone-specific modulation of subsequent nuclear-directed events, including cytoplasmic protein synthesis. Furthermore, each of the two steroids has the ability to regulate the synthesis of not only its own receptors but those of the other steroid as well. Increasing estrogen (as in proestrus) causes increased synthesis of estrogen receptors and progesterone receptors, preparatory for subsequent progesterone action, effects reversed by estrogen withdrawal. Increasing progesterone (as in estrus) causes a suppression of estrogen receptor synthesis and a diminished synthesis of progesterone receptor as well, effects reversed by progesterone withdrawal. Thus, estrogen facilitates subsequent progesterone action, progesterone facilitates estrogen withdrawal, and progesterone withdrawal facilitates estrogen action. Effects on estrogen and progesterone receptors are rapidly becoming the focus of research seeking to develop antiestrogens and antiprogestogens as regulators of reproductive function.

PREGNANCY

Pregnancy in the bitch is often misleadingly reported to last 63 days. The estimated gestation length, normally expressed as the interval from a first or single mating to parturition, is highly variable. Furthermore, the observed variability or the mean length can differ among kennels and among breeds. The interval from first mating to parturition in bitches permitted multiple matings can range from 57 to 72 days. Gestation length following fertile single matings can range from 58 to 71 days. The mean gestation length in the author's beagle colony increased from 64 to 66 days during a program of breeding each bitch at the earliest possible opportunity. The actual gestation length is far less variable based on recent findings in the same colony. Each of 60 bitches whelped from 64 to 66 days after the day of the LH peak, whereas the intervals from first mating to whelping ranged from 57 to 71 days.

The variation in apparent gestation length is due to variation in the time of breeding in relation to the time of fertilization. Recall that the normal onset of estrus can range from three days before to four days after the LH peak. In extreme cases matings may be obtained as early as five days before the LH peak, and some bitches may not accept a mating until five to six days after the LH peak. With certain breeding practices, such as waiting until 9, 11, or 13 days after the first evidence of proestrus, or with the need to transport the bitch some distance for breeding, mating might not take place until late in estrus, seven to eight days after the LH peak. Regarding the time of fertilization, canine spermatozoa can retain their fertility in the estrous tract for up to six to seven days. Canine ova are ovulated from follicles as primary oocytes, about 36 to 48 hours after the LH peak. The time required for the oocytes to undergo maturation in the oviducts is not known but may be as long as two to three days, and fertilization probably occurs no earlier than three days after the LH peak. The fertile life span of oocytes after maturation (germinal vesicle breakdown and extrusion of the first polar body) is not known because the exact time of maturation is not known. It may be two to three days, since in some bitches fertilization and pregnancy resulted from mating as late as seven days after the LH peak. The *in vivo* requirement for sperm capacitation in the dog is not known. Mahi and Yanagamachi (1976) found that dog sperm can penetrate oocytes after seven hours of incubation *in vitro* and that they can penetrate immature or degenerated oocytes as well as mature oocytes. Oocyte maturation to the stage of germinal vesicle breakdown usually required 48 to 72 hours of *in vitro* incubation following removal from follicles, providing indirect evidence that the process may take as long as two to three days *in vivo* as well.

In Table 1 the approximate timing of events involved in the establishment and progression of pregnancy in the bitch are estimated in relation to the day of the LH peak as well as to other potential times of mating. Diagnosis of pregnancy by palpation of uterine swellings at implantation sites may be possible as early as 17 or 18 days after mating when mating occurs late in estrus but may not be possible until 26 days after a mating occurring 3 days before the LH peak. Implantation swellings of the uterine horns may initially be difficult to differentiate from the bends of the uterine horns of early metestrus in the nonpregnant bitch, and several days of rapid enlargement are often needed to ensure an accurate diagnosis. The uterine swellings are about 1.0 cm in diameter at 19 to 20 days after the LH peak, about 1.5 cm at 23 to 24 days, 2.0 cm at 27 to 28 days, and 3.0 cm at 31 to 32 days. By days 30 to 35 the uterine swellings become more confluent and often are no longer palpable as individual entities, particularly in obese bitches or bitches with a distended or unrelaxed abdomen. Thus, at approximately the same stage of the luteal phase that nonpregnant bitches may be first presented with signs of pseudopregnancy, mucometra, or pyometra, a differential diagnosis of pregnancy is often impossible. Radiography can be used to diagnose pregnancy only during the last three weeks of gestation. Studies conducted with Rendano demonstrated that fetal skeletons do not become sufficiently radiopaque for a pregnancy diagnosis until about 46 days after the LH peak or 19 to 20 days prior to parturition (see page 947). Thus, depending on the time of mating in relation to the LH peak, a radiographic diagnosis of pregnancy might be possible as early as 38 days after mating in some cases but not until 50 days after mating in others.

The endocrine mechanisms required for, or specific to, the establishment and maintenance of pregnancy in the dog have not been examined to any great extent. There appears to be little or no difference between nonpregnant and pregnant bitches in the secretion or blood levels of progesterone and estrogen prior to the time of implantation. Following implantation, however, there are secondary elevations in progesterone levels during the fourth and fifth weeks of pregnancy that are not seen at the corresponding time in the nonpregnant bitch. Mean levels of progesterone are higher in pregnant than in nonpregnant bitches between days 35 and 60, but reports vary as to the extent of the difference and its significance. The difference cannot be used diagnostically because of the large variation encountered in progesterone levels. However, assays to detect progesterone levels above 5 ng/ml can be used to retrospectively confirm the occurrence of ovulation in bitches that fail to conceive and are suspected of failing to ovulate.

The additional progesterone in pregnant bitches may represent a pregnancy-specific increase in luteal progesterone secretion caused by placental gonadotropic activity. However, such activity has yet to be demonstrated in the dog. One factor that may affect the extent to which circulating hormone levels reflect secretion rate in pregnant bitches could be the hemodilution that most likely accompanies the rather dramatic anemia of pregnancy in the bitch. The mean hematocrit (PCV) falls below 40 per cent following implantation and by term reaches 30 to 35 per cent. If a significant increase in blood volume does accompany the pregnancy anemia, it may also account for the limited nature of the increase in circulating estrogen levels in late pregnancy. Estrogen levels increase slightly as term approaches but

Table 1. *Approximate Times of the Events of Canine Pregnancy*

Event	Days After the Preovulatory LH Peak*	Potential Range of Days After a Fertile Mating†
Onset of proestrus	−20 to −3	−25 to −2
Full vaginal cornification	−4 to +2	
Onset of estrus	−3 to +5	
Estradiol peak	−3 to −1	
Decreased vaginal edema	−1 to 0	
LH surge and sharp rise in progesterone	−1 to 0	
LH peak	0	−7 to +3
First mating	−5 to +10	
First fertile mating	−3 to +7	
Crenation of vaginal mucosa	0 to 1	
Ovulation of primary oocyte	2	−5 to +5
Oviductal oocytes		
Resumption of meiosis	3 (?)	
Extrusion of first polar body	4 (?)	
Sperm penetration	3 to 5	0 to 7
Fertilization/pronucleus formation	5 to 7	1 to 8
Degeneration of unfertilized ova	6 to 8 (?)	
Two-cell embryo	6 to 8	
Loss of vaginal crenulation	6 to 8	0 to 9
End of complete vaginal cornification	6 to 9	
Return of leukocytes to vaginal smear	7 to 12	
Morulae (8 to 16 cells) in oviduct	8 to 10	
Blastocyst (32 to 64 cells) entry into uterus	9 to 11	3 to 14
Intracornual migration (1-mm blastocysts)	10 to 13	
Transcornual migration (2-mm blastocysts)	12 to 15	
Attachment sites established, zona pellucidae shed	16 to 17	
Swelling of implantation sites, primitive streak formation	18 to 19	
Palpable uterine swellings of 1-cm diameter	20 to 25	17 to 27
Onset of pregnancy anemia	30	
Reduced palpability of 3-cm swellings	32	26 to 38
Hematocrit below 40 % PCV	40	
Hematocrit below 35 % PCV	50	
Fetal skeleton becomes radiopaque	43 to 46	
Radiographic diagnosis of pregnancy	45 to 48	39 to 50
Prepartum luteolysis and hypothermia	63 to 65	
Parturition	64 to 66	58 to 70

*Conservative estimates based on literature reports and unpublished observations.
†Based on fertile single matings from three days before to seven days after the LH peak.

do not reach values comparable to those seen in proestrus.

Pregnancy maintenance in the bitch is considered to be dependent on luteal progesterone secretion throughout gestation, and the corpora lutea of pregnancy appear to have the same pituitary luteotropic requirements as in the nonpregnant bitch. Pregnancy can be terminated by ovariectomy at any stage of gestation. Pregnancy termination following ovariectomy is prevented if a long-lasting depot of progestin is injected prior to extirpation of the ovaries. Pregnancy was also terminated following the limited number of hypophysectomies that have

been reported. As in the nonpregnant bitch, interference with LH action by the administration of anti-LH serum or suppression of prolactin secretion by the administration of bromoergocryptine reduces progesterone secretion in pregnant bitches. Repeated administration of bromoergocryptine or prostaglandin $F_{2\alpha}$ can induce luteolysis and cause abortion, albeit at the risk of undesirable side effects. Thus, in pregnant as well as nonpregnant bitches, LH and prolactin are required luteotropins and $PGF_{2\alpha}$ is luteolytic.

Between days 30 to 35 and day 60 of pregnancy, progesterone levels slowly but progressively decline from peak values of 15 to 80 ng/ml to a prepartum plateau of 4 to 16 ng/ml, which is maintained for one to two weeks until one to two days prior to parturition. Concomitant with this approximately 80 per cent decline in progesterone levels, there is a two- to fivefold increase in serum prolactin levels. Although the fall in progesterone is not unlike that seen at this time in the nonpregnant cycle, the considerable rise in radioimmunoassayable prolactin activity reported appears to be pregnancy specific. A corresponding but less pronounced increase in prolactin during the period of declining progesterone secretion in the luteal phase of the nonpregnant cycle may also occur. The broad rise in prolactin levels as progesterone levels slowly decline during the second half of pregnancy and the sharp rise in prolactin during the rapid prepartum fall in progesterone have led to the speculation that declining progesterone may be a stimulus for prolactin release in the bitch. Perhaps, in turn, elevations in prolactin activity provide the stimulus for the broader profiles of progesterone secretion seen in pregnant versus nonpregnant bitches and thereby ensure the maintenance of progesterone secretion throughout the course of gestation. However, the potential for prolactin to increase progesterone secretion in the bitch has not been demonstrated.

A pregnancy-specific, postimplantation increase in FSH has also been reported. The twofold increase in FSH was observed as early as day 28 of pregnancy and was present one week ante partum. Such increases in FSH might account for the slight increase in estrogen and increased follicular activity that have been observed in the second half of pregnancy. Regarding the reported pregnancy-specific increases in both FSH and prolactin activity, the possibility that some or all of these increases might involve placental factors that have immunologic cross-reactivity in the assays utilized has not been adequately addressed.

The endocrine changes that have been demonstrated, reported, or suggested to date are summarized schematically in Figure 4. It must be emphasized, however, that composite schematics such as these are compilations of published and unpublished data from a variety of sources and may not adequately provide for the considerable variability that can be encountered among individual bitches or the inconsistencies among various reports.

PARTURITION AND LACTATION

The onset of parturition and delivery of the first pup occurs 64 to 66 days after the preovulatory LH peak but can range from 58 to 71 days after mating. Gestation length is reportedly increased in bitches bearing small litters. The trigger for parturition in the bitch probably involves a maturation of the fetal pituitary-adrenal axis near term as proposed for several other species. A prepartum luteolysis and progesterone withdrawal are required for normal parturition in the bitch. Serum progesterone levels are maintained at a plateau of 4 to 16 ng/ml during the last week of pregnancy and then rapidly decline 24 to 36 hours ante partum to reach 0.5 to 1.5 ng/ml at the time of parturition. The administration of subcutaneous implants of progesterone, which prevents the decline in progesterone, prevents normal parturition. The elevated levels of estrogen still present immediately ante partum probably facilitate the effects of progesterone withdrawal, one of which may be to increase the number of oxytocin receptors in the myometrium, thereby increasing uterine contractility.

Variable increases in maternal circulating levels of cortisol were observed during the week prior to parturition, and cortisol levels were consistently elevated 24 hours ante partum at the time of the steepest decline in progesterone levels. The prepartum luteolysis can be monitored by recording rectal temperature twice daily and observing the transient prepartum hypothermia that parallels the decline in progesterone with a delay of about 12 hours. Rectal temperature falls about 1°C between 12 and 36 hours ante partum. This is followed by a rapid rise in temperature during, or immediately after, parturition, with temperatures being slightly above normal for several days. The prepartum rise in cortisol may play some role in the transient hypothermia. However, the transient hypothermia observed during $PGF_{2\alpha}$-induced luteolysis has prompted the suggestion that the prepartum hypothermia reflects a transient inability of thermoregulatory mechanisms to compensate for the rapid withdrawal of the hyperthermic effects of progesterone.

The mechanism of prepartum luteolysis in the dog has not been detailed. The rise in cortisol may reflect fetal cortisol secretion, which in turn is involved in a placental or uterine release of luteolytic activity. Although $PGF_{2\alpha}$ is luteolytic in the bitch, the role of prostaglandins in prepartum luteolysis has not been adequately studied and no conclusion can be made. Gerber and coworkers (1979) found that the pregnant uterus produces considerable PGE_2 and PGI_2 but no $PGF_{2\alpha}$. The high PGE_2:$PGF_{2\alpha}$ ratio in the products of arachidonic acid may represent a protective mechanism for the maintenance of corpora lutea function as well as the maintenance of myometrial and vascular tone during late pregnancy. Perhaps the ratio is altered in favor of $PGF_{2\alpha}$ by the mechanism that subsequently triggers parturition.

During the week prior to parturition, prolactin levels are clearly elevated above baseline. Prolactin then surges during and following the decline in progesterone, reaching peak levels 0 to 24 hours ante partum. Prolactin levels decline following parturition and remain relatively low for one to two

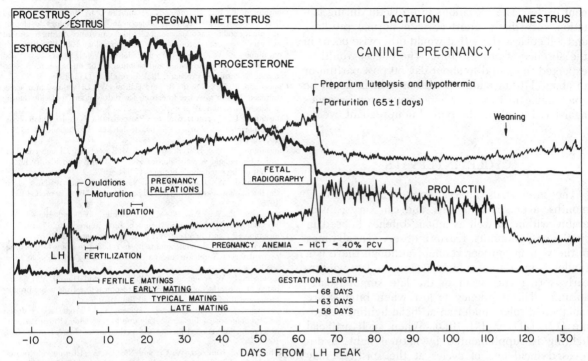

Figure 4. A schematic representation of typical endocrine changes reported or presumed to occur during the course of a fertile canine ovarian cycle, including pregnancy and lactation, and their relation to events critical to breeding protocols, pregnancy diagnosis, and estimation of gestation length.

days before obvious increases are observed in response to suckling. Prolactin levels remain high during lactation and decline following weaning. The elevations are suckling dependent and are absent in bitches not nursing pups.

Measurements of oxytocin levels at parturition and during lactation have not been reported for the bitch. It is likely, however, as in other species studied, that neural reflex release of oxytocin occurs in response to cervical and vaginal distention during delivery of pups and suckling during lactation. The administration of oxytocin will hasten delivery of a litter, but its routine use for such purpose hardly seems justified, as overt stimulation of uterine contractions might compromise the survival of remaining pups. The normal delivery of average or large litters may be rapid or may take 12 to 18 hours. There is ample, albeit incidental, evidence that bitches can actively postpone the onset of labor or the delivery of subsequent pups when nervous, frightened, or placed in strange surroundings. Therefore, if the bitch is to be moved to a specific whelping area and provided a nesting box this should be done a week or so prior to parturition.

The prepartum decline in progesterone is probably responsible for the relaxation and dilation of the cervix that occurs at that time. The abrupt prepartum rise in prolactin may play a role in the increased restlessness, panting, scratching, chewing, and nesting behavior usually observed 12 to 24 hours prior to parturition. The elevated levels of prolactin at the time of delivery may promote

normal maternal activities such as removal of membranes, eating of the placenta, chewing of the umbilical cord, and licking of each pup as it is born. It is not known if variations in endocrine events at parturition account for the variability in delivery times seen within and among bitches. The total delivery time for a bitch can vary from litter to litter; it is usually completed within 6 hours but can take up to 24 hours. The interval between deliveries of individual pups may be two to three hours, particularly between the first and second pup, after which intervals between pups are usually shorter. Intervals of relaxation prior to delivery of a pup do not appear to be a matter of concern, but more than two hours of active straining and attempts at labor are indicative of the need for intervention.

The role of oxytocin release during labor and/or lactation in the process of normal, post-partum uterine involution and hemostasis has not been investigated. Preliminary observations on normal post-partum periods suggest that some uterine bleeding and vaginal discharge of blood is common during lactation and may increase in association with weaning. The routine administration of oxytocin following the completion of delivery in one large commercial breeding colony is thought to result in the absence of any obvious blood discharge during or following lactation.

The six- to nine-week lactation in the dog probably functions as a lactational anestrus. There is little or no difference in the mean interestrus interval (seven months) between pregnant and nonpregnant cycles. The elevations in prolactin during lactation very likely interfere with normal pituitary and follicular activity that would otherwise occur in the absence of progesterone. The effects would be expected to extend to about day 50 post partum or to about 110 days after ovulation, which would be comparable in time to when progesterone reaches near-basal levels in the typical nonpregnant cycle.

CYCLE INTERVALS

The interestrus interval ranges from 3 to 12 months, averages 7 months, and can vary considerably within as well as among bitches housed in similar environments. Estrus is observed at all times of the year in outdoor kennels, although there is a tendency for a greater incidence in the late winter-early spring and again in the late summer-early autumn. This tendency is lost when bitches are maintained solely under an artificial lighting schedule (12L:12D or 14L:10D). When such artificial lighting is supplemented by natural light, a decreased incidence of cycles at the solstices may occur. Although the photoperiod may influence the onset of proestrus and interestrus intervals, other factors are probably equally effective in influencing cycle length, including season of birth, breed, age, duration of progesterone secretion in nonpregnant cycles, duration of lactation in pregnant cycles, and proximity of other cycling bitches. Termination of luteal function and pregnancy with prostaglandin treatment was reported to reduce the interestrus interval by about one month. Interestrus intervals are reported to increase with age after four to five years. It is a common practice in commercial kennels to move anestrous bitches close to estrous bitches to hasten the imminent cycle. The tendency for some dogs to cycle at nearly six-month intervals, spring and autumn, is very likely facilitated by the annual photoperiod. Photoperiod effects are probably mediated via modulation of pineal secretions. Indolamines, including melatonin, and argine vasotocin have been shown to have an inhibitory effect on LH release in the dog.

REFERENCES AND SUPPLEMENTAL READING

Albassam, M. A., Thomson, R. C., and O'Donnell, L.: Normal postpartum involution of the uterus in the dog. Can. J. Comp. Med. 45:217, 1981.

Andersen, A. C.: Reproduction. *In* Andersen, A. C. (ed.): *The Beagle as an Experimental Animal.* Ames, IA: Iowa State University Press, 1970, pp. 31–39.

Andersen, A. C., and Simpson, M. E.: *The Ovary and Reproductive Cycle of the Dog (Beagle).* Los Altos: Geron-X, 1973.

Chakraborty, P. K., Panko, W. B., and Fletcher, W. S.: Serum hormone concentrations and their relationships to sexual behavior at the first and second estrous cycles of the Labrador bitch. Biol. Reprod. 22:227, 1980.

Concannon, P. W.: Effects of hypophysectomy and of LH administration on luteal phase plasma progesterone levels in the beagle bitch. J. Reprod. Fert. 58:407, 1980.

Concannon, P. W., Altszuler, N., Hampshire, J., Butler, W. R., and Hansel, W.: Growth hormone, prolactin and cortisol in dogs developing mammary nodules and an acromegaly-like appearance during treatment with medroxyprogesterone acetate. Endocrinology 106:1173, 1980.

Concannon, P. W., Butler, W. R., Hansel, W., Knight, P. J., and Hamilton, J. M.: Parturition and lactation in the bitch: serum progesterone, cortisol and prolactin. Biol. Reprod. 19:1113, 1978.

Concannon, P. W., Cowan, R., and Hansel, W.: LH release in ovariectomized dogs in response to estrogen withdrawal and its facilitation by progesterone. Biol. Reprod. 20:523, 1979.

Concannon, P. W., and Hansel, W.: Prostaglandin $F_{2\alpha}$ induced luteolysis, hypothermia and abortions in beagle bitches. Prostaglandins 13:533, 1977.

Concannon, P. W., Hansel, W., and McEntee, K.: Changes in LH, progesterone and sexual behavior associated with preovulatory luteinization in the bitch. Biol. Reprod. 17:604, 1977.

Concannon, P. W., Hansel, W., and Visek, W. J.: The ovarian cycle of the bitch: plasma estrogen, LH and progesterone. Biol. Reprod. 13:112, 1975.

Concannon, P. W., Powers, M. E., Holder, W., and Hansel, W.: Pregnancy and parturition in the bitch. Biol. Reprod. 16:517, 1977.

Concannon, P., and Rendano, V.: Radiographic diagnosis of pregnancy: the onset of fetal skeletal radiopacity in relation to times of breeding, preovulatory LH release and parturition. Am. J. Vet. Res. in press 1983.

Concannon, P. W., Weigand, N., Wilson, S., and Hansel, W.: Sexual behavior in ovariectomized bitches in response to estrogen and progesterone treatments. Biol. Reprod. 20:799, 1979.

Eigenmann, J. E., and Venker-van Hagen, A. J.: Progestagen-induced and spontaneous canine acromegaly due to reversible growth hormone overproduction: clinical picture and pathogenesis. J.A.A.H.A. 17:813, 1981.

Gerber, J. G., Hubbard, W. C., and Nies, A. S.: Uterine vein prostaglandin levels in late pregnant dogs. Prostaglandins 17:623, 1979.

Ginther, O. J.: Comparative anatomy of uterovarian vasculature. Vet. Scope 20:2, 1976.

Graf, K.-J.: Serum oestrogen, progesterone and prolactin concentrations in cyclic, pregnant and lactating beagle dogs. J. Reprod. Fert. 52:9, 1978.

Holst, P. A., and Phemister, R. D.: The prenatal development of the dog: preimplantation events. Biol. Reprod. 5:194, 1971.

Holst, P. A., and Phemister, R. D.: Onset of diestrus in the beagle bitch: definition and significance. Am. J. Vet. Res. 35:401, 1974.

Holst, P. A., and Phemister, R. D.: Temporal sequence of events in the estrous cycle of the bitch. Am. J. Vet. Res. 36:705, 1975.

Jochle, W., and Andersen, A. C.: The estrous cycle in the dog: a review. Theriogenology 7:113, 1977.

Knight, P. J., Hamilton, J. M., and Hiddleston, W. A.: Serum prolactin during pregnancy and lactation in the beagle bitch. Vet. Rec. 101:202, 1977.

Lessey, B. A., and Gorell, T. A.: Nuclear progesterone receptors in the beagle uterus. J. Steroid Biochem. 14:585, 1981.

Lessey, B. A., Wahawisan, R., and Gorell, T. A.: Hormonal regulation of cytoplasmic estrogen and progesterone receptors in the beagle uterus and oviduct. Mol. Cell. Endocrinol. 21:171, 1981.

Lindsay, F. E. F.: An introduction to endoscopy of the canine bitch—post uterine tract. Pedigree Dig. 5(3):8, 5(4):8, 1980.

Mahi, C. A., and Yanagimachi, R.: Maturation and sperm penetration of canine ovarian oocytes in vitro. J. Exper. Zool. 196:189, 1976.

Olson, P.N.S.; The ovary, ovarian hormones and contraceptives (canine). *In* Kirk, R. W. (ed.): *Current Veterinary Therapy VII.* Philadelphia: W. B. Saunders, 1980, pp. 1030–1034.

Phemister, R. D.: Abnormal estrous activity (bitch). *In* Morrow, D. A. (ed.): *Current Therapy in Theriogenology.* Philadelphia: W. B. Saunders, 1980, pp. 620–622.

Phemister, R. D., Holst, P. A., Spano, J. S., and Hopwood, M. L.: Time of ovulation in the beagle bitch. Biol. Reprod. 8:74, 1973.

Reimers, T., Phemister, R., and Niswender, G.: Radioimmunological measurement of follicle stimulating hormone and prolactin in the dog. Biol. Reprod. 19:673, 1978.

Roszel, J. F.: Genital cytology of the bitch. Vet. Scope XIX:3, 1975.

Shille, V. M., and Stabenfeldt, G. H.: Clinical reproductive physiology in dogs. *In*: Morrow, D. A. (ed.): *Current Therapy in Theriogenology.* Philadelphia: W. B. Saunders, 1980, pp. 571–574.

Shille, V. M., and Stabenfeldt, G. H.: Current concepts in reproduction of the dog and cat. Adv. Vet. Sci. Comp. Med. 24:211, 1980.

Smith, M. S., and McDonald, L. E.: Serum levels of luteinizing hormone and progesterone during the estrous cycle, pseudopregnancy and pregnancy in the dog. Endocrinology 94:404, 1974.

Sokolowski, J. H.: Normal events of gestation in the bitch and methods of pregnancy diagnosis. *In* Morrow, D. A. (ed.): *Current Therapy in Theriogenology.* Philadelphia, W. B. Saunders, 1980, pp. 590–595.

Sokolowski, J. H., Stover, D. G., VanRavenswaay, F.: Seasonal incidence of estrus and interestrous interval for bitches of 7 breeds. J.A.V.M.A. 171:271, 1977.

Vickery, B., and McRae, G.: Effect of synthetic PG analogue on pregnancy in beagle bitches. Biol. Reprod. 22:438, 1980.

Wildt, D. E., Levinson, C. J., and Seager, S. W. J.: Laparoscopic exposure and sequential observation of the ovary of the cycling bitch. Anat. Rec. 189:443, 1977.

Wildt, D. E., Panko, W. B., Chakraborty, P., and Seager, S. W.: Relationship of serum estrone, estradiol-17β and progesterone to LH, sexual behavior and time of ovulation in the bitch. Biol. Reprod. 20:648, 1979.

Yamashita, E., and Mieno, M.: Melatonin and arginine vasotocin inhibition on the action of LHRH in the release of LH. IRCS Med. Sci. 8:652, 1980.

FERTILITY REGULATION IN THE BITCH: CONTRACEPTION, STERILIZATION, AND PREGNANCY TERMINATION

P. W. CONCANNON, Ph.D.

Ithaca, New York

The options available for preventing estrus cycles or pregnancy in bitches remain decidedly limited, particularly to practitioners in the United States (Table 1). Surgical intervention, in the form of ovariohysterectomy, is the most obvious approach if permanent sterility is desired. However, reversible contraception by pharmacologic means is often requested as a means of postponing litter bearing or preventing estrus behavior without precluding subsequent cycles and fertility. In such cases, the administration of available synthetic progestogens or androgens, if properly timed in relation to the cycle, can be used for either long- or short-term prevention of estrus and ovulation. Following unintentional matings, antinidatory doses of an estrogen preparation are often used when "mismating shots" are requested, despite the well-known problems that can be caused by inappropriate selection of preparation or dose. Methods of nonsurgically terminating an established, post implantation pregnancy are limited to experimental protocols involving prostaglandins, corticosteroids, or ergot alkaloid treatments, all of which have yielded inconsistent results.

SURGICAL STERILIZATION

Bilateral ovariectomy accomplished via panoophorohysterectomy (complete spaying) is the usual and recommended approach to surgical sterilization in the bitch and has advantages over other approaches that have been described, including tubal ligation, ovariectomy alone, salpingectomy, or subtotal hysterectomy. Removal of the uterus (and cervix) as well as the ovaries precludes any subsequent development of uterine disease. Estrus cycles following spaying, although most often probably due to incomplete removal of one of the ovaries, may also result from accessory ovarian tissue located at some distance from the ovaries. The standard approach involves a single mid ventral incision. Time spent "loosening" the ovarian ligaments to gain full exposure of the ovaries is well spent, for it allows for clamping and placement of ligatures well proximal to the ovaries, thus decreasing the chance of leaving behind ovarian tissue. The increased ovarian and uterine vascularity associated with proestrus and estrus can be avoided by delaying the spaying of bitches in heat until mid metestrus. A transient pseudocyesis is not uncommon following ovariectomy during the luteal phase and probably results from the subsequent fall in progesterone, which mimics the fall that occurs at parturition.

During the last decade there has been an increased tendency to carry out spaying operations on young prepubertal or pubertal bitches for several reasons. The infantile tract can be located and removed with a minimum of trauma. There is epidemiologic evidence that ovariectomy prior to the first cycle reduces the incidence of mammary tumors to a greater extent than spaying after the first heat. However, puberty may occur as early as five months of age, can be expected any time after six months, and may occur without obvious external signs. The possible complications of spaying for the

Table 1. *Approaches and Methods for Regulation of Fertility in the Bitch*

Approach and Method	Duration of Effect	Status of Method
Prevention of Cycles or Ovulation		
Surgical		
Ovariohysterectomy	Permanent	
Steroid therapy with progestogens or androgens		
Oral administration		
Megestrol acetate (MGA)		
Proestrus treatment	1 or 2 cycles	1, 2
Anestrus treatment	1 or 2 cycles	1, 2
Combined treatments	2 cycles	1, 2
Mibolerone		
Medium-term	2 to 9 months	1, 2
Long-term	1 to 2 years	1, 2
	3 to 5 years	3
Depo injections		
Medroxyprogesterone acetate (MPA)	6 to 18 months	2, 3
Proligestone	6 to 18 months	2, 3
Subcutaneous implants		
Progesterone	12 months	3
Testosterone	15 months	3
Immunization		
Against gonadotropins (LH, HCG)	variable	3
Against GnRH	variable	3
Prevention of Copulation		
Isolation of bitch		
Intravaginal devices		
Prevention of Implantation		
Antinidatory estrogen treatment		
Oral stilbestrol DES		2, 4
Repositol DES injection		2, 3
Oral mestranol		3
Estradiol cypionate (ECP)		2, 4
Estradiol valerate (EV)		2, 4
Estradiol benzoate (EB)		2, 4
Estrone		2, 4
Termination of Pregnancy		
Prostaglandins		
PGF$_{2\alpha}$		3
PGF analogs		3
Bromoergocryptine		3

Note: 1 = Available, marketed, and approved in US.
        2 = Available, marketed, or approved outside US.
        3 = Not marketed, not approved, or experimental in US.
        4 = Availability, approval, or indication limited in US.

most part are likely to be no more severe following a prepubertal spaying than following spaying carried out after the first cycle. Mann, however, has suggested that perivulvar dermatitis is more likely to occur and to be of greater severity following prepubertal spaying (1971). The extent to which prepubertal spaying might effect bone development, epiphyseal closure, or adult body conformation has not been adequately addressed.

Complications of spaying include a susceptibility to severe obesity for some bitches, although the majority of spayed bitches either experience no change in weight or size or can be regulated by exercise and restricted feeding. In a small study more bitches experienced a permanent weight loss than a weight gain following spaying, although obesity, when observed, was considerable and difficult to control by food intake alone. The latter probably involved reduced spontaneous activity in addition to any endocrine "imbalance" resulting from spaying. Other complications associated with ovariectomy include perivulvar dermatitis and bilateral miliary dermatoses.

The need to exercise care in the handling of viscera and the reproductive tract, in the selection of suture and ligature materials, and in the placement of clamps and ligatures should not be minimized. Okkens and colleagues recently reported on 109 cases of single or multiple complications after ovariohysterectomy. Of these, 40 per cent involved incomplete removal of ovarian tissue; 20 per cent involved inflammatory (usually fistulated) reactions to suture material in the upper flank; 15 per cent involved adhesions to or around intestines or colon causing enterologic problems; 10 per cent involved granulomas or adhesions affecting kidney or ureter function; and 5 per cent involved ligation of a ureter, with resulting urologic disturbances. Inflamed and infected uterine stumps were seen in 20 per cent of cases.

STEROID HORMONE SUPPRESSION OF CYCLES

Various steroid hormones have been shown to suppress or inhibit normal ovarian cyclicity in the bitch during the course of their administration. They include the naturally occurring steroids, progesterone and testosterone, and a variety of synthetic steroids derived from testosterone or progesterone. The latter include medroxyprogesterone acetate, megestrol acetate, delmadinone acetate, melengestrol acetate, proligestone, norethisterone acetate, and mibolerone. Their mechanism of action in the dog is not fully understood. Since they suppress the recurrence of ovarian cyclicity, the primary mode of action probably involves a suppression or modification of gonadotropic hormone secretion by interfering with or mimicking the normal feedback effects of endogenous ovarian steroids on the hypothalamus and/or pituitary. All the previously mentioned steroids can prevent ovarian cyclicity in the bitch, and some of them are approved for use and are marketed as canine contraceptives. However, there is a tendency for progestin administration to promote uterine disease and other problems in the dog and for androgens to have masculinizing effects, so particular attention must be given to appropriate doses and appropriate timing during the cycle when initiating administration.

At present, only two products are commercially available and approved for use as canine contraceptives in the U.S. They are the progestin megestrol acetate (Ovaban*) and the androgen derivative mibolerone (Cheque Drops†). Both are for oral administration and are discussed hereafter, along with other contraceptive steroid treatments.

ORAL CONTRACEPTIVE STEROIDS

MEGESTROL ACETATE

The progestin megestrol acetate is marketed as a canine contraceptive in 5- and 20-mg tablets for oral administration. The trade names are Ovaban* in the United States and Ovarid‡ in the United Kingdom and Europe. The recommended doses and treatment regimens vary somewhat among suppliers. Daily doses and duration of treatment depend on whether administration is started during anestrus or proestrus (Table 2). Diabetes mellitus is a contraindication to the use of megestrol acetate. Treatment can be started during anestrus to postpone the next estrus cycle or during proestrus to prevent the continuation of proestrus and the onset of estrus. Megestrol acetate tablets can be administered intact or crushed and mixed into food.

OVABAN

Proestrus Treatment. Ovaban treatment started in proestrus to prevent the imminent estrus should begin during the first three days of proestrus, assuming that the proestrus would have lasted the normal duration of six to ten days or longer. However, in some bitches the first external signs of proestrus may not be observed until shortly before the onset of estrus. Harding has indicated that a bitch with a proestrus period of less than 4 days or more than 20 days is not a candidate for oral megestrol acetate therapy (1981). The occurrence of proestrus should be verified by examination of the vaginal smear prior to initiation of treatment. The recommended dosage for administration in proestrus is 1 mg/lb body weight (approx. 2 mg/kg) daily for eight days. It is also recommended that the bitch be confined for three to eight days or until the cessation of bloody discharge, as bitches may attract and accept males until the cessation of the proestrus discharge. A suppression of proestrus occurs within three to eight days. A subsequent return to proestrus and estrus can be expected about four to six months later in most bitches. A range of one to seven months was observed in clinical trials. If treatment is started too early in proestrus, the bitch may return to proestrus shortly after treatment. If treatment is started too late in proestrus, a fertile estrus may occur during treatment.

Anestrus Treatment. In anestrous bitches a longer course of lower dosage is recommended for postponement of the next proestrus and estrus. The recommended Ovaban dose for anestrous bitches is 0.25 mg/lb body weight for 32 days. The next cycle may occur any time after cessation of the treatment initiated in anestrus. The return to estrus in clinical trials ranged from one to seven months after treatment and averaged four to six months. If treated too early in anestrus the effect may be lost too soon to result in an obvious postponement of the cycle. It is recommended that the time for initiating treatment during anestrus be selected based on the bitch's history of interestrus intervals and be at least one or two weeks prior to the next expected proestrus. If started too late the bitch may enter proestrus while on the 0.25-mg dose and may require a change to the proestrus dosage. If Ovaban treatment is started immediately prior to the onset of a proestrus the treatment may only temporarily prevent "heat," with a return to proestrus two to four weeks after treatment.

---

*Schering Corp., Kenilworth, NJ.
†The Upjohn Co., Kalamazoo, MI.
‡Glaxovet Ltd., Greenford, Middlesex (U.K.).

Table 2. *Suggested Applications of Oral Megestrol Acetate for Estrus Cycle Regulation in the Bitch*

Application	Ovaban	Ovarid
Anestrus Treatment for cycle postponement in normal cycling adults	Dose: 0.25 mg/lb/day for 32 days Start: Begin at least 1 week before expected proestrus Limit: No more than 2 consecutive treatments	Dose: 0.5 mg/kg/day for 40 days Start: Begin 2 or more weeks before expected proestrus Limit: No more than 2 times a year
Extended anestrus regimen for cycle postponement	No indication	Dose: 0.5 mg/kg/day for 40 days, then 0.2 mg/kg twice weekly for up to 4 months Limit: Allow normal cycle before treatment
Proestrus treatment for estrus suppression in cycling bitches	Dose: 1 mg/lb/day for 8 days Start: During first 3 days of proestrus confirmed by vaginal smears	Dose: 2 mg/kg/day for 8 days Start: During early proestrus after both bleeding and vulval swelling
Proestrus regimen for estrus suppression in pubertal, problem, or kennel bitches	No indication	Dose: 2 mg/kg/day for 4 days, then 0.5 mg/kg/day for 16 days
Post-treatment return to estrus	Approximately 4 to 6 months after end of treatment; range from 1 to 7 months	About 3 months after end of anestrus regimen; 1 to 2 months earlier than if not treated, for proestrus treatment

Precautions on the use of Ovaban indicated by the manufacturer should be noted. Ovaban should not be administered for more than two consecutive treatment periods. It must not be used in bitches with reproductive tract disease, pregnant bitches, or bitches with mammary tumors. Overdosage or prolonged treatment may cause cystic endometritis. Ovaban is not recommended prior to or during the first estrus of pubertal dogs. However, Ovaban has been reported to be safe and effective for suppression of estrus when administered during proestrus in first-heat bitches when the onset of proestrus is accurately determined.

OVARID

Ovarid dosages and regimens recommended for use in the United Kingdom are similar to those for Ovaban in the United States but provide for alternative protocols as well. For prevention of estrus in normal proestrus bitches, the recommended dose of Ovarid is 2 mg/kg (approximately 1 mg/lb) daily for eight days. However, in cases involving a potentially abnormal proestrus, a first cycle, a bitch housed with other bitches, or a bitch with a history of pseudopregnancy, a protracted protocol is suggested. This protracted proestrus protocol is 2 mg/kg for 4 days followed by 0.5 mg/kg for 16 days. Both schedules involve the same total dose of 16 mg/kg. The next cycle can be expected four to six weeks earlier than would be expected if the bitch had not been treated. The recommended Ovarid schedule for postponing the onset of the next cycle in anestrus bitches is 0.5 mg/kg (approximately 0.25 mg/lb) daily for 40 days, beginning at least 1 week, but preferably 2 weeks, before an expected proestrus. This may be followed by 0.2 mg/kg twice a week for a maximum of 4 months after the 40-day

treatment regimen. Following such an extended estrus-postponement treatment started in anestrus, a subsequent normal cycle should be permitted before retreating. Otherwise, the normal 40-day anestrus treatment can be followed by an estrus-prevention treatment given early in the next observed proestrus if a further period of infertility is desired. Ovarid schedules should not be initiated more than twice a year in any case.

MIBOLERONE

Mibolerone, an orally active androgen-derived steroid, is approved and marketed for long-term estrus prevention in dogs in the form of Cheque Drops* in the United States and as Matenon in the United Kingdom. Cheque is supplied as a liquid solution to be added to the feed. Administration is recommended for up to two years, starting in early or mid anestrus, to prevent the onset of the next anticipated proestrus and estrus. Clinical trials have shown efficacy for up to five years of continuous treatment. Administration should begin at least 30 days prior to the expected estrus. Approval has recently been obtained to market mibolerone-containing canned dog food as a prescription diet in the United States.

The return to estrus following cessation of mibolerone administration is usually two to three months (range one to seven months). Verification of the stage of the cycle is important when starting treatment. Initiation of treatment in very late anestrus may not be effective because of the inability of mibolerone to prevent estrus in bitches about to enter proestrus, and such bitches may express es-

---

*The Upjohn Co., Kalamazoo, MI.

Table 3. *Dosages of Mibolerone Recommended for Long-Term Estrus Prevention in Anestrus Bitches*

Body Weight Range		Dosage
lb	kg	μg/day
1–25	0.5–12	30
26–50	12–23	60
51–100	23–45	120
≥101	> 45	180
Any German shepherd or shepherd-origin bitch		180

Notes: Return to estrus after end of treatment expected in 1 to 7 months, average 2.5 months.
Up to 24 months continuous treatment approved. Efficacy to 5 years demonstrated.

trus during the first 30 days of treatment. Dosage is dependent on body weight and breed, with a two-year maximum period of treatment (Table 3). The reason for the requirement of higher doses by dogs of German shepherd origin is not known, but the exception applies to both pure bred and mixed-breed bitches with Alsatian lineage. In addition to vaginal discharge, an obvious enlargement of the clitoris to various degrees may be expected in 15 to 20 per cent of treated bitches and to a minor extent in most bitches. Overdosing can result in anal gland inspissation and resulting odors. Mibolerone should not be given to bitches that might possibly be pregnant, as it causes masculinization of female fetuses.

PARENTERAL CONTRACEPTIVE STEROIDS

STEROID IMPLANTS

Silastic capsules filled with either testosterone or progesterone release the hormone for long periods of time, as the hormones are slightly soluble in the Silastic. Progesterone implants placed subcutaneously in bitches inhibited cycles for 15 to 20 months without having to be replaced. Such implants are unlikely to be made available commercially, as they are not biodegradable and their insertion and removal require minor surgery that may not be acceptable to many owners for cosmetic reasons.

DEPOT INJECTABLE STEROIDS

MEDROXYPROGESTERONE ACETATE (MPA)

This progestin is poorly soluble in aqueous solutions, and a single intramuscular injection of a suspension of MPA maintains effective circulating levels of the hormone for several months. MPA is widely used as a human contraceptive in many countries, but not in the United States. It is marketed for human use other than contraception in

the U.S. as Depo-Provera.* MPA was marketed as a canine contraceptive (Promone*) in the U.S. until 1969, but the preparation was removed from the market because of a high incidence of cystic endometrial hyperplasia in many treated bitches. The adverse effects may have been related to overdosing and/or administration during stages of the cycle other than anestrus. High doses of MPA in the dog, in addition to causing cystic endometrial hyperplasia and pyometra, may also cause mammary tumors, adrenal suppression, and acromegaly. However, MPA is widely used in other countries as a canine contraceptive (Depopromone, Perlutex, Anovulin). MPA should only be administered in deep anestrus, prior to any evidence of proestrus. The minimum effective contraceptive dose is approximately 2 mg/kg for three months. Extreme care should be taken never to exceed doses or injection schedules recommended by the supplier.

PROLIGESTONE

A unique progestin, proligestone (14α, 17α propylidene-dioxy progesterone), is available in suspension as an injectable canine contraceptive in Europe (Delvosterone from Mycofarm and Gist-Brokades). Doses of 10 to 30 mg/kg are injected subcutaneously at zero, three, and seven months of treatment, followed by the same doses given at five-month intervals thereafter. Reports of clinical trials suggested that this treatment regimen did not promote development of uterine disease or mammary tumors and may, in fact, decrease their incidences. They further suggested little or no need to restrict usage to any particular stage of the cycle. Proligestone is not currently marketed in the United States.

NONSTEROIDAL CONTRACEPTION

Devices. Vaginal devices developed as blocks to copulation have been marketed, but problems with fitting, retention, perforation, and inflammatory reactions have resulted in an unacceptable failure rate and dissatisfaction on the part of owners and practitioners.

Pilocarpine. The oral administration of two to four drops of 1 per cent solution of pilocarpine has been reported to suppress estrus in dogs, but the method has not been subjected to controlled investigation.

Immunization. Bitches (as well as studs) can be immunized against endogenous luteinizing hormone (LH) by injection of bovine LH mixed with adjuvant. However, adjuvants used have produced unsightly skin lesions, and the duration of immunologic contraceptive efficacy has been highly variable.

---

*The Upjohn Co., Kalamazoo, MI.

A recent study has provided evidence that immunization against GnRH (gonadotropin-releasing hormone) has a contraceptive effect (Faulkner et al., 1975).

Several reports indicate the potential to suppress fertility by immunization with antigens prepared from whole ovaries or the zona pellucida of oocytes. However, as of this writing no contraceptive immunization protocol for dogs has warranted clinical trials.

Gonadotropin Injections. There is some contention whether LH administration during proestrus has any antifertility effect, and there are no reliable data available. Mann has suggested that normal proestrus can be curtailed by injection of LH (20 units/kg, IV) with a second injection given after two or three days if proestrus signs have not subsided (1971). Efficacy may depend on timing administration early enough in follicular development to ensure that the LH injection does not induce estrus and ovulation but also late enough to ensure that the LH causes premature luteinization of follicles rather than stimulation of further follicular growth.

POST-COITAL, ANTINIDATORY ESTROGEN TREATMENTS

Large doses of estrogen are often used to prevent implantation following misalliance. The efficacy is related to the inhibition of oviductal transport and/or direct embryotoxic action by pharmacologic doses of estrogen. However, many bitches so treated subsequently develop cystic endometrial hyperplasia leading to mucometra and pyometra. Therefore, post-coital estrogen administration is considered contraindicated for valuable breeding bitches.

FORMULATIONS, SIDE EFFECTS, DOSE SELECTION

A variety of estrogen treatments have been suggested for the prevention of nidation in the bitch. These include oral administration of diethylstilbestrol (DES), injection of DES, or a combination of injected and oral DES therapy; and estradiol injections in the forms of estradiol benzoate, estradiol valerate, or the long-acting estradiol cyclopentanopropionate (ECP or estradiol cypionate). The doses administered (Table 4) are clearly supraphysiologic, but there appears to be no reliable information on the minimum effective doses required for any of the various preparations used. The need to exercise considerable precaution in selecting preparations and doses is clear from reports of bone marrow suppression, aplastic anemia, internal hemorrhaging, and death following estrogen administration to prevent implantation.

The potential for inappropriate estrogen dosages to cause uterine disease that can progress to a life-threatening pyometra cannot be overemphasized.

Although there are no data available on the incidence of uterine complications following estrogen therapy for misalliance, the relationship appears clear. Jochle has reported on the history of bitches submitted for uterine disease problems in two European clinics (1974; 1975). In one instance, 92 of 164 bitches presented with endometritis had received estrogen for prevention of nidation within the previous six months. In the other survey, involving about 400 cases of uterine disease, nearly 25 per cent had recently received antinidatory estrogen treatments.

The problems of preparation and dose selection are also complicated by the lack of dose versus efficacy data for any preparation and the limitation of dosage recommendations to dose per animal or a small dose range per animal rather than dosage per unit body weight. Furthermore, many practitioners are finding it necessary to use preparations with unfamiliar formulations, concentrations, or pharmacodynamics. This is particularly true in the U.S. because of the withdrawal of injectable preparations of DES from the market, the limited availability of veterinary preparations of DES tablets for oral administration, and variations in DES content of various marketed DES tablets. Furthermore, the recommended indications for veterinary usage of ECP preparations are changing and the concentration of ECP varies among the available formulations. One major pharmaceutical firm has removed misalliance in bitches (as well as all other applications in small animals) from the indications for its veterinary ECP product.

It is important to remember that so-called estradiol preparations vary widely in duration of action following intramuscular injection in oil owing to the differing solubilities among estradiol and its esters in oil vehicles. Thus, mEq doses of "estradiol" can result in very high levels of estradiol for short periods (estradiol benzoate) or less extreme levels for protracted periods (ECP), depending on formulation. Although total dose affects the duration of action, it appears from available data that estradiol benzoate is released over 2 to 3 days, estradiol valerate over 10 to 20 days, and ECP over 20 to 40 days. Data specific to the dog are not available. There is also no information on the blood levels of estradiol or the timing or duration of estradiol therapy needed to prevent subsequent implantation in the bitch.

ESTRADIOL CYPIONATE (ECP)

ECP, because of its long duration of action, is commonly used in cases of misalliance. Lacking information on the critical time and/or amount of estrogen needed, its use is probably justified. Every effort should be made to use a minimal efficacious dose to reduce the subsequent incidence of uterine

Table 4. *Antinidatory Injectable Estrogen Treatments Indicated for Mismated Bitches Without Data on Safety or Side Effects*

Dosage (per bitch)	Comment	Reference
	Repositol Stilbestrol (DES)	
0.4 mg/kg	Within 36 to 48 hours	Mann, 1971
1.0 mg/kg	Safety questioned	Jochle, 1975
1.1 mg/kg	Within 5 days	Merck Veterinary Manual, 5th ed., 1980
2.0 mg/kg	Maximum dosage 25 mg	Jackson and Johnston, 1980
	Estradiol Cypionate (ECP)	
0.25 mg/30 kg	Maximum dosage 0.5 mg	Okin et al., 1976
0.125 to 1.0 mg		Jackson and Johnson, 1980
0.25 mg	For toy breeds	Merck Veterinary Manual, 5th ed., 1980
0.5 to 2.0 mg	Within 5 days	Merck Veterinary Manual, 5th ed., 1980
1.0 to 2.0 mg	Within 5 days	Jochle, 1975
1.0 to 2.0 mg	If after 5 days	Jochle, 1975
	Estradiol Valerate	
3.0 to 7.0 mg	Once, days 4 to 10	Jochle, 1975
	Estradiol Benzoate	
0.5 to 3.0 mg every other day	Three injections, days 4 to 10	Jochle, 1975
	Estrone	
2.0 to 5.0 mg	Within 5 days	Okin et al., 1976

or other complications. Important in this regard is the fact that there are no reported instances of a stated dose of ECP having failed to prevent pregnancy. Doses of 0.125 to 1.0 mg ECP have been suggested by Jackson and Johnston as sufficient, with optimum time for injection three to five days after the onset of estrus (1980). Mandell has reported 0.25 mg ECP/30 lb, with 0.5 mg ECP being the maximum dose, as being consistently antinidatory when given within 48 hours after breeding (see Okin et al., 1976). Considering the prolonged duration of ECP release following a single injection of ECP, a second injection, often suggested for bitches presented more than four to five days after mating, is probably not warranted. The selection of dose based on time after observed mating is difficult to justify. A bitch can be bred as early as three days before her LH peak (five days before ovulation and ten days before oocytes are destined to be released from the oviduct). In such a case, an immediate injection might delay the LH surge and permit subsequent fertility. An injection six days later would be the optimum time to block oocyte transport and prevent conception. A bitch might be bred as late as six days after the LH peak (four days after ovulation and only one to two days before oocytes are destined to be released into the uterus), and although an immediate injection would be most opportune, the bitch might not be presented until three to four days later. Therefore, if there is concern about the possibility of mistiming or underestimating the dose, examination of the vaginal smear is recommended. Holst and Phemister have shown that the oocytes remain in the oviducts, and thus remain most susceptible to a transport-delaying effect of estrogen, until one to three days after the vaginal smear is no longer fully cornified and begins to contain some nonsuperficial epithelial cell types (1974). Thus, if the smear is still of the estrous type,

only a most conservative dose of ECP should be considered. If it is not yet fully cornified, as in late proestrus or early estrus, a delay of one to three days before estrogen administration might be considered. If the smear is of the very late estrus or early metestrus type (containing nonsuperficial cells such as parabasals and small intermediates with healthy nuclei and usually small to large numbers of leukocytes), then an immediate injection of a possibly less conservative dose might be warranted. Table 5 lists conservative doses for antinidatory ECP injections based on prior reports that doses from 0.5 to 1.0 mg are maximal and doses from 0.5 to 0.125 mg are minimal. Maintaining a dilution of the commercial preparation (mixing stock with additional oil vehicle such as castor, sesame, or cottonseed oil) to a strength of 1.0 and/or 0.5 mg/cc might facilitate injection of small doses.

STILBESTROL (DIETHYLSTILBESTROL, DES)

Repositol DES or DES in oil is no longer marketed in the U.S. DES tablets are still commercially available in formulations of 0.1 to 5.0 mg/tablet. Doses of injectable DES that have been used for misalliance are listed in Table 4.

ESTRADIOL BENZOATE (EB) AND ESTRADIOL VALERATE (EV)

Injectable preparations of EB and EV are commercially available. Recommended doses of EV are not available. Since EV has a considerable duration of action, single-dose injections suggested for ECP are likely to be sufficient as "mismating shots," despite the higher doses that have been suggested (see Table 4). Since EB has a relatively short

Table 5. *Conservative Doses of Antinidatory Estradiol Cypionate Following Mismating in the Bitch*

Status of Vaginal Smear	Dosage Level	Dose of ECP* (mg/10 lb, IM)	Maximum Dose for Any Bitch (mg)
Estrus (fully cornified)	Conservative	0.1	≤0.5
Metestrus (Noncornified superficial cells present)	Less conservative	0.2	≤1.0

*Estradiol valerate, at the same doses, is also probably sufficient (see text).

duration of action, repeated injections might be justified (see Table 4), but the danger of inducing toxic effects or pyometra will likewise be increased.

ESTRONE

A veterinary preparation of estrone is commercially available. The supplier recommends a single injection of 2.5 to 5.0 mg for misalliance. As with all the estrogens, there are no reliable data on efficacy or safety based on a dose per unit body weight for the dog.

TERMINATION OF ESTABLISHED PREGNANCIES IN THE BITCH

There are no preparations approved, marketed, or recommended for termination of canine pregnancy following implantation. Injectable estrogens have probably been used but no reports are available. All potential protocols reported to date are experimental in nature, with numbers of animals insufficient to permit conclusions on either efficacy or safety. These have included estrogen implants and treatments with prostaglandin, bromocriptine (an ergot alkaloid), and dexamethasone.

Estrogen Implants. Silastic capsules containing crystalline estradiol, sufficient to maintain blood levels of estradiol at proestrus values, were inserted subcutaneously during midpregnancy. All bitches treated either resorbed or aborted their litters. Apparently, the level of estrogen needed to interfere with pregnancy is not very great.

Prostaglandins. $PGF_{2\alpha}$ (THAM salt) is luteolytic in the bitch if administered repeatedly. Doses of 30 μg/kg twice daily for three days after day 30 of pregnancy caused complete luteolysis and abortion in one half the bitches tested but failed to do so in the remaining bitches. PGF causes uterine contractions in addition to affecting luteal function, and its uterine effects may play a role in its action as an abortifacient. Limited trials of PGF at doses of 50 to 100 μg/kg once or twice daily to and beyond effect have routinely aborted mid- to late-pregnant bitches. However, cessation of treatment at the initiation of abortion can result in incomplete abortion, with the remainder of the litter going to term.

PGF side effects can be considerable and may include salivation, emesis, diarrhea, hypothermia, and lethargy. PGF can be lethal in high doses, and single doses that are abortifacient can be debilitating. The LD_{50} is about 5 mg/kg, not greatly different from the single dose of 1 mg/kg that is routinely luteolytic. A PGF analog (TPT) has been reported to routinely induce luteolysis and terminate pregnancies following a single injection, but it is not commercially available.

Corticosteroids. Adrenal steroids have the potential to terminate established pregnancies in the bitch, but the duration of treatment required and mechanisms of action are not known. Dexamethasone, 5 mg IM twice daily for ten days, starting on day 30 caused resorption and starting on day 45 resulted in abortion *after* the end of the ten days of treatment. Neither the effects of natural corticosteroids nor the effects of corticoid and prostaglandin combined (as used in cattle) have been tested for abortifacient efficacy in the bitch.

Ergot Alkaloids. Bromoergocryptine, a dopamine agonist that reduces prolactin secretion in the dog, is luteolytic and thus abortifacient following multiple administrations. However, doses of 0.1 mg/kg daily for six to ten days terminated pregnancy in only 60 per cent of the bitches studied.

REFERENCES AND SUPPLEMENTAL READING

Austad, R., Lunde, A., and Sjaastad, Ø. U.: Peripheral plasma levels of oestradiol-17β and progesterone in the bitch during the oestrous cycle, in normal pregnancy and after dexamethasone treatment. J. Reprod. Fertil. 46:129, 1976.

Bigbee, H. G., and Hennessy, P. W.: Megesterol acetate for postponing estrus in first heat bitches. V.M./S.A.C. 72:1727, 1977.

Bryan, H. S.: Parenteral use of medroxyprogesterone acetate as an antifertility agent in the bitch. Am. J. Vet. Res. 34:659, 1973.

Burke, T. J., and Reynolds, H. A., Jr.: Megestrol acetate for estrus postponement in the bitch. J.A.V.M.A. 167:285, 1975.

Castrodale, D., Bierbaum, O., Helwig, E. B., and Macbryde, C. M.: Comparative studies of the effects of estradiol and stilbestrol upon the blood, liver and bone marrow. Endocrinology 2:356, 1941.

Concannon, P. W., Altszuler, N., Hampshire, J., Butler, W. R., and Hansel, W.: Growth hormone, prolactin and cortisol in dogs developing mammary nodules and an acromegaly-like appearance during treatment with medroxyprogesterone acetate. Endocrinology 106:1173, 1980.

Concannon, P. W., and Hansel, W.: Prostaglandin F2α-induced luteolysis, hypothermia and abortions in Beagle bitches. Prostaglandins 13:533, 1977.

Eigenmann, J. E., and Venker-van Hagen, A. J.: Progestogen-induced and spontaneous canine acromegaly due to reversible growth hormone over production: clinical picture and pathogenesis. J.A.A.H.A. 17:813, 1981.

Faulkner, L., Pineda, M., and Reimers, T.: Immunization against gonadotropins in dogs, *In* Nieschlag, E. (ed.): *Immunization with Hormones in Reproduction.* New York: American Elsevier, 1975, pp. 199–214.

Harding, R. B.: The use of megesterol acetate in oestrus control in dogs. Post. Acad. Onder. 13:30, 1981.

Holst, P. A., and Phemister, R. D.: Onset of diestrus in the Beagle bitch: definition and significance. Am. J. Vet. Res. 35:401, 1974.

Holst, P. A., and Phemister, R. D.: Temporal sequence of events in the estrous cycle of the bitch. Am. J. Vet. Res. 36:705, 1975.

Jackson, W., and Johnston, S.: Pregnancy prevention and termination. *In* Kirk, R. W. (ed.): *Current Veterinary Therapy VII.* Philadelphia: W. B. Saunders, 1980, pp. 1239–1241.

Jochle, W.: Planned parenthood for pets. Bull. Atom. Sci. 73:10, 1973.

Jochle, W.: Pet population control: chemical methods. Canine Pract. 1:8, 1974.

Jochle, W.: Hormones in canine gynecology: a review. Theriogenology 3:152, 1975.

Kennelly, J.: The effect of mestranol on canine reproduction. Biol. Reprod. 1:282, 1969.

Legendre, A. M.: Estrogen-induced bone marrow hypoplasia in a dog. J.A.A.H.A. 12:525, 1976.

Mahi, C. A., and Yanagimachi, R.: Prevention of in vitro fertilization of canine oocytes by antiovary antisera: a potential approach to fertility control in the bitch. J. Exp. Zool. 210:129, 1979.

Mann, C. J.: Some clinical aspects of problems associated with oestrus and with its control in the bitch. J. Small Anim. Pract. 12:391, 1971.

McDonald, L. E.: Hormones affecting reproduction. *In* Jones, L., Booth, N. and McDonald, L. (eds.): *Veterinary Pharmacology and Therapeutics.* Ames, IA: Iowa State University Press., 1977, pp. 629–658.

Okin, R., Mullican, M., LaDu, R., Mandell, M., Nugent, T., Wells, C., and Durr, J.: Preventing pregnancy after mismating in dogs (panel report). Mod. Vet. Prac. 57:1041, 1976.

Okkens, A., Dielman, S., and Gaag, I.: Gynaecological complications after ovariohysterectomy in the dog. Post. Acad. Onder. 13:56, 1981.

Olson, P. N. S.: The ovary, ovarian hormones and contraceptives (canine). *In* Kirk, R. W. (ed.): *Current Veterinary Therapy VII.* Philadelphia: W. B. Saunders, 1980, pp. 1030–1034.

Pyle, R. L., Hill, B. L., and Johnson, J. R.: Estrogen toxicity in a dog. Canine Pract. 3:39, 1976.

Shille, V. M., and Stabenfeldt, G. H.: Current concepts in reproduction of the dog and cat. Adv. Vet. Sci. Comp. Med. 24:211, 1980.

Shivers, C. A., Sieg, P. M., and Kitchen, H.: Pregnancy prevention in the dog: potential for an immunological approach. J.A.A.H.A. 17:823, 1981.

Siegmund, O. (ed.): *The Merck Veterinary Manual,* 5th ed. Rahway, NJ: Merck & Co., Inc., 1979, p. 835.

Sokolowski, J. H.: Pharmacological control of fertility in small domestic animals. Friskies Res. Dig. 10:1, 1974.

Sokolowski, J. H., and Geng, S.: Biological evaluation of mibolerone in the female beagle. Am. J. Vet. Res. 38:1371, 1977.

Sokolowski, J. H., and Geng, S.: Effects of prostaglandin F2α-THAM in the bitch. J.A.V.M.A. 170:536, 1977.

Sokolowski, J. H., and Kasson, C. W.: Effects of mibolerone on conception, pregnancy, parturition and offspring in the beagle. Am. J. Vet. Res. 39:837, 1978.

Sokolowski, J. H., and Zimbelman, R. G.: Evaluation of selected compounds for estrus control in the bitch. Am. J. Vet. Res. 37:939, 1976.

Steinberg, S.: Aplastic anemia in a dog. J.A.V.M.A. 157:966, 1970.

van Os, J. L., and Oldenkamp, E. P.: Oestrus control in bitches with proligestone, a new progestational steroid. J. Small Anim. Pract. 19:521, 1978.

van Os, J. L., and Oldenkamp, E. P.: Proligestone—a safe, injectable progestational steroid for oestrus regulation (bitch). Kleintierpraxis 24:225, 1979.

Vickery, B., and McRae, G.: Effect of a synthetic PG analogue on pregnancy in beagle bitches. Biol. Reprod. 22:438, 1980.

Vickery, B., McRae, G., Kent, J., and Tomlinson, R. V.: Manipulation of duration of action of a synthetic PG analogue (TPT) assessed in the pregnant beagle bitch. Prostaglandins Med. 5:93, 1980.

Wildt, D. E., Kinney, G. M., and Seager, S. W. J.: Reproduction control in the dog and cat: an examination and evaluation of current and proposed methods. J.A.A.H.A. 13:223, 1977.

EXAMINATION OF THE BITCH FOR BREEDING SOUNDNESS

D. H. LEIN, D.V.M.

Ithaca, New York

A detailed history, thorough urogenital tract examination, and general physical examination of the bitch are all indicated for a thorough fertility examination.

The history should include fertility records of the bitch, littermates, and other related animals in the environment of the patient. The record of the stud dog used on this bitch should also be examined. Pedigrees should be examined to determine inbreeding or known genetic defects. Information on the number of estrus cycles, pregnancies, parturitions, previous urogenital problems, breedings, litters whelped, condition of puppies, and general health should be closely examined. Information concerning vaccinations, medications for treatment or prophylaxis, especially use of sex hormones, and diet and management practices should be studied.

A general examination should be carried out to detect problems or diseases of other systems that may affect fertility. An estimate of the psychologic stability of the bitch should be made. Highly nervous, shy bitches frequently have reproductive behavioral and cycling problems. All breeding dogs should be blood tested for *Brucella canis*. Positive rapid slide test sera should be confirmed by a standard laboratory tube test, agar gel immunodiffusion, and blood culture.

Hormone profiles and/or vaginal cytology may be helpful in determining the stage of cycle, presence of luteal tissue, and irregular patterns of the estrus cycle. Blood serum levels of estrogens and progesterone are followed and interpreted (see Reproductive Physiology and Endocrine Patterns of the Bitch; Infertility in the Bitch; and Endocrine Testing for

Infertility in the Bitch). Infertile bitches and stud dogs should also have thyroid and adrenocortical blood serum hormone level and function tests performed and interpreted, since dysfunction of these two endocrine glands can cause infertility (see Endocrine Testing for Infertility in the Bitch).

Examination of the urogenital tract should include the following:

1. *Vulva* (lips and vestibule): conformation, size, dischargers, inflammation, tumors. The size and condition of the clitoris and the clitoral fossa should be examined with a speculum and light.

2. *Urethra:* The urethral opening should be viewed with the aid of a speculum. A sterile catheterized urine sample may be collected at this time for culture, cytology, and urinalysis. The bladder should be examined via abdominal palpation. The close proximity of the urinary and genital tracts warrants consideration of dual involvement when considering anatomic abnormalities, inflammation, and neoplasia.

3. *Vagina:* A sterile spreading vaginal speculum should be carefully passed in the closed position without lubrication (causes artifacts in vaginal smear) over the urethra and brim of the pelvis (dorsal direction) into the vagina (horizontal). Cleansing of the vulva, perineum, and surrounding hair, if needed, should be done 12 to 24 hours prior to obtaining specimens for culture, since a wet skin surface frequently causes heavy contamination of the area. The long feather hair of the legs should be pinned to the side of the dog with a hair clip, and long tail hair can be covered with a tail wrap of 2- to 3-inch gauze roll bandage. Sterile cranial vaginal cultures can be obtained with a sterile guarded Tiegland swab (used in the mare for endometrial specimens) or a sterile swab (Culturette). Care should be taken not to contaminate the specimen while passing through the vestibule or caudal vagina for microbiologic examination.

The cytology of the *vaginal smear* is highly reflective of estrus cycle changes and can be useful in diagnosing inflammatory and neoplastic disorders of the upper genital tract. The cells of the cranial vagina are most reflective of the ovarian changes. The smear should not be contaminated with less reflective cells from the vestibule or caudal vagina.

Utilizing one or more assistants, a closed, sterile, expanding vaginal speculum is passed dorsally over the urethral opening and brim of the pelvis and is then directed horizontally to the cranial vagina and opened. A guarded swab for culture or a sterile saline–moistened 6-inch cotton swab applicator stick is passed along the open inside blade of the speculum, taking care to avoid vestibule and caudal vaginal surfaces. Cells are taken from the anterior surface. Smears are made by rolling the swab and cells onto clean glass slides and either air drying or fixing immediately, depending on the stain desired or the degree of drying artifact that will be tolerated.

For quick interpretation, a wet mount new methylene blue stain with a coverslip works well, but for permanent stains and later comparison studies any of the hematologic or cytologic stains may be used (see Reproductive Physiology and Endocrine Patterns of the Bitch).

The following estrous changes are viewed by microscopic study of the smear:

1. Proestrus: predominantly erythrocytes, leukocytes, and noncornified rounded epithelial cells with a few cornified polyhedral cells; by the end of proestrus most epithelial cells are cornified and leukocyte numbers are decreased markedly; background contains debris and sometimes bacteria.

2. Estrus: predominantly cornified polyhedral epithelial cells, called squames; cell edges may be curled or rolled, with small pyknotic nuclei or loss of nuclei; variable amounts of erythrocytes; no leukocytes or noncornified epithelial cells; background appears *clear* and *lacks debris.*

3. Metestrus: decrease in cornified cells; increase in ratio of smaller, round noncornified cells containing larger round nuclei, cellular debris, and increasing presence of leukocytes; erythrocytes may still be present in some dogs.

4. Anestrus: noncornified round small epithelial cells, usually in nest or clusters; few leukocytes with variable debris in the background.

The vaginal smear is constantly changing during proestrus, estrus, and early metestrus and must be carefully followed daily or every other day to see the comparative cell changes for that individual and predict the stage of the cycle. The smears are valuable diagnostic aids when behavioral changes cannot be studied or the bitch does not show behavioral changes. It is important to breed during early estrus. The return of leukocytes and noncornified epithelial cells indicates that ovulation has taken place and metestrus is present.

Deep vaginal cultures taken via a guarded swab should be submitted directly to a microbiology laboratory; if a delay in transit time is necessary, a transport media should be used (Amies Modified Transport Medium with Charcoal*). Bacteria, mycoplasma, and ureaplasma isolations should be attempted. Deep vaginal cytology for evidence of active inflammation, vaginoscopic examination and number of organisms isolated, and purity of cultures should all be used to interpret the significance of deep vaginal cultures. Using the previously mentioned swab technique to obtain a specimen from normal bitches will give a more definitive diagnosis of a "clean" bitch with negative cultures, an infected bitch with active inflammation, or a bitch with commensal or opportunist microorganisms without evidence of an active inflammation.

---

*BBL Microbiology System, Div. of Becton, Dickinson, and Co., Cockeysville, MD.

The vestibule and caudal vagina should next be palpated by digital examination, using a sterile surgery glove lubricated with sterile jelly. Strictures, stenosis, tumors, and abnormalities of the birth canal may be found at this time. Next, a digital rectal palpation should be performed with the same lubricated gloved hand. The free hand may be used to manipulate the urogenital tract per abdomen.

The entire vagina should next be viewed with a sterile small human proctoscope or sigmoidoscope (Welch-Allen) or other fiberoptic instrument, in both noninflated and insufflated stages. Anatomic abnormalities, tumors, inflammation (local or uterine), and stage of estrus cycle can be ascertained from this examination (see Endoscopy of the Bitch Reproductive Tract).

The cervix cannot be easily viewed, and the anterior vaginal folds are frequently mistaken for the cervix by some veterinarians during speculum examination. The dorsal median anterior vaginal fold, which extends caudally from the edge of the vaginal portion of the cervix, is largest during estrus and pregnancy. The caudal portion of the fold and the constriction of the lateral and ventral walls present the misleading appearance of the vaginal portion of the cervix, with a ventral fissure simulating the external uterine ostium. The true external os is approximately 2 to 3 cm cranial in adult beagle bitches and opens on the ventral surface of the dorsal anterior vaginal fold. The external os is best viewed when the vagina is insufflated with air. The vaginoscope can be used as a probe and the cervix identified by palpation per abdomen by passing the scope to the limits of the cranial vagina. Evidence of abnormal uterine drainage, cervical abnormalities, cervicitis, and tumors may be found during this examination.

The cervix, dorsal to the bladder and the caudal uterus, can usually be examined via abdominal palpation in the relaxed fasted bitch. Radiographs, intrauterine contrast media (hysterosalpingography), pneumoperitoneal contrast radiography, ultrasonic (Doppler) and density-amplitude ultrasonic examination, laproscopic examination, and laparotomy are all means of examining the uterus for anatomic abnormalities, neoplasia, and inflammation and obtaining uterine specimens for biopsy to confirm a diagnosis.

Vaginal smears and/or sex hormone profiles will predict the state of ovarian activity: follicular, luteal, or inactive. Palpation per abdomen may be possible if the ovary is greatly enlarged (tumors, cyst, anomalies, inflammation). Laparotomy and peritoneal scopic examination are used to view the ovaries. Remember that a fatty bursa completely encloses the ovary of the bitch except for a ventral slit, which contains the fimbrial portion of the oviduct. The slit will have to be opened further to remove the ovary from the bursa. The oviduct is difficult to view, as it passes through the mesosalpinx.

The infertile bitch may need several examinations during the estrus cycle to make a diagnosis of physiologic dysfunction or inflammatory conditions and to follow the animal's response to therapy and management. An orderly, systematic examination is essential to adequately identify any reproductive disorder or assure reproductive soundness in the bitch.

SUPPLEMENTAL READING

Concannon, P. W., Hansel, W., and Visek, W. J.: The ovarian cycle of the bitch: plasma estrogen, L.H. and progesterone. Biol. Reprod. 13:112, 1975.

Johnston, S. D.: Diagnostic and therapeutic approach to infertility in the bitch. J.A.V.M.A. 176:1335, 1980.

Olson, P. N. S.: Canine vaginitis. *In* Kirk, R. W. (ed.): *Current Veterinary Therapy VII.* Philadelphia: W. B. Saunders, 1980, pp. 1219–1222.

Pineda, M. H., Kainer, R. A., and Faulkner, L. C.: Dorsal median postcervical fold in the canine vagina. Am. J. Vet. Res. 34:1487, 1973.

ENDOSCOPY OF THE REPRODUCTIVE TRACT IN THE BITCH

FLORA E. F. LINDSAY, M.R.C.V.S.

Glasgow, Scotland

Modern endoscopic equipment is useful when examining the interior of a bitch's reproductive tract. It permits assessment of the physiologic status and/or patency of the tract and is a valuable aid in many reproductive tract procedures and in the diagnosis of pathologic conditions of the tract.

Plasma hormone assays and evaluation of the exfoliative vaginal cytology are laboratory methods recommended to determine the phase of the bitch's sexual cycle and are necessary in the full investigation of normal or abnormal estrus cycles. Endoscopy should also be considered for bitches assumed to be endocrinologically normal. In the normal cycling bitch, changes in the external genitalia and behavioral observations are very useful but may not be totally satisfactory or sufficiently precise. Some bitches have vulvar changes that may not be distinctive, some may not exhibit a reflex deviation of the tail, and some may exhibit an acceptance stance before or after conception is likely. Temperamental bitches may never allow mating. Postuterine endoscopy is a relatively simple and rapid technique that, with a little experience, offers satisfactory detection of several phases of the sexual cycle in the bitch and consequently aids the clinician in advising the client on the optimum time for natural or artificial insemination.

INSTRUMENTATION

Modern endoscopic equipment consists of a cold light source, i.e., light-transmitting flexible glass fibers that transport the light to the viewing system or endoscope (Fig. 1). The fiberoptic viewing system may be either a rigid or a flexible endoscope. In a flexible fiberoptic viewing system, the image is transferred along a bundle of coherent glass fibers; each fiber is suitably coated or clad to achieve maximal internal reflection of the light beam along the fiber to the viewer. The light-transmission and image-transporting fibers are enclosed in a common sheath. In a rigid endoscope, a series of specially coated glass rods are arranged by computer calculation within a metal sheath to form a series of air lenses in glass. Endoscopes are available with the distal lens oriented in a direct-forward, side, or oblique-forward viewing angle. Both flexible and rigid viewing systems have ancillary equipment allowing lavage, insufflation, collection of biopsy material, grasping, polypectomy, and so on. In the flexible system, channels for this equipment are included within the common outer sheath; in the rigid system ancillary equipment may be housed in accessory stainless steel sheaths. Attachments for a still camera allow the collection of permanent objective records, which can be attached to the patient record card. Attachments for cine and video cameras are also available. The rigid telescope system has the following advantages: it is often cheaper, it allows miniaturization of the scope without loss of optical quality, it can be introduced entirely by the operator, and it has been found quite suitable for endoscopic examinations that do not require considerable maneuverability, including laparoscopy, vaginoscopy, and hysteroscopy.

A rigid pediatric telescope (30.0 cm in length, 4.7 mm in outside diameter, an oblique-forward viewing angle of 30°) is most suitable for endoscopic examination of the reproductive tract of bitches of all sizes. A useful adjunct is a removable stainless steel cystoscope sheath with an outside diameter of 5.0 mm, and a connecting post with a valve allows the introduction of gas or liquid. A speculum previously inserted into the vagina serves to protect and support the scope and test the reaction of the unanesthetized bitch to the examination procedure. Specula should have the minimum outside diameter that allows passage of the scope and causes the least trauma and disturbance to the bitch. Specula need only be long enough to pass beyond the vestibulovaginal junction. Disposable plastic tubes, 12 to 20 cm in length and 10 mm in diameter, have been found adequate. For vaginal insufflation, an insufflation bulb or an automatic insufflator with a hose connection to a commercial carbon dioxide cylinder is attached to the removable sheath of the scope. Air insufflation channels are also built into many flexible scopes.

STERILIZATION OF ENDOSCOPES

Complete sterilization of endoscopes is probably not feasible in either veterinary practices or many

912

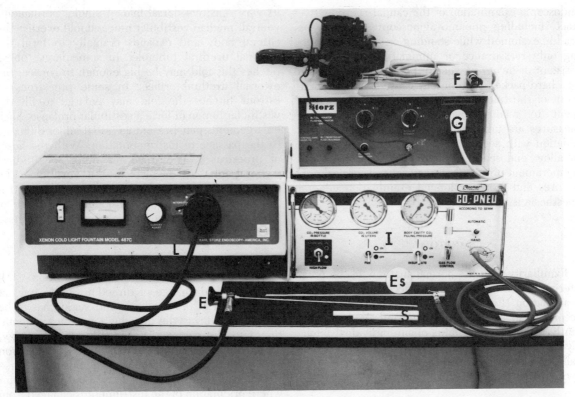

Figure 1. Endoscopic equipment. L = Cold light source; E = pediatric endoscope with fiberoptic cable attached; Es = endoscope sheath with insufflator tube attached; S = plastic specula; G = flash generator; F = flash box attachments for camera.

veterinary hospitals. Some antiseptic solutions in common use may be harmful to endoscopic equipment, and advice should be sought from the manufacturer of the particular instrument. After-use care of flexible scopes is described in specialist literature. Rigid scopes and any ancillary sheath can be immersed briefly in, or washed through with, a 10 per cent w/v benzalkonium chloride solution immediately after use. For reasonable bacterial sterilization, immersion of the scope and sheaths for 15 minutes in a mixture of equal parts of methanol and hypochlorite followed by rinsing in saline has been recommended.

POSTUTERINE ENDOSCOPY: ENDOSCOPY OF THE CAUDAL REPRODUCTIVE TRACT

The bitch's reproductive tract essentially consists of a uterine component and a caudal or "postuterine" component, which includes the vaginal cervix as well as the vagina, vestibule, and vulva. This "postuterine" component forms a functional unit as a copulatory organ and birth canal. Endoscopy of the reproductive tract can thus include endoscopy of the uterus, or hysteroscopy, and "postuterine" endoscopy, i.e., endoscopic examination of the vaginal cervix, vagina, and vestibule.

INDICATIONS

Endoscopic examinations of the postuterine tract can be used to detect phases of the sexual cycle; determine the optimum time for natural and artificial insemination; and program and monitor the effect of exogenous hormonal treatment. Vaginoscopy can be used to detect or inspect congenital abnormalities and abnormal or traumatic conditions, including ectopic ureters, vestibular prolapse, vaginal prolapse, vaginitis, tumors, internal uterine prolapse through the cervix, and rape or postpartum surgical instrument trauma. Vaginoscopy is also useful in determining the source of abnormal vulvar discharge in suspected cases of open pyometra.

In the parturient bitch, endoscopy can be used to ascertain if the cervix is open; to determine the presence, condition, and position of pups; and to obtain visual control over the removal of pups. Postuterine endoscopy can also facilitate retrieval of vaginal foreign bodies, catheterization of the bladder, and intracervical cannulations.

PROCEDURES

If care is taken when introducing the vaginal speculum or scope, most bitches are indifferent to endoscopic examination of the caudal reproductive tract, including pneumovaginoscopy, and can be readily examined while standing on a table, requiring only reassurance or minimal restraint by an assistant or owner. A very full bladder or abdomen or a hard-packed rectum may cause some displacement of the tract and may provoke minor resentment to manipulative procedures; appropriate measures are taken in these circumstances. Light sedation with acetylpromazine is usually adequate to allow endoscopic examination of bitches with temperament problems. For associated surgical procedures and more prolonged examination general anesthesia is required.

ANATOMY

Familiarity with the normal anatomy of the postuterine tract is essential for its successful endoscopic examination (Fig. 2). The vagina varies in length according to breed, body size, and, most importantly, the hormonal status of any individual bitch. Cyclic variations, which are observable endoscopically, are described in the section on detection of cyclical changes (*vide infra*).

VESTIBULE

In all bitches the vestibule slopes steeply in a dorsocranial direction from the vulva to the vestibulovaginal junction. The slope varies among and within breeds. Two or three centimeters from the ventral vulvar commissure is the clitoral fossa with its very sensitive dorsal fold. A single, permanent, ventral, median vestibular mucosal fold overlies the clitoral body and expands cranially to form the external urethral tubercle. In some large, obese bitches this fold may be big enough to conceal the external urethral orifice. In some proestrous or estrous bitches the fold may enlarge to fill the vestibular lumen or form a vestibular prolapse. Such enlargements may present an initial minor difficulty to the passage of instrumentation. With the onset of proestrus it is normal for other longitudinal mucosal folds to develop in the vestibule. The vulvar labia enlarge and become turgid in proestrus and soften during estrus, although the degree of labial tumescence varies among individual bitches.

VESTIBULOVAGINAL JUNCTION: CINGULUM

The marked change of direction of the tract at the junction of the vestibule and vagina has to be considered during the introduction of instrumentation into the vagina. The cingulum is a narrow, smooth annular band that constricts the junction and "gathers in" the caudal vaginal folds like a purse string. It overlies the ischial arch and is the point where orientation of the instrument is changed from an upward angle to a horizontal position (Fig. 3). The cingulum serves as a functional sphincter to the vagina and in most bitches presents some resistance to manipulative procedures. Vestigial remnants of the hymen on the ventral wall of the cingulum are not uncommon but functionally are often of little significance.

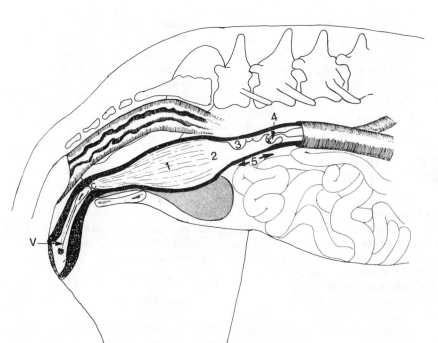

Figure 2. A schematic view of the canine postuterine or caudal reproductive tract. 1 = Plicate area of vagina; 2 = rugose area of vagina; 3 = dorsal median fold of paracervix (number is placed on caudal tubercle of the dorsal median fold); 4 = vaginal cervix; 5 = paracervix; V = ventral median fold in vestibule; C = cingulum at the vestibulovaginal junction.

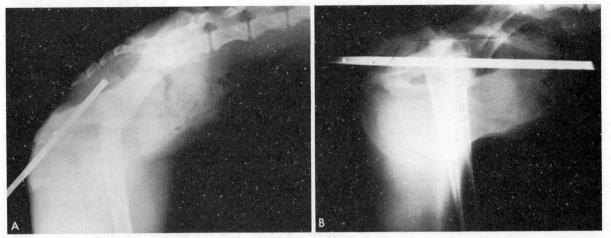

Figure 3. Radiographs of endoscope *in situ*. *A*, Scope in the vestibule; distal end at the vestibulovaginal junction. *B*, Scope advanced almost to the vaginal cervix. Observe the steep slope of the vestibule and the change of direction of the scope required at the vestibulovaginal junction.

VAGINA

The vagina can be considered as bottle-shaped, with the cervix projecting caudally into the neck of the bottle. The vaginal mucosa has four morphologically and functionally distinct regions: a plicate area; a rugose or intermediate area; a paracervical area; and the vaginal cervix. Recognition of these areas enables the practitioner to guide the scope with expertise within the vagina and to appreciate the mucosal changes that occur during the cycle. The plicate area corresponds to the caudal three-fifths of the body of the "bottle," the widest part of the vagina. It has *permanent longitudinal* mucosal folds (plicae). In the estrous bitch, the longitudinal plicae adapt to accommodate the transverse expansion of the bulbus glandis of the penis during coition. Cranial to the plicate area and forming the shoulders of the "bottle" is an intermediate or rugose area. During anestrus the rugose area is virtually devoid of mucosal folds, but during proestrus it develops many rugae-mucosal folds oriented predominantly obliquely and transversely and accommodates the elongation of the pars longa of the penis. The paracervical area corresponds to the short narrow neck of the "bottle"; its lumen appears as a narrow tunnel into which the cranial end of the vaginal cervix projects. The distinctive features of the paracervix are its narrow, crescent-shaped lumen and the permanent, single, longitudinal mucosal fold on its dorsal median wall, i.e., the dorsal median fold (dmf). Cranially, the dmf attaches to the cervix. A caudal tubercle demarcates the fold from the rugose area behind; there is a less well-developed cranial tubercle immediately behind the vaginal cervix (Fig. 4). Changes in the dmf and its tubercles are particularly sensitive indicators of the stage of the cycle. Caution must be exercised so as not to mistake the dmf and the tunnel-like paracervical lumen for the vaginal cervix and its canal. The caudal aspect of the paracervical area can

present as a pseudocervix. The internal dimensions of the paracervix vary among individual bitches. The paracervical "tunnel" is 20 to 50 mm in length and seldom exceeds 5 to 7 mm in intraluminal diameter. In the proestrous bitch additional mucosal folds develop on the ventrolateral walls of the paracervix and accommodate the penile urethral process during coition. The vaginal cervix with its external os projects caudoventrally or ventrally into the cranial end of the paracervical lumen. Furrows in the mucous membrane around the os present a star shape. The cervix is attached by the dmf to the cranial roof of the paracervix (Fig. 5).

TECHNIQUES

The vulva is routinely examined, and the appearance of the labia and evidence of any discharge are noted. The labia are parted to ascertain the presence of any obvious vulvar or vestibular abnormality such

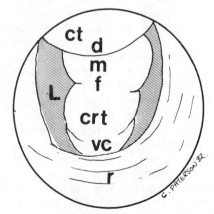

Figure 4. Canine anterior vagina, drawn from endophotograph showing paracervix and dorsal median fold (dmf). ct = Caudal tubercle; crt = cranial tubercle of the dorsal median fold; vc = vaginal cervix; L = paracervical lumen; r = rugose area.

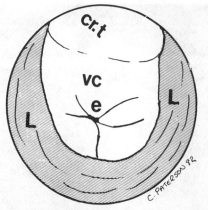

Figure 5. Canine cervix within paracervical lumen, drawn from endophotograph. L = Lumen of paracervix; vc = vaginal cervix; e = external os; cr.t = cranial tubercle of the dorsal median fold.

as a vestibular prolapse. The commonest cause of resentment to vaginoscopic procedures in an otherwise placid bitch is the careless passage of instrumentation through the vestibule and vestibulovaginal junction. The following procedure avoids unnecessary trauma and ensures the cooperation of the bitch. Excess hair is clipped or parted to the side, and the perineum and labia are suitably cleansed. A speculum previously moistened in warm saline or distilled water is inserted through the vulvar cleft, taking care to avoid the sensitive clitoral fold just within the ventral vulvar commissure. To accommodate the slope of the vestibule and the change of direction of the tract at the vestibulovaginal junction, the speculum is first directed dorsocranially (see Fig. 3A) from the vulvar cleft until its tip is felt within the vestibule by a finger placed just below the anus. When light digital pressure on the vestibular wall adjusts the speculum to the correct angle, it can be readily advanced under gently increased pressure through the vestibulovaginal junction into the vaginal lumen (see Fig. 3B). Normally a slight "give" at the cingulum indicates that the instrument has passed through the vestibulovaginal junction into the vaginal lumen. Resistance by the cingulum to the passage of even one finger is normal in many bitches and is always greater, and therefore resented more, during anestrus and in spayed bitches. In bitches with an enlarged vestibular fold, the small-diameter speculum is readily introduced if guided over a finger depressing the enlarged fold. If considerable resistance is encountered to the passage of the speculum, the vestibule should be re-examined for the presence of an imperforate hymen or a vestibular tumor not found on the preliminary external examination.

Moistening the distal end of the rigid scope with warm distilled water just before its introduction obviates fogging due to differences in ambient and intravaginal temperatures. Advancement of the scope within the vaginal lumen is always monitored visually. If guided properly, little resistance to the scope is encountered until it arrives at the narrower paracervix. In early proestrus, vaginal folds obscure the lumen and the scope may have to be partially withdrawn and readvanced. Increasing steady pressure is required to advance the scope into the paracervical lumen, and a distinct "give" is often experienced. Controlled pneumovaginoscopy, although not essential, is helpful in guiding the scope through the vaginal lumen in bitches with very long postuterine tracts or during the early proliferative phase of the cycle. If using an automatic insufflator, gas is allowed to flow freely into and out of the tract at the minimum pressure and volume required to open the lumen while viewing. In all bitches it is essential to observe the presence and character of any mucus membrane folds or fluids before insufflation causes pallor of the tissues. In some longbacked breeds, such as basset hounds, in which the vagina falls steeply over the pubic brim into the abdomen, it may be necessary to have an assistant support the ventral abdominal wall to bring the cranial part of the tract into view and avoid bending of the scope. During all endoscopic examinations viewing must be continuous throughout advancement or withdrawal of the instrument to avoid trauma and ensure a thorough examination. Retraction of the dmf with grasping forceps facilitates intracervical procedures.

DETECTION OF CYCLICAL CHANGES

Clinicians are often consulted concerning the failure of a bitch to reproduce. A common reason for lack of conception is that many bitches are not presented for mating at the correct stage of the estrus cycle. Detection of the phases of the cycle is essential to enable prediction of the optimum time for natural or artificial insemination. Endoscopically observable cyclic changes in the postuterine tract that are useful in assessing the stage of the cycle involve the development of new mucosal folds; alterations in length, height, complexity, character, and color of the folds; and the presence and consistency of fluids in the tract.

ANESTRUS

During anestrus the postuterine tract of any individual bitch is shortest in length and simplest in structure. All mucosal folds present are, on viewing, low, simple, and rounded in outline. The vestibule has only its single permanent, median, ventral fold. Cranial to the cingulum, plicate mucosal folds do not fill the vaginal lumen. The intermediate or rugose area is featureless and almost totally devoid of folds. The round caudal tubercle of the dmf forms

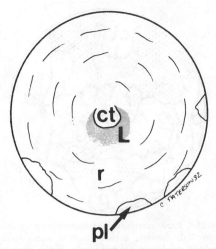

Figure 6. Anestrous bitch's vaginal mucosa, drawn from endophotograph and containing: low, simple plicate folds (pl); featureless rugose area (r); small, round, caudal tubercle (ct) forming obvious landmark at the entrance to the lumen of the paracervix (L). pl = Plicate folds.

an obvious landmark at the junction of the intermediate and paracervical areas (2 distinct areas) (Fig. 6).

The vaginal mucosa has a scant, transparent mucous coating and a translucent, diffuse, pink-red color. In anestrus the mucosa is thin and susceptible to trauma; minor scope contact can cause local submucosal hemorrhaging.

PROESTRUS

During proestrus two stages of changes in the mucosa are observable. The first stage is an early proliferative and edematous phase during which new folds develop and all folds become edematous (Fig. 7). In late proestrus this stage is succeeded by a "shrinking" phase in which the folds lose their edematous appearance.

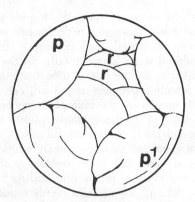

Figure 8. Early-proestrous bitch's vaginal mucosa, drawn from endophotograph. r = Balloon-like edematous folds of the rugose area; p = large, round, edematous folds of plicate area; p¹ = large, sacculated, edematous fold. These general vaginal folds fill the lumen during this stage.

The onset of proestrus is identifiable by an obvious edematous enlargement of the plicate vaginal folds and the dmf. This change from anestrus to proestrus is endoscopically identifiable several days before any external evidence of bleeding, although serosanguineous fluid may be seen intravaginally. Edematous enlargement of the plicate folds is followed rapidly by the development of new, radiating, broad folds in the vestibule; by balloon-like folds in the rugose area; and by annular folds in the ventral and lateral walls of the paracervix (Fig. 8). All mucosal folds appear edematous, soft, rounded, and symmetric in outline; the general vaginal folds fill the adjacent lumen. Within about five days of the onset of external discharge of blood, many vaginal folds acquire a round, "sacculated" appearance while the dmf and its tubercles still present an even, rounded outline. Commonly a clear, bright-red fluid is seen among the folds or flooding through the external os of the soft, prominent, flaccid, tubular cervix.

As proestrus progresses toward estrus the shrinking stage becomes evident. The endoscopic picture

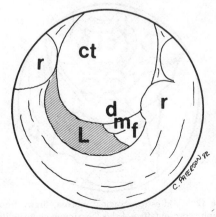

Figure 7. Early-proestrous bitch's anterior vagina, drawn from endophotograph and showing onset of edematous/proliferative change in mucosa. dmf = Edematous, round, dorsal median fold; L = lumen of paracervix; ct = large, round, edematous caudal tubercle; r = balloon-like edematous folds developing in the rugose area.

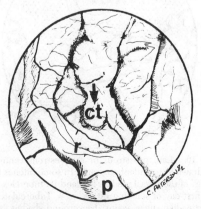

Figure 9. Late-proestrous bitch's "shrinking" vaginal mucosa, drawn from endophotograph. Tubercle and folds still have rounded profiles. p = Complex, wrinkled, some tuberculate plicae; r = transverse folds or rugae; ct = caudal tubercle.

becomes one of many narrow, simple, radiating vestibular folds; a vagina with lower, wrinkled, increasingly elongated, and complexly crumpled plicate folds that no longer totally fill the vaginal lumen (Fig. 9). By the end of proestrus, the transversely oriented complex rugae adjacent to the paracervix emphasize the crumpled concertina-like picture; some of the more cranial plicate folds are now tuberculate. However, careful observation will show that almost all these complexly wrinkled general vaginal folds still have *rounded* profiles. By contrast, the surfaces of the dmf and its tubercles begin to "flatten," losing their evenly rounded outlines. This change frequently signals the imminent onset of estrus (Fig. 10). The vaginal cervix shows much less shrinkage. Uterine fluid is often still quite profuse in the lumen.

ESTRUS

During estrus, the "shrinking" of the mucosal folds begun in proestrus progresses and intensifies. A sharp, peaked, or angulated profile for all general vaginal mucosal folds becomes the outstanding feature of estrus. During this period of "total" or "maximum" angulation, the vaginal folds appear as a series of pale, angular peaks, diminishing in height cranially to low angular mounds or tubercles. Areas that are shadowed from the light beam may not appear as pale as other areas. The vaginal lumen is wider. The dmf and its tubercles become increasingly shrunken and distorted. The vaginal cervix shows little further shrinkage and remains obviously tubular, but with deepening furrows radiating from the external os. The simple radiating vestibular folds have sharp, even profiles.

Endoscopically, estrus is characterized by several recognizable stages. Its onset is signalled by the

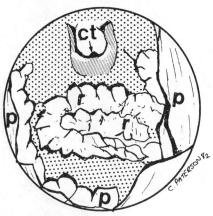

Figure 11.   Early-estrous canine vaginal mucosa, drawn from endophotograph showing a pseudocervix. Some vaginal folds show peaking/angulation; ventral border of the caudal tubercle (ct) is notched (arrow). p = Plicate folds; r = rugose folds with wrinkled edges showing against background shadow (stippling). The caudal tubercle forms a "pseudocervix."

initial angulation of the dmf and its tubercles (Fig. 11); this precedes the period of total or maximum angulation and peaking of the vaginal and vestibular folds by approximately 48 hours (Fig. 12). The initial angulation of the dmf is most easily seen in the profile of its tubercles (Fig. 13). In early estrus some bitches develop a ventral notch in the caudal tubercle. This notched appearance accentuates the pseudocervix appearance of the region such that it actually might be readily mistaken for the cervix.

Toward the end of estrus all folds are in their most shrunken and angular stage. During the last two days of estrus, the rugose area adjacent to the paracervix often has a very wide lumen lined by a characteristic "crepe paper," i.e., crinkled mucosa of very low, fine folds. This area contrasts sharply with the narrow paracervical lumen and a very shrunken caudal tubercle and dmf (Fig. 14). An inconsistent ring-like construction at the plicate/

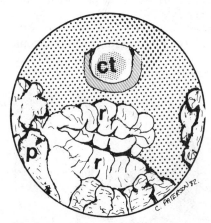

Figure 10.   Late proestrous or early-estrous canine vaginal mucosa, drawn from endophotograph. In some bitches the initial "flattening" of the dorsal median fold and its tubercles coincides with the first day of standing estrus. p = Tuberculate plicae; r = concertina-like rugae against background shadow (stippling); ct = caudal tubercle beginning to flatten, outlined by paracervical lumen.

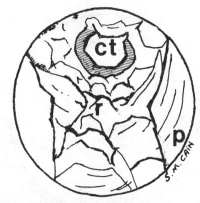

Figure 12.   Mid-estrous vaginal mucosa, drawn from endophotograph representative of this "maximum angulated/peaked" period. The vaginal lumen is wide. p = Plicate folds forming a series of higher caudal peaks diminishing in height to low angular mounds in rugose area (r); ct = smaller and obviously angular outline of caudal tubercle.

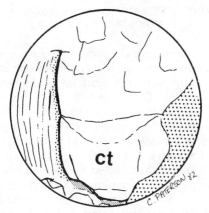

Figure 13.   Close-up view of very angular caudal tubercle (ct) of dorsal median fold in anterior vagina of an estrous bitch, drawn from endophotograph.

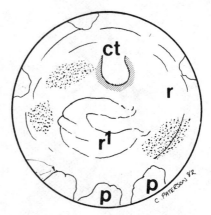

Figure 15.   Early-diestrous (metestrous) canine vaginal mucosa, drawn from endophotograph. Stippled areas represent patchy, hyperemic appearance of mucus membranes. ct = Rounded out caudal tubercle; p = low, simple, rounded plicate folds; r = almost fold-free rugose area.

rugose junction is seen in late estrus in otherwise apparently normal bitches. Fluid in the vaginal lumen, typical of estrus in many bitches, is scanty, clear, and straw-colored or, less frequently, a clear bright-red and may be observed endoscopically throughout estrus. The onset of diestrus is signalled when a "rounding out" of the mucosal folds commences.

METESTRUS/DIESTRUS

A characteristic feature of diestrus (i.e., metestrus) is a patchy or banded hyperemic appearance of the general vaginal mucosa, giving it an overall tigroid appearance when viewed endoscopically. The dmf and plicate vaginal folds are low, simple, rounded, and even. The intermediate area is almost free of folds except, characteristically, for one oblique, soft fold adjacent to the paracervix. In

response to stimulation by the endoscope, this fold and the adjacent area will frequently form a "rosette" of soft, moist, pink folds, which often subsides quite quickly (Fig. 15). This "rosette" of folds around the central lumen forms another pseudocervix, which might be mistaken for the cervix by the inexperienced viewer (Fig. 16). The vaginal mucus is often more abundant, slightly thicker, and clear or slightly opalescent in color.

DIFFERENTIAL DIAGNOSES AND APPLICATION

When examining a bitch endoscopically to determine its sexual status, the clinician should consider the following: the relatively *featureless appearance of anestrus, the edematous phase of proestrus, the banded or patchy hyperemia, and the "rosette" of diestrus* are endoscopically characteristic of the respective stages and enable the clinician to advise on mating times for the bitch.

The maximum *"peaked/angulated" period and relative pallor of the mucosal folds in estrus* are also endoscopically distinctive and characteristic of estrus. Although some bitches will accept the dog when the tubercles of the dmf begin to "flatten," the total or maximum "peaked/angulated" period coincides closely with the period of the "estrous" vaginal smear and should be recommended as the optimum period for mating, especially if only one service is available. Although most bitches will readily accept the dog throughout the maximum "peaked/angulated" period, it is the author's experience that a few bitches will *only* accept the stud in the last 48 hours of the "peaked period," when the cranial vagina has a wide lumen with very low crinkled mucosa; yet they conceive successfully.

The clinician should also take into account that some bitches with the typical "peaked/angulated"

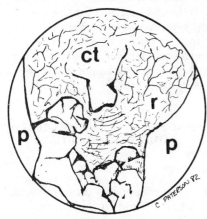

Figure 14.   Late-estrous vaginal mucosa, drawn from endophotograph. All folds are very shrunken, low, and very angular. Note the very low, crinkled "crepe paper" appearance of the mucosa of the rugose area (r). The caudal tubercle (ct) is very distorted, small, shrunken. The vaginal lumen is very wide. Plicate folds (p) are still angular in outline. In some bitches this presentation is typical of the last 48 hours of standing estrus.

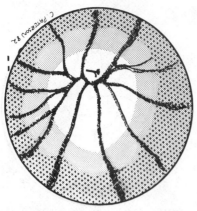

Figure 16. Diestrous vaginal "rosette" forming a pseudocervix, drawn from endophotograph. r = Rosette of soft, round folds, which forms at rugose/plicate area junction.

estrus endoscopic profile may lack pheromonal attraction for the stud. Others may have temperamental or physical problems, so-called humanized bitches, and will not stand for the stud. As an alternative to artificial insemination, such bitches can be lightly sedated with acetylpromazine to obtain acceptance of the stud. However, the clinician *must* be satisfied that the endoscope profile in these bitches is appropriate and there are no significant physical abnormalities. If a bitch has to be sent some distance to a stud dog, the crumpled concertina-like appearance typical of the end of proestrus and the *initial* angulation of the dmf, seen first as a "flattening" of the tubercle surfaces, serve as guides to the onset of estrus. The termination of standing estrus, the first refusal, is usually related endoscopically to either the first or second day that the dmf tubercles lose their angular profiles and "round out," and the rugose area becomes almost fold-free or presents a soft "rosette" appearance. These changes signal the onset of metestrus and therefore occur near the end of any likely conception time. If absent in estrus, the return of a bright-red fluid often accompanies the onset of metestrus but is not constant or precise.

To allow for variations in the duration of the estrus cycle or particular phases in individual bitches, endoscopic examination to detect estrus should be begun as early as possible in proestrus. Likewise, the frequency of endoscopic examination depends on the experience of the clinician with the method, the history of the bitch, and the needs of the client. Examination at 48-hour intervals is advisable. When detection of the onset of estrus is critical, daily examination is necessary. Daily endoscopic examination is well tolerated without anesthesia in almost all bitches, provided care is taken to avoid trauma during the introduction of suitable instrumentation.

ENDOSCOPIC MONITORING OF EXOGENOUS HORMONAL CONTROL

Several commercially available exogenous hormonal compounds are recommended for suppression or temporary or permanent postponement of heat in bitches. The correct timing of the administration of these drugs in relation to the sexual status of the bitch is necessary for their success. For temporary postponement of heat, a drug course given in anestrus is generally recommended, with repeat dosing in the induced anestrus for permanent postponement. For suppression of heat, a drug course is begun as soon as possible after external signs of proestrus are observed. However, the external signs of proestrus (vulvar swelling, vulvar bleeding) are inconstant between bitches and variable in time of onset, duration, and intensity and may be overlooked initially by the owner. Furthermore, there are no reliable external signs to indicate the onset, duration, or termination of metestrus. All of these phases of the cycle are identifiable endoscopically, and a suitable regimen of endoscopic examination could be usefully implemented in bitches on a regular program of estrus control, such as kennelled greyhounds, to reduce the incidence of "breakthrough" estrus. The endoscopically observable "silent changeover" period from anestrus to proestrus often coincides with the initial increased interest of the male dog in the bitch's urine. Owners of pet bitches may be advised to be observant of these circumstances and present a bitch for endoscopic confirmation of the onset of proestrus to ensure correct timing of estrus-suppressing regimens. Bitches may be presented by owners unsure of the onset of proestrus. Current endoscopic studies indicate that, with most courses, successful estrus suppression should commence no later than the early, simple, sacculated, edematous phase to avoid a "rebound" estrus. Furthermore, in many contraceptive courses the vaginal mucosa changes directly from proestrus to a metestrus appearance. This change can be monitored endoscopically to indicate the success or failure of the regimen and its earliest termination.

POSTUTERINE ENDOSCOPY OF POST-TRAUMATIC OR PATHOLOGIC CONDITIONS

VAGINAL TEARS

Probably the commonest cause of vaginal tear is the inexpert and "blind" use of surgical instrumentation during whelping. Another cause is rape. Rape most commonly occurs in pedigree bitches as a result of deliberate forced mating when the bitch is not in physiologic estrus and refusal of the bitch to stand is wrongly attributed to "temperament." Vaginal tears frequently result from mating of bitches with locomotor dysfunction. Following genital or iatrogenic trauma, bruising of the vestibule wall, tears in the vaginal mucosa with whole blood in the lumen, or clotted blood in the vaginal tear is seen. Whatever the cause, most vaginal mucosal tears, provided with suitable antibiotic cover, will repair completely. However, healing may take several months, and a breeding bitch should be endoscopically examined before its next mating. Surgical repair should be considered for a complete perforating tear of the vaginal wall.

VESTIBULITIS AND VAGINITIS

The normally patchy or striped hyperemia of the metestrous vagina or the overall pink/red coloration of the thin, nonedematous, and readily traumatized anestrous vagina must not be mistaken for vaginitis. In cases of vaginitis or vestibulitis, the anestrous mucosa is often a dense cherry-red or dark-red color, is frequently *edematous,* and hemorrhages readily into the lumen; careful examination often reveals enlarged *vestibular* lymph nodules. The presence of tumors or foreign bodies giving rise to secondary vaginitis or ulcerative vaginitis can be confirmed by postuterine endoscopy.

ABNORMAL VULVAR DISCHARGE AND VAGINAL FLUIDS

Postuterine endoscopy is of considerable value in the differential diagnosis of the source of "abnormal" vulvar discharges that may be due to a secondary vaginitis, an "open" pyometra, or prolonged proestral bleeding. When ectopic ureters are a cause of urine leakage and positional changes due to pooling of urine in the vagina, endoscopy combined with IV injection of methylene blue is diagnostic.

In many of the previously mentioned conditions, pneumovaginum is extremely helpful and improves ease of visualization of the mucus membrane and lumen during endoscopy. It should, however, always be used with caution and under visual control and should be discontinued when there is evidence of vaginal tears or mucosal erosion.

ENDOSCOPY AND HYSTEROSCOPY OF THE PREGNANT BITCH

Postuterine endoscopy has been used in several pregnant bitches without any visibly adverse effects. Bitches have been examined at several stages of pregnancy, including first- and second-stage labor and within a few hours post partum. Post-partum clots that obscure viewing can be removed by careful use of sterile vaginal swabs. The endoscopic examination of bitches during parturition has been conducted in the same room as the whelping box, with any pups and the owner present. In these circumstances the examination has been well tolerated by the bitch and certainly seems no more stressful than other more common manipulative obstetric procedures. In the immediate post-partum period the endoscope can be advanced easily through the open cervix to examine the uterine body and horns.

TRANSCERVICAL INTRAUTERINE CATHETERIZATIONS

The vaginal cervix in the bitch lies at the cranial end of the narrow paracervix and is not as readily accessible to catheterization as in the larger domestic species. Endoscopy with pneumovaginum allows good visualization of the paracervical area. Retraction of the dmf with grasping forceps placed as near the cervix as possible helps to "fix" the cervix and allows a plastic catheter to be directed through the cervix and into the uterus. Such intrauterine catheterization has been recommended for contrast hysterography to determine pathologic changes in the uterus and for nonsurgical treatment of pyometra with chemotherapeutic or antibiotic agents.

SUPPLEMENTAL READING

Hollanders, D.: *Gastrointestinal Endoscopy.* London: Bailliere Tindal, 1979, pp. 77–83.
Kelsey, J. C., Mackinnon, I. H., and Maurer, I. M.: Sporicidal activity of hospital disinfectant. J. Clin. Path. 27:632, 1974.
Lindsay, F. E. F.: The normal endoscopic appearance of the caudal reproductive tract of the cyclic and non-cyclic bitch; post uterine endoscopy. J. Small Anim. Pract. 24:1, 1983.
Pineda, M. H., Kainer, R. A., and Faulkner, L. C.: Dorsal median postcervical fold in the canine vagina. Am. J. Vet. Res. 34:1487, 1973.

ENDOCRINE TESTING FOR INFERTILITY IN THE BITCH

T. J. REIMERS, Ph.D.

Ithaca, New York

Long interestrous intervals or failure of a bitch to show a reproductive cycle may be associated with ovarian disorders, hypothyroidism, or hyperadrenocorticism. The development and validation of specific and sensitive radioimmunoassays for quantifying hormones make possible direct evaluation of endocrine function of the ovaries and thyroid and adrenal glands. Radioimmunoassays allow measurement of hormones in nanogram (ng, 10^{-9}gm), picogram (pg, 10^{-12}gm), and even femtogram (fg, 10^{-15}gm) units in as little as 0.1 cc of serum or plasma. This article describes uses and interpretations of hormone measurements relevant to infertility in the bitch.

OVARY

Two classes of ovarian hormones (progestins and estrogens) are quantified by radioimmunoassay to evaluate reproductive status. Either total estrogens or estradiol-17β are measured; progesterone is usually the progestin that is measured. Estrogen levels are elevated only for a brief period of 24 to 72 hours around the onset of estrus (Table 1). Concentrations of estrogen have been reported to be higher during pregnancy than during diestrus and pseudopregnancy and to decrease rapidly to low levels by the day of parturition. However, not all investigators have found higher levels of estrogen during pregnancy.

Estradiol is very difficult to measure consistently in canine blood. This is probably because of the extremely low concentrations present, 1000 times less than progesterone. This has led to quite variable reference values among different testing laboratories and researchers studying canine reproduction. Because estrogen measurements are so variable among and within dogs, their usefulness in evaluating abnormal estrus cycles in the bitch is questionable.

Quantification of progesterone is useful in the diagnosis of various reproductive disorders (see Table 1). In the normal bitch, progesterone secretion is related to secretory activity of corpora lutea. Proestrus and anestrus are characterized by low concentrations of progesterone in blood (less than 1.0 ng/ml). Progesterone concentrations increase during estrus, corresponding to the developing corpora lutea. During diestrus, pregnancy, and pseudopregnancy, concentrations of progesterone in serum or plasma are between 10 and 50 ng/ml.

Whether or not concentrations of progesterone differ among diestrous, pregnant, and pseudopregnant bitches remains controversial. Several investigators reported that concentrations of progesterone were similar in pregnant and nonpregnant bitches, whereas others have reported that the concentrations of progesterone in the serum of pregnant bitches are twice as high as those in nonpregnant bitches beginning 20 to 25 days after the onset of estrus. Although these differences have been reported, quantification of progesterone in a sample of serum or plasma is not a test for pregnancy in the bitch. A high progesterone level in a sample only indicates that luteal tissue is present on the ovaries. Therefore, it is useful for confirming ovulation, missed heats, silent heats, and luteinized cysts, but not pregnancy.

THYROID GLAND

A common cause of long interestrous intervals in the bitch is hypothyroidism, although its relationship to reproductive disorders is poorly understood. Diagnosing hypothyroidism by quantifying total thyroid hormones (T_3, T_4) in serum or plasma is fairly simple. However, interpretation of baseline concentrations of T_3 and T_4 in single blood samples often is difficult, particularly in samples with borderline concentrations of these hormones. Several factors account for this difficulty. T_3 and T_4 levels are increased or decreased by certain normal physiologic conditions, drugs, and nonthyroidal illnesses regardless of functional status of the thyroid gland. Puppies generally have higher levels and dogs over six years of age generally have lower levels of thyroid hormones than young, adult dogs. The normal thyroid gland secretes mostly T_4 and very little T_3. The latter, which is the biologically active form of the hormone, is produced by conversion of T_4 to T_3 in muscle, liver, kidneys, and other peripheral tissues. More than 99 per cent of T_3 and T_4 in

Table 1. *Reference Values for Some Endocrine Tests in the Bitch as Determined by Radioimmunoassay**

Endocrine gland	Test	Reference Values
Thyroid	T_3 baseline	1–2 ng/ml
	T_4 baseline	1.5–3 µg/dl
	TSH baseline	1–4 ng/ml
	Thyroid-response test	
	T_3: pre-TSH	1–2 ng/ml
	post-TSH	2–4 ng/ml
	T_4: pre-TSH	1.5–3 µg/dl
	post-TSH	3–6 µg/dl
Adrenal	Cortisol baseline	1.8–4 µg/dl
	ACTH-response test	
	Cortisol: pre-ACTH	1.8–4 µg/dl
	post-ACTH	7–16 µg/dl
	Dexamethasone-suppression test	
	Cortisol: pre-dexamethasone	1.8–4 µg/dl
	post-dexamethasone	<0.5 µg/dl
	Dexamethasone suppression/ACTH-stimulation test	
	Cortisol: pre-dexamethasone	1.8–4 µg/dl
	post-dexamethasone	<0.5 µg/dl
	post-ACTH	7–16 µg/dl
Ovary	Progesterone baseline	
	Anestrus	< 1 ng/ml
	Proestrus	< 1 ng/ml
	Late estrus (metestrus)	1–10 ng/ml
	Diestrus	10–50 ng/ml
	Pregnancy	10–50 ng/ml
	Pseudopregnancy	10–50 ng/ml
	Estradiol baseline	
	Late proestrus/early estrus	25–70 pg/ml
	Diestrus	15–30 pg/ml
	Pregnancy	15–30 pg/ml
	Pseudopregnancy	15–30 pg/ml

*Because different laboratories may use different techniques for measuring hormones, practitioners should use reference values given by their own reference laboratory.

the blood is bound to the serum proteins thyroid-binding globulin (TBG), thyroid-binding prealbumin (TBPA), and albumin. Exogenous or endogenous hormones, such as estrogens, may increase TBG levels, and glucocorticoids and androgens may decrease TBG levels, thereby causing corresponding increases and decreases in T_3 and T_4 concentrations. Higher levels of TBG during pregnancy may account for higher levels of T_3 and T_4 during this reproductive state.

Interpretation of baseline levels of thyroid hormones may be improved by quantifying TBG and other binding proteins, free (unbound) T_3 and T_4, or binding capacity of T_3 to TBG (T_3 uptake test) in conjunction with total T_3 and T_4. These parameters are examined extensively in human medicine to evaluate thyroid status. However, none of these tests has been validated adequately for the dog, and preliminary studies suggest that they are of little value in diagnosing canine hypothyroidism.

Currently, the most useful means of evaluating thyroid function in the dog is by quantifying T_3 and T_4 before and after stimulation of the thyroid gland with exogenous thyroid-stimulating hormone (TSH). The TSH-response test can distinguish between a defect in the thyroid gland (primary hypothyroidism), a defect in the pituitary gland (secondary hypothyroidism), and subnormal thyroid function due to nonthyroidal illness (e.g., Cushing's syndrome). Although hypothyroidism resulting from insufficient secretion of thyrotropin-releasing hormone by the hypothalamus has been described in humans, the existence of this form of hypothyroidism (tertiary hypothyroidism) has not been described in dogs.

One procedure for the TSH-response test is as follows:

1. Collect a pre-injection, baseline blood sample.
2. Inject 5 IU of TSH intravenously.
3. Collect a postinjection blood sample four hours later.
4. Allow samples to clot in the refrigerator, centrifuge, and submit serum samples to a laboratory for T_3 and T_4 radioimmunoassays.

In normal dogs (see Table 1), the baseline concentration of T_4 is between 1.5 and 3.0 µg/dl; T_3 is between 1.0 and 2.0 ng/ml (100 to 200 ng/dl). Four hours after TSH stimulation, T_4 and T_3 levels are increased two to three times. Dogs with primary hypothyroidism have subnormal (often undetectable) or low normal baseline levels of T_4; after TSH, levels of T_4 change very little, if at all. Baseline and post-TSH levels of T_3 are more variable and less predictable. T_3 levels may be within the normal range, whereas T_4 is severely depressed. In humans, T_3 levels in early stages of hypothyroidism may be within the normal range. The thyroid gland appears to compensate by secreting more T_3 directly. Further research is needed to elucidate the relationship between T_3 levels and the degree of hypothyroidism; duration of hypothyroidism; and the roles of diet, age, breed, size, and so on in dogs.

Dogs with secondary hypothyroidism also have subnormal or low baseline levels of T_4. These patients show some increase in T_4 after administration of TSH, but not as much as in normal dogs. Dogs with certain chronic, nonthyroidal illnesses may have low baseline T_4 levels but show a response to TSH that falls within the normal range. Confirmation of this pattern needs further study.

ADRENAL GLAND

Adrenocortical hyperfunction (Cushing's syndrome) also may lead to infertility in the bitch. Persistent anestrus may be seen in over 75 per cent of bitches with hyperadrenocorticism. A significant proportion of these may have clitoral enlargement, suggesting that some reproductive disorders associated with Cushing's syndrome may be the result of abnormal secretion of androgens as well as glucocorticoids.

Assessment of adrenal function is best done by quantification of corticosteroids (i.e., cortisol) either by fluorometry, competitive protein-binding assay, or radioimmunoassay. Because fluorometry and competitive protein-binding assays measure other corticosteroids besides cortisol, levels obtained from these assays are usually higher than those determined by the more specific radioimmunoassay.

Because cortisol is released episodically into the circulation and is significantly affected by stress, phase of the reproductive cycle, and certain drugs and hormones (barbiturates, dexamethasone, diphenylhydantoin, estrogens, prostaglandins), determination of the concentration of cortisol in a single sample of serum or plasma is of little or no value in diagnosing Cushing's syndrome. Frequently, baseline cortisol values may be within the normal range.

Quantification of cortisol in blood before and after injection of adrenocorticotropin (ACTH) can more accurately identify dogs with Cushing's syndrome than can measurement of cortisol in a single baseline sample. The procedure for the ACTH-response test is as follows:

1. Collect a baseline, pre-ACTH blood sample.

2. Inject 2.2 IU/kg of aqueous ACTH intravenously or ACTH gel intramuscularly.

3. Collect a postinjection blood sample two hours later.

4. Allow samples to clot in the refrigerator, centrifuge, and submit serum samples to a laboratory for cortisol determination.

In normal dogs (see Table 1), concentrations of cortisol increase three to five times after injection of ACTH from a baseline of 1.8 to 4.0 µg/dl. Dogs with Cushing's syndrome will likely have high-normal or above-normal baseline cortisol levels regardless of the etiology. In a dog with idiopathic adrenal hyperplasia or adrenal hyperplasia secondary to an ACTH-secreting pituitary tumor, the concentration of cortisol after injection of ACTH will be elevated to exaggerated levels, frequently above 30 µg/dl. In both cases, the exaggerated secretion of cortisol after administration of ACTH is due to hyperplasia of the adrenal cortices caused by excessive secretion of ACTH from the pituitary gland. Administration of exogenous ACTH will not affect cortisol levels in the blood of dogs with autonomous adrenocortical tumors. Lack of an increase in cortisol after injection of ACTH is an excellent indication of an adrenocortical tumor. However, not all adrenocortical tumors are autonomous, and these may show normal or exaggerated increases.

Although the ACTH-response test works well in diagnosing hyperadrenocorticism, it often does not accurately identify the cause of the disease. An exaggerated response to ACTH may be seen in dogs with idiopathic adrenal hyperplasia, a pituitary tumor, and a nonautonomous adrenocortical tumor. The combination of dexamethasone suppression and ACTH stimulation frequently is more discerning. Unfortunately, results of the dexamethasone-suppression/ACTH-stimulation test also may be ambiguous. One protocol for the dexamethasone-suppression/ACTH-stimulation test is as follows:

1. Collect a baseline, pre-dexamethasone blood sample.

2. Inject dexamethasone intravenously in a dose of 0.1 mg/kg of body weight at 9:00 AM.

3. Collect a post-dexamethasone blood sample at 12:00 noon.

4. Inject 2.2 IU/kg of aqueous ACTH intravenously or ACTH gel intramuscularly.

5. Collect a post-ACTH blood sample at 1:30 PM.

6. Allow samples to clot in the refrigerator, centrifuge, and submit serum samples to a laboratory for cortisol determination.

In normal dogs (see Table 1), cortisol is suppressed to very low levels (less than 0.5 µg/dl) three hours after administration of this dose of dexamethasone. After injection of ACTH, cortisol values increase three to five times above the baseline level. In dogs with idiopathic adrenal hyperplasia, the previously mentioned dose of dexamethasone is sufficient to suppress cortisol to low levels (less than 0.8 μg/dl). Because the glands are functionally hyperplastic, very high levels of cortisol, frequently above 30 μg/dl, are elicited by exogenous ACTH.

If an autonomous pituitary tumor is present and secreting excess ACTH, dexamethasone will not suppress ACTH secretion, and, as a result, cortisol levels will remain unchanged. After injection of ACTH, very high levels of serum cortisol will be observed. Further tests may be required for pituitary tumors that are not autonomous.

When a functional adrenocortical tumor is the cause of hyperadrenocorticism, the level of cortisol in serum is usually unchanged after dexamethasone administration. After ACTH administration, the response may be normal or exaggerated or there may be no increase at all.

A brief comment on proper collection and handling of blood samples for hormone measurements is in order. Some hormones (e.g., progesterone) deteriorate rapidly in blood samples, whereas others (e.g., T_4) are more stable. Before collecting a sample, check with your reference laboratory for the correct type and volume of sample to collect, the proper means of storage, and the best way to deliver the sample. Additionally, your laboratory may have different normal reference values than those shown in Table 1.

SUPPLEMENTAL READING

Belshaw, B. E., and Rijnberk, A.: Hypothyroidism. *In* Kirk, R. W. (ed.): *Current Veterinary Therapy VI*. Philadelphia: W. B. Saunders, 1977, pp. 1017–1019.

Belshaw, B. E., and Rijnberk, A.: Radioimmunoassay of plasma T_4 and T_3 in the diagnosis of primary hypothyroidism in dogs. J. Am. Anim. Hosp. Assoc. 15:17, 1979.

Concannon, P. W., Hansel, W., and Visek, W. J.: The ovarian cycle of the bitch: plasma estrogen, LH and progesterone. Biol. Reprod. 13:112, 1975.

Johnston, S. D.: Diagnostic and therapeutic approach to infertility in the bitch. J.A.V.M.A. 176:1335, 1980.

Johnston, S. D., and Mather, E. C.: Canine plasma cortisol (hydrocortisone) measured by radioimmunoassay: clinical absence of diurnal variation and results of ACTH stimulation and dexamethasone suppression tests. Am. J. Vet. Res. 39:1766, 1978.

Kallfelz, F. A.: Thyroid function in the dog. Vet. Clin. North Am. 7:497, 1977.

Larsen, P. R., Silva, J. E., and Kaplan, M. M.: Relationships between circulating and intracellular thyroid hormones: physiological and clinical implications. Endocrinol. Rev. 2:87, 1981.

Lubberink, A. A. M. E., Rijnberk, A., der Kinderen, P. J., and Thijssen, J. H. H.: Hyperfunction of the adrenal cortex: a review. Aust. Vet. J. 47:504, 1971.

Martin, S. L., Murdick, P. W., and Capen, C. C.: Laboratory evaluation of adrenocortical function in dogs. In Kirk, R. W. (ed.): *Current Veterinary Therapy IV*. Philadelphia: W. B. Saunders, 1971, pp. 589–592.

Nett, T. M., Akbar, A. M., Phemister, R. D., Holst, P. A., Reichert, Jr., L. E., and Niswender, G. D.: Levels of luteinizing hormone, estradiol and progesterone in serum during the estrous cycle and pregnancy in the Beagle bitch. Proc. Soc. Exp. Biol. Med. 148:134, 1975.

Owens, J. M., and Drucker, W. D.: Hyperadrenocorticism in the dog: canine Cushing's syndrome. Vet. Clin. North Am. 7:583, 1977.

Reimers, T. J.: Radioimmunoassays and diagnostic tests for thyroid and adrenal disorders. Comp. Cont. Educ. Pract. Vet. 4:65, 1982.

Scott, D. W.: Hyperadrenocorticism (hyperadrenocorticoidism, hyperadrenocorticalism, Cushing's disease, Cushing's syndrome). Vet. Clin. North Am. 9:3, 1979.

INFERTILITY IN THE BITCH

P. N. OLSON, D.V.M.,
T. M. NETT, Ph.D.,
Ft. Collins, Colorado

and S. F. SODERBERG, D.V.M.
Detroit, Michigan

An increasing number of owners of infertile show dogs, rescue dogs, security dogs, cattle dogs, and canine pets are seeking help from veterinarians in an attempt to produce offspring from their animals. Veterinarians are often reluctant to work with these owners; because of the many causes of infertility in bitches only a few have been described in detail. Therefore, the clinician lacks a valid basis for making differential diagnoses upon which decisions concerning treatment must be based. Additionally,

details of past estrus cycles and breedings are often difficult to obtain, especially if the bitch has had multiple owners. Frequently there is little information concerning the males used in past breedings. If the males were not proven fertile, it may be necessary to advise the owner that the bitch not be subjected to an extensive or costly infertility examination until the males' fertility is known.

The veterinarian is also hampered by the inaccessibility of the ovaries, oviducts, and uterus on physical examination. Although laparoscopic evaluation of the canine reproductive tract has been described, the ovaries cannot be directly visualized until the ovarian bursa is incised. Although the bursa can be easily incised via laparoscopy, no critical studies have been performed to evaluate the effects of incising the bursa on the development of adhesions and subsequent infertility. Uterine biopsies should not be performed via laparoscopy, since one cannot suture the uterus after a biopsy has been obtained. This could result in abdominal contamination if an infected uterus was biopsied. Laparotomy remains the method of choice for evaluating the uterus if a biopsy or culture is needed, since uterine biopsies and cultures cannot be obtained by passing a biopsy instrument or culture unit per vagina, as the canine cervix is usually impossible to cannulate.

By assaying concentrations of sex hormones in the serum of cycling bitches, recent advances have been made in understanding the hormonal events of the normal canine estrous cycle (Figs. 1 and 2); however, the cost of quantitating hormones in serum samples of infertile bitches can be prohibitive, especially if several samples, obtained at various times throughout an estrous cycle, are to be assayed. Therefore, owners may be reluctant to pursue a precise diagnosis if an endocrine-related infertility is suspected. Lacking a precise diagnosis, the veterinarian may be forced to administer hormones empirically, frequently without success.

The veterinarian approaching an infertility case must carefully explain the aforementioned limitations to the owner. Because the bitch optimally cycles only one to three times a year, the veterinarian can only evaluate the diagnosis and treatment

a few times a year. Thus, the owner must realize that several months to years may be required to solve some infertility cases and that others will remain undiagnosed. If the owner and veterinarian are both aware of the current limitations of solving an infertility case and both are willing to proceed, the potential results can be extremely rewarding. An occasional healthy litter of puppies encourages us to continue pursuing the problem of infertility.

CLINICAL APPROACH TO EVALUATING THE INFERTILE BITCH WITH NORMAL ESTROUS CYCLES

EVALUATION OF MALE FERTILITY

The fertility of the males used in previous breedings must be established before subjecting the bitch to an extensive infertility work-up (see page 962). The best evidence of fertility in the male dog is normal litters sired with other bitches during the same time that a pregnancy failure occurred with the bitch being presented for infertility. Evaluation of semen can also aid in evaluating male fertility, since ranges for concentration of spermatozoa in an ejaculate, percentage of spermatozoa with progressive motility, and percentage of spermatozoa with normal gross morphology have been established for the male dog (Table 1). A semen evaluation must be critically made and a male should not be condemned on the basis of a single semen sample. Occasionally fertile males may not ejaculate the sperm-rich fraction during a manual collection, although some presperm and prostatic fluid are passed. Therefore, one must be careful not to

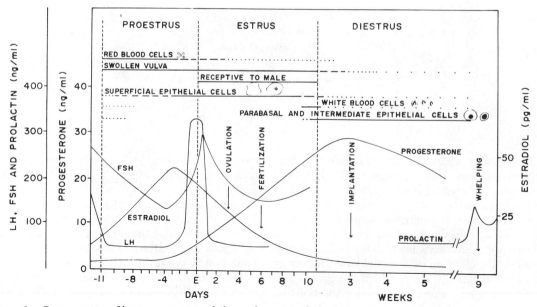

Figure 1.   Concentrations of hormones in serum; behavioral events and physiologic changes during the canine estrous cycle.

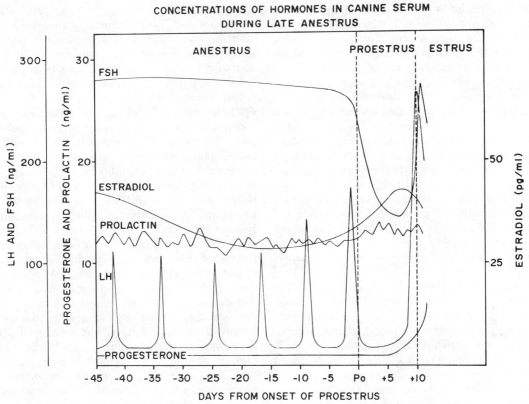

Figure 2.   Concentrations of hormones in canine serum during late anestrus, proestrus, and estrus.

condemn a male because of incomplete ejaculation. Conversely, an occasional stud dog may have normal-appearing semen but the spermatozoa are incapable of fertilizing ova. Because stud dogs are usually presented for semen evaluation after a pregnancy failure has been diagnosed (usually at least one month following a mating), the semen evaluation may not be an accurate picture of the quality of semen at the time of breeding.

EVALUATION OF BREEDING MANAGEMENT

The relationship between hormonal events, behavioral events, and physiologic changes of the reproductive tract has been established for "average" bitches (see Fig. 1).

Proestrus is defined as the stage of the reproductive cycle during which the bitch attracts males but is not receptive to mating. The average length of proestrus is 9 days but can range from 3 to 17 days. During proestrus concentrations of estradiol in serum rise as ovarian follicles mature. This results in proliferation of the vaginal epithelium and diapedesis of red blood cells through uterine capillaries. Vaginal proliferation and uterine diapedesis account for the vaginal epithelial cells and red blood cells in vaginal smears taken during proestrus. In early and mid proestrus, neutrophils may be present as well as red blood cells and parabasal, intermediate, and superficial vaginal epithelial cells (see Fig. 1). By late proestrus the predominant cell types on a vaginal smear are red blood cells and superficial epithelial cells.

Table 1.   *Parameters for Normal Canine Semen*

	Volume (ml)	Range (ml)	Time for Ejaculation	pH
First fraction (presperm)	0.8	0.25–2.8	30–50 sec	6.1
Second fraction (sperm-rich)	0.6	0.30–4.0	50–80 sec	6.3
Third fraction (prostatic)	3.0+	1.1–16.0	3–30 min	6.6

Notes: Percentage of sperm with progressive motility: 75 to 80
Percentage of normal sperm: >70
Total sperm per ejaculate (concentration per ml × ml collected): 300,000,000

Estrus is defined as that stage of the reproductive cycle during which the bitch is sexually receptive to the male. The average length of estrus is 9 days, but a range of 3 to 21 days is not uncommon. Often the serosanguineous discharge of proestrus clears during estrus, but occasionally it may persist into diestrus. The turgid vulva observed during proestrus softens, and when a male attempts to mount the estrous bitch will lift her tail (flag), present her perineum, and stand to be bred. Vaginal smears taken during estrus usually contain no neutrophils and fewer red blood cells, but these indications may persist into early diestrus. Large numbers of bacteria may be present in vaginal smears of estrous bitches even though no inflammation exists and leukocytic infiltration is absent. Greater than 90 per cent of the vaginal epithelial cells observed on vaginal smears taken during estrus are of the superficial type.

Diestrus may be defined behaviorally as the first day after a period of estrus when the bitch refuses a male. During diestrus the bitch's reproductive tract is under the primary influence of progesterone produced by corpora lutea. The duration of diestrus, based on luteal function, is similar for nonpregnant and pregnant bitches, with serum concentrations of progesterone being greater than 2.0 ng/ml for approximately two months after the onset of diestrus.

There is a sharp decline in superficial cell numbers from the vaginal epithelium about three days prior to the onset of behavioral diestrus in most bitches. It has been suggested that the onset of diestrus be defined by this event rather than by behavior. There is some merit to this suggestion since the luteinizing hormone (LH) peak, ovulation, and oocyte maturation can be timed more accurately using the disappearance of superficial cells from the vaginal smear than by using breeding times or the end of behavioral estrus. The number of superficial cells decreases by at least 20 per cent, with the numbers of parabasal and intermediate cells increasing to more than 10 per cent and often greater than 50 per cent on the first day of diestrus when defined cytologically. The appearance of neutrophils on the vaginal smear usually coincides with the time of increased numbers of parabasal and intermediate cells but occasionally precedes or lags behind changes.

Anestrus is the period extending from the end of diestrus to the beginning of a new follicular phase. This stage can last from two to ten months in individual bitches. The hormonal events during late anestrus have been recently reported for the bitch (see Fig. 2). Parabasal and intermediate epithelial cells are the predominant cell types in vaginal smears taken during anestrus. Neutrophils may be present or absent but are generally fewer in number than during early diestrus.

Although the relationship between hormonal events, behavioral events, and physiologic changes of the reproductive tract has been established for "average" bitches (see Fig. 1), many fertile bitches vary from the "norm." Some bitches have a very short proestrus and will allow a male to mate soon after the owner observes vulvular swelling or a serosanguineous discharge passing from the vestibule. Vaginal smears obtained from these bitches reveal greater than 90 per cent of the vaginal epithelial cells to be of the superficial type. Serum concentrations of progesterone of such bitches are soon elevated, also suggesting that the bitch enters estrus sooner than most female dogs. If the owner is unaware of this possibility, the bitch may not be presented to a stud dog until she is in diestrus and unreceptive to mating. The owner may request that the nonreceptive bitch be artificially inseminated. Inseminating such diestrous bitches will generally not result in pregnancy, as the ova are no longer capable of being fertilized. The duration of proestrus in pubertal cycles may frequently be less than five days. Although the mean duration of proestrus in mature bitches is 9 days, ranges of 3 to 17 days are common for normal dogs. Similarly, the average length of estrus is 9 days, but a range of 3 to 21 days has been reported for mature bitches. Therefore, determining when a bitch is in estrus and capable of conceiving is extremely important when evaluating "infertile" bitches. Although acceptance of a male provides a reliable indicator of estrus, many bitches are shipped to male dogs and cannot be evaluated daily for receptivity prior to shipment. Daily evaluation of vaginal smears should enable the veterinarian or owner to determine when estrus is occurring or about to occur.

Normal canine spermatozoa are capable of inducing maximal conception rates following a single breeding that occurs any time during the interval from four days prior to ovulation until three days after ovulation. Similarly, motile spermatozoa in undiminished concentrations may be present in the canine uterus for four to six days after a single mating. Therefore, breeding a bitch every fourth day beginning at the onset of receptivity (or when more than 90 per cent of the vaginal epithelial cells are of the superficial type) is a better breeding plan than breeding a female dog on days 9 and 11 after the onset of visual signs of proestrus. This would be especially true for bitches that vary from the norm and could be in proestrus or diestrus on days 9 and/or 11. Many breeders may want to breed their bitches every 48 hours. Although this plan appears to offer no advantage over breedings every fourth day, it is an acceptable approach as long as the bitch is covered at least every fourth day throughout her *entire* receptive period (or during the time when more than 90 per cent of the vaginal epithelial cells are of the superficial type).

EVALUATION OF THE NONRECEPTIVE BITCH

Vaginal-vestibular strictures, vestibular strictures, persistent hymen, and bands in the posterior vagina from failure of müllerian duct fusion are common causes of reproductive failure in the bitch with normal estrous cycles. The bitch will usually stand to be mounted but will wince in pain when the male attempts to insert the penis into the vestibule and/or vagina. Likewise, the male may become reluctant to mate a bitch with strictures or bands, especially if pain has been experienced during a previous attempt at intromission. Diagnosis is usually achieved by digital examination of the vagina but is frequently missed using vaginoscopy. The vaginoscope may pass along one side of the band, or the band may be occluded by folds of vaginal epithelium and may therefore elude visualization. Likewise, a vaginoscope may pass through a circular stricture without the examiner being aware of the confining nature of the stricture. Injecting a radiopaque dye into the vagina may aid in evaluating the exact location and magnitude of a stricture or band. Manual dilation, surgical correction, or artificial insemination may be used to manage these problems. If artificial insemination is performed, the owner must be cautioned that a dystocia could result when a puppy enters the birth canal and that a natural delivery may not be possible. Vestibular or vaginal-vestibular strictures should only be diagnosed during proestrus or estrus, as palpable strictures during anestrus or prior to puberty may relax when serum concentrations of estradiol increase and stimulate a target-tissue response in the vagina and vestibule.

Rarely, a bitch may be unreceptive to mating during estrus even though no physical or endocrinologic abnormality can be identified. Artificially inseminating these bitches frequently results in conception.

EVALUATION OF THE UTERUS AND OVIDUCTS FOR OCCLUSIONS

As previously mentioned, it is impossible to critically evaluate the uterus and oviducts on routine physical examination. Bilateral segmental aplasia of the proximal uterine horns or occlusion of both oviducts could result in a bitch that cycles normally but fails to conceive.

Hysterosalpingography has been used to evaluate the uterus and oviducts in normal bitches. A radiopaque, nonirritating dye is injected under pressure into the vagina. Passage of the dye through the cervix and into the uterus and oviducts is variable. The dye generally passes through the cervix in estrous bitches when the cervical os is dilated. However, the dye rarely passes through the uterotubal junction during estrus, so evaluating the patency of the oviducts at this time is impossible. In contrast, the uterotubal junction relaxes during diestrus but at this time the cervical os is tight so that one must be careful not to rupture the vagina when attempting to force dye through a closed

cervix. Therefore, the clinician may have to resort to laparotomy and dye injection to demonstrate uterine and oviductal patency. This should be considered only after other causes of infertility in the cycling bitch have been eliminated.

EVALUATION OF INFECTIOUS CAUSES OF INFERTILITY

Although bacterial infections have been frequently implicated as causing vaginitis, metritis, endometritis, abortion, and neonatal septicemia, it is difficult to establish the role of bacterial infections in canine infertility. Because similar types of aerobic bacteria are present in the vaginas of infertile and fertile bitches, it is difficult to associate a positive vaginal culture with infertility. The canine uterus does not appear to harbor bacteria, so a positive uterine culture may be clinically significant. Since the canine cervix cannot be cannulated in most instances, cultures of the uterus must be obtained during laparotomy. Obtaining a positive culture from the anterior vagina during proestrus or estrus when the cervix is open does not enable one to conclude that the bacteria cultured are from the uterus.

Brucella canis has been reported to cause canine infertility as well as abortions and stillborn and sick puppies. All bitches presented for infertility should be evaluated for canine brucellosis. A rapid slide agglutination test* can provide a presumptive diagnosis. However, owing to occasional false positives with this test, additional tests (tube agglutination, gel immunodiffusion, and culture) should be performed before a definite diagnosis is made.

Herpesvirus infection characteristically causes neonatal deaths but has also been reported to cause placentitis, abortion, and stillborn and runted puppies. Infected bitches may have a vesicular vaginitis and mild rhinitis but are frequently asymptomatic. Periodic shedding of the virus in nasal secretions of clinically asymptomatic animals has been reported. Similarly, clinical herpes infection causing neonatal death, stillborn or runted puppies, and placentitis has been reported to recur in the bitch.

Chronic endometritis could potentially cause infertility in the bitch by preventing implantation. However, to date endometritis has not been documented as a cause of infertility in the bitch. This may be due, in part, to the fact that uterine biopsies and cultures are difficult to obtain and many owners are reluctant to subject their animals to exploratory surgery as part of the infertility examination. The length of the estrous cycle may be altered in some species with endometritis, as the diseased endometrium releases prostaglandin (PG) $F_{2\alpha}$, which can decrease the life span of the corpora lutea. Although

---

*Pitman-Moore Inc., Washington Crossing, NJ.

the normal canine endometrium contains little $PGF_{2\alpha}$, no critical studies have examined concentrations of $PGF_{2\alpha}$ in inflamed endometrium. Reportedly, concentrations of $PGF_{2\alpha}$ are elevated in purulent material assayed from pyometritic uteruses of bitches. However, the luteal phase of bitches with pyometra appears normal. Clearly, more research is needed to demonstrate the role, if any, of subclinical uterine infections on fertility in the bitch.

CLINICAL APPROACH TO EVALUATING THE INFERTILE BITCH WITH ABNORMAL ESTROUS CYCLES

FAILURE TO CYCLE

Occasionally an owner may present a bitch for infertility that has not had an observed estrus. Some bitches of larger breeds may not reach a growth plateau or exhibit estrus until they are nearly two years old. If a bitch has not cycled by the time the growth plateau has been reached plus six months, an infertility examination should begin. Bitches that have never cycled should be carefully evaluated for an intersex condition. Clitoral hypertrophy, abnormal positioning of the urethral orifice, abnormal positioning of the vulva, the presence of a phallus-like structure, and elevated concentrations of testosterone in serum (> 0.5 ng/ml) may be present in some but not all intersexes. Chromosomal analysis or determining the presence of the male-specific histocompatibility antigen (HY antigen) may aid in diagnosing intersexes. Although most intersexes fail to cycle, an intact true hermaphrodite American cocker spaniel reportedly whelped a litter of three puppies, representing the first such report involving a mammal. However, if estrous cycles do occur in intersexes they usually occur at irregular intervals and are variable in duration.

Primary ovarian or pituitary dysfunction should also be considered as a cause for cycle failure. Abnormally low serum concentrations of pituitary gonadotropins (follicle-stimulating hormone, FSH; luteinizing hormone, LH) might be associated with pituitary dysfunction. Conversely, abnormally high concentrations of pituitary gonadotropins might suggest ovarian dysfunction with lack of ovarian feedback to inhibit the release of FSH or LH.

If a bitch that fails to cycle has had more than one owner, previous ovariohysterectomy should be considered. Careful examination of the skin covering the abdominal midline may reveal a surgical scar. Concentrations of LH in the serum of ovariohysterectomized bitches are consistently elevated in repeated serum samples and not merely transiently increased, such as occasionally occurs during anestrus in the bitch (see Fig. 2).

Occasionally a bitch may be cycling but the clinical signs of estrus are so slight that they go unnoticed by the owner. These cycles are referred to as *silent heats*. The reason for the attenuated estrus is unknown, but conception can occur if the estrus can be identified and the bitch bred at appropriate times. These bitches appear to have normal luteal function, since serum concentrations of progesterone will be elevated during diestrus.

Sometimes a bitch will cease cycling after being fertile. Failure of a bitch that once had normal interestrous intervals to cycle could be due to hypothyroidism, hypoadrenocorticism, or hyperadrenocorticism. The exact cause for infertility in bitches with these diseases is unknown, but treating the disease usually results in resumption of normal estrous cycles.

Occasionally a bitch may cease cycling and no abnormality can be identified. Induction of estrus can be attempted in these cases by using diethylstilbestrol (DES), 1 mg orally for four days, and gonadotropins. On day 8 the bitch begins receiving 2 mg FSH subcutaneously twice daily until greater than 90 per cent of the vaginal epithelial cells observed on a vaginal smear are of the superficial type. This usually occurs by the eighth day of FSH injections or day 15 after starting the induction protocol. If maximal stimulation of the vagina (> 90 per cent superficial epithelial cells) has not occurred by the tenth day of FSH injections or day 17 after starting the induction protocol, the treatment is considered a failure and further injections of FSH are not warranted. Twenty four hours after maximal stimulation of the vagina has occurred, 500 IU of human chorionic gonadotropin (HCG) are given intravenously. Bitches will usually accept a male 48 to 72 hours post HCG. Although this protocol has produced a few litters with small numbers of puppies in bitches presented for prolonged anestrus, it has not produced pregnancies in normal bitches when begun during anestrus. An ideal method for inducing a fertile estrus in the bitch remains to be developed.

PROLONGED INTERESTROUS INTERVALS

An interestrous interval is the length of time from the onset of one proestrus to the next. An abnormally long interestrous interval is defined as one that is twice the normal interestrous interval for an individual bitch or breed. Thyroid, adrenal, and pituitary dysfunction can all delay the onset of the next estrus. Older bitches tend to have more irregular cycles than younger females and generally cycle fewer times per year even when no physical abnormality can be identified. However, a critical study evaluating ovarian and pituitary function in these older bitches has not been performed.

SHORTENED INTERESTROUS INTERVALS

Occasionally an infertile bitch is presented to the veterinarian with a history of cycling more frequently than in the past or more frequently than is accepted for that particular breed. Unfortunately, little work has been published suggesting causes for shortened interestrous intervals in the bitch.

"Split heats" may be observed in pubertal bitches and occasionally in adults. The bitch exhibits vulvar swelling and a serosanguineous discharge for a few days as follicles develop. This is followed by declining target-tissue responsiveness for a few weeks until the bitch enters her "true" season and ovulates. Normal bitches may have elevations in serum concentrations of estradiol four to six weeks before proestrus begins (see Fig. 2). However, during the weeks immediately prior to the onset of proestrus, concentrations of estradiol decline before the ovulatory follicular phase begins. Although most dogs show no overt signs in response to the increased concentrations of estradiol present four to six weeks before proestrus, it is possible that some bitches may exhibit signs of proestrus during this period of transient follicular growth. Although "split heats" are not associated with infertility, bitches that repeatedly cycle every few weeks without conceiving should be considered abnormal, and the cause for the abbreviated cycles should be determined, if possible. Through assaying serum concentrations of estradiol and progesterone in such bitches at least weekly, the veterinarian can identify which stages of the estrous cycle are abnormally shortened. Bitches failing to ovulate might be expected to have no luteal phase in their estrous cycle, thereby shortening the interestrous interval by approximately two months. However, there have been no critical studies evaluating the length of anestrus following ovulation failure in the bitch. If ovulation failure is suspected, 500 IU HCG can be given intravenously to the bitch when greater than 90 per cent of the vaginal epithelial cells on a vaginal smear are of the superficial type. If given prior to observing maximal stimulation on a vaginal smear, follicles may be luteinized prior to ovulation and an ovarian cyst may result.

Premature regression of corpora lutea has not been documented in the bitch. Although serum concentrations of progesterone may be less than 2.0 ng/ml at the time of an abortion, it is difficult to determine if this was due to premature regression of the corpora lutea or secondary to the initiation of parturition as a result of some other disease process (fetal death, placentitis, etc.). Therefore, administering progesterone to an aborting bitch may be contraindicated, especially if the abortion is occurring because of uterine or fetal disease.

Uterine biopsies may be taken from bitches with shortened interestrous intervals to determine if the endometrium is normal. Although endometritis has been associated with altered cycle lengths in some species, it has not been reported to cause shortened cycles in the bitch.

PROLONGED ESTRUS

Although the mean duration for estrus is 9 days, a range of 3 to 21 days has been given for normal bitches. Estrus may be considered prolonged when a bitch accepts a male for longer than three weeks. Prolonged receptivity can occur with follicular cysts. Although the causes of spontaneously occurring follicular cysts in the bitch are unknown, a nymphomaniac-like behavior with persistent estrus has been observed in some bitches receiving estradiol as an abortifacient. These bitches will continually stand to be bred for several weeks to months following the administration of the abortifacient. Treatment consists of 500 IU HCG intravenously in an attempt to luteinize cystic follicles. It is important to terminate cystic conditions as soon as possible when serum concentrations of estradiol are elevated. Prolonged elevations of estradiol can lead to bone marrow suppression and an aplastic anemia in the dog.

CONCLUSIONS

The clinical approach to infertility is a systematic one. Yet many questions raised during the evaluation remain unanswered owing to lack of information on the etiologies of infertility. It is hoped that these questions can someday be answered as research funding becomes available to study reproductive disorders in the bitch.

SUPPLEMENTAL READING

Johnston, S. D.: Diagnostic and therapeutic approach to infertility in the bitch. J.A.V.M.A. 176:1335, 1980.

Nett, T. M., and Olson, P. N. Reproductive physiology of dogs and cats. *In* Ettinger, S. J. (ed.).: *The Textbook of Veterinary Internal Medicine,* Vol. II. Philadelphia: W. B. Saunders, 1982.

Senior, D. F.: Infertility in the cycling bitch. Comp. Cont. Ed. 1:17, 1979.

FELINE REPRODUCTION

P. W. CONCANNON, PH.D.,
and D. H. LEIN, D.V.M.

Ithaca, New York

BREEDING SEASONS

The adult female cat is seasonally polyestrous. The breeding season in temperate zones usually begins 20 to 60 days after the winter solstice and may end any time after the summer solstice. The length of the breeding or estrous season varies with latitude. In the northern temperate zones the breeding season usually begins in January or February. The greatest incidence of estrus occurs in February and March. Termination of the breeding season in experimental colonies has been reported to be as early as August and as late as October or November. In most colonies October to mid December is considered the anestrous period. In colonies maintained under artificial light schedules of 12L:12D or 14L:10D many cats cycle throughout the year. In the authors' colony of cats exposed to a natural photoperiod supplemented with a 14L:10D artificial light schedule, most queens cycled year-round, and, surprisingly, some queens in the colony still experienced a winter anestrus during November and December. In addition, in the summer months, during periods of very warm weather, a decreased incidence of estrus has been observed. Since house cats may experience a wide range of supplemental lighting conditions, little can be said regarding an average or typical breeding season in pet queens.

ESTROUS CYCLES

The queen is an induced ovulator. Most reports suggest that spontaneous ovulation rarely occurs.

However, one report has indicated that spontaneous ovulation may not be uncommon. Nevertheless, in the absence of coitus (or other vaginal stimulation) most queens will continue to undergo nonovulatory estrous cycles throughout the breeding season. The cycles reflect repeated sequential waves of follicular growth (and estrogen secretion) and follicular atresia (Fig. 1). This results in periods of behavioral estrus interrupted by periods of sexual nonreceptivity.

Periods of estrus are usually characterized by overt displays of sexual behavior in the absence of a male as well as by receptivity to mounting attempts and coitus when a male is present. Reports on mean and range for durations of estrus, interestrous periods, and cycle intervals differ considerably. Some, but not all, of the variations encountered may be due to differences in recognizing preferences among queens for certain males, in considering a nonreceptive proestrus period in some cycles when testing with a tom was not performed, or in criteria for full estrous behavior in the absence of a tom.

In some cycles (about 20 per cent), estrus may be preceded by a 0.5- to 2-day proestrus in which many of the behaviors characteristic of estrus are observed but the queen will not allow mounting and copulation. Proestrus can only be characterized clearly in the presence of a male. During an observed proestrus the queen usually is less sexually demonstrative than during the subsequent estrus.

Fully estrous behavior is characterized by persistent spontaneous episodes of vocalization, rolling, rubbing against inanimate objects, and, often, repetitive treading in place. During estrus, the re-

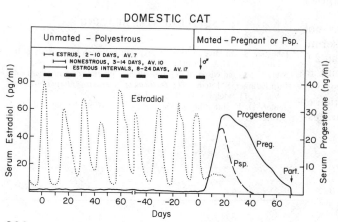

Figure 1. A schematic representation of endocrine changes typically observed during polyestrus cyclic activity in unmated queens and during pregnancy or pseudopregnancy (Psp.) following fertile matings or vaginal stimulation resulting in ovulation. Solid bars indicate periods of estrus; open portions indicate potential proestrous periods.

sponse to an acceptable tom includes treading or standing in place when approached and remaining still during neck biting and mounting. The intensity of the estrous display can vary considerably within and among queens. In the absence of a male a fully estrous queen will normally display a full complement of estrous behavior if grasped firmly by the skin on the back of the neck and stroked on the back, tailhead, and/or genitalia.

Estrus may last 3 to 20 days under normal circumstances. Some queens display estrus for as little as two days. Estrus lasting longer than ten days is considered prolonged. The average duration of estrus reported in several studies ranged from five to eight days. In the authors' colony the average was seven days. The duration of estrus is not greatly influenced by mating and induced ovulation. Some reports indicate that estrus may be one or two days shorter in average duration in mated queens. Although this has been the case in our colony, decidedly contrary results have also been reported.

The nonestrous interval between periods of estrus in unmated queens normally ranges from 3 to 14 days during the breeding season but may be as long as 30 days. The mean durations reported for the nonestrous interval (interestrus interval) range from 9 to 13 days; in our cats the average was about 11 days. The length of the cycle (interval from onset of one estrus to the onset of the next) can range from 7 to 40 days. Most cycles are between 12 and 22 days long. Mean cycle lengths reported ranged from 16 to 20 days; in our colony the average was about 18 days.

In cycling queens follicle growth and development associated with increased secretion of estradiol occurs rapidly over a two- to three-day period just prior to the onset of estrus. The onset of estrus in most instances occurs as estradiol levels attain peak levels or during the subsequent rapid decline. Basal serum estradiol levels range from 5 to 20 pg/ml; peaks of 40 to 100 pg/ml are attained by or before the onset of estrus. In most cycles, estradiol levels decline during estrus as the fully mature follicles begin to undergo atresia. The follicles retain the capacity to ovulate in response to a sufficient copulatory stimulus, at least for the first four to five days of estrus. There appears to be no report on fertility in late estrus during either average or protracted periods of estrus. Serum progesterone levels remain low (≤ 0.5 ng/ml) throughout polyestrous periods.

INDUCED OVULATION

Ovulation of matured follicles depends on the release of sufficient amounts of luteinizing hormone (LH) from the anterior pituitary, as in other species. In the cat, however, LH release is dependent on a neural reflex initiated by vaginal-cervical stimulation during coitus. Ovulation occurs 25 to 30 hours after a mating or series of matings that cause release of sufficient LH.

A typical mating sequence involves neck biting, mounting, positioning, pelvic thrusting, and intromission by the male. The estrous queen remains stationary in an inviting position and permits neck biting. She has the elbows, chest, and abdomen on the floor; the pelvis elevated and often the tail deviated; and may spontaneously tread the hind feet. Following the neck bite the queen treads and raises the vulvular area further, to nearly a horizontal position as the male treads backwards and mounts. When both are positioned the male begins pelvic thrusting. Upon intromission the female emits a dramatic vocalization.

The time from neck bite to intromission can vary from 0.5 to 5 minutes. Intromission itself is brief, about 4 seconds, but may be prolonged to 15 to 20 seconds by a forceful male. During intromission, following or during the coital "scream," the queen attempts to break the male's hold by turning, rolling, and striking at him with her paws. The experienced male rapidly withdraws and stands or sits watchfully as the queen displays the coital afterreaction. The afterreaction includes periods of rolling and thrashing and obsessive licking of the vulval area. The afterreaction may last for one to nine minutes following a copulation. A subsequent mating sequence may occur immediately following the completion of the afterreaction, or the female may refuse mounting attempts for several minutes to some hours following copulation. Intervals between initial matings are usually brief (5 to 30 minutes) and become longer as time increases. A queen may permit up to 30 copulations in a day, up to 36 copulations in 36 hours (Concannon and Lein, unpublished data). The number of copulations that may be experienced throughout a typical four- to eight-day estrus have not been reported.

The initial copulation causes LH release, which may or may not be sufficient to cause ovulation. Less than 50 per cent of fully estrous queens ovulate after a single copulation. Most, but not necessarily all, queens ovulate after four or more copulations (Fig. 2). Although repeated copulations may continue for one or two days (or more), additional LH release becomes negligible after the first two to four hours. Ovulation occurs about 24 hours after the rapid rise in LH.

LH release (and subsequent ovulation) can also be induced by artificial stimulation of the vaginal cervix. This can be accomplished by probing the vagina with a smooth glass rod, repeated several times at 5- to 15-minute intervals. Some queens may not release adequate LH or may not ovulate following repeated matings or stimulation early in estrus but will do so later in estrus. Data on the cause and incidence of this phenomenon are not

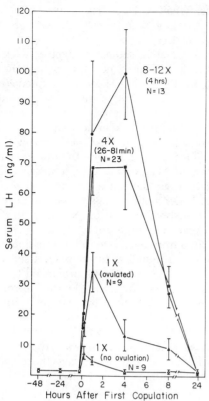

Figure 2. Serum LH levels in estrus queens permitted single (1 ×) or multiple (4 and 8 to 12 ×) copulations. Single copulations induced LH release sufficient to cause ovulations in only one-half the queens. Multiple copulations caused a greater release of LH, and all queens ovulated. (Reprinted with permission from Concannon et al.: Biol. Reprod. 23:111, 1980.)

sufficient to make a generalized statement. Sterile matings or artificial stimulation sufficient to cause ovulation results in a pseudopregnancy. Following ovulation the corpora lutea form and become luteinized within one to three days and persist for three to seven weeks. Progesterone levels rise over 1 ng/ml by day 3 after mating or stimulation, reach peak levels of 15 to 90 ng/ml by day 15 to 25, and decline thereafter. Progesterone levels fall below 1 ng/ml within 30 to 50 days. This is followed, in four to ten days, by a follicle phase ending in estrus a few days later. The duration of pseudopregnancy, as the interval from mating to the next estrus, ranges from 35 to 70 days; the average is around 45 days. (Late in the breeding season a pseudopregnancy may be followed by a seasonal anestrus, yielding an apparent duration of up to several months.)

PREGNANCY

Gestation length in the domestic cat, as the interval from a fertile mating to parturition, lasts 64 to 69 days according to most recent reports. In the authors' colony pregnancy averaged 66 days. Earlier reports of pregnancy lasting an average of 63 days

may have been based on studies timed from the last of multiple matings taking place over several days. The possibility also exists that there are strain, breed, or colony differences in mean gestation length.

Cat sperm require about one to two hours for capacitation in the female reproductive tract. The duration of sperm fertility has not been determined; if brief, a reason for prolonged bouts of mating, in addition to providing for hybrid vigor, would emerge. Following ovulation, 25 to 30 hours after mating and LH release, oocytes remain fertile for up to 48 hours and probably no longer. Oviductal transport of fertilized oocytes takes four to five days. Blastocysts migrate in the uterine horns for six to eight days. Implantation occurs around days 12 to 14.

The corpora lutea persist and produce progesterone for 40 to 50 days, but their capacity to secrete progesterone thereafter is not clear. By day 50 placental production of progesterone is adequate to maintain pregnancy. Pregnancy has been reported to be maintained following ovariectomy performed after, but not before, the forty-ninth day of pregnancy.

Progesterone levels in early pregnancy are not different from those seen in pseudopregnancy prior to implantation. After day 20 progesterone levels are, on the average, higher in pregnant queens, and the difference is significant and obvious by day 30. The pregnancy-specific increases may reflect increased luteal progesterone secretion in addition to placental progesterone production. Estradiol levels increase in late pregnancy and fall near term.

Parturition is accompanied by a decline in progesterone to basal levels. Whether the fall in peripheral progesterone precedes or follows placental dislocation has not been studied in detail. Measurements of serum prolactin levels in the queen have only recently been accomplished. Prolactin levels remain basal during the first half of pregnancy (day 35), increase to reach three- to five-fold higher levels by day 63, and rise to peak levels just prior to parturition. Levels are elevated in response to suckling during lactation, albeit at somewhat reduced levels late in lactation. Prolactin declines to basal levels about two weeks after weaning.

Estrous behavior displays and matings may occur during late pregnancy or pseudopregnancy but apparently are related to only minor excursions in estrogen levels. A brief post-partum estrus has been reported in some cats. Lactation, however, suppresses normal estrus cycles (Fig. 3). Lactation lasts six to eight weeks, with nursing activity declining after five weeks. Results on the residual effects of lactation on the post-weaning interval to estrus vary. In our colony, weaning at seven weeks was followed by a 15- to 60-day nonestrual period before the next cycle; following early weaning at three days post

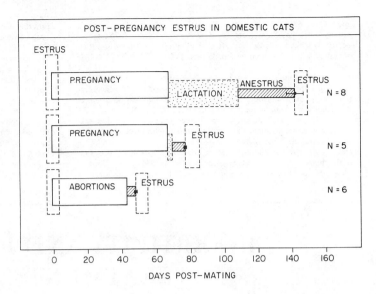

Figure 3. Diagrammatic representation of durations of estrus, pregnancy, lactation, and nonestrous intervals prior to the post-pregnancy estrus following lactation (or pregnancy) in queens allowed a normal seven-week lactation, queens weaned three days post partum, and queens that aborted their kittens. The respective intervals from the end of pregnancy to the next estrus averaged 12 weeks, 1 week, and less than 1 week.

partum the interval to estrus was only six to eight days. Abortion usually results in a return to estrus within one week. In most colonies for which reports are available, return to estrus following normal lactation and weaning takes an average of two to three weeks. In our colony the average has been about four weeks.

LUTEAL FUNCTION AND PREGNANCY MAINTENANCE

The contribution of luteal versus placental secretion to progesterone levels during the second half of pregnancy is not known, but the ovaries are apparently not needed for pregnancy maintenance after day 50. The luteal requirements for tropic hormone support from the pituitary have not been examined, but LH is probably required as in most other species, including the dog. Prolactin is luteotropic in some carnivores, including the dog and mink, and may be important for normal luteal function in the cat as well. However, doses of ergocryptine sufficient to reduce prolactin levels in the dog and cause luteolysis did not result in luteolysis in preliminary trials conducted on pseudopregnant cats (Concannon, unpublished data).

Feline corpora lutea are very resistant to the luteolytic effects of prostaglandin. Repeated administration of $PGF_{2\alpha}$ during the second week of pseudopregnancy caused only a nonsignificant reduction in progesterone levels. Repeated $PGF_{2\alpha}$ injections during the fourth week of pseudopregnancy caused a significant decline in progesterone levels but did not cause a complete luteolysis and did not reduce the length of pseudopregnancy. $PGF_{2\alpha}$ (5000 to 1000 μg) administered during pregnancy caused abortion when given after day 40 but not before. The extent to which the abortive effect

is due to suppression of placental progesterone secretion, suppression of ovarian progesterone secretion, stimulation of uterine contractions, or induction of placental detachment has not been determined.

SUPPLEMENTAL READING

Banks, D., and Stabenfeldt, G.: Prolactin activity during pregnancy and lactation in the cat. Biol. Reprod. 24(Suppl. 1):63, 1981.
Bareither, M. L., and Verhage, H. G.: Control of the secretary cell cycle in cat oviduct by estradiol and progesterone. Am. J. Anat. 162:107, 1981.
Breeding and reproduction in cats. Feline Pract. 11:35, 1981.
Burke, T. J., Reynolds, H. A., and Sokolowski, J. H.: A 180-day tolerance efficacy study with mibolerone for suppression of estrus in the cat. Am. J. Vet. Res. 38:469, 1977.
Cline, E. M., Jennings, L. L., and Sojka, N. J.: Analysis of the feline vaginal epithelial cycle. Feline Prac. 10:47, 1980.
Colby, E. D.: The estrous cycle and pregnancy (feline). *In* Morrow, D. (ed.): *Current Therapy in Theriogenology.* Philadelphia: W. B. Saunders, 1980, pp. 832–839.
Colby, E. D.: Infertility and disease problems (cat). *In* Morrow, D. (ed.): *Current Therapy in Theriogenology.* Philadelphia: W. B. Saunders, 1980, pp. 869–874.
Concannon, P., Hodgson, B., and Lein, D.: Reflex LH release in estrous cats following single and multiple copulations. Biol. Reprod. 23:111, 1980.
Concannon, P., Lein, D., and Hodgson, B.: Sexual behavior and self-limiting reflex LH release during extended periods of adlibitum copulatory activity in domestic cats. J. Anim. Sci. 55(Suppl. 1):344, 1982.
Dawson, A. B.: The domestic cat. *In* Ferris, E. (ed.): *Care and Breeding of Laboratory Animals.* New York: Wiley and Sons, 1952, pp. 202–233.
Dawson, A. B., and Friedgood, H. B.: The time and sequence of preovulating changes in the cat ovary after mating or mechanical stimulation of the cervix uteri. Anat. Rec. 76:411, 1940.
Hammer, C. E., Jenning, L. L., and Sojka, N. J.: Cat (*Felis catus* L.) spermatozoa require capacitation. J. Reprod. Fertil. 23:477, 1970.
Herron, M. S., and Sis, R. F.: Ovum transport in the cat and the effect of estrogen administration. Am. J. Vet. Res. 35:1277, 1974.
Herron, M. A., and Stein, B.: Prognosis and management of feline infertility. *In* Kirk, R. (ed.): *Current Veterinary Therapy VII.* Philadelphia: W. B. Saunders, 1980, pp. 1231–1237.
Johnson, M. L., and Gay, V. L.: Luteinizing hormone in the cat: I. Tonic secretion. Endocrinology 109:240, 1981.
Johnson, M. L., and Gay, V. L.: Luteinizing hormone in the cat: II. Mating-induced secretion. Endocrinology 109M:247, 1981.

Paape, S. R., Shille, V. M., Seto, H., and Stabenfeldt, G. H.: Luteal activity in the pseudopregnant cat. Biol. Reprod. 13:470, 1975.

Rees, H. D., Switc, G. M., and Michael, R. P.: The estrogen-sensitive neural system in the brain of female cats. J. Comp. Neurol. 193:789, 1980.

Shille, V. M., Lundstrom, K. E., and Stabenfeldt, B. H.: Follicular function in the domestic cat as determined by estradiol-17β concentrations in plasma: Relation to estrous behavior and cornification of exfoliated vaginal epithelium. Biol. Reprod. 21:953, 1979.

Shille, V. M., and Stabenfeldt, G. H.: Luteal function in the domestic cat during pseudopregnancy and after treatment with prostaglandin $F_{2\alpha}$. Biol. Reprod. 21:1217, 1979.

Shille, V. M., and Stabenfeldt, G. M.: Current concepts in reproduction of the dog and cat. Adv. Vet. Sci. Comp. Med. 24:211, 1980.

Verhage, H. G., Beamer, N. B., and Brenner, R. M.: Plasma levels of estradiol and progesterone in the cat during polyestrus, pregnancy and pseudopregnancy. Biol. Reprod. 14:579, 1976.

Wildt, D. E., Chan, S. Y. W., Seager, S. W. J., and Chakraborty, P. K.: Ovarian activity, circulating hormones, and sexual behavior in the cat. 1. Relationships during the coitus-induced luteal phase and the estrous period without mating. Biol. Reprod. 25:15, 1981.

Wildt, D. E., Guthrie, S. C., and Seager, S. W. J.: Ovarian and behavioral cyclicity of the laboratory maintained cat. Horm. Behav. 10:251, 1978.

Wildt, D. E., and Seager, S. W. J.: Laparoscopic determination of ovarian and uterine morphology during the reproductive cycle (cat). In Morrow, D. (ed.): Current Therapy in Theriogenology. Philadelphia: W. B. Saunders, 1980, pp. 828–832.

Wildt, D. E., Seager, S. W., and Chakraborty, P.: Effect of copulatory stimuli on incidence of ovulation and on serum luteinizing hormone in the cat. Endocrinology 107:1212, 1980.

INFERTILITY AND FERTILITY TREATMENTS AND MANAGEMENT IN THE QUEEN AND TOM CAT

D. H. LEIN, D.V.M.,
and P. W. CONCANNON, Ph.D.

Ithaca, New York

FELINE REPRODUCTIVE PHYSIOLOGY

The queen attains puberty at 4 to 12 months of age, with a minimum body weight of usually 2.3 to 2.5 kg. Puberty depends on growth rate and season of birth. Adequate nutrition, freedom from disease, late winter or early spring birth, and the companionship of other sexually active queens and toms are necessary for early puberty. The tom cat is usually fertile at six to eight months of age, with a minimal body weight of 3.5 kg. The reproductive life may be 14 or more years, with a period of 8 to 10 years most suitable for continuous breeding of a queen. The litter size is reduced if the queen conceives on the first estrus or as an aged cat. The average litter size is about four kittens (range one to eight). Siamese cats average about six kittens.

Implantation occurs about day 13 to 14 of gestation, with a "band" or zonary placentation formed.

Estrus behavior is estimated to occur in about 10 per cent of pregnant queens, with acceptance of a male, copulation, and post-coital rolling occurring at about 21 or 42 days of pregnancy. It is believed that some queens may conceive on this breeding, resulting in a second litter, a phenomenon called *superfetation*.

SELECTION OF QUEENS FOR BREEDING

Queens and tom cats should not be selected only by pedigree, conformation, or show performance.

Both sexes should also be selected from parents that show good sexual aggression and normal sexual cycles. Both cats should come from a litter of good size and a queen that delivered easily and reared a healthy litter. These desirable characteristics are genetically based and therefore can be inherited. Individuals selected for breeding should have a complete physical examination, including the reproductive tract, mammary glands, and all other body systems, for evidence of any abnormalities. Records of all heats, breeding dates, queenings, litter size, and rearing information should be strictly maintained and utilized when making decisions about breeding.

ESTRUS CONTROL

Estrus control in the queen using progestins has been successful in Europe and Australia. Medroxy-progesterone acetate (Perlutex* and Anobulin†) has been used successfully in oral and injectable forms, but neither is available in the United States. Megestrol acetate (Ovaban‡) has been released for use only in dogs but has been used successfully in the queen. The progestin is believed to act as a viable corpus luteum, causing negative feedback on the

---

*Leo Laboratories Ltd., Middlesex, England.
†Berk Pharmaceuticals Ltd., Surrey, England.
‡Schering Corp., Kenilworth, NJ.

hypothalamic nuclei so that gonadotropin-releasing factors are not released.

Megestrol acetate, 5 mg/day for three days, then 2.5 to 5 mg/week, has effectively suppressed estrus for two years in young queens. Estrus returns after withdrawal of megestrol acetate. Queens expressing estrus are reported to go out of heat after three days with 5 mg/day of megestrol acetate. This drug has been used to control urine spraying in toms and queens (5 mg/day until spraying is controlled, then 5 mg/week) and in the treatment of miliary dermatitis and control of eosinophilic granulomas. Progestin therapy may cause an increasing appetite with a resultant increase in body weight, a calming effect, and an increase in the affection of some cats. Prolonged and indiscriminate use may produce Cushingoid cats.

Progestins should not be used in cats with genital tract infections. Prolonged or indiscriminate use of progesterone or progestins may lead to cystic endometrial hyperplasia-pyometra complex, hypertrophy and hyperplasia of mammary glands, and possible mammary gland neoplasia.

MISMATING

Mismating in the queen has been successfully treated with estrogens. It has been found that as little as 0.125 to 0.25 mg of estradiol cypionate (ECP) given 40 hours after coitus retarded egg transport through the oviduct to at least six days instead of the normal four to five days and caused degeneration of the eggs. ECP appears to be effective at this single dose between days one to six after cessation of estrus. The client should be advised that signs of estrus may be prolonged following estrogen therapy. Indiscriminate estrogen usage in the cat or dog can lead to bone marrow depression, thrombocytopenia, and rapid death. It is reported that the cat should not be given more than 8 mg of estrogen-equivalent within a four-month period.

INDUCTION OF ESTRUS

Estrus followed by successful mating can be induced by using a daily intramuscular injection of pregnant mare's serum gonadotropin (PMSG) for eight days, the dosage depending on time of the year (Table 1) as reported by Colby (1970, 1980).

Estrogens (50 mcg of estradiol benzoate or 0.25 mg of ECP given intramuscularly and repeated in 48 hours) will induce estrus in most queens. Estrus will occur within two to five days and may last two to four weeks unless mating occurs.

Follicle-stimulating hormone–pituitary (FSH-P) has recently been used to induce estrus in the queen. A dose of 2 mg of FSH-P injected daily intramuscularly until the queen exhibits estrus is recommended. It should not be administered any longer than five days. Most queens exhibit estrus between 4 and 5 days, with the entire period lasting an average of 6.2 days. On days 1 and 2 of estrus, 250 IU of human chorionic gonadotropin are given intramuscularly to enhance ovulation. Mean litter size is normal. Queens should be bred at least twice on each day of estrus for a period of up to four days.

CYTOLOGIC EXAMINATION

Cytologic examination of the vaginal epithelium can be used to reflect ovarian activity and stage of cycle. No diapedesis of red blood cells is seen in the queen during proestrus and estrus, as in the bitch.

1. *Anestrus or prepuberty:* numerous small, round epithelial cells with high nuclear/cytoplasmic ratio; increased debris.

2. *Proestrus:* fewer but larger nucleated epithelial cells with a low nuclear/cytoplasmic ratio; increased debris.

3. *Estrus:* numerous large, polyhedral cornified cells with curled edges; small, dark, pyknotic nuclei or loss of nuclei; markedly less debris.

4. *Early metestrus* (following ovulation): cornified cells; margin ragged and hazy; none to numerous leukocytes appear and, possibly, numerous bacteria; increased debris.

5. *Late metestrus:* proportion of smaller basophilic cells increases; leukocytes are still present.

PROCEDURE FOR VAGINAL CYTOLOGY

1. Vaginal cells are collected with a moistened sterile cotton swab either by inserting the swab 2 cm into the vagina of a restrained cat or by inserting a clean glass eyedropper containing a few drops of sterile water 1.5 to 2.0 cm into the vagina and

Table 1. Dosage Schedule for Inducing Estrus With PMSG*

	Day							
Time of Year	1	2	3	4	5	6	7	8
Dec to Jan	100	50	50	50	50	50	50	50
Feb to Aug	100	50	50	50	50	25	25	25
Sept to Nov	100	50	50	50	50	50	50	50

*Dosage in IU, IM, for cats in Northern hemisphere.

flushing the cavity. This procedure may trigger ovulation in some queens at estrus.

2. Roll the swab on a clean glass slide or place fluid from the eyedropper on a slide and either fix immediately or air dry, depending on stain procedure. Stain with any good cytologic or hematologic process. Keep slides for reference of changes throughout the estrus cycle.

REPRODUCTIVE PROBLEMS IN THE QUEEN

Lactation anestrus is common in queens until the kittens are weaned. A few queens will show estrus seven to ten days post partum and may conceive. Most queens show signs of estrus three to four weeks after weaning their kittens.

Precociousness has been seen in well-grown kittens, although this is usually within the four-month age range and is quite acceptable. Good nutrition, late winter or early spring litters, adequate light, and contact with older cycling queens are effective stimuli for early cycling. Some cycling queens are still nursing their previous litter, and one may wonder if the milk during estrus may contain enough natural estrogens to "mimic" estrus in these kittens.

Precocious mammary gland development or hyperplasia has occasionally been seen in supposedly prepubertal queens. These conditions have been misdiagnosed clinically as extensive neoplasia of the individual glands or the complete mammary chain. The enlarged mammary glands are usually firm and may or may not be secreting. In severe cases the mammary tissue may perforate, but there is no purulent drainage. Histopathologic examination reveals a fibroadenomatous hyperplasia of the gland. Examination of the genital tract of these affected queens usually reveals estrus, undiagnosed pregnancy, or an early involuting uterus following an undetected parturition with cannibalism or abortion. A hormonal cause involving combinations of estrogen and/or progesterone following a sterile mating, possible spontaneous ovulation, and prolonged nursing of a cycling queen with transfer of steroids via milk to the prepubertal offspring are other possible causes if ovarian activity or uterine pathology is not found. Regression to normal will usually take place with time. If the condition recurs with each estrus, ovariohysterectomy is recommended.

Nymphomania has been encountered in females with apparent cystic follicular degeneration. These are usually older nulliparous queens with cystic hyperplasia-endometritis-pyometra complex. Ovariohysterectomy is recommended. Nymphomania has also been seen following ovariohysterectomy when an ovary or a portion of an ovary has been left intact or when a possible accessory ovary is present. In those individuals with no ovarian tissue,

estrogen blood levels would be revealing. A possible adrenocortical source or a psychic state may be involved in this behavioral problem. Progestin therapy may be beneficial in these conditions.

Pseudocyesis or *pseudopregnancy* can be induced by pseudocopulation, a sterile mating, luteinizing hormone (LH) therapy, and, possibly, spontaneous ovulation. Spontaneous ovulation has been reported in isolated caged cats and is thought to be caused by handling, stroking, or examining of the cat in estrus. Estrogens, androgens, and progestins have been used to suppress any clinical manifestations of overt pseudocyesis. Testosterone (2 mg, IM), given once and repeated in one week if needed, has been reported to be effective.

Cystic hyperplasia-endometritis-pyometra complex is a condition seen in queens ranging from 3 to 14 years of age but especially in nulliparous queens over 5 years of age. The incidence is decreased in free-roaming queens that have consecutive pregnancies. Dow (1962) showed that this feline syndrome is similar to that in the bitch, starting with cystic hyperplasia induced by estrogen and progesterone of consecutive periods of pseudocyesis followed by acute, subacute, and chronic endometritis and pyometra. *Escherichia coli* is most frequently isolated. *Pseudomonas* spp., staphylococci, and streptococci have also been found.

Pyometra and degrees of endometritis have been diagnosed in virgin kittens at puberty and in breeding queens housed in catteries. This complex is frequently associated with infertility characterized by poor conception, early embryonic death and reabsorption, abortion, mummification, maceration, stillborn fetuses, and early neonatal death. Various bacteria (previously mentioned) have been isolated. The syndrome appears different from that described by Dow (1962) and has been associated with the presence of feline leukemia complex and feline infectious peritonitis. Whether these viral diseases are the primary factor in this form of pyometritis has not been proved. Post-partum endometritis and pyometritis may follow retained placenta, dystocias, and manipulations to relieve dystocia.

The affected queen may appear normal or may show various degrees of clinical signs resulting in a possible fulminating septic acute endometritis with a bloody discharge, depression, toxic bone marrow depression, and septicemia with rapid death. Pyometras may be closed or open with drainage and discharge. The uterus is frequently paper thin in the closed condition, and rupture with extensive peritonitis and rapid death is possible. The total white blood cell count may be in the high-normal range, i.e., 20,000 to 100,000+/mm^3, or may appear depressed with toxic bone marrow depression. This demands immediate treatment and carries a grave prognosis. About 50 per cent of cats with pyometra have a normocytic, normochromic anemia. Antibiotic sensitivities, supportive therapy, and ovario-hysterectomy are indicated.

Queens intended for future breeding should be given sexual rest as soon as signs of vaginal discharge or septic pyometritis are observed. A deep vaginal culture and cytologic smears are obtained by using a sterile saline-moistened swab or by flushing with sterile saline via a sterile bovine teat cannula and syringe or eyedropper. The use of a sterile otoscope head as a speculum may decrease contamination of the specimen from the perineum and vestibule. Prolonged systemic treatment with antibiotics effective against the cultured organisms is indicated. Increased drainage from a filled uterus may be accomplished with estrogen or prostaglandin ($PGF_{2\alpha}$, 25 mcg/kg body weight b.i.d. IM for three to five days). Remember that low doses of estrogen should be given (0.125 to 0.25 mg of ECP since the bone marrow may already be depressed from chronic infections. A flexible plastic catheter may be inserted through the cervix to establish drainage and treat the uterus daily. Exploratory laparotomy may be indicated to examine the female genital tract and also aid in passing a catheter through the cervix. A hysterotomy may be performed to evacuate the uterus and flush it with antibiotics or chemotherapeutic agents such as nitrofurazone solution.

Sexual rest, normal estrus without vaginal discharge, normal hemograms, and negative vaginal cultures with normal vaginal cytology are necessary before attempting rebreeding. If breeding is successful, systemic antibiotics should be administered again during the last ten days of pregnancy and the first week after parturition. Following weaning, deep vaginal-cervical specimens should be cultured and cytologic smears examined to determine if treatment is needed. The prognosis for future breeding of queens with pyometritis or chronic endometritis should be guarded to poor.

Teratogenic effects in kittens throughout the pregnancy period have been linked to griseofulvin; therefore, this drug should not be used during this time. Medications, worm medication, dietary additives, and possible toxic substances should be avoided or carefully scrutinized before use during pregnancy.

Inherited congenital defects or inherited causes of infertility should be suspected in registered breeding cats that are line bred or in isolated household cats that are constantly inbreeding. All other causes of these defects should be eliminated by history, clinical examination, and laboratory tests. Study of pedigrees or possible successful outcrossing may be adequate proof of inherited defects.

Habitual or chronic abortion, recurring at the same time of gestation, is thought to be due to progesterone insufficiency (when all other causes have been eliminated). Treatment consisting of intramuscular injections of 0.5 to 1.0 mg/lb body weight of progesterone in oil every seven days should begin about a week before the anticipated abortion and should end seven to ten days prior to the anticipated parturition. Prolonged gestation will follow continued use of progesterone. Endogenous progesterone blood levels of chronic aborters should be studied, and the possible inheritance of this condition should be considered.

Uterine torsion of one whole gravid horn or, more likely, of one fetus within a horn does occur and may result in dystocia, uterine hemorrhage, acute abdominal pain, rupture, or peritonitis. In many cases, no clinical signs are observed and the twisted portion tears and may separate completely, allowing one or more fetuses with their placentas to drop into the peritoneal cavity. The fetus may disintegrate into small pieces and become embedded in the omentum, or the entire fetus may mummify and become attached to the omentum or abdominal organs. The affected uterine horn may straighten after rupture and heal with a slight scar. *Secondary extrauterine pregnancy* can occur following uterine rupture. *Primary extrauterine pregnancy* is rare in the queen.

Chronic cervicitis and vaginitis can be seen in the queen. A discharge may be difficult to detect. It may be caused by trauma or infection following a dystocia. Stenosis may follow, with closure of the vagina at the vestibule, or there may be fibrosis of the cervix. Diagnosis may be possible using sedation and a sterile otoscope cone. A differential diagnosis from a draining pyometra can usually be made by clinical examination and vaginal cytology. Cultures for organisms and antibiotic sensitivities are required for proper treatment.

Prolonged anestrus may be caused by several factors: debility, nutrition, endocrine imbalance, genetics, or disease. An adequate history and examination are needed to determine the cause. Simple problems such as improper illumination (less then 12 hours of light per day) and lack of exposure to other cats can cause anestrus.

PREGNANCY DIAGNOSIS

Pregnancy should be determined as early as possible following mating. Early diagnosis ensures proper care and use of the queen through the gestation period, and plans can be made for queening and rearing of the kittens. Pregnancy diagnosis can be accomplished by the following methods: (1) abdominal palpation of the pregnant uterus, individual fetuses, and their fetal membranes from 20 to 30 days (the beaded effect of the pregnant uterus can be detected as early as 16 days in a very relaxed queen); (2) x-ray of the abdomen from about 45 days to term; (3) ultrasonic Doppler detection of placental circulation and fetal heart beat from about the fourth week to term; (4) enlargement and pink color of the teats and mammary glands from about day 18 to term.

CARE DURING PREGNANCY

The pregnant queen needs a well-balanced diet, and food should be provided so that as fetal growth causes increased weight food intake can increase automatically. Overfeeding and excessive weight gain should be avoided. Feeding recommendations of quality commercial cat food manufacturers for pregnant and nursing queens should be followed. Advice and discretion should be sought before supplements of vitamins, minerals, proteins, or fats are given.

Nonstrenuous daily exercise to keep good muscle tone may promote easy queening. Obesity and poor muscle tone can result in low conception rates and difficult queening.

Medication, vaccination, and worming should be avoided during pregnancy. Treatment should be planned and performed prior to breeding, if possible. A clean, warm, dry, secluded, comfortable area with a large nesting box should be provided at least ten days before queening. Near term the enlarged abdomen may cause restricted physical activity. A few days prior to queening, the mammary glands enlarge further and milk is present. The excessive hair in long-haired breeds should be removed from around the teats and vulva, and the vulvar area, if soiled, should be cleansed just prior to queening.

Evidence of abnormal vulvar discharges, fetal resorption, abortions, premature or stillborn kittens, mummified fetuses, or weak kittens that die during the neonatal period should be carefully evaluated. Specimens of the vulvar discharge, blood, and any fetal or placental tissue or dead kittens should be submitted to a veterinary diagnostic laboratory for examination in the hope that a definitive diagnosis can be made and meaningful treatment, control, and/or preventive measures instituted. The queen and any remaining kittens should be strictly isolated from other cats, especially pregnant queens, since a contagious agent may be involved.

Feline viral rhinotracheitis, panleukopenia, toxoplasmosis, and bacterial agents can cause fetal loss. Feline leukemia virus and feline infectious peritonitis virus have also been associated with this syndrome.

Diseases that primarily affect other body systems may secondarily affect the pregnant uterus. These must be properly diagnosed and treated.

QUEENING

Nesting may be exhibited 12 to 24 hours before queening. The rectal temperature falls in the first stage of labor. Normal presentation of the fetuses can be either forward or backward as they enter the birth canal. Thirty- to sixty-minute intervals are frequently seen between the delivery of one or two kittens. During this time the queen removes the placenta and cord from the kitten and ingests them and cleans and stimulates the kitten to breathe and move. The queen also cleanses her vulvar area during this time. The kittens may be nursed before delivery of the next fetus. Occasionally there may be a 12- to 24-hour delay following the delivery of two or three kittens before the rest are born. This is most commonly seen when a queen's labor is interrupted. If free she may move her litter to another secluded spot.

The first litter of a queen with only one or two large kittens may be difficult, and assistance may be needed. Healthy queens seldom have difficulty with delivery. Queens that are inbred or that have nutritional deficiencies or the stress of a disease may have poor uterine contractions (inertia) and may require assistance. Trauma or a nutritional deficiency may result in a pelvic deformity, causing difficult delivery. Assistance for surgical intervention or medication with uterine muscle stimulating and contracting agents will be needed for difficult births (5 units of oxytocin IM, repeated at 15- to 20-minute intervals).

Stillborn kittens and placentas are usually eaten by the queen. Cannibalism is seen, but it is more likely at the first queening and with highly nervous queens. These queens should not be used for breeding.

Post-partum hemorrhage, retained fetal membranes, dead kittens, and uterine inversion are uncommon in the queen. Oxytocin, 5 to 10 units IM, may be used to control hemorrhage. Treatment of shock, systemic antibiotics, and abdominal surgery with possible removal of the reproductive tract may be needed following uterine prolapse. A brown vaginal discharge and enlarged segments of the uterine horns indicate a retained fetus and/or placentas. Medical or surgical removal of the material will be needed to correct this condition.

It is desirable to observe the vulva and surrounding areas of the queen daily for evidence of abnormal discharges. A bloody discharge is usually present for seven to ten days post queening. Persistent discharges that are odorous or bloody indicate uterine infections. The mammary glands should also be examined for evidence of mastitis.

Queens with the previously mentioned post-partum problems may be listless and unable to nurse or care for their kittens. Immediate diagnosis, treatment, and supplemental care for the kittens are required or loss of both the queen and kittens may occur. Both the queen and the kittens may need antibiotic and supportive therapy. Antibiotic sensitivity tests for organisms cultured from vulvar discharges or mastitic milk are important. Separation of the queen and kittens may be needed but will depend on the severity and contagiousness of the infection and the queen's ability to care for the kittens.

MATERNAL CARE AND LACTATION

The queen usually remains continuously with her kittens for a period of 24 to 48 hours. About 2 to 3 ml of milk are taken by the kittens three times an hour. Kittens double their weight in seven days and open their eyes at eight to ten days. They are able to take 5 to 7 ml of milk at a feed in the second week. At this time, the queen will leave the nest for several hours. In her absence normal kittens will sleep quietly. After feeding, the queen washes each kitten, especially around its head and anal region. She consumes the urine and feces voided in response to grooming. By three weeks of age the kittens have increased their activity to exploring and playing. The queen then teaches the kittens to urinate and defecate away from the nest. Lactation is supplemented with solid food beginning in the fourth week, and weaning is completed by the seventh or eighth week.

Queens with a strong maternal instinct and a good milk supply are capable of fostering orphaned kittens or will allow kittens from their previous litters to nurse. Alternatively, orphaned kittens can be raised on commercial replacement diets (follow manufacturer's instructions for amount and frequency of feeding). Stimulation and cleaning of orphaned kittens with warm, wet cotton swabs must follow each feeding to stimulate urination and defecation. A warm area must be provided for very young kittens to maintain body temperature. Daily weights should be recorded. Kittens that are not gaining daily or that are losing weight should be examined and treated immediately.

REPRODUCTIVE PHYSIOLOGY AND INFERTILITY OF THE TOM

The male is born with descended testes. A cryptorchid or ectopic testis should not be corrected; rather, both testes should be removed when the tom has reached appropriate age, size, and maturity, since this condition may be inherited.

Spermatozoa are present in the seminiferous tubules of well-grown toms by 24 to 36 weeks of age. The average volume of an ejaculate is about 0.05 ml (0.03 to 0.3 ml) and contains from 60×10^6 to 12 or 15×10^8 sperm/ml. Approximately 80 to 90 per cent motility is present. The pH of fresh semen is 7.4. Normal ejaculate contains less than 10 per cent abnormal sperm.

Semen can be collected with an artificial vagina or by electroejaculation while the tom is anesthetized. The tom must be trained for more than three weeks to ejaculate into an artificial vagina, which consists of a 2-ml rubber bulb with the end cut off and fitted over a 3×44 mm test tube. The unit is placed into a small polyethylene bottle with warm water to produce a temperature at collection of 45°C. A female in estrus or an ovariectomized female that has been estrogenized should be used as a teaser and mount. Collection takes one to four minutes. Semen can be obtained by flushing the vagina of a queen immediately following copulation, but the quality of the specimen is poor.

A tom will defend and mark a territory. The territory will be marked by an exudate from the anal glands that produces the characteristic penetrating "catty" urine odor. Urine spraying may be inhibited by castration in the complete male or controlled by progesterone therapy in the complete or castrated tom.

Infertility in the tom is infrequently seen or reported, although purebred or inbred toms should be examined closely. The role of the tom in possible venereal spread of infectious diseases is unknown. A negative status for toxoplasmosis, feline leukemia, and feline infectious peritonitis is important when obtaining a breeding tom. Adequate vaccination prior to breeding is also important.

Bite wounds of the scrotum and testes are frequently found following territorial fights. A febrile response and scrotal abscessation should be treated, but the affected testis may have to be removed to save the nonaffected testis from heat degeneration and extension of the infection.

A hair ring may form around the base of the glans penis following several matings, resulting in difficult intromission and mating. If the tom does not remove this ring during routine cleaning, it must be removed by retracting the preputial sheath and sliding the hair ring over the penis. Successful mating is then possible.

Psychological infertility may be seen in tom cats undergoing environmental or territorial changes or in young novice males placed with aggressive experienced queens. Time and acclimation may result in acceptance and a return of fertility. If not, the tom may have to be removed to a less hostile environment.

Congenital testicular hypoplasia may be a consequence of fetal or neonatal panleukopenia. Poor libido and variable testicular degeneration leading to aspermatogenesis have been associated with malnutrition, obesity, hypothyroidism, and hypervitaminosis A caused by diets containing excessive liver. Proper diagnosis of the condition and treatment of the cause usually eventually result in normal fertility.

The tortoiseshell male cat is reportedly sterile, but a few are reported to be fertile. The orange and black color genes are in the X chromosome and are sex-linked. The white gene is a dominant gene S for the piebald trait and may mix with orange and black, producing the "calico" or "tricolor" pattern. Tortoiseshell cats should be heterozygous for two sex-linked alleles and should therefore have two X chromosomes. They are usually female, but male tortoiseshell cats occasionally occur. Blood, bone marrow, and skin cultures of these males show a karyotype of XXY or XX/XY/XXY mosaicism. These male cats have small testicles, lack libido, are sterile, and contain a Barr body at the nuclear membrane in smears from buccal cells or drumstick polymorphonuclear leukocytes (expressions of extra X chromosome). This syndrome is homologous to the Klinefelter's syndrome in humans. Fertile tortoiseshell males may have an XX/XY mosaic karyotype or possibly a normal XY component, with somatic mutation occurring in the X cells so that some express orange and others black.

SUPPLEMENTAL READING

Bittle, J. L., and Peckham, J. C.: Comments: genital infection induced by feline rhinotracheitis virus and effects on newborn kittens. J.A.V.M.A. 58:927, 1971.

Burges, D.: The collection of vaginal smears from the bitch. Vet. Rec. 89:127, 1971.

Burke, T. J.: Feline reproduction. Paper presented at the annual meeting of the American Association of Feline Practitioners, Cincinnati, 1975.

Carlson, J. N.: Feline panleukopenia. In Kirk, R. W. (ed.): Current Veterinary Therapy VI. Philadelphia: W. B. Saunders, 1977, pp. 1292–1296.

Colby, E. D.: Induced estrus and timed pregnancies in cats. Lab. Anim. Care 20:1075, 1970.

Colby, E. D.: Suppression/induction of estrus in cats. In Morrow, D. (ed.): Current Therapy in Theriogenology. Philadelphia: W. B. Saunders, 1980, pp. 861–864.

Colby, E. D.: Infertility and disease problems. In Morrow, D. (ed.): Current Therapy in Theriogenology. Philadelphia: W. B. Saunders, 1980, pp. 869–874.

Cotter, S. M., Hardy, W. D., and Essex, M.: Association of feline leukemia virus with lymphosarcoma and other disorders in the cat. J.A.V.M.A. 166:449, 1975.

Csiza, C. K., de Lahunta, A., Scott, F. W., and Gillespie, J. N.: Pathogenesis of feline panleukopenia virus in susceptible newborn kittens. I. Clinical signs, hematology, serology and virology. II. Pathology and immunofluorescence. Infect. Immun. 3:833, 1971.

Dow, K.: The cystic hyperplasia-pyometra complex in the cat. Vet. Rec. 74:141, 1962.

Gilbride, A. P.: A quick review of the genetics of the male calico cat. Feline Prac. 2:33, 1972.

Herron, M. A.: Feline vaginal cytologic examination. Feline Prac. 3:36, 1977.

Herron, M. A., and Sis, R. F.: Ovum transport in the cat and the effect of estrogen administration. Am. J. Vet. Res. 35:1277, 1974.

Hoover, E. A., and Griesemer, R. D.: Comments: pathogenicity of feline viral rhinotracheitis virus and effect on germfree cats, growing bone and the gravid uterus. J.A.V.M.A. 159:929, 1971.

Houdeshell, J. W., and Hennessey, P. W.: Megestrol acetate for control of estrus in the cat. V.M.S.A.C. 72:1013, 1977.

Kowali, N. L.: Feline toxoplasmosis. In Kirk, R. W. (ed.): Current Veterinary Therapy V. Philadelphia: W. B. Saunders, 1974, pp. 976–980.

McEntee, K.: Personal communication, 1975.

Mowrer, R. T., Conti, P. A., and Rossow, C. F.: Vaginal cytology, an approach to improvement of cat breeding. V.M. S.A.C. 70:691, 1975.

Paape, S. R., Shille, V. M., Seto, H., and Stabenfeldt, G. H.: Luteal activity in the pseudopregnant cat. Biol. Reprod. 13:470, 1975.

Post, J. E.: Feline leukemia and related viruses. Feline Information Bulletin 1:1, 1975, Cornell Feline Research Laboratory, Ithaca, NY.

Povey, R. C.: Feline respiratory disease complex. In Kirk, R. W. (ed.): Current Veterinary Therapy VI. Philadelphia: W. B. Saunders, 1977, pp. 1281–1287.

Roberts, S. J.: Infertility in the bitch and queen. In Veterinary Obstetrics and Genital Diseases. Michigan: Edwards Brothers, Inc., 1971, pp. 584–595.

Scott, F. W.: Personal communication, 1975.

Scott, P. O.: Cats. In Hafez, E. S. E. (ed.): Reproduction and Breeding Techniques for Laboratory Animals. Philadelphia: Lea & Febiger, 1970, pp. 192–208.

Seager, S. W. J.: Semen collection, evaluation, and artificial insemination of the domestic cat. In Kirk, R. W. (ed.): Current Veterinary Therapy VI. Philadelphia: W. B. Saunders, 1977, pp. 1252–1254.

Smith, H. A., Jones, T. C., and Hunt, R. D.D.; The tortoiseshell male cat. In Veterinary Pathology, 4th ed. Philadelphia: Lea & Febiger, 1972, p. 328.

Sojka, N. J., Jennings, L. L., and Hamner, C. E.: Artificial inemination in the cat (Felis catus). Lab. Anim. Care 20:2, 1970.

Stein, B.: The genital system. In Catcott, E. J. (ed.): Feline Medicine and Surgery, 2nd ed. Santa Barbara, CA: American Veterinary Publications, Inc., 1975, pp. 303–354.

Verhage, H. G., Beamer, N. B., and Brenner, R. M.: Plasma levels of estradiol and progesterone in the cat during polyestrus, pregnancy and pseudopregnancy. Biol. Reprod. 14:579, 1976.

PYOMETRITIS IN THE BITCH AND QUEEN

D. H. LEIN, D.V.M.

Ithaca, New York

CAUSES

Pyometritis in the bitch and queen can occur spontaneously; secondary to an infectious disease process, a post-partum metritis, or a mismating injection of estrogen, especially estradiol; as a postcopulation or postinsemination infection; and as the final sequela of cystic endometrial hyperplasia-endometritis-pyometritis complex. This complex most commonly occurs in bitches starting at three to four years of age. The incidence increases with age and is increased in bitches with several nonpregnant cycles. This complex also affects the intact queen and increases in occurrence with age following repeated nonproductive matings, pseudocopulation, and spontaneous ovulation. Bitches and queens with this syndrome have a poor prognosis for treatment and future breeding because of endometrial degeneration as well as inflammation.

The ideal breeding age of the bitch and queen is prior to three years of age. Once started, continuous production of litters is desirable. Bitches and queens that are not intended for breeding should be oophorohysterectomized, since virtually every aged intact bitch and queen can develop cystic endometrial hyperplasia-endometritis-pyometritis complex.

Spontaneous pyometritis usually occurs in the prepubertal bitch or queen. These cases may be secondary to a septicemia from another infectious disease process.

Acute endometritis and metritis in the bitch or queen are usually diseases of the post-partum period following retained placentas or fetuses, obstetric manipulations, dystocias, or abortions. They may occasionally follow mating or artificial insemination. The post-partum uterus is frequently enlarged, friable, and flaccid. The bitch or queen is usually depressed, febrile, agalactous, and anoretic and has a malodorous vaginal discharge, which may be sanguineous to brown and thick. Frequently the bitch or queen will ignore her newborn.

Estrogen therapy, especially estradiol cypionate, is used in both the bitch and queen for mismating within five days of copulation. A single dose of 0.25 mg in the cat and small dog has been successful in preventing pregnancy. Dosages as high as 2 mg have been recommended for large-breed dogs. Following this treatment, some animals have developed pyometritis, especially if the dosage of estradiol is excessive. Owners should be warned that pyometritis can be a sequela of the mismating injection if estradiol is used.

Cystic endometrial hyperplasia-endometritis-pyometritis complex has been shown to result from the cyclic stimulation of estrogens and, more importantly, the strong progesterone influence during metestrus or the luteal phase in the nonpregnant bitch and queen. Following repeated nonproductive cycles, the uterus undergoes cystic endometrial hyperplasia with an eventual superimposed endometritis and, finally, pyometritis or chronic endometritis with *Escherichia coli* infecting the endometrium. Clinical signs of septicemia and toxemia are usually seen in metestrus or the luteal phase of the cycle and are not necessarily associated with behavioral pseudopregnancy.

DIAGNOSIS

The early syndrome, cystic endometrial hyperplasia with or without superimposed endometritis, may be associated with a blood-tinged discharge.

Frequently there are no clinical signs, but infertility is demonstrated by poor conception, small litter size, early embryonic death, abortion, stillborn fetuses, and neonatal death. Frank endometritis-pyometritis may be indicated by a purulent to brown vaginal discharge or, in closed pyometritis, no discharge. Severe septicemia and bacteremia are associated with a closed pyometritis. The total white blood cell count ranges from 20,000 to 100,000 +/ cu mm. Higher counts are associated with a closed cervix. Normal to subnormal counts and thrombocytopenia are seen in toxic bone marrow depression, and the prognosis should be grave. A normocytic, normochromic anemia is present in a large number of cases. Marked hyperproteinemia (increased serum glubulin) and elevated BUN concentration may be present.

Extragenital lesions of this chronic syndrome include membranoproliferative glomerulonephropathy, caused by *E. coli* antigen-antibody complexes; extramedullary myelopoiesis, especially involving the liver, spleen, kidney, lymph nodes, lungs, and adrenal glands; bone marrow depression; bilateral adrenol cortical collapse; and medullary hemorrhage.

Nonbacterial cystic endometrial hyperplasia and endometritis are difficult to diagnose. History, age of the bitch or queen, and, possibly, a vaginal discharge may suggest a hysterosalpingography. This is performed with a sterile soluble radiopaque preparation infused via a Foley catheter placed in the anterior vagina. Hysterosalpingography should be done when the cervix is not in the luteal phase so that cystic hyperplasia can be demonstrated. An exploratory laparotomy may be needed to obtain a uterine specimen for biopsy. A macroscopic cyst may be seen in the endometrium or may be palpated per abdomen if it is 1 cm or larger in diameter. Chronic endometritis associated with *E. coli* and a closed or open pyometra is easier to diagnose. History, vaginal discharge, vaginal cultures, physical examination of the genital tract, hematologic studies, radiographs, and laparotomy examination may all be used. Hysterosalpingography should not be attempted when the uterus is infected. This procedure may result in a fulminating peritonitis.

Frequently, pyometras may create a sacculated uterus. *Do not* confuse a *normal pregnancy* with pyometra and remove the uterus. Always palpate the suspicious uterus before removal, even if the owner is sure that the bitch has not been in estrus and mated. A pregnant bitch may show the same abdominal distention but will not be as depressed. Radiographs after 45 days gestation will reveal the fetuses. Hemograms throughout the pregnancy should differentiate closed pyometra from pregnancy anemia seen in the last month of pregnancy (see page 886).

TREATMENT

Oophorohysterectomy with supportive therapy and administration of antibiotics, fluids, and blood is the best treatment for the nonbreeding bitch and queen. Surgical-risk patients, i.e., those with severe toxicity, high BUNs, anemia, and leukopenia, may be treated more conservatively with antibiotics, blood, and fluid. It may be wise to promote drainage with prostaglandin therapy. With tranquilization and local anesthesia the uterus can be marsupialized by suturing the uterus to the ventral abdomen and creating a fistula for drainage and local treatment until the bitch's condition improves for oophorohysterectomy.

Deep or cranial vaginal or uterine swabs for culture should always precede treatment. Frequently *E. coli* or beta-hemolytic streptococci are isolated. Use antibiotic sensitivity tests and give specific antibiotics for treatment. Breeding bitches and queens should be hospitalized and treated with specific antibiotics and prostaglandin for expulsion of exudate. Antibiotic therapy should precede prostaglandin therapy by 24 hours so that adequate blood levels are established prior to uterine contractions and expulsion of exudate. Antibiotic therapy should continue for at least 10 to 14 days. Prostaglandin $F_{2\alpha}$ ($PGF_{2\alpha}$) is administered at the rate of 25 to 50 mcg/kg of body weight IM only b.i.d. for three to five days. The lower dose is given during the first few days and is increased only if needed for maximal uterine contraction. During the luteal phase, five days of therapy are usually needed to complete luteolysis and reduce the serum level of progesterone to 1 ng/ml or less. Increased vulvar drainage should be noted in 24 hours, with abundant drainage, maximal uterine contraction, and decreased uterine size in three days. Side effects are frequently seen in the first 15 minutes after administration of $PGF_{2\alpha}$. These consist of vomition, salivation, anxiety, bradycardia, dyspnea, and diarrhea and may be more common after a few days of therapy. These reactions last for only a few minutes. Dogs or cats with lung, liver, or kidney disease should not be treated with $PGF_{2\alpha}$. Pregnant bitches or queens accidentally misdiagnosed as having pyometras will usually abort with this therapy.

Others report treatment of pyometras with $PFG_{2\alpha}$, 200 mcg/kg of body weight IM, given once or possibly repeated the second day. Side effects are much more drastic, and recurrence of pyometras and incomplete evacuation of the exudate from the uterus appears to be more prevalent. PGF_2 (Lutalyse*) is commercially available and approved for

cattle use only. It is marketed in a concentration of 5 mg or 5000 mcg/ml and must be diluted for appropriate administration in small animals.

Older animals with endometrial polyps are poor candidates for prostaglandin therapy because blockage of exudate evacuation from the uterus may cause reflux of the exudate via the oviducts, resulting in fulminating peritonitis. Surgical removal is the choice for animals with endometrial polyps.

Systemic treatment with fluids and/or blood may be necessary. It is desirable to use gravity to lavage the deep vaginal-cervical area with a treatment pipette and a solution containing warmed high volumes (100 to 500 ml) of tamed iodine solution (1 per cent Betadine solution†). This should be done daily while vulvar drainage is maximal.

PROGNOSIS

The prognosis for medical treatment of this condition should always be guarded. The success rate decreases with age and degree of degeneration and inflammation in the uterus. Successfully treated bitches and queens should always be bred on the next estrus, since recurrence following nonproductive cycles is common. Deep vaginal swabs for culture and cytology should be obtained early in proestrus to interpret the success of treatment and guide possible management and treatment for this breeding. Bitches and queens not intended for breeding should have surgery for oophorohysterectomy prior to the next estrus period.

Research in the prevention and treatment of this syndrome in the bitch and queen is needed. Prevention of nonproductive cycles, hygienic breeding, whelping care, and routine genital tract examination will decrease the incidence of this disease.

---

†The Purdue Frederick Co., Norwalk, CT.

SUPPLEMENTAL READING

Dow, C.: The cystic hyperplasia-pyometra complex in the bitch. Vet. Rec. 69:1, 1957.

Dow, C.: The cystic hyperplasia-pyometra complex in the bitch. J. Comp. Pathol. Therapeut. 69:237, 1959.

Dow, C.: Experimental reproduction of the cystic hyperplasia-pyometra complex in the bitch. J. Pathol. Bacteriol. 78:267, 1959.

Dow, C.: The cystic hyperplasia-pyometra complex in the cat. Vet. Rec. 74:141, 1962.

Fidler, I. J., Brodey, R. S., Howson, A. E., and Cohen, D.: Relationship of estrogen irregularity, pseudopregnancy, and pregnancy to canine pyometra. J.A.V.M.A. 149:1043, 1966.

Hardy, R. M., and Osborne, C. A.: Canine pyometra—a polysystemic disorder. *In* Kirk, R. W. (ed.): *Current Veterinary Therapy VI.* Philadelphia: W. B. Saunders, 1977, pp. 1229–1234.

Larsen, R. E., and Wilson, J. W.: Acute metritis. *In* Kirk, R. W. (ed.): *Current Veterinary Therapy VI.* Philadelphia: W. B. Saunders, 1977, pp. 1227–1229.

---

*The Upjohn Company, Kalamazoo, MI.

ABORTIFACIENTS

S. F. SODERBERG, D.V.M.,

Detroit, Michigan

and P. N. OLSON, D.V.M.

Ft. Collins, Colorado

Unwanted pregnancies frequently occur in the bitch despite conscientious preventive efforts by the owner. The contraceptive drugs approved for use in the female dog have limitations that may prevent their widespread use in bitches not intended for breeding. These drugs are not recommended for use until after the first estrus and have not been approved for use in the brood bitch. Physical barriers such as tall fencing, indoor confinement, or britches are frequently inadequate in preventing contact between an estrous bitch and her overeager suitors. Therefore, veterinarians continue to receive requests to terminate pregnancy in mismated bitches.

A careful history is necessary to determine when and if copulation occurred. Although the tie is not essential for a fertile mating, this observation establishes that a breeding occurred. Likewise, the presence of sperm on a vaginal smear also confirms that mating occurred. Vaginal smears should also be examined to establish the stage of the estrus cycle. If greater than 90 per cent of the vaginal epithelial cells are of the superficial type, the bitch is likely to be in estrus and is, therefore, susceptible to breeding and conception. If the bitch is not in estrus, the use of an abortifacient is unnecessary. The bitch will ovulate approximately three days after the onset of estrus. Ova are capable of being fertilized approximately six days after the onset of estrus or three days after ovulation has occurred. Because canine sperm are viable in the female reproductive tract for six to eight days, a single mating during estrus may result in conception.

OVARIOHYSTERECTOMY

An ovariohysterectomy performed during the first month of pregnancy is generally safe in the bitch. Ovariohysterectomy is the preferred method of pregnancy termination if future reproductive function need not be maintained. This procedure has the advantages of being a permanent contraceptive measure and eliminating future disease of the uterus and ovaries. Bitches that have been ovariohysterectomized prior to their first estrus also have a decreased incidence of mammary disease.

MEDICAL ABORTIFACIENTS

A medical abortifacient that is both safe and effective has not been developed. The owner should be carefully counseled about the potential side effects of medical abortifacients before administering these drugs to terminate a pregnancy.

The drug dosages in this article are correct in the authors' experience but are not FDA approved. Prostaglandin $F_{2\alpha}$ is not yet licensed for use in dogs. The estrogenic compounds are not licensed for use as abortifacients in bitches, although estrogens have been used in practice as abortifacients for many years.

ESTROGENS

The exact mechanisms by which estrogens act to prevent pregnancy in companion animals are still unknown. Estrogens appear to delay ova transport through the oviducts, possibly by stimulating contraction of smooth muscle at the uterotubal junction. If transit is delayed, the ova degenerate and are no longer capable of implantation when they finally reach the uterus. The dog is especially vulnerable to this type of abortifacient owing to the long transit time of the ova through the oviducts. Estrogens may also act by interfering with implantation, since investigators have found histologic alterations of endometrial implantation sites after estrogen administration.

The optimum time to administer estrogens to terminate a pregnancy is three to five days after the onset of standing behavior. By this time the ova are usually in the oviduct and are susceptible to the delayed transit caused by maintaining elevated concentrations of estrogens in the serum. A *single* dose of 0.125 to 1.0 mg of estradiol cypionate is given intramuscularly on the third to fifth day after the onset of estrus. Diethylstilbestrol tablets may be used orally at a dose of 1 to 2 mg daily for five days beginning on the third day after the onset of estrus.

Persistence of estrual behavior for seven to ten days often occurs following therapy. If subsequent mating occurs during the extended receptive period, estrogen therapy should not be repeated. The previous therapy should have resulted in degenerating ova, and further treatments can only increase the incidence of toxic side effects. Myelosuppression owing to estrogen toxicity can lead to severe thrombocytopenia and aplastic anemia. There is great individual variation among dogs as to the severity of a toxic response after estrogen treatment. Although most of the reports of myelosuppression have been associated with dosages exceeding those

945

just described, the authors have identified dogs that have developed aplastic anemia after receiving the previously mentioned recommended doses of estrogen. There is also an increased incidence of pyometra one to six weeks following estrogen administration. Estrogens can stimulate the synthesis of progesterone receptors in the canine endometrium and may potentiate the effect of the endogenous progesterone, which is secreted by the corpus luteum for two months after estrus. Dow demonstrated experimentally that cystic endometrial hyperplasia can occur following progesterone treatment and can develop more rapidly in dogs pretreated with estrogen (1959). Although the exact incidence of cystic endometrial hyperplasia and pyometra after estrogen administration has not been established, owners should be cautioned about this potential sequela. The effects of estrogen therapy on future fertility likewise have not been critically evaluated. Because most dogs presented for medical therapy following mismating are brood bitches, it may be best to allow the pregnancy to continue to term if further reproductive capabilities are desired. The owners should also be warned that estrogens are not always efficacious in terminating the pregnancy.

PROSTAGLANDINS

Bitches require functional corpora lutea for maintenance of pregnancy. Prostaglandin $F_{2\alpha}$ reportedly is luteolytic in several domestic species and also results in decreased concentrations of progesterone when administered to dogs in late pregnancy. Abortions occurred in four of seven beagle bitches treated between 31 and 53 days of gestation with 60 mcg/kg divided b.i.d. or t.i.d. for three days. A single dose of prostaglandin $F_{2\alpha}$ resulting in luteolysis reportedly is 1 mg/kg. Severe side effects were observed with this dose, which is near the LD_{50} of 5.13 mg/kg. Signs of prostaglandin toxicity in dogs include hyperpnea, tachycardia, vomiting, diarrhea, ataxia, and possible death 90 to 120 minutes after treatment. At present prostaglandins are not approved for use in companion animals.

ABORTIFACIENTS OF THE FUTURE

An immunocontraceptive measure using active immunization with zona pellucida antigens is being studied. The zona pellucida is an acellular, gelatinous-like layer that surrounds and protects the mammalian egg. Inhibition of fertilization *in vitro* of canine oocytes has been demonstrated using antisera containing antizona antibodies. These antibodies may act by blocking sperm attachment and penetration. The exact antibody titer and immunization schedule required to establish and maintain a critical titer necessary to prevent pregnancy needs to be established. Pregnancy was prevented when immunizations were performed during the preceding anestrus period or as late as the first day of proestrus. Once the immunizations stopped, the titers dropped and pregnancy occurred during the next estrus. Side effects were not observed, and ovarian pathology was not detected. Further studies may prove immunizations to be effective when given later in estrus. Antizona pellucida antibodies may also prevent the hatching of fertilized eggs, since implantation does not occur until approximately three weeks after the onset of estrus.

Efficacious abortifacients with fewer toxicities need to be developed for the bitch. Perhaps such abortifacients can be developed as we come to understand the normal events surrounding conception and pregnancy in companion animals.

REFERENCES AND SUPPLEMENTAL READING

Concannon, P. W., and Hensel, W.: Prostaglandin $F_{2\alpha}$-induced luteolysis, hypothermia and abortions in beagle bitches. Prostaglandins 13:533, 1977.
Concannon, P. W., Powers, M. E., Holder, W., and Hansel, W.: Pregnancy and parturition in the bitch. Biol. Reprod. 16:517, 1977.
Dow, C.: Production of the cystic hyperplasia-pyometra complex in the bitch. J. Pathol. Bacteriol. 78:267, 1959.
Herron, M. A., and Sis, R. F.: Ovum transport in the cat and the effect of estrogen administration. Am. J. Vet. Res. 35:1277, 1974.
Holst, P. A., and Phemister, R. D.: The prenatal development of the dog: preimplantation events. Biol. Reprod. 5:194, 1971.
Jochle, W., Lamond, D. R., and Anderson, A. C.: Mestranol as an abortifacient in the bitch. Theriogenology 4:1, 1975.
Legendre, A. M.: Estrogen-induced bone marrow hypoplasia in a dog. J. Am. Anim. Hosp. Assoc. 12:525, 1976.
Pineda, M. H., and Faulkner, L. C.: Immunologic control of reproduction in dogs. Canine Pract. 1:11, 1974.
Shivers, C. A., Sieg, P. M., and Kitchen, H.: Pregnancy prevention in the dog: potential for an immunological approach. J. Am. Anim. Hosp. Assoc. 17:823, 1981.
Sokolowski, J. H.: The effect of ovariectomy on pregnancy maintenance. Lab. Anim. Sci. 21:696, 1971.
Sokolowski, J. H.: Effect of prostaglandin $F_{2\alpha}$-THAM in the bitch. J.A.V.M.A. 170:536, 1977.
Vickery, B., and McRae, G.: Effect of a synthetic prostaglandin analogue on pregnancy in beagle bitches. Biol. Reprod. 22:438, 1980.

RADIOGRAPHIC EVALUATION
OF FETAL DEVELOPMENT IN
THE BITCH AND FETAL DEATH
IN THE BITCH AND QUEEN

VICTOR T. RENDANO, JR., V.M.D.

Ithaca, New York

NORMAL CANINE INTRAUTERINE DEVELOPMENT

Radiographic evidence of pregnancy is unequivocal when fetal mineralization can be identified. Prior to fetal mineralization, the uterus can be visualized as an enlarging homogeneous soft tissue structure in the caudal abdomen that may show sacculations; however, other disease processes, such as pyometra, mucometra, uterine enlargement associated with pseudocyesis, uterine torsion with hemorrhage, and neoplasia, can cause similar changes.

The determination of when to radiograph a bitch to detect pregnancy is difficult because of the potential time lag between breeding and ovulation-fertilization. Work by Concannon has shown that there can be as much as a seven-day difference between the time of breeding and the time of ovulation and fertilization; thus, if gestation is based on breeding date rather than preovulatory luteinizing hormone (LH) peak, the detection of fetal mineralization may be mistakenly timed (1982). The gestation ages presented in this article are based on the time when the preovulation surge in circulating levels of LH occurred and a mean gestation length of 65 days, counting the day of the LH peak as day 0. Ovulation was assumed to occur two days after the preovulatory LH peak, and fertilization probably occurs four to five days after the LH peak. If times were presented based on mating dates, then gestation length could vary from 58 to 71 days. Several beagle bitches were serially radiographed in the study used to obtain the dates stated in this article.

Implantation of the embryo occurs around 19 days after the LH peak (16 to 18 days after ovulation). Radiographs taken 28 days after the LH peak do not show uterine enlargement associated with pregnancy. As the conceptus grows, the uterus enlarges, radiographically changing from pear-shaped (30 days after the LH peak, range 28 to 34 days) to spherical (35 days after the LH peak, range 31 to 38 days) to ovoid (41 days after the LH peak, range 38 to 44 days) (Table 1). The spherical shapes can usually be detected radiographically between days 31 and 38 after the LH peak, and their presence is highly suggestive, but not definitive, of pregnancy rather than a pathologic condition. The time following the LH peak at which the spherical shapes can be seen radiographically will vary, depending on the shape and size of the maternal abdomen, fullness of the intestines and bladder, radiographic technique, and patient motion. The spherical uterine masses are seen earlier in thin quiet animals using high-detail radiographic techniques following evacuation of the bowel and bladder. Radiographic definition can also be increased by applying pressure to the caudal abdomen with a radiolucent paddle during the radiographic procedure. From the time the uterine swellings become ovoid (41 days after the LH peak, range 38 to 44 days) until fetal mineralization is detected (45 days after the LH peak, range 43 to 46 days), one cannot radiographically determine whether the enlarged "sausage-shaped uterus" is due to pregnancy or a disease process.

In utero radiographic detection of fetal mineralization lags behind *ex utero* radiographic or staining techniques for detection of bone by 7 to 18 days. Thus, whereas *ex utero* mineralization may be seen as early as day 33, *in utero* mineralization is usually not seen until day 45 after the LH peak in the bitch. The discrepancy in times between *ex utero* and *in utero* detection of mineralization suggests that, with refinement of radiographic technique and with animals of thin body configuration, earlier *in utero* detection may occur. Likewise, if technique is inadequate or if the animal is large, detection may be delayed even longer. In the same animal, fetal mineralization is usually seen earlier in the lateral radiograph than in the dorsoventral radiograph.

Acknowledgement: Dr. P. W. Concannon, Ithaca, NY, assisted in the collection of data on normal canine intrauterine development.

947

Table 1. *Radiographic Detection of Uterine Enlargement and Fetal Mineralization in the Bitch*

Radiographic Finding	Days After Preovulatory LH Peak	Days Ante Delivery
Uterus first seen	30 (28–34)*	35 (32–36)*
Spherical uterine swellings	35 (31–38)	30 (27–33)
Ovoid uterine swellings	41 (38–44)	24 (22–27)
Mineralized fetus first seen: spine, skull, and ribs	45 (43–46)	21 (20–22)
Scapula, humerus, and femur seen	48 (46–51)	17 (15–18)
Radius, ulna, and tibia seen	52 (50–53)	11 (9–13)
Pelvis seen	54 (53–57)	11 (9–13)
13 pairs ribs countable	54 (52–59)	11 (7–12)
Caudal vertebrae, fibula, calcaneus, and paws seen	61 (55–64)	5 (2–9)
Teeth seen	61 (58–63)	4 (3–8)
Whelping	65 (64–66)	0

*Numbers in parentheses indicate range.

At 45 days after the LH peak, it is possible to observe fetal ossification in the bones of the head, bodies of the vertebrae, and ribs. At 48 days after the LH peak (range 46 to 51 days), the scapula, humerus, and femur become visible. At 52 days after the LH peak (range 50 to 53 days), the radius, ulna, and tibia are seen; and at 54 days after the LH peak (range 53 to 57 days), the ilium and ischium are visualized. All 13 pairs of ribs are usually seen distinctly enough to be counted on day 54 after the LH peak (range 53 to 57 days). The caudal vertebrae, fibula, calcaneus, and paws can be seen on day 61 (range 55 to 64 days).

A rapid transition from inability to visualize fetal skeletons to the ability to clearly visualize a large number of osseous structures (within five days) reflects the rapid growth of the fetus during this period of mid gestation (Fig. 1). *Ex utero* crown-rump measurements of beagle fetuses indicated that the average increase in length between days 35 and 40 is 30.5 mm, or 6.1 mm/day. In the last three weeks of gestation, fetal mineralization continues to progress, with the bones becoming more promi-

nent, larger, and better defined. Calcification of deciduous teeth is initiated by day 55. Deciduous teeth are usually seen radiographically on day 61 after the LH peak (range 58 to 63 days). The ability to clearly visualize deciduous teeth is an indication that the fetuses are near term. The anatomic structures previously mentioned and listed in Table 1 will not be seen in every fetus at each radiographic examination but will be detectable in at least one fetus at the stated times.

When evaluating an animal for pregnancy determination, it is important to limit patient motion. Fetal detection can be obscured by motion, especially during the early stages of mineralization. In addition, it is advantageous to withhold food from the bitch for several hours prior to radiographic evaluation and to have the animal defecate and urinate prior to being radiographed. When fetal skeletons are identified, counting the skulls and spinal columns is used to help determine the minimum number of fetuses present. The exact number of fetuses present may not always be detected radiographically, especially if the fetuses are in the

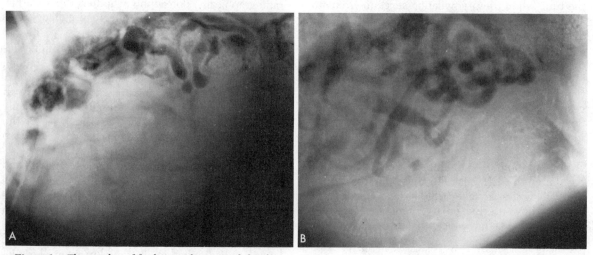

Figure 1.   The rapidity of fetal mineralization and development can be seen in these two radiographs of a beagle bitch. *A*, 49 days after LH peak; 16 days ante partum. *B*, 54 days after LH peak; 11 days ante partum.

early stage of mineralization, if there is fetal motion during the radiographic exposure, or if the fetuses are overlying prominent maternal abdominal viscera, the spinal column, ingesta-filled stomach, a distended stomach, or fecal-filled colon. Thus, the minimum number of fetuses present can be stated, whereas the exact number may not be determined. An animal that does not deliver the minimum number of fetuses should be re-evaluated radiographically; however, it is also important to realize that additional fetuses may be present even though the number of fetuses initially detected have been delivered. Once fetal mineralization is detected, the extent of mineralization progresses rapidly so that within a five-day period fetal mineralization is overt. Radiographic re-evaluation is indicated in five days if early fetal mineralization is only suspected in the initial radiograph.

RADIOGRAPHIC SIGNS OF FETAL DEATH IN THE BITCH AND QUEEN

Prior to fetal mineralization, the radiographic signs of intrauterine death are based on alterations in the size and shape of the uterus rather than on the appearance of the fetus. Failure of the uterus to continue to enlarge between days 28 and 44 of gestation, rapid decrease in size of the uterus during this period, and gas within the uterus are all signs of abnormal intrauterine development and usually signify intrauterine death, abortion, or resorption. Prior to day 30 after the LH peak, the uterus is not discernible radiographically, and thus most cases of early embryonic death go misdiagnosed as infertility.

Once the fetus becomes mineralized and detectable radiographically (day 45 after the LH peak), direct statements about the status of the fetus can be made rather than inferred from the appearance of the uterus. Most animals that are being evaluated for possible intrauterine fetal death are examined during the post-maturity period rather than during the prematurity period. These animals usually have surpassed their anticipated whelping dates, have delivered some young but not the number as determined from previous radiographic evaluation, are in duress but are not delivering additional young, have a fetus palpable in the abdomen, or have a fetus that can be seen or felt in the birth canal but is not being delivered. In the human literature, more than 20 radiographic signs have been described to help determine if a fetus is viable when viewed in the survey radiograph. Of those 20 methods, three are seen with sufficient frequency, are sufficiently reliable, and are practical enough to be seriously considered when evaluating companion animals for intrauterine fetal death. These signs are (1) alteration of fetal skull bone alignment: overrid-

ing of the fetal skull bones or extreme deformity of the fetal skull; (2) intra- and perifetal gas collections: gas subcutaneously; in the cardiovascular system, central nervous system, body cavities, amniotic space; around the conceptus; (3) abnormal fetal posture: ball sign of increased fetal flexion or straightening of hind limbs.

Radiographic signs indicating the absence of fetal life that are based on absence of change in fetal position on two identical radiographs made at different times, failure to observe fetal motion by a double exposure technique or during fluoroscopy, or disproportion between fetal size and expected delivery date are too unreliable or impractical to consider as serious signs of fetal death. Lack of continued fetal growth and demineralization of the fetal skeleton are reliable signs of fetal death but require repeat radiographic examination.

Overriding of the fetal skull bones or skull collapse is a positive radiographic sign of fetal death when the fetus is not in the birth canal (Fig. 2). Once the fetus dies, compression by the uterus results in skull collapse. Once the collapse occurs, it is a persistent sign of fetal death; however, to detect the collapse, the x-ray beam must intersect the overriding bones tangentially. This radiographic sign of fetal death may be missed because of this technical reason. *Ex utero* radiographs of a dead fetus will often show this sign despite the inability to visualize it *in utero*, suggesting that the sign may be obscured by overlying soft tissue structures *in utero*.

The presence of gas in or around the fetus is also a reliable sign of fetal death (Fig. 3). If the gas is carbon dioxide or oxygen formed or liberated shortly after death, then it may be transitory; it may be detectable within 12 hours after fetal death but then may dissipate and no longer be visualized radiographically. However, if the gas is produced by bacteria, it persists as long as the bacteria are present and producing the gas. Gas should not be seen surrounding the fetus even when it is in the birth canal. The detection of intra- or perifetal gas is made difficult by the presence of gas in the intestinal tract of the bitch or queen, which may overlie the fetus and mimic a pathologic state. Gas should be detectable in or around the fetus in two radiographic views to help make this a more reliable sign of fetal death, especially if only a small volume of gas is present. If the amount of gas is voluminous and clearly outlines the fetus or intrafetal structures, then only one radiographic view is required for diagnosis.

Abnormal fetal posture relative to the orientation of the appendicular skeleton to the spine and increased fetal vertebral column flexion are reliable radiographic signs of fetal death. When the hind limbs of the fetus are extended (straight-leg appearance) or if the fetus is "rolled" into a ball, fetal

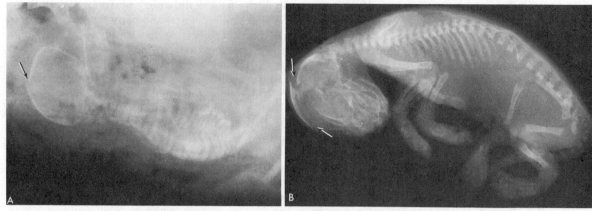

Figure 2.   Overriding of fetal skull bones (arrows). *A*, Dead canine fetus *in utero*. *B*, Dead feline fetus *ex utero*.

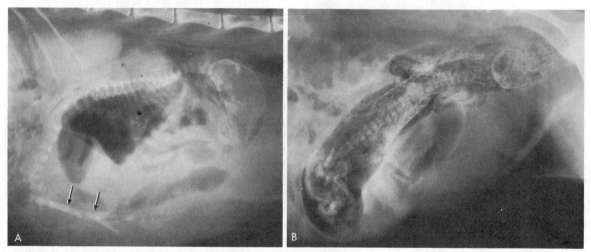

Figure 3.   Intra- and perifetal gas. *A*, Dead feline fetus. Gas is seen intrafetally. This fetus also has its hind limbs extended (arrows). *B*, Dead canine fetus. Gas is seen intra- and peri-fetally.

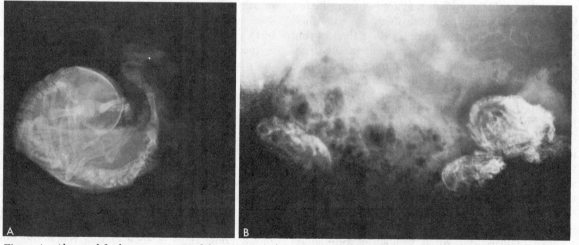

Figure 4.   Abnormal fetal posture. *A*, Dead fetus *ex utero* shows hyperflexion of the vertebral column (ball sign), extension of the hind limbs, and overriding of the skull bones. *B*, Mummified fetuses show loss of definition, increased vertebral column flexion, and increased radiodensity.

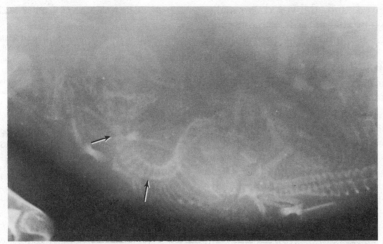

Figure 5.   Prominent angulation of the vertebral column (arrows) is seen in this viable feline fetus.

death is indicated (Fig. 4; see Fig. 3A). Increased radiodensity of the fetus as it collapses or mummifies and loss of ability to visualize the extremities as the fetus collapses are also reliable signs of fetal death. As the fetus becomes mummified or macerated, its appearance as a distinctive fetal entity will become obscure. Alterations in the neck and head-neck angles can look abnormal radiographically; however, the fetus can still be viable (Fig. 5), and thus these are not good radiographic indicators of fetal death.

Although the previously mentioned radiographic signs of fetal death are reliable when seen, they are not always present. In evaluating 13 cases of known fetal death, overriding of the skull bones was seen in 38 per cent, gas in or around the fetus was seen in 61 per cent, and abnormal fetal posture (straight hind limbs, "ball" sign) was seen in 61 per cent of the cases. In one case, none of the reliable signs of fetal death was identified. As the time interval between fetal death and radiographic evaluation decreases, so does the ability to detect fetal death.

GENERAL OBSERVATIONS

There are situations that may mimic intrauterine fetal death and that should be considered when evaluating a bitch or queen; such conditions as bones within the gastrointestinal tract (especially chicken bones and birds), a consumed fetus in the stomach, mummified intra-abdominal fetus, mineralized neoplasm, omental cyst, hematoma, or teratoma can mimic intrauterine fetal death. Superfetation can result in fetuses in different stages of development being seen in the radiographs and mimicking fetal death. Fetal monsters are sometimes seen, especially when two bodies are cojoined to one head.

A pregnant animal with a diaphragmatic hernia may show overt clinical signs of respiratory distress as the uterus enlarges and viscera are displaced into the thoracic cavity. Fetuses may be identified free within the thoracic cavity following uterine rupture or within the thoracic cavity and confined within the uterus in animals with a diaphragmatic hernia, especially if trauma occurred during pregnancy. Fetuses may also be seen outside the abdominal cavity in animals with abdominal wall hernias when the uterus has become displaced through the rent. As the conceptus enlarges, so does the size of the soft tissue mass in the hernia.

Mummified fetuses have been identified in animals that have been ovariohysterectomized. Presumably these masses were present but undetected when the spay was performed.

The hazard of radiation damage to the conceptus should always be considered when deciding to evaluate a pregnant or potentially pregnant animal radiographically. The conceptus is most sensitive to the effects of ionizing radiation during the first trimester of pregnancy and is more sensitive to the effects of ionizing radiation throughout pregnancy when compared with the adult. Therefore, a pregnant animal should not be radiographed for frivolous reasons but only when there is a clear medical indication, such as an animal with a history of dystocia in which knowledge of the number of fetuses present is desired prior to the delivery date to help determine appropriate management of the bitch, evaluation of the pelvic canal and caudal lumbar vertebrae when there is a suspected or known deformity of these areas, cases of planned abortion, suspected cases of fetal death, or following cessation of meaningful labor to assess that all pups or kittens have been delivered. Six bitches were radiographed thrice weekly beginning on day 20 of pregnancy until term. Each bitch delivered a normal litter, and two of the bitches were subsequently rebred and conceived and delivered normally. Thus, although the potential hazards of radiographing a pregnant bitch are known, the probability of inducing a lesion with one or two radiographic exposures seems small.

Techniques other than routine radiography have been used to evaluate fetal development and viability. Aortography, aminography, and fetal pyelography have all been used to determine fetal viability; however, these techniques are generally not practical or are not sufficiently reliable when dealing with companion animals to be recommended. Other diagnostic techniques, especially ultrasound, have been used for determining pregnancy and fetal viability and offer an alternate method of diagnosis without using ionizing radiation.

Finally, it should be remembered that a pregnant animal may become ill for reasons unassociated with pregnancy; in these cases, a thorough examination is always indicated.

REFERENCES AND SUPPLEMENTAL READING

Boyd, J. S.: The radiographic identification of the various stages of pregnancy in the domestic cat. J. Small Anim. Pract. 12:501, 1971.

Concannon, P.: Personal communication, 1982.

Evans, H. E.: Prenatal development of the dog. Paper presented at the Gaines Veterinary Symposium, 18, Cornell University, 1974.

Evans, H. E., and Sack, W. O.: Prenatal development of domestic and laboratory mammals. Zentralbl. Veterinaermed. [A] 2:11, 1973.

Farrow, C. S., Morgan, J. P., and Story, E. C.: Later term fetal death in the dog: early radiographic diagnosis. J. Am. Vet. Rad. Soc. 17:11, 1976.

Holst, P. A., and Phemister, R. D.: The prenatal development of the dog: preimplantation events. Biol. Reprod. 5:194, 1971.

Nelson, N. S., and Cooper, J.: The growing conceptus of the domestic cat. Growth 39:435, 1975.

Smith, D. M., and Kirk, G. R.: Detection of pregnancy in the dog. J.A.A.H.A. 11:201, 1975.

Stewart, A. M.: The study of free gas in the foetus as a sign of intrauterine death. Br. J. Radiol. 34:187, 1961.

Thomas, C. R., Lang, E. K., and Lloyd, F. P.: Fetal pyelography—a method for detecting fetal life. Obstet. Gynecol. 22:335, 1963.

Tiedemann, K., and Henschel, E.: Early radiographic diagnosis of pregnancy in the cat. J. Small Anim. Pract. 14:567, 1973.

Waldman, I., Berlin, L., and McLain, C. R.: Amniography in the diagnosis of fetal death. Radiology 84:1066, 1965.

Zeit, R. M.: Sonographic demonstration of fetal death in the absence of radiographic abnormality. Obstet. Gynecol. 48:49S, 1976.

MANAGEMENT OF PREGNANCY DISORDERS IN THE BITCH AND QUEEN

SHIRLEY D. JOHNSTON, D.V.M.

St. Paul, Minnesota

ABNORMAL VAGINAL DISCHARGE

The pregnant or nonpregnant diestrual bitch and queen may show occasional mucous discharge from the vagina. Hemorrhagic or purulent discharge, however, is abnormal, and bacterial culture and cytology of the discharge and evaluation of a complete blood count are indicated when either of these is present.

Occasionally a bitch or queen will discharge a small amount of blood during a normal gestation, but more commonly hemorrhage is a sign of impending pregnancy loss. When hemorrhage is present without evidence of infection, the patient should be kenneled to enforce rest and permit monitoring (rectal temperature, hemorrhage observed) until the hemorrhage ceases or abortion occurs.

The diestrual female with purulent discharge should be evaluated radiographically or ultrasonographically if possible to distinguish a purulent discharge in pregnancy from open-cervix pyometra. Prior to 45 days gestation, when fetal skeletons are

calcified, all bitches and queens with purulent discharge should be treated with specific antibiotics; after 45 days gestation the pregnant female is similarly treated with antibiotics and supportive treatment, and the pyometra female is ovariohysterectomized or given medical/surgical treatment to cause uterine evacuation.

EARLY PREGNANCY LOSS/SPONTANEOUS ABORTION

The incidence of early pregnancy loss and spontaneous abortion in the bitch and queen is unknown. Causes of pregnancy loss in these species include fetal defects; abnormal maternal environment (hypothyroidism, hypoluteoidism); viral, bacterial, and protozoal infectious causes; and trauma. Early abortion in women is usually associated with chromosomal abnormalities (polyploidy, autosomal monosomy, sex chromosome abnormality), and aging of human ova and spermatozoa before fertilization is significantly associated with increased incidence of abortion. Chromosomal abnormalities have been identified in feline but not canine pregnancy loss. Hypoluteoidism, or insufficient progesterone production, a hypothetical cause of abortion in the bitch, which needs luteal progesterone throughout gestation, and the queen, which needs it through days 42 to 45, was incriminated as a cause of abortion in the veterinary literature before progesterone assays were developed; this cause of pregnancy loss has not been documented in companion animals. There is evidence, however, that queens may cycle and conceive during gestation (superfetation), and the feline ovary is not refractory to exogenous gonadotropin stimulation during mid gestation. This suggests that the queen may cycle and abort during gestation, producing insufficient luteal progesterone to maintain negative feedback inhibition on gonadotropin release. Hypothyroidism, which is frequently diagnosed in the dog, may be associated with increased risk of early pregnancy loss and/or abortion. The common viral diseases of the dog and cat (canine distemper, canine herpesvirus, feline leukemia, feline infectious peritonitis, feline respiratory diseases) have all been demonstrated to cause spontaneous abortion with or without concurrent fetal infection. Canine herpesvirus, usually associated with respiratory disease and death in puppies and mild vaginitis in the bitch, was reported to cause abortion of nearly full-term puppies in a kennel of German shepherd bitches. Feline leukemia virus may cause abortion of fetal tissue and a bloody vaginal discharge at four to seven weeks gestation; the discharge persists for five to six days and the cat appears otherwise normal. The cat may cycle four to six weeks after aborting and may conceive but will abort again. Abortion due to bacterial infection with *Brucella canis*, *Brucella abortus*, *Streptococcus* β-hemolyticus type L, *Escherichia coli*, and *Leptospira* spp. has been reported in the bitch. Although classic *B. canis* abortion occurs between days 45 and 55 of pregnancy, infected bitches may also appear infertile owing to early embryonic death of their fetuses. *Toxoplasma gondii* can cause experimental abortion in both the bitch and the queen. Traumatic abortion is uncommon in human patients but occurs occasionally during laparotomy when surgery is near the pelvic organs.

Diagnosis of abortion is made by inspection of aborted tissues or by demonstration of pregnancy loss in the female. When fetal death occurs without abortion, radiographic examination of the bitch may demonstrate gas within the fetal tissues, overlapping of cranial bones, or collapse of the spinal column of the fetuses.

Management of the aborting patient is directed toward establishing the cause of abortion and providing rest and supportive care until uterine contents are completely expelled or the pregnancy is completed. The bitch and queen may abort one or more fetuses and carry the rest to normal parturition at term. Aborted fetal tissue should be submitted for karyotyping (available at many veterinary colleges) if possible, histopathology, and bacterial culture. The vaginal discharge of the dam is submitted for bacterial culture. Blood is drawn from the dam for a complete blood count, *Toxoplasma gondii* serology, serum thyroxine assay, *B. canis* serology (bitch), feline leukemia virus test (queen), and feline infectious peritonitis serology (queen). Abdominal radiographs are taken to evaluate number of fetuses, if any, remaining and to look for radiographic evidence of fetal death. The dam is hospitalized or kenneled to enforce rest and permit close observation. If the patient is toxic or in shock, appropriate supportive therapy is instituted. Antibiotics are indicated if the hemogram and/or rectal temperature is consistent with the presence of infection. Oxytocic agents (oxytocin, 5 to 20 U IM; ergonovine maleate, 0.2 mg/30 lb IM; or prostaglandin $F_{2\alpha}$, 0.25 mg/kg IM) are given to aid uterine evacuation *if all fetuses have been aborted* and if membranes are retained or there is severe hemorrhage. Progesterone should not be given; this hormone promotes uterine quiescence, which is undesirable if a dead or abnormal fetus or infection is present.

Prevention of pregnancy loss/abortion is empirical unless the cause of the problem is understood. Optimum health, good vaccination history, negative *B. canis* titer, negative feline leukemia test, and normal thyroid function are desirable prior to breeding. Prevention of recurrent abortion in the bitch/queen when fetal defect, hypothyroidism, and infection have been ruled out may be attempted with repositol progesterone therapy (2 mg/kg IM on days 35, 45, and 55); however, masculinization of the external genitalia of female puppies and kittens has been observed after administration of progestogens during pregnancy.

ECTOPIC PREGNANCY

Ectopic or extrauterine pregnancy has been reported in both the dog and cat, although the distinction has not been made between fetuses developing outside the uterus and uterine rupture followed by expulsion of the fetus into the peritoneal cavity. Encapsulated mummified fetuses with mesenteric attachments have been removed from both bitches and queens months after parturition and from one bitch with pyometra but no evidence of fetal infection. No signs of uterine rupture have been observed, but such scars may be hard to detect. Diagnosis is by inspection (incidental) at laparotomy, and treatment is surgical removal.

UTERINE TORSION

Torsion of one or both uterine horns has been reported in eight bitches (five pregnant) and eight queens (eight pregnant) in the veterinary literature. The cause of uterine torsion in these species is unknown; torsions are attributed to presence of uterine tumors, uterine anomalies, fetal anomaly, excessive fetal movement and weight, and uterine adhesions in women, cows, and mares. Torsions of gravid horns most often occur at term but have been reported as early as six weeks gestation. Torsions may occur in females with previous normal pregnancies. Torsions of 180° to 2,160° (six rotations) have been reported in the bitch and queen.

Presenting signs vary from signs of shock and acute abdomen (abdominal pain, prolonged capillary refill time, tachycardia, hyperpnea, weak pulse, hypothermia) to dystocia; and some females with uterine torsion are asymptomatic.

Diagnosis is based on inspection at exploratory laparotomy. Radiographic examination of the uterus after induction of a pneumoperitoneum may also be diagnostic.

Treatment requires surgical correction of the torsion. Both hysterotomy and hysterectomy have been performed successfully on pregnant patients.

HYPOCALCEMIA (ECLAMPSIA/PUERPERAL TETANY)

Hypocalcemia in the pre- or post-partum bitch or queen is associated with serum calcium concentrations of less than 7 mg/dl. The condition is most frequently observed in small bitches nursing large litters two to four weeks following whelping, but it may occur in any breed bitch or in the queen during lactation or prior to parturition. Hypocalcemia has been reported in concert with hyperkalemia and oliguric renal failure in a bitch 59 days pregnant. The cause of prepartum hypocalcemia is unknown, although parathyroid gland dysfunction has been suggested.

Clinical signs of the prepartum hypocalcemic bitch are those of trembling and weakness, which may proceed to tonic-clonic convulsions. The temperature and pulse rate may be elevated. Uterine inertia may be present in the hypocalcemic bitch at term. Total serum calcium is usually less than 7 mg/dl.

Treatment of hypocalcemia in the prepartum bitch is 10 per cent gluconate given slowly IV to effect (usually 3 to 20 cc), followed by 1 to 3 gm calcium lactate or gluconate and 10,000 to 25,000 U vitamin D PO once daily throughout the remaining gestation and lactation.

HYPOGLYCEMIA AND KETONEMIA

Several cases of hypoglycemia associated with ketonemia and ketonuria have been reported in bitches in late pregnancy. Inadequate food consumption and influence of serum progesterone on glucose metabolism via serum insulin concentrations and glucose tolerance were suggested as etiologic factors. Presenting complaints are convulsions or coma associated with serum glucose concentrations of less than 40 mg/dl.

These patients respond to IV glucose administration to effect and undergo remission following delivery of the puppies. In one bitch tested subsequent to delivery, serum glucose concentrations were comparable to those of normal healthy dogs following starvation (48 hours); carbohydrate-free diet (2 weeks); and glucose, glucagon, and progesterone tolerance tests.

PROLONGED GESTATION

Parturition occurs approximately 63 days following ovulation in the bitch and queen. Because dog sperm may survive and be capable of fertilizing eggs in the estrogen-sensitized female tract for 7 to 8 days prior to ovulation, bitches bred that early may have apparent gestations of 70 to 71 days if timed from the first breeding. Because the bitch ovulates primary oocytes, which must undergo two meiotic divisions before fertilization can be completed (approximately 3 days), dogs bred several days after ovulation may conceive and undergo gestations of 58 to 59 days. Therefore, normal gestation length may vary from 58 to 71 days, depending on the day of the cycle at which the bitch was bred. Not all bitches should be allowed to go 71 days, however. Clinicians should use date (of the cycle) of breeding, rectal temperature drop, and evidence of cervical dilation to determine when parturition has started and how it should be managed (see following section). True prolonged gestation unassociated with primary uterine inertia in the bitch has not been documented.

Because the queen is an induced ovulator, breeding date is a better indicator of ovulation date in the queen than in the bitch. However, cats bred a single time may not release sufficient luteinizing hormone to induce ovulation; if these females are bred repeatedly several days later, gestation may need to be timed from the later breedings.

DYSTOCIA

Dystocia, or difficult birth, may be caused by an inadequate maternal birth canal, an abnormal fetus, or insufficient uterine expulsive efforts. An inadequate birth canal is most often due to the presence of a bony callus formed subsequent to pelvic/acetabular fracture; other causes include vaginal tumors, vaginal hyperplasia, and breed predisposition. Fetal causes of dystocia may include a small number of disproportionately large fetuses, a developmental abnormality ("monsters"), fetal anasarca, fetal death, and cephalopelvic disproportion in the brachioce-phalic breeds. Uterine inertia may be primary (cause unknown) or secondary (owing to uterine fatigue).

Diagnosis of dystocia is based on gestation length, drop in rectal temperature to less than 100°F and often less than 99°F in the 24 hours prior to onset of whelping, and progress of the bitch in stage II labor. Gestation length and rectal temperature drop are of special interest with primary uterine inertia when the cervix dilates but uterine contractions are absent or ineffectual and puppies die *in utero* without being expelled. Rectal temperature drop and a dilated cervix are key factors of primary uterine inertia in the bitch. Failure to progress in stage II labor forms the basis for diagnosis of maternal and fetal dystocias and secondary uterine inertia. In normal canine parturition, stage I labor lasts 6 to 12 hours and is characterized by uterine contractions (not visible externally) and gradual cervical dilation; external signs of stage I labor include restlessness and panting. Stage II labor occurs when fetuses move through the dilated cervix and birth canal to be born. Stretching of the cervix by the fetus causes oxytocin release, which strengthens the uterine contractions and often causes the bitch to strain and contract her voluntary abdominal musculature. Such straining or presence of fetal membranes at the vulva signals that the bitch is in stage II labor. If four hours pass after the onset of stage II labor without birth of a puppy or if more than two hours pass between puppies, the client should seek veterinary assistance. If the stage II bitch is showing nonproductive but constant severe straining she should be examined after no more than one hour.

Clinical management of dystocia includes a complete physical examination; digital or vaginoscopic examination of the birth canal; serum calcium and glucose assays, if possible; and abdominal radiography to determine size and number of remaining fetuses and to look for signs of fetal death.

Treatment of nonobstructive dystocias characterized by failure to progress consists of feathering the vagina and administering 5 to 20 U oxytocin IM (repeated two to three times at 30-minute intervals) and 3 to 5 cc 10 per cent calcium gluconate given once, IV, slowly over five to ten minutes. Bitches that fail to progress after three to four injections of oxytocin or those with obstructive dystocias are then managed surgically with cesarean section.

Dystocia in the queen is fortunately less common than in the bitch. Although guidelines used in evaluating dystocia in the queen may be similar to those used in the bitch, feline patients are more difficult to stage, as a prepartum rectal temperature drop has not been reported in this species and the vagina is often too small for adequate digital examination. Queens have also been observed to deliver live, normal, healthy kittens one to three days apart, a situation that does not occur in the bitch.

SUPPLEMENTAL READING

Acland, B. M., and Butcher, D. R.: Habitual abortion in cats. Austr. Vet. J. 50:179, 1974.

Arañez, J. B., and Lapuz, G. R.: Dystocia in a native bitch. J.A.V.M.A. 944:416, 1955.

Austad, R., and Bjerkas, E.: Eclampsia in the bitch. J. Small Anim. Pract. 17:793, 1976.

Benirschke, K., Edwards, R., and Low, R. J.: Trisomy in a feline fetus. Am. J. Vet. Res. 35:257, 1974.

Bennett, D.: Canine dystocia—a review of the literature. J. Small Anim. Pract. 15:101, 1974.

Carmichael, L. E.: Canine brucellosis: an annotated review with selected cautionary comments. Theriogenology 6:105, 1976.

Carmichael, L. E., and Kenney, R. M.: Canine abortion caused by *Brucella canis*. J.A.V.M.A. 152:605, 1968.

Chan, S. Y. W., Chakraborty, P. K., and Wildt, D. E.: Ovarian-endocrine-behavioral function in domestic cats treated with exogenous gonadotropins during midgestation. Biol. Reprod. 24(Suppl. 1):122A, 1981.

Concannon, P. W., Hodgson, B., and Lein, D.: Reflex LH release in estrous cats following single and multiple copulations. Biol. Reprod. 23:111, 1980.

Concannon, P. W., Powers, M. E., Holder, W., and Hansel, W.: Pregnancy and parturition in the bitch. Biol. Reprod. 16:517, 1977.

Curwen, P.: Anasarca as a cause of dystocia in the bitch. Vet. Rec. 61:572, 1949.

Farrow, C. S., Morgan, J. P., and Story, E. C.: Late term fetal death in the dog: early radiographic diagnosis. J. Am. Vet. Rad. Soc. 17:11, 1976.

Freak, M. J.: Abnormal conditions associated with pregnancy and parturition in the bitch. Vet. Rec. 74:1323, 1962.

Handcock, W. J.: Hypoglycemia in a pregnant bitch. J. South Afr. Vet. Med. Assn. 49:69, 1978.

Irvine, C. H. G.: Hypoglycaemia in the bitch. N. Z. Vet. J. 12:140, 1964.

Jackson, R. F., Bruss, M. L., Growney, P. J., and Seymour, W. G.: Hypoglycemia-ketonemia in a pregnant bitch. J.A.V.M.A. 177:1123, 1980.

Morgan, A. F.: Extrauterine mummified fetus in a Burmese. Feline Pract. 6:55, 1976.

Nava, G. A.: Cases of abortion due to *Brucella*, *Leptospira* and *Toxoplasma* in bitches. Atti. Soc. Ital. Sci. Vet. 23:376, 1969.

Peck, G. K., and Badame, F. G.: Extrauterine pregnancy with fetal mummification and pyometra in a Pomeranian. Can. Vet. J. 8:136, 1967.

Poste, G., and King, N.: Isolation of a herpesvirus from the canine genital tract: association with infertility, abortion, and stillbirths. Vet. Rec. 88:229, 1971.

Schlotthauer, C. T., and Wakim, K. G.: Ectopic pregnancy in a dog. J.A.V.M.A. 127:213, 1955.

Shull, R. M., Johnston, S. D., Johnston, G. R., Caywood, D., and Stevens, J. B.: Bilateral torsion of the uterine horns in a nongravid bitch. J.A.V.M.A. 172:601, 1978.

Stein, B. S.: Abortion in cats. Mod. Vet. Pract. 55:597, 1974.

Taylor, D. J., Renton, J. P., and McGregor, A. B.: *Brucella abortus* biotype I as a cause of abortion in the bitch. Vet. Rec. 96:428, 1975.

Todd, A. J., and Lonsdale, T.: Prolonged gestation. Vet. Rec. 98:100, 1976.

Wolfersteig, D., Schaer, M., and Kirby, R.: Hypocalcemia, hyperkalemia and renal failure in a bitch at term pregnancy. J. Am. Anim. Hosp. Assn. 16:845, 1980.

BREEDING SOUNDNESS EXAMINATION OF THE MALE DOG

ROLF E. LARSEN, D.V.M.

Gainesville, Florida

A breeding soundness examination of the stud dog is most often conducted if a bitch or series of bitches bred by the dog has failed to conceive. Other indications for examination include concern by the owner about possible exposure to infectious venereal disease, a seller or buyer seeking evidence of breeding soundness, change in sexual behavior, and questionable reproductive maturity in a young male.

The owner should prepare a written history of breeding dates and results. Complete medical records, including all prior medications, should be evaluated. An estrous teaser bitch of the same breed or size should be available for use as a mount animal. The examination schedule should be planned so that a mount of a teaser animal, observation of sexual reflexes, and semen collection are given priority. Unsuccessful semen collection results in an inconclusive examination, and re-evaluation is necessary. In most cases it is advisable to perform semen collection and semen laboratory evaluation before the physical examination and other procedures that may reduce the animal's willingness to cooperate with semen collection attempts. Therefore, semen evaluation will be described first.

SEMEN COLLECTION AND EVALUATION

The following items are needed for semen collection: (1) artificial vagina; a rubber end cone of a bovine AV is typically used; (2) plastic calibrated 10- to 15-cc centrifuge tubes; (3) sterile aqueous lubricant. Semen evaluation requires the following items: (1) slide warmer; (2) microscope; (3) slides; (4) coverslips; (5) hemocytometer; (6) 1/100 blood dilutor kit for white blood cells or other dilution method; (7) isotonic diluent, pH 7.0 (physiologic saline or 2.9 per cent sodium citrate); (8) sperm morphology stain (e.g., eosin-nigrosin)

COLLECTION PROCEDURE

Masturbation of the dog during a mount of an estrous bitch is preferred. Alternatively, a secured anestrous bitch may be used. Some dogs, when accustomed to manipulation of the external genitalia, will allow masturbation while standing with no teaser present. If the male is not an experienced breeder a certain amount of foreplay and tentative mounting attempts should be allowed. The teaser bitch may be left unmuzzled for a brief period during the initial contacts. Both the stud dog and the bitch should be kept on leads. After the first contacts the bitch should be muzzled. The male will often make initial mounting attempts that are brief and unsuccessful. If the teaser is not in heat she should be held in a standing position.

When the male appears ready for a strong effort at mating, the bitch should be held in a steady position. As the male mounts he will thrust the penis and his hips forward, searching for the vulva. When the vulva or artificial vagina is encountered the dog will start to thrust violently, pushing the complete shaft of the nonerect penis into the vagina, or artificial vagina, and sliding the prepuce behind the bulbus glandis. The os penis provides sufficient rigidity to the penis to permit intromission prior to complete erection. When collecting an ejaculate it is important to slide the prepuce back early in the thrusting process so that the bulbus glandis will engorge outside of the prepuce.

Manual pressure to stimulate a dog with poor libido should be applied with the hand cradling the shaft of the penis within the prepuce. The penis should be massaged only through the prepuce before thrusting exposes the shaft and only through the artificial vagina after protrusion. Care must be taken to prevent forcing of the penis through the length of the artificial vagina against the attached tube, which may traumatize the penis. As the erection proceeds the bulbus glandis will become two to three times the diameter of the shaft of the penis, and the artificial vagina is then backed off the shaft of the penis and bulbus slightly to prevent pressure and trauma to the penile surface.

During the most rapid pelvic thrusting a few drops of clear *presperm fraction (fraction 1)* are ejaculated. Toward the end of the thrusting phase the ejaculate becomes cloudy with 0.5 to 5.0 cc of *sperm-rich fraction (fraction 2)*. The only manual pressure necessary at this stage is gentle pressure around the circumference of the penis, proximal to the bulbus glandis. At this point most dogs will dismount and attempt to step over the bitch and the operator's arm with one hind leg and stand with the penis directed caudally. This position may play a role in maintaining the erection and fluid flow and should be encouraged in the inexperienced male. The fibroelastic base of the penis is turned 180° in a horizontal plane when the dog steps over the bitch, so that the dorsal surface of the penis remains dorsal. (If the bulbus glandis is inadvertently trapped within the prepuce this turn is impossible.) During manual semen collection the dog may remain in a mounted position and the penis alone (inside the artificial vagina) may be turned 180° under one (lifted) hind leg.

Ejaculated semen will become clear again after one to three minutes and 1 to 5 cc of the ejaculate. This clear fluid is the third fraction and is prostatic fluid, which can be ejaculated for 5 to 45 minutes and which ranges from 1 to 40 cc in volume. Usually only a portion of this fluid need be collected. Collection tubes may be changed at this point so that prostatic fluid can be collected separately if prostatic function is to be evaluated. For insemination with raw semen only the small amount of prostatic fluid necessary to bring total semen volume to a sufficient quantity to minimize sperm loss due to syringe and pipette wetting (usually 3 to 6 cc) is collected. The stud dog will lean forward during this phase and let the bulb of the penis support a portion of his weight. Continued pressure and support by the operator around the circumference of the penis proximal to the bulb will generally maintain the flow of prostatic fluid for the same interval as with a normal tie. When the penis is released by the operator the erection is usually lost within a few minutes. The dog should be kept on a lead by an observer until the erection has been lost and the penis is completely inside the prepuce. The penis and prepuce should always be checked for paraphimosis following loss of erection.

SEMEN EVALUATION

VOLUME

Volume is read directly from the calibrated collection tube. Normal volume in the dog may range from 0.5 to more than 30 cc, depending on the quantity of prostatic fluid (third fraction) collected. Semen should be collected for at least four to five minutes or a time sufficient to observe the ejaculation of each of the three fractions; most normal dogs over 30 lb will ejaculate at least 5 cc in the first ten minutes. The tube on the artificial vagina can be changed after the ejaculate starts to clear. Volume is not correlated with fertility.

COLOR

The normal color of dog semen is white to opalescent. Yellow semen usually indicates contamination with urine, which is toxic to sperm. When blood is observed in the ejaculate, it is important to determine immediately whether the source is from the penile surface or from within the urethra and, if possible, whether blood is emitted early or late in the ejaculation process. Most blood observed in the ejaculate of dogs is prostatic in origin or is due to abrasions of the highly vascular surface of the glans penis.

MOTILITY

A fraction of a drop of semen diluted with 1 drop of 37°C 2.9 per cent sodium citrate or 0.9 per cent sodium chloride is placed on a microscope slide, coverslipped, and examined at 200 to 400× magnification to estimate percentage of progressively motile cells. Normal canine spermatozoa are highly motile. A drop of raw sperm-rich semen may show swirl patterns. It is always preferable to estimate individual motility in a diluted sample. Dogs of high fertility commonly have over 80 per cent progressively motile sperm. Motility of less than 60 per cent is considered unsatisfactory.

TOTAL SPERM NUMBERS

Sperm cells are easily counted on a hemocytometer after dilution with a 1/100 Unopette white blood cell dilutor kit or with 1/100 dilution accomplished by pipetting an appropriate volume of semen into diluent. Sperm cells can also be counted using a calibrated spectrophotometer or a Coulter counter.

Sperm concentration varies tremendously among dogs and ejaculates because of the variable quantity of prostatic fluid ejaculated in this species. Therefore, total number of sperm cells per ejaculate (concentration × volume) is the parameter that must be determined. Total number of spermatozoa in the adult dog should be at least 200×10^6 in the sexually rested animal, and numbers greater than 500×10^6 are commonly encountered. Testicular size and interval since the last ejaculate influence total sperm cell numbers in the ejaculate. For artificial insemination a minimum of 50×10^6 live cells are needed to routinely achieve pregnancy. In general, when sexually rested dogs have fewer than 100×10^6 total cells in the ejaculate, a high number of morphologically abnormal spermatozoa are also present.

MORPHOLOGY

The eosin-nigrosin morphology stain is commonly used for evaluation of sperm defects. A drop of stain is mixed gently with a fraction of a drop of sperm-rich semen on a warmed microscope slide, and this mixture is then drawn slowly across the slide in the manner of a blood smear and allowed to air dry. Sperm morphology is observed at 1000× magnification (oil immersion). Head-shape abnormalities, proximal droplets, and middle-piece and tail (principal piece) defects should be quantitated by percentage of incidence. Doubled structures and detached heads should be tabulated separately.

Head-shape abnormalities, acrosomal defects, and presence of proximal cytoplasmic droplets in more than 20 per cent of the sperm cells are generally associated with reduced conception rates. Kinked tails and detached heads are the earliest and most common abnormalities seen following inflammation and heating of the scrotum.

Smears of raw semen should also be stained for evaluation of inflammatory cells (Wright's stain, new methylene blue stain). Diagnostic numbers of inflammatory cells are not always present in the ejaculate when bacterial infection is present. Semen or prostatic fluid from infertile dogs with a high incidence of morphologically defective sperm should be cultured bacteriologically. Sperm morphology has not been quantitatively related to fertility in the dog; however, it is very rare to find an infertile dog with normal sperm numbers (over 200×10^6) and morphology (over 75 per cent normal).

PHYSICAL EXAMINATION

A complete general physical examination should be performed to rule out interactions of the reproductive system with other systems. The reproductive examination should be thorough and systematic and, where possible, both quantitative and qualitative. The examination of the penis is generally done during the collection process when it is erect. This examination should be repeated when the penis is in a flaccid state if any abnormalities are noted.

PENIS AND PREPUCE

The penis of the dog is structured in a way that makes possible a unique coital pattern: intromission without erection, coital lock, and a 180° change of the male's position during coitus.

The os penis lies within the ventral portion of the shaft of the penis, extending from the area of the bulbus glandis almost to the tip of the glans penis. During a mount of a female the initial thrusts of the nonerect penis result in protrusion from the prepuce and penetration of the vulva only because the os penis holds the penis stiff and directs it forward. Dogs with a short os penis or with the bone terminating distally too far from the tip will have a flaccid

portion of the distal glans penis and may not be able to direct the penis into the vulva, even though complete erection is possible.

The bulbis glandis is the proximal portion of the shaft of the penis and is capable of engorging to two to three times the diameter of the long portion of the shaft. The proximal two-thirds of the bulb is covered by the prepuce, which reflects back along the shaft when the penis is retracted. The circumferential line of attachment is seen as a white band around the bulb in the engorged state. The bulbus glandis does not generally engorge until intromission is complete. In most animals it is large enough to prevent withdrawal through the vulvar orifice. Early engorgement will prevent intromission of the bulb and coital lock.

The prepuce consists of an outer cutaneous sheath and an inner lamina that covers the proximal portion of the penis during erection and creates the inner lining of the preputial cavity when the penis is retracted. The inner lamina contains lymphoid follicles, which are often observed as swollen or hemorrhagic when the penis is protruded for examination. These are most easily observed during a complete erection. Enlargement of these follicles is a common response to local irritants and infections. A congenitally shortened cutaneous portion of the prepuce may result in the tip of the penis protruding from the sheath for long periods with resultant trauma. Abnormal musculature of the preputial lining has been noted to cause a similar syndrome.

SCROTUM, TESTES, EPIDIDYMIS

The scrotal skin is palpated and visualized over its entire surface for evidence of trauma or inflammation. Testicular size is measured and consistency evaluated. Measurements of scrotal width may provide an indication of total parenchyma and sperm cell production potential.

The testes normally lie horizontally in the scrotum. The spermatic cord leaves the craniodorsal aspect of the testis and angles cranially and dorsally so that the cranial pole of the testis can be identified.

The epididymis in many dogs is identifiable by palpation along its entire length. The ductus deferens passes cranially along the dorsomedial surface of the testis, running on the medial aspect of the pampiniform plexus as it leaves the testicle. Granulomas, spermatoceles, and segmental aplasia within the epididymis or ductus deferens are difficult to identify on palpation unless they produce an enlarged, indurated mass. Normal texture and anatomic location do not ensure an intact duct system. The spermatic cords should be palpated to their entrance at the inguinal ring. Scrotal enlargement or spermatic cord thickening should always suggest inguinal hernia as a differential diagnosis.

PROSTATE GLAND

The prostate gland is the only significant accessory sex gland in the dog, although the terminal portion of the ductus deferens is sometimes called an ampulla owing to its slight widening. The prostate lies on the pelvic floor close to the pelvic brim. As dogs get older it enlarges and extends over the pelvic brim into the abdominal cavity. This means that for effective palpation of the prostate per rectum two hands must be used. With one finger in the rectum over the prostate the other hand can be used to lift the prostate up against the rectal finger by pressure on the abdominal wall. Physical examination of the prostate can reveal abnormal size, asymmetry, texture, fluid-filled structures, or pain.

Sperm-free prostatic fluid can be collected during ejaculation after passage of the sperm-rich fraction. This allows cytologic, bacteriologic, and chemical analysis.

SATISFACTORY POTENTIAL BREEDING SOUNDNESS

Stud dogs are generally considered to have satisfactory potential breeding soundness when semen parameters fall within the normal ranges, when physical examination reveals no abnormality of the reproductive tract or of other systems, and when *Brucella canis* serology is negative. In addition, the dog should be capable of and willing to mate.

MANAGEMENT OF THE POST-PARTUM BITCH AND QUEEN

SHIRLEY D. JOHNSTON, D.V.M.

St. Paul, Minnesota

CARE OF THE DAM

Rectal temperature of the post-partum bitch and queen should be monitored twice daily for two weeks following parturition; temperature elevations greater than 103.5°F may signal early mastitis or metritis. Each mammary gland should be inspected daily by the owner for signs of inflammation (erythema, swelling, pain, heat), and milk should be expressed from each gland to look for abnormal discharge. The vaginal discharge is also examined daily by the owner for evidence of pus or foul odor. Oxytocin is not given routinely post partum unless the dam is known to have retained placental tissue or hemorrhage or is not nursing any puppies. The dam may eat soon after parturition is complete and, as lactation progresses, may consume two to three times her normal maintenance ration to maintain milk production and normal body weight.

Lochia (green to red to brown endometrial breakdown products expelled as vaginal discharge) may be discharged in small amounts for two to four weeks.

The bitch will next come into heat at her regular interval, usually four to five months after whelping. The queen usually cycles three to four weeks after weaning her kittens but may cycle, be bred, and become pregnant as early as seven days post partum.

CARE OF THE NEONATES

Neonatal puppies and kittens require colostrum, daily milk intake, maternal stimulation of urination/defecation reflexes, and an environmental temperature of approximately 85°F, which the mother may help provide. Neonates should be weighed daily and their diet supplemented with commercial bitch/queen milk replacer if they fail to gain weight daily. Puppies' tails are docked and dewclaws removed at about three days of age. Depending on the breed, puppies and kittens are weaned onto a petfood/milk/water gruel between three and six weeks of age.

PUERPERAL MATERNAL DISEASES

HEMORRHAGE

Severe post-partum hemorrhage is first treated with oxytocin (5 to 20 U IM) or ergonovine maleate (0.2 mg/30 lb). If hemorrhage persists, transfusion and ovariohysterectomy must be considered (see

Subinvolution of Placental Sites). Average packed cell volumes of the normal bitch and queen at term are 30 and 28 per cent respectively.

RETAINED PLACENTA

Retained placental tissue is not uncommon in the bitch and queen, and it usually breaks down and passes as lochia without causing clinical disease. If the owner has counted placentas at parturition and knows that one or more are retained, the dam should be treated once with oxytocin (5 to 20 U IM). Use of a sponge forceps holding a gauze square inserted into the uterus and rotated so as to engage and draw out the retained placenta has been described. The bitch is then sent home without further treatment until the tissue breaks down and is passed. The owner is instructed to take the animal's rectal temperature two to three times daily and observe the character of the vaginal discharge. If elevated temperature, depression, or purulent discharge occurs, she is treated immediately for metritis.

UTERINE PROLAPSE

Prolapsed uterus is rare in the dog and cat, but it may occur at or soon after parturition; one horn may prolapse while fetuses are present in the other. Diagnosis is made by visual inspection and digital examination of the vagina. The owner is instructed to prevent drying and mutilation of the prolapsed tissue while the patient is transported to the clinic, where the uterus is replaced and retracted anteriorly via laparotomy. Recommendations have been made for surgical excision of the prolapsed tissue without laparotomy. If the broad ligament has torn the patient may be compromised by intra-abdominal bleeding.

HYPOCALCEMIA (ECLAMPSIA/PUERPERAL TETANY)

Hypocalcemia occurs most frequently in small bitches with large litters two to four weeks post partum, but it may occur in any breed or in cats at any time during lactation or even ante partum. Presenting signs include weakness and trembling and may proceed to tonic-clonic convulsions. Pulse rate and temperature are usually elevated during convulsions.

Diagnosis is based on clinical signs in a lactating female, and treatment is usually started before results of serum calcium assay (values less than 7 mg/dl are diagnostic) have been received.

Treatment includes removing the puppies/kittens for 12 to 24 hours, treating the dam (to effect) with slow IV administration of 10 per cent calcium glu-conate (usually 3 to 20 cc), and sending the dam home on 1 to 3 gm calcium lactate or gluconate and 10,000 to 25,000 U vitamin D PO daily. Recurrence in the same or subsequent lactations is common, and the young should be weaned if more than one attack occurs.

METRITIS

Metritis is a post-partum disease of bacterial origin that occurs following abortion, fetal infection, obstetric manipulations, or ascending infection following normal birth. Clinical signs include fever, foul-smelling and purulent vaginal discharge, anorexia, depression, and neglect of the neonates. Occasionally, signs of septicemia, toxemia, and shock occur.

Diagnosis is based on the presence of clinical signs and an immature leukocytosis in the hemogram. Careful abdominal palpation and radiographs may be used to rule out the presence of retained fetal tissue. The vaginal discharge should be cultured.

Treatment of metritis includes antibiotic therapy, fluid and supportive therapy if necessary, and use of drugs to evacuate the uterus. The patient is started on a broad spectrum antibiotic until culture and sensitivity testing has been completed. If the uterus is enlarged, uterine evacuation may be accomplished by administration of 5 to 20 U oxytocin IM (early post partum), two injections of 0.25 mg/kg prostaglandin $F_{2\alpha}$ SQ given 24 hours apart, or 0.2 mg/30 lb ergonovine maleate IM. Occasionally hysterotomy and uterine lavage are necessary. In general, pups/kittens may be returned to the dam after she is started on therapy if no signs of toxemia are present.

MASTITIS

Infection of the lactating mammary gland of the bitch and queen results from ascending or hematogenous bacterial infection. Coliforms, streptococci, and staphylococci are most commonly cultured from mastitic milk. Clinical signs include the presence of one or more enlarged, painful, hot, reddened mammary glands; elevated rectal temperature; and neglect of the young.

Diagnosis is based on inspection of the affected glands and a smear of the mastitic milk or on the presence of an immature leukocytosis in the hemogram and on culture and sensitivity of the mastitic milk.

Treatment of acute mastitis in the absence of abscessation or gangrene consists of the use of broad spectrum antibiotics, followed by specific antibiotics when culture results are available. Nursing may continue if the mother is on antibiotics and no abscessation or gangrene is present. Abscessed/

gangrenous tissue should be drained surgically if necessary and the tissue treated as an open wound with frequent warm soaks, standing the patient to mid abdomen in a basin or bathtub of hot water and Betadine. Puppies/kittens should be removed from mastitic mothers and fed commercial milk replacer when abscessation/gangrene is present.

SUBINVOLUTION OF PLACENTAL SITES

Post-partum subinvolution of sites of fetal placental attachment has been described in the bitch. Typical clinical signs include the presence of a serosanguineous vaginal discharge containing blood and mucus for 4 to 12 weeks post partum. Occasional bitches lose enough blood to require transfusion and ovariohysterectomy. Others show persistent scanty blood-tinged discharge for up to five months until onset of the next proestrus. This condition can be distinguished clinically from metritis by the fact that the discharge is not purulent or foul-smelling and the bitch does not appear to be systemically ill.

Diagnosis is based on clinical signs and the absence of signs of infection in a smear of the discharge. Culture of the discharge may reveal no growth or mixed vaginal flora.

Treatment is unnecessary if the bitch does not suffer severe blood loss. Ergonovine maleate (0.2 mg/30 lb, IM) may cause a decline in bleeding owing to its vasoconstrictor effects. Antibiotics may be used prophylactically, but they will not alter the course of the bleeding.

POST-PARTURIENT HYSTERIA

Post-parturient hysteria is associated with the mother's savaging of normal, healthy puppies or kittens. Most dams respond well to a low oral dose of tranquilizer given once daily in the morning.

Some breeders believe this is a manifestation of hypocalcemia and treat their bitches with injections of calcium.

AGALACTIA

Agalactia is a poorly documented disorder in the bitch and queen that should be diagnosed only after careful examination of all of the mammary glands with failure to express milk. The young should be encouraged to suckle and should be supplemented only if they fail to gain weight daily. The mother should be given food and water *ad libitum* to provide adequate fluid and calories. An oxytocin nasal spray for humans is available by prescription in pharmacies to facilitate milk letdown. It will not, however, aid in milk production.

SUPPLEMENTAL READING

Austad, R., and Bjerkas, E.: Eclampsia in the bitch. J. Small Anim. Pract. 17:793, 1976.

Beck, A. M., and McEntee, K.: Subinvolution of placental sites in a postpartum bitch. Cornell Vet. 66:269, 1966.

Devereaux, W. P.: Acute puerperal mastitis. Am. J. Obstet. Gynecol. 108:78, 1970.

Glenn, B. L.: Subinvolution of placental sites in the bitch. Paper presented at the 18th Gaines Veterinary Symposium, 7, 1968.

Gray, S. J.: A case of feline eclampsia. Austr. Vet. Pract. 5:182, 1975.

Hosek, J. J.: Syntocinon: a treatment for agalactia in the dog. V.M./S.A.C. 67:405, 1972.

Kitzman, L. M.: Endometritis and uterine rupture in a bitch. Mod. Vet. Pract. 59:535, 1978.

Marshall, B. R., Hepper, J. K., and Zirbel, C. C.: Sporadic puerperal mastitis: an infection that need not interrupt lactation. J.A.M.A. 233:1377, 1975.

Reid, J. S., and Frank, R. J.: Double contrast hysterogram in diagnosis of retained placentae in the bitch: a case report. J. Am. Anim. Hosp. Assn. 9:367, 1973.

Roudebush, P., and Wheeler, K. G.: Peracute gangrenous mastitis in a cat. Feline Pract. 9:35, 1979.

Schall, W. D., Duncan, J. R., Finco, D. R., and Knecht, C. D.: Spontaneous recovery after subinvolution of placental sites in a bitch. J.A.V.M.A. 159:1780, 1971.

THE INFERTILE STUD DOG

FRANCES SMITH, D.V.M.,
St. Paul, Minnesota

and ROLF E. LARSEN, D.V.M.
Gainesville, Florida

HISTORY

Before presentation, the clinician should request that the owner gather a complete breeding history, including numbers of females bred, number whelping, and frequency of breedings. Mating behavior should be noted, especially libido and willingness to mount. The client should also gather a complete medical history, including inherited disorders such as epilepsy and hip dysplasia. The client should be prepared to list medications administered, including steroids and reproductive hormones. Dates of negative *B. canis* serology tests should be noted. A complete history is helpful in determining whether the infertility is congenital or acquired, permanent or temporary.

SEMEN EVALUATION

Semen collection is best accomplished in the presence of a bitch in standing heat. Although an estrous teaser bitch may be used, an experienced stud dog may not deliver his optimum quality semen in this situation. The semen is best collected in an artificial vagina with a calibrated plastic centrifuge tube attached. The artificial vagina allows the clinician to assess the ability to ejaculate, the ability to copulate, and the volume of ejaculate obtained. Ordinarily, only the first two fractions of semen (the presperm and the sperm-rich) are collected for semen evaluation. The semen is evaluated for volume, color, motility, total numbers, morphology, and presence of foreign matter.

Volume. Volume may be read directly from the calibrated tube, is variable, and may range from 0.5 to more than 30 cc. Volume is greatly affected by the volume of prostatic fluid collected. There is no correlation between volume and fertility.

Color. Color of normal canine semen is opalescent to white. Canine semen is not the heavy creamy white seen in bovine semen owing to a lower concentration of sperm. Yellow semen indicates urine contamination, and red semen is due to blood, generally of prostatic origin.

Motility. A drop of semen diluted with a drop of 2.9 per cent sodium citrate or 0.9 per cent sodium chloride is placed on a warmed slide (37°C), coverslipped, and examined at 400× magnification for an estimate of progressively motile sperm. Dogs of normal fertility generally have over 80 per cent progressively motile sperm.

Total Sperm Numbers. Sperm can be counted by use of a calibrated spectrophotometer, a Coulter counter, or a hemacytometer after dilution in a commercially available dilutor kit. Sperm concentration varies tremendously because of differences in the volume of prostatic fluid collected. Total numbers of sperm per ejaculate (concentration × volume) must be determined to assess fertility. The total number of sperm in the sexually rested adult male should be at least 300×10^6. Numbers as high as 1×10^9 are sometimes encountered. The minimum insemination dose for the dog is unknown, but 100×10^6 live, normal sperm are considered necessary for routine impregnation by artificial insemination. Dogs with less than 100×10^6 live sperm are considered oligospermic.

Morphology. An accurate assessment of sperm morphology requires the use of an oil immersion objective (1000×) and an appropriate stain. Sperm are examined for primary abnormalities (head and midpiece abnormalities), which are associated with problems in the testes, and secondary abnormalities (tail abnormalities), which are associated with sperm maturation in the epididymis. A normal male will have no more than 20 per cent abnormal sperm.

PHYSICAL EXAMINATION

A complete physical examination is then performed, with special emphasis on the genitourinary and musculoskeletal systems. It is best to perform the physical examination following semen collection. The spermatic cords should be carefully palpated and their symmetry and uniformity noted. The testes should be evaluated for size, texture, and consistency; the epididymides should be examined for palpable evidence of aplasia or enlargement. The prostate is palpated per rectum for size and uniformity.

962

CLASSIFICATION OF MALE INFERTILITY

A male may be classified by history as always infertile, once fertile, and subfertile.

CONGENITAL INFERTILITY

The always infertile dog is congenitally infertile. Congenital infertility encompasses diseases that result in anatomic defects that mechanically prevent the sperm cell from reaching and moving through the penile urethra, conditions resulting in lack of sperm cell formation, and permanent functional abnormalities that result in the formation of defective spermatozoa, such as testicular hypoplasia, segmental aplasia of the deferent ducts or epididymis, bilateral cryptorchidism, chromosomal abnormalities (Klinefelter's syndrome XXY), errors in androgen metabolism, the immotile cilia syndrome, inguinal hernia, sperm cell formation defects, and behavioral or physical abnormalities resulting in the inability to mate or ejaculate.

ACQUIRED INFERTILITY

Acquired infertility may be due to testicular degeneration, a blockage in the duct system, changes in morphology or motility of sperm, or conditions that prevent mating and ejaculation. Examples include neoplasia, sperm granulomas (spermatoceles), trauma to the testes and scrotum, infections of the testes and/or epididymides, predisposition to testicular degeneration at an early age, toxic reactions, systemic or metabolic disease, improper hormone therapy, pain on ejaculation, inguinal hernia, and hormonal dysfunctions. Senile atrophy of the testes occurs commonly in males over ten years old. The American Kennel Club does not recognize litters sired by males over 12 years of age unless breeding soundness is verified by a veterinarian.

It should be noted that the common notion that a male may breed a bitch every other day indefinitely without a decrease in sperm numbers may be a misconception. Individual dogs vary widely in their ability to tolerate frequent use. Recovery may occur after a period of sexual rest.

Environmental stress may result in temporary infertility. Recovery may occur within six months. Spermatozoa are antigenic and are not recognized as self by immune-competent cells, thus disease or trauma exposing testicular tissue or spermatozoa to the immune system may result in antibody formation and the development of sensitized white blood cells. Certain strains of beagles, cocker spaniels, and corgis exhibit an autoimmune lymphocytic thyroiditis. The disease has also been associated with lymphocytic orchitis, as lymphocytic infiltrates are present throughout all portions of the testes and in the epididymis.

Any agent resulting in an inflammatory response may disrupt duct wall integrity and result in the release of spermatozoa and the accompanying foreign antigen response. Sperm granuloma may result in complete blockage of sperm to the epididymis if the granuloma occurs at the level of the efferent duct.

SUBFERTILITY

Subfertility results in very small litters or in a poor conception rate compared with other studs of the same breed. Subfertility may be due to poor breeding management or to poor fertility in the bitch. A stud dog with good libido and normal semen quality is rarely infertile. Causes of subfertility include low sperm numbers, high incidence of morphologic or motility abnormalities, and chronic prostatitis. Inguinal hernia with omentum or intestine in the scrotum may be associated with poor morphology, motility, and concentration of sperm. Semen abnormalities include proximal droplets, detached heads, and tail defects, with an incidence of greater than 20 per cent for any one defect resulting in infertility.

EPIDIDYMITIS

Bacteria, especially *Escherichia coli*, *Proteus* spp., *Streptococcus* spp., and *Staphylococcus* spp. are commonly isolated from acute suppurative epididymitis and/or orchitis. Prostatic disease is also associated with epididymitis and may be either a primary site of infection or may contribute to retrograde infections from the urinary tract. The epididymis is a specific target for *Brucella canis*, and bacteria are housed in this organ.

Distemper virus is also associated with epididymitis. During infection with distemper, a dog may lose the ability to produce any fluid during ejaculation. Neither sperm nor prostatic fluid is ejaculated.

Orchitis follows the same routes of infection as those causing epididymitis. Many of the same organisms are responsible for the infectious disease. Additionally, trauma often results in orchitis. Testicular tumors (seminomas, Sertoli cell tumors, and interstitial cell tumors) reduce sperm production and fertility.

DIAGNOSIS

Diagnosis is based on complete history and physical examination and semen evaluation. Testicular biopsy is of additional use to determine the etiology and severity of the degeneration in acquired infertility. Biopsy techniques have been previously described. These require meticulous technique and asepsis to avoid trauma. Several hormones can be assessed in the infertile dog. Serum testosterone can be measured, but owing to the wide range of values over a given day, it is difficult to associate testosterone concentration with testicular function. Thyroid function should be assessed, especially in males of low libido or low sperm production. Pituitary gonadotropins are major controlling mechanisms in spermatogenesis and testosterone production. Luteinizing hormone (LH), which controls the Leydig cells and thus testosterone production, is of interest in fertility, but a commercial assay for LH or follicle-stimulating hormone (FSH) in dogs is not available. If available, the FSH:LH ratio and response to chemical stimuli provide better diagnostic information than do basal values. Karyotyping of congenitally infertile dogs can be done at many veterinary schools and may help diagnose intersex states such as Klinefelter's syndrome (XXY).

TREATMENT

Many infectious causes of orchitis and/or epididymitis can be treated. Culture and sensitivity should indicate correct antibiotic therapy. Therapy of *B. canis* is uniformly unrewarding, and euthanasia or castration should be considered. Inguinal hernia can be repaired, with return to normal semen quality within 10 to 12 weeks. As there is a heritable component to hernia formation, herniorrhaphy for the sole purpose of return to breeding soundness involves questionable ethics.

In cases of idiopathic infertility, many hormones and old folk mixtures have been used as treatment. Occasional success occurs, but little or no documentation of success is available.

Pregnant mare's serum gonadotropin (PMSG) is the most commonly used therapy for azoospermic or oligospermic dogs. Although PMSG does have a stimulatory effect on spermatogenic cells, there have been no documented returns to fertility. Azoospermic males do not respond to PMSG; however, oligospermic males may respond to 200 to 500 IU PMSG IV at three- to six-day intervals. FSH at 25 mg SQ once weekly has also been used. In human medicine, clomiphene citrate has been used at a dose of 25 mg/day for 25 days; the patient is then rested for 5 days and then treatment is reinstituted. In men without elevated FSH levels, semen quality improved and pregnancies resulted. Comparable work has not been done in the dog. Testosterone cannot be used to improve spermatogenesis. Hormones that combine FSH and LH activity are often used with questionable results. Human chorionic gonadotropin (HCG) may be used if LH activity is desired. HCG is antigenic, but antibodies against it are not as likely to cross react with the dog's endogenous LH as are pituitary LH products.

In humans, synthetic androgens such as mesterolone and fluoxymesterone have been used with improvements in sperm motility.

PROGNOSIS

In general, azoospermic males remain azoospermic despite therapy. Prognosis is related to the etiology of the condition. The prognosis is very guarded for return or acquisition of fertility in an infertile male.

SUPPLEMENTAL READING

Evans, J., and Renton, J. P.: A case of azoospermia in a previously fertile dog with subsequent recovery. Vet. Rec. 92:198, 1973.

Fritz, T. E., Lombard, L. S., Tyler, S. A., et al.: Pathology and familial incidence of orchitis and its relationship to thyroiditis in a closed Beagle colony. Exp. Morphol. Pathol. 24:142, 1976.

Hadley, J. C.: Spermatogenic arrest with azoospermia in two Welsh Springer Spaniels. J. Small Anim. Pract. 13:135, 1972.

Harrop, A. E.: The infertile male dog. J. Small Anim. Pract. 7:723, 1966.

Larsen, R. E.: Evaluation of fertility problems in the male dog. Vet. Clin. North Am. 7:735, 1977.

Larsen, R. E.: Testicular biopsy in the dog. Vet. Clin. North Am. 7:747, 1977.

Mauss, J., Mohnfeld, G., and Borsch, G.: Synthetic L.H. releasing factor and clomiphene stimulation in oligospermic males with normal FSH excretion. J. Reprod. Fertil. 40:171, 1974.

Paulson, D. F., Wacksman, J., Hammond, C. B., and Wiebe, H. R.: Hypofertility and clomiphene citrate therapy. Fertil. Steril. 26:982, 1975.

Roberts, S. J.: Veterinary Obstetrics and Genital Disease. Ann Arbor, MI: Edwards Brothers, Inc., 1971.

Taha, M. B., Noakes, D. E., and Allen, W. E.: The effects of some exogenous hormones on seminal characteristics, libido and peripheral plasma testosterone concentrations in the male Beagle. J. Small Anim. Pract. 22:587, 1981.

Wright, P. J., Stelmasiak, T., Black, D., and Syber, D.: Medroxyprogesterone acetate and reproductive processes in male dogs. Austr. Vet. J. 55:437, 1979.

Continued

Diseases of the Lower Urinary Tract

Diseases of the Kidneys

IMMUNE-MEDIATED RENAL DISEASE

RICHARD C. SCOTT, D.V.M.

New York, New York

Diseases of the kidney can be caused by abnormalities of the immune system. Collectively, two major categories have been described: glomerulonephritis (GN) and immune-mediated tubulointerstitial disease. In immune-mediated GN the initial target of damage is the glomeruli. Once severe damage occurs, reduced perfusion through peritubular capillaries causes ischemic damage to the tubules and interstitium. In tubulointerstitial disorders, the initial insult is directed at the tubules, with subsequent involvement of glomeruli.

GLOMERULONEPHRITIS

PATHOGENESIS

Reports show that three major mechanisms may result in GN. With the first, antibodies produced by B-lymphocytes react with antigens located in glomerular basement membranes (GBM). This form of anti-GBM glomerulonephritis is typified by Goodpasture's syndrome, a disorder in which antibodies are formed against lung basement membrane antigens following respiratory disease. These antibodies cross react with kidney GBM to cause progressive GN (Lewis et al., 1971). Anti-GBM disease has been reported in horses in association with equine infectious anemia (Banks and Henson, 1972) and may occur in dogs (Osborne et al., 1977).

With the second mechanism, B-lymphocytes form antibodies against circulating soluble antigens. If an insufficient amount of antibody is produced so that immune complexes are formed in antigen excess, soluble, biologically active immune complexes are formed that may induce immune injury. If they become trapped in glomerular capillary walls, they may initiate GN. This is a common form of GN in human patients (Wilson, 1977). It is recognized that the size, solubility, and biologic activity of immune complexes are determined by a number of factors (Barnett et al., 1979; Inman and Day, 1981). The concentration and valence of antibodies and antigens are especially important. Insoluble, biologically inactive complexes are formed when multivalent antibodies and antigens interact at equivalence or in antibody excess. Very small and less active complexes are formed with a large excess of antigen, especially when such antigens are monovalent.

Cell-mediated immunity may be important in initiating immune complex GN, especially in human patients with systemic lupus erythematosus (SLE) (Schwartz, 1981). T-lymphocytes exist in two major subsets: helper T-lymphocytes and suppressor T-lymphocytes. Each subset has different functions that regulate the activity of antibody-producing B-lymphocytes. Dysfunction of suppressor T-lymphocytes has been theorized to cause excessive antibody production by B-lymphocytes in immune complex GN. According to one theory, deficiency of the number and/or function of suppressor T-lymphocytes unleashes B-lymphocytes to produce antibody. In a second theory, B-lymphocytes are unresponsive to the regulatory signals of normal T-lymphocytes. Finally, a theory has been advanced wherein "outlaw" B-lymphocytes produce antibodies directed against suppressor T-lymphocytes. Subsequent interaction with these antibodies impairs suppressor T-lymphocyte activity, which results in the unleashing of additional B-lymphocytes to produce antibody. T-lymphocytes have also been implicated in the production of lymphokines, which are toxic to the GBM in minimal change nephrotic syndrome in humans (Shalhoub, 1974).

Immune complex GN has been well-documented in animals (Osborne et al., 1973, 1977; Slauson and Lewis, 1979). Various morphologic classes of GN have been described including membranoproliferative GN (Osborne et al., 1973; Slauson and Lewis, 1979) and membranous GN (Osborne et al., 1973; Slauson and Lewis, 1979; Wright et al., 1981). Less commonly reported morphologic classes include mesangial proliferative GN (Murray and Wright, 1974) and sclerosing GN (Slauson and Lewis, 1979).

The third mechanism that may produce GN is similar to the second and thus far has been recognized primarily in experimental forms of GN (Couser et al., 1978; Teusher and Donaldson, 1979). In this mechanism there is local formation of antibody-antigen complexes in tissues. Fixed antigen is present in the GBM. Circulating antibody is filtered and combines with fixed antigen, resulting in immune complex formation and damage. The importance of this mechanism in naturally occurring GN in humans and animals requires further clarification (Douglas et al., 1981; Naruse et al., 1973).

ETIOLOGY

Antigens in the proper concentration relative to antibodies are necessary to produce GN. Identification of specific antigens and/or recognition of alterations or abnormalities in humoral and/or cellular immunity may permit identification of the cause of GN. Unfortunately, such abnormalities have not been recognized in most naturally occurring forms of GN. Most cases are therefore referred to as idiopathic GN.

Idiopathic membranous GN (Osborne et al., 1973; Slauson and Lewis, 1979; Wright et al., 1981) has been reported in dogs and cats. Idiopathic membranoproliferative GN has also been reported in dogs (Osborne et al., 1977; Slauson and Lewis, 1979) and cats (Slauson and Lewis, 1979). Membranous GN has been reported in association with *Dirofilaria immitis* infection in dogs (Casey and Splitter, 1975), with SLE in dogs and cats (Osborne et al., 1973; Slauson and Lewis, 1979), and with leukemia in cats (Osborne et al., 1977; Slauson and Lewis, 1979). Membranoproliferative GN has been reported in dogs with pyometra (Obel et al., 1964) and SLE (Osborne et al., 1973; Slauson and Lewis, 1979). Specific antigens have been linked to membranoproliferative GN in sheep with *Vibrio fetus,* in horses with equine infectious anemia, and in swine with African swine fever (Slauson and Lewis, 1979). The other less commonly seen forms of GN that have been reported are idiopathic (Slauson and Lewis, 1979).

CLINICAL SIGNS AND LABORATORY FINDINGS

Glomerular damage caused by immune mechanisms result in at least two major abnormalities. Changes in glomerular morphology and ultrastructure produce various morphologic forms of GN. In addition, changes in the normal electrical charge of glomerular walls alter their selective permeability to various solutes. Normal glomeruli have a fixed negative charge, which is important in the maintenance of normal glomerular permeability to anionic molecules such as albumin (Hunsicker et al., 1981). This negative charge is generated primarily by glycosialic acids called glomerular polyanion (GPA). In GN, loss of GPA results in loss of albumin in urine. In addition to loss of charge-dependent permeability, a change in pore size results from loss of GPA (Hunsicker et al., 1981). This can lead to loss of globulins in urine. Loss of GPA is also associated with epithelial foot process fusion commonly associated with proteinuria (Hunsicker et al., 1981).

The hallmark of GN is sustained albuminuria.

The magnitude of albuminuria may vary during the course of disease; however, large amounts of albumin are usually present in urine. Varying degrees of albuminuria persist even during resolution of glomerular lesions. In randomly collected urine samples the magnitude of albuminuria varies from trace to more than 1000 mg/dl. However, disorders other than GN can cause albuminuria and should be considered when interpreting the significance of proteinuria. Nonglomerular forms of proteinuria include hematuria and pyuria resulting from urinary tract infection, hematuria following urinary tract trauma, fever, and congestive heart failure. Twenty four–hour urine samples obtained from animals with GN typically reveal albumin excretion above the normal level of 150 to 200 mg (Barsanti and Finco, 1979). It is our experience that most animals with GN produce in excess of 0.75 gm of protein in 24 hours.

Concomitant low serum albumin concentrations associated with proteinuria support a diagnosis of GN. Since serum albumin can wax and wane throughout the course of GN, some animals have normal serum albumin concentrations for long periods. The severity of hypoalbuminemia is determined by disease activity and albumin synthesis by the liver, which can match or exceed urinary losses for variable periods of time. Cachexia and anorexia may also influence the magnitude of hypoalbuminemia.

When the degree of hypoalbuminemia is severe (below 1 gm/dl), edema can occur. Proteinuria, hypoproteinemia, hypoalbuminemia, and edema are collectively termed the nephrotic syndrome. This syndrome is frequently associated with hypercholesterolemia. Edema is caused primarily by loss of plasma osmotic pressure owing to hypoalbuminemia, but other factors are also involved. Edema can undergo remission and exacerbation during the course of GN. Some animals never develop edema. The reader is referred to an excellent discussion of these factors in *Current Veterinary Therapy VII* (pages 1053–1062).

When evaluating patients with GN, a search for antigens should be initiated. Antinuclear antibody (ANA) and microfilaria (millipore technique) tests should be done, and thoracic and abdominal radiography should be performed. The ANA test is convenient for detecting SLE, whereas the microfilaria test and thoracic radiographs are diagnostic for heartworm disease. Thoracic and abdominal radiography can also give information about the presence of neoplasia or pyometra. If heartworms are suspected, a heartworm antibody test should be performed. In cats suspected of having GN, a feline leukemia virus test is indicated. Appropriate cultures and serologic tests should be done if bacterial or viral infection is suspected. If the ANA test is negative it should be repeated every two to four months. In some animals with SLE the results of the SLE test are initially negative but subsequently become positive as the disease progresses.

Less specific clinical and laboratory findings that may occur in dogs and cats with GN are related to uremia, which can occur in animals after progression to end-stage GN. Hematuria and red blood casts are rare in dogs and cats with GN.

DIAGNOSIS

Although results of clinical and laboratory testing may aid in the diagnosis of GN, detection of the underlying cause usually requires renal biopsy. Histologic examination of biopsy specimens by light microscopy using special stains typically reveals glomerular morphology consistent with one of the various types of GN. This confirms the diagnosis. Detection of ultrastructural abnormalities typical of those found in GN provides further confirmation. Immunofluorescent microscopy may permit identification of immune complex or anti-GBM GN.

THERAPY

If specific antigens known to cause GN have been identified (e.g., *D. immitis*, neoplasia, pyometra), appropriate steps should be taken to eliminate them. It is emphasized, however, that a persistent abnormality in humoral or cellular immunity may result in recurrence of GN with any of a variety of antigens that normally do not cause immune-mediated injury. Amyloidosis should be eliminated from the differential diagnosis of GN.

Specific treatment of mild edema may not be necessary; however, in my opinion severe edema should be controlled inasmuch as more than mild accumulation of fluid beneath the skin may produce discomfort. Diuretics may be used for this purpose. The loop diuretics are satisfactory, particularly furosemide (Lasix*). The initial dosage is 2.2 to 4.4 mg/kg, b.i.d. to t.i.d., PO, IV, or IM. Oral medication at this dosage can be continued for up to 14 days or until the animal is free of edema. Thereafter, the dosage should be gradually tapered to alternate-day therapy for 14 days. If this dosage is sufficient to maintain the animal free of edema, the dosage can be reduced to every third day for 14 days. If the animal is still edema free, furosemide can be discontinued. The same dosage schedule can be used if relapse occurs. If edema persistently recurs, then lower dose, alternate-, or every-third-day therapy can be maintained for long periods of time without ill effect. Periodic re-examination is indicated to determine any need for dosage change. In the process of controlling edema with diuretics, care must be exercised not to further compromise

blood vascular volume, which is already compromised as a result of reduction in colloidal osmotic pressure.

Broad spectrum systemic antibiotics should be administered during episodes of severe edema, since infections tend to be more common with edema. We prefer to use drugs that can be administered orally so that treatment can be continued at home until the edema is resolved.

A high-quality protein diet should be given to replace persistent urinary protein loss unless contraindicated by severe uremia. Many animals with GN are intermittently anorexic, which aggravates hypoproteinemia unless a high-quality protein diet is given. If signs of uremia worsen while the animal is consuming a high-protein diet, the amount of dietary protein should be reduced.

If dehydration associated with uremia is encountered, an appropriate amount of parenteral fluid should be administered. The total amount of fluid administered per 24 hours must be monitored closely to prevent exacerbation of edema. When hypoalbuminemia and edema are present, the extracellular fluid compartment is contracted because fluid is lost from the plasma space into the tissues. In this situation, diuretics should be administered with fluids so that parenteral fluids do not move from the extracellular compartment into tissues, aggravating edema. In this fashion a better fluid balance may be achieved while the effective extracellular space is adequately restored. The total quantity of parenteral fluids may be estimated by skin turgor provided edema does not preclude this evaluation. The principles used in estimating the quantity of fluid necessary to replace deficits are identical to those conventionally used for nonedematous dehydrated animals.

In addition to deficit fluid replacement, total daily fluid replacement volume should include a sufficient quantity to provide for insensible fluid loss (22 ml/kg/day) and urine output. The latter is either measured continuously, or estimated from representative hourly urine volumes. If edema occurs or worsens during fluid therapy, fluid volume should be reduced appropriately and diuretics should either be administered or increased in dosage (if already being given). The choice of fluid is dependent on the presence or absence of edema. If edema is present, the fluid should be isotonic but lower in sodium than normal saline. Hypotonic fluids should be avoided, since they further dilute the effective extracellular fluid compartment and aggravate fluid loss into tissues. Hypertonic saline solutions should not be used, since sodium retention can aggravate fluid retention. The best fluids are Ringer's lactate or other balanced isotonic solutions (e.g., Plasma-Lyte†).

---

*Hoechst-Roussel Pharmaceuticals Inc., Somerville, NJ.

†Travenol Laboratories, Inc., Deerfield, IL.

Other general supportive measures that may be considered in animals with or without edema include administration of B vitamins, rest, and avoidance of stress. If edema is present, it is advisable to avoid administration of large quantities of oral medications containing sodium.

Immunosuppressive therapy may be considered after a diagnosis of GN is established by renal biopsy and an immune-mediated mechanism is documented or strongly suspected. Such therapy remains controversial in veterinary clinical practice (Osborne and Jeraj, 1980). The immune-mediated nature of most GN in animals has been established (Osborne et al., 1977; Slauson and Lewis, 1979; Wright et al., 1981). It is conceivable that suppression of the immune system with drugs can aggravate the disease by creating a greater excess of antigen and thus more biologically active immune complexes capable of fixing complement and causing damage to glomeruli. In addition, it is possible that clearance of immune complexes by the reticuloendothelial system could be impaired by immunosuppressive therapy. Although these possibilities exist, it is also possible that immunosuppressive therapy can cause formation of smaller, less biologically active immune complexes by creating a large antigen excess as antibody formation is suppressed. There is growing evidence that some forms of GN in human patients respond to immunosuppressive treatment. Such patients frequently have rapidly progressive, proliferative GN (Bolton and Couser, 1979; Kimberly et al., 1981; O'Neil et al., 1979; Oredugba et al., 1980). Recently, human patients with chronic forms of GN have responded to immunosuppressive therapy (Collaborative Study, 1979; Jarrett et al., 1981). The salutary effects of corticosteroids in the management of lipoid nephrosis of children have also been reported (Cameron, 1975).

It therefore is justifiable to consider a trial of immunosuppressive therapy in animals with GN; however, care must be exercised in choosing patients for such a trial. There must be strong evidence that immune-mediated disease is present and that immunosuppressive therapy has a potential for success. Patients likely to develop serious complications at the outset of immunosuppressive therapy are not good candidates. Therefore, pneumonia, sepsis, and bone marrow suppression should be treated prior to treatment with immunosuppressive agents. Therapy is only indicated when results of biopsy suggest that the glomerular lesions are reversible. If results of renal function tests worsen after biopsy has been performed and there is no evidence that a second renal disease is the cause of deterioration, the potential value of a trial of immunosuppressive therapy is further supported.

It is difficult to site guidelines for the treatment of canine and feline GN with immunosuppressive drugs, inasmuch as no clinical trials have been reported. The following recommendations are based on clinical observations at the Animal Medical Center. A trial of therapy should include appropriate follow-up evaluations to determine the outcome of treatment.

Oral prednisone therapy can be initiated at a dosage of 2.2 mg/kg body weight divided b.i.d. This dosage should be continued for four weeks. Thereafter the dosage should be reduced by 50 per cent every two weeks until a dosage of 0.12 mg/kg body weight divided b.i.d. is reached. Determinations of 24-hour urinary albumin excretion and serum albumin and creatinine concentrations should be obtained at least 4 and 12 weeks following initiation of therapy. Endogenous creatinine clearance can also be calculated if urine creatinine concentration is determined.

Complete response to therapy is defined as diminution in 24-hour albumin excretion to less than 150 mg. A partial response is defined as diminution to 150 to 750 mg. A rise in serum albumin concentration should be expected in either case. In addition, abnormal serum creatinine and urea nitrogen concentrations and endogenous creatinine clearance may stabilize or improve. If complete or partial response is observed, these evaluations (serum electrophoresis, 24-hour albumin excretion, serum creatinine, and, optionally, endogenous creatinine clearance) should be repeated about every four to six months or more frequently if necessary. Recurrence of GN should prompt consideration of a second trial of corticosteroid therapy.

Lack of response is defined as little or no diminution in 24-hour albumin excretion (> 750 mg). In such an event the serum albumin concentration will frequently remain abnormally low, and azotemia may gradually or quickly become more severe. If no response is observed, further corticosteroid therapy is inadvisable.

During prednisone therapy animals should be given antacids (Amphogel*) to prevent gastric ulcer formation. Antacid therapy should be continued for the first six to eight weeks of glucocorticoid therapy. It may be discontinued thereafter.

The dosage of prednisone should be reduced rapidly if serious complications develop. These include severe symptomatic uremia with escalating serum creatinine and urea nitrogen values, manifestations of iatrogenic Cushing's syndrome (including severe myopathy and thromboembolism), psychotic manifestations of steroid administration (such as panting and alopecia induced by fur chewing), and bleeding from gastrointestinal ulcers. If one or more of these complications occur, the dosage of prednisone should be reduced by 50 per cent every three to five days to a dosage of 0.12 mg/kg body weight divided b.i.d. This dosage should be main-

---

*Wyeth Laboratories, Philadelphia, PA.

tained on alternate days for two weeks, after which time prednisone should be discontinued.

If rapidly progressive proliferative GN is encountered, administration of a combination of other immunosuppressive agents with prednisone may be considered. However, the use of such drug combinations has not been very successful in humans (Cameron, 1975). We have had insufficient experience with a combination of prednisone and azathioprine (Imuran*) to recommend specific protocols and dosage regimens. Preliminary trials of IV pulse doses of methylprednisolone given to human patients with rapidly progressive GN have yielded promising results, but long-term trials are still needed (Bolton and Couser, 1979; Kimberly et al., 1981; O'Neil et al., 1979; Oredugba et al., 1980). This form of therapy has not been evaluated in dogs or cats with GN.

Anticoagulants (e.g., heparin and warfarin), antiplatelet drugs (dipyridamole and indomethacin), and anti-inflammatory agents (prednisone and azathioprine) have been used in combination to treat aggressive forms of GN in human patients with some beneficial results (Cameron, 1975). However, the long-term outcome of such treatment awaits further investigation. This form of therapy has not been evaluated in animals.

Plasmapheresis has been reported to offer promise for rapidly progressive forms of GN in humans (Lockwood et al., 1979). The rationale for this treatment is that plasma exchange removes immune complexes and perhaps other, as yet unidentified, factors that impair the normal clearance of immune complexes by the reticuloendothelial system. Even though plasmapheresis induces only a transient decline in immune complex concentrations in human patients, they remain in clinical remission as these concentrations return to pretreatment values. Thus, some further unidentified correction of reticuloendothelial function may occur (Lockwood et al., 1979). For further information, consult the article on plasmapheresis in this textbook (page 442).

IMMUNE-MEDIATED TUBULOINTERSTITIAL RENAL DISEASE

PATHOGENESIS

Immune-mediated tubulointerstitial lesions have been produced experimentally in animals and have been identified in humans (McCluskey and Colvin, 1978). Three major mechanisms have been shown to cause such lesions. One involves the production of antibodies directed against tubular basement membrane (TBM) antigens (McCluskey and Colvin,

---

*Burroughs Wellcome Co., Research Triangle Park, NC.

1978). This form of anti-TBM disease has been reported in human patients with Goodpasture's syndrome, in which antibodies cross react with antigens in the GBM and TBM (McPhaul and Dixon, 1970). In addition, human anti-TBM antibodies and interstitial nephritis have been reported in association with immune complex GN following exposure to methicillin and diphenylhydantoin, following renal transplantation, and in association with idiopathic interstitial nephritis (McCluskey and Colvin, 1978).

Another mechanism involves the formation of immune complexes that accumulate in TBM. They remain there because of saturation of normal mechanisms for immune complex removal. Another possible mechanism involves the local formation of immune complexes (McCluskey and Colvin, 1978). In humans, this localized formation of immune complexes has been reported in patients with SLE and idiopathic interstitial nephritis and following renal transplantation (McCluskey and Colvin, 1978).

The third mechanism involves T-lymphocytes and cell-mediated immunity, both of which have been reported to induce experimental disease (McCluskey and Colvin, 1978). It is suspected that this mechanism is associated with naturally occurring renal diseases in humans including pyelonephritis and renal failure induced by methicillin and penicillin (McCluskey and Colvin, 1978).

Results of experiments in laboratory animals and studies of naturally occurring disease in humans suggest that immune-mediated mechanisms may be a cause of naturally occurring chronic tubulointerstitial disease (CTID) in dogs and cats. Further studies, however, are required to prove this hypothesis.

ETIOLOGY

No etiologic agents have been identified in naturally occurring immune-mediated tubulointerstitial renal disease in dogs and cats. However, it is noteworthy that this disorder may be readily induced in laboratory animals (McCluskey and Colvin, 1978).

CLINICAL SIGNS, LABORATORY FINDINGS, AND THERAPY

The clinical signs and laboratory findings of CTID have been described in detail in *Current Veterinary Therapy VII* (pages 1076–1079).

Inasmuch as no clinically recognized forms of immune-mediated CTID have been reported, recommendations cannot be made regarding immunosuppressive therapy. Treatment of uremia resulting from CTID of the kidney has been discussed in *Current Veterinary Therapy VII* (pages 1076–1079).

REFERENCES AND SUPPLEMENTAL READING

Banks, K. L., and Henson, J. B.: Immunologically mediated glomerulitis of horses. II. Antiglomerular basement membrane antibody and other mechanisms in spontaneous disease. Lab. Invest. 26:708, 1972.

Barnett, E. V., Knutson, D. W., Abrass, K. C., et al.: Circulating immune complexes: Their immunochemistry, detection and importance. Ann. Intern. Med. 91:430, 1979.

Barsanti, J. A., and Finco, D. R.: Protein concentration in urine of normal dogs. Am. J. Vet. Res. 40:1583, 1979.

Bolton, W. K., and Couser, W. G.: Intravenous pulse methylprednisolone therapy of acute crescentic rapidly progressive glomerulonephritis. Am. J. Med. 66:495, 1979.

Cameron, J. S.: Drug treatment of chronic glomerulonephritis. Kidney 8:14, 1975.

Casey, H. W., and Splitter, G. A.: Membranous glomerulonephritis in dogs infected with Dirofilaria immitis. Vet. Pathol. 12:111, 1975.

Collaborative Study of the Adult Idiopathic Nephrotic Syndrome. A controlled study of short-term prednisone treatment in adults with membranous nephropathy. N. Engl. J. Med. 301:1301, 1979.

Couser, W. G., Steinmuller, D. R., Stilmant, M. M., et al.: Experimental glomerulonephritis in the isolated perfused rat kidney. J. Clin. Invest. 62:1275, 1978.

Douglas, M. F., Rabideau, D. P., Schwartz, M. M., et al.: Evidence for autologous immune complex nephritis. N. Engl. J. Med. 305:1326, 1981.

Hunsicker, L. G., Schearer, T. P., and Shaffer, S. J.: Acute reversible proteinuria induced by infusion of the polycation hexadimethrine. Kidney Int. 20:7, 1981.

Inman, R. D., and Day, N. K.: Immunologic and clinical aspects of immune complex disease. Am. J. Med. 70:1097, 1981.

Jarrett, M. P., Sablay, L. B., Walter, L., et al.: The effect of continuous normalization of serum hemolytic complement on the course of lupus nephritis. Am. J. Med. 70:1067, 1981.

Kimberly, R. P., Lockshin, M. D., Sherman, R. L., et al.: High dose intravenous methylprednisolone pulse therapy in systemic lupus erythematosus. Am. J. Med. 70:817, 1981.

Lewis, E. J., Cavallo, T., Harrington, J. T., et al.: An immunopathologic study of rapidly progressive glomerulonephritis in the adult. Human Pathol. 2:185, 1971.

Lockwood, C. M., Worlledge, S., Nicholas, A., et al.: Reversal of impaired splenic function in patients with nephritis or vasculitis (or both) by plasma exchange. N. Engl. J. Med. 300:524, 1979.

McCluskey, R. T., and Colvin, R. B.: Immunologic aspects of renal tubular and interstitial disease. Ann. Rev. Med. 29:191, 1978.

McPhaul, J. J., and Dixon, F. J.: Characterization of human antiglomerular basement membrane antibodies elevated from glomerulonephritic kidneys. J. Clin. Invest. 49:308, 1970.

Murray, M., and Wright, N. G.: A morphologic study of canine glomerulonephritis. Lab. Invest. 30:213, 1974.

Naruse, T., Kitamura, K., Miyakawa, Y., et al.: Deposition of renal tubular epithelial antigen along the glomerular capillary walls of patients with membranous glomerulonephritis. J. Immunol. 110:1163, 1973.

Obel, A. L., Nicander, L., and Asheim, A.: Light and electron microscopal studies of the renal lesion in dogs with pyometra. Acta Vet. Scand. 5:146, 1964.

O'Neil, W. M., Jr., Etheridge, W. B., and Bloomer, H. A.: High dose corticosteroids: Their use in treating idiopathic rapidly progressive glomerulonephritis. Arch. Intern. Med. 139:514, 1979.

Oredugba, O., Mazumdar, D. C., Meyer, J. S., et al.: Pulse methylprednisolone therapy in idiopathic, rapidly progressive glomerulonephritis. Ann. Intern. Med. 92:504, 1980.

Osborne, C. A., Hammer, R. F., Stevens, J. B., Resnick, J. S., and Michael, A. F.: The glomerulus in health and disease: a comparative review of domestic animals and man. Adv. Vet. Sci. Comp. Med. 21:207, 1977.

Osborne, C. A., and Jeraj, K.: Glomerulonephropathy and the nephrotic syndrome. In Kirk, R. W. (ed.): Current Veterinary Therapy VII. Philadelphia: W. B. Saunders, 1980, pp. 1053–1062.

Osborne, C. A., Stevens, J. B., McLean, R., et al.: Membranous lupus glomerulonephritis in a dog. J. Am. Anim. Hosp. Assoc. 9:295, 1973.

Osborne, C. A., and Vernier, R. L.: Glomerulonephritis in the dog and cat. A comparative review. J. Am. Anim. Hosp. Assoc. 9:101, 1973.

Schwartz, R. S.: Immunologic and genetic aspects of systemic lupus erythematosus. Kidney Int. 19:474, 1981.

Scott, R. C.: Chronic tubular-interstitial disease of the kidney. In Kirk, R. W. (ed.): Current Veterinary Therapy VII. Philadelphia: W. B. Saunders, 1980, pp. 1076–1079.

Shalhoub, R. J.: Pathogenesis of lipoid nephrosis: A disorder of T-cell function. Lancet 2:556, 1974.

Slauson, D. O., and Lewis, R. N.: Comparative pathology of glomerulonephritis in animals. Vet. Pathol. 16:135, 1979.

Teuscher, C., and Donaldson, D. M.: The deposition and formulation of immune complexes in collagenous tissues. Clin. Immunol. Immunopathol. 13:56, 1979.

Wilson, C. B.: Recent advances in the immunological aspects of renal disease. Fed. Proc. 36:1271, 1977.

Wright, N. G., Nash, A. S., and Cornwell, H. J.: Experimental canine adenovirus glomerulonephritis: persistence of glomerular lesions after oral challenge. Br. J. Exp. Pathol. 62:183, 1981.

RENAL DYSPLASIA IN LHASA APSO AND SHIH-TZU DOGS

CARL A. OSBORNE, D.V.M.,
and TIMOTHY D. O'BRIEN, D.V.M.

St. Paul, Minnesota

Clinical observations of veterinarians and breeders throughout the United States during the past 15 years indicate the widespread occurrence of a potentially life-threatening progressive, chronic irreversible generalized renal disease in Lhasa apso and Shih-Tzu dogs. Both breeds have been incorporated into this discussion because of the similarity of their physical appearance and genealogy and because the renal disorder appears to be identical in each.

Pending further studies, the renal disorder in young dogs of these breeds has been called *renal dysplasia*. Renal dysplasia is defined as malformation of the kidneys marked by microscopic abnormalities variously attributed to developmental arrest or failure to differentiate, with persistence of fetal structures, mesonephric tissue, or both.

CLINICAL FEATURES

SEX AND AGE

This disorder affects male and female dogs. In a retrospective survey of 21 Lhasa apso and 14 Shih-

Table 1. *Summary of Age Data* of 21 Lhasa Apsos and 14 Shih-Tzus with Chronic Progressive Generalized Renal Disease at the Time of Diagnosis*

	Lhasa Apso	Shih-Tzu
Mean	13	9.6
Mode	6	6
Median	6	6
Range	0.75–60	1–36

*In months.

Tzu dogs with clinical evidence of renal dysfunction evaluated at the University of Minnesota, most were immature or young adults at the time of diagnosis (Table 1). Of 20 affected Lhasa apso dogs for which the age at diagnosis was recorded, 16 were less than 18 months old. None were older than five years of age. Of 12 affected Shih-Tzu dogs for which age at diagnosis was recorded, 11 were less than 12 months old. None were older than three years of age.

HISTORY AND PHYSICAL EXAMINATION

In our series of symptomatic dogs, the most commonly reported clinical abnormalities were vomiting, polydipsia, weight loss, and diarrhea. Less frequently observed signs were polyuria, anorexia, dehydration, and depression. Other abnormalities that were detected in some dogs included pale mucous membranes, small irregular kidneys detected by abdominal palpation, and ascites. No individual dog developed the entire spectrum of clinical abnormalities.

LABORATORY FINDINGS

Common laboratory abnormalities observed at the time of diagnosis in our series included nonregenerative anemia, azotemia, and impaired ability to concentrate urine despite dehydration. Less common abnormalities included hyperphosphatemia, hypocalcemia, metabolic acidosis, hypoproteinemia, hypercholesterolemia, hyperamylasemia, and mild hyperkalemia. Two dogs were mildly hypercalcemic. Proteinuria and glucosuria (characteristic features of familial renal disease in Norwegian elkhounds, so-called renal cortical hypoplasia of cocker spaniels, and familial renal disease of Samoyeds) were not commonly observed in affected Lhasa apsos and Shih-Tzus.

RADIOGRAPHIC FINDINGS

The kidneys are usually of normal size during earlier phases of renal dysplasia. In our studies, chronic renal failure was typically associated with bilateral reduction in renal size detected by survey and/or contrast radiography (Fig. 1). The surface

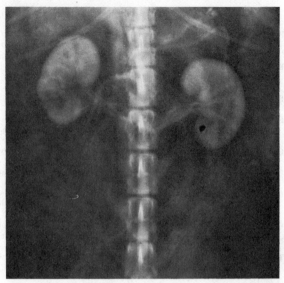

Figure 1. Ventrodorsal view of the abdomen of a one-year-old male Lhasa apso with renal dysplasia. Radiographs obtained approximately ten seconds after injection of radiopaque contrast material reveal that both kidneys are small and have thin cortices. Note poor opacification of the caudal pole of the right kidney. The serum urea nitrogen concentration was 27 mg/dl. (Courtesy of Dr. Daniel A. Feeney, College of Veterinary Medicine, University of Minnesota.)

contour of the kidneys was sometimes irregular. Varying degrees of skeletal demineralization associated with renal osteodystrophy were also detected.

GROSS AND MICROSCOPIC FINDINGS

Gross and microscopic lesions of dogs evaluated in our series were typical of chronic generalized irreversible progressive renal disease. Gross lesions were characterized by small kidneys, irregular capsular surfaces, thin cortices, and capsular adhesions. Polysystemic lesions consistent with chronic renal failure included gastritis, uremic mineralization, osteodystrophy, and enlarged parathyroid glands. Less frequently observed lesions included ascites, hepatomegaly, and renal cortical cysts.

Microscopic lesions of varying degrees are seen in various severely affected components of nephrons in the cortex and medulla. Renal cortical lesions were often segmental in distribution (Fig. 2); medullary lesions were consistently diffuse and generally more severe than those in the cortex. The segmental distribution of lesions in many dogs was suggestive of interruption of blood supply, apparently at the level of glomeruli. Lesions in both the renal cortex and medulla resulted in destruction of nephrons, with subsequent replacement with collagenous connective tissue.

Glomeruli. Glomerular atrophy and fetal glomeruli were characteristic microscopic lesions. Other glomerular lesions included mild, focal, seg-

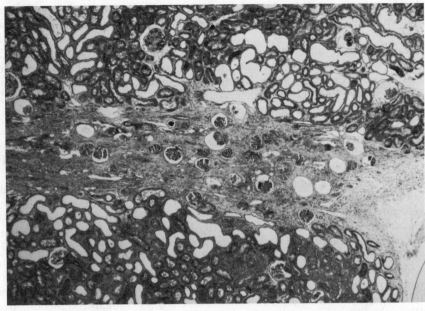

Figure 2. Photomicrograph of the renal cortex of a two-year-old female Lhasa apso with renal dysplasia, illustrating segmental distribution of lesions. Note shrunken glomeruli surrounded by collagenous connective tissue and absence of inflammatory cells. Trichrome stain × 125. (Reprinted with permission from O'Brien et al.: J.A.V.M.A. in press.)

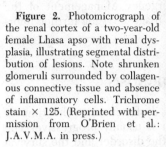

mental glomerular basement membrane thickening; hypercellularity; decreased capillary lumen size; and sclerosis. Decreased glomerular number, thickened Bowman's capsules, and mineralization of Bowman's capsules were also observed in some kidneys. Glomerular lesions, especially atrophy, were most severe in segmental areas of cortical interstitial fibrosis.

Tubules. Tubular lesions were characterized by moderate to severe tubular dilatation, tubular basement membrane mineralization, decreased tubular numbers, and flattened epithelium. Cortical tubular lesions were most severe in zones of segmental interstitial fibrosis.

Interstitium. Diffuse interstitial fibrosis was the most commonly observed lesion in the medulla and was typically severe. Diffuse infiltrates of interstitial mononuclear cells were conspicuously absent.

Vessels. Renal arteries were generally normal; however, intimal or medial calcification and adventitial fibrosis were observed in some cases. Afferent and efferent arterioles in severely affected areas of the cortex occasionally had hyalinized or thickened hypercellular walls.

ETIOPATHOGENESIS

The etiology of renal dysplasia in young Lhasa apso and Shih-Tzu dogs cannot be ascertained from available clinical, laboratory, radiographic, and light microscopic findings. Sufficient data are available to exclude primary hypercalcemia, bacterial and mycotic infections, obstruction to urine outflow, renal amyloidosis, and neoplasia as primary causes, however. Although the numbers of nephrons in affected dogs' kidneys at the time of death from uremia were

reduced, gross and microscopic lesions suggest that this was an acquired rather than a congenital phenomenon. The underlying disorder is not renal cortical hypoplasia. Similar observations have been reported in young Norwegian elkhounds with chronic, irreversible generalized renal disease.

There is a general consensus of opinion that renal dysplasia in young Lhasa apso and Shih-Tzu dogs is the most common (but not the only) renal disorder of these breeds. The high incidence of progressive irreversible renal disease in Lhasa apsos and Shih-Tzus prompts the hypothesis that the disorder is familial. Although the exact genetic mode of inheritance is unknown, pilot studies have been interpreted to suggest that it is not a simple autosomal recessive trait. Carefully conducted breeding trials must be performed before meaningful conclusions can be established. The possibility that the etiology of this disorder is related to viral infection of the dam during prenatal development of fetuses has been neither proved nor disproved.

DIAGNOSIS

Because the kidneys of normal puppies continue to undergo functional maturation for several months following birth, recognition of impaired ability to concentrate urine in affected Lhasa apso or Shih-Tzu puppies before they are placed in homes may be very difficult. Appropriate caution must be used when interpreting urine specific gravity and osmolality values of immature animals, since they probably have different average, minimum, and maximum values than those of mature dogs. In severely affected dogs, marked polydipsia, poor growth, and varying degrees of anorexia may be indicative of the disorder. In some instances these dogs may develop sudden dehydration and may succumb within a few days.

Less severely affected dogs may not develop clinical signs of renal dysfunction until they are at least five to six months of age. At that time, clinical and laboratory findings and radiographic abnormalities are typical of chronic progressive renal failure due to any cause.

Irrespective of the underlying cause, detection of bilateral reduction in renal size is indicative of an irreversible lesion. Renal biopsy of patients with small kidneys does not provide information that will aid in formulating a prognosis already known to be associated with an irreversible disease. Morphologic evaluation of kidney tissue obtained by biopsy or necropsy may be of value to breeders, however.

Early detection of characteristic renal lesions by needle biopsy may be difficult because of the segmental distribution of renal lesions. Investigators at the College of Veterinary Medicine, University of Pennsylvania, recommend surgical wedge biopsies to detect characteristic abnormalities in asymptomatic dogs being considered for breeding stock. It has been suggested that biopsies be performed when the dogs are approximately 3 to 12 months of age, before the development of other types of renal disease complicates biopsy interpretation. Further studies comparing age-matched renal biopsy specimens in normal and affected pups are needed to permit identification of the disease in asymptomatic dogs being considered for pets or breeding stock.

Characteristic morphologic features of the disease include (1) glomerular atrophy, (2) abnormal numbers or persistence of fetal glomeruli, (3) segmental or radial distribution of severe cortical lesions, (4) a paucity of inflammatory cell infiltrate, and (5) a disproportionate severity of medullary tubular lesions and medullary interstitial fibrosis compared with concurrent lesions in the renal cortex.

It is essential to avoid overdiagnosis of renal dysplasia in Lhasa apso and Shih-Tzu dogs. As with any breed, they may develop renal disease and renal dysfunction as a result of a variety of other congenital and/or acquired disorders.

TREATMENT

Because the underlying cause of renal dysplasia in Lhasa apsos and Shih-Tzus is unknown, specific therapy is unavailable. Current management is limited to appropriate supportive and symptomatic therapy designed to minimize deficits and excesses in fluid, electrolyte, acid-base, endocrine, and nutrient balance caused by renal dysfunction. Consult the articles entitled "Conservative Medical Management of Canine Chronic Polyuric Renal Failure" (page 991) and "Emergency Management of the Acute Uremic Crisis" (page 981) for further information.

PROGNOSIS

In dogs with renal dysfunction at the time of diagnosis, the disorder is usually progressive. The rate of progression of the disorder and the survival time are dependent on the degree of renal dysfunction at the time of diagnosis, the presence or absence of concomitant but unrelated diseases, and the initiation of appropriate supportive and symptomatic therapy. In our series of affected dogs with renal dysfunction, death occurred during the first year of life or shortly thereafter. Affected dogs occasionally survived until they were two or three years old; one dog died at the age of five years.

Recommendations regarding prevention of this disease await further characterization of its etiopathogenesis. Findings thus far support the hypothesis that the disease is familial and probably inherited. Further studies are required to determine if breeding stock may be asymptomatic carriers of this disorder. Pending the availability of controlled breeding trials and further evaluation of clinical cases, we recommend that affected dogs not be used for breeding.

SUPPLEMENTAL READING

Bernard, M. A., and Valli, V. E.: Familial renal disease in Samoyed dogs. Can. Vet. J. 18:181, 1977.

Finco, D. R., Duncan, J. R., Crowell, W. A., and Hulsey, M. L.: Familial renal disease in Norwegian elkhound dogs: Morphologic examinations. Am. J. Vet. Res. 38:941, 1977.

Finco, D. R., Kurtz, H. J., Low, D. G., and Perman, V.: Familial renal disease in Norwegian elkhound dogs. J.A.V.M.A. 156:747, 1970.

Finco, D. R., Thrall, D. E., and Duncan, J. R.: The urinary system. *In* Catcott, B. J. (ed.): *Canine Medicine*, Vol. 1. 4th ed. Santa Barbara, CA: American Veterinary Publications, Inc., 1979.

Johnson, M. E., Denhart, J. D., and Graber, E. R.: Renal cortical hypoplasia in a litter of cocker spaniels. J. Am. Anim. Hosp. Assoc. 8:268, 1972.

Krook, L.: The pathology of renal cortical hypoplasia in the dog. Nord. Vet. Med. 9:161, 1957.

O'Brien, T., Osborne, C. A., Yano, B., and Barnes, D. M.: Clinicopathologic manifestations of progressive renal disease in Lhasa Apso and Shih Tzu dogs. J.A.V.M.A. in press.

Osborne, C. A., Low, D. G., and Finco, D. R.: *Canine And Feline Urology*. Philadelphia: W. B. Saunders, 1972.

FAMILIAL RENAL DISEASE IN DOBERMAN PINSCHER DOGS

DENNIS J. CHEW, D.V.M.,
and STEPHEN P. DiBARTOLA, D.V.M.

Columbus, Ohio

Familial renal disease in dogs has been reported to occur in cocker spaniels, Norwegian elkhounds, Lhasa apsos, and Samoyeds. Recently, progressive renal disease has been described in related Doberman pinscher dogs. Over the past ten years, 22 young Doberman pinschers with renal failure have been evaluated at The Ohio State University. The cause of this disease is unknown.

CLINICAL FINDINGS

The average age of these Doberman pinschers at the time of diagnosis of renal disease has been about two years. There is no apparent sex predilection, but males were evaluated for renal disease at a slightly younger age than females. About one-third of the dogs were admitted to our hospital for evaluation at less than one year of age.

In over one-half of the dogs, client complaints were anorexia, weight loss, vomition, lethargy, polydipsia, and polyuria. These findings are suggestive of, but not specific for, advanced renal failure. Less commonly reported complaints were diarrhea, epistaxis, and nocturia. The duration of the clinical signs prior to evaluation was highly variable.

The most common physical findings were emaciation and dehydration. The average weight of adult Doberman pinschers with this disease was 24 kg. Other physical abnormalities were hypothermia (< 100.5°F), pallor of the mucus membranes, foul oral odor, oral ulceration, ascites or edema, small kidneys, and retinal lesions. Fundic abnormalities were characterized by retinal edema, retinal hemorrhage, and retinal detachment. These physical abnormalities, like the historical findings, are suggestive of but not specific for advanced renal failure. Some dogs less than one year of age had severe fibrous osteodystrophy with deformable maxilla and mandible (so-called "rubber jaw").

DIAGNOSIS

Routine laboratory evaluation provides confirmation of advanced renal disease. Azotemia, hyperphosphatemia, nonregenerative anemia, lymphopenia, hypercholesterolemia, mild hyperglycemia, and isosthenuria were typical findings. Serum calcium values were variable; affected dogs may be hypocalcemic, normocalcemic, or hypercalcemic. Normochloremic metabolic acidosis with an increased anion gap was observed in some affected dogs. Elevation of serum sodium and total plasma protein levels was associated with dehydration. Serum albumin concentration was normal to subnormal, unless animals were dehydrated.

Urinalysis findings were characterized by moderate proteinuria and, occasionally, glucosuria. Determinations of 24-hour urine protein excretion in a few dogs revealed moderate loss (2 to 5 gm/day). Although hematuria and pyuria were occasionally observed, urine cultures were usually negative. Hyaline and granular cylindruria occurred in about one-half of the cases.

Survey abdominal radiographs revealed reduction in kidney size, poor visceral detail owing to lack of abdominal fat, and reduced bone density owing to osteoporosis. Coagulation studies including prothrombin time, partial thromboplastin time, and platelet numbers were normal. Fibrin degradation products were not detected. In one dog, marked reduction in platelet retention was indicative of abnormal platelet function caused by uremia.

Confirmation of the diagnosis requires renal biopsy. Renal lesions were characterized by increased mesangial matrix, glomerular sclerosis, cystic glomerular atrophy, periglomerular fibrosis, tubular atrophy, tubular dilatation, hyperplasia of medullary collecting-duct epithelium, interstitial fibrosis, interstitial infiltrates of lymphocytes and plasma cells, and focal interstitial mineralization. Occasionally, segmental glomerular hyaline nodular deposits and crescent formation were observed.

The histologic lesions can be classified into three categories: predominantly glomerular sclerosis (25 per cent of cases), predominantly cystic glomerular atrophy (25 per cent of cases), and a mixture of these two glomerular lesions (50 per cent of cases). Tubular dilatation, tubular atrophy, and interstitial infiltrates of lymphocytes and plasma cells were similar in severity among these three categories, but interstitial fibrosis appeared to be most severe in dogs with cystic glomeruli. It is possible in these dogs that severe interstitial fibrosis led to tubular obstruction and consequent cystic glomerular atrophy. Interstitial mineralization and collecting-duct hyperplasia also were more common in dogs with cystic glomerular change. The importance of these observations with regard to the pathogenesis of the disease remains to be determined.

Immunofluorescent microscopic examination of a limited number of affected dogs revealed glomerular deposits of immunoglobulins and complement. These findings are compatible with immune complex glomerulonephritis. Preliminary electron microscopic studies in one dog revealed electron-dense deposits in the glomerular capillary wall. Additional studies utilizing immunofluorescence and electron microscopy will be needed to further characterize these glomerular lesions.

Gross pathologic findings were typical of advanced renal failure. The kidneys were smaller than normal, pale, and had irregularly pitted surfaces. A small number of affected female Doberman pinschers had unilateral renal aplasia. Extrarenal lesions, including hemorrhagic gastritis, gastric mineralization, secondary hyperparathyroidism, and fibrous osteodystrophy, were typical of uremia. Fibrous osteodystrophy was most severe in dogs less than one year of age.

THERAPY

There is no specific therapy. Symptomatic and supportive therapy should consist of restoration of hydration with appropriate fluid therapy. When the patient has been stabilized, nutritional management can be initiated. A low-protein diet (0.6 to 2.0 gm/lb/day) consisting of high-quality protein with adequate nonprotein calories to spare protein catabolism should be initiated. Guidelines for institution of a low-protein diet are a stable BUN > 80 mg/dl, a stable creatinine level > 2.5 mg/dl, and a stable serum phosphorus level > 6 mg/dl. Changes in dietary sodium should be made gradually and should be adjusted to levels similar to those consumed by the dog prior to starting the low-protein diet.

Administration of a phosphorus-binding gel such as Amphojel or Basalgel is recommended to bind phosphorus in the intestine and enhance its elimination from the body. Supplementation of water-soluble vitamins is advisable. Administration of sodium bicarbonate is recommended if metabolic acidosis has been documented, but this source of sodium should be considered when planning the patient's daily sodium requirement. Anabolic steroids such as oxymetholone, testosterone, or nandrolone decanoate are used to stimulate protein anabolism and promote erythropoiesis. The animal should always have fresh water available. Stress should be avoided.

PROGNOSIS

The prognosis is dependent on the extent of disease at the time of diagnosis. The long-term prognosis for survival is poor owing to the progressive nature of the disease. Affected animals should not be used for breeding. Experimental breeding trials and further light, immunofluorescent, and electron microscopic studies are needed to determine the pattern of inheritance of this disease and to characterize the nature of early renal lesions.

SUPPLEMENTAL READING

Chew, D. J., DiBartola, S. P., Boyce, J. T., Hayes, H. M., and Brace, J. J.: Juvenile renal disease in Doberman pinscher dogs. J.A.V.M.A. In press, 1983.
Wilcock, B. P., and Patterson, J. M.: Familial glomerulonephritis in Doberman pinscher dogs. Can. Vet. J. 20:244, 1979.

FELINE RENAL AMYLOIDOSIS

DENNIS J. CHEW, D.V.M.,
and STEPHEN P. DiBARTOLA, D.V.M.

Columbus, Ohio

Amyloidosis represents a variety of disease processes that have in common the extracellular deposition of biochemically unique fibrillar proteins. The beta-pleated sheet configuration of these fibrils leads to their characteristic microscopic staining and optical properties. Amyloidosis is not an inflammatory disease; however, accumulation of this inert material in vital organs may impair their function and may ultimately lead to death. Amyloidosis may involve many organs including the liver, kidney, spleen, thyroid, adrenal, pancreas, and intestine. Progressive renal involvement leading to failure is usually responsible for clinical signs in dogs and cats.

PATHOGENESIS

A recent classification of amyloidosis divides acquired systemic amyloidosis into immunoglobulin-associated, reactive, heredofamilial, and localized syndromes. The major fibrillar protein of immunoglobulin-associated amyloidosis (primary and myeloma-associated amyloidosis) is an N-terminal fragment from the variable region of immunoglobulin-light chains, often of the lambda variety. The immunocyte is the origin of these light chains. Such amyloid deposits are designated as amyloid L or AL.

Reactive systemic amyloidosis (secondary amyloidosis) may be associated with chronic infectious, inflammatory, or neoplastic diseases. The amyloidogenic precursor is a serum alpha globulin, which is elevated in many inflammatory and neoplastic conditions by virtue of its behavior as an acute-phase reactant. The source of this precursor, known as serum amyloid A–related protein (SAA), appears to be the liver. In patients with this form of amyloidosis, tissue deposits are composed of N-terminal fragments of SAA and are called amyloid A or AA. Almost all experimental animal models of amyloidosis are examples of reactive systemic amyloidosis. These include murine models of amyloidosis induced by casein injections and the amyloidosis that occurs in gray collie dogs with cyclic hematopoiesis. There is some evidence that amyloidosis of low leukocyte count (LLC) mice may result from kappa-light chains and thus may be an example of immunoglobulin-associated amyloidosis.

Serum precursors of amyloid are known for two heredofamilial syndromes in humans. In familial Mediterranean fever, the precursor is SAA; in familial Portuguese neuropathy it is a variant of serum prealbumin. In some forms of localized amyloidosis that occur in the pancreas and thyroid gland, deposits may be derived from hormone precursors of insulin and calcitonin. Amyloid deposits in the pancreatic islets of older cats have been described, and, although their amino acid sequence has not been determined, their resistance to potassium permanganate treatment indicates that they do not contain amyloid A.

One hypothesis concerning the pathogenesis of amyloidosis is defective proteolysis of amyloidogenic precursor proteins by phagocytic cells in predisposed individuals (Fig. 1). The inciting event may be excessive production of light chains associated with plasma cell dyscrasias including multiple myeloma, or it may be an elevated level of SAA in chronic inflammatory or neoplastic disorders. Elastase-like proteases associated with the cell membrane of monocytes degrade SAA. At least two steps in the process have been identified: initial breakdown of SAA to an AA-like protein and subsequent degradation to smaller peptides. In human patients with amyloidosis, the breakdown of AA to smaller peptides is prolonged. Individuals whose phagocytic cells are abnormally slow in degradation of AA may

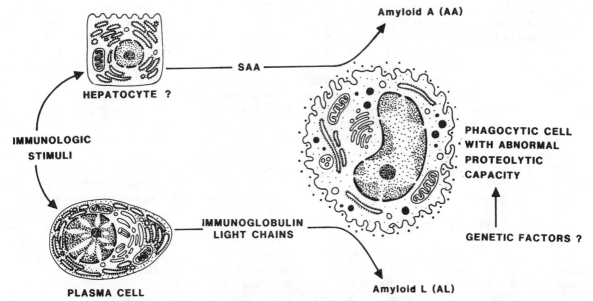

Figure 1. Pathogenesis of reactive and immunoglobulin-associated amyloidosis based on proteolysis of amyloidogenic precursors by altered phagocytic cells. (Modified from Glenner: N. Engl. J. Med. 302:1283, 1333, 1980.)

be predisposed to reactive systemic amyloidosis if they develop inflammatory or neoplastic disorders that cause prolonged elevation of SAA. Fibrils identical to amyloid also have been produced by proteolytic degradation of Bence Jones light chains.

In dogs, renal amyloidosis occurs secondary to many chronic inflammatory and neoplastic disorders. Examples include abscesses, osteomyelitis, pyometra, pyothorax, systemic mycoses, tuberculosis, lupus erythematosus, cyclic hematopoiesis, septic arthritis, dirofilariasis, pyelonephritis, multiple myeloma, and lymphosarcoma. In 25 per cent of canine cases a predisposing disorder can be found; in the remaining 75 per cent of cases none can be detected. Amyloidosis in the cat is less commonly detected. Most cases have been idiopathic in nature. Hypervitaminosis A causes diffuse reticuloendothelial hyperplasia and was incriminated as a predisposing factor in a series of feline amyloidosis cases from Australia. The diagnosis of hypervitaminosis A was based on characteristic histologic lesions and elevated levels of vitamin A in the liver of some affected cats. We have recently observed idiopathic renal amyloidosis in related Abyssinian cats.

The distribution of amyloid in the kidney of cats often differs from that in dogs. In dogs, renal amyloidosis is primarily a glomerular disease with early involvement of the mesangium. As the disease progresses to involve the capillary tuft and efferent arteriole, there may be interference with blood supply to the tubules, leading to tubular atrophy, interstitial fibrosis, and interstitial infiltration of lymphocytes and plasma cells. Renal failure and uremia occurs when sufficient renal parenchyma has been affected. In cats, renal amyloidosis is primarily a disease of the medullary interstitium. Glomerular involvement is variable. The most severe lesions found in the inner medulla are characterized by amyloid deposition between tubular cells and in tubular basement membranes. Interference with the vasa recta results in ischemia of the inner medulla and papillary necrosis. Progressive nephron destruction is associated with medullary interstitial fibrosis and interstitial infiltrates of mononuclear cells. The end result is renal failure and uremia. The magnitude of glomerular deposition of amyloid is variable in cats. Amyloid may accumulate in the mesangium, basement membranes, and/or subendothelial spaces.

CLINICAL FINDINGS

There is no sex predilection for renal amyloidosis in dogs; 90 per cent of cases occur in dogs five years of age and older. Feline renal amyloidosis has been reported in older cats. The disease has been reported to affect equal numbers of males and females by some investigators and predominantly males by others. We recently encountered renal amyloidosis in six related young adult Abyssinian cats from two catteries.

Historical findings in dogs and cats with renal amyloidosis are typical of those associated with renal insufficiency. The owner may become concerned because of signs such as polydipsia and polyuria, weight loss, lethargy, anorexia, poor haircoat, subcutaneous edema, or abdominal distention due to ascites. Vomiting or diarrhea may be present if the animal is uremic. If predisposing infectious, inflammatory, or neoplastic diseases are present, the predominant clinical signs may be related to them. In dogs, thromboembolism may complicate amyloidosis and may cause major clinical signs. Pulmonary thromboembolism associated with dyspnea has been the most commonly encountered clinical finding, but thrombosis may occur in other vessels. Physical findings in cats with advanced renal amyloidosis include depression, poor condition, and dehydration. Uremic odor of the breath and stomatitis may occur. .

Results of urinalysis in dogs and cats with amyloidosis include proteinuria, cylindruria, impaired urine concentration, and, occasionally, mild hematuria. When there has been an approximately 67 per cent loss of functional nephrons, polyuria and defective urinary concentrating ability are expected. When glomerular disease is more severe than medullary interstitial disease in dogs (and presumably cats), glomerulotubular imbalance characterized by higher urine specific gravity values than expected with azotemia may occur. Severe proteinuria is common in dogs owing to the glomerular nature of the disease. In one study, dogs with glomerular amyloidosis lost an average of 10.3 grams urinary protein per day. In cats, severe proteinuria may not be a major feature, and early interference with urinary concentrating ability may occur owing to medullary interstitial deposition of amyloid. Severe glomerular involvement in cats, however, may be associated with marked proteinuria.

Dogs with renal amyloidosis may develop hypoalbuminemia, hypercholesterolemia, and hyperglobulinemia owing to elevations of alpha, beta, and gamma globulins. Severe hypoalbuminemia may result in subcutaneous edema. Ascites may develop owing to secondary hyperaldosteronism in the presence of inadequate levels of albumin to maintain oncotic pressure. The classic nephrotic syndrome is characterized by proteinuria, hypoalbuminemia, hypercholesterolemia, and subcutaneous edema or ascites. Dogs with advanced glomerular disease frequently have all of these features except for ascites or edema. Similar findings would be expected in cats with marked proteinuria due to severe glomerular involvement.

With progression of renal amyloidosis, nephron

destruction in excess of 75 per cent leads to laboratory findings typical of renal failure. Azotemia, hyperphosphatemia, metabolic acidosis, mild hyperglycemia, and nonregenerative anemia typically occur. All of these findings were present in Abyssinian cats with advanced renal amyloidosis. However, their serum albumin concentrations were normal or slightly reduced. These cats had hyperglobulinemia, which in two animals was due to elevations of alpha-2 and gamma fractions. One cat had hyperamylasemia and two had hypercholesterolemia. Proteinuria, cylindruria, mild hematuria, and low urine specific gravity values were detected by routine urinalysis. At necropsy, marked accumulations of medullary interstitial amyloid associated with papillary necrosis, interstitial fibrosis, and interstitial mononuclear inflammatory cell infiltrates were observed. The glomeruli of these cats contained variable quantities of amyloid.

DIAGNOSIS

If renal amyloidosis is suspected as a cause of renal failure, detection of predisposing inflammatory or neoplastic disorders provides added support for this diagnosis. If a plasma cell dyscrasia is suspected, serum protein electrophoresis, immunoelectrophoresis, and radial immunodiffusion for quantitation of immunoglobulins may be helpful in characterizing abnormal immunoglobulins. Evaluation of bone marrow aspirates may reveal abnormal numbers of plasma cells in patients with plasma cell dyscrasias.

Ultimately, the diagnosis of renal amyloidosis requires renal biopsy. Keyhole techniques are adequate in dogs with glomerular involvement. In cats with inner medullary rather than glomerular involvement, open wedge biopsy may be superior to percutaneous punch biopsy techniques.

Amyloid stained with hematoxylin and eosin appears homogenous and eosinophilic. Amyloid stained with crystal violet often appears metachromatic. Periodic acid–Schiff reagent usually has a high affinity for amyloid owing to a minor nonfibrillar glycoprotein component present in amyloid deposits (P-component). A diagnosis of amyloidosis by light microscopy is dependent upon detection of typical bright green birefringence when sections of kidney are stained with Congo red and observed with the aid of polarized light. This characteristic feature is associated with the beta-pleated sheet configuration of amyloid deposits. Feline amyloid deposits may not stain as well with Congo red as canine amyloid deposits but brilliantly fluoresce when stained with thioflavine-T and examined with the aid of ultraviolet light. The ultrastructure of amyloid deposits is characterized by nonbranching fibrils 10 nm in diameter. In the medulla, the fibrils are typically located between tubular cells and below tubular basement membranes. In glomeruli they are found in the mesangium, basement membranes, and subendothelial spaces.

Potassium permanganate oxidation often allows differentiation of reactive amyloidosis from immunoglobulin-associated and localized amyloidosis. In reactive amyloidosis, deposits containing AA lose their affinity for Congo red after permanganate oxidation. In contrast, immunoglobulin-associated and localized forms of amyloidosis retain their Congo red staining qualities after permanganate treatment. In Abyssinian cats we have studied, loss of Congo red staining of kidney sections following permanganate oxidation suggests that their renal amyloid deposits may be reactive amyloid.

TREATMENT

Treatment of amyloidosis should ideally be designed to prevent further deposition of amyloid and accelerate the removal of existing deposits. However, at the present time therapy is limited to attempts to resolve underlying inflammatory or neoplastic stimuli of amyloid deposits and supportive care of renal failure. In the majority of canine and feline cases of amyloidosis, an underlying disease has not been identified. Likewise, the Abyssinian cats we have studied had no discernible predisposing disease. By the time renal amyloidosis is recognized in dogs and cats, advanced renal disease often has already led to uremia. At this point it is unlikely that removal of a predisposing cause would result in resolution of renal lesions.

Experimental therapy for amyloidosis includes corticosteroids, antineoplastic agents, D-penicillamine, colchicine, and dimethyl sulfoxide (DMSO). Use of corticosteroids has been shown to accelerate amyloid deposition in experimental reactive amyloidosis. In addition, the catabolic effects of corticosteroids could aggravate the severity of uremia. For these reasons, their use is not recommended in dogs or cats with amyloidosis unless they are required for management of a predisposing inflammatory disease. If an overt plasma cell dyscrasia with monoclonal gammopathy can be documented, chemotherapy with melphalan or cyclophosphamide may be considered. DMSO is thought to denature noncovalently bound amyloid fibrils and promote their removal. Because these treatments have not been carefully evaluated in dogs or cats with amyloidosis, recommendations for their use cannot be formulated at this time.

PROGNOSIS

If a diagnosis of renal amyloidosis is made after the disease has progressed to renal failure, the prognosis is very poor. However, with supportive care, comfortable survival for up to a year may be expected, depending on the severity of the renal disease at the time of diagnosis. The Abyssinian cats we have encountered were in an advanced state of uremia, and therefore therapy was not initiated.

SUPPLEMENTAL READING

Chew, D. J., DiBartola, S. P., Boyce, J. T., and Gasper, P. W.: Renal amyloidosis in related Abyssinian cats. J.A.V.M.A. 181:139, 1982.

Clark, L., and Seawright, A. A.: Amyloidosis associated with chronic hypervitaminosis A in cats (letter to the editor). Aust. Vet. J. 44:584, 1968.

Clark, L., and Seawright, A. A.: Generalized amyloidosis in seven cats. Pathol. Vet. 6:117, 1969.

Crowell, W. A., Goldston, R. T., Schall, W. D., et al.: Generalized amyloidosis in a cat. J.A.V.M.A. 161:1127, 1972.

DiBartola, S. P., Spaulding, G. L., Chew, D. J., et al.: Urinary protein excretion and immunopathologic findings in dogs with glomerular disease. J.A.V.M.A. 177:73, 1980.

Eisenbud, L. E., Lerner, C. P., and Chai, C. K.: The effect of dimethyl sulfoxide (DMSO) upon spontaneous amyloidosis in mice. Proc. Soc. Exp. Biol. Med. 168:172, 1981.

Glenner, G. G.: Amyloid deposits and amyloidosis. The beta fibrilloses. N. Engl. J. Med. 302:1283, 1333, 1980.

Lavie, G., Zucker-Franklin, D., and Franklin, E. C.: Degradation of serum amyloid A protein by surface-associated enzymes of human blood monocytes. J. Exp. Med. 148:1020, 1978.

Lucke, V. M., and Hunt, A. C.: Interstitial nephropathy and papillary necrosis in the domestic cat. J. Pathol. Bacteriol. 89:723, 1965.

Osborne, C. A., Johnson, K. H., Perman, V., et al.: Renal amyloidosis in the dog. J.A.V.M.A. 153:669, 1968.

Slauson, D. O., and Gribble, D. H.: Thrombosis complicating renal amyloidosis in dogs. Vet. Pathol. 8:352, 1971.

Slauson, D. O., Gribble, D. H., and Russell, S. W.: A clinicopathological study of renal amyloidosis in dogs. J. Comp. Pathol. 80:335, 1970.

Yano, B. L., Johnson, K. H., and Hayden, D. W.: Feline insular amyloid: histochemical distinction from secondary amyloid. Vet. Pathol. 18:181, 1981.

PERIRENAL CYSTS (PSEUDOCYSTS) IN THE CAT

JAMES J. BRACE, D.V.M.

Knoxville, Tennessee

Perirenal fluid accumulation in the cat is an uncommon disorder that results in progressive abdominal enlargement and palpable cyst-like masses that completely surround one or both kidneys. This condition has been given various names, including perinephric pseudocyst, perirenal pseudocyst, renal capsular cyst, capsulogenic renal cyst, capsular hydronephrosis, and retroperitoneal perirenal cyst. Because these masses could be mistaken for enlarged kidneys, this disorder should be considered in the differential diagnosis of suspected renomegaly.

Perirenal cysts have been reported only in male or neutered male cats and, with one exception, have occurred in cats eight years of age and older. Historically, the cats are generally healthy except for asymptomatic progressive abdominal enlargement of 1 to 16 weeks duration. Abdominal palpation reveals a large, nonpainful, firm mass in the region of one or both kidneys. Complete blood counts and serum biochemical determinations are either normal or reveal only mild azotemia (BUN < 40 mg/dl). Azotemia is probably the result of underlying primary renal disease (e.g., interstitial nephritis) but may occasionally be due to a large cyst obstructing the renal pelvis or ureter. Urinalyses have not been performed with sufficient fre-

quency in cats with this disorder to make any conclusions. Abdominal radiographs reveal large, soft-tissue–dense unilateral or bilateral masses in the region of the kidneys. Excretory urography may suggest the diagnosis. Normal-sized kidneys with either normal or irregular cortical margins may be seen surrounded by smooth, soft-tissue–dense masses. The renal pelves do not appear dilated, and extravasation of contrast material into the perirenal cystic structures has not been seen. However, contrast of the kidneys may be so poor that renal size and contour cannot be evaluated. Laboratory evaluation of fluid aspirated from these masses typically reveals a transudate. In one cat, the urea nitrogen concentration in the transudate was 50 mg/dl compared with the BUN of 6 mg/dl, suggesting that escape of urine into perirenal tissues may have played some role in the pathogenesis of the disorder.

The etiology and pathogenesis of these fluid-filled perirenal sacs are unknown. Fluid may accumulate between the renal parenchyma and renal capsule, with the renal capsule comprising the outer wall of the sac. Fluid accumulation may also be completely extracapsular, surrounded by a thin-walled sac attached to the kidney at various sites (hilus, posterior pole, and so on). Microscopic examination of perirenal sacs in one cat revealed that they were composed of fibrous connective tissue with focal aggregates of lymphocytes. Because the sacs were not lined by epithelium, a characteristic of true cysts, they were more correctly termed *pseudocysts*. Histologic examination of these structures in cats has been infrequent, however, and whether all such structures should be called pseudocysts is unknown.

In humans, perinephric pseudocysts (cysts) occur most often following trauma to the renal parenchyma, renal pelvis, or upper ureter that results in chronic extravasation of urine into surrounding tissues. Other possible causes are extravasation of urine following urinary tract obstruction or renal biopsy. If extravasated urine is not absorbed, it can stimulate an inflammatory reaction that may result in the formation of a fibrous sac without an epithelial lining that completely surrounds the urine. Other possible causes of perirenal pseudocyst (cyst) formation in humans are resolution of perirenal hematomas, perirenal lymphocele formation following renal transplantation, and idiopathic disorders. Significant bleeding into perirenal tissues may stimulate a severe inflammatory response similar to extravasation of urine. Perirenal lymphocele formation is due to leakage of lymph fluid by the renal transplant recipient because of inadequate lymphostasis, and is characterized by accumulation of protein-rich fluid around the kidney. It has been suggested that one possible cause of perirenal cysts

in cats is obstruction of lymphatic drainage of the renal capsule. However, the protein-poor nature of the cystic fluid in cats does not support this hypothesis.

Current therapy of perirenal cysts (pseudocysts) in cats is surgical. The cysts should be drained and as much of the cyst wall resected as possible. If there is evidence of primary renal dysfunction or if the kidneys appear grossly normal, a renal biopsy obtained at the time of celiotomy should be considered. If an underlying etiology can be determined, it should be corrected if possible. On the basis of the few reports in the literature, prognosis for recovery appears to be good.

SUPPLEMENTAL READING

Abdinoor, D. J.: Perinephric pseudocysts in the cat. J.A.A.H.A. 16:763, 1980.

Arnold, M. B.: Pararenal pseudocyst. Br. J. Urol. 44:40, 1972.

Chastain, C. B., and Grier, R. L.: Bilateral retroperitoneal perirenal cysts in a cat. Feline Pract. 5:51, 1975.

Elkin, M.: *Radiology of the Urinary System*, Vol. 2. Boston: Little, Brown and Co., 1980.

Kraft, A. M., and Kraft, C. G.: Renal capsular cyst. V.M./S.A.C. 65:692, 1970.

Mitten, R. A.: Pararenal pseudocysts in a cat. Iowa State Univ. Vet. 2:65, 1978.

Ticer, J. W.: Capsulogenic renal cyst in a cat. J.A.V.M.A. 143:613, 1963.

Witten, D. M., Myers, G. H., and Utz, D. C.: *Emmett's Clinical Urography*, Vol. 3, 4th ed. Philadelphia: W. B. Saunders, 1977.

EMERGENCY MANAGEMENT OF THE ACUTE UREMIC CRISIS

DONALD G. LOW, D.V.M.,
and LARRY D. COWGILL, D.V.M.

Davis, California

Prompt diagnosis is essential in managing the acute uremic crisis if the patient is to have the maximum chance of survival. Signs associated with uremic crises are similar regardless of underlying cause. Therefore, the clinician must consider at least the following diagnostic possibilities: (1) prerenal azotemia with normal kidneys, (2) prerenal azotemia complicating chronic renal failure, (3) acute renal failure, (4) acute renal failure associated with pre-existing chronic renal failure, (5) post-renal azotemia, and (6) terminal chronic renal failure. Depression, anorexia, vomiting, dehydration, fetid breath, scleral injection, and oral ulcers or erosions may occur in association with all of these situations;

therefore, other clinical and laboratory signs must be evaluated if serious errors are to be avoided. Oliguria and/or anuria may also occur in patients with any of these disorders; conversely, polyuria may be associated with both acute and chronic renal failure.

DIAGNOSIS

PRERENAL AZOTEMIA AND PRERENAL AZOTEMIA COMPLICATING CHRONIC RENAL FAILURE

Prerenal azotemia is associated with hypoperfusion of the kidneys and may be caused by dehydration, septic or hypovolemic shock, hypotension, severe heart failure, cardiac tamponade, or hypoadrenocorticism. Any problem that causes marked hypoperfusion of the kidneys has the potential to induce prerenal azotemia. During prerenal azotemia the kidneys are usually normal, but if severe hypoperfusion persists, prolonged ischemia may cause acute renal failure.

Since prerenal azotemia frequently complicates pre-existing chronic renal failure, this combination of disorders must be carefully considered and promptly treated if the remaining renal function is to be preserved. In fact, patients with chronic renal failure are among the most susceptible to the development of prerenal azotemia. Severe dehydration can rapidly develop as a result of vomiting and/or diarrhea, or deliberate or accidental water restriction. This is especially true in hot weather when insensible fluid losses are high and because of the obligatory polyuria associated with chronic renal failure. Under these conditions the BUN will rapidly increase from 40 to 80 mg/dl (commonly found in patients with early chronic renal failure) to values between 100 and 200 mg/dl. Prompt therapy often reverses the uremic crisis, and the BUN concentration typically returns to the 40 to 80 mg/dl range.

Prerenal azotemia associated with normal kidneys can usually be recognized by detecting the primary disease that is causing hypoperfusion of the kidneys. The clinician's suspicion is aroused by evidence of marked dehydration, shock, hypovolemia and circulatory inadequacy. If a urine sample is evaluated before therapy is initiated, it usually is concentrated distinctly above the fixed specific gravity range of 1.007 to 1.015, thereby eliminating primary renal failure as the predominating problem. Animals with chronic renal failure complicated by prerenal azotemia will have a urine specific gravity within the fixed range. Prerenal azotemia complicating chronic renal failure is often accompanied by a long-standing history of polyuria and polydipsia or other clinical findings suggestive of chronic renal failure. Reduced renal size, renal osteodystrophy, and the onset of nonregenerative anemia may be additional signs suggesting the chronic nature of the underlying problem. As in prerenal azotemia with normal kidneys, prerenal azotemia complicating chronic renal failure may follow gastrointestinal upsets or water deprivation, resulting in dehydration and renal hypoperfusion. Absence of severe renal osteodystrophy and marked nonregenerative, normochromic, normocytic anemia helps distinguish this problem from terminal chronic renal failure (Tables 1 and 2).

ACUTE RENAL FAILURE

Acute renal failure (ARF) must be considered in patients with anuria or oliguria. Urine specific gravity levels evaluated before therapy and restoration of fluid volume will reveal impaired ability to concentrate or dilute urine (see Tables 1 and 2 for distinguishing features of various causes of uremic crises). It is emphasized that some patients with ARF have polyuria at the time of initial evaluation rather than oliguria or anuria. Polyuria is often associated with ARF caused by aminoglycoside antibiotics, especially gentamicin. Polyuria is also encountered in some patients during the early recovery stages of ARF. At this stage tubular epithelial cells lack the ability to respond to antidiuretic hormone (ADH) and to reabsorb a normal quantity of solute and water. Patients poisoned by ethylene glycol are often anuric at the time of initial evaluation, as are many patients with ARF due to ischemia.

Historical evidence of exposure to common nephrotoxins (Table 3) or conditions that may result in renal ischemia is important in establishing a diagnosis of ARF. The onset is usually sudden and without previous evidence of polyuria or polydipsia. Renal pain may be evident but must be interpreted cautiously. The clinician should carefully evaluate the patient for other causes of sublumbar pain before ascribing it to the kidneys.

Infectious agents, including leptospira serotypes, *E. coli*, streptococci, staphylococci, *Proteus*, and others, may cause ARF by inducing an acute non-suppurative interstitial nephritis (leptospirosis), or an acute, generalized pyelonephritis. Patients with these disorders are often febrile, have a marked leukocytosis, and, in the case of pyelonephritis, usually have bacteriuria and pyuria.

Acute renal failure due to renal ischemia may be associated with trauma, extensive surgery, prolonged anesthesia, renal artery occlusion, rhabdomyolysis and myoglobinuria, sepsis, incompatible blood transfusions, peritonitis, gastric torsion, disseminated intravascular coagulapathy, or pancreatitis. Advanced age and pre-existing renal disease probably increase the animal's susceptibility to ARF.

A diagnosis of ARF should not be made until extracellular fluid volume is restored and shock or hypotension is corrected. Renal biopsies are of great value in helping to establish the diagnosis and prognosis in ARF. Infection as in acute pyelonephritis, is a relative contraindication to a biopsy.

ARF due to ischemia is associated with a poorer prognosis in humans than ARF due to nephrotoxins or infectious agents, even when uremia is controlled by hemodialysis. Mortality in humans with ARF due to ischemia is approximately 50 per cent, whereas ARF associated with nephrotoxins is about 15 per cent. There are no comparable statistics available in veterinary medicine, although clinical impressions suggest that the prognosis in ARF due to nephrotoxins may carry a less unfavorable prog-

Table 1. *Differentiating Features Among Causes of Uremic Crises*

Cause	Renal Osteo-dystrophy	Kidney Size	Potassium (mEq/L)	Urine Specific Gravity	PCV	BUN (mg/dl)	Creatinine (mg/dl)	PO$_4$ (mg/dl)	History of PU/PD*	History of Anuria/ Oliguria	Urine Sediment
Prerenal azotemia with normal kidneys	NO	Normal	3.5–5.5	>1.030	35–60	60–100	1.8–4.5	4.5–7.0	NO	YES	Normal; −casts
Prerenal azotemia complicating chronic renal failure	YES No	SMALL Normal	3.5–6.5	1.007–1.015	25–45	100–250	4.5–15.0	7.5–12.0	YES	Yes NO	Usually little sediment
Acute renal failure	NO	Large NORMAL	6–9	1.007–1.015	25–45	75–250	5–15	7–20	NO	YES No	Maybe casts, >RBC, >WBC
Acute renal failure complicating chronic renal failure	YES No	SMALL Normal	6–9	1.007–1.015	25–45	75–250	5–15	7–20	YES	Yes NO	Maybe casts, >RBC, >WBC
Post-renal azotemia	NO	NORMAL Large	4–10	1.015–1.060	35–60	50–300	2–25	6–20	NO	YES	Variable; often >WBC and >RBC
Terminal chronic renal failure	YES	SMALL	4.0–7.5	1.007–1.015	10–20	150–250	12–20	12–25	YES	NO Yes	Usually little sediment

*PU/PD = polyuria/polydipsia.

Notes: Usual or commonly encountered laboratory values are listed.
Results outside of these ranges may be found.
Answer in capital letters indicates most common situation.

Table 2. *Changes in Some Differentiating Features Among Causes of Uremic Crises Following Treatment for Hypotension and Hypovolemia**

Cause	Potassium (mEq/L)	Urine Specific Gravity	PCV	BUN (mg/dl)	Creatinine (mg/dl)	PO$_4$ (mg/dl)	Increased Urine Volume	Biopsy
Prerenal azotemia with normal kidneys†	3.5–5.0	1.010–1.035	30–45	10–20	1.0–1.5	3.5–5.0	YES	Not necessary
Prerenal azotemia complicating chronic renal failure	3.5–5.0	1.007–1.015	20–40	50–120	1.8–6.0	4.5–10.0	YES	Not necessary
Acute renal failure	6–9	1.007–1.015	20–40	75–250	5–15	7–20	NO Yes	Very useful
Acute renal failure complicating chronic renal failure	6–9	1.007–1.015	20–40	75–250	5–15	7–20	NO Yes	Very useful
Post-renal azotemia†	3.5–5.0	1.007–1.035	30–45	10–20	1.0–1.5	3.5–5.0	YES	Not necessary
Terminal chronic renal failure	4.5–7.5	1.007–1.015	9–18	100–200	10–20	10–25	Slight increase	Not necessary

*Compare with pretreatment values in Table 1.
†After relief of primary problem plus restoration of fluid balance.
Notes: Usual or commonly encountered laboratory values are listed.
　　　Results outside of these ranges may be found.
　　　Answer in capital letters indicates most common situation.

Table 3. *A Partial List of Nephrotoxins*

I. Metals and their compounds	D. *Anticonvulsants*
Antimony	Phenurone
Arsenic	Trimethadione
Beryllium	E. *Pesticides*
Bismuth	Chlorinated hydrocarbons
Cadmium	Phosphorus
Chromium	**III. Miscellaneous**
Copper	A. *Organic Solvents*
Gold	Carbon tetrachloride
Iron	Chloroform
Lead	Methanol
Mercury	Tetrachlorethylene
Phosphorus	B. *Glycols*
Silver	Diethylene glycol
Thallium	Ethylene dichloride
Uranium	Ethylene glycol
II. Therapeutic Agents	Ethylene glycol dinitrate
A. *Antimicrobials*	C. *Normal electrolytes at*
Amikacin	*abnormal concentrations*
Bacitracin	Hypercalcemia
Cephalosporins	Hypokalemia
Gentamicin	D. *Miscellaneous*
Kanamycin	Cantharides
Neomycin	Cyclophosphamide
Penicillins	Hemolysins
Streptomycin	Iodinated radiographic
Sulfonamides	contrast media
Tetracycline	Methotrexate
Tobramycin	Snake venom
B. *Antifungals*	Thiacetarsamide sodium
Amphotericin B	
C. *Analgesics*	
Phenacetin	
Phenylbutazone	
Salicylates	

nosis than that associated with ischemia. If anuria is present after volume correction, the prognosis is unfavorable.

ACUTE RENAL FAILURE COMPLICATING CHRONIC RENAL FAILURE

Acute renal failure complicating pre-existing chronic renal failure may be difficult to diagnose. There may be a prior history of chronic renal failure. Additional history may indicate exposure to potential nephrotoxins, especially nephrotoxic drugs; clinical states that predispose to renal ischemia; or infection resulting in sudden further deterioration of renal function. A biopsy is useful but not always necessary to establish a diagnosis.

POST-RENAL AZOTEMIA

A diagnosis of post-renal azotemia is usually easy to confirm. The diagnostic possibilities include urethral obstruction due to calculi, mucous plugs in male cats, strictures, constriction of the bladder neck caused by malposition of the urinary bladder into perineal hernias or inguinal hernias, traumatic injuries, urethral neoplasms, and, rarely, prostatic disease. Traumatic rupture of the urinary bladder

and transection of the urethra by a fractured pubis are additional causes. Bilateral ureteral obstruction or rupture can also cause post-renal azotemia, as can unilateral ureteral obstruction or rupture if the contralateral kidney is seriously diseased or absent.

Urethral obstruction can usually be recognized by finding a distended bladder, by attempts to pass a catheter and, if necessary, by urethrography. Malposition of the bladder into an inguinal or perineal hernia can usually be detected by palpation. Radiographs may be useful but are usually not necessary to establish this diagnosis.

Rupture of the bladder is most readily confirmed by a positive contrast cystogram, whereas ureteral rupture or obstruction can be recognized by an excretory urogram. Ureteral ruptures and obstructions are uncommon in small domestic animals.

TERMINAL CHRONIC RENAL FAILURE

Terminal chronic renal failure is usually easy to detect. Many times the patient has been treated for renal failure for months or even years before progressing to a point where functional capability is inadequate. Terminal chronic renal failure may be differentiated from prerenal azotemia complicating chronic renal failure and from acute renal failure complicating chronic renal failure by detection of *severe* nonregenerative normochromic normocytic anemia, which characterizes terminal chronic renal failure. Renal osteodystrophy will also be more pronounced in terminal chronic renal failure. Marked bilateral reduction in renal size combined with a long-standing history of polyuria and polydipsia may be present. Biochemical changes become more abnormal in terminal chronic renal failure despite all attempts to correct these parameters through various management practices and treatments. There is considerable wasting and chronic debilitation associated with terminal chronic renal failure.

THERAPY

The first steps in the treatment of a uremic crisis, regardless of cause are: (1) treat shock if present, and (2) rehydrate the patient if volume expansion is needed. Before any fluid replacement (other than emergency treatment of shock or hemorrhage) is given, samples for diagnostic tests should be taken. The patient should be accurately weighed to provide an initial weight and to help estimate the replacement volume of fluid that may be needed. Most patients in an acute uremic crisis require fluid to replace deficits associated with vomiting, diarrhea, insensible fluid losses, and, in some instances, obligatory polyuria. Other fluids such as blood, plasma, or dextran may be needed, depending on the cause of the uremic crisis. In the absence of pre-existing anemia or hypoproteinemia, measurement of the packed cell volume or total proteins may be helpful in evaluating the fluid deficit. Clinically detectable dehydration is assumed to represent at least a 5 per cent deficit. Severe, potentially fatal dehydration is usually estimated as a 12 to 15 per cent deficit. The rehydration needs should be estimated and replaced by the intravenous route. Unless contraindicated by congestive heart failure or pulmonary edema, an attempt should be made to rehydrate the patient within four to six hours. If hyperkalemia is a serious problem, 0.9 per cent saline should be used as the rehydrating solution; otherwise a polyionic solution such as lactated Ringer's solution is usually preferable (see Fluid Therapy in the Uremic Patient, page 989, for further information). The volume of fluid needed to rehydrate the patient is estimated by the following formula: per cent dehydration × weight in kg × 1000 = volume of fluid to be administered in ml. If a vigorous program of fluid administration is being pursued, the patient should be weighed at least two or three times daily to avoid either overhydration or inadequate fluid replacement. The weight obtained immediately after rehydration is used as the basis for future comparison to evaluate whether too much or too little fluid is being administered.

After fluid administration is established, an indwelling catheter should be introduced into the urinary bladder and secured in place. Urine output should be carefully monitored to help determine the response to fluid administration. This is best accomplished by attaching the catheter to a closed collection system. Production of at least 0.5 to 1.0 ml of urine/kg body weight/hr is commonly used to indicate adequate diuresis during fluid therapy, but this volume is probably inadequate for most patients in any of the six categories of uremic crisis discussed herein. The necessary or desired urine volume has not been established and obviously will vary among the different categories. In patients with prerenal or post-renal azotemia, a lower urine output will be more adequate than it would be in the other four categories. If a larger urine output can be attained without inducing overhydration, this is highly desirable.

Overhydration represents a serious therapeutic error. If overhydration occurs, as evidenced by pulmonary edema and/or peripheral pitting edema, administration of all fluids should be discontinued. An attempt should be made to increase urine flow with diuretics. Furosemide (Lasix*), 2 to 4 mg/kg, may be given intravenously and repeated at twice or triple this dose if diuresis does not occur within one hour. If there is still no response, dialysis must be instituted to remove the excess fluid. If the patient has a normal packed cell volume, some reduction in fluid load can be attained by removing 10 ml of blood/kg body weight. When the blood is collected aseptically it may be saved for later readministration.

If there is no improvement in urine flow as the result of rehydration, a test dose of mannitol combined with furosemide may be attempted. Mannitol at a dose of 0.25 to 0.5 gm/kg body weight should be given intravenously as a 20 to 25 per cent solution to well-hydrated patients, accompanied by 2 to 4 mg/kg body weight of furosemide given intravenously. If urine flow increases, additional diuretics (both mannitol and furosemide) can be given along with an appropriate volume of saline or balanced electrolyte solution to replace fluid losses and maintain urine output. Hypertonic dextrose can be used in lieu of mannitol to induce osmotic diuresis. A dose of 4 ml of 20 per cent dextrose/kg body weight may be infused over 15 to 20 minutes. The urine formed can be tested for glucose, or the blood sugar concentration can be measured a few minutes after completion of the infusion. The blood sugar concentration should be more than 200 mg/dl so that the renal threshold for glucose is exceeded.

If there is no response after one hour and if overhydration is not a problem, the dose of mannitol or dextrose can be repeated along with a double or

---

*Hoechst-Roussel Pharmaceuticals Inc., Somerville, NJ.

triple dose of furosemide. Studies in humans indicate that a slow infusion of dopamine (Intropin*) at the rate of 5 mcg/kg body weight/min may also be beneficial. If there is no response the dose can be increased to 10 or 20 mcg/kg/min. The dopamine is diluted in 0.9 per cent saline or 0.9 per cent saline and 5 per cent dextrose. Increased urine output is an indication for continued fluid and diuretic administration with or without additional dopamine. Use of dopamine as described previously in human patients has been minimally evaluated in dogs and cats.

If there is no response to the therapy previously described, the patient probably has ARF. Few private veterinary hospitals are able to adequately handle this problem because of the great need for intense monitoring of electrolyte and acid-base balance and the necessity of obtaining prompt laboratory results. There is also an extremely high probability that the patient will have to be treated by either hemodialysis or peritoneal dialysis. Both of these techniques are expensive, labor-intensive procedures that require close supervision and frequent monitoring. To proceed beyond the initial therapy requires a dedicated owner who is willing and able to finance an intensive program of dialysis. In addition to the close monitoring, it is usually highly desirable to obtain a renal biopsy to confirm the diagnosis of ARF and help establish the prognosis. For all of these reasons, referral of such a patient to a center that provides specialized care and resources is in order.

If a response to therapy is obtained, as evidenced by increased urine flow, it is still necessary to monitor acid-base balance, electrolytes, and BUN or creatinine often, preferably twice daily, until the uremic crisis subsides. The prognosis is grave to unfavorable even under the best of circumstances when anuria or oliguria has persisted following these corrective measures.

ELECTROLYTE IMBALANCES

Therapy for electrolyte and acid-base balance should be based on measurement of deviations from normal whenever possible. If anuria or oliguria does not respond to correction of hypovolemia and hypotension, it must be assumed that ARF and some degree of hyperkalemia are present. It is preferable to measure serum potassium whenever possible, but the electrocardiogram (ECG) can be used to demonstrate the cardiotoxic effects of hyperkalemia in an emergency as well as progress in alleviation of hyperkalemia during therapy. Tall, peaked T waves associated with missing or reduced-amplitude P waves are commonly found along with heart rates

of less than 60/min. Hyperkalemia of 8 mEq/liter or greater in association with ECG abnormalities is an indication for immediate administration of 10 per cent calcium gluconate as a slow bolus at a dose of approximately 0.5 ml/kg body weight. Calcium provides immediate improvement of the arrhythmias, but its effect is transient. Therefore, more lasting therapy must be used. Intravenous glucose solution (20 per cent) with or without insulin may be used. If insulin is used, it should be added to the intravenous solution at the rate of 1 unit of regular insulin for each 3 grams of glucose. This therapy will help move potassium into the cells and reduce its toxicity. If acidosis is present, intravenous 0.5 to 1.0 mEq/kg body weight administration of sodium bicarbonate, may help to alleviate the hyperkalemia. But, just as the response to glucose and calcium therapy, the effect is transitory. For a longer-term effect, the clinician must usually resort to peritoneal dialysis or hemodialysis.

A cation exchange resin, sodium polystyrene sulfonate (Kayexalate†), is available to reduce the severity of hyperkalemia by exchanging sodium ions for potassium ions in the bowel. The resin can be administered orally at a dose of 25 to 50 grams three times daily if the patient can retain it. The sodium polystyrene sulfonate can also be administered by retention enema. The resin should be retained for 30 to 45 minutes for best results, a serious drawback to its use. Because sodium is exchanged for potassium, one must also be alert for evidence of sodium overload.

Infrequently, hypokalemia rather than hyperkalemia may develop in patients with high urine volume renal failure or following intense diuresis. This possibility should be considered in unusually weak and depressed animals that are anorectic. Potassium should be cautiously given to such patients if their serum potassium is below 3.5 mEq/liter. Oral supplementation is preferred when vomiting is not a problem; potassium gluconate tablets or elixir can be used for this purpose. Potassium gluconate tablets (Kaon Tablets‡) may be used at the rate of 2.2 mEq of potassium per 100 calories of required energy intake. Potassium chloride may be added to intravenous solutions when necessary, but the rate of administration should not exceed 0.5 mEq/kg/hr.

SODIUM CHLORIDE

Serum sodium and chloride concentrations are usually normal in patients with oliguric or anuric renal failure but may be low in patients with prerenal azotemia associated with Addison's disease, when 5 per cent dextrose is used as a rehydrating

---

*Arnar-Stone Laboratories, Inc., Mount Prospect, IL.

†Breon Laboratories Inc., New York, NY.
‡Adria Laboratories Inc., Dublin, OH.

solution, or when severe vomiting is present. Administration of 0.9 per cent saline is usually adequate to replace the deficits.

CALCIUM

Hypocalcemic tetany is occasionally encountered in association with ethylene glycol poisoning. A slow intravenous infusion of approximately 0.5 ml/ kg of 10 per cent calcium gluconate is usually adequate to control hypocalcemic tetany.

Hypercalcemia is a recognized cause of ARF and is associated with a variety of problems including primary hyperparathyroidism, malignancies (especially lymphosarcoma), osteolytic bone lesions, and hypervitaminosis D. Hypercalcemia should be treated when the calcium concentration exceeds 13 mg/dl. Infusions of normal saline along with furosemide (thiazide diuretics are contraindicated) at 5 mg/kg have been recommended for lowering the serum calcium, since both enhance its excretion. If this treatment is ineffective, prednisone at a dose of 1 mg/kg b.i.d. is generally effective in lowering the serum calcium concentration. Its use should be delayed until the cause of hypercalcemia is determined unless the hypercalcemia is itself causing serious renal failure as suggested by a rapidly increasing serum urea nitrogen or creatinine concentration associated with polyuria.

ACID-BASE BALANCE

Whenever possible, the acid-base status of uremic patients should be measured. Most animals in uremic crisis develop moderate to severe metabolic acidosis. Infrequently, a patient may develop metabolic alkalosis, and somewhat more often their acid-base state will be normal. If the serum bicarbonate is known, the amount of sodium bicarbonate necessary to replace the deficit can be calculated by using the following formula: body weight in kg $\times$ 0.3 $\times$ bicarbonate deficit = mEq of replacement bicarbonate required. Unless the serum bicarbonate is 18 mEq/liter or lower, no therapy is usually administered. When bicarbonate or blood gases cannot be measured, one can estimate the degree of bicarbonate deficit based on the magnitude of elevation of BUN. Mild uremic states are assumed to be associated with a bicarbonate deficit of 5 mEq/ liter and usually are not treated. The deficit in moderate and severe uremia is estimated at 10 and 15 mEq/liter, respectively. One-half of the calculated bicarbonate deficit is given over the first hour, and the remaining half is administered over the next five to six hours. The acid-base status should be evaluated after the deficit of bicarbonate has been replaced and daily thereafter if possible.

MAINTENANCE THERAPY

Maintenance fluid, electrolyte, and acid-base therapy is continued as long as necessary provided adequate urine output is attained to control or eliminate the uremic crisis. Input and output of fluid must be in close balance as determined by measurement of urine production and, especially, maintenance of body weight. If oliguria or anuria persists, survival is dependent on initiation of peritoneal dialysis or hemodialysis. With the onset of polyuria, larger quantities of fluid and close electrolyte surveillance are necessary to avoid serious deficits (see Parenteral Nutrition During a Uremic Crisis, page 994). Administration of 5 per cent dextrose in saline or lactated Ringer's solution alternated with 10 per cent dextrose may relieve the catabolic state to some degree by providing a portion of the required daily calories.

A diuretic phase may develop in some patients during the recovery stage from ARF and in other patients during early stages of ARF, especially when ARF is due to use of aminoglycosides. The magnitude of the diuresis is variable and may be more extreme if the patient was volume overloaded initially. Therefore, it is important to follow the patient's weight frequently and accurately. Electrolytes should be measured at least daily during severe diuresis to detect deficits or excesses. Potassium replacement may be necessary if urine flow is extremely high. Sodium-containing fluids are used to replace urinary losses. Lactated Ringer's solution or similar fluids usually are appropriate. Insensible losses, usually estimated at about 20 ml/kg/day, are replaced with 5 or 10 per cent dextrose solution.

PREVENTION

Causes of uremic crises that the veterinarian can influence center mainly around nephrotoxic drugs and chemicals, extensive surgery, and prolonged and deep anesthesia, especially in aged patients. Clinicians should monitor renal function regularly in all patients receiving nephrotoxic drugs. At the first sign of nephrotoxicity, the drug should be withdrawn and an effort made to induce greater urine flow by carefully monitored fluid administration. When using potent nephrotoxic drugs such as amphotericin B, the drug should be administered slowly by the intravenous route. A high urine output should be maintained and monitored during therapy. Mannitol administration and salt loading have been helpful in reducing the nephrotoxicity of amphotericin B. The concomitant use of nephrotoxic antimicrobials and diuretics is strictly contraindicated, since the combination may potentiate renal damage.

The dosage of drugs excreted by the kidney, and especially nephrotoxic drugs, given to patients with renal dysfunction should be reduced by an amount related to the severity of renal impairment. Dosage may be reduced either by using the standard dose but decreasing the frequency of administration or by using the usual maintenance interval but reducing the dose. Drugs should not be given to animals in renal failure unless there is an indication for their use. Whenever possible, drugs that are excreted by alternate routes should be used. Renal function should be evaluated before using drugs that have marked nephrotoxicity. The clinician can then compare pretreatment BUN or serum creatinine concentrations with those that may become distinctly abnormal following administration of the drug. The drug can then be withdrawn, the interval between doses increased, or the dose reduced, as may be appropriate. Extensive information on excretion of drugs in renal failure has been tabulated for humans. Although this information is intended for modifying drug use in humans, it may be of some benefit to veterinarians (Bennett et al., 1980). Unfortunately, there is no comparable information available suggesting appropriate modification of drug dosages in animals (see "Checklist of Hazardous Drugs in Patients With Renal Failure," page 1036, for further details).

Extensive surgery or prolonged anesthesia may cause ARF, especially in aged or debilitated animals. Intravenous fluids, usually balanced polyionic solutions, should be administered during these procedures to support adequate urine flow. This precaution may reduce the frequency with which ARF develops following surgery. Urine production should be monitored by placing an indwelling catheter in the bladder. If urine flow is poor, diuresis may be induced with osmotic agents such as mannitol or dextrose.

REFERENCES AND SUPPLEMENTAL READING

Bennett, W., et al.: Drug therapy in renal failure: dosing guidelines for adults. Part I: Antimicrobial agents, analgesics. Ann. Intern. Med. 93:62, 1980.
Bennett, W. M., et al.: Drug therapy in renal failure: dosing guidelines for adults. Part II: Sedatives, hypnotics, and tranquilizers; cardiovascular, antihypertensive, and diuretic agents; miscellaneous agents. Ann. Intern. Med. 93:286, 1980.

FLUID THERAPY IN THE UREMIC PATIENT

LARRY M. CORNELIUS, D.V.M.

Athens, Georgia

Fluid therapy is especially important in the treatment of uremic dogs and cats, since alternative techniques for maintaining the normal volume and composition of body fluids (i.e., peritoneal dialysis, hemodialysis, renal transplantation) are expensive, time-consuming, and not well developed in veterinary medicine. General principles of fluid therapy have been outlined in another article. The purpose of this discussion is to present specific details of fluid and electrolyte therapy in uremic dogs and cats.

It is helpful to categorize uremic patients into those with anuria, oliguria, or polyuria. Differentiation into prerenal, primary renal, and post-renal causes has been discussed previously (Finco et al., 1975). Combinations of these categories of azotemia are sometimes present.

ANURIC UREMIA

Anuria is usually caused by obstructive uropathy or rents in the lower urinary tract (Finco et al., 1975). Uremia develops owing to accumulation of waste products normally eliminated in urine. Life-threatening metabolic abnormalities associated with anuric uremia include hypothermia, dehydration, hyperkalemia, and metabolic acidemia (see Emergency Management of the Acute Uremic Crisis, page 981, for further information). Dehydration occurs despite lack of urine outflow because of sequestration of fluid in the bladder or abdominal cavity, lack of water intake, and continued water loss by nonrenal routes.

TREATMENT

Animals with anuric uremia may be markedly depressed or moribund and must be treated quickly and effectively. Urinary tract obstruction should be relieved before or immediately after initiating fluid therapy. With rupture of the urinary tract, fluid administration should be begun prior to repair of the rent. Peritoneal drainage using a peritoneal dialysis catheter is helpful in alleviating uremia prior to surgical correction of a ruptured bladder.

The composition of the solutions used for therapy depends on the patient's clinical condition and the severity of hyperkalemia and metabolic acidemia. A serum potassium concentration of 6.0 to 8.0 mEq/liter and an arterial pH of 7.2 to 7.4 are mild to moderate disturbances. Electrocardiographic changes are usually minimal (prolonged P-R interval; tall, peaked T waves) and the patient's clinical condition is not critical. Lactated Ringer's solution, in sufficient quantities to alleviate dehydration, will usually correct both the hyperkalemia and metabolic acidemia. The volume of fluid needed should be determined from the estimated percentage of dehydration (existing deficit) and administered intravenously at the rate of 90 ml/kg/hr (assuming cardiac function is adequate).

Additional fluid to supply maintenance needs and continuing nonrenal losses may be required (see Fluid Therapy, page 28). Lactate is converted to bicarbonate by the liver (1 mEq of lactate = 1 mEq of bicarbonate), thus alkalinizing body fluids. The quantity of lactate needed can be estimated from the following formula: mEq of lactate (or bicarbonate) = 0.5 × body weight (kg) × plasma bicarbonate deficit (normal bicarbonate-patient bicarbonate). In the absence of plasma bicarbonate data, one may estimate lactate (bicarbonate) needs as 1 to 2 mEq/kg.

Hyperkalemia is usually corrected by fluid therapy with lactated Ringer's solution because alkalinization of extracellular fluid causes transfer of extracellular potassium ions into cells in exchange for hydrogen ions. Also, serum potassium is decreased by dilutional effects as extracellular fluid volume is increased. The small quantity of potassium in lactated Ringer's solution (4 mEq/liter) will not worsen hyperkalemia. Once urine flow is re-established, potassium will be excreted in the urine owing to diuresis and correction of metabolic acidemia. Adequacy of response to therapy should be assessed frequently by clinical evaluation of the patient's state of hydration and by periodic determination of serum bicarbonate and potassium concentrations.

More severe hyperkalemia (serum potassium > 8.0 mEq/liter) and metabolic acidemia (arterial pH < 7.20) occasionally may require different treatment. Each patient's condition must be evaluated individually before making a decision concerning more intensive therapy. If cardiac dysfunction is severe, the lactated Ringer's treatment regimen described previously may cause heart failure owing to volume overload before the cardiotoxic effects of hyperkalemia and metabolic acidemia are reversed. Evidence of severe cardiac abnormalities (bradycardia, EKG changes such as atrial standstill with idioventricular rhythm) is usually an indication for immediate correction of hyperkalemia and metabolic acidemia.

Initially, sodium bicarbonate solution (0.5 to 1.0 mEq of bicarbonate/kg) is infused intravenously over three to five minutes. This is followed by intravenous administration of 20 per cent dextrose solution (0.5 to 1.0 gm of dextrose/kg) infused over five to ten minutes. Regular insulin may be given as an intravenous bolus at a dosage of 1 unit/3 gm of glucose administered; however, the need for insulin is unproved. Bicarbonate, dextrose, and insulin cause transfer of potassium ions from the extracellular fluid to the intracellular fluid and lessen cardiotoxity. It is best to evaluate response to treatment with the aid of an EKG while administering these drugs. The benefits of bicarbonate and glucose-insulin therapy occur within a few minutes but are relatively short in duration.

Calcium ions directly counteract the cardiotoxic effects of hyperkalemia and can be administered intravenously as 10 per cent calcium gluconate solution. Since the effective dosage of calcium gluconate is variable (usually 0.5 ml/kg), the heart rate or EKG should be carefully monitored while slowly injecting calcium gluconate. The infusion should be stopped when the heart rate increases or the EKG becomes more normal.

Correction of dehydration should be accomplished by slow intravenous infusion of lactated Ringer's solution. Deficit requirements are estimated and replaced over four to six hours, with careful observation of the patient for signs of cardiac failure and pulmonary edema (see the following section on oliguric uremia).

These measures must be considered temporary emergency procedures; efforts to correct the cause of anuria should proceed without delay. Peritoneal dialysis or hemodialysis may be necessary for longer-term control of the metabolic abnormalities of uremia associated with prolonged anuria (see Continuous Ambulatory Peritoneal Dialysis, page 1028, and Current Status of Veterinary Hemodialysis, CVT VII, page 1111, for further information).

Postobstruction diuresis occurs in some patients with obstructive uropathy and can cause dehydration and electrolyte losses. Oral administration of water and electrolytes (water and food if the patient will drink and eat) should be supplemented with parenteral fluids. Lactated Ringer's solution administered subcutaneously is generally sufficient, but extra potassium may be required to replace the potassium being lost in urine. Potassium chloride solution can be added to lactated Ringer's solution in amounts sufficient to yield a final concentration of 35 mEq of potassium/liter and administered subcutaneously. Daily potassium dosage should be a minimum of 1 to 3 mEq/kg. Serum potassium concentration should be determined daily to assess the adequacy of potassium replacement. The total daily fluid volume required is variable (minimum of 50 to 60 ml/kg), and therefore frequent assessment of the patient's state of hydration (including body weight) is essential.

OLIGURIC UREMIA

PHYSIOLOGIC VERSUS PATHOLOGIC OLIGURIA

Oliguria is defined as the formation of a reduced quantity of urine and may be either physiologic or pathologic. Physiologic oliguria occurs when normal kidneys conserve water in excess of solute in response to dehydration. Physiologic oliguria is characterized by a small volume of urine of high specific gravity (Finco et al., 1975). Azotemia associated with physiologic oliguria is classified as prerenal. It is essential that the clinician determine whether oliguria is physiologic or pathologic, because appropriate fluid therapy for each is markedly different (see hereafter).

TREATMENT OF PHYSIOLOGIC OLIGURIA

For prerenal azotemia associated with physiologic oliguria, correction of dehydration with lactated Ringer's solution should promptly alleviate the mild metabolic acidosis occasionally present and normalize the BUN concentration. The volume of lactated Ringer's solution needed should be estimated from the patient's percentage of dehydration (see Fluid Therapy, page 28). At least one-half of the estimated fluid deficit requirements should be administered intravenously over four to six hours. The remaining fluid can be administered subcutaneously. Periodic re-evaluation of the patient's state of hydration and BUN concentration should be done while attempts are made to correct the cause of the prerenal azotemia.

CHARACTERISTICS OF PATHOLOGIC OLIGURIA

Pathologic oliguria occurs during the early stages of acute renal failure, terminally in chronic renal failure, and occasionally when dehydration is superimposed on chronic polyuric renal failure (Finco et al., 1975). In any case, it is characterized by a small urine volume of low specific gravity (Finco et al., 1975).

The mechanisms responsible for the reduction in renal function during the generation and maintenance phases of oliguric renal failure have not been fully explained (Stein et al., 1978). Renal vasoconstriction with marked reduction in renal blood flow

and glomerular filtration rate (GFR) have been found consistently in the initial phase of experimentally induced acute renal failure (Lindner et al., 1979). Other factors, such as a decrease in the glomerular capillary ultrafiltration coefficient, back leakage of filtrate across damaged tubular epithelium, and tubular obstruction caused by swelling of damaged tubular epithelial cells, may contribute to acute oliguric renal failure (Lindner et al., 1979).

Abnormalities of fluid, electrolyte, and acid-base balance in patients with oliguric renal failure are similar to those described in the previous section on anuric uremia. Dehydration, hyperkalemia, and metabolic acidemia are common.

TREATMENT OF PATHOLOGIC OLIGURIA

Treatment given as soon as possible after the initiating insult improves the chances for successful management of oliguric renal failure. A word of caution: fluid administration must be undertaken with the awareness that iatrogenic volume overload and subsequent fatal pulmonary edema are distinct possibilities.

FLUID AND ELECTROLYTE THERAPY

After estimation of the fluid volume deficit (see Fluid Therapy, page 28), lactated Ringer's solution should be administered intravenously. It is advisable to use an indwelling jugular catheter for fluid infusion to allow periodic measurement of central venous pressure. The rate of infusion depends on the severity of dehydration, the presence or absence of hypotension, and the state of cardiac function. If dehydration is mild to moderate and hypotension is absent, 10 to 20 ml/kg/hr is an appropriate rate. If dehydration is severe, the infusion rate should be 90 ml/kg/hr, assuming cardiac function is good. Urine output should be quantitated with the aid of an indwelling urinary catheter. The quantity of fluid input and urine output should be recorded on a flow sheet. Totals should be summarized, preferably every three or four hours. Other parameters that should be periodically monitored and recorded on the flow sheet are body temperature; heart rate; respiratory rate; body weight; PCV; and plasma protein (determined by refractometry), serum potassium, and serum bicarbonate (total CO_2) concentrations.

Response to therapy is indicated by significant urine flow (1 to 2 ml/kg/hr) noted after replacement of the estimated volume deficit. If oliguria persists, the volume deficit was underestimated, or (more likely) renal damage is severe and other measures are needed. The decision to administer more lactated Ringer's solution should be made only after careful consideration of the patient's cardiovascular status. Central venous pressure should be added to the list of parameters monitored and recorded on the flow sheet, and lung sounds should be periodically evaluated for evidence of pulmonary edema.

Hyperkalemia and metabolic acidemia may occur with oliguric renal failure. These complications and their treatment were discussed previously.

Other drugs that may be beneficial in oliguric renal failure are diuretics and vasodilators. The benefits of these drugs in prophylaxis and during the early stages (first few hours) of acute oliguric renal failure have been well documented, but their benefits in later phases of the disorder have not yet been established.

DIURETICS

Both osmotic (hypertonic dextrose and mannitol) and loop (furosemide and ethacrynic acid) diuretics have been advocated for the treatment of acute oliguric renal failure. Their precise beneficial effects are not well defined, but they appear to modify early mechanisms that initiate acute oliguric renal failure. Osmotic diuretics may increase blood volume, renal blood flow, and GFR. By their osmotic effects in renal tubular filtrate, they inhibit tubular reabsorption of water and may reduce swelling of tubular epithelial cells. Decreased intratubular obstruction and enhanced urine flow may occur. I prefer 20 per cent dextrose solution over mannitol because it is (1) just as effective, (2) less expensive, (3) readily detected in urine when its effects begin, and (4) metabolized by body cells for energy (see the article that follows).

For a trial of osmotic diuresis, administer 20 per cent dextrose intravenously at a total dosage of 25 to 65 ml/kg and a rate of 2 ml/min for 10 to 15 minutes. Then reduce the infusion rate to 1 ml/min. Test newly formed urine (if any) for glucose. If positive, anuria does not exist. The procedure can only be safely continued if urine volume increases to 1 to 4 ml/min. If adequate urine flow is not observed by the time one-half the 20 per cent glucose solution is administered, the infusion must be discontinued, since overhydration and hyperosmolality will occur. If adequate diuresis occurs, a maintenance infusion of 10 per cent dextrose solution can be continued to promote diuresis for the next 12 to 24 hours. Lactated Ringer's solution should be alternated with 10 per cent dextrose to correct any detectable dehydration. The total quantity of fluid administered should only slightly exceed urine output.

Loop diuretics such as furosemide may sometimes initiate diuresis in oliguric renal failure, but the results have been better in the early stages of experimental acute renal failure than in clinical cases. Use of these agents should always be accompanied by adequate fluid volume replacement. Otherwise, decreased blood volume and GFR induced by furosemide may result in worsening of uremia. Patients who fail to develop diuresis after initial fluid therapy may be given furosemide intravenously as a bolus (2 to 4 mg/kg). If no significant diuresis is noted in one hour, the dosage may be doubled or tripled.

VASODILATORS

As discussed previously, renal vasoconstriction is a consistent part of the initial phase of acute oliguric renal failure. Constriction of the preglomerular afferent arteriole causes decreased renal blood flow and GFR. Reduced surface area of glomerular capillaries caused by glomerular capillary constriction may cause a decreased glomerular ultrafiltration coefficient (Lindner et al., 1979).

Dopamine, a precursor of norepinephrine, is useful as a renal vasodilator in both experimental and clinical cases of acute oliguric renal failure, especially during the early phases (Lindner et al., 1979). For treatment, 50 mg of dopamine is diluted in 500 ml of lactated Ringer's solution (final concentration = 100 μg of dopamine/ml) and administered slowly intravenously at the rate of 1 to 3 μg/kg/min. At this dosage, dopamine also slightly increases cardiac output. With higher dosage rates, dopamine causes undesirable effects similar to those of isoproterenol (beta-adrenergic stimulation), such as tachycardia and cardiac arrhythmias. A pediatric minidrip infusion set must be used to regulate the slow rate of dopamine infusion. If significant diuresis develops, the dopamine infusion is continued until urine flow can be maintained with fluid therapy alone.

Results of a recent study of experimental acute toxic nephropathy in dogs indicated that early intravenous administration (within 15 minutes of toxin administration) of a *combination* of dopamine (3 μg/kg/min) and furosemide (1 mg/kg as a bolus followed by 1 mg/kg/hr) was more effective in preventing oliguric renal failure than either drug used alone (Lindner et al., 1979). It was concluded that the mechanisms of the synergistic effects of dopamine and furosemide were multifactorial and possibly included increased delivery of furosemide to a critical intrarenal location as a result of dopamine-induced renal vasodilation (Lindner et al., 1979). The clinical applicability for oliguric renal failure of combination diuretic-vasodilator therapy remains to be proved. This therapy is more likely to be effective when a renal insult is of short duration (e.g., intraoperative hypotension or hypovolemia).

If these measures are ineffective in sustaining adequate urine production or in controlling uremia, peritoneal dialysis or hemodialysis must be considered (see Continuous Ambulatory Dialysis, page 1028, for details).

PARENTERAL NUTRITION

Evidence in uremic people and experimentally nephrectomized dogs suggests that parenteral administration of glucose and amino acid solutions during the uremic crisis is beneficial. Once the critical abnormalities of fluid, electrolyte, and acid-base balance are corrected, consideration should be given to parenteral nutrition (see the article that follows).

PROGNOSIS

With appropriate monitoring of the previously mentioned laboratory parameters and careful supportive therapy, the ultimate outcome of oliguric renal failure usually depends on the severity and potential reversibility of the underlying cause of renal failure. Failure to sustain diuresis with conservative treatment indicates severe disease and suggests an unfavorable outcome. Intensive peritoneal dialysis or hemodialysis is time-consuming and expensive but may occasionally be successful in acute oliguric renal failure (see the article that follows).

POLYURIC UREMIA

Polyuria begins during the early stages of chronic renal failure and during the late or recovery phase of acute renal failure (Finco et al., 1975). With progression of chronic renal failure, other signs characteristic of uremia (depression, anorexia, and vomiting) may develop.

Uremic patients with primary renal failure are usually dehydrated as a result of anorexia and vomiting. Dehydration results in decreased renal blood flow and GFR, thereby superimposing a prerenal factor on primary renal failure. Serum potassium concentration is usually normal until the terminal or oliguric phase of chronic renal failure, at which time hyperkalemia may be present. Serum sodium concentration is usually normal. Deficits of both potassium and sodium are usually present but are masked by transfer of potassium ions from cells into the extracellular fluid and by isotonic dehydration. The patient's blood acid-base status varies, depending on the severity of renal failure as well as the presence or absence of concurrent abnormalities that may also affect acid-base balance. For example, severe vomiting may cause significant loss of hydrogen ions (metabolic alkalosis) and tends to offset the retention of hydrogen ions (metabolic acidosis) caused by renal failure. It is best to measure either arterial blood gases and pH or plasma total CO_2 content. If this is not possible, one should assume that mild to moderate metabolic acidosis is present. Hyperphosphatemia is characteristic of polyuric renal failure. Serum calcium concentration is usually normal but may be either decreased or increased.

TREATMENT

Fluid therapy for polyuric chronic renal failure may encompass both initial rehydration and osmotic diuresis.

INITIAL REHYDRATION

Lactated Ringer's solution is the fluid of choice to initially correct dehydration and mild to moderate metabolic acidosis. Estimation of fluid volume and bicarbonate requirements have been discussed previously (see section on anuric uremia). The estimated fluid deficit should be administered intravenously over four to six hours. Additional lactated Ringer's solution to supply maintenance needs and continuing losses may be required.

OSMOTIC DIURESIS

Osmotic diuretics increase renal blood flow, GFR, and urine flow within minutes of intravenous administration (as contrasted with hours for balanced electrolyte solutions) (Finco and Low, 1980). Osmotic diuresis should be considered whenever correction of volume depletion with lactated Ringer's solution does not promptly reduce the BUN concentration significantly and alleviate signs of uremia. The following technique of osmotic diuresis has been described previously (Finco and Low, 1980).

1. Use a flow sheet to frequently record body temperature, heart and respiratory rates, body weight, fluid input, urine output, PCV, plasma total protein concentration, and BUN concentration.

2. Hydrate the patient with lactated Ringer's solution as previously described.

3. After rehydration, catheterize the patient and empty the bladder.

4. Accurately weigh the patient and record this baseline weight.

5. Administer 20 per cent dextrose solution intravenously at a total dosage of 25 to 65 ml/kg at a rate of 2 ml/min for 10 to 15 minutes. Then reduce the infusion rate to 1 ml/min.

6. Test newly formed urine for glucose with a urine dipstick. If the test is positive, sufficient glucose to exceed the renal threshold has been administered, and anuria does not exist. Continue treating only if urine volume increases to 1 to 4 ml/min.

7. If adequate urine flow is not present by the time one-half of the calculated quantity of glucose solution has been given, stop the infusion, since overhydration and hyperosmolality may occur.

8. If adequate urine flow is obtained, the entire calculated amount of 20 per cent glucose solution should be administered. Lactated Ringer's solution (3 to 5 per cent of body weight), followed by 20 per cent glucose solution is repeated as described previously. Two or three cycles of glucose and lactated Ringer's solutions are administered every 24 hours.

9. After 24 hours, the patient is re-evaluated by physical examination and determination of BUN concentration and body weight. If necessary, the entire procedure is repeated.

10. Weight gain indicates fluid retention and obviates the administration of lactated Ringer's solution prior to osmotic diuresis. Weight loss indicates the need for additional fluid therapy with lactated Ringer's solution to correct dehydration prior to osmotic diuresis.

11. Care must be taken to prevent hypokalemia and hypoalbuminemia.

12. If serum potassium concentration decreases to < 3.0 mEq/liter, potassium chloride solution should be added to lactated Ringer's solution in amounts sufficient to yield 25 to 35 mEq of potassium/liter. It is safest to administer this fluid subcutaneously (total daily potassium dosage at least 1 to 3 mEq/kg). If given intravenously, the rate of administration should not exceed 0.5 mEq of potassium/kg/hr.

13. If plasma protein concentration decreases to < 3.5 gm/dl, serum albumin should be periodically measured. If the serum albumin concentration decreases to < 1.0 gm/dl, osmotic diuresis should be stopped to avoid generalized edema from low plasma colloid osmotic pressure. Plasma administration may help correct hypoalbuminemia.

14. Generally, response to osmotic diuresis, indicated by a decrease in BUN concentration, occurs in two to four days. Failure to respond indicates severe functional impairment and dictates the use of other measures such as peritoneal dialysis or hemodialysis. Furosemide and dopamine may be tried if 20 per cent dextrose fails to induce adequate diuresis (see previous section on oliguric uremia).

PARENTERAL NUTRITION

Intravenous administration of calories and protein in the form of 20 per cent dextrose and amino acid solutions may be helpful in uremic patients (see the article that follows).

Whenever clinical and laboratory response is good, oral treatment should be gradually substituted for parenteral therapy (see Conservative Management of Canine Chronic Polyuric Renal Failure, page 997).

REFERENCES

Finco, D. R., and Low, D. G.: Intensive diuresis in polyuric renal failure. *In* Kirk, R. W. (ed.): *Current Veterinary Therapy VII*. Philadelphia: W. B. Saunders, 1980, pp. 1091–1093.

Finco, D. R., Osborne, C. A., and Low, D. G.: Physiology and pathophysiology of renal failure. *In* Ettinger, S. J. (ed.): *Textbook of Veterinary Internal Medicine*. Philadelphia: W. B. Saunders, 1975, pp. 1453–1534.

Lindner, A., Cutler, R. E., and Goodman, W. G.: Synergism of dopamine plus furosemide in preventing acute renal failure in the dog. Kidney Int. 16:158, 1979.

Stein, J. H., Lieschitz, M. D., and Barnes, L. D.: Current concepts on the pathophysiology of acute renal failure. Am. J. Physiol. 234:F171, 1978.

PARENTERAL NUTRITION DURING A UREMIC CRISIS

DELMAR R. FINCO, D.V.M.,
and JEANNE A. BARSANTI, D.V.M.

Athens, Georgia

Considerable attention has been given to dietary management of renal failure in the dog. This attention has been motivated by the belief that a diet is beneficial to the azotemic dog if it (1) fulfills the dog's need for calories from nonprotein sources; (2) contains "adequate" vitamins, minerals, and essential fatty acids; and (3) has a protein content that maintains nitrogen balance without leading to catabolism of ingested amino acids (i.e., protein) to nitrogenous wastes. The character, formulation, and controversy concerning such diets are discussed elsewhere (see the article that follows).

Paradoxically, nutrition in the azotemic dog during periods of anorexia and vomiting (i.e., a uremic crisis) has received little attention despite the probability that nutritional therapy during uremia is more important than most other causes of anorexia.

EFFECTS OF ANOREXIA ON THE NORMAL DOG

To evaluate the benefits and limitations of parenteral nutritional therapy during a uremic crisis, conceptual understanding of metabolism during uremia and starvation is required. With lack of food intake, body components are utilized to provide nutrients necessary for metabolic processes and muscular activity. Glycogen stores are sufficient only for the first few days of anorexia. Thereafter, caloric requirements must be fulfilled by protein and fat catabolism. Most tissues can use fatty acids for their energy needs, but the brain, peripheral nerves, and RBCs require glucose or ketone bodies. Fatty acids cannot be utilized for net synthesis of glucose, and the glycerol from triglyceride provides inadequate glucose for maintenance of adequate blood glucose concentrations. Body proteins are used for glucose synthesis to fulfill basal needs. In muscle, protein provides glucose precursors, particularly by catabolism of branched-chain amino acids. Thus, protein catabolism accompanies fat catabolism early in the course of complete anorexia.

DELETERIOUS EFFECTS OF ANOREXIA ON THE UREMIC DOG

Catabolic processes occur during anorexia in both normal and uremic animals. However, the consequences are more devastating in uremic animals because of several factors. Anorexia in combination with metabolic derangements of chronic uremia results in gradual tissue wasting prior to a uremic crisis. Both protein and fat reserves available for catabolism are reduced in these patients once a uremic crisis supervenes. In addition, the products of protein catabolism are believed to be deleterious, and such products accumulate during uremia. Although the exact identity of uremic toxins is not known, there is a good clinical correlation between signs of uremia and retention of nitrogenous wastes. Catabolism of tissues with a high-protein content has the same effect on production of nitrogenous wastes as oral intake of a meat diet. The obvious difference is that the tissue in the case of the uremic crisis is a component of the patient's own body. Consequently, the end result of anorexia in uremic dogs in an increase in production of uremic toxins during the period of catabolism. A phenomenon occurs in which uremic toxin production, anorexia, and catabolism create a self-perpetuating cycle.

CAPABILITIES OF THE UREMIC PATIENT TO REVERSE THE CATABOLIC STATE

Since catabolism and weight loss occur prior to anorexia and vomiting associated with uremic crises in chronic uremia, it is reasonable to question whether reversal of catabolism can be achieved even when appropriate nutrients are supplied. It is known that certain metabolic alterations exist during the uremic state, including glucose intolerance and altered lipid and amino acid metabolism. Despite these formidable adversities, nutritional treatment of uremic humans has resulted in reversal of catabolism to such a degree that an anabolic state is achieved. During nutritional therapy, BUN values decreased coincident with the administration of amino acids. An experimental study in nephrectomized dogs revealed that life could be prolonged by providing nutritional therapy with dextrose and amino acids. Dogs given food and water *ad libitum* survived three to five days. Dogs infused with 50 ml/kg/24 hr of 5 per cent dextrose survived four to six days. Dogs that received 50 ml/kg/24 hr of 56 per cent dextrose survived 5 to 11 days. Dogs given 50 ml/kg/24 hr of a solution containing 56 per cent dextrose and 0.525 gm/kg of essential L-amino acids survived 6 to 14 days. Serum creatinine levels increased at the same rate in all the dogs, but dogs receiving amino acids had markedly lower BUN values than dogs in the other three groups. These data clearly demonstrate the benefits of nutritional therapy during uremia and emphasize the deleterious effects of ignoring nutritional therapy.

METHODS OF CORRECTING NUTRITIONAL DEFICIENCIES DURING THE UREMIC CRISIS

OBJECTIVES

The objectives of parenteral nutritional therapy are nearly the same as those for oral therapy prior to the uremic crisis. Fulfillment of the maintenance caloric requirements of the dog from nonprotein sources is probably the most important step. In addition, it is beneficial to provide just enough amino acids in the correct proportion for nitrogen balance or anabolism. Administration of water-soluble vitamins is also important, but giving essential fatty acids and trace minerals is indicated only if therapy is conducted for several weeks.

SOURCES OF NONPROTEIN CALORIES

Dextrose solutions are available for use from numerous manufacturers. Five per cent dextrose is an inadequate source of calories unless massive volumes of fluid are used (see CVT VI, pp. 3–12).

Solutions of 20 to 25 per cent are sufficiently concentrated to fulfill caloric requirements in reasonable volumes of fluid.

A lipid emulsion (Intralipid 10%*) is now available in the United States for use in humans. This product is apparently safe for dogs, although other lipid emulsions sold in Europe have caused fatalities in dogs. Lipid emulsions have the advantage of being a concentrated source of calories without the hyperosmotic property of concentrated glucose solutions. Their current cost prohibits their routine use in veterinary medicine.

SOURCES OF AMINO ACIDS

Protein (casein, fibrin) hydrolysate solutions (Aminosol 5 and 10%,† Amigen 5 and 10%‡) have been available for years. The hydrolyzed solution is supplemented with essential amino acids to provide a reasonably balanced product. Because hydrolysis of the protein is not complete, however, only about 75 per cent of the contents are actually retained for anabolism after injection.

More recently, parenteral preparations of essential "semisynthetic" amino acids (Aminosyn,† Freamine§) have become available. These products are devoid of unutilizable polypeptide chains, but their cost is nearly twice that of protein hydrolysates. It has been stated that administration of essential amino acids alone is advantageous since the nonessential amino acids can be synthesized by the body.

Keto and hydroxy acids have recently attracted considerable attention for use in uremic humans. Studies revealed that some analogs of essential amino acids that are devoid of nitrogen could be converted to amino acids in uremic individuals. Species variations exist in the ability to convert and in the efficiency of the conversion. These compounds have potential advantages over amino acids, since nitrogen that could otherwise be retained as harmful wastes is used to convert the keto or

hydroxy to an amino acid, which can then be used for anabolism.

PROGRAMS FEASIBLE FOR THE DOG

The first priority for nutrition of dogs during uremic crises is to provide nonprotein calories in adequate quantities to minimize catabolism. The daily caloric requirements of dogs are determined; 20 or 25 per cent dextrose is used to provide these calories. The solution is given slowly via jugular catheter to avoid complications of extracellular hyperosmolality. The program can be conveniently combined with one of intensive diuresis (see Intensive Diuresis in Renal Failure, CVT VII, pp. 1091–1094). Since about 20 per cent of the glucose may be lost during the diuresis program, daily requirements should be increased by this increment. Precautions listed for intensive diuresis should be strictly followed. Since dextrose is relatively inexpensive, this procedure is economically feasible. A minor negative nitrogen balance will exist with this program because nitrogen losses are inevitable.

Use of amino acids in addition to dextrose increases the cost of the procedure but provides the potential for establishing nitrogen balance. Data are not available in the dog concerning the superiority of semisynthetic preparations over hydrolysates. Likewise, the amino acid requirements of the uremic dog are not known. Until more specific data are available, it is recommended that 0.3 gm/kg/24 hr of a balanced amino acid solution be provided to dogs in a uremic crisis. Thus, for a 20-kg dog, 6 gm, or 125 ml, of a 5 per cent amino acid solution would be required each day. Since amino acids may spill over in the urine, slow administration over the course of each day is advisable.

---

*Cutter Laboratories, Berkeley, CA.
†Abbott Laboratories, North Chicago, IL.
‡Baxter Laboratories, Morton Grove, IL.
§McGaw Laboratories, Glendale, CA.

SUPPLEMENTAL READING

Kopple, J. D., and Swendseid, M.D.: Amino acids and keto acid diets for therapy in renal failure. Nephron 18:1, 1977.

Kopple, J. D., et al.: Symposium on nutrition in renal disease. Am. J. Clin. Nutrit. 33:1363, 1980.

Van Buren, C. T., et al.: Effects of intravenous essential L-amino acids and hypertonic dextrose on anephric beagles. Surg. Forum 23:83, 1972.

Walzer, M.: Keto acid therapy in chronic renal failure. Nephron 21:57, 1978.

CONSERVATIVE MEDICAL MANAGEMENT OF CANINE CHRONIC POLYURIC RENAL FAILURE

DAVID J. POLZIN, D.V.M.,
and CARL A. OSBORNE, D.V.M.

St. Paul, Minnesota

INDICATIONS

Chronic primary polyuric renal failure is often associated with varying degrees of uremia. Uremia is a polysystemic clinical syndrome that results from severe impairment of renal function. Therapy of chronic primary polyuric renal failure should be directed toward correction of signs associated with renal failure and uremia and should include various combinations of the following: (1) unlimited access to water, (2) avoidance of conditions associated with body stress, (3) dietary regulation, (4) oral administration of multiple vitamins and sodium bicarbonate, (5) consideration of oral administration of sodium chloride, (6) administration of anabolic agents, and (7) control of hyperphosphatemia and hypocalcemia. All of these therapeutic manipulations are directed toward correcting deficits and excesses in fluid, electrolyte, acid-base, endocrine, and nutrient balance and toward minimizing retention of metabolic waste products.

Conservative medical management primarily encompasses symptomatic and supportive therapy of chronic polyuric renal failure. However, the importance of determining an etiologic/pathologic diagnosis and formulating specific therapy should not be overlooked, since patients may benefit from specific treatment designed to modify, destroy, or eliminate the primary cause of renal disease (Table 1). Examples of specific treatment include correc-

Table 1. *Examples of Renal Diseases Classified by Primary Site of Involvement*

Glomeruli	Tubules	Interstitium	Vessels
Amyloidosis	Congenital disorders	Amyloidosis (cats)	Atherosclerosis (uncommon)
Diabetic glomerulopathy (?)	Hypercalcemia	Drugs	Embolic disorders
Disseminated intravascular coagulation	Immune complex and antitubular basement membrane disorders (?)	Heavy metals	Polyarteritis nodosa (uncommon)
Embolic disorders	Ischemia	Immune disorders (?)	Hypertension
Immune complex disorders	Nephrotoxins	Leptospirosis	Others
Bacterial endocarditis (?)	Drugs		
Dirofilaria immitis	Heavy metals		
Drugs (haptens)			
Feline leukemia			
Lupus erythematosus			
Neoplasia			
Pyometra (?)			
Idiopathic forms			
Antiglomerular basement membrane disorders	Neoplasia	Pyelonephritis	
Dirofilaria immitis (?)			
Idiopathic forms			
Others	Obstructive disorders	Systemic mycoses	
	Tubular transport disorders	Others	
	Fanconi's syndrome		
	Renal tubular acidosis		
	Primary renal glucosuria		
	Others		

tion of hypercalcemia that has caused calcium ne-phropathy, administration of antibiotics to eliminate bacterial infections, removal of obstructive lesions causing post-renal azotemia, and correction of abnormal renal perfusion that has caused renal ischemic lesions.

The objective of this article is to summarize current recommendations for conservative medical management of dogs with compensated chronic polyuric renal failure. Conservative medical management and the therapy and practice of nutritional management of chronic polyuric renal failure in the dog have been recently reviewed in detail (Osborne and Polzin, 1979; Polzin and Osborne, 1979, 1980). The therapy discussed herein is designed for patients that are not vomiting or anorexic and for uremic patients in which vomiting and anorexia have been controlled so that oral therapy is feasible. For information concerning treatment of uremic dogs that are vomiting, anorexic, severely depressed, oliguric, or unable to tolerate oral therapy

owing to some other complication of uremia, consult the article entitled "Emergency Management of the Acute Uremic Crisis" (page 981). Recommendations included in this article are suitable for most recompensated patients following successful treatment of the uremic crisis.

DIAGNOSIS

An algorithm to aid in the diagnosis of chronic primary polyuric renal failure is summarized in Figure 1. Polyuria has been used as the key sign prompting consideration of this type of renal failure because it is a commonly encountered early manifestation of chronic primary polyuric renal failure. Polyuria should be verified by observation or by quantitation of 24-hour urine output. In general, normal urine production should not exceed 50 ml/kg body weight/24 hr. Urine specific gravity may be used as an index of polyuria. Verification of

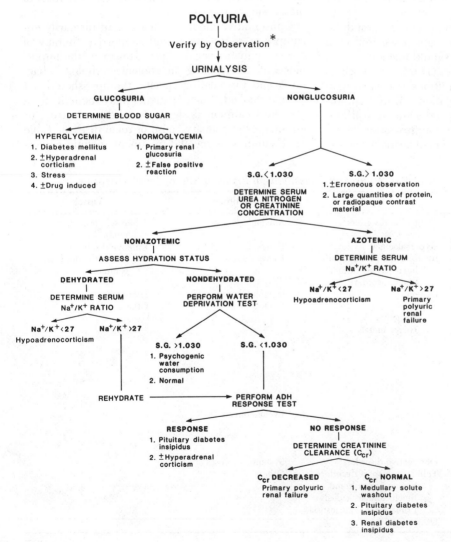

Figure 1. Diagnostic algorithm for chronic polyuric renal failure. The algorithm is based on probabilities. Exceptions to these generalities may occur.

*Measurement of 24-hour urine volume is recommended. See text for methods and normal values.

polyuria is supported by a urine specific gravity of less than 1.030, whereas a urine specific gravity of greater than 1.030 is a reliable index of urine concentration (Hardy and Osborne, 1980).

Dogs with chronic polyuric renal failure typically are nonglucosuric and have a urine specific gravity of less than 1.030 (see Fig 1). Dogs with concurrent azotemia and urine specific gravity values of less than 1.030 usually have primary renal failure. In our experience, the disease most likely to be confused with azotemic primary renal failure is hypoadrenocorticism (see Fig. 1). Although characteristically associated with oliguria, hypoadrenocorticism may be characterized by polyuria, azotemia, and a urine specific gravity of less than 1.030. However, hypoadrenocorticism differs from primary polyuric renal failure in that the ratio of serum sodium concentration to serum potassium concentration is usually less than 27:1. Unfortunately, the ratio of serum sodium concentration to serum potassium concentration may not invariably differentiate hypoadrenocorticism from primary renal failure. Therefore, clinical signs, electrocardiographic changes, hematologic findings, results of an adrenocorticotropic hormone (ACTH) response test, and response to therapy should be used to confirm the diagnosis of hypoadrenocorticism. Other polyuric diseases may be associated with azotemia and urine specific gravity values of less than 1.030 but only if the azotemia has a prerenal cause (e.g., pituitary diabetes insipidus with dehydration).

Diagnosis of primary renal failure in nonazotemic dogs is based on (1) inability to concentrate urine in response to dehydration or exogenous administration of antidiuretic hormone, and (2) reduced renal function in the absence of identifiable prerenal causes. Specific recommendations for water deprivation and vasopressin concentration tests are beyond the scope of this article but have been described elsewhere (Hardy and Osborne, 1979, 1980; Osborne et al., 1972). It must be emphasized that water deprivation tests are contraindicated in dehydrated and/or azotemic patients.

Renal function (glomerular filtration rate—GFR) may be determined by endogenous or exogenous creatinine clearance. The concept of clearance and details concerning performance of creatinine clearance (C_{cr}) studies are not described in this discussion but have been reviewed elsewhere (Bovee and Joyce, 1979; Finco, 1980, 1981). Determination of endogenous C_{cr} requires collection of a blood sample and an accurately timed urine collection. The procedure for performing endogenous C_{cr} studies is summarized in Table 2.

Major factors that influence the results of endogenous C_{cr} studies include (1) completeness of urine collection, (2) method of determination of serum creatinine concentration (S_c), (3) systemic hemodynamics, and (4) the status of renal function. Failure

Table 2. *Method for Performing Endogenous Creatinine Clearance Studies in Dogs*

1. Catheterize and empty the urinary bladder. Rinse the bladder with several ml of sterile saline. Discard urine and saline.
2. Collect *all* urine produced during a timed period. If an extended collection period is used, place the patient in a metabolism cage or frequently collect voluntarily voided urine.
3. At the midpoint of the timed urine collection, obtain a blood sample for determination of serum creatinine concentration (S_c).
4. At the end of the timed urine collection, catheterize and empty the bladder. Rinse the bladder with several ml of sterile saline. Urine *and* saline should be added to the urine already collected. Record the total time elapsed during urine collection (T). The total urine volume produced (including the final saline rinse) should be measured (V). A well-mixed aliquot of urine should be submitted for determination of urine creatinine concentration (U_c).
5. Accurately determine the dog's body weight (BW).
6. Calculate C_{cr} using the following formula:

$$C_{cr} = \frac{U_c V}{S_c \cdot T \cdot BW}$$

   a. C_{cr} = ml/min/kg
   b. U_c and S_c = mg/dl
   c. V = milliliters
   d. T = minutes
   e. BW = kilograms

to empty the bladder completely at the beginning of the study will result in an erroneously high C_{cr} value, whereas failure to empty the bladder at the end of the study will result in an erroneously low C_{cr} value. The potential magnitude of these errors progressively increases as collection times become shorter. A word of caution: care in emptying and rinsing the bladder is mandatory for accurate 20-minute urine collections.

The method of determination of S_c influences C_{cr} because of serum noncreatinine chromogens. The most commonly used methods of S_c determination (including automated techniques) cannot differentiate between true creatinine and noncreatinine chromogens and therefore overestimate S_c. Noncreatinine chromogens do not appear in urine. Determination of C_{cr} by methods that are influenced by serum noncreatinine chromogens underestimate C_{cr}. This error is greatest when S_c is within the normal range because serum noncreatinine chromogen concentrations are not substantially elevated as a result of reduced glomerular filtration. Exogenous C_{cr} techniques are likely to be more accurate than endogenous C_{cr}, especially in nonazotemic patients, because the influence of noncreatinine chromogens is minimized. A clinically applicable method for determination of exogenous C_{cr} using a subcutaneous injection of sterile, pyrogen-free creatinine has been described (Finco, 1981).

Normal 20-minute and 24-hour endogenous creatinine clearance values have been reported. Studies of 20-minute C_{cr} determinations performed on 29 normal dogs of both sexes revealed values of 2.8 ± 0.96 ml/min/kg (range 1.7 to 5.0 ml/min/kg) (Finco, 1971). The results of 24-hour C_{cr} determinations performed on 36 normal female beagle dogs were 3.7 ± 0.77 ml/min/kg (approximate range 1.7 to 4.5 ml/min/kg) (Bovee and Joyce, 1979). Noncreatinine chromogens were included in the determination of S_c for the 24-hour study but not the 20-minute study.

Because creatinine clearance may be influenced by prerenal factors as well as by primary renal failure, prerenal factors should be carefully considered when interpreting the results of C_{cr} studies.

Chronic primary renal failure may be differentiated from acute primary renal failure on the basis of (1) history (onset and duration of clinical signs), (2) nonregenerative anemia, (3) radiographic evidence of renal osteodystrophy, and (4) bilateral reduction in kidney size.

TREATMENT OVERVIEW

GOALS

The goals of conservative medical management of dogs with chronic primary renal failure are to (1) ameliorate the clinical signs of uremia, (2) minimize electrolyte, vitamin, mineral, and acid-base disturbances, and (3) supply daily nutritional requirements. Best results are achieved when therapy is individualized for each patient.

RECOMMENDATIONS

Recommendations based on clinical and laboratory abnormalities that may be used to provide conservative medical management to patients are summarized in Table 3. Recommended therapeutic plans for the most common clinical/laboratory patterns of chronic primary polyuric renal failure are summarized in Table 4. Refer to the section entitled "Summary of Therapeutic Regimens" in this article for specific details about each component of therapy.

DESCRIPTION OF SPECIFIC THERAPEUTIC COMPONENTS

AVOIDANCE OF STRESS

Damaged kidneys have reduced capacity to compensate for stress imposed by changes in external environment, dietary indiscretion, or newly acquired nonrenal diseases. Prevention is the best treatment; stress should be minimized so that diseased kidneys can maintain homeostasis. We rec-

ommend that dogs with compensated renal failure be treated as outpatients whenever possible.

UNLIMITED ACCESS TO WATER

Fluid balance in patients with polyuric renal failure is maintained by compensatory polydipsia. If water consumption is insufficient to balance excessive water loss associated with polyuria, dehydration and decreased renal blood flow may precipitate a uremic crisis. If dehydration and decreased renal blood flow persist, additional renal damage may occur. For these reasons, fresh, clean water should be available in adequate quantities at all times.

In our experience, dogs with renal failure frequently consume inadequate quantities of fluid during periods of hospitalization. If insufficient thirst leads to negative body water balance characterized by rapid loss in body weight, loss of skin pliability, and/or hemoconcentration, supplemental fluids should be given orally or parenterally.

DIET THERAPY

OVERVIEW

The rationale, objectives, and specific recommendations for diet therapy as a component of conservative medical management of chronic polyuric renal failure in dogs have been reviewed in detail (Polzin and Osborne, 1979, 1980; Osborne and Polzin, 1979). Although exceedingly important, dietary management represents only one component of the overall conservative medical management of dogs with chronic polyuric renal failure. Optimum therapeutic response is best achieved by selection of essential conservative management designed for the needs of each patient (see Table 3).

DIETARY PROTEIN

The adverse effects of consumption of excessive quantities of protein during renal failure are common knowledge. However, studies performed in our laboratory revealed that uremic dogs fed 1.25 gm/kg body weight/day (0.6 gm/lb body weight/day) of cooked egg protein developed malnutrition characterized by hypoalbuminemia, anemia, weight loss, and reduced body tissue mass (Polzin and Osborne, 1981). These results, and results of similar studies in humans, suggest that uremic patients have higher dietary protein requirements than normal individuals. The point is that diets either deficient in protein or with excessive protein may adversely effect uremic patients.

Optimum dietary protein requirements for dogs with varying degrees of chronic polyuric renal fail-

Table 3. *Recommendations for Use of Various Components of Conservative Medical Management in Dogs With Chronic Primary Polyuric Renal Failure*

Clinical or Laboratory Sign	Avoidance of Stress	Free Access to Water	Diet Therapy	B Vitamins	Oral NaCl	Oral $NaHCO_3$	Phosphate Binders	Calcium Supplements	Vitamin D Supplements	Anabolic Steroids	Antihypertensive Agents	Consider Pharmacokinetics of Drugs
Polyuria/polydipsia	+	+	0	?	0	0	0	0	0	0	0	+
Azotemia	+	+	+	+	+/0	0	0	0	0	?	0	+
Hyperphosphatemia	+	+	+	0	0	±	+	0	x	0	0	+
Hypocalcemia w ↑PO_4	+	0	0	0	0	±	0	x	x	0	0	+
Hypocalcemia w/o ↑PO_4*	+	0	0	0	0	+	0	+	+	0	0	+
Acidosis	+	0	±?	0	0	+	0	0	0	0	0	+
Anemia	0	0	?	+/0	0	0	0	0	0	+	0	+
Renal osteodystrophy	0	0	+	0	0	+/0	+	+/x	+/x	+/0	0	+
Infections	+	0	?	0	0	0	0	0	0	0	0	+
Hypertension	+	0	?	0	–	x	0	0	0	0	+	+

*This occurs when hyperphosphatemia is controlled by therapy.

Key: + = indicated   x = see Description of Specific Therapeutic Components
   0 = of no benefit or harm   ? = unknown
   – = contraindicated   ± = variable effects

Table 4. *Recommended Treatment of Chronic Primary Polyuric Renal Failure*

Clinical Category	Recommended Treatment
Polyuric, nonazotemic, normophosphatemic, normocalcemia, nonacidotic, and nonanemic	Avoid stress Permit free access to water Consider pharmacokinetics of drugs
Polyuric, nonazotemic, normophosphatemic, hypercalcemic, nonacidotic, and nonanemic	Correct hypercalcemia Avoid stress Permit free access to water Consider pharmacokinetics of drugs
Polyuric, azotemic, normophosphatemic, normocalcemia, nonacidotic, and nonanemic	Avoid stress Permit free access to water Establish diet therapy Administer B vitamins Consider pharmacokinetics of drugs
Polyuric, azotemic, normophosphatemic, hypercalcemic, nonacidotic, and nonanemic	Correct hypercalcemia Avoid stress Permit free access to water Establish diet therapy Administer B vitamins Consider pharmacokinetics of drugs
Polyuric, azotemic, hyperphospatemic, normocalcemic, acidotic, and anemic	Avoid stress Permit free access to water Establish diet therapy Administer B vitamins Administer oral phosphate binders Administer oral sodium bicarbonate Administer anabolic agents Consider pharmacokinetics of drugs
Polyuric, azotemic, hyperphosphatemic, hypercalcemic, acidotic, and anemic	Correct hypercalcemia Avoid stress Permit free access to water Establish diet therapy Administer B vitamins Administer oral phosphate binders Administer oral sodium bicarbonate Administer anabolic agents Consider pharmacokinetics of drugs
Polyuric, azotemic, hyperphosphatemic, hypocalcemic, acidotic, and anemic	Avoid stress Permit free access to water Establish diet therapy Administer B vitamins Administer oral phosphate binders Administer oral calcium supplements Administer oral vitamin D supplements Administer oral sodium bicarbonate Administer anabolic agents Consider pharmacokinetics of drugs

ure have not been established. However, the intrinsic variability of dietary requirements in normal dogs and the varied influence of uremia on protein requirements indicate that protein requirements of individual uremic patients are probably variable. Therefore, attempts should be made to individualize dietary protein requirements to patient needs. In general, patients should receive that quantity of dietary protein which is consistent with control of their biochemical and clinical uremic manifestations and yet maintains adequate nutrition. If clinical or laboratory evidence of protein malnutrition develops, dietary protein may be gradually increased until the best attainable compromise between dietary control of the biochemical and clinical manifestations of uremia and prevention of protein depletion is achieved.

We currently recommend that dogs with a mild to moderate degree of chronic polyuric renal failure be fed approximately 2.0 to 2.2 gm/kg body weight/day (0.9 to 1.0 gm/lb/day) of high biologic value protein.* If evidence of protein malnutrition (hypoalbuminemia, anemia, weight loss, or loss of body tissue mass) occurs, dietary protein should gradually be increased until these abnormalities are corrected. On the other hand, if diets designed to provide 2.0 gm/kg body weight/day of high biologic value protein do not result in amelioration of clinical and biochemical manifestations of uremia, dietary protein intake may be further reduced. One protein-restricted diet has been designed to provide 1.3 gm protein/kg body weight to patients with severe renal dysfunction (Prescription Diet u/d†). Greater reductions in dietary protein intake (at least to the level of 0.66 gm/kg body weight/day of cooked egg protein) are associated with progressively reduced blood urea nitrogen concentrations and may result in amelioration of clinical signs in dogs with severe renal dysfunction. However, as dietary protein intake is reduced, clinical and biochemical evidence of protein malnutrition may become more pronounced.

CALORIES

Determination of caloric requirements must be individualized on the basis of clinical evaluation of the patient, including serial determination of body weight. The following recommendations have been adopted from those reported by the National Research Council. Dogs should consume approximately 70 to 110 kcal/kg body weight/day (30 to 50 kcal/lb/day). Since the caloric requirement per kilogram body weight tends to vary inversely with the total body weight, small adult dogs should receive approximately 110 kcal/kg body weight, whereas large dogs should receive approximately 70 kcal/kg body weight. At least 1.32 gm/kg body weight/day should consist of fat. A minimum dietary require-

*This quantity of protein is provided in Prescription Diet k/d, Hills Division, Riviana Foods, Topeka, KS.
†Hills Division, Riviana Foods, Topeka, KS.

ment for carbohydrate has not been established in dogs. Additional modifications of caloric intake may be required to compensate for the nutritional status and activity of the patient. Steady body weight over a period of weeks or months is usually a reliable index of adequate caloric intake.

PRESCRIPTION DIETS

Controlled studies to determine the benefits and risks associated with the use of prescription diets for the treatment of renal failure in dogs have been performed at the University of Minnesota (Polzin and Osborne, 1981). The influence of two reduced protein renal prescription diets containing 8 (Prescription Diet u/d*) and 17 per cent (Prescription Diet k/d*) dry weight protein on the clinical and biochemical abnormalities associated with moderate renal failure were compared with a maintenance diet containing 44 per cent dry weight protein. The beneficial effects observed in dogs fed either Prescription Diet k/d or Prescription Diet u/d included (1) reduced mortality, (2) amelioration of clinical signs, (3) reduced SUN concentration, (4) reduced serum phosphorus concentration, (5) minimized development of renal osteodystrophy (8 per cent protein diet only), (6) reduced serum magnesium concentration, and (7) reduced severity of anemia and tissue wasting (17 per cent protein diet only). Undesirable effects of the 8 per cent Prescription Diet u/d included: varying degrees of body protein depletion (weight loss, reduced tissue mass, hypoalbuminemia, and anemia) and hyperchloremic metabolic acidosis. The hyperchloremic metabolic acidosis associated with feeding the 8 per cent protein diet was readily corrected with orally administered sodium bicarbonate.

The glomerular filtration rate of dogs fed both prescription diets was reduced compared with dogs fed the maintenance diet. Although reduction in glomerular filtration rate has generally been regarded as an undesirable effect of reduced protein diets, recent studies have suggested that the renal hemodynamic effects of high protein diets (glomerular hyperfiltration) may lead to progressive deterioration of renal structure and function (Hostetter et al., 1982). Dietary protein restriction and subsequent prevention of glomerular hyperfiltration may be of benefit in minimizing the progressive deterioration of renal function characteristic of chronic renal failure. In our study, no adverse effects resulting from a diet-associated reduction in GFR were detected.

Although a more ideal homemade diet may be formulated to meet an individual patient's needs, results of our study indicate that prescription diets are often superior to regular commercially prepared

*Hills Division, Riviana Foods, Topeka, KS.

Table 5. *Sample Calculation of Dietary Requirements for a Uremic 25-G Dog*

Caloric Density of Foods:
1. Carbohydrates   4 cal/gm
2. Proteins   4 cal/gm
3. Fat   9 cal/gm

Calculation:
1. 25-kg dog × 70 cal/kg/day = 1750 calories required per day
2. 25-kg dog × 2.0 gm protein/kg/day = 50 gm protein required per day
3. Addition of 33 gm dietary fat per day   = 297 cal/day
4. Addition of 363 gm dietary carbohydrates per day   = 1452 cal/day
5. Total calories excluding protein   = 1749 cal/day

dog foods in minimizing signs of primary renal failure. Advantages of prescription diets include convenience and elimination of error in diet preparation. A disadvantage of prescription diets is that individualization to patient needs is more difficult. Failure to adapt a diet to a patient's needs may result in suboptimum therapeutic response.

HOMEMADE DIETS

Homemade diets may be formulated for patients with polyuric renal failure (Table 5). Natural proteins of high biologic value include cooked eggs, lean meats, chicken, and dairy products. Proteins of low biologic value that should be avoided include most plant proteins, meat by-products, gelatin, and dehydrated meat and fish meal. Sources of nonprotein calories include commercially prepared products, butter, margarine, vegetable oils, jellies, sugar, honey, and candy. High calorie value foods with a minimum quantity of protein include spaghetti, macaroni, pancakes, rice, cake, bread, cookies, crackers, potato chips, and pretzels.

INITIATION OF TREATMENT

When to initiate a low protein diet remains a matter of personal opinion. As long as the serum urea nitrogen concentration, serum phosphorus concentration, and fractional excretion of phosphorus in urine remain within normal limits, it is probably unjustified to initiate therapy. However, once serum phosphorus concentrations exceed normal limits it seems logical to recommend initiation of dietary therapy on the assumption that the associated reduction of dietary phosphorus intake will help to minimize renal secondary hyperparathyroidism and the rate of self-perpetuating renal dysfunction. In fact, it may be advisable to initiate therapy to control hyperparathyroidism prior to the onset of hyperphosphatemia. Renal secondary hyperparathyroidism may be recognized prior to the onset of hyperphosphatemia by detection of increased fractional excretion of phosphorus in urine (see Treatment of Mineral Imbalances of Chronic Renal Failure for additional details). Further studies are required to clarify the benefit of this tentative recommendation, however. When serum phosphorus and SUN concentrations exceed normal limits and polysystemic abnormalities associated with the uremic syndrome become evident, initiation of appropriate modifications in diet is clearly justified.

PALATABILITY

Protein-restricted diets may be less palatable to some patients than higher protein diets. Palatability may be enhanced by (1) warming the food to create an appetizing odor, (2) flavoring the food with small quantities of meat or animal fat (i.e., chicken or turkey fat), and (3) dividing the diet into three to four meals daily.

FEEDING FREQUENCY

Uremic dogs, especially those with inappetance or intermittent emesis, should be given several smaller meals daily rather than one large meal. Feeding small meals frequently may enhance palatability and consumption of food. In addition, shortening periods of fasting may reduce body catabolism (uremic animals have an enhanced catabolic response during fasting).

WATER-SOLUBLE VITAMINS

Minimum daily requirements of water-soluble vitamins (B and C) have not been established for dogs with renal failure. Because of the likelihood of impaired tubular reabsorption of these vitamins in patients with polyuric renal failure and because of reduced intake of these vitamins caused by varying degrees of anorexia, we recommend that supplemental vitamins be given to such patients. A single high-potency capsule containing B complex vitamins and vitamin C given daily is probably sufficient supplementation for most patients. Since prescription diets are supplemented with additional vitamins, patients consuming them may not require additional vitamin supplements.

ORAL SODIUM CHLORIDE

OVERVIEW

In past years, oral administration of sodium chloride was recommended for dogs with chronic polyuric renal failure on the basis of the following hypotheses: (1) subsequent diuresis minimizes tubular reabsorption of potential uremic toxins, and (2) obligatory urinary sodium loss predisposed uremic patients to negative sodium balance. However, it has recently been shown that increased fractional excretion of sodium in urine in dogs with one form of experimentally induced chronic polyuric renal failure is a compensatory response to sodium intake. Whether or not this data can be extrapolated to dogs with all forms of naturally occurring renal failure has not yet been determined. Nonetheless, the question of the advantages and disadvantages of administration of oral sodium chloride must be re-examined in light of this new information.

SODIUM CONTENT OF DOG FOODS

Recommended dietary sodium allowance for normal adult dogs is approximately 132 mg/kg body weight/day (Hamlin and Ettinger, 1976). However, a minimum dietary requirement for sodium has not been established in dogs. On the average, (1) commercial canned dog foods contain approximately 750 mg sodium/100 gm dry diet, (2) semimoist dog foods contain approximately 580 mg sodium/100 gm dry diet, and (3) dry dog foods contain approximately 440 mg sodium/100 gm dry food. When canned or semimoist foods are fed at a rate of 70 kcal/kg body weight, they supply approximately 105 mg sodium/kg body weight. Dry dog foods fed at the same level supply about 80 mg sodium/kg body weight. In the past, Prescription Diet k/d contained approximately 250 mg sodium/100 mg dry weight, whereas Prescription Diet u/d contained approximately 1,200 mg sodium/100 gm dry weight. Currently, both prescription diets have been modified so that they contain approximately 250 mg sodium/100 gm dry diet. At this level, they supply approximately 35 mg sodium/kg body weight/day when consumed at a rate of 70 kcal/kg body weight/day.

RECOMMENDATIONS

The optimum sodium intake for dogs with chronic polyuric renal failure has not been established. However, high-sodium diets may contribute to hypertension in dogs with renal failure. In humans, hypertension is an established cause of renal dysfunction and may aggravate the polysystemic manifestations of uremia. Recent experimental and clinical studies suggest that hypertension occurs in dogs with some types of chronic polyuric renal failure.

Results of studies performed in our laboratory revealed that dogs with experimental chronic renal failure (remnant kidney model induced by infarction) were able to maintain sodium balance for periods of up to 40 weeks when fed diets containing approximately 35, 200, or 220 mg sodium/kg body weight/day.

Pending availability of results of controlled experimental and clinical studies designed to evaluate sodium balance in dogs with primary renal failure, specific recommendations for dietary sodium intake cannot be made. Therefore, dietary sodium intake should be individualized on the basis of knowledge of concurrent disease processes (e.g., hypertension, congestive heart failure, hypoproteinemia, edema, and so on) and response to modulation of dietary sodium intake.

Patients with chronic polyuric renal failure are usually able to adapt to a wide range of dietary sodium consumption patterns; however, renal adaptation occurs gradually. Abrupt changes in dietary sodium may be associated with a transient imbalance between intake and urinary loss. A sudden reduction of sodium intake in dogs with chronic polyuric renal failure may cause a reduction of extracellular fluid volume, which in turn may lead to poor renal perfusion and further reduction in renal function. Therefore, abrupt alterations in dietary sodium intake should be avoided. We recommend that such changes be made gradually over a period of two or more weeks. Because some prescription diets (k/d and u/d) are lower in sodium content than commercially available maintenance diets, caution should be used to avoid a sudden reduction in sodium intake. The change from a normal diet to a protein-restricted prescription diet may be made by mixing the two in varying proportions over a period of one to two weeks.

For further details concerning sodium intake in patients with chronic polyuric renal failure, consult the article that follows.

ORAL SODIUM BICARBONATE

Chronic polyuric renal failure is typically associated with varying degrees of metabolic acidosis. However, there is no consistent relationship between the severity of metabolic acidosis and the magnitude of renal dysfunction. Because severity of metabolic acidosis cannot be reliably determined on the basis of knowledge of the magnitude of renal dysfunction (i.e., serum urea nitrogen or creatinine concentrations), blood pH and bicarbonate concentration (or total CO_2 or CO_2 content) should be obtained to assess the need for supplemental therapy.

The dosage of oral sodium bicarbonate should be individualized for each patient. Patients with substantial metabolic acidosis (blood bicarbonate concentration less than 18 mEq/L) should be given oral sodium bicarbonate at a dose of 5 to 30 grains three times daily. The dosage of sodium bicarbonate may subsequently be altered to maintain blood bicarbonate concentration between 18 and 26 mEq/L. Care should be taken to avoid iatrogenic metabolic alkalosis. Until the appropriate dosage of oral sodium bicarbonate is determined, blood bicarbonate concentration should be monitored at 10- to 14-day intervals. If blood bicarbonate concentration is less than 18 mEq/L, the dosage of sodium bicarbonate

should be increased. If blood bicarbonate concentration exceeds 26 mEq/L, the dosage should be reduced.

In the event that the plasma bicarbonate concentration is unknown, urine pH may be used as a crude index to titrate bicarbonate dosage. Uremic dogs that consistently have a urine pH of 5.5 or lower usually have metabolic acidosis of sufficient magnitude to warrant sodium bicarbonate therapy. A sufficient quantity of sodium bicarbonate should be given to maintain urine pH between 6.5 and 7.0. Urine pH values of 7.5 or greater suggest excessive administration of sodium bicarbonate; urine pH values of 6.0 or lower suggest that an inadequate quantity of sodium bicarbonate is being given.

Sodium bicarbonate should be used with caution. Because hydrogen ions compete with calcium ions for protein binding sites, rapid correction of acidemia may decrease the concentration of ionized calcium and result in hypocalcemic tetany. This event may be avoided by correcting the metabolic acidosis associated with renal failure over a period of several days. Large quantities of sodium should not be administered to patients with hypertension, congestive heart failure, hypoproteinemic edema, or oliguria. Calcium lactate or calcium carbonate may minimize the severity of acidosis with less danger of aggravating hypernatremia and body fluid accumulation in these situations.

INTESTINAL PHOSPHORUS BINDERS

Hyperphosphatemia in dogs with chronic primary polyuric renal failure may be minimized by (1) maintaining body water balance, blood vascular volume, and renal perfusion; (2) feeding reduced protein diets; (3) enhancing gastrointestinal loss of phosphorus by administration of nonabsorbable phosphorus binding agents; and/or (4) a combination of these treatments. We prefer to utilize reduced protein diets in properly hydrated patients, supplemented with phosphorus-binding agents if they fail to adequately control hyperphosphatemia. Our preference for dietary management is related to the fact that most oral phosphate binding agents (except capsules) are poorly tolerated by dogs and owners. In addition, the use of oral phosphate binding agents requires greater patient monitoring to prevent hypophosphatemia and other complications.

Available oral phosphate binding agents include aluminum hydroxide (Amphojel Tablets and Suspension*; Dialume Capsules†) and aluminum carbonate (Basaljel Tablets, Capsules, and Suspension*). Capsules are generally preferred over tablets and liquid suspensions because their contents can

---

*Wyeth Laboratories, Philadelphia, PA.
†Armour Pharmaceutical Co., Tarrytown, NY.

be mixed with food and are more likely to be dispensed throughout ingesta. Tablets are less convenient because they must be crushed to achieve maximum benefit in dogs. In our experience, liquid suspensions are unpalatable and therefore must be administered with the aid of a dose syringe or stomach tube.

Dosage of intestinal phosphate binding agents must be individualized. The goal is to reduce serum phosphorus concentration to normal (3.0 to 4.5 mg/dl). If reduced protein diets fail to reduce serum phosphorus concentration to the desired level, oral administration of phosphate binding agents with meals at an initial dose of 300 to 500 mg given three times daily is recommended. Serial evaluation of serum phosphorus concentration is required to determine efficacy of therapy and to detect hypophosphatemia. Serum phosphorus concentration should be evaluated at 10- to 14-day intervals until the proper dose of phosphate binding agent is determined. Constipation, a common side effect of therapy, may require treatment with laxatives. For additional information concerning the use of intestinal phosphate binding agents, consult the article entitled "Treatment of Mineral Imbalances of Chronic Renal Failure."

CONTROL OF HYPOCALCEMIA

OVERVIEW

Varying degrees of hypocalcemia may occur in dogs with advanced chronic primary renal failure. Treatment of uremic hypocalcemia consists of (1) control of hyperphosphatemia, (2) vitamin D therapy, and (3) oral administration of calcium supplements. A word of caution: vitamin D and calcium supplements should only be given to hypocalcemic dogs that are normophosphatemic (serum phosphorus concentration = 3.0 to 4.5 mg/dl). Administration of vitamin D and/or calcium to hyperphosphatemic patients may result in deposition of calcium and phosphorus in soft tissues including the kidneys. Renal mineralization may be associated with progressive irreversible renal damage. In human patients with renal failure, vitamin D and calcium supplementation are not initiated unless the product of serum calcium and phosphorus is below 70. The applicability of this recommendation for uremic dogs has not been examined but is presumed to be similar.

Because of potential nephrotoxicity of vitamin D and calcium supplements, their use should be limited to dogs proven to be hypocalcemic. Some dogs with chronic renal failure may develop hypercalcemia rather than hypocalcemia. In addition, hypercalcemia may be the cause of renal failure in some dogs. When considering vitamin D and/or calcium supplements in hypoproteinemic uremic

dogs, remember that total serum calcium concentration may be reduced without substantial reduction in serum ionized calcium concentration. Changes in total serum calcium concentration associated with hypoalbuminemia in dogs may be corrected by using the following formula: adjusted serum calcium concentration (mg/dl) = serum calcium concentration (mg/dl) − serum albumin concentration (gm/dl) + 3.5 (Meuten, 1982). However, this calculation must be used with caution until its validity in dogs with renal failure is confirmed.

VITAMIN D

Hypercalcemia is a potential complication of vitamin D therapy. Because of potential adverse consequences associated with the use of vitamin D, selection of rapidly acting and rapidly metabolized agents is preferred. One form of vitamin D (Rocaltrol Capsules, 0.25 mg*) that is chemically and clinically identical to naturally occurring 1,25-dihydroxycholecalciferol is commercially available. This drug has a short duration of action (peak serum concentration in four hours; duration of pharmacologic activity three to five days), permitting control of unwanted hypercalcemia.

Dosage for 1,25-dihydroxycholecalciferol has not yet been determined for dogs. The suggested dosage for humans is 0.25 mcg given daily or every other day. Optimum dosage must be determined for each patient on the basis of serial evaluation of serum calcium and phosphorus concentrations. Initially, serum calcium and phosphorus concentrations should be evaluated at 24- to 48-hour intervals until an appropriate dosage is determined. We do not recommend the use of vitamin D if serum calcium and phosphorus concentrations cannot be monitored. Consult the article that follows for additional information concerning the use of vitamin D therapy in patients with renal failure.

ORAL CALCIUM SUPPLEMENTS

Calcium carbonate may be given at an initial dosage of 100 mg/kg body weight/day. Calcium gluconate and calcium lactate may also be considered. Dosage must be individualized for each patient on the basis of serial evaluation of serum calcium and phosphorus concentrations.

ANABOLIC AGENTS

Anabolic steroids may be of value in promoting positive nitrogen balance (anabolism) and calcium deposition in bones. However, the primary indication for the use of anabolic agents in patients with

---

*Roche Laboratories, Nutley, NJ.

renal failure is related to control of anemia. The most effective erythropoietic androgens for the treatment of uremic anemia in dogs have not been determined. Available products include testosterone propionate (Oreton*), given at a dosage of 10 to 15 mg/per day, and nandrolone decanoate (Deca-Durabolin†), given at a dosage of 1.0 to 1.5 mg/kg body weight/week by intramuscular injection. Other products include testosterone enanthate (Delatestryl‡), stanazolol (Winstrol-V§), and oxymethalone (Adroyd‖). Beneficial effects in humans have been reported to require two to three months of therapy. Consult the article that follows for additional information concerning the treatment of uremic anemia.

ANTIHYPERTENSIVE AGENTS

Treatment of hypertension involves dietary sodium restriction and drug therapy. Drug therapy includes the administration of diuretics, sympatholytic agents, and vasodilators. For specific recommendations concerning the treatment of hypertension, consult Recognition and Management of Hypertension in the Dog, page 1025.

PHARMACOKINETICS OF DRUGS

Nonspecific use of corticosteroids, antibiotics, diuretics, and other drugs likely to be associated with adverse reactions should be avoided. Consult Checklist of Hazardous Drugs in Patients With Renal Failure, page 1036, for additional information.

MONITORING THERAPEUTIC RESPONSE

Adequacy of therapy can be determined only by re-evaluation of patients at appropriate intervals. Re-evaluation will permit alteration of diets and other components of conservative medical management according to individual needs. In addition to evaluation of the owner's impression of therapeutic response and the results of a physical examination including hydration and body weight, certain laboratory evaluations should be performed. Because restriction of dietary protein may reduce the concentration of serum urea nitrogen without any significant improvement in glomerular filtration rate, it is recommended that both serum urea nitrogen and creatinine concentrations be evaluated as indices of therapeutic response. Evaluations of serum albumin concentration and packed cell volume may be of value in determining the need for additional dietary protein. Control of metabolic acidosis may be assessed by evaluation of blood pH and bicarbonate concentration, whereas control of hypocalcemia and hyperphosphatemia may be assessed by serial evaluation of serum calcium and phosphorus concentrations.

REFERENCES AND SUPPLEMENTAL READING

Bovee, K. C., and Joyce, B. A.: Clinical evaluation of glomerular function: 24 hour creatinine clearance in dogs. J.A.V.M.A. 174:488, 1979.

Finco, D. R.: Simultaneous determination of phenolsulfonphthalein excretion and endogenous creatinine clearance in the normal dog. J.A.V.M.A. 159:336, 1971.

Finco, D. R.: Kidney function. *In* Kaneko, J. J. (ed.): *Clinical Biochemistry of Domestic Animals*, 3rd ed. New York: Academic Press, 1980.

Finco, D. R.: Simple, accurate method for clinical estimation of glomerular filtration rate in the dog. Am. J. Vet. Res. 42:1874, 1981.

Hamlin, R. L., and Ettinger, S. J.: *Congestive Heart Failure in Dogs: An Update.* Somerville, NJ: National Laboratories Corp., 1976.

Hardy, R. M., and Osborne, C. A.: Water deprivation test in the dog: Maximal normal values. J.A.V.M.A. 174:479, 1979.

Hardy, R. M., and Osborne, C. A.: Water deprivation and vasopression concentration tests in the differentiation of polyuric syndromes. *In* Kirk, R. W. (ed.): *Current Veterinary Therapy VII.* Philadelphia: W. B. Saunders, 1980.

Hostetter, T. H., Rennke, H. J., and Brenner, B. M.: Compensatory renal hemodynamic injury: A final common pathway of residual nephron destruction. Am. J. Kidney Dis. 1:310, 1982.

Meuten, D. J., Chew, D. J., Capen, C. C., and Kociba, G. J.: Relationship of serum total calcium to albumin and total protein in dogs. J.A.V.M.A. 180:63, 1982.

Osborne, C. A., Low, D. G., and Finco, D. R.: *Canine And Feline Urology.* Philadelphia: W. B. Saunders, 1972.

Osborne, C. A., and Polzin, D. J.: Strategy in the diagnosis, prognosis, and management of renal disease, renal failure, and uremia. Proceedings of the 46th Annual Meeting of the American Animal Hospital Association. 559, 1979.

Polzin, D. J., and Osborne, C. A.: Management of chronic primary polyuric renal failure with modified protein diets: Concepts, questions, and controversies. Proceedings of the 29th Annual Gaines Veterinary Symposium, White Plains, NY, 24, 1979.

Polzin, D. J., and Osborne, C. A.: Conservative management of polyuric primary renal failure. Diet therapy. *In* Kirk, R. W. (ed.): *Current Veterinary Therapy VII.* Philadelphia: W. B. Saunders, 1980, pp. 1097–1101.

Polzin, D. J., Osborne, C. A., Hayden, D. W., and Stevens, J. B.: Experimental evaluation of reduced protein diets in the management of primary polyuric renal failure: Preliminary findings and their clinical significance. Minn. Vet. 21:16, 1981.

---

*Schering Corp., Kenilworth, NJ.
†Organon Pharmaceuticals, West Orange, NJ.
‡E. R. Squibb & Sons, Inc., Princeton, NJ.
§Winthrop Laboratories, New York, NY.
‖Parke-Davis, Morris Plains, NJ.

CONSERVATIVE MEDICAL MANAGEMENT OF FELINE CHRONIC POLYURIC RENAL FAILURE

CARL A. OSBORNE, D.V.M.,
and DAVID J. POLZIN, D.V.M.

St. Paul, Minnesota

In recent years, improved knowledge of the pathophysiology of renal failure and uremia in humans and dogs has resulted in significant advancements in specific, supportive, and symptomatic treatment of renal failure in these species. In contrast to humans and dogs, the causes, metabolic consequences, and biologic behavior of renal failure in cats have been less well characterized. With few exceptions, current recommendations for formulation of supportive and symptomatic therapy of cats with renal failure represent extrapolations from those for the dog. Although these recommendations appear to be conceptually logical, species-related differences must be evaluated before they are adopted.

Many of the following recommendations are based on the therapy of renal failure in humans and dogs and on logic rather than results of controlled experimental and clinical trials. Therefore, their validity should be viewed as tentative pending further studies. Individualization of therapy within the guidelines outlined herein is essential. Therapeutic efficacy should be assessed by frequent re-evaluation of the patient's physical condition and metabolic status.

SPECIFIC VERSUS SUPPORTIVE AND SYMPTOMATIC TREATMENT

Signs of uremia are not directly caused by renal lesions but are related to varying degrees of fluid, acid-base, and electrolyte imbalances, vitamin and endocrine alterations, and retention of products of protein catabolism that develop as a result of lesions. Although this article pertains primarily to the supportive and symptomatic treatment of primary polyuric renal failure in cats, the importance of specific therapy should not be overlooked. Specific treatment should be designed to modify, destroy, or eliminate the primary cause of a disease process. Examples of specific treatments of renal disease include administration of antibiotics to eliminate bacterial infections, use of antidotes to counteract nephrotoxins, removal of obstructive lesions causing post-renal azotemia, correction of abnormal renal perfusion that has caused renal ischemic lesions, and correction of hypercalcemia that has caused calcium nephropathy.

Once primary renal failure has developed, no regimen will eliminate the renal lesions.

Although precipitating causes must be eliminated if further renal damage is to be prevented, the renal damage that has occurred must heal spontaneously over a period of days to weeks and/or the remaining viable nephrons must undergo compensatory adaptation if survival is to occur. The following principles should guide the therapy of primary renal failure:

1. There is no therapy that will eliminate renal lesions; renal lesions must heal spontaneously. The polysystemic metabolic and biochemical disorders caused by generalized renal lesions, however, may be modified or eliminated by appropriate therapy.

2. Detect and eliminate reversible nonrenal disorders that may have precipitated or aggravated a uremic crisis.

3. Evaluate the potential reversibility of renal disease and renal dysfunction with the knowledge that adequate renal function is not synonymous with total renal function.

4. Formulate specific therapy to eliminate or control the underlying cause with the objective of preventing further renal destruction.

5. Formulate supportive and symptomatic therapy that will minimize alterations in fluid, electrolyte, acid-base, endocrine, and nutrient balance and, therefore, sustain life until the processes of regeneration, repair, and compensatory adaptation allow the kidneys to regain adequate function to re-establish homeostasis. Formulate supportive and symptomatic therapy according to whether the patient has oliguric or nonoliguric primary renal failure.

6. Drugs should be administered to patients with

renal failure only after consideration of their routes and rates of metabolism and elimination and their potential to induce adverse reactions in the uremic environment.

7. Avoid overtreatment. The Miraclemycins of our medical armamentarium are Mother Nature and Father Time. We must strive to be children that augment rather than hinder their efforts.

There is a significant conceptual difference between the irreversibility of renal lesions and the reversibility of polysystemic metabolic and biochemical disorders caused by varying degrees of renal failure. The fact that dysfunction caused by generalized renal lesions can be modified or eliminated is the basis for the formulation of symptomatic and supportive therapy of primary renal failure.

It is obvious that an effective form of specific therapy may be ineffective if not combined with appropriate supportive and symptomatic therapy. All forms of supportive and symptomatic therapy help to minimize deficits and excesses in fluid, electrolyte, acid-base, endocrine, and nutrient balance that have developed as a result of loss of renal function (Table 1). Although these metabolic deficits and excesses are qualitatively similar in patients with renal dysfunction, they are often quantitatively dissimilar. Because there are significant differences in the type and magnitude of excesses and deficits

Table 1. *Summary of Conservative Medical Management of Polyuric Chronic Renal Failure*

Component	Purpose
Unlimited access to water	Maintain body water balance
Avoidance of conditions associated with body stress	Minimize alterations in body homeostasis
Dietary regulation	See Table 2
Administration of vitamins B and C	Compensate for inefficient conservation by diseased kidneys
Oral administration of sodium bicarbonate	Control metabolic acidosis of renal failure
Administration of anabolic agents	Promote positive nitrogen balance; beneficial effect on anemia; enhance calcium deposition in bones
Control of hyperphosphatemia	Control renal secondary hyperparathyroidism and renal osteodystrophy; prevent soft tissue calcification; possibly delay self-perpetuating progression of renal dysfunction
Control of hypocalcemia	Prevent consequences of hypocalcemia including renal secondary hyperparathyroidism
Avoidance of medications that are nephrotoxic or likely to produce adverse drug reactions	Prevent further reduction of renal function; prevent adverse drug reactions

of fluids and electrolytes that develop in patients with oliguric and nonoliguric primary renal failure, it is imperative to divide candidates for therapy of renal failure into two groups: those with oliguria and those with polyuria.

Polyuric primary renal failure tends to be associated with greater deficits; oliguric primary renal failure tends to be associated with greater excesses. The following guidelines for supportive and symptomatic therapy are designed for cats with primary chronic polyuric renal failure. Consult Emergency Management of the Acute Uremic Crisis, page 981, for further information on the treatment of oliguric renal failure.

THIRST

Obligatory polyuria associated with chronic polyuric renal failure is induced, at least in part, by (1) impaired ability to maintain a hypertonic medullary interstitium and, therefore, a functional countercurrent system, and (2) excretion of abnormally large quantities of solute through viable nephrons as a result of generalized nephron destruction and retention of metabolic wastes in the body. Compensatory polydipsia is essential for maintenance of body fluid balance. For this reason, an unrestricted supply of water should be available at all times. Except in instances of significant vomiting, the amount of water consumed should be dictated by the patient's thirst.

In patients unable to maintain water balance by compensatory polyuria, body water balance must be maintained by parenteral administration of appropriate fluids.

AVOIDING STRESS

Because severely damaged kidneys have a diminished ability to compensate for stresses imposed by concomitant disease states, uremic signs may be precipitated by a variety of prerenal or post-renal factors that develop in patients with previously compensated renal failure. Treatment should be directed toward prevention. To prevent precipitation of a uremic crisis or aggravation of abnormalities already present, every effort should be made to keep body stresses to a minimum so that the diseased kidneys can maintain homeostasis. Prolonged changes in environment should be avoided by treating compensated uremic animals as outpatients. Uremic patients that require surgery should receive adequate preoperative fluid therapy and renoprotective therapy. In addition, clients should be educated about the importance of supportive and symptomatic therapy.

DIET

OVERVIEW

The rationale for reduction of dietary protein in cats with renal failure has been reviewed elsewhere (Osborne et al., 1982). Although a direct cause-and-effect relationship has not been proved in many instances, it is generally accepted that protein catabolites (including nitrogenous substances, hydrogen ions, sulfur, potassium, and phosphorus) contribute significantly to the production of uremic signs in patients with renal failure.

Patients with primary renal failure have an impaired ability to excrete many protein catabolites because of a marked reduction in glomerular filtration rate. Retention of metabolic wastes may be further aggravated by alterations in tubular reabsorption and tubular secretion and by extrarenal factors that cause a reduction in renal perfusion and/or increased catabolism of body tissues.

One of the basic premises that currently influences nutritional management of patients with primary renal failure is that controlled reduction of excess dietary proteins will result in decreased production of nitrogenous wastes, with consequent amelioration of some clinical signs. Clinical, biochemical, and pathologic features of the uremic syndrome that are likely to be partially or completely corrected by appropriate dietary manipulations are summarized in Table 2. By formulating diets that contain reduced quantities of high biologic-value protein sufficient to provide daily requirements and adequate quantities of nonprotein

calories to prevent catabolism of protein for energy, many of the signs associated with uremia may be reduced in severity or eliminated, even when renal function remains unchanged.

A wide variety of therapeutic benefits have been proposed to result from the use of low-quantity, high-quality protein diets in the therapy of chronic primary polyuric renal failure (see Table 2). Although many of these proposed benefits have been reported to occur in humans and dogs, their occurrence in cats remains unproved in many instances. Because of numerous physiologic and nutritional differences among humans, dogs, and cats, benefits noted in one species cannot be assumed to occur in another. Because of numerous unanswered questions, controlled studies of modified protein diets in the therapy of chronic primary polyuric renal failure are needed to better define the benefits and risks of these diets in cats.

PROTEIN REQUIREMENTS

NORMAL

Cats have a significantly higher requirement for dietary protein than dogs and most other mammals. The minimum requirement of high-quality protein (quality equivalent to that derived from unprocessed mammalian, avian, or fish muscle) of growing kittens (29 per cent of diet calories) is approximately two and one-half times that of growing puppies (12 per cent of diet calories), whereas the protein requirement of adult cats (19 per cent of diet calories) is

Table 2. *Hypothesized Benefits of Low-Quantity, High-Quality Protein Diets in Chronic Polyuric Primary Renal Failure*

	Proved		
	In Humans	*In Dogs*	*In Cats*
Clinical manifestations of uremia			
eliminated	sometimes	sometimes	unknown
improved	usually	usually	unknown
Retained nitrogenous waste products reduced	usually	usually	probably
Uremic acidosis			
eliminated	sometimes	unknown	unknown
improved	usually	unknown	unknown
Renal secondary hyperparathyroidism			
eliminated	sometimes	sometimes	unknown
improved	sometimes	sometimes	unknown
Anemia of renal failure			
corrected	seldom or never	unknown	unknown
improved	sometimes	sometimes	unknown
Progressive, irreversible dysfunction minimized	probably	unknown	unknown
Prolonged survival	sometimes	sometimes	unknown
Hemorrhagic diathesis			
corrected	sometimes	unknown	unknown
improved	sometimes	unknown	unknown
Neurologic disturbances			
corrected	seldom or never	unknown	unknown
improved	sometimes	sometimes	unknown
Malnutrition prevented	unknown	unknown	unknown

almost five times that of adult dogs (4 per cent of diet calories) (Ullrey et al., 1978). The higher protein requirements for cats is apparently not solely the result of a higher requirement for one or more essential amino acids (Rogers et al., 1977). Rather, it appears to be associated with a reduced efficiency of utilization of dietary protein for body protein anabolism in cats compared with dogs and many other mammals. A significant quantity of protein in their diet is used as a source of calories (Rogers et al., 1977).

Although the minimum requirement of an ideal protein for kittens is reported to be approximately 29 per cent of the diet calories and that for adult cats is approximately 19 per cent of the diet, Smalley, Rogers, and Morris (unpublished data) have obtained maximum growth in weanling kittens fed a 25 per cent fat diet containing 18 per cent of an "ideal" amino acid mixture. Based on the assumption that the daily caloric requirement of adult cats is approximately 70 to 80 Kcal/kg (32 to 36 kcal/lb) body weight/day, the minimum protein requirement of high-quality natural protein (19 per cent of the dietary calories) would be approximately 3.3 to 3.8 gm/kg (1.5 to 1.7 gm/lb) body weight/day. If an ideal amino acid mixture were utilized instead of high-quality natural protein, the minimum daily protein requirement for adult cats (12 per cent of dietary calories*) would be approximately 2.1 to 2.4 gm/kg (1.0 to 1.1 gm/lb) body weight/day.

REQUIREMENTS IN RENAL FAILURE

Controlled restriction of dietary protein in humans and dogs may result in amelioration of many manifestations of the uremic syndrome. Presumably the same phenomenon occurs in cats. Unfortunately, optimal protein and amino acid requirements for uremic cats have not been established. However, there is evidence in humans, rats, and dogs that protein requirements for uremic animals may be greater than those for normal individuals. This is not surprising, since uremia is characterized by a catabolic state induced by a variety of endocrine and metabolic derangements including hyperglucagonemia, hypersomatotropinemia, hyperparathormonemia, insulin resistance, acidosis, potassium depletion, and hyperkalemia (Osborne and Polzin, 1979). Protein and amino acid requirements of uremic cats may be increased by pathophysiologic disturbances associated with the uremic syndrome, including any combination of the following: (1) endocrine alterations; (2) impaired intestinal absorption of amino acids; (3) impaired tubular reabsorption of amino acids; (4) impaired distribution of specific amino acids; (5) impaired metabolism of specific amino acids; and (6) decreased activity of intestinal dipeptidases and disaccharidases, which may result in impaired digestion of proteins and carbohydrates. Protein requirements may also be increased by external losses of protein (i.e., albuminuria, hematuria, or gastrointestinal hemorrhage) and/or the catabolic effects of concurrent illness.

Although great emphasis has been placed on the adverse effects of high-protein diets in patients with uremia, it becomes obvious from the preceding discussion that protein-deficient diets may also be detrimental. Protein deficiency may produce impaired resistance to infection through, at least in part, decreased complement activity, decreased cell-mediated immunity, and decreased antibody production (Ritz et al., 1978). Infection may be particularly detrimental to the patient if it further increases protein requirements. Other proposed effects of protein depletion include reduced hemoglobin production with resultant anemia, retardation of growth (in uremic rats and children), altered plasma protein binding of drugs, reduced plasma protein concentrations, and muscle protein depletion.

On the basis of current knowledge, the concept of maximal protein reduction in uremic patients to the limit of protein requirements for normal cats must be questioned. Either protein-deficient diets or high-protein diets may have adverse effects. Based on the results of recent experimental studies performed on normal cats that indicate that they are unable to adapt to a marked reduction of dietary protein, formulation of beneficial diets for cats in renal failure poses unique problems. Inadequate protein intake would lead to malnutrition (even if low-protein diets were palatable), whereas excessive protein consumption would enhance the production of potentially toxic metabolic waste products and might cause detrimental hyperfiltration. It seems logical, however, to recommend that cats with renal failure be offered as much protein as control of uremic manifestations will permit. Considering intrinsic variability in protein requirements of normal cats and the large number of variables with the potential to influence protein requirements in the uremic state, it is difficult to predict the protein requirements of uremic cats. Pending further studies, an effort should be made to individualize dietary protein intake according to patient response, aiming toward the minimal adult protein requirement.

CALORIC REQUIREMENTS

NORMAL

Cats not only have the capacity to tolerate and utilize high levels of dietary fat, they prefer high levels of dietary fat and perform better nutritionally when fed a high-fat diet. Cats are dependent on a

---

*Based on the unproven assumption that an adult cat would require two-thirds of the ideal amino acid mixture shown to be adequate for kittens (see text).

dietary source of arachadonic and linoleic fatty acids (Ullrey et al., 1978). Although linoleic acid is present in animal fats and vegetable oils, arachadonic acid is present only in animal fats. Dietary fat serves as a concentrated energy source, a carrier for fat-soluble vitamins, and a source of essential fatty acids and influences the palatability of food. Fats commonly compose 15 to 40 per cent of cat diets (Ullrey et al., 1978).

Whereas carbohydrates compose a major source of calories in many diets consumed by dogs, fats and proteins are the major energy sources in many cat foods (Ullrey et al., 1978). Cats can digest considerable quantities of dietary carbohydrates but apparently do not require dietary carbohydrates per se (Ullrey et al., 1978).

REQUIREMENTS IN RENAL FAILURE

Dietary energy is as important as dietary protein for maintenance of nitrogen balance and prevention of protein malnutrition. Modification of diets for the treatment of chronic primary polyuric renal failure should be based on reduction of protein intake and provision of adequate quantities of nonprotein calories (i.e., fats and carbohydrates). Caloric intake should be regulated to optimize protein anabolism.

Unfortunately, the minimum daily requirement of calories (fats and carbohydrates) for cats has not been established under conditions of renal failure. Because this information is unavailable, it has been necessary to make the unproved assumption that the minimum requirement for these nutrients in uremic animals is the same as that for normal animals. Accordingly, it seems logical to recommend that cats receive 70 to 80 Kcal/kg (32 to 36 cal/lb) body weight/day. Because glucose intolerance, intestinal maldigestion, elevated serum insulin and glucagon concentrations, and other pathophysiologic disturbances associated with the uremic syndrome may alter carbohydrate, fat, and caloric requirements, these values should be used only as guidelines. Determination of caloric requirements must be individualized on the basis of serial body weight determinations and clinical evaluation of the patient. Unless the patient is markedly obese and weight reduction is deemed necessary, an attempt should be made to maintain stable body weight. If the animal is malnourished, caloric intake should be increased for an appropriate period.

DIET RECOMMENDATIONS

Pending information based on controlled studies utilizing cats with a known degree of renal dysfunction, the following guidelines are recommended.

PROTEINS

Diets should be formulated so that uremic cats will consume a minimum of 3.3 to 3.8 gm/kg (1.5 to 1.7 gm/lb) body weight/day of high-quality natural protein. This is equivalent to approximately 20 per cent of the total diet calories. The amount of protein given should approach the maximum (rather than the minimum) that the patient can tolerate at each level of renal dysfunction. Conceptually, none of the protein should be catabolized for energy. However, this may be impossible to attain in cats because they normally catabolize substantial quantities of protein for energy. Additional quantities of high-quality protein may be required to balance protein loss caused by severe proteinuria (i.e., addition of 1 gram of protein in diet for each gram of protein lost in urine per day). This recommendation is especially applicable to patients with significant hypoproteinemia. The number of grams of protein lost in the urine per unit of time may be determined with the aid of a metabolism cage and should be correlated with the serum protein concentration.

CALORIES

Diets should be formulated so that uremic cats consume approximately 70 to 80 Kcal/kg (32 to 36 Kcal/lb) body weight/day. Since fat is a good source of calories (9 Kcal/gm) and since fat increases the palatability of food for most cats, a large percentage of the diet may be added to achieve the desired caloric balance.

Additional modifications of caloric intake may be required to compensate for the nutritional status and activity of the patient. Steady body weight over a period of weeks or months is usually a reliable index of adequate caloric intake.

HOMEMADE DIETS

Homemade diets may be formulated for the management of polyuric renal failure (Table 3). Potential advantages associated with homemade renal failure diets include individualization of the diet to meet the needs and palatability of the patient (protein and fat content, caloric density, and so on), and selection and manipulation of high-quality proteins. Potential disadvantages of homemade diets include client error in the preparation of a nutritionally adequate diet and inconvenience.

Cats are often accused of being finicky eaters and prefer high-fat, high-protein diets, especially from animal sources (i.e., liver, fish, and muscle). Protein-deficient diets are especially unpalatable to cats unless they contain high levels of animal fat. Cold food may also be less appetizing to cats. Therefore, refrigerated food should be allowed to warm to

Table 3. *Sample Calculation of Dietary Requirements for a Uremic 10-Lb Cat*

Caloric Density of Foods:

Carbohydrates	= 4 cal/gm
Proteins	= 4 cal/gm
Fats	= 9 cal/gm

Calculations:

10-lb cat × 35 cal/lb/day = 350 Kcal/day

10-lb cat × 1.5 gm protein/lb/day = 15 gm protein = 60 Kcal/day

Addition of 20 gm dietary fat/day = 180 Kcal/day

Addition of 28 gm dietary carbohydrate/day = 112 Kcal/day

Total calories = 352 Kcal/day

room temperature or should be heated prior to feeding.

Controlled studies comparing the therapeutic efficacy of homemade diets with that of prescription diets in cats with primary renal failure have not been reported. Until the results of such studies become available, the decision to use prescription diets or homemade diets must be based on personal opinion and the desires of the client.

PRESCRIPTION DIETS

One commercially available diet (Feline k/d) recommended for cats with renal failure contains 20 per cent of dietary calories as protein (equivalent to approximately 8 per cent protein for canned food and 20 to 22 per cent protein for dry food). The diet contains less dry-weight protein than most commercially available dry (32 to 36 per cent), semimoist (34 to 40 per cent), canned (35 to 41 per cent), and gourmet (40 to 65 per cent) cat foods (Ullrey et al., 1978). The manufacturers have reported that the diet is capable of supporting long-term maintenance of normal adult cats. Reduction of the protein content of the diet below 18 per cent of total dietary calories was reported to have resulted in reduced intake and weight loss in normal cats (Morris, 1975). Controlled studies of the diet in cats with experimental and naturally occurring renal failure have not been performed. Empirical clinical observations indicate that the diet is palatable.

Because of significant differences in the protein requirements of cats and dogs and significant differences in the composition of canine and feline prescription diets, cats should not be fed diets designed for canine patients with renal failure.

INITIATION OF THERAPY

There have been no controlled studies in humans or animals that define when during the evaluation of progressive renal failure dietary therapy should

be initiated. Therefore, the decision when to begin a low-protein diet remains a matter of personal opinion. Lack of a consensus of opinion as to the appropriate time to begin to restrict protein intake is in part related to an inability to quantitate the degree of uremic toxicity. Modified protein diets will not prevent renal failure nor will they reverse established renal lesions. Furthermore, studies in dogs with a mild degree of experimentally induced renal dysfunction demonstrated that high-protein diets fed for over one year did not adversely affect renal function (Bovee et al., 1979). However, more recent studies in rats and dogs with a greater degree of renal dysfunction indicate that excessive protein in the diet may cause glomerular hyperfiltration, which could lead to progressive glomerular sclerosis (Hostetter et al., 1982). Recent information derived from experimental studies in rats suggests that control of hyperphosphatemia and hyperparathormonemia during the early phases of progressive renal failure *may* be of value in minimizing the development of polysystemic clinical signs and self-perpetuating progression of generalized renal disease (Ibele et al., 1978). Similar studies performed in cats revealed that consumption of low-phosphorus diets minimized the degree of mineralization of the renal parenchyma (consult Treatment of Mineral Imbalances of Chronic Renal Failure for additional information).

As long as the serum urea nitrogen concentration, serum phosphorus concentration, and fractional excretion of phosphorus in urine remain within normal limits, it is probably unjustified to initiate therapy. Once serum phosphorus concentrations exceed normal limits, it seems logical to recommend initiation of dietary therapy on the assumption that the associated reduction of dietary phosphorus intake will help minimize renal secondary hyperparathyroidism and the rate of self-perpetuating renal dysfunction. In fact, it may be advisable to initiate therapy to control hyperparathyroidism prior to the onset of hyperphosphatemia. Renal secondary hyperparathyroidism may be recognized prior to the onset of hyperphosphatemia by detection of increased fractional excretion of phosphorus in urine. Further studies are required to clarify the benefit of this tentative recommendation, however. When serum phosphorus and SUN concentrations exceed normal limits and polysystemic abnormalities associated with the uremic syndrome become evident, initiation of appropriate modifications in diet is clearly justified.

FREQUENCY OF FEEDING

Cats are frequent eaters and normally require access to food for longer periods than dogs. Based on experience with uremic dogs, it seems logical to recommend feeding of several small meals daily rather than one large meal.

VITAMINS

WATER-SOLUBLE VITAMINS

Minimum daily requirements of water-soluble vitamins (B and C) have not been established for cats with renal failure. Because of the possibility of impaired tubular reabsorption of these vitamins in patients with polyuric renal failure and because of reduced intake of these vitamins caused by varying degrees of anorexia, we recommend that supplemental vitamins be given to such patients. A single high-potency tablet or capsule containing these water-soluble vitamins given daily is probably sufficient supplementation for most patients.

Although vitamin C (ascorbic acid) has the potential to aggravate metabolic acidosis in patients with renal failure, empirical clinical observations in our hospital indicate that therapeutic dosages of this substance are not likely to enhance acidosis in patients with mild to moderate renal failure.

VITAMIN A

Cats must ingest a preformed source of vitamin A because they are unable to convert β-carotene to vitamin A (Ullrey et al., 1978). Although the minimum daily requirement of vitamin A has not been established for cats under conditions of renal failure, human patients with renal failure often develop an excess of vitamin A. Excess vitamin A may directly or indirectly increase parathormone release and therefore aggravate renal osteodystrophy and acidosis. Pending further studies, *we do not recommend* supplementation of diets with vitamin A.

VITAMIN D

Progressive loss of renal parenchyma is associated with impaired conversion of vitamin D precursors to their most active form (1,25-dihydroxycholecalciferol). Even though the need for 1,25-vitamin D increases as renal function decreases, oral or parenteral administration of vitamin D without consideration of serum and dietary concentrations of calcium and phosphorus is extremely hazardous. Therapeutic elevation of the plasma concentration of calcium in patients with hyperphosphatemia may result in soft-tissue calcification and further deterioration of renal function. Therefore, supplementation of the diet with vitamin D must be carefully individualized to the patient. Specific recommendations have been reviewed elsewhere (Osborne and Polzin, 1979) (see the section on Control of Hypocalcemia in this article and Treatment of Min-

eral Imbalances of Chronic Renal Failure for additional information).

CORRECTION OF METABOLIC ACIDOSIS

CAUSES

Factors that may contribute to metabolic acidosis in patients with primary renal failure include (1) catabolism of exogenous (dietary) or endogenous (body) protein for energy, (2) impaired tubular reabsorption of filtered bicarbonate (and perhaps other buffer ions) caused by hyperparathormonemia and renal tubular dysfunction, (3) impaired tubular secretion of hydrogen ion, and (4) decreased renal tubular production of ammonia.

The onset and severity of metabolic acidosis in patients with primary renal failure vary. Most patients do not become severely acidotic until they develop polysystemic signs associated with uremia because the kidneys have not totally lost their capacity to excrete nonvolatile acids, and buffer systems are capable of compensating for the acidosis.

TREATMENT

AGENTS AND DOSAGE

Although orally administered sodium bicarbonate, calcium lactate, calcium carbonate, or sodium acetate may be considered for conservative management of metabolic acidosis, our clinical experience has been limited to the use of sodium bicarbonate.

Ideally, the dosage of $NaHCO_3$ should be titrated on the basis of serial measurement of plasma bicarbonate concentration and blood pH. Alternatively, the dosage may be guesstimated on the basis of urine pH, the severity of uremic signs, and the degree of azotemia. In general, patients with mild degrees of uremia may be expected to require about 3 mEq/kg body weight, those with moderate uremia about 6 mEq/kg body weight, and those with severe uremia about 9 mEq/kg body weight. A sufficient dosage of $NaHCO_3$ should be given to maintain plasma bicarbonate between 18 and 24 mEq/L and/or urine pH between 6 and 7. This usually requires between 5 and 15 grains per day (1 grain of $NaHCO_3$ = approximately ¾ mEq). A more precise dosage is difficult to establish because of unpredictable losses of bicarbonate in the gastrointestinal tract.

INITIATION OF THERAPY

Ideally, the need for alkalinizing therapy should be determined on the basis of the plasma bicarbonate concentration and blood pH. Alternatively, it may be estimated on the basis of clinical signs and other laboratory parameters. In humans, administration of alkalinizing agents is usually not recommended until plasma bicarbonate concentration falls below 15 to 18 mEq/L. Uncontrolled clinical observations suggest that similar recommendations for cats would be appropriate.

PRECAUTIONS

Care must be taken not to cause metabolic alkalosis. Large quantities of sodium should not be administered to patients with hypertension, congestive heart failure, hypoproteinemic edema, or oliguria. When administration of large quantities of sodium is undesirable, calcium lactate or calcium carbonate may be useful in minimizing the severity of acidosis with less danger of aggravating hypernatremia and body fluid accumulation.

Metabolic acidosis in severely hypocalcemic patients should be corrected with caution, since it has been reported that rapid correction of acidosis may decrease the concentration of ionized calcium and predispose to hypocalcemic tetany.

MAINTENANCE OF SODIUM BALANCE

The question of sodium balance in patients with renal failure is extremely important, since negative sodium balance would result in negative water balance, contraction of extracellular fluid volume, reduction in renal blood flow, and, ultimately, reduction in glomerular filtration rate. The resulting prerenal azotemia would aggravate the reduction in renal function caused by generalized renal lesions. In contrast, positive sodium balance would lead to positive water balance, expansion of fluid volume in various body compartments, and a variety of undesirable sequelae (hypertension, edema, release of potentially toxic quantities of biologic substances to maintain sodium balance, and so on).

In past years, it was generally accepted that patients with polyuric renal failure lose or "waste" sodium to a varying degree. Carefully performed clinical studies in dogs and cats that document this assumption have not been performed, however. The problem is compounded by the fact that the serum concentration of sodium is not a reliable index of total body sodium concentration. Measurement of the quantity of sodium lost in urine compared with sodium intake would help to solve this problem. Experimental studies performed in dogs have suggested that increased excretion of sodium in urine by functioning nephrons may represent an adaptive rather than an obligatory phenomenon (Bricker and Fine, 1981). If oral intake of a solute normally excreted in urine (such as sodium) remains unaltered while renal function declines, body balance can be maintained only if fractional excretion

of the solute increases in proportion to reduction in nephron numbers. A biologically active substance that induces natriuresis in rats and inhibits sodium transport by the frog skin and toad bladder has been identified in the serum of uremic dogs and humans. A factor with the same characteristics has been found in the urine of uremic humans; its natriuretic action appears to be related to concurrent patterns of sodium excretion. It has been hypothesized that this factor is a "natriuretic hormone" that serves as a modulator for sodium excretion.

Care must be used in evaluating urine sodium excretion in uremic animals or humans following reduction of sodium intake. Abrupt reductions of sodium intake caused sodium wasting in human patients with severe renal insufficiency, whereas a gradual reduction of sodium intake resulted in much improved adjustment of sodium excretion to equal intake. A proportional reduction of salt intake to match a proportional reduction in nephrons in dogs allowed sodium balance to be maintained without a detectable rise in natriuretic factor.

Further studies are required before dogmatic generalities influence formulation of therapeutic maneuvers designed to maintain sodium homeostasis in patients with renal failure and uremia. It seems logical that sodium balance in patients with primary renal failure would vary with (1) location of lesions within nephrons, (2) volume of urine produced (oliguria or polyuria), (3) severity and extent of nephron dysfunction, and (4) each individual patient. Patients with primary tubulointerstitial forms of renal failure are more likely to have impaired renal conservation of sodium than patients with primary glomerular forms of renal failure.

These statements should not be interpreted as indicating that administration of sodium chloride is of no value, nor should they be interpreted as suggesting that salt restriction is in order. However, pending availability of results of experimental and clinical studies designed to evaluate sodium balance in cats with various forms of primary polyuric renal failure, we do not recommend that oral sodium chloride be routinely supplemented or withheld from uremic patients. Dosage recommendations for administration of sodium chloride to salt-deficient dogs with primary renal failure have been described elsewhere.

MANAGEMENT OF ANEMIA

CAUSES

The kidneys are involved in red cell production by way of synthesis and release of erythropoietin when the oxygen tension of blood perfusing the kidneys is reduced. Unlike dogs, whose kidneys are apparently the sole site of erythropoietin production, erythropoietin is produced by the kidneys and the carotid bodies in cats (Tramezzani et al., 1971).

Anemia, which is typically nonregenerative, is a common manifestation of chronic uremia. It may also occur in patients with acute uremia, however. Causes of anemia associated with primary renal failure and uremia include (1) decreased production of erythropoietin by damaged kidneys, (2) inhibition of erythroblasts in marrow by toxic substances in uremic serum, (3) shortened RBC survival, (4) iron deficiency caused by chronic blood loss (associated with coagulation factor defects), impaired gastrointestinal absorption, and repeated blood sampling, (5) myelofibrosis secondary to renal osteodystrophy, and (6) chronic infection and malnutrition. Because multiple etiologic factors may underlie the anemia of uremia, the potential significance of each should be accounted for when considering therapy for severe anemia.

TREATMENT

OVERVIEW

The exact therapeutic regimen should be individualized for each patient. Blood transfusions are usually unnecessary, even in severely anemic patients. Because restoration of red cell numbers is short-lived, use of blood transfusions to correct the anemia of uremia is not recommended as a routine therapeutic procedure.

Administration of erythropoietin would logically appear to be of value in the treatment of uremic anemia, but quantities in excess of those normally released by the kidneys might be required, since bone marrow cells are less responsive to erythropoietin in an uremic environment. Unfortunately, contamination with endotoxins has interfered with commercial production of erythropoietin.

To date, androgenic anabolic hormones appear to be the most useful nonspecific stimulus of red cell production in uremic patients.

ANABOLIC AGENTS

Testosterone and synthetic derivatives of testosterone have anabolic effects. In humans, synthetic derivatives are commonly used because their androgenic masculinizing effect has been minimized, whereas their anabolic effect has been maximized. Anabolic steroids should not be confused with corticosteroids. Corticosteroids have a catabolic effect and are not routinely recommended for the supportive and symptomatic management of patients with primary renal failure.

Anabolic steroids have been reported to be of benefit in humans with primary renal failure because (1) they promote positive nitrogen balance (anabolism) provided the patient is not in a state of negative caloric balance, (2) they have a beneficial effect on anemia associated with uremia, and (3) they may enhance calcium deposition in bones. Although subjective clinical evaluation of the therapeutic efficacy of anabolic steroids in dogs and cats with renal failure has been favorable, data that document that anabolic agents exert effects in these species similar to those described in humans have not been reported.

Postulated beneficial effects of anabolic agents on the anemia of uremia include (1) direct stimulation of red cell precursors in bone marrow by 5-beta-hydroxy metabolites, (2) increased renal production of erythropoietin by 5-alpha-hydroxy compounds, and (3) increased production of RBC 2,3-diphosphoglycerate with an associated shift of the oxygen-hemoglobin dissociation curve to the right. Erythrocyte 2,3-DPG facilitates the release of oxygen from hemoglobin to tissues by decreasing the affinity of hemoglobin for oxygen. This action is of benefit even if the number of RBCs is not increased. Studies in humans indicate that two to three months may be required to detect an increase in packed cell volume following administration of anabolic agents.

The most effective erythropoietic androgens for treatment of uremic anemia in cats have not been determined. Available products include stanazolol (Winstrol-V*), nandrolone decanoate (Deca-Durabolin†), testosterone proprionate (Oreton‡), oxymethalone (Adroyd§), and testosterone enanthate (Deletestryl‖).

CONTROL OF HYPERPHOSPHATEMIA

Consult the article entitled "Management of Uremic Hyperphosphatemia" for details pertaining to the causes and detrimental effects of uremic hyperphosphatemia.

Methods of controlling hyperphosphatemia may include (1) enhancing glomerular filtration rate by correcting dehydration and/or maintaining sodium and water balance, (2) reducing dietary phosphorus via the use of high quality, low-quantity protein diets or specially formulated low-phosphorus diets, and (3) enhancing gastrointestinal nonabsorbable phosphorus binding agents. Most contain aluminum hydroxide or aluminum carbonate. Following ingestion, aluminum phosphate forms and passes through the intestinal tract unabsorbed.

---

*Winthrop Laboratories, New York, NY.
†Organon Pharmaceuticals, West Orange, NJ.
‡Schering Corp., Kenilworth, NJ.
§Parke-Davis, Morris Plains, NJ.
‖E. R. Squibb & Sons, Inc., Princeton, NJ.

A variety of oral phosphorus binding agents are commercially available including aluminum hydroxide gel (Amphojel Tablets and Suspension,* Dialume Capsules,†) and aluminum carbonate gel (Basaljel Tablets, Capsules, and Suspension.*) Aluminum carbonate has been reported to be a more potent phosphorus binding agent than aluminum hydroxide because it is more completely ionized than aluminum hydroxide.

In general, tablets may be less satisfactory for use in cats than in humans because cats do not voluntarily chew them. Liquid suspensions may be very difficult to administer to cats. In our hands, capsules containing aluminum carbonate gel in powder form have been most satisfactory for cats. The powder may be mixed with food.

Nonabsorbable phosphate binding agents should be given to effect. Strive to maintain a serum phosphorus concentration between 3.0 and 4.5 mg/dl. Until further data regarding the use of these drugs in cats become available, it is cautiously suggested that initial daily dosages of 150 mg/lb/day of aluminum carbonate or aluminum hydroxide be given, divided three times per day at meal time (consult Treatment of Mineral Imbalances of Chronic Renal Failure for information pertaining to initiation of therapy and precautions associated with use of oral phosphorus binding agents).

CONTROL OF HYPOCALCEMIA

CAUSES

Varying degrees of hypocalcemia is a common, but not consistent, finding in patients with chronic primary renal failure. Mechanisms of hypocalcemia associated with primary renal failure include (1) hyperphosphatemia caused by decreased renal clearance of phosphorus and lesser degrees of hyperphosphatemia induced by tissue catabolism; hyperphosphatemia results in induction of a reciprocal decrease in serum ionized calcium concentration, (2) impaired renal production of 1,25-vitamin D, (3) impaired tubular reabsorption of filtered calcium caused by lesions in nephrons, and (4) reduced consumption of dietary calcium. The severity of hypocalcemia in patients with chronic renal failure is variable. Variable degrees of hyperphosphatemia usually occur prior to the onset of clinical hypocalcemia. Because of mobilization of large reserves of calcium stored in the skeleton, the serum concentration of calcium does not become detectably decreased until the late stages of the disease.

TREATMENT

DIET AND NONABSORBABLE PHOSPHORUS BINDING AGENTS

Hypocalcemia may be controlled during the earlier stages of chronic progressive renal failure with oral administration of nonabsorbable phosphorus binding agents and low-protein diets. These mechanisms will not correct disturbances caused by impaired renal production of 1,25-vitamin D, however (consult the sections on Diet and Control of Hyperphosphatemia for specific recommendations).

VITAMIN D

Administration of 1,25-vitamin D or vitamin D analogues in conjunction with therapy to minimize hyperphosphatemia in humans with naturally occurring chronic renal failure and in dogs with experimentally induced chronic renal failure has been of benefit in controlling renal secondary hyperparathyroidism and associated abnormalities. Although similar results would be expected in cats, this hypothesis has not been confirmed by experimental or clinical trials.

Extreme caution must be used when considering administration of vitamin D or oral calcium. Under no circumstances should vitamin D and oral calcium supplements be administered to hyperphosphatemic patients, since increased intestinal absorption of calcium and increased skeletal mobilization of calcium will result in precipitation of calcium phosphate salts in various body tissues including the kidneys. This sequela is very undesirable for many reasons including the fact that it produces renal lesions. In humans, it is recommended that vitamin D and calcium supplements not be administered to hypocalcemic patients with renal failure unless the product of serum phosphorus and calcium concentration is less than 70 mg/dl. Preferably, the serum concentration of phosphorus should be less than 6.0 mg/dl. Pending studies in uremic cats, these recommendations may be used as guidelines for vitamin D therapy.

A form of vitamin D (Rocaltrol capsules, 0.25 mcg‡) that is chemically and clinically identical to naturally occurring 1,25-dihydroxycholecalciferol is commercially available for use in humans. Provided that intake of calcium is adequate and hyperphosphatemia has been properly controlled, administration of 1,25-vitamin D to hypocalcemic humans with chronic renal failure results in increased intestinal absorption of calcium, increased serum calcium concentration, and reduced serum parathormone concentration. The drug has a short duration of

*Wyeth Laboratories, Philadelphia, PA.
†Armour Pharmaceutical Co., Tarrytown, NY.

‡Roche Laboratories, Nutley, NJ.

action, permitting control of unwanted hypercalcemia. It is rapidly absorbed from the intestines, reaches a peak concentration in serum after four hours, and exerts pharmacologic activity for three to five days. Although the optimum dose must be determined for each patient, the suggested dosage for humans is 0.25 mcg daily or every other day. The manufacturers of the drug suggest appropriate serial evaluation of serum calcium concentration, serum calcium-phosphorus products, and serum alkaline phosphatase activity. They indicate that a decrease in serum alkaline phosphatase activity usually precedes the occurrence of hypercalcemia. Because the drug may be associated with enhanced intestinal absorption of magnesium, it should not be used in combination with nonabsorbable phosphate binding agents that contain magnesium.

Dosages of 1,25-vitamin D have not been determined for hypocalcemic cats with primary renal failure. Administration of 120 to 240 ng/kg body weight to dogs with normal renal function and normal serum calcium concentration resulted in hypercalcemia. Other products advocated for use in humans include (1) 25-hydroxycholecalciferol (calcifediol) at a dosage of 100 mcg given three times per week (administration of 20 mcg/day to dogs with chronic renal failure and receiving low phosphorus diets resulted in hypercalcemia), (2) dihydrotachysterol: the starting dosage for crystalline DHT is 40,000 U/day, and (3) 1α-hydroxycholecalciferol at an initial dose of 0.04 to 0.08 mcg/kg/day.

ORAL CALCIUM SUPPLEMENTATION

Oral calcium supplements include calcium carbonate, calcium glucanoate, and calcium lactate. Calcium carbonate may be given at an initial dosage of 50 mg/lb body weight/day. Dosage must be individualized for each patient based on serial evaluation of serum calcium and phosphorus concentrations.

PRECAUTIONS

It is emphasized that calcium supplements and vitamin D must not be given to hyperphosphatemic patients. It is also important to recall that total serum calcium concentration may be decreased in hypoproteinemic patients, even though ionized serum calcium concentration is normal.

A word of caution: some patients with chronic renal failure may be hypercalcemic rather than hypocalcemic. In addition, some patients may have renal failure caused by hypercalcemia (so-called hypercalcemic nephropathy).

MONITORING RESPONSE

Re-evaluation of patients at appropriate intervals will permit alteration of various components of conservative medical management according to individual needs. In addition to evaluation of the owner's impression of therapeutic response, hydration, body weight, and the results of a physical examination, certain laboratory evaluations should be considered. Because restriction of dietary protein may reduce the concentration of serum urea nitrogen without any significant improvement in glomerular filtration rate, it is recommended that both serum urea nitrogen and creatinine concentrations be evaluated as indices of dietary adherence and therapeutic response. Reduction of urea nitrogen concentration associated with a stable creatinine concentration suggests a favorable therapeutic response.

Evaluation of serum albumin concentrations may be of value in determining the need for additional dietary protein. The usefulness of serum albumin as an index of dietary protein adequacy is limited, however, because physiologic adaptations sustain serum albumin concentrations within the normal range at the expense of the extravascular protein pool. Hypoalbuminemia may also be induced or aggravated by abnormalities not directly related to dietary protein intake.

Periodic evaluation of blood pH, plasma bicarbonate concentration (or total CO_2 or CO_2 content), and serum phosphorus concentration may indicate the need for and/or efficacy of supplemental forms of therapy to control metabolic acidosis and hyperphosphatemia.

SUMMARY OF RECOMMENDATIONS

1. Provide unlimited access to water.
2. Avoid conditions associated with body stress.
3. Formulate diets with a low quantity of high-quality protein. A suggested value for high-quality protein is 1.5 to 1.7 gm/lb body weight/day. Be sure that caloric intake is adequate to prevent catabolism of proteins for energy.
4. Supplement low-protein diets with vitamins B and C.
5. Consider administration of sodium bicarbonate for patients with moderate or severe acidosis.
6. Consider the use of anabolic agents to help minimize the consequences of uremic anemia.
7. Consider the use of nonabsorbable phosphorus binding agents in addition to low-protein diets to control hyperphosphatemia and its consequences.
8. Cautiously consider the use of vitamin D and oral calcium supplements to control hypocalcemia and its consequences in patients in which hyperphosphatemia has been controlled.
9. Avoid the use of corticosteroids, antibiotics, and other drugs likely to be associated with adverse reactions. Avoid the use of diuretics in nonedematous patients.
10. Use urinary catheters with great caution to avoid iatrogenic urinary tract infections.

REFERENCES AND SUPPLEMENTAL READING

Bovee, K. C., Abt, D. A., and Kronfeld, D. S.: The effects of dietary protein intake on renal function in dogs with experimentally reduced renal function. J. Am. Anim. Hosp. Assoc. 15:9, 1979.

Bricker, N. S., and Fine, L. G.: The renal response to progressive nephron loss. In Brenner, B. M., and Rector, F. C. (eds.): The Kidney, Vol. 1, 2nd ed. Philadelphia: W. B. Saunders, 1981.

Hostetter, T. M., Rennke, H. G., and Brenner, B. M.: Compensatory renal hemodynamic injury. A final common pathway of residual nephron destruction. Am. J. Kid. Dis. 1:310, 1982.

Ibele, L. S., Alfrey, A. C., Haut, L., and Huffer, W. E.: Preservation of function in experimental renal disease by dietary restriction of phosphate. N. Engl. J. Med. 298:122, 1978.

Morris, M. L.: Feline dietetics. Feline Pract. 5:39, 1975.

Osborne, C. A., and Polzin, D. J.: Strategy in the diagnosis, prognosis, and management of renal disease, renal failure, and uremia. Proceed-ings of the 46th Annual Meeting of the American Animal Hospital Association. 559, 1979.

Osborne, C. A., Polzin, D. J., Abdullahi, S., Klausner, J. S., and Rogers, Q. R.: Role of diet in management of feline chronic polyuric renal failure: Current status. J. Am. Anim. Hosp. Assoc. 18:11, 1982.

Ritz, E., Mehls, O., Gilli, J., and Heuck, C. C.: Protein restriction in the conservative management of uremia. Am. J. Clin. Nutr. 31:1703, 1978.

Rogers, Q. R., Morris, J. G., and Freedland, R. A.: Lack of hepatic enzymatic adaptation to low and high levels of dietary protein in the adult cat. Enzyme 22:348, 1977.

Tramezzani, J. H., Morita, E., and Chiocchio, S. R.: The carotid body as a neuroendocrine organ involved in control of erythropoiesis. Proc. Nat. Acad. Sci. 68:52, 1971.

Ullrey, D. E., Kealy, R. D., Mehring, J. S., and Smith, R. E.: Nutrient Requirements of Cats. Washington, DC:: National Research Council, National Academy of Sciences, 1978.

TREATMENT OF MINERAL IMBALANCES OF CHRONIC RENAL FAILURE

DELMAR R. FINCO, D.V.M.,
and JEANNE A. BARSANTI, D.V.M.

Athens, Georgia

Abnormal blood concentrations of calcium (Ca), phosphorus (P), vitamin D metabolites, and parathormone (PTH) occur during chronic renal failure in the dog and cat. The following discussion summarizes the pathogenesis of these imbalances, contemporary knowledge concerning their deleterious effects, and therapeutic approaches to minimizing their degree.

PATHOGENESIS OF IMBALANCES

When consuming common commercial diets, normal dogs ingest quantities of minerals in excess of daily requirements. Ca absorption from the gut is partially regulated by need, whereas absorption of P is conducted in a less discriminating manner. Consequently, large amounts of P are excreted in urine of dogs and cats by their relatively unimpeded passage through the glomerular filtration barrier into tubular lumens. However, the quantity of P filtered (glomerular filtration rate [GFR] × plasma P concentration) is enormous and would result in body depletion were it not for reabsorption of most of the filtered P by renal tubular cells. Because tubular reabsorption of P (TRP) is normally greater than 90 per cent of the quantity filtered, normal plasma P concentration is maintained.

In animals with developing renal dysfunction, a decrease in GFR and the amount of P filtered leads to retention of P in plasma. Because of a physicochemical relationship between Ca and P, a small elevation of plasma P leads to a small decrease in plasma Ca concentration. Decreased plasma Ca concentration stimulates the release of PTH by the parathyroid glands. PTH has several effects that correct the hypocalcemia. By inhibiting renal tubular reabsorption of P (i.e., TRP decreases) so that more P is excreted in the urine, normal plasma P concentration is re-established. PTH also increases blood Ca concentration by mobilizing Ca from bone and by stimulating the kidneys to produce 1,25-dihydroxy-vitamin D from its 25-OH-vitamin D precursor. 1,25-Dihydroxy-vitamin D, the biologically active form of this vitamin, stimulates intestinal absorption and bone accretion of Ca after a lag period of 24 to 48 hours. The result of these responses to hyperphosphatemia is re-establishment of normal plasma Ca and P concentrations. However, plasma PTH and TRP deviations persist as long as GFR is decreased. This mechanism of elevation of plasma PTH levels is called *renal secondary hyperparathyroidism*, since renal dysfunction is the precipitating factor. Although the aforementioned alterations in plasma Ca and P levels are of sufficient magnitude to be detected by the sensitive parathyroid glands, which subsequently release PTH, they cannot be detected by clinical laboratory determinations of Ca and P.

With progression of disease and a further decrease in GFR, the events previously outlined continue. However, increased quantities of PTH are required to re-establish normocalcemia and normophosphatemia. Only when GFR is reduced to about 25 per cent of normal do these compensatory mechanisms fall short. At this time TRP is suppressed maximally. Hyperphosphatemia occurs, however, because of decreased filtration of P. In addition, moderate to severe renal failure is associated with impaired intestinal absorption of Ca because of impaired production of 1,25-dihydroxy-vitamin D. Since Ca mobilization from bones continues, blood Ca concentration is maintained near normal after hyperphosphatemia supervenes. However, decreased plasma Ca concentration eventually occurs in most patients with chronic, severe uremia.

EFFECTS OF IMBALANCES

There are proven consequences of the aforementioned sequence of events. Bone disease (collectively referred to as renal osteodystrophy) has been detected and characterized by histologic and radiologic studies. The extreme clinical manifestation of the bone disease is the "rubber jaw" syndrome. Neurologic disease has also been detected. In one study, experimental induction of acute uremia in dogs was associated with abnormal EEG patterns and increased brain tissue concentration of Ca. However, these abnormalities were prevented if the dogs were thyroparathyroidectomized prior to induction of uremia. These results suggest that PTH is the factor responsible for the abnormalities.

A plethora of other abnormalities have been attributed to PTH excess, including bone marrow inhibition; abnormal myocardial function; peripheral neuropathy; altered lipid, carbohydrate, and acid-base metabolism; soft tissue calcification; pruritus; myopathy; and impotence. However, the role of PTH in the genesis of these abnormalities associated with uremia awaits further clarification.

Progression of renal failure has been attributed to the mineral imbalance associated with uremia. Results of studies in rats with surgically reduced renal mass revealed that dietary restriction of P and protein prevented renal mineralization and progression of renal failure. Both of these abnormalities occurred in rats fed a normal diet. A study of cats with surgically reduced renal mass demonstrated that severe renal mineralization occurred if normal dietary levels of P were fed. However, only mild renal mineralization occurred if dietary P was restricted. In contrast to the results of the rat study, progression of renal failure was not observed in cats consuming either diet during the period of study.

Studies have not yet been conducted in azotemic dogs to establish whether P restriction is beneficial to renal function. This point is emphasized because of contrary statements by some food manufacturers.

In summary, some beneficial effects (bone, CNS) can be anticipated if renal secondary hyperparathyroidism is prevented. The effects of prevention of renal secondary hyperparathyroidism on other signs of uremia and on progression of renal failure in the dog and cat remain to be established. On the presumption that there are benefits to be gained by minimizing the degree of renal secondary hyperparathyroidism, treatment of this disorder in patients with renal dysfunction should be considered. Limited studies indicate that blood levels of PTH will decrease with appropriate therapy.

THERAPY OF MINERAL IMBALANCES OF UREMIA

Despite normal plasma Ca and P concentrations, renal secondary hyperparathyroidism and mineral imbalances already exist at the time of diagnosis of renal failure. At this time TRP is decreased. The single most important factor in therapy is a decrease in intestinal P absorption. Maximum benefit is most likely to be attained if efforts to reduce P absorption are initiated early in the course of renal failure. Since we do not believe that protein restriction is required for other purposes until the BUN exceeds 75 mg/dl, normal diets can be supplemented with P binders (aluminum gels) used to decrease P absorption. Several therapeutic agents (Amphojel*, AlternaGEL†, Basaljel*) are available. Alternative products may also be used, but any containing magnesium (Mg) should be avoided, since this element is retained in the body during renal failure.

It is very important to administer P binders at the time of food intake to maximize binding of P in the gut lumen. Animals previously given food "free choice" should be fed at set times; and P binder should be administered with or at the conclusion of the meal. The dosage of this drug is to effect. An initial dose of 30 to 90 mg/kg/day may be instituted and the effect monitored by appropriate laboratory evaluations.

Unfortunately, simple tests that indicate when P restriction is adequate are not available. Plasma PTH levels and TRP are the most accurate indices of response to therapy but are relatively time-consuming and expensive. Measurement of plasma P concentration provides an indication of gross inadequacy of P restriction because elevated P concentrations are a definite indication of mineral imbalance. This method is crude because normal plasma P concentration does not assure absence of

---

*Wyeth Laboratories, Philadelphia, PA.
†Stuart Pharmaceuticals, Wilmington, DE.

Table 1. *Ingredients for Preparation of a Low-Phosphorus Diet for Dogs**

Food	Amount	Protein	Fat	Ca	P	Calories
				Composition (gm)		
Ground beef†	100 gm (3½ oz)	16.0	28.0	0.009	0.172	316
White rice‡	90 gm (2¼ cups cooked)	6.9	0.3	0.009	0.084	315
Table sugar	1 tbs	—	—	—	—	60
Vegetable oil	1 tsp	—	3.0	—	—	30
Calcium carbonate§		—	—	0.500	—	—
Totals		22.9	31.3	0.518	0.256	721
KD Prescription Diet (can)		18.8	32.0	0.608	0.304	642

*A maintenance vitamin and trace mineral preparation should be administered with this diet.
†Fat from cooked ground beef must be included in the mixture.
‡Ground corn (90 gm, 2 cups cooked) may be used, as it has a composition equivalent to that of white rice.
§Available as OsCal, 500 mg Ca/tablet, Marion Labs Inc., Kansas City, MO.

renal secondary hyperparathyroidism. The timing of measurement of plasma P concentration in relation to eating must be controlled because an increase in P of several mg/dl occurs in normal and azotemic animals following oral P intake. To ensure that serial measurements are not affected by recent P ingestion, blood samples should be obtained after a 12-hour fast. Since RBCs are rich in P, hemolysis should be avoided and RBCs should be separated from plasma soon after blood samples are obtained. We presently interpret fasting plasma P concentrations above 6 mg/dl in adult dogs and cats as indicative of inadequate P restriction. Further studies are needed to evaluate the validity of this arbitrary choice.

Constipation is one side effect that may be associated with administration of P binders. Some concern about increased tissue concentrations of aluminum has been cited in human patients with renal failure, but its importance in dogs is unknown.

In addition to P binders, reduced P intake may be achieved by feeding diets with a low P content. Once protein restriction is indicated, P restriction can be achieved by providing a high-quality, low-quantity protein diet in which the bulk of the calories is obtained from fat and carbohydrate sources low in P. A palatable low-P diet can be formulated by dog owners (Table 1). Prescription diets for patients with renal failure are lower in P than commercial foods and also may be utilized when BUN concentration exceeds 75 mg/dl (see Table 1).

One trap to be avoided when using special diets or binders for control of P absorption is the assumption that a single formulation suffices for all patients. Since control of renal secondary hyperparathyroidism depends on reduction of P intake proportionate to the reduction in GFR, patients with different levels of GFR require different levels of P restriction. Likewise, if GFR continues to decrease in the same patient, a further decrease in P intake is required. Adjustments in P intake can be made for the formulated diet (see Table 1) by increasing caloric density with vegetable oil and table sugar. However, there are limits to which this can be done without causing protein depletion. Phosphate binders may be used in conjunction with special diets if further P restriction is required.

Uremic human patients often are given supplemental dietary Ca and vitamin D metabolites to increase intestinal Ca absorption and bone mineral accretion. We hesitate to recommend either of these treatments because indiscriminant use of vitamin D products without adequate P restriction may lead to soft-tissue mineralization and possibly overt hypercalcemia. In addition, commercial pet foods are already high in Ca content.

SUPPLEMENTAL READING

Arieff, A. I., et al:: Calcium metabolism of brain in acute renal failure. J. Clin. Invest. 53:387, 1974.
Coburn, J. W.: Renal osteodystrophy. Kidney Int. 17:677, 1980.
Rutherford, E., et al.: Use of a new phosphate binder in chronic renal insufficiency. Kidney Int. 17:528, 1980.
Slatopolsky, E., et al.: Parathyroid hormone metabolism and its potential as a uremic toxin. Am. J. Physiol. 239:F1, 1980.

CONTROL OF VOMITING IN THE UREMIC PATIENT

JERRY A. THORNHILL, D.V.M.

West Lafayette, Indiana

Vomiting may be defined as the reflex act of ridding an overdistended or irritated stomach and upper duodenum of their contents. The reflex is mediated through the bilateral vomiting center in the medulla. Vomiting may also occur as a result of stimulation of the vomiting center by impulses arising from the chemoreceptor trigger zone (CTZ) on the floor of the fourth ventricle. Uremia stimulates centrally mediated vomition through activation of the CTZ. However, evidence incriminating irritation of the upper gastrointestinal tract from hyperacidity as the principle cause of vomition in renal failure is mounting.

ROLE OF HYPERGASTRINEMIA

Naturally secreted gastrin from the antral mucosa of the stomach containing predominately heptadecapeptide gastrin (17 amino acids, G17) and from the duodenal mucosa containing big gastrin (33 amino acids, G33) stimulates gastrin receptors on parietal cells. This leads to stimulation of histamine H_2-receptors on the same cells, followed by synthesis and release of hydrochloric acid (Fig. 1). Gastrin may also indirectly stimulate mast cells near parietal cells to release histamine, which directly stimulates H_2-receptors. Regardless of cause, increased and prolonged stimulation of H_2-receptors leads to gastric hyperacidity, mucosal irritation, destruction of the mucosal barrier, and diffusion of acid back into mucosal cells. Acid-induced mast cell damage results in the release of histamine, creating further stimulation of H_2-receptors, capillary fragility, and hemorrhage.

This sequence of events (Fig. 2) leading to upper gastrointestinal tract irritation and hemorrhage is thought to occur in patients with significantly reduced renal function. Normally, up to 40 per cent of gastrin per minute is cleared from the plasma by renal uptake and excretion. When gastrin clearance is diminished, prolonged H_2-receptor stimulation results. Elevated plasma gastrin levels have been well-documented by radioimmunoassay (RIA) in acute and chronic renal failure in humans. In a study at Purdue (Fig. 3), resting RIA plasma gastrin* levels in four nonazotemic dogs averaged 41.15

---

*Cambridge Nuclear Radiopharmaceutical Corp. Billerica, MA.

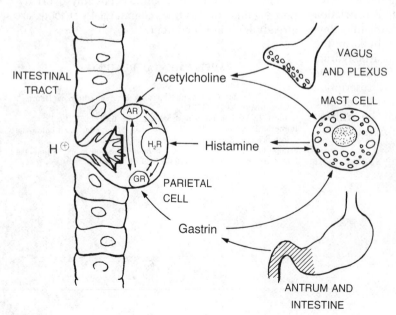

Figure 1. Parietal cell with relationship of H_2, gastrin, and acetylcholine receptors. (Adapted from Baron *in* Creutzfeldt: *Cimetidine—Proceedings of an International Symposium on Histamine H_2-Receptor Antagonists.* Amsterdam: Excerpta Medica, 1977.)

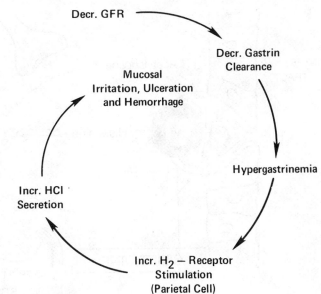

Figure 2. Circle of decreased glomerular filtration rate (GFR), hypergastrinemia, and mucosal irritation and hemorrhage.

Fasting Plasma Gastrin in the Dog

	Serum Creatinine	*Plasma Gastrin*
Control No. 1	<1.5 mg/dl	42 pg/ml
Control No. 2	<1.5 mg/dl	34 pg/ml
Control No. 3	<1.5 mg/dl	44.4 pg/ml
Control No. 4	<1.5 mg/dl	41.2 pg/ml

Range = 34 — 44.4, Mean = 41.15 (± 3.08)

Figure 3. Fasting plasma gastrin concentration in four control dogs.

	Serum Creatinine mg/dl	C_{CR} ml/min/kg	Plasma Gastrin pg/ml
1. Beagle, 11 yrs., male, ESRD	7.7	0.23	63
2. Min. Poodle, 13 yrs., female (S), ESRD	17.4	0.17	492
3. Min. Schnauzer, 8 yrs., male, ESRD	8.0	0.20	85.2

Figure 4. Fasting plasma gastrin concentration in three dogs with advanced chronic end-stage renal disease. C_{CR} = endogenous creatinine based on 24-hour urine collection.

ESRD = End Stage Renal Disease

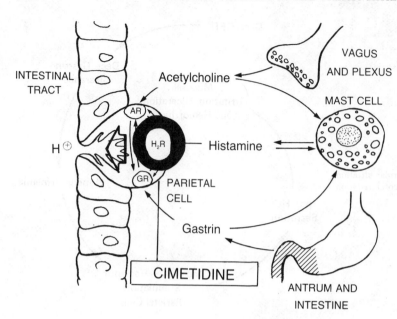

Figure 5. Cimetidine antagonism of the H_2-receptor of the parietal cell.

pg/ml (range = 34.0 to 44.4). Hypergastrinemia was documented in three dogs with gastrointestinal signs due to end-stage renal failure (Fig. 4).

CONTROL OF VOMITING WITH CIMETIDINE

In light of knowledge that hypergastrinemia is a cause of vomiting, mediated through gastrin receptor and H_2-receptor stimulation in parietal cells leading to upper bowel irritation and hemorrhage from hyperacidity, the beneficial role of agents that block H_2-receptor sites is apparent. Cimetidine was developed in the late 1970s as an H_2-receptor antagonist to curb duodenal ulcers in humans. Cimetidine has a biochemical structure similar to that of histamine, differing only in substitution of the side chain with cyanoquanidine. It prevents H_2-receptor stimulation by histamine or gastrin and acetylcholine, which feed through the H_2-receptor (Fig. 5). In studies of dogs infused with pentagastrin and histamine, greater than 75 per cent of acid secretion was inhibited 60 to 90 minutes following oral doses of cimetidine. In our hospital, cimetidine has provided symptomatic relief to dogs with uremic gastroenteritis.

CIMETIDINE DOSAGE

Cimetidine (Tagamet*) is supplied as tablets (200 and 300 mg), oral liquid (300 mg/tsp), and injectable liquid (300 mg/2 ml). The initial intravenous dose for uremic gastropathy is 10 mg/kg body weight, followed by 5 mg/kg given intravenously twice daily for the duration of hospitalization. At the time of hospital discharge, patients are given oral cimetidine at a dosage of 5 mg/kg twice daily for two to

three weeks. The dosage is reduced to 5 mg/kg given once daily for two to three weeks before being withdrawn. In humans, cimetidine dosage adjustments are made when the glomerular filtration rate (GFR) is less than 50 per cent. No less than one-half of the total dosage is given if GFR is between 0 and 50 per cent of normal. In dogs, dosage adjustments for reduced kidney function have not been determined. Although cimetidine is a dialyzable compound, only a small portion of the administered dose is removed by dialysis. The recommended dosage adjustments for patients being dialyzed are as follows: (1) administer standard dose following hemodialysis, or (2) maintain a three-times-a-day dose during continuous ambulatory peritoneal dialysis (CAPD).

SUPPLEMENTAL READING

Baron, J. H.: Round table discussion: Implications of cimetidine research for the understanding of gastric physiology and pathogenesis of peptic ulcer diseases. *In* Creutzfeldt, W. (ed.): *Cimetidine—Proceedings of an International Symposium on Histamine H_2-Receptor Antagonists*. Amsterdam: Excerpta Medica, 1977, pp. 169–171, 178–179.

Brimblecombe, R. W., Duncan, W. A. M., Durant, G. J., Emmett, J. C., Ganellin, C. R., Leslie, G. B., and Parsons, M. E.: Characterization and development of cimetidine as a histamine H_2-receptor antagonist. Gastroenterology 74:339, 1978.

Christensen, C. K., Nielsen, H. E., Kamstrup, O., Olsen, K. J., Brandsborg, M., and Brandsborg, O.: Serum gastrin and serum calcitonin in patients with chronic renal failure. Acta Endocrinol. 91:564, 1979.

Clendinnen, B. G., Davidson, W. D., Reeder, D. D., Jackson, B. M. and Thompson, J. C.: Renal uptake and excretion of gastrin in the dog. Surg. Gynecol. Obstet. 132:1039, 1971.

Davenport, H. W.: Salicylate damage to the gastric mucosal barrier. N. Engl. J. Med. 276:1307, 1967.

Dubb, J. W., Stote, R. M., Familiar, R. G., Lee, K., and Alexander, F.: Effect of cimetidine or renal function in normal man. Clin. Pharmacol. Ther. 24:76, 1978.

Hallgren, R., Landelius, J., Fjellstrom, K. E., and Lundquist, G.: Gastric acid secretion in uremia and circulating levels of gastrin, somatostatin, and pancreatic polypeptide. Gut 20:763, 1979.

*Smith Kline & French Co., Carolina, PR.

Hansky, J.: Clinical aspects of gastrin physiology. Med. Clin. North Am. 58:1217, 1974.

Hirschowitz, B. I., and Gibson, R. G.: Effect of cimetidine on stimulated gastric secretion and serum gastrin in the dog. Am. J. Gastroenterol. 70:437, 1978.

Korman, M. G., Laver, M. C., and Hansky, J.: Hypergastrinaemia in chronic renal failure. Br. Med. J. 1:209, 1972.

Krempien, B., Ritz, E., Wanke, M., and Wegener, K.: Gastropathy in uremia. In Kluthe, R., Berlyne, G., and Burton, B. (eds.): Uremia. London: Churchill Livingstone, 1972.

Larsson, R., Bodemar, G., Kagedal, B., and Walan, A.: The effects of cimetidine (Tagamet) on renal function in patients with renal failure. Acta Med. Scand. 208:27, 1980.

Larsson, R., Bodemar, G., and Norlander, B.: Oral absorption of cimetidine and its clearance in patients with renal failure. Europ. J. Clin. Pharmacol. 15:153, 1979.

Luk, G. D., Luk, W. J., and Hendrix, T. R.: Cimetidine and impaired renal function. Ann. Intern. Med. 90:991, 1979.

Ma, K. W., Brown, D. C., Masler, D. S., and Silvis, S. E.: Effects of renal failure in blood levels of cimetidine. Gastroenterology 74:473, 1978.

Munshid, H. A. E., Hakanson, R., Liedberg, G., Rehfeld, J. F., and Sundler, F.: Importance of the kidneys for gastrin elimination and gastric function. J. Physiol. 299:157, 1980.

Shepherd, A. M. M., Stewart, W. K., and Wormsley, K. G.: Peptic ulceration in chronic renal failure. Lancet 1:1357, 1973.

Taylor, D. C., Cresswell, P. R., and Bartlett, D. C.: The metabolism and elimination of cimetidine, a histamine H$_2$-receptor antagonist, in the rat, dog, and man. Drug Metab. Dispos. 6:21, 1978.

Vaziri, D., Ness, R. L., and Barton, C. H.: Hemodialysis clearance of cimetidine. Arch. Intern. Med. 138:1685, 1978.

RECOGNITION AND MANAGEMENT OF HYPERTENSION IN THE DOG

LARRY D. COWGILL, D.V.M.,
and ANDREW J. KALLET, D.V.M.

Davis, California

Routine and systematic assessment of arterial blood pressure has been ignored in veterinary practice despite the significant incidence of hypertension in human medicine. Arterial hypertension plays a direct role in organ damage and is a major cause of morbidity and mortality in humans. Despite the lack of attention given to the routine diagnosis of hypertension in the dog, numerous surveys have documented its frequent association with some diseases. There is little epidemiologic information to substantiate the clinical significance of sustained hypertension in dogs. However, available data suggest that hypertension in dogs must be held in the same clinical regard as is hypertension in humans. Therefore, veterinarians must be able to readily and accurately measure blood pressure, recognize diseases that predispose to hypertension, and therapeutically intervene to prevent or correct established hypertension.

INCIDENCE OF HYPERTENSION

Normal canine blood pressure values have not been clearly established owing to the variety of measurement techniques used and the variable physiologic status of animals during measurement. Lack of suitable and convenient methods of measuring blood pressure in dogs has also prevented its routine determination in clinical settings.

Blood pressure can be accurately measured by the percutaneous placement of a needle, coupled to a pressure-sensitive transducer, directly into a peripheral artery. However, this technique suffers from the disadvantages of invasiveness, mild pain, and the need for specialized equipment. In most dogs, direct recordings from the femoral artery are well-tolerated and easily performed with the patient in lateral recumbency. Stable pressures can be recorded over several minutes with no appreciable change in heart rate and without chemical restraint. Lidocaine may be infiltrated into the puncture site with a 25-gauge needle to reduce the pain associated with cutaneous puncture. With this technique, single or repeated assessment of arterial pressure has become a routine procedure for dogs and cats at the Veterinary Medical Teaching Hospital (VMTH) of the University of California.

Indirect and noninvasive methods of assessing blood pressure have been described for dogs and have variable applications in clinical practice. Auscultation techniques that utilize Korotkoff sounds have generally been unsatisfactory and imprecise for clinical purposes because of the acoustic properties of the canine vasculature and the difficulty of applying occlusive cuffs to canine extremities.

The most applicable indirect technique for measuring blood pressure utilizes ultrasonic Doppler principles. Arterial wall movements at the point of arterial reflow following partial release of an occlusive cuff transform ultrasonic signals applied over the artery to audible sounds. When properly performed, this indirect measuring technique correlates well with direct methods and can be a safe and convenient means of monitoring blood pressure in a variety of clinical situations.

At the VMTH, normal systolic pressure in conscious dogs using direct techniques was 148 ± 16 mm Hg, the diastolic pressure was 87 ± 8 mm Hg, and mean pressure was 102 ± 9 mm Hg. These values are consistent with reported values in conscious or slightly sedated dogs using both direct and ultrasonic Doppler techniques.

Hypertension is diagnosed when sustained systolic pressures exceed 180 mm Hg or when diastolic pressures exceed 95 mm Hg. These values exceed the upper limits of blood pressures generally found in normal dogs. The incidence of spontaneous or essential hypertension in the dog is unknown. Surveys in large research colonies suggest an incidence of less than 2 per cent. The incidence of secondary hypertension is higher and more predictable. It has been recognized in dogs with a variety of metabolic and degenerative diseases but occurs most frequently in association with renal diseases. In a recent survey of dogs with a variety of renal dis-

eases, more than 60 per cent were found to be hypertensive by the criteria previously described (Fig. 1). The systolic pressure for dogs with hypertension averaged 174 ± 33 mm Hg, the diastolic pressure was 108 ± 24 mm Hg, and the mean pressure averaged 129 ± 27 mm Hg. These pressures are significantly greater than those for normal dogs and are independent of the degree of azotemia. Dogs with glomerular diseases are at even greater risk. An 80 per cent incidence of hypertension was identified in dogs with confirmed glomerulopathies or persistent proteinuria. Although preliminary, these observations complement previous observations and document a close association between renal disease and arterial hypertension. They also emphasize the need to consider hypertension as a consistent clinical sequela of renal injury.

SIGNIFICANCE OF SUSTAINED HYPERTENSION

Prospective studies documenting the clinical significance of hypertension in the dog are unavailable, and only predictions based on clinical experience in humans can be utilized for guidance. Epidemiologic investigations in humans clearly document the risks of cardiac enlargement, heart failure, vascular disease, stroke, and renal failure with sustained hypertension. Even though the occurrence of stroke appears insignificant in dogs, the manifestation, development, or progression of renal and cardiac insufficiency is of major concern. Necrosis, sclerosis, fibrinoid lesions, hyalinization, and capillary occlusion have been described in glomeruli of hypertensive dogs. Fibrinoid lesions, hyalinization, and myoarteritis have been observed in arterioles (renal and cardiac) of dogs in association with tubular degeneration and interstitial fibrosis. The importance of hypertension in the progression of renal injury, erosion of residual renal function, or development of other systemic disturbances is unknown for dogs. Until information is available to correlate hypertension-induced changes in renal morphology with changes in function, it is reasonable to regard hypertension as a harmful process. As in humans, the resultant arteriosclerosis, glomerular and tubular atrophy, and nephrosclerosis should be considered as significant factors in reducing residual renal mass in dogs.

Left ventricular hypertrophy is a consistent feature of renal insufficiency and is attributed to sustained hypertension in humans and dogs. Cardiovascular stress induced by hypertension may progress to ventricular dilatation. It is likely to reduce cardiac reserve and predisposes the myocardium to ischemia.

Retinal vascular pathology, hemorrhage, and ret-

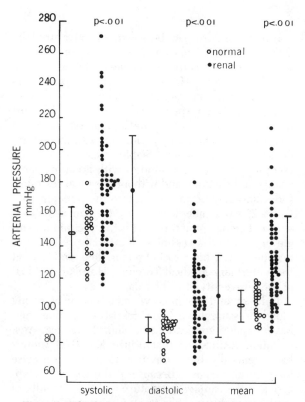

Figure 1. Individual values plus the means and SD for systolic, diastolic, and mean arterial pressures obtained directly from the femoral artery of 21 normal dogs (open circles) and 56 dogs with renal disease (closed circles).

inal detachment are less frequent but dramatic manifestations of hypertension. An acute onset of blindness secondary to retinal detachment or hemorrhage may be the first recognizable indication of hypertension.

The pathogenesis of hypertension involves a variety of factors that act singularly or in combination to deregulate pressor and volume hemostatic mechanisms. Arterial hypertension develops from an increased blood flow and cardiac output, greater resistance to blood flow secondary to increased peripheral vascular resistance, or a combination of both. Major factors initiating or sustaining the hypertensive state include (1) failure to excrete a normal quantity of salt or fluid at normotensive pressures; (2) stiffening of the venous capacitance system; (3) alterations of adrenergic activity; (4) activation of the renin-angiotensin-aldosterone axis, leading to increased vascular resistance and salt retention; (5) stimulation of renopressor systems; and (6) suppression of renodepressors or prostaglandins.

TREATMENT

Treatment of hypertension consists of nonpharmacologic control and use of a hierarchy of drugs commensurate with the severity of the hypertension. Reduction of dietary salt intake to counteract the tendency for positive sodium and water balance is the mainstay of nondrug therapy. Sodium intake should be reduced to 0.1 to 0.3 per cent of the diet to provide a daily intake of approximately 200 to 600 mg for a 15-kg dog. Since the majority of commercial dog foods provide sodium at approximately 0.8 to 1.0 per cent of the diet, special dietary products or formulated diets must be instituted. In patients with moderate or advanced renal insufficiency, the transition from a high- to a lower-sodium diet should be made gradually. The two diets can be mixed initially, with gradual reduction of the high-salt diet over a two- to four-week period. However, sodium restriction should be stopped temporarily or moderated if the patient becomes dehydrated. Sodium supplements should not be given to dogs with renal insufficiency and hypertension to promote an increase in water turnover, since they will exaggerate hypertension.

Drug therapy for hypertension consists of diuretics, sympatholytic agents, and vasodilators administered in sequence to provide pressor control. Specific protocols for drug therapy are empirical and inadequately tested in dogs, but similarities in the pathogeneses of canine and human hypertension warrant a treatment program similar to that used for humans. Drug therapy is generally initiated with a thiazide diuretic such as chlorothiazide (Diuril), given at a dose of 20 to 40 mg/kg once or twice daily to provide mild natriuresis. These agents are ineffective in patients with advanced renal insufficiency. For these patients, furosemide (Lasix), given at a dose of 2 to 4 mg/kg body weight once or twice daily, should be administered.

If arterial pressure is not controlled by sodium restriction and diuretic administration, a sympatholytic drug alone or in combination with a vasodilator should be included with the previously mentioned recommendations. In mild hypertension, propanolol (a β-adrenergic blocking agent), administered at a dosage of 5 to 20 mg twice or three times daily, may provide pressor control. This dose can be increased two to three times if the initial dose is ineffective. Propanolol may also reduce renin production, which is important in the later stages of renal parenchymal disease. Alpha-adrenergic blocking drugs such as clonidine hydrochloride (Catapres) and methyldopa (Aldomet) may also be used to control heart rate, cardiac output, and arteriolar and venous tone, but experience with these drugs in dogs has been limited. The major side effects of sympatholytic agents include sedation, gastrointestinal distress, dizziness, and hypotension.

Vasodilator drugs compose a third class of pharmaceuticals that may be used to treat hypertension. Vasodilators enhance venous compliance and reduce arteriolar tone. If the previously mentioned therapy does not result in an adequate response, it may be combined with hydralazine, given at a dosage of 1 to 2 mg/kg every 8 to 12 hours, or prazosin, given at a dosage of 0.5 to 1.0 mg twice daily. Since vasodilators tend to activate the sympathetic nervous system, their effects may be offset without adequate sympathetic blockade. Prazosin represents an exception to this generalization, since it can produce an effective antihypertensive response when utilized as the sole agent.

Hypertensive emergencies are rarely encountered, but may be induced by the pressor episodes of pheochromocytoma, acute renal failure, or acute glomerulonephritis. Signs of retinal detachment or hemorrhage, enecphalopathy, intracranial hemorrhage, or acute heart failure are indications for rapid correction of hypertension. Intravenous injections of 0.25-mg boluses of acepromazine can be tried initially. If ineffective, the boluses may be repeated up to a maximum of 3.0 mg. If an adequate response does not occur, sodium nitroprusside (Nipride) can be infused by continuous intravenous drip at a rate of approximately 3 μg/kg/min. Larger doses up to 10 μg/kg/min may be used in refractory patients. In patients receiving antihypertensive therapy, a lower dosage may be effective. Simultaneous with nitroprusside infusion, attempts should be made to effect more prolonged control with sympatholytic and vasodilator drugs as described previously. In patients with acute renal failure, fluid administration should be carefully regulated to prevent excessive extracellular fluid (ECF) volume expansion.

SUPPLEMENTAL READING

Spangler, W. L., Gribble, D. H., and Weiser, M. G.: Canine hypertension: A review. J.A.V.M.A. 170:995, 1980.
Weiser, M. G., Spangler, W. L., and Gribble, D. H.: Blood pressure measurement in the dog. J.A.V.M.A. 171:364, 1977.

CONTINUOUS AMBULATORY PERITONEAL DIALYSIS

JERRY A. THORNHILL, D.V.M.

West Lafayette, Indiana

The technique of peritoneal dialysis in the dog has improved considerably as a result of the development of a functionally reliable catheter, better control of peritonitis, and a new dialysis method called *continuous ambulatory peritoneal dialysis* (CAPD). In CAPD, the peritoneum serves as a dialysis membrane 24 hours a day. Dialysate fluid that has been stored in a plastic bag is instilled into the peritoneal cavity, where it is allowed to remain for a prescribed period. It is then drained back into the original bag by gravity flow and discarded. While the dialysate is in the peritoneal cavity between exchanges (dialysate dwell), the empty bag and its tubing (which remains attached to the peritoneal catheter) are rolled up and wrapped against the patient's side, allowing complete freedom of movement during the procedure.

Dialysis consists of diffusion of solutes from one solution to another across a semipermeable membrane. Dialysis of blood may be performed by transferring the blood out of the body (hemodialysis) or by transferring fluid into the peritoneal cavity (peritoneal dialysis). In peritoneal dialysis, the peritoneum is utilized as a semipermeable exchange surface. Dialysate, the fluid into which plasma solutes are transferred, is a physiologic solution that contains varying concentrations of dextrose (1.5 or 4.25 per cent) to induce osmotic fluid removal from the patient. Because dialysate does not contain urea, creatinine, or other uremic waste solutes, these substances diffuse from plasma into the dialysate along concentration gradients.

Peritoneal dialysis is a slower process than hemodialysis. The time needed for development of equilibrium of solutes between the interstitial fluid and dialysate varies from one to eight hours. For example, only a portion of the total unwanted solutes are removed following hourly exchanges. Therefore, up to two days of frequent exchanges of

dialysate fluid may be required to adequately stabilize patients in acute uremic crises. Following the initial frequent dialysis exchanges, many patients can be supported with only a few exchanges each day.

Dialysate placed in the abdominal cavity may be allowed to remain there for up to four to six hours prior to removal. Periodic exchanges throughout the day result in continuous dialysis (CAPD). This technique is currently used to manage human patients with acute renal failure or end-stage chronic renal failure.

Patients with acute oliguric renal failure must be supported by dialysis if diuresis cannot be stimulated with fluid and/or diuretic therapy or if the patient's clinical status does not improve once diuresis has been initiated. Because most patients with acute renal failure have an unfavorable short-term/favorable long-term prognosis, the effort and expense of peritoneal dialysis are justified.

On the other hand, patients with chronic renal failure often have a favorable short-term prognosis with proper conservative management but an unfavorable long-term prognosis as renal function steadily deteriorates. Such patients may undergo acute decompensation from prerenal causes (i.e., vomiting, diarrhea, fever, sepsis, congestive heart failure, and so on) or subtle decompensation as a result of progressive destruction of nephrons. Such patients may be recompensated by chronic maintenance dialysis.

THE COLUMN DISC CATHETER

The technique of peritoneal dialysis in humans was greatly improved in 1968 by the development of the Tenckhoff catheter. This catheter allows chronic dialysis to be performed without the necessity of repeated punctures of the peritoneum. The Tenckhoff catheter is a soft Silastic tube designed so that its distal end floats freely in the abdominal cavity. Unfortunately, the use of Tenckhoff and other straight tube catheters in dogs has been associated with failure to remove significant quantities of dialysate from the abdomen, limiting the usefulness of peritoneal dialysis. Although inflow of fluid was unimpeded, outflow obstruction characterized by inability to recover administered dialysate from the abdominal cavity occurred as a result of plugging of the catheter holes by omentum or involvement of the catheter in intestinal loops.

Owing to inconsistent reliability of available peritoneal catheters to drain the abdominal cavity after one to three days of dialysis, we developed a dialysis catheter that could be used in dogs with negligible outflow obstruction. The catheter, called the "column disc catheter," has excellent inflow and outflow characteristics owing to the fact that the disc portion of the catheter rests against the peritoneum and does not float freely in the abdominal cavity. An anephric dog was supported for 78 days by CAPD using a column disc catheter and bagged dialysate. Even though the dialysate was exchanged four to six times each day, the column disc catheter remained patent throughout the study.

The column disc catheter* is composed of a terminal disc (approximately 2¾ inches in diameter and 5⁄16 inch thick), which consists of silicone sheets separated by numerous pillars, each ¼ inch tall (Fig. 1). Silastic tubing (outside diameter ¼ inch, inside diameter ⅛ inch) enters the ventral portion of the disc and communicates with the space between the Silastic sheets. Two Dacron velour cuffs, one next to the base of the catheter and one near the free end, are positioned so that they may be placed preperitoneally and subcutaneously. The cuffs stimulate fibroblastic ingrowth to wall off the

catheter and to prevent bacterial migration along the wall of the tubing.

DIALYSATE FLUID AND CONTAINERS

The recent availability of dialysate in plastic bags (Dianeal 137 with 1.5% Dextrose-Viaflex†) facilitates the administration of dialysate fluids. The bag with transfer-set tubing (Dianeal-Viaflex Transfer-Set Tubing†) can be rolled up and secured to the patient's side with bandage material during the dwell time and unrolled and refilled by gravity flow during outflow (Fig. 2). The tube connection at the bag site is only touched when the bag is exchanged for a new one. Therefore, one set of tubing can be used for many bags.

Although commercially prepared dialysate fluid is currently available only in 2-liter bags, dialysate bags in 1000-, 500-, and 250-ml sizes will soon be available. This will facilitate peritoneal dialysis in small dogs and cats.

Commercially prepared dialysate fluid contains either 1.5 or 4.25 per cent dextrose. Solutions containing 1.5 per cent dextrose are recommended for routine use, since 4.25 per cent dextrose solutions produce a potent osmotic draw of extracellular fluid, which is lost during each outflow exchange.

TECHNIQUE

CATHETER PLACEMENT

The catheter should be placed into the lower abdominal quadrant (Fig. 3). A paramedial incision should be made in the skin, and the external and internal abdominal oblique and rectus abdominis muscles should be bluntly dissected to expose the

---

*Physio Control Corp., Redmond, WA.

†Travenol Laboratories, Inc., Deerfield, IL.

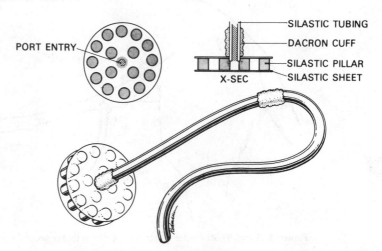

PORT ENTRY

SILASTIC TUBING
DACRON CUFF
SILASTIC PILLAR
SILASTIC SHEET
X-SEC

Figure 1. Purdue column disc catheter with double-layered disc separated by pillars and dacron velour cuffs around Silastic tubing.

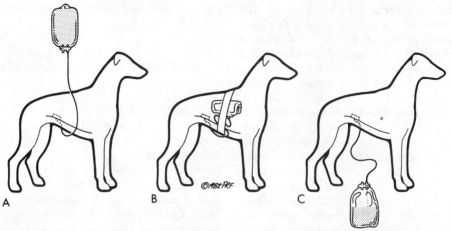

Figure 2. Schematic illustration of bag. *A*, During instillation of fluid to the peritoneal cavity. *B*, Rolled up against patient's side during dwell time. *C*, Unrolled during outflow for gravity drainage.

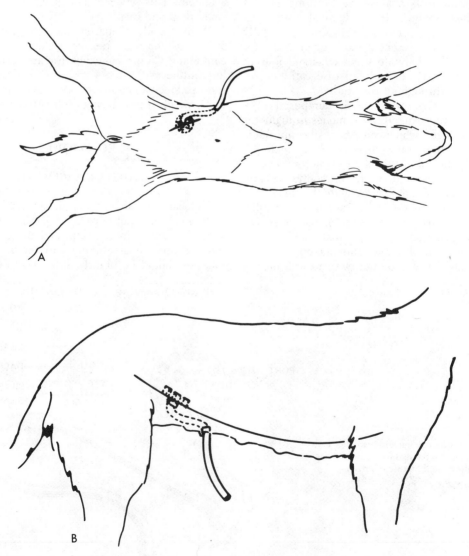

Figure 3. *A* and *B*, Schematic illustration of disc catheter properly positioned in the abdominal cavity.

peritoneum. After penetration of the peritoneum, the foldable disc should be collapsed and placed through the surgical opening into the peritoneal cavity. The disc should then be pulled firmly against the parietal peritoneum, which is then sutured over the base of the catheter. Muscle layers should be sewn tightly around the first Dacron velour cuff, but sutures need not enter the cuff to create a good seal. The free end of the catheter should be placed through a subcutaneous tunnel so that it exits through a skin stab incision at a point beyond the second Dacron velour cuff, which is buried. All patients with peritoneal access catheters should be given cephalosporin for five days following surgery (preferably started the day before surgery).

HOURLY PERITONEAL DIALYSIS

1. Following induction of anesthesia with appropriate agents, surgically place the disc catheter in the caudal quadrant of the abdomen in a paramedial position.

2. Using sterile technique (see Technique for CAPD), attach a prewarmed dialysate solution bag to the peritoneal catheter via transfer-set tubing (note: transfer-sets spike the bag at one end and couple with the catheter at the other end via an adapter [Beta-Cap Adapter*] that has been permanently affixed to the distal catheter end). Select the appropriate size of plastic dialysate bag for the patient. A sufficient volume of fluid should be instilled into the peritoneal cavity to mildly distend the abdomen.

3. Clamp the tubing with a Beta-Cap clamp*, roll up the tubing and bag, and secure them against the patient's body wall with bandage material.

4. The dialysate solution should be allowed to remain in the peritoneal cavity for 45 to 50 minutes (dwell time). (The techniques for outflow drainage, old bag discard, new bag hookup, and so on are described in the section that follows.)

5. Dialysis cycles should be repeated hourly until the uremic crisis subsides. This may require 12 to 36 hours for patients with acute renal failure or decompensated end-stage renal failure.

6. Maintain records of the volume of solution instilled and removed from the abdominal cavity during each exchange. During the first few exchanges there will be less fluid recovered from the abdomen than delivered as the peritoneal cavity becomes "primed." Subsequently, outflow should approximate inflow. In fact, outflow may exceed inflow as the osmotic influence of dextrose in the dialysate exerts its influence.

---

*Quinton Instruments Co., Seattle, WA.

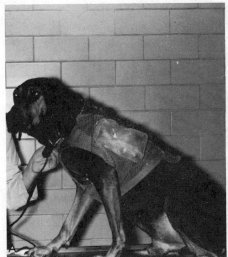
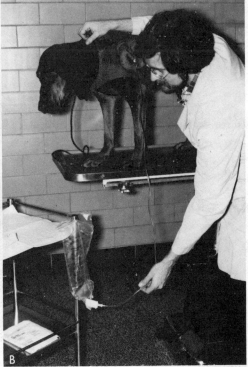

Figure 4. *A*, Dialysis patient wearing harness and satchel for carrying empty Viaflex bag during dialysate dwell time. *B*, Bag attached to table during outflow cycle (gravity drainage).

CONTINUOUS AMBULATORY PERITONEAL DIALYSIS

Patients that are compensated but that still require dialysis for 10 to 14 days for acute renal failure and for life for end-stage chronic renal failure may be successfully managed by maintenance dialysis. The schedule for maintenance peritoneal dialysis is spread out compared with that for intense hourly dialysis. Patients can be maintained in a compensated state with as few as four to six exchanges per day.

The following procedure is recommended for CAPD:

1. Following intense hourly dialysis, increase the dwell time to four to six hours.

2. To remove the dialysate fluid, place the patient (shown with harness and satchel, facilitating storage of empty bag during dwell period) in a sitting position on a table to establish better drainage of dialysate fluid (Fig. 4A).

3. Unwrap the empty bag, unroll the tubing, and straighten the bag.

4. Attach the bag to a hook on a table of lesser height and open the Beta clamp to permit drainage of dialysate fluid (Fig. 4B). The bag should fill within five to seven minutes.

5. Clamp the Beta clamp on the Viaflex tubing and place the used bag on the table alongside of a new bag of warmed dialysate (usually positioned to the left). Using a CAPD prep kit*, put on a surgical mask and sterile exam gloves (to keep hands clean) and place Port Outlet clamps* over the ports of used and new bags (Fig. 5A).

6. Pull off the protective covering over the port of the new bag. With a brisk motion pull the spike from the old bag holding the Port Outlet clamp for stability and spike the new bag port holding its Port Outlet clamp for stability (Fig. 5B and C).

7. Remove the Port Outlet clamp on the new bag. Remove the povidone-iodine swab from the CAPD prep kit and wrap the spike-port coupling (Fig. 5D).

8. Remove the sterile 4" × 4" gauze sponges from the CAPD prep kit, and wrap the povidone-iodine swab around the spike-port coupling.

9. Remove two tape strips from the prep kit, and secure the gauze overwrap of the iodine swab.

---

*Travenol Laboratories, Inc., Deerfield, IL.

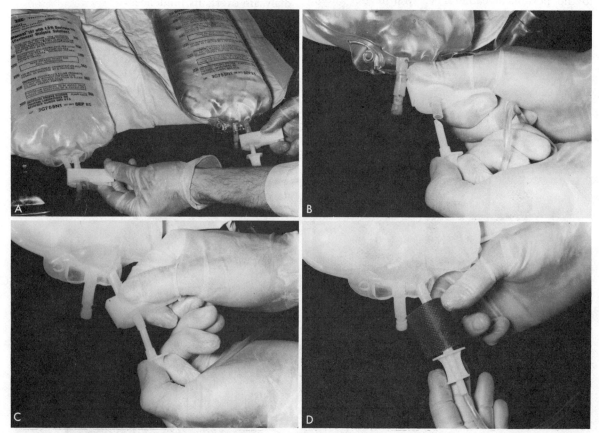

Figure 5. *A*, Used bag placed on table alongside new bag (to left). "Port Outlet" clamp applied to each bag. *B* and *C*, Spike pulled from discarded bag to be introduced into new bag at port. Note "outlet" clamp firmly held to give spike introduction stability. *D*, Application of povidone-iodine swab around spike-port coupling after "outlet" clamp removed. New cycle initiated by introduction of dialysate fluid to abdominal cavity.

10. Hang the new bag above the patient and instill the dialysate fluid into the peritoneal cavity.

11. After fluid inflow, clamp the Beta clamp, roll the tubing around the bag, and place it into the satchel or under a suitable elastic bandage wrap for storage. The fluid remains in the peritoneal cavity for 4 to 6 hours or even 8 to 12 hours, depending on patient response.

12. Repeat the cycle.

PERITONITIS

Peritonitis is a serious potential complication of peritoneal dialysis. Although procedures to prevent infection are technically demanding, prevention of infection through sterilization of materials, use of aseptic technique, and use of Betadine on all connections is far easier than attempting to treat iatrogenic infection. Despite these precautions, peritonitis may still occur.

A new technique utilizing a "saline–saline plus iodine" wash of the abdominal cavity has proved to be very effective in curbing bacterial peritonitis in dogs receiving peritoneal dialysis at Purdue University and the University of Minnesota. Iodine reacts with water in the following manner to form hypoiodous acid:

$$I_2 + H_2O \rightleftarrows HOI + H^+ + I^-$$

Both I_2 and HOI are microbicidal. Dextrose should be removed from the abdominal cavity with a saline flush prior to instillation of the saline-iodine solution because iodine is converted to inactive iodide in the presence of dextrose. The technique should be performed as follows:

1. Once each day following removal of dialysate, instill and then immediately remove 1 liter of physiologic saline into the peritoneal cavity.

2. Instill 1 liter of physiologic saline to which has been added 0.2 ml of 2 per cent solution of iodine USP. Allow the solution to remain in the abdominal cavity for four minutes. Remove the iodine-saline solution.

3. Initiate the next peritoneal dialysate exchange.

Daily saline–saline plus iodine washes may be used prophylactically until attendants become well schooled in the technique of CAPD. They may also be used as the initial treatment of peritonitis. If the saline–saline plus iodine wash proves to be inadequate, the procedure may be used twice each day, or the concentration of 2 per cent iodine can be increased to 0.4 cc/liter rather than 0.2 cc/liter. However, if this fails, antimicrobial therapy must be initiated. A standard solution of 16 mg tobramycin/2 liter dialysate and 250 mg cephalothin sodium/2 liter dialysate during each exchange (four to six/day) should clear all forms of bacterial peritonitis. Also, the patient should be given systemic cephalexin at a dosage of 20 mg/kg t.i.d. during the crisis.

Treatment after peritonitis has developed should be based on identification of bacteria in the effluent and determination of their susceptibility to antimicrobial agents. Dialysate effluent should be cultured for bacterial growth as often as once a day when a patient is on intense hourly dialysis and weekly in cases of less intense long-term dependency. Peritonitis is usually caused by bacteria. However, aseptic peritonitis associated with signs typical of peritoneal infection have been reported in 15 to 30 per cent of human patients with this problem.

CLINICAL RELEVANCE

The availability of dialysate solution in collapsible bags and the promising performance of the column disc catheter have renewed interest in the technique of peritoneal dialysis in veterinary medicine. Clinicians at Purdue University and the University of Minnesota have been encouraged by the applications of the new catheter and dialysate bag system for the treatment of patients with primary oliguric renal failure. Although the use of a saline–saline plus iodine wash has greatly curbed the incidence of peritonitis, it is still not the final solution. Work is currently under way at Purdue to develop an "inline" filter to prevent entry of bacteria into the peritoneal cavity. Studies to date have been encouraging, and the application of the filter to standard dialysis procedures in the future appears axiomatic.

SUPPLEMENTAL READING

Ash, S. R., Johnson, H., Hartman, J., Granger, J., Koszuta, J., Sell, L., and Thornhill, J. A.: The immobilized disc peritoneal catheter. A peritoneal access device with improved drainage. Trans. Am. Soc. Artif. Intern. Organs 3:109, 1980.

Blumenkrantz, M. J.: Maintenance peritoneal dialysis as an alternative for the patient with end-stage renal failure. Clin. Digest. 6:1, 1977.

Moncrief, J. W.: Continuous ambulatory peritoneal dialysis. Dial. Transplant. 8:1077, 1165, 1979.

Moncrief, J. W., Nolph, K. D., Rubin, J., and Popovich, R. P.: Additional experience with continuous ambulatory peritoneal dialysis (CAPD). Trans. Am. Soc. Artif. Intern. Organs 24:476, 1978.

Nolph, K. D., Popovich, R. P., and Moncrief, J. W.: Theoretical and practical implications of continuous ambulatory peritoneal dialysis. Nephron 21:117, 1978.

Oreopoulos, D. G.: Renewed interest in chronic peritoneal dialysis. Kidney Int. 13:S117, 1978.

Stephen, R. L., Kablitz, C., Kitahara, M., Nelson, J. A., Duffy, D. P., and Kolff, W. J.: Peritoneal dialysis: Peritonitis: Saline-iodine flush. Dial. Transplant. 8:584, 1979.

Tenckhoff, H., and Schecter, H.: A bacteriologically safe peritoneal access device. Trans. Am. Soc. Artif. Intern. Organs 14:181, 1968.

Thornhill, J. A.: Peritoneal dialysis in the dog and cat: An update. Comp. Cont. Ed. Pract. Vet. 3:20, 1981.

Thornhill, J. A., Ash, S. R., Dhein, C. R., Polzin, D. J., and Osborne, C. A.: Peritoneal dialysis with the Purdue column disc catheter. Minn. Vet. 20:27, 1980.

Thornhill, J. A., Dhein, C. R., Kaufman, G. M., Knab, W., and Ash, S. R.: Successful support of an anephric dog for 78 days with continuous ambulatory peritoneal dialysis and a new peritoneal access catheter design. J.A.V.M.A. in review.

Valk, T. W., Swartz, R. D., and Hsu, C. H.: Peritoneal dialysis in acute renal failure: Analysis of outcome and complications. Dial. Transplant. 9:48, 1980.

TREATMENT OF CANINE DIROFILARIASIS IN PATIENTS WITH RENAL FAILURE

DAVID F. SENIOR, B.V.Sc.

Gainesville, Florida

Dirofilaria immitis infection in dogs frequently appears concurrently with compromised cardiopulmonary and hepatic function. In many cases renal function may also be impaired. Before treating dogs for heartworm, the following questions should be considered: (1) What is the nephrotoxic potential of the drugs used? and (2) Will pre-existing impaired renal function cause abnormally high drug accumulation with exacerbation of renal and extrarenal toxic effects?

THIACETARSEMIDE

The toxic ingredient of thiacetarsemide (Caparsolate*) is arsenic, which is distributed widely in many tissues following intravenous administration. Trivalent arsenic in thiacetarsemide is excreted very slowly via many routes including feces, urine, skin, milk, hair, and lungs. After a single dose, only 10 to 15 per cent of the total dose is excreted in the urine during the first 24 hours.

The toxicity of thiacetarsemide appears to be directly proportional to its arsenic content. At normal therapeutic doses arsenic does not accumulate to any significant extent. At higher doses a wide range of organs are affected, especially the liver and kidneys. The toxicity is related to uncoupling of oxidative phosphorylation by competitive substitution of arsenic for organic phosphate and to arsenic binding to sulfhydryl groups in enzymes, thereby inactivating them. Although a minor deleterious effect on renal function may be expected following thiacetarsemide treatment, changes in renal function have never been accurately documented. In toxicity studies, dogs given 5.4 to 9.0 mg/kg/day of arsenic died within 5 days; however, dogs given 0.9 mg/kg/day of arsenic for 30 days showed no ill effects. In contrast, during a standard treatment (normal dose 2.2 mg/kg IV b.i.d. for two days), dogs receive only about 0.8 mg/kg/day for two days.

Veterinarians have observed showers of renal tubular epithelial cells, moderate proteinuria, and increased numbers of granular casts in urine during and for the first few days following arsenical treatment. It is difficult to separate the direct effect of arsenic on the kidney from its more dramatic effect on liver function and the effect of dead and dying heartworms on hemodynamics. If a severe reaction occurs, reduced extracellular fluid volume may induce prerenal azotemia. However, pre-existing reduced renal function probably has minimal effect on arsenic retention at normal therapeutic doses.

Routine assessment of liver and kidney function prior to commencement of thiacetarsemide treatment should include CBC, SUN and/or serum creatinine, SGPT, and urinalysis. A BSP clearance test is optional if reduced liver function is suspected. Absence of emesis, anorexia, icterus, bilirubinuria, and cylindruria after 24 hours is an indication that treatment can be continued to conclusion with reasonable safety.

DITHIAZANINE IODIDE

Dithiazanine iodide (Dizan†) is a cyanine dye that is very insoluble in water and poorly absorbed from the gastrointestinal tract. Most of an oral dose is excreted unchanged in the feces. In humans, inflammatory bowel disease with enhanced phagocytosis of dye particles is thought to enhance drug absorption and induce toxic symptoms. Even though little is absorbed under normal circumstances, sufficient drug is distributed systemically to be effective as a microfilaricide.

The most commonly observed toxic side effects in the dog include anorexia, emesis, and diarrhea. The manufacturer's literature includes a warning against the use of the drug in the face of pre-existing renal disease. In rare instances, use of dithiazanine in human patients with renal disease was reported to accelerate the disorder. In acute toxicity studies, the LD_{50} for dogs was 200 mg/kg. In chronic oral toxicity studies in dogs, administration of 9.2 mg/kg/day for 147 days and 61.5 mg/kg/day for 19 days induced diarrhea and weight loss with fatty liver. Nephrotoxicity was not observed. By contrast, the usual normal microfilaricidal dose is 6 to 11 mg/kg PO given daily for seven to ten days.

---

*Abbott Laboratories, Inc., North Chicago, IL.

†Pitman-Moore Inc., Washington Crossing, NJ.

At present there appears to be no clinical evidence of dithiazanine-induced nephrotoxicity in dogs when the drug is given at therapeutic doses. However, controlled studies have not been performed. The common side effects of emesis and diarrhea could induce prerenal azotemia, which may be life-threatening in animals with pre-existing reduced renal function.

Pending results of controlled studies, microfilaremic patients with marginal renal function may be identified by routine test procedures. Owners of such dogs should be educated about the possible consequences of vomiting and diarrhea during therapy. Administration of tablets following or with meals tends to reduce gastrointestinal disturbances.

LEVAMISOLE

Levamisole (Levasole*) is the L-isomer of DL-tetramisole. Although not an approved microfilaricide for use in dogs in the United States, it is widely used, particularly since the availability of dithiazanine has become sporadic. Following oral administration, levamisole is rapidly absorbed from the gastrointestinal tract. In rats, 50 per cent of a single oral dose is excreted by the kidneys, whereas 30 per cent is excreted in the stool in 24 hours.

Although levamisole is not an organophosphate, toxic levels have predominantly nicotinic action, with some muscarinic action. In acute toxicity studies in dogs, single oral doses of tetramisole at 20 mg/kg were well-tolerated, whereas dogs given 37.4 mg/kg of levamisole developed emesis, salivation, muscular tremor, and apprehension. These signs resolved within three hours following supportive treatment.

Reduced appetite and moderate weight loss occurred in dogs given 6 mg/kg/day orally for 12 weeks and 30 mg/kg/day orally for 16 weeks. Necropsies performed on dogs given 6 mg/kg/day revealed no abnormalities. Transient reticuloendothelial proliferation was observed throughout the central nervous system in 44 of 58 dogs given 11 mg/kg for 7 to 120 days. Hemolytic anemia has been observed in two of six dogs after repeated doses of levamisole given for an extended period. Although many questions concerning the safety of this drug remain unanswered, nephrotoxicity has not been observed. The only regularly observed signs associated with the commonly used normal microfilaricidal dose (11 mg/kg PO daily for six to ten days) are emesis and mild depression.

As the major route of excretion is the urinary system, reduced renal function could delay the clearance of levamisole and its metabolites and could lead to their accumulation within the body during the six- to ten-day period of treatment.

Enhanced extrarenal toxic signs may occur, but a nephrotoxic effect per se should not be anticipated. Emesis with dehydration could induce prerenal azotemia, an important consideration if pre-existing renal function is marginal.

DIETHYLCARBAMAZINE CITRATE

Diethylcarbamazine citrate (Caricide†) is a derivative of piperazine. It is rapidly absorbed from the gastrointestinal tract. After a single dose, peak plasma levels occur at 3 hours, and the drug is eliminated by 48 hours. The drug is distributed throughout all tissues except fat. Excretion is almost entirely by the kidneys; 70 per cent is eliminated in urine by 24 hours. Only 10 to 25 per cent enters the urine unchanged; the remainder is eliminated as four different metabolites.

Diethylcarbamazine citrate is relatively nontoxic at doses used to prevent heartworm infection (normal dose 6 mg/kg given daily), although emesis occasionally occurs. The major side effect at higher doses appears to be gastric irritation. Emesis has been frequently observed in dogs treated for ascariasis with 50 to 100 mg/kg. Unusually high levels would be expected to accumulate in patients with reduced renal function; however, this has not been reported. Reductions in dose proportional to reduced renal function would be necessary to achieve the same plasma level as that of an animal with normal renal function.

Severe hypovolemic shock secondary to anaphylaxis is a frequent occurrence when diethylcarbamazine is given to microfilaremic dogs. Such a reaction could initiate acute renal failure and may induce a crisis in patients with compensated chronic renal failure.

STYRYLPYRIDIUM

Styrylpyridium (Styrid-Caricide†) is frequently given in combination with diethylcarbamazine. Although absorption, fate, and excretion data are not readily available, oral administration at 80 mg/kg/day for six months and 20 mg/kg/day for two years did not change SUN levels or induce histologic changes in the kidneys. Because the normal dose is 2.5 mg/kg given daily, this drug has a wide therapeutic index.

CONCLUSION

The direct nephrotoxic effect of drugs routinely used in the treatment of dirofilariasis in dogs has minimal or undocumented renal effects in healthy animals. The direct effect on renal function in patients with reduced renal reserve secondary to

---

*Pitman-Moore Inc., Washington Crossing, NJ.

†American Cyanamid, Princeton, NJ.

advanced heartworm disease is unknown. Certainly, side effects that reduce extracellular fluid volume may induce life-threatening prerenal azotemia in dogs with pre-existing compromised renal function. Precautions should be taken to prevent this adverse reaction.

SUPPLEMENTAL READING

Alford, B. T., and Burkhart, R. L.: Safety studies of levamisole in dogs. In American Heartworm Society, Morgan, H. C. (ed.): *Proceedings of the Heartworm Symposium 1974.* Bonner Springs, KS: VM Publishing, Inc., 1974.

Gilman, A. G., Goodman, L. S., and Gilman, A.: *The Pharmacological Basis of Therapeutics,* 6th ed. New York: Macmillan Publishing Co., Inc., 1980.

Hue, W. T.: Toxicity and drug interactions of levamisole. J.A.V.M.A. 176:1166, 1980.

Jones, L. M., Booth, N. H., and McDonald, L. E.: *Veterinary Pharmacology and Therapeutics,* 4th ed. Ames, IA: The Iowa State University Press. 1977.

Osborne, C. A., Hammer, R. F., O'Leary, T. P., Pomeroy, K. A., Jeraj, K., Barlough, J. E., and Vernier, R. L.: Renal manifestations of canine dirofilariasis. In American Heartworm Society: *Proceedings of the Heartworm Symposium 1980.* Edwardsville, KS: VM Publishing Co., 1980, pp. 67–92.

Vandevelde, M., Boring, J. G., Hoff, E. J., and Gingerich, D. A.: The effect of levamisole on the canine central nervous system. J. Neuropath. Exp. Neur. 37:165, 1978.

CHECKLIST OF HAZARDOUS DRUGS IN PATIENTS WITH RENAL FAILURE

J. EDMOND RIVIERE, D.V.M.

Raleigh, North Carolina

The kidney is the primary excretory route for many drugs commonly used in veterinary medicine. Unfortunately, renal insufficiency often results in changes in drug disposition that may lead to toxicosis. To compound this problem, the kidney itself is often the target of drug toxicity because of its relatively large blood supply and its ability to concentrate substances within its parenchyma or tubular system. These facts emphasize the difficulty of safely administering drugs to patients with renal insufficiency. It has been estimated that 9 per cent of all human nephrologic consultations involve a nephrotoxic cause. The purpose of this article is to define the conditions under which drug toxicity occurs in patients with renal insufficiency, to list drugs that should be avoided in patients with renal insufficiency, to indicate how dosage regimens should be constructed to minimize toxicity, and to summarize diagnostic criteria used to detect drug-induced nephrotoxicosis.

The decision to administer any drug to a patient with renal insufficiency should be carefully considered. Because of the increased risk of drug-induced toxicity in renal patients, it is wise to avoid drug therapy unless definite and specific indications for its use are present. This article encompasses only those drugs that should be avoided in renal failure or whose dose should be reduced in proportion to the severity of renal dysfunction.

MECHANISMS FOR ENHANCED DRUG TOXICITY IN RENAL INSUFFICIENCY

Unmetabolized, pharmacologically active drugs normally eliminated by renal excretion accumulate when renal function is impaired. Renal clearance of drugs is dependent on glomerular filtration rate (GFR), active tubular secretion and/or reabsorption, and passive flow-dependent reabsorption. Glomerular filtration is an unidirectional process that removes non–protein-bound free drug from the blood by bulk flow. Active tubular secretion and/or reabsorption is a bidirectional process independent of the extent of drug protein binding. The active secretory process is a saturable, carrier-mediated system located in the pars recta of proximal tubules and has two distinct components: one for organic acids and one for organic bases. Passive flow-dependent nonionic back-diffusion is a mechanism for tubular reabsorption of lipid-soluble, nonionized weak acids and bases. Depending on the partition coefficient of the nonionized form, weak acids will be absorbed at low urine pH and weak bases at high urine pH. Increasing the rate of urine flow (e.g., by diuresis) will decrease the rate of reabsorption.

Renal insufficiency characterized by decreased creatinine or inulin clearance would be expected to result in decreased clearance of drugs eliminated by glomerular filtration. Similarly, renal insufficiency will also decrease tubular secretion of drugs secondary to decreased renal blood flow or direct toxic damage to tubules. The subsequent reduction in drug clearance and prolongation of drug half-life result in accumulation of drugs within the body. The mathematical relationship between GFR and drug half-life is not linear; it is a hyperbolic function. This means that the half-life of drugs eliminated primarily by the kidney remains relatively stable until GFR is 30 to 40 per cent of normal, after which point half-life rapidly increases. However, dosage reduction may be necessary even when GFR is only 50 per cent of normal, if the drug has a narrow therapeutic safety margin. Polyuric renal failure may increase renal clearance of drugs that undergo passive flow-dependent tubular reabsorption owing to the increased rate of urine flow. However, it is likely that this disease-induced increase in clearance would be offset by the concomitant decrease in GFR. The acidosis of polyuric renal failure would tend to decrease the clearance (increased reabsorption) of weak acids and increase the clearance (decreased reabsorption) of weak bases. Weak acids such as salicylates are an example of the phenomenon. Therefore, the effect of decreased renal function on drug disposition is generally one of decreased drug clearance unless extensive passive tubular reabsorption occurs. In the latter situation, the rate of urine flow and the urine pH become important.

Renal insufficiency can also affect the disposition of drugs that undergo hepatic biotransformation. Renal failure does not appear to alter microsomal oxidation, reduction, glucuronide or sulfate conjugation, or methylation pathways. However, glycine conjugation, acetylation, and hydrolysis reactions are slowed. Notably, the biotransformation of cephalothin, cortisol, insulin, isoniazid, procaine, procainamide, salicylate, succinylcholine, and some sulfonamides may be decreased. Marked species differences exist. In addition, the canine kidney can conjugate salicylate with glycine and can metabolize insulin, catecholamines, morphine, serotonin, and other substances. Renal failure may adversely influence these processes. Finally, pharmacologically active products of biotransformation eliminated primarily by the kidney may accumulate in patients with renal insufficiency as a result of decreased renal clearance. Examples of drugs whose active metabolites accumulate and induce intoxication in this situation include adriamycin, allopurinol, amobarbital, cephalothin, chlorpropamide, clofibrate, daunorubicin, digitoxin, lidocaine, meperidine, mephobarbital, naltrexone, primidone, procainamide, and some sulfonamides.

Marked reduction in serum protein binding of some drugs has been documented in patients with renal failure. Decreased protein binding results in increased free drug concentration and may be associated with an enhanced pharmacologic effect. An increased concentration of free drug will also result in increased renal clearance if GFR is the primary route of its elimination. The mechanisms of this binding defect is not fully understood, although accumulation of "uremic toxins" may alter albumin conformation or may compete with the drug for binding sites, thereby displacing the bound drug. Displacement is pharmacologically significant only if a substantial fraction of the drug is normally bound to serum proteins. Examples encountered in veterinary medicine are benzylpenicillin, clofibrate, diazepam, diazoxide, dicloxacillin, fluorescein, pentobarbital, phenobarbital, phenylbutazone, phenytoin, salicylate, sulfonamides, thiopental, thyroxine, triamterene, valproic acid, and warfarin.

The volume of distribution (Vd) of a drug, the proportionality constant relating drug dose to expected blood concentration, may also change in renal insufficiency. Vd is defined as the hypothetical volume of fluid required to contain the total amount of drug in the body uniformly distributed at a concentration equal to that in blood. As previously mentioned, decreased serum protein binding increases Vd in renal failure. Digoxin Vd decreases in renal failure, whereas gentamicin Vd increases in acute canine glomerulonephritis. The relationship of altered Vd to drug efficacy or toxicity is not known for most drugs; however, the loading dose of digoxin should be reduced in the presence of decreased GFR.

Numerous other adverse drug effects can also occur in patients with renal dysfunction as a result of fluid, electrolyte, and metabolic disturbances. The blood-brain barrier appears to be abnormal in the presence of renal dysfunction, resulting in increased sensitivity to opiates, barbiturates, and tranquilizers. Decreased protein binding and acidemia accentuate these effects. Insulin sensitivity is decreased in the uremic patient. The rate and extent of oral drug absorption can also be impaired. The antianabolic activity of tetracycline and the catabolic activity of corticosteroids can worsen azotemia associated with renal failure. Drug toxicity can be potentiated if the drug's action is synergistic with uremic complications; examples include administration of anticoagulants to patients with uremia-induced bleeding disorders and administration of urinary acidifiers or buffered acetic acid solutions (for the removal of urethral plugs) to patients with metabolic acidosis. Administration of antibiotics containing sodium (ampicillin 3 mEq/gm; carbenicillin 4.7 mEq/gm; cephalothin 2.5 mEq/gm; penicillin G 1.7 mEq/gm) could result in electrolyte overload. High ceiling loop diuretics (furosemide, ethacrynic acid) have been shown to enhance the toxicity of aminoglycosides and cephaloridine in some species. Drug interactions not normally observed in patients with normal renal function may occur when decreased renal elimination of drug occurs, an example being carbenicillin and ticarcillin inactivation in vivo by gentamicin in human patients with end-stage kidney disease.

Diseased kidneys may also be inherently more sensitive to nephrotoxic drugs. In an animal with chronic renal failure, Bricker's intact nephron hypothesis and magnification hypothesis predict that each individual nephron will be exposed to a greater concentration of drug per unit GFR than a nephron in a normal animal. Therefore, even if drug dose is adjusted for decreased GFR, the tubular load of the drug could be greater and the nephrotoxic potential of the drug increased. By contrast, in patients with prerenal azotemia, the kidneys may actually be protected from potential tubular nephrotoxicity because the decrease in GFR in this situation will reduce the tubular load of drug at the site of toxicity in the proximal tubules. These situations would be expected to alter the nephrotoxic potential of drugs such as aminoglycosides. Altered distribution of intrarenal blood flow in renal disease might also modify the toxic potential of some drugs. Intrarenal antibiotic concentration is decreased in chronic renal failure, probably secondary to decreased renal mass, making the treatment of conditions such as pyelonephritis more difficult. Finally, the combination of decreased drug clearance and polyuria may result in subinhibitory concentrations of antimicrobial drugs in urine and failure to eradicate urinary tract infections.

DRUGS TO BE AVOIDED IN RENAL INSUFFICIENCY

Controversy exists as to which drugs should be avoided in patients with renal failure because specific drug therapy may be essential for survival in spite of the toxic risk. Examples include administration of aminoglycosides to patients with renal failure for treatment of life-threatening sepsis and cancer chemotherapy in the face of severe renal insufficiency. However, certain drugs should be avoided in patients with renal failure (Table 1). These drugs may be administered if judged absolutely essential; however, the clinician must be prepared for the onset of toxicity, marked worsening of the renal dysfunction, and/or therapeutic failure.

DOSE REGIMENS IN RENAL FAILURE

Doses of drugs primarily eliminated by the kidney must be reduced when renal insufficiency is present to avoid accumulation (Table 2). This is especially important when drugs are nephrotoxic, because exacerbation of the underlying renal disease may occur. For drugs eliminated primarily by hepatic routes (e.g., chloramphenicol, isoxazolyl penicillins), dose adjustment is not necessary. In the case of relatively safe drugs such as penicillin, halving the normal dose or doubling the normal dose interval suffices in patients with severe renal failure. Dosage adjustment is not necessary for other drugs eliminated by the kidney, but they should not be used in patients with severe renal failure because of the increased likelihood of toxicity or lack of efficacy.

Total daily drug dose of the majority of drugs listed in Table 2 should be reduced in direct proportion to decreased GFR. This can be accomplished by administering either a normal dose at an increased dose interval or by giving a reduced dose at the normal interval. The following equations allow one to calculate reduced doses rapidly by either method. Both equations are based on the assumption that renal failure is stable and that the volume of distribution is normal.

Equation 1: Interval Extension Method

$$^T\text{renal failure} = {^T}\text{normal} \times \frac{\text{normal Cl}_{cr}}{\text{patient Cl}_{cr}}$$

Equation 2: Dose Reduction Method

$$^D\text{renal failure} = {^D}\text{normal} \times \frac{\text{patient Cl}_{cr}}{\text{normal Cl}_{cr}}$$

Table 1. *Drugs to be Avoided in Patients with Severe Renal Failure*

Drug	Pharmacologic Class	Adverse Signs
Methenamine mandelate	Urinary tract antiseptic	GI distress, crystalluria, systemic acidosis
Nalidixic acid*	Urinary tract antiseptic	Nausea, vomition, neurotoxicity, dermatotoxicity
Neomycin	Antibiotic	Renal failure, ototoxicity
Nitrofurantoin	Urinary tract antiseptic	Polyneuritis, GI disturbances, rapid emergence of bacterial resistance, pulmonary infiltrates
Polymyxin B	Antibiotic	Renal failure, neurotoxicity
Tetracyclines (except doxycycline)	Antibiotics	Vomition, diarrhea, antianabolic effect, renal sodium wasting
Thiacetarsamide	Antiparasitic (dirofilariasis)	Vomition, anorexia, thromboembolism, hepatic and renal failure

*Editor's Note: This drug is contraindicated in *any* dog or cat.

Table 2.   *Drugs Whose Dose Should be Reduced in Patients with Renal Failure*

Drug	Dosage Adjustment	Adverse Signs
Antimicrobials		
Amikacin Gentamicin Kanamycin Netilmicin Sisomicin Tobramycin Streptomycin	Interval extension* Double or triple interval with severe renal failure	Aminoglycoside toxicity: renal failure, ototoxicity, neuromuscular blockage
Cephaloridine Cephalexin Cephazolin	Interval extension*	Renal failure
Cephalothin Cefamandole	Double interval With severe One-half dose renal failure	Anaphylaxis (cephalosporins may potentiate aminoglycoside nephrotoxicity)
Methicillin Penicillin Ampicillin Amoxicillin Carbenicillin Ticarcillin	Mild dose adjustment with severe renal failure†	Anaphylaxis, neurotoxicity (methicillin has been associated with interstitial nephritis more than other penicillins)
Sulfisoxazole	Double or triple interval with severe renal failure	Renal failure
Trimethoprim/ sulfamethoxazole	Avoid in *severe* renal failure	Vomition, diarrhea
Colistimethate Lincomycin	Dose reduction* Triple interval in severe renal failure	Renal failure Diarrhea, vomition, enterocolotoxic reaction
Vancomycin	Interval extension*	Ototoxicity, possible renal toxicity
Antifungals		
Amphotericin B	One-half dose in severe renal failure	Renal failure, hypokalemia
5-Fluorocytosine	Interval extension*	Hepatic and bone marrow toxicity
Cardioactive Drugs		
Digoxin	Decrease dose 50 per cent for each 50 mg/dl elevation in SUN	Vomition, weakness, arrhythmias
Procainamide	Double interval with severe renal failure	Hypotension, myocardial depression
Antineoplastics		
Bleomycin	Decrease dose	Dermatotoxicity, pulmonary fibrosis
Cyclophosphamide	Double interval in severe renal failure	Vomition, diarrhea, cystitis, bone marrow depression, hyponatremia
Methotrexate	One-half dose in severe renal failure	Renal failure, vomition, bone marrow depression
Cis-platinum	Increase interval	Renal failure
Azothioprine	Double interval in severe renal failure	Renal failure, bone marrow and immunosuppression
Miscellaneous Drugs		
Phenobarbital Primidone	Double interval with severe renal failure Double or triple interval with severe renal failure	Excessive sedation
Methoxyflurane	Avoid in severe renal failure	Renal failure

*Use formula (see text).
†Half dose or double interval.

where T is the dosage interval, D is the dose, and Cl_{cr} is the creatinine clearance used to estimate GFR. With the interval extension method, the dose interval may become unduly prolonged with very low CL_{cr}. To prevent this, one should multiply the dose and calculated ^{T}renal failure by a constant fraction (e.g., ½, ⅓) to shorten the dose interval to a more realistic value.

The selection of one method over another has been extensively reviewed in the literature. For antibiotics, some authors advocate Equation 1 for bacteriostatic drugs and Equation 2 for bacteriocidal drugs because of their relative half-lives. However, microbiologic arguments can be made in favor of both techniques in that dose reduction maintains effective drug concentrations for prolonged periods, whereas interval extension results in high peak concentrations. Both methods may be effective in killing bacteria. In our opinion, the primary consideration for dose reduction is the avoidance of drug toxicity. Therefore, toxicologic criteria should be considered in the selection of the method of dose reduction.

For aminoglycoside antibiotics, the interval extension method appears to be safer than dose reduction. This method also results in improved penetration of drug into tissues. In addition, aminoglycosides bind to receptors in susceptible bacteria and continue to exert bacteriocidal activity even after drug removal from medium. This indicates that sustained blood levels of drugs may not be necessary and that the increased risk of toxicity is not warranted. However, when treating serious cases of sepsis with aminoglycosides, very long dose intervals may result in "breakthrough" bacteremias. Therefore, dose intervals should not be excessively long. In the case of digoxin, dose reduction based on SUN is the preferred technique, since effective serum concentrations of drugs must always be maintained. Normal loading doses of drug should always be administered so that therapeutically effective concentrations are immediately attained. If a loading dose is not administered, the prolonged half-life in renal failure would cause excessive delays in reaching steady-state drug levels. The loading dose of digoxin should be slightly reduced in patients with renal insufficiency because of its decreased volume of distribution in renal disease. Consult supplementary readings for an in-depth discussion of these concepts.

Finally, selection of dose adjustment methods must be based on an initial clinical assessment of the patient followed by serial evaluations for signs of therapeutic efficacy or drug-induced toxicity. Recommendations in Table 2 for initiation of therapy are only guidelines to be followed until clinical feedback dictates change. If Cl_{cr} is not available, guesstimates based on serum creatinine can be used.

Table 3. *Clinical Signs of Aminoglycoside-Induced Toxic Nephropathy*

Reduced glomerular filtration rate reflected by elevated serum creatinine and serum urea nitrogen concentrations or decreased creatinine clearance
Polyuria and decreased urine osmolarity
Cylindruria (casts)
Enzymuria, proteinuria
Glycosuria, aminoaciduria
Increased fractional sodium excretion

DETECTION OF NEPHROTOXICITY

Differentiation between progression of the primary renal disease process and loss of renal function secondary to drug-induced nephrotoxicosis may be a major problem when treating a patient with renal failure. This problem is particularly common with administration of aminoglycoside antibiotics. Table 3 provides a summary of clinical signs associated with aminoglycoside-induced toxic nephropathy. Elevations of serum creatinine or SUN are relatively late indicators of drug-induced toxicity. The other parameters listed may permit earlier detection of toxicosis because they are more sensitive to proximal tubular insults. Early detection of toxicosis is essential in patients with pre-existing renal insufficiency because their renal reserve has already been exhausted. Further insult could easily precipitate an acute uremic crisis in a patient with stable chronic renal insufficiency. Drug therapy in patients with acute renal failure is especially difficult, since renal functional indices are neither accurate nor stable and signs of toxic nephropathy may be masked by the primary active renal disease process.

SUPPLEMENTAL READING

Anderson, R. J., Bennett, W. M., Gambertoglio, J. G., and Schrier, R. W.: Fate of drugs in renal failure. *In* Brenner, B. M., and Rector, F. C. (eds.): *The Kidney*, 2nd ed. Philadelphia: W. B. Saunders, 1981.

Anderson, R. J., Gambertoglio, J. G., and Schrier, R. W.: Fate of drugs in renal failure. *In* Brenner, B. M., and Rector, F. C. (eds.): *The Kidney*. Philadelphia: W. B. Saunders, 1976.

Benet, L. Z. (ed.): *Effects of Disease States on Drug Pharmacokinetics*. Washington, DC: Academy of Pharmaceutical Sciences, 1976.

Chennavasin, P., and Brater, D. C.: Nomograms for drug use in renal disease. Clin. Pharmacokinet. 6:193, 1981.

Davis, L. E.: Drug therapy in renal disorders. *In* Kirk, R. W. (ed.): *Current Veterinary Therapy VII*. Philadelphia: W. B. Saunders, 1980, pp. 1114–1117.

Davis, L. E., Baggot, J. D., Neff-Davis, C. A., and Powers, T. E.: Elimination kinetics of pentobarbitol in nephrectomized dogs. Am. J. Vet. Res. 34:231, 1973.

Gibson, T. P.: Influence of renal disease on pharmacokinetics. *In* Evans, W. E., Schentag, J. J., and Jusko, W. J. (eds.): *Applied Pharmacokinetics*. San Francisco: Applied Therapeutics, Inc., 1980, pp. 32–56.

Gierke, K. D., Perrier, D., Mayersohn, M., and Marcus, F. I.: Digoxin disposition kinetics in dogs before and during azotemia. J. Pharmacol. Exp. Ther. 205:459, 1978.

Klausner, J. S., Meuner, P. C., Osborne, C. A., Stevens, J. B., and Stowe, C. M.: Half-life of cephaloridine in dogs with reduced renal function. Am. J. Vet. Res. 38:1191, 1977.

Osborne, C. A., and Klausner, J. S.: Adverse drug reactions in the uremic patient. *In* Kirk, R. W. (ed.): *Current Veterinary Therapy VI.* Philadelphia: W. B. Saunders, 1977, pp. 1152–1158.

Reidenberg, M. M., and Drayer, D. E. Drug therapy in renal failure. Ann. Rev. Pharmacol. Toxicol. 20:45, 1980.

Reiner, N. E., Bloxham, D. D., and Thompson, W. L.: Nephrotoxicity of gentamicin and tobramycin given once daily or continuously in dogs. J. Antimicrob. Chemother. 4(Suppl. A):85, 1978.

Riviere, J. E., and Coppoc, G. L.: Dosage of antimicrobial drugs in patients with renal insufficiency. J.A.V.M.A. 178:70, 1981.

Riviere, J. E., and Coppoc, G. L.: Selected aspects of aminoglycoside antibiotic nephrotoxiciosis. J.A.V.M.A. 178:508, 1981.

Riviere, J. E., Coppoc, G. L., Hinsman, E. J., and Carlton, W. W.: Gentamicin pharmacokinetic changes in induced, acute canine nephrotoxic glomerularnephritis. Antimicrob. Agents Chemother. 20:387, 1981.

Riviere, J. E., and Davis, L. E.: Renal handling of drugs in renal failure. *In* Bovee, K. C. (ed.): *Canine Nephrology.* Media, PA: Harwal Publishing, in press.

Senior, D. F.: Drug therapy in renal failure. Vet. Clin. North Am. 9:805, 1979.

Thornhill, J. A.: Toxic nephropathy. *In* Kirk, R. W. (ed.): *Current Veterinary Therapy VII.* Philadelphia: W. B. Saunders, 1980, pp. 1047–1052.

Diseases of the Upper and Lower Urinary Tract

VESICOURETERAL REFLUX

JEFFREY S. KLAUSNER, D.V.M.,
and DANIEL A. FEENEY, D.V.M.

St. Paul, Minnesota

Vesicoureteral reflux is the retroflow of urine from the bladder into the ureters through an incompetent vesicoureteral junction. It occurs in dogs, cats, and humans and provides a means of spread of urinary tract infection from the lower urinary tract to the kidneys.

THE VESICOURETERAL JUNCTION

The ureters curve in a cranial direction as they enter the bladder. Following penetration of the serosa, the ureters tunnel through the bladder musculature and submucosa before terminating at mucosal orifices at the trigone. Although a well-defined vesicoureteral valve is not present, urine reflux is prevented during bladder filling and voiding by the unique anatomic arrangement of the vesicoureteral junction, which forms a "flap valve." Detrusor muscle fibers pass above and below the submucosal ureter. When these muscle fibers are stretched during bladder contraction, pressure placed on the ureter closes its lumen and prevents urine reflux.

PATHOGENESIS OF VESICOURETERAL REFLUX

The etiology of vesicoureteral reflux may be classified as primary or secondary. Primary reflux, the most common type, occurs in otherwise normal young animals and usually disappears as the animal matures. Primary vesicoureteral reflux can be demonstrated by a voiding cystourethrogram in approximately 50 per cent of dogs less than six months of age but occurs in less than 10 per cent of adult dogs (Christie, 1971). It occurs more frequently in female dogs than in male dogs and is more often bilateral (65 per cent) than unilateral (35 per cent).

The submucosal ureter must be of a critical length in relation to its diameter for reflux to be prevented (Lenaghan and Cassen, 1968). In young animals with reflux, the length of the submucosal ureter tends to be short compared with its diameter. Primary vesicoureteral reflux is thought to result from delayed maturation of the vesicoureteral junction, resulting in weakness of the terminal ureteral musculature attachments to the trigone. As a result, the submucosal ureter becomes shorter and is displaced. With maturity, the ratio of ureteral length to diameter increases and reflux usually ceases.

Secondary vesicoureteral reflux has been related to urinary tract infection, urethral or bladder neck obstruction, neurogenic bladder disease, congenital ureteral defects, and iatrogenic causes. Although urinary tract infection and vesicoureteral reflux commonly occur together, controversy exists regarding the importance of urinary tract infection as a cause of vesicoureteral reflux. In an experimental study, reflux occurred in 4 of 8 dogs infected with *E. coli* and in 16 of 17 dogs infected with *Proteus* spp. (Sommer and Roberts, 1966). Reflux ceased following antibiotic cure of the urinary tract infections. In other canine studies, however, a causal relationship between infection and reflux could not be clearly demonstrated (Harrison et al., 1974).

Urinary tract infection may predispose to vesicoureteral reflux in an animal with an already incompetent vesicoureteral junction. Trigonal inflammation caused by infection could predispose to vesicoureteral reflux by decreasing ureteral compliance or by altering the course of the submucosal ureter. A less oblique and shortened submucosal ureter would be more likely to reflux than a normal ureter. In addition, increased intravesical pressure associated with infection might increase the likelihood of vesicoureteral reflux.

Damage to nerves innervating the bladder results in secondary vesicoureteral reflux in humans. Neurologic diseases predispose to reflux by altering trigonal tone and predisposing to urinary tract infection. The frequency of secondary vesicoureteral reflux in dogs and cats with neurogenic bladder disease has not been determined. Increased intravesicular pressure secondary to partial urethral obstruction has been suggested as a cause of secondary vesicoureteral reflux, but supportive evidence is lacking (Stamey, 1980). Congenital anomalies of the urinary bladder and ureter are known to predispose humans to vesicoureteral reflux (Cook and King, 1979). Anomalies associated with reflux include ectopic ureters, ureteral duplication, and bladder diverticula in the region of the trigone. These conditions are associated with an abnormal anatomic arrangement of the vesicoureteral junction.

Studies at the University of Minnesota have revealed that manual expression of the urinary bladder in normal dogs and cats can result in reflux. Reflux occurred more often in dogs in which a great deal of pressure was required to express urine from the bladder. These results suggest that techniques other than manual expression should be used to collect urine from animals with urinary tract infections to avoid iatrogenic spread of infection from the lower to upper urinary tract.

SIGNIFICANCE OF VESICOURETERAL REFLUX

Opinions vary regarding the significance of vesicoureteral reflux. Present evidence suggests that reflux is important because it permits the spread of lower urinary tract infections to the kidneys and can increase tissue damage caused by established upper urinary tract infections. Experimental canine studies have revealed that vesicoureteral reflux in the absence of urinary tract infection is probably not significant. However, when reflux and urinary tract infection occur together, pyelonephritis and renal scarring result. In one study it was clearly demonstrated that spontaneous and surgically induced vesicoureteral reflux without persistent urinary tract infection did not result in gross or microscopic renal abnormalities. However, in dogs with reflux and urinary tract infections, pyelonephritis and decreased renal function developed (Newman et al., 1974). For unknown reasons, young animals appeared especially susceptible to renal damage.

Whether vesicoureteral reflux can predispose to recurrent lower urinary tract infections remains unknown. Reflux increases residual bladder urine, but studies in humans have not revealed a definite association between reflux and an increased susceptibility to recurrent infection (Stamey, 1980).

DIAGNOSIS OF VESICOURETERAL REFLUX

The diagnosis of vesicoureteral reflux must be established radiographically. Reflux can be influenced by the type of anesthetic used, the depth of anesthesia, patient positioning, and the degree of bladder distention. Many of these variables have not been controlled in clinical studies.

Reflux can occur during bladder filling, voiding, or both. In adult dogs, reflux occurs near the time of maximal bladder distention; in puppies it tends to occur earlier during the course of bladder filling (Christie, 1971). Although unilateral reflux has been reported in the dog, it is usually bilateral. Contrast medium generally reaches the renal pelves. Depending on the cause of reflux, other radiographic abnormalities may also be noted.

Radiographic techniques used to identify vesicoureteral reflux include voiding cystourethrography, retrograde (maximum distention) cystourethrography, and compression cystourethrography. We currently recommend either voiding or retrograde cystourethrography (maximum distention). Voiding cystourethrography has been the technique most often used in canine studies to demonstrate vesicoureteral reflux but is technically cumbersome.

Voiding cystourethrography is performed as follows. With the dog lightly anesthetized and in lateral recumbency, the bladder is catheterized and urine is removed. An iodinated radiocontrast agent is allowed to enter the bladder by gravity flow. The receptacle containing the contrast medium should be approximately 3 ft above the patient. A radiograph is exposed, or the urinary tract is visualized fluoroscopically as spontaneous voiding occurs around the catheter (Christie, 1973).

Retrograde cystourethrography is performed by infusing an iodinated radiocontrast agent into the urinary bladder following catheterization of the membranous or prostatic urethra. A higher frequency of reflux is observed if the urinary bladder is distended to the point of trigone-urethral dilation prior to the urethral injection. This modified technique, termed maximum distention cystourethrography, demonstrated a 50 per cent incidence of reflux in adult male beagle dogs studied at the University of Minnesota. Care should be used to prevent urinary bladder rupture, especially if balloon catheters are used to prevent spontaneous voiding.

Compression cystourethrography is performed with the dog or cat under a light plane of anesthesia. The patient's urinary bladder is filled with an iodinated radiocontrast agent. After the patient is placed in a lateral recumbent position, external pressure is applied to the patient's bladder to express urine. When urine flow is observed, an abdominal radiography is exposed or the vesicoureteral junction is observed fluoroscopically. In humans, manual expression cystourethrography has been found to be less sensitive in the detection of vesicoureteral reflux than voiding cystourethrography. Comparison of voiding cystourethrography and manual expression cystourethrography has not been performed in dogs.

TREATMENT OF VESICOURETERAL REFLUX

Therapeutic approaches to vesicoureteral reflux include medical therapy to eradicate urinary tract infection and surgical therapy to correct an abnormal vesicoureteral junction. Since primary vesicoureteral reflux is common in young dogs and since reflux will usually cease as the dogs mature, therapy is not indicated in young dogs with reflux without

urinary tract infection. If urinary tract infection and reflux coexist, antibiotic therapy should be administered to sterilize the urine. It is important to maintain sterile urine as long as reflux persists to prevent pyelonephritis. Quantitative urine cultures should be obtained to ensure that infection has been eradicated. Techniques other than manual expression should be used to collect urine.

Although surgical procedures have been developed to correct primary reflux in humans, their value is uncertain at the present time. If reflux occurs secondary to some other urologic abnormality, therapy should be directed at the underlying problem. The urine should be kept sterile by use of appropriate antibiotic therapy.

REFERENCES AND SUPPLEMENTAL READING

Christie, B. A.: Incidence and etiology of vesicoureteral reflux in apparently normal dogs. Invest. Urol. 10:184, 1971.
Christie, B. A.: Vesicoureteral reflux in dogs. J.A.V.M.A. 162:772, 1973.
Cook, W. A., and King, L. R.: Vesicoureteral reflux. In Harrison, J. M., Gittes, R. F., Perlmutter, A. D., Stamey, T. A., and Walsh, P. C. (eds.): Campbell's Urology, Vol. 2. Philadelphia: W. B. Saunders, 1979, pp. 1596–1633.
Harrison, L., Cass, A., Cox, C., and Boyce, W.: Role of bladder infection in the etiology of vesicoureteral reflux in dogs. Invest. Urol. 12:123, 1974.
Lenaghan, D., and Cassen, L. J.: Vesicoureteral reflux in pups. J. Urol. 5:449, 1968.
Newman, L., Buey, J. G., and McAlister, W. H.: Experimental production of reflux in the presence and absence of infected urine. Radiology 111:591, 1974.
Sommer, J. L., and Roberts, J. A.: Ureteral reflux resulting from chronic urinary infections in dogs: long term studies. J. Urol. 95:502, 1966.
Stamey, T. A.: Pathogenesis and Treatment of Urinary Tract Infections. Baltimore: Williams & Wilkins, 1980.

CANINE AND FELINE URETERAL ECTOPIA

ROY T. FAULKNER, D.V.M.,

St. Petersburg, Florida

CARL A. OSBORNE, D.V.M.,
and DANIEL A. FEENEY, D.V.M.

St. Paul, Minnesota

Ureteral ectopia is a congenital abnormality in which either one or both ureters do not normally terminate in the trigone of the urinary bladder. In females, ectopic ureters may terminate in the vagina (70 per cent), urethra (20 per cent), neck of the bladder (8 per cent), or uterus (3 per cent) (Owen, 1973b). In males, ectopic ureters are most commonly recognized when they terminate in the cranial portion of the pelvic urethra.

Although the underlying cause of ureteral ectopia in dogs and cats has not been determined, the high predisposition to it in certain canine breeds and the observation of two littermates with unilateral right ectopic ureter suggest a familial tendency (Johnston et al., 1977a). The embryologic pathogenesis of ectopic ureters is related to abnormal origin or migration of metanephric ducts that become ureters (Owen, 1973a). Because of the close relationship between the metanephric duct system and the development of other urogenital organs, ureteral ectopia may be associated with other anomalies such as agenesis of the urinary bladder and urethra, persistent hymen, and abnormalities of the urethra (Osborne et al., 1972; Pearson and Gibbs, 1971).

DIAGNOSTIC CONSIDERATIONS

INCIDENCE

Dogs. Ureteral ectopia is a common cause of urinary incontinence in female dogs. The risk of this clinical manifestation in females is approximately 20 times greater than that in males (Hayes, 1974). Breeds at high risk for ureteral ectopia in females include the Siberian husky, Labrador retriever, collie, West Highland white terrier, fox terrier, Skye terrier, and toy miniature poodle (Hayes, 1974; Johnston et al., 1977a). Although the majority of cases reported in male dogs have been in mixed breeds, Labrador retrievers, Welsh corgis, and fox terriers have been reported to be affected more frequently than other breeds. Ectopic ureters in approximately two-thirds of female dogs have been unilateral; there has been an equal distribution of right and left ureters. In male dogs, an almost equal occurrence of bilateral and unilateral ureteral ectopia has been recognized. The left ureter has more frequently been ectopic in unilateral cases.

Cats. Three clinical cases of ureteral ectopia have been reported in cats. One was a female and two were males (Bebko et al., 1977; Biewenga et al., 1978). Both ureters were ectopic in all three cases and terminated in the urethra.

Age. Since ureteral ectopia is a congenital anomaly, associated urinary incontinence is usually recognized in younger animals. The majority of female dogs have been recognized before they are one year old; many are recognized between the sixth and sixteenth weeks of age. However, recognition of urinary incontinence due to ureteral ectopia has been reported in adult female dogs following ovariohysterectomy (Brodeur, 1977; Greene et al., 1978). Although male dogs with urinary incontinence caused by ectopic ureters are usually recognized when they are immature, cases have been encountered in which the diagnosis was not established until the patients were three years old (Lane, 1973; Lennox, 1978).

Ectopic ureters in the three cats with urinary incontinence were recognized when they were 12 to 16 weeks of age.

CLINICAL SIGNS

Clinical signs of ureteral ectopia are dependent on the site of termination of the ectopic ureters and the presence of other congenital or acquired abnor-malities. Other causes of urinary incontinence (neurogenic disorders, hormonal imbalances, neoplasia, cystitis, urethritis, psychologic dribbling, or other congenital abnormalities) should be considered. We have found a problem-specific data base useful in this regard (Table 1).

Female Dogs and Cats. The most common clinical sign in affected females is continuous involuntary dribbling of urine, which may be noticed by the client at birth but which is usually not recognized until the animal is weaned. The severity of incontinence may vary from continuous dribbling from the vulva to intermittent incontinence associated with vaginal pooling of urine that gravitates out of the vulva when body position is changed. Incontinent patients with unilateral ureteral ectopia usually micturate normally because urine continues to pass into the urinary bladder through the unaffected ureter. Although patients with bilateral ureteral ectopia may not micturate normally, reflux of a sufficient quantity of urine from the urethra into the bladder may be associated with normal micturition if the ureters terminate in the urethra. Persistent dribbling of urine that accumulates around the perivulvar area and caudal thighs may produce discoloration of the hair in this area, especially if it is white or a light color. If severe and/or prolonged, incontinence may lead to so-called urine scald dermatitis.

Progressive destruction of renal parenchyma of the associated kidney as a result of ascending bacteriuria and pyelonephritis may be associated with a progressive decrease in the severity of urinary incontinence. We have observed one female dog with a unilateral ectopic ureter in which complete destruction of the associated kidney resulted in remission of incontinence.

Table 1.   *Problem-Specific Data Base for Urinary Incontinence*

Owner's definition of incontinence
Duration of incontinence
Status of reproductive tract and relationship to incontinence
Hemogram
Urinalysis
Observation of micturition
Evaluation of bladder size
   Before micturition
   After micturition
Verification of incontinence
Appropriate neurologic examination
Evaluation of survey radiographs (if patient is dysuric or if urine cannot be expelled readily from the bladder by manual compression); catheterization to evaluate patency of the urethral lumen may be considered*
Contrast radiography
   High-dose intravenous urography
   Retrograde contrast vaginography or urethrocystography (if excretory urography is not diagnostic)

*Caution: such patients are predisposed to catheterization-induced urinary tract infection.

Male Dogs and Cats. Like females, continuous involuntary dribbling of urine detected at a young age is the most common sign associated with ureteral ectopia in males. Additional clinical findings that have been observed in male cats include a constricted preputial opening (phimosis) with dilatation of the sheath due to accumulation of urine, urine staining of the perineum and hindlimbs, and inflammation of the perineal skin. As with females, unilateral ureteral ectopia in males is usually associated with sufficient filling of the urinary bladder to initiate normal micturition. In male patients with bilateral ectopia, insufficient urinary bladder filling associated with reduced size of the urinary bladder may prevent normal micturition. However, reflux of urine from the urethra into the bladder may permit distention of the urinary bladder and normal micturition in addition to incontinence (Smith et al., 1980).

ENDOSCOPIC FINDINGS

Examination of the vagina with a speculum may permit identification of an ectopic ureteral orifice if the anomalous ureter enters the vagina. However, radiographic techniques are usually more rewarding than endoscopy. Satisfactory visualization of the entire mucosal surface of the vagina is dependent on the use of a vaginoscope that eliminates mucosal infoldings by distention of the vaginal wall. We prefer to use glass (Pyrex) test tubes from which the bottoms have been removed and the ends fire polished, pediatric proctoscopes, disposable plastic syringe cases (Monoject*) from which a large rectangular section has been removed from the wall, or fiberoptic endoscopes. Otoscopic cones and nasal specula are less satisfactory alternatives. Injection of air into the vaginal lumen during endoscopy may enhance visualization of the mucosa by causing distention of the vaginal wall. Caution: unless two ureteral openings can be found, a definitive diagnosis of bilateral ureteral ectopia cannot be made by this method.

In our experience, many female dogs with ectopic ureters have had a persistent hymen. Visual inspection of the vagina of such patients revealed a fleshy piece of tissue that was attached to the dorsal and ventral walls of the vagina. The lateral aspects of the structure often formed slit-like openings with the vaginal wall. Care must be used not to mistake such openings for ectopic ureteral openings.

RADIOGRAPHIC FINDINGS

Excretory Urography. A standard technique and normal findings of excretory urography have been described (Feeney et al., 1981). Excretory urograms may permit confirmation of a diagnosis of

ectopic ureter. In addition, the position, size, and shape of the kidneys; the size of the ureters; and the site of termination of the ureters may be evaluated.

In our experience, localization of the exact site of termination of ectopic ureters by excretory urography is difficult. Poor visualization may occur if the ectopic ureter tunnels through the bladder wall for several centimeters before opening into the urethra or vagina. In addition, the ectopic orifice may be obscured by accumulation of contrast material in the bladder lumen. Poor visualization of the ureter may also occur as a result of reduced excretion of contrast medium by pyelonephritic kidneys. Interference with visualization of the distal portion of ectopic ureters caused by accumulation of contrast medium within the bladder lumen may be minimized by exposure of films before it becomes distended with contrast material, by a combination of pneumocystography with intravenous urography, and/or by exposure of oblique radiographic views in addition to lateral and ventrodorsal views. Megaureter (ureteroectasis) characterized by dilation of the ureteral lumen and abnormal peristalsis is a common finding in dogs with ectopic ureters. This abnormality has not been as consistently observed in cats with ureteral ectopia. Although the cause of megaureter has not been established, developmental abnormalities of the distal portion of the ureter have been cited as a cause of megaureter in humans (Belman, 1974). However, since the distal end of an ectopic ureter has no functional valve, the pathogenesis of megaureter might be related to vesicoreflex. Urinary tract infection caused by organisms (*Escherichia coli* and *Pseudomonus* spp.) known to impair ureteral peristalsis by release of bacterial products and/or stimulation of biologically active substances by the host may also be a contributing factor in dogs (Boyarsky et al., 1971).

Dilation and irregular margins of the renal pelvis (pyelectasis) accompanied by shortened or blunted renal pelvic diverticula are characteristic of chronic pyelonephritis that often occurs in dogs with ectopic ureters. Progressive reduction in renal size also commonly occurs in patients with ureteral ectopia. The abnormal ureteral function is conducive to ascending bacterial infection of the kidneys. In our experience, contracted kidneys of patients with ectopic ureters typically have had gross, microscopic, and bacteriologic findings typical of those of chronic generalized pyelonephritis.

Positive or negative contrast cystography is required to confirm abnormal reduction in the size and distensibility of the urinary bladder. Although this finding has been associated with embryologic cystic hypoplasia, it is most likely to occur in patients with bilateral ureteral ectopia as a consequence of disuse.

Retrograde Ureteropyelography. When an abnormal orifice is detected on endoscopic examina-

---

*Sherwood Medical Industries, Inc., St. Louis, MO.

tion, catheterization of the orifice with a radiopaque catheter followed by retrograde ureteropyelography may be performed. This technique should not be used as a substitute for intravenous urography, since it will not permit evaluation of other portions of the urinary system for concomitant abnormalities. It also may prevent recognition of bilateral ureteral ectopia.

Retrograde Contrast Urethrography or Vaginography. We have found these techniques to be extremely helpful in localizing the site of termination of ectopic ureters. Either pediatric Foley catheters* or Swan-Ganz flow-directed balloon catheters† may be used (Johnston et al., 1977b). Care must be used so as not to occlude the openings of ectopic ureteral orifices with inflated balloons of these catheters, especially those that terminate in the distal urethra.

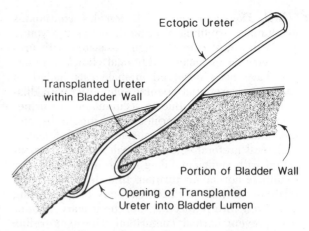

Figure 1. Schematic diagram of ureterovesicular anastomosis illustrating a submucosal antireflux tunnel. Distention of the bladder lumen with urine will compress that portion of the ureteral lumen located within the bladder wall and thus will minimize reflux of urine from the bladder into the ureter.

MANAGEMENT

There is no effective medical treatment for urinary incontinence caused by an ectopic ureter; surgical correction is the only viable alternative. Choice of surgical technique is dependent on the number of ectopic ureters and their location, the functional status of the kidneys, and the presence or absence of concomitant abnormalities.

PREOPERATIVE CONSIDERATIONS

A physical examination and evaluation of a hemogram and urinalysis to assess the general health of the animal and radiographic evaluation (excretory urography, urethrocystography) to detect concomitant congenital abnormalities and localize the termination sites of the ectopic ureters are essential. The serum concentration of urea nitrogen or creatinine should be determined to assess glomerular filtration rate. Since persistent urinary tract infection is common, bacterial culture of urine and determination of the antimicrobial susceptibility of pathogens are recommended. If significant bacteriuria is present, appropriate antimicrobial therapy should be initiated prior to surgery.

URETEROVESICAL ANASTOMOSIS

Reconstructive surgery designed to direct urine flow from the ectopic ureter into the urinary bladder should be seriously considered when there is (1) normal function of the kidney drained by the ectopic ureter, (2) extravesical termination of both ureters, or (3) reduced functional capacity of both kidneys. If generalized renal disease is present, removal of

*American Cystoscope Makers, Sullivan, IN.
†Edwards Laboratories, Santa Ana, CA.

an ectopic ureter and associated kidney may result in removal of a sufficient quality of renal parenchyma to precipitate renal failure.

The most widely accepted method of ureterovesicular anastomosis involves transection of the abnormal ureter near the bladder and reimplantation into the urinary bladder through a submucosal antireflux tunnel formed in the bladder wall (Fig. 1) (Greene and Greiner, 1975; Owen, 1973b; Tarvin, 1979). Ureterovesicular anastomosis without transection of the ectopic ureter may also be considered (Fig. 2) (Dingwall et al., 1976). In our experience, dilation of ectopic ureters has not interfered with the success of their reimplantation. With either technique, a ventral cystotomy should be performed. This surgical approach facilitates corrective surgery of the anomalous ureter and allows one to determine whether or not one or both ureters enter the dorsolateral aspect of the bladder lumen at the trigone. The fact that a ureter enters the bladder lumen usually, but not invariably, indicates that it is not ectopic. However, we have observed a female Siberian husky with an ectopic ureter that entered the bladder lumen at its normal trigonal position but continued caudally and terminated in the urethra. Insertion of a catheter through the ureteral orifice in a caudal direction confirmed this unusual variation.

NEPHRECTOMY-URETERECTOMY

Nephrectomy and removal of as much of the abnormal ureter as possible should be performed in patients with a unilateral ectopic ureter when the associated kidney is affected by generalized disease or when intractable infection is present. Nephrectomy and ureterectomy may be considered in patients with unilateral ureteral ectopia provided the

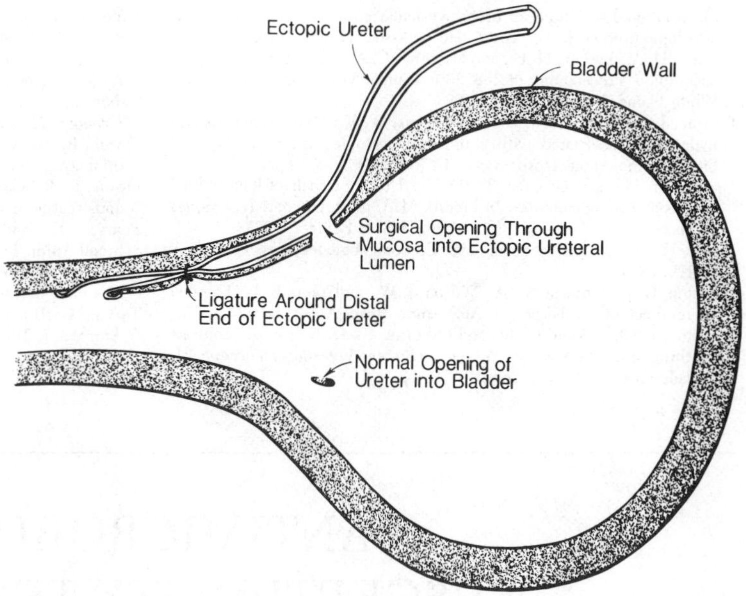

Figure 2. Schematic illustration of a technique of ureterovesicular anastomosis in which the ectopic ureter is not transected. Urine is prevented from passing from the ureter into the urethra by ligating the distal portion of the ectopic ureter. Urine from the ectopic ureter is diverted into the bladder lumen by placing an opening between the transmural section of the ureter and the bladder mucosa.

contralateral kidney has a normal appearance and function.

POSTOPERATIVE RECOMMENDATIONS

Following ureterovesicular anastomosis, a stent is usually placed in the distal portion of the ureter for several days to minimize obstruction to urine outflow caused by post-surgical inflammation. If there is concern about the patency of the ureter following removal of the stent, an excretory urogram should be performed approximately five to seven days later. If complete obstruction of the ureteral lumen is not corrected within one week following its occurrence, irreversible damage to the associated kidney is probable. Evaluation of an excretory urogram four to six weeks following surgery is also recommended to assess the status of the urinary tract.

Every effort should be made to avoid the use of catheters to collect urine samples or to obtain retrograde radiographic studies, since they predispose patients to urinary tract infections. Samples for urinalysis and urine culture should be collected by cystocentesis. Urinalyses should be assessed at appropriate intervals following surgery to monitor the patient for urinary tract infection.

In patients with bacterial urinary tract infection, antimicrobial therapy selected on the basis of urine culture and antimicrobial susceptibility tests should be continued until clinical signs of infection have subsided, the results of urinalysis are normal, and urine is sterile. Consult Treatment of Urinary Tract Infections With Antimicrobial Agents (page 1051) for specific details.

PROGNOSIS

Female dogs with unilateral or bilateral ectopic ureters that terminate in the urethra may continue to have some degree of urinary incontinence following ureterovesicular anastomosis or extirpation of the affected ureter and kidney. This may be related to concomitant abnormalities of the urethra. A better prognosis is associated with a ureter that terminates in the vagina or uterus. Reimplantation of ectopic ureters that terminate in the urethra has been associated with a higher rate of continence in males than in females. Reimplantation of dilated ureters into the urinary bladder may be associated with varying degrees of vesicoureteral reflux. This phenomenon is of clinical significance, since it predisposes the patient to ascending infection of the kidney. Even though a better long-term result may be obtained when the ureters have some degree of peristalsis and are not extremely dilated, we have obtained satisfactory long-term results in several dogs in which markedly dilated ureters were reimplanted into the urinary bladder.

REFERENCES AND SUPPLEMENTAL READING

Bebko, R. L., Prier, J. E., and Biery, D. N.: Ectopic ureters in a male cat. J.A.V.M.A. 171:738, 1977.
Belman, A. B.: Megaureter: Classification, etiology, and management. Urol. Clin. North Am. 1:497, 1974.
Biewenga, W. J., Rothuizen, J., and Voorhout, G.: Ectopic ureters in the cat: A report of two cases. J. Small Anim. Pract. 19:531, 1978.
Boyarsky, S., et al.: *Urodynamics: Hydrodynamics Of The Ureter And Renal Pelvis.* New York: Academic Press, 1971.
Brodeur, G. Y.: Diagnosis of ectopic ureter. Canine Pract. 4:25, 1977.
Dingwall, J. S., Eger, C. E., and Owen, R. R.: Clinical experiences with

the combined technique of ureterovesicular anastomosis for treatment of ectopic ureters. J. Am. Anim. Hosp. Assoc. 12:406, 1976.

Feeney, D. A., Barber, D. L., and Osborne, C. A.: Advances in excretory urography. Proceedings of the 30th Gaines Veterinary Symposium, White Plains, N.Y., 1981, pp. 8–22.

Greene, J. A., Thornhill, J. A., and Blevins, W. E.: Hydronephrosis and hydroureter associated with a unilateral ectopic ureter in a spayed bitch. J. Am. Anim. Hosp. Assoc. 14:708, 1978.

Greene, R. W., and Greiner, T. P.: The Ureter: Repair of longitudinal defects and reimplantation. In Bojrab, M. J. (ed.): Current Techniques In Small Animal Surgery. Philadelphia: Lea & Febiger, 1975.

Hayes, H. M.: Ectopic ureter in dogs. Epidemiologic features. Teratology 10:129, 1974.

Johnston, G. R., Osborne, C. A., Wilson, J. W., and Yano, B. L.: Familial ureteral ectopia in the dog. J. Am. Anim. Hosp. Assoc. 13:168, 1977a.

Johnston, G. R., Jessen, C. R., and Osborne, C. A.: Retrograde contrast urethrography. In Kirk, R. W. (ed.): Current Veterinary Therapy VI. Philadelphia: W. B. Saunders, 1977b.

Lane, J. G.: Canine ectopic ureter: Two further case reports. J. Small Anim. Pract. 14:555, 1973.

Lennox, J. S.: A case report of unilateral ectopic ureter in a male Siberian husky. J. Am. Anim. Hosp. Assoc. 14:331, 1978.

Osborne, C. A., Low, D. G., and Finco, D. R.: Canine And Feline Urology. Philadelphia: W. B. Saunders, 1972.

Owen, R. R.: Canine ureteral ectopia: A review. I. Embryology and etiology. J. Small Anim. Pract. 14:407, 1973a.

Owen, R. R.: Canine ureteral ectopia: A review II. Incidence diagnosis and treatment. J. Small Anim. Pract. 14:419, 1973b.

Pearson, H., and Gibbs, C.: Urinary tract abnormalities in the dog. J. Small Anim. Pract. 12:67, 1971.

Smith, C. W., Stowater, J. L., and Kneller, S. H.: Bilateral ectopic ureter in a male dog with urinary incontinence. J.A.V.M.A. 177:1022, 1980.

Tarvin, G. B.: Surgical treatment of ectopic ureters. Vet. Clin. North Am. 9:277, 1979.

ANTIMICROBIAL SUSCEPTIBILITY TESTS FOR URINARY TRACT PATHOGENS

GERALD V. LING, D.V.M.,
and DWIGHT C. HIRSH, D.V.M.

Davis, California

The antimicrobial susceptibility testing techniques described in this article are used to determine minimum inhibitory concentration (MIC), which may be defined as the least amount of an antimicrobial agent that inhibits growth of a specific species or strain of bacteria in a defined and reproducible set of in vitro conditions. All standard methods of susceptibility testing used in veterinary medicine determine MIC values whether they are reported as such or not. However, in occasional clinical situations higher antimicrobial concentrations than those merely inhibiting bacterial growth may be desirable. This may be especially true in the treatment of infections in immune-compromised patients. In these situations it may be desirable to know the minimum bacteriocidal concentration (MBC) of the therapeutic agent. The MBC is defined as the least amount of an antimicrobial agent that results in the in vitro death of at least 99.9 per cent of the test bacteria within a standard period of time. In urinary bacterial infections, the MIC and MBC values of bacteriocidal antimicrobials are similar. Therefore, measurement of MBC often is not necessary for successful chemotherapy, nor is it practical because of the additional time and expense involved.

The terms "sensitive" and "resistant" are used daily by veterinarians when discussing antimicrobial therapy. A clear understanding of what the two terms mean is basic to successful use of antimicrobials in the treatment of infectious diseases. The two terms are relative. They have been simply defined as the ability or lack of ability of a specific species or strain of bacteria to multiply (grow) in the presence of a certain concentration of a specific antimicrobial agent. The terms are relative to the concentrations of antimicrobial agents attainable at the site of the infection. For example, a certain bacterial species for which growth is inhibited at 10 μg/ml may be "resistant" to the drug in the lung but "sensitive" to the same drug given at the same dose by the same route in the urinary bladder. It may be possible to achieve a maximum of 8 μg/ml of this drug in lung tissue (a value less than that needed to inhibit growth of these bacteria). Using the same dose, however, it may be possible to achieve a level of 300 μg/ml of urine of this drug, a value 30 times that needed for inhibition of growth of these bacteria.

A basic goal of antimicrobial therapy is to provide the appropriate antibacterial activity at the site of the infection in excess of that needed to inhibit growth of, or to kill, infecting organisms. Although achieving this goal in patients with diseases of various organs and tissues of the body is sometimes difficult, it is not difficult to achieve in the urinary tract.

All common antimicrobial agents that have been recommended for use in urinary tract infections in animals develop very high urine concentrations of active drug following administration of oral or injected doses. Urine concentrations of active antimicrobial agents may attain as much as 100 times the corresponding peak serum concentration owing to rapid elimination of the drug from serum into urine. To illustrate, suppose that 8 per cent of a dose of a hypothetical antimicrobial agent is eliminated in active form into the urine of a dog during the first eight hours following oral administration (the remaining 92 per cent is inactivated and excreted or is eliminated in the feces). The dog weighs 25 lbs; the recommended oral dose of the antimicrobial is 20 mg/lb every eight hours. At this dosage a maximum *serum* concentration of 10 µg/ml is reached one hour after administration. By multiplying 20 mg by 25 lbs, the calculated antimicrobial dose for a dog of this weight is 500 mg given every eight hours. If the eight-hour dose is divided by the percentage of active drug eliminated in the urine in eight hours (8 per cent), 40 mg of active antimicrobial may be expected to be present in the total eight-hour urine output. The average dog produces about 20 ml of urine/lb body weight/day; 20 ml × 25 lbs = 500 ml urine output/day from this dog; 500 ml ÷ 3 = 167 ml of urine produced in eight hours. Since the 40 mg of active antimicrobial is dissolved in this volume of urine, we divide 40 mg by 167 ml and find that 0.240 mg (240 µg) of active antimicrobial is present per ml of urine. As noted previously, the maximum serum concentration achieved during this time was 10 µg/ml, which means that the urine concentration achieved in this case was 24 times greater than the maximum serum concentration.

It is possible, and in fact desirable, to make use of this phenomenon when treating urinary tract infections, since antimicrobial concentrations in urine have been shown to be an important factor (along with bacterial susceptibility) in the success or failure of therapy.

The percentages of active antimicrobial agent eliminated in canine urine in eight hours for several commonly used antimicrobial agents are listed in Table 1. Using these percentages it is possible to calculate (as in the previous example) the approximate eight-hour accumulated urine concentration of any of the antimicrobial agents listed for any dog with normal water intake and normal renal function. Remember: as the volume of urine produced per unit time increases (regardless of the reason), the concentration of the antimicrobial agent in the urine decreases (assuming constant dose and treatment intervals). Therefore, dogs that produce massive

Table 1. *Percentage of Active Antimicrobial Agent in Urine Collected from Dogs with Normal Renal Function and Hydration for Eight Hours Following Administration of Therapeutic Doses*

Antimicrobial Agent	Percentage (± S.D.)
Penicillin G	8.0 (± 3.4)
Penicillin V	6.7 (± 2.1)
Ampicillin	19.2 (± 3.8)
Hetacillin	12.4 (± 2.1)
Amoxicillin	22.5 (± 3.1)
Chloramphenicol	6.3 (± 2.6)
Oxytetracycline	11.2 (± 2.0)
Sulfisoxazole	68.5 (± 2.1)
Gentamicin	75.8 (± 8.2)
Tobramycin	82.2 (± 11.5)
Amikacin	69.5 (± 30.0)

volumes of urine may need an increased amount of antimicrobial agent to maintain an effective urine concentration. The reverse is also true; dogs that produce abnormally small volumes of urine per unit time may have abnormally high urine concentrations of antimicrobial in the urine (even toxic amounts). Therefore, the amount of antimicrobial agent administered in each dose may have to be reduced or the interval between doses may have to be lengthened when treating urinary infections in oliguric dogs.

LABORATORY METHODS FOR TESTING BACTERIAL SUSCEPTIBILITY TO ANTIMICROBIAL AGENTS

DIFFUSION METHOD

The diffusion method of antimicrobial susceptibility testing, first reported nearly 20 years ago, is used by many commercial laboratories. The method is performed on a 15-cm Mueller-Hinton agar plate onto which is streaked test bacteria that have been grown in pure culture in a nutrient broth to a standard concentration.

Commercially available paper discs that are 6 mm in diameter and that have been impregnated with a specified amount of an antimicrobial agent are then pressed gently but firmly onto the surface of the agar to assure uniform contact. With the 15-cm plate, 12 antimicrobial agents, 1 per disc, may be tested simultaneously. Discs must be stored at − 14°C or lower over a desiccant, which is supplied with the discs. A small number of discs may be stored in a refrigerator over a desiccant but for no longer than one week. Potency of the antimicrobial agent in the disc may be reduced or lost if this guideline is not strictly followed.

During incubation at 37°C for 18 to 24 hours, each antimicrobial agent diffuses through the agar from the paper disc. The distance that each antimicrobial agent diffuses into the Mueller-Hinton agar and the concentration that it attains in the diffusion zone is unique and is dependent, in part, on the type and depth of the agar and its water content. Therefore, the following variables must be standardized to ensure proper interpretation of results: (1) the type of agar used, (2) the age of the agar as it relates to water content, (3) the depth of the agar (4 mm is standard), (4) the incubation time, and (5) the number of bacteria per ml of inoculum.

The method is based on a straight line relationship, called the regression line, that exists between the size of the zone of bacterial growth inhibition in the agar around each disc after incubation and the concentration (MIC in μg/ml) of each antimicrobial agent that will completely inhibit growth of the test bacterial strain or species. The angle of slope of the regression line is different for each antimicrobial agent. Therefore, it is necessary to test each drug that may be useful in therapy on each bacterial isolate. Based on the attainable concentration of each antimicrobial agent in the body following administration of standard doses, sensitive (S), intermediate (I), and resistant (R) limits have been established along the regression line for each antimicrobial agent.

The standard agar-disc diffusion method used in most laboratories is the Kirby-Bauer method. It is based on attainable concentrations of antimicrobial agents in human *serum* but has been used to test bacterial isolates from animals on the assumption (not always correct) that blood levels of antimicrobial agents are similar in all species. Four or five colonies of test bacteria are transferred from an agar plate to a test tube containing tryptose soy broth and are incubated for four to six hours. After incubation, the numbers of bacteria per ml of this inoculum are compared with a McFarland 0.5 standard. If necessary, the turbidity of the test inoculum is adjusted to that of the McFarland 0.5 standard by dilution with broth. This standard inoculum is then streaked with a sterile cotton swab onto the surface of the Mueller-Hinton agar plate and allowed to dry. Discs are aseptically placed on the agar, and the plate is incubated overnight in air at 37°C. The next day, the diameter of the clear zone around each disc is measured across the center of the disc with calipers to the nearest millimeter. The susceptibility of the test bacteria is determined with the aid of a zone size interpretive chart designed for use with the Kirby-Bauer test.

An agar overlay modification of this test, first reported about 12 years ago, is now widely used to test rapidly growing organisms. In this modification, four to five colonies of the test bacteria are transferred to a tube containing 0.5 ml of brain-heart infusion broth and are incubated for four to five hours at 37°C. At the end of this time, 0.001 ml is transferred with a calibrated loop to 10 ml of melted Mueller-Hinton agar. The agar and inoculum are mixed and poured onto the surface of a standard 15-cm Mueller-Hinton agar plate. Discs are placed on the surface of the overlay after solidification occurs. The plate is incubated, and results are obtained by the same method as that described for the standard Kirby-Bauer test.

One additional modification of the agar-disc diffusion method was developed as the result of an international collaborative study published ten years ago. In this modification, the bacterial inoculum is made by transferring a 0.001 ml calibrated loopful of bacteria (five to ten colonies) from an agar plate to 1 ml of sterile lactated Ringer's solution. Following mixing, one drop of the inoculum is transferred with a 1-ml pipette to a tube containing 5 ml of sterile lactated Ringer's solution and is mixed. If the test bacteria are gram positive cocci, this mixture becomes the inoculum. If the test bacteria are gram negative rods, one drop of the mixture from the test tube containing 5 ml of sterile lactated Ringer's solution is transferred to a second test tube containing 5 ml of sterile lactated Ringer's solution and is mixed. The mixture in this second test tube becomes the inoculum. The surface of a 15-cm Mueller-Hinton agar plate is flooded with 5 ml of the appropriately diluted inoculum, which is spread evenly by gentle rotation of the plate. The excess inoculum is removed with a pipette, and the surface of the agar is allowed to dry. Discs are then applied and the plates are allowed to stand face up for 30 minutes at room temperature before overnight incubation at 37°C. The results are obtained by comparing the diameter of the clear zone around each disc with the appropriate chart of MIC zone size relationships for each antimicrobial agent.

Two obvious advantages of this modification are the ability to record the results in terms of MIC (μg/ml) of each agent tested and the ability to extend the MIC/zone size charts to include attainable urine concentrations of antimicrobials in addition to the standard serum concentrations.

DILUTION METHOD

This method involves direct measurement of the MIC from a series of dilutions of each antimicrobial agent (usually serial twofold dilutions) in broth or agar. A standard number of test bacteria are inoculated into each dilution. After incubation, the MIC is recorded as the test tube, well, or agar plate containing the least amount of the antimicrobial agent that prevented growth of the test organism.

Recent developments based on this method include machinery that automatically dilutes and inoculates broth in disposable plastic trays containing 96 tiny wells aligned in rows. Serial dilutions of each of 8 to 12 antimicrobial agents are prepared automatically in many trays, which are then stored at −60°C until they are used.

Each bacterial inoculum is grown in broth to a predetermined density, and an entire tray is inoculated in a single operation. After incubation, a magnification system is used to visualize the wells to determine the MIC of each agent. The MIC is read as the clear well in each row that contains the least amount of that antimicrobial agent.

Because of these and other automated advances in micro well dilution hardware and techniques, this method of susceptibility testing will undoubtedly become widely adopted by commercial laboratories in the future. The ability to conduct many tests quickly and accurately makes this method highly suitable for commercial use. However, the initial cost of these systems is currently so great that the volume of testing must be very large to offset the investment in equipment.

DETERMINATION OF MINIMUM BACTERIOCIDAL CONCENTRATION

MBC is determined by dilution methods. One accurate method involves the broth microdilution (tray) method. After determination of MIC values, the automatic inoculating apparatus is inserted into the wells containing broth and test bacteria, and an inoculum is passed to a blood agar plate. After incubation, the MBC is determined by noting the least amount of each antimicrobial agent that has no bacterial growth in the blood agar.

DISCUSSION

It is not necessary to routinely conduct susceptibility tests on all urinary bacterial isolates. In cases of canine urinary tract infections involving any one of the common bacterial species (*E. coli, Staphylococcus aureus, Proteus mirabilis, Streptococcus* spp., *Klebsiella pneumoniae,* and *Pseudomonas aeruginosa*), data are available that may be used to select an appropriate antimicrobial agent with at least an 80 per cent chance of cure, *provided that the species of the causative agent has been identified* (see the article that follows for additional information).

Susceptibility testing is mandatory (1) in cases of urinary tract infection in which two or more bacterial species are isolated simultaneously from the urine, (2) in instances in which a drug selected by methods mentioned previously has failed, and (3) in cases in which the bacteria causing the urinary tract infection are uncommon, or have unpredictable antimicrobial susceptibility.

SUPPLEMENTAL READING

Barry, A. L.: *The Antimicrobic Susceptibility Test: Principles and Practices.* Philadelphia: Lea & Febiger, 1976.
Bauer, A. W., Kirby, W. M. M., Sherris, J. C., and Turck, M.: Antibiotic susceptibility testing by a standardized disk method. Am. J. Clin. Pathol. 45:493, 1964.
Ericsson, H. M., and Sherris, J. C.: Antibiotic sensitivity testing. Acta Pathol. Microbiol. Scand. [B] 217:Suppl. 217:1, 1971.
Stamey, T. A.: Antimicrobial sensitivity testing. *In Urinary Infections.* Baltimore: Williams & Wilkins, 1972, pp. 31–53.

TREATMENT OF URINARY TRACT INFECTIONS WITH ANTIMICROBIAL AGENTS

GERALD V. LING, D.V.M.

Davis, California

Bacterial infection of the urinary tract is one of the most common infectious diseases in dogs but is rare in cats. Between 5 and 10 per cent of the canine patients seen in veterinary hospitals for any reason have a urinary tract infection. Unlike the signs of fever, malaise, back ache, increased frequency of urination, and so on that accompany urinary tract infections in women, dogs seldom have any clinical signs or physical findings that indicate to the owner or veterinarian that a urinary infection is present. Cats with dysuria, pollakiuria, and pink urine, which has been characterized as *feline urologic syndrome,* usually have bacteriologically sterile bladder urine. Therefore, the bulk of this article is related to dogs.

The consequences of urinary tract infections are

similar regardless of whether clinical signs are present. Pyelonephritis leading to scarring and renal failure is a major sequela to long-standing urinary tract infection. In addition, urinary tract infection caused by *Staphylococcus aureus* is an initiating factor that results in struvite urolithiasis in dogs. Urinary infections may spread to the prostate and other areas of the male and female reproductive systems and may cause infertility in both sexes. Extension of urinary tract infection to other parts of the body (septicemia) occurs occasionally for unknown reasons. Septicemia is a significant hazard when large doses of steroids are given to dogs with undiagnosed urinary tract infections. There are many reasons, therefore, to recognize and properly manage urinary tract infections in dogs. Because they are so common and because serious consequences of urinary infections can be prevented, use of proper procedures for diagnosis and management of these patients is essential.

DIAGNOSTIC METHODS

URINE COLLECTION AND HANDLING

Whenever urine is obtained for microbial culture or sediment examination, it should be collected in a manner that does not allow contamination of the specimen with bacteria from the lower urogenital tract. The urethra, prepuce, and vagina of dogs have resident microbial populations (bacteria, mycoplasma, yeasts, and so on) that vary with the species and numbers of organisms present. These organisms contaminate voided and catheterized urine specimens, since it is generally not possible to completely cleanse the external genitalia and the external urethral orifice before specimen collection. Therefore, it is often difficult to reliably distinguish between true bacteriuria and bacterial contamination if specimens for sediment examination or culture are obtained by catheterization or during micturition. Reliability of results is greatly enhanced by collection of the specimen by antepubic cystocentesis, since identification of any bacteria in specimens collected by this method constitutes firm evidence of urinary tract infection (see the supplemental reading list).

If urinalysis or culture is not conducted within 30 minutes following collection, urine specimens should be cooled to about 4°C within minutes after collection. Bacteria in urine may double their numbers as often as every 45 minutes if the specimen is allowed to remain at room temperature. Refrigeration temperatures prevent this *in vitro* event. False negative results (failure of bacteria to grow) may occur if the specimen is refrigerated for an extended period of time (12 to 24 hours or more, depending on the bacterial species present). Bacterial culture of the specimen, therefore, should be performed within six hours of collection if possible.

Diagnosis of urinary tract infection by urine sediment examination is based primarily on finding increased numbers of white blood cells and bacteria during examination of the sediment with the aid of the high dry or oil immersion lens of a microscope. Rod-shaped bacteria may be seen in unstained preparations of urine sediment if more than 10,000 bacteria/ml are present but are difficult to visualize consistently if their numbers are less than 10,000/ml. Cocci are difficult to visualize consistently if their numbers are less than 100,000/ml. It is important to recognize these two limitations, since about 25 per cent of all dogs with urinary tract infections have bacterial counts below these figures at the time of specimen collection.

An increased number of white blood cells in the sediment (more than three white blood cells per high dry microscopic field in urine collected by antepubic cystocentesis) strongly suggests bacteriuria. When bacteria, increased number of white blood cells, or both are seen in urine sediment, the bacteria can be cultured from about 90 per cent of such specimens.

Gram stains of smears of active sediment (visible bacteria and white blood cells) may add greatly to accumulated information. Differentiation of gram positive, gram negative, or gram mixed bacterial pathogens can aid in early selection (before culture results are available) of an antimicrobial agent.

URINARY MICROBIOLOGY

All species of bacteria commonly associated with canine urinary tract infections grow rapidly enough on standard culture media (blood agar and MacConkey agar) that recognizable colonies are present after overnight incubation at 37°C. In addition, common urinary pathogens (with few exceptions) can be recognized by characteristic changes produced after overnight growth on blood agar, MacConkey agar, or eosin–methylene blue (EMB) agar. Therefore, information that will aid in making a treatment decision (identification of the infecting organism) will often be available at this time. This is not true if differentiation between *E. coli*, *Klebsiella* spp., and *Enterobacter* spp. is necessary or in situations in which more than one infecting bacterial species is present (about 18 per cent of the time). One or more extra days and additional biochemical testing of the isolates may be necessary in these cases for the laboratory to be able to provide definitive information (see supplemental reading list).

It may not be possible to obtain reliable susceptibility test results to aid in selection of appropriate therapy. The information obtained from the Kirby-Bauer susceptibility test, available from most commercial laboratories, is of limited value, since only antibiotics that test in the sensitive (S) and intermediate (I) ranges may be considered appropriate choices. Drugs that test resistant (R) by this method may or may not actually be effective at easily attainable urine concentrations, since the test is standardized to blood concentrations.

It is generally accepted that urine concentrations of antimicrobial agents are more important than blood concentrations in the successful treatment of urinary tract infections. All of the antimicrobials commonly used in the treatment of urinary tract infections will be present in urine in active form at concentrations that may exceed up to 100 times their peak blood concentrations. The critical antimicrobial concentration in the treatment of any urinary tract infection is called the minimum inhibitory concentration (MIC), defined as the least amount of an antimicrobial agent that causes complete inhibition of growth of the infecting species or strain of bacteria under controlled and reproducible laboratory conditions. Understanding the relationship of bacterial MIC to the concentration of each antimicrobial agent in the urine is of prime importance, since it is the basis for effective use of drugs such as penicillin in the treatment of many gram negative infections (*E. coli, Proteus mirabilis,* and others) encountered in the urinary tract that are typically "resistant" to penicillin in other organs or tissues of the body.

If antimicrobial susceptibility test results that reflect high antimicrobial concentrations attainable in urine are not available, it is often possible to select an appropriate antimicrobial agent if the species of the infecting bacteria is known (Table 1).

SELECTION OF AN ANTIMICROBIAL AGENT

When planning treatment of urinary tract infections, one should choose an antimicrobial agent that (1) is easy for the client to administer, (2) has few (if any) undesirable or toxic side effects, (3) is relatively inexpensive, and (4) will result in urine concentrations that exceed the MIC for the infecting species or strain of bacteria at least fourfold. The drug should be administered frequently enough to maintain inhibitory urine concentrations (usually three times daily for oral antimicrobial agents) and long enough to rid the urinary tract of the infecting agent (usually 7 to 14 days).

Common bacterial species (those causing more than 3 per cent of the infections) associated with canine urinary tract infections and their predictable antimicrobial susceptibility, based on results of clinical trials in dogs, are summarized in Table 1. The MIC of oral penicillin G, ampicillin, and other penicillins for virtually all urinary streptococci and

Table 1. In Vivo *Susceptibility of Common Canine Urinary Tract Bacterial Pathogens to Certain Oral Antimicrobial Agents*

Approaching 100 Per Cent Susceptibility
  Staphylococcus spp. (penicillin)*
  Streptococcus spp. (penicillin)

About 80 Per Cent Susceptibility
  Escherichia coli (trimethoprim/sulfa)†
  Proteus mirabilis (penicillin)
  Pseudomonas aeruginosa (tetracycline)‡
  Klebsiella pneumoniae (cephalexin)§

*Penicillin G given orally at the rate of 110,000 U/kg (50,000 U/lb) in three divided doses daily. Ampicillin given orally at the rate of 77 mg/kg (35 mg/lb) in three divided doses daily.

†Tribrissen, Septra, or Bactrim given orally at the rate of 26.4 mg/kg (12 mg/lb) in two divided doses daily.

‡Tetracycline given orally at the rate of 55 mg/kg (25 mg/lb) in three divided doses daily.

§Keflex given orally at the rate of 30 mg/kg (13.6 mg/lb) in two divided doses daily.

staphylococci, including penicillinase-producing strains, is less than 10 μg/ml, whereas the mean eight-hour urine concentration of these agents is about 350 μg/ml at recommended urinary dosages. It may be assumed with almost 100 per cent confidence, therefore, that these antimicrobials will be effective in the treatment of urinary tract infections caused by *Streptococcus* spp. and *Staphylococcus* spp.

Approximately 80 per cent of urinary tract infections caused by *E. coli* may be treated successfully with oral trimethoprim-sulfa based on information obtained by testing the product against urinary isolates of *E. coli* and testing in dogs with urinary infections caused by *E. coli*. Using similar information, oral penicillin G or ampicillin may be used to successfully treat about 80 per cent of canine urinary tract infections caused by *Proteus mirabilis,* oral cephalexin may be used to successfully treat about 80 per cent of canine urinary tract infections caused by *Klebsiella pneumoniae,* and oral tetracycline may be used in the treatment of urinary tract infections caused by *Pseudomonas aeruginosa* with a success rate of about 80 per cent. The surprising success of oral tetracycline is due to the fact that the MIC of tetracycline for most canine urinary isolates of *Pseudomonas* spp. is less than 40 μg/ml, whereas the mean eight-hour urine concentration of tetracycline given orally at standard dosage to dogs is about 150 μg/ml.

Daily doses and recommended frequency of administration of penicillin G, ampicillin, trimethoprim-sulfa, cephalexin, and tetracycline are listed in Table 1. There are many other antimicrobial agents available for treatment of urinary tract infections in animals. These five drugs are mentioned specifically because they seem to offer the best chance of therapeutic success at the least cost to the client and the least risk to the patient and because clinical trials substantiating their efficacy have been conducted in dogs.

It may be tempting at times to initiate treatment by administering two or more antimicrobial agents simultaneously, especially when two or more causative bacterial species are isolated from the urine of a single animal. When two antimicrobials are indiscriminately administered simultaneously, the effect of the combination on the infecting bacterial population may be additive, synergistic, antagonistic, or one of indifference and may vary unpredictably with the antimicrobials administered, the bacterial species involved, and the site of infection in the body. Therefore, combining two or more antimicrobial agents without in-depth knowledge of their interaction in each specific set of circumstances for which therapy is being given is contraindicated. Mixtures of antimicrobial agents have been shown to be superior to a single agent on the basis of controlled clinical trials in only a few instances.

The use of aminoglycoside antimicrobials (e.g., gentamicin, tobramycin, and amikacin) should be limited to urinary tract infections that have persisted in spite of appropriate therapy with other antimicrobials or when two or more bacterial species with widely differing antimicrobial susceptibilities are present during a single episode.

MANAGEMENT OF URINARY TRACT INFECTIONS

SINGLE EPISODES

Since virtually all gram positive bacteria isolated from the urinary tract (*Streptococcus* spp. and *Staphylococcus* spp.) are susceptible to penicillin and many of the gram negative bacteria found there are susceptible to trimethoprim-sulfa, it may be possible to select an antimicrobial agent and begin therapy one to two days earlier than would be possible if one waited for the culture results. This practice is risky, however, especially when dealing with gram negative bacterial infections. Therefore, the treatment selected should be modified, if necessary, after culture (organism identification) and susceptibility test results are known.

After identification of the infecting bacteria, an appropriate antimicrobial agent may be selected on the basis of results of antimicrobial susceptibility tests or by using the information presented in Table 1. Most oral antimicrobial agents should be given in three daily doses to maintain effective drug concentrations in urine.

A urine specimen for bacterial culture should routinely be taken between the fourth and seventh days of therapy. If bacterial growth is not observed, the medication should be continued for a total of 14 days. A second follow-up urine culture should be conducted on a urine specimen collected two to four days after completion of the therapeutic course.

If growth of the same or a different species of bacteria is observed in a urine specimen taken between the fourth and seventh days of therapy, the treatment has failed and another antimicrobial agent must be substituted immediately, using a new susceptibility test as a guideline for selection. Culture of urine should then be conducted four to seven days after beginning the substitute antimicrobial and two to four days after completion of the therapeutic course.

Culture of all follow-up urine specimens in patients with urinary tract infection is strongly recommended over urine sediment examination for two reasons. First, if the numbers of infecting bacteria in a follow-up specimen are less than 10,000/ml, a false impression of cure may be given, since bacteria cannot usually be demonstrated in sediment examination if their numbers are below this figure. Second, the number of white blood cells may unpredictably decrease to normal during treatment of a urinary tract infection, even when the antimicrobial agent used is ineffective in eradicating the infecting organism. Therefore, examination of urine sediment is unreliable for assessment of success or failure of antimicrobial therapy of urinary tract infections.

About 18 per cent of canine urinary tract infections are associated with more than one bacterial species. In these situations, selection of an antimicrobial agent depends on the bacterial pathogens and their susceptibilities. For instance, if *E. coli* or *Proteus mirabilis* occurs in any combination with *Streptococcus* spp. or *Staphylococcus* spp. (a gram negative and a gram positive species), trimethoprim-sulfa is a logical choice. If *Streptococcus* spp. and *Staphylococcus* spp. are the associated organisms (two gram positive species), penicillin is a logical choice. If two gram negative species (e.g., *E. coli*, *Proteus mirabilis*, *Enterobacter* spp. or *Klebsiella pneumoniae*) occur together, trimethoprim-sulfa or cephalexin is the logical choice. Penicillin is a poor choice since only about 20 per cent of *Klebsiella pneumoniae* isolates are susceptible to penicillin at urine concentrations.

If the combination of infecting bacteria includes *Pseudomonas aeruginosa*, an effective oral antimicrobial may not be available. In this situation, two options are available: treat the non-*Pseudomonas* isolates with the most effective agent and then treat the *Pseudomonas* spp. isolate with tetracycline after the other isolate is eliminated, or use one of the injectable aminoglycoside antimicrobials (gentamicin, tobramycin, or amikacin). I favor the first option because of the risk of nephrotoxicity, higher cost, and inconvenience associated with the use of aminoglycosides.

Recurrent Urinary Tract Infections

Preliminary evidence indicates that recurrence of urinary tract infections in dogs is caused by bacterial reinfection (a different strain or species) rather than bacterial relapses (the same strain or species) in about 80 per cent of cases. When reinfection occurs only once or twice each year, administration of the appropriate oral antimicrobial agent for 7 to 14 days as described previously is the best approach to management. When reinfection occurs more than four times in a single year, long-term antimicrobial administration may be necessary to prevent reinfection.

Use of trimethoprim-sulfa or nitrofurantoin in dogs with histories of gram negative or gram mixed infections and penicillin G or ampicillin in dogs with histories of gram positive infections is effective in reducing the incidence of reinfection to about one-tenth its former frequency. The dosage given is about one-third of the total daily dose administered once daily at bedtime for six months. Urine specimens collected only by cystocentesis are cultured once each month. If bacteria cannot be cultured from urine collected during follow-up evaluation, the regimen should be continued unchanged. If bacteria are cultured from follow-up urine samples, the appropriate oral antimicrobial agent should be given three times daily as previously described for individual infections. If, at the end of two weeks of this type of therapy, urine is once again culture-negative, the nighttime regimen is resumed with monthly follow-ups for six months. At the end of six consecutive months of bacteria-free urine cultures, the nighttime antimicrobial therapy is discontinued. The majority of animals receiving this regimen have not had additional episodes of bacteriuria.

It is very important to prevent nighttime urination in dogs receiving antimicrobials at bedtime, since this regimen is only effective if a high concentration of drug is present during the entire nighttime sleep period. If the dog is permitted to urinate during the night, the post-void urine may have insufficient antimicrobial concentration to prevent colonization of the bladder wall by bacteria ascending the urinary tract. This regimen will not be effective, therefore, if the patient has continuous access to areas where it is allowed to urinate.

As noted above, follow-up urine specimens taken from these patients should be collected only by cystocentesis. Introduction of a urinary catheter in these patients, regardless of how carefully and aseptically the procedure is conducted, will introduce urethral bacterial contaminates that may colonize in the urothelium and initiate an infection in the bladder.

SUPPLEMENTAL READING

Ling, G. V.: Antepubic cystocentesis in the dog: An aseptic technique for routine collection of urine. Calif. Vet. 30:50, 1976.

Ling, G. V., Biberstein, E. L., and Hirsch, D. C.: Bacterial pathogens associated with urinary tract infections. Vet. Clin. North Am. 9:617, 1979.

Stamey, T. A., Fair, W. R., Timothy, M. M., Millar, M. A., Mihara, G., and Lowery, Y. C.: Serum versus urinary antimicrobial concentrations in cure of urinary tract infections. N. Engl. J. Med. 291:1159, 1974.

TREATMENT OF URINARY TRACT CANDIDIASIS

DAVID J. POLZIN, D.V.M.,
and JEFFREY S. KLAUSNER, D.V.M.

St. Paul, Minnesota

Candidial urinary tract infections are uncommon in dogs and cats. Candiduria (the presence of *Candida* organisms in urine) was detected in only 6 of 851 (0.71 per cent) canine and 1 of 326 (0.31 per cent) feline urine specimens in a recent study (Wooley and Blue, 1976). However, no information relating these results to clinical or laboratory evidence of urinary tract infection was reported.

Candida albicans and other *Candida* species are normal saprophytic inhabitants of the gastrointestinal tract in dogs, cats, and humans but are not normally present in the urinary tract. Studies in human patients have suggested that the patient's own intestinal flora is the most common source of urinary tract candidiasis. Infection may result from penetration of the intestinal wall and transport via lymphatic or hematogenous pathways to the kidneys (hematogenous infection), or fecal contamination via the urethra (ascending infection).

Candiduria may develop because conditions are

Table 1. *Factors Predisposing to Candiduria*

Increased intestinal *Candida* population
　Antibiotic administration
Decreased cellular defense mechanisms
　Administration of corticosteroids or immunosup-
　　pressive drugs (e.g., cyclophosphamide)
　Radiation therapy
　Underlying diseases that alter cellular immunity
　　(e.g., certain blood dyscrasias)
Impaired fungicidal properties of prostatic secretions
Local conditions in the urinary tract
　Diabetes mellitus
　Acid urine pH (optimum pH 5.1 to 6.4)
　Indwelling urinary catheters

favorable for growth of the fungus or because the patient's defense mechanisms are depressed. Several factors are known to predispose to candiduria in humans (Table 1). Diabetes mellitus, long-term use of antibiotics or corticosteroids, and indwelling urinary catheters have been associated with urinary candidiasis in dogs in our hospital.

Candiduria may be symptomatic or asymptomatic (Table 2). Symptomatic candiduria may be associated with signs of cystitis, pyelonephritis, or septicemia. The clinical signs of candidial cystitis and pyelonephritis are the same as those of bacterial cystitis and pyelonephritis. *Candida* septicemia may result from candidial urinary tract infection, particularly in immunodeficient patients. Normal cell-mediated immunity and polymorphonuclear neutrophilic phagocytic activity are important in preventing systemic candidiasis. Because the kidneys are the principal target organ in systemic candidiasis, *Candida* septicemia not originating from the urinary tract may induce candidial pyelonephritis and candiduria.

Symptomatic candiduria may also result from bezoar formation. Bezoars are aggregates of *Candida* organisms that form in the renal pelvis or urinary bladder. When located in the renal pelvis, bezoars may be associated with urinary tract obstruction, progressive deterioration of renal function, or acute anuria. Bezoars located in the bladder may be associated with pollakiuria.

Table 2. *Clinical Manifestations of Candiduria*

Symptomatic candiduria
　Classical symptoms
　　Cystitis
　　Pyelonephritis
　　Septicemia
　Bezoar formation
　　Progressive renal failure
　　Anuria
Asymptomatic Candiduria
　Spontaneous recovery
　Long-term persistence
　Symptomatic candiduria

The clinical significance of asymptomatic candiduria in dogs and cats is unknown. In humans, asymptomatic candiduria may persist for months to years, despite substantial pyuria, without causing discernible harm. It is usually associated with one or more predisposing factors (see Table 1) and often resolves spontaneously following removal of the predisposing factor. However, symptomatic infection may develop if the patient's general condition deteriorates as a result of some other disease process. We observed one dog in which asymptomatic candiduria spontaneously resolved after ten months of infection.

DIAGNOSIS

The diagnosis of candiduria is based on the results of urinalysis and urine culture. These laboratory findings must be interpreted in light of the clinical findings.

Urinalysis. Examination of urine sediment is important in the diagnosis of urinary tract candidiasis. Urine sediment examination may reveal *Candida* organisms, pyuria, and sometimes hematuria. *Candida* organisms usually appear as budding unicellular yeasts that measure about $3 \times 7\ \mu$, but they may also appear in a pseudomycelial form, measuring up to $600\ \mu$ in length.

When seen, yeasts are commonly considered to be contaminants. However, urinary tract candidiasis should be considered when yeasts are observed in serial urinalyses or in patients with (1) known predisposition to candiduria (see Table 1), (2) debilitating disease, or (3) bacteriologically "sterile" pyuria.

Pyuria may occur in patients with symptomatic or asymptomatic candiduria. Absence of pyuria does not assure that *Candida* is not a pathogen; fatal renal candidiasis has been observed in the absence of pyuria in humans. It has been proposed that pyuria may not occur in patients in which the *Candida* infection is explosive and body defenses are impaired.

Urine Culture. A definite diagnosis of candiduria is based on results of urine culture. Most common fungal and bacterial culture media, including Sabouraud's dextrose agar and blood agar, are saitsfactory for isolation of *Candida* species; however, media that contain cycloheximide inhibit growth of some species.

Unlike bacteriuria, the clinical significance of candiduria in humans cannot be reliably predicted by the number of colony-forming units per milliliter of urine. Although significant bacteriuria is defined as greater than 10^5 colony-forming units/ml of urine, fewer than 10^5 *Candida* organisms/ml of urine are commonly observed in clinically significant infections. Since the appearance of any *Candida* organisms is abnormal in a properly collected specimen, candiduria should be tentatively regarded as pathologic, regardless of the size of the colony count. This finding should be confirmed by culture of a subsequent sample, preferably obtained by cystocentesis. Because true candiduria may occur in low numbers, cystocentesis is usually required to differentiate true candiduria from contamination. Identification of *Candida* organisms on two properly collected serial urine specimens should be considered significant.

Because significant candiduria may be associated with low numbers of organisms, urine sediment cultures have been recommended to increase diagnostic sensitivity. Cultures are performed on sediment obtained by centrifugation of 10 ml of urine at 3000 revolutions per minute for three minutes. It is recommended that samples for urine sediment cultures be obtained by cystocentesis.

TREATMENT

A rational therapeutic approach for candiduria must be based on the patient's clinical history, physical examination, and laboratory findings. Because candiduria may be transient and benign, aggressive therapy should probably be reserved for those cases in which clinical evidence suggests that candiduria may be of pathologic significance.

Asymptomatic candiduria should be treated by correcting identifiable predisposing factors (see Table 1; e.g., cessation of antibiotic or corticosteroid administration, removal of indwelling urinary catheters) and by alkalinizing the urine. Alkalinization of urine is helpful because *Candida* grows best when urine pH is in the range of 5.1 to 6.4. Urine alkalinization may be accomplished by oral administration of sodium bicarbonate in a dose sufficient to increase urine pH to greater than 7.5. Five grains of sodium bicarbonate administered orally every eight hours may be used initially. Dosage should be increased until the desired urine pH is achieved.

A more aggressive therapeutic approach is indicated for patients with symptomatic candiduria and patients that are debilitated, have a grave underlying illness, or whose condition has suddenly deteriorated. In addition to correcting identifiable predisposing factors and alkalinizing the urine, treatment with 5-fluorocytosine (flucytosine, 5-FC; Ancobon*) should be initiated. Flucytosine should be administered orally at a dosage of 200 mg/kg/day in three or four daily doses. Flucytosine is an ideal drug for the treatment of candiduria because it can be given orally, is excreted in urine in the active form, and is of low toxicity. Toxic side effects include reversible bone marrow depression, mild hepatic toxicity, and dermatitis. Because excretion of 5-FC is almost entirely renal, toxicity is most likely to

occur when renal function is compromised. Dosage of 5-FC must be adjusted in patients with renal failure. The major disadvantage of 5-FC is resistance. Although resistance may be intrinsic, it usually develops after initiation of treatment, particularly when low doses of 5-FC are being given.

Amphotericin B is also effective in the treatment of *Candida* infections. However, it must be administered parenterally or as a local irrigant, is associated with substantial toxicity (primarily nephrotoxicity), and is not excreted in active form in the urine. Although some strains of *Candida albicans* have been resistant to amphotericin B, this is less of a problem than with 5-FC. Amphotericin B should be considered in patients with systemic candidiasis, candidial septicemia, or infections unresponsive to treatment with 5-FC. Amphotericin B is effective in the treatment of candiduria only when used as a local irrigant in the urinary tract. We have no experience with this method of treatment in dogs and cats. Amphotericin B and 5-FC appear to be synergistic when used in combination.

Response to treatment should be monitored by urine culture at weekly intervals. Treatment should be continued until two successive negative urine cultures are obtained. It has been recommended that urine sediment cultures be used to monitor response to treatment because of their greater sensitivity. As a general rule, patients with renal or systemic candidiasis should be treated for at least four to six weeks.

Acute onset of abdominal pain, oliguria, or anuria in patients with candiduria may suggest bezoar formation in the urinary tract. An intravenous urogram should be performed to rule out this possibility. If radiographic procedures support the diagnosis of bezoar formation, surgical removal should be considered.

PROGNOSIS

The prognosis for patients with asymptomatic candiduria appears to be good to excellent. Patients with renal or systemic candidiasis and candiduria have a guarded prognosis. Early detection and treatment are important in the successful management of these cases.

SUPPLEMENTAL READING

Michigan, S.: Genitourinary fungal infections. J. Urol. 116:390, 1976.
Schönebeck, J.: Studies on *Candida* infection of the urinary tract and on the antimycotic drug 5-fluorocytosine. Scand. J. Urol. Nephrol. Suppl. 11:7, 1972.
Stamey, T. A.: *Pathogenesis and Treatment of Urinary Tract Infection*, 2nd ed. Baltimore: Williams & Wilkins, 1981.
Wise, J. G., Goldberg, P., and Koznin, P. J.: Genitourinary candidiasis: Diagnosis and treatment. J. Urol. 116:778, 1976.
Wooley, R. E., and Blue, J. L.: Bacterial isolations from canine and feline urine. Mod. Vet. Pract. 57:535, 1976.

*Roche Laboratories, Nutley, NJ.

FELINE URINARY TRACT INFECTIONS

GEORGE E. LEES, D.V.M.,
College Station, Texas

and CARL A. OSBORNE, D.V.M.
St. Paul, Minnesota

Unlike the case in dogs and humans, bacterial infections are an uncommon cause of urinary tract disease in cats. Although inflammatory disorders of the bladder and urethra occur frequently in each of these species, bacteria play a prominent primary etiologic role only in the disorders of dogs and humans. In fact, simple (uncomplicated) bacterial cystitis characterized by dysuria, hematuria, pyuria, and bacteriuria ($\geq 10^5$ organisms/ml) is one of the most common causes of lower urinary tract inflammation in humans and dogs. Cats are commonly affected by lower urinary tract disease (so-called feline urologic syndrome) characterized by dysuria, hematuria, and, in male animals, urethral obstruction. However, the feline urologic syndrome (FUS) is so infrequently associated with pyuria and bacteriuria that neither can be considered characteristic of the condition. Bacterial infection is not an important primary etiologic factor in FUS. However, cats may develop bacterial urinary tract infection (UTI) as a complication of pre-existing urinary tract disease including FUS.

There are two plausible explanations for the infrequent occurrence of primary bacterial urinary tract infections in cats. First, UTI may be uncommon because cats have host defense mechanisms that are more effective in preventing UTI than those in dogs or humans. Second, UTI might occur in cats but remain undiagnosed because it often fails to produce the specific features that veterinarians have been trained to expect when UTI is present. This hypothesis implies that criteria that should be used to diagnose UTI in cats are different than those used for other species. There is evidence to support each of these hypotheses, but neither one has been proved. Further studies must be performed before meaningful generalities about the significance of bacterial infections in feline urinary tract disorders can be formulated.

ETIOPATHOGENESIS OF UTI

In most instances, bacteria that cause UTI ascend or are propelled into the bladder through the ure-
thra. Bacteria may infect the urinary tract via vascular channels or by extension from surrounding tissues, but infection by these routes is uncommon. Ascent of bacteria and their persistence in any part of the urinary tract except the distal urethra are prevented by urinary tract defense mechanisms. There are numerous specific components to this defense that operate synergistically to protect the urinary tract from colonization by bacteria. Normally these mechanisms are so effective that even gross bacterial contamination of the bladder will not result in UTI. However, when there is urinary tract disease, the associated compromise in defense mechanisms permits even a minor degree of bacterial contamination to cause UTI.

Lower urinary tract defenses consist primarily of (1) anatomical and functional components that produce unidirectional urine flow and complete emptying of the bladder at frequent intervals, (2) mucosal barriers and bacteriocidal actions, and (3) antibacterial properties of urine. In humans, the antimicrobial properties of urine are thought to be relatively unimportant, because human urine is typically an excellent medium for bacterial growth. However, cats usually excrete urine that appears to be a poor medium for bacterial growth. Characteristics of feline urine that have been hypothesized to inhibit bacterial growth include (1) high osmolality (some bacteria have limited tolerance to osmotic stress), (2) high concentrations of specific solutes (urea, organic acids, and so on) that have antibacterial action, and (3) acidity.

Once the urinary bladder is colonized by bacteria, integrity of the vesicoureteral junctions is an important factor protecting the kidneys from infection. In comparison with lower urinary tract defenses, renal medullary defense mechanisms are relatively ineffective. Thus, reflux of infected bladder urine to the renal pelvis is likely to produce renal infection.

Host urinary tract defenses against UTI are compromised during episodes of FUS, particularly in the aftermath of urethral obstruction. Cystitis and urethritis alter mucosal integrity, whereas urethral obstruction produces urine retention. Relief of ure-

1058

thral obstruction often requires catheterization, which may cause further tissue injury and/or propel bacteria to the bladder. Subsequently, urine retention may continue if micturition is impaired by persistent or recurrent urethral obstruction (partial or complete) or by detrusor hypotony resulting from overdistention. Use of indwelling catheters to maintain urine outflow and to keep the bladder empty is associated with an increased risk of catheter-induced trauma and bacterial invasion of the bladder. Postobstructive diuresis that may occur following relief of obstruction or that is induced with parenteral fluids may be associated with increased risk of infection because less concentrated urine is a more favorable medium for bacterial survival and growth. Finally, inflammation of the bladder wall can extend into the confluent tissues of the distal ureter and produce vesicoureteral junction incompetence, especially if forces generated in an effort to expel urine from the bladder are excessive (consult Vesicoureteral Reflux, page 1041, for further details).

The development of UTI is characterized by sequential phases. The first of these, the contamination phase, begins when bacteria arrive in any part of the urinary tract that is normally sterile. In most circumstances it is likely that contamination occurs with several types of organisms, but bacterial numbers are initially low. If local conditions are favorable, bacteria survive, grow, and initiate the colonization phase. Initially, colonization may involve only tissues of the urinary tract or urine, but ultimately both are usually involved. Colonization by a single type of bacteria usually occurs, but occasionally several species may be involved. Bacteria may multiply to produce large numbers in their new habitat, particularly in bladder urine, where they have the opportunity to multiply during urine storage prior to micturition. Bacteria will only multiply, however, if urine provides a favorable medium for their growth. To the extent that urine restricts the rate or magnitude of their growth, bacteria will be less abundant. It is even conceivable that bacteria that have succeeded in colonizing tissues of the urinary tract could be killed as they are shed into urine contained in the urinary space.

The final symptomatic phase of UTI occurs when inflammation develops in urinary tract tissues because of infection. Pain, altered patterns of micturition, and inflammatory debris in the urine (i.e., hematuria, pyuria, and proteinuria) characterize this phase. A word of caution: urinary tract inflammation has many potential causes other than bacterial infection.

Urinary tract infections do not always produce clinical signs of inflammation. Bacterial growth confined to urine may produce little or no inflammation in surrounding tissues. This phenomenon is called asymptomatic bacteriuria. It has been observed in humans and dogs but has not yet been documented in cats.

DIAGNOSIS OF UTI

Definitive diagnosis of UTI is based on isolation of bacteria from urine or tissue obtained from portions of the urinary tract that are normally sterile. Urine culture is the principal technique used for this purpose, but microscopic examination or bacteriologic culture of affected urinary tract tissue may also be considered.

Urine cultures must be properly performed and interpreted. Quantitative urine culture techniques should be used because the abundance of organisms found in a urine sample is of diagnostic value. Interpretation of urine culture results should include knowledge of the method of sample collection, clinical signs, results of urinalysis and other laboratory tests, medications being administered (particularly antibacterial agents), and the possibility of spurious results induced by *in vitro* changes in the sample before it was cultured.

Because the distal urethra normally contains bacteria, voided urine samples and those obtained by catheterization may contain bacteria even when bladder urine is sterile *in vivo*. In humans, the number of contaminating bacteria is consistently low ($\leq 10^3$ organisms/ml). However, in dogs (particularly females), urine samples that are carefully collected during voiding or by catheterization may contain large numbers of bacteria ($\geq 10^5$ organisms/ml) even though samples concomitantly obtained by cystocentesis are sterile. Although $\geq 10^5$ bacteria/ml of urine is a reliable index of UTI in humans, similar conclusions are not as consistently reliable for dogs.

There are no set guidelines for interpreting urine culture results for cats because there are few data regarding levels of bacteriuria to be expected in samples obtained by various means from normal animals. Some experimental studies of urine culture obtained from normal male cats by cystocentesis or by catheterization have been performed. All samples obtained by cystocentesis were sterile, as were 91 per cent of samples obtained by catheterization. Samples obtained by catheterization that were not sterile contained 10^3 to 10^4 organisms/ml. There are no reported data for urine samples obtained by any means from normal female cats or for voided urine samples obtained from male cats.

It has been suggested that cats with UTI often do not have high levels of bacteriuria (i.e., $\geq 10^5$ organisms/ml). Experimental studies of UTI in male cats following indwelling urethral catheterization and/or perineal urethrostomy have consistently shown that urine samples obtained from animals with bacteriuria usually contain 10^2 to 10^4 organisms/ml. Thus, the degree of bacteriuria associated with UTI in cats may often be similar to that produced by contamination of initially sterile urine samples collected from dogs or humans by voiding or catheterization.

Although bacteria isolated from urine obtained by cystocentesis are abnormal, caution must be used when interpreting the significance of a few organisms. Low levels of bacteriuria might represent the contamination phase of UTI; colonization of the urinary tract by the bacteria may or may not have occurred. Furthermore, detection of bacteria in urine removed from a cat with lower urinary tract disease does not necessarily prove that bacterial infection is the cause of the disease. Although it is important to eliminate the bacteria by administration of appropriate antimicrobial agents, the infection may be a secondary phenomenon.

Pyuria should arouse suspicion of UTI in cats, even though lack of pyuria does not rule out UTI. Results of experimental studies and empirical clinical observations indicate that pyuria ($\geq$ 8 WBC/HPF) is usually associated with bacteriuria in cats. In this situation, low numbers of bacteria are indicative of UTI, especially if the urinary sample was obtained by cystocentesis.

It is emphasized that lack of pyuria is not a reliable index of lack of UTI. Clinical and experimental studies have revealed that significant bacteriuria can occur in cats without pyuria. In fact, this situation occurs more often than does bacteriuria with pyuria. Because bacterial numbers are frequently low when pyuria is absent, diagnosis of an established infection is often questionable. Nonetheless, we recommend that appropriate antimicrobial agents be administered to such patients.

OCCURRENCE OF UTI

In the last 15 years no less than a dozen clinical investigations have encompassed microbiologic studies of urine samples obtained from cats with urinary tract disease, primarily FUS. Because most affected cats lacked bacteriuria, it has been generally accepted that FUS is not a primary bacterial disease. It is also apparent from these studies, however, that many cats with FUS do have bacteriuria. In some studies it has been difficult to discriminate between bacteriuria that might be spurious (i.e., due only to contamination) and bacteriuria that is abnormal. However, evaluation of these studies indicates that about 25 to 50 per cent of the cats with FUS have noteworthy bacteriuria. For example, samples obtained by cystocentesis contained bacteria in 29 and 55 per cent of the cats in two studies. Other studies using voided urine samples revealed $\geq 10^4$ bacteria/ml in 27, 15, and 0 per cent of the cats examined. A further 25 per cent of

cats in each of the two last-mentioned studies had $\leq 10^3$ bacteria/ml of urine. Additionally, 33 per cent of cats with cystic calculi and 43 per cent of cats scheduled for perineal urethrostomy had UTI.

Several experimental studies have revealed that indwelling urinary catheterization frequently induces bacteriuria in normal male cats. Cats with FUS are more likely to develop UTI as a result of indwelling catheters because of abnormalities in local host defense mechanisms. Clinical and experimental studies have also shown that cats frequently develop bacteriuria following perineal urethrostomy and that postoperative use of indwelling catheters is associated with increased risk of persistent infection.

On occasion, UTI has been diagnosed in cats even though urine cultures have not revealed bacteriuria. For example, a female cat had hematuria for three weeks. Although two preoperative urine cultures were negative, bladder tissue obtained by cystotomy yielded a pure culture of *E. coli*, and the hematuria subsided following administration of antibiotics. These observations suggest that bacteria may colonize urinary tract tissues in cats even though viable organisms are not found in the urine. In this situation, bacteria might not be shed into the urine or the urine might kill bacteria shed from adjacent tissues.

Feline UTI is usually caused by bacteria of the following genera: *Staphylococcus, Streptococcus, Escherichia, Proteus, Klebsiella, Enterobacter, Pseudomonas,* and *Pasteurella*. With the exception of *Pasteurella*, this assortment of bacteria also causes most UTI in dogs. In some studies, *E. coli* was found more often than any other type of bacteria, whereas in other studies staphylococci and streptococci were most commonly isolated from feline urine. Highly concentrated urine commonly produced by cats provides a plausible explanation for the preponderance of cocci in cats with UTI compared with dogs and humans.

TREATMENT OF UTI

The principles of therapy of UTI in cats are the same as those in other species. The propensity of cats to form highly concentrated urine makes attainment of effective levels of antimicrobial drugs in feline urine comparatively easy. Although data regarding the efficacy of specific antimicrobial drugs for particular pathogens causing UTI in cats are not available, it is likely that the general guidelines that have been developed for use in dogs would be appropriate for use in cats (consult Treatment of Urinary Tract Infections with Antimicrobial Agents, page 1051, and Feline Urologic Syndrome: Medical Therapy, page 1108, for additional details).

Results of bacterial culture and antimicrobial susceptibility tests provide the most reliable data base for selection and monitoring efficacy of antimicrobial agents (consult Antimicrobial Susceptibility Tests for Urinary Tract Pathogens, page 1048, for additional details). Prophylactic use of antimicrobial agents in cats with sterile urine or symptomatic use of antimicrobial agents in cats with clinical signs may be justified for several reasons. However, administration of an antibiotic does not assure prevention or cure of UTI. In one study, more than 40 per cent of cats that underwent perineal urethrostomies had UTI preoperatively. In another study, at least 55 per cent of cats with recurrent urethral obstructions developed UTI. Because the cats were previously given antibiotics, these results emphasize the fact that nonspecific antimicrobial therapy is frequently ineffective in cats with FUS.

It is emphasized that infections that develop or persist while antibiotics are being given are resistant to the drug being used. If an infection develops during concomitant use of an indwelling urinary catheter and an antibiotic, it is irrational to remove the catheter and continue use of the same antibiotic. In one experimental study, catheter-induced bacteriuria developed in 25 per cent of normal male cats given ampicillin during catheterization. All of the organisms were resistant to that drug. When prolonged use of an antibiotic (e.g., for two to four weeks) is contemplated, urine cultures should be used to verify that the drug has successfully prevented or eradicated bacteriuria.

SUPPLEMENTAL READING

Lees, G. E., Osborne, C. A., and Stevens, J. B.: Antibacterial properties of urine: Studies of feline urine specific gravity, osmolality, and pH. J. Am. Anim. Hosp. Assoc. 15:135, 1979.

Lees, G. E., Osborne, C. A., Stevens, J. B., and Ward, G. E.: Adverse effects of open indwelling urethral catheterization in clinically normal male cats. Am. J. Vet. Res. 42:825, 1981.

Smith, C. W., and Schiller, A. G.: Perineal urethrostomy in the cat: A retrospective study of complications. J. Am. Anim. Hosp. Assoc. 14:225, 1978.

Smith, C. W., Schiller, A. G., Smith, A. R., Wells, S. K., and Kissil, M.: Effects of indwelling urinary catheters in male cats. J. Am. Anim. Hosp. Assoc. 17:427, 1981.

ANALYSIS OF CANINE AND FELINE UROLITHS

CARL A. OSBORNE, D.V.M.,
JEFFREY S. KLAUSNER, D.V.M.,
St. Paul, Minnesota

and CHRIS W. CLINTON, M.T.
Houston, Texas

OVERVIEW

Uroliths are polycrystalline concretions that typically contain greater than 95 per cent organic or inorganic crystalloids and less than 5 per cent organic matrix (weight versus weight ratio). They may also contain a number of minor constituents. A variety of different types of uroliths may occur in dogs and cats. Uroliths may be named according to mineral composition (Table 1), location (nephroliths, renoliths, ureteroliths, cystoliths, vesical calculi, urethroliths), or shape (smooth, faceted, pyramidal, laminated, mulberry, jackstone, staghorn, and so on).

The most common mineral types of calculi encountered in dogs are magnesium ammonium phosphate, ammonium urate, calcium oxalate, and cystine. Less common types of calculi encountered in dogs include calcium phosphate, silica, carbonate, xanthine, tetracycline, and matrix uroliths. The most common types of calculi encountered in cats include magnesium ammonium phosphate, calcium phosphate, calcium oxalate, ammonium urate, and uric acid. Matrix uroliths occur more frequently in cats than in dogs. To date, uroliths composed primarily of cystine or silica have not been reported in cats.

Trace elements including iron, copper, zinc, tin, lead, and aluminum have been identified in human uroliths. It is logical to suspect that they may also occur in canine and feline uroliths. These elements appear to be incorporated into calculi by adsorption during growth. They do not appear to play an important role in the initiation or growth of calculi.

Table 1.   *Crystalline Substances That May Be Detected in Uroliths*

Chemical Name	Crystal Name	Formula
Oxalates		
Calcium oxalate monohydrate	Whewellite	$CaC_2O_4 \cdot H_2O$
Calcium oxalate dihydrate	Weddellite	$CaC_2O_4 \cdot 2H_2O$
Phosphates		
β-tricalcium phosphate (calcium ortho- phosphate)	Whitlockite	$\beta\text{-}Ca_3(PO_4)_2$
Carbonate-apatite	Carbonate-apatite	$Ca_{10}(PO_4 \cdot CO_3 \cdot OH)_6 \, (OH)_2$
Calcium hydrogen phosphate dihydrate	Brushite	$Ca \, HPO_4 \cdot 2H_2O$
Calcium phosphate	Hydroxyapatite	$Ca_{10}(PO_4)_6 \, (OH)_2$
Magnesium ammonium phosphate hexa- hydrate	Struvite	$Mg \, NH_4 \, PO_4 \cdot 6H_2O$
Magnesium hydrogen phosphate trihy- drate*	Newberyite	$Mg \, HPO_4 \cdot 3H_2O$
Uric Acid and Urates		
Anhydrous uric acid	Same	$C_5 \, H_4 \, N_4 \, O_3$
Uric acid dihydrate	Same	$C_5 \, H_4 \, N_4 \, O_3 \cdot 2H_2O$
Ammonium acid urate	Same	$C_5 \, H_3 \, N_4 \, O_3 \cdot NH_4$
Sodium acid urate monohydrate	Same	$C_5 \, H_3 \, N_4 \, O_3 \, Na \cdot H_2O$
Cystine	Same	$(SCH_2CHNH_2COOH)_2$
Silicone Dioxide	Same	$Si \, O_2$
Xanthine	Same	$C_5 \, H_4 \, N_4 \, O_2$

*Not a primary constituent; forms as a result of decomposition of struvite.

Knowledge of the actual frequency with which various types of minerals and metabolites occur in uroliths of dogs and cats has been severely hampered by widespread use of relatively insensitive qualitative methods of urolith analysis.

Urolithiasis should not be thought of as a single disease, but rather as a sequela of one or more underlying abnormalities. Although a particular mineral usually predominates, the mineral composition of calculi is frequently mixed. On occasion the center of a urolith may be composed of one type of crystalloid (e.g., cystine), whereas outer layers are composed of a different crystalloid (especially struvite). Detection, treatment, and prevention of the causes underlying urolithiasis are dependent on knowledge of the composition and structure of uroliths.

METHODS OF UROLITH ANALYSIS

A variety of methods have been used to determine the composition of uroliths including gross appearance, crystalluria, radiographic appearance, qualitative analysis, quantitative analysis, and urolith culture. Of these, quantitative analysis provides the most definitive diagnostic, prognostic, and therapeutic information. With the exception of qualitative chemical analysis, information gained by other methods of evaluation may also be of clinical value.

GROSS APPEARANCE

COLOR

Following removal of surface debris and blood, most uroliths, including struvite, are white, cream,

or light yellow in color. Cystine and urate stones are often light yellow or light brown. Oxalate stones are often white or cream colored. The yellow color of calculi may be associated with urochrome pigment in urine.

SHAPE

The manner in which crystals aggregate determines the basic shape of calculi. Because some calculogenic crystalloids have a characteristic mode of deposition (so-called habit), the mineral composition of calculi can sometimes be inferred from their shape. Under no circumstances, however, should the shape of calculi be used as a substitute for appropriate analyses to determine their mineral composition.

Uroliths may be round, elliptical, wafer-like, pyramidal, jackstonelike, or cylindrical or they may assume the shape of the lumen in which they were formed. Many uroliths are basically spherical in shape, implying more or less uniform deposition or accumulation of calculogenic material around their circumference. When calculi become of sufficient size to restrict or prevent motion, they may become faceted as a result of rapid growth on surfaces not in contact with neighboring calculi.

Rapidly growing uroliths, especially those composed of struvite, may form a cast of the lumen in which they were formed. In humans, rapidly growing renal calculi sometimes assume the configuration of the multipyramidal renal pelvis. They are commonly referred to as branched or staghorn calculi. Because the renal pelvis of dogs and cats is unipyramidal rather than multipyramidal like that of humans, true staghorn calculi do not develop in canine and feline kidneys. Rapidly growing canine and feline calculi may assume the shape of funnels, mushrooms, doorknobs, or umbrellas, however. On occasion such calculi may also have surface projections corresponding to renal pelvic diverticula.

Struvite may assume a wide variety of shapes but in dogs are commonly round, elliptical, or pyramidal. In cats, struvite crystoliths are often wafer-like in shape. Struvite uroliths often contain a greater quantity of matrix than other types of calculi. On occasion, gelatinous-crystalline accumulations or sludge-like deposits may occur in patients with urinary tract infections caused by urease-producing bacteria.

Canine cystine uroliths are usually small and round. Urate uroliths are usually round or elliptical but may assume a variety of shapes including funnel (renal pelvis), jackstone, and wafer-like (feline cystolith). Oxalate uroliths frequently have a rough, jagged, quartz-like appearance. They may form mulberry shapes or jackstones. Silica uroliths in dogs are typically, but not invariably, jackstone in shape.

NUCLEI AND LAMINATIONS

Examination of cross sections of calculi often reveals a nucleus and adjacent peripheral laminations. Nuclei of calculi are focal points (or cores) that differ in appearance from more peripheral portions of the stone. They are usually, but not invariably, located in the center of uroliths. Nuclei may be of crystalline composition, or they may be composed of foreign material, tissue debris, blood clots, bacteria, and so on. The mineral composition of crystalline nuclei may be identical or different from the remainder of the calculus. Nuclei surrounded by well-defined layers (or lamellae) of solid material suggest that they represent an early phase of stone evolution. Centrally located nuclei suggest that the urolith was freely accessible to urine from all sides and that growth proceeded at a similar rate on all sides.

Laminated calculi are common and may represent (1) alternating bands of different mineral types, (2) periods during which stone growth occurred without interruption, and (3) alternating periods of precipitation of minerals and gel. Although a difference in appearance between two consecutive layers should prompt suspicion of a difference in composition, this is not always the case.

RADIOGRAPHIC CHARACTERISTICS

OBJECTIVE

The primary objective of radiographic evaluation of patients suspected of having uroliths is to determine the site, number, density, and shape of calculi. Once urolithiasis has been confirmed, radiographic

evaluation also is an important technique to detect predisposing abnormalities.

APPEARANCE

The radiographic appearance of uroliths is dependent on their size and mineral composition. Very small calculi may not be visualized. Most canine and feline uroliths have varying degrees of radiodensity and therefore can be detected by survey abdominal radiography (Table 2). Oxalate, phosphate, and silica calculi are typically, but not invariably, more radiodense than cystine and urate calculi. This may be related to their calcium content. Urate uroliths may be radiolucent but usually are radiodense. Because of significant variation, the radiodensity of uroliths is not a reliable index of mineral composition.

Uroliths must be differentiated from (1) nephrocalcinosis associated with dystrophic or metastatic calcification of the renal parenchyma, (2) radiodense medications or ingesta in the gastrointestinal system, (3) calcified mesenteric lymph nodes, (4) osseous metaplasia of transitional epithelium or mineralization of a neoplasm, and (5) radiodensities in the gallbladder (uncommon in dogs and cats). Calcifications of the renal parenchyma will typically be in the proximity of, but not within, the renal pelvis. Radiodense calculi within the excretory pathway may disappear or become radiolucent following excretion of radiopaque contrast agents. Radiodense objects outside the excretory pathway remain radiodense.

In our experience, radiolucent uroliths are very uncommon in dogs and cats. Uric acid uroliths of humans are typically radiolucent. However, in our experience, most (but not all) ammonium acid urate uroliths of dogs are radiodense. This may be related to the presence of a variable quantity of phosphates

Table 2. Radiographic Characteristics of Uroliths Commonly Occurring in Dogs and Cats

Mineral Type	Degree of Radiopacity	Shape
Cystine	+ to + +	Smooth; usually small; round to oval
Oxalate	+ + + +	Usually rough; round to oval
Phosphate (struvite)	+ + to + + + +	Smooth; round or faceted; sometimes assume shape of renal pelvis, ureter, bladder, or urethra; sometimes laminated
Phosphate (apatite)	+ + + +	Smooth; round or faceted
Urate	0 to + +	Smooth; round or oval; sometimes jackstone
Silica	+ + to + + + +	Typically jackstone

in urate uroliths of dogs. Matrix uroliths may be radiolucent. They have not been commonly recognized in dogs but do occur in cats. Blood clots may be mistaken for radiolucent uroliths.

Calculi that appear radiodense by survey radiography may appear to be radiolucent when evaluated by positive contrast radiography. This is related to the fact that many calculi are more radiodense than body tissue but less radiodense than the contrast material. A diagnosis of radiolucent stones should be based on their radiodensity compared with body tissues and not their radiodensity compared with positive contrast material.

CRYSTALLURIA

Crystalluria is a common, but not invariable, phenomenon in patients with uroliths. Identification of some crystals (especially cystine and sometimes ammonium urate or calcium oxalate) may provide a clue as to the type of urolith present. However, identification of urine crystals should not be relied upon as definitive identification of the mineral composition of uroliths.

Crystals in urine may be normal or abnormal; therefore, caution must be used in interpreting their significance. Crystal formation in urine is influenced by several variables including (1) *in vitro* temperature, (2) *in vivo* and *in vitro* pH, (3) solubility, (4) concentration of the crystalloid, and (5) administration of medications. When interpreting the significance of crystalluria, a fresh sample must be evaluated, since *in vitro* changes that occur following collection may significantly change the spectrum of crystals observed. Ideally, fresh samples should be examined when they are at body temperature rather than room or refrigeration temperature.

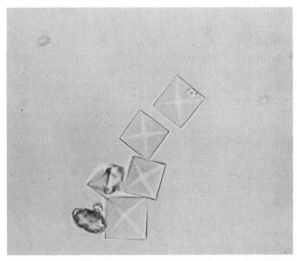

Figure 2. Calcium oxalate dihydrate crystals. Unstained × 160 = original magnification.

Cystine crystalluria is not a normal event. Cystine uroliths are usually associated with cystinuria; however, not all patients with cystine crystalluria have cystine uroliths. Cystine crystals have a characteristic hexagon (benzene ring) shape and are most often present in concentrated acid urine (Fig. 1). Addition of glacial acetic acid followed by refrigeration and centrifugation may aid in detection of typical crystals in alkaline urine samples.

Calcium oxalate dihydrate crystals have a characteristic octahedral or envelope shape (Fig. 2).

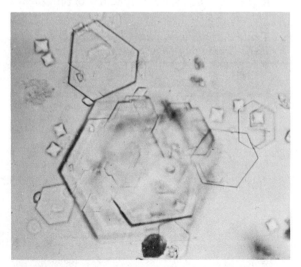

Figure 1. Cystine crystals surrounded by white cells and occasional calcium oxalate dihydrate crystals. Unstained × 100 = original magnification.

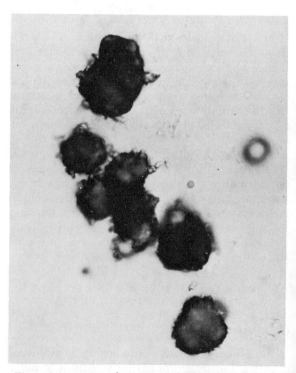

Figure 3. Ammonium biurate crystals (thornapple form). Unstained × 40 = original magnification.

They may occur in normal or abnormal urine. In humans with oxalate urolithiasis, there is a tendency for oxalate crystals to occur in increased numbers and for them to aggregate. There have been no quantitative studies of crystalluria or crystal aggregation in dogs or cats with urolithiasis.

Struvite crystals may be observed in (1) normal dogs and cats, (2) dogs and cats with struvite urolithiasis, and (3) dogs and cats with non-struvite uroliths. Ammonium urate crystals (Fig. 3) may be observed in (1) normal dogs and cats, (2) dogs and cats with urate uroliths, and (3) dogs and cats with nonurate uroliths. They have been commonly observed in dogs with portal vascular anomalies and concomitant ammonium urate urolithiasis (see Urate Calculi Associated with Portovascular Anomalies, page 1073).

ANALYSIS OF CALCULI

OVERVIEW

Following removal of uroliths, compare the number removed with the number detected by radiography. If there are too many calculi (as determined by radiography) to count, post-surgical radiography is indicated to detect uroliths that have been inadvertently allowed to remain in the urinary tract. Immediate detection of calculi remaining in the urinary tract following surgery is important, since it has prognostic significance. If uroliths inadvertently missed during surgery to remove them are not detected for several weeks following surgery, it may be erroneously assumed that the patient is highly predisposed to recurrent urolithiasis.

Record the location of the uroliths removed from the urinary tract in addition to their size, shape, color, and consistency. Save all uroliths in a container (preferably a sterile one) for future analysis. One or more uroliths may be placed into a container of 10 per cent buffered formalin if microscopic examination is desired.

Because many uroliths contain more than one mineral component, it is important to examine representative portions of them. The mineral composition of crystalline nuclei may be identical or different from the remainder of calculi. The nuclei of uroliths should be analyzed separately from outer zones when possible, since the underlying cause of its presence may be suggested by the mineral composition of the nuclei.

QUALITATIVE ANALYSIS

We do not recommend analysis of uroliths by single qualitative chemical analysis. The major disadvantage of this procedure is that only some of the chemical radicals and ions can be detected. In addition, the proportions of the different chemical

Table 3. *Comparison of Results of Qualitative and Quantitative Analyses of a Urolith Removed from the Urinary Bladder of an Adult Female Miniature Schnauzer*

Qualitative Analysis	Quantitative Analysis	
Magnesium	Struvite	80%
Ammonium	Apatite	10%
Phosphate	Ammonium urate	10%
Calcium		
Urate		

constituents in the urolith cannot be quantified. One kit commonly used by veterinarians and veterinary laboratories is the Oxford Stone Analysis Set.* In our hands, this chemical kit is unreliable in the accurate detection of the composition of mixed uroliths (Table 3). It is not designed to detect infrequently occurring uroliths, including those composed of silica or xanthine. The kit is also unreliable in consistently detecting calcium in calculi.

QUANTITATIVE ANALYSIS

In contrast to chemical methods of analysis, physical methods have proved to be far superior in identification of crystalline substances. They also permit differentiation of various subgroups of minerals (e.g., calcium oxalate monohydrate and calcium oxalate dihydrate or uric acid and ammonium acid urate) and allow semiquantitative determinations of various mineral components (see Table 3). Physical methods commonly used by laboratories that specialize in quantitative urolith analysis† include combinations of polarizing light microscopy, x-ray diffractometry, infrared spectroscopy, and thermogravimetry. Some laboratories are also equipped to perform elemental analysis with an energy-dispersive type of x-ray microanalyzer (EDX). On occasion, chemical methods of analysis and paper chromatography may be used to supplement information provided by the physical methods mentioned.

We recommend that veterinarians utilize the services provided by laboratories equipped to provide quantitative urolith analysis. At this time, most (but not all) veterinary clinical pathology laboratories are not equipped to provide quantitative urolith analysis. Caution must be used to avoid irrevocable loss of uroliths by unreliable qualitative chemical studies. If qualitative studies are performed, representative uroliths should be saved for subsequent quantitative analysis. Although the cost of routine

---

*Oxford Laboratories, San Mateo, CA.

†Urolithiasis Laboratory, P.O. Box 25475, Houston, TX; Louis C. Herring and Co., Orlando, FL; Beck Analytical Services, Bloomington, IN.

quantitative urolith analysis is about double that of routine qualitative analysis (approximately $10 versus $20), it is minute compared with the costs caused by mismanagement based on erroneous results.

UROLITH CULTURE

Bacteria harbored inside uroliths are not always the same as those present in urine. Bacteria detected within uroliths probably represent those present at the time the stone was formed and may serve as a source of recurrent urinary tract infection. Bacteria may remain viable within the uroliths for long periods. In a pilot study, we were able to culture viable staphylococci from struvite uroliths removed from a miniature schnauzer up to three months following surgery. When all the uroliths cannot be removed from the patient, knowledge of the type of associated bacterial pathogens and their antimicrobial susceptibility may be of therapeutic significance.

We use the following procedure to sterilize the outside of uroliths so that their inside may be cultured.

1. Place uroliths in an alcoholic solution of 3 per cent iodine for two hours.

2. Wash uroliths with 1000 ml of sterile physiologic saline solution.

3. Culture the last portion of the saline in contact with the surface of the urolith by inoculating 1 ml into 9 ml of trypticase soy broth.

4. Crush the uroliths with a sterile mortar and pestle and add a small quantity of sterile physiologic saline solution to the crushed crystalline material.

5. Inoculate 1 ml of the saline-calculi suspension into 9 ml of trypticase soy broth.

6. Incubate the broth tubes at 37° C for 48 hours.

7. Make appropriate subcultures utilizing blood agar and MacConkey agar plates.

Detection of bacterial growth in the saline that contacted the surface of the uroliths indicates inadequate sterilization and invalidates the results of culture of the crushed calculi. Bacterial growth in saline mixed with crushed calculi, but not in saline in contact with the surface of calculi, indicates that the organisms were within the calculi. Antimicrobial susceptibility tests may be performed on bacteria isolated from the inside of calculi, especially if they are different from those isolated from urine.

SUPPPLEMENTAL READING

Dyer, R., and Nordin, B. E. C.: Urinary crystals and their relation to stone formation. Nature 215:751, 1967.

Kennoki, F., Mizuhira, V., Konjiki, T., and Kawai, H.: Elemental analysis of urinary tract calculi using an electron microscope with electron probe x-ray microanalyzer. Acta Histochem. Cytochem. 11:387, 1978.

Otnes, B., and Montgomery, O.: Method and reliability of crystallographic stone analysis. Invest. Urol. 17:314, 1980.

Sutor, D. J.: Crystallographic analysis of urinary calculi. In Williams, D. I., and Chisholm, G. D. (eds.): Scientific Foundations Of Urology, Vol. 1. Renal Disorders, Infections and Calculi. London: William Heinemann Medical Books, 1976.

MEDICAL DISSOLUTION AND PREVENTION OF CANINE STRUVITE UROLITHS

CARL A. OSBORNE, D.V.M.,
JEFFREY S. KLAUSNER, D.V.M.,
St. Paul, Minnesota

SHEHU ABDULLAHI, D.V.M.,
Zaria, Nigeria

and DONALD R. KRAWIEC, D.V.M.
Urbana, Illinois

CHARACTERISTICS OF STRUVITE UROLITHS

Struvite uroliths are predominantly composed of magnesium ammonium phosphate (Table 1). They are found more frequently in the urinary tract of dogs than are other types of uroliths. Struvite uroliths also have been called MAP (magnesium ammonium phosphate) calculi, phosphate calculi, "infection stones," "urease stones," and triple phosphate stones. Triple phosphate is a misnomer that originated because chemical analyses of uroliths revealed calcium, magnesium, ammonium, and phosphate (three cations and one anion). The name is incorrect, since struvite does not contain calcium. Struvite uroliths frequently contain calcium phos-

Table 1. *Characteristics of Canine Struvite Uroliths*

Chemical name
  Magnesium ammonium phosphate hexahydrate
Crystal name
  Struvite
Formula
  $MgNH_4PO_4 \cdot 6H_2O$
Variations in composition
  Struvite only
  Struvite and apatite (calcium phosphate)
  Nucleus of different mineral surrounded by struvite
Physical characteristics
  Color: Usually white, cream, or light yellow
  Shape: Variable; commonly round, elliptic, or pyramidal; rapidly growing uroliths with a large quantity of matrix may form a cast of the lumen (renal pelvis, ureter, bladder, urethra) in which they are formed
  Number: Single or multiple
  Nuclei and laminations: Common
  Density: May be very soft if they contain a large quantity of matrix; sometimes dense and hard to cut; radiodense compared with nonskeletal tissue on survey radiographs
  Location: Usually located in the urinary bladder; occasionally in the bladder and urethra; uncommonly in the renal pelvis; less commonly in the renal pelvis and ureter
Predisposing factors
  Urinary tract infections with urease-producing bacteria
  Alkaline urine pH
  Genetic
  Unidentified causes
Characteristics of affected canine patients
  Mean age: 6 years (range < 1 to > 15 years)
  Especially common in miniature schnauzers, dachshunds, poodles, Scottish terriers, beagles, Pekingese, and Welsh corgis; any breed may be affected
  More common in females (60 per cent) than males (40 per cent)

phate (apatite), however, and may contain calcium carbonate.

ETIOPATHOGENESIS

OVERVIEW

Urine must become supersaturated with magnesium ammonium phosphate before struvite uroliths can form. Several factors appear to play a role in supersaturation of urine with struvite, including bacterial urinary tract infections, alkaline urine, and genetics. Of these factors, urinary tract infections appear to be most important in dogs.

BACTERIAL URINARY TRACT INFECTIONS

The solubility of struvite decreases in alkaline urine. Conversion of urea to ammonia as a result of bacterial urease appears to play an important role in causing urine to become supersaturated with magnesium ammonium phosphate as well as with calcium phosphate and carbonate-apatite crystals. Urease produced by bacteria catalyzes the formation of ammonia (NH_3), carbon dioxide (CO_2), and, subsequently, carbonate (CO_3). Hydroxyl (OH^-) and ammonium (NH_4^+) ions are then produced from hydrolysis of ammonia. The results of these reactions include (1) alkalinization of urine, (2) increased availability of ammonium ions for formation of struvite crystals, and (3) an increase in the concentration of phosphate ion ($PO_4^{\equiv}$) because of increased dissociation of phosphorus. Both urea and urease are required for alkalinization, supersaturation, and subsequent precipitation of struvite and apatite crystals. Because of the importance of urease in the etiopathogenesis of struvite uroliths, the name "urease stones" has been proposed.

Staphylococci and *Proteus* spp. are both potent urease producers. For reasons that are unexplained, staphylococci are far more commonly associated with struvite uroliths in dogs than *Proteus* spp., whereas *Proteus* spp. are most commonly associated with struvite uroliths in humans. Evaluation of struvite uroliths removed from dogs revealed that staphylococci produce phosphatase in addition to urease. Bacterial phosphatase might increase the concentration of inorganic phosphorus by action on organic phosphates. Although other organisms such as *Klebsiella* spp. and *Pseudomonas* spp. have the potential to produce varying quantities of urease, they are not commonly associated with initiation of struvite urolith formation. Likewise, *Escherichia coli* organisms are not associated with initiation of struvite uroliths because they rarely produce urease.

Infection of male or female dogs with urease-producing bacteria, primarily staphylococci, precedes the development of struvite uroliths. In one study, cystic calculi were detected by abdominal survey radiography approximately two to eight weeks following infection of the urinary tract. Staphylococci have been cultured from the inside of canine struvite uroliths, suggesting their presence at the time of urolith formation. In contrast, bacteria have been uncommonly cultured from the inside of nonstruvite uroliths. After formation of struvite uroliths as a result of staphylococcal urinary tract infection, the bacterial flora of urine may change. The change in bacterial flora may be associated with damage to local host defense mechanisms by uroliths, iatrogenic infection induced by urinary catheters, or administration of antimicrobial agents.

A small percentage of dogs with struvite urolithiasis have sterile urine. In some of these cases, however, bacteria have been isolated from the inside of calculi. This observation indicates that bacterial infection of the urinary tract may undergo spontaneous remission after initiating urolith formation in some patients.

In contrast to struvite uroliths, bacterial infection of the urinary tract is not a consistent finding in dogs with nonstruvite uroliths (e.g., ammonium urate, calcium oxalate, cystine, silica). When infection does occur in association with these so-called metabolic uroliths, it is a sequela rather than a predisposing cause of urolith formation. If by chance staphylococci are the cause of the secondary urinary tract infection, however, layers of struvite may form around a nucleus composed of the metabolic calculus.

ALKALINE URINE

Factors that produce persistently alkaline urine decrease the solubility of struvite. It is doubtful that alkaline urine per se will cause struvite urolithiasis, however. Alkaline urine appears to be only a predisposing cause of struvite urolith formation.

In addition to bacterial urease, factors that may produce reduced acidity or inappropriate alkalinity of urine include medications (such as sodium bicarbonate and sodium lactate) and disorders associated with impaired ability to secrete hydrogen ion in urine (i.e., renal tubular acidosis). Although cells lining the gastrointestinal tract are capable of producing urease, this enzyme apparently cannot be produced by uroepithelium.

GENETIC FACTORS

The high incidence of struvite uroliths in some breeds such as miniature schnauzers suggests a familial tendency. We hypothesize that susceptible miniature schnauzers inherit some abnormality of local host defenses of the urinary tract that increases their susceptibility to urinary tract infections. Hereditary factors thought to be associated with inbreeding have been reported to increase the incidence of struvite uroliths in beagles.

OTHER FACTORS

Abnormal urinary excretion of minerals as a result of enhanced glomerular filtration, reduced tubular reabsorption, or enhanced tubular secretion does not appear to play a role in the initiation and formation of struvite uroliths. As yet there are no data to support the theory that dietary factors play a specific role in the etiopathogenesis of struvite urolithiasis. As will be discussed, however, dietary factors play an important role in the management of struvite uroliths. Metabolic and anatomic abnormalities may play an indirect role in the formation

of struvite uroliths by predisposing to urinary tract infections.

On occasion we have encountered dogs in which urine and the inside of struvite uroliths have been sterile. Bacteriologically sterile urine and struvite uroliths have been encountered much more frequently in cats (see "Feline Urolithiasis," page 1076). The significance of these observations and their relationship to the hypothesis that struvite uroliths are initiated by bacterial infection are unknown.

DIAGNOSIS

Uroliths are usually suspected on the basis of typical findings obtained by history and physical examination. Urinalyses, quantitative urine culture, and radiography often are required to confirm urolithiasis and to determine if uroliths are associated with concomitant disorders of the urinary system. Since most struvite uroliths in dogs occur as sequelae to urinary tract infections and since urinary tract infections occur as sequelae to abnormalities in local or systemic host defense mechanisms, appropriate effort should be directed toward defining the underlying problem.

A definitive diagnosis of magnesium ammonium phosphate urolithiasis is dependent on an analysis of the mineral composition of calculi (see preceding article for further details).

MANAGEMENT OF STRUVITE UROLITHIASIS

OVERVIEW

Therapy of struvite urolithiasis encompasses (1) relief of obstruction to urine outflow when necessary, (2) elimination of existing calculi, (3) eradication or control of urinary tract infections, and (4) prevention of recurrence of uroliths. As with all forms of therapy, cautious and careful judgment is in order. The unpredictable and erratic rate at which canine uroliths form, grow, recur following removal, and undergo dissolution mandates carefully designed and controlled experimental trials before a particular regimen of therapy is judged to be of benefit. The following recommendations should not be used as a standardized approach to treatment, since no two patients have identical therapeutic needs. Within the guidelines outlined herein, individualization of therapy is essential.

Textbooks of veterinary surgery and reference materials provide detailed information on surgical and nonsurgical methods of re-establishing urine outflow (see Nonsurgical Removal of Urethral Calculi from Female Dogs, page 1081).

MEDICAL MANAGEMENT

INDICATIONS

Circumstances occasionally preclude surgical removal of struvite uroliths, including recurrence of calculi following repeated surgical procedures to remove them, factors that enhance the adverse consequences of general anesthesia or surgery, and situations in which owners will not consent to surgical therapy but will consider medical therapy. Medical management that would induce struvite urolith dissolution or minimize further urolith growth is also of value when calculi or fragments of calculi remain within the urinary tract following surgery. The fact that the underlying cause may persist despite surgery is also of significance.

The results of several experimental and clinical investigations support the feasibility of dissolution of struvite uroliths by nonsurgical methods. To reduce the concentration of specific calculogenic crystalloids in urine, knowledge of the composition of uroliths is important. When uroliths are not available for analysis and consideration is being given to medical therapy, one may be forced to make an educated guess about their composition (Table 2).

OBJECTIVES

The objectives of medical management of struvite uroliths are to arrest further urolith growth and/or promote urolith dissolution by correcting or controlling underlying abnormalities. For therapy to be effective it must induce undersaturation of urine with calculogenic crystalloids by (1) increasing the solubility of crystalloids in urine, (2) increasing the volume of urine in which crystalloids are dissolved or suspended, and (3) reducing the quantity of calculogenic crystalloids in urine.

INCREASING SOLUBILITY OF CRYSTALLOIDS IN URINE

Because acidification of urine increases the solubility of struvite, it is an important therapeutic goal in the medical management of struvite urolithiasis. The dosage of urine acidifiers should be titrated for each patient on the basis of urine pH. The pH of the first voided morning sample is least likely to be affected by post-prandial alkaline tide. However, if the pH of urine obtained a few hours after eating is acidic, it is likely that the urine will be acidic throughout the entire day. The most reliable data may be obtained by periodically monitoring pH throughout the day. Ideally, urine acidifiers should be administered three to four times per day to maintain a consistently acid environment within the

Table 2. *Factors That May Aid in Guesstimation of Mineral Composition of Uroliths*

Radiographic density and physical characteristics of uroliths
Urine pH
    Struvite and apatite uroliths: usually alkaline
    Ammonium urate uroliths: variable
    Cystine uroliths: acid
    Calcium oxalate uroliths: variable
    Silica uroliths: variable
Identification of crystals in urine sediment
Type of bacteria, if any, isolated from urine
    Urease-producing bacteria, especially staphylococci, are commonly associated with struvite uroliths
    Urinary tract infections often are absent in patients with calcium oxalate, cystine, ammonium urate, and silica uroliths
    Calcium oxalate, cystine, ammonium urate, and silica uroliths may predispose patients to urinary tract infections; if infections are caused by urease-producing bacteria, struvite may precipitate around them
Serum chemistry evaluation
    Hypercalcemia may be associated with calcium-containing uroliths
    Hyperuricemia may be associated with urate uroliths
Breed of dog and history of occurrence of uroliths in patient's ancestors or littermates
Analysis of uroliths fortuitously passed and collected during micturition

urinary tract (see Urinary Acidifiers, page 1095, for further information).

INCREASING VOLUME OF URINE

Diuresis induced by augmenting water consumption appears to be a logical way to decrease the urine concentration of struvite and other calculogenic substances. Depending on the size of the patient, the quantity of urine produced, the status of the cardiovascular system, and the composition of the diet, we recommend oral administration of 0.5 to 10 gm sodium chloride/day to stimulate thirst (obviously contraindicated in patients with congestive heart failure). It is desirable to encourage water consumption throughout the day. The success of this procedure mandates the availability of drinking water at all times. Alternatively, water, gravy, or other liquids can be mashed into food.

A satisfactory compensatory increase in urine volume is indicated by the formation of urine with a specific gravity < 1.030. Provided that administration of sodium chloride is effective in augmenting water consumption and the formation of less concentrated urine, we recommend that it be continued indefinitely, especially for patients with recurrent urolithiasis. Sodium chloride–induced diuresis should only be discontinued if it is certain that the underlying cause of urolithiasis has been eliminated.

ROLE OF AHA IN REDUCING CALCULOGENIC CRYSTALLOIDS IN URINE

Studies of a urease inhibitor, acetohydroxamic acid (AHA; Urostat*), in dogs with infection-induced struvite urolithiasis indicate that the drug is of value in the medical management of this disorder. AHA is rapidly and completely absorbed from the gastrointestinal tract of dogs and is excreted and concentrated in urine. When given orally at pharmacologic doses, AHA retards alkalinization of urine caused by growth of urease-producing bacteria. Its urease-inhibiting activity is effective in the urine pH range of 5 to 9 but is most effective at pH 7. AHA appears to have a dose-related bacteriostatic effect against gram positive and gram negative bacteria and may potentiate the antimicrobial effect of antibiotics.

Experimental studies performed at the University of Minnesota revealed that struvite uroliths experimentally induced in dogs were prevented from further growth or underwent dissolution following oral administration of AHA at a dosage of 100 mg/kg/day divided into two doses. The dogs had normal renal function. Unfortunately, administration of the drug at a dosage sufficient to induce dissolution of uroliths (100 mg/kg/day) resulted in a mild hemolytic anemia (mean PCV 37 per cent compared with a pretreatment value of 47 per cent). The anemia rapidly underwent amelioration when the daily dosage of AHA was reduced from 100 to 25 mg/kg/day. Although urolith growth was retarded at this dosage, dissolution did not occur. Similar results were obtained when AHA was administered at a dosage of 50 and 75 mg/kg/day. Studies in progress to evaluate

*Mission Pharmaceutical Company, San Antonio, TX.

the efficacy of AHA in causing stone dissolution when combined with antimicrobial agents and/or calculolytic diets have revealed that these combinations substantially reduce the time required to cause litholysis.

ROLE OF CALCULOLYTIC DIETS IN REDUCING CALCULOGENIC CRYSTALLOIDS IN URINE

Knowledge that inhibition of bacterial urease with AHA was effective in inhibiting canine struvite urolith growth and in some instances induced struvite urolith dissolution led to the hypothesis that reduction of the urine concentration of urea (the substrate of urease) would provide similar results. To test this hypothesis, a calculolytic diet (S/D†) was formulated that contained a reduced quantity of high-quality protein (1.6 per cent) and reduced quantities of phosphorus (0.048 per cent) and magnesium (0.006 per cent). The diet was supplemented with salt to stimulate thirst and induce compensatory polyuria.

This calculolytic diet was found to be highly effective in inducing struvite urolith dissolution in experimental dogs despite persistent infection with urease-producing bacteria. The uroliths underwent dissolution in about 3.5 months (range 8 to 20 weeks). When fed to dogs with experimental sterile struvite urolithiasis, all uroliths underwent dissolution within one month.

When a combination of the calculolytic diet and antimicrobial agents was given to dogs with naturally occurring urease-positive urinary tract infections and uroliths presumed to be composed of struvite, similar results were obtained (Figs. 1 and

†Hills Division, Riviana Foods, Inc., Topeka, KS.

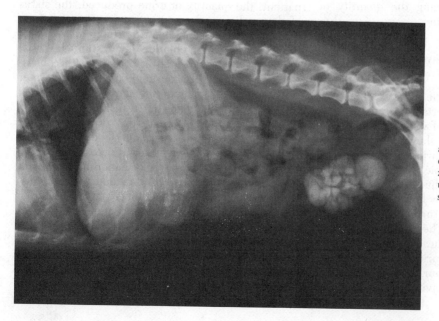

Figure 1. Lateral view of a survey abdominal radiograph of a 12-year-old spayed female miniature schnauzer with numerous urinary bladder uroliths likely to be composed of struvite.

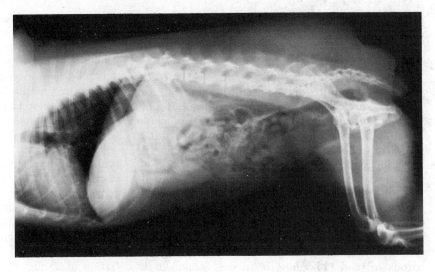

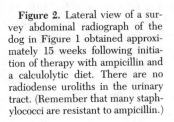

Figure 2. Lateral view of a survey abdominal radiograph of the dog in Figure 1 obtained approximately 15 weeks following initiation of therapy with ampicillin and a calculolytic diet. There are no radiodense uroliths in the urinary tract. (Remember that many staphylococci are resistant to ampicillin.)

2). A combination of calculolytic diet, antimicrobial agent, and AHA given to dogs with experimentally induced staphylococcal urinary tract infection and struvite urolithiasis induced stone dissolution within six weeks.

Because calculolytic diets stimulate thirst and promote diuresis, owners should be informed that dogs with uroliths located in the urinary bladder may develop pollakiuria for a short time following initiation of dietary therapy. The pollakiuria will subside as the infection is controlled and the uroliths decrease in size.

CURRENT RECOMMENDATIONS FOR MEDICAL DISSOLUTION OF CANINE STRUVITE UROLITHS

ADULT DOGS WITH URINARY TRACT INFECTION AND UROLITHS

1. Eradicate or control urinary tract infections with appropriate antimicrobial therapy (consult other articles in this section). Maintain antimicrobial therapy during and for two to three weeks following urolith dissolution.

2. Initiate therapy with calculolytic diets. No other food should be fed to the patient. Compliance with dietary recommendations is suggested by a reduction in the serum concentration of urea nitrogen (usually below 10 mg/dl). Maintain affected animals on the diet for one month following disappearance of uroliths as detected by survey radiography. Avoid retrograde radiographic studies requiring catheterization.

3. Induce diuresis only if polyuria does not occur while the patient is consuming the calculolytic diet.

4. Administer urine acidifiers if antimicrobial agents and calculolytic diets do not result in formation of acid urine.

5. Administer AHA (25 mg/kg per day divided into two doses) to patients with persistent urease-producing bacteriuria despite use of antimicrobial agents and calculolytic diets.

ADULT DOGS WITH STERILE STRUVITE UROLITHS

1. Follow the same procedure recommended for dogs with concomitant urinary tract infections and uroliths but do not administer antimicrobial agents or AHA.

2. Periodically culture urine samples obtained by cystocentesis to detect secondary bacterial urinary tract infections. If they develop, eliminate them with appropriate antimicrobial agents.

IMMATURE DOGS WITH STRUVITE UROLITHS

1. Calculolytic diets have not been evaluated in normal growing pups or in a large number of immature dogs with struvite urolithiasis. Although they will induce struvite urolith dissolution, if consumed for prolonged periods these low-protein diets would probably impair normal growth. Pending further studies, we recommend that they be avoided unless the alternative is no treatment or euthanasia.

2. AHA has not been evaluated in growing pups.

3. Pending further studies, surgical removal of uroliths provides the safest means of removing uroliths from immature dogs.

SURGICAL MANAGEMENT

Studies are currently in progress at the University of Minnesota to compare the effects of various combinations of calculolytic diets, AHA, and antimicrobial agents in inducing struvite urolith dissolution. Our goal is to reduce the time required to induce dissolution of struvite uroliths by medical management. A successful outcome of these studies will allow noninvasive elimination of canine struvite uroliths.

Despite the development of effective medical regimens to induce dissolution of struvite uroliths in dogs, surgical intervention will continue to play a role in some patients. Surgical candidates include those with obstruction to urine outflow that cannot be corrected by nonsurgical techniques and patients with anatomic defects of the urogenital tract that predispose to urinary tract infection. Eradication or control of infections of the urinary tract with urease-producing bacteria is the most important factor in preventing recurrence of most struvite uroliths. Development of urinary tract infections is dependent on the balance between infectious agents (analogous to seeds) and host resistance (analogous to soil). In order for microbial "seeds" to grow, a suitable "soil" must be present. Although pathogenic bacteria must gain access to the urinary tract to induce infection, entrance of bacteria into the urinary tract is not synonymous with infection. Current evidence indicates that host defense mechanisms must be transiently or persistently abnormal for bacterial colonization of the urinary tract to occur. Although antimicrobial agents remain the cornerstone of therapy, the status of host defense mechanisms appears to be the most important factor in the pathogenesis of urinary tract infections. Permanent eradication of infection often is impossible unless the abnormality in host defense mechanisms is identified and eliminated. Examples of surgical disorders that predispose to urinary tract infections by altering local host defense mechanisms include diverticula of the bladder, strictures that impede urine outflow, metabolic uroliths (silica, ammonium urate, calcium oxalate, and so on) that damage the mucosal lining of the urinary tract, and neoplasms that damage the mucosal lining and/or impede urine outflow. Consult other appropriate articles in this section for additional information.

PREVENTION OF RECURRENCE OF STRUVITE UROLITHIASIS

Because of the frequent (21 per cent) but unpredictable rate of recurrence of struvite uroliths in dogs, long-term success is usually dependent on effective prophylactic therapy. A persistent state of undersaturation of urine with struvite is the goal of preventive therapy.

Eradication or control of infections of the urinary tract with urease-producing bacteria is the most important factor in preventing recurrence of most struvite uroliths. Consult appropriate articles in this section for additional information.

In addition to administration of antimicrobial agents, appropriate use of urine acidifiers and induction of diuresis by stimulating thirst should be considered.

Studies to evaluate the effectiveness of AHA in the prevention of struvite urolithiasis in dogs with persistent urinary tract infection with urease-producing bacteria have been encouraging. Administration of 25 mg AHA/kg/day to dogs with urinary bladder foreign bodies (zinc discs) and experimentally induced urease-positive staphylococcal urinary tract infections has been effective in preventing urolith formation in most dogs and minimizing the rate of urolith growth in others.

In light of the effectiveness of diets in inducing struvite urolith dissolution, dietary modification to prevent recurrence of uroliths would appear to be both logical and feasible. However, further studies must be performed to evaluate the long-term effects of low-protein calculolytic diets in dogs before reliable recommendations can be established.

SUPPLEMENTAL READING

Kasper, L. V., Poole, C. M., and Norris, W. P.: Incidence of struvite urinary calculi in two ancestral lines of beagles. Lab. Animal Sci. 28:545, 1978.

Klausner, J. S., Osborne, C. A., O'Leary, T. P., Gebhart, R. N., and Griffith, D. P.: Struvite urolithiasis in a litter of miniature schnauzer dogs. Am. J. Vet. Res. 40:712, 1980.

Klausner, J. S., Osborne, C. A., O'Leary, T. P., Muscoplat, C. M., and Griffith, D. P.: Experimental induction of struvite uroliths in miniature schnauzer and beagle dogs. Invest. Urol. 18:127, 1980.

Krawiec, D. R., Osborne, C. A., Leininger, J. R., and Griffith, D. P.: Effect of acetohydroxamic acid on dissolution of canine struvite uroliths. Am. J. Vet. Res., in press.

Osborne, C. A., and Klausner, J. S.: War on canine urolithiasis: problems and solutions. Proceedings of the 45th Annual Meeting of the American Animal Hospital Association, South Bend, IN, 1978.

Osborne, C. A., Klausner, J. S., Krawiec, D. R., and Griffith, D. P.: Canine struvite urolithiasis: problems and their dissolution. J.A.V.M.A. 1979:239, 1981.

Osborne, C. A., et al.: Medical dissolution of canine struvite uroliths. Minn. Vet. 22:14, 1982.

URATE CALCULI ASSOCIATED WITH PORTAL VASCULAR ANOMALIES

ROBERT M. HARDY, D.V.M.,
and JEFFREY S. KLAUSNER, D.V.M.

St. Paul, Minnesota

Numerous reports of congenital portal vascular anomalies in both dogs and cats have appeared since 1974. This disorder is one of the most fascinating clinical entities in all of internal medicine. Each month it seems a different clinical syndrome secondary to hepatic vascular shunts is reported. Because the spectrum of disease induced by these anomalies is very diverse, clinicians must be constantly alert to avoid missing portal systemic shunts (PSS) in clinical practice. Congenital shunts between the portal and major systemic veins divert blood from the intestinal tract away from hepatic parenchyma and into the systemic circulation. Diversion of portal blood around or through (patent ductus venosus) the liver leads to hepatic atrophy. The severity of clinical signs depends on the volume of blood shunted and the location of the shunting vessels.

HISTORY AND PHYSICAL FINDINGS

Clinical signs in dogs with PSS are highly variable, but all result from hepatic encephalopathy or the consequences of progressive hepatic functional impairment. In many cases the clinical signs have an episodic nature, being present for a few hours or a day or two, the animal then appearing to "recover" for a variable period of time. The association of clinical signs with eating, particularly high-protein meals, is a helpful but inconsistent diagnostic sign. The majority of dogs with PSS have been diagnosed under one year of age, but congenital anomalies of the portal vascular system have been first diagnosed in dogs over eight years of age. No breed or sex predisposition has been identified. Many dogs have difficulty gaining weight and are stunted, depressed or weak, and in poor physical condition. One term used to describe these animals is "chronic poor doer."

Gastrointestinal signs are often noted but usually are mild. These include vomiting, diarrhea, and anorexia. Central nervous system involvement may be the best diagnostic clue for the clinician. When present, CNS signs are almost pathognomonic for these anomalies. Particularly bizarre behavioral changes or dementia characterized by hysteria, unpredictable bouts of aggression, staggering, head pressing, circling or pacing, amaurotic (cortical) blindness, or coma should put PSS high on a differential diagnosis list. Grand mal seizures and intermittent ataxia or incoordination have also been reported. Signs of less localizing value include polydipsia and polyuria, ascites, and anesthetic/tranquilizer intolerance.

Physical examination of these animals is usually not indicative of the underlying problem. The most severely affected dogs are stunted, thin to the point of cachexia, and may have ascites. These signs are not exclusively indicative of hepatic involvement, however.

Recurrent urinary calculi is one additional sign of PSS (Maretta et al., 1981). Signs referable to lower urinary tract disease (i.e., dysuria, pollakiuria, and hematuria) may also be present. In a few cases, urinary tract signs were the primary reason for the physical examination. Occasionally, solitary or multiple cystic calculi may be palpated in dogs with PSS. It is particularly important to note that many dogs with urate uroliths associated with PSS were several years old when the hepatic disorder was first identified, and several dogs had undergone multiple surgeries for calculi removal before hepatic disease was recognized.

A review of ten reported cases of urinary calculi in dogs with PSS (Barrett et al., 1976; Campbell et al., 1980; Ewing et al, 1974; Maretta et al., 1981) plus an additional four cases observed at the University of Minnesota indicates that all the calculi have been composed primarily of ammonium urate or ammonium magnesium phosphate (Table 1). Because of the metabolic derangements associated with PSS, such a finding would be expected.

URATE UROLITHS—AN OVERVIEW

Urinary calculi containing uric acid or its major salt, ammonium urate, occur infrequently in the dog. Urate calculi comprise approximately 5 per

Table 1. *Clinical, Radiographic, and Laboratory Data of 14 Dogs with Congenital Portal Vascular Anomalies and Urinary Calculi*

Age (yrs)	Sex	Breed	Clinical Signs	Location of Calculi			Radiographic Appearance	Calculi Composition	Reference
				Kidney	Bladder	Urethra			
0.9	M	Miniature schnauzer*	Recurrent cystic calculi, dysuria, seizure in hospital	-	+	+	Opaque	Ammonium urate, ammonium magnesium phosphate, uric acid	Maretta et al., 1981
4	F	Pekingese*	Hepatic encephalopathy, cortical signs	-	+	+	Opaque	Ammonium urate	Maretta et al., 1981
8	M	Pekingese	Weight loss, diarrhea, polydipsia, polyuria, weakness	+	-	-	Opaque	Ammonium magnesium phosphate	Maretta et al., 1981
3	F	Yorkshire terrier	Hematuria, ataxia, head tremor	-	+	-	Opaque	Uric acid, ammonium magnesium phosphate	Maretta et al., 1981
2.5	F	Yorkshire terrier	Intermittent stupor, responsive to oral dextrose	+	+	-	Opaque	Uric acid, ammonium magnesium phosphate	Maretta et al., 1981
3	M	Miniature poodle	Ataxia, weakness	-	+	+	Radiolucent	Uric acid	Maretta et al., 1981
0.5	M	Miniature schnauzer	Polyuria, polydipsia, lethargy, vomiting, ataxia, disoriented	+	+	-	?	Ammonium urate	Barrett et al., 1981
?	?	?	Not reported	+†	++†	++	?	Ammonium urate	Ewing et al., 1974
?	?	?	Not reported	+†	++†	++	?	Ammonium urate	Ewing et al., 1974
2	M	Old English sheepdog	Anorexia, weakness, vomiting	-	++†	-	?	Ammonium urate	Campbell et al., 1980
9	M	Miniature poodle	Dysuria	-	-	+	Opaque	Uric acid, ammonium magnesium phosphate	Univ. of MN
5	M	Yorkshire terrier*	Dysuria, urethral obstruction	-	+	+	Opaque	Ammonium urate	Univ. of MN
1.2	F	Yorkshire terrier*	Encephalopathy and dysuria, hematuria	+	+	-	Opaque	Ammonium urate	Univ. of MN
1	F	Miniature schnauzer	Hematuria	+	+	-	Opaque	Ammonium urate, magnesium ammonium phosphate, calcium apatite	Univ. of MN

*Multiple surgeries for removal of calculi.

†Heavy deposits of aggregated crystals identified at necropsy.

cent of all canine uroliths (range 2 to 18 per cent) (Osborne and Klausner, 1978). They are frequently found in combination with ammonium magnesium phosphate. Calculi may be located in the kidney, bladder, and/or urethra in a given dog. In 90 to 95 per cent of reported cases calculi were in the bladder or urethra, although renal calculi may have been present but overlooked in some cases. The Dalmatian is the most common breed with reported urate calculi. However, at least ten other breeds have been identified with urate uroliths. Males predominate over females, probably owing to the high frequency of urethral obstruction in male dogs with small urate uroliths. Factors considered to predispose dogs to urate calculi include increased urinary excretion of uric acid, a negative water balance, which promotes supersaturation of urine with uric acid, and urine pH.

ETIOPATHOGENESIS

Uric acid is the end-product of purine metabolism and has limited solubility in urine. In dogs, uric acid is oxidized by the intrahepatic enzyme uricase to allantoin and then excreted in urine. Allantoin is a much more soluble compound than uric acid.

Dalmatians have a significantly reduced hepatic oxidation of uric acid to allantoin despite normal concentrations of hepatic uricase. It has been hypothesized that a membrane transport defect impairing hepatocellular uptake of uric acid is responsible for the reduced allantoin formation. Serum uric acid concentrations for Dalmatians are consistently elevated, i.e., 2 to 4 mg/dl, and urinary excretion of uric acid is massively increased over that of non-Dalmatians (i.e., 400 to 600 mg/24 hr in Dalmatians versus 10 to 60 mg/24 hr in non-Dalmatians).

Urate uroliths in dogs are composed primarily of ammonium urate, in contrast to humans in whom uric acid calculi predominate. The high ammonia excretion of the canine coupled with the very low solubility of ammonium urate probably accounts for its prevalence in dogs. The solubility of ammonium urate calculi is less pH dependent than uric acid calculi, which are much more soluble in alkaline than acid urine.

The predisposition for dogs with congenital PSS to develop ammonium urate calculi is presumably due to a number of factors. Hepatic encephalopathy secondary to congenital PSS is typically associated with elevated blood ammonia concentrations. Although confirmatory quantification of 24-hour urinary ammonia excretion has not been reported, one would expect urinary ammonia concentrations to reflect blood levels. Increased urinary ammonia would favor the formation of ammonium urate uroliths. In addition, severe hepatic atrophy and/or portal shunting is likely to impair the ability of the liver to convert circulating uric acid to allantoin for secretion in urine. This is supported by consistent elevations in serum uric acid concentrations in these dogs. Uric acid levels in 13 dogs with PSS evaluated at the University of Minnesota were increased (i.e., > 1.0 mg/dl, range 1.2 to 4.0). Increased serum concentrations of uric acid would be expected to result in an increase in renal excretion and thus increased urinary concentrations. No information regarding urinary uric acid concentrations in dogs with PSS is available, however.

DIAGNOSIS

The diagnosis of urate uroliths is based on data obtained from the history, physical exam, and survey and/or contrast radiographs of the urinary tract. The majority of the urate calculi identified in dogs with congenital PSS have been radiopaque and were identified on survey radiographs of the abdomen. Because these calculi are of lesser radiographic density than struvite uroliths, good radiographic detail is essential for their visualization. Retrograde or intravenous positive contrast radiography may be necessary to identify some calculi, especially those located in the kidney. Ultimately, quantitative or qualitative analysis of the calculi following their removal is necessary to determine their mineral composition.

THERAPY

Traditional therapy of urate uroliths usually involves a combination of medical and surgical approaches. Qualitative and/or quantitative analysis of all urinary calculi is essential for optimal medical management. Because many of the stones found in dogs with PSS were composed of both ammonium urate and ammonium magnesium phosphate, the urate component may be overlooked and the dogs treated as if they were uncomplicated struvite formers. Medical therapy involves dietary changes, drugs to reduce uric acid excretion, changing urine pH, enhancing production of dilute urine, and controlling urinary tract infections. Attempts to reduce the purine intake of dogs by feeding them an all-vegetable diet have not been successful in reducing the incidence of urate uroliths in Dalmatians.

Allopurinol (Zyloprim*) is an effective drug for reducing the urinary excretion of uric acid. Allopurinol is a synthetic isomer of isoxanthine, which inhibits the hepatic conversion of hypoxanthine to xanthine and xanthine to uric acid. Utilizing allopurinol to reduce the urinary concentration of uric acid has been reported to significantly reduce the recurrence of urate uroliths in Dalmatians. No

---

*Burroughs Wellcome Co., Research Triangle Park, NC.

reports of its use in dogs with PSS and urate uroliths have appeared.

Adjusting urine pH is primarily of value in dogs with uroliths composed principally of uric acid. Alkalinizing urine to a pH range of 6.5 to 7.0 significantly enhances the solubility of uric acid. Altering urine pH has a minimal effect on ammonium urate solubility, however. Augmenting water intake to induce the formation of dilute urine should reduce the concentration of crystalloids in urine and make conditions necessary for calculus formation less optimal. Sodium chloride given in divided doses of 0.5 to 10 gm/day will induce increased water intake and diuresis. The urine specific gravity should be maintained below 1.030. Adequate supplies of fresh water must be available at all times. In some cases urinary tract infections may be identified in dogs with urate calculi. They are considered secondary to the presence of the calculi and are treated with appropriate antibiotics based on culture and sensitivity information.

Surgical therapy involves removing all calculi within the urinary tract.

Medical therapy for dogs with urate uroliths and PSS is a complex problem. Because of our recent awareness of the incidence of urate uroliths in non-Dalmatian dogs with PSS, we are of the opinion that *all* non-Dalmatians with ammonium urate calculi should be evaluated for PSS. We see relatively few urate uroliths in our clinical practice. Of the last four non-Dalmatians with urate uroliths we have seen, all proved to have congenital PSS (see Table 1). Two of these dogs had had multiple surgeries for calculi. Since metabolic derangements associated with the hepatic disease are likely to be responsible for the urate urolith formation, surgical ligation of identified anomalous vessels should be considered. In one of our patients with renal and cystic calculi, the renal calculus dissolved over a six-month period following shunt ligation. During the same time the cystic calculus remained the same size and therefore was removed three months following shunt surgery. Many non-Dalmatian dogs with recurrent urate calculi have no other typical PSS signs of hepatic encephalopathy. Although these cases represent diagnostic challenges, the ability to prevent recurrent urate calculi is critically dependent on identification of predisposing metabolic abnormalities (hepatic atrophy).

REFERENCES

Barrett, R. E., DeLahunta, A., Roenick, W. J., Hoffer, R. E., and Coons F. H.: Four cases of congenital portacaval shunt in the dog. J. Small Anim. Pract. 17:71, 1976.

Campbell, T. M., Lording, P. M., Wrigley, R. H., and Lavelle, R. B.: Portal vein anomaly and hepatic encephalopathy in three dogs. Aust Vet. J. 56:593, 1980.

Ewing, E. O., Suter, P. F., and Baily, C. S.: Hepatic insufficiency associated with congenital anomalies of the portal vein in dogs J.A.A.H.A. 10:463, 1974.

Maretta, S. M., Pask, A. J., Greene, R. W. and Liu, S. K.: Urinary calculi associated with portosystemic shunts in six dogs. J.A.V.M.A 178:133, 1981.

Osborne, C. A., and Klausner, J. S.: War on canine arolithiasis: Problems and solutions. Scientific Proceedings of the 45th Annual Meeting of the American Animal Hospital Association. 569, 1978.

FELINE UROLITHIASIS

CARL A. OSBORNE, D.V.M.,
GARY R. JOHNSTON, D.V.M.,
St. Paul, Minnesota

and SHEHU ABDULLAHI, D.V.M.
Zaria, Nigeria

FELINE URETHRAL PLUGS

Although urethral obstruction with plugs presumably composed primarily of struvite has been reported to occur in 1 to 10 per cent of all male cats, the composition of most plugs appears to be dissimilar to struvite uroliths in other species and struvite uroliths in cats. Urethral plugs appear to lack a definite structural organization. Most are thought to contain varying quantities of proteinaceous material, cellular debris, and crystals. The general consensus of opinion is that the crystals in most plugs are composed of struvite, although there have been very few documented studies of quantitative evaluation of the mineral and matrix components of plugs. In addition, there have been few documented studies of the radiodensity of feline urethral plugs. Pilot studies performed in our hospital indicate that they are usually not radiodense, which may be related to their relatively small diameter and/or the large quantity of radiolucent matrix that they contain.

Gelatinous plugs frequently retain the shape of the urethral lumen when they are forced out the

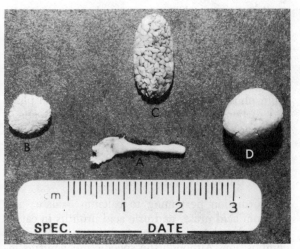

.**Figure 1.** Urethral plugs removed from the urinary tracts of male cats. *A*, Urethral plug. *B* and *C*, Two wafer-like sterile struvite uroliths. *D*, An infected struvite urolith.

Table 1. *Quantitative Mineral Composition of Uroliths Removed from the Urinary Tract of 103 Male and Female Cats**

Mineral Composition	Number
100% Magnesium ammonium phosphate	68
> 70% Magnesium ammonium phosphate with calcium phosphate and/or ammonium urate	20
60% Magnesium ammonium phosphate; 40% ammonium urate	1
60% Calcium phosphate; 40% magnesium ammonium phosphate	1
100% Calcium phosphate	3
> 90% Calcium oxalate	3
100% Ammonium acid urate	2
100% Uric acid	2
Matrix	3
Cystine	0
Silica	0

*Mineral composition determined by crystallographic methods.

external urethral orifice (Fig. 1). Their shape is probably influenced by their rapid rate of formation and/or growth. It is tempting to hypothesize that their rapid formation is somewhat analogous to the formation of renal tubular casts. A slower rate of growth similar to that of a vascular thrombus is another possibility.

Unlike most struvite uroliths in dogs, humans, and mink, infection with urease-producing bacteria is uncommonly associated with struvite urethral plugs in cats. A variety of factors, including viruses and dietary imbalances of calcium, phosphorus, and magnesium, have been incriminated as etiologic agents.

FELINE UROLITHS

PHYSICAL AND CHEMICAL CHARACTERISTICS

Uroliths are polycrystalline concretions that typically contain greater than 95 per cent organic or inorganic crystalloids and less than 5 per cent organic matrix (weight versus weight ratio). They may also contain a number of minor constituents. Although a particular mineral usually predominates, the mineral composition may be mixed (Table 1). Unlike urethral plugs, uroliths are not disorganized precipitates of crystalline material. They are typically composed of organized crystal aggregates with a complex internal structure. Cross sections of uroliths often reveal nuclei, laminations, and, occasionally, radial striations.

Uroliths similar in appearance to those in dogs and humans have been observed in the urinary system of male and female cats. In contrast to urethral plugs, most are radiodense. Struvite calculi comprise the most common mineral form of feline

uroliths; ammonium acid urate, uric acid, and calcium oxalate calculi have been encountered much less frequently (see Table 1). Uroliths composed primarily of cystine and silica have not been observed in cats.

In a study of 103 uroliths obtained from cats and submitted to the University of Minnesota for analysis, the mean age of occurrence was 5.8 years (range 2 months to 15 years). In 83 cats in which their sex was specified, 19 occurred in intact males, 22 occurred in castrated males, 20 occurred in intact females, and 22 occurred in spayed females. In 53 cats in which location of the uroliths was specified, 43 occurred in the urinary bladder, 9 occurred in the urethra, and 1 occurred in the kidneys (Fig. 2). Although ureteroliths are apparently rare in cats, they have been reported. Breeds affected were domestic short-haired (35), domestic long-haired

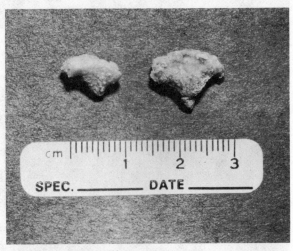

Figure 2. Photograph of infected struvite uroliths removed from the renal pelves of a five-year-old female cat. (Courtesy of Dr. Lyle Hanson, Fond Du Lac, WI.)

(11), Persian (6), Siamese (9), Himalayan (2), Burmese (1), and unknown (39).

Calculi located in the urinary bladders of cats are frequently shaped like a wafer or disc; they typically are somewhat thicker at the center than at the periphery (see Fig. 1). The factors responsible for this unusual shape are unknown.

ETIOPATHOGENESIS

STRUVITE UROLITHIASIS

Results of our clinical studies suggest that two different populations of struvite uroliths occur in cats: sterile and infected.

In most cats, especially those with wafer-shaped struvite calculi, urolith initiation and growth does not appear to be related to bacterial urinary tract infections, since affected patients typically have bacteriologically sterile urine. The mechanisms that lead to supersaturation of urine with magnesium ammonium phosphate in this group of patients have not been conclusively established. It is tempting to speculate that formation of highly concentrated urine, inappropriately high urine pH, and renal excretion of high concentrations of calculogenic minerals are involved. Lack of substances called *crystallization inhibitors* in the urine of affected cats is also a distinct possibility.

Infection-induced struvite uroliths are uncommon in cats because bacterial urinary tract infections are uncommon in cats. However, if cats develop urinary tract infections with urease-producing bacteria (especially staphylococci), struvite uroliths that are similar in radiographic, gross, and microscopic appearance to those that occur in dogs with similar types of urinary tract infections may occur (Figs. 3 and 4). Conversion of urea to ammonia as a result of bacterial urease plays an important role in the supersaturation of urine with magnesium ammonium phosphate as well as with calcium phosphate and carbonate-apatite crystals (see Medical Dissolution and Prevention of Canine Struvite Uroliths for further details).

OTHER UROLITHS

Information pertaining to calcium oxalate, ammonium acid urate, and uric acid uroliths in cats is limited to isolated case reports and studies of urolith composition. Although the specific mechanisms involved in initiation and growth of these types of uroliths have not been defined, they are presumed to be similar to those involved in other species.

BIOLOGIC BEHAVIOR

Like canine uroliths, feline uroliths have a tendency to recur. In a recent survey of uroliths in cats, there were 25 known recurrences in 131 patients. Twenty-one cats had two episodes of recurrence, three cats had three episodes, and one cat had four episodes. Recurrence may be related to persistence of the underlying cause of urolithiasis and/or failure to remove all uroliths from the urinary tract, especially those that are subvisible.

Although spontaneous dissolution of uroliths has been observed in dogs with struvite urolithiasis, to

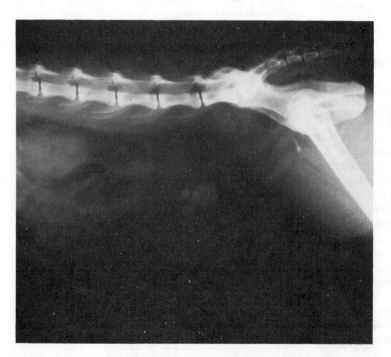

Figure 3. Lateral view of a survey abdominal radiograph of a seven-year-old male cat with multiple uroliths in the urinary bladder. The cat had a urinary tract infection caused by urease-producing staphylococci.

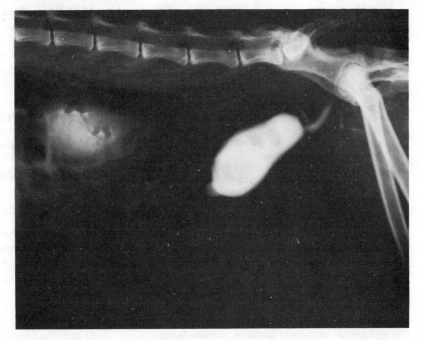

Figure 4. Lateral view of an intravenous urogram of the cat in Figure 3. The uroliths appear to be less radiodense than the contrast medium in the bladder lumen. There is a urachal diverticulum at the vertex of the bladder wall. It is probable that the diverticulum was the predisposing cause of staphylococcal urinary tract infection, which in turn predisposed the cat to struvite urolithiasis.

date it has not been detected in cats. This is undoubtedly related to the fact that the two most common choices of management of urolithiasis in cats have been surgical removal and euthanasia. Based on knowledge of the biologic behavior of uroliths in other species, it is logical to assume that feline uroliths may on occasion undergo spontaneous dissolution.

DIAGNOSIS

Perhaps the most important factor in the diagnosis of feline urolithiasis is a high index of suspicion of their presence. So much attention has been focused on the formation of urethral plugs in male cats and the ill-defined feline urologic syndrome in male and female cats that classical uroliths are frequently overlooked as diagnostic possibilities. The fact that many uroliths located in the urinary bladder of cats are too small to be palpated per abdomen has also played an important role in their lack of recognition. Any cat with persistent dysuria, pollakiuria, and/or hematuria should be suspected of having uroliths.

It is emphasized that feline vesical uroliths are difficult and sometimes impossible to detect by abdominal palpation. Their detection will be hindered if the bladder is distended or overdistended. In the latter situation, the bladder should be repalpated after urine has been eliminated by voiding, manual compression, cystocentesis, or (if absolutely necessary) catheterization.

Survey and contrast radiography are the most reliable methods of detecting the number, size, and location of radiodense and radiolucent uroliths (see

Analysis of Canine and Feline Uroliths). Radiography should also be considered to detect concomitant abnormalities of the urinary tract that are contributing to urinary tract dysfunction (see Localization of Male Feline Urethral Lesions Prior to Urethrostomy).

It is emphasized that uroliths are a sequela of some underlying disorder. In addition to radiography, urinalysis, quantitative urine culture, and serum chemistries may be required to detect the underlying cause. A sufficient quantity of urine for routine urinalysis and quantitative bacterial culture should be collected (preferably by cystocentesis) prior to administration of radiopaque contrast agents or therapeutic agents. Evaluation of a hemogram and serum chemistry profile prior to corrective surgery should be routine. Uroliths voided through the urethra or removed by surgery should always be analyzed by quantitative techniques (see Analysis of Canine and Feline Uroliths). We have developed a problem-specific data base for evaluation of patients with uroliths (Table 2).

MANAGEMENT

OVERVIEW

Therapy of struvite urolithiasis encompasses (1) relief of obstruction to urine outflow when necessary, (2) elimination of existing calculi, (3) eradication or control of urinary tract infection (when present), and (4) prevention of recurrence of uroliths (see Table 2). The following recommendations should not be used as a standardized approach to

Table 2.   *Problem-Specific Data Base for Urolithiasis*

1. Obtain appropriate history and perform physical examination
2. Perform complete urinalysis
3. Perform complete blood count
4. Freeze aliquot of serum collected at time of venipuncture to obtain complete blood count for possible determination of urea nitrogen, creatinine, or calcium concentrations
5. Obtain quantitative urine culture; obtain antimicrobial susceptibility if pathogens are identified
6. Obtain radiographs
   a. Take survey radiographs of entire urinary system
   b. Consider IV urography for patients with renal or ureteral calculi
   c. Consider IV urography or contrast cystography for patients with bladder calculi
   d. Consider contrast urethrography for patients with urethral calculi
7. Remove bladder or kidney biopsy specimens during nephrotomy or cystotomy for potential microscopic examination
8. Correct anatomic defects during surgical procedures performed to remove uroliths
9. Compare number of uroliths removed during surgery with number of uroliths identified by radiography; if necessary, post-surgical radiographs should be obtained to evaluate completeness of urolith removal
10. Save all uroliths for quantitative analysis
11. Initiate therapy to promote dissolution of uroliths or to arrest growth of uroliths, if necessary
12. Initiate therapy to eradicate urinary tract infection
13. Initiate therapy to prevent recurrence of uroliths
14. Formulate follow-up protocol with clients

treatment, since no two patients have identical therapeutic needs. Within the guidelines outlined herein, individualization of therapy is essential.

ELIMINATION OF EXISTING CALCULI

With our present knowledge concerning feline urolithiasis, surgical removal remains the most consistently reliable way to remove uroliths from the kidneys, ureters, and urinary bladder. Lack of knowledge of the underlying causes of various types of uroliths in cats has prevented the development of consistently effective nonsurgical methods to induce urolith dissolution. However, with the advent of effective methods to induce struvite urolith dissolution in dogs, development of equally effective methods for cats with struvite uroliths is probable. The following list of suggestions may help to minimize post-surgical complications and may help to prevent recurrence of uroliths.

1. Remove and save all uroliths for analysis. Thoroughly flush the operative area with an isotonic polyionic solution (e.g., lactated Ringer's solution) to remove subvisible uroliths that may serve as a nidus for recurrent urolithiasis.

2. Obtain appropriate biopsy samples of urinary bladder and/or kidney at the time of cystotomy and/or nephrotomy.

3. Do not allow suture material to become entrapped within the lumen of the excretory pathway of the urinary system, since it may serve as a nidus for urolith formation.

4. Avoid the use of indwelling urethral catheters whenever possible, since they serve as a common source of iatrogenic urinary tract infection.

5. Formulate appropriate therapy to eradicate or control urinary tract infections, especially in patients with struvite uroliths caused by urease-producing bacteria (see Medical Dissolution and Prevention of Canine Struvite Uroliths).

PREVENTION OF RECURRENCE

Because of the unpredictable tendency of uroliths to recur, long-term success is usually dependent on effective prophylactic therapy. Effective forms of prophylactic therapy create an undersaturated concentration of calculogenic crystalloids in urine by (1) increasing the solubility of crystalloids in urine, (2) increasing the volume of urine in which crystalloids are dissolved or suspended, and/or (3) reducing the quantity of calculogenic crystalloids in urine.

For nonuremic patients with sterile struvite uroliths prophylactic therapy involves (1) acidifying inappropriately alkaline urine (see Urinary Acidifiers), (2) promoting diuresis by stimulating thirst with salt and/or providing foods with a high moisture content, and (3) considering the use of diets with reduced quantities of magnesium and phosphorus (Prescription Diet C/D*).

Implantation of copper coils into the lumen of the urinary bladder has been suggested to prevent feline urolith formation, although convincing data to support this form of therapy were not documented. Because foreign material within the lumen of the urinary tract is known to enhance rather than prevent urolith formation by the phenomenon of heterogeneous nucleation, in our opinion this form of therapy is questionable. Pending controlled studies in naturally occurring cases, its use should not be adopted.

For nonuremic patients with struvite uroliths induced by infection with urease-producing bacteria, prophylactic therapy involves (1) eradicating or controlling the urinary tract infection (see Feline Urinary Tract Infections), (2) acidifying inappropriately alkaline urine, (3) promoting diuresis by stimulating thirst with salt and/or providing foods with a high moisture content, and (4) considering the use of diets that contain reduced quantities of protein, phosphorus, and magnesium (see Medical Dissolution and Prevention of Canine Struvite Uroliths). Use of the urease inhibitor acetohydroxamic acid has not been evaluated in cats.

We have had insufficient experience in prophy-

---

*Hills Division, Riviana Foods, Inc., Topeka, KS.

lactic management of cats with urate, calcium oxalate, and calcium phosphate urolithiasis to provide
meaningful recommendations. It seems logical to
suggest that calcium-containing uroliths in cats with
hypercalcemia would be prevented by correcting
the underlying cause of hypercalcemia. The same
line of logic would apply to cats with uric acid
uroliths and hyperuricemia. Pending further clinical
and experimental studies, consult information suggested for dogs with these types of uroliths.

SUPPLEMENTAL READING

Bohonowych, R. O., Parks, J. L., and Greene, R. W.: Features of cystic
calculi in cats in a hospital population. J.A.V.M.A. 173:301, 1978.
Osborne, C. A., and Klausner, J. S.: War on canine urolithiasis: Problems
and solutions. *In* Proceedings 45th Annual Meeting Am. Anim. Hosp.
Assn. A.A.H.A., South Bend, Indiana, 1978. pp 569–620.
Osborne, C. A., and Lees, G. E.: Feline cystitis, urethritis, urethral
obstruction syndrome. Mod. Vet. Pract. 59:173, 349, 513, 669, 1978.
Ryan, C. P.: Feline uroliths. Feline Pract. 11:21, 1981.
Suter, D. J., and Wooley, S. E.: Crystalline material from the feline
urinary bladder. Res. Vet. Sci. 2:298, 1970.

NONSURGICAL REMOVAL OF URETHRAL CALCULI FROM FEMALE DOGS

CARL A. OSBORNE, D.V.M.

St. Paul, Minnesota

The fact that uroliths frequently become lodged
in the urethra of male dogs is common knowledge.
A nonsurgical technique utilizing urohydropropulsion has been very effective in removing uroliths
from male dogs; it has been described in previous
editions of *Current Veterinary Therapy* (Piermattei
and Osborne, 1977).

Uroliths may also become firmly lodged in the
urethra of female dogs. In some patients, uroliths
become lodged at the junction of the bladder neck
and ureters in addition to the urethra (Fig. 1).
Although this phenomenon is less common than
lodged uroliths in male dogs, the relative inaccessibility of the female urethra to urethrotomy mandates the use of nonsurgical methods to remove
obstructing uroliths from females. Because urethral
obstruction may cause life-threatening renal dysfunction and because urinary tract infection associated with obstruction to urine outflow frequently
leads to life-threatening bacterial nephritis and septicemia, prompt restoration of urine outflow is essential.

DIAGNOSIS

The most common clinical sign associated with
uroliths lodged in the urethra of female dogs is an
abrupt onset of persistent dysuria. Owners often
indicate that intermittent dysuria of variable duration preceded the current episode. Gross hematuria
may also be observed.

Complete obstruction of the urethra is typically
associated with an inability to micturate and marked
distention of the urinary bladder. Rectal or vaginal
palpation is the best mechanism to localize the site
of obstruction in dogs large enough to permit this
technique. Overdistention of the urinary bladder
with urine often prevents detection of bladder uroliths by abdominal palpation. Spontaneous rupture
of the urethra or urinary bladder may occur in some
patients.

Although inability to catheterize a patient is
suggestive of urethral calculi, survey or retrograde
contrast urethrography is the preferred method of
detection, since the vast majority of uroliths are
radiodense (see Analysis of Canine and Feline Uroliths). Once uroliths have been identified in the
urethra, the entire urinary tract should be thoroughly evaluated via radiography to determine if
uroliths are also present in the kidneys, ureters, or
urinary bladder.

Results of urinalyses are usually typical of those
of urinary tract inflammation. Patients with struvite
uroliths usually have bacteriuria. In patients with
persistent obstruction, varying degrees of azotemia,
hyperphosphatemia, and metabolic acidosis usually
occur. Acute generalized pyelonephritis caused by
ascending urinary tract infection is typically associated with fever and immature neutrophilic leukocytosis.

TREATMENT

Persistent obstruction of the urethra or both
ureters will cause the demise of the patient; re-

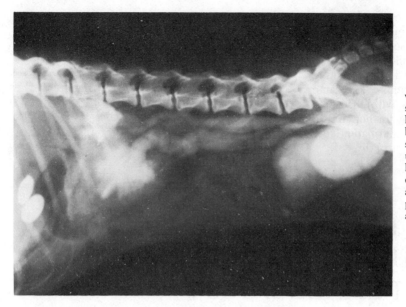

Figure 1. Lateral view of the abdominal wall of a 21-month-old female miniature schnauzer during intravenous urography. A large urolith lodged at the junction of the bladder neck with the urethra has obstructed the outflow of urine through the ureters and the urethra. A diverticulum is located at the vertex of the bladder. The dog died as a result of post-renal azotemia, acute pyelonephritis, and septicemia. (Reprinted with permission from Osborne et al.: J.A.V.M.A. 182:47, 1983.)

establishment of urine outflow should receive emergency priority. Regardless of the technique employed, care must be used to avoid severe trauma to the urethra.

CYSTOCENTESIS

If obstruction to urine outflow has been present for a sufficient period of time to cause marked overdistention of the urinary bladder, it is advisable to decompress the urinary tract by cystocentesis. This technique has been described in previous editions of *Current Veterinary Therapy* (Osborne et al., 1980).

PALPATION

Unidirectional massage of the urethral urolith with a finger inserted into the vagina or rectum has frequently been effective in dislodging urethral uroliths (Figs. 2 and 3). Prior to palpation, a liberal quantity of a 1:1 mixture of sterilized physiologic saline (or a comparable nonirritating physiologic solution) and aqueous lubricant (Lubafax Surgical Lubricant*) should be injected through a catheter into the urethral lumen adjacent to the urolith. This maneuver will help to lubricate the urethral mucosa, which is often inflamed and swollen, and the urolith. We recommend that this mixture be prepared by connecting the tips of two large-capacity syringes, one partially filled with aqueous lubricant and the other partially filled with saline, with a three-way valve (Fig. 4). Injection of these materials back and forth between the syringes will allow rapid mixing without loss of sterility.

Aqueous lubricants should not be injected into the urinary tract of patients known to have large tears in the wall of the urethra or urinary bladder, since they may cause granulomas.

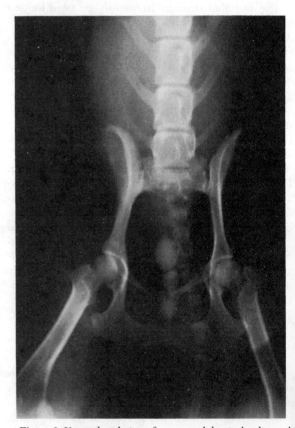

Figure 2. Ventrodorsal view of a survey abdominal radiograph of a nine-year-old female miniature poodle illustrating multiple radiodense uroliths lodged in the urethral lumen. (Reprinted with permission from Osborne et al.: J.A.V.M.A. 182:47, 1983.)

*Burroughs Wellcome Co., Research Triangle Park, NC.

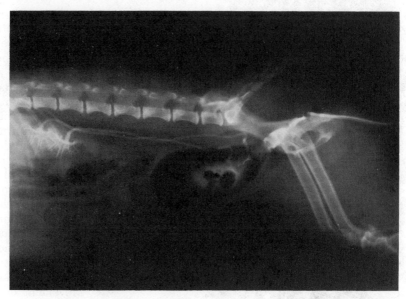

Figure 3. Lateral view of a double contrast retrograde urethrocystogram of the dog described in Figure 2. One urolith was pushed back into the bladder lumen by digital palpation. Two uroliths remain lodged within the lumen of the proximal urethra. Both uroliths were forced back into the urinary bladder by urohydropropulsion. (Reprinted with permission from Osborne et al.: J.A.V.M.A. 182:47, 1983.)

UROHYDROPROPULSION

Uroliths firmly lodged in the urethra of female dogs have frequently been moved back into the lumen of the urinary bladder by a form of urohydropropulsion developed for use in male dogs. The technique is based on dilatation of a portion of the urethra with fluid under pressure.

Depending on the disposition of the patient, sedation or general anesthesia may be required. Pharmacologic agents that are dependent on renal metabolism or excretion for inactivation and elimination from the body should be avoided (see Checklist of Hazardous Drugs in Patients with Renal Failure). If an uncooperative patient is an anesthetic risk because of a uremic crisis, topical application of lidocaine gel (Anestacon*) to the urethral mucosa in combination with parenteral administration of low dosages of analgesics may provide adequate patient restraint.

General anesthesia should be used whenever possible if calculi cannot be removed from the urethra of nonanesthetized patients by urohydropropulsion. As yet, we have not encountered any urethral calculi that could not be removed by this technique following general anesthesia. Short-acting barbiturates (e.g., thiamylal) may be used, since they are primarily inactivated by the liver. Appropriate caution should be used, since patients in

---

*Conal Pharmaceuticals Inc., Chicago, IL.

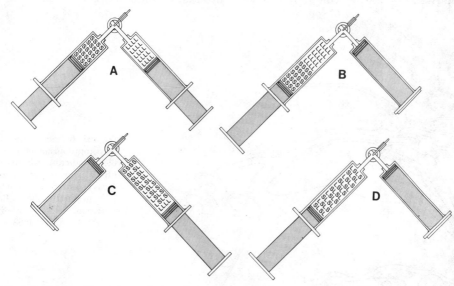

Figure 4. Schematic diagram illustrating technique for mixing sterilized aqueous lubricant (L) with physiologic saline (S) in two syringes connected by a three-way valve. (Reprinted with permission from Osborne et al.: J.A.V.M.A. 182:47, 1983.)

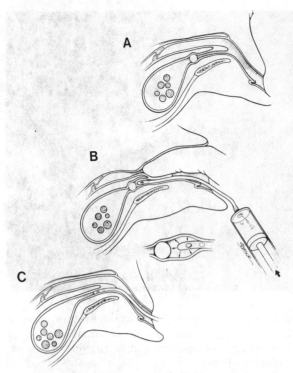

Figure 5. Schematic illustration of urohydropropulsion in a female dog with a solitary urethral urolith using a conventional urinary catheter. *A,* A urolith originating from the urinary bladder has become lodged in the urethra. *B,* A small portion of the urethral lumen distal to the urolith and proximal to a site occluded by digital pressure applied through the vaginal wall has been expanded by injecting saline through a catheter. *C,* The urolith has been forced back into the bladder lumen, eliminating obstruction to urine outflow. (Reprinted with permission from Osborne et al.: J.A.V.M.A. 182:47, 1983.)

renal failure are more sensitive to general anesthetics than normal patients. Inhalant anesthetics such as halothane may also be considered, since

they are not dependent on the kidneys for inactivation and excretion from the body.

To remove urethral uroliths by urohydropropulsion, inject a liberal quantity of a 1:1 mixture of sterilized saline and aqueous lubricant (described in the section on palpation) into the urethral lumen adjacent to the uroliths via a flexible catheter. With an index finger either in the rectum or, preferably, in the vagina, firmly occlude the lumen of the distal urethra around the catheter (Fig. 5). This will create a closed system between the occluding urolith and the site of digital compression of the urethra. Next, inject saline through the lumen of the catheter to distend the urethra to its maximum capacity. Dilation of the urethra combined with pressure generated by the intraluminal saline will usually cause the urolith to move back into the bladder lumen. It may be necessary to aid movement of the urolith by gentle digital manipulation.

Movement of large uroliths that have become firmly lodged in the neck of the bladder and proximal urethra may require application of digital pressure per abdomen by an assistant when saline is injected through the catheter.

Because of the reflux of saline through the external urethral orifice, it may be necessary to repeat the procedure several times before the uroliths reach the urinary bladder. The position of the uroliths may be monitored by digital palpation, attempts to advance the catheter, or radiography. If difficulty is encountered in occluding the external urethral orifice around the catheter, a 4 to 7 French Swan-Ganz balloon catheter or pediatric Foley catheter may be used (Fig. 6). Inflation of the balloon after it has been inserted into the distal urethra combined with firm digital pressure is often effective in minimizing reflux of saline through the external urethral orifice.

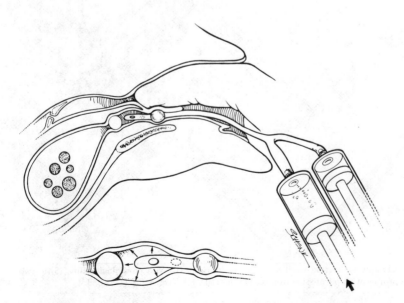

Figure 6. Schematic illustration of urohydropropulsion utilizing a Swan-Ganz balloon catheter. Inflation of the balloon with air helps to prevent reflux of saline injected through the catheter out the external urethral orifice. (Reprinted with permission from Osborne et al.: J.A.V.M.A. 182:47, 1983.)

CATHETERIZATION

Although urethral uroliths may be pushed back into the bladder with the aid of a catheter, this technique is often unsuccessful and is associated with the risk of urethral trauma. If the urolith can be easily moved by inserting a catheter into the urethral lumen, our experience has been that it can also be readily moved by digital pressure applied through the vaginal or rectal wall.

Judicious use of a catheter to attempt to dislodge urethral uroliths may be justified as a last resort. The diameter of the catheter should be as large as is consistent with atraumatic technique. A rigid catheter is more likely to be associated with success than a flexible one; it is also more likely to cause urethral trauma. The catheter should be liberally coated with sterilized, water-soluble lubricant. Unless there is a tear in the urethral wall, a liberal quantity of a 1:1 mixture of saline and water-soluble lubricant should be injected through the catheter as the urolith is being advanced toward the urinary bladder. This mixture may be prepared according to the directions summarized in the discussion about palpation. If a tear in the urethra is present, only a nonirritating isotonic solution such as physiologic saline or lactated Ringer's should be used. Appropriate caution must be used to avoid trauma to the urethra; excessive force should never be used.

Stone baskets have been designed to retrieve small calculi from the ureters of humans. The Mitchell Stone Basket* has been used for removal of urethral uroliths from male dogs. They may be of value in small female dogs with urethral uroliths; however, we have had no clinical experience with this technique.

---

*C. R. Bard Co.

FOLLOW-UP

If uroliths lodged in the urethra cannot be removed by nonsurgical techniques and the patient is severely azotemic, intermittent cystocentesis should be performed to reduce the severity of the biochemical abnormalities caused by urethral obstruction. Surgical correction of the problem may then be accomplished via cystotomy.

If uroliths are returned to the urinary bladder by nonsurgical techniques, further management may involve surgical or nonsurgical techniques. Consult textbooks of veterinary surgery and reference materials for detailed information on surgical methods of urolith management. Combinations of modified diets, antimicrobial agents, and drugs that inhibit bacterial urease have been effective in causing dissolution of canine struvite uroliths (see Medical Dissolution and Prevention of Canine Struvite Uroliths).

REFERENCES AND SUPPLEMENTAL READING

Drach, G. W.: Stone manipulation. Modern usage and occasional mishaps. Urology 12:286, 1978.

Osborne, C. A., Abdullahi, S., Klausner, J. S., Johnston, G. R., and Polzin, D. J.: Nonsurgical removal of uroliths from the urethra of female dogs. J.A.V.M.A. 182:47, 1983.

Osborne, C. A., and Klausner, J. S.: War on canine urolithiasis: Problems and solutions. Proceedings of the 45th Annual Meeting of the American Animal Hospital Association. 569, 1980.

Osborne, C. A., Lees, G. E., and Johnston, G. R.: Cystocentesis. *In* Kirk, R. W. (ed.): *Current Veterinary Therapy VII.* Philadelphia: W. B. Saunders, 1980, pp. 1150–1153.

Piermattei, D. L., and Osborne, C. A.: Urohydropropulsion—nonsurgical removal of urethral calculi in male dogs. *In* Kirk, R. W. (ed.): *Current Veterinary Therapy VI.* Philadelphia: W. B. Saunders, 1977, pp. 1194–1196.

Diseases of the Lower Urinary Tract

HORMONAL RESPONSES TO URINARY INCONTINENCE

JEANNE A. BARSANTI, D.V.M.,
and DELMAR R. FINCO, D.V.M.
Athens, Georgia

APPLIED PHYSIOLOGY OF CONTINENCE

Urinary continence is the ability to voluntarily control micturition. In order for an animal to be continent, the neurologic and urinary systems must act in concert in the following manner: (1) the ureters must empty into the bladder; (2) the bladder must be able to expand normally without increasing intravesicular pressure to accommodate the urine inflow; (3) the urethra must exert sufficient resting pressure to oppose the movement of urine out of the bladder; (4) when the bladder reaches normal capacity, afferent neurons must transmit a signal to the spinal cord and brain; (5) the brain must institute an appropriate efferent response; (6) impulses must travel down the spinal cord to efferent neurons that initiate contraction of the abdominal and bladder detrusor muscles; and (7) as the bladder contracts, the bladder neck must open and a spinal reflex that decreases urethral tone must occur.

CAUSES OF INCONTINENCE

Urinary incontinence is the involuntary passage of urine and is associated with a long list of potential causes. In order to obtain a correct diagnosis, one should first determine if there is neurologic dysfunction. This is done by obtaining an appropriate history, performing a thorough physical examination, and, if a possible neurologic abnormality is detected, performing a complete neurologic examination. Depending on the location of the neurologic lesion, other diagnostic tests such as radiography and spinal fluid analysis may be required to ascertain its underlying cause.

If neurologic abnormalities are not associated with the incontinence, non-neurogenic causes should be considered. If continuous incontinence was first noted during house breaking, a congenital defect is likely. A persistent urachus can be diagnosed on physical examination; an ectopic ureter is more

difficult to confirm. Ectopic ureters more commonly cause incontinence in female puppies because of their shorter urethral length. The ectopic ureter may open into the distal urethra or vagina. The diagnosis can be confirmed by detecting an abnormal orifice during vaginal endoscopy or by contrast radiography. Although an excretory urogram will allow visualization of the ureters, their termination sites may be difficult to determine. A combination of excretory urography and pneumocystography may increase the contrast so that the distal ureters are easier to visualize. In some cases, the ureters enter the bladder serosa at the proper site but tunnel subserosally before they open into the urethra. In these cases, detection of contrast material in the vagina may aid in establishing the correct diagnosis. Surgical correction of an ectopic ureter does not eliminate incontinence in all dogs; some dogs seem to have an associated defect in urethral tone.

If incontinence develops acutely and is associated with dysuria, a partial urethral obstruction should be considered. Palpation of a distended bladder, inability to pass a urethral catheter, and visualization of an obstruction by survey or contrast urethrography will help to confirm urethral obstruction. If overdistention of the bladder leads to detrusor damage and atony, incontinence may persist after the obstruction is relieved. This may also occur in animals with no physical urethral obstruction (such as those with severe pelvic trauma) but that have been unwilling or unable to urinate. Keeping these animals' bladders empty for several days by means of indwelling catheterization will often allow the detrusor muscle to regain normal function.

Inability of the bladder wall to expand as a result of severe chronic cystitis or neoplastic infiltration of the bladder wall may also cause incontinence. Urination of only small volumes and palpation of a thickened bladder wall are suggestive of this abnormality. The diagnosis can be confirmed by finding a thickened, nondistensible bladder wall via cystography, by finding detrusor contractions at low intravesicular volumes on cystometrography, and by bladder wall biopsy.

Normal urethral tone is also important for maintenance of continence, since it prevents urine leakage as the bladder fills. In cases of urethral incompetence, affected individuals urinate normally because bladder function is normal. However, when an increase in intra-abdominal pressure occurs (such as with standing or laughing in humans), urine dribbles through the urethra. In older women, inability of the urethra to maintain normal resting pressure is a major cause of incontinence. Less is known about the contribution of the urethra to naturally occurring incontinence in animals because of the inability (until recently) to measure urethral function. Development of the technique of urethral pressure profilometry will permit more accurate detection of urethral causes of incontinence. One common type of incontinence that may be due to decreased urethral resting tone is hormone-responsive incontinence.

HORMONE-RESPONSIVE INCONTINENCE

DIAGNOSIS

If incontinence, typified by urine leakage while a dog is at rest but normal urination when the dog is awake, develops in a neutered dog, hormone-responsive incontinence is the most likely cause. Evaluation of these dogs by physical examination, urinalysis, and micturition reveals no abnormalities. Residual bladder volume, determined by bladder palpation or catheterization, is also normal (less than a few milliliters). This condition is so named because it is confirmed by response to therapy.

The cause of hormone-responsive incontinence in dogs is unknown. Four of five female dogs and the only male dog we have evaluated by cystometrography and urethral pressure profilometry have had decreased resting urethral resistance. We have not had the opportunity to re-evaluate any of the five dogs while they were on therapy and continent.

TREATMENT—FEMALE DOGS

In neutered female dogs the drug of choice is diethylstilbestrol (DES), available by prescription at pharmacies. The recommended dose is 0.1 to 1.0 mg/day for three to five days and as needed thereafter. The minimum dose and frequency of administration to control incontinence should be determined for each dog. Only the minimum amount needed to achieve continence should be used. Potential side effects include signs of estrus and bone marrow toxicity, varying from thrombocytopenia with leukocytosis to aplastic anemia. However, bone marrow failure is unlikely with minimal dosage. Longer-acting estradiol cypionate is more likely to result in this potentially life-threatening complication. Another side effect that we have seen in one dog with long-term daily DES administration was an endocrine-type alopecia.

TREATMENT—MALE DOGS

In the past three years, we have evaluated two neutered male dogs and one neutered male cat with incontinence similar to that seen in neutered female dogs. These animals became continent following intramuscular injection of testosterone at a dosage of 2.2 mg/kg. Parenteral administration is best, since testosterone administered orally is subject to rapid hepatic degradation. Approximately ten times more testosterone must be administered orally to reach the serum concentration that occurs following parenteral injection.

Various testosterone esters are available for parenteral therapy. Testosterone propionate has a duration of action of 48 to 72 hours. Occasionally one dose will be effective for several weeks. If multiple doses are required per week, one can change to testosterone cypionate (Depo-testosterone). This drug is slowly absorbed over at least a month. No direct side effects have been reported in dogs given this dosage. However, if male dogs are neutered for treatment of prostatic disease or perianal adenomas, administration of testosterone could worsen these conditions. If such complications are possible, shorter-acting testosterone esters should be used. Then if adverse effects occur, the drug can be withheld, and testosterone concentrations will decrease within a few days.

SUPPLEMENTAL READING

Barsanti, J. A., Edwards, P. D., and Losonsky, J.: Testosterone responsive urinary incontinence in a castrated male dog. J. Am. Anim. Hosp. Assoc. 17:117, 1981.

Johnsen, S. G., Bennett, E. P., and Jensen, V. G.: Therapeutic effectiveness of oral testosterone. Lancet 2 (7895):1473, 1974.

Rosin, A., Rosin, E., and Oliver, J.: The canine urethral pressure profile. Am. J. Vet. Res. 41:1113, 1980.

DYSURIA CAUSED BY REFLEX DYSSYNERGIA

JOHN E. OLIVER, D.V.M.

Athens, Georgia

Normal micturition requires a coordinated contraction of the smooth muscle of the bladder (detrusor) and relaxation of smooth and striated muscle of the urethra. The complex series of reflexes involving parasympathetic, sympathetic, and somatic neurons is organized in the sacral spinal cord and regulated by descending pathways from the brain.

Detrusor/urethral dyssynergia occurs when bladder contraction (detrusor reflex) is initiated without relaxation of the urethra. Either the smooth or striated muscle of the urethra may be involved. The dyssynergia is presumed to arise from lack of coordination caused by a lesion of the nervous system cranial to the sacral spinal cord. Upper motor neuron paralysis with no detrusor reflex and increased tone in the urethra is not reflex dyssynergia, because the reflex is absent. The condition has only been encountered in male dogs.

DIAGNOSIS

Dogs with reflex dyssynergia have the sensation and desire to void. Attempts to micturate are often associated with straining, and are typically characterized by small interrupted spurts of urine that subsequently stop completely. Large residual volumes of urine in the bladder are common. Overdistention of the bladder can occur, resulting in the loss of detrusor contractility.

Confirmation of the diagnosis is difficult. Mechanical obstruction to outflow should be ruled out by catheterization and/or radiography. Cystometry should indicate a normal or hyperactive detrusor reflex. The resting urethral pressure profile is normal. There is no denervation of perineal or periurethral striated muscle when evaluated by electromyography (EMG). Simultaneous bladder and urethral pressures or bladder pressure and urethral EMG recordings are required to verify dyssynergia. Anal sphincter EMG is not an adequate substitute.

When reflex dyssynergia is suspected, trials with pharmacologic agents may be used to relieve the signs and establish the diagnosis.

TREATMENT

The objective of therapy is to relax the urethra without blocking contraction of the detrusor muscle. If it can be determined whether the smooth or striated muscle is the problem, therapy can be specific. In most cases, trials with relaxants for both muscles will be necessary.

For smooth muscle dyssynergia, an alpha-adrenergic blocking agent is used. Phenoxybenzamine (Dibenzyline*) is the preferred drug. It is supplied in 10-mg capsules. Treatment is started at 10 mg once daily. If there is no benefit after four days, the dosage is increased to 10 mg twice daily. If there is no response after four more days, dosage is increased to a total of 30 mg daily. During treatment the bladder must not be allowed to become overdistended. Aseptic catheterization three times daily is necessary if the animal cannot void. Before each catheterization the animal should be given the opportunity to void, preferably outside. Side effects of the drug include hypotension, weakness, dizziness, and vomiting. If these signs occur, dosage should be reduced or discontinued. The animal should be kept quiet and should be monitored for shock.

For striated muscle dyssynergia, diazepam (Valium†) or dantrolene (Dantrium‡) is recommended. Diazepam acts centrally, may produce sedation at higher doses, and has been reported to depress detrusor reflex excitability in humans. Dosage ranges from 2 to 10 mg three times daily. Dantrolene is a skeletal muscle relaxant. Starting at 1 mg/kg three times daily, the dose may be increased to 5 mg/kg t.i.d. The primary side effect of generalized muscle weakness indicates that the dose is too high.

Combinations of smooth and striated muscle relaxants may be tried if neither is effective alone.

Failure in treatment is usually a result of the wrong diagnosis. A poor or absent detrusor reflex is the most common problem. The desire to void and straining to void do not necessarily mean that the detrusor reflex is present. Cystometry is the only positive diagnostic test for detrusor function.

SUPPLEMENTAL READING

Awad, S. A., and Downie, J. W.: Sympathetic dyssynergia in the region of the external sphincter: A possible source of lower urinary tract obstruction. J. Urol. 118:636, 1977.

*Smith Kline & French Laboratories, Philadelphia, PA.
†Roche Laboratories, Nutley, NJ.
‡Norwich-Eaton Pharmaceuticals, Norwich, NY.

International Continence Society Committee on Standardization of Terminology: Standardization of terminology of lower urinary tract function. Urology 17:618, 1981.

Krane, R. J., and Siroky, M. C.: Clinical Neuro-urology. Boston: Little, Brown and Co., 1979.

McGuire, E. J., and Brady, S.: Detrusor-sphincter dyssynergia. J. Urol. 121:774, 1979.

Oliver, J. E., Jr.: Neurology of visceral function. Vet. Clin. North Am. 4:517, 1974.

Oliver, J. E., Jr., and Osborne, C. A.: Neurogenic urinary incontinence. In Kirk, R. W. (ed.): Current Veterinary Therapy VII. Philadelphia: W. B. Saunders, 1980.

Oliver, J. E., Jr., and Young, W. O.: Air cystometry in dogs under xylazine-induced restraint. Am. J. Vet. Res. 34:1433, 1973.

Rosin, A. H., and Barsanti, J. A.: Diagnosis of urinary incontinence in dogs: role of the urethral pressure profile. J.A.V.M.A. 178:814, 1981.

Rosin, A. H., and Ross, L.: Diagnosis and pharmacological management of disorders of urinary continence in the dog. Comp. Cont. Ed. Pract. Vet. 3:601, 1981.

URINARY INCONTINENCE ASSOCIATED WITH MALPOSITION OF THE URINARY BLADDER

STEPHEN P. DiBARTOLA, D.V.M.,
Columbus, Ohio

and W. M. ADAMS, D.V.M.
Madison, Wisconsin

The neck of the canine bladder is normally located cranial to the pecten of the pubic bone during contrast radiography. Occasionally the urinary bladder has been observed in a more caudal location. In affected dogs, the bladder neck lies in the pelvic canal caudal to the pecten, and its caudal pole is more abruptly blunted than normal (Fig. 1). The portion of the bladder located within the pelvic canal may vary from less than 10 to more than 30 per cent of the total bladder, depending on the amount of bladder filling and the degree of bladder distensibility. The term *pelvic bladder* has been used to describe this radiographic abnormality. Urinary incontinence, urinary tract infection (UTI), or structural abnormalities may occur in dogs with pelvic bladder. Uncommonly it may be an asymptomatic radiographic finding.

CLINICAL FEATURES (Table 1)

Pelvic bladder has been observed in dogs with congenital and acquired structural abnormalities of the lower urinary tract. It has been observed in young dogs with urinary incontinence due to ectopic ureters and in dogs with urachal diverticuli. Acquired anatomic abnormalities that have been detected in association with pelvic bladder include adhesions in the area of the bladder neck due to previous trauma and uterine stump granulomas. The relationship of congenital abnormalities of the lower urinary tract to pelvic bladder is not known.

Acquired adhesions in the area of the bladder neck may contribute to fixation of the bladder in a caudally displaced position. However, radiographic studies have not been performed to determine whether correction of the acquired problems has any effect on the position of the bladder in the abdomen.

Urinary tract infection and/or urinary incontinence frequently occur in dogs with pelvic bladder. The significance of radiographic detection of a pelvic location of a portion of the bladder in dogs with UTI and/or urinary incontinence is not clear. Increased urge to empty an inflamed bladder may predispose to caudal displacement of the bladder from straining and should be considered in cases of pelvic bladder with UTI. On the other hand, pelvic location of the bladder may predispose to lower UTI. Whether pelvic bladder predisposes to bacterial invasion or whether bladder irritation and inflammation predispose to the appearance of pelvic bladder is unknown.

The organisms isolated from the urine of dogs with pelvic bladder and UTI are similar to isolates from other dogs with UTI (e.g., *E. coli, Staphylococcus aureus, Streptococcus, Proteus, Klebsiella, Pseudomonas*).

Urinary incontinence occurs in over 50 per cent of dogs with radiographically demonstrable pelvic bladder. Caudal displacement of a portion of the bladder into the pelvic canal may alter normal pressure relationships in the bladder and urethra

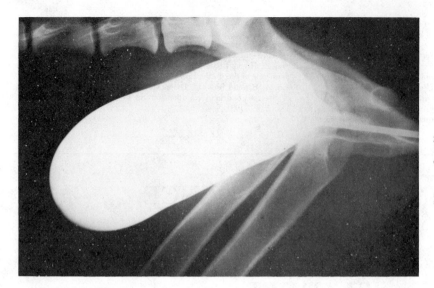

Figure 1. Positive contrast cystogram of a four-year-old spayed female Doberman pinscher with a pelvic bladder and urinary incontinence.

and may lead to incontinence. In human females with stress incontinence, abnormal anatomic support of the bladder neck and proximal urethra may lead to displacement of the proximal urethra outside the pelvic diaphragm so that sudden increases in abdominal pressure are not transmitted to the proximal urethra. During sudden increases in abdominal pressure (e.g., coughing) intravesical pressure may exceed intraurethral pressure and may lead to urinary incontinence. Urethral pressure profiles obtained before and after effective therapy of dogs with pelvic bladder and urinary incontinence would be valuable in defining pressure relationships in this disorder.

The frequency of occurrence of urinary incontinence in dogs with pelvic bladder is similar regardless of the presence of UTI. Some dogs with pelvic bladder that had UTI and urinary incontinence were incontinent when urine was sterile as well as when it was infected. Also, dogs with pelvic bladders that do not have urinary incontinence frequently have UTI. None of the few male dogs seen with pelvic bladder had urinary incontinence, but most had UTI with or without structural abnormalities. These findings suggest that UTI is not a necessary factor in the pathogenesis of urinary incontinence in dogs with pelvic bladder. It is emphasized, however, that urge incontinence may occur in dogs with UTI.

Some dogs with pelvic bladder have urinary incontinence but do not have UTI or structural abnormalities. These are often large-breed, adult spayed female dogs. Doberman pinschers appear to be overrepresented in this group. In some instances, UTI or structural abnormalities have been detected, but urinary incontinence has persisted after appropriate antibiotic therapy or surgical correction of structural abnormalities. In these dogs there may be an incomplete response to diethylstilbestrol but a favorable response to ephedrine.

DIAGNOSIS

Evaluation of dogs with urinary incontinence begins with an appropriate history. Loss of voluntary control should be differentiated from polyuria. With polyuria, the animal may urinate in the house because it is not allowed out frequently enough to accommodate its large daily production of urine. Some owners misinterpret this as urinary incontinence. It is important to ask the owner if dribbling of urine has been observed while the animal is sleeping.

The owner should be questioned about the animal's posture during micturition. If the animal can be interrupted during micturition, this suggests voluntary control. It is important to determine if dysuria, pollakiuria, and hematuria have occurred, since these signs suggest lower UTI. The owner should be asked about the dog's normal house training and frequency of urination. The age at ovariohysterectomy in spayed females is of importance in the diagnosis of estrogen-responsive urinary incontinence. A history of previous trauma or surgery that may have affected the region of the bladder neck is also of significance. If initiation of urination is followed by a poor stream of urine or by dribbling of urine, functional bladder outlet obstruction due to failure of urethral relaxation (reflex dyssynergia) or partial mechanical obstruction should be considered. Normal urination at inappropriate times and in inappropriate places may suggest a cerebral lesion associated with loss of learned behavior.

Appropriate general and neurologic examinations of the patient should be performed. Special attention should be given to abnormal bladder tone, size, thickness, and masses (e.g., calculi, tumors). The pelvic urethra can be palpated per rectum. Examination of the bulbocavernosus and perineal reflexes

Table 1.   *Clinical Findings in Dogs with Pelvic Bladder*

Breed	Sex	Age	UTI*	Anatomic Abnormality	Urinary Incontinence	Therapy and Response
Doberman pinscher	F	4 mo	Yes	Inverted vulva	Yes	UTI responsive to antibiotics; not incontinent after control of UTI
Boxer	F	5 mo	Yes	No	Yes	Response to antibiotics and DES unknown†
Miniature poodle	FS	15 yr	Yes	Bladder polyp, adhesions	Yes	UTI response to antibiotics unknown; surgery revealed bladder polyp and adhesions
Doberman pinscher	FS	1 yr	No	Urachal diverticulum	Yes	Urachal diverticulum surgically removed, but control of incontinence required ephedrine
Doberman pinscher	FS	6 yr	No	No	Yes	Partial response to DES
Doberman pinscher	FS	4 yr	No	No	Yes	No therapy attempted
Old English sheepdog	FS	5 yr	Yes	No	Yes	UTI responsive to antibiotics; incontinence partially responsive to DES; good response to ephedrine
German shepherd	FS	2 yr	Yes	No	Yes	UTI response to antibiotics unknown; good response of incontinence to DES for 4 to 5 months; further therapy not required
German shepherd	FS	2 yr	Yes	No	Yes	UTI responsive to antibiotics; incontinence poorly responsive to DES; good response to ephedrine
Collie	FS	6 yr	No	No	Yes	No response to antibiotics or DES
Akita-Labrador mix	F	2 mo	Yes	No	No	UTI responsive to antibiotics
Afghan	M	5 yr	Yes	Urachal diverticulum	No	UTI responsive to antibiotics and surgical removal of urachal diverticulum
Australian shepherd	M	2 yr	Yes	Urachal diverticulum	No	UTI responsive to antibiotics and surgical removal of urachal diverticulum
Great Dane	M	5 yr	Yes	No	No	UTI responsive to antibiotics
Mix	F	5 yr	No	Rectal vaginal fistula	No	Surgical repair successful
German shepherd	M	2 yr	No	No	No	Asymptomatic
Boxer	F	7 mo.	Yes	No	No	UTI responsive to antibiotics

*UTI = urinary tract infection.
†DES = diethylstilbestrol

allows evaluation of the sacral spinal cord. The animal should also be observed during micturition. Catheterization performed after micturition may help to rule out mechanical obstruction or retention of an excessive residual volume. The normal residual volume in the urinary bladder should be less than 10 ml.

Laboratory evaluation should include urinalysis and quantitative urine culture to rule out UTI. If UTI is present, it should be treated by appropriate antibiotic therapy before any pharmacologic manipulation of micturition is attempted. If urge incontinence is present, it should resolve with eradication of UTI.

Survey and contrast radiographs (excretory urography and cystography) may be used to detect anatomic abnormalities, calculi, or neoplasms. These disorders are corrected surgically if present.

The cystometrogram and urethral pressure profile are potentially useful in the evaluation of dogs with micturition disorders, but these tests are presently only available at teaching institutions.

If urine culture is negative and there are no radiographic abnormalities other than a pelvic bladder, pharmacologic control of urinary incontinence should be attempted. If the patient is an older spayed female, the clinician may elect to try a course of diethylstilbestrol. Caution must be exercised with estrogen therapy because of the potential bone marrow toxicity of estrogens. Therapy with alpha-adrenergic agents may be considered to eliminate the risk of marrow toxicity or to treat patients unresponsive to diethylstilbestrol.

THERAPY

Adrenergic receptors in the bladder and urethra play an important role in the filling phase of micturition and in the maintenance of urinary continence. Beta receptors predominate in the body of the bladder and aid in receptive relaxation to accommodate increasing volumes of urine. Alpha receptors predominate in the bladder neck and in the urethra, where they play a major role in the maintenance of resting urethral tone. Stimulation of alpha-adrenergic receptors in the bladder neck and urethra of female dogs results in increased resting urethral pressure, sphincter closure, and increased bladder capacity.

Sympathomimetic drugs that stimulate alpha receptors may increase urethral pressure and facilitate urinary continence. This has been shown in female dogs by stimulation of alpha-adrenergic receptors with imipramine hydrochloride. In humans, ephedrine sulfate has been used successfully to manage individuals with mild urinary incontinence regardless of cause. Urethral pressures increased along the entire length of the urethra in patients responsive to ephedrine.

Ephedrine stimulates both alpha- and beta-adrenergic receptors. It stimulates the release of norepinephrine from sympathetic nerve terminals and has a direct action on adrenergic effector cells. Ephedrine increases urethral pressure by causing contraction of urethral smooth muscle through stimulation of urethral alpha receptors and facilitates filling and increased bladder capacity by stimulation of beta receptors in the body of the bladder. Urethral pressure profiles of affected dogs before and after treatment with alpha-adrenergic agents are needed to determine if ephedrine induces similar responses in incontinent dogs.

Ephedrine is effective orally and has a long duration of action. It is available as 25- and 50-mg capsules and as a syrup in concentrations of 4 and 11 mg/ml. In humans, it is used at a dosage of 50 to 200 mg/day divided t.i.d. to q.i.d. We have effectively used ephedrine in a small number of large-breed dogs with urinary incontinence and malposition of the urinary bladder at a dosage of 50 mg b.i.d. or q.i.d. The recommended initial dosage is 4 mg/kg body weight given t.i.d.*

Ephedrine may have cardiovascular and central nervous system side effects. As a positive inotrope, it may increase blood pressure. Heart rate usually does not increase unless vagal reflexes have been blocked. The drug may cause restlessness, hyperexcitability, and anxiety. In humans, tachyphylaxis may develop, and repeated doses frequently become less effective owing to depletion of norepinephrine stores. In our experience with dogs, clients have not complained about restlessness, and the effectiveness of the drug has not decreased with time.

SUPPLEMENTAL READING

Benson, G. S., Jacobowitz, D., Raezer, D. M., et al.: Adrenergic innervation and stimulation of canine urethra. Urology 7:337, 1976.

Diokno, A. C., Taub, M.: Ephedrine in treatment of urinary incontinence. Urology 5:624, 1975.

Khanna, O. P.: Disorders of micturition: Neuropharmacologic basis and results of drug therapy. Urology 8:316, 1976.

Khanna, O. P., Heber, D., Elkouss, G., et al.: Imipramine hydrochloride: Pharmacodynamic effects on lower urinary tract of female dogs. Urology 6:48, 1975.

Oliver, J. E., and Osborne, C. A.: Neurogenic urinary incontinence. *In* Kirk, R. W. (ed.): *Current Veterinary Therapy VII.* Philadelphia: W. B. Saunders, 1980, pp. 1122–1127.

Oliver, J. E., and Young, W. D.: Air cystometry in dogs under xylazine-induced restraint. Am. J. Vet. Res. 34:1433, 1973.

Raezer, D. M., Wein, A. J., Jacobowitz, D., et al.: Autonomic innervation of canine urinary bladder. Urology 2:211, 1973.

Raz, S., and Caine, M.: Adrenergic receptors in the female canine urethra. Invest. Urol. 9:319, 1972.

Rosin, A., Rosin, E., and Oliver, J. E.: Canine urethral pressure profile. Am. J. Vet. Res. 41:1113, 1980.

---

*Use of ephedrine first suggested by Dr. Lloyd Davis, Urbana, IL.

DIVERTICULA OF THE URINARY BLADDER

JEFFREY S. KLAUSNER, D.V.M.,
GARY R. JOHNSTON, D.V.M.,
and CARL A. OSBORNE, D.V.M.

St. Paul, Minnesota

CLINICAL SIGNIFICANCE

Congenital or acquired evaginations of the bladder wall, called *diverticula,* may occur anywhere along the urinary tract but are especially common in the urinary bladder. They are of clinical significance because they predispose to recurrent bacterial urinary tract infections by permitting urine stasis and/or by harboring pathogenic bacteria in tissues of which they are composed. They may or may not be related to the ill-defined feline urologic syndrome. Although they have been associated with carcinomas in human patients, neoplasms of the urachus have not been reported in animals.

CONGENITAL DIVERTICULA

Congenital diverticula result from malformation of the urinary bladder. In humans, bladder diverticula often occur because the mucosa herniates through a weakened wall caused by abnormal development of muscular layers (Cook and King, 1979). Obstruction to urine outflow predisposes to mucosal herniation in such patients by increasing intravesical pressure.

Most congenital bladder diverticula in dogs and cats appear to result from urachal anomalies. To date it has not been established whether urachal anomalies in dogs and cats have a familial tendency. The urachus, an embryonic structure that arises from the urinary bladder, provides a channel of communication between the urinary bladder and the allantoic sac. In most animals, the urachus closes and atrophies after birth, leaving only a scar at the bladder apex. However, in humans the urachus persists as a nonfunctional fibromuscular cord called the middle umbilical ligament that connects the bladder apex to the umbilicus. Although it is normally not patent, the middle umbilical ligament has a small lumen lined by transitional cell epithelium. In dogs and cats, the middle umbilical ligament is a double fold of peritoneum that connects the ventral wall of the bladder to the ventral abdominal wall.

Vesicourachal diverticula located at the vertex of the urinary bladder result from failure of urachal segments in close proximity to the bladder to completely atrophy after birth. The result is a blind diverticulum that protrudes from the serosal surface of the bladder apex. In our experience, vesicourachal diverticula have varied in diameter from a few millimeters to several centimeters (Fig. 1). Small diverticula may not extend beyond the serosal margin of the bladder; large diverticula may be up to one-third the size of an empty urinary bladder. The frequency of occurrence of vesicourachal diverticula in dogs and cats has not been established; however, in our hospital population they have been very common.

In the dog, vesicourachal diverticula are a significant predisposing factor to recurrent urinary tract infections, especially in young animals (Wilson et al., 1979). Retention of urine and bacteria within diverticula probably alters the ability of normal host defense mechanisms to remove bacteria from the urinary tract. Although urine may be sterilized by administration of an appropriate antibiotic, urinary tract infection often recurs soon after the antibiotic is discontinued. Recurrences typically continue until the diverticulum is removed.

By predisposing to urinary tract infections, vesicourachal diverticula may directly contribute to the formation of struvite uroliths. Failure to remove diverticula at the time of urolith removal may result in recurrence of urinary tract infection and calculi.

The significance of vesicourachal diverticula in cats is more difficult to assess. In a study performed at the University of Minnesota, 60 per cent of male and female cats evaluated for signs of lower urinary tract disease had vesicourachal diverticula detected by contrast cystography. Surprisingly, only 40 per cent of these cats had bacterial urinary tract infections. This finding may be related to the inherent resistance of the cat's urinary tract to bacterial infection, or it may suggest that vesicourachal diverticula in cats are less likely to predispose to bacterial urinary tract infection than in dogs.

A relationship between feline urachal remnants and feline urologic syndrome (FUS) has been suggested (Hansen, 1977). Clinical studies performed at the University of Minnesota also revealed that many male and female cats with FUS have radio-

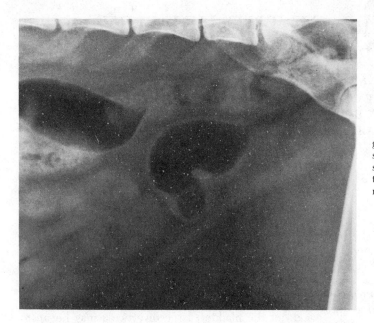

Figure 1. Lateral radiograph of a pneumocystogram of a nine-year-old neutered male domestic short-haired cat with intermittent lower urinary tract signs of five years duration. Note a cyst-like diverticulum and adjacent uroliths. The urine was bacteriologically sterile.

graphically demonstrable vesicourachal diverticula. However, the significance of these observations cannot be assessed until the frequency of diverticula in normal cats and cats with FUS has been determined.

In our experience, canine vesicourachal diverticula have not been associated with clinical signs of lower urinary tract disease unless bacterial infection is also present. In the latter situation, dysuria, hematuria, and increased frequency of urination are only indicative of lower urinary tract disease. There are no clinical signs indicative of vesicourachal diverticula; they cannot be palpated. However, signs of lower urinary tract disease in animals less than two years of age should arouse a high index of suspicion of this abnormality. Occasionally a vesicourachal diverticulum develops because of increased intravesical pressure due to obstruction of urine outflow, an abnormality that can occur at any age.

Urinalyses from animals with infected diverticula usually reveal varying degrees of pyuria, hematuria, proteinuria, and bacteriuria. Significant numbers of bacteria may be isolated by quantitative urine culture. In our experience, *Proteus* spp. are most frequently isolated from the urine of dogs with infected diverticula. In dogs that have diverticula without urinary tract infection, urinalyses have been normal and urine cultures sterile.

A definitive diagnosis of vesicourachal diverticulum can only be established by contrast radiography or laparotomy. Diverticula are best identified by positive contrast cystography. They typically appear as convex or triangular protrusions from the vertex of the bladder. Overdistension of the urinary bladder with contrast material may obscure small diverticula that do not extend beyond the serosal margin. To minimize this hazard, radiographs of the bladder

should be exposed following different degrees of bladder distention with contrast material.

Diverticulectomy is the treatment of choice for vesicourachal diverticula associated with bacterial urinary tract infections. Visualization of the diverticulum at the time of surgery can sometimes be enhanced by distending it with urine forced into the bladder vertex via digital pressure applied to

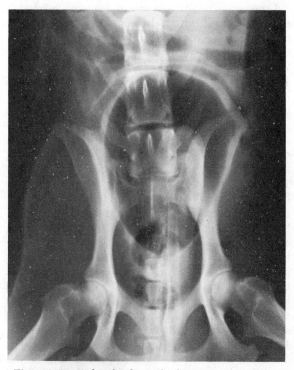

Figure 2. Ventrodorsal radiograph of a pneumocystogram of a one-year-old male malamute with recurrent urinary tract infection. The diverticulum located on the left lateral aspect of the urinary bladder wall was removed surgically, resulting in a resolution of the patient's urinary tract infection.

the bladder. The diverticulum may be excised by making a serosal-to-mucosal elliptical incision around its margin.

Microscopic examination of the diverticulum and adjacent tissue typically reveals inflammation characterized by ulceration of the urothelium, formation of fibrous connective tissue, and diffuse accumulations of mononuclear cells. In some instances, lymphoid follicles may be observed. Postoperative care should include a 14-day course of antibiotic therapy selected on the basis of susceptibility testing. Response to therapy should be evaluated by urine culture performed at appropriate intervals during and following antimicrobial therapy (see Treatment of Urinary Tract Infections with Antimicrobial Agents for further details). In our experience, removal of vesicourachal diverticula combined with appropriate therapy to eradicate urinary tract infections has significantly reduced the frequency of recurrent urinary tract infection.

ACQUIRED DIVERTICULA

Acquired diverticula are uncommon in dogs and cats (Fig. 2). They have been associated with traumatic injury to the bladder and bladder outflow obstruction. In many instances, they occur without a detectable underlying cause. Management of an acquired diverticulum is similar to that described for vesicourachal diverticula.

REFERENCES AND SUPPLEMENTAL READING

Cook, W. A., and King, L. R.: Vesicoureteral reflux. In Harrison, J. M., Gittes, R. F., Perlmutter, A. D., Stamey, T. A., and Walsh, P. C. (eds.): Campbell's Urology, Vol. 2. Philadelphia: W. B. Saunders, 1979, pp. 1596–1633.
Hansen, J. S.: Urachal remnant in the cat: Occurrence and relationship to feline urological syndrome. V.M./S.A.C. 72:1735, 1977.
Wilson, J. W., Klausner, J. S., Stevens, J. B., and Osborne, C. A.: Canine vesicourachal diverticula. Vet. Surg. 8:63, 1979.

URINARY ACIDIFIERS

DELMAR R. FINCO, D.V.M.,
and JEANNE A. BARSANTI, D.V.M.

Athens, Georgia

Urinary acidifiers represent one of the most overused classes of drugs in small animal practice. Knowledge of their strengths and limitations is imperative for rational use. Acidifiers are commonly used in the treatment of: urinary tract infection (UTI), feline urologic syndrome (FUS), and urolithiasis. They also may be used to adjust urine pH for modifying urinary excretion of drugs or for altering drug activity in urine.

URINARY TRACT INFECTION

There is little dispute that the growth of certain urinary pathogens is inhibited in acidic urine. Prior to the discovery of sulfonamides and antibiotics, adjusting urine pH was one of the few tools available for therapy of UTI. On the other hand, it is our opinion that the efficacy of urinary acidifiers in the eradication of urinary infections is generally poor compared with that of antibiotics, sulfonamides, and nitrofurantoins. Our disenchantment with acidifiers for the treatment of urinary infection stems from several factors. First, other available antibacterial agents have a high rate of in vitro success in inhibiting bacterial growth by bacteriostatic or bacteriocidal mechanisms of action. Administration of these drugs is associated with reliably high urine concentrations because many are excreted exclusively or predominantly by the kidney. Many are available as inexpensive generic products that cost the owner little more than urinary acidifiers. By contrast, the degree and duration of urine acidification after administration of urinary acidifiers are highly variable and are dependent on factors other than administration of the acidifier. In order to be certain that the desired degree of acidification has occurred, evaluation of serial urine samples and subsequent adjustments of dosage may be indicated. In addition, acidifiers are less likely to eliminate the infection than other antibacterial agents and are more likely to require a longer period of administration if success is to be expected.

For these reasons it is our opinion that urinary acidifiers are not indicated for their antibacterial properties in the treatment of urinary infection unless: (1) all other antibacterial agents are shown to be ineffective by in vitro testing or clinical use, or (2) all other agents are contraindicated because of undesirable side effects.

In cases of chronic UTI that are resistant to antibiotics, sulfonamides, and nitrofurantoins, we believe that the combination of a urinary antiseptic (methenamine) and an acidifier (Mandelamine*) is superior to an acidifier alone. In urine of low pH (below 6.0), methenamine is slowly converted to formaldehyde, which has bacteriocidal activity against many organisms. Methenamine is more effective in treating bladder infections than renal infections, since about one hour is required for conversion of methenamine to formaldehyde. This conversion may take place in residual bladder urine but is less likely to occur in the kidney unless urine outflow is restricted. Methenamine is available alone or in combination with mandelic acid or other acidifiers. The oral dose of methenamine mandelate for dogs is 20 mg/kg every six hours. Urine pH must be monitored to be assured of adequate acidity. If urine pH is not below 6.0, additional acidifier must be administered. We have had no experience with the use and safety of this drug in cats.

URINARY ACIDIFIERS AND FUS

The cause of FUS is unknown, but it is not due to bacterial infection. Acidifiers are commonly used in the treatment of FUS on the presumption that they decrease formation of struvite crystals. However, no objective studies have been performed to prove or disprove efficacy of acidifiers in the treatment of FUS. Our position on the use of acidifiers for the treatment of FUS differs from that for UTI, because alternate, effective forms for therapy of FUS are unknown. For this reason we neither condemn nor advocate their use in cats with FUS. We use them sparingly (see Role of Diet in Feline Urologic Syndrome), rationalizing that they usually do no harm and sometimes may be beneficial.

URINARY ACIDIFIERS AND UROLITHIASIS

Magnesium ammonium phosphate calculi are the most common uroliths found in dogs. They usually are associated with urinary infection due to urease-producing staphylococci or *Proteus* spp. We believe that urinary acidifiers are contraindicated in the management of most patients with this type of calculus for the following reasons: (1) Acidifiers are poor tools for eradication of infection when compared with other antibacterial agents. Eradication of infection and maintenance of the dog in an infection-free state are essential for the prevention of recurrence of calculi. (2) Acidifiers are ineffective or only partially effective in acidifying the urine in patients with infection with urea-splitting organisms. (3) Use of acidifiers provides a false sense of security to both the client and the veterinarian.

Following surgery for removal of uroliths, it has been popular to combine short-term antibiotic therapy with long-term acidifier therapy. Since infection may be suppressed but not eradicated by antibiotic therapy, acidifiers may mask residual infection for variable periods, with eventual exacerbation and stone recurrence. When infection is eradicated, acidifiers may not have adequate antibacterial effects to prevent recurrence of both infection and stones.

We believe a more rational approach to phosphate urolith prophylaxis is the use of a sound initial program to eradicate infection with antibiotics, followed by a lifelong re-examination program to detect recurrence of infection. Because calculi may form in a matter of a few weeks, re-examination must be performed at frequent intervals. Our re-examination program includes at least weekly urine pH measurements by the client. A first-voided morning sample is checked with a sensitive pH paper spanning the range of 6.0 to 8.0.† Any pH value above 7.5 prompts three measurements on consecutive days to establish the consistency of the finding. Consistently alkaline urine demands investigation and appropriate therapy. This program makes lifelong re-examination for infection with urea-splitting organisms economically feasible and reasonably practical for the client. Obviously the use of urinary acidifiers would interfere with this program.

Since uroliths (e.g., cystine, urate) are less soluble in acid urine than in alkaline urine, composition of calculi should be established for rational therapy. Obviously urinary acidifiers are contraindicated for these types of calculi.

ADJUSTING URINE pH FOR MAXIMAL DRUG ACTIVITY

Urine pH may alter renal drug excretion by altering diffusion between the tubular lumen and the contents of renal tubular cells. Activity of various drugs within urine may also be influenced by urine pH and is the strongest indication for the use of urinary acidifiers. Since the activity of many antibiotics is related to pH, the concomitant use of specific antibiotics and acidifiers is justified. On the other hand, many antibiotics are excreted in urine in concentrations far in excess of the minimal inhibitory concentration for a particular infection, and the pH range for activity is fairly broad. In such instances, adjusting urine pH to the point of maximum efficiency for that antibiotic may do little to enhance antibiotic efficacy. Drugs requiring acid urine for maximal activity include nitrofurantoin, penicillin G, and tetracyclines. Drugs requiring alkaline urine for maximal activity include chloramphenicol, erythromycin, gentamicin, streptomycin, neomycin, and kanamycin (see *Current Veterinary Therapy VI*, page 25).

---

*Parke-Davis, Morris Plains, NJ.

†Micro Essential Labs Inc., Brooklyn, NY.

PRODUCTS AVAILABLE AND DOSES

Consult the approximate appendix for doses of DL-methionine, ascorbic acid, and ammonium chloride. However it must be emphasized that there is no correct dose for any urinary acidifier. Each should be given in an amount sufficient to cause the desired change in urine pH. Since there are limits to the kidneys' ability to excrete H^+, overdosage with acidifiers can lead to metabolic acidosis, particularly in patients with compromised renal function.

SUPPLEMENTAL READING

Hamilton-Miller, J.M.T., and Brumfitt, W.: Methenamine and its salt as urinary tract antiseptics. Invest. Urol. 14:287, 1977.
Hardy, R. M.: Urinary acidifiers and their clinical applications. *In* Kirk, R. W. (ed.): *Current Veterinary Therapy* V. Philadelphia: W. B. Saunders, 1974, pp. 889–891.

USE AND MISUSE OF INTERMITTENT AND INDWELLING URINARY CATHETERS

GEORGE E. LEES, D.V.M.,
College Station, Texas

and CARL A. OSBORNE, D.V.M.
St. Paul, Minnesota

Urinary catheters have numerous specific uses, many of which are essential for optimum patient care. However, certain risks to the patient's welfare are associated with urinary catheterization. Although the nature and magnitude of risk vary with the clinical circumstances, the possibility of an adverse outcome exists whenever a urinary catheter is used. In light of this fact, veterinarians should carefully weigh decisions about the use of urinary catheters so that wise choices are made initially and remain vigilant when catheters are used so that adverse consequences are recognized promptly and treated appropriately.

To accomplish these two tasks, veterinarians must consider numerous variables and be guided by the particular facts in each case. Legitimate exceptions to general principles make dogmatic advocacy of any statement unwise. Rather than promulgate a list of rules regarding use of urinary catheters, we have summarized potential advantages and disadvantages of catheterization. With this information informed decisions can be made about the use of urinary catheters.

INDICATIONS FOR URINARY CATHETERIZATION

Specific uses for urinary catheters can be categorized as diagnostic or therapeutic (Table 1). The intended purpose of catheterization largely determines which of the three general types of catheterization will be useful. Single brief catheterization is appropriate when a catheter can serve its purpose in a few hours or less. However, when the need for catheterization spans longer periods, intermittent or indwelling catheterization is required.

COMPLICATIONS OF URINARY CATHETERIZATION

OVERVIEW

Urinary catheters may produce two general types of adverse effects: (1) trauma to the urinary tract caused by insertion or continued presence of the catheter, and (2) initiation of bacterial urinary tract

Table 1. *Indications for Urinary Catheterization*

Diagnostic
    Collection of a urine sample for analysis or bacterial
        culture
    Collection of accurately timed volumes of urine for
        renal function studies
    Measurement of urine output
    Measurement of post-micturition residual urine volume
    Instillation of contrast material for radiographic studies
        of the bladder, urethra, or prostate gland
    Verification and localization of urethral obstruction
    Catheter aspiration biopsy of urethral, prostatic, or
        bladder lesions
Therapeutic
    Relief of urethral obstruction to urine flow
    Relief of urine retention
    Instillation of medications into the urinary bladder
    Facilitation of surgery of the bladder, urethra, or sur-
        rounding structures

infection (UTI). The risk of these adverse effects varies from patient to patient because it is affected by numerous factors.

STATUS OF THE URINARY TRACT

Foremost among the variables that affect the risk of catheter-induced complications is the physical and functional status of the patient's urinary tract (especially the urethra and bladder) during and following catheterization. When diseases of the urinary tract make catheterization mechanically difficult, poor technique that leads to bacterial contamination and urinary tract trauma is likely. In addition, local urinary tract defense mechanisms are usually compromised by urinary tract diseases. Thus, animals with urinary tract disorders have the greater risk of catheter-induced complications. Unfortunately, it is these patients for which catheterization is most often indicated.

PATIENT PROFILE

Risk of catheter-induced complications is also associated with species, sex, size, temperament, and general health status. Cats are generally more difficult to catheterize than dogs. However, dogs may be more susceptible to UTI than cats (see Feline Urinary Tract Infections). Regardless of species, males are more easily catheterized than females. Perhaps this and other sex-related factors are associated with the greater risk of catheter-induced UTI in females as compared with male dogs. Because veterinary patients vary greatly in size and cooperativeness, equipment and techniques that work optimally for some are less satisfactory for others. Failure to use methods that are appropriate for each patient can be detrimental. Catheter-induced UTI can lead to episodes of bacteremia, particularly when a catheter is removed from an infected urinary tract.

General health status and concomitant disorders also influence the risk of catheter-associated complications. For example, dogs with Cushing's syndrome or diabetes mellitus have increased susceptibility to UTI. In addition, animals with valvular cardiac disease have increased risk of developing bacterial endocarditis as a result of bacteremia.

TECHNIQUE

Techniques of catheterization influence the frequency and nature of adverse sequelae. Abrasion, contusion, laceration, and even puncture of the urethra and bladder can occur during catheterization. Prevention of these undesirable effects, in addition to control of catheter-induced UTI, is dependent on selection and careful use of an appropriate catheter.

Frequency and duration of catheterization also influence the risk of catheter-induced complications. Iatrogenic infection is least likely to occur as a consequence of a single brief catheterization. Studies of repeated intermittent brief catheterization have revealed that the risk of inducing infection is similar following each catheterization. Thus, the cumulative risk of catheter-induced UTI is proportional to the number of catheterizations.

Risk of iatrogenic infection is greatest during indwelling catheterization, especially when the portion of catheter protruding from the urethra is not connected to a receptacle (i.e., it is open). In general, the risk of infection during indwelling catheterization is proportional to the duration of catheterization. When there is need for long-term catheterization, intermittent catheterization is often safer because it is less likely to induce UTI than indwelling catheterization. In addition, indwelling catheters may cause continuous trauma to the urinary tract and may elicit a foreign body reaction in surrounding tissue. In some situations, however, risk of urethral trauma caused by repeated insertion of a catheter is sufficient to make indwelling catheterization the safer alternative.

It is often difficult to maintain closed indwelling catheter systems in ambulatory patients. Although this difficulty is minimized when patients are severely injured or moribund, such patients may have increased susceptibility to infection.

PREVENTION OF CATHETER-INDUCED COMPLICATIONS

The best cure is prevention. Unnecessary use of urinary catheters should be avoided. Urinary catheters should not be indiscriminately used to obtain urine samples for urinalysis or bacterial culture, especially in high risk patients. Collection of samples during voluntary voiding or by cystocentesis is preferred because of technical ease and safety to the patient. Catheterization for the sole purpose of obtaining a urine sample should be reserved for situations in which it is the safest available alternative and the clinical importance of the sample justifies the risk of catheter-induced complications.

When use of urinary catheters is unequivocal, precautions should be taken to minimize physical damage to the urinary tract. In general, the smallest diameter and most pliable catheter that can be used successfully should be selected. Although soft flexible catheters are more difficult to insert into the urethra, the extra time and effort required are worthwhile, particularly if they are used as indwelling catheters. In one study of male cats catheterized for three days, polyvinyl catheters (Sovereign Disposable Infant Feeding Tube and Urethral Catheter*) were much less damaging to the lower urinary tract than polypropylene catheters (Sovereign Tom Cat Catheter*). Because commercial polyvinyl catheters are 30 cm long, they can also be used in many male dogs. Latex rubber Foley catheters marketed for use in humans are too short and/or too large in diameter for use in most males but can be effectively used in many female dogs. Because Foley catheters have an inflatable balloon surrounding their proximal ends, they are technically easier to use as indwelling catheters than those that must be sutured or taped to the patient.

Urinary catheters should be in good physical condition without sharp edges or abrasive surfaces. They should be liberally coated with sterile aqueous lubricant before use. Catheters should be gently inserted to minimize damage to the delicate epithelial lining of the urethra and bladder. A word of caution: overinsertion of excessive lengths of catheter should be avoided to minimize trauma to the bladder and to prevent the catheter from becoming knotted or entangled within the bladder and/or urethra. If an indwelling catheter is used, it should be removed as soon as it has served its purpose.

Precautions must also be used to minimize bacterial contamination of the urinary tract during catheterization. Because the distal portion of the urethra normally contains bacteria, it is impossible to aseptically catheterize a patient. Nonetheless, other potential sources of bacterial contamination should be avoided. Catheters, lubricants, irrigating solutions, specula, and other instruments should be sterilized. Contamination by genitalia or surrounding hair should be minimized. Hair that cannot otherwise be excluded from the operative field should be removed, and the tissue surrounding the distal urethra should be cleansed prior to catheterization.

When indwelling catheters are used, bacterial contamination following their insertion must be minimized. There are two primary routes by which bacteria may gain access to the urinary bladder during indwelling catheterization: through catheter lumens, and around the outside of catheters through the urethral lumen. Bacterial ascent through the catheter is prevented primarily by use of closed urine drainage systems that prevent reflux of urine from the collection receptacle back into the urinary tract. In humans, closed urine drainage systems have been the most effective method of preventing indwelling catheter-induced UTI. To be maximally effective, the catheter, drainage tubing, and collection reservoir must form a sealed sterile system that communicates only with the bladder lumen. Urine that enters the reservoir through a one-way inlet is intermittently removed through a separate outlet. Bacterial colonization of the reservoir is prevented by addition of a disinfectant (e.g., 30 ml of 3 per cent hydrogen peroxide). This is an important step, since colonization of the reservoir with bacteria is often the first step in the development of UTI during closed indwelling catheterization. Although it is frequently difficult to maintain closed indwelling urinary drainage systems in dogs and cats, principles of good medical practice demand that closed catheter drainage be used whenever possible.

Although closed drainage greatly reduces the incidence of indwelling catheter–induced UTI, bacteria may still enter the bladder through the urethral lumen adjacent to the catheter. Frequent cleaning of the urethral meatus–catheter junction and application of antimicrobial creams or ointments to this area have been advocated to minimize bacterial contamination via this route. However, controlled studies of human patients have revealed that this procedure is ineffective. In fact, bacteriuria was acquired at significantly higher rates in treated groups than in untreated groups, probably because urethral manipulation induced bacterial contamination. Although the aforementioned meatal care regimens have dubious value, efforts to keep the catheter and surrounding hair and skin free of gross contamination (e.g., feces) are warranted.

Local or systemic administration of antimicrobial agents may also be useful for the prevention of catheter-induced UTI. The rationale for this approach is to kill bacteria that enter the bladder before they can establish infection. It is emphasized that antimicrobial therapy is an adjunct to, and not a substitute for, efforts to control bacterial contamination during catheterization.

Antimicrobial therapy following brief catheterization may be considered for high risk patients, including females, and patients with urinary tract abnormalities, diabetes mellitus, Cushing's syndrome, and so on. In these situations, two approaches can be considered. One is instillation of an antiseptic solution into the bladder just prior to removal of the catheter. The solution infused should

_____
*Sherwood Medical Industries, St. Louis, MO.

be sterile. Although this approach may be effective, there are several pitfalls that may lead to its failure. Retrograde injection of the antiseptic solution could wash contaminating bacteria into the bladder from the distal portion of the catheter. In addition, solutions of antimicrobial drugs in multiple-dose containers may become colonized by bacteria during storage; infusion of such solutions may cause infection. Furthermore, dilution of the drug in urine that remains or accumulates in the bladder following the procedure may reduce the drug's concentration to an ineffective level and/or urination may remove the drug before it can complete its intended action. Most of these pitfalls may be avoided by the use of systemic antimicrobial agents. Oral or parenteral administration of one or more doses of antibiotics primarily excreted by the kidneys may produce sufficiently high urinary drug levels for a short period following catheterization to prevent bacterial colonization of the urothelium. Drugs of the penicillin group (penicillin G, ampicillin, and so on) are recommended because they are safe, bacteriocidal, and effective against most bacteria found in the microbial flora of the urethra (i.e., streptococci and staphylococci) that contaminate urinary catheters.

Antimicrobial therapy cannot be relied upon to prevent indwelling catheter–induced UTI. Rather than preventing or substantially delaying onset of infections, such therapy often predisposes to resistant infections that are less susceptible to many chemotherapeutic agents. Administration of ampicillin during indwelling catheterization was beneficial in an experimental study of normal male cats because catheter-induced infections occurred less frequently and were less severe in cats given this drug. However, 25 per cent of cats given ampicillin developed catheter-induced bacteriuria with pathogens that had reduced susceptibility to ampicillin and several other antimicrobial agents. In another study, use of indwelling catheters in cats following perineal urethrostomy was associated with a higher risk of postoperative complications than perineal urethrostomy of cats that were not catheterized.

INDICATIONS FOR INDWELLING CATHETERS

Indwelling catheters should generally be reserved for use during (1) intensive care of critically ill patients when continuous measurement of urine production is required, and (2) the initial management period following relief of urethral obstruction. In this situation, the purpose of the catheter is to assure urethral patency and prevent continued urine retention. The three main indications for use of indwelling catheters following initial relief of urethral obstruction are as follows: (1) lack of a relatively normal urine stream, (2) persistence of intraluminal material or extraluminal compression likely to cause reobstruction, and (3) loss of detrusor muscle contractility and overdistention of the bladder that has induced ineffective micturition despite urethral patency. If these abnormalities do not exist following relief of urethral obstruction, indwelling catheterization is usually unnecessary and should be avoided.

If indwelling catheters are employed, closed drainage systems should be used. Even if an antimicrobial drug is administered, UTI may still develop. Therefore, the catheter should be removed as soon as it has served its purpose, and bacterial urine culture should be obtained to detect iatrogenic infection.

Urine retention caused by neurogenic disorders of urinary tract function (e.g., spinal cord disease, reflex dyssynergia, and so on) is optimally managed by manual compression of the bladder to expel the urine or by intermittent catheterization. Indwelling catheterization is the least desirable method of combating urine retention in these situations because of the likelihood of iatrogenic infection and trauma.

SUPPLEMENTAL READING

Biertuempfel, P. H., Ling, G. V., and Ling, G. A.: Urinary tract infection resulting from catheterization in healthy adult dogs. J.A.V.M.A. 178:989, 1981.

Lees, G. E., and Osborne, C. A.: Urinary tract infections associated with the use and misuse of urinary catheters. Vet. Clin. North Am. 9:713, 1979.

Lees, G. E., Osborne, C. A., Stevens, J. B., and Ward, G. E.: Adverse effects caused by polypropylene and polyvinyl feline urinary catheters. Am. J. Vet. Res. 41:1836, 1980.

Lees, G. E., Osborne, C. A., Stevens, J. B., and Ward, G. E.: Adverse effects of open indwelling urethral catheterization in clinically normal male cats. Am. J. Vet. Res. 42:825, 1981.

Smith, C. W., Schiller, A. G., Smith, A. R., Wells, S. K., and Kissil, M.: Effects of indwelling urinary catheters in male cats. J. Am. Anim. Hosp. Assoc. 17:427, 1981.

TREATMENT OF BACTERIAL PROSTATITIS

JEANNE A. BARSANTI, D.V.M.,
and DELMAR R. FINCO, D.V.M.

Athens, Georgia

Antibiotics are the primary mode of therapy of bacterial prostatitis in dogs. Effective use of antibiotic therapy is dependent on knowledge of the causative bacterium and its antibiotic susceptibility, and whether the prostatic infection is acute or chronic.

The prostate gland is composed of glandular acini and interstitial stroma. Prostatic epithelium surrounding acini produces prostatic fluid, which is more acidic than interstitial tissue or blood. This pH differential and the epithelial cells themselves form a blood–prostatic fluid barrier that influences entrance of antibiotics into prostatic fluid. This barrier is disrupted during acute prostatitis, allowing antibiotic diffusion from blood. In chronic prostatitis, this barrier remains intact and restricts antibiotic diffusion.

TECHNIQUES FOR DETECTION OF PROSTATIC INFECTION

Prostatic infection is often difficult to diagnose, especially when it is chronic. An appropriate history and physical examination, including rectal and caudal abdominal palpation of the prostate gland, are essential. Urinalysis and quantitative urine culture should be performed on a urine sample collected by cystocentesis. Prostatic infection should always be suspected in male dogs with urinary tract infection. Infections may be localized to the prostate gland by examination of (1) urethral discharges, (2) semen, (3) material obtained by post-prostatic massage, (4) urethral or bladder contents, and (5) biopsy samples.

If a urethral discharge is to be examined, the penis should be cleaned gently and wiped dry with sterile sponges. The discharge should be collected in a sterile tube. An aliquot should be examined microscopically, and an aliquot should be used for quantitative bacterial culture. Discharge culture results should be compared with urine culture results. Urethral discharges are unavoidably contaminated with resident gram positive urethral flora, creating problems when interpreting examination results. Detection of large numbers of gram negative organisms is often indicative of prostatic or urethral infection. Large numbers ($>10^5$/ml) of gram positive organisms or small numbers ($<10^5$/ml) of gram negative organisms may be associated with infection or contamination. Comparison of urethral culture results with urine culture results obtained by cystocentesis may help to differentiate microbial pathogens from contaminants.

Semen samples may also be contaminated by the resident preputial and urethral flora. Preputial contamination can be minimized by careful collection and by gently removing discharges from the penis with a sterile sponge. Urethral contamination may also be minimized (but probably not eliminated) by allowing the dog to urinate prior to collection. To aid in the detection of urethral contaminants, a urethral swab (Calgiswab*) may be cultured directly, or it can be placed in 5 ml of saline and subsequently cultured by quantitative methods. An ejaculate should then be collected and evaluated by quantitative culture and cytology. Comparison of ejaculate culture results with urethral culture results may allow one to determine whether the organisms identified were present in the urethra.

Collection of a sample from the urethra or bladder after prostatic massage may help to minimize distal urethral contaminants and organisms in the testicles or epididymis. However, urine contamination cannot be prevented in dogs, since all collection methods involve aspiration of a sample at the level of the prostatic urethra and bladder with or without flushing the prostatic urethra with a sterile solution. In the majority of dogs with prostatic disease, aspiration of prostatic fluid without flushing is not possible. If the urine contains large numbers of bacteria ($>10^5$/ml), prostatic fluid culture results obtained following massage cannot be interpreted if urine contamination occurs. To circumvent this problem, patients may be given antimicrobials (e.g., nitrofurantoin or ampicillin), which do not penetrate prostatic fluid but which reach high urine concentrations. Prostatic massage is then performed after the patients have been given the drug for 24 to 48 hours. Since this maneuver usually sterilizes the urine, organisms present in fluid obtained by pros-

---

*American Can Company, Glenwood, IL.

tatic massage can be identified. The sample must be cultured immediately, however, to avoid killing of bacteria by high concentrations of the antibiotic in urine.

Prostatic biopsy samples can be obtained by perineal punch biopsy or caudal celiotomy. It should be emphasized that histologic evidence of inflammation is not synonymous with infection. The sample must be cultured to prove prostatic infection. Since bacterial numbers may be low or the infection may be focal, the tissue should be ground prior to culture to increase the likelihood of detecting bacteria. If the infection is focal, a biopsy may yield false negative results.

ACUTE BACTERIAL PROSTATITIS

DIAGNOSIS

A presumptive diagnosis of acute bacterial prostatitis is usually based on results of the history, physical examination, urinalysis, and urine culture. An acute onset of a hemorrhagic or purulent urethral discharge, caudal abdominal tenderness, fever, and lethargy are suggestive of acute bacterial prostatitis. Clinical signs in some patients may be limited to urethral discharge. The prostate may be painful. Changes in size and symmetry are variable. Infection is often superimposed on prostatic hyperplasia in older male dogs. Results of urinalysis are typically characterized by hematuria, pyuria, and bacteriuria, indicating urinary tract infection, and culture of urine often reveals bacteria in large numbers, most often *E. coli*.

Typical findings obtained by history, physical examination, and urinalysis provide presumptive evidence of acute bacterial prostatitis. Evaluation of prostatic fluid often provides more definitive information. Urethral discharges collected cleanly in a sterile container and evaluated by light microscopy and quantitative culture probably reflect the character of prostatic fluid. Prostatic fluid may also be obtained by ejaculation; however, many dogs with acute prostatitis will not ejaculate. Even if an ejaculate is collected, the testicles and epididymis must be ruled out as points of origin of any abnormality found.

Prostatic massage may also be used to collect prostatic fluid. Since this fluid must usually be retrieved from the urethra and bladder via a catheter, results are difficult to interpret if concomitant urinary tract infection is present. When large numbers ($>10^5$/ml) of bacteria are present in the urine, it is impossible to determine whether the massage produced any additional increase in bacterial numbers. This technique is more useful when urine bacterial numbers are low.

TREATMENT

An antibiotic should be chosen on the basis of susceptibility of organisms isolated by culture of urine, urethral discharge, or ejaculate or after prostatic massage. An antibiotic that results in high blood, tissue, and urine concentrations is preferable. The blood–prostatic fluid barrier is apparently not intact during acute inflammation. The route by which the antibiotic is given depends on the severity of the dog's illness. Once an antibiotic is chosen, it should be continued for a minimum of 14 days. Supportive care may be necessary if the dog has systemic signs.

RE-EXAMINATION

Dogs with acute bacterial prostatitis should be re-evaluated after therapy to determine if the infection has been eliminated. Failure to eradicate the causative agent may result in an unresolvable chronic infection associated with intermittent episodes of generalized urinary infection. The dog should be rechecked about 17 to 20 days after the onset of illness (3 to 5 days after discontinuing antibiotics). Because remission of clinical signs provides no assurance that infection has been eliminated, physical examination, urinalysis, and urine culture should be performed. Prostatic fluid obtained by ejaculation or prostatic massage should be evaluated by bacterial culture and cytology. Persistent infection is indicative of chronic bacterial prostatitis and should be managed accordingly.

CHRONIC BACTERIAL PROSTATITIS

DIAGNOSIS

A presumptive diagnosis of chronic bacterial prostatitis may be established by results obtained from history, physical examination, and examination of prostatic fluid by cytology and bacterial culture. Prostatic fluid can be obtained by prostatic massage or ejaculation. The history is usually characteristic of recurrent urinary tract infections caused by the same organism. Recurrent hemorrhagic or purulent urethral discharges may also have been noted. Palpation of the prostate gland may reveal that it is normal or may indicate a change in its consistency or symmetry. Areas of increased firmness or softness may be noted. Changes in size are variable and may be related to concomitant prostatic disease such as hyperplasia. The prostate is usually not painful; the dog has no signs of systemic illness.

Urinalysis and urine culture may or may not indicate urinary tract infection at the time of examination. Whether or not urinary tract infection is present, an effort should be made to localize the problem to the prostate. An ejaculate should be collected, evaluated cytologically, and cultured quantitatively. The results should be compared with culture results from a urethral swab. If an ejaculate cannot be collected, a prostatic massage sample should be obtained. If the dog does not have a urinary tract infection, prostatic fluid should be collected for analysis immediately. If the dog has a significant ($>10^5$ bacteria/ml) urinary tract infection, an antibiotic that reaches high levels in the urine but not in the prostatic fluid (e.g., ampicillin) should be given for a few days. Antibiotics should not be given on the morning the prostatic massage is performed. The sample must be cultured immediately to prevent any antibiotic remaining in urine from killing the organisms introduced after massage.

A definitive diagnosis of chronic bacterial prostatitis can be made by culture of prostatic tissue obtained by biopsy. The biopsy should also be examined histologically.

TREATMENT

Current information suggests that prostatic fluid is acidic in normal dogs and dogs with bacterial prostatitis. Thus, to penetrate the blood–prostatic fluid barrier, which is intact during chronic prostatitis, a lipid-soluble antibiotic or one with a basic pKa is needed. Antibiotics that meet these criteria include chloramphenicol, trimethoprim, erythromycin, oleandomycin, and tetracycline. The susceptibility of the organism cultured to these antimicrobial agents should be carefully reviewed. Once an antibiotic is chosen, it should be continued for at least four weeks. Three to five days after the antibiotic is discontinued, prostatic fluid should be cultured and examined cytologically. If infection persists, treatment should be reinstituted with the same or a different antibiotic, depending on the number of choices available. After a few weeks, prostatic fluid should be collected while the dog is receiving antibiotics. If infection persists, the antibiotic should be changed or adjunctive therapy should be considered. If the infection is under control, the antibiotic should be continued for at least another four weeks. Prostatic fluid should be checked again prior to, and five days after, discontinuing antibiotic therapy.

ADJUNCTIVE THERAPY

Adjunctive therapy for bacterial prostatitis is designed to reduce the mass of tissue available to be infected (hormonal therapy) or improve prostatic defense mechanisms (zinc supplementation).

Hormonal therapy is the most widely used adjunctive therapy for canine prostatic diseases. Castration, administration of antiandrogens (e.g., flutamide), and administration of estrogens will reduce the size of the prostate. Administration of estrogens may be associated with adverse side effects including prostatic abscessation, squamous metaplasia with obstruction of prostatic ducts, and aplastic anemia. These adverse effects may be avoided by using low doses of estrogens administered at infrequent intervals. Reduction in prostatic size alone will not eliminate infection. It has been presumed but not proved that reduction in prostatic size will improve the efficacy of appropriate antibiotic therapy. Hormonal therapy plus antibiotics cannot be relied upon to cure the patient. Persistent followup is essential to ensure that the infection has been eliminated.

The canine and human prostate is known to produce a zinc protein antibacterial factor. Reduced concentrations of zinc have been observed in the prostatic fluid of humans with prostatic infection. Supplemental oral zinc has been recommended to increase the concentration of this antibacterial factor. Although some data suggest clinical improvement after oral administration of zinc sulphate, most studies have shown no increase in prostatic fluid zinc concentrations following oral administration of zinc.

RE-EXAMINATION

Dogs with chronic bacterial prostatitis should be persistently re-evaluated if the infection is to be controlled and/or eliminated. Once prostatic fluid cultures are negative, the dog should be rechecked at 30 and 60 days to detect recurrences. In some dogs, the prostatic infection may not be cured by antibiotic and hormonal therapy. Total prostatectomy should be considered in these dogs. The alternative is antibiotic therapy given to control secondary urinary tract infection rather than to eliminate prostatic infection.

PROSTATIC ABSCESSATION

DIAGNOSIS

Prostatic abscessation is a form of chronic bacterial prostatitis in which pockets of pus of variable size develop. Prostatic abscesses may be associated with signs of systemic illness similar to those associated with acute bacterial prostatitis including fever, depression, anorexia, and vomiting (probably from visceral pain or localized peritonitis). Signs of lower urinary tract infection or a hemorrhagic or purulent urethral discharge are also often present. In some cases only urinary tract signs occur. Abscesses may be palpable as fluctuant areas within or on the surface of the gland. In other cases, only an irregular surface may be palpable because abscess pockets are within the gland. The gland may or may not be enlarged. In some cases, leukocytosis, with or without immaturity, may occur. Urinalysis and urine culture usually indicate urinary tract infection. Evaluation of an ejaculate usually reveals infection of the reproductive tract. Prostatic massage may help to localize the infection to the prostate if urinary tract infection is not severe. If an abscess is suspected, a needle aspiration biopsy should be performed prior to a perineal punch biopsy. Suspicion of prostatic abscess is a contraindication for percutaneous punch biopsy. We have identified prostatic abscesses by aspirating pus from needles directed to prostate glands via abdominal or perineal approaches. Immediately following identification of prostatic abscesses by aspiration, the patients were given antibiotics and scheduled for surgery, usually within 24 hours. A surgical wedge may be obtained to confirm the diagnosis.

TREATMENT

Prostatic abscesses should be incised and drained or removed. Comparison of various surgical procedures at the University of Georgia has revealed that all procedures are associated with significant complications. Periprostatic and intraprostatic drains have resulted in recalcitrant bacterial infections. Marsupialization is often technically difficult and may be associated with infection of surrounding tissues. Prostatectomy has been associated with the fewest complications but is technically difficult and can result in urinary incontinence.

Concomitant castration is recommended as adjunctive therapy to reduce prostatic size. However, castration alone is not recommended, since the abscess remains.

FOLLOW-UP

After surgery, patients should be managed in a fashion identical to that recommended for dogs with chronic bacterial prostatitis. Periodic follow-up evaluation of the patient for urinary tract infection is essential.

SUPPLEMENTAL READING

Barsanti, J. A., and Finco, D. R.: Canine bacterial prostatitis. Vet. Clin. North Am. 9:679, 1979.

Barsanti, J. A., Shotts, E. B., Prasse, K., and Crowell, W.: Evaluation of diagnostic techniques for canine prostatic diseases. J.A.V.M.A. 177:160, 1980.

Baumueller, A., Kjair, T. B., and Madsen, P. O.: Prostatic tissue and secretion concentrations of rosamicin and erythromycin. Invest. Urol. 15:158, 1977.

Finco, D. R.: Prostate gland biopsy. Vet. Clin. North Am. 4:367, 1974.

Hornbuckle, W. E., MacCoy, D. M., Allan, M. S., et al.: Prostatic disease in the dog. Cornell Vet. 68:284, 1978.

Ling, G. V., and Ruby, A. C.: Aerobic bacterial flora of the prepuce, urethra and vagina of normal adult dogs. Am. J. Vet. Res. 39:695, 1978.

Stamey, T. A., Meares, E. M., and Winningham, D. C.: Chronic bacterial prostatitis and the diffusion of drugs into prostatic fluid. J. Urol. 103:187, 1970.

Stone, E. A., Thrall, D. E., and Barber, D. L.: Radiographic interpretation of prostatic disease in the dog. J. Am. Anim. Hosp. Assoc. 14:115, 1978.

LOCALIZATION OF MALE FELINE URETHRAL LESIONS PRIOR TO URETHROSTOMY

GARY R. JOHNSTON, D.V.M.,
DANIEL A. FEENEY, D.V.M.,
and CARL A. OSBORNE, D.V.M.

St. Paul, Minnesota

Disorders of the feline lower urinary tract characterized by dysuria, hematuria, crystalluria, and/or urethral obstruction are well known to all veterinarians in companion animal practice. Most describe varying combinations of these clinical signs as the feline urologic syndrome (FUS). Although the terminology lacks specificity, it parallels the current lack of understanding of the cause of these signs.

Differences in the anatomy of the male and female feline urethra are undoubtedly related to the higher incidence of obstruction in males compared with females. The difference appears to be related to the length of the male urethra and the fact that the diameter of the penile urethra is much smaller than the diameter of the pelvic and preprostatic urethra (Fig. 1). The urethra of females is shorter, wider, and more distensible than the urethra of males.

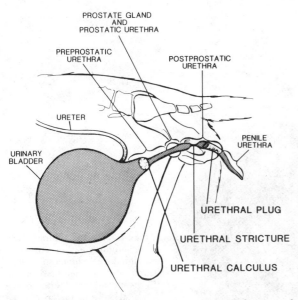

PROSTATE GLAND
AND
PROSTATIC URETHRA

PREPROSTATIC
URETHRA

POSTPROSTATIC
URETHRA

URETER

PENILE
URETHRA

URINARY
BLADDER

URETHRAL PLUG

URETHRAL STRICTURE

URETHRAL CALCULUS

Figure 1. Schematic illustration of some potential causes of urethral obstruction in male cats.

THE SITE OF URETHRAL OBSTRUCTION IN MALE CATS

Clinical experience and knowledge of the anatomy of the male urethra of cats has led to a general consensus of opinion that the penile urethra is the most common site of urethral obstruction. This opinion has led to the widespread use of perineal and preputial urethrostomy rather than antepubic urethrostomy to control recurrent urethral obstruction in male cats. Although this theory is logical, the site and degree of urethral obstruction have not been carefully documented in a large series of cats with naturally occurring disease. Survey radiography has not been of value in detecting the location and size of urethral plugs because the plugs are not radiopaque. Lack of information about the site of obstruction of the urethra in a suitable number of male cats with urethral obstruction is a conspicuous void in our knowledge, especially considering the frequency with which surgical removal of the penile urethra is recommended to treat this disorder.

Clinical studies performed at the University of Minnesota Veterinary Teaching Hospital have revealed that several patients with FUS had one or more of a variety of abnormalities, including (1) urethral strictures at sites other than, or in addition to, the penile urethra, (2) urethral and/or bladder uroliths, (3) bladder wall thickening with or without mucosal erosions and/or ulcerations, (4) bladder (urachal) diverticula, (5) vesicoureteral reflux, and (6) various other anomalies of the urethra and/or urinary bladder (Figs. 2, 3, and 4). These lesions were detected by a combination of positive contrast cystography, double contrast cystography, and retrograde positive contrast urethrocystography. These preliminary results suggest that surgical procedures designed to minimize urethral obstruction in male cats by amputation of the penile urethra may be partially or totally ineffective in some patients. In addition, these abnormalities may contribute to the recurrent nature of lower urinary tract disease in male cats.

TECHNIQUE OF LOCALIZATION OF URETHRAL LESIONS

Prior to perineal, preputial, or antepubic urethrostomy, verification of urethral lesions and their sites should be considered. Although urethral catheters may be used as urethral "sounds," this method of localization is crude at best. We recommend radiographic evaluation of the lower urinary tract. The technique or combination of techniques utilized

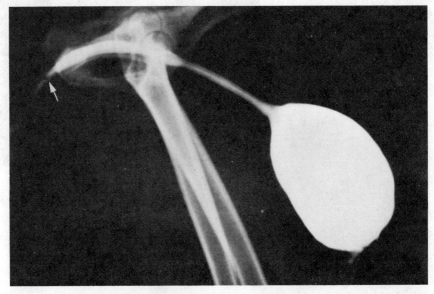

Figure 2. Positive contrast retrograde urethrocystogram of a five-year-old castrated male domestic short-haired cat illustrating an obstructing urolith in the lumen of the penile urethra (arrow) and a diverticulum located at the vertex of the bladder wall.

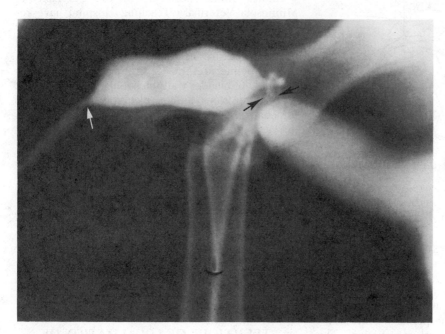

Figure 3. Positive contrast retrograde urethrogram of an eight-month-old male domestic shorthaired cat illustrating a stricture in the penile urethra (white arrow), and a stricture in the area of the prostatic urethra (black arrows).

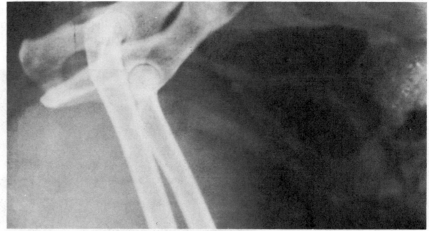

Figure 4. Negative contrast retrograde urethrocystogram of a two-year-old male Persian cat illustrating multiple uroliths in the bladder lumen and an obstructing urolith in the lumen of the preprostatic urethra.

depends on whether the urethra is partially or totally obstructed at the time of surgery.

Irrespective of the technique used, survey radiographs should be exposed in two projections for evaluation of patient preparation, radiographic technique, and lesions that may be distorted or obscured by contrast radiography.

RETROGRADE CONTRAST URETHROGRAPHY

Several techniques for retrograde contrast urethrography may be considered; however, retrograde studies utilizing balloon or nonballoon catheters are recommended for male cats. The technique is the same for obstructed and nonobstructed cats. A 4 French balloon catheter (Swan-Ganz*) (Fig. 5), and a 3.5 French tom cat urethral catheter (Sovereign Open End Tom Cat Catheter†) have produced satisfactory studies. Balloon-tipped catheters have a distinct advantage over other types of urethral catheters in preventing reflux of contrast medium through the external urethral orifice, thus ensuring proper filling of the urethral lumen proximal to the inflated balloon. Retrograde urethrography in male cats in which a urethral catheter is secured in the penile urethra by external digital compression is not recommended because of the potential exposure to ionizing radiation.

Meglumine diatrizoate (Hypaque Meglumine 60%‡) and meglumine iothalamate (Conray§) are contrast agents that we recommend, although other aqueous organic tri-iodinated compounds utilized for intravascular injections may be considered. The contrast medium should be diluted 1:3 with sterile distilled water or saline. Reduction of the radiodensity of the contrast material will aid in the detection of filling defects that may be obscured by undiluted contrast agents. Sterile aqueous lubricants (e.g., K-Y Jelly, Lubrafax, Xylocaine Jelly 2%)

*Edwards Laboratories, Santa Ana, Calif.
†Sherwood Medical Industries, Inc., St. Louis, MO.
‡Winthrop Laboratories, NY.
§Mallinckrodt, Inc., St. Louis, MO.

may be mixed with contrast medium to increase its viscosity, thus promoting distention of the urethral lumen.

The lumen of the balloon catheter should be filled with contrast medium prior to its placement in the urethra to prevent artifacts caused by air bubbles. Care should also be used to prevent iatrogenic trauma and infection of the urinary tract with balloon catheters.

To perform retrograde positive contrast urethrocystography in male cats, exteriorize the penile urethra and insert a 4 French balloon catheter into the urethral lumen for approximately 1.5 cm. Lubrication of the catheter tip with an aqueous lubricant will facilitate catheter placement. Inflation of the balloon with 0.5 ml of air will help to stabilize the catheter in this location. Placement of the balloon just inside the urethral orifice should be avoided if possible, because the small diameter of the penile urethra at this site will prevent sufficient inflation of the balloon to maintain it in this position.

The volume of contrast medium that can be injected into the urethral lumen depends on whether or not complete obstruction of the lumen is present. If the urethral lumen is patent, injection of 2 to 3 ml of contrast medium will usually opacify the urethral lumen but may not cause maximal distention. Moderate distention of the urinary bladder with positive contrast medium is required to provide sufficient intraluminal pressure to ensure maximum distention of the proximal portion of the preprostatic urethra. The volume of contrast medium required to distend the bladder lumen of normal cats is approximately 3 ml/lb body weight. However, smaller volumes may be tolerated in cats with lower urinary tract disease.

POSITIVE CONTRAST ANTEGRADE (VOIDING) URETHROGRAPHY

NONOBSTRUCTED CATS

Use of balloon catheters for retrograde contrast urethrography prevents radiographic evaluation of the urethra occupied by, and distal to, the balloon. This portion of the urethra may be visualized by

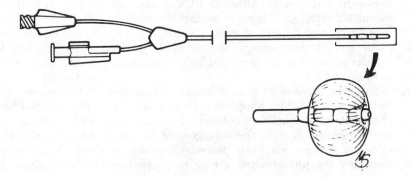

Figure 5. Schematic illustration of a Swan-Ganz balloon catheter. Air injected into the valve (lower arm) will inflate the balloon (inset).

antegrade contrast urethrography if necessary. The bladder lumen should be distended with an appropriate quantity of aqueous contrast material injected via a urinary catheter. Contrast material can be forced into the urethra with the aid of a wooden spoon placed over the abdomen at a site adjacent to the bladder. Abdominal compression can be induced at the appropriate time by pressing on the handle. Exposure of the lateral view of the entire lower urinary tract at the time of induced micturition will permit evaluation of the distal urethra. External compression with a wooden spoon may produce some distortion to the bladder and proximal urethra and may cause vesicoureteral reflux.

OBSTRUCTED CATS

Antegrade contrast urethrocystography may also be considered for evaluation of the urethral lumen of cats that are difficult to catheterize or whose urethral lumens are obstructed. The technique does not require the use of balloon catheters. The urinary bladder may be distended with contrast medium by excretory urography or percutaneous transabdominal bladder infusion following cystocentesis with a 22-gauge, 3-inch spinal needle. Following distention of the bladder, antegrade urethrography can be performed in a manner identical to that described for patients without urethral obstruction. Contrast medium may be forced into the urethral lumen by external bladder compression or by spontaneous micturition induced by gradual distention of the urinary bladder during light anesthesia of the patient. External compression of the bladder with a wooden spoon is preferred but may result in some degree of distortion of the bladder and proximal urethra. Appropriate caution should be used to prevent iatrogenic bladder rupture.

FELINE UROLOGIC SYNDROME:
MEDICAL THERAPY

JEANNE A. BARSANTI, D.V.M.,
and DELMAR R. FINCO, D.V.M.

Athens, Georgia

As of this writing, feline urologic syndrome (FUS) is not a specific disease but rather a complex of clinical signs, the etiology of which is still unknown. Even the complex of clinical signs associated with the term FUS varies with different authors, especially in regard to the inclusion of cats without urethral obstruction. We define FUS as hematuria and dysuria in male or female cats, unassociated with bacteriuria. Urethral obstruction due to a conglomeration of mucus and struvite crystals may be present in males. We admit that this definition is as flawed as the current understanding of FUS. It is a diagnosis by exclusion of other causes of hematuria and dysuria. Although FUS is the most commonly recognized cause of urethal obstruction, hematuria, and dysuria in cats, bacterial cystitis, cystic and urethral calculi, and neoplasia of the bladder and urethra can occur and have signs similar to those of FUS.

Since the cause of FUS is not known, no specific treatment is possible. Supportive therapy for the obstructed cat is fairly well defined, although some controversy exists as to the management of these cats. No therapy has been proved efficacious in managing the unobstructed cat or in preventing recurrent episodes of obstruction or hematuria and dysuria without urethral obstruction. To summarize our current knowledge, the following discussion has been divided into three parts: (1) management of cats with urethral obstruction, (2) management of cats without urethral obstruction, and (3) prevention of recurrent episodes of FUS.

FELINE URETHRAL OBSTRUCTION

Relief of obstruction and supportive fluid therapy are required for cats with urethral obstruction. Which is instituted first depends on the severity of the post-renal uremia that has resulted. If the cat is not markedly depressed, the obstruction is generally relieved first. If the cat is depressed and weak, intravenous fluid therapy is instituted immediately.

Correction of urethral obstruction is most often accomplished by retrograde flushing of the urethra with a sterile solution such as saline or lactated Ringer's solution through a lubricated urethral catheter. Many instruments are available for urethral catheterization. One must remember that the urethra of an obstructed male cat has already been damaged as the result of the pressure of the obstructing material and the retained urine and the pressure exerted during the cat's attempts to micturate. Gentle technique is necessary to avoid further urethral trauma. Polyethylene catheters such as tom cat catheters (Sovereign Open End Tom Cat Catheter*) or intravenous catheters (Sovereign Indwelling Catheter*) are probably less traumatic than metal instruments such as a blunt lacrimal cannula or a silver abscess needle.† However, the gentle technique of the operator is more important than the instrument in preventing urethral trauma.

Sufficient sedation should be used to facilitate catheterization. The degree of sedation required depends on the cat's condition and temperament. Intravenous short-acting barbiturates, inhalant anesthetics, or low doses of ketamine (2 to 6 mg/kg IM or IV) can be used. Since ketamine is excreted by the kidneys, prolonged recovery may occur if the obstruction is not relieved or if renal function does not rapidly improve after relief of obstruction.

If the obstruction cannot be dislodged by initial retrograde flushing of the urethra, the bladder should be emptied by cystocentesis with a 22-gauge needle, a three-way valve, and a syringe. Gentle manipulation of the bladder should be used to avoid bladder rupture, since the distended bladder wall is often damaged by the increased intravesicular pressure. Once bladder pressure has been relieved, material that is occluding the urethral lumen can often be flushed out with the aid of a urethral catheter.

After the obstruction is relieved, a flexible 3.5F rubber catheter (Sovereign Sterile Disposable Feeding Tube and Urethral Catheter*) should be inserted into the bladder to collect a urine sample for urinalysis and bacterial culture. Flexible catheters are preferred because of their longer length (10-cm polypropylene catheters often do not reach the bladder (Lees and Osborne, 1980) and because they produce less bladder and urethral trauma. The catheter should be inserted just far enough to reach the bladder neck as determined by the point at which urine is first obtained by aspiration. Overinsertion of the catheter can result in trauma to the bladder. The bladder is repeatedly flushed with a sterile isotonic solution until the returning flushing solution is clear.

Whether the catheter is removed or sutured in place is an individual clinician's decision. Leaving the catheter in place prevents immediate reobstruction but also leads to bacterial urinary tract infection and urethral irritation (Lee et al., 1981; Smith et al., 1981). Administration of a broad spectrum bacteriocidal antibiotic (e.g., ampicillin, amoxicillin)

while the catheter is in place will reduce the incidence of infection, but infection can still develop, and the bacteria will be resistant to the drug being used (Lees et al., 1981). If the urethral catheter is left in place, a closed drainage system should be established by connecting the urethral catheter via extension tubing to a recently emptied sterile fluid bottle or bag. An Elizabethan collar may be necessary to prevent the cat from removing the urethral catheter or disconnecting the drainage system.

At present, the best recommendation seems to be to leave the catheter in place only if one of the following three conditions is present: (1) the obstruction was relieved only with difficulty; (2) the urine stream is weak and small after relief of the obstruction; (3) the cat is uremic (depressed, dehydrated, vomiting, hypothermic, and so on) and hyperkalemic (weak, cardiac arrhythmias present). In uremic cats, rapid reobstruction must be prevented and urine output monitored. The catheter is left in place until the uremic signs abate and the cat again begins to eat and drink. A urine sample is collected for urinalysis and culture when the catheter is removed. If bacterial infection is present, antibiotic therapy is instituted for seven to ten days. A urine culture should be performed again three to five days after the antibiotic regimen is completed to ensure that the infection is eliminated.

Uremic cats are often hypothermic. Support of normal body temperature with blankets or a heating pad is recommended. The cat should not be placed directly on a cold examining table during urinary and intravenous catheterization. Temperature support should be continued until the cat's temperature reaches the low-normal range and the cat's activity increases.

Cats that are uremic at the time of examination are usually also hyperkalemic and acidemic (Burrows and Bovee, 1978). For survival of these cats, intravenous fluid therapy is required in addition to relief of obstruction (Finco, 1976). Alkalinizing electrolyte solutions (Multisol‡) have been shown to reverse acidemia and hyperkalemia in experimentally induced urethral obstruction, even though these fluids do contain a small amount of potassium (Finco, 1976; Finco and Cornelius, 1977). Solutions containing dextrose and insulin have been recommended (Schaer, 1975), but no evidence exists that such therapy is more beneficial than alkalinizing electrolyte solutions alone. Adding sodium bicarbonate to the treatment regimen will more rapidly reverse the acidemia of obstructed cats (Burrows and Bovee, 1978), but there is no benefit in terms of survival over cats treated with electrolyte solutions containing the equivalent of 53 mEq/L NaHCO$_3$ (Finco, 1976; Finco and Cornelius, 1977).

---

*Sherwood Medical Industries, St. Louis, MO.
†Becton-Dickinson, Rutherford, NJ.

‡Abbott Laboratories, North Chicago, IL.

The volume of fluids administered is based on the severity of dehydration, uremic signs, and hyperkalemia. A quantity of fluid equivalent to approximately 5 per cent body weight should be given if the signs are mild, 8 per cent if moderate, and 12 per cent if severe. This amount of fluid should be administered over one to two hours. These are only general guidelines; actual volume replacement must be individualized for each cat on the basis of vital signs, changes in hydration status, mental attitude, and urine output. Pulmonary edema may result from too rapid fluid replacement. Hyperkalemia, acidemia, and uremia will not be rapidly reversed if the rate of fluid administration is too slow. No evidence of pulmonary edema developed when experimentally obstructed cats were given a balanced electrolyte solution at a rate of 50 to 60 ml/kg/hr (Finco et al., 1976).

After the initial therapy with fluids, the cat's mental attitude is usually improved, urine output is often sustained, and severe hyperkalemia is frequently reversed (as shown by biochemical measurement, improved attitude, or reversal of electrocardiographic abnormalities). If such improvement occurs, the rate of fluid administration can be reduced. Sufficient volume should be given over 24 hours to provide insensible water losses (estimated at 20 ml/kg/day) and replace urine losses. If urine output is not measured, sufficient fluids should be given to provide maintenance needs (estimated at 60 ml/kg/day) and to correct any dehydration detected by changes in skin turgor or moisture of the mucous membranes.

Fluid therapy should be continued until azotemia is resolved or minimized sufficiently. Subcutaneous fluids can be substituted for intravenous fluids once uremic signs abate and serum potassium is normal (usually within 24 hours). Postobstructive diuresis that leads to renal water and electrolyte losses necessitates continued fluid therapy. The cause of postobstructive diuresis is unknown, but decreased renal tubular function and the need to excrete solutes retained during obstruction may be involved. The percentage of cats predisposed to dehydration by a diuretic phase of recovery from obstruction is unknown.

Fluid therapy in cats with partial or total anorexia may lead to hypokalemia a few days after obstruction is relieved. Recurrent or worsening weakness and lethargy may be the only clinical signs of this abnormality. If hypokalemia is suspected, it should be confirmed by measurement of serum potassium concentration. If present, potassium supplementation can be given orally if the cat is not vomiting. Alternatively, 20 mEq KCl can be added to each liter of balanced electrolyte solution. Hypokalemia is not a frequent consequence of fluid therapy, since most previously obstructed cats begin to eat as soon as uremia is reversed (Finco, 1976; Finco and Cornelius, 1977).

Bladder detrusor muscle dysfunction during prolonged urethral obstruction may occur owing to bladder overdistention. This dysfunction is manifested clinically as bladder atony. The bladder becomes distended, the cat may or may not attempt to void without success, but the bladder can easily be expressed manually. Bladder atony is an indication for the use of an indwelling urethral catheter. The bladder should be kept empty for several days to allow tight junctions of the detrusor muscle to re-form. Bethanechol (Urecholin*, 2.5 mg every eight hours) can also be tried after a few days of maintaining the bladder in an empty state. If this drug is not effective after the first few doses, it should be discontinued. The urethra must be patent during use of parasympathomimetic drugs, or rupture of the bladder may occur.

FELINE UROLOGIC SYNDROME WITHOUT OBSTRUCTION

Cats with FUS without obstruction typically arouse owner concern because of the presence of hematuria, dysuria, and/or urination in inappropriate places. The cats otherwise act normally. Both male and female cats can be affected. The bladder is empty, but palpation may induce spasm, causing the cat to void a small amount of blood-tinged urine. Results of urinalysis are characterized by hematuria and, occasionally, mild pyuria, but bladder urine is bacteriologically sterile.

Antibiotics, smooth muscle relaxants, and fluid diuresis have been recommended as treatment for these cats. The rationale of antibiotic therapy is questionable in the face of negative urine cultures. We recently completed a prospective study of the efficacy of chloramphenicol versus a placebo in 20 cats. No difference in response to therapy was noted. Most cats were normal within five days regardless of therapy.

The cats in the aforementioned study were also treated with subcutaneous fluids (100 ml lactated Ringer's) and a smooth muscle relaxant (probantheline bromide [Pro-Banthine†], 7.5 mg PO) to facilitate urine collection. In a second study of 29 cats, all cats were hospitalized for 24 hours. Each cat received subcutaneous fluids (100 ml lactated Ringer's), probantheline (7.5 mg PO), or nothing. The cats were then discharged and the owners contacted after five days. Again, there was no difference in response to the various treatments. In the majority of cats, clinical signs had resolved.

Based on the results of four pilot studies, FUS without obstruction appears to be a self-limiting condition in the majority of cats. If the signs do not abate within five to seven days, a diagnostic plan to

---

*Merck, Sharp and Dohme, West Point, PA.
†Searle & Co., San Juan, PR.

rule out other causes of hematuria and dysuria should be instituted, including urine culture and survey and contrast radiography. Future studies to determine efficacious therapy for cats with FUS without obstruction will have to be placebo-controlled because of the high rate of spontaneous resolution of clinical signs.

Urinary products that contain methylene blue or phenazopyridine *should not be used in cats* because of their potential for causing methemoglobinemia and Heinz body anemia (Osborne and Lees, 1978).

PREVENTION OF RECURRENCE OF FUS

One of the most frustrating features of FUS is the high rate of recurrence of clinical signs (Bovee et al., 1979; Walker et al., 1977). Various recommendations have been made to reduce this recurrence rate, including long-term use of urinary acidifiers, low-mineral diets, and increasing water intake and urine output. None of these recommendations has been evaluated objectively.

Only one acidifier has been evaluated in clinical cases of urethral obstruction. Ethylenediamine dihydrochloride (Chlorethamine*) given for 21 days after obstruction did not prevent recurrent obstruction (Bovee et al., 1979). Whether obstruction would have been as likely if the acidifier had been continued was not answered by this study. Ethylenediamine hydrochloride has also been found to be only a weak urinary acidifier in cats (Finco, 1981). DL-Methionine slowed, but did not prevent, the development of urethral obstruction in cats fed an experimental calculogenic diet (Chow et al., 1976). However, the obstructing material in cats fed this diet is different from that in clinical cases of obstruction. In normal cats, ammonium chloride (15 grains/day) is the only acidifier shown to prevent the post-prandial alkaline tide (Chow et al., 1978). Other than the mild alkalinity that occurs in the first few hours after eating, normal cat urine is acidic (Chow et al., 1978). The majority of cats with FUS with and without obstruction also have acidic urine (Bovee et al., 1979; Taussig, 1975). Thus, the efficacy of acidifiers in preventing recurrence of FUS in the majority of cats with acidic urine is questionable.

Dietary recommendations have also been made for cats with FUS, based on reducing mineral intake and increasing water intake. Although a calculogenic diet has been formulated experimentally, no commercially available cat food has been shown to be calculogenic. Nor has any low-mineral cat food been objectively shown to prevent recurrence of FUS.

Increasing water intake and thus urine output has also been recommended for cats with FUS. Feeding moist cat foods, moistening dry cat foods, salting the food (0.25 to 1.0 gm salt/day), and giving diuretics have been recommended to increase water turnover. Although one case-controlled study found a higher incidence of an initial episode of urethral obstruction in cats eating more than 50 per cent dry food (Burrows and Bovee, 1978), the risk of recurrence of obstruction was not associated with the percentage of dry food intake (Bovee et al., 1979). And although oral salt increases water consumption and urine output in cats, the addition of 4 per cent NaCl to a calculogenic diet did not prevent calculi formation (Hamar et al., 1976). Again, this experimental model may not duplicate clinical FUS. The results of one clinical study, which was not well controlled, suggested a decreased risk of recurrence of FUS following the addition of salt and fluids to a cat's food for life (Bernard, 1978). DL-Methionine was also administered to affected cats for at least a month.

Efficacy of crystallization inhibitors such as tripolyphosphate (CureCal†) and of chelators of calcium and magnesium (Curecal†) is unknown, but limited work has not demonstrated any efficacy (Rich, 1971). Addition of 15 per cent alanine to calculogenic diets prevented the formation of magnesium phosphate uroliths in cats (Chow et al., 1976). A high concentration of alanine in urine was postulated to increase the solubility of magnesium phosphate and to impair the aggregation of the proteinaceous matrix. No studies of the efficacy of alanine in preventing recurrence of urethral obstruction in clinical cases of FUS have been reported.

At the present time there is no therapy proved to prevent recurrence of FUS. Prospective clinical trials are needed. Owners should be advised that recurrence is probable and that there is no therapy proved to prevent such a recurrence. If the cat's urine is alkaline, acidifiers can be tried. After starting acidifiers, urine pH should be rechecked at various times in relation to eating to be sure the urine is consistently acidic. Increasing water intake is recommended for cats that have had urethral obstruction.

REFERENCES AND SUPPLEMENTAL READING

Bernard, M. A.: Feline urological syndrome: A study of seasonal incidence, frequency of repeat visits, and comparison of treatments. Can. Vet. J. 19:284, 1978.
Bovee, K. C., Rief, J. S., Maguire, T. G., Gaskell, C. J., and Batt, R. M.: Recurrence of feline urethral obstruction. J.A.V.M.A. 174:93, 1979.
Burrows, C. F., and Bovee, K. C.: Characterization and treatment of acid-base and renal defects due to urethral obstruction in cats. J.A.V.M.A. 172:801, 1978.
Chow, F. C., Dysart, I., Hamar, O. W., Lewis, L. O., and Rich, L. J.: Effect of dietary additives on experimentally produced feline urolithiasis. Feline Pract. 9:51, 1976.
Chow, F. C., Taton, G. F., Lewis, L. D., and Hamar, D. W.: Effect of

---

*Pitman-Moore, Washington's Crossing, NJ.

†Albion Laboratories, Inc., Clearfield, UT.

dietary ammonium chloride, DL-methionine, sodium phosphate and ascorbic acid on urinary pH and electrolyte concentrations of male cats. Feline Pract. 8:29, 1978.

Finco, D. R.: Induced feline urethral obstruction: Response of hyperkalemia to relief of obstruction and administration of parenteral electrolyte solution. J. Am. Anim. Hosp. Assoc. 12:198, 1976.

Finco, D. R.: Efficacy of ethylenediamine dihydrochloride in dogs and cats. Am. J. Vet. Res. 42:670, 1981.

Finco, D. R., and Cornelius, L. M.: Characterization and treatment of water, electrolyte, and acid-base imbalances of induced urethral obstruction in the cat. Am. J. Vet. Res. 38:823, 1977.

Hamar, D., Chow, F. H. C., Dysart, M. I., and Rich, L. J.: Effect of sodium chloride in prevention of experimentally produced phosphate uroliths in male cats. J. Am. Anim. Hosp. Assoc. 12:514, 1976.

Lees, G. E., and Osborne, C. H.: Feline urologic syndrome: Removal of urethral obstructions and use of indwelling urethral catheters. In Kirk, R. W. (ed.): Current Veterinary Therapy VII, Philadelphia: W. B. Saunders, 1980, pp. 1191–1195.

Lees, G. E., Osborne, C. A., Stevens, J. B., and Ward, G. E.: Adverse effects of open indwelling urethral catheterization in clinically normal male cats. Am. J. Vet. Res. 42:825, 1981.

Osborne, C. A., and Lees, G. E.: Feline cystitis, urethritis and urethral obstruction syndrome. Mod. Vet. Pract. 59:513, 1978.

Reif, J. S., Bovee, K., Gaskell, C. J., Batts, C. M., and Maguire, T. G.: Feline urethral obstruction: A case-control study. J.A.V.M.A. 170:1320, 1977.

Rich, L. J.: Urethral obstruction and urolithiasis in cats. In Kirk, R. W. (ed.): Current Veterinary Therapy IV. Philadelphia: W. B. Saunders, 1971, pp. 705–706.

Schaer, M.: The use of regular insulin in the treatment of hyperkalemia in cats with urethral obstruction. J. Am. Anim. Hosp. Assoc. 11:106, 1975.

Smith, C. W., Schiller, A. G., Smith, A. C., Wells, S. K., and Kissil, M.: Effects of indwelling urinary catheters in male cats. J. Am. Anim. Hosp. Assoc. 17:427, 1981.

Taussig, R. A.: Cystitis in the female cat: Therapy and prophylaxis. Feline Pract. 3:52, 1975.

Walker, A. D., Weaver, A. D., Anderson, R. S., Crighton, G. W., Fennell, C., Gaskell, C. J., and Wilkinson, G. T.: An epidemiological survey of the feline urological syndrome. J. Small Anim. Pract. 18:283, 1977.

Welleberg, P., and Priester, W. A.: Feline urological syndrome: Associations with some time, space and individual patient factors. Am. J. Vet. Res. 37:975, 1976.

ROLE OF DIET IN FELINE UROLOGIC SYNDROME

DELMAR R. FINCO, D.V.M.,
and JEANNE A. BARSANTI, D.V.M.

Athens, Georgia

The feline urologic syndrome (FUS) is a disease of unknown etiology. Diet is one of many factors incriminated as causative or contributory. Surveys indicate that most veterinarians recommend specific dietary regimens for cats with FUS. Yet a retrospective study of the relationship of diet to recurrence of FUS found no correlation. It is becoming apparent that designating direct cause-and-effect relationships between diet and FUS may be overly simplistic. It is also apparent that much more study is required to unravel the many mysteries of this disease.

The objective of this article is not to provide simple, absolute answers for immediate application; those answers do not exist at present. Our objective is to outline our opinions concerning existing knowledge of diet and FUS so that one viewpoint is available for scrutiny, criticism, and further thought by the veterinary profession.

SOME DEFICITS IN EXISTING KNOWLEDGE OF FUS

For want of more specific data, it has been assumed that the role of diet in FUS can be related to composition. Thus, the percentage of minerals, particularly magnesium (Mg), in the diet is deemed significant. Such data suffer from several presumptions that warrant consideration. The total quantity of any suspected component such as Mg ingested per unit time (i.e., daily intake) is likely to be more relevant than composition percentage. Two diets of the same Mg concentration but different caloric densities would very likely result in greater Mg ingestion by cats eating the low-caloric food, since more of it would be ingested. Total intake would also depend on the digestibility of the macromolecular components and possibly the protein quantity and quality. Because of these factors, judgements of diets on the basis of mineral percentage are somewhat misleading and should be formulated with caution.

It often has been presumed that intake of minerals is synonymous with intestinal absorption and eventual excretion in urine. Several factors related to these processes warrant close consideration. The form of mineral components in the diet may affect this absorption. Organic minerals may be absorbed less readily than inorganic salts. Complexing of ions with one another also may affect their absorption. If in fact urinary mineral excretion is related to

FUS, little attention has been directed to the possibility of susceptible cats having different intestinal absorptive capabilities than nonsusceptible cats. Perhaps it is as much the individual cat's mineral absorptive efficiency as it is dietary mineral content that is responsible for disease.

Also related to diet and absorption is the matter of peak versus trough blood levels of mineral. It is known that post-prandial plasma phosphorus (P) concentration increases markedly. Would a single, massive meal combined with efficient, rapid absorption cause elevated blood P or Mg levels so that a "urinary mineral shower" occurs? Does post-prandial alkaline urine production by cats, combined with a mineral shower, precipitate FUS? This unstudied possibility may be relevant.

Little consideration has been given to the possibility that cats prone to FUS have a primary renal reabsorptive defect for minerals incriminated in the etiopathogenesis of FUS. Loss of these minerals in urine could cause secondary enhancement of intestinal mineral absorption as a mechanism of homeostasis.

All previous considerations are based on the assumption that increased urinary mineral excretion is a significant factor in the genesis of FUS. Yet few data are available to substantiate this assumption. In some studies, the quantity of crystal formed by cats was no greater after obstruction than before. A few preliminary studies have been directed toward the hypothesis that urinary mineral content is of secondary importance in FUS and that the primary problem is a urinary factor that facilitates precipitation of minerals. Such a factor could be produced by the body independent of the nature of the diet, or it could be a dietary component. The presence of such a nondietary factor would relegate diet to a minor or insignificant role in the pathogenesis of the disease.

The influence of diet on body water turnover has been proposed as a significant factor in FUS. Decreased urine volume with constant urinary mineral excretion will increase urine mineral concentration. Decreased urine volume was documented in cats fed dry food manufactured in England but was not observed in cats fed dry food manufactured in the United States. Thus, the interrelationship between diet, urine volume, and FUS remains vaguely defined.

EXPERIMENTALLY PRODUCED OBSTRUCTION

Urethral obstruction can be induced in cats by feeding diets with a Mg content 40 to 200 per cent greater than that in commercial foods. Two questions arise as a consequence of these studies. One

is whether the levels of Mg in calculogenic diets are close enough to those of commercial diets to allow extrapolation of data from the experimental disease to the natural one. The other is whether the induced disease is the same as the naturally occurring one. The first question remains unanswered because of lack of data. With regard to the second question, comparison of data collected from cats obstructed as a consequence of the calculogenic diet with findings from cats with the natural disease reveals significant differences. Consumption of the calculogenic diet resulted in obstructing material that is different in composition from the obstructing material found in the natural disease. Struvite crystals (13 per cent ammonium) are present in most cats with the natural disease but were almost absent from the experimentally induced deposits. In addition, serum Mg concentrations were markedly elevated in cats with induced blockage, but hypermagnesemia is absent in the natural disease. Both of these observations raise serious doubts about the validity of this model as a prototype for FUS. Unfortunately, the distinction between the natural disease and the experimental one has not always been made in reports in the veterinary literature; publications exist in which the induced disease is called FUS. Until more convincing proof is provided, FUS and experimentally induced obstruction should be clearly differentiated.

EFFICACY OF LOW-MINERAL DIETS IN FUS

The fact that urethral obstruction can be induced in cats by feeding high-Mg diets has led to the hypothesis that low-Mg diets are helpful in its prophylaxis. Unfortunately, this hypothesis has not been tested by objective study, and claims of efficacy by prescription diet food manufacturers have not been substantiated. Valid studies are needed to resolve this issue.

DIETARY RECOMMENDATIONS FOR FUS

From the preceding discussion it is readily apparent that few specific dietary recommendations based on scientific fact can be made for cats with FUS. Present recommendations are the product of opinions and prejudices.

Our recommendations are made in an attempt to balance client and cat inconvenience factors with presumed benefit from the regimen.

1. At present, we see no justification for the use of prescription diets in cats with FUS because proof of efficacy in preventing the disorder is lacking and their use imposes a considerable financial burden on the client.

2. Regardless of the type of food (dry, intermediate, or moist) given, we recommend a liberal salt diet (0.25 to 1.0 gm daily) to increase water turnover rate. Since salt adheres more easily to semidry and moist foods, these types are more convenient for client use. Alternatively, dry food may be moistened and salt subsequently added.

3. Urinary acidifiers have not been proved effective in treating FUS, but there is some theoretical basis for their use. We recommend that they be used if urinary pH values are repeatedly 7.0 or above or if recurrence of signs is frequent.

4. Cold, clean water should be available at all times.

DISEASES OF THE CANINE URETHRA

ALAN J. LIPOWITZ, D.V.M.

St. Paul, Minnesota

CONGENITAL ANOMALIES

Congenital anomalies of the canine urethra are uncommon. However, the male dog is more frequently affected than the female. Anomalies that have been reported include imperforate urethra, urethral aplasia, ectopic urethra, duplicated urethra, hypospadias, urethral diverticulum, and urethrorectal fistula. In some cases lower urinary tract anomalies may be associated with genital system abnormalities such as pseudohermaphroditism or true hermaphroditism (Schwartz et al., 1974). Signs of these conditions may include dysuria, incontinence, flow of urine through abnormal orifices, and dermatitis due to urine scald. Imperforate urethra and urethral aplasia (agenesis) have been reported in female dogs and hypospadias in male dogs, whereas urethrorectal fistulas have been reported in both sexes (Archibald and Owen, 1974).

Hypospadias is a developmental anomaly in which the urethra opens on the ventral surface of the penis at any locus between the ischial arch and the normal urethral orifice at the tip of the penis. The condition may be amenable to surgical correction, depending on the location of the abnormal opening and the presence of other anomalies (Adler and Hobson, 1978; Johnston and Archibald, 1974).

Urethrorectal fistula is a developmental anomaly of the embryonic cloaca that results in a persistent communication between the urethra and the rectum. The condition has been reported in both sexes. During urination (micturition), urine passes from the anal orifice of these animals as well as from the normal urethral orifice. Bacterial cystitis is often an associated complication. Treatment involves surgical removal or ligation of the abnormal communication between the urethra and the rectum (Goulden et al., 1973; Osborne et al., 1975).

URETHRAL NEOPLASIA

Primary tumors of the urethra are uncommon. Female dogs are far more commonly affected than males. Squamous cell carcinoma is the most common tumor type. This is not surprising, since the distal two-thirds of the female canine urethra is lined with squamous epithelium, whereas the proximal one-third is lined with transitional cell epthelium. In males, the entire urethra is lined with transitional cell epithelium, except for a small segment at the external orifice (Tarvin et al., 1978). Transitional cell carcinoma, adenocarcinoma, hemangiosarcoma, and embryonic rhabdomyosarcoma have also been reported.

As mentioned previously, females are more commonly affected, especially with squamous cell carcinoma. Age at the time of diagnosis averages 10.9 years. When metastasis of squamous cell carcinomas occurs, regional tissues, including lymph nodes, are more likely to be affected than distal organs such as the lung.

Signs of urethral tumors are usually those common to lower urinary tract disease, with stranguria a consistent finding. Hematuria has been reported to occur in less than one-half of the cases. Exfoliative cytology of urine may aid in establishing a diagnosis. Double contrast and voiding contrast urethrography are most useful in localizing the lesion to the urethra and delineating the extent of urethral involvement. Survey radiographs of the thorax and caudal abdomen assist in determining pulmonary metastasis or iliac lymph node involvement.

Complete surgical removal was not feasible in reported cases because of the extent of urethral involvement at the time of exploratory surgery. Perhaps earlier recognition of the problem would allow tumor removal and urethroplasty if necessary.

Chemotherapy, either alone or in combination with therapeutic radiation, might be beneficial.

PROLAPSE OF THE MALE URETHRA

Prolapse of the urethra, or eversion of the urethral mucosa through the urethral orifice, is a rare condition. It has been reported only in young male English bulldogs and Boston terriers. Sexual excitement and/or urethritis is thought to play a significant role in its occurrence. In addition, a congenital or genetic defect has been postulated because of the predominance in English bulldogs (Sinibaldi and Greene, 1973).

Signs include urine dribbling, urine blood clots, and blood dripping from the penis. In addition, persistent licking of the lesion may be noted. On examination, a small, red, pea-shaped mass will be noted at the urethral orifice of the glans penis. Although manual reduction of the prolapse along with tranquilization and cage rest may be attempted, surgical removal is the treatment of choice (Johnston and Archibald, 1974; Sinibaldi and Greene, 1973). After insertion of a urinary catheter, the distal 4 to 5 mm of the penis including the mass is amputated. The urethral orifice must be recreated by carefully suturing the cut edge of the urethral mucosa to the squamous epithelium of the penis. Postoperative care should include a neck brace or collar to prevent the patient from licking the surgical site and systemic antibiotics. Tranquilizers, topical medicaments, and anti-inflammatory drugs may also be advisable.

If sexual excitement was instrumental in precipitating the prolapse, estrogen therapy or castration may be needed to prevent recurrence.

URETHRITIS

Inflammation of the urethra may be infectious or noninfectious. Infectious urethritis may occur as an isolated clinical entity or in association with bacterial cystitis, vaginitis, or prostatitis. Clinical data are not available regarding the etiology of primary infectious urethritis. It is assumed that the etiologic agents are the same as those of the associated diseases just mentioned (Greene and Scott, 1975; Polzin and Jeraj, 1979).

Noninfectious urethritis of dogs and cats is most frequently associated with urethral catheterization (Lees and Osborne, 1979). Calculi and trauma may also cause urethral inflammation. Occasionally, nonspecific urethritis with no identifiable etiologic agent may be found (Greene and Scott, 1975; Polzin and Jeraj, 1979).

Because of the frequency with which urinary catheters are used, it is important to recognize the adverse effects of intermittent and indwelling catheterization (Lees et al., 1981). Since trauma to the urethral mucosa during catheterization will cause inflammation and since lower urinary tract infection is a common sequela to urethral catheterization, careful, gentle technique to minimize trauma and contamination is mandatory during catheterization.

The composition of the catheter may play a part in the degree of inflammation, especially that produced by indwelling catheterization. In one study in dogs, however, significant differences were not found in urethral reactions to six different catheter materials in the absence of bacterial infection. In normal cats, indwelling catheters were found to produce varying degrees of urethral inflammation (Lees et al., 1981). Indwelling urethral catheters increase the likelihood of the development of bacterial urethritis and cystitis.

CLINICAL MANIFESTATIONS OF URETHRITIS

Clinical signs of urethritis include stranguria and increased frequency of micturition. If gross hematuria is present, it is most frequently seen at the onset of micturition. Dribbling of blood independent of micturition may also occur. However, if an abnormal urethral discharge is present it must be differentiated from problems involving the penis, prepuce, prostate, and vagina. Complete urethral obstruction due to uncomplicated urethritis is rare.

Analysis and bacterial culture of urine should be performed whenever urethritis is suspected. Results must be interpreted in light of the method of urine collection and the normal bacterial flora of the urethra. Microscopic examination of urine sediment should not be overlooked. If a urethral discharge is present, it should also be cultured and examined microscopically. All samples must be collected aseptically.

The prostate and intrapelvic urethra should be evaluated by digital palpation per rectum in male dogs. Retrograde contrast urethrography and cystography or voiding contrast urethrography will aid in diagnosing structural abnormalities, urolithiasis, neoplasms, strictures, or loss of urethral continuity.

Because primary isolated urethritis is so rarely diagnosed, the urethritis that is seen clinically may be considered a secondary problem. Resolution of secondary urethritis would therefore require accurate diagnosis and successful therapy for the primary problem. Urethritis associated with cystitis, vaginitis, or prostatitis should subside if these conditions are effectively treated. Likewise, urethral inflammation accompanying urolithiasis, trauma, and neoplasia should resolve with successful therapy for the initial problem (Polzin and Jeraj, 1979).

Antimicrobial therapy is indicated in all types of urethritis. Agents should be selected on the basis of results of urine culture and bacterial susceptibility tests. Trimethoprim appears to be a good choice because it attains a high local concentration and has a broad spectrum of antimicrobial activity (Polzin and Jeraj, 1979).

URETHRAL INJURY

Injuries to the urethra may be due to a variety of causes. The most severe result in loss of urethral continuity and urine leakage. Lacerations of the urethra are frequently associated with pelvic fractures (Brown, 1975). Complete transection of the urethra or avulsion of the urethra from the bladder may also be seen in cases of severe trauma (Archibald and Owen, 1974). Urethral trauma may also be caused by rough handling of urethral catheters.

Hematuria or blood at the external urethral orifice is frequently associated with small urethral tears or lacerations. If the tear is large or if the urethra has become completely transected, blood and urine will escape into the surrounding tissues and will produce swelling, erythema, edema, and eventually tissue necrosis (Archibald and Owen, 1974). These patients may still have the ability to void urine, although in decreased amounts. Stranguria is commonly observed.

Injury to the prostatic and intrapelvic portions of the urethra may allow intra-abdominal or retroperitoneal leakage of urine. Urine leakage into the abdominal cavity may produce signs typical of peritonitis. Within 24 hours following injury, these patients often become azotemic. Although azotemia may also occur with retroperitoneal leakage of urine, it will usually take longer to manifest itself than if urine were leaking into the abdominal cavity.

Minor lacerations of the urethra may be difficult to diagnose because the clinical signs are frequently associated with other urethral or lower urinary tract problems. Positive retrograde contrast urethrography is the method of choice when diagnosing urethral trauma (Johnston et al., 1977). Catheters can be easily advanced across the laceration site.

Major lacerations and complete transection of the urethra are usually obvious from the history and clinical signs. In many cases of major lacerations and in some cases of complete transection, a catheter can be passed across the injury site into the urinary bladder. Therefore, successful catheterization of the bladder should not be interpreted as irrefutable evidence of complete urethral continuity.

The canine urethra has great regenerative capacity. Regeneration of all components of the urethral wall can be expected even if the two-thirds of the urethral diameter has been transected. The mucosa regenerates within days, but complete regeneration of the entire wall may require up to five weeks (Archibald and Owen, 1974).

Because of its regenerative capacity, lacerations of the urethra may be treated by urinary diversion through a urethral catheter. The sterile catheter must be placed aseptically and must traverse the injury site with its tip in the urinary bladder. To reduce the potential of urinary tract infections, a closed sterile urine drainage system must be used (Lees and Osborne, 1979). In addition, both patient and catheter must be kept as clean as possible. Although an indwelling catheter may cause some inflammation of the urethra and may potentiate the possibility of bacterial urethritis, it is a fair exchange if surgical repair of the urethra, particularly the prostatic or intrapelvic portion, can be avoided.

Complete transection of the urethra will not heal spontaneously, even if a urinary diverting urethral catheter is used. Urethral transection must be treated by surgical anastomoses or creation of an artificial orifice by transposing the proximal undamaged portion of the urethra outside the body (Archibald and Owen, 1974; Brown, 1975).

Urethral injury may also occur in association with fractures of the os penis. Although relatively uncommon, displacement of the fractured bone can result in urethral stenosis and urinary obstruction (Johnston et al., 1977).

Other injuries to the penis may also involve the urethra. Rubber bands or other objects maliciously applied to the penis or urethra may cause urethral injury (Archibald and Owen, 1974).

URETHRAL CALCULI

Calculi are the most common cause of urethral obstruction in male dogs. Struvite stones are the most common calculi seen, followed by cystine or urate calculi and then those composed of oxalates and silica (Greene and Scott, 1975). Cystine calculi have not been reported in the bitch. Infection is a predisposing factor in the genesis, growth, and recurrence of struvite calculi. In patients with oxalate, urate, cystine, and silica calculi, infection is frequently a secondary complication (Klausner and Osborne, 1979). Eradication of urinary tract infection is often difficult until the uroliths are removed.

Clinical signs of urethral calculi vary with the sex of the animal, anatomic location of the urolith within the urinary tract, and the degree of obstruction. The female urethra is short, wide, and relatively straight and rarely becomes obstructed. The long urethra of the male dog decreases in diameter from the bladder to the penis and must curve over the ischium. Urethral calculi not associated with renal or cystic calculi are extremely rare in females but are occasionally found in male dogs. However, urethral calculi in males are usually associated with cystic calculi. When calculi are located in the bladder and urethra they are most frequently composed of cystine and urate. This is not surprising, as calculi of these two types are more common in males than in females (Brown et al., 1977; Greene and Scott, 1975).

Signs of urethral calculi include anuria, dysuria, tenesmus, and abdominal distention. Azotemia will occur in patients with complete obstruction. Although calculi may lodge anywhere in the urethra, they are often found at the ischial arch or more commonly at the caudal end of the os penis (Archibald and Owen, 1974; Greene and Scott, 1975). Inability to pass a catheter along the entire length of the urethra frequently reveals the point of obstruction. However, in some cases a catheter of small diameter may pass beyond the calculi. In these situations a "gritty" sensation may be felt as the catheter first encounters and then passes the calculi. Because the incidence of isolated urethral calculi is low, all male dogs with urethral obstruction should be considered as having cystic calculi as well as urethral calculi until proved otherwise.

Diagnosis is based on the patient's history, particularly regarding urinary habits, clinical signs, and the ability to pass a urethral catheter. The differential diagnosis should include those conditions previously discussed that may also produce urethral obstruction.

Radiographs may not be necessary to confirm the presence of calculi at the caudal end of the os penis. However, abdominal radiographs to detect calculi elsewhere in the urinary tract should be obtained. It is important to cleanse fecal material from the rectum by enema prior to radiography so that radiodense feces will not be superimposed on the bladder and urethra. In addition, the entire urethra must be included in the radiograph. It is helpful to pull the patient's legs as far forward as possible so that they do not obscure the urethra on the lateral radiographic views (Johnston et al., 1977). A true ventrodorsal projection may not be as diagnostic as an oblique ventrodorsal projection because of superimposition of vertebrae between the urethra and the radiographic film and of the penile urethra over the membranous and prostatic urethral segments (Johnston et al., 1977).

TREATMENT

Any patient with obstruction of the urinary tract should be treated as an emergency. Treatment of urethral urolithiasis should be directed first at relieving the obstruction and then at surgical removal of the calculi if necessary. If complete obstruction has been present for some time, fluid, acid-base, and electrolyte disturbances associated with prerenal azotemia may also necessitate immediate attention (Greene and Scott, 1975).

A catheter should be placed into the urethra to identify the location of the calculi. A topical anesthetic may be flushed into the urethra via the catheter to aid in reducing urethral spasms. In most cases patient sedation or general anesthesia will be required for complete patient relaxation and cooperation. Nonsurgical relief of the obstruction should be attempted first. One technique is to flush a sterile saline solution through a well-lubricated catheter that has been positioned adjacent to the obstructing calculi while applying gentle pressure around the catheter at the distal end of the penis. The flushing will dilate the urethra and hopefully propel the calculi into the urinary bladder. Once this occurs, the catheter is advanced into the bladder. The cystic calculi may then be removed by cystotomy (Greene and Scott, 1975).

Repeatedly advancing and retracting the catheter while continually forcing fluid through it may be necessary to dislodge the stones. Care must be used to prevent iatrogenic urethral rupture.

If the calculi cannot be dislodged, a modification of this technique may be tried. Instead of a catheter, a teat cannula is inserted into the urethra, to which is attached to a 60-cc syringe filled with sterile saline. An assistant inserts a gloved index finger into the rectum and firmly occludes the intrapelvic urethral lumen by applying digital pressure against the ischium through the ventral wall of the rectum. With pressure maintained around the cannula, saline is injected, dilating the urethra and increasing its intraluminal pressure. Sudden release of the digital pressure on the urethra while continuing to inject solution will force the calculi into the bladder (Piermattei and Osborne, 1977). This maneuver may need to be repeated several times before success is achieved.

Excessive pressure should not be generated within the urethral lumen using these techniques, particularly in long-standing cases of obstruction, to avoid rupture of the urethra.

A variation of the preceding technique has also been described (Piermattei and Osborne, 1977). Instead of releasing digital pressure on the saline-dilated urethra, the rectally placed finger pressure is maintained and the teat cannula quickly removed. This promotes antegrade flushing of the calculi; if they are small enough to pass the caudal end of the os penis they will be carried with the saline through the external urethral orifice. Repeated attempts may be needed to dislodge all the calculi.

If obstruction has been present for some time, the urinary bladder may be quite distended with urine, making retrograde flushing of calculi difficult. A catheter small enough to bypass the obstruction may be passed to relieve the urinary distention. Alternatively, cystocentesis can be performed.

If the obstruction cannot be removed nonsurgically, a urethrostomy or a cystotomy will be necessary. Calculi lodged in the intrapelvic portion of the urethra may in some cases be removed by retrograde flushing of the urethra during the cystotomy procedure. Those calculi close to the bladder may be grasped and extracted with forceps placed through the cystotomy incision into the proximal urethra. In the rare case in which the calculi are firmly lodged in the intrapelvic portion of the urethra, a urethrotomy via pelvic symphysiotomy will be necessary.

External urethrotomy may be performed if the calculi cannot be removed nonsurgically. The procedure is commonly performed at one of three separate urethral locations, depending on the position of the calculi (Greene and Scott, 1975). Prepubic (prescrotal) and scrotal urethrotomies are recommended when calculi have accumulated at the caudal end of the os penis. The prepubic technique involves a midline approach to the urethra through an incision made between the caudal end of the os penis and the cranial limit of the scrotum. Scrotal urethrotomy involves castration and scrotal ablation to approach the urethra. Permanent urethrostomy by this technique has been recommended to prevent reobstruction in chronic stone formers, because the portion of the urethra dorsal to the scrotum has a larger diameter than the urethra just caudal to the os penis.

For stones lodged at the ischial arch, a perineal urethrotomy is recommended. It is performed on the midline of the perineum over the ischium midway between the ischial arch and the caudal limit of the scrotum.

Although surgical closure of the urethrotomy incision is possible, it is recommended that permanent urethrostomies be created by suturing the cut edge of the urethral mucosa to the cut edge of the skin. This is particularly desirable in chronic stone formers. Scrotal urethrostomies should always be permanent.

REFERENCES AND SUPPLEMENTAL READING

Ader, P. L., and Hobson, H. P.: Hypospadias: A review of the veterinary literature and report of three cases in the dog. J. Am. Anim. Hosp. Assoc. 14:721, 1978.

Archibald, J., and Owen, R. R.: Urinary systems. *In* Archibald, J. (ed.): *Canine Surgery*, 2nd ed. Santa Barbara, CA: American Veterinary Publications, Inc., 1974.

Brown, N. O., Parks, J. L., and Greene, R. W.: Canine urolithiasis: Retrospective analysis of 438 cases. J.A.V.M.A. 170:414, 1977.

Brown, S. G.: Surgery of the canine urethra. Vet. Clin. North Am. 5:457,, 1975.

Goulden, B., Bergman, M. M., and Wyburn, R. S.: Canine urethrorectal fistulae. J. Small Anim. Pract. 14:143, 1973.

Greene, R. W., and Scott, R. C.: Lower urinary tract disease. *In* Ettinger, S. J. (ed.): *Textbook of Veterinary Internal Medicine*. Philadelphia: W. B. Saunders, 1975.

Greene, R. W., and Scott, R. C.: Diseases of the urethra. *In* Kirk, R. W. (ed.): *Current Veterinary Therapy VI*. Philadelphia: W. B. Saunders, 1977.

Johnston, D. E., and Archibald, J.: Male genital system. *In* Archibald, J. (ed.): *Canine Surgery*, 2nd ed. Santa Barbara, CA: American Veterinary Publications, Inc., 1974.

Johnston, G. R., Jessen, C. R., and Osborne, C. A.: Retrograde contrast urethrography. *In* Kirk, R. W. (ed.): *Current Veterinary Therapy VI*. Philadelphia: W. B. Saunders, 1977.

Klaussner, J. S., and Osborne, C. A.: Urinary tract infection and urolithiasis. Vet. Clin. North Am. 9:701, 1979.

Lees, G. E., and Osborne, C. A.: Urinary tract infections associated with the use and misuse of urinary catheters. Vet. Clin. North Am. 9:713, 1979.

Lees, G. E., Osborne, C. A., Stevens, J. B., and Ward, G. E.: Adverse effects of open indwelling urethral catheterization in clinically normal male cats. Am. J. Vet. Res. 42:825, 1981.

Osborne, C. A., Engen, M. H., Yano, B. L., Brasmer, T. H., Jessen, C. R., and Blevins, W. E.: Congenital urethrorectal fistula in two dogs. J.A.V.M.A. 166:999, 1975.

Pearson, H., and Gibbs, C.: Urinary tract abnormalities in the dog. J. Small Anim. Pract. 12:67, 1971.

Piermattei, D. L., and Osborne, C. A.: Urohydropropulsion—Nonsurgical removal of urethral calculi in male dogs. *In* Kirk, R. W. (ed.): *Current Veterinary Therapy VI*. Philadelphia: W. B. Saunders, 1977.

Polzin, D. J., and Jeraj, K.: Urethritis, cystitis, and ureteritis. Vet. Clin. North Am. 9:661, 1979.

Schwartz, A., Lipowitz, A. J., and Burt, J.: Urinary incontinence due to multiple urogenital anomalies in a mature dog. J.A.V.M.A. 164:1021, 1974.

Sinibaldi, K. R., and Greene, R. W.: Surgical correction of prolapse of the male urethra in three English bulldogs. J. Am. Anim. Hosp. Assoc. 9:450, 1973.

Tarvin, G., Patnaik, A., and Greene, R. W.: Primary urethral tumors in dogs. J.A.V.M.A. 172:931, 1978.

MANAGEMENT OF TRANSITIONAL CELL CARCINOMAS OF THE URINARY BLADDER

STEVEN E. CROW, D.V.M.,

East Lansing, Michigan

and JEFFREY S. KLAUSNER, D.V.M.

St. Paul, Minnesota

Neoplasms of the canine urinary bladder are diagnostic and therapeutic challenges for the veterinary clinician. Diagnosis is frequently delayed owing to a lack of observation of clinical signs by the owner or prolonged empirical treatment. Successful therapy may be impaired by these delays.

Most neoplasms of the canine urinary bladder are malignant. Transitional cell carcinoma (TCC) is the predominant neoplasm. Squamous cell carcinomas, leiomyosarcomas, rhabdomyosarcomas, and other sarcomas are occasionally seen in dogs. Benign tumors reported include papilloma, fibroma, and leiomyoma. Bladder neoplasms are rare in cats.

Several studies have revealed a greater frequency of canine bladder tumors in females than in males. This tendency is the reverse of a male sex predilection in human bladder cancer.

CLINICAL SIGNS

Clinical signs of urinary bladder neoplasms include stranguria, pollakiuria, and hematuria. Urine dribbling following micturition and incontinence at rest are sometimes noted. Signs of systemic illness are rare. Dehydration, anorexia, and vomiting may be observed when urine flow is obstructed by a large, infiltrating tumor in the bladder trigone.

Urinalysis frequently reveals evidence of hematuria and/or urinary tract infection (pyuria, hematuria, bacteriuria, and proteinuria). The specific gravity may vary from very dilute to concentrated. Some dogs with TCC voluntarily drink large amounts of water; this polydipsia appears to be psychogenic, because concentrated urine is usually produced following water deprivation. Hemogram and serum chemistry determinations are usually normal, except that serum urea nitrogen and creatinine concentrations are elevated in dogs with lower urinary tract obstruction. Examination of stained urine sediment may reveal clusters of anaplastic epithelial cells. Caution is advised in making a definitive diagnosis by cytology alone, because atypical transitional cells may appear in some dogs with cystitis.

Survey radiographs of the abdomen are rarely contributory when bladder neoplasia is present but may help to rule out other problems including radiodense uroliths and prostatic disease. Contrast radiographs are needed to demonstrate a mass in the urinary bladder. We recommend a double contrast technique. An excretory urogram to identify the size and location of the renal pelves and ureters should be followed by a negative contrast cystogram. Double contrast is most effective in delineating masses in the urinary bladder lumen and wall. Radiographic findings include bladder wall thickening, ulceration, and space-occupying masses.

Hypertrophic osteopathy (i.e., painful swelling and periosteal bone proliferation of the long bones) is a paraneoplastic syndrome occasionally seen in dogs with bladder tumors. This debilitating complication has been associated with embryonal rhabdomyosarcomas and transitional cell carcinomas.

DIAGNOSIS

Diagnosis is rendered by correlating history, physical examination, urine sediment cytology, and radiographic evidence. Exploratory surgery is sometimes required to obtain a definitive diagnosis; however, percutaneous cystocentesis/bladder wall–fine needle aspiration will occasionally yield strong evidence of neoplasia. When surgery is required, other therapeutic possibilities should be considered before operating.

Prognosis and treatment of TCC are dependent on the location and extent of the neoplasm. Clinical staging of each neoplasm should be performed (Ta-

Table 1. *Clinical Stages of Canine Bladder Tumors**

T Primary Tumor
 T0 No evidence of primary tumor
 T1S Carcinoma *in situ*
 T1 Superficial papillary tumor
 T2 Tumor invading the bladder wall with induration
 T3 Tumor invading neighboring organs (prostate, uterus, vagina, anal canal)
N Regional Lymph Nodes (RLN)†
 N0 No RLN involved
 N1 RLN involved
 N2 RLN and juxta RLN involved
M Distant Metastasis
 M0 No evidence of metastasis
 M1 Distant metastasis present; specify site(s)

---

*Approved by the World Health Organization, 1979.
 †The RLN are the internal and external iliac lymph nodes. The juxta RLN are the lumbar lymph nodes.
 Notes: The following information is necessary for the determination of the categories (if unavailable, the symbols Tx, Nx, and Mx should be used).
  T categories: Clinical examination, cystoscopy, urography or cystography, laparotomy.
  N categories: Surgical examination (laparotomy or laparoscopy).
  M categories: Clinical examination, radiography of the thorax, laparotomy.
 No Stage grouping is recommended at present.

ble 1). Preinvasive carcinoma and small invasive lesions should be treated by partial cystectomy. Excision should be as complete as possible.

Unfortunately, TCC is usually very advanced by the time a diagnosis is made. In addition, the majority of neoplasms arise in the trigone area. Consequently, partial cystectomy is rarely feasible. On the positive side, regional lymph node or distant metastases usually have not occurred at the time of diagnosis. When such metastases are observed (usually months after diagnosis), the iliac and sublumbar lymph nodes and lungs are most often involved.

TREATMENT

The goals of treatment of TCC are regional control of neoplastic growth and prevention of distant me-

tastases. Specific objectives of regional control include relief of urinary discomfort, maintenance of urinary continence, and prevention of hydronephrosis and hydroureter. Many different surgical techniques have been tried in humans with TCC. A majority of these involve total or radical cystectomy with urinary diversion. Total cystectomy entails complete removal of the bladder and urethra in females and the bladder, prostate, and urethra in males. Radical cystectomy combines pelvic lymph node dissection with total cystectomy.

Several methods of urinary diversion have been attempted in dogs following cystectomy, including ureteral or trigonal colostomy, ureteroileostomy, and gastrocystoplasty. Although we have had limited experience with these procedures, none have been notably successful for bladder tumor management. Abnormal defecation and azotemia are frequent complications, but fecal continence is usually preserved. Other complications include hyperchloremic acidosis and pyelonephritis. Gastrocystoplasty, which involves formation of a substitute bladder from a portion of stomach, is technically difficult and requires frequent emptying by the owner. Following transplantation of ureters into the gastric pouch, an intussuscepted segment of ileum is attached to the pouch and exteriorized in the abdominal flank. This conduit is positioned so that intestinal peristalsis away from the abdominal stoma minimizes leakage. The substitute bladder is emptied by catheter. Postoperative complications include azotemia, ascending urinary tract infection, and peritonitis. At the present time we cannot recommend any surgical procedure on the basis of unacceptable quality of life produced.

Whereas curative therapy may be unattainable in most dogs with TCC, symptoms may be minimized in many patients. Treatment of urinary tract infection with antibacterial drugs or removal or dissolution of urinary calculi may relieve straining and discomfort for weeks to months. When urinary tract infection is present, bacterial culture and antimicrobial susceptibility tests should be performed. Treatment with appropriate antibiotics should be contin-

Table 2. *Dosage, Route, and Frequency of Administration of Anticancer Drugs Used for Treatment of Transitional Cell Carcinoma of the Urinary Bladder in Dogs*

Agent	Dose	Route	Frequency of Administration
Systemic Agents			
Cyclophosphamide (Cytoxan, Mead Johnson)	50 to 75 mg/m^2*	PO	4 times weekly
	200 to 300 mg/m^2	IV	q7d
Doxorubicin HCl (Adriamycin, Adria)	30 mg/m^2	IV	q21d
5-fluorouracil (Fluorouracil, Roche)	200 mg/m^2	IV	q7d
Intravesicular Agents			
5-fluorouracil	300 mg/m^2	—	q7d
Triethylene thiophosphoramide (Thiotepa, Lederle)	15 to 30 mg	—	q7 to 14d

*m^2 = square meters of body surface.

ued as long as required to eliminate or control infection.

When marked hematuria is present, chemical cauterization should be considered. Moderate bleeding may be minimized by treatment with methenamine mandelate (10 mg/kg orally every six hours to effect). Severe hematuria may require intravesicular instillation of a dilute formalin solution.

Tumor progression may be delayed in some cases by radiation therapy or chemotherapy. Anticancer drugs have not caused objective reduction of TCC in our experience, but subjective responses consisting of apparent growth arrest and partial relief of symptoms have been seen in four of seven dogs treated with combinations of intravesicular instillation of triethylene thiophosphoramide or 5-fluorouracil and systemic administration of doxorubicin, cyclophosphamide, and/or 5-fluorouracil (Table 2).

External beam irradiation is generally not indicated owing to excessive scatter radiation; however, investigators at several veterinary schools have been evaluating intraoperative radiation. Doses of 1500 to 2000 rads have been given directly to the tumor following surgical exposure of the neoplasm. Preliminary results have been encouraging, with partial regression of tumor in more than one-half of the cases.

Additional treatment methods that warrant further study include radiation via radon or cesium implants and development of prosthetic bladders. It is hoped that these newer techniques will bring improved results.

In summary, treatment for TCC remains palliative in most cases, but there is reason for optimism in the future. Prognosis is guarded to unfavorable for remission but fair to good for partial relief of symptoms.

SUPPLEMENTAL READING

Osborne, C. A., Low, D. G., and Finco, D. R.: Neoplasms of the urinary bladder. *In* Osborne, C. A. (ed.): *Canine and Feline Urology.* Philadelphia: W. B. Saunders, 1972, pp. 374–385.

Strafuss, A. C., and Dean, M. J.: Neoplasms of the canine urinary bladder. J.A.V.M.A. 166:1161, 1975.

Section
14

INFECTIOUS DISEASES

FREDRIC W. SCOTT, D.V.M.
Consulting Editor

Immunization

CANINE IMMUNIZATION

LARRY J. SWANGO, D.V.M.

Auburn, Alabama

Immunization practices are reviewed periodically by committees and panels that recommend vaccination schedules that maximize immunization in the largest percentage of the population. The Panel Report of the Symposium on Immunity to Selected Canine Infectious Diseases (1970); periodic reports by the AVMA Council on Biologic and Therapeutic Agents (Synopsis of vaccination procedures, 1973; Canine and feline immunization guidelines, 1982); the Compendium of Animal Rabies Vaccines (1983), prepared annually by the National Association of State Public Health Veterinarians, Inc.; and recent research reports constitute the basic guidelines for canine immunization. Recommendations are changed or modified as new information is obtained concerning the safety and efficacy of vaccines. The United States Department of Agriculture has established licensing requirements for vaccines. All vaccines licensed by the USDA must meet strict requirements and regulations for production and marketing as well as for safety and efficacy. Some vaccines not licensed by the USDA may be licensed by individual states for intrastate use only. These vaccines may or may not comply with the standards established by the USDA. Manufacturer's recommendations for the use of vaccines are in accord with established requirements and immunization practices based on the results of studies determining safety and efficacy (Table 1).

RABIES

Modified live virus (MLV) and inactivated virus vaccines are available for immunizing dogs against rabies. All rabies vaccines should be administered by intramuscular injection. Several vaccines, both MLV and inactivated, have been shown to induce immunity against rabies for three years after the initial vaccination series (see page 1138). It is recommended that the first dose of vaccine be given at three to four months of age, a second dose one year later, and booster doses at three-year intervals thereafter. State and local laws may require rabies vaccination annually or biennially.

Some rabies vaccines, both MLV and inactivated, require annual booster doses to maintain adequate immunity (see page 1138). It is recommended that the first dose of vaccine be given at three to four months of age and booster doses given annually. Because inactivated rabies vaccines contain nonviable virus, they do not carry the risk of vaccine-induced rabies. In recent years, some MLV rabies vaccines have been withdrawn from use because they were shown to occasionally induce clinical rabies.

There are no rabies vaccines approved for use in wild animals. Vaccine-induced rabies has occurred in several species of wild animals given MLV rabies vaccine. Inactivated rabies vaccines do not induce rabies, but they have not been proved effective for use in wild animals. Administration of vaccines to animals for which they have not been approved involves calculated risks.

CANINE DISTEMPER

There have been no major changes in canine distemper virus (CDV) vaccines or in recommended vaccination schedules during the last several years (Synopsis of vaccination procedures, 1973; Schultz et al., 1980; Canine and feline immunization guidelines, 1982). The currently available CDV vaccines are all MLV vaccines, but there are different strains of CDV used in manufacturing the vaccines and different degrees of attenuation of virulence among the vaccine viruses. Attenuation of virulence is usually based on safety testing in young dogs or pups of weaning age. Evidence suggests that MLV canine distemper vaccines may occasionally induce disease in susceptible pups vaccinated at less than four weeks of age. CDV viruses adapted to embryonating eggs and chicken tissue culture are more highly attenuated than vaccine viruses adapted to canine cell cultures. The egg-adapted CDV vaccines appear to be as immunogenic as the canine cell culture vaccines and may be safer for use in orphan pups less than four weeks of age.

Only one dose of MLV canine distemper vaccine

1123

Table 1. *Summary of Vaccination Procedures for Dogs*

Disease	Type of Vaccine	Recommended Vaccination Schedule
Rabies	Modified live virus or inactivated virus	First vaccination at 3 to 4 months of age; second dose one year later; revaccinate annually, biennially, or triennially, depending on licensed approval of vaccine for duration of immunity and state or local laws
Distemper	Modified live virus distemper or measles	First vaccination at 5 to 7 weeks of age; additional doses at three-week intervals until 14 to 16 weeks of age; revaccinate annually with a single dose of vaccine Alternatively, vaccinate with a single dose at 4 to 10 weeks of age followed by a single dose at 14 to 16 weeks of age; revaccinate annually with a single dose.
Hepatitis	Modified live virus CAV-1 or CAV-2	Vaccinate according to distemper schedule using combination vaccine for distemper and hepatitis
Tracheobronchitis	Parenteral vaccines: MLV CAV-1 or CAV-2 with MLV canine parainfluenza	Vaccinate according to distemper schedule using combination vaccine for distemper, hepatitis, and parainfluenza virus
	Intranasal vaccines: MLV canine parainfluenza and live, avirulent *Bordetella bronchiseptica*	Administer a single dose of combination parainfluenza–*Bordetella bronchiseptica* vaccine as early as four weeks of age or any time thereafter; repeat annually
Parvovirus	MLV or inactivated CPV vaccine or MLV feline panleukopenia vaccine licensed for dogs	First vaccination at 6 to 9 weeks of age; additional doses at three-week intervals until 18 weeks of age or older; revaccinate annually; vaccine may be given in combination with distemper, hepatitis, and parainfluenza vaccines
Leptospirosis	Bacterin of *Leptospira canicola* and *Leptospira icterohemorrhagica*	Two doses of bacterin three weeks apart beginning at 9 to 12 weeks of age in combination with distemper and other vaccines; revaccinate annually

Note: Vaccines for other infectious diseases of dogs are not currently available.

is needed to induce immunity in dogs free of antibody and susceptible to infection with CDV. Passive immunity acquired from colostral and placental transfer of antibody interferes with active immunization of pups and is the primary cause of vaccine failures. Pups cannot be immunized until they become susceptible to infection with CDV. Inasmuch as the duration of maternally derived immunity is proportional to the titer of antibody in the dam's serum and colostrum, some litters will become susceptible to infection and can be immunized by four to five weeks of age, whereas other litters may be more than three months old before they can be immunized. Approximately 50 per cent of pups from random litters can be immunized at six weeks of age with a single dose of MLV canine distemper vaccine. By 13 to 14 weeks of age, a single dose of vaccine would induce immunity in 95 per cent or more of pups. Because the immune status of a given pup or litter is unknown unless virus neutralization titers have been determined on serums from the dam and/or pups, it is recommended that a series of vaccinations be given at three-week intervals beginning at 5 to 7 weeks of age and continuing until 13 to 16 weeks of age. If a dog is over three months of age when first presented, only one dose of MLV canine distemper vaccine is recommended. Immunity will usually persist for more than a year in dogs vaccinated in this manner. Dogs with protective titers of antibody will not respond to booster doses of vaccine. How-

ever, annual revaccination is recommended because of the few dogs that may have become susceptible within a year after vaccination.

As a general rule, pregnant bitches should not be vaccinated with MLV vaccines because of potential hazards to developing fetuses. There is a lack of specific information on both the risks and safety of MLV canine distemper vaccines in pregnant bitches.

Attenuated strains of measles virus have been shown to induce "heterotypic" immunity to CDV. Measles virus is not neutralized by low levels of antibody to CDV and provides temporary protection against CDV. The immunity induced in young pups vaccinated with MLV measles vaccine is predominantly cell-mediated immunity. Older pups and dogs that are fully susceptible to CDV will develop titers of antibody to measles virus. Measles vaccine given singly or in combination with distemper and canine parainfluenza vaccines is indicated only in young pups four to ten weeks of age. If a pup is ten weeks of age or older when first vaccinated, MLV canine distemper vaccine is preferred over measles vaccine. Measles vaccine is not indicated in pups over 12 weeks of age and is contraindicated in breeding bitches. Although concerns have been expressed over possible human health hazards associated with the use of MLV measles vaccines in dogs, there is a lack of definitive evidence for such concerns. The MLV measles vaccines licensed for use in dogs are not the same as measles vaccines for humans, and the latter should not be used in dogs.

INFECTIOUS CANINE HEPATITIS

Canine adenovirus type 1 (CAV-1) is the agent of infectious canine hepatitis (ICH). Canine adenovirus type 2 (CAV-2), a respiratory adenovirus of dogs, has antigens in common with CAV-1. Antibodies against either CAV-1 or CAV-2 cross protect against the heterologous virus. Because of this serologic cross reaction, either CAV-1 or CAV-2 vaccines can be used to immunize dogs against ICH. Both MLV and inactivated virus vaccines are available. The MLV vaccines appear to induce immunity of longer duration. MLV CAV-2 and inactivated vaccines circumvent the occasional uveitis and "blue eye" associated with some strains of MLV CAV-1 vaccines. The MLV CAV-1 vaccines have been shown to protect against respiratory disease associated with CAV-2. Annual revaccination for ICH is commonly combined with distemper vaccination; however, the necessity for annual boosters with MLV CAV vaccines is questionable. The recommended immunization schedule for ICH is the same as that for canine distemper, since the vaccines are usually administered in combination.

INFECTIOUS TRACHEOBRONCHITIS ("KENNEL COUGH")

Several viruses, bacteria, and mycoplasmata have been determined to be involved in the etiology of "kennel cough." Canine parainfluenza (CPI) virus, CAV-2, and *Bordetella bronchiseptica* are the most important etiologic agents of infectious tracheobronchitis, and vaccines have been developed for all three agents (Appel, 1981). Vaccines are not available for other viruses, bacteria, or mycoplasmata associated with kennel cough.

Immunity against infections of the respiratory tract is of shorter duration than immunity against disseminated systemic infections such as CDV and ICH. Immunologic protection of the respiratory tract against infections is dependent upon the presence of antibody in respiratory secretions. Antibodies of the IgG class of immunoglobulins will be present in secretions of the lower respiratory tract (bronchial-bronchiolar secretions) in proportion to the titer of circulating antibody. Very little antibody will be present in secretions of the upper respiratory tract (nasopharyngeal secretions) regardless of the titer of circulating antibody unless there has been stimulation of secretory antibodies of the IgA class (S-IgA) of immunoglobulins (Bey et al., 1981). Infection of the respiratory tract will stimulate the production of S-IgA, resulting in high concentrations of antibody in secretions of both the upper and lower respiratory tract.

Clinical signs of kennel cough are usually related to irritation at the tracheobronchial-bronchiolar level of the respiratory tract. Infection with CAV-2, CPI virus, and *B. bronchiseptica* all result in lesions in the bronchi, bronchioles, and/or alveolar interstitial tissue. Thus, infectious tracheobronchitis, kennel cough, is pathologically a disease of the lower respiratory tract. Parenteral vaccines induce immunity in the lower respiratory tract via IgG in bronchial-bronchiolar secretions, although infection of the respiratory tract may occur. Subclinical infection of the respiratory tract in vaccinated dogs stimulates the production of S-IgA, resulting in enhanced immunologic protection against respiratory infections and disease. Intranasal vaccines provide better protection than parenteral vaccines because they stimulate local immunity in both the upper and lower respiratory tract (Appel, 1981; Bey et al., 1981; Chladek, 1981). The intranasal vaccines also have the advantage of being effective in pups with titers of maternally derived antibody, which interferes with parenteral vaccines.

CANINE ADENOVIRUS TYPE 2

The MLV CAV-1 and CAV-2 vaccines have been found to protect dogs against respiratory disease associated with CAV-2. If dogs are seronegative for CAV, a single dose of vaccine will immunize against CAV-2. Since the MLV CAV-1 and CAV-2 vaccines are also used for immunization against ICH, dogs should be vaccinated according to the schedule recommended for ICH and canine distemper. Intranasal vaccines have been considered for CAV-2, but they are not yet available. Experimental studies have shown excellent results, and the vaccine is not affected by maternally derived antibody.

CANINE PARAINFLUENZA (CPI) VIRUS

Attenuated CPI virus vaccines are available for parenteral vaccination and intranasal administration. Unlike CAV vaccines, a single dose of MLV CPI vaccine given parenterally does not provide adequate immunity. At least two doses of parenteral CPI vaccine must be given initially regardless of the age of the dog when first vaccinated. Annual revaccination with a single dose of vaccine is recommended. Parenteral CPI vaccines are available in combination with vaccines for canine distemper and infectious canine hepatitis. Vaccination according to the canine distemper schedule provides adequate immunity. A combination MLV CPI and measles virus vaccine is available.

Intranasal vaccines for CPI virus have been shown to induce immunity with a single application, and they are effective in pups with maternal antibody

(Appel, 1981; Chladek et al., 1981). Intranasal CPI virus vaccines are available in combination with live avirulent *B. bronchiseptica*. They have been shown to be effective and free of adverse reactions. Annual revaccination is recommended.

Bordetella bronchiseptica

Bacterins have been used in attempts to immunize dogs against bordetellosis. The bacterins available in the 1970s provided a degree of protection against disease, but they did not prevent infection. Adverse reactions were common at the site of injection, and systemic reactions occurred occasionally. Until improved bacterins free of adverse reactions become available, parenteral vaccines for bordetellosis will have limited use.

Avirulent strains of *B. bronchiseptica* are available as a live vaccine for intranasal immunization. They are essentially devoid of side effects, and a single administration provides effective immunity against bordetellosis, although vaccinated dogs become infected with *B. bronchiseptica* (Bey et al., 1981; Chladek et al., 1981). Intranasal vaccines available in combination with attenuated CPI virus have been found to significantly decrease clinical signs of kennel cough in both experimental studies and clinical trials (Appel, 1981). In experimental studies, the addition of MLV CAV-2 to the combined *B. bronchiseptica*–CPI virus intranasal vaccine resulted in further reduction in clinical signs of kennel cough. At the present time an intranasal vaccine with CAV-2 is not available.

It is recommended that pups be inoculated intranasally with a combined CPI virus–*B. bronchiseptica* vaccine two weeks prior to weaning. Since maternal antibody does not interfere with intranasal vaccines, one intranasal inoculation of nursing puppies will provide immunity in one to two weeks, i.e., by the time they are weaned. Annual revaccination is recommended.

VIRAL ENTERITIS

Canine coronavirus, a rotavirus, and canine parvovirus have all been found to be associated with acute enteritis in dogs. Vaccines are currently available only for canine parvovirus.

Immunity to infection with canine parvovirus (CPV) has been found to correlate directly with titers of circulating antibody (Pollock and Carmichael, 1982). Maternally derived passive immunity and vaccine-induced active immunity provide protection against infection with CPV and CPV-associated disease. As with other parenteral vaccines, antibody interferes with immunization; maternally derived antibody is the primary cause of vaccine failure in young dogs.

Between 1979 and 1982, there was marked improvement in the immunogenic quality of vaccines for CPV. The original inactivated vaccines containing feline panleukopenia virus were safe but induced immunity of short duration. Inactivated CPV and MLV feline panleukopenia vaccines were only somewhat better. The MLV CPV vaccines that became available in 1981 and 1982 provide good immunity that lasts for at least a year, provided that existing antibody does not interfere with immunization at the time of vaccination. Titers of antibody in dogs immunized with MLV CPV vaccines approach titers in dogs that have recovered from infections with street strains of CPV. Pups from a bitch that has recovered from infection frequently do not respond to vaccine until four months of age or older because of the high level of maternally derived antibody. If a bitch has a low titer of protective antibody, her pups may become susceptible to infection with CPV before six weeks of age. Without knowing the antibody status of each litter, it is difficult to recommend a practical vaccination schedule that will result in immunity in nearly all dogs. There is the additional problem of pups becoming susceptible to infection with virulent strains of CPV a week or more before they can be immunized with vaccine.

To maximize the probability of immunizing the individual dog, it is recommended that pups of unknown immune status be vaccinated at 6, 9, 12, 15, and 18 weeks of age, followed by annual revaccination. The MLV CPV vaccines are preferred over the inactivated CPV or MLV feline panleukopenia vaccines. Vaccines in combination with CDV, CAV, and CPI virus are available and appear to be as effective as MLV CPV by itself.

LEPTOSPIROSIS

Bacterins for *Leptospira canicola* and *L. icterohemorrhagica* provide immunity that persists for at least one year after primary immunization. Two doses of bacterin should be given three weeks apart beginning at 9 to 12 weeks of age. Annual revaccination is recommended. The bacterins currently available contain fewer nonprotective antigenic components and induce fewer adverse reactions than the first bacterins used. However, risks are inherent with repeated injection of antigenic substances, and provisions for treatment and observation of patients after vaccination should be available in the event that anaphylaxis should occur.

REFERENCES AND SUPPLEMENTAL READING

Appel, M. J.: Canine infectious tracheobronchitis (kennel cough): A status report. Comp. Cont. Ed. 3:70, 1981.

Bey, R. F., Shade, F. J., Goodnow, R. A., and Johnson, R. C.: Intranasal vaccination of dogs with live avirulent *Bordetella bronchiseptica:* Correlation of serum agglutination titer and the formation of secretory IgA with protection against experimentally induced infectious tracheobronchitis. Am. J. Vet. Res. 42:1130, 1981.

Canine and feline immunization guidelines—1982. J.A.V.M.A. 18:332, 1982.

Chladek, D. W., Williams, J. M., Gerber, D. L., et al.: Canine parainfluenza–*Bordetella bronchiseptica* vaccine: Immunogenicity. Am. J. Vet. Res. 42:266, 1981.

Compendium of animal rabies vaccines, 1983. J.A.V.M.A. 182:16, 1983.

Panel report of symposium on immunity to selected canine infectious diseases. J.A.V.M.A. 156:1661, 1970.

Pollock, R. V. H., and Carmichael, L. E.: Maternally derived immunity to canine parvovirus infection: Transfer, decline, and interference with vaccination. J.A.V.M.A. 180:37, 1982.

Schultz, R. D., Appel, M., Carmichael, L. E., and Farrow, B.: Update on canine immunization. *In* Kirk, R. W. (ed.): *Current Veterinary Therapy VII.* Philadelphia: W. B. Saunders, 1980, pp. 1252–1255.

Synopsis of vaccination procedures for dogs. J.A.V.M.A. 162:228, 1973.

FELINE IMMUNIZATION

FREDRIC W. SCOTT, D.V.M.

Ithaca, N.Y.

An effective immunization schedule is an integral part of a preventive medicine program for cats. The type of vaccine used, the route of administration, the effect of maternal antibody derived from colostrum, and the age of the cat vaccinated can affect the immune response (or lack thereof) that occurs following vaccination.

NATURE OF THE VACCINE

Both inactivated and modified live virus (MLV) vaccines are available. The MLV vaccines must be handled and stored according to the manufacturer's instructions to maintain potency. MLV vaccines should not be administered to pregnant cats.

ROUTE OF ADMINISTRATION

The route by which the vaccine is administered may affect the degree of protection provided. Feline panleukopenia (FP) vaccine can be given intramuscularly (IM) or subcutaneously (SC) with equal effect. The MLV FP vaccines can also be given by the intranasal or aerosol route but not the oral route.

Rabies vaccine must be given by the IM route at one site in the thigh. Although extensive studies on the route of administration of rabies vaccine in cats have not been reported, studies in dogs have shown that the IM route is at least 100 times more effective than the SC route. The same should hold true for the cat.

The MLV respiratory vaccines appear to be slightly more effective when given by the IM route, but they can be given SC. Aerosol vaccination with injectable vaccines may result in mild signs of illness.

The intranasal (IN) respiratory vaccines are administered by allowing the cat to inhale drops of recently reconstituted lyophilized viral rhinotracheitis–caliciviral disease (FVR-FCV) or FVR-FCV-FP vaccine into the nostrils. One or two drops are also placed in each conjunctival sac. These vaccines produce rapid local as well as systemic immunity. Clients should be warned that cats vaccinated by the IN route may sneeze and develop mild ocular and/or nasal discharge four to seven days after vaccination. Occasionally, ulcers develop on the tongue. Vaccinated cats shed FVR and FCV viruses for long periods after IN vaccination.

AGE OF THE CAT

The most frequent cause of vaccine failure with FP vaccines is interference caused by maternally derived immunity. These cats become susceptible later after the passive immunity wanes. The level and duration of passive immunity following nursing are determined by the antibody titer of the queen at parturition, assuming that the kitten nurses. Although the majority of cats can be immunized successfully at 8 to 10 weeks of age, occasional kittens may not be susceptible to vaccination until 12 weeks of age. Therefore, if FP vaccines are given to kittens less than 12 weeks of age, they should be repeated at three- to four-week intervals until the cat is at least 12 weeks old.

Little is known about maternal antibody interference in FVR and FCV vaccines. The same principles of colostral transfer, antibody half-life, and vaccine virus neutralization should apply to these viruses as well as to FP. Therefore, we can predict that there will be interference if the maternal titers are high enough. Generally, the FVR and FCV titers are much lower than the FP titer, and therefore the duration of interference (and passive protection) should be much shorter. It is doubtful that this will be longer than five to six weeks for FVR and seven to eight weeks for FCV. By nine to ten weeks of age, the vast majority of cats should be susceptible to FVR and FCV vaccination.

FELINE PANLEUKOPENIA VACCINES

There are many excellent vaccines available for immunization of cats against FP (Scott and Gillespie, 1971). If these are used correctly and given at the proper age, cats should be completely protected against this very severe viral infection. It behooves veterinarians to immunize as many cats as possible in their practice.

Several slightly different programs for the immunization of cats against FP have been presented during the past few years. The safest recommendation is to start the immunization program at an early age and vaccinate kittens at frequent intervals until they are at least 16 weeks of age. This might prove beneficial in certain circumstances, such as in catteries or colonies, in which kittens could be vaccinated at 6 weeks of age, followed by repeated vaccinations at two-week intervals until the cats are 16 weeks old. However, most kittens presented to the practitioner must be immunized with a minimum of two or possibly three vaccinations. Therefore, the clinician must attempt to immunize the maximum number of cats with a reasonable number of vaccinations per cat.

Most recommendations indicate that the kittens should be vaccinated starting at eight, nine, or ten weeks of age. A single vaccination will immunize the cats if they are susceptible at the time of vaccination. It interference occurred at the time of the first vaccination, chances are much greater that the cat will be susceptible to vaccination four weeks later, instead of seven to ten days later. If the first vaccination was successful, the increase in titer following the second vaccination will be comparable whether it is given at four or two weeks if inactivated vaccines are used. For MLV vaccines, the second vaccination would have no effect on a previously immunized kitten owing to the high titer.

In reviewing the different programs for immunization of cats, the report of the Panel for the Colloquium on Selected Feline Infectious Diseases (1971) suggested a two-week interval as opposed to a four-week interval, since fewer cats would be returned for revaccination four weeks later. After evaluating all the available information, the panel recommended that two doses of inactivated vaccine be given at two-week intervals, starting at nine to ten weeks of age. For maximum protection, especially in areas of high concentration of street virus, a third vaccination is recommended at 16 weeks of age. For MLV vaccines, the first dose should be administered at 9 to 10 weeks of age, followed by a second dose between 14 and 16 weeks of age. If the cat is older than 12 weeks at the time of the first vaccination with MLV vaccine, a repeat vaccination is not indicated.

With the advent of respiratory vaccines, for which there is good evidence for revaccination at three- to four-week intervals instead of two-week intervals, and since one should try to immunize the maximum number of cats with the minimum number of office visits, it now seems advisable to recommend the three- to four-week interval between vaccinations, as outlined in Table 1 and as suggested in the 1982 Current Canine and Feline Immunization Guidelines from the Council on Biologic and Therapeutic Agents, American Veterinary Medical Association (see Current Canine and Feline Immunization Guidelines, page 1134).

Table 1. *Feline Vaccine Recommendations*

Disease	Type of Vaccine	Age at First Vaccination (Weeks)	Age at Second Vaccination (Weeks)	Revaccination	Route of Administration
Panleukopenia (FP)	Inactivated	8 to 10	12 to 14	Annual	SC or IM
	MLV	8 to 10	12 to 14	Annual	SC or IM
	MLV IN	8 to 10	12 to 14	Annual	IN
Viral rhinotracheitis (FVR)	MLV	8 to 10 (or earlier)	12 to 14	Annual	SC or IM
	MLV IN	8 to 10	—	Annual	IN
	Inactivated	8 to 10 (or earlier)	12 to 14	Annual	SC or IM
Caliciviral disease (FCV)	MLV	8 to 10 (or earlier)	12 to 14	Annual	SC or IM
	MLV IN	8 to 10	—	Annual	IN
	Inactivated	8 to 10 (or earlier)	12 to 14	Annual	SC or IM
Pneumonitis	MLV	8	—	Annual	SC or IM
Rabies	Inactivated	12	—	Annual	IM
	MLV*	12	—	Annual	IM

*Approved for use in cats (only one vaccine as of January 1983). Use of nonapproved MLV vaccines in cats can result in vaccine-induced rabies.

FELINE VIRAL RHINOTRACHEITIS (FVR) VACCINES

FVR vaccines should be given in combination with FCV vaccine or as a triple FP-FVR-FCV vaccine. The FVR vaccines produce significant immunization following vaccination and as such should be part of the routine vaccination program, as outlined in Table 1. As a result of local viral replication, vaccinated cats develop a rapid anamnestic response when exposed to virulent virus. Some vaccinated cats may sneeze, and an occasional cat may have watery eyes for one to two days. Severe systemic disease does not occur in properly immunized cats, as it does in unvaccinated cats.

FELINE CALICIVIRUS (FCV) VACCINE

It was originally thought that multiple serotypes of FCV existed and, therefore, that an effective vaccine would not be possible. However, most but not all isolates fall into a single serotype of FCV. Most strains of FCV tested exhibit good protection against other strains of FCV. The same parameters that apply to FVR vaccines (i.e., route of vaccination, anamnestic response when challenged, and good clinical protection against virulent virus exposure but not protection against local viral replication) also apply to FCV vaccines. These vaccines are produced in combination with FVR vaccine, and immunization recommendations are the same as those for FVR (see Table 1).

FELINE PNEUMONITIS (FPn) VACCINE

Although FPn is not as prevalent as FVR or FCV disease, it is evident that in some cat populations a severe, chronic respiratory disease is produced by the FPn agent, a chlamydial organism. According to recent studies, the vaccines currently available appear to produce significant protection following a single IM vaccination. As with other respiratory vaccines, complete protection is not afforded, but clinical signs, if they do occur, are restricted to a very short course and are mild and local. Chronic disease (characteristic of natural infection in susceptible cats) does not occur in vaccinated cats.

Although there are many unknown parameters concerning immunity to FPn, it appears that, if FPn is a problem in a particular area, the FPn vaccine should be part of the routine vaccination program. The age at which to vaccinate is not critical, since there appears to be little interference with maternal antibody by the time kittens would normally be old enough to be vaccinated. A single injection appears to afford adequate protection.

RABIES VACCINES

Rabies vaccine recommendations are included in the 1983 Compendium of Animal Rabies Vaccines, page 1137. Only inactivated vaccines or MLV vaccines specifically licensed for use in cats should be given.

REFERENCES AND SUPPLEMENTAL READING

Kolar, J. R., and Rude, T. A.: Clinical evaluation of a commercial feline pneumonitis vaccine. Feline Pract. 7:47, 1977.
Report of the Panel for the Colloquium on Selected Feline Infectious Diseases. J.A.V.M.A. 158:835, 1971.
Schultz, R. D.: Theory and practice of immunization. In Kirk, R. W. (ed.): Current Veterinary Therapy VII. Philadelphia: W. B. Saunders, 1980, pp. 1248–1251.
Scott, F. W.: Evaluation of an experimental vaccine against feline viral rhinotracheitis and feline calicivirus disease. Am. J. Vet. Res. 38:229, 1977.
Scott, F. W. et al: Current canine and feline immunization guidelines. In Kirk, R. W. (ed.): Current Veterinary Therapy VIII. Philadelphia: W. B. Saunders, 1983, pp. 1134–1142.
Scott, F. W., and Gillespie, J. H.: Immunization for feline panleukopenia. Vet. Clin. North Am. 1:231, 1971.

IMMUNOPROPHYLAXIS IN NONDOMESTIC CARNIVORES

MURRAY E. FOWLER, D.V.M.

Davis, California

Prevention of viral diseases in carnivores is a pressing concern for zoo veterinarians, but practitioners with less exposure to nondomestic carnivores are no less concerned. Numerous vaccination regimens have been devised. There is little agreement within the veterinary profession as to the protocol for a safe, effective program. The diversity of opinion is caused by the lack of sound experimental data. Veterinarians are compelled to rely on empirical experience.

Some basic principles must be understood when planning vaccination of valuable wild carnivores. A major decision involves the selection of either a modified live virus (MLV) or a killed virus (KV) vaccine. When choosing one or the other, it must be fully understood that the live agents of MLV vaccines have been attenuated only for a specific host (the species for which the vaccine was developed) and a specific route of administration. If either of these factors is altered, there is no assurance that the product is either safe or effective.

Since it is usually desirable to avoid rehandling of a wild species, if protection against multiple diseases is planned, the tendency is to administer all the antigens at the same time. Such a practice may inhibit normal antigen-antibody response in the host as a result of antigenic competition. One antigen may stimulate the antibody-forming system so powerfully that response to a second and/or third antigen is suppressed.

The inefficacy of immunization may result from the failure of the animal to mount an immune response following vaccination or, following the use of MLV vaccine, the development of a vaccine-induced infection.

Any of the following factors may contribute to an inadequate immune response: (1) inability of a particular antigen to respond, (2) destruction of a MLV vaccine by careless handling, (3) improper balance of a multiple-antigen vaccine for that species, or (4) inhibition of antigen response in a neonate by passive maternal antibodies. One cannot rely on a protective immune response to domestic animal vaccines in nondomestic species nor can one predict the persistence of immunity. Annual or more frequent booster vaccinations in nondomestic animals are indicated, even with the supposedly single-injection, lifetime protection vaccines.

Canine distemper and feline panleukopenia affect a broad spectrum of wild carnivores. It is important to recognize that the disease syndrome exhibited by wild carnivores may vary widely from that seen in the domestic dog and cat. A wild felid with panleukopenia may not exhibit the classic hemogram response seen in domestic species. Furthermore, both viral agents (i.e., canine distemper and feline panleukopenia) may produce a similar syndrome in certain species, e.g., raccoon, *Procyon lotor*. Many references of these diseases in wild carnivores in veterinary literature have been based on clinical signs and, possibly, gross necropsy lesions. A definitive diagnosis cannot be made on this basis. Virus isolation, histopathology, or a rise in antibody titers with acute and convalescent serum is required for a definitive diagnosis. Veterinarians only complicate the problem when they report the incidence of disease in wild carnivores without obtaining precise diagnoses.

Recognizing these inherent difficulties, an attempt must still be made to provide a sound immunoprophylactic program for wild carnivores. Information can be gleaned from the vaccination of domestic carnivores in addition to the experiences reported on disease outbreaks in wild species. The documentation for statements made in this discussion is found in another publication. A complete reference list will be supplied by the author upon request.

The primary diseases of concern in nondomestic carnivores are feline panleukopenia (FP), canine distemper (CD), infectious canine hepatitis (ICH), canine parvovirus infection (CPI), rhinotracheitis (upper respiratory syndrome of cats [RCS]), and rabies.

FELINE PANLEUKOPENIA (FP)

All felids are considered susceptible to panleukopenia. No canid cases have been reported. The only mustelid with a confirmed diagnosis is the mink, *Mustela vison*. Raccoons and coatimundi, *Nasua nasua*, in the procyonid group are also susceptible.

Both MLV and KV vaccines are available and effective in domestic cats. Definitive protocols for wild felids are not known, but based on a review of the literature and personal experience the author recommends the following.

MLV vaccine should never be given to a pregnant felid. Fetal infection of the germinal layer of the cerebellum prevents formulation of the granular layer of the cerebellar cortex. Cerebellar hypoplasia results, and the kitten is ataxic.

Colostrum-deprived neonates should be given KV vaccine at 2, 4, 8, 12, and 16 weeks of age. MLV vaccine may be given after initial use of the KV vaccine. Annual boosters are recommended. Follow the manufacturer's directions as to the injection site.

Neonates from dams known to be immune should be vaccinated with KV at 8, 12, and 16 weeks of age. Annual boosters can be KV or MLV. Neonates from dams of unknown immune status should be vaccinated according to the protocol for colostrum-deprived neonates.

Adults with a known history of FP vaccination should be vaccinated with either KV or MLV vaccine at first handling and annually thereafter.

Adults with no history of vaccination should be given KV vaccine at first handling and either KV or MLV vaccine annually thereafter.

Dosages of vaccine are based strictly on conjecture. In large adult felids, such as the tiger, as much as three to five times the domestic cat dose of KV vaccine may be appropriate, but no studies have correlated dosage with animal size, titer response, or persistence of immunity.

CANINE DISTEMPER (CD)

Canine distemper has been definitively diagnosed in numerous carnivore species. The veterinarian is faced with a serious dilemma in that KV CD vaccines do not confer permanent immunity unless the animal is subsequently challenged with an exposure to the street virus. In a zoo or home setting, such an exposure may not occur soon enough after vaccination or may not occur at all. Only MLV CD vaccines are available commercially in the United States and Canada. Vaccine-induced canine distemper has been confirmed in black-footed ferrets, *Mustela nigripes;* lesser pandas, *Ailurus fulgens;* gray foxes, *Urocyon cinereoargenteus;* and kinkajous, *Potos flavus.* Those species sensitive to MLV vaccines present special problems. Special KV vaccines must be obtained from experimental facilities. Theoretically, MLV vaccine is safe to use following administration of KV vaccine, but no sound data have been collected to support such a decision.

MLV CD vaccine should be used in all nonsensitive species, following the same vaccination protocol as that recommended for FP.

INFECTIOUS CANINE HEPATITIS (ICH)

Infectious canine hepatitis disease has been confirmed in domestic dogs, foxes, skunks, and bears. In one incident, young brown bears developed an encephalitis shortly after being vaccinated with MLV ICH vaccine. The signs and necropsy findings in the bears were similar to those seen in fox encephalitis. The presence of jaundice and bilirubinemia in a sick canid is an indication of ICH. However, it has been demonstrated that raccoons and ferrets with canine distemper virus infections also exhibit similar signs.

An outbreak of ICH occurred in zoo canids that had been vaccinated regularly with MLV vaccines. Vaccination had failed to protect these animals from a highly pathogenic strain of the virus.

Only MLV ICH vaccines are available. Foxes should definitely be vaccinated, as they are susceptible to ICH.

CANINE PARVOVIRUS INFECTION (CPV)

Parvovirus infections in domestic dogs and wild carnivores have recently complicated the diagnostic picture of enteric diseases in carnivores. CPV infection has been definitively diagnosed in bush dogs, *Speothos venaticus;* maned wolves, *Chrysocyon brachyurus;* crab-eating foxes, *Cerdocyon thous;* and coyotes, *Canis latrans.* A parvovirus isolated from raccoons closely resembles the canine parvovirus. The host range of canine and raccoon parvoviruses is unknown, but infections caused by these viruses must be considered in differential diagnoses of enteric diseases of wild carnivores.

Parvovirus infection produces macro- and microscopic lesions that are indistinguishable from those of FP. It may be possible to distinguish between these viruses by the results of serologic tests (hemagglutination, serum neutralization), fluorescent antibody tests, cytopathic effects on tissue culture, and electron microscopy.

Canine parvovirus vaccines are being used on wild canids, but there are no data to support statements on efficacy or safety.

RHINOTRACHEITIS (UPPER RESPIRATORY SYNDROME OF CATS)

Rhinotracheitis is a serious and potentially fatal disease complex in wild felids. The inflammatory response of the oropharyngeal mucous membranes and the conjunctiva induces total anorexia. Secondary infections develop. Feeding by gastric intubation may be crucial to recovery. Parenterally administered MLV vaccines have been tested for safety and efficacy in a variety of wild felids (Laughlin, 1980), but apparent vaccine-induced infection has been reported by others (Boever, 1982).

RABIES

Vaccination of wild carnivores against rabies is sometimes warranted. It is wise to ascertain the legality of vaccinating wild carnivores in a given area before administering the vaccine.

No MLV rabies vaccine should be used on nondomestic species. Numerous examples of vaccine-induced rabies in coyotes, skunks, and raccoons have been reported.

REFERENCES AND SUPPLEMENTAL READING

Boever, W.: Personal communication, 1982.
Fowler, M. E.: Preventive medical planning. *In* Jones, D. M. (ed.): *Recent Advances in Zoo Animal Medicine, Symposium.* London: Zoological Society of London, 1982, in press.
Laughlin, D. C.: Immunization of exotic cats. *In* Kirk, R. W. (ed.): *Current Veterinary Therapy VII.* Philadelphia: W. B. Saunders, 1980, pp. 1258–1261.

IMMUNIZATION AGAINST
FELINE LEUKEMIA

RICHARD G. OLSEN, Ph.D.,
and LAWRENCE E. MATHES, Ph.D.

Columbus, Ohio

Historically, the development of practical vaccines to prevent naturally occurring cancer in humans or animals has been frustrated by failures. The major problems associated with cancer vaccines have been insufficient knowledge about the causative agents (carcinogens) for specific cancers and a lack of a clear understanding of the cancer cell neoantigens that play an important role in inducing protective immunosurveillance mechanisms.

The feline leukemia virus (FeLV) diseases in the domestic cat present an ideal opportunity to the scientist to develop and evaluate cancer vaccines. This is due, in part, to various aspects of FeLV disease. First, FeLV (synonyms: feline retrovirus, feline oncornavirus) is the confirmed etiologic agent of the multiple clinical forms of FeLV disease (Hoover et al., 1981). The clinical manifestations of the FeLV diseases include lymphosarcoma, leukemia, thymic lymphosarcoma, fibrosarcoma, nonregenerative anemias, and fetal resorption. An associated disease entity of FeLV disease in cats is generalized immunosuppression. This factor increases the mortality and morbidity in cats to other infectious disease such as feline infectious peritonitis.

Second, a single species of feline retrovirus (carcinogen) induces all of the previously mentioned diseases (Schaller and Olsen, 1981).

Third, the immunogens associated with FeLV disease have been well characterized (Schaller and Olsen, 1981). FeLV is comprised of three serotypes (A, B, C), and the major envelope glycoprotein (70 K daltons) that elicits virus-neutralizing antibody has been identified. The tumor-associated neoantigen in FeLV disease referred to as FOCMA (feline oncornavirus–associated cell membrane antigen) is common to all forms of FeLV disease (Rice and Olsen, 1981).

Fourth, unlike most other known cancer viruses of animals, FeLV is horizontally transmitted. In other words, the cancer virus is contagious and spreads by cat-to-cat contact (Hoover et al., 1981).

Fifth, the FeLV disease begins with a productive virus infection that may culminate months later with the formation of clinical disease including cancer. The resistance to FeLV disease depends on the development of at least two immunologic responses: one toward the infectious virus and one toward FOCMA of the cancer cell (Mathes and Olsen, 1981). Because the antigens of the infectious virus are distinct from FOCMA, a FeLV vaccine should contain both components.

EXPERIMENTAL VACCINES

The approaches to producing a FeLV vaccine have included killed FeLV, attenuated FeLV, and feline leukemia tumor cells (both killed and alive). Killed FeLV vaccine was shown to induce virus-neutralizing antibodies in adult cats but not in young kittens. Administration of killed FeLV to young kittens, in fact, rendered the kittens more susceptible to FeLV disease than nonvaccinated controls (Olsen and Lewis, 1981).

The use of attenuated (live) FeLV vaccine involves several serious problems. Since attenuated FeLV is infectious, the site of and events in the infection are similar to those seen in the infection caused by the wild (street) unattenuated FeLV. This means that attenuated FeLV infects bone marrow cells, potentially leading to the insertion of the virus genetic material into the genome of the host chromosomes. Eventually derepression of host cell transformation genes due to upstream inserting of the virus genome may culminate in the phenotypic expression of transformation-specific protein and cell transformation (cancer). It is thought that FOCMA may be the transformation-specific protein of feline leukemia. It is now clear that, for attenuated FeLV vaccine to express FOCMA, the previously described infectious events must take place. In addition to this problem it has been clearly shown that FeLV attenuated for adult cats may be oncogenic in younger kittens. Needless to say, the risk factor of an infectious cancer-causing vaccine is unacceptable.

Attempts have been made to develop tumor cell vaccines against FeLV. Killed FeLV tumor cell vaccines were effective in producing tumor immunity (FOCMA) and protecting the cats against tumor development. However, those vaccines did not prevent the initial FeLV infection or the subsequent FeLV carrier state.

Table 1. *Efficacy Testing of FeLV Soluble Tumor Vaccine (STAV)*

Adjuvant Used	Number of Cats Vaccinated	Per Cent Producing Antibody to FOCMA	Per Cent Protected From FeLV Disease
SPF Cats			
None	13	92	54
CFA	16	100	81
Household Cats			
None	45	100	73*

*These cats remained FeLV-disease free 52 weeks post vaccination.

A dual vaccine composed of killed FeLV tumor cell and killed FeLV was tested in hopes of preventing both the FeLV infectious state and ensuing cancer. Cats given dual vaccine were more susceptible to FeLV disease than controls. Moreover, the combining of FeLV with tumor vaccine interfered with the protective tumor immunity.

From these studies, it was found that a low molecular weight protein (FeLV p15E) from the FeLV (living or killed) was immunotoxic (Olsen et al., 1981). That is, FeLV p15E molecule was immunosuppressive for cat lymphocyte functions. The presence of FeLV p15E interfered with the cat's ability to immunologically respond to FeLV virus or tumor antigen (FOCMA); therefore, FeLV p15E abrogated the prophylactic properties of killed FeLV or killed tumor antigens.

Our goal has been to produce a subunit FeLV vaccine free of FeLV p15E immunotoxic properties that will bestow protective immunity on cats of all age groups.

PREPARATION OF A SOLUBLE TUMOR ANTIGEN VACCINE (STAV) FOR FELINE LEUKEMIA

The method for the preparation of soluble FeLV-induced cell surface antigen was described by Lewis and associates (1981). This technique relied upon the natural release of antigens from tumor cells during their maintenance at 37°C in serum-deficient medium.

EFFICACY TESTING OF STAV

Table 1 summarizes the results of vaccinating and challenging specific-pathogen free (SPF) cats with STAV (either alone or emulsified in complete Freund's adjuvant [CFA]). For each experiment, approximately the same number of vaccinated and nonvaccinated control cats were used. The control cats and the vaccinated cats were treated similarly (i.e., administered adjuvant or cell culture media) and were challenged with oncogenic FeLV. All control cats developed FeLV viremia after FeLV challenge. By contrast, 81 per cent of the cats that received STAV plus CFA and 54 per cent of cats that received STAV alone were completely resistant to FeLV disease.

Forty-five household cats that possessed little or no tumor immunity but yet were free of determinable FeLV infection were vaccinated with STAV (see Table 1). These cats developed FOCMA antibody. Seventy-three per cent of these animals remained free of FeLV disease 52 weeks post STAV vaccination. Ten SPF control cats were introduced into the colony, and after ten weeks nearly half of these showed evidence of being infected with FeLV, indicating that FeLV is still prevalent in the colony.

RECOMMENDATIONS AND SUMMARY

The subunit feline leukemia vaccine (STAV) reported in this article fulfills the criteria for an efficacious FeLV vaccine. First, when properly administered, it elicits protective antibody to both virus and FOCMA. Second, STAV does not have a deleterious effect on the immune system of young kittens. Third, and most important, STAV protects kittens and adult cats from becoming viremic and developing FeLV disease.

Work in progress with adjuvants other than CFA suggests that comparable protection can be achieved with STAV without the inflammatory effects induced by CFA.

Additional work in progress indicates that two vaccinations with STAV spaced two weeks apart followed by a booster one month later induced high FOCMA titers and affords solid protection.

The STAV for feline leukemia is used like any killed virus vaccine. The shelf life is quite long (many months to years), and the veterinarian can be assured that this vaccine confers few allergenic problems. The vaccine is prepared in the absence of fetal calf serum, the major allergin in most conventional vaccine preparations.

REFERENCES AND SUPPLEMENTAL READING

Hoover, E. A., Rojko, J. L., and Olsen, R. G.: Pathogenesis of feline leukemia virus infection. *In* Olsen, R. G., (ed.): *Feline Leukemia.* Boca Raton, FL: CRC Press, 1981, pp. 31–52.

Lewis, M. G., Mathes, L. E., and Olsen, R. G.: Protection against feline leukemia by vaccination with a subunit vaccine. Infect. Immun. 34:888, 1981.

Mathes, L. E., and Olsen, R. G.: Immunobiology of feline leukemia virus disease. *In* Olsen, R. G. (ed.): *Feline Leukemia.* Boca Raton, FL: CRC Press, 1981, pp. 77–88.

Olsen, R. G., and Lewis, M. G.: Immunoprophylaxis: Experimental vaccine, development, and testing. *In* Olsen, R. G. (ed.): *Feline Leukemia.* Boca Raton, FL: CRC Press, 1981, pp. 135–148.

Olsen, R. G., Mathes, L. E., and Nichols, W. S.: FeLV-related immunosuppression. *In* Olsen, R. G. (ed.): *Feline Leukemia.* Boca Raton, FL: CRC Press, 1981, pp. 149–165.

Rice, J. B., and Olsen, R. G.: FeLV/FeSV-associated transformation specific protein(s). *In* Olsen, R. G. (ed.): *Feline Leukemia.* Boca Raton, FL: CRC Press, 1981, pp. 553–568.

Schaller, J. S., and Olsen, R. G.: Virology of feline leukemia. *In* Olsen, R. G. (ed.): *Feline Leukemia.* Boca Raton, FL: CRC Press, 1981, pp. 1–30.

CURRENT CANINE AND FELINE IMMUNIZATION GUIDELINES*

FREDRIC W. SCOTT, D.V.M.,
Ithaca, New York

WILLIAM GRANT, D.V.M.,
Garden Grove, California

and JAMES BITTLE, D.V.M.
La Jolla, California

There have been a number of significant advances made in the field of canine and feline immunization since the last guidelines were issued by the AVMA in 1973. The most current information available on the most common diseases affecting the dog and cat has been assembled and summarized along with recommendations for immunization to control these diseases. It is recommended that only products licensed by the United States Department of Agriculture be used in immunization procedures.

DEFINITIONS RELATING TO VACCINES AND IMMUNIZATION

Adjuvant. A substance that, when mixed with antigen, enhances the immune response.

Cell Culture. Growth or maintenance of cells *in vitro* so that the cells are no longer organized into tissues.

Cell Line. A group of cells arising from a primary culture at the time of the first subculture.

Diploid Cell Line. A cell line in which, arbitrarily, at least 75 per cent of the cells have the same karyotype as the normal cells of the species from which the cells were originally obtained.

Established Cell Line. A cell line that can be subcultured indefinitely *in vitro.* The ability to grow indefinitely usually is acquired only after numerous (e.g., 70) subcultures *in vitro.*

Heterotypic Vaccine. A vaccine developed to immunize against an antigenically distinct but immunologically related virus (e.g., measles-canine distemper, feline panleukopenia–canine parvovirus).

Homotypic Vaccine. A vaccine developed to immunize against the same antigenic strain of virus.

Inactivated Vaccine. A vaccine containing an agent that has been treated so that it no longer is infectious or capable of replication in the host.

Interference. A phenomenon that may occur when susceptible cells are exposed to two or more viruses at the same time, or within a short interval, whereby one virus blocks or excludes the replication of the second virus.

Maternal Antibody (Maternally Derived Antibody). Passive antibody in neonatal animals acquired from their mother by transuterine passage of antibody or intestinal absorption of antibody from colostrum.

Modified Live Virus (MLV). (1) Synonymous with attenuated virus. (2) A virus that is reduced in natural virulence to the point at which it multiplies in the host but does not produce serious disease.

Monolayer. A single layer of cells growing on a surface.

Monovalent Vaccine. Vaccine containing only one virus.

*These guidelines are based on the report prepared by the authors for the A.V.M.A. Council on Biologic and Therapeutic Agents and published in J.A.V.M.A. 181:332–335, 1982.

The 1983 Compendium of Animal Rabies Vaccines, prepared by the National Association of State Public Health Veterinarians Inc., is appended to this article as a separate section.

Multivalent (Polyvalent) Vaccine. Vaccine containing a mixture of viruses (e.g., canine distemper, canine adenovirus II, canine parainfluenza, canine parvovirus) or viral types (e.g., canine adenovirus I and II).

Passage. (1) Synonymous with subculture. (2) The transfer of supernatant culture fluid for virus isolation, propagation, or attenuation.

Primary Culture. A culture started from cells, tissues, or organs taken directly from an animal.

Secondary Culture. A subculture of cells passaged or transferred from a primary culture. The second passage or transfer results in a tertiary culture.

Subculture. The transplantation of cells from one culture vessel to another.

Suspension Culture. A type of culture in which cells multiply while suspended in medium.

Tissue Culture or Organ Culture. (1) Maintenance or growth of tissues, organ primordia, or the whole or parts of an organ *in vitro* in a way that may allow differentiation and preservation of the architecture and/or function. (2) The term "tissue culture" is often used synonymously with "cell culture."

Titer. A measure of the quantity of virus (or antibody) present. Usually determined by serial dilution of the test sample until the particular activity of the virus (or antibody) being assayed is lost.

GENERAL IMMUNOLOGIC CONSIDERATIONS

An animal reacts to an invading organism by mounting an immunologic response to it. If the animal has been previously exposed to the organism, either naturally or by immunization (immunogen), it will usually be protected. The degree of protection depends on a number of factors, but humoral antibody is one of the most important defense mechanisms. This antibody may be of several types including IgM (rapid-responding antibody), IgA (local antibody), or IgG (long-acting antibody), all offering various means of protection. The antibody will usually combine with the infectious agent to render it noninfectious. The degree of protection is often dependent on the level of specific antibody present. Therefore, it is important to maintain a high level of antibody. This may be accomplished by occasional exposure of the animal to the antigen. Thus, following an initial immunization regimen, booster vaccinations are very important.

Animals are exposed to a number of infectious agents throughout their life, but they are most susceptible in early life (first six months). Thus, providing early protection through maternal antibody by immunization of the dam prior to breeding and vaccination of offspring at the proper time (when the maternal antibody has been depleted) is essential to a good immunization program. It is difficult to predict exactly when the maternal antibody will be depleted, so the initial immunization regimen is divided into a number of doses beginning as early as possible. It is also difficult to predict the kind of infectious agents to which an animal will be exposed. For this reason, *multivalent vaccines* containing immunogens for most of the common infectious diseases have been developed. These vaccines have been proved to be effective and safe; therefore, *their widescale use is recommended*.

In rare instances, the immune system of an animal may fail to respond following immunization to the immunogen. Conversely, the *occasional reaction* seen following the injection of an immunogen is due to an over-response of the immune system. Both of these defects in the immune system are usually genetically controlled.

Vaccines have been developed to control the major infectious diseases affecting the dog and cat, and rigorous licensing requirements regulate their manufacture.

The benefits, in most instances, of any vaccine far outweigh the risks. General contraindications for most vaccines include animals that are (1) obviously ill, (2) pregnant, or (3) undergoing a course of immunosuppressant therapy.

CANINE DISEASES AND RECOMMENDATIONS FOR IMMUNOPROPHYLAXIS (Table 1)

CANINE DISTEMPER

Canine distemper is a widespread disease caused by a paramyxovirus. The virus is highly contagious, causing a generalized infection and microscopic lesions but few distinct macroscopic lesions. The symptoms are mainly respiratory, but intestinal and neurologic signs are common.

MLV vaccines are highly effective in controlling the disease. Maternal antibody may interfere with immunization. This, of course, depends on the amount of antibody transmitted to puppies from the dam; since this is usually not known, multiple vaccinations at prescribed intervals are recommended.

INFECTIOUS CANINE HEPATITIS (ICH)

ICH is caused by the canine adenovirus type 1 and should be distinguished from canine adenovirus type 2, which causes a respiratory tract infection. The virus spreads from dog to dog mainly by infected urine. ICH virus infects many tissues but it primarily attacks the parenchymal cells of the liver, often causing a severe hepatitis. A corneal opacity is often an aftermath of infection, and this is due to an acute anterior uveitis with corneal edema. On rare occasions, vaccines may also cause this corneal opacity.

Both inactivated and MLV vaccines are available, but the MLV vaccines appear to induce a longer duration of immunity.

CANINE PARVOVIRUS INFECTION (CPV)

Canine parvovirus (CPV) infection is apparently a new disease caused by a parvovirus related to feline panleukopenia virus (FPV). The virus causes an enteritis in dogs of all ages and a myocarditis in young puppies. Animals that recover from natural infection are immune for at least two years.

Inactivated and MLV vaccines containing the feline panleukopenia virus are available as well as inactivated and MLV vaccines prepared from the canine parvovirus. Inactivated FPV and CPV vaccine viruses do not replicate in the dog, and therefore their efficacy is related to the quantity of antigen in the vaccines. Canine MLV parvovirus vaccines are also available, and the vaccine virus replicates and may spread from dog to dog. The MLV FPV vaccine viruses replicate in lymphoid tissues of the dog but do not spread to other dogs. The duration of immunity is longer with the canine MLV vaccine.

Coronaviruses and rotaviruses have also been implicated in canine viral enteritis. The need for vaccines for these infections has not been determined.

CANINE ADENOVIRUS TYPE 2 INFECTION (CAV-2)

CAV-2 is a respiratory tract disease caused by a virus closely related to CAV-1. The virus produces tracheobronchitis, the severity depending on conditions under which dogs are kept. The disease is much more severe when animals are kept in close quarters (poor ventilation).

A modified strain of CAV-2 immunizes dogs against this disease. Modified CAV-1 vaccines will also cross protect.

CANINE BORDETELLOSIS

Bordetella bronchiseptica is a common bacterial inhabitant of the respiratory tract of many animals.

It has been incriminated in the dog as a serious respiratory pathogen and one of the primary causes of tracheobronchitis (kennel cough). The bacteria colonize in the upper respiratory tract, often producing severe chronic cough.

Inactivated bacterins are effective when given parenterally, and live modified organisms may be given intranasally to control the disease.

CANINE PARAINFLUENZA

The canine parainfluenza virus causes a mild respiratory tract infection in dogs but has been associated with other respiratory agents, such as CAV-2 and *Bordetella bronchiseptica*, causing a more severe respiratory disease.

A MLV vaccine protects against this virus, and the antigen has been combined with other immunogens to give a broader range of protection.

CANINE LEPTOSPIROSIS

Canine leptospirosis is an acute infection in dogs caused by *L. canicola* and/or *L. icterohemorrhagica*. These spirochetes enter the body primarily through the mucous membranes and cause a leptospiremia, affecting a number of organs with ensuing symptoms. The organism may impair renal function, causing kidney failure with a resulting uremia. The usual source of infection is from the urine of infected dogs or rats.

Inactivated bacterins containing immunogens to both *L. canicola* and *L. icterohemorrhagica* are available and immunize for periods of up to one year. Booster vaccinations are required annually.

CANINE RABIES

Rabies is an acute encephalomyelitis caused by a rhabdovirus. All warm-blooded animals are affected, and the virus is mainly transmitted by a bite introducing saliva-borne virus. Strains of the virus have become established in wild animal populations, affecting mainly shunks, foxes, raccoons, and bats.

Mass vaccination of dogs has been effective in preventing the spread of the disease from wild animals to dogs and cats and also to humans.

Both inactivated and MLV vaccines are available, and immunity varies. Protection from some vaccines may last as long as three years. One inoculation is required via the intramuscular route. The initial vaccination is given at three to four months of age.

Text continued on page 1141

COMPENDIUM OF ANIMAL RABIES VACCINES, 1983*

PART I: RECOMMENDATIONS FOR IMMUNIZATION PROCEDURES

The purpose of these recommendations is to provide information on rabies vaccines to practicing veterinarians, public health officials, and others concerned with rabies control. This document will serve as the basis for animal rabies vaccination programs throughout the United States. Its adoption by cooperating organizations will result in standardization of procedures among jurisdictions, which is necessary for an effective national rabies control program. These recommendations are reviewed and revised as necessary prior to the beginning of each calendar year. All animal rabies vaccines licensed by the USDA and marketed in the United States are listed in the table, and Part II describes the principles of rabies control.

Vaccine administration.   It is recommended that all animal rabies vaccines be restricted to use by or under the supervision of a veterinarian.

Vaccine selection.   While recognizing the efficacy of vaccines with the one-year duration of immunity, the Committee recommends the use of vaccines with three-year duration of immunity, because their use constitutes the most effective method of increasing the proportion of immunized dogs and cats in comprehensive rabies control programs.

Route of inoculation.   All rabies vaccines must be administered intramuscularly at one site in the thigh.

High-risk rabies area.   An area (town, city, or county) where a high incidence of rabies exists in wildlife or domestic species as determined by state health officials may be declared a high-risk rabies area. In such areas the public should be alerted to the risk and urged to make sure that their dogs and cats have current rabies vaccinations. State health officials may wish to consider temporarily altering revaccination schedules.

Wildlife vaccination.   It is recommended that neither wild nor exotic animals be kept as pets. Since no rabies vaccine is licensed for use in wild animals and since there is no evidence that animal rabies vaccines produce acceptable levels of immunity in wild animals, vaccination is not recommended.

Accidental human exposure to vaccine.   Accidental inoculation may occur in individuals during administration of animal rabies vaccine. Such exposures to inactivated vaccines constitute *no known* rabies hazard. There have been no cases of rabies resulting from needle or other exposure to a licensed modified live virus vaccine in the United States.

Identification of vaccinated dogs.   It is recommended that all government agencies and veterinarians adopt the standard tag system. This will aid the administration of local, state, national, and international procedures. Dog license tags should not conflict in shape and color with rabies tags.

RABIES TAGS

Calendar Year	Color	Shape
1983	Green	Bell
1984	Red	Heart
1985	Blue	Rosette
1986	Orange	Fireplug

RABIES CERTIFICATE.   Government agencies and veterinarians should use the NASPHV form #50, Rabies Vaccination Certificate, which can be obtained from vaccine manufacturers.

*Prepared by the National Association of State Public Health Veterinarians, Inc. Reprinted with permission from J.A.V.M.A. 182:16, 1983.

Vaccine: Generic Name	Produced by	Marketed by (Product Name)	For Use In*	Dosage†	Age at Primary Vaccination‡	Booster Recommended
Modified live virus						
Canine cell line origin	Norden License No. 189	Norden (Endurall-R)	Dogs	1 ml	3 mo and 1 yr later	Triennially
High egg passage			Cats	1 ml	3 months	Annually
			Dogs	1 ml	3 mo and 1 yr later	Triennially
Porcine cell line origin High cell passage	Wellcome (Jensen-Salsbery) License No. 107	Wellcome (Jensen-Salsbery) (ERA Strain Rabies Vaccine)	Cattle	1 ml	4 months	Annually
			Horses	1 ml	4 months	Annually
			Sheep	1 ml	4 months	Annually
			Goats	1 ml	4 months	Annually
Canine tissue culture origin High cell passage	Philips Roxane License No. 124	Bio-Ceutic (Neurogen-T-C)	Dogs	1 ml	3 mo and 1 yr later	Triennially
Canine tissue culture origin High cell passage	Philips Roxane License No. 124	Bio-Ceutic (Unirab)	Dogs	1 ml	3 months	Annually
Inactivated vaccines						
Murine origin	Rolynn License No. 165-B (Prev. No. 266)	Ft. Dodge (Trimune)	Dogs	1 ml	3 mo and 1 yr later	Triennially
			Cats	1 ml	3 months	Annually
Murine origin	Rolynn License No. 165-B (Prev. No. 266)	Ft. Dodge (Annumune)	Dogs	1 ml	3 months	Annually
			Cats	1 ml	3 months	Annually
Murine origin	Douglas License No. 165-B (Prev. No. 266)	Not specified (Biorab-1)	Dogs	1 ml	3 months	Annually
			Cats	1 ml	3 months	Annually
Murine origin	Douglas License No. 165-B (Prev. No. 266)	Not specified (Biorab-3)	Dogs	1 ml	3 mo and 1 yr later	Triennially
			Cats	1 ml	3 months	Annually
Murine origin	Wildlife Vaccines, Inc. License No. 277	Wildlife Vaccines (Dura-Rab 1)	Dogs	1 ml	3 months	Annually
			Cats	1 ml	3 months	Annualy
Hamster cell line origin	Beecham License No. 225	Beecham (Rabcine)	Dogs	1 ml	3 months	Annually
			Cats	1 ml	3 months	Annually
Hamster cell line origin	Beecham License No. 225	Beecham (Rabcine-Feline)	Cats	1 ml	3 months	Annually
Hamster cell line origin	Vaccines, Inc. License No. 227	Guardian (Rabies Vacc)	Dogs	1 ml	3 months	Annually
Hamster cell line origin	Jackson License No. 288	Schering (Rabmune)	Dogs	1 ml	3 months	Annually
			Cats	1 ml	3 months	Annually
Porcine cell line origin	Norden License No. 189	Norden (Endurall-K)	Dogs	1 ml	3 months	Annually
			Cats	1 ml	3 months	Annually
Porcine cell line origin	Norden License No. 189	Norden (Rabguard-TC)	Dogs	1 ml	3 mos and 1 yr later	Triennially
			Cats	1 ml	3 mos and 1 yr later	Triennially
Monkey cell line origin	Wellcome License No. 107	Wellcome (Cytorab)	Dogs	1 ml	3 months	Annually
			Cats	1 ml	3 months	Annually
Monkey cell line origin	Wellcome License No. 107	Wellcome (Trirab)	Dogs	1 ml	3 mos and 1 yr later	Triennially
			Cats	1 ml	3 months	Annually
Feline cell line origin	Fromm License No. 195-A	Fromm (Rabvac)	Dogs	1 ml	3 months	Annually
			Cats	1 ml	3 months	Annually
Combination						
Murine origin	Douglas License No. 165-B (Prev. No. 266)	Douglas (Pan-Rab)	Cats	1 ml	3 months	Annually
Feline cell line origin	Fromm License No. 195-A	Fromm (Eclipse III KP-R)	Cats	1 ml	3 months	Annually
Feline cell line origin	Fromm License No. 195-A	Fromm (Eclipse IVKP-R)	Cats	1 ml	3 months	Annually

*Refers only to domestic species of this class of animals.

†All vaccine must be administered intramuscularly at one site in the thigh.

‡Three months is the earliest age recommended. Dogs vaccinated between 3 and 12 months of age should be revaccinated one year later.

PART II: PRINCIPLES OF RABIES CONTROL, 1983

These guidelines were prepared by the National Association of State Public Health Veterinarians (NASPHV*) for use by government officials, practicing veterinarians, and others who may become involved in certain aspects of rabies control. It is intended that the NASPHV will annually review and revise these recommendations as necessary. Standardized control procedures are needed to effectively deal with the public health aspects of rabies.

Principles of Rabies Control

THE DISEASE IN HUMANS. Rabies in humans can be prevented by eliminating exposure to rabid animals and by prompt local wound treatment and immunization when exposed. Current recommendations of the Public Health Service Advisory Committee on Immunization Practices are suggested for consideration by attending physicians. The recommendations, along with the current status of animal rabies in the region and information concerning the availability of rabies biologics, are available from state health departments.

DOMESTIC ANIMALS. Local governments should initiate and maintain effective programs to remove strays and unwanted animals and vaccinate all dogs and cats. Since cat rabies cases now equal the annual incidence in dogs, immunization of cats should be emphasized. Such procedures in the U.S. have reduced laboratory-confirmed rabies cases in dogs from 8000 in 1947 to 216 in 1981. The recommended vaccination procedures and the licensed animal vaccines are specified in Part I and in the table of the Compendium.

RABIES IN WILDLIFE. The control of rabies in foxes, skunks, raccoons, and other terrestrial animals is very difficult. Selective reduction of these populations when indicated may be useful, but the utility of this procedure depends heavily on the circumstances surrounding each rabies outbreak.

Control Methods in Domestic and Confined Animals

PRE-EXPOSURE VACCINATION

Animal rabies vaccines, because of species limitations, techniques, and tolerances, should be administered only under the direct supervision of a veterinarian. Within one month after vaccination, a peak rabies antibody titer is reached and the animal can be considered to be immunized. See Part I and the table of the Compendium for recommended vaccines and procedures.

1. *Dogs and cats:* All dogs and cats should be vaccinated against rabies commencing at three months of age and revaccinated in accordance with the table of the Compendium.
2. *Livestock:* It is not economically feasible, nor is it justified from a public health standpoint, to vaccinate all livestock against rabies. Owners of valuable animals and veterinary clinicians may consider immunizing certain breeding stock located in areas where wildlife rabies is epizootic.
3. *Other animals:*
   a. Animals maintained in exhibits and zoologic parks: Captive animals not completely excluded from all contact with local vectors of rabies can become infected with rabies. Moreover, such animals may be incubating rabies when captured. Exhibit animals, especially those carnivores and omnivores having contact with the viewing public, should be quarantined for a minimum of 180 days. Since there is no rabies vaccine licensed for use in wild animals, vaccination even with inactivated vaccine is not recommended. Pre-exposure rabies immunization of animal workers at such facilities is recommended and reduces the need for euthanasia of valuable animals for rabies testing after they have bitten a handler.
   b. Wild animals: Because of the existing risk of rabies in wild animals such as raccoons, skunks, and foxes, the AVMA, the NASPHV, and the Conference of State and Territorial Epidemiologists strongly recommend the enactment of state laws prohibiting the interstate and intrastate importation, distribution, and relocation of wild animals. Further, these same organizations continue to recommend the enactment of laws prohibiting the distribution and/or ownership of wild animals as pets.

STRAY ANIMAL CONTROL

Stray animals should be removed from the community, especially in rabies epizootic areas. Local health department and dog control officials can enforce the pick-up of strays more efficiently if owned animals are confined or kept on leash when not confined. Strays should be impounded for at least three days to give owners sufficient time to reclaim animals apprehended as strays.

---

*THE NASPHV COMPENDIUM COMMITTEE FOR 1983: Kenneth L. Crawford, DVM, MPH, Chairman; Melvin K. Abelseth, DVM, DVPH, PhD.; John I. Freeman, DVM, MPH; Robert F. Goldsboro, DVM, MPH; Grayson B. Miller, Jr., MD; James M. Shuler, DVM, MPH; R. Keith Sikes, DVM, MPH; CONSULTANTS TO THE COMMITTEE: Bernard LaSalle, DVM, Veterinary Biologics Staff, APHIS, USDA; William G. Winkler, DVM, MS: CDC, PHS, HHS; Dale E. Bordt, PhD, Vet. Biologics Section, Animal Health Inst.; Lowell W. Hinchman, DVM: AVMA, Council on Public Health and Regulatory Veterinary Medicine; ENDORSED BY: Conference of State and Territorial Epidemiologists; AVMA, Council of Public Health and Regulatory Veterinary Medicine; REPRODUCED BY: Maryland State Dept. of Health and Mental Hygiene.

QUARANTINE

1. *International:* Present regulations (CFR No. 71154) governing the importation of wild and domesticated felines, canines, and other potential vectors of rabies are minimal for preventing the introduction of rabid animals into the United States. All dogs and cats imported from countries with endemic rabies should be vaccinated against rabies at least 30 days prior to entry into the United States. The Centers for Disease Control (CDC) are responsible for these animals imported into the United States. Their requirements should be coordinated with interstate shipment requirements. The health authority of the state of destination should be notified within 72 hours of any animal conditionally admitted into its jurisdiction.

    The conditional admission into the United States of such animals must be subject to state and local laws governing rabies. Failure to comply with these requirements should be promptly reported to the director of the CDC.

2. *Interstate:* Prior to interstate shipment, dogs and cats should be vaccinated against rabies according to the Compendium's recommendations and preferably shall be vaccinated at least 30 days prior to shipment. While in shipment, they should be accompanied by a currently valid NASPHV Form #50 *Rabies Vaccination Certificate.* One copy of the certificate should be mailed to the appropriate Public Health Veterinarian or State Veterinarian of the state of destination.

3. *Health Certificates:* If a certificate is required for dogs and cats in transit, it must not replace the NASPHV rabies vaccination certificate.

ADJUNCT PROCEDURES

Methods or procedures that enhance rabies control include the following:

1. *Licensure:* Registration or licensure of all dogs and cats may be used as a means of rabies control by controlling the stray animal population. Frequently a fee is charged for such licensure and revenues collected are used to maintain a rabies or animal control program. Vaccination is usually recommended as a prerequisite to licensure.

2. *Canvassing of area:* This includes house-to-house calls by members of the animal control program to enforce vaccination and licensure requirements.

3. *Citations:* These are legal summonses issued to owners for violations including failure to vaccinate or license their animals.

4. *Leash Laws:* All communities should adopt leash laws, which can be incorporated in their animal control ordinances.

POST-EXPOSURE MANAGEMENT

ANY DOMESTIC ANIMAL THAT IS BITTEN OR SCRATCHED BY A BAT OR A WILD CARNIVOROUS MAMMAL THAT IS NOT AVAILABLE FOR TESTING SHOULD BE REGARDED AS HAVING BEEN EXPOSED TO A RABID ANIMAL.

1. When bitten by a rabid animal, unvaccinated dogs and cats should be destroyed immediately. If the owner is unwilling to have this done, the unvaccinated animal should be placed in strict isolation for six months and vaccinated one month before being released. Dogs and cats that are currently vaccinated should be revaccinated immediately and leashed and confined at home for 90 days.

2. *Livestock:* All species of livestock are susceptible to rabies infection; cattle appear to be among the most susceptible of all domestic animal species. Livestock known to have been bitten by rabid animals should be destroyed (slaughtered) immediately. If the owner is unwilling to have this done, the animal should be kept under very close observation for six months.

    With regard to management of livestock exposed to rabid animals, the following recommendations and considerations are suggested:

    a. If slaughtered within seven days of being bitten, tissues may be eaten without risk of infection providing liberal portions of the exposed area are discarded. Federal meat inspectors will reject any animal that has been exposed to rabies within eight months.

    b. No tissues or secretions from a clinically rabid animal should be used for human or animal consumption; however, pasteurization temperatures will inactivate rabies virus. Therefore, drinking pasteurized milk or eating meat from a rabid animal that has been completely cooked does not constitute a rabies exposure.

Control Methods in Wild Animals

TERRESTRIAL MAMMALS. Since there is no evidence that control programs reduce either wildlife reservoirs or rabies incidence on a statewide basis, persistent, continuous, and routine trapping or poisoning campaigns as a means of wildlife rabies control should be abolished. However, limited control in high contact areas (picnic grounds, camps, suburban areas) may be indicated for the removal of selected high-risk species of wild animals. The public should be warned not to handle wild animals. The state game department should be consulted early to manage any elimination programs when requested to do so by the state health department.

BATS. Rabid bats have been reported from every state except Hawaii and have caused human rabies infections in the United States. It is neither feasible nor practical, however, to control rabies in bats by areawide bat population reduction programs.

Bats should be eliminated from houses and surrounding structures to prevent direct association with people. Such structures should then be made bat-proof by sealing routes of entrance with screen or other means.

A person bitten by a bat or any wild animal should immediately report the incident to a physician or hospital emergency persons, who will evaluate the need for antirabies treatment according to the Rabies Prophylaxis Recommendation of the Public Health Service Advisory Committee on Immunization Practices. Bats and other wild carnivorous mammals that bite people should be killed and sent to the laboratory for examination for rabies.

CANINE BRUCELLOSIS

This disease is caused by *Brucella canis,* a newly recognized member of the Brucella family. The organism causes abortion from the middle of gestation on and is directly transmitted from infected dogs or infected tissues or discharges. Infected dogs are often persistently infected and, therefore, are long-term carriers.

Infected male dogs show mild signs, i.e., enlarged epididymides and testicles. A slide or tube agglutination test may be used to identify infected dogs.

No adequate means of immunization or treatment are available for this disease. Therefore, control is based on identification and quarantine of infected animals.

CANINE HERPESVIRUS INFECTION

Canine herpesvirus causes a fatal disease in young dogs less than one month of age. Milder respiratory symptoms are seen in older dogs through weaning age. The disease may cause heavy losses in puppies raised in kennels. Although persistent infection in dams may occur, dams that have lost puppies usually do not lose their offspring on subsequent whelping because of maternal antibody protection during the critical neonatal period.

No vaccine is available for this disease, and at the present time the need does not appear great enough to warrant its development.

FELINE DISEASES AND RECOMMENDATIONS FOR IMMUNOPROPHYLAXIS (See page 1128)

FELINE PANLEUKOPENIA (FP)

Feline panleukopenia is a highly contagious and devastating viral disease of cats caused by the feline parvovirus (FPV). Producing cytologic effects on actively mitotic cells, FPV produces severe leukopenia, enteritis, dehydration, and a high mortality. Recovery from natural infection results in lifelong immunity.

Inactivated and MLV vaccines of cell culture origin are available for parenteral vaccination, and certain MLV strains may be administered by the intranasal route. If administered after maternally derived immunity has waned, these vaccines result in rapid and sustained protection for at least one year and probably longer.

FELINE VIRAL RHINOTRACHEITIS (FVR)

Feline viral rhinotracheitis is a common, highly contagious upper respiratory disease of cats caused by feline herpesvirus I.

Recovery from natural infection results in immunity against systemic disease but not necessarily against local infection. A latent infection with intermittent periods of viral shedding frequently occurs.

Table 1. *Canine Vaccine Recommendations*

Disease	Type of Vaccine	Route of Administration	Age at First Vaccination (Weeks)	Age at Second Vaccination (Weeks)	Age at Third Vaccination (Weeks)	Revaccination
Distemper	MLV	SC or IM	6 to 8	10 to 12	14 to 16	Annual
Infectious	MLV	SC or IM	6 to 8	10 to 12	14 to 16	Annual
canine hepatitis CAV-1 or CAV-2	Inactivated	SC or IM	6 to 8	10 to 12	14 to 16	Annual
Parvovirus	MLV	SC or IM	6 to 8	10 to 12	14 to 16	Annual
infection	Inactivated	SC or IM	6 to 8	10 to 12	14 to 16	Annual
Bordetellosis	Inactivated	SC or IM	6 to 8	10 to 12	14 to 16	Annual
	Live attenuated	IN	>2	—	—	Biannual
Parainfluenza	MLV	SC, IM or IN	6 to 8	10 to 12	14 to 16	Annual
Leptospirosis	Inactivated	SC or IM	10 to 12	14 to 16	—	Annual
Rabies*	MLV	IM	12 to 16	—	—	Annual/triennial
	Inactivated	IM	12 to 16	—	—	Annual/triennial

*To comply with state laws.

Inactivated and MLV parenteral vaccines as well as intranasal MLV vaccines of cell culture origin are available for vaccination. Parenteral vaccines given in two doses at least three weeks apart or in a single dose of intranasal MLV produce significant protection for at least one year. The cat should be revaccinated annually. A rapid anamnestic immune response occurs in vaccinated cats after exposure to virulent FVR virus. Intranasal vaccination may result in mild sneezing and oculonasal discharge four to seven days after vaccination.

FELINE CALICIVIRUS (FCV)

Feline calicivirus infection is an acute respiratory and/or ulcerative disease of cats caused by one of several strains of FCV. Recovery results in good immunity against all strains, but a persistent infection occurs with continuous shedding of a small amount of virus from the oral pharynx.

Inactivated and MLV cell culture origin vaccines in combination with FVR are available for parenteral vaccination, and combination MLV intranasal vaccines are also available. The same parameters as described previously for FVR vaccines apply to FCV vaccines.

FELINE PNEUMONITIS (FPn)

Feline pneumonitis is an acute to chronic respiratory infection of cats caused by a strain of *Chlamydia psittaci.*

Live attenuated vaccines of embryonated egg or cell culture origin are available for parenteral vaccination, either as individual vaccines or in combination with other feline vaccines. A single vaccination appears to afford adequate protection for at least one year.

RABIES

Feline rabies, an acute encephalomyelitis caused by a rhabdovirus, results primarily from exposure of cats to virus-infected wildlife such as skunks, raccoons, foxes, and bats. There is a high geographic correlation between shunk rabies and feline rabies. Since there are approximately 200 feline rabies cases per year in the United States and since these cases pose significant risks to humans, cats should be routinely vaccinated for rabies annually, especially in areas of endemic wildlife rabies.

Inactivated vaccines of mouse brain and cell culture origin are available. A high egg passage cell culture adapted MLV strain is also approved for use in cats. Other MLV strains not approved for use in the cat should not be given, since vaccine-induced rabies may result.

FELINE LEUKEMIA VIRUS (FeLV)

Feline leukemia virus infection is a contagious oncornaviral disease that may result in a non-neoplastic FeLV-related disease (i.e., anemia, immunosuppression, panleukopenia-like disease) as well as neoplastic disease (i.e., lymphosarcoma, fibrosarcoma, leukemia). Although some cats develop an effective immune response, infection of other cats results in a persistent viremia with viral shed and/or the development of neoplastic disease.

There is a great need for an efficacious and safe vaccine for this disease. Accurate tests are available to detect infected animals, and those cats found to be infected should be quarantined.

FELINE INFECTIOUS PERITONITIS (FIP)

Feline infectious peritonitis is a prevalent, usually fatal disease of cats caused by a coronavirus. Subclinical infections with FIP virus or a closely related enteric coronavirus stimulate antibody but do not provide protection against clinical FIP. Rather, coronaviral antibody appears to enhance clinical disease if re-exposure to virulent FIP virus occurs. Although there is a great need for a vaccine against FIP, traditional approaches to vaccine development for FIP do not appear promising.

Diagnostic Procedures

PRACTICAL DIAGNOSTIC PROCEDURES FOR VIRAL DISEASES

RICHARD C. WEISS, V.M.D.

Mountain View, California

Laboratory methods for the diagnosis of specific viral diseases are becoming increasingly useful to the small animal practitioner for several reasons. When the clinical signs of disease are nonspecific, laboratory procedures are invaluable in establishing an etiologic diagnosis, prognosis, and rational approach to clinical management as well as in influencing control measures (i.e., in catteries and kennels). For example, the identification of feline leukemia virus (FeLV) in the blood of a cat with severe anemia living in a breeding cattery would indicate a different prognosis, therapeutic approach, and isolation procedure than those for an FeLV-negative cat with anemia and a chronic nonspecific infection. Similarly, rapid identification by electron microscopy of parvovirus in the feces of a depressed puppy with severe enteritis would necessitate a different therapy and prognosis than those for a puppy with intestinal parasitism and diarrhea. Although of limited use at present, chemotherapy with specific antiviral drugs (e.g., iododeoxyuridine and adenine arabinoside in cases of herpetic keratitis) may be beneficial once a viral diagnosis is established.

The identification of specific viral pathogens (e.g., feline panleukopenia virus, canine distemper virus) in disease outbreaks in catteries or kennels is essential for proper control measures, including vaccination schedules, isolation procedures, and choice of effective disinfectants. Naked (nonenveloped) viruses, such as canine parvovirus or feline panleukopenia virus, are more resistant to disinfectants in general than are enveloped viruses such as canine distemper virus or feline rhinotracheitis virus (feline herpesvirus 1); a timely change to a more effective virucide may be required to adequately control viral disease outbreaks in the cattery or kennel. Lastly, diagnostic virology is essential for control of important zoonotic diseases and public health hazards, particularly rabies. Considering that a rabid dog or cat may expose and infect numerous individuals, rapid diagnosis of rabies virus infection is crucial for proper immunoprophylaxis of exposed persons and animals.

As the number of laboratories providing services for diagnostic virology increases, there will be correspondingly more opportunity for veterinarians to diagnose and control specific viral diseases in the feline and canine population. The purpose of this article is to provide the small animal practitioner with a brief outline of the various laboratory techniques used to diagnose viral infection; to recommend practical procedures for the selection, collection, and submission of specimens; and to summarize the available diagnostic tests and preferred clinical materials used in diagnosis of specific virus diseases of dogs and cats.

VIRAL DIAGNOSTIC TECHNIQUES

There are many similarities between the laboratory diagnosis of viral and bacterial diseases: the suspected agent is cultured in a growth medium or cells and identified by morphologic, biochemical, or immunologic criteria; and specific serologic host responses against the pathogen are demonstrated. Compared with diagnostic bacteriology, however, diagnostic virology is expensive and requires substantially more time to process fewer samples.

In addition to clinical signs and clinicopathologic changes, diagnosis of viral infection may be confirmed in the laboratory on the basis of one or more of five methods: (1) viral isolation (tissue culture, embryonated eggs, animal inoculation); (2) electron microscopy (tissues, fluids, feces, infected cell cultures); (3) histopathology (tissue, cell imprints); (4) identification of viral antigens or virus-induced antigens by serologic methods (immunofluorescence, virus neutralization, gel diffusion, complement fixation, hemagglutination, enzyme-linked immunosorbent assay [ELISA]); (5) demonstration of specific antiviral antibody responses (serum neutralization, indirect fluorescent antibody test, hemagglutination inhibition, plaque reduction test, complement fixation, ELISA).

The particular method employed in the diagnosis of viral disease depends on several factors, including the suspected virus, type and condition of the specimen, and the technical capabilities of available diagnostic laboratories. Each method has inherent advantages and disadvantages (Table 1). For example, virus isolation is a sensitive technique that is available at most laboratories; however, identification of the agent may be difficult and time-consuming, nonviable virus cannot be detected, noncytopathogenic viruses may be overlooked, and nonpathogenic viruses unrelated to the disease may be inadvertently isolated from clinical material. In contrast, electron microscopic (EM) examination of clinical specimens is rapid and detects nonviable or noncultivable viruses. However, EM is costly, not available in many areas, and not as sensitive as virus isolation (i.e., numerous virus particles, approximately several hundred thousand to one million per milliliter of sample, must be present to be visualized by EM).

In clinical practice, the decision to utilize a particular method depends on the urgency for diagnosis, cost to the client, and availability and condition of clinical specimens. To optimize the chances for successful viral diagnosis, it is beneficial to use several techniques: submission of frozen, unfixed material for virus isolation and/or serologic identification of viral antigens (e.g., fluorescent antibody test); formalin-fixed tissues for histopathology; serum for antibody tests; and, in cases of enteric

disease (e.g., suspected canine coronavirus or parvovirus infection), feces for negative-staining electron microscopy.

SELECTION OF SAMPLES

When selecting clinical specimens for diagnosis of suspected viral disease, several general points concerning viral pathogenesis should be considered:

1. Virus titers are usually highest during the acute stage of disease and at affected tissue sites. Specimens for viral isolation should, therefore, be obtained from affected tissues early in the course of disease, e.g., feces or rectal swabs in acute enteritis; ocular, oral, or nasopharyngeal swabs in acute upper respiratory infections.

2. Peak virus titers may develop before the onset of clinical signs and may coincide with the initial febrile episode in viremic diseases. In cases of multiple exposure it is often useful to sample asymptomatic contacts, superficially affected animals, and clinically ill animals early in the course of disease.

3. Primary viral infections may often be accompanied by secondary bacterial infections. Samples taken postmortem or during chronic stages of disease may not contain viable virus necessary for successful virus isolation.

4. In demonstrating serologic evidence of virus infection, it is imperative that paired (i.e., acute and convalescent) serum samples be taken at least 10 to 14 days apart, if possible, since only a significant (fourfold or greater) rise in antibody titer is meaningful. Occasionally, the demonstration of a markedly elevated antiviral antibody titer in a single serum sample (e.g., in clinical cases of feline infectious peritonitis) will support the diagnosis when

Table 1. *Comparison of Viral Diagnostic Methods**

Diagnostic Method	Advantages	Disadvantages
Virus isolation	Available in most laboratories Sensitive	Cannot detect nonviable virus Adventitious agents may confuse diagnosis Time-consuming Field virus may not be cell adapted
Electron microscopy	Rapid Detects nonviable or noncultivable virus Can identify mixed infections	Expensive Not readily available Not as sensitive as virus isolations
Histopathology	Rapid Available in most laboratories Handling and storage of specimens not as critical as with other methods	Not sensitive; many viruses do not produce specific tissue changes
Serologic identification of viral antigens	Rapid Available in most laboratories Sensitive Can identify viral serotypes	Not applicable to some viruses May over look mixed infections
Demonstration of specific antibody responses (paired samples)	Supportive evidence that isolated virus was related to disease Serum easily collected and stored	Not rapid Antibody responses may be to other unrelated viruses

*Modified from Gibbs: In. Pract. 1:21, 1979.

characteristic clinical signs and clinicopathologic findings are present. Elevated antibody levels in very young animals may be difficult to interpret, especially during the transition between passive and active immunity when significant increases in antibody titer to unrelated viruses may occur. Demonstration of an elevated IgM antibody response against a specific virus probably indicates recent infection with the virus and as such may be useful in correlating a virus with recent disease outbreaks in patients where only a single serum sample is available.

In general, the appropriate selection of samples frequently depends on whether antemortem or post-mortem samples are used and on the suspected disease itself (e.g., blood, tumor, pleural fluids in suspected feline leukemia; nasal or throat swabs in suspected feline rhinotracheitis or caliciviral disease; feces or rectal swabs in suspected canine parvovirus enteritis). When a specific virus is not suspected, samples should generally be taken from the major organs affected, especially where lesions are present. In systemic diseases without gross lesions, it is advisable to submit samples from blood, lymph nodes, spleen, lung, and tonsils.

COLLECTION AND SUBMISSION OF SAMPLES

SPECIMENS FOR VIRAL ISOLATION

The ideal time to collect clinical material for virus isolation is during the acute stage of disease, prior to the formation of antibodies, when viral titers in affected tissues or blood are highest. Various materials, such as blood; nasal, conjunctival, and oral swabs; urine; feces; and biopsy or necropsy tissue samples are used for virus isolations. Specimens for viral isolation should be fresh and collected aseptically. No fixatives or preservatives should be used. When gross lesions are present, the sample should include the outer margins of the lesion and adjacent healthy tissue.

Since the biochemical and biophysical properties of viruses vary markedly (i.e., many viruses are heat- and acid-sensitive), fresh tissues should be frozen to $-60°$ to $-70°C$ immediately after harvesting. Alternatively, tissue specimens may be placed in a deep freeze at $-20°C$ until dry ice is obtained for packaging and shipment to the nearest diagnostic laboratory. For transport, especially when long-distance land or air transportation is required, the frozen specimens should be shipped in labelled, sealed jars or plastic bags surrounded by dry ice (and insulated with newspaper) in styrofoam cartons; the dry ice should be of sufficient quantity to last for at least 48 hours. If dry ice is not available, small pieces of tissue, fecal material,

or mucus may be placed in vials completely filled with 50 per cent glycerol and stored at 6°C. A special charcoal transport medium for viruses is commercially available and does not require freezing or refrigeration.* This medium is particularly useful when dry ice and low-temperature freezers are not available or when shipping is delayed; many viruses will apparently survive in this medium for up to three weeks at room temperature.

Small pieces of tissue and swabs should be placed in a suitable viral transport medium, frozen, and shipped in dry ice as described previously. These specimens should be submitted in labelled screw-cap vials containing 2 ml of the transport medium ("culturette" swabs or Ames bacterial transport medium should not be used, as it contains thioglycolate, which inhibits certain viruses). A suitable virus transport medium is sterile Hank's balanced salt solution with 10 per cent bovine albumin or 0.5 per cent lactalbumin hydrolysate; antibiotics (e.g., gentamycin, 500 µg/ml) and antifungals (e.g., Nystatin, 25 U) may be added to inhibit bacterial and fungal growth, respectively. In an emergency, 10 per cent boiled skim milk solution may be substituted for the virus transport medium.

SPECIMENS FOR ELECTRON MICROSCOPY (EM)

Tissue samples for transmission EM should immediately be cut into very small (1 mm³) pieces and fixed 24 hours in ten times their volume of 2 to 4 per cent glutaraldehyde at 20°C. If the vials cannot be taken directly to the EM laboratory, they should be transferred after 24 hours in glutaraldehyde to vials containing 0.1 M cacodylate buffer and refrigerated. Formalin-fixed tissue sections can be processed for EM if necessary, but formalin is not an adequate fixative for EM. Samples (feces, fluids) for negative-staining EM should be refrigerated when shipped to the laboratory.

SPECIMENS FOR HISTOPATHOLOGY

Samples for histologic examination should not be frozen. Small 3.0- to 5.0-mm thick tissue sections should be fixed and stored in ten times their volume of 10 per cent neutral-buffered formalin. Where specific lesions are observed, sections should include both the periphery of the lesion and surrounding healthy tissue.

SPECIMENS FOR IMMUNOFLUORESCENCE (FA)

Fresh tissue samples for FA testing should not be fixed. For maximum preservation of virus and viral antigens, the samples should be placed in

---

*Colab Laboratories, Chicago Heights, IL.

Table 2. *Laboratory Diagnosis of Feline Viral Diseases*

Virus	Disease	Diagnostic Tests*	Preferred Specimens
Panleukopenia	Feline distemper	VI	Ileum, spleen, lymph nodes, rectal swab
		EM	Feces
		FA	Ileum, thymus, lymph nodes
		H	Ileum, thymus, liver
		SN	Serum
Herpesvirus 1	Feline viral rhinotracheitis	VI	Nasal, oral, ocular swabs; lung, trachea
		H	Nasal turbinates, lung, trachea
		FA	Nasal scrapings
		SN, PRT	Serum
Calcivirus	Feline calciviral disease	VI, VN, CF	Nasal, oral, ocular swabs; lung, trachea
		FA, H	Lung, trachea; oral ulcers
		SN, PRT	Serum
Feline leukemia	Lymphoma; FeLV-related diseases	IFA	Blood smears
		ELISA	Blood, serum, plasma
		H	Tumor, lymph nodes, bone marrow
		Cyt	Blood, fluid, bone marrow
		VI	Tumor, blood, bone marrow
Feline coronavirus	Feline infectious peritonitis; enteric disease; kitten mortality (?)	H, (FA)	Kidney, liver, lymph nodes, lung, peritoneum, CNS
		AI	Tissue homogenates (lesions), fluids, blood
		IFA	Serum, fluids
		EM	Feces
Rabies virus	Rabies	H, FA, AI	Brain, salivary glands
		VN	Serum
Reovirus	Conjunctivitis	VI	Ocular swab

Notes:
VI	= virus isolation	EM	= electron microscopy
FA	= direct fluorescent antibody test	H	= histopathology
SN	= serum neutralization	PRT	= plaque reduction test
VN	= virus neutralization	CF	= complement fixation
IFA	= indirect immunofluorescent test	ELISA	= enzyme-linked immunosorbent assay
Cyt	= cytology	( )	= not very commonly applied
AI	= animal inoculation		

small, screw-top polyethylene vials, frozen immediately in a thermos containing liquid nitrogen or in a container containing dry ice, and stored either in a deep freeze (−20°C) or, preferably, at −70°C prior to shipment under dry ice. Tissue imprints or blood smears should be air dried and shipped by regular mail with or without refrigeration.

SPECIMENS FOR SEROLOGY

In preparing serum samples for submission, a recommended procedure is to allow the blood sample (collected in tubes without anticoagulant) to clot overnight at room temperature, then rim and remove the clot, centrifuge, and transfer the serum to labelled sterile vials. If a centrifuge is unavailable, the blood should be left overnight at room temperature to allow the clot to shrink; the serum is then removed with a sterile pipette or disposable syringe. If shipment to the laboratory is delayed, the serum samples should be frozen and stored at −20°C;

otherwise, they may be refrigerated and then shipped under wet-ice refrigeration.

SUMMARY OF DIAGNOSTIC TESTS AND PREFERRED SPECIMENS FOR DIAGNOSIS OF FELINE AND CANINE VIRAL DISEASES

The various methods and preferred clinical specimens used in diagnosing feline and canine viral diseases are presented in Tables 2 and 3. It is important to remember that the isolation of a virus or viral antigens from clinical material does not in itself establish a specific diagnosis. This is particularly true when mixed infections with unrelated agents or persistent infections with nonpathogenic agents may occur. It is therefore imperative that the clinician correlate the clinical symptoms, course of disease, and supportive clinicopathologic findings with results of viral isolations and/or demonstration of significant serologic responses when relating a viral agent to a specific disease syndrome.

Table 3. *Laboratory Diagnosis of Canine Viral Diseases*

Virus	Disease	Diagnostic Tests*	Preferred Specimens
Canine distemper virus	Canine distemper	H	Intestine, bladder, lung, brain (conjunctiva)
		FA	As above; also footpad biopsy and conjunctival scrapings
		SN	Serum, CSF
		VI	Intestine, bladder, lung, brain (conjunctiva)
Canine adenovirus 1	Infectious canine hepatitis	VI, VN, FA, CF	Liver, urine
		H	Liver, gallbladder
		SN	Serum
Canine adenovirus 2	Respiratory disease complex	VI, VN, FA	Lung, nasal swabs
Parinfluenza 2 virus (SV-5)	Parainfluenza	VI, VN, HI	Nasal swabs
Canine parvovirus	Viral gastroenteritis	H, FA	Small intestine, heart
		EM, VI, HA	Feces, rectal swab
		IFA, SN, HI	Serum
Canine coronavirus	Viral gastroenteritis	EM	Feces
		H	Small intestine
		VI	Small intestine, feces, rectal swab
Canine herpesvirus	Neonatal mortality, reproductive disease	H	Lung, kidney, liver
		VI, VN, FA	Same as above
		SN	Serum
Canine reovirus 1 (2)	Upper respiratory infection (pneumonia); enteritis	VI	Nasal swab, lung, feces
Canine rotavirus	Viral gastroenteritis	EM	Feces
		VI	Feces, small intestine
Rabies virus	Rabies	see Table 2	

Notes: HA = hemagglutination test; HI = hemagglutination inhibition. Other abbreviations are identified in Table 2.

REFERENCES AND SUPPLEMENTAL READING

Gibbs, E. P. J.: Veterinary laboratory; collecting specimens for Virus disease diagnosis. In. Pract. 1:21, 1979.

Gillespie, J. H., and Timoney, J. F. (eds.): *Hagan and Bruner's Infectious Diseases of Domestic Animals.* Ithaca: Cornell University Press, 1981, pp. 447–483.

Lennette, D. A., and Schmidt, N. J.: *Diagnostic Procedures for Viral and Rickettsial Infections,* 4th ed. New York: American Public Health Association, 1969.

Roberts, A. W., and Carter, G. R.: *Essentials of Veterinary Virology.* East Lansing: Michigan State University Press, 1981.

Weiss, R. C., and Scott, F. W.: Feline diagnostic virology. Feline Pract. 11:31, 1981.

PRACTICAL DIAGNOSTIC PROCEDURES FOR BACTERIAL DISEASES

SANG J. SHIN, D.V.M.,
and PATRICK L. McDONOUGH, M.S.

Ithaca, New York

Diagnosis of bacterial disease in the small animal practitioner's laboratory has become increasingly important because of the problems associated with referral (often distant) laboratories, i.e., slow turnover time and expense. Also, the recent availability of commercially prepared media and bacterial culturing kits has made it possible for practitioners to perform bacterial cultures in their own office laboratory with a minimum of equipment (Table 1). Unlike viral culture techniques, which require elaborate equipment and reagents, bacterial cultures can be performed confidently by properly trained laboratory personnel with a minimum of equipment and reagents.

Textbook information concerning the selection of antimicrobial agents is quickly outdated because of the emergence of drug resistance in pathogenic

Table 1. Equipment and Suppliers for Practitioner's Laboratory

Small incubator (Forma Scientific, Marietta OH)
CO₂ (candle jar) or Gas Pak Anaerobic System (BBL Microbiology Systems, Cockeysville, MD; check local hospital suppliers); Campylobacter Systems (BBL Microbiology Systems)
Gram staining kit (Difco Laboratories, Detroit, MI; check local hospital suppliers)
Other staining kit (methylene blue, acid–fast staining kit) (Difco Laboratories)
Loops: plain loop (Jorgensen inoculating loop) (Scientific Products, McGraw, IL); needle inoculating loop (Scientific Products); calibrated loop, size 0.01 ml (Scientific Products)
Frosted slides, cover glasses (Scientific Products)
Gas or alcohol Bunsen burner
Strikers and flints
Spatulas
Microscope with 10x, 45x, and 100x objectives
Amies transport media with charcoal (BBL Microbiology Systems; REMEL, Regional Media Laboratories, Lenox KS)
Port-A-Cul (for anaerobic transport media) (BBL Microbiology Systems)
Ice packs
Whirl-pack bags
Double-tube mailer
Grease pencils

Note: Most supplies can be obtained through local scientific suppliers (VWR, Fisher Scientific, Inc., etc.).

bacteria involved in small animal bacterial disease. Therefore, sensitivity testing performed in the practitioner's laboratory can provide excellent information regarding the drug of choice for the treatment of certain bacterial diseases of small animals.

However, one should realize there are limitations as to what can be accomplished in a practitioner's laboratory; certain fastidious bacteria require special conditions and equipment, selective media, and reagents with a short shelf life, which are impossible to maintain in small laboratories but which are needed for isolation and characterization. Also one must use good judgement in determining when to refer samples to outside laboratories, for example, in suspicious cases of leptospirosis, canine brucellosis, unknown abortions, mycoplasmosis, anaerobic bacterial diseases, systemic fungal disease, and so on.

The purpose of this article is to discuss the microbiologic isolation and identification procedures that may be successfully used by the practitioner in a small clinical laboratory (Table 2). For the more demanding isolation procedures (which are best referred to diagnostic laboratories) requiring a range of incubation conditions and selective media, details are given for the proper transport of specimens to optimize the chances of identifying a potential etiologic agent.

LABORATORY DIAGNOSIS OF URINARY TRACT INFECTION

Urinary tract infection (UTI) in the small animal is one of the most common bacterial diseases seen by veterinarians in daily practice. One should have an understanding of the etiologic agents and should know the number of bacteria in the urine when UTI is suspected. Thus, the quantitative bacterial examination of urine can be a valuable aid in the diagnosis and treatment of UTI.

Urine samples should be examined for bacteria within two hours of collection for several reasons. First, normal urine samples taken by catheterization

1148

contain more than 300 bacteria/ml. Second, most of these organisms have a 15- to 20-minute generation time. Third, urine is an enriched medium for bacterial growth. Urine samples always should be kept under refrigeration until cultured or referred to a laboratory. Urine samples on the bench for more than two to three hours should not be cultured for bacteria. Generally, urine samples should not be sent for bacterial culture by mail to distant laboratories; if this is necessary, extreme caution should be taken by using sterile containers and packing them well in a refrigerated box.

The most frequently involved bacteria in UTI are *Escherichia coli*, *Klebsiella* spp., *Pseudomonas* spp., *Proteus* spp., *Staphylococcus* aureus, and *Streptococcus* spp. (beta-hemolytic streptococci, enterococci).

ISOLATION SCHEME

The preferred methods for obtaining samples (in descending order of choice) are cystocentesis, midstream catheterization, and expressed or voided sample.

INTERPRETATION

1. If the sample is obtained by *cystocentesis*, more than 10^3 organisms/ml should be considered significant. If fewer than 10^3 organisms/ml are counted, refer to other clinical signs, e.g., pus cells in urine, before working on the organisms. If other clinical signs indicate UTI, even though fewer than 10^3 organisms/ml are present, organisms should be considered significant.

2. If the sample is from *mid-stream catheterization*, more than 10^5 organisms/ml should be considered significant. A count of 10^4 to 10^5 organisms/ml should be considered significant if there are no more than two different species of organisms. If 10^2 to 10^4 organisms/ml of one species of organism (pure culture) are counted, refer to clinical symptoms.

3. If the sample is from *expressed or voided urine*, only more than 10^5 organisms/ml should be considered significant.

LABORATORY DIAGNOSIS OF DIARRHEA OF BACTERIAL ORIGIN IN SMALL ANIMALS

When diagnosing acute infectious diarrhea of bacterial origin, one is faced with the task of isolating and identifying from among the microbial flora of the intestinal tract those bacteria most likely to be involved in the disease process. Most of the common pathogens are members of the *Enterobacteriaceae* (e.g., *E. coli*, *Salmonella* spp.), and their isolation is facilitated by growth on the available enteric media such as Levine eosin–methylene blue agar (EMB), MacConkey agar (MAC), and brilliant green agar (BG), along with enrichment procedures using selenite F broth (SF) and gram negative broth (GN), Hajnu (Table 3). However, with the recent finding of additional bacterial etiologies of diarrhea such as *Clostridium difficile* (pseudomembranous colitis associated with antibiotic usage), *Yersinia enterocolitica* (acute gastroenteritis), *Campylobacter fetus* subs. *jejuni* (enteritis), and *Aeromonas hydrophila* (enteritis), the laboratory diagnosis of diarrhea is becoming more complicated, requiring the use of various selective media, incubation temperatures, and atmospheres to successfully isolate and determine the causative agent of the disease.

ETIOLOGIC AGENTS OF BACTERIAL DIARRHEA

Table 4 lists the microorganisms that cause diarrhea in mammalian species. Since many of these bacteria are found as part of the resident flora of the intestinal tract and since healthy carrier hosts (animals not showing clinical signs of disease but shedding bacteria from time to time, especially when stressed) exist in any animal population, one should be cautious in linking the mere *isolation of a microorganism* with *causation of disease*. However, a more definitive interpretation of laboratory results may be possible when considering the overall clinical signs, treatment history (especially antimicrobials), vaccination history, and feeding practices of the animal under evaluation.

ISOLATION SCHEME

Samples should be taken in the acute stage of disease before the institution of antimicrobial therapy and must be plated out onto isolation media (Table 5) as soon as possible. If the specimen is not culturable in a reasonable amount of time, it should be refrigerated and transport media should be con-

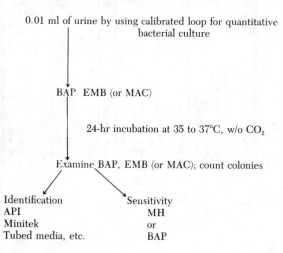

0.01 ml of urine by using calibrated loop for quantitative
bacterial culture

BAP   EMB (or MAC)

24-hr incubation at 35 to 37°C, w/o CO₂

Examine BAP, EMB (or MAC); count colonies

Identification   Sensitivity
API   MH
Minitek   or
Tubed media, etc.   BAP

Table 2.   Selected Biochemical Tests for Common Bacteria Isolated From Small Animals

BACTERIA	Gas from glucose	Glucose	Lactose	Mannitol	Citrate	Urea	H₂S production	Indole	Motility	Malonate	Phenylalanine	Arginine	Lysine	Ornithine	Oxidase
Salmonella	+ or −	A	□	A	Var +	−	⊞ (−)	−	+	−	−	+ (L)	⊞ (−)*	⊞†	−
Arizona	+	A	Var	A	⊞	−	⊞ (w)	−	+	⊞	−	+ (L)	⊞	⊞	−
Citrobacter freundii	+	A	A(L)	A	⊞	+, W, −	⊞	−	+	Var	−	Var	□	Var	
C. diversus	+	A	+ or −	A	⊞	+ or −	□	⊞	+	+ or −	−	+ or +(L)	⊞	⊞	
C. amalonaticus	+	A	+(+) or −	A	⊞	+ or −	□	⊞	+	−	−	+	□	⊞	
Escherichia	+ or −	A	A/−	A	□	□	−/w	⊞ (−)	⊞	−	−	Var	Var	Var	−
Shigella	□‡	A	□§	Var	−	−	−	Var +	−	−	−	+ (L)	□	∥	
Eduardsiella	+	A	□	−	−	−	⊞	⊞	+	−	−	−	⊞	⊞	
Serratia	□ (+)	A	□ (A)	A	⊞	− (+)	−	−	+	−	−	−	⊞	⊞	
Proteus vulgaris,	Var⁷	A	□	−	Var	⊞	⊞	⊞	+	−	⊞		□	□	
P. mirabilis	+⁷	A	□	−	+(L)	⊞	⊞	−	+	−	⊞		□	⊞	
Morganella morganii	Var⁷	A	□	−	−	⊞	−	⊞	+	−	⊞		□	⊞	
Providenciaalcali faciens	+ or −	A	□	−	+	−	−	⊞	+	−	⊞		□	□	
P. stuartii	−	A	□	Var	+	−	−	⊞	+	−	⊞		□	□	
P. stuartii (urea +)	−	A	□	Var	+	−	−	⊞	+	−	⊞		□	□	
P. rettgeii	Var⁷	A	□	Var	+	⊞	−	⊞	+	−	⊞		□	□	
Klebsiella pneumoniae	+	A,G	A	A	⊞	⊞	−	−	□	+	−		⊞	□	
K. oxytoca	+	A,G	A	A	⊞	⊞	−	⊞	−	+	−		⊞	□	
K. ozaenae	Var	A	Var	A	Var	Var	−	−	−	+	−		□ or +	□	
K. rhinoscleromatis	−	A	A,L, or −	A	Var	−	−	−	−	+	−		− or +	−	

Enterobacter sakazakii (formerly *E. cloacae*)	+	A	A	A	⊞	Var	−	Var	+	⊞	⊡
E. aerogenes	+	A	A	A	⊞	−	−	−	+	⊞	⊞
E. liquefaciens	+	A	22° Var, L 35° Var	A	⊞	Var	−	−	−	⊞	22° + 35° + or − / ⊡
E. agglomerans	Var −	A,G	A	A	A(−),L	− or +	− or −	− or +	−	⊡	⊞
Hafnia alvei (formerly *E. hafniae*)	+	A	− orA,L	A	22° Var 35° L, +, −	−	−	Var	−	⊡	⊞
Aeromonas (Plesiomonas) shigelloides	⊡	+	⊞(−)	−	⊞(−)	−	⊞(−)	+	+(−)	+	+(−)
A. hydrophila	+ or −	+	⊞(+)	+	−(+)	−	+	+	−(+)	−(+)	−
Yersinia enterocolitica	⊡	+	+(L)	+	−	−	Var +	22° + 37° −	−	−	⊞
Pasteurella multocida	⊞(−)	+	⊡	+ or −	−	−	⊡	⊡	⊡	⊡	+(−)
P. aerogens (multocida gas +)	+	− (+ L)	⊡	−	⊞⊞	−	⊞⊞	−	−	−	+(−)
Brucella canis	−	−	−	−	⊞(−)	−	−	−	+	−	−
Bordetella bronchiseptica	⊡	⊞	−	+(−)	+(−)	−	⊞⊞	⊞⊞	+	−	−
Pseudomonas aeruginosa											

S. paratyphi A is lysine negative.
†*S. typhi* is ornithine negative.
‡*S. flexneri* 6: some biotypes positive.
§§*S. sonnei* A:L.
‖*S. sonnei* and *S. boydii* 13 are positive.
Notes: + = 90 per cent or more positive; − = 90 per cent or more negative.
L = late.
Numbers in parentheses indicate small percentage.
Var = variable.
⊡ = key biochemical reactions.
Boxed symbols indicate key biochemical tests for bacterial species.
A = acid.
W = weak reaction.
G = gas.
° = degrees centigrade.
⁷ = seven days after.

Table 3. *Media for Practitioner's Laboratory*

Isolation
- Blood agar plate (BAP) (trypticase soy 5% sheep blood agar plate)*
- Chocolate agar (CHOC)†
- Levine eosin–methylene blue agar (EMB)*
- MacConkey agar (MAC)*
- Brilliant green agar (BG)†
- Selenite F (SF)†
- Gram negative broth (GN broth)†
- Phosphate-buffered saline (PBS)
- Campylobacter blood agar plate (Campy)†
- Blood culture bottle

Sensitivity
- Mueller-Hinton agar plate (MH) (100 × 15 mm)
- Blood agar plate (BAP)*
- Sensi-discs*
- Cotton swabs*

Identification
- API: recommended for small and large laboratories
- Minitek: recommended for large laboratories
- Other commercial sources

Transport
- Amies transport medium with charcoal
- 0.067 M phosphate-buffered saline (PBS), pH 7.6 (*Yersinia* transport media only)
- Port-A-Cul anaerobic transport systems

Tissues from necropsy
- Whirl-pack bags or sterile container

*Essential.
†Optional.

Table 4. *Bacterial Agents of Acute Diarrhea*

Agent	Lactose Fermentation*
Escherichia coli	+
Salmonella spp. (nontyphoidal)	−
Yersinia enterocolitica	−
Aeromonas hydrophila	+
Staphylococcus aureus	NA
Campylobacter fetus subsp. *jejuni*	NA
Clostridium difficile	NA
Clostridium perfringens	NA
Other: *Pseudomonas* spp.	−
Candida spp. (yeast)†	NA

*+ = lactose fermenter; − = lactose nonfermenter; NA = not applicable.

†Note: Although fungal agents are not included here, *Candida* spp. are mentioned because of their frequent isolation on bacterial media, especially from patients receiving antibiotic therapy in which there may be an overgrowth of yeast in the intestinal tract.

LABORATORY DIAGNOSIS OF RESPIRATORY BACTERIAL INFECTION

If bacteria are considered either primary or secondary etiologic agents in lower respiratory tract infection, one should carefully consider the proper samples before attempting bacterial culture. Since the oropharyngeal area of the small animal is known to be heavily populated with normal bacterial flora, only tracheal or *bronchial washings* from the sick animal should be examined for bacterial culture; *throat swabs* for suspect pneumonia or bronchitis should never be cultured for bacteria. Throat swabs should be considered only for tonsilitis and pharyngitis cases. Even though most of the common bacterial pathogens in lower respiratory tract infec-

sidered. The specimen of choice for enteric disease is a *freshly passed fecal sample* or *rectal swab* received in good condition in the laboratory. The specimens of choice from necropsied animals are a tied-off *loop of ileum and colon*, a *gallbladder swab*, and *mesenteric lymph nodes*. Laboratory work must be performed systematically for the most economical and rapid recovery of bacterial agents.

Fecal sample, ileum/colon contents
↓
Wet mount in NB* (rapidly motile organism, comma-shaped: *Campylobacter*)
↓
Gram/Giemsa-stained smear (leukocytes; large, round-ended gram positive rods: *Clostridium perfringens*)

If referred to diagnostic laboratory: *feces* in Amies transport media with charcoal and PBS vial (keep on ice); *necropsy specimen* on ice
If *anaerobic culture* (for *Clostridia* spp.) use Port-A-Cul anaerobic vial

BAP†: (note hemolysis, colony types: *E. coli*, *Aeromonas* spp., *Staphylococcus aureus*)
MAC†: (*must* be used for *Yersinia*, LAC− colony‡: see PBS below)
EMB§: LAC +/− colonies
BG§:LAC − colonies to TSI slant→API identify: *Salmonella*

Campy (check tiny colonies: catalase, wet mount, oxidase; refer to diagnostic laboratory to confirm as *Campylobacter*)
§SEL F→BG: check LAC− on TSI slant→API etc. *Salmonella*
§GN→EMB: *Salmonella*
§PBS→MAC: check LAC− on TSI slant→API strip etc., *Yersinia*

---

*NB = nutrient broth.
†Essential media.
‡LAC = lactose.
§Optional media.

Table 5. *Isolation Media Used in the Diagnosis of Diarrhea of Bacterial Origin*

Media	Incubation Conditions*
Primary Plated Media (streak for isolated colonies)	
Trypticase soy agar with 5% sheep blood (BAP)	18 to 24 hrs, 35°C, O_2
Levine EMB agar (EMB)	18 to 24 hrs, 35°C, O_2
MacConkey agar (MAC)	24 to 48 hrs, 35°C or 22°C (see PBS below)
Campylobacter (BAP) (Campy)	48 hrs, 42°C, microaerophilic
Brilliant green agar (BG)	18 to 24 hrs, 35°C, O_2
Enrichment Media (inoculate 10% feces [w/v])	
Selenite F broth (SF)	48 hrs, 35°C, O_2, subculture to BG
Gram negative broth (GN), Hajnu	24 hrs, 35°C, O_2, subculture to EMB
0.067 M phosphate-buffered saline, pH 7.6 (PBS)	1 to 3 wks, 5°C, O_2, subculture to MAC at weekly intervals

*Notes: Room temperature: 22°C (72°F); 35°C (95.5°F). Microaerophilic atmospheres: 10% CO_2, 10% H_2, 80% N_2 (must be less than 6% O_2). O_2: no added gases.

Miscellaneous Bacterial Isolation Schemata

Infection	Media; Incubation Conditions	Common Bacteria
Vaginitis	BAP, MAC; 24 to 48 hrs, 35 to 37°C, CO_2	*E. coli; Staph. aureus;* beta-strep.; *Hemophilus* spp.; *Mycoplasma* spp.*
Metritis	BAP, MAC, 24 to 48 hrs, 35 to 37°C, CO_2	*Staph. aureus; E. coli;* beta-strep.; *Pseudomonas* spp.; *Proteus* spp.; *Klebsiella* spp.; *Mycoplasma* spp.*
Conjunctivitis	BAP, MAC; 24 to 48 hrs, 35 to 37°C, CO_2	*Staph. aureus; Hemophilus* spp.; beta-strep.; *Pseudomonas* spp.
Otitis	BAP, MAC; 48 to 72 hrs, 35 to 37°C, CO_2	*Staph. aureus.; Proteus* spp.; *Pseudomonas* spp.; beta-strep.; *Malessezia pachydermatis*
Pyoderma	BAP, MAC; 48 to 72 hrs, 35 to 37°C, CO_2	*Staph. aureus; Proteus mirabilis; Pseudomonas aeruginosa*
Bite wound	BAP, MAC; 48 to 72 hrs, 35 to 37°C, CO_2	*Pasteurella multocida; Staph. aureus;* beta-strep.; anaerobic bacteria*
Abscess	BAP, MAC; 48 to 72 hrs, 35 to 37°C, CO_2	*Staph. aureus;* beta-strep.; *Pasteurella multocida; Nocardia* spp.*; *Actinomyces* spp.*; Anaerobic bacteria*

*Referral tests: leptospirosis, brucellosis, mycoplasmosis, campylobacteriosis, yersiniosis, anaerobic infection (including clostridial infection).

tions are relatively slow growing, e.g., *Bordetella bronchiseptica, Hemophilus* spp., *Pasteurella multocida (aerogenes)*, their growth can be enhanced by incubating in CO_2 on special media. However, in the veterinarian's laboratory, one can perform bacterial cultures very effectively with minimal media.

ISOLATION SCHEME

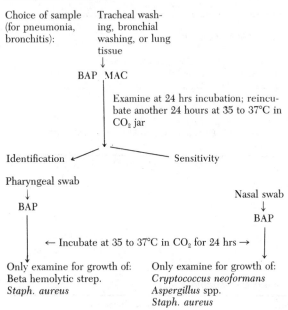

The most frequently involved bacteria in lower respiratory tract infection are as follows:

1. *Bordetella bronchiseptica*: grow on BAP, MAC; most common pathogen.
2. *Mycoplasma* spp.: no growth on BAP, MAC; refer to reference lab.
3. *Pasteurella multocida (aerogenes)*: grow on BAP; common pathogen.
4. *Staph. aureus*: grow on BAP; common pathogen.
5. Beta-hemolytic streptococci: grow on BAP; common pathogen.
6. *Hemophilus canis*: only on BAP and CHOC; common pathogen.
7. Others: *Pseudomonas aeruginosa, E. coli, Klebsiella pneumonia* (all rare to common pathogens).

Normally no more than two bacterial agents are involved in acute pneumonia or bronchitis; in clinical cases, bacterial growth of the pathogen from the sample is profuse. If there are few isolates, one should interpret culture results very carefully, since small numbers of any of the previously mentioned organisms isolated from tracheal washings could represent normal flora.

COLONY APPEARANCE OF SELECTED BACTERIAL SPECIES

The following is a guide to the colony morphology on plated media of some of the bacterial species mentioned as etiologic agents of disease in small animals.

BAP

Most gram negative bacteria are difficult to differentiate on blood agar, especially the agents of bacterial diarrhea. However, there are some clues that can be used to help the clinician distinguish between the various bacteria.

1. Some *E. coli* are beta-hemolytic (complete clearing) colonies and are oxidase −, indole + (quick test).
2. *Aeromonas hydrophilia* (oxidase +, indole +) also forms beta-hemolytic mucoid colonies.
3. In cases of enterotoxemia, *Clostridium perfringens* sometimes appears as small white hemolytic colonies growing beneath faster-growing *E. coli* colonies that have provided an anaerobic atmosphere. A gram-stained smear made from such hemolytic areas would reveal short, fat, round-ended, relatively uniform size gram positive rods (*Clostridium* spp.) amidst smaller gram negative rods (*E. coli*).
4. *Pseudomonas aeruginosa* also forms beta-hemolytic, flat, spreading colonies (oxidase +) with a fruit-like odor and a "metallic sheen."
5. *Bordetella bronchiseptica* grows well by 48 hours incubation. Organisms appear as gray colonies (oxidase +, rapid urease +) with small (2 to 3 mm diameter), gram negative coccobacilli.
6. *Hemophilus canis (hemoglobinophilus)* grows in 48 to 72 hours on BAP as tiny pinpoint colonies. It requires X factor (hemin) but not V factor. It is oxidase +.
7. *Staphylococcus aureus* on BAP forms small- to medium-sized, usually white-yellowish colonies surrounded by a double zone of hemolysis (inner zone of complete hemolysis, outer zone of incomplete hemolysis). *Staphylococcus* spp. are catalase +. Beta-hemolytic streptococcus (usually *Strep. canis*) is a small, white, beta-hemolytic colony on BAP; it is catalase −. Other *Streptococcus* spp., i.e., enterococci (group D streptococci), viridans streptococci, may be alpha- (incomplete), beta- (complete), or gamma- (non) hemolytic on BAP and are catalase −.
8. *Cryptococcus* spp. (yeast) grow very well on BAP as very mucoid, whitish colonies that tend to run together.

9. *Pasteurella multocida (aerogenes)* appears as small gray colonies with gram negative coccobacilli. It has a characteristic musty or dried-sputum smell and is nonhemolytic, oxidase +, and indole +.

Levine EMB agar

1. Lactose-fermenting (LAC +) enteric bacteria, e.g., *E. coli*, usually have dark purple to black centers with or without a green metallic sheen.
2. *A. hydrophila* (LAC +) is a more mucoid colony than most *E. coli*, with a dark center but no green metallic sheen.
3. *Salmonella* spp. are clear, uncolored colonies without centers. They are non-lactose-fermenting (LAC −) enteric bacteria.
4. *Proteus vulgaris* and *P. mirabilis* may appear as LAC −, spreading colonies on EMB. (These colonies do not spread as much on EMB as they do on BAP.)
5. *Pseudomonas* spp. appear on EMB as flat LAC −, slightly spreading colonies with irregular edges.
6. Most gram positive bacteria, e.g., *Staphylococcus* and *Streptococcus*, are inhibited from growing on EMB agar.
7. *Candida* spp. (yeast) may grow on EMB agar as small, creamy, pinkish-white, star-shaped colonies.
8. *Malessezia pachydermatis (Pityrosporum canis)* from ear swabs will grow on EMB, forming blackish, dry, small colonies after 48 hours incubation.

MacConkey (MAC) agar

1. LAC + bacterial colonies (*E. coli*, *Aeromonas* spp.) at 24 hours incubation at 35°C are a brick-red color in the center and 2 to 3 mm in diameter.
2. LAC − colonies (*Salmonella*) are clear and uncolored.
3. *Bordetella bronchiseptica* appears as grayish colonies 2 to 3 mm in diameter at 24 hours incubation at 35°C.
4. *Yersinia enterocolitica* at 24 hours incubation at 22°C appears as small, light-pink to peach colored colonies 1 to 2 mm in diameter. By 48 hours they may be 2 to 3 mm in diameter.
5. Gram positive bacteria are inhibited on MAC agar.

BG Agar

1. BG is a very highly selective media for *Salmonella* spp.

2. LAC + colonies (*E. coli*) are usually greenish-yellow and are surrounded by a yellow-green zone.
3. LAC − colonies (*Salmonella*, *Proteus*, *Pseudomonas*) are pinkish to red in color and are surrounded by an intense red zone. *Proteus* spp. and *Pseudomonas* spp. do not spread very much on BG agar.

Campy agar

Most enteric bacteria are inhibited on this highly selective medium containing antibiotics. Also, many organisms will not grow at the temperature recommended for Campy plates (42°C). *Campylobacter* spp. are very small, pinpoint colonies at 24 hours; by 48 hours, gray colonies are 2 to 3 mm in diameter, sometimes spreading out along the streaking line. For quick screening, perform a wet mount in nutrient broth from one to two similar-appearing colonies to check for the characteristic darting motility of *Campylobacter* spp. *Campylobacter fetus* subs. *jejuni* is oxidase + and catalase +.

DECONTAMINATION OF CONTAMINATED TISSUE SURFACES FOR BACTERIAL CULTURE

Before internal tissues, e.g., lymph node, liver, spleen, intestines, and lung, may be cultured, surface-contaminating bacteria and fungi must be eliminated. This is accomplished by touching an area of tissue with a hot spatula (heated to redness in Bunsen burner flame); the heated area of the tissue is then incised with a sterile scalpel and a sterile swab inserted. The swab is then either placed into transport medium or plated onto appropriate culture medium. The aim of this procedure is to decontaminate the tissue surface, *not cook* the tissue; therefore, the hot spatula is not left in place for a long time. Pieces of tissue too small to sear can be quickly dipped in 70 per cent alcohol and flamed with a match; in this way surface bacteria are destroyed and the tissue itself is not harmed. Note that intestinal samples should first be tied off with a length of string before incisions are made to isolate the section and remove it from the abdominal cavity.

REFERRAL TESTS

Fastidious organisms and organisms requiring unusual incubation temperatures and/or atmospheres, expensive selective media with a short shelf life, and much technical expertise for identification, e.g., *Clostridium* spp., perhaps *Campylobacter* spp., and *Yersinia* spp., are best sent to a reference diagnostic facility for isolation and identification. *Transport media* (see Table 3) are useful for sending specimens for referral tests and are also useful when specimens cannot be quickly plated onto appropriate solid and/ or enrichment media. In such cases there is danger of overgrowth of pathogenic baceteria, which might be present in small numbers, by other bacteria. Transport media hold the bacterial population at a stationary level, preventing overgrowth or decreased viability of the desired microorganism.

Swabs taken from nasopharyngeal areas, eyes, skin lesions, necropsy tissues, and so on are inserted into the transport media and broken off. Both transport media and whirl-pack bags should be *ice packed, not frozen*. Necropsy tissues themselves should not be placed into Amies transport media or Port-A-Cul. Abscess material, thoracic or peritoneal fluid material, and other fluids for anaerobic culture should be soaked onto a swab and inserted into the Port-A-Cul tube. Fluid material may also be retained in the syringe into which it was first aspirated (syringe barrel and needle must be *taped* firmly in place) and the syringe packed in ice for shipment to the referral laboratory.

All specimens must be shipped by the fastest, most economical means possible, e.g., first class mail, United Parcel Service, to the referral laboratory.

SUPPLEMENTAL READING

Carter, G. R.: *Diagnostic Procedures in Veterinary Microbiology*, 3rd ed. Springfield, IL: Charles C Thomas, 1979.

Edwards, P. R., and Ewing, W. H.: *Identification of Enterobacteriaceae*, 3rd ed. Minneapolis: Burgess Publishing Co., 1972.

Lennette, E. H., et al. (eds.): *Manual of Clinical Microbiology*, 3rd ed. Washington, DC: American Society of Microbiology, 1980.

MacFaddin, J. F.: *Biochemical Tests for Identification of Medical Bacteria*, 2nd ed. Baltimore: Williams & Wilkins, 1980.

Sack, R. B., Tilton, R. C., and Weissfeld, A. S.: *Cumitech 12: Laboratory Diagnosis of Bacterial Diarrhea*. Washington, DC: American Society for Microbiology, 1980.

Suppliers of Plated Media, Tubed Media, Sensitivity Testing Equipment, and Identification Kits

BBL Microbiology Systems, Cockeysville, MD: plated, tubed media; sensitivity testing discs; transport media (Amies, Port-A-Cul); Minitek Enteric Set, Nonfermenter Set; swabs

Gibco Diagnostics, Madison, WI: Plated, tubed media

Difco Laboratories, Deteroit, MI: staining kits, dehydrated media, sensitivity testing discs

Remel, Regional Media Laboratories, Manhattan, KS: plated, tubed media; transport media (Amies, PBS)

Scott Laboratories, Fiskville, RI: plated media

Inolex Biomedical Operations, Inolex Division, Glenwood, IL: Amies transport media; swabs

API, Analytab Products, Plainview, NY: API 20E System for *Enterobacteriaceae* and other gram negative bacteria, Staphase coagulase test system

PRACTICAL DIAGNOSTIC PROCEDURES FOR MYCOTIC DISEASES

MARIE H. ATTLEBERGER, D.V.M.

Auburn, Alabama

The majority of mycotic infections can be diagnosed in the practitioner's office. The practitioner should, however, have a basic knowledge of mycology so that he can recognize fungal elements (yeasts, hyphae, or spherules).

Obtaining the proper specimen is essential for making a diagnosis using direct smears or culture methods. The following equipment is needed to obtain a specimen:

Microscope with oil immersion lens

10 to 20 per cent potassium hydroxide in glycerol or dimethylsulfoxide (a commercial kit containing clearing and staining solutions is available*)

Parker's ink (optional)

Gram stain, hematologic stain, India ink

Glass slides, cover slips

Medical mycology textbook

COLLECTION OF CLINICAL SPECIMENS

HAIR

1. If the animal is very dirty, clean it with soap and water. If not, wash and thoroughly rinse the collection area and dry it completely.

2. With forceps, epilate many hairs from the edge of an *active* lesion. The hair should be pulled in the direction of growth, not "snapped off," as the root is needed for culture. Look for broken, stubby hairs, which are often infected.

3. If a sample is to be sent to a laboratory, place a sufficient amount of hair in a clean envelope labelled with the patient's data, including any therapy.

4. Animals under treatment should have any therapy withheld for at least one week before obtaining specimens.

5. Examine hairs in wet mounts for hyphae, arthrospores, or both.

SKIN

1. If necessary, clean the skin with an alcohol gauze sponge (cotton leaves too many fibers).

2. Scrape the periphery of the lesion with a scalpel. If more than one lesion is present, several should be scraped. Pool scrappings and place in a clean envelope or between clean glass slides.

3. Animals under treatment should have any therapy withheld for at least one week before obtaining specimens.

4. Examine scrapings in wet mounts for hyphae, arthrospores, or both.

5. Dermatophytes will live for several weeks in the specimen. Specimens from lesions due to *Candida* or other yeasts should be sent to the laboratory as soon as possible in some type of transport medium to prevent drying.

NAILS

1. *Proven* nail infections in animals are rare.

2. Diseased nails should be scraped with a scalpel blade so that fine pieces are collected.

3. Place the scrapings in paper or between slides for submission to the laboratory or for direct microscopic examination for hyphae, arthrospores, or both.

4. Debris under nails also should be cultured.

5. An avulsed nail should be placed in a Petri dish or envelope.

6. A nail micronizer† is available to reduce the nail to a fine powder.

BIOPSY SPECIMEN

1. Surgical biopsies: place tissue specimen between two moistened gauze squares, which are then placed in a Petri dish.

2. Node biopsies: follow the previous step if the entire node is being used. For needle biopsy of the node, media should be inoculated immediately at the patient's side. Alternatively, a small amount of sterile water or broth can be used to keep the specimen moist.

3. Punch biopsy: place the sample in a small sterile tube in sterile water or broth.

4. If there is enough material, prepare a wet mount and/or slide for hematologic staining.

---

*Dermassay, Pitman-Moore, Washington Crossing, NJ.

†Micro Labs, Inc., W. Freed, IN.

FLUIDS

Collect all fluids as aseptically as possible, and send them to lab at once. Contaminating bacteria and saprophytic fungi can prevent recovery of pathogenic fungi.

1. Urine: place sample in sterile tube, centrifuge, and use sediment for culture and direct smears.

2. Cerebrospinal fluid: place sample in small sterile tube. If cryptococcosis is suspected, make India ink preparation.

3. Pleural or abdominal fluid: place sample in small sterile tube. If fluid from thoracic cavity contains flakes or granules, be sure to include these as well. Stain granules with Gram stain and/or hematologic stain. Granules are frequently seen in nocardiosis and actinomycosis. When culturing granules, first wash them in sterile saline. A wet mount may be useful.

4. Transtracheal or bronchial washing: place sample in sterile tube. Washings should be centrifuged and the sediment cultured and examined in a wet mount.

5. Nasal flush: centrifuge and examine sediment in a wet mount for hyphae.

6. Fluid from anterior chamber of eye (used primarily for culturing for ocular blastomycosis: place sample in small sterile tube or inoculate media at patient's side. Make wet mount.

7. Prostatic fluid (for blastomycosis): place sample in small sterile tubes. Make wet mount.

EXUDATES

1. If possible, aspirate from unopened lesions and place sample in small sterile tube. If necessary, saline can be added to prevent specimen from drying out.

2. Exudates from open draining lesions, ulcers, fistulous tracts, and so on are usually contaminated with bacteria and, possibly, saprophytic fungi.

EARS

A swab from each ear, properly labelled, is needed. If direct smears are needed in addition to culture, two swabs from each ear should be submitted. Since yeasts are frequently incriminated in ear infections, some hematologic stain should be used. These stains do not distort the yeast morphology, as does the gram stain.

EYE

1. For mycotic infection of the cornea, aseptically remove small pieces of the diseased area. Some of these pieces should immediately be placed directly on the culture medium. Some should be directly placed into a drop of potassium hydroxide for microscopic examination.

2. If exudate is present, a swab moistened in sterile water or broth may be used. Immediate culturing is recommended. Culturettes are satisfactory. Platinum spatulas are also available for obtaining specimens.

NASAL POLYPS

If nasal polyps show small white specks, some of the material should be crushed and examined in a wet mount for spherules with endospores, suggestive of rhinosporidiosis.

DIRECT EXAMINATION OF CLINICAL SPECIMENS

WET MOUNT

Most specimens suspected of containing fungi are examined in wet mounts to prevent distortion of the morphology. It is strongly recommended that this examination be performed by the practitioner in his office when the animal's history so indicates. A fungus infection should be considered in all chronic conditions that fail to respond to an accepted treatment or for which there is an uncommon etiology.

Put one or two drops of potassium hydroxide or other clearing solution on a slide. Place some of the material to be examined in this solution and cover. The preparation may be warmed if desired and examined under the $10\times$ and $40\times$ objectives. Oil is not needed.

If no fungi (hyphae, yeasts, spherules) are seen in the first examination, the slide should be held overnight and re-examined. The thickness and type of specimen influence the time needed for adequate clearing. If the clearing agent is in glycerol or dimethylsulfoxide, slides may be kept for several days.

When a drop or two of Parker's ink (blue black) is added to the clearing solution on the slide, it will outline the fungus, making it easier to find. Other inks may precipitate (Table 1).

HEMATOLOGIC STAINS

Any hematologic stain is suitable for staining exudates and will demonstrate the fungus without distorting it. These stains are especially recommended for demonstrating yeasts and the filaments and zoospores seen in dermatophilosis. The practitioner usually has one of these stains in his office and should follow manufacturer's directions for its use (see Table 1).

Table 1. *Microscopic Appearance of Fungi in the Tissue*

Disease	Microscopic Examination	Appearance in Tissue
Aspergillosis	Wet mount	Septate hyphae; sometimes mature fruiting heads may be seen
Candidiasis and other yeast infections	Wet mount	Budding and nonbudding yeasts; pseudohyphae may be present
	Hematologic stain	Best for smears of yeasts from dog's ears
Dermatophytosis (ring-worm)	Wet mount	Hair: arthrospores, hyphae, or sheath of spores around hair; skin and nails: arthrospores, hyphae
Mycetoma (eumycotic)	Wet mount	Crush granules, observe for dark brown chlamydospores and clear (hyaline) hyphae
Phaeohyphomycosis	Wet mount	Dark hyphae
Rhinosporidiosis	Wet mount	Spherules (some very large) with and without endospores
Sporotrichosis	Fluorescent antibody	Yeasts
	Gram or hematologic stain	These stains may demonstrate yeasts occasionally
Zygomycosis (phycomycosis)	Wet mount	Broad, relatively nonseptate hyphae
Fungi Causing Systemic Infection		
Blastomycosis	Wet mount	Thick-walled budding yeast; bud has broad base at attachment to mother cell
Coccidioidomycosis	Wet mount	Spherules with and without endospores
Cryptococcosis	India ink and water	Encapsulated yeast
Histoplasmosis	Hematologic stain	Small yeast with narrow neck where bud attaches; found in macrophages and other RE cells
Actinomycetes Causing Infection		
Actinomycosis	Gram stain (view under oil)	Gram positive, branching filaments; some show beading; clubs may be seen
	Water mount of flakes or granules (40×)	Clubs
Nocardiosis	Gram stain (view under oil)	Same as Actinomycosis
	Hank's or cold Kinyoun acid-fast stain with 1% Aq H_2SO_4 as decolorizer (oil)	Some nocardiae are totally to partially acid fast; lack of acid fastness does not rule out *Nocardia*
Dermatophilosis	Hematologic stain (view under oil)	Branched tapered filaments that divide transversely and longitudinally to form packets of coccoid cells; sometimes only packets of cells or sparsely scattered cells are found

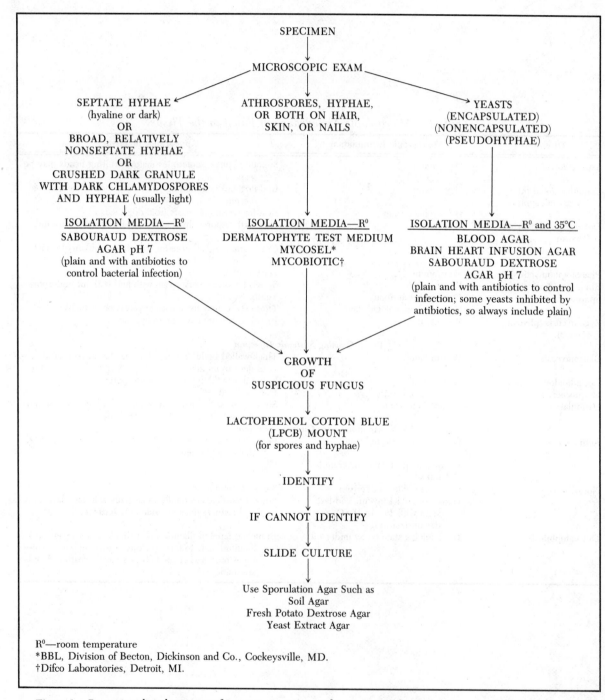

Figure 1.   Processing clinical specimens for yeasts, ringworm, and opportunistic fungus infections in veterinary medicine.

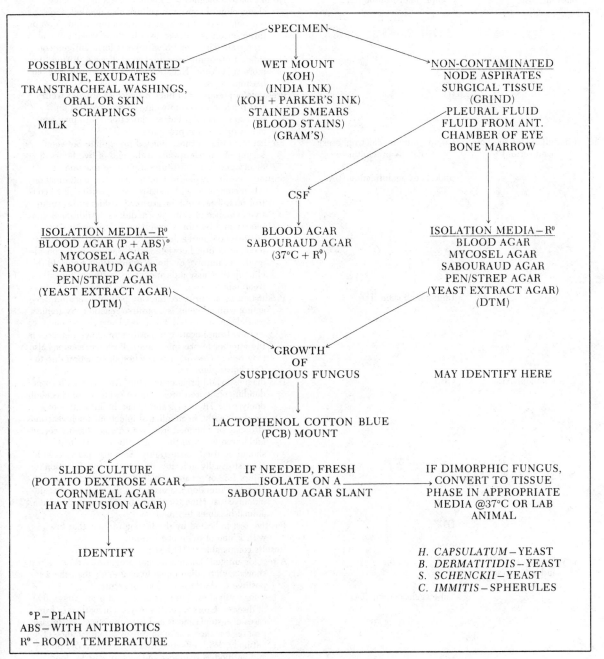

Figure 2. Processing clinical specimens for systemic fungus infections in veterinary medicine.

Table 2.* *Fungal Serology

Disease	Serologic Tests	Remarks
Aspergillosis	Immunodiffusion (ID) (agar-gel test, precipitin test)	Presence of one or more precipitin bands interacting with the antigen is indicative of some form of aspergillosis.
Blastomycosis	Complement fixation (CF)	Do not make a diagnosis of blastomycosis on serology alone; clinical signs and culture also needed. Cross reactions with other mycotic infections occur. Two or three serum samples at two- to three-week intervals preferred. Titers of 1:8 with yeast form antigen considered presumptive evidence of disease. Rising titers more significant. Negative reaction does not rule out blastomycosis.
	ID	Presence of precipitin in lines A (close to antigen well) and B (close to serum well) is a positive test and indicates recent or current infection. Sera may contain A or A and B precipitins.
Candidiasis (nonhemolized serum)	Counterimmunoelectrophoresis (CEP) (A precipitin test)	Formation of one or more lines of precipitate between serum and antigen walls at the end of two hours of electrophoresis constitutes a positive reaction.
	Slide latex agglutination (LA)	Serum is positive when it demonstrates 2+ agglutination when compared with negative and positive (2+) control sera. Titers of 8 or greater considered presumptive evidence of systemic candidiasis. Additional samples should be run. Conversion from negative to positive (1:4) for agglutinins or a fourfold or greater increase in titer between serum specimens is considered presumptive evidence of infection. Fourfold decline in titer may indicate success with antifungal treatment.
	Immunodiffusion (ID)	Production of one or more lines by patient's serum interacting with antigens is a positive reaction. Systemic candidiasis suspected when serial serum specimens convert from negative to positive or show increases in the number of precipitin lines. Positive reactions also may reflect *Candida* colonization or infection due to *Torulopsis glabrata*.
Coccidioidomycosis	CF	Has diagnostic and prognostic value. Any titer with coccidioidin considered presumptive evidence of coccidioidomycosis. Titers of 2 and 4 may be indicative of residual, early, or meningeal infection. Such reactions also may be obtained from patients not having coccidioidomycosis. With titers of 1:8 or less, ID test should be used concurrently. Sera also positive with ID test usually indicates recent or active infection. Titers 1:32 or greater usually indicate dissemination. Negative titers do not exclude a diagnosis of coccidioidomycosis. High titers may become negative when animal becomes terminal.
	ID	Positive test indicated by production of lines that fuse with F line of reference serum.
	CEP	Results comparable to ID test but more rapid.
Cryptococcosis (CSF and urine in addition to serum)	LA	A test for antigen. Diagnostic and prognostic. Positive test shows agglutination equal to or greater than the 2+ positive *C. neoformans* control serum.
	Tube agglutination (TA)	A test for antibodies. Titers of 2 or greater are suggestive of disease. Cross reactions may occur with sera from cases of histoplasmosis and blastomycosis. As disease progresses, excess antigen causes disappearance of antibody. With effective therapy, antigen disappears and antibodies reappear and may persist for long periods after cessation of therapy. A negative test does not exclude cryptococcosis.
	Indirect fluorescent antibody IFA	Staining intensity of 2+ or greater is presumptive evidence of active cryptococcosis or may reflect past infection or a cross reaction. Negative test does not exclude cryptococcosis.

Table 2. *Fungal Serology (Continued)*

Disease	Serologic Tests	Remarks
Histoplasmosis	CF	Two antigens used; histoplasmin from mycelial form and the yeast form of *H. capsulatum.* Yeast form more sensitive. Interpretation may be difficult because of cross reactions or nonspecific reactions with the antigens. A titer of 1:8 is usually considered presumptive evidence of histoplasmosis. More than one serum sample should be run, and rising titers are more significant. ID tests should also be performed.
	ID	Test based on development of H and M lines. The H line develops nearest the antiserum wall and occurs less frequently than M lines. H line seen most in patients with active histoplasmosis and may be detected a year or more after apparent clinical recovery. The M line is closest to the antigen well and is seen in patients with acute and chronic histoplasmosis. The M lines may be indicative of active or past infection or antibody induced by a recent skin test with histoplasmin.
	CEP	Results comparable to ID test but more rapid.
Sporotrichosis	LA	Titers of 4 or greater considered presumptive evidence of sporotrichosis.
	TA	Titers of 8 or greater with the yeast form antigen considered presumptive evidence of sporotrichosis if clinical signs present. Because false positives occasionally occur in the range between 8 and 16 with sera from patients with nonfungal infections, a minimum titer of 16 would be needed in the absence of clinical evidence of the disease.

GRAM STAIN

This stain is recommended when examining a specimen for gram positive, branching filaments seen in nocardiosis and actinomycosis. It is generally too heavy a stain for filaments and zoospores seen in dermatophilosis and tends to distort yeast morphology (see Table 1).

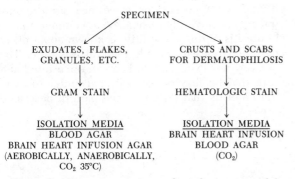

Figure 3. Processing specimens for infections caused by some actinomycetes.

CULTURE

The practitioner can successfully culture for ringworm fungi in his office. Other fungi, however, are probably best cultured in a laboratory equipped for this purpose.

Commercially prepared media are available, and Figures 1, 2, and 3 may be referred to when culturing for pathogenic and opportunistic fungi, yeasts, and actinomycetes.

SEROLOGY

Table 2 shows the tests available and all require nonhemolyzed serum. Only the tests generally in use are mentioned here.

SUPPLEMENTAL READING

Palmer, D. F., Kaufman, L., Kaplan, W., and Cavallaro, J. J.: *Serodiagnosis of Mycotic Diseases.* Springfield, IL: Charles C Thomas, 1977.

Enteric Infections

CANINE VIRAL ENTERITIS

ROY V. H. POLLOCK, D.V.M.

Ithaca, New York

Identifying the cause of emesis and diarrhea in dogs is always a diagnostic challenge; a wide variety of physical, chemical, and infectious agents can produce a similar clinical syndrome (see Clinical Management of Acute Gastroenteritis Including Virus-Induced Enteritis, page 1171). Fortunately, appropriate therapy can usually be initiated without a definitive diagnosis.

In 1978 it was recognized that viral enteritis needed to be included in the differential diagnosis of vomiting and diarrhea in dogs. In the spring of that year, the first clinical outbreak of canine coronaviral enteritis in the United States was described; and in the fall canine parvovirus was isolated. Although canine coronavirus (CCV) had apparently been present in the dog population for at least a decade, canine parvovirus (CPV) is truly a new pathogen; retrospective serologic studies have failed to identify antibodies to CPV in serum samples collected prior to 1977.

Nevertheless, canine viral enteritis is now recognized as a significant cause of morbidity and mortality, especially among puppies. Although the true incidence of viral enteritis and the percentage of virus-induced gastrointestinal illnesses seen in practice are not known, viral enteritis must always be considered when a dog is presented with an acute onset of emesis and diarrhea. Parvoviral enteritis, in particular, continues to cause significant morbidity and mortality, especially among 6- to 16-week-old pups. The present incidence is lower now, however, than in the first three years following its introduction (1978 to 1980). This is because all dogs were initially susceptible, favoring rapid and wide spread of infection; now, however, the great majority of dogs are immune by virtue of vaccination or previous infection. Hence, largescale outbreaks are unlikely to recur.

CAUSAL AGENTS

The two most important causes of viral enteritis in dogs are canine coronavirus (CCV) and canine parvovirus (CPV). Both are widespread in the world's canine population. Serologic surveys indicate that subclinical infection is common; in kennels, 50 to 90 per cent of dogs may have serologic evidence of previous infection with one or both viruses.

A canine rotavirus has also been observed in the feces of neonatal dogs with diarrhea, but its etiologic role has not been clearly established. Again, serologic evidence suggests that subclinical infection is common. Although rotaviruses have been shown to be important causes of neonatal diarrhea in other species, including humans, it remains to be demonstrated whether this is also true for dogs.

Canine distemper virus can, on rare occasions, also produce a hemorrhagic diarrhea, and other, as yet unidentified, viruses have been observed in stool samples from dogs with enteritis. Undoubtedly, additional viral causes of enteritis will be discovered as researchers further examine diarrheic dog feces.

The possibility of other viral pathogens notwithstanding, this article will confine its discussion to CPV and CCV enteritides, since these are the only viral agents currently recognized as common causes of enteritis in dogs. Too little is known about other viral enteritides to include them at this time. The clinician, however, should keep an open mind and recall that he may occasionally encounter cases of viral enteritis that do not fit the pattern described here.

CLINICAL SIGNS

The clinical signs accompanying CCV or CPV infection vary from undetectable to severe and rapidly fatal. Dogs of all ages can be infected, but typical cases now seem to occur primarily among 6- to 16-week-old pups.

Often the pup has been very recently acquired, either from a pet shop or a private breeder. The owner has usually noticed that the pup was lethargic or inappetent the evening before more overt clinical signs appeared. On presentation, the pup is usually febrile, depressed, dehydrated, and vomiting or passing diarrheic stool. The feces may be simply watery, tinged with blood, or frankly hemorrhagic.

Other physical findings are usually unremarkable, although about one dog in ten displays abdominal guarding, which might lead the clinician to suspect pancreatitis or intestinal obstruction. Pyrexia is usually more marked with CPV enteritis than with CCV infection. Indeed, dogs with CCV enteritis generally have normal or even subnormal temperatures. Complete blood counts are usually normal with CCV enteritis but may help to establish a diagnosis in cases of CPV infection. About one-third of dogs with clinical CPV infection are leukopenic at the time of admission. Serial hemograms will detect transient leukopenia in an additional 50 per cent and lymphopenia in most. Atypical "reactive" lymphocytes are frequently present and support the diagnosis of a viral etiology. Severe leukopenia warrants a guarded to grave prognosis. In general, leukopenia accompanying other signs of enteritis is strong presumptive evidence of CPV infection. Leukocytosis is usually observed during recovery.

Noncontrast radiographic changes are nonspecific. Barium sulfate studies, however, reveal several abnormal findings that are highly suggestive of CPV enteritis. These include flocculation of contrast material, scalloping of the luminal margin, and a cobblestone pattern at the contrast-mucosa interface (Farrow, 1982). Care must be exercised when interpreting radiographic studies in dogs that may have viral enteritis, however. Many of the radiographic signs mimic those of an intestinal obstruction, including small bowel dilatation, gas-capped fluid levels, and greatly prolonged transit time.

The clinical course of the disease is usually five to ten days, although intermittent diarrhea may persist in some dogs with CCV enteritis for up to three weeks. Recovery appears to be complete in dogs that survive. Long-term debilities resulting from viral enteritis have not been documented in dogs.

A myocardial form of CPV infection has also been described in very young pups. The usual manifestation was sudden unexpected death among otherwise healthy pups. Post-mortem examination revealed a nonsuppurative myocarditis, which was eventually shown to be caused by the same virus (CPV) that causes enteritis in older dogs. Fairly frequent initially, the myocardial form is becoming increasingly rare. Fatal myocarditis apparently results only when pups are infected within a very few days of birth. Since maternally derived antibody protects pups against parvoviral infection and since most adults have been either vaccinated or previously infected, almost all puppies are now immune to infection during this critical period.

DIAGNOSIS

A diagnosis of viral enteritis should be considered in all acute cases of vomiting and diarrhea in dogs, especially if more than one animal has been affected simultaneously or sequentially (see Clinical Management of Acute Gastroenteritis Including Virus-Induced Enteritis, page 1171). A history of vaccination is not sufficient to rule out CPV enteritis in young dogs; maternally derived antibody may have suppressed the development of an active immune response to vaccination.

A definitive diagnosis of viral enteritis cannot be established from the history and clinical signs alone. However, although a definitive diagnosis may be important for epidemiologic or other reasons, it is not a prerequisite for the initiation of appropriate therapy. In fact, it is essential to begin vigorous supportive therapy immediately, long before virologic assays could be completed.

A definitive diagnosis can be established in several ways. Parvoviral, coronaviral, or rotaviral virions can be identified by electron microscopy in stool samples collected during the acute phase of illness. This method is relatively insensitive, however, and false negatives may be common. Furthermore, CCV may be difficult to distinguish from artifacts in the specimen. Direct isolation of CPV or CCV from feces, intestinal contents, or mesenteric lymph nodes can be attempted by many diagnostic laboratories. A positive stool hemagglutination test may suggest CPV, but false positives are common unless known antiserum is used to perform a simultaneous blocking test. Thus, the results of in-office tests (HA) must be interpreted with caution. A sensitive ELISA test for CPV in stool samples has been described recently. All fecal tests are applicable only during the period of most active viral shed (i.e., during clinical illness).

In fatal cases, the microscopic lesions of CPV enteritis are usually sufficiently distinct to permit definitive diagnosis, even when gross lesions were not obvious. A pathologic diagnosis of coronaviral enteritis, however, cannot usually be made with surety. Fluorescent antibody staining of frozen sections can be used for diagnosis of both CPV and CCV.

Serologic tests are rapid, relatively inexpensive, and widely available, but their shortcomings must be kept in mind. Dogs infected with CPV usually have high levels of circulating antibody at the time of hospitalization. Thus, although a marked rise in titer between acute and convalescent samples is a diagnostic criterion for CCV infection, it is seldom observed in cases of CPV. Moreover, the mere presence of a high anti-CPV titer is not diagnostic of active infection either, since antibody titers remain high for months after initial infection. Thus, in order to establish a diagnosis it is important to demonstrate that the anti-CPV antibody is predominantly of the IgM class, indicating recent infection. This is less important in puppies; a very high titer in a pup with diarrhea would be strongly suggestive of active infection. Low titers in such pups would likely be of maternal antibody origin. Finding no or only a low titer suggests that there is some other cause for the enteritis.

TREATMENT

The treatment of acute diarrhea is discussed in detail elsewhere (see page 1171). A few points will be repeated here. Treatment of viral enteritis is supportive only; there are no effective antiviral agents. The primary objective of therapy is to replace fluid and electrolyte losses, since dehydration and electrolyte imbalances themselves may be fatal. Lactated Ringer's solution is a good basic replacement fluid. Potassium, bicarbonate, or other supplementation may be indicated (see page 1171).

Broad spectrum antibiotics should be administered to control secondary bacterial infection, particularly in animals with suspected parvoviral enteritis in which some compromise of the immune system is presumed. The oral route is contraindicated, certainly during the acute phase of illness, because of the delayed gastric emptying time and the possibility of emesis. The value of other oral medications is moot, particularly those containing antibiotics intended to suppress intraluminal bacterial growth; such preparations may even be contraindicated (see page 1171). Intestinal motility modifiers may partially control the diarrhea but may also increase absorption of endotoxins. Bismuth subsalicylate (Pepto-Bismol) is more effective than kaolin-pectin preparations in the treatment of viral enteritis.

Disseminated intravascular coagulation may develop as a terminal event in some dogs; attempts at treatment have been uniformly unsuccessful. Good nursing care is indispensable.

TRANSMISSION

Both CPV and CCV are highly contagious. The primary route of infection is apparently fecal-oral. Clinically ill dogs shed prodigious amounts of infective virus for at least one to two weeks. Virus then persists as an environmental contaminant. Canine parvovirus, in particular, is extremely hardy; virus has been shown to remain infectious in dog feces for more than six months at room temperature.

Good hygienic measures, such as thorough and frequent cleansing with detergent/chlorine bleach solutions, will help to reduce the amount of virus in the hospital or kennel environment. It has *not* been possible, however, to control either of these infections by sanitation alone or even by typical isolation procedures. The emphasis, then, must be on prophylactic immunization.

IMMUNIZATION

There is no vaccine against CCV at the present time. Efforts to develop one are hampered by apparent antigenic differences among strains and by the fact that parenteral inoculation failed to provide immunity to oral challenge. Thus, little can be done at the present time to prevent CCV infection besides maintaining good hygienic practices and using care when introducing or regrouping dogs. As previously noted, however, even scrupulous hygiene is seldom sufficient to contain these highly contagious viruses. Prophylactic immunization for CPV (and CCV if effective vaccines can be developed) should be part of the routine health program for dogs.

Four general types of vaccine are available for immunization of dogs against CPV: inactivated (killed) or live virus vaccines containing either CPV or the closely related feline panleukopenia virus (feline parvovirus [FPV]). Representatives of each type have been licensed by the USDA for use in dogs. The following is a generic discussion of each type based on available research findings. Performance data on individual vaccines should be requested from the manufacturer, and unsupported claims or generalizations should be viewed skeptically.

In general, inactivated CPV and inactivated FPV vaccines behave similarly. The antigenic cross reactivity between FPV and CPV is sufficiently great that reciprocal cross-protection occurs. The magnitude of the response to an inactivated vaccine is proportional to its antigenic mass, which varies considerably among different lots of vaccine. Some adjuvants may help ensure vigorous and sustained responses.

The humoral immune response to inactivated vaccines decays with time; antibody titers usually fall to low levels within two to four months. In our studies, killed vaccines provided protection against *clinical* disease for at least six months, but subclinical infections, which included active shedding of virulent virus, occurred as early as five weeks after vaccination. Thus, most killed parvovirus vaccines appear to adequately protect the individual dog from clinical illness, but they fail to prevent infection and spread of infection in the population.

Live vaccines generally stimulated greater and more durable immune responses than did killed vaccines. The response to live FPV vaccine was extremely variable, however, apparently depending upon whether viral replication (productive infection) occurred. Dogs in which there was apparently no FPV replication responded to the antigen in a manner similar to that observed following inoculation with inactivated virus; the immune response was proportional to the antigenic mass and decayed rapidly with time. Dogs in which FPV replication was demonstrated had antibody responses that paralleled those observed after CPV infection; such dogs were completely refractory to CPV infection for at least 13 months. The number of dogs responding in this fashion appears to be related to the amount of living FPV in the vaccine and perhaps also to the FPV strain employed.

Dogs immunized with an adequately attenuated strain of CPV developed antibody responses identical to those observed after natural infection: very high titers that persisted for more than two years. Dogs immunized with attentuated live CPV were completely refractory to infection for at least two years.

Vaccinal CPV is shed from inoculated dogs and immunizes contacts. No evidence of reversion to virulence could be demonstrated in the sequential back passages required for licensure. Speculations about the dangers of further mutations of vaccinal CPV have been greatly overemphasized. The safety of live parvovirus vaccines for pregnant bitches has not yet been conclusively demonstrated, however. Therefore it would seem prudent not to immunize pregnant dogs with live vaccines until further information is available.

In summary, when used according to manufacturer's directions, all four types of parvovirus vaccine licensed for use in dogs have generally performed adequately in the field, especially in adults. Immunization of puppies, as discussed hereafter, has been less successful. Annual revaccination is recommended by the manufacturers of all four types, but this interval has not been demonstrated directly by experiment in all cases. Live CPV vaccines appear to engender a more durable barrier to infection and subsequent viral shed.

VACCINATION OF PUPS

Puppies receive antibody from an immune dam through the placenta and colostrum. Absorption from the colostrum accounts for about 90 per cent of the pup's total maternally derived antibody. Since nearly all breeding bitches have been either vaccinated or previously infected, nearly all pups born nowadays receive some antibody. The amount is proportional to the dam's titer.

Initially, when the pups' maternal antibody titers are high, they are refractory to infection. Hence, CPV enteritis is now rarely encountered in pups younger than six weeks of age, and the myocardial form of the disease (which apparently results only from perinatal infection) is now very rare. As pups grow, however, their maternal antibody titers decline as a result of dilution and catabolism. The half-life is approximately nine days. Thus, all pups eventually become susceptible. The age of susceptibility depends on the amount of antibody they received initially, which, in turn, depends on the antibody titer of the dam. Most pups become susceptible between 6 and 16 weeks of age.

Unfortunately, during the period in which pups are refractory to infection they are also refractory to active immunization. In fact, it appears that pups may not respond to vaccination for one to three weeks after they become susceptible to field challenge. That is, there is a critical period during which we are unable to provide protection for puppies. Normally, this would not be a cause for concern (a similar situation exists for panleukopenia in cats), since the risk of exposure during the period of susceptibility is usually slight. In certain situations, however, like very large breeding colonies or puppy broker/pet shop operations, exposure is almost assured during this period.

Under such conditions, it has been virtually impossible to completely prevent infection and morbidity among puppies, even with rigorous vaccination schedules. Live CPV vaccines are more effective in such problem kennels; they apparently are able to immunize pups at a somewhat younger age than live FPV or inactivated virus vaccines. Even so, complete control is not always achieved.

It is not yet possible to predict with surety at what age a given pup will respond to vaccination. Efforts to develop a predictive nomograph, similar to that available for distemper, have been thwarted by the variety of vaccines in use and the lack of a standardized serologic test.

Thus, the most prudent recommendation at this time is to give a series of vaccinations beginning at the time of first presentation (typically 6 to 8 weeks) and continuing until 16 weeks of age. The timing and number of vaccinations will depend on the professional assessment of the risk, the value of the animals, and the expense involved. In most cases, a two to four week interval will be selected. Regardless of the timing, number, and type of vaccine used, the owners should be warned that no program is an absolute guarantee against infection; pups might be exposed at a time when they have not yet responded to vaccination.

SUMMARY

Viruses were only recently recognized as important causes of vomiting and diarrhea in dogs. Future research will likely identify other viral enteritides besides those caused by CPV and CCV, and, despite the availability of effective CPV vaccines, viral enteritis will continue to be a significant clinical problem in dogs.

REFERENCES AND SUPPLEMENTAL READING

Carmichael, L. E., and Binn, L. N.: New enteric viruses in the dog. Adv. Vet. Sci. Comp. Med. 25:1, 1981.
Carmichael, L. E., Joubert, J. C., and Pollock, R. V. H.: A modified live canine parvovirus strain with novel plaque characteristics. I. Viral attenuation and dog response. Cornell Vet. 71:408, 1981.
Farrow, C. S.: Radiographic appearance of canine parvovirus enteritis. J.A.V.M.A. 180:43, 1982.
Glickman, L. T., and Appel, M. J. G.: A controlled field trial of an attenuated canine origin parvovirus vaccine. Comp. Cont. Ed. Vet. Pract. 4:888, 1982.
Kramer, J. M., Meunier, P. C., and Pollock, R. V. H.: Canine parvovirus: Update. V.M./S.A.C. 75:1541, 1980.
Moreau, P. M.: Canine viral enteritis. Comp. Cont. Educ. Vet. Pract. 2:540, 1980.
Pollock, R. V. H., and Carmichael, L. E.: Dog response to inactivated feline panleukopenia virus and canine parvovirus vaccines. Cornell Vet. 72:1, 1982.
Pollock, R. V. H., and Carmichael, L. E.: Maternally derived immunity to canine parvovirus infection: Transfer, decline and interference with vaccination. J.A.V.M.A. 180:37, 1982.
Pollock, R. V. H., and Carmichael, L. E.: Use of modified live virus feline panleukopenia vaccine to immunize dogs against canine parvovirus. Am. J. Vet. Res. 44:169, 1982.
Weirup, M., Olson, P., Hedhammar, A., Klingeborn, B., and Karlsson, K. A.: Evaluation of a killed feline panleukopenia virus vaccine against parvoviral enteritis in dogs. Am. J. Vet. Res. 43:2183, 1982.

FELINE ENTERIC VIRUSES

SANDY BALDWIN, D.V.M.

Ithaca, New York

This article will briefly discuss the viruses that have been shown to produce diarrhea in cats as well as those viruses that are, for now, only associated with disease. Several of the viruses are presumed to be possible etiologic factors in feline diarrhea only because similar viruses have been found to produce diarrhea in other species, including humans. It will be assumed that other well-known causes of diarrhea, such as bacteria (e.g., *Salmonella* and *Clostridium*), foreign bodies (string), endoparasites, intussusception, and allergic responses, have all been excluded as possible causes of enteric disease.

Viral diarrhea, particularly chronic diarrhea, is difficult to definitively diagnose, especially if one does not have access to an electron microscope or viral isolation techniques. Both of these techniques are expensive, and, in the case of viral isolation, the outcome of immediate treatment would probably have "decided" the case long before the laboratory results returned. This also holds true for serologic tests, such as paired serum samples.

This article deals with the growing list of enteric viruses found in cats, and some comparisons will be made to the viral diseases that exist in humans and other animals. These viruses include feline parvovirus (panleukopenia virus), feline rotavirus, feline astrovirus, feline enteric coronavirus, feline calicivirus, and feline leukemia virus. Feline leukemia virus is covered on page 1193 and will not be discussed here. In addition, much information on the therapy of diarrhea is discussed in the article that follows.

FELINE PARVOVIRUS (FELINE PANLEUKOPENIA VIRUS)

Feline parvovirus produces an acute, severe, watery diarrhea in all Felidae as well as in raccoons, coatimundis, and mink. Parvoviruses are one of the smallest of the known viruses, measuring about 20 to 22 nm, and contain a single DNA strand surrounded by a protein capsid. The viruses are non-enveloped and are resistant to most chemicals. However, Clorox at a 1/32 dilution is a good virucidal mixture. The virus can remain viable and infectious for more than one year at room temperature. Parvoviruses are known to cause severe diarrhea in several species, including the dog, cat, mink, and humans. The lesions and site of action are identical in the dog and cat. This is also true for mink enteritis virus, which is thought to be antigenically identical to, but a variant of, feline parvovirus. Canine parvovirus may be another variant of feline parvovirus. In humans, a small, 22- to 25-nm virus particle (the Norwalk agent), is known to cause diarrhea. It can be transmitted via fecal extracts and is thought to be either a parvovirus or a calicivirus.

Since the virus requires help in replicating, it infects rapidly dividing cells. This replication requirement explains the clinical signs. *In utero* infection produces many kinds of reproductive failures, ranging from resorption, stillbirth, mummification, and abortion to weak kittens (fading kittens). Infection at the time of parturition and up to about ten days postnatally produces cerebellar hypoplasia, thymic atrophy, and possible blindness due to retinal dysplasia. Mild intestinal lesions may develop, since cellular turnover rate in the crypt epithelium is minimal in this neonatal period. After 10 to 14 days, the cerebellum is no longer dividing as rapidly as before. However, the bone marrow and small intestinal crypt cells are, so clinical signs are referable to these sites of viral infection.

In the intestines, the virus infects the rapidly dividing crypt cells. Normally, crypt cells divide in the basal area. As they mature, they migrate up to the tips of the villi and are eventually sloughed off, a process enhanced by the abrasive action of food passing the tips of the villi. This migrating process takes approximately two to three days. When parvovirus infects the crypt cells, the cells die and become necrotic; no replacement cells migrate up the villi, and they progressively become blunted and denuded and may completely collapse. No absorption of water and/or nutrients will then occur, and severe watery diarrhea, malnutrition, and dehydration are the end results.

Since the bone marrow cells are also infected, the leukocytes, another cell type with a rapid turnover rate, become depleted in peripheral blood. This is the origin of the name feline panleukopenia.

The severity of the disease varies with the age of the cat and, obviously, with the virulence of the virus. The cat may be affected peracutely and may be presented to the practitioner either dead or dying. Frequently, the onset is so rapid that the owner thinks that the cat has been poisoned. In its acute form, the cat is depressed, anorectic, and vomiting, and dehydration, abdominal pain, and diarrhea are evident. White blood cell (WBC) counts taken at this time may be normal or severely depressed, often less than 1000 WBC/mm^3. In mild cases, the cat may be noticed to be slightly "off," but it may not show any signs referable to specific disease and many times will never be seen by the practitioner.

The differential diagnosis list would include such diseases as salmonellosis (which also frequently produces leukopenia and a fetid diarrhea), feline leukemia virus (discussed hereafter), clostridial diseases, and giardiasis, among others. A diagnosis of salmonellosis is made on the basis of a positive fecal culture for *Salmonella,* although positive results must be viewed with caution, since some cats are carriers. Salmonellosis usually responds to intensive fluid therapy and antibiotics, such as Tribrissen, Amoxicillin, and Chloromycetin. Antibiotics should not be used in any animal with salmonellosis *unless* systemic disease is present. If only enteric disease is present and antibiotics are used, the disease may become systemic, resistant forms emerge more rapidly, and the period of fecal shed becomes more prolonged.

Treatment of parvoviral infections consists of supportive therapy, since there is no specific antiviral therapy currently available. This therapy should include high levels of intravenous fluids and broad spectrum antibiotics. Nothing should be given orally, particularly if the cat is vomiting, since little can be absorbed very well through a denuded, injured mucosa and since oral medication may induce further vomiting, dehydration, and electrolyte imbalance. Antibiotics are given prophylactically for bacterial infections, since many cats will die from the severe septicemia associated with bacterial absorption and penetration across an injured intestinal mucosa.

Feline parvovirus is not seen as commonly as previously owing to the excellent vaccines now available. Kittens acquire a high level of immunity from immune queens. This colostral antibody will decrease over a period of 4 to 12 weeks, depending on the level of passive antibodies received in the colostrum. Since it is not known when this level is low enough to produce a response to vaccination, the kitten should be vaccinated at the first office visit and at four-week intervals until it is 12 to 14 weeks of age. If the cat is 12 to 14 weeks old at the first visit, only one dose of a MLV is necessary to protect against feline parvovirus. Two doses are needed for adequate protection if an inactivated vaccine is used or to provide protection against any respiratory viruses with polyvalent vaccines. Periodic booster protection is then indicated for feline parvovirus.

FELINE LEUKEMIA VIRUS

A single-strand RNA virus, feline leukemia virus, also infects rapidly dividing cells. In fact, one stage of the pathogenesis of leukemia virus infection has been shown to include infection of the crypt epithelial cells. As in parvovirus infection, the crypt epithelial cells and the villi are lost and diarrhea results. If the diarrhea persists beyond one week, parvovirus is an unlikely diagnosis, and thoughts should turn to other causative agents, particularly the panleukopenia-like syndrome of feline leukemia. Prognosis in leukemia is poor, and long-term infection is probable. Diagnosis can be made based on a positive Feleuk test coupled with a chronic nonresponsive diarrhea. Histopathology would not be of any benefit, since the results would be similar to those of parvovirus infection.

One should also remember that feline leukemia virus can produce large tumors in the gastrointestinal tract, and this condition may also present as a chronic diarrhea due to the space-occupying lesion.

CORONAVIRUS

Coronavirus, another single-strand RNA virus, is an important pathogen in many species of animals.

Notable coronaviruses producing diarrhea include calf coronavirus, porcine coronavirus, and the recently reported canine coronavirus. There appear to be two or three possible coronaviruses in the cat. One is known to be the etiologic factor in feline infectious peritonitis (FIP). A second coronavirus, found in approximately 10 per cent of cats in a virologic survey of enteric viruses in cats, is feline enteric coronavirus (FEC-1). It is morphologically distinct from the FIP virus, particularly in the size and shape of the surface projections. FEC can also be found in the feces of both coronavirus–antibody positive and negative cats, regardless of the magnitude of the titer. Work is presently under way to clinically and serologically determine the difference between FIP virus and FEC-1.

A second FEC (FEC-2) has also been described and has been determined to be indistinguishable from FIP virus. It is reported to produce a mild to inapparent diarrhea and fever in young kittens 4 to 12 weeks of age. Cats will appear to seroconvert to a coronaviral–antibody positive status following infection. It has been proposed that this second enteric coronavirus is ubiquitous in nature, prevalent in virtually all catteries, and possibly the reason that many cats have coronavirus antibody titers. It has been further suggested that FIP is a virulent variant of this mild enteric coronavirus.

Finally, another coronavirus also related antigenically to FIP virus has been found in a cat with fatal hemorrhagic enteritis. How this virus is related to the other feline coronaviruses is unknown at this time. It may possibly be a third enteric coronavirus.

In general, coronaviruses infect the tips of intestinal villi. The diarrhea usually is not as profuse or severe as is seen in parvovirus. This naturally varies with the virulence of the particular virus and how much of the villus tip becomes eroded. Some resorption of water does occur in the lower villi and crypt region, resulting in a milder diarrhea.

Further research is needed to clarify the confusion concerning the coronaviruses. This endeavor will be aided greatly by the ability to grow all of the viruses in tissue culture.

FELINE ASTROVIRUS

Astroviruses are small RNA viruses that present as either five- or six-pointed stars, as seen on electron microscopy. These new and unclassified viruses are known to produce profuse diarrhea in sheep, turkeys, humans, and possibly dogs. Reinoculation of fecal extracts containing astrovirus particles produces diarrhea in sheep. Astrovirus was found in the feces of one cat with diarrhea, but its role in feline diarrhea needs further evaluation. Until recently, research had been hampered by the inability to grow astrovirus in the laboratory.

FELINE CALICIVIRUS

Feline calicivirus (FCV) is another single-strand RNA virus that has been identified in the feces of cats with diarrhea. On electron microscopy, FCV appears to be similar to the astrovirus; however, FCV presents only as a five-pointed star, and the capsomers are more cup shaped. Many practitioners know FCV as a cause of upper respiratory infections, ulcerations, and pneumonia in cats. It appears that a variant may also be a cause of diarrhea and, possibly, malabsorption. In humans, several epidemics of gastrointestinal disease caused by caliciviruses have been reported in school environments in both England and Japan. Another intestinal virus in humans thought to be either a calicivirus or, more likely, a parvovirus is the Norwalk agent.

Further work is needed to grow the intestinal caliciviruses in cell cultures, inoculate specific pathogen-free cats, and follow the disease progression, if one exists. Also, until the virus can be cultured in the laboratory, any cross reaction with respiratory strains of calicivirus can only be speculated upon.

FELINE ROTAVIRUS

Rotaviruses have been isolated from several cats, but they have not been definitively linked to disease. In all species from which they have been isolated, rotaviruses have been a cause of severe diarrhea, particularly in the neonate. Rotavirus is known to be a major cause of the neonatal calf diarrhea complex and of diarrhea in mice, horses, goats, sheep, poultry, deer, antelope, and humans. It is estimated that more than 50 per cent of the children hospitalized with viral gastroenteritis have rotavirus disease. As with astrovirus and coronavirus, the rotavirus infects the tips of the villi, but perhaps not enough of the cells are infected to produce a disease state in cats. Recently, a cat with severe diarrhea was seen from which a rotavirus was tentatively isolated. This cat was also positive for leukemia. Perhaps an immunosuppressed cat may show signs referable to rotavirus infections; however, there may have been other factors involved in this case of fatal gastroenteritis, and no conclusions concerning rotavirus should be drawn until future research can provide more definitive answers.

CONCLUSIONS

Several new viruses have been described that may be implicated in feline enteric disease. The primary viral disease remains parvovirus. Several of the viruses are resistant, and contamination of the environment is an important disease factor. More definitive information about enteric viral diseases would be helpful to practitioners but will only be possible when the viruses can be grown in the laboratory and when more pathogenic studies are completed. For the present, references and comparisons to viruses of like type in other species can be used as possible guides, but much is only speculation.

SUPPLEMENTAL READING

Hoshino, Y., and Scott, F.W.: New insights in gastrointestinal viruses of cats. Cornell Vet. Submitted for publication, 1983.

McKeirnan, A. J., Evermann, J. F., Hargis, A., Miller, L. M., and Ott, R. L.: Isolation of feline coronaviruses from two cats with diverse disease manifestations. Feline Pract. 11:16, 1981.

Pedersen, N. C., Boyle, J. F., Floyd, K., Fudge, A., and Barker, J.: An enteric coronavirus infection of cats and its relationship to feline infectious peritonitis. Am. J. Vet. Res. 42:368, 1981.

CLINICAL MANAGEMENT OF ACUTE GASTROENTERITIS INCLUDING VIRUS-INDUCED ENTERITIS

JAMES F. ZIMMER, D.V.M.

Ithaca, New York

The past few years have seen a dramatic increase in the interest in and diagnosis of acute infectious gastroenteritis in dogs. Since its recognition in 1978, canine parvovirus enteritis has become established as a worldwide clinical disease of significant incidence. As a result of the interest generated in the parvovirus-induced disease in dogs, the canine coronavirus agent was rediscovered and its clinical significance recognized. More recently, rotavirus- and astrovirus-like agents have been found in the feces of dogs. The pathogenicity and clinical importance of these agents are yet to be determined.

Many cases of acute gastroenteritis that would have been attributed to nonspecific causes prior to the recognition of these viral agents are now diagnosed as viral in origin. In recent surveys of dogs manifesting clinical signs of acute gastroenteritis, these enteric viral agents were indeed the most frequently encountered enteropathogens and caused about one-third of such cases. Despite extensive bacteriologic and virologic examinations of these cases, however, the presence of these potential enteropathogens was identified in less than one-half of the patients. Conversely, no definitive identification of an infectious agent was made in the majority of the patients. Thus, within the population of dogs presenting with clinical signs of an acute gastroenteritis, those animals with an identifiable infectious disease could not be readily distinguished from those patients with signs caused by other disease processes. In that regard, the results of these surveys parallel the anecdotal experiences of clinical veterinarians. Also, on the basis of both theoretical and pragmatic considerations, these cases of acute gastroenteritis, both infectious and noninfectious in origin, can be managed with the same diagnostic and therapeutic protocols. In the following sections of this article, a differential diagnosis for acute gastroenteritis in the dog, a diagnostic protocol, and a therapeutic regimen are described.

CLINICAL CHARACTERIZATION AND DIFFERENTIAL DIAGNOSIS

The clinical manifestations of acute gastroenteritis, regardless of the cause, vary greatly. The severity of the most common clinical signs, vomiting and diarrhea, range from relatively mild and innocuous to severe and life-threatening. Other signs may or may not be present. The clinical signs documented in 40 confirmed cases of parvovirus enteritis and their frequencies are listed in Table 1. Recent serologic surveys, however, have demonstrated that the majority of dogs infected with parvovirus, especially those older than six months of age, had mild or inapparent infections not requiring veterinary care. It must also be remembered that disease processes other than virus-induced enteritis can produce this cluster of clinical signs. Table 2 contains a partial list of the differential diagnoses for

Table 1. *Clinical Signs in 40 Confirmed Cases of Canine Parvovirus Enteritis**

Clinical Sign	Frequency (%)
Diarrhea	100
Hemorrhagic	55
Nonhemorrhagic	45
Vomiting	85
Depression	48
Anorexia	48
Pyrexia	45
Dehydration	43
Leukopenia (by only one hemogram)	28
Tender abdomen	18

*Data from Pollock and Carmichael: 30th Gaines Veterinary Symposium, 1981.

acute gastroenteritis in the dog. Although this list does not include all the possible causes of signs of acute gastroenteritis in dogs, it does include those clinical problems that should be considered and ruled out first by the veterinarian. The results generated by applying the diagnostic protocol described in the next section of this article may enable the veterinarian to establish a definitive diagnosis and administer specific therapy.

DIAGNOSTIC PROTOCOL

The severity of the clinical signs present at the onset or that develop during the course of the disease determines the degree of effort to be applied in establishing a definitive diagnosis. Concurrent with any diagnostic evaluation of a patient with signs of acute gastroenteritis and integral to that diagnostic plan is the clinical assessment of the animal's response to symptomatic and supportive therapy. The steps in a thorough diagnostic plan for acute gastroenteritis in the dog are listed in Table 3.

The clinical history, signalment, and results of physical examination may indicate the underlying cause of the signs. In many cases, the diagnostic conclusions or even suspicions that develop from information gathered from the history and physical examination may warrant only symptomatic therapy

Table 2. *Differential Diagnoses for Acute Gastroenteritis in the Dog*

Dietary indiscretion	Gastrointestinal foreign bodies
Viral enteritis	Gastrointestinal parasites
Parvovirus	Intussusception
Coronavirus	Ingestion of toxins
Canine distemper	Acute pancreatitis
Others?	Hemorrhagic gastroenteritis
Bacterial enteritis	Hypoadrenocorticism
Salmonellosis	Various combinations of the above
Colibacillosis	
Others?	

Table 3. *Diagnostic Protocol for Acute Gastroenteritis in Dogs*

History and signalment
Physical examination
Response to treatment
Laboratory evaluation
    Fecal direct smears and flotation
    Hemogram
    Blood chemistry determinations
    Fecal hemagglutination
    Titers for canine parvovirus
    Fecal electron microscopy
    Fecal cultures (aerobic and anaerobic)
    Blood cultures (aerobic and anaerobic)
Radiographic examination
    Plain films
    Contrast studies
Endoscopic examination
Exploratory laparotomy

and subsequent assessment to response without further diagnostic intervention. Simple dietary management and the administration of oral medications may suffice in most patients presented with a brief history of moderate vomition and/or diarrhea and no clinical dehydration or other marked systemic signs.

More aggressive supportive therapy and further diagnostic evaluation may be warranted for patients that do not respond to treatment and those in which the history and physical findings suggest a more serious problem. For animals suffering from a severe and/or persistent diarrhea, the first logical step is examination of feces. The gross characteristics of the stool often indicate whether the small or large bowel is primarily affected. Microscopic examination of a saline slurry of a small amount of fresh fecal material may demonstrate the presence of motile protozoal pathogens such as *Giardia* or trichomonads. However, even repeated fresh, direct fecal smears will not identify all cases of protozoan infestation. Microscopic examination of the supernatants of several fecal specimens may be necessary to identify a parasitic infestation. The sediment should also be examined for parasitic larvae. However, parasitic infestation may not be the direct cause of the diarrhea. The clinical response to anthelmintic and/or antiprotozoal medications should indicate the significance of the parasitosis.

The results of a complete hemogram can be informative and can aid in the evaluation of a patient. Monitoring serial hemograms allows the veterinarian to follow the progress of a patient and assess response to treatment. The packed cell volume and concentration of plasma total solids reflect the degree of dehydration of the animal and may indicate excessive loss of blood or plasma proteins into the intestinal tract. The presence of a leukopenia may suggest a parvovirus-induced or severe bacterial enteritis. The severity of the leukopenia roughly correlates with the mortality of such cases.

As noted in Table 1 and as reported in other studies, most dogs with parvovirus enteritis did not have a leukopenia when assessed by only one hemogram. When followed sequentially, however, nearly 90 per cent of the dogs had a significant leukopenia. The duration of this leukopenia ranged from one to six days and averaged two days. Dogs recovering from parvovirus enteritis developed neutrophilic leukocytosis with a left shift. Several of the other diseases among the differential diagnoses (see Table 2) can produce a nonspecific leukocytosis in various stages of their courses. Therefore, to glean the greatest amount of information from the hemogram with the best accuracy, the veterinarian should perform sequential hemograms and evaluate their results in light of the clinical course of the disease.

Blood chemistry determinations provide a rapid, economic assessment of the animal's metabolic status and a rapid screen for the presence of azotemia, active hepatic disease, adrenocortical insufficiency, other electrolyte imbalances, and alkalosis. These results should help identify any underlying metabolic disorder that might be contributing to, causing, or resulting from the signs of acute gastroenteritis. Measurement of the serum concentrations of amylase and lipase aids in establishing the diagnosis of acute pancreatitis.

During the acute phase of viral enteritis, infected dogs shed large numbers of viral particles. A hemagglutination assay has been described to test for the presence of parvovirus virions in the feces. A positive result may suggest parvovirus infection, but false positive results are possible unless proper controls are run. Because the period of fecal shedding of virus particles is brief, spanning the period of approximately three to nine days after infection, false negative results are also possible.

Virus-induced enteritis can be confirmed by serologic tests in many cases (see page 1164). Electron microscopic examination of feces can substantiate a diagnosis in some cases of viral enteritis. However, both false positive and false negative results are possible.

Bacterial culture of the feces may be of benefit in the diagnosis and management of some patients. The growth of *Salmonella*, *Shigella*, or *Campylobacter* species would have public health significance but may not affect the clinical management of the case, since dogs can carry these organisms. Similarly, the growth of coliforms is expected, but enteropathogenic strains can be identified only by *in vivo* testing. Thus, the interpretation of the results of fecal cultures is difficult at best, if not impossible.

In animals showing clinical signs of septicemia, i.e., fever and malaise, repeated blood cultures may allow identification of the causative bacterium and may indicate antibiotic sensitivity. Septicemia may be an extension of a primary bacterial enteritis, a complication of a viral enteritis, or a sequela of an erosive enteritis of any cause. If a septicemia is seriously suspected, parenteral antibiotic therapy should be started before the results of blood cultures are reported.

The radiographic appearance of the gastrointestinal tract of a dog with acute gastroenteritis varies according to the cause and severity of the problem. Plain radiographs of the abdomen may show distended or thickened loops of small bowel, gas and fluid patterns suggestive of obstruction, or obvious foreign bodies. Regardless of the cause, moderate to severe enteritis can result in delayed gastric emptying due to altered gastric motor function. This delay may be marked enough to mimic pyloric outflow disease, including foreign body obstruction of the pyloric canal. Uncoordinated, ineffective intestinal peristalsis may also be apparent in contrast studies on patients with severe enteritis. Alternatively, contrast studies may demonstrate a markedly rapid transit of material through the bowel.

The last two steps in the diagnostic evaluation of acute gastroenteritis are endoscopic examination of the upper gastrointestinal tract and exploratory laparotomy. These steps should be applied to those patients that do not respond to treatments indicated by the other diagnostic procedures and when there are indications that these procedures would help the diagnostic effort.

THERAPEUTIC REGIMEN

The intensity of symptomatic and supportive therapy is also determined by the gravity of the presenting signs. Most patients with acute gastroenteritis are presented to the veterinarian with a brief history of vomiting and diarrhea without historical evidence of more serious clinical signs. Physical examination of most of these animals will not detect significant primary abnormalities. Usually these patients can be managed successfully with simple, symptomatic therapy. Even with the relatively high incidence of virus-induced enteritis, approximately 90 to 95 per cent of the cases of acute gastroenteritis can be managed effectively in this way. More aggressive therapy is needed for those animals showing more severe clinical signs and for those with serious abnormalities detected on physical examination.

Following the gathering of the history and completion of the physical examination and after consideration of further diagnostic steps, the veterinarian must formulate a specific plan of treatment for each case. General guidelines for the therapy of acute gastroenteritis are presented in Table 4.

The first question to be answered in treating acute gastroenteritis is Should the animal be hospitalized or not? A number of factors must be

Table 4. *Therapeutic Regimen for Acute Gastroenteritis in Dogs*

Outpatient	In Hospital
Fast	Fast
Bland diet	Fluid therapy
Pepto-Bismol	Intravenous
Fluid therapy	Parenteral antibiotics
Oral	(Motility modifiers)
Subcutaneous	Bland diet
Follow-up	Pepto-Bismol
	Follow-up

considered by the veterinarian and the owner before this question can be resolved. The severity of clinical signs and the general condition of the animal, e.g., state of hydration, degree of depression or lethargy, and body temperature, should be the major determinants. Intractable or bloody vomiting and/or diarrhea, marked dehydration, fever, or severe depression are indications for hospitalization. The extremely contagious nature of the viral enteritides may preclude hospitalization unless adequate isolation facilities are available. Such animals could be treated on an outpatient basis with daily or more frequent visits. Other factors that bear on the decision to hospitalize an animal include the temperament of the animal, the availability of nursing care, the owner's ability to care for the animal at home, and the cost of in-hospital care.

OUTPATIENT MANAGEMENT

For animals that can be treated symptomatically as outpatients, clinical management includes (1) dietary restriction, (2) administration of locally acting gastrointestinal medications, (3) fluid therapy, orally and/or subcutaneously, and (4) follow-up re-evaluation.

DIETARY RESTRICTION

Dietary restriction is perhaps the single most effective tool in the symptomatic treatment of acute gastroenteritis. The goal is to rest the inflamed intestinal tract. During this stage of treatment, all food is withheld for 12 to 24 hours or longer, depending on the age and size of the animal. If vomiting has been severe, water is also withheld. Warm electrolyte solutions may be given by mouth if vomition is not a problem. During this fast, the animal's activity and accessibility to food, garbage, and foreign bodies must be restricted. Dogs with gastrointestinal upsets often develop pica and ingest materials that exacerbate their problem. This restricted activity should also facilitate closer observation for further clinical signs.

At the end of this fast, small amounts of a warm bland diet should be offered frequently. This diet should be low in fat, low in fiber, and easily digested and absorbed. The diet must also be palatable to the patient and acceptable to the owner. Commercially available bland diets (e.g., Prescription Diet i/d) meet most of these criteria and are convenient to prescribe. A homemade bland diet of cottage cheese and boiled rice can also be used (see *Current Veterinary Therapy VII*, pages 919–929). When the patient is to be fed, a small amount of either a warm, salted meat broth or a warm puree of the bland diet should be offered. If the animal ingests this meal and does not show a recrudescence of signs, frequent small meals of the bland diet should be offered for the next two or three days. If the animal continues to do well, the regular diet can be reintroduced gradually over an additional three to five days. At the end of that time, the patient should be back on a normal diet on a normal schedule. If clinical signs do appear again during this process, re-examination and re-evaluation of the patient may be warranted. After such reconsideration, starting the fast again and repeating the previously mentioned steps may suffice. Alternatively, further diagnostic evaluation and more intensive supportive therapy may be necessary.

LOCALLY ACTING GASTROINTESTINAL MEDICATIONS

Although there is a wide spectrum of commercial medications available to treat acute gastroenteritis, most have not been shown to be of benefit. In reasonably well-controlled clinical studies, the commonly recommended kaolin-pectin mixture has not produced significant clinical effects. A proprietary compound containing bismuth subsalicylate (Pepto-Bismol) shortened the duration of gastrointestinal signs and reduced the duration and severity of abdominal cramps in humans with an experimental viral enteritis. Although its gastrointestinal coating action may help reduce irritation, the principle benefit of bismuth subsalicylate is thought to arise from salicylate inhibition of prostaglandin synthesis. Since prostaglandins function as mediators in the pathogenesis of diarrhea, affecting both motility and secretion, the local antiprostaglandin effect of the salicylate moiety is felt to be the major mechanism by which Pepto-Bismol produces its clinical benefit. The dose of Pepto-Bismol for the dog is empirical; 1 ml/lb body weight three to four times daily has been recommended.

FLUID THERAPY

For those animals that are mildly dehydrated or that may be subclinically dehydrated at the time of presentation, some form of supportive fluid therapy should be instituted and continued either at home or on an outpatient basis. The oral administration of balanced electrolyte solutions is one means of providing fluid therapy to animals that are not vomiting severely but are in need of fluids. Since intestinal absorptive capacity often is unaffected in animals with acute gastroenteritis, oral fluid therapy can often effectively replace water and electrolytes. Commercially available (Gatorade and similar products) and homemade oral fluids are inexpensive and easy to administer. They can be used at home and often eliminate the need for more aggressive fluid therapy. One recommended formula consists of sodium chloride (3.5 gm), sodium bicarbonate (2.5 gm), potassium chloride (1.5 gm), and glucose (20 gm) added to 1 liter of water. Approximately 30 ml/lb body weight/day is needed to meet maintenance requirements. Depending on the clinical signs and the severity of those signs, the oral administration of fluids may replace the previously described fast or may be begun at the end of the fast.

Subcutaneous fluid administration is generally effective in animals that are mildly to moderately dehydrated and vomiting. The advantages of this route include rapid and easy administration and continuous absorption of fluids over several hours. These advantages enable the veterinarian to use this route to manage animals as outpatients. Subcutaneous fluid administration also helps prevent the progression or development of dehydration that might otherwise occur as a result of withholding food and water during the recommended period of fasting. Lactated Ringer's solution supplemented with potassium chloride (10 to 20 mEq/L of fluids) and sodium bicarbonate (1 to 4 mEq/kg body weight) is generally recommended; 10 to 20 ml/lb body weight can be instilled subcutaneously at multiple sites.

Animals that are markedly dehydrated owing to severe vomiting and/or diarrhea should be hospitalized and treated with intravenous fluids.

FOLLOW-UP RE-EVALUATION

The most important aspect of the clinical management of animals with acute gastroenteritis treated as outpatients may well be the follow-up evaluation. This may take the form of a simple, brief telephone call or may entail re-examination of the animal, depending on the response of the patient to symptomatic therapy. Developing and maintaining close client contact until recovery is complete not only helps build one's practice but also enables the veterinarian to evaluate the success of the prescribed treatment.

HOSPITALIZATION AND MANAGEMENT

Hospitalization, more aggressive diagnostic evaluation, and more intense supportive therapy are needed by animals showing more serious clinical signs, especially signs not attributable to acute gastroenteritis or not responsive to symptomatic therapy. The diagnostic procedures for such patients have been mentioned earlier. The intensity of the supportive therapy in the hospital varies with the spectrum and severity of the clinical signs. Withholding food and water from animals with severe vomiting and/or diarrhea should help quiet the inflamed intestinal tract. The fast should be continued until the underlying problem has been identified and treated effectively or until the animal's clinical signs have subsided.

Many patients with signs of severe acute gastroenteritis will require intravenous fluid therapy to correct dehydration and minimize dependence on the alimentary canal. Indwelling intravenous catheters facilitate the administration of the volumes of fluids needed to treat these patients effectively. Animals that have suffered from persistent or severe vomiting may have developed metabolic alkalosis, hyponatremia, and hypochloridemia. Either physiologic saline or lactated Ringer's solution supplemented with potassium chloride should be administered. The consequences of severe diarrhea include metabolic acidosis, impaired renal function, and shock. The two last-mentioned conditions result from dehydration and diminished tissue perfusion. Volume expansion with a balanced electrolyte solution is recommended. Serial monitoring of serum electrolyte concentrations and acid-base status enables more accurate management with fluid therapy.

The parenteral administration of broad spectrum antibiotics may be warranted in animals with signs of severe gastroenteritis. Dogs (and cats) with clinical signs of parvovirus-induced enteritis may have compromised integrity of the mucosal barrier of the intestines and ineffective intestinal peristalsis. These intestinal tract changes and reduced systemic resistance due to associated leukopenia predispose these animals to bacteremia and septicemia. Patients with similar pathologic lesions of the intestinal tract due to other etiologic agents (i.e., primary bacterial enteritis) suffer similar risks. These animals should be treated with effective doses of broad spectrum antibiotics administered without dependence on intestinal absorption. One combination of parenterally administered antibiotics that has been effective in such cases consists of ampicillin (5 to 10 mg/lb body weight every six to eight hours intramuscularly, subcutaneously, or intravenously) and gentamicin (1 mg/lb body weight every eight hours intramuscularly or subcutaneously). The penicillin family of antibiotics (ampicillin) is effective against the anaerobic bacteria, which are the predominant organisms in the lower alimentary canal. The aminoglycoside antibiotics (gentamicin) are effective against the coliform organisms, which constitute the aerobic flora of the gut. However, caution must be exercised in the administration of gentamicin to animals that are or may be dehydrated. The urine sediment should be monitored frequently to detect granular casts, which herald the development of tubular nephrosis from this aminoglycoside antibiotic.

Oral administration of antibiotics or other medications to animals with severe acute gastroenteritis is not recommended. Vomiting, delayed gastric emptying, ineffective intestinal peristalsis, and altered intestinal mucosal integrity make the effects of oral medications unpredictable and unreliable. The oral administration of the aminoglycoside antibiotics (neomycin, kanamycin, gentamicin, and streptomycin), often given in hopes of "sterilizing" the gut, may be contraindicated. Antibiotics of this family have been shown to produce deleterious effects on the intestinal mucosa in some species. Also, the overuse of antimicrobial agents can have marked effects on the microflora of the intestinal tract (see *Current Veterinary Therapy VII*, pages 901–914). Patients with primary bacterial enteritis should not receive oral antibiotics unless signs of systemic involvement are present. The administration of oral antibiotics can alter the microflora of the intestinal tract in favor of pathogens that may be present. Oral antibiotics can also prolong the persistence of bacterial infection and shedding of the pathogen. In summary, orally administered antibiotics rarely have a place in the treatment of acute gastroenteritis. Appropriate doses of parenterally administered antibiotics should be given to animals showing signs of severe gastroenteritis and/ or systemic involvement.

Medications that alter the motility of the intestinal tract have been used individually or in combination with other medications (often orally administered aminoglycoside antibiotics) in the treatment of acute gastroenteritis. Recent improvements in our understanding of the physiology and pathophysiology of intestinal motility indicate that the use of such medications may not be in the best interests of the patient. The commonly prescribed anticholinergics block the effect of acetylcholine on both the nicotinic receptors of the intrinsic myenteric plexus ganglia and the muscarinic receptors on the intestinal smooth muscle cells. This blockade reduces both circular and longitudinal smooth muscle contractions. The reduction in intestinal smooth muscle activity, however, is asymmetric so that peristaltic activity usually is not decreased to the same extent as segmental activity. Thus, anticholi-

nergics result in a marked reduction in the resistance to intestinal flow normally provided by segmental contractions. Therefore, the usefulness and efficacy of anticholinergics in the treatment of acute gastrointestinal upsets are highly questionable.

Narcotic analgesics, including morphine, meperidine, and paregoric, as well as the synthetic opiate agonists increase rhythmic segmental smooth muscle contractions and decrease propulsive contractions. These effects decrease the functional diameter of the bowel lumen and increase resistance to the flow of ingesta. However, a major disadvantage in the use of the narcotic analgesics is the associated depression of the central nervous system. The synthetic opiate agonists diphenoxylate (Lomotil) and loperamide (Imodium) have greater gastrointestinal activity than the narcotic analgesics with less effect on the central nervous system. Although the narcotic analgesics and synthetic opiate agonists may be effective in slowing the flow of intestinal contents in acute gastroenteritis, they should be used cautiously because of their potential complications. In some types of invasive bacterial and viral enteritis, spastic, disorganized, segmental contractions of the intestine occur. Opiate motility modifiers would be of dubious benefit in restoring normal segmental coordination in such cases. Also, inefficient propulsive activity caused by spasmodic contractions in these cases allows colonization of the small intestine by pathogenic bacteria. Reduction in small intestinal propulsion resulting from the opiate motility modifiers may further inhibit clearance of intestinal toxins and potentiate pathogen infiltration of the bowel wall by prolonging contact time. Additionally, opiate motility modifiers should not be used unless intestinal obstruction can be ruled out. The increased segmental pressures produced by these drugs can result in rupture of the compromised, obstructed bowel. Therefore, the use of the opiate motility modifiers should be reserved for more chronic and severe cases of diarrhea that are unresponsive to conservative management.

During the course of hospitalization and therapy, when the patient's condition has progressed to the point at which clinical signs have subsided, the previously described bland diet, Pepto-Bismol, and oral fluid therapy may be administered. Hospitalization and observation are continued if necessary. After discharge from the hospital, follow-up evaluation can proceed as described for the management of the outpatient.

SUPPLEMENTAL READING

Hirsch, D. C.: Microbiology of the gastrointestinal tract: Microflora and immunology. *In* Kirk, R. W. (ed.): *Current Veterinary Therapy VII*. Philadelphia: W. B. Saunders, 1980, pp. 901–912.

Hirsch, D. C., and Enos, L. R.: The use of antimicrobial drugs in the treatment of gastrointestinal disorders. *In* Kirk, R. W. (ed.): *Current Veterinary Therapy VII.* Philadelphia: W. B. Saunders, 1980, pp. 913–914.

Jacobs, R. M., Weiser, M. G., Hall, R. L., and Kowalski, J. J.: Clinicopathological features of canine parvoviral enteritis. J. Am. Anim. Hosp. Assoc. 16:809, 1980.

Neill, S. D., McNulty, N. S., Bryson, D. G., and Ellis, W. A.: Microbiological findings in dogs with diarrhoea. Vet. Rec. 109:538, 1981.

Pietrusko, R. D.: Drug therapy review: Pharmacotherapy of diarrhea. Am. J. Hosp. Pharm. 36:757, 1979.

Pollock, R. V. H., and Carmichael, L. E.: Newer knowledge about canine parvovirus. Presented at the 30th Gaines Veterinary Symposium, 1981, pp. 36–40.

Strombeck, D. R.: Management of diarrhea: Motility modifiers and adjunct therapy. *In* Kirk, R. W. (ed.): *Current Veterinary Therapy VII.* Philadelphia: W. B. Saunders, 1980, pp. 914–919.

Strombeck, D. R.: Diet and nutrition in the management of gastrointestinal problems. *In* Kirk, R. W. (ed.): *Current Veterinary Therapy VII.* Philadelphia: W. B. Saunders, 1980, pp. 919–929.

Zimmer, J. F.: Examination of the gastrointestinal tract. Vet. Clin. North Am. 11:561, 1981.

Mycoses and Mycosis-Like Diseases

SUBCUTANEOUS AND OPPORTUNISTIC MYCOSES

MARIE H. ATTLEBERGER, D.V.M.

Auburn, Alabama

The subcutaneous mycoses develop in the host at the site of inoculation. Entry is usually through an injury, and the fungus remains localized or may spread slowly via the lymphatics. Most of the fungi involved are soil saprophytes.

The opportunistic fungi are usually thought of as contaminants. Under certain conditions, these fungi invade the tissue and produce disease. Immunosuppressants, long-term antibiotic therapy, certain debilitating diseases, steroids, and immune deficiencies are some of the factors that play a role in their pathogenicity. Before these opportunistic fungi can be incriminated as the etiologic agent of infection, active tissue invasion must be demonstrated and the fungus should be isolated from the diseased tissue two or more times. Attempts to transmit the invading fungus to other animals are usually unsuccessful.

SPOROTRICHOSIS

Definition. Sporotrichosis is a chronic infection characterized by nodules, shallow ulcers, and granulomatous lesions frequently involving the skin and often the lymphatics. It may disseminate.

Etiology and Epidemiology. The infection is caused by *Sporothrix schenckii*, a dimorphic fungus that exists in nature in the saprophytic form and in the tissue or parasitic form as an oval or elongated budding yeast. It is found in soil and on plants and wood and has been isolated from spaghnum moss, humus, grasses, water, horse hair, fleas, ants, and even frankfurters in cold storage. Environmental temperature may have some effect on the organism's growth in nature as well as in the host. The fungus usually enters the body through an injury to the skin, but it may be inhaled or even ingested.

Animal-to-human transmission has been known to occur, especially following handling of infected cats. In three of these cases there was no record of the cat biting or scratching the person. Care should be taken when handling any infected animal, especially cats, and the owner should be informed of the possibility of transmission. Fomites may also transmit infection.

Clinical Signs. In the dog with cutaneous involvement, nodules, ulcers, and granulomas may be found in a random pattern over the body or may follow the lymphatics of the extremities. Nodules may be firm and tender and may ulcerate or show evidence of healing. Wart-like lesions may occur. Nodules, crusty circular lesions, ulcers, abscesses, granulomas, and areas of necrosis are seen on the cat. Dissemination may occur in both the dog and cat but appears to be more frequent in the cat, involving the lungs, liver, and possibly other organs.

Diagnosis and Culture. Direct examination of the usual stained smears or wet mounts generally is fruitless, as the organism is difficult to demonstrate on smears. Special fungal stains or fluorescent antibody stains will give better results. Culture is the most effective method of diagnosis (see page 1161), and the fungus appears in 5 to 14 days. Refer to a text on medical mycology for a description of the fungus.

Treatment. Inorganic iodides are the preferred treatment in the dog. Good results have been experienced using 1 ml of 20 per cent NaI per 10 lbs body weight orally b.i.d. Other drugs and doses are 0.5 gm KI daily for six weeks in the feed and 25 to 30 drops of saturated KI b.i.d. for four to six weeks or until all signs of infection have disappeared. Treatment should continue for at least one month following the disappearance of clinical signs to avoid recurrence. Amphotericin B may be tried in the cat following the regimen for cryptococcosis.

RHINOSPORIDIOSIS

Definition. Rhinosporidiosis is characterized by polypoid growths on the mucous membranes of the nasal cavity. Occasionally these growths appear on the conjunctiva and skin. This infection is chronic and benign.

Etiology and Epidemiology. *Rhinosporidium seeberi* appears in the tissue as spherical, thick-walled sporangia (up to 350μ) with endospores (7 to 9μ). The fungus has not been grown in a mycelial form. Its natural habitat is unknown, and its association with water has not been documented. Trauma may be a predisposing factor in the infection, but attempts to transmit it to other animals have been unsuccessful.

Clinical Signs. The dog usually has a history of sneezing, and there may be epistaxis or a mucopurulent, blood-stained discharge. The nasal passage should be examined for sessile, pedunculate, or cauliflower-like polyps. These polyps are pinkish, bleed easily, and contain white specks, which are the sporangia. Usually only one nostril is involved. The infection has not been known to disseminate in animals.

Diagnosis. Crush a small piece of polyp and examine it in water or 10 to 20 per cent KOH under the 10× or 45× objective for sporangia with endospores. Culturing is not done.

Treatment. Surgical excision of the polyps is the most effective treatment. Surgery must be extensive and complete to prevent recurrence. The area may be cauterized following surgery.

ASPERGILLOSIS

Definition. Aspergillosis is a broad spectrum of diseases involving members of the genus *Aspergillus*. They involve the respiratory tract, digestive tract, skin, eyes, and other structures.

Etiology and Epidemiology. *Aspergillus fumigatus* is probably the most frequently isolated species. The aspergilli are found worldwide, are one of the most common fungi in the environment, and are frequently seen as laboratory contaminants. Therefore, their isolation on plates must be evaluated. Most are secondary invaders to some debilitating condition, but many are also the primary cause of infection. Overexposure to large amounts of spores can stress the body's defenses and lead to infection. In some respiratory infections, it is difficult to determine if the aspergilli isolated are invading or merely colonizing. Birds are the most frequently affected animals. Infection is not normally transmitted from animal to animal or animal to human. The long-term use of antibiotics, steroids, and immunosuppressants as well as immune deficiencies and debilitating diseases contribute to infections by the aspergilli.

Clinical Signs. Nasal aspergillosis in the dog is not infrequent, and the animal is usually presented with a history of sneezing for several weeks duration. There usually is a nasal discharge. Often only one of the nasal passages is involved, and the fungi are found growing high in the frontal sinus. In severe cases the fungi erode through the bone and may invade the brain. Neurologic signs are evident, and the temperature may rise to 104 or 105°F. Prognosis is very poor at this stage and should be guarded in the early stage of infection. *Pseudomonas* infection can present an additional problem. Signs are often vague in other forms of aspergillosis, and many are diagnosed at necropsy. Some signs that may be seen in other forms of the infection are weight loss, diarrhea, eye involvement, and granulomas on the skin. In cats, aspergillosis may be secondary to infectious feline enteritis. Respiratory infections, although rare, do occur in the cat.

Diagnosis and Culture. Nasal washings, biopsies, and scrapings of infected areas should be examined in 10 to 20 per cent KOH for septate hyphae and heads of the aspergilli. It should be remembered that heads frequently are not found and that other fungi show septate hyphae when invading tissue. Culture assures a positive diagnosis. Material must be collected as aseptically as possible and cultured at room temperature on Sabouraud dextrose agar with and without antibiotics. Bacterial cultures are also necessary. Nasal swabs are unsatisfactory because they do not reach the area of infection. Tissue invasion must be demonstrated either by direct smears or histopathology.

Treatment. Surgery plus a course of amphotericin B is the usual treatment for nasal aspergillosis. Other treatments that may prove effective in other forms of aspergillosis, if diagnosed in time, are potassium iodide, nystatin, and natamycin. Aerosol administration of natamycin or nystatin, as is done in humans, is not always possible in animals.

PHYCOMYCOSIS (ZYGOMYCOSIS)

Definition. Phycomycosis in animals is mostly a granulomatous disease caused by a variety of fungi in the class Phycomycetes.

Etiology and Epidemiology. Members of the genera *Mucor, Rhizopus, Absidia, Hypnomyces, Entomophthora, Basidiobolus,* and others have been isolated from infections in humans and animals. These organisms are associated with soil, water, and decaying vegetation. The *Mucor* and *Rhizopus* species are common laboratory contaminants. As with the aspergilli, tissue invasion and repeated isolation must be demonstrated to incriminate them in infection. Attempts to transmit them to other animals are usually unsuccessful. Factors predisposing animals to these infections are not known.

Clinical Signs. In the dog, abdominal masses, granulomas, draining fistulous tracts, and subcutaneous nodules are some of the signs presented. Chronic vomiting is present in some cases of abdominal involvement. At necropsy, the fungi have been found invading the intestinal tract and other organs. Occasionally they may invade blood vessels.

Diagnosis and Culture. Biopsies and exudates should be examined in 10 to 20 per cent KOH for wide, relatively nonseptate hyphae. Specimens for culture should be obtained as aseptically as possible and cultured at room temperature on Sabouraud agar with and without antibiotics.

Treatment. Surgery is recommended when possible and can be followed by a course of amphotericin B if deemed necessary. *Basidiobolus* sp. and *Entomophthora* sp. have been treated successfully in humans using 30 mg/kg of KI daily for one month or more.

PROTOTHECOSIS

Definition. Protothecosis is a cutaneous or systemic infection caused by various species of *Prototheca*, which are considered to be achloric algae.

Etiology and Epidemiology. *Prototheca wickerhamii* has been isolated from gross lesions in dogs and cats and *P. zopfii* from other animals. *Prototheca* spp. are found worldwide and have been isolated from soil, sewage, water, human feces in cases of sprue, and lesions on potato skin and from cases of bovine mastitis in addition to infections in humans, dogs, and a cat. The infection is usually cutaneous in humans and systemic in animals, although cutaneous infections in animals do occur. In the tissue, the organisms appear as hyaline, globose to oval cells 1.3 to 13.4 to 1.3 by 16.1μ in size. The cells contain two or more autospores. Budding does not occur. The colony is yeast-like in appearance and consistency. The mode of transmission to animals has not been established, but ingestion, inhalation, and injury should be considered. Only a few cases of protothecosis have been reported, and there has been no evidence of transmission among individuals.

Clinical Signs. Small sores, dry crusty lesions, granulomas, and nasal exudate have been observed superficially in the dog. Pain, chronic nephritis, bloody diarrhea, polyuria, polydypsia, polyphagia, and iritis followed by blindness have occurred in the dog with systemic infection. Organisms have been isolated from heart, liver, kidneys, para-adrenal connective tissue, eyes, and brain.

The cat had a soft, fluctuant, subcutaneous mass on the plantar surface of the left tarsus.

Diagnosis. Exudates and other material should be examined microscopically in 10 to 20 per cent KOH under the 45× objective for oval to globose structures containing two or more autospores. The *Prototheca* organisms are easily cultured on blood agar or Sabouraud dextrose agar with and without antibiotics. Yeast-like colonies are visible in 48 hours. Fluorescent antibody conjugate is also available for direct smears.

Treatment. No therapeutic treatment has proved effective for protothecosis. Surgical excision is recommended for localized lesions.

PHAEOHYPHOMYCOSIS

Definition. Phaeohyphomycosis is an infection caused by dematiaceous fungi that form dark-walled, septate hyphae in the host's tissue.

Etiology and Epidemiology. *Drechslera spicifera* is the fungus most frequently isolated in animals. It is widespread in the environment and has been recovered from soil and air. At the present time, cases have been reported only in cats and horses. The disease in animals has so far been limited to the subcutaneous tissue.

Clinical Signs. A cat at Auburn with the infection had a draining lesion on the tail and a larger, swollen area with a draining tract on the footpad. The infection may begin as a nodule, and fistulous tracts may or may not develop.

Diagnosis and Culture. Direct examination of the exudate or pieces of tissue in 10 to 20 per cent KOH reveal black, septate hyphae, some of which may show unusual dilatations. The specimen should be cultured on Sabouraud dextrose agar, with and without antibiotics, at room temperature.

Treatment. Complete surgical excision of the lesion has proved to be successful.

MYCETOMA

Definition. Mycetoma refers to tumefactions with draining tracts and granules in the exudate.

Etiology and Epidemiology. There are two groups of etiologic agents: (1) actinomycotic, which include various species of *Actinomyces, Nocardia,*

Actinomadura, and *Streptomyces,* and (2) eumycotic, which include *Allescheria boydii, Curvularia geniculata, Maduralla* spp., and others. Most are soil saprophytes or plant pathogens and gain entry to the host through injury. Most of the mycetomas in lower animals contain black granules, although white or yellow grains have been reported.

Clinical Signs. The extremities are frequently involved, but, regardless of the location, the triad of signs—tumefaction, draining tracts, and granules in the exudate—is present.

Diagnosis and Culture. The granules, which are colonies of the organism, should be crushed and examined in 10 to 20 per cent KOH for the presence of hyphae and chlamydospores, which are seen in eumycotic mycetoma. A Gram stain also should be performed and examined under oil for gram positive filaments found in acintomycotic mycetoma. For culture the granules should be washed several times in sterile saline, crushed, and streaked onto Sabouraud agar without antibiotics and on blood agar. A duplicate set of plates should be incubated at room temperature and at 37°C. The group to which the etiologic agent belongs should be determined, because treatment depends on which group is involved.

Treatment. Complete surgical excision of the lesion is recommended for eumycotic mycetoma. Actinomycotic mycetoma may be treated with sulfa drugs, as in nocardiosis.

SUPPLEMENTAL READING

Anderson, N. V., et al.: Cutaneous sporotrichosis in a cat: A case report. J. Am. Anim. Hosp. Assoc. 9:526, 1973.

Barsanti, J. A., Attleberger, M. H., and Henderson, R. A.: Phycomycosis in a dog. J.A.V.M.A. 167:293, 1975.

Bolton, G. R., and Brown, T. T.: Mycotic colitis in a cat. V.M./S.A.C. 67:978, 1972.

Brodey, R. S., et al.: Mycetoma in a dog. J.A.V.M.A. 151:442, 1967.

Heller, R. A., et al.: Three cases of phycomycosis in dogs. V.M./S.A.C. 66:472, 1971.

Jang, S. S., and Popp, J. A.: Eumycotic mycetoma in a dog caused by *Allescheria boydii.* J.A.V.M.A. 157:1071, 1970.

Kaplan, W., et al.: Prototheocosis in a cat: First recorded case. Sabouraudia 14:281, 1976.

Koehne, M. A., Powell, H. S., and Hail, R. I.: Sporotrichosis in a dog. J.A.V.M.A. 159:892, 1971.

Kurtz, H. J., Finco, D. R., and Perman, V.: Maduromycosis (*Allescheria boydii*) in a dog. J.A.V.M.A. 157:917, 1970.

Muller, G. H., et al.: Phaeohyphomycosis caused by *Drechslera spicifera* in a cat. J.A.V.M.A. 166:150, 1975.

Rippon, J. W.: *Medical Mycology: The Pathogenic Fungi and the Pathogenic Actinomycetes.* Philadelphia: W. B. Saunders, 1974.

Scott, D. W., Bentinck-Smith, J., and Haggerty, G. F.: Sporotrichosis in three dogs. Cornell Vet. 64:416, 1974.

Sudman, M. S., Majka, J. A., and Kaplan, W.: Primary mucocutaneous prototheocosis in a dog. J.A.V.M.A. 163:1372, 1973.

Werner, R. E., et al.: Sporotrichosis in a cat. J.A.V.M.A. 159:407, 1971.

Wood, G. L., et al.: Disseminated aspergillosis in a dog. J.A.V.M.A. 172:704, 1978.

SYSTEMIC MYCOSES

MARIE H. ATTLEBERGER, D.V.M.

Auburn, Alabama

Excluding humans, the dog appears to be the natural host for the systemic fungus infections histoplasmosis, blastomycosis, and coccidioidomycosis, whereas cryptococcosis occurs in the dog and cat. Infections in other animals are rare. Following the inhalation of spores, the infections are usually pulmonary in origin and may heal spontaneously or may worsen and spread to the skin, nodes, other organs, and bone via the blood or lymphatics.

Animals with a systemic fungus infection present a wide variety of signs such as granulomatous lesions, abscesses, ulcers, fistulous tracts, enlarged and/or draining nodes, and even areas of necrosis. Most signs develop slowly and elicit little pain except for lameness. Usually the animal has a history of "going downhill for some time."

Rarely are these infections acute. However, when they are acute they are usually diagnosed at necropsy. Since most of these infections can be diagnosed on direct smears of infected material, it is essential that clinicians be able to obtain correct specimens and be familiar with the organism's appearance in tissue.

With the exception of *Cryptococcus neoformans,* the other fungi causing the deep mycoses are dimorphic, growing in the mycelial or saprophytic form at 25°C and in the tissue or parasitic form at 37°C as a yeast (histoplasmosis and blastomycosis) or as a spherule with endospores (coccidioidomycosis).

Resistance to fungal infections appears to reside with cellular immunity, whereas humoral antibodies are useful in the diagnosis and prognosis of an infection. Any agents that suppress the immune system are contraindicated in fungus infections.

Although serologic tests are an aid in diagnosing fungus infections, one should not make a positive diagnosis based on serology alone. There are cross reactions as well as false negatives and false positives in these tests. In addition to serology, there should be some clinical signs suggestive of a fungal infection or a positive direct smear or culture.

Animal-to-animal, animal-to-human, and human-to-human transmission of the systemic fungi does not occur naturally. Most of the infections in animals occur in those under five years of age.

BLASTOMYCOSIS

Definition. Blastomycosis is a chronic granulomatous and suppurative infection that is primarily pulmonary in origin but that may disseminate to the skin, eyes, bone, and other organs.

Etiology and Epidemiology. *Blastomyces dermatitidis*, a dimorphic fungus, appears in the tissue phase as a large, thick-walled, budding yeast (8 to 20μ) and exists in nature in the mycelial or saprophytic phase, where it needs high humidity (85 to 88 per cent) to grow. Although it has been isolated a few times from soil rich in organic matter during the cool wet months and from tree bark, its true habitat is still unknown. Soil microorganisms (bacilli and streptomycetes) have been shown to destroy both the mycelial and yeast forms. An association with cedar trees has been noticed in some of the dogs hospitalized at the Auburn University Small Animal Clinic. Although infection usually occurs following inhalation of the spores, cases in humans have occurred following the handling of fomites. The organism is endemic in the eastern United States and parts of southern Canada, especially in areas drained by rivers. It also has been reported in countries outside of the North American continent. It is not a contagious disease.

Clinical Signs. In dogs, the infection usually begins in the lung and then disseminates to other areas of the body. Dogs usually are depressed, debilitated, and thin and may or may not show pyrexia. A cough may or may not be present with the respiratory involvement, which may be severe or mild. Skin lesions are usually present and consist of cutaneous and subcutaneous abscesses, ulcers, draining tracts, and granulomas. These lesions may be seen in various stages of healing and breakdown. Occasionally, hair has a greasy feeling, which disappears following treatment. Frequently, the prescapular and/or popliteal nodes are enlarged and draining.

The eyes are very often affected, and permanent blindness is not uncommon. If exophthalmia is present, this usually can be corrected with treatment and the eye returns to normal. The eyes are especially sensitive to sunlight, but this will disappear as treatment progresses.

Lameness may occur, especially in the large breeds, and the hind legs are often swollen, probably as a result of lymphatic stasis. In male dogs, there may be an orchitis, as the prostate and testicles are often infected.

Radiographs of the lung usually reveal a dense mass at the bifurcation of the trachea due to enlargement of the bronchial and mediastinal nodes. Local or diffuse pulmonary consolidation is frequently present.

COCCIDIOIDOMYCOSIS
(VALLEY FEVER)

Definition. Coccidioidomycosis (valley fever) is a fungus infection that is usually pulmonary in origin. It may be asymptomatic and self-limiting or may disseminate to bone and other organs.

Etiology and Epidemiology. *Coccidioides immitis* is endemic in the arid southwestern United States, northern Mexico, and various areas of Central and South America. The organism is dimorphic and exists in nature in the mycelial form and occurs in tissue as a thick-walled spherule (20 to 60μ) with endospores (2 to 5μ). Immature spherules with no endospores may be seen.

C. immitis is frequently found in association with rodent burrows, and dogs digging in these or disturbing infected soil become infected. The organism remains viable in the soil during the hot, dry weather and appears to grow following periods of rainfall. When conditions become windy and dusty, animal infection is more prevalent. Animals inhale spores in the dust. Fomite transmission can occur also. The disease is not contagious. Infection usually appears in a few days to a few weeks following exposure. Dogs are very susceptible, and it is reported that boxers and Doberman pinschers are especially sensitive to the disseminated form.

Clinical Signs. Infection may be asymptomatic or benign, showing only respiratory illness, or it may disseminate to bones and other organs. The dogs presented for treatment are usually under two years of age and have the disseminated form. There are episodes of coughing, and the temperature may be normal or may rise to 106°F. Other signs include anorexia, dyspnea, listlessness, loss of weight, episodes of diarrhea, and even ascites. Difficulty in swallowing has been observed. Nodes may be enlarged and draining.

Between the pulmonary infection and dissemination (frequently to bone), the dog may experience periods of good health, or dissemination may occur soon after the pulmonary infection. Lameness and swollen joints occur, and, when bone is involved, radiographs frequently show proliferative osteomyelitis with lesions near the epiphyseal junction.

Less frequently, a meningitis manifested by incoordination or eye involvement may occur.

HISTOPLASMOSIS

Definition. Histoplasmosis is a systemic fungus infection usually contracted by inhaling spores from infected soil. Both the pulmonary and intestinal forms are seen in the dog. Histoplasmosis is rare in cats.

Etiology, Ecology, and Epidemiology. *Histoplasma capsulatum* is a dimorphic fungus that appears in the tissue or parasitic phase as tiny, intracellular oval bodies (2 to 4μ in diameter) found in cells of the reticuloendothelial system. The mycelial or saprophytic form occurs in nature, and it is the small microaleuriospores (2 to 5μ) that, when inhaled into the alveolar spaces, transform into yeasts and begin the tissue phase.

The fungus is found in the Eastern United States, the Central Mississippi Valley, the Ohio Valley, and along the Appalachian Mountains. The highly endemic areas of the United States are in Kentucky, Tennessee, Missouri, southern Illinois, Arkansas, Indiana, Ohio, and some parts of North Carolina, Minnesota, and Iowa. Isolated areas are also found in the St. Lawrence River Valley and Lake Champlain areas. It is also found in other parts of the world.

The organism is frequently associated with soil contaminated with chicken, bat, starling, and other bird droppings. Temperature, soil type, humidity, and other factors also influence its presence in the soil. If one wishes to disinfect contaminated soil in a confined area, a 3 per cent formaldehyde or 3 per cent cresol solution should be used. Nine gallons should be disseminated over a 25 square foot area daily for three days.

Although the fungus has been cultured from a dog tick allowed to feed on a dog with a known positive blood culture, the role of insects in the transmission is unknown.

Histoplasmosis is not a contagious disease.

Clinical Signs. Most dogs are seen in an advanced stage of the disease and are emaciated, lethargic, and depressed; show dyspnea and anorexia; and have an elevated temperature. A nasal or ocular discharge and a cough may or may not be present. Nodes are frequently enlarged, and hepatomegaly, splenomegaly, ascites, and anemia may be present. Often there is a diarrhea of unexplained origin, which may be persistent or intermittent, resulting in dehydration. Any persistent enteritis should be cultured for fungi (*H. capsulatum*). Radiographs show a granulomatous pneumonia.

CRYPTOCOCCOSIS

Definition. Cryptococcosis is a systemic fungal infection, usually pulmonary in origin, that may remain in the respiratory tract or spread to the brain, skin, nodes, other organs, and bone, possibly by the blood and lymphatics.

Etiology and Epidemiology. *Cryptococcus neoformans* is soil-borne and worldwide in distribution and exists in nature in the yeast form. It is 4 to 7μ

in diameter, and most of the yeast cells are surrounded by a polysaccharide capsule. It is found in association with pigeon nests and excreta as well as with excreta from other birds and bats. Natural infection in birds does not appear to occur. Cryptococcosis is not a contagious disease.

Clinical Signs. These vary greatly among individually infected animals. Ulcerated areas may occur on the oral, pharyngeal, or nasal mucosa. The turbinates, facial sinuses, and surrounding bony structures may be invaded. Ulcerative and granulomatous skin lesions and, occasionally, abscesses may be present. These abscesses often contain a mucoid exudate. Even though the initial involvement is usually pulmonary, respiratory involvement may not be seen. Lameness due to septic arthritis may occur.

If the nervous system is visibly involved, there may be incoordination, various eye lesions, or even blindness. A head tilt also occurs in advanced cases. Lymph nodes are usually enlarged, and bones and other organs may be involved.

In cats, a respiratory problem is usually evident, and granulomas occluding the nasal cavity are often seen. If no external lesions are visible, the cat's mouth should be examined for ulcerated areas. Sometimes there is no evidence of respiratory involvement, and only a single lesion or abscess may be present.

DIAGNOSIS OF THE SYSTEMIC MYCOSES

DIRECT SMEARS

Exudate, node aspirates, direct scrapings from skin lesions, and granulomas are suitable for direct smears. Urine, cerebrospinal fluid, and transtracheal washings should be centrifuged and the sediment examined. Diagnosis by direct microscopic examination of clinical specimens in 10 to 20 per cent KOH under the low and high dry objectives can be made in blastomycosis and coccidioidomycosis. Large, thick-walled, budding yeasts with internal structure are seen in blastomycosis. Thick-walled spherules with endospores as well as smaller spherules devoid of spores are found in coccidioidomycosis. Parker ink added to the KOH will outline the fungi (1 drop of ink/2 drops KOH).

For cryptococcosis, the specimen is placed in a mixture of Pelican or India ink and water. Only enough ink to make the water dark gray in color is used. Typically, a small, round, budding yeast surrounded by a capsule is seen under 45×. The capsule appears as a halo around the yeast because it holds back the carbon particles in the ink. Occasionally no capsules are present and only nonencapsulated yeasts are seen. Culture and identification are then necessary.

Histoplasmosis is not easily diagnosed by direct

smears. Node aspirates or biopsies may be tried and should be stained with a hematologic stain. Small, intracellular, oval bodies (yeast cells) are found within the macrophages. Biopsies from the liver, spleen, or sternal bone marrow may be useful. Except in very advanced cases, yeasts are difficult to demonstrate in peripheral blood.

CULTURE

Plates should be heavily streaked with the correct specimens and held at least six weeks. Although most of the systemic fungi grow slowly, *Coccidioides immitis* may be visible in three to four days and may be mistaken for a contaminant. The mycelial phase is usually easier to recover, and one should wet down the mycelia of *Histoplasma capsulatum* and *C. immitis* with sterile saline or water before removing any of the fungi for microscopic study in lactophenol cotton blue. Refer to a textbook of medical mycology for descriptions of the fungi.

HISTOPATHOLOGY

Specimens should be submitted to pathology laboratories in 10 per cent buffered formalin. In addition to the hematoxylin-and-eosin stain, fungal stains such as Gridley, Grocott-Gomori methenamine-silver, or periodic acid–Schiff should be used.

TREATMENT AND PROGNOSIS OF THE SYSTEMIC MYCOSES

In deciding which dogs to treat, it is felt that those that are eating and able to stand are most likely to benefit. Amphotericin B (Fungizone*) is the drug of choice, and each dog should be treated on an individual basis depending on the severity of the infection.

The drug should be diluted according to the manufacturer's directions, and 0.15 mg/kg is given intravenously in 25 to 30 ml of 5 per cent dextrose in water over a 20- to 30-minute period. Avoid saline, as it causes the drug to precipitate. The dosage may be increased gradually over the second or third week until 0.20 to 0.25 mg/kg is reached. Only in exceptionally severe cases is a higher dose needed. Treatment is administered every other day. Because amphotericin B is nephrotoxic, the blood urea nitrogen (BUN) should be determined before treatment is begun and at least once a week, and preferably twice a week, during treatment. It is best to keep the BUN under 30 mg/100 ml, and it should not be allowed to exceed 40 mg/100 ml. If higher, treatment should be stopped until the BUN decreases and then resumed at a slightly lower dosage so that the BUN falls into acceptable limits.

No nephrotoxic effects on dogs using this dosage have been encountered at the Auburn University Small Animal Clinic. Treatment may be given on an outpatient basis and in most cases should be continued for six to eight weeks; 20 to 22 injections are usually sufficient but more can be given if needed. Dogs should be fed a high-caloric diet and should have at least six weeks rest following treatment. Owners should be advised that dogs may become reinfected if allowed access to old areas of infection. Treatment failures, although few, may occur, and the animal may be retreated.

If bone is involved, treatment should continue until there are no signs of infection as indicated by radiography or culture.

For coccidioidomycosis, 1 mg of amphotericin B per 4 lbs twice a week for six to eight weeks has been used with good results (Graham, 1982). Graham states that this dosage is effective in bone involvement.

For cats, the following procedure using amphotericin B has been found successful. The dry amphotericin B powder should be diluted with 20 ml of diluent (water). Each adult cat is given 0.8 mg in 10 ml of 5 per cent dextrose in water every three to four days. Using a 25-gauge needle, administer this solution intravenously as rapidly as possible. Monitor the BUN as for dogs. The BUN may reach 40 to 80 mg/100 ml following administration of the first two or three treatments and may be decreased by therapy with lactated Ringer's solution. Treatment is continued until the cat is asymptomatic and cultures are negative. The cat may be treated as an outpatient.

Ketoconazole (Nizoral†) a water-soluble experimental antifungal drug, is administered orally and is well absorbed from the gastrointestinal tract. It is relatively free of toxic side effects and is currently being evaluated in the treatment of fungal infections in humans and animals. The dose for dogs treated for coccidioidomycosis at the University of California School of Veterinary Medicine (Wolfe and Pappagianis, 1981) is 10 mg/kg given orally t.i.d. for six months. Studies at the College of Veterinary Medicine at Mississippi State University (Pyle et al., 1981) on canine blastomycosis showed no adverse reactions in dogs treated with doses ranging from 10 to 30 mg/kg for up to 62 days. The higher dose appeared to be more effective. In Alabama, two dogs with blastomycosis were treated with ketoconazole. Recovery occurred in one dog following treatment for three weeks, and the other has shown improvement and is still undergoing treatment. Additional studies with this drug on other fungal infections and in other animals are needed.

The prognosis for most systemic fungus infections should be guarded. When treating bone lesions, it will probably be necessary to treat the animal for a longer period of time and possibly with higher doses

*E. R. Squibb & Sons, Inc., Princeton, NJ.

†Janssen Pharmaceutica Inc., New Brunswick, NJ.

longer period of time and possibly with higher doses of amphotericin B; therefore, nephrotoxicity may be a problem. Prognosis is poor if the central nervous system is involved. Canine blastomycosis occurs more frequently in Alabama than any of the other deep mycoses, and favorable results using the previously described regimen of therapy have been experienced. Resistance by the deep fungi to amphotericin B and severe side effects such as those seen in humans have not occurred in dogs treated at the Auburn University Small Animal Clinic. Anemia may occur and should be treated symptomatically.

REFERENCES AND SUPPLEMENTAL READING

Ausherman, R. J., Sutton, H. H., and Oakes, J. T.: Clinical signs of blastomycosis in dogs. J.A.V.M.A. 130:541, 1957.

Barrett, R. E., and Scott, D. W.: Treatement of feline cryptococcosis: Literature review and case report. J. Am. Anim. Hosp. Assn. 11:511, 1975.

Graham, L. P.: Personal communication, 1982.

Jungerman, P. F., and Schwartzman, R. M.: *Veterinary Medical Mycology.* Philadelphia: Lea & Febiger, 1972.

Pyle, R. L., Dunbar, M., Nelson, P. D., Hawkins, J. A., and Turner, L. W.: Canine blastomycosis. Comp. Cont. Ed. Pract. Vet. 3:963, 1981.

Rippon, J. W.: *Medical Mycology: The Pathogenic Fungi and The Pathogenic Actinomycetes.* Philadelphia: W. B. Saunders, 1974.

Rhoades, H. E., Helper, L. C., and Fritz, T. E.: Canine histoplasmosis with intestinal involvements. J.A.V.M.A. 136:171, 1960.

Wolfe, A. M., and Pappagianis, D.: Canine coccidioidomycosis—treatment with a new antifungal agent: ketoconazole. Calif. Vet. 5:25, 1981.

ACTINOMYCOSIS, NOCARDIOSIS AND DERMATOPHILOSIS

MARIE H. ATTLEBERGER, D.V.M.

Auburn, Alabama

Actinomycosis and nocardiosis are caused by bacteria that show a tendency to branch as well as to break up into coccobacillary forms. These bacteria belong to the Actinomycetales order. Lesions are similar in both infections, and animals show abscesses, draining tracts, raw ulcers, granulomas, necrosis, fibrosis, and respiratory involvement.

Dermatophilosis is included in this group, as the etiologic agent is also an actinomycete. The clinical signs in this infection consist of crusts and scabs. Infections are rare in the dog and cat.

ACTINOMYCOSIS

Definition. Actinomycosis is a localized or systemic infection characterized by suppurative and granulomatous lesions. Draining sinuses may be present.

Etiology and Epidemiology. Actinomycosis is found worldwide, and many species of actinomycetes are involved in infection. The organisms are gram positive filaments that usually branch and break up into coccobacillary forms. They are non-acid-fast and are anaerobic and microaerophilic in their oxygen requirements. They appear to be endogenous in humans and animals and seem to need other bacteria to produce infection. Injury may be a predisposing factor in their pathogenicity. Animal-to-human transmission does not occur.

Clinical Signs. Numerous clinical syndromes appear in dogs and cats infected with *Actinomyces* species, and they are very similar to those described for nocardiosis. The following signs have been observed in dogs and cats in the Auburn, Alabama area: localized abscesses with elevated temperature, deep abscesses, abdominal masses, vertebral osteomyelitis, severe respiratory conditions with pleuritis, and draining tracts.

Diagnosis. Follow the same diagnostic procedure as for nocardiosis using the gram stain and cultural methods. Although *Actinomyces* spp. are non–acid-fast, this should not be the sole characteristic used for diagnosis, since some nocardia are non–acid-fast. The flecks or granules present in the exudates are colonies of the organisms and should be used for staining and culture. Blood agar and brain heart infusion agar should be streaked and incubated at 37°C under aerobic, anaerobic, and microaerophilic conditions. The clubs seen in granules of *A. bovis* are not always present in exudates from dogs and cats. Culture and identification are necessary to differentiate *Nocardia* spp., as treatment differs. *Actinomyces viscosus* and other unidentified species have been isolated from dogs.

Treatment and Prognosis. Surgery to establish drainage or remove localized infected areas plus antibiotics and other chemotherapeutic agents is the recommended treatment. Penicillin is the drug of choice. High doses (40,000 to 50,000 units/lb intramuscularly) should be given daily. Treatment should be continued until clinical signs are absent and cultures are negative. For systemic infections, it is necessary to continue treatment for several months. For dogs allergic to penicillin, chloramphenicol may be tried. Iodine preparations applied topically to localized lesions are helpful. Prognosis is poor in systemic infections, many of which are diagnosed at necropsy. It is usually good in localized infections.

NOCARDIOSIS

Definition. The infection may be acute or chronic and may be limited to the skin and show ulcers, abscesses, or draining tracts. The lungs and possibly other organs may be involved. Mycetoma-type lesions may also occur.

Etiology and Epidemiology. *Nocardia asteroides* and *N. brasiliensis* are the two species most frequently isolated from animals, and infections with *N. caviae* have been reported. *N. asteroides* has often been isolated from soil and the other two less frequently. The organisms may be inhaled or ingested but often enter through an injury site. In humans, they frequently disseminate to the brain. The infection is not transmitted from animal to animal or animal to human.

Clinical Signs. In the dog or cat with the localized form of infection there is usually a history of some injury with a lesion that does not respond to treatment. There are often draining fistulous tracts and a raw, ulcerated lesion. Subcutaneous abscesses, granulomas, and enlarged nodes also occur. In the primary pulmonary form, the dog and cat show pleural effusion and empyema along with signs of respiratory distress and usually weight loss. The systemic form closely resembles distemper and is characterized by dyspnea, coughing, anorexia, pyrexia, emaciation, and possibly nasal and ocular discharge. Neurologic disturbances are seen when the brain is involved.

Diagnosis and Culture. For the cutaneous form, a scraping of the ulcer or pus can be gram stained and observed under oil for gram positive, branching, beaded filaments. As many of the *Nocardia* spp. are acid-fast or partially acid-fast, a Hank's acid-fast stain should also be done. When the thickened, rusty fluid is removed from the chest, it should be examined for flecks or granules, which are clumps of the organism. These granules should be stained as previously described. The importance of the granules in making a diagnosis cannot be overstressed, for the organism often is not found in the fluid alone. These granules may be found in the fistulous tracts and pus and may be seen in infections other than nocardiosis.

Obtain pus, exudates, and granules as aseptically as possible for culture. Blood agar and plain Sabouraud dextrose agar plates should be inoculated in duplicate with the flakes or granules. One set of plates should be incubated at 37°C and the other at 25°C and held for at least two weeks. The nocardias grow as rough, adhering colonies and may show a variety of colors with age. Colonies should be examined early for filaments, as these organisms break up into coccobacillary forms, which may be mistaken for bacteria, thus resulting in an incorrect diagnosis. The Hank's acid-fast stain should be made on colonies also.

Treatment and Prognosis. Sulfa drugs, especially sulfamerazine and sulfadiazine, are preferred. Triple Sulfa #4* has been used successfully at the Auburn University Small Animal Clinic; 60 mg/lb is given intravenously as the initial dose, then 30 mg/lb b.i.d. is given for as long as needed and as long as the dog is able to tolerate the drug. This drug may be diluted 1:10 and used to flush fistulous tracts. If preferred, oral sulfadiazine, 40 mg/lb t.i.d., may be used. Tribrissen† has proved effective in some cases. In the pulmonary and systemic forms treatment may be needed for two to three months. Cultures and radiographs may be helpful in determining the length of treatment. In one instance a dog in the clinic was unable to tolerate sulfa drugs, and, as a last resort, surgical removal of the granulomatous lesion proved effective. Chest drains are needed with empyema, and a daily lavage with physiologic saline should be carried out until the thoracic fluid is clear. Proteolytic enzymes and penicillin may be added to the lavage if needed. Prognosis is usually good, and recovery is rapid in localized lesions. In the systemic and pulmonary forms the prognosis should be guarded to poor.

DERMATOPHILOSIS

Definition. Dermatophilosis is an exudative dermatitis characterized by crusts and scabs that may be localized or widespread over the entire body.

Etiology and Epidemiology. *Dermatophilus congolensis,* an actinomycete, appears as branching filaments that swell and divide longitudinally, then transversely, to form parallel rows of coccoid zoospores. Injury to the skin and excessive prolonged moisture are predisposing factors. The exact habitat of the organism is unknown, and it has not been isolated from soil. Experimentally, flies have been shown to transmit the infection. As healing occurs, crusts and scabs fall away and can contaminate the premises. There are a few reported cases of humans contracting the infection following the handling of infected animals. These cases are rare, and self-healing occurs.

Clinical Signs. The crusts and scabs on the dog

---

*Vet Products Corp., Kansas City, MO.
†Burroughs Wellcome Co., Research Triangle Park, NC.

are thickened owing to the build-up of the exudate and, when removed, contain unbroken intact hair. The area beneath the scab may contain a yellowish pus or the skin may appear normal to slightly eythematous. Removal of the scabs leaves areas of alopecia, and some scabs are found clinging to the hair. Two cases have been reported in cats, and the lesions appeared as glossal granulomas or tumors on the tongue and resulted in dysphagia and dyspnea. An embedded feather in one case suggested entry through injury.

Diagnosis.   Crush scabs in a small amount of water and prepare a heavy smear. Stain with a blood stain (Diff Quick* or Camco Quick Stain†) and examine under oil for filaments and parallel rows of spores.

Treatment and Prognosis.   Daily bathing with an iodine shampoo and gentle removal of the loosened scabs is usually sufficient treatment. It is best not to remove tightly adhering scabs, as bleeding

---

*Harleco Co., Gibbstown, NJ.
†American Scientific Products Co., Stone Mountain, GA.

frequently occurs. Following bathing, the animal should be dried and kept in dry quarters until all skin lesions have healed. If secondary bacterial infection occurs, topical applications of furacin may be applied, but the furacin has no effect on the actinomycete. Spontaneous healing may occur. Prognosis is usually good in the dog. Procaine penicillin, 300,000 units daily for five days, was used to treat the cat in one of the reported cases.

SUPPLEMENTAL READING

Baker, G. J., Breeze, R. G., and Dawson, C. O.: Oral dermatophilosis in a cat: a case report. J. Small Anim. Pract. 13:649, 1972.
Campbell, B., and Scott, D. W.: Successful management of nocardial empyema in a dog and cat. J. Am. Anim. Hosp. Assn. 11:769, 1975.
Georg, L. K., Brown, J. M., Baker, H. J., and Cassell, G. H.: *Actinomyces viscosus* as an agent of actinomycosis in the dog. J.A.V.M.A. 33:1457, 1972.
Jungerman, P. F., and Schwartzman, R. M.: *Veterinary Medical Mycology*. Philadelphia, Lea & Febiger, 1972.
Maderazo, E. G., and Quintilani, R.: Treatment of nocardial infection with trimethoprim and sulfamethoxazole. Am. J. Med. 57:671, 1974.
Rippon, J. W.: *Medical Mycology: The Pathogenic Fungi and the Pathogenic Actinomycetes*. Philadelphia: W. B. Saunders, 1974.

Viral Diseases

FELINE INFECTIOUS PERITONITIS

JEFFREY E. BARLOUGH, D.V.M.,
Ithaca, New York

and RICHARD C. WEISS, V.M.D.
Mountain View, California

Feline infectious peritonitis (FIP) is an important and complex infectious disease of domestic and exotic cats. It is characterized by a nonsuppurative fibrinous peritonitis and/or pleuritis, disseminated pyogranulomatous inflammation, or both. Lesions are present within serous membranes, abdominal and thoracic viscera, lymph nodes, central nervous system, and eyes. Three forms of the disease are recognized: (1) effusive ("wet") FIP, characterized by abdominal and/or thoracic effusion; (2) noneffusive ("dry") FIP, with minimal effusion and marked pyogranulomatous lesions involving especially the kidneys, liver, central nervous system, and/or eyes; and (3) combinations of the two.

Reports indicate that FIP has apparently been observed since the early 1950s although it had not been previously recognized as a separate disease entity. In the United States, FIP has been reported in California since at least 1954, in the New York City area since 1956, and in the Midwest since 1962. The disease is worldwide in occurrence.

ETIOLOGIC AGENT

The causative agent of FIP is a virus belonging to the family Coronaviridae, a closely related group of single-strand RNA viruses characterized morphologically by radiating surface projections (peplomers) resembling the solar corona. Coronaviruses are important causes of upper respiratory and enteric disease, hepatitis, peritonitis, and encephalitis in several species of birds and mammals. FIP virus (FIPV) is closely related to certain other animal and human coronaviruses, including transmissible gastroenteritis virus (TGEV) of swine, canine coronavirus (CCV), and human respiratory coronavirus 229E (HCV 229E), that share one or more antigenic determinants (Pedersen et al., 1978). Certain coronaviral antibodies in cats will cross react with these viruses, and this phenomenon has been exploited serodiagnostically in several laboratory assays.

Studies of FIPV have been hampered for many years by failure to cultivate the virus in conventional monolayer cell cultures. The feline mononuclear phagocyte was originally believed to be the only cell type capable of supporting FIPV growth and replication, and early studies of the virus involved propagation in autochthonous peritoneal cell (macrophage) cultures from infected cats (Pedersen, 1976a). The first successful *in vitro* isolation and propagation of FIPV in intestinal ring organ cultures (Hoshino and Scott, 1978) was followed by isolation in several feline monolayer cell cultures, including embryonic lung cells (O'Reilly et al., 1979; Hitchcock et al., 1981), fetal fibroblasts and primary whole fetus cells (Pedersen et al., 1981a), and Crandell kidney cells (Black, 1980; Evermann et al., 1981; McKeirnan et al., 1981). *In vivo* propagation of FIPV in the brains of suckling mice, rats, and hamsters was reported (Osterhaus et al., 1978a, 1978b). The isolates identified in these reports are apparently pathogenic field strains that had undergone adaptation for growth and continued passage outside the host. In this respect they are quite different from the majority of FIPV field strains, and each is uniquely suited to propagation in its respective cell culture system. Routine virus isolation from field cases (a common procedure with other feline viruses such as panleukopenia virus, calicivirus, herpesvirus, and feline leukemia virus) is currently not possible with FIPV.

FIPV is heat-labile, ether-sensitive, and inactivated by most detergents and disinfectants. Maintenance of the virus at room temperature results in complete loss of infectivity within 24 to 48 hours. Viral particles are destroyed by formaldehyde and quaternary ammonium compounds but are apparently resistant to phenol. Household bleach (sodium hypochlorite, Clorox) diluted 1:32 in water or in combination with A–33 (Airkem) to give a final concentration of 1:32 Clorox and 1:64 A–33 has been recommended for removal of FIPV from contaminated premises (Scott et al., 1979).

DIAGNOSIS

The clinical diagnosis of FIP is made by evaluation of history and presenting signs and the results of supportive laboratory tests. Clinicopathologic and serologic procedures important in FIP diagnosis include analysis of pleural or peritoneal fluids, hemogram (including total serum protein), serum protein electrophoresis, clinical chemistry profiles, serum coronaviral antibody titer, and biopsy.

Considering the grave prognosis associated with a clinical diagnosis of FIP and the lack of curative therapy, it is essential to differentiate this disease from other conditions with similar symptoms. Differential diagnosis of thoracic fluid accumulation should include cardiac insufficiency (cardiomyopathy, cardiac neoplasia, dirofilariasis), lymphosarcoma and other neoplasms, pyothorax, chylothorax, diaphragmatic hernia, hemothorax (trauma, clotting disorders, vascular neoplasms, thrombosis), cryptococcosis, and tuberculosis. Peritoneal fluid accumulation may be associated with hypoalbuminemia (hepatic failure, renal failure, protein-losing enteropathy, intestinal maladsorption), septic peritonitis, diaphragmatic hernia, chlamydial or mycoplasmal peritonitis, organ rupture, pancreatitis, hemoperitoneum (trauma, clotting disorders, vascular neoplasms, thrombosis, torsion of stomach or spleen), ruptured abscess, pansteatitis, toxoplasmosis, and tuberculosis. Noneffusive FIP may resemble other systemic diseases depending on the organ affected. Differential diagnosis of this form should include lymphosarcoma and other neoplasms, toxoplasmosis, cryptococcosis, and chronic bacterial infections.

CLINICAL SIGNS

Effusive FIP is characterized by chronic weight loss, dehydration, depression, anorexia, refractory fever, and progressive abdominal enlargement due to ascites. Icterus may be seen in cases with severe liver involvement. Pleural effusion with clinical signs of respiratory insufficiency occurs in less than 25 to 30 per cent of cases. The onset of noneffusive FIP is more insidious and is frequently associated with organ-specific signs resulting from disseminated pyogranulomatous lesions in various organs. Clinical signs of renal and/or hepatic insufficiency, pancreatic disease, and central nervous system disease (meningitis, meningoencephalitis, myelitis) may be observed in cats with severe organ impairment. Neurologic signs may include posterior paresis, ataxia, nystagmus, behavioral changes, increased muscle rigidity, paralysis, and seizures, Ocular lesions, which occur in 25 per cent or more of cases of noneffusive FIP, include iritis, hyphema, keratic precipitates, retinal hemorrhage or detachment, chorioretinitis, and panophthalmitis. Ophthalmoscopic examination of cats that show signs of systemic disease is therefore an important diagnostic procedure.

The volume of fluid present in cases of effusive FIP varies and is generally a reflection of disease chronicity. In chronic cases a liter or more of fluid may accumulate within the abdominal cavity. Typically, this fluid is clear or slightly opaque, straw-colored to yellow, and viscous; contains fibrin strands or flakes; and often clots upon exposure to air. The fluid is an exudate of high specific gravity (1.017 to 1.047) and protein content (5 to 10 gm/dl) and variable cell numbers (1600 to 25,000 cells or more per µl); it probably represents leakage of fibrin-rich serum constituents directly out of damaged or inflamed blood vessels. In the acute form of FIP, the differential leukocyte count consists of neutrophils (predominantly), with smaller numbers of mononuclear cells. In the more chronic cases, mononuclear inflammatory cells (macrophages, lymphocytes, plasma cells) and mesothelial cells predominate. In contrast to cases of septic peritonitis, the majority of the leukocytes are intact (i.e., nondegenerate). Fungal, bacterial, mycoplasmal, and chlamydial isolations are usually negative.

Changes in the hemogram are variable and not specific for FIP. Commonly observed changes in affected cats are leukocytosis due to an absolute neutrophilia (which may be accompanied by either a regenerative or a degenerative left shift), moderate monocytosis, and eosinopenia. There is usually an absolute lymphopenia, which may be profound (0 to 250 cells/µl in some experimentally induced cases). Occasionally leukopenia may develop, especially in more fulminating or terminal cases. Nearly half of all cats with FIP develop a mild-to-moderate normocytic, normochromic anemia, which may be exacerbated by coinfection with feline leukemia virus and/or *Hemobartonella felis* (approximately 40 to 50 per cent of cats with FIP are also infected with feline leukemia virus). An increase in the icterus index may occur when the inflammatory process involves the liver. In noneffusive cases, total plasma proteins may exceed 8 gm/dl. The hyperproteinemia of FIP is frequently the result of a polyclonal hypergammaglobulinemia (elevations in IgG_1 and IgG_2 subclasses), with variable elevations of α_2 and β_2 globulins. However, FIP may also be associated with a monoclonal gammopathy (MacEwen and Hurvitz, 1977). Frequently there is a reversal of the A:G ratio (i.e., A:G < 0.6). Although these changes are suggestive of FIP, they are not diagnostic; hypergammaglobulinemia may also occur in other chronic inflammatory conditions associated with persistent antigenic stimulation of antibody-producing cells.

Experimentally, disseminated intravascular coagulation (DIC) has been observed in cats with FIP (Weiss et al., 1980). Multiple *in vitro* clotting abnormalities, including prolonged prothrombin and partial thromboplastin times; depression of coagulation factors VII, VIII, IX, X, and XII; elevation of fibrinogen and fibrin-fibrinogen degradation products; and thrombocytopenia, were documented in these cases. Severe vascular inflammation and thrombosis were reported in cats that developed DIC. Prolonged thromboplastin times, hyperfibrinogenemia, and elevation of fibrin-fibrinogen degradation products have also been seen in FIP field cases. The development of DIC is probably secondary to vascular damage, which is due to either virus-induced inflammation or deposition of immune complexes (which activate complement); DIC itself represents an important pathophysiologic mechanism in FIP.

Single or multiple acidophilic intracytoplasmic inclusion bodies, morphologically similar to canine and equine *Ehrlichia* structures, have been observed within a small number of circulating neutrophils in both natural and experimental cases. It has been suggested that they represent phagocytosed FIPV immune complexes rather than replicating virus (Horzinek and Osterhaus, 1979).

In general, abnormalities in clinical chemistry profiles reflect the extent of involvement of different organ systems in the disease process. Extensive liver involvement may produce hyperbilirubinemia and mild or moderate elevations in serum glutamic pyruvic transaminase (SGPT), serum glutamic oxaloacetic transaminase (SGOT), sorbitol dehydrogenase (SDH), and urobilinogenuria. A proteinuria with or without increased blood urea nitrogen (BUN) and serum creatinine and electrolyte disturbances may be seen in cases of renal involvement. Generalized peritoneal lesions involving the pancreas may result in clinical pancreatitis with elevations in serum lipase and/or amylase; severe cases may lead to diabetes mellitus (Pedersen, 1976b). Analysis of cerebrospinal fluid from cats with extensive meningeal lesions may reveal a nonseptic fluid high in protein (90 to 2000 mg/dl or more) and leukocytes (90 to 9000 cells/µl), the latter predominantly neutrophils. Similar changes may occur in aqueous humor from cats with anterior chamber involvement.

Histopathologic examination of suitable biopsy samples (the kidneys and mesenteric lymph nodes are most commonly involved in dry FIP) fixed in 10 per cent neutral-buffered formalin remains the most definitive technique for reliable antemortem diagnosis of noneffusive (and early effusive) FIP. Exploratory laparotomy and organ punch biopsy are the preferred methods (Abel and Johnson, 1975). Percutaneous needle biopsy is not recommended owing to the friability of affected viscera and the potential for serious hemorrhage, especially in cases with clotting abnormalities. Light general anesthesia with an inhalant such as halothane is preferred over barbiturates or ketamine, as these agents may further jeopardize hepatic and renal function in an already compromised patient.

Fibrinous peritonitis and/or pleuritis, with areas of focal necrosis in the omentum, liver, spleen, kidneys, and other organs, is the principal histologic feature of FIP. Necrotic foci are often subcapsular in location but may also be distributed throughout the organ parenchyma. Lesions contain necrotic neutrophils and debris surrounded by mononuclear cells (predominantly macrophages). The necrotic foci in FIP have a perivascular orientation, and there is a proliferative and necrotizing vasculitis, which is associated with the development of these necrotic lesions. In acute lesions both direct and indirect immunofluorescence microscopy may be useful for detection of coronaviral antigen in tissues. In more chronic lesions, viral antigen is less easily identified.

Coronaviral antibody titers in serum and exudates are also useful in the diagnosis of FIP in clinically ill animals (Scott, 1979; Barlough et al., 1981b). Feline coronaviral serology is discussed in the following section.

SEROLOGY AND SEROEPIDEMIOLOGY

The humoral response of the cat to FIPV has been studied by several immunologic techniques, including indirect immunofluorescent assay (IFA), enzyme linked–immunosorbent assay (ELISA), virus neutralization, and passive hemagglutination. Although IFA is the only one of these procedures to have been widely utilized thus far in clinical situations, ELISA has shown excellent potential as a more rapid and sensitive method for detection of feline coronaviral antibodies.

IFA

Indirect IFAs for feline coronaviral antibodies are either *homologous* or *heterologous,* depending on the source of antigen. In the homologous IFA, FIPV-infected tissue sections from cats with FIP are dried onto microscope slides and reacted with different dilutions of test serum. In the heterologous IFA, a cross reacting coronavirus grown in tissue culture serves as target antigen. The cross reacting virus most frequently used is TGEV, although CCV has also received attention. Reactions observed with HCV 229E are generally weak and are not acceptable for diagnostic purposes.

Serologic surveys using the IFA have indicated that coronaviral infections in cats are much more widespread than was once believed, especially in certain selected populations of cats. In the general feline population, excluding cats in catteries and isolated closed breeding colonies and cats with FIP, approximately 10 to 40 per cent will be seropositive for coronaviral antibodies. Titers in breeding catteries that have not experienced cases of FIP are either absent or present in 80 to 90 per cent of animals. Catteries in which FIP has occurred in general have a slightly higher prevalence of antibodies, in the range of 90 per cent or greater. Virtually 100 per cent of cats with clinical FIP are seropositive, whereas antibodies are absent in many specific pathogen-free (SPF) cats from closed colonies.

The presence of coronaviral antibodies in a healthy cat is indicative only of prior exposure to coronavirus (probably FIPV, but perhaps certain enteric coronaviruses or other cross reactive viruses, such as TGEV or HCV 229E). A positive coronaviral antibody titer in a healthy animal therefore does not diagnose clinical FIP, latent FIP, or viremia. Because the underlying basis of FIP is an immunopathologic mechanism involving virus, antibodies, and complement, a positive titer in a cat does not necessarily signal protection against the development of lethal FIP. Considering that FIP occurs sporadically in the general population and that most cats in FIP-problem catteries are seropositive yet do not contract FIP, it seems that a certain percentage of cats with coronaviral antibodies are protected against the development of FIP following natural exposure. The question remains whether these antibodies actually confer immunity or whether other humoral and/or cellular factors are involved in resistance.

Seropositive cats may shed virus from either the gastrointestinal or respiratory tract (or both); cats with persistently high titers apparently shed more FIPV than do cats with persistently low titers. Experimentally, seropositive cats develop a more rapid onset of FIP when compared with seronegative cats, and there is little difference in disease susceptibility among seropositive cats regardless of the magnitude of the coronaviral antibody titer. Presently there is no way to differentiate the cat with immunity to FIP from the asymptomatic chronic carrier, nor is there any way of predicting whether a seropositive cat will ever develop FIP.

In the general feline population, asymptomatic seropositive cats usually have titers ranging from 1:25 to 1:400 or greater. Titers in healthy cats may vary with time; some cats with titers of 1:1600 have shown a decrease in titer to less than 1:25 within one year (Post et al., 1978). A low or negative titer in an animal with clinical signs suggestive of FIP does not altogether eliminate the possibility of FIP, even though almost all cats with clinical disease have moderate to high titers. Antibody titers of 1:400 and above are consistent with *but not diagnostic of* FIP; fulminating effusive FIP may occasionally be associated with lower titers. The magnitude of the antibody titer is proportional to the chronicity of the disease; i.e., cats with noneffusive FIP generally have higher titers than cats with the more acute, effusive form.

There are several situations in which the immunofluorescent coronaviral antibody test is valuable to the general practitioner and the cat owner.

1. As an *aid* in the diagnosis of FIP in a symptomatic cat with signs suggestive of FIP.

2. To determine the presence or absence of antibodies (i.e., coronavirus exposure) in a previously untested household.

3. To detect potential virus carriers when introducing new cats into FIPV-free households or catteries.

4. To monitor treatment of FIP. Decreasing titers over time (except during the terminal stages of the disease) are indicative of clinical remission.

Virus Neutralization

Virus neutralization tests have been developed for detection of TGEV-, CCV-, and FIPV-neutralizing antibodies in feline serum and body fluids. Microtiter and plaque reduction assays have been used for measurement of TGEV- and CCV-neutralizing antibody titers, whereas FIPV-neutralizing antibody titers have been determined using *in vivo* propagation of FIPV in the brains of suckling mice. However, the results of virus neutralization tests have been conflicting and have not yet resolved important questions regarding humoral immunity to FIPV.

ELISA

A microtiter-based ELISA using TGEV as antigen has been reported (Osterhaus et al., 1979). ELISA titers in this system were found to correlate well with heterologous IFAs performed in parallel. A computer-assisted kinetics-based ELISA has recently been developed in our laboratory at Cornell University that has also shown good correlation with the heterologous IFA (Barlough et al., 1981a, 1983). Either TGEV or CCV can be used as antigens in these assays, and both produce essentially equivalent results.

IMMUNOPATHOGENESIS OF FIP

Experimental studies have shown that initial exposure to FIPV may result in localized upper respiratory disease in approximately 25 per cent of cats from two to six weeks later (Pedersen, 1978). This "primary" stage of disease manifests clinically as a mild to severe conjunctivitis and/or rhinitis, which may persist for one to four weeks. During this period, exposed cats develop low to moderate coronaviral antibody titers. Although the vast majority of cats undergoing the primary form of FIP recover, many cats will probably remain chronically infected (i.e., they will be chronic virus carriers). A very small number of exposed cats will develop the lethal disseminated ("secondary") form of the disease weeks to months (or years) after their primary

infection. The factors involved in susceptibility to fatal FIP are probably multiple: dose and strain of virus, route of exposure, age at time of exposure, concurrent viral infections (e.g., FeLV), genetic predisposition (e.g., inheritable abnormalities in immune response genes, genetically programmed macrophage dysfunction), administration of immunosuppressive drugs, and adverse environmental influences such as stress, overcrowding, and so on.

Although mechanisms of disease in FIP have been discussed for many years, recent evidence indicates that clinical FIP is the result of Arthus-like antigen-antibody-complement interactions across blood vessel walls and viral persistence within mononuclear phagocytes.

The basic lesion in FIP is a perivascular pyogranulomatous reaction consisting of a central area of necrotic cell debris and neutrophil infiltration surrounded by a thickened ring of mononuclear cells. FIP viral antigen, IgG, and the third component of complement (C3) have been demonstrated in these lesions by immunofluorescent microscopy (Weiss et al., 1980; Pedersen and Boyle, 1980; Weiss and Scott, 1981a, 1981b, 1981c). Circulating immune complexes and renal glomerular deposits of IgG and C3 have also been observed in both natural and experimental cases (Jacobse-Geels et al., 1980).

Studies have shown that when kittens with coronaviral antibody titers are challenged with FIPV, either by intraperitoneal inoculation or by exposure to live virus aerosols, a more fulminating form of FIP is produced than when seronegative kittens are similarly challenged (Weiss et al., 1980; Pedersen and Boyle, 1980; Weiss and Scott, 1981a, 1981b, 1981c). In addition, administration of either anti-FIPV immune serum or highly purified anti-FIPV IgG to seronegative cats prior to challenge has produced a rapidly fatal disease after exposure to FIPV (Pedersen and Boyle, 1980; Weiss and Scott, 1981b). A chronology for development of lesions and disease in FIPV-challenged seropositive and seronegative kittens is presented in Table 1.

TREATMENT

Presently there is no curative therapy for FIP. There are no antiviral agents or prophylactic vaccines that are effective against the virus, nor is there any way to eliminate the virus from asymptomatic chronic carrier cats. However, some treatment regimens may induce temporary remissions in a small percentage of carefully selected patients (Table 2).

The basic aim of therapy in FIP is to alleviate the disseminated inflammatory reactions resulting from deposition of antigen-antibody complexes. The most effective treatment protocols combine high levels of corticosteroids, cytotoxic drugs, and broad spectrum antibiotics and maintenance of nutrient intake and

Table 1. *Pathogenesis of Feline Infectious Peritonitis in Kittens Challenge Exposed by Virus Aerosol**

Sequence of Events	Time of Onset (Days Post Challenge)	
	Seropositive Kitten	Seronegative Kitten
1. Inhalation of virus	1	1
2. Phagocytosis (infection?) by macrophages in upper respiratory tract, tonsils, lung	1	1
3. Lymphatic drainage to pulmonary lymph nodes	1	1
4. Primary viral replication in lymph nodes	1 to 2	4 to 5
5. Primary viremia	1 to 2	4 to 5
6. Infection of blood monocytes; fixed macrophages in liver, spleen, vessel adventitia	2 to 3	6 to 11
7. Secondary viremia (persistent, cell associated)	2 to 3	6 to 11
8. Vascular inflammation	2 to 3	6 to 11
9. Perivascular necrosis, pyogranulomatous inflammation (complement mediated?)	3 to 4	11 to 13
10. Severe clinical disease, death	7 to 9	16 to 23

*Reprinted with permission from Weiss and Scott: Am. J. Vet. Res. 42:382, 1981.

fluid and electrolyte balance. Drainage of exudate followed by instillation of fibrinolytic enzymes (e.g., Varizyme,* 10,000 units) twice daily may be of benefit in some cases of effusive FIP. Cats receiving cytotoxic drugs should be routinely monitored (weekly intervals) for evidence of severe myelosuppression (leukopenia, thrombocytopenia, anemia).

The best candidates for therapy are cats in good physical condition that do not show severe anemia, neurologic signs, or other significant organ dysfunction. If the patient shows a positive response to therapy over the first few weeks, treatment can be continued for at least three months. If the cat is in complete remission at this time, therapy may be discontinued. Treatment should be reinstituted if signs recur or if the coronaviral antibody titer begins to show a significant elevation. Progressive deterioration of physical condition and persistence of high coronaviral antibody levels in the face of treatment are generally poor prognostic signs. Coinfection

*American Cyanamid Co., Princeton, NJ.

Table 2. *Chemotherapeutic Protocol for Feline Infectious Peritonitis*

Drug	Dosage
1. Prednisolone	4 mg/kg, PO once daily in the evening
2. Cyclophosphamide (Cytoxan*)	2 mg/kg PO once daily for four consecutive days of each week OR
Melphalan (Alkeran†)	1 mg PO every third day
3. Ampicillin	20 mg/kg PO three times daily
4. Stanozolol (Winstrol-V‡)	1 mg PO twice daily

*Mead Johnson Pharmaceutical, Evansville, IN.
†Burroughs Wellcome Co., Research Triangle Park, NC.
‡Winthrop Laboratories, New York, NY.

with feline leukemia virus is a significant complicating factor, and the FeLV status of all suspected FIP cats should be determined prior to commencing treatment.

Research into other treatments for FIP is continuing. Complement depletion, anticoagulant therapy, and interferon are possible areas of investigation, representing new therapeutic approaches based on recent understanding of FIP pathogenesis.

IMMUNIZATION

Routine immunization against FIP is not currently possible. Experiments thus far with various preparations of FIPV and TGEV have been unsuccessful in conferring protective immunity against FIP. Owing to the immunologic nature of the disease, parenteral coronavirus immunization with existing virus strains may paradoxically predispose cats to lethal, disseminated FIP. Further research involving the immunogenicity of individual viral proteins of tissue culture-adapted FIPV strains may yield information necessary for the development of an effective subunit vaccine.

CONTROL OF FIPV INFECTIONS

General recommendations for the management of coronaviral antibody-positive and antibody-negative catteries are given in Table 3.

A test-and-removal program for asymptomatic coronaviral antibody–positive cats similar to that utilized for FeLV infection *is not currently recommended.* Since there is no available diagnostic test that differentiates actively infected cats from immune seropositive cats, there is no indication at the present time for destroying healthy seropositive cats.

Table 3. *General Recommendations for Control of FIPV Infection in Catteries**

Coronaviral Antibody–Positive Catteries
1. Maintain cats in as good health as possible. Provide adequate air circulation, but keep temperature conditions warm. Avoid stress by providing good nutrition, vaccinating against other viruses, eliminating feline "psychosomatic" conditions, and so on.
2. Isolate or remove any FeLV-positive cats.
3. Remove breeding queens with repeat problems of bloody vaginal discharge, reproductive failure, neonatal deaths.
4. Wean all kittens as early as possible and hand rear them away from other cats.
5. Keep premises thoroughly cleaned with an effective virucidal disinfectant, such as standard bleach diluted 1:32 in water.

Coronaviral Antibody–Negative Catteries
1. Keep premises clean and sanitary.
2. New cats should come from catteries without a past history of FIP diagnosis and should have tested negative for coronaviral antibodies within the past 30 days. All new cats should be kept in quarantine for two to three weeks before entering the cattery and then retested for coronaviral antibodies. Cats testing negative both times can be allowed to enter the cattery.
3. Cattery cats should not be sent to coronaviral antibody–positive catteries for breeding and should not be allowed to contact coronaviral antibody–positive cats in any way.
4. All cats returning from shows should be kept in quarantine for at least two weeks. If signs of upper respiratory infection are noted, quarantine should be continued and a coronaviral antibody titer determined after three to four weeks.

*From Scott et al.: Feline Info. Bull. No. 4, 1978; Scott et al.: Proceedings of the 46th Annual A.A.H.A. Meeting, 1979; Scott: J.A.V.M.A. 175:1164, 1979.

FELINE ENTERIC CORONAVIRUSES (see also Feline Enteric Viruses, page 1168)

Another coronavirus, morphologically distinct from FIPV, has been observed by electron microscopy in feces from healthy kittens and adult cats from two different minimal-disease feline breeding colonies (Hoshino and Scott, 1980). This enteric coronavirus is morphologically similar to enteric coronaviruses of humans, monkeys, and dogs. Both coronaviral antibody-positive and negative cats can excrete viral particles, and there appears to be little correlation between serum coronaviral antibody titer and the presence of this virus. Electron microscopic examination of feces indicates that virus excretion may persist for up to four months. This virus has also been detected in fecal samples from cats hospitalized at the small animal clinic of the Veterinary Medical Teaching Hospital, Cornell University. Both clinically normal cats and cats with enteric disease may shed viral particles in their feces.

A second feline enteric coronavirus, morphologically indistinguishable from FIPV, has been reported from cats reared in a conventional feline breeding colony (Pedersen et al., 1981b). This virus was detected in feces of healthy cats and produces mild pyrexia, leukopenia, and diarrhea when experimentally fed to young kittens. Exposure to this virus is followed by the appearance of coronaviral antibodies in serum. It was suggested that this second enteric coronavirus is responsible for a major proportion of the coronaviral antibody titers present in the general feline population and that FIPV possibly represents an uncommon pathogenic variant.

A coronavirus has recently been isolated in tissue culture from a cat with fatal hemorrhagic enteritis (McKeirnan et al., 1981). This virus was related antigenically to both FIPV and CCV. It is not known whether this virus represents an enteric-adapted FIPV strain or another distinct enteric coronavirus.

REFERENCES AND SUPPLEMENTAL READING

Abel, D. L., and Johnson, J. J.: Parenchymal feline infectious peritonitis: antemortem diagnosis by punch biopsy. Feline Pract. 5(3):44, 1975.

Barlough, J. E., Jacobson, R. H., Downing, D. R., Marcella, K. L., Lynch, T. J., and Scott, F. W.: Evaluation of a computer-assisted, kinetics based enzyme-linked immunosorbent assay for detection of coronavirus antibodies in cats. J. Clin. Microbiol., in press, 1983.

Barlough, J. E., Jacobson, R. H., Marcella, K. L., and Scott, F. W.: Semiautomated kinetics-based ELISA for detection of feline coronaviral antibodies. Cornell Feline Health Center News 5:1, 1981a.

Barlough, J. E., Weiss, R. C., and Scott, F. W.: Interpretation of serum antibody titers to feline infectious peritonitis virus. Minnesota Vet. 21;28, 1981b.

Black, J. W.: Recovery and *in vitro* cultivation of a coronavirus from laboratory-induced cases of feline infectious peritonitis (FIP). V.M./S.A.C. 75:811, 1980.

Evermann, J. F., Baumgartener, L., Ott, R. L., Davis, E. V., and McKeirnan, A. J.: Characterization of a feline infectious peritonitis virus isolate. Vet. Pathol. 18:256, 1981.

Hitchcock, L. M., O'Reilly, K. J., and Beesley, J. E.: In vitro culture of feline infectious peritonitis virus. Vet. Rec. 108:535, 1981.

Horzinek, M. C., and Osterhaus, A. D. M. E.: The virology and pathogenesis of feline infectious peritonitis. Arch. Virol. 59:1, 1979.

Hoshino, Y., and Scott, F. W.: Brief communication: Replication of feline infectious peritonitis virus in organ cultures of feline tissue. Cornell Vet. 68:411, 1978.

Hoshino, Y., and Scott, F. W.: Coronavirus-like particles in the feces of normal cats. Arch. Virol. 63:147, 1980.

Jacobse-Geels, H. E. L., Daha, M. R., and Horzinek, M. C.: Isolation and characterization of feline C3 and evidence of the immune complex pathogenesis of feline infectious peritonitis. J. Immunol. 125:1606, 1980.

MacEwen, E. G., and Hurvitz, A. I.: Diagnosis and management of monoclonal gammopathies. Vet. Clin. North Am. 7:119, 1977.

McKeirnan, A. J., Evermann, J. F., Hargis, A., Miller, L. M., and Ott, R. L.: Isolation of feline coronaviruses from two cats with diverse disease manifestations. Feline Pract. 11(3):16, 1981.

O'Reilly, K. J., Fishman, B., and Hitchcock, L. M.: Feline infectious peritonitis: Isolation of a coronavirus. Vet. Rec. 104:348, 1979.

Osterhaus, A. D. M. E., Horzinek, M. C., and Wirahadiredja, R. M. S.: Feline infectious peritonitis virus. II. Propagation in suckling mouse brain. Zentralbl. Veterinaermed. [B]25:301, 1978a.

Osterhaus, A. D. M. E., Horzinek, M. C., Wirahadiredja, R. M. S., and Kroon, A.: Feline infectious peritonitis (FIP) virus. IV. Propagation in suckling rat and hamster brain. Zentralbl. Veterinaermed. [B]25:816, 1978b.

Osterhaus, A., Kroon, A., and Wirahadiredja, R.: ELISA for the serology of FIP virus. Vet. Quart. 1:59, 1979.

Pedersen, N. C.: Morphologic and physical characteristics of feline infectious peritonitis virus and its growth in autochthonous peritoneal cell cultures. Am. J. Vet. Res. 37:567, 1976a.

Pedersen, N. C.: Feline infectious peritonitis: Something old, something new. Feline Pract. 6(3):42, 1976b.

Pedersen, N. C.: Feline infectious diseases. Proceedings of the 45th Annual A.A.H.A. Meeting, 125, 1978.

Pedersen, N. C., and Boyle, J. F.: Immunologic phenomena in the effusive form of feline infectious peritonitis. Am. J. Vet. Res. 41:868, 1980.

Pedersen, N. C., Boyle, J. F., and Floyd, K.: Infection studies in kittens, using feline infectious peritonitis virus propagated in cell culture. Am. J. Vet. Res. 42:363, 1981a.

Pedersen, N. C., Boyle, J. F., Floyd, K., Fudge, A., and Barker, J.: An enteric coronavirus infection of cats and its relationship to feline infectious peritonitis. Am. J. Vet. Res. 42:368, 1981b.

Pedersen, N. C., Ward, J., and Mengeling, W. L.: Antigenic relationship of the feline infectious peritonitis virus to coronaviruses of other species. Arch. Virol. 58:45, 1978.

Post, J. E., Wellenstein, R. C., and Clarke, R. D.: Serological tests for feline infectious peritonitis using TGE virus antigen. Proceedings of the 21st Annual Meeting of the American Association of Veterinary Laboratory Diagnosticians, 427, 1978.

Scott, F. W.: FIP antibody test—interpretation and recommendations. J.A.V.M.A., 175:1164, 1979.

Scott, F. W., Hoshino, Y., and Weiss, R. C.: Feline infectious peritonitis. Feline Info. Bull. No. 4, 1978.

Scott, F. W., Weiss, R. C., and Hoshino, Y.: Feline infectious peritonitis. Proceedings of the 46th Annual A.A.H.A. Meeting, 109, 1979.

Weiss, R. C., Dodds, W. J., and Scott, F. W.: Disseminated intravascular coagulation in experimentally induced feline infectious peritonitis. Am. J. Vet. Res. 41:663, 1980.

Weiss, R. C., and Scott, F. W.: Pathogenesis of feline infectious peritonitis: nature and development of viremia. Am. J. Vet. Res. 42:382, 1981a.

Weiss, R. C., and Scott, F. W.: Antibody-mediated enhancement of disease in feline infectious peritonitis: Comparisons with dengue hemorrhagic fever. J. Comp. Immunol. Microbiol. Infect. Dis. 4:175, 1981b.

Weiss, R. C., and Scott, F. W.: Pathogenesis of feline infectious peritonitis: pathologic changes and immunofluorescence. Am. J. Vet. Res. 42:2036, 1981c.

DIAGNOSIS AND MANAGEMENT OF FELINE LEUKEMIA VIRUS INFECTIONS

JEFFREY E. BARLOUGH, D.V.M.

Ithaca, New York

Feline leukemia virus (FeLV) is the causative agent of the most important fatal infectious disease complex of American domestic cats today. It is a horizontally transmitted, enveloped, single-strand ribonucleic acid (RNA) virus of the family Retroviridae. Retroviruses causing lymphoproliferative neoplasia have been identified in a number of species, including cats, cattle, swine, domestic fowl, certain nonhuman primates, and rodents. Other retroviruses are associated with nonmalignant disease processes, such as the agents of visna/maedi of sheep, arthritis-encephalitis of goats, and equine infectious anemia.

Replication-competent retroviruses possess an enzyme, *reverse transcriptase*, that permits viral replication by way of a deoxyribonucleic acid (DNA) intermediate. A single-strand complementary DNA (cDNA) copy of the retroviral genome is synthesized by reverse transcriptase in the cytoplasm, converted to double-strand (duplex) DNA, and transported to the nucleus. There it is integrated into the genome of the host cell as a *provirus*, where it can code for the synthesis of new virions. The mechanism of integration is unknown. New viral RNA synthesis from proviral DNA is initiated by a polymerase of host cell origin. Virus assembly occurs in the cyto-

plasm, with budding of mature virions from the plasma membrane.

Excretion of FeLV occurs primarily by way of salivary secretions, although virus is also present in respiratory secretions, feces, and urine. Healthy FeLV-infected cats excrete levels of virus in their saliva that are as high or higher than levels found in the general circulation (10^3 to 10^6 infectious virions/ml). Infection probably occurs primarily by ingestion of the virus. In addition, *in utero* transfer across the placenta and colostral excretion are known to occur. Thus, the social grooming habits of cats, licking and biting, sneezing, and the urban practice of sharing litter boxes and feeding bowls probably represent the major methods of spread of FeLV among pet cats. Kittens may become infected either through an infected queen or by close contact with other infected cats. Prolonged close contact among cats is necessary for the most efficient transmission of the virus. The latent period between initial exposure to FeLV and the development of either infection or immunity is quite variable and may be dependent, in part, on the route of virus transmission.

Studies have demonstrated that age at time of exposure to FeLV and the amount and strain of infective dose are important determinants of the outcome of a FeLV challenge. Whereas most kittens experimentally infected with FeLV become persistently viremic, most adult cats over six months of age resist FeLV infection, suggesting that age-related maturational changes in lymphoreticular and hematopoietic tissues are involved. Evidence indicates that these changes occur between two and four months of age, a period during which maternal immunity is waning and active immunity is developing.

Following experimental infection of kittens with FeLV, a low-grade viremia involving small numbers of circulating mononuclear cells occurs within two weeks (Rojko et al., 1979). In this way the virus is transported to other regions of the body, especially to systemic lymphoid tissue, intestinal crypt epithelium, and bone marrow, areas that contain populations of rapidly dividing cells where viral replication can be enhanced. Infection of neutrophil and platelet precursor cells and their subsequent release into the circulation result in a second, more profound viremia. In those cats that resist widespread infection and replication of FeLV, virus containment occurs in the early lymphoreticular stage of infection. In those animals that become persistently viremic, there is extensive infection of bone marrow and epithelial tissues of the pharynx, esophagus, stomach, bladder, respiratory tract, and salivary glands.

FeLV infection has been associated with thymic atrophy, depletion of peripheral blood lymphocytes and secondary lymphoid tissue, especially lymph nodes, and an impairment of cell-mediated immunity (CMI), thought to be the result of a local and/or generalized loss of T lymphocyte responsiveness. Both intact and disrupted viral particles are capable of inducing CMI suppression. One mediator of FeLV immunosuppression has been identified as a viral envelope-associated protein, $p15(E)$ (Mathes et al., 1978). The significance of FeLV-induced immunosuppression is especially apparent when one considers the array of secondary diseases associated with FeLV infection. In addition, immunosuppression mediated by $p15(E)$, even from disrupted virus, is an important consideration in the design of an effective FeLV vaccine.

DIAGNOSTIC AIDS FOR FeLV INFECTION

There are currently three basic laboratory procedures commercially available to assist the practitioner in determining the FeLV and FeLV-immune status of an animal: (1) detection of viral antigens; (2) detection of virus-neutralizing antibodies (VNA); and (3) detection of antibodies to the feline oncornavirus cell membrane–associated antigen (FOCMA).

DETECTION OF VIRAL ANTIGENS

A 27,000-dalton protein moiety, $p27$, is a structural component of the viral core shell and is the major FeLV group-specific antigen. It can be found in great abundance in the cytoplasm of infected leukocytes and platelets and in soluble form in plasma and serum of infected cats. This protein provides the major antigenic basis for both the indirect immunofluorescence assay (IFA) and the enzyme-linked immunosorbent assay (ELISA) for FeLV. The significance of the immunologic response to $p27$ itself is at present uncertain, because antibodies directed against it are not protective and prevent neither viremia nor FeLV-related disease. Indeed, some studies suggest that immune complex disease can result from the humoral response to $p27$.

For the IFA procedure (FeLeuk Test*), at least three unfixed, air-dried blood smears made on clear glass microscope slides should be submitted. Two to three drops of freshly drawn blood should be placed in the center of each slide and then smeared in a single smooth motion with the edge of another slide held at an oblique angle. Smears can also be made from recently drawn heparinized or EDTA-treated blood. Smears made from partially clotted or traumatized blood samples are difficult to interpret and should not be submitted.

In the laboratory the blood smears are fixed with acetone or alcohol and overlaid with rabbit antibodies directed against disrupted FeLV (Hardy et al., 1973. FeLV-infected cells present in the smears will bind to and retain these antibodies. After the excess antiserum has been removed, a conjugate composed of fluorescein-labelled antibodies to rabbit immunoglobulin G is applied. After final washing and counterstaining, the slides are viewed with a fluorescent microscope. The presence of multiple fluorescing apple-green granules within the cytoplasm of leukocytes and/or platelets is indicative of the presence of FeLV and constitutes a positive test.

In the ELISA kit test (Leukassay-F†), either whole blood, serum, or plasma is added to test plate wells that have been coated with antibody to FeLV $p27$ (Mia et al., 1981). If soluble FeLV or FeLV released from damaged cells is present in a test sample, it will be immunologically bound at the surface of the well. A second antibody, which also recognizes $p27$ and which is linked to an enzyme (peroxidase), is then added and complexes with $p27$ already bound. After appropriate washing, a substrate solution containing hydrogen peroxide and orthophenylenediamine (OPD) is added. Immunologically bound peroxidase will hydrolyze the hydrogen peroxide, releasing oxygen, which con-

---

*National Veterinary Laboratory, Franklin Lakes, NJ.
†Pitman-Moore, Inc., Washington Crossing, NJ.

verts the OPD into a colored form. Development of an amber color distinctly more intense than that of a negative reference well is indicative of the presence of FeLV p27 in the test sample.

Virus isolation in monolayer cell cultures is a common procedure in research laboratories studying the biology of FeLV and is used for the diagnosis of FeLV infection in certain other countries, such as Scotland (Jarrett, 1980). Isolation of infectious FeLV from blood is well correlated with salivary excretion of virus and usually indicates persistent viremia.

DETECTION OF VNA

FeLV virions consist of two distinct components: an electron-dense inner core or *nucleoid*, and an outer envelope containing an immunologically important 70,000-dalton glycoprotein, *gp70*. This glycoprotein is the principal antigen present in the projecting knobs (peplomers) of the viral envelope. It is also expressed on the plasma membrane of infected cells. Attachment and penetration by FeLV are mediated by this antigen in cooperation with host cell–surface receptors. VNA directed against gp70 of the appropriate FeLV subgroup is an essential component of a successful immunologic response to FeLV. A number of commercial and university veterinary laboratories currently perform focus inhibition assays for VNA.

DETECTION OF FOCMA ANTIBODIES

A certain percentage of cats exposed to FeLV will develop complement-dependent antibodies directed against FOCMA, a tumor-specific virus-specified antigen complex in the plasma membrane of both FeLV-producing and FeLV-nonproducing transformed cells. Detection of FOCMA antibodies is accomplished by reacting test serum in an immunofluorescence procedure with cultured FeLV-producing feline lymphoma (FL-74) cells. The presence of distinct flecks or bands of plasma membrane fluorescence in these cells is indicative of the presence of FOCMA. Although it has been generally accepted that only *transformed* FeLV-infected cells express FOCMA at their surface, there is recent *in vitro* evidence that some FeLV-infected nontransformed cells can also express FOCMA (Rice et al., 1981).

INTERPRETATION OF FeLV TEST RESULTS

VIRAL ANTIGENS

A positive test for FeLV by IFA indicates the presence of FeLV-infected blood cells in a cat at the time the sample was taken. Additionally, a positive IFA test implies that a cat is shedding virus and is a potential health hazard to uninfected, susceptible cats, especially kittens and immunosuppressed animals. A positive test does not diagnose an FeLV-related disease. A negative test indicates that no detectable infected blood cells are present. It does not exclude the possibility that a cat is incubating FeLV at the time of testing, nor does it imply that a cat has developed immunity to FeLV. Virus-nonproducing lymphosarcomas and leukemias, representing variably 10 to 50 per cent of all feline lymphoid tumors, will test negatively for FeLV. Almost invariably, cats that test positive by IFA are persistently viremic; reversion to negative status is a rare occurrence (Lester and Searcy, 1981; Hardy, 1981). A positive test by ELISA can indicate either transient or persistent FeLV infection. Because viral replication in transiently viremic cats is limited to lymphoreticular tissue and does not involve extensive invasion of neutrophil and platelet precursor cells in bone marrow, viral antigen is found only in soluble form (serum, plasma) and in small amounts in circulating mononuclear cells. Soluble FeLV in both transiently and persistently viremic cats can be detected by the ELISA.

Transiently viremic cats characteristically test positive by ELISA and then revert to negative status several weeks later. It is thus important that ELISA-positive tests be either repeated in three to four weeks or confirmed by IFA to determine whether the infection is transient or persistent. Recently, comparison studies of IFA and ELISA methods have identified some cats with persistence of soluble p27 (ELISA-positive) for extended periods of time without expression of cell-associated p27 (IFA-negative) or with only transient ($\leq$ 1 week) expression (Lutz et al., 1980). Experimentally, some IFA-negative cats have low levels of circulating p27, which are detectable by ELISA for many months (Rice and Olsen, 1981). These findings suggest that a persistent, low-level FeLV infection, with release of either infectious virus or a form of soluble p27 from as yet unidentified cells, may be responsible for some persistently ELISA-positive, IFA-negative test results.

VNA

Cats with protective levels of VNA ($\geq$ 1:10 by focus inhibition assay) have resisted widespread FeLV infection and in most cases are protected against subsequent development of persistent viremia. Thus, most cats with protective levels of VNA will not develop any of the FeLV-associated diseases. However, because a duplex DNA copy of the retroviral genome stably integrates into the host cell chromosomal DNA during viral infection and replication, latent FeLV proviral infection with possible transformation at some time in the future cannot be excluded in cats with VNA. Moreover, previously exposed FeLV-negative cats treated with synthetic corticosteroids may experience a reactivation of their infection, presumably owing to the continued presence of integrated FeLV proviral sequences (Post and Warren, 1980).

FOCMA ANTIBODIES

There is currently some discussion concerning interpretation of antibody titers to FOCMA. FOCMA antibody titers appear to be higher in cats that resist FeLV infection and cellular transformation and in persistently viremic healthy cats and lower in cats with FeLV-induced neoplasms. In general, the higher the FOCMA antibody titer, the greater the probability that a cat is protected against the oncogenic effects of FeLV. Titers of 1:32 and above are probably protective for most cats in the general population (Hardy, 1981). However, recent research suggests a more complex situation, involving numerous FOCMA antigenic determinants with a constellation of specific antibodies comprising the anti-FOCMA immune response. Cats with FeLV-induced tumors have a restricted capacity to respond to many FOCMA determinants, suggesting that their tumors may have arisen because FOCMA antibodies were directed against specific FOCMA determinants different from those present on the tumor cells (Grant and Michalek, 1981).

CONTROL OF FeLV INFECTIONS

Elimination of FeLV from an infected household can be achieved by adherence to the FeLV IFA test-and-removal protocol, as outlined hereafter.

All cats in the household should be tested, regardless of age or condition. *All* infected cats should be removed and the household premises thoroughly cleaned with a commercial product such as sodium hypochlorite (Clorox bleach) diluted 1:32 in water. All litter boxes and food and water bowls should be replaced. Cats that initially tested negative should be retested several times over a period of 8 to 12 months in the event that they were infected just before the first test or prior to the onset of detectable viremia or are cycling in their level of detectable viremia. The latent period between exposure and viremia is extremely variable, and an infected cat that tested negative initially may be positive when tested again later. During this period of testing no new cats should be allowed to enter the household. If any FeLV-positive cats are found, they should be removed and another quarantine period imposed.

All new cats entering an FeLV-negative household should be tested prior to entry. Those that test negative should be quarantined in separate quarters for three to five months and retested negative two to three times before being allowed to intermix with the established FeLV-negative household population. New cats should ideally be obtained only from other households or catteries practicing FeLV test-and-removal.

Routine yearly or twice yearly testing for FeLV is suggested for all cats in catteries owing to the variable latent period of infection. Viremic cats should never be used for breeding purposes, because infected queens will transmit virus to their viable offspring *in utero* and by colostral and salivary excretion.

FeLV test-and-removal has been highly effective in eliminating FeLV from infected multiple-cat households. In a survey of 45 households from which 159 FeLV-infected cats were removed, 561 of 564 (99.5 per cent) FeLV-negative cats remained negative upon subsequent testing (Hardy et al., 1976). Multiple-cat households in which FeLV test-and-removal has not been implemented have experienced an infection rate over 40 times greater than that experienced by catteries in which the program has been successfully introduced.

In solitary-cat households, an FeLV-infected cat should be removed, the litter box and feeding dishes replaced, and the premises thoroughly cleaned with an agent such as sodium hypochlorite. A "waiting period" of approximately three months should then be observed prior to repopulation with one or more FeLV-negative cats.

It is not uncommon for owners of asymptomatic (and often symptomatic) FeLV-positive cats in both solitary- and multiple-cat households to decline implementation of FeLV test-and-removal. Under these circumstances, certain modifications of the program may serve as a reasonable compromise. FeLV-positive cats in these households should be isolated from contact with all other cats. This will not only prevent the spread of infectious FeLV to susceptible animals but will also decrease exposure of immunosuppressed, viremic cats to other infectious agents. No new cats should be introduced at any time, and FeLV-positive cats should not be allowed to breed. Separate litter boxes and feeding dishes should be maintained for positive and negative cats. Cleanliness and personal hygiene should be observed at all times, and it has been suggested that separate clothing be kept for contact with FeLV-positive cats to minimize mechanical transmission of virus. FeLV is relatively labile in the environment, however, and the degree of virus transmission under these circumstances is uncertain.

REFERENCES AND SUPPLEMENTAL READING

Grant, C. K., and Michalek, M. T.: Feline leukemia—unique and crossreacting antigens on individual virus-producing tumors identified by complement-dependent antibody. Int. J. Cancer 28:209, 1981.

Hardy, W. D., Jr.: The feline leukemia virus. J. Am. Anim. Hosp. Assoc. 17:951, 1981.

Hardy, W. D., Jr., Hess, P. W., MacEwen, E. G., McClelland, A. J., Zuckerman, E. E., Essex, M., Cotter, S. M., and Jarrett, O.: Biology of feline leukemia virus in the natural environment. Cancer Res. 36:582, 1976.

Hardy, W. D., Jr., Hirshaut, Y., and Hess, P.: Detection of the feline leukemia virus and other mammalian oncornaviruses by immunofluorescence. Bibl. Haemat. 39:778, 1973.

Jarrett, O.: Feline leukaemia virus diagnosis. Vet. Rec. 106:513, 1980.

Lester, S. J., and Searcy, G. P.: Hematologic abnormalities preceding apparent recovery from feline leukemia virus infection. J. A. V. M. A. 178:471, 1981.

Lutz, H., Pedersen, N. C., Harris, C. W., Higgins, J., and Theilen, G. H.: Detection of feline leukemia virus infection. Feline Pract. 10(4):13, 1980.

Mathes, L. E., Olsen, R. G., Hebebrand, L. C., Hoover, E. A., and Schaller, J. P.: Abrogation of lymphocyte blastogenesis by a feline leukaemia virus protein. Nature 274:687, 1978.

Mia, A. S., Kahn, D. E., Tierney, M. M., and Post, J. E.: A micro-enzyme-linked immunosorbent assay (ELISA) test for detection of feline leukemia virus in cats. Comp. Immun. Microbiol. Infect. Dis. 4:111, 1981.

Post, J. E., and Warren, L.: Reactivation of latent feline leukemia virus. In Hardy, W. D., Jr., Essex, M., and McClelland, A. J. (eds.): Feline Leukemia Virus. New York: Elsevier North Holland, Inc., 1980, pp. 151–155.

Rice, J. B., and Olsen, R. G.: Feline oncovirus-associated cell membrane antigen and feline leukemia virus group-specific antigen expression in bone marrow and serum. J. Natl. Cancer Inst. 66:737, 1981.

Rice, J. B., Schaller, J. P., Lewis, M. G., Mathes, L. E., Hoover, E. A., and Olsen, R. G.: Infection of feline embryo adherent cells with feline leukemia virus: feline oncornavirus-associated cell membrane antigen expression and morphologic transformation. J. Natl. Cancer Inst. 66:89, 1981.

Rojko, J. L., Hoover, E. A., Mathes, L. E., Olsen, R. G., and Schaller, J. P.: Pathogenesis of experimental feline leukemia virus infection. J. Natl. Cancer Inst. 63:759, 1979.

Rickettsial and Protozoal Diseases

CANINE EHRLICHIOSIS

JENNIFER E. PRICE, B.V.M.,
and PAUL D. SAYER, B.V.M.S.

Nairobi, Kenya

In the past 20 years, canine ehrlichiosis has been described in many areas of the world. Its manifestations can be surprisingly varied. Synonyms include tropical canine pancytopenia, canine hemorrhagic fever, tracker dog disease, canine rickettsiosis, canine tick typhus, and Nairobi bleeding disease.

Ehrlichia canis, the causative agent of canine ehrlichiosis, is an intracellular, tick-borne rickettsial organism that passes transstadially but not transovarially through the tick and is found in the mononuclear series of dog leukocytes. Lewis and Huxsoll (1977) have reviewed the epidemiology of canine erhlichiosis, which has been reported from most zones where *Rhipicephalus sanguineus*, the brown dog tick, is found, Australia being a notable exception. No reports of natural transmission by any other vector have been confirmed. The infection is restricted to the Canidae.

Although differences in the incidence of canine ehrlichiosis are to be expected from one endemic area to another and at different seasons of the year in relation to changing vector densities, greater awareness of the disease and improved diagnostic technique have increased identification. Canine ehrlichiosis is often found in association with, or as a result of, other stress or disease entities and for this reason may be overlooked.

CLINICAL SIGNS

A wide variety of clinical syndromes is associated with *Ehrlichia canis* infection, ranging from asymptomatic cases through those showing only mild malaise and inappetance to severe and sometimes fatal cases. Signs commonly seen in naturally occurring canine ehrlichiosis are selective appetite, lethargy, weight loss, pallor or congestion of mucous membranes, pyrexia, splenomegaly, and lymph node enlargement. Other signs include blood in feces, hematuria, hematemesis, epistaxis, petechiation or ecchymosis of the visible mucous membranes or skin, abortion, and eye lesions. In spite of a considerable degree of overlap, classification may usefully be attempted according to major clinical, hematologic, or serum biochemical changes. The following broad groups of cases may be distinguished: acute, chronic, hemorrhagic, neurologic, those with breeding disorders, uremic, subclinical, and carrier state. Babesiosis may be present concurrently with ehrlichiosis in some areas.

There is no evidence of any age, sex, or breed predisposition in our series of 1,500 clinical cases.

Acute Cases. Dogs with acute ehrlichiosis may present with a sudden onset of depression, anorexia, pyrexia, and emesis. Pale or congested mucous membranes, splenomegaly, and lymph node enlargement may be detected on physical examination. Since many of these signs are also seen in dogs with babesiosis, it is essential that a Giemsa-stained peripheral blood smear from such animals be carefully examined for the presence of *Babesia* parasites and/or *E. canis*.

Chronic Cases. Animals with chronic ehrlichiosis show either repeated hemorrhage or progressive weakness until death. The hemorrhage may be in the form of epistaxis and hemorrhage into body cavities or organs and subcutaneously. All dogs in this group are anemic, leukopenic, and thrombocytopenic. This state of pancytopenia is associated with hypoplasia of the bone marrow. Once dogs reach this chronic stage, they are refractory to treatment, and the course is likely to be brief, terminating in death.

There is a difference in the pathogenesis of acute and severe chronic ehrlichiosis. In acute ehrlichiosis, there is increased sequestration or destruction of blood cells, which results in a transitory pancytopenia, whereas the bone marrow remains normal (Buhles et al., 1974). Treatment of this stage of disease results in rapid recovery. However, in chronic ehrlichiosis, pancytopenia is associated with bone marrow hypoplasia. Treatment of these cases is not usually successful.

Hemorrhagic Cases. Dogs with hemorrhagic ehrlichiosis exhibit the classic signs for which canine ehrlichiosis acquired its notorious reputation as a severe bleeding disease in parts of Africa, India, and Southeast Asia. Few hemorrhagic cases, however, are seen in the chronic, bone marrow hypoplastic state. Petechial and ecchymotic hemorrhages may be visible on the mucous membranes of the mouth, eye, prepuce, or vulva or in the relatively hairless areas of the skin on the abdomen and pinna of the ears or on the iris. Frank bleeding may occur in the form of epistaxis, hematuria, hematemesis, and blood in the feces (either melena or fresh blood). Bleeding may occur into one or more joints, which may result in a sudden onset of lameness. Prolonged bleeding from injection sites or from minor surgical procedures (e.g., claw clipping) and during routine surgery is a possible feature in this group. These signs may either appear suddenly with no other complaint or detectable abnormality or may be present in dogs that are in a state of collapse.

Thrombocytopenia is present in both acute (sometimes it may be transitory) and chronic ehrlichiosis.

Hemorrhage is due to a rapid decrease in platelets and not to a coagulation factor abnormality (Huxsoll et al., 1970). Only a bone marrow biopsy establishes the difference between the two forms of ehrlichiosis and aids in prognosis.

Neurologic Cases. Animals with neurologic ehrlichiosis show involvement of the central nervous system, probably owing to hemorrhage. One or more of the following signs may be noted: arched back, severe pain in the neck or back, unilateral or bilateral hind leg paresis, paraplegia, or sudden collapse. No abnormalities of the spinal column will be detectable by plain radiography. Spinal hemorrhage has proved difficult to confirm in the cases we have seen because it was not always justifiable to subject the patient to the risk of general anesthesia for cerebrospinal fluid collection and because none of the cases with neurologic involvement were submitted for autopsy. In the animals from which cerebrospinal fluid was collected, the erythrocyte count was equivocal. The presence of frank blood in the fluid suggested a sampling fault, whereas negligible changes in erythrocytes merely indicated that any hemorrhage or capillary leak might be within the parenchyma of the cord and not into the subarachnoid space. Xanthochromic yellow cerebrospinal fluid was not detected. Attempts to culture the causal organism in cells from the cerebrospinal fluid were not successful; however, *E. canis* could be cultured from the blood of these animals, and improvement occurred after treatment.

Breeding Disorders. A number of problems associated with breeding have been found in *Ehrlichia*-positive bitches; these include prolonged bleeding during the estrous cycle, inability to conceive, abortion, and neonatal death. Confirmation of *Ehrlichia* as a causative factor was only circumstantial, in that improvement occurred following therapy.

Uremic Cases. Ehrlichiosis results in a variable degree of cell infiltration in the kidney. The range of signs shown in uremic cases includes polyuria, polydipsia, depression, anorexia, emesis, pale or congested mucous membranes, edema of limbs, halitosis, and oral ulceration. Serum analysis reveals increased blood urea nitrogen and inorganic phosphorus levels. After treatment of uncomplicated cases of ehrlichiosis, the blood urea nitrogen and inorganic phosphorus levels can be expected to return to normal. Dogs with irreversible kidney damage, on the other hand, resulting from ehrlichiosis or other causes continue to have high blood urea nitrogen levels but may be maintained for a period of time on a low-protein diet.

Subclinical Cases. This term is applied to those animals in which there is evidence that stressful factors such as major surgery, malnutrition, pregnancy, extensive neoplasia, or other concomitant disease are observed to precipitate obvious clinical ehrlichiosis. Presenting signs include weight loss, selective appetite, and intermittent lethargy, and the dog is often described by the owner as "not being in good condition." The term *selective appetite* is used to describe the situation in which the dog will not eat all of its food every day, eats one day but not the next, or merely picks at its food, whereas previously it has been in the habit of eating all the food offered. It may be difficult or impossible to find morulae of *E. canis* in peripheral blood smears from these cases, but the organism can be identified by the cell culture test.

Carrier State. Dogs in the healthy carrier state differ from those with subclinical ehrlichiosis. When dogs in this state are stressed, no clinical disease develops. Similarly, in the healthy carrier state, *E. canis* can rarely be found on peripheral blood smear examination but may be readily identified by the cell culture test.

Concomitant Babesiosis. In areas where simultaneous ehrlichiosis and *Babesia* infection are common, the signs generally seen are typical of canine babesiosis, namely, pyrexia, anorexia, depression, lethargy, emesis, pallor, splenomegaly, and accelerated pulse rate. Hemorrhagic signs are seen occasionally. If *Babesia* infection is diagnosed and treated while the ehrlichiosis remains untreated, the dog is likely to respond initially, but recovery will be considerably slower than if both diseases are treated simultaneously or if babesiosis is the only disease present. When ehrlichiosis remains untreated in dual infections, some dogs suffer from acute ehrlichiosis a week or so after *Babesia* treatment, whereas others may be presented weeks to months later with acute ehrlichiosis or subclinical infection, i.e., weight loss and the development of a selective appetite.

DIAGNOSIS

Diagnosis is usually based on clinical signs, as identification of *E. canis* in blood smears is often difficult or impossible (Ewing, 1969). Thin blood smears, preferably made from a peripheral capillary bed (e.g., ear tip) rather than a venous blood sample, or buffy coat smears are stained with Giemsa stain. Microscopic examination of the smear under oil immersion reveals morulae of *E. canis* in the cytoplasm of mononuclear cells (Fig. 1). These morulae need to be distinguished from azurophilic granules, although some reports suppport the impression that an increase in visible granules within the rather extended cytoplasm of a monocyte may be strongly linked with *Ehrlichia*-positive cases.

An indirect fluorescent antibody test has been developed (Ristic et al., 1972), but this test may not always be readily available.

A simple modification of an *in vitro* culture technique based on that of Nyindo and colleagues (1971) can be used in laboratories with limited facilities as an aid to diagnosis and to confirm clearance of the organism after treatment. In this test, 10 ml of whole blood are drawn from the animal directly into a sterile heparin-coated plastic syringe; the needle is then discarded. After attachment of a new needle, the syringe is taped immediately to the wall in an upright position. Approximately half way up, the shaft of the needle is bent at an acute angle using the sterile needle cover (see Fig. 1). Particular care is taken to allow the blood-filled syringe to remain undisturbed for 30 to 60 minutes (in most *Ehrlichia* cases the erythrocyte sedimentation rate is accelerated). Without disturbing the syringe, 2 ml of plasma are carefully transferred through the bent needle into each of two sterile Leighton tissue culture tubes containing glass coverslips (5 × 22 mm). These tubes are incubated horizontally at 37°C. During incubation, mononuclear cells settle on to the coverslips, and, if present, the organism begins to replicate rapidly. After 48 hours one Leighton tube is removed from the incubator and the cells on the coverslip are washed with 0.9 per cent saline, fixed with methanol, and stained with Giemsa stain. All these procedures are carried out within the Leighton tube. The coverslip is then removed from the tube and mounted on a glass microscopic slide. The mononuclear cells are examined for the presence of purple-staining morulae of *E. canis* in the cytoplasm of the cells, using an oil immersion lens at 1000× magnification. If this proves negative, the cells on the coverslip from the second tube are examined following incubation for a total of 96 hours. The same procedure is used. Culture medium or antibiotics are not added to the Leighton tubes during incubation, but great care is taken to avoid contamination of the culture tubes.

Laboratory investigation in experimentally induced *Ehrlichia canis* infection reveals that thrombocytopenia is dramatic and occurs as early as 14 days after infection and may persist for a long period of time. Leukopenia is detected later (three to four weeks post infection) and is followed by anemia; thereafter the leukocytes and erythrocytes increase in number. In the acute disease, eosinopenia and monocytosis are also present.

Coagulation and prothrombin times are unaltered, but bleeding time is prolonged. The erythrocyte sedimentation rate is increased. Blood urea nitrogen levels are increased in prolonged cases or those with renal impairment. In the later stages of ehrlichiosis, gammaglobulin levels rise whereas albumin levels decrease.

Studies of the pathology indicate that there is generalized activation and enlargement of the lymphoid organs. Gastrointestinal lesions are frequent, ranging from slight congestion to large ser-

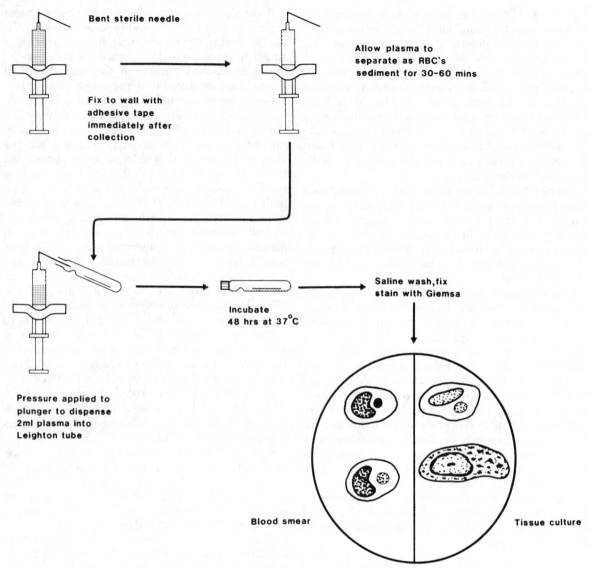

Figure 1. A simple method of monocyte culture from suspect dog plasma for the detection of *Ehrlichia canis*.

osal and mucosal hemorrhages with free blood in the intestinal lumen. The liver may be pale and enlarged. Petechiation and ecchymoses can be found in the wall of the gallbladder.

The kidneys may be mottled in appearance, with numerous scattered pale areas. Subcapsular and focal hemorrhages near the corticomedullary junction are seen. They are also commonly found on the mucosal and serosal surfaces of the urinary bladder and may be present in the prostate, testicle, and epididymis.

Cardiac hemorrhages are present on both the epicardium and endocardium and in the lungs, which may be edematous. Hyphema and corneal opacity are found in a few dogs.

Evidence of bleeding may be observed in the cranial and spinal dura mater. Microscopically,

there is proliferative, disseminated panencephalitis with distinct swelling and proliferation of vascular endothelium and the perivascular tissue. There is perivascular plasma cell and lymphocyte infiltration of the meninges, lungs, spleen, lymph nodes, kidneys, and retina. With prolonged disease, centrilobular necrosis of the liver and bone marrow hypoplasia occur.

TREATMENT

Three effective drugs are available for the therapy of canine ehrlichiosis: tetracycline hydrochloride, doxycycline, and imidocarb diproprionate. The standard treatment is oral tetracycline hydrochloride at 33 mg/kg every 12 hours for 14 consecutive days (Davidson et al., 1972). Although most animals respond clinically to this regimen, 75 per cent still show the presence of *E. canis* organisms using the cell culture test. Many of these animals show a recurrence of signs within a month or two of treatment. Discoloration of the decidous teeth in young puppies or of the permanent teeth in older puppies has been noted in dogs given tetracycline hydrochloride when their teeth were erupting. At this high dose level, some dogs may vomit after tetracycline therapy, especially those with renal disease.

Doxycycline (Vibramycin*) is a broad spectrum, semisynthetic tetracycline analogue that attains effective blood concentrations after a single daily oral dose of 10 mg/kg for 14 consecutive days. Since doxycycline is less nephrotoxic than tetracycline hydrochloride, it is the treatment of choice in animals with evidence of renal insufficiency.

More recently, a good response has been achieved with imidocarb dipropionate (Imizol†). The drug is administered as a single, deep intramuscular injection at a dosage of 5 mg/kg, repeated after an interval of two weeks. Imidocarb dipropionate may elicit a marked but brief pain response during injection but does not cause lameness or swelling at the site of injection. Within ten minutes of the injection, a number of dogs may show the following transitory signs: profuse salivation, serous ocular discharge, diarrhea, and tremors. After 30 minutes, no further effects are seen in these dogs. The subcutaneous route of administration of this drug has been found occasionally to cause sterile abscesses at the injection site.

The use of imidocarb dipropionate avoids the need for daily oral treatment, and it rids the dog of the causative organism in 80 per cent of cases (Price and Dolan, 1980). In our opinion, it is the drug of choice in most cases. However, the clinician has a choice of three drugs for treatment of the different syndromes, and the advantages and disadvantages of each drug should be carefully assessed for each case.

It is believed that the hemorrhagic manifestations of canine ehrlichiosis are the result of an immunologic phenomenon (Scott, 1978). Treatment of these cases (hemorrhagic, neurologic, and breeding) with high levels of corticosteroid in combination with either tetracycline hydrochloride, doxycycline, or imidocarb dipropionate has been found to be successful. Corticosteroid should be administered intravenously at 1 to 2 mg/kg as a single initial dose and thereafter reduced progressively over five to seven days. After the initial dose, the corticosteroid may be administered orally or by intramuscular injection. Blood transfusions, if necessary, should be preceded by corticosteroid therapy to reduce platelet sequestration, and only fresh, whole blood that is rich in platelets should be used. Intravenous fluids may also be used.

PREVENTION

There is no evidence to suggest that the dog will be resistant to reinfection after any of the previously mentioned treatments. Prophylactic oral use of tetracycline hydrochloride at 3 mg/kg/day has been reported to be successful (Davidson et al., 1978), but strict tick control using acaricides at regular intervals appears to be the only really effective means of preventing this disease in an *Ehrlichia canis* endemic area.

REFERENCES AND SUPPLEMENTAL READING

Buhles, W. C., Huxsoll, D. L., and Ristic, M.: Tropical canine pancytopenia: Clinical, hematologic and serologic response of dogs to *Ehrlichia canis* infection, tetracycline therapy, and challenge inoculation. J. Infect. Dis. 130:357, 1974.

Davidson, D. E., Hill, G. S., Tingpalapong, M., Premabutra, S., Nguen, P. L., Stephenson, E. H., and Ristic, M.: Prophylactic and therapeutic use of tetracycline during an epizootic of ehrlichiosis among military dogs. J.A.V.M.A. 172:697, 1978.

Ewing, S. A.: Canine ehrlichiosis. Adv. Vet. Sci. Comp. Med. 13:33, 1969.

Huxsoll, D. L., Hildebrandt, P. K., Mins, R. M., and Walker, J. S.: Tropical canine pancytopenia. J.A.V.M.A. 157:1627, 1970.

Lewis, G. E., and Huxsoll, D. L.: Canine ehrlichiosis. *In* Kirk, R. W.: *Current Veterinary Therapy VI.* Philadelphia: W. B. Saunders, 1977.

Nyindo, M. B. A., Ristic, M., Huxsoll, D. L., and Smith, A. R.: Tropical canine pancytopenia: *in vitro* cultivation of the causative agent— *Ehrlichia canis.* Am. J. Vet. Res. 32:1651, 1971.

Price, J. E., and Dolan, T. T.: A comparison of the efficacy of imidocarb diproprionate and tetracycline hydrochloride in the treatment of canine ehrlichiosis. Vet. Rec. 107:275, 1980.

Ristic, M., Huxsoll, D. L., Weisiger, R. M., Hildebrandt, P. K., and Nyindo, M. B. A.: Serological diagnosis of tropical canine pancytopenia by indirect immunofluorescence. Infect. Immun. 6:226, 1972.

Scott, G. R.: *In* Wilde, J. H. K. (ed.): *Tick-Borne Diseases and their Vectors.* Edinburgh: University of Edinburgh: Centre for Tropical Veterinary Medicine, 1978, pp. 451–473.

---

*Pfizer Laboratories Ltd., N.Y.

†The Wellcome Foundation, London, England.

ROCKY MOUNTAIN SPOTTED FEVER

BARRY A. LISSMAN, D.V.M.

Stony Brook, New York

Rocky Mountain spotted fever (RMSF) is a disease affecting dogs as well as humans. The disease has been identified in dogs in areas that are considered endemic for the disease in humans, including the eastern end of Long Island and areas in Virginia and North Carolina. The causative organism, *Rickettsia rickettsii*, is transmitted to the dog through the bite of an infected *Dermacentor variabilis* tick, (the American dog tick). For infection to occur, the tick usually must be on the host long enough to become fully engorged.

The incubation period is five to ten days. The clinical signs may vary among dogs but usually include a high fever, anorexia, and lethargy. Other signs may include abdominal tenderness, nystagmus, dehydration, weight loss, lymphadenitis, edema of the limbs, and edema of the sheath and scrotum in male dogs. Hyperemia and petechiae may also be seen on the oral, ocular, and genital mucous membranes and nonpigmented skin. Death of untreated experimentally infected dogs has been reported. Dogs may also have increased serum alkaline phosphatase activity and serum cholesterol content and hyponatremia and hypochloremia.

The diagnosis of RMSF can be confirmed by a rising titer based on the microimmunofluorescence test for rickettsial antibodies, using an anti-dog IgG fluorescein-labelled conjugate. The hemolymph test may be used to determine if ticks are harboring a rickettsia of the spotted fever group.

Tetracycline should be started immediately at a dosage of 10 mg/lb t.i.d. for approximately one week. Appropriate supportive therapy is important, too. A favorable response can be expected a few days after tetracycline therapy is initiated.

Veterinarians should be alert to the occurrence of RMSF in humans in their practice area. During the active tick season, RMSF should be suspected in dogs with intractable fever and a combination of the signs described here. Veterinarians and their staff also should be aware that dogs have been reported to be rickettsemic during the acute phase of the infection; thus, care must be exercised to prevent exposure when obtaining blood samples or necropsying dogs.

SUPPLEMENTAL READING

Burgdorfer, W.: Hemolymph test: A technique for detection of rickettsiae in ticks. Am. J. Trop. Med. Hyg. 19:1010, 1970.

Keenan, K. P., Buhles, W. C., Jr., Huxsoll, D. L., et al.: Studies on the pathogenesis of *Rickettsia rickettsii* in the dog: Clinical and clinicopathologic changes of experimental infection. Am. J. Vet. Res. 38:851, 1977.

Lissman, B. A., and Benach, J.: Rocky Mountain spotted fever in dogs. J.A.V.M.A. 10:994, 1980.

Philip, R. N., Casper, E. A., Ormsbee, R. H., et al.: Microimmunofluorescence test for the serological study of Rocky Mountain spotted fever and typhus. J. Clin. Microbiol. 3:51, 1976.

APPENDICES

ROBERT W. KIRK, D.V.M.

Consulting Editor

TABLES OF NORMAL PHYSIOLOGIC DATA

ELECTROCARDIOGRAPHY*

It is recognized that normal and abnormal electrocardiographic measurements overlap and that the criteria for the normal electrocardiogram serve only as a guide for the clinician. Deviations from normal in an individual electrocardiogram suggest but are not always diagnostic of heart disease. As additional statistical data become available for the electrocardiograms of dogs of each breed, body type, age and sex, the data herein may require revision and "normal" may be more precisely defined. The *value of serial electrocardiograms* from an individual cannot be overemphasized, since serial changes best demonstrate electrocardiographic abnormalities.

Criteria for the Normal Canine Electrocardiogram†

Heart rate – 60 to 160 beats per minute for adult dogs; up to 180 beats per minute in toy breeds, and 220 beats per minute for puppies.

Heart rhythm—Normal sinus rhythm; sinus arrhythmia; and wandering sinoatrial pacemaker.

P wave—Up to 0.4 millivolt in amplitude; up to 0.04 second in duration; always positive in leads II and aVF; positive or isoelectric in lead I.

P-R interval — 0.06 to 0.14 second duration.

QRS complex—Mean electric axis, frontal plane, 40 to 100 degrees.

Amplitude—Maximum amplitude of R wave 2.5 to 3.0 millivolts in leads II, III, and aVF. Complex positive in leads II, III, and aVF; negative in lead V_{10}.

Duration – To 0.05 second (0.06 second in dogs over 40 lbs).

Q-T 0.15 to 0.22 seconds duration.

S-T segment and T wave – S-T segment free of marked coving (repolarization changes).

S-T segment depression not greater than 0.2 millivolt.

S-T segment elevation not greater than 0.15 millivolt.

T wave negative in lead V_{10}.

T wave amplitude not greater than 25 per cent of amplitude of R wave.

Criteria for the Normal Feline Electrocardiogram†

Heart rate—240 beats per minute maximum.

Heart rhythm—Normal sinus rhythm or, infrequently, sinus arrhythmia.

P wave – Positive in leads II and AVF: may be isoelectric or positive in lead I; should not exceed 0.03 second in duration.

P-R interval – 0.04 to 0.08 second duration (inversely related to the heart rate).

QRS complex—More variable than in the canine; the mean electric axis in the frontal plane is often insignificant. Often the QRS complex is nearly isoelectric in all frontal plane limb leads (so-called horizontal heart).

Amplitude—The amplitude of the R wave is usually low; marked amplitude of R waves (over 0.8 millivolt) in the frontal plane leads may suggest ventricular hypertrophy.

Duration – Less than 0.04 second.

Q-T segment – 0.16 to 0.18 second duration.

S-T segment and T wave – S-T segment and T wave should be small and free of repolarization changes as well as marked depression of elevation.

---

*From Ettinger, S. J., and Suter, P. F.: *Canine Cardiology*. Philadelphia, W. B. Saunders Co., 1970, pp. 102–169.

†From Ettinger, S. J.: *Textbook of Veterinary Internal Medicine*, 2nd ed., Vol. I. Philadelphia, W. B. Saunders Co., 1983, p. 984.

TABLES FOR CONVERSION OF WEIGHT TO BODY-SURFACE AREA IN SQUARE METERS FOR DOGS

KG.	M.²	KG.	M.²
0.5	0.06	26.0	0.88
1.0	0.10	27.0	0.90
2.0	0.15	28.0	0.92
3.0	0.20	29.0	0.94
4.0	0.25	30.0	0.96
5.0	0.29	31.0	0.99
6.0	0.33	32.0	1.01
7.0	0.36	33.0	1.03
8.0	0.40	34.0	1.05
9.0	0.43	35.0	1.07
10.0	0.46	36.0	1.09
11.0	0.49	37.0	1.11
12.0	0.52	38.0	1.13
13.0	0.55	39.0	1.15
14.0	0.58	40.0	1.17
15.0	0.60	41.0	1.19
16.0	0.63	42.0	1.21
17.0	0.66	43.0	1.23
18.0	0.69	44.0	1.25
19.0	0.71	45.0	1.26
20.0	0.74	46.0	1.28
21.0	0.76	47.0	1.30
22.0	0.78	48.0	1.32
23.0	0.81	49.0	1.34
24.0	0.83	50.0	1.36
25.0	0.85		

(From Ettinger, S. J.: Textbook of Veterinary Internal Medicine. Philadelphia, W. B. Saunders Co., 1975.)

*Nomogram for the Estimation of Surface Area of the Dog**

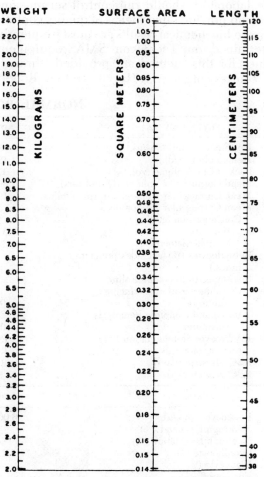

°Length = Nose to anus measured along abdomen.
From Smith, H. W.: Principles of Renal Physiology, 3rd ed. New York, Oxford University Press, 1957.

A ROSTER OF NORMAL VALUES FOR DOGS AND CATS

JOHN BENTINCK-SMITH, D.V.M.

Mississippi State, Mississippi

Age, sex, breed, diurnal periodicity, and emotional stress at the time of sampling can be expected to cause variation in normal values. The methodology will also affect the biologic parameters.

For these reasons practitioners are well advised to employ the normal values supplied by the laboratory that they patronize. However, this laboratory must have determined their normal ranges and means by a sufficient number of normal samples to provide statistical validity. The laboratory should run control serum samples and provide other means of quality control.

Since biochemical results are most frequently determined on Technicon SMA, equipment values for this method are provided (through the courtesy of Dr. A. I. Hurvitz and Dr. Robert

J. Wilkins of the Animal Medical Center). Other data are derived from the New York State College of Veterinary Medicine, the Ralston Purina Corp., Biozyme Veterinary Laboratory (a division of Biozyme Medical Laboratories, Inc.), standard texts, and the literature. References are cited as footnotes within the tables and appear in full at the end of this appendix. Values for reptiles and exotic animals can be found in *Current Veterinary Therapy VII*, pages 748 and 749, and in *Current Veterinary Therapy VI*, page 795.

Inappropriate collection and preparation, prolonged storage, hemolysis, lipemia, and hyperbilirubinemia may invalidate the laboratory results.

NORMAL BLOOD VALUES[31]

ERYTHROCYTES	ADULT DOG	AVERAGE	ADULT CAT	AVERAGE
Erythrocytes (millions/μl.)	5.5–8.5	6.8	5.5–10.0	7.5
Hemoglobin (g./dl.)	12.0–18.0	14.9	8.0–14.0	12.0
Packed Cell Volume (vol. %)	37.0–55.0	45.5	24.0–45.0	37.0
Mean Corpuscular Volume (femtoliters)	66.0–77.0	69.8	40.0–55.0	45.0
Mean Corpuscular Hemoglobin (picograms)	19.9–24.5	22.8	13.0–17.0	15.0
Mean Corpuscular Hemoglobin Concentration (g./dl.)				
Wintrobe	31.0–34.0	33.0	31.0–35.0	33.0
Microhematocrit	32.0–36.0	34.0	30.0–36.0	33.2
Reticulocytes (%) (excludes punctate retics.)	0.0–1.5	0.8	0.2–1.6	0.6
Resistance to hypotonic saline (% saline solution producing)				
Minimum	0.40–0.50	0.46	0.66–0.72	0.69
initial and complete hemolysis				
Maximum	0.32–0.42	0.33	0.46–0.54	0.50
Erythrocyte Sedimentation Rate (mm. at 60 min.)	PCV 37 PCV 50	13 0	PCV 35–40	7–27
RBC life span (days)	100–120		66–78	
RBC diameter (μ)	6.7–7.2	7.0	5.5–6.3	5.8

LEUKOCYTES	ADULT DOG	AVERAGE	ADULT CAT	AVERAGE
Leukocytes (no./μl.)	6,000–17,000	11,500	5,500–19,500	12,500
Neutrophils—Bands(%)	0–3	0.8	0–3	0.5
Neutrophils—Mature (%)	60–77	70.0	35–75	59.0
Lymphocyte (%)	12–30	20.0	20–55	32.0
Monocyte (%)	3–10	5.2	1–4	3.0
Eosinophil (%)	2–10	4.0	2–12	5.5
Basophil (%)	Rare	0.0	Rare	0.0
Neutrophils—Bands (no./μl.)	0–300	70	0–300	100
Neutrophils—Mature (no./μl.)	3,000–11,500	7,000	2,500–12,500	7,500
Lymphocytes (no./μl.)	1,000–4,800	2,800	1,500–7,000	4,000
Monocytes (no./μl.)	150–1,350	750	0–850	350
Eosinophils (no./μl.)	100–1,250	550	0–1,500	650
Basophils	Rare	0	Rare	0

CANINE BLOOD PARAMETERS AT DIFFERENT AGES—AVERAGE VALUES[1]

Age	millions/μl. RBC	Retic. % *	Nucl. RBC/ 100 WBC *	g./dl. Hb	Vol. % PCV	/dl. WBC	/dl. Neut.	/dl. Bands	/dl. Lymph.	/dl. Eos.
Birth	5.75	7.1	1.8	16.70	50	16,500	1,300	400	2,500	600
2 weeks	3.92	7.1	1.8	9.76	32	11,000	6,500	100	3,000	300
4 weeks	4.20	7.1	1.8	9.60	33	13,000	8,600	0	4,000	40
6 weeks	4.91	3.6	1.8	9.59	34	15,000	10,000	0	4,500	100
8 weeks	5.13	3.9	0.3	11.00	37	18,000	11,000	234	6,000	270
12 weeks	5.27	3.9	Rare	11.60	36	15,300	9,400	115	4,600	322

*See reference 13.

CANINE BLOOD PARAMETERS AT DIFFERENT AGES[26]

	Sex	Birth to 12 mo.	Average	1–7 yr.	Average	7 yr. and Older	Average
Erythrocytes (million/μl)	Male	2.99–8.52	5.09	5.26–6.57	5.92	3.33–7.76	5.28
	Female	2.76–8.42	5.06	5.13–8.6	6.47	3.34–9.19	5.17
Hemoglobin (gm/dl)	Male	6.9–16.5	10.7	12.7–16.3	15.5	14.7–21.2	17.9
	Female	6.4–18.9	11.2	11.5–17.9	14.7	11.0–22.5	16.1
Packed Cell Volume (vol. %)	Male	22.0–45.0	33.9	35.2–52.8	44.0	44.2–62.8	52.3
	Female	25.8–55.2	36.0	34.8–52.4	43.6	35.8–67.0	49.8
Leukocytes (thousands/μl)	Male	9.9–27.7	17.1	8.3–19.5	11.9	7.9–35.3	15.5
	Female	8.8–26.8	15.9	7.5–17.5	11.5	5.2–34.0	13.4
Neutrophils	Male	63–73	68	65–73	69	55–80	66
Mature (%)	Female	64–74	69	58–76	67	40–80	64
Lymphocytes (%)	Male	18–30	24	9–26	18	15–40	29
	Female	13–28	21	11–29	20	13–45	29
Monocytes (%)	Male	1–10	6	2–10	6	0–4	1
	Female	1–10	7	0–10	5	0–4	1
Eosinophils (%)	Male	2–11	3	1–8	4	1–11	4
	Female	1–9	5	1–10	6	0–19	6

FELINE BLOOD PARAMETERS AT DIFFERENT AGES[31]

Age	millions/μl. RBC	g./dl. Hb	Vol. % PCV	/dl. WBC	/dl. Neut.	/dl. Lymph.
Birth	4.95	12.2	44.7	7,500		
2 weeks	4.76	9.7	31.1	8,080		
5 weeks	5.84	8.4	29.9	8,550		
Average*	4.80	7.5	26.2	11,770	4,600	6,970
Range*	3.90–5.70	6.6–8.4	21.0–33.5	7,500–14,500		4,500–9,400
6 weeks	6.75	9.0	35.4	8,420		
8 weeks	7.10	9.4	35.6	8,420		
Average*	5.90	7.5	26.2	12,400	7,500	4,900
Range*	3.30–7.30	7.6–15.0	22–38	6,900–23,100		1,925–10,100

*See reference 2.

FELINE BLOOD PARAMETERS AT DIFFERENT AGES[25]

	Sex	Birth to 12 mo.	Average	1–5 yr.	Average	6 yr. and Older	Average
Erythrocytes (millions/μl)	Male	5.43–10.22	6.96	4.48–10.27	7.34	5.26–8.89	6.79
	Female	4.46–11.34	6.90	4.45–9.42	6.17	4.10–7.38	5.84
Hemoglobin (gm/dl)	Male	6.0–12.9	9.9	8.9–17.0	12.9	9.0–14.5	11.8
	Female	6.0–15.0	9.9	7.9–15.5	10.3	7.5–13.7	10.3
Packed Cell Volume (vol. %)	Male	24.0–37.5	31	26.9–48.2	37.6	28.0–43.8	34.6
	Female	23.0–46.8	31.5	25.3–37.5	31.4	22.5–40.5	30.8
Leukocytes (thousands/μl)	Male	7.8–25.0	15.8	9.1–28.2	15.1	6.4–30.4	17.6
	Female	11.0–26.9	17.7	13.7–23.7	19.9	5.2–30.1	14.8
Neutrophils	Male	16–75	60	37–92	65	33–75	61
Mature (%)	Female	51–83	69	42–93	69	25–89	71
Lymphocytes (%)	Male	10–81	30	7–48	23	16–54	30
	Female	8–37	23	12–58	30	9–63	22
Monocytes (%)	Male	1–5	2	1–5	2	0–2	1
	Female	0–7	2	0–5	2	0–4	1
Eosinophils (%)	Male	2–21	8	1–22	7	1–15	8
	Female	0–15	6	0–13	5	0–15	6

EFFECT OF PREGNANCY AND LACTATION ON BLOOD PARAMETERS OF THE DOG[1]

	GESTATION				TERM	LACTATION		
	2 Weeks	4 Weeks	6 Weeks	8 Weeks	0 Weeks	2 Weeks	4 Weeks	6 Weeks
RBC (millions/dl.)	8.85	7.48	6.73	6.26	4.53	5.13	5.65	6.15
PCV (Vol. %)	53	47	44	37	32	34	38	42
Hb (g./dl.)	19.6	16.4	14.7	13.8	11.0	11.7	12.8	13.4
Sedimentation Rate (mm. at 60 min.)	0.6	11.0	31.0	14.0	12.0	14.0	14.0	13.0
WBC (thousands/dl.)	12.0	12.2	15.7	19.0	18.9	16.9	17.1	15.9

EFFECT OF PREGNANCY AND LACTATION ON BLOOD PARAMETERS OF THE CAT[6]

		GESTATION				TERM	LACTATION	
	1 Day Past Conception	*2 Weeks*	*4 Weeks*	*6 Weeks*	*8 Weeks*	*0 Weeks*	*2 Weeks*	*4 Weeks*
RBC (millions/dl.)	8.0	7.9	7.1	6.7	6.2	6.2	7.4	7.4
PCV (Vol. %)	36.1	37.0	33.0	32.0	28.0	29.0	33.0	33.0
Hb (g./100 ml.)	12.5	12.0	11.0	10.8	9.5	10.0	11.5	11.2
Reticulocytes (%) (includes punctate retics.)	9	11	9	10	20.1	15	9	6

	ADULT DOG	AVERAGE	ADULT CAT	AVERAGE[31]
Thrombocytes $\times 10^5/\mu$l.	2–5	3–4	3–8	4.5
Icterus Index	2–5 units		2–5 units	
Plasma Fibrinogen (g./l.)	2.0–4.0		0.50–3.00	

NORMAL BONE MARROW (Percentage)

ERYTHROCYTIC CELLS	DOG[31]	CAT[23]
Rubriblasts	0.2	1.71
Prorubricytes	3.9	12.50
Rubricytes	27.0	
Metarubricytes	15.3	11.68
Total Erythrocytic Cells	46.4	25.89

GRANULOCYTIC CELLS		
Myeloblasts	0.0	1.74
Progranulocytes	1.3	0.88
Neutrophilic Myelocytes	9.0	9.76
Eosinophilic Myelocytes	0.0	1.47
Neutrophilic Metamyelocytes	7.5	7.32
Eosinophilic Metamyelocytes	2.4	1.52
Band Neutrophils	13.6	25.80
Band Eosinophils	0.9	—
Neutrophils	18.4	9.24
Eosinophils	0.3	0.81
Basophils	0.0	0.002
Total Granulocytic Cells	53.4	58.542
M:E Ratio—Average	1.15:1.0	2.47:1.0
M:E Ratio—Range (Schalm)	0.75–2.50:1.0	0.60–3.90:1.0

OTHER CELLS		
Lymphocytes	0.2	7.63
Plasma Cells	0	1.61
Reticulum Cells	0	0.13
Mitotic Cells	0	0.61
Unclassified	0	1.62
Disintegrated Cells	0	4.60

BLOOD, PLASMA, OR SERUM CHEMICAL CONSTITUENTS
(B) = Blood, (P) = Plasma, (S) = Serum

Chemical constituents are liable to show markedly different values, depending on the methodology employed.

CONSTITUENT	ADULT DOG		ADULT CAT	
	Coulter Chemistry[34]	*Technicon SMA*[36]	*Coulter Chemistry*[34]	*Technicon SMA*[36]
Urea N(S) (mg/dl)	8–23	10–22	18–32	5–30
Glucose (S) (mg/dl)	71–115	50–120	66–95	70–150
Total bilirubin (S) (mg/dl)	0.1–0.6	0–0.6	0.15–0.3	0–0.8
Total protein (S) (gm/dl)	5.2–7.0	5.4–7.8	5.9–7.3	5.5–7.5
Albumin (S) (gm/dl)	2.7–3.8	2.2–3.4	2.2–3.0	2.2–3.5
Alkaline phosphatase (S) (IU/l)	10–82	20–120	7–30	10–80
Calcium (S) (mg/dl)	9.8–11.4	9–11.6	8.9–10.6	7.6–11.0
Inorganic phosphorus (S) (mg/dl)	2.8–5.1	3.9–6.3	4.3–6.6	3.2–6.3
LDH (S) (IU/l)	8–89	40–200	33–99	10–200
AST or SGOT (S)	13–93[*]	5–80[†]	32–58[*]	10–60[†]
ALT or SGPT (S)(IU/l)	15–70	5–25	10–50	10–60
Total CO_2 (S) (mEq/l)	18–25	17–25[‡]	18–25	16–25[‡]
Creatinine (S) (mg/dl)	0.5–1.2	0 4–1.5[‡]	0.5–1.7	1.3–2.1[‡]
Uric acid (S) (mg/dl)		0.2–0.8[‡]		0.1–0.7[‡]
Total cholesterol (S) (mg/dl)	82–282	156–294[‡]	41–225	116–126[‡]
Triglycerides (S) (mg/dl)		10–42[‡]		6–58[‡]
CPK (S) (IU/l)	12–84	27–93[‡]	6–130	62–262[‡]

CHEMICAL PARAMETERS AFFECTED BY AGE	DOG < 6 MO–SMA[36]	CAT < 6 MO–SMA[36]
Inorganic phosphorus (S) (mg/dl)	3.9–9.0	3.9–8.1
Calcium (S) (mg/dl)	7.0–11.6	7.0–11.0
Alkaline phosphatase (S) (IU/l)	20–200	10–120
LDH (S) (IU/l)	40–400	10–300

	SEX	DOGS[26] AND CATS[25]					
		Birth to 12 mo.	*Average*	*1–5 yr.*	*Average*	*6 yr. and Older*	*Average*
Total Protein (S) (gm/dl)	Male	3.90–5.90	5.15	4.90–9.60	6.33	5.5–7.3	6.4
(Dogs)	Female	4.00–6.40	5.58	5.50–7.80	6.34	4.7–7.5	6.2
Total Protein (S) (gm/dl)	Male	4.3–10.0	6.4	6.8–10.0	8.1	6.2–8.5	7.2
(Cats)	Female	4.8–9.1	6.4	6.6–8.9	7.4	6.0–9.0	7.3

ELECTROPHORESIS	DOG	CAT
Albumin (S) (gm/dl)	2.3–3.4	2.3–3.5
Globulin (S) (gm/dl)	3.0–4.7	2.6–5.0
Alpha 1 (S) (gm/dl)	0.3–0.8	0.3–0.5
Alpha 2 (S) (gm/dl)	0.5–1.3	0.4–1.0
Beta (S) (gm/dl)	0.7–1.8	0.6–1.9
Gamma (S) (gm/dl)	0.4–1.0	0.5–1.5
Albumin/globulin ratio, A/G (S)	0.7–1.1	0.5–1.0

[*] Trans Act Units/liter (General Diagnostics). 1 Trans Act Unit of GOT activity is the amount of enzyme in 1 liter of sample that will form 1 mM of oxalic acid in 1 minute under specified conditions.

[†] IU/liter.

[‡] See reference 7.

BLOOD, PLASMA OR SERUM CHEMICAL CONSTITUENTS—*Continued*
(B) = Blood, (P) = Plasma, (S) = Serum

Chemical constituents are liable to show markedly different values depending on the methodology employed.

OTHER CONSTITUENTS	ADULT DOG	ADULT CAT
Lipase (S)		
(Sigma Tietz Units/ml)	0–1	0–1
Roe Byler Units (5)	0.8–12	0–5
IU (5)	13–200	0–83
Amylase (S)		
Harleco Units/dl	0–800	0–800
Harding Units/dl	1600–2400	0–2700 (5)
Dy Amyl (General Diagnostics)	<3200 (5)	0–2600 (5)
Caraway Units/dl[24]	330–1530	170–1170
Lactic acid (S) (mg/dl)	3–15	
Pyruvate (B) (mEq/l)	0.1–0.2	
Cholesterol esters (S) (mg/dl)	84–168	45–120
Free cholesterol (S) (mg/dl)	28–84	15–60
Total lipid (P) (mg/dl)	47–725	145–607
Free glycerol (S) 24-hr fast (mg/dl)[28]	14.2–23.2	
Bromsulfalein retention test (P) (%)	<5	
Iron (S) (μg/dl)	94–122	68–215
Total iron-binding capacity (S) (μg/dl)	280–340	170–400
Lead (B) (μg/dl)	0–35	0–35

	DOGS		CATS	
ELECTROLYTES	*Coulter*[34]	*Technicon*[7]	*Coulter*[34]	*Technicon*[7]
Sodium (S) (mEq/l)	143–151	144–154	150–162	147–161
Potassium (S) (mEq/l)	4.1–5.7	3.8–5.8	3.7–5.5	3.7–4.9
Magnesium (S) (mEq/l)	1.4–2.4	1.07–1.73	2.2	1.92–2.28
Chloride (S) (mEq/l)	103–115	93–121	114–124	80–158
Sulfate (S) (mEq/l)	2.0			
Osmolality (S) (mOsm/kg)	280–310		280–310	
pH (Corning)	7.31–7.42		7.24–7.40	

BLOOD GASES	ADULT DOG	ADULT CAT
P_{O_2} (B) mm Hg (arterial)*	85–95	—
(B) mm Hg (venous)*	40–60	—
P_{CO_2} (B) mm Hg (arterial)*	29–36	—
(B) mm Hg (venous)*	29–42	—
Base excess (B) (mEq/l)	±2.5	±2.5
Bicarbonate (P) (mEq/l)	17–24	17–24

*Standard temperature and pressure.

	ADULT DOG		ADULT CAT	
ENDOCRINE SECRETIONS	*Resting Level*	*Post-ACTH**	*Resting Level*	*Post-ACTH**
Cortisol (S) (RIA) (μg/dl)[27]	1.8–4	3–4× Pretreatment	1–3	3–4× Pretreatment
Cortisol (S) (CPB) (μg/dl)[35]	2–6	3–4× Pretreatment[32]	2–5	3–4× Pretreatment[32]
Cortisol (S) (fluorometric) (μg/dl)	5–10	10–20		

	Resting Level	*Post-TSH*†	*Resting Level*	*Post-TSH*
T_4 (P) (RIA) (μg/dl)[4]	1.52–3.60	At least 3–4 fold	1.2–3.8	
T_3 (P) (RIA) (ng/dl)[4]	48–154	More than 10 ng increase		
Protein-bound iodine[3] (μg/dl)	1.6–3.0	Increase of 3 μg/dl (mean)		

BLOOD, PLASMA OR SERUM CHEMICAL CONSTITUENTS—*Continued*
(B) = Blood, (P) = Plasma, (S) = Serum

Chemical constituents are liable to show markedly different values depending on the methodology employed.

T$_4$ CHANGES WITH AGE	DOG	CAT
T$_4$ (S) (RIA)	Decrease of 0.07 μg/dl per year of age[4]	No values for cat
T$_4$ (S) (CPB) (μg/dl)		
10–12 wk[15, 16]	3.24 ± 0.51	2.82 ± 0.73
1 yr[15, 16]	2.25 ± 0.33	2.43 ± 0.55
	Adult Dog	*Adult Cat*
Thyroid uptake of radioiodine (^{131}I) (%)[15, 16]	17–30	
Insulin (S) (RIA) (μU/ml)[37]	0–30	0–50

*2 μ ACTH gel IM 2 hours after injection.
†5 μ TSH IV 4–6 hours after injection.

HEMOSTATIC PARAMETERS (No test should be interpreted without an accompanying normal control.)

	ADULT DOG	ADULT CAT
Bleeding time		
Dorsum of nose (min)	2–4	1–5[33]
Lip (sec)	85–110	
Ear (min)	2.5–3	
Abdomen (min)	1–2	
Whole blood coagulation time		
Glass (Lee and White) (min)	6–7.5	8[33]
Silicone (Lee and White) (min)	12–15	
Capillary tube (min)[11]	3–4	5.2 ± 0.2[21]
Activated coagulation time of whole blood		
Room temp. (sec)	60–125[10]; 83–129[19]	A limited number of cats have shown a range similar to that of the dog.
37°C (sec)	64–95[19]	
Prothrombin time (sec)[11]	6–10	8.6 ± 0.5[21]
Puppies 1–4 hours old (sec)[5]	42.2	
6–12 hours old (sec)	49.1	
16–48 hours old (sec)	36.8	
48 hours old (sec)	24.5	
Russell's viper venom time (sec)[29]	11	9
Partial thromboplastin time (sec)	15–25	
Prothrombin consumption (sec)[29]	20.5	20
Fibrin degradation products (μg/ml)	<10	

BASENJI DOGS[13]		CATS[31]
Plasma Proteins (g./dl.)		*Plasma Proteins (g./dl.)*
6–8 weeks	5.33 ± 0.29	Lower values for younger animals
9–12 weeks	5.87 ± 0.46	Adults 6–8
4–6 months	6.6 ± 0.25	
1–2 years	7.03 ± 0.33	

NORMAL RENAL FUNCTION AND URINE PARAMETERS

Urine[22]	Adult Dog	Adult Cat
Specific Gravity		
Minimum	1.001	1.001
Maximum	1.060	1.080
Usual Limits (normal water and food intake)	1.018–1.050	1.018–1.050
Volume (ml./kg. body weight/day)	24–41	22–30
Osmolality Urine (m osm./kg.)		
Usual Range	500–1200	
Maximal Limits	2000–2400	
Osmolality Plasma	300	

Urine Constituents[37] (Values markedly affected by degree of concentration.)	Adult Dog	Adult Cat
Creatinine (mg/dl)	100–300	110–280
Urea (gm/dl)	1.0–2.5	1.0–3.0
Protein (mg/dl)	0–30	0–20
Amylase (Somogyi units)	50–150	30–120
Sodium (mEq/l)	20–165	
Potassium (mEq/l)	20–120	
Calcium (mEq/l)	2–10	
Inorganic phosphorus (mEq/l)	50–180	

Urinalysis — Semiquantitative Values	Adult Dog	Adult Cat
Protein sulfosalicylic acid	0–trace	0–trace
Protein Multistix[12a]	0–1+	0–1+
Glucose	0	0
Ketones	0	0
Bilirubin	0	0
10–20% Dogs – high specific gravity	1+	
5% Cats – high specific gravity		1+
Urobilinogen (Ehrlich unit)	0–1	0–1
(Wallace and Diamond)	<1:32	<1:32

Urine Total Protein Excretion (24 hr) in the Dog (Trichloroacetic Acid Ponceau Method)

N	Range (mg)	$\overline{X}$	SD
17[12a]	48–1040	333 mg	± 309 mg
10[3a]	8–151	38 mg	

*TM Ames Corp., Miles Laboratories, Inc., Elkhart, IN.

Renal Function – Dog[22]	
Effective renal plasma flow	266 ± 66 ml/min/m² body surface
	13.5 ± 3.3 ml/min/kg body weight
Glomerular filtration rate	84.4 ± 19 ml/min/m² body surface
	4 ml/min/kg body weight

Renal Function Tests – Dog	
Phenolsulfonphthalein	
Excretion in urine at 20 min, 6-mg dose[11]	21–66%
Clearance (P) 1 mg/kg at 60 min[17]	<80 μ/ml
$T_{1/2}$ clearance 5 mg/kg[9]	19.6 min
Creatinine, endogenous clearance[22]	60 ± 22 ml/min/m² body surface
	2.98 ± 0.96 ml/min/kg body weight

CEREBROSPINAL FLUID AND SYNOVIAL FLUID

CEREBROSPINAL FLUID[12]	ADULT DOG	ADULT CAT
Color	Clear, colorless	Clear, colorless
Pressure (mm H_2O)	<170	<100
Cells/μl	<5 lymphocytes	<5 lymphocytes
Protein (ml/dl)	<25	<20
Glucose (mg/dl)	61–116	85

CEREBROSPINAL FLUID AND SYNOVIAL FLUID—*Continued*

NORMAL SYNOVIAL FLUID—CARPAL, ELBOW, SHOULDER, HIP, STIFLE, AND HOCK JOINTS[30]	ADULT DOG	
	Range	*Mean*
Amount (ml)	0.01–1.00	0.24
pH	7–7.8	7.33
Leukocytes ($\times 10^3/\mu$l)	0–2.9	0.43
Erythrocytes ($\times 10^3 \mu$l)	0.320.0	12.15
Neutrophils/μl	0–32	3.63
Neutrophils(%)[20]	10	
Monocytes/μl	0–838	230.77
Lymphocytes/μl	0–2436	245.6
Clasmatocytes/μl	0–166	14.69
Mononuclear cells(%)[20]	90	
Mucin clot	Tight ropy clump Clear supernate	

CANINE SEMEN[14]

Regular collection by hand manipulation with a teaser (125 ejaculates from small dogs, mostly beagles).[8]

	Mean	*Standard Deviation*	*Range*
Volume (ml.)	5	4.3	0.5-20.4
% Motile Sperm	75	7.5	30-90
% Normal Sperm	86	14.7	34-97
pH	6.72	0.19	6.49-7.10
Concentration/cu. mm. (10^3)	148	84.6	27.2-388.8
Total Sperm per Ejaculate (10^6)	528	321.0	94-1428

FRACTIONATED EJACULATES (BASED ON 65 EJACULATES)

	Mean	*Range*	*pH*
1st Fraction	0.8 ml.	0.25-2.00	6.37
2nd Fraction	0.6 ml.	0.40-2.00	6.10
3rd Fraction	0.4 ml.	1.0-16.3	7.20

PUREBRED LABRADOR RETRIEVERS, 18 TO 48 MONTHS OLD[33]

	Mean	*Range*
Volume (ml.)	2.2*	0.5-6.5
% Motile Sperm	93	75-99
% Unstained Sperm (Eosin Nigrosin)	84	61-99
Concentration/cu. mm. (10^3)	564	103-708

*Only the first two fractions were collected, resulting in smaller volume and higher concentration of sperm/cu. mm. than would result if all the prostatic fluid (3rd fraction) were obtained.

SUPPLEMENTAL READING AND REFERENCES

1. Andersen, A. C., and Gee, W.: Normal values in the beagle. Vet. Med., 53:135–138, 156; 1958.
2. Anderson, L., Wilson, R., and Hay, D.: Haematological values in normal cats from four weeks to one year of age. Res. Vet. Sci., 12:579–583, 1971.
3. Baker, H. J.: Laboratory evaluation of thyroid function. In Kirk, R. W. (ed.): *Current Veterinary Therapy IV*. Philadelphia, W. B. Saunders Co., 1971.
3a. Barsanti, J. A., and Finco, D. R.: Protein concentration in urine of normal dogs. Am. J. Vet. Res., 40:1583, 1979.
4. Belshaw, B. E., and Rijnberk, A.: Radioimmunoassay of plasma T_4 and T_3 in the diagnosis of primary hypothyroidism in dogs. J. Am. Anim. Hosp. Assoc., 15:17–23, 1979.
5. Benjamin, M.: *An Outline of Veterinary Clinical Pathology*, 3rd ed. Ames, Iowa, Iowa State University Press, 1978.

6. Berman, E.: Hemogram of the cat during pregnancy and lactation and after lactation. Am. J. Vet. Res., 35:457–460, 1974.
7. Biozyme Veterinary Laboratory (a division of Biozyme Medical Laboratories, Inc.): *Normal Ranges Chemistry*. Olean, N.Y., Bioenzyme Vet. Lab., 1978.
8. Boucher, J. H.: Evaluation of semen quality in the dog and the effects of frequency of ejaculation upon semen quality, libido and restoration of sperm reserves. M.S. Thesis, Cornell University, Ithaca, N.Y., 1957.
9. Brobst, D. F., Carter, J. M., and Horron, M.: Plasma phenolsulfonphthalein determination as a measure of renal function in the dog. 17th Gaines Veterinary Symposium, University of Minnesota, 1967, p. 15.
10. Byars, T. D., Ling, G. V., Ferris, N. A., and Keeton, K. S.: Activated coagulation time (ACT) of whole blood in normal dogs. Am. J. Vet. Res., 37:1359–1361, 1976.

11. Coles, E. H.: *Veterinary Clinical Pathology*, 2nd ed. Philadelphia, W. B. Saunders Co., 1974.
12. deLahunta, A.: New York State College of Veterinary Medicine, Cornell University, Ithaca, New York 14853. Personal communication.
12a. DiBartola, S. P., Chew, D. J., and Jacobs, G.: Quantitative urinalysis including 24-hour protein excretion in the dog. J. Am. Anim. Hosp. Assoc., *16*:537, 1980.
13. Ewing, G. O., Schalm, O. W., and Smith, R. S.: Hematologic values of normal Basenji dogs. J. Am. Vet. Med. Assoc., *161*:1661, 1972.
14. Revisions and corrections courtesy of Dr. R. H. Foote, Professor of Animal Physiology, Department of Animal Science, New York State College of Life Sciences, Cornell University, Ithaca, New York 14853.
15. Kallfelz, F. A.: Associate Professor of Clinical Nutrition, Department of Large Animal Medicine, Obstetrics and Surgery, New York State College of Veterinary Medicine, Ithaca, New York 14853. Personal communication.
16. Kallfelz, F. A., and Erali, R. P.: Thyroid function tests on domesticated animals. Am. J. Vet. Res., *34*:1449, 1973.
17. Kaufman, C. F., and Kirk, R. W.: The 60-minute plasma phenolsulfonphthalein concentration as a test of renal function in the dog. J. Am. Anim. Hosp. Assoc., *9*:66, 1973.
18. Kraft, W.: Schielddrusenfunktionsstörunge. beim Hund. (Thyroid function disturbances in the dog.) Thesis, Justus Liebig University, Giessen, West Germany, 1964. (Cited by Belshaw.)
19. Middleton, D. J., and Watson, A. D. J.: Activated coagulation times of whole blood in normal dogs and dogs with coagulopathies. J. Small Anim. Pract., *19*:417–422, 1978.
20. Miller, J. B., Perman, V., Osborne, C. A., Hammer, R. F., and Gambardella, P. C.: Synovial fluid analysis in canine arthritis. J. Am. Anim. Hosp. Assoc., *10*:392, 1974.
21. Osbaldiston, G. W., Stowe, E. C., and Griffith, P. R.: Blood coagulation: Comparative studies in dogs, cats, horses and cattle. Br. Vet. J., *126*:512, 1970.
22. Osborne, C. A., Low, D. G., and Finco, D. R.: *Canine and Feline Urology*. Philadelphia, W. B. Saunders Co., 1972.
23. Penny, R. H. C., Carlisle, C. H., and Davidson, H. A.: The blood and marrow picture of the cat. Br. Vet. J., *126*:459–464, 1970.
24. *Chemassay Amylase*. Pitman-Moore, Inc., Washington Crossing, N.J. 08560.
25. *1975 Normal Blood Values for Cats*. Ralston Purina Co., Professional Marketing Services, Checkerboard Square, St. Louis, Missouri 63188.
26. *1975 Normal Blood Values for Dogs*. Ralston Purina Co., Professional Marketing Services, Checkerboard Square, St. Louis, Missouri 63188.
27. Reimers, Thomas J.: Assistant Professor and Director of the Endocrinology Laboratory, New York State College of Veterinary Medicine, Cornell University, Ithaca, N.Y. 14853. Personal communication.
28. Rogers, U. A., Donovan, E. F., and Kociba, G. J.: Lipids and lipoproteins in normal dogs and dogs with secondary hyperlipoproteinemia. J. Am. Vet. Med. Assoc., *166*:1092–1100, 1975.
29. Rowsell, H. C.: Blood coagulation and hemorrhagic disorders. In: Medway, W., Prier, J. E., and Wilkinson, J. S. (eds.): *Textbook of Veterinary Clinical Pathology*. Baltimore, Williams & Wilkins Co., 1969, p. 247.
30. Sawyer, D. C.: Synovial fluid analysis of canine joints. J. Am. Vet. Med. Assoc., *143*:609, 1963.
31. Schalm, O. W., Jain, N. C., and Carroll, E. J.: *Veterinary Hematology*, 3rd ed. Philadelphia, Lea & Febiger, 1975.
32. Scott, D. W.: Assistant Professor of Medicine, Dept. of Clinical Sciences, New York State College of Veterinary Medicine, Cornell University, Ithaca, N.Y. 14853. Personal communication.
33. Seager, S. W. J., and Fletcher, W. S.: Collection, storage, and insemination of canine seman. Lab. Anim. Sci., *22*:177–182, 1972.
34. Tasker, J. B.: Reference values for clinical chemistry using the Coulter Chemistry System. Cornell Vet. *68*:460–479, 1978.
35. Wallace, R.: Research Support Specialist, New York State College of Veterinary Medicine, Cornell University, Ithaca, N.Y. 14853. Personal communication.
36. Wilkins, R. J., and Hurvitz, A. I.: *Profiling in Veterinary Clinical Pathology*. Tarrytown, New York, Technicon Instruments Corp., 1978, pp. 17, 19.
37. Wilkins, R. J.: Animal Medical Center, 510 East 62nd St., New York, New York 10021. Personal communication.

TABLE OF COMMON DRUGS: APPROXIMATE DOSES *

DRUG NAME	DOG	CAT
Acetazolamide	10 mg/kg q6h PO	Same
Acetylcysteine (Mucomyst)	*Eye*: Dilute to 2% soln with artificial tears and apply topically q2h to eye for maximum of 48 hours *Respiratory*: 50 ml/hr for 30–60 min every 12 hr by nebulization	Same
Acetylpromazine (acepromazine)	0.055–0.11 mg./kg IV, IM, SC	0.055–0.11 mg/kg IM, SC
Acetylsalicylic acid (aspirin)	*Analgesia*: 10 mg/kg PO q12h *Antirheumatic*: 40 mg/kg PO q18h or 25 mg/kg q8h	*Analgesia*: 10 mg/kg PO q52h *Antirheumatic*: 40 mg/kg q72h
ACTH	2 units/kg/day IM (therapeutic) or 40 units/dog IM (response test; take post sample in 2 hr)	Same
Actinomycin D (Cosmegan)	0.015 mg/kg/once daily for 5 days	None
Aldactone (spironolactone)	1–2 mg/kg q12h	Same
Allopurinol (Zyloprim)	10 mg/kg PO q8h, then reduce to 10 mg/kg PO daily	None
Amforol	2–6 tablets/9 kg initially. Maintenance: 1–3 tabs/9 kg q8h	None
Amikacin	5 mg/kg q 8 h IM, IV	None
Aminophylline	10 mg/kg q8h PO, IM, IV	Same
Ammonium chloride	100 mg/kg q12h PO	20 mg/kg q12h PO
Amoxicillin	11 mg/kg q12h PO for 5–7 days	11–22 mg/kg q24h PO for 5–7 days
Amphetamine	4.4 mg/kg IV, IM	Same
Amphotericin B	0.15–1.0 mg/kg dissolved in 5–20 ml 5% dextrose and water given rapidly IV 3× weekly for 2–4 mo. Do not exceed 2.0 mg/kg. Pretreat with antiemetics if needed. Monitor BUN.	Same
Ampicillin (Polyflex, Princillin)	10–20 mg/kg q6h PO, or 5–10 mg/kg q6h IV, IM, SC	Same
Amprolium	100–200 mg/kg/day in food or water for 7–10 days	None
Anterior pituitary gonadotropin	*Bitches*: 100–500 units once daily to effect	None
Apomorphine	0.02 mg/kg IV or 0.04 mg/kg SC	None
Aqua-B (vitamin B complex)	0.5–2.0 ml q24h IV, IM, SC	0.5–1.0 ml q24h IV, IM, SC
Aquamephyton (vitamin K_1)	5–20 mg q12h IV, IM, SC	1–5 mg q12h IV, IM, SC
Ascorbic acid (vitamin C)	100–500 mg/day (maintenance) or 100–500 mg q8h (urine acidifier)	100 mg/day (maintenance) or 100 mg q8h (urine acidifier)
L-Asparginase	10,000–20,000 IU/M² weekly IP or 400 IU/kg weekly	Same
Atropine	0.05 mg/kg q6h IV, SC, IM or 1% soln in eye *Organophosphate poisoning*: 0.2–2.0 mg/kg IV, SC, IM. Give ¼ dose IV and remainder IM or SC prn.	Same
Aurothioglucose (Solganol)	First week 5 mg IM, second week 10 mg IM, then 1 mg/kg once a week IM decreasing to once a month	First week 1 mg IM, second week 2 mg IM, then 1 mg/kg once a week IM decreasing to once a month
Azathioprine	2 mg/kg q24h PO	None
BAL	4 mg/kg q4h IM until recovered	None
Betamethasone (Betasone®)	0.028–0.055 ml/kg IM. Give only once.	None
Bethanechol (Urecholine)	5–25 mg q8h PO	2.5–5.0 mg q8h PO
Bismuth, milk of	10–30 ml q4h PO	Same
Bismuth (subnitrate, subgallate, or subcarbonate)	0.3–3.0 gm q4h PO	Same
Bleomycin (Blenoxane®)	10 mg/M² daily IV or SC for 4 days, then 10 mg/M² weekly to a maximum total dose of 200 mg/M²	None
Blood	20 ml/kg IV or IP or to effect	Same
Brewer's yeast	0.2 gm/kg once daily PO	Same

Table compiled by Richard Johnson, Reg Ph.

*See page 1205 for Tables for Conversion of Weight to Body-surface Area in Square Meters for Dogs.

DRUG NAME	DOG	CAT
Bromsulphalein (BSP) (5% solution)	*Test only*: 5 ml/kg IV; post sample in 30 min	None
Bunamidine (Scolaban)	25–50 mg/kg PO. Fast 3 hr before and after administration.	Same
Busulfan (Myleran®)	4.0 mg/M² daily PO or 0.1 mg/kg daily	None
Butorphanol	0.055–0.11 mg/kg q6 to 12h SC up to 7 days	None
Caffeine	0.1–0.5 gm IM	None
Calcium	500 mg/kg/day PO	150 mg/kg/day PO
Calcium carbonate	1–4 gm/day PO	Same
Calcium EDTA	100 mg/kg diluted to 10 mg/ml in 5% dextrose and given SC in 4 divided doses; continue for 5 days	Same
Calcium gluconate (10% solution)	10–30 ml IV (slowly)	5–15 ml IV (slowly)
Calcium lactate	0.5–2.0 gm PO	0.2–0.5 gm PO
Canine distemper-hepatitis vaccine	1 vial SC at 8, 12, and 16 weeks of age; annual booster	None
Canopar	500 mg PO for dogs heavier than 4.55 kg; 250 mg bid for those 2.27–4.55 kg. Repeat in 2–3 weeks.	None
Carbenicillin	15 mg/kg q8h IV	Same
Cardioquin	10–20 mg/kg q8h PO	Same
Castor oil	8–30 ml PO	4–10 ml PO
Cephalexin (Keflex)	30 mg/kg q12h PO	Same
Cephalothin sodium	35 mg/kg q8h IM, IV	Same
Cephapirin	10–20 mg/kg q6h IM, IV	Same
Charcoal, activated (Requa)	0.3–5 gm q8–12h PO *Poisoning*: 1–2 tsp/10–15 kg in 200 ml tap water. Administer by stomach tube.	Half the canine dose
Cheracol	5 ml q4h PO	3 ml q4h PO
Chlorambucil (Leukeran)	0.2 mg/kg PO once daily 1.5 mg/M² PO as single dose; decrease for repeated dosage	Same
Chloramphenicol	50 mg/kg q8h PO, IV, IM, SC	Same, except q12h
Chlordane	0.5% solution on dog or premises	None
Chlorethamine	0.2–1.0 gm q8h PO	100 mg q8h PO
Chlorpheniramine	4–8 mg q12h PO	2 mg q12h PO
Chlorpromazine (Thorazine)	3.3 mg/kg PO sid to qid; 1.1–6.6 mg/kg IM sid to qid; 0.55–4.4 mg/kg IV sid to qid	Same
Chlortetracycline	20 mg/kg q8h PO	Same
Chlorthiazide (Diuril)	20–40 mg/kg q 12h PO	Same
Cimetidine (Tagamet)	5–10 mg/kg q6–12h	None
Cloxacillin	10 mg/kg q6h PO, IV, IM	Same
Cod liver oil	1 tsp/10 kg once daily PO	Same
Codeine	*Pain*: 2 mg/kg q6h SC *Cough*: 5 mg/dose q6h PO	None
Colistimethate (Coly-Mycin)	1.1 mg/kg q6h IM	Same
Colistin	1 mg/kg q6h IM	Same
Cyclophosphamide (Cytoxan)	6.6 mg/kg PO for 3 days, then 2.2 mg/kg PO once daily; 10 mg/kg q7–10 days IV; 50 mg/M² PO, IV once daily for 3–4 days/wk; repeat prn.	Same
Cyclothiazide	0.5–1.0 mg/PO once daily	None
Cytarabine (Cytosar)	5–10 mg/kg once daily for 2 wk, or 30–50 mg/kg IV, IM, SC once/wk; 100 mg/M² once daily IV, IM for 4 days, then 150 mg/M².	Same
Dapsone	1.1 mg/kg q8h PO	None
Darbazine	0.14–0.22 ml/kg q12h SC 2–7 kg: 1 #1 capsule q12h PO 7–14 kg: 1–2 #1 capsules q12h PO Over 14 kg: 1 #3 capsule q12h PO	0.14–0.22 ml/kg q12h SC
Delta albaplex	3–7 kg: 1–2 tablets/day PO 7–14 kg: 2–4 tablets/day PO 14–27 kg: 4–6 tablets/day PO Over 27 kg: 6–8 tablets/day PO	1 tablet q12h PO
Depo-penicillin	15,000–30,000 units/kg q48h IM, SC	Same
Desoxycorticosterone acetate (Doca)	1–5 mg q24h IM	0.5–1.0 mg q24h IM

DRUG NAME	DOG	CAT
Desoxycorticosterone pivalate	Each 25 mg releases 1 mg Doca/day for 1 month. IM dose: 5–50 mg once/month to effect.	Same
Dexamethasone (Azium)	0.25–1.0 mg IV, IM once daily; 0.25–1.25 mg PO once daily *Shock*: 5 mg/kg IV	0.125–0.5 mg once daily PO, IV, IM *Shock*: same
Dextran	20 ml/kg IV to effect	Same
Dextrose solutions (5% in water, saline, or Ringer's)	40–50 ml/kg q24h IV, SC, IP	Same
D.F.P. (Floropryl)	0.1% solution for eyes, topically	Same
Diazepam (Valium)	2.5–20 mg IV, PO; 10-mg bolus IV (slowly) if in status epilepticus; repeat if no effect	2.5–5.0 mg IV, PO
Dichlorphenamide	50 mg/15 kg tid PO	10–25 mg tid PO
Dichlorvos (Task)	26.4–33 mg/kg PO; in risk animals divide dose; give remaining half 8–24 hr later	None
Dicloxacillin (Dicloxin)	11–55 mg/kg q8h PO	Same
Diethylcarbamazine (Caricide, Cypip, Filaribits)	*Treatment of ascarids*: 55–110 mg/kg PO *Prevention of ascarids* (Cypip): 3.3 mg/kg PO once daily *Prevention of heartworms* (Caricide, Filaribits): 6.6 mg/kg PO once daily	*Treatment of ascarids*: 55–110 mg/kg PO
Diethylstilbestrol (DES)	0.1–1.0 mg/day PO or 2 mg/kg up to 25 mg total IM (repositol) *once*.	0.05–0.10 mg/day PO (Caution)
Di-Gel (liquid)	30–60 ml PO	Half the canine dose
Digitoxin (Foxalin-Vet)	0.033–0.11 mg/kg PO, divided bid	None
Digoxin (Lanoxin, Cardoxin)	*Digitalization*: 0.028–0.055 mg/kg q12h PO for 2 days *Maintenance*: 0.0055–0.011 mg/kg q12h PO 0.044 mg/kg IV to digitalize, then switch to oral maintenance; *or* 0.01–0.02 mg/kg IV q1h to digitalize, then switch to oral maintenance	0.0055 mg/kg q12h (tablet only)
Dihydrocodeinone	5 mg q6h PO	None
Dihydrostreptomycin	20 mg/kg q6h PO; 10 mg/kg q8h IM, SC	Same
Dihydrotachysterol	0.01 mg/kg/day	None
Diphenhydramine (Benadryl)	2–4 mg/kg q8h PO; 5–50 mg q12h IV	Same
Dimenhydrinate (Dramamine)	25–50 mg q8h PO	12.5 mg q8h PO
Dioctyl sulfosuccinate (Surfak, Permeatrate)	10–15 ml of 5% soln with 100 ml water q12h PO, per rectum prn; 1 or 2 50-mg capsules q12–24h PO	2 ml of 5% soln with 50 ml water q12h PO, per rectum prn 1 50-mg capsule q12h–24h PO
Diphenthane 70	200 mg/kg PO after 12-hr fast; repeat in 3 weeks	Same
Diphenylhydantoin (Dilantin). See *Phenytoin*		
Diphenylthiocarbazone	60 mg/kg q8h PO for 5 days beyond recovery	None
Disophenol (D.N.P.)	10 mg/kg SC; may be repeated in 2–3 weeks	None
Dithiazanine (Dizan)	6.6–11 mg/kg PO once daily for 7–10 days	None
Dobutamine HCl (Dobutrex®)	250 mg in 500 ml saline; give IV to effect	None
Domeboro's solution	1–2 tablets/pint water; apply topically q8h; store soln no longer than 7 days	Same
Dopamine HCl (Intropin®)	200 mg in 500 ml saline; give IV to effect	Same
Doxapram (Dopram)	5–10 mg/kg IV *Neonate*: 1–5 mg SC, sublingual or umbilical vein	5–10 mg/kg IV *Neonate*: 1–2 mg SC, sublingual vein
Doxorubicin (Adriamycin)	30 mg/M² IV q 3 weeks	None
Doxylamine succinate	1–2 mg/kg q8h IM	Same
D-Penicillamine (Cuprimine)	10–15 mg/kg q12h	None

DRUG NAME	DOG	CAT
Edrophonium	0.11–0.22 mg/kg IV	None
Emetrol	4–12 ml q 15 min PO until emesis ceases	Same
Enflurane (Ethrane)	*Induction*: 2–3% *Maintenance*: 1.5–3%	Same
Ephedrine	5–15 mg PO	2–5 mg PO
Epinephrine (1:1000 soln)	0.1–0.5 ml SC, IM, IV, or intracardiac	0.1–0.2 ml SC, IM, IV, or intracardiac
Erythromycin	10 mg/kg q8h PO	Same
Estradiol cyclopentyl propionate (ECP)	0.25–2.0 mg IM *once*	0.25–0.5 mg IM *once*
Ether	0.5–4.0 ml (Induction: 8%; Maintenance: 4% Inhalant to effect.	Same
Ethoxzolamide (Cardrase)	4 mg/kg q12h PO	Same
Feline panleukopenia vaccine	Used, but not FDA-approved	1 vial SC at 8, 12, and 16 weeks of age; annual booster
Fenbendazole	50 mg/kg/day for 3 days	None
Fentanyl (Sublimaze)	0.02–0.04 mg/kg (preanesthetic) IM, IV, SC	Same, but use with tranquilizer to prevent excitation
Ferrous sulfate	100–300 mg q24h PO	50–100 mg q24h PO
Festal	1–2 tablets PO with or immediately after feeding	1 tablet PO with or immediately after feeding
Flucytosine (Ancobon)	100 mg/kg q12h PO	Same
Fludrocortisone (Florinef)	0.2–0.8 mg once daily PO	0.1–0.2 mg once daily PO
Flumethasone (Flucort)	0.06–0.25 mg once daily PO, IV, IM, SC	0.03–0.125 mg once daily PO, IV, IM, SC
5-Fluorouracil	5 mg/kg IV q 5–7 days; 200 mg/M² IV once daily for 3 days followed by 100 mg/M² IV on alternate days until signs of toxicity appear; then 200–400 mg/M² IV weekly	None
Folic acid	5 mg/day PO	2.5 mg/day PO
Framycetin	20 mg/kg q6h PO	Same
Furosemide (Lasix)	2–4 mg/kg q8–12h PO; no more than 40–50 mg total IV to any dog, q12h	2–3 mg/kg bid or tid IV, IM (5–10 mg total IV); 2–4 mg/kg q8–12h PO
Gentamicin	4 mg/kg IM, SC q12h first day, then q24h	Same
Glucagon	*Tolerance test*: 0.03 mg/kg IV	None
Glycerin	0.6 ml/kg q8h PO	Same
Glycobiarsol (Milibis-V)	220 mg/kg PO once daily for 5 days with food; repeat in 3 months	None
Glycopyrrolate	0.01 mg/kg IM or SC	None
Griseofulvin	50 mg/kg PO once daily with fat for 6 weeks	Same
Halothane (Fluothane)	*Induction*: 3% *Maintenance*: 0.5–1.5%	Same
Heparin	Initial IV dose: 200 units/kg; continue by SC administration q8h	Same
Hetacillin (Hetacin)	10–20 mg/kg q8h PO	Same
Hydralazine	1 mg/kg q8h PO	None
Hydrochlorothiazide (Hydrodiuril)	2–4 mg/kg q12h PO	Same
Hydrocortisone (Solu-Cortef)	4.4 mg/kg q12h PO *Shock*: 50 mg/kg IV	Same
Hydrogen peroxide (3%)	5–10 ml q 15 min PO until emesis occurs	Same
Hydroxyurea (Hydrea)	80 mg/kg q 3 days PO; 40–50 mg/kg divided twice daily PO; 20–30 mg/kg PO as a single daily dose	Same
Imidazole (DTIC)	200 mg/M² for 5 days IV; repeat 5-day cycle q 3 weeks	None
Innovar-Vet	0.1–0.14 ml/kg IM; 0.04–0.09 ml/kg IV; Administer with atropine to minimize bradycardia and salivation	CNS excitation Do not use.
Insulin (regular)	2 units/kg q2–6h IV (ketoacidosis), modified to effect *Hyperkalemia*: 0.5–1.0 units/kg with 2 gm dextrose per unit of insulin	3–5 units SC q6h, modified to effect

DRUG NAME	DOG	CAT
Insulin (intermediate)	0.5–1.0 units/kg q24h SC, modified as needed	3–5 units q24h SC, modified as needed
Isuprel	0.1–0.2 mg q6h IM, SC; 15–30 mg q4h PO; 1 mg in 200 ml 5% dextrose IV to effect	Same
Isuprel	Elixir: 0.44 ml/kg q8H PO	
Jenotone	2 mg/kg q12h IM, SC	Same
Kanamycin (Kantrim)	10 mg/kg q6h PO; 7 mg/kg q6h IM, SC	Same
Kaopectate	1–2 ml/kg q2–6h	Same
Ketamine (Vetalar)	None	*Restraint*: 11 mg/kg IM *Anesthesia*: 22–33 mg/kg IM; 2.2–4.4 mg/kg IV
Ketoconazole	10 mg/kg q8h PO	Same
Lactated Ringer's solution	40–50 ml/kg/day IV, SC, IP	Same
Laxatone	*Laxative*: 2–4 ml PO 2–3 days/week	*Laxative*: 1–2 ml PO 2–3 days/week *Hairballs*: 2–4 ml/day PO for 2–3 days; then 1–2 ml 2–3 days/week
Leucovorin	3 mg/M² within 3h of methotrexate administration	None
Levallorphan (Lorfan)	0.02–0.2 mg/kg IV prn	1 mg/kg IV prn
Levamisole (L-tetramisole)	*Microfilariae*: 10 mg/kg once daily PO for 6–10 days	*Lungworms*: 20–40 mg/kg PO every other day for 5–6 treatments
Levo-Thyroxin	22 mcg/kg q12h PO	0.05–0.1 mg PO once daily
Lidocaine (without epinephrine) (Xylocaine)	1–2 mg/kg IV bolus, followed by IV drip, 0.1% soln at 30–50 μg/kg/min	Do *not* use as antiarrhythmic.
Lime sulfur (Vlem-Dome) (1:16–1:40 dilution of concentrate)	Topical	Same
Lincomycin	15 mg/kg q8h PO; 10 mg/kg q12h IV, IM	Same
Lindane	0.025–0.1% aqueous soln topically	None
Liothyronine	4 mcg/kg q8h PO	None
Lomotil	2.5 mg q8h PO	None
Magnesium hydroxide (milk of magnesia)	*Antacid*: 5–30 ml PO *Cathartic*: 3–5 times the antacid dose	*Antacid*: 5–15 ml PO
Magnesium sulfate (Epsom salts)	8–25 gm PO	2–4 gm PO
Mannitol (20% soln)	1.0–2.0 gm/kg q6h IV	Same
Measles vaccine	1 vial SC to dogs between 6 and 8 weeks of age	None
Mebendazole (Telmintic)	22 mg/kg with food q24h for 3 days	None
Meclizine (Bonine)	25 mg once daily PO	12.5 mg once daily PO
Megestrol acetate (Ovaban®)	*Skin*: 1 mg/kg/day PO *Behavior*: 2–4 mg/kg once daily; reduce to half dose at 8 days for maintenance *To postpone estrus*: In proestrus: 2 mg/kg PO daily for 8 days In anestrus: 0.5 mg/kg PO daily for 32 days False pregnancy: 2.0 mg/kg PO daily for 8 days	*Skin*: 5 mg/day PO for one week, then twice weekly. *Behavior*: 2–4 mg/kg once daily; reduce to half dose at 8 days for maintenance. None
Melatonin	1–2 mg once daily SC for 3 days; repeat monthly as needed	None
Melphalan (Alkeran)	0.05–0.1 mg/kg PO once daily; 1.5 mg/M² PO once daily for 7–10 days, then no therapy for 2–3 weeks	Same
Meperidine (Demerol)	10 mg/kg IM prn	3 mg/kg IM prn
6-Mercaptopurine (6-MP)	50 mg/M² daily PO or 2 mg/kg daily	None
Metamucil	2 to 10 gm q12 to 24h in wetted or liquid food	2 to 4 gm q12 to 24h in wetted or liquid food
Metaraminol (Aramine)	2–10 mg SC, IM; 10–50 mg/500 ml saline infused IV to effect	None
Methenamine mandelate (Mandelamine)	10 mg/kg q6h PO to effect	None
Methicillin	20 mg/kg q6h IV, IM	Same

DRUG NAME	DOG	CAT
DL-Methionine	0.2–1.0 gm q8h PO	0.2 gm q8h PO
Methischol	1 capsule/15 kg q8h PO	1 capsule q12h PO
Methocarbamol	44.4–222.2 mg/kg IV 44.4 mg/kg q8h PO first day, then 22.2–44.4 mg/kg q8h	Same
Methohexital (Brevital)	11 mg/kg IV (2.5% soln)	Same
Methotrexate	0.06 mg/kg once daily PO; 0.3–0.8 mg/kg IV weekly; 2.5 mg/M² once daily PO, IV, IM	Same
Methoxyflurane (Metofane)	*Induction*: 3% *Maintenance*: 0.5–1.5%	Same
Methylprednisolone (Medrol®) (Depomedrol®)	See *prednisolone* 1.0 mg/kg IM every 2 weeks	Same 20 mg/cat IM once
Methyltestosterone	0.5 mg/kg q24h PO	Same
Metronidazole	60 mg/kg q24h PO for 5 days	Same
Metropine	0.5–1.0 mg q8h PO	None
Mibolerone	30 mcg/0.45–11.3 kg, 60 mcg/11.8–22.7 kg, 120 mcg/23–45.3 kg, 180 mcg/45.8 kg and over daily PO German Shepherd and German Shepherd mix: 180 mcg all weights daily PO	None
Milk of magnesia. See *Magnesium hydroxide*		
Mineral oil	2–60 ml PO	2–10 ml PO
Mithramycin	2 µg/kg IV once daily for 2 days	Same
Morphine	1 mg/kg SC, IM prn	0.1 mg/kg SC, IM prn
Nafcillin	10 mg/kg q6h PO, IM	Same
Nalorphine	1.0 mg/kg IV, IM, SC	None
Naloxone (Narcan)	0.04 mg/kg IV, IM, SC	None
Neo-Darbazine	1 #1 capsule q12h PO (4.5 to 9 kg) 2 #1 capsules q12h PO (9 to 13.6 kg) 3 #1 capsules or 1 #3 capsule q12h PO (13.6 to 27.3 kg) 1 or 2 #3 capsules q12h PO (over 27.3 kg)	None
Neomycin (Biosol)	20 mg/kg q6h PO; 3.5 mg/kg q8h IV, IM, SC	Same
Neostigmine (Stiglyn)	1–2 mg IM prn; 5–15 mg PO prn	None
Nikethimide (Coramine)	7.8–31.2 mg/kg IV, IM, SC	Same
Nitrofurantoin (Dantefur)	4 mg/kg q8h PO; 3 mg/kg q12h IM	Same
Novobiocin	10 mg/kg q8h PO	Same
Nystatin	100,000 units q6h PO	Same
Octin	0.5–1.0 ml IM; 1 tablet q8–12h PO	0.25–0.5 ml IM; ½ to 1 tablet q12h PO
o,p-DDD(Lysodren)	50 mg/kg once daily PO to effect (approx. 5–10 days), then once every 2 weeks	None
Orgotein	5 mg once weekly SC	None
Ouabain	0.04 mg/kg total dose IV; give half of dose stat, ⅛ of dose q 30 min (maintenance dose: ¼ of total q3h)	Same
Oxacillin	10 mg/kg q6h PO, IV, IM	Same
Oxymorphone (Numorphan)	0.1–0.2 mg/kg SC, IM, IV prn	Same
Oxytetracycline	20 mg/kg q8h PO; 7 mg/kg q12h IV, IM	Same
Oxytocin	5–10 units IM, IV; repeats q 15–30 min	0.5–3.0 units IM, IV
2-PAM	40 mg/kg IV over 2-minute period, q12h as needed (may be given IM or SC)	None
Pancreatin	2–10 tablets with food	1–2 tablets with food
Pancuronium	0.1 mg/kg IV	None
Paregoric	3–5 ml q6h PO	None
Penicillin G, benzathine	40,000 units/kg q 5 days IM	Same
Penicillin G (Na or K)	40,000 units/kg q6h PO (not with food); 20,000 units/kg q4h IV, IM, SC	Same

DRUG NAME	DOG	CAT
Penicillin G, procaine	20,000 units/kg q12–24h IM, SC	Same
Penicillin V	10 mg/kg q8h PO	Same
Pentazocine (Talwin)	0.5–1.0 mg/kg IM maximum. **Never IV.**	None
Pentobarbital	*Sedation*: 2–4 mg/kg IV *Anesthesia*: 30 mg/kg IV to effect	Same
Pepto-Bismol	2.2 ml/kg PO	None
Phenethicillin	10 mg/kg q8h	Same
Phenobarbital	*Status epilepticus*: 6 mg/kg q6–12h IM, IV prn *Less severe conditions*: 2 mg/kg PO bid	Same
Phenoxybenzamine	0.25–0.5 mg/kg q6 to 8h PO	Same
Phenylbutazone (Butazolidin)	22 mg/kg q8h IV; total dose not to exceed 0.8 gm/day	None
Phenylephrine (Neo-Synephrine)	0.15 mg/kg IV; 10% soln topically in eye	Same
Phenytoin (Dilantin)	*Antiepileptic*: 2–6 mg/kg q8–12h PO *Antiarrhythmic*: 24 mg/kg PO stat, then 3–5 mg/kg q6–8h	None
Phthalofyne (Whipcide)	180 mg/kg PO after 24-hr fast; repeat in 3 months	None
Phthalylsulfathiazole (Sulfathaladine)	50 mg/kg q6h PO; 100 mg/kg q12h PO	Same
Phytonadione. See *Aquamephyton*		
Piperacetazine (Psymod)	*Tranquilization*: 0.11 mg/kg PO bid to qid; 0.11 mg/kg IV, IM, SC *Sedation*: 0.44 mg/kg IV, IM, SC	Same
Piperazine	62 mg/kg PO; may be repeated in 30 days	Same
Pitressin (ADH)	10 units IV, IM (aqueous) or 0.5–1.0 ml IM every other day (oil)	Same
Polymyxin B	2 mg/kg q12h IM; 1–2 mg/kg q12h PO Aerosol: Nebulize 300,000 units in 2.5 ml saline q8–12h	Same
Potassium chloride	1–3 gm/day PO IV: maximum 10 mEq/hr and 40 mEq/day/dog	0.2 gm/day PO
Praziquantel (Droncit)	½ tablet/2.3 kg and under 1 tablet/2.7–4.5 kg 1½ tablets/5–6.8 kg 2 tablets/7.3–13.6 kg 3 tablets/14–20.5 kg 4 tablets/20.9–27.3 kg 5 tablets maximum over 27.3 kg	½ tablet/1.8 kg and under 1 tablet/2.3–5.0 kg 1½ tablets/5 kg and over
Prednisolone	*Allergy*: 0.5 mg/kg bid PO or IM	1.0 mg/kg bid PO or IM
	Immune suppression: 2.0 mg/kg bid PO or IM	3.0 mg/kg bid PO or IM
	Prolonged use: 0.5–2.0 mg/kg every other morning PO	2.0–4.0 mg/kg every other evening PO
(Solu-Delta-Cortef®)	*Shock*: 5.5–11.0 mg/kg IV, then q 1,3,6, or 10 hours prn	Same
Primidone	55 mg/kg PO sid	None
Procainamide (Pronestyl)	50 mg/kg/day *total* PO q3–6h; 11–22 mg/kg IM q3–6h; 100-mg bolus IV, followed by IV drip at 10–40 µg/kg/min	Not recommended
Promazine (Sparine)	2.2–4.4 mg/kg IV, IM	Same
Promethazine (Phenergan)	0.2–1.0 mg/kg q8–12h PO, SC	None
Propantheline (Pro-Banthine)	Small: 5–7.5 mg q8h PO Medium: 15 mg q8h PO Large: 30 mg q8h PO	5–7.5 mg q8h PO
Propiopromazine (Tranvet)	1.1–4.4 mg/kg PO sid to bid	None
Propranolol (Inderal)	5–40 mg PO tid; 1–3 mg IV (1 mg q 1–2 min); total dose not to exceed 1.5 mg/kg	None
Prussian blue	0.1 gm/kg/day PO q8h	None
Pyrantel pamoate	5 mg/kg PO, repeat in 3 weeks	10 mg/kg PO, repeat in 3 weeks

DRUG NAME	DOG	CAT
Pyrimethamine	1 mg/kg q24h PO for 3 days, then 0.5 mg/kg q24h PO	Same
Quadrinal	¼ to ½ tablet q4–6h PO	¼ tablet q4–6h PO
Quibron	1–3 capsules q8h PO Elixir: 5 ml/15 kg q8h PO	½ capsule q8h PO Elixir: 2 ml q8h PO
Quinacrine (Atabrine)	50–100 mg q12h PO for 3 days; repeat in 3 days	None
Quinaglute	6–20 mg/kg q8–12h PO	Same
Quinidine (Cardioquin, Quinaglute)	10–20 mg/kg PO, IM tid to qid	Not recommended
Rabies vaccine (CEO)	1 vial IM (as per state regulations)	Same
Rabies vaccine (TCO)	1 vial IM (as per state regulations)	Same
Riboflavin	10–20 mg/day PO	5–10 mg/day PO
Ringer's solution	40–50 ml/kg/day IV, IP, SC	Same
Rompun. See *Xylazine*		
Septra	30 mg (combined)/kg q24h PO or 15 mg/kg q12h	None
Sodium bicarbonate	50 mg/kg q8–12h PO (1 tsp powder equals 2 gm)	Same
Sodium chloride (0.9% soln)	40–50 ml/kg/day IV, IP, SC	Same
Sodium dioctyl sulfosuccinate	100–300 mg q12h PO	100 mg q12–24h PO
Sodium iodide (20% soln)	1 ml/5 kg q8–12h PO, IV	Same
Sodium sulfate (Glauber's salt)	*Purgative*: 10–25 gm PO *Laxative*: ⅕ the purgative dose	*Purgative*: 2–4 gm PO
Spectinomycin	5.5–11 mg/kg q12h IM	None
Stanozolol (Winstrol-V)	½ to 2 tablets q12h PO	½ tablet q12h PO
Streptomycin	20 mg/kg q6h PO; 10 mg/kg q8h IM, SC	Same
Styrid-Caricide	1 ml/10 kg once daily PO for heartworm prevention	None
Sulfonamides:		
Phthalylsulfathiazole	100 mg/kg q12h PO (not absorbed)	Same
Sulfadiazine	220 mg/kg initial dose, then 110 mg/kg q12h	Same
Sulfadimethoxine	25 mg/kg q24h PO, IV, IM	Same
Sulfamethazine, sulfamerazine, sulfadiazine	50 mg/kg q12h PO, IV	Same
Sulfasalazine (Azulfidine)	10–15 mg/kg q6h PO	None
Sulfathalidine	100 mg/kg q12h PO (not absorbed)	Same
Sulfisoxazole, sulfamethizole	50 mg/kg q8h PO	Same
Tannic acid (Tannalbin)	1 tablet/5 kg q12h PO; decrease dose for several days after diarrhea is under control	Same
Tan-Sal (5% tannic acid, 5% salicylic acid, and 70% ethyl alcohol)	Topical, q8h; no more than 2 treatments	Same
Temaril-P	1 capsule PO q24h (up to 5 kg) 2 capsules PO q24h (5–10 kg) 4 capsules PO q24h (10–20 kg) 6 capsules PO q24h (over 20 kg)	Same
Testosterone	2 mg/kg once daily q 2–3 days PO up to 30 mg total; 2 mg/kg (up to 30 mg total) IM (repositol) q 10 days	Same
Tetracycline	20 mg/kg q8h PO; 7 mg/kg q12h IV, IM	Same
Thiabendazole	50 mg/kg once daily PO for 3 days; repeat in 1 month	None
Thiarcetamide (Caparsolate)	2.2 mg/kg IV bid for 2 days	None
Thiamine	10–100 mg/day PO	5–30 mg/day PO
Thiamylal (Surital, Bio-Tal)	17.5 mg/kg IV (4% soln)	Same, but use 2% soln
6-Thioguanine (6-TG)	1 mg/kg/day PO	Same
ThioTEPA	0.5 mg/kg once daily for 10 days IV or intralesionally; 9 mg/M² as single dose or in 2–4 divided doses on successive days IV or intracavitary	Same
Thyroid (desiccated)	10 mg/kg/day PO	Same
L-Thyroxine	20 µg/kg (0.02 mg/kg) OD PO	Same
Toluene (methylbenzene)	200 mg/kg PO	Same
Tresaderm	Topically, q12h; maximum duration of treatment 7 days	Same

DRUG NAME	DOG	CAT
Triamcinolone (Vetalog)	0.25–2 mg once daily PO for 7 days; 0.11–0.22 mg/kg IM, SC	0.25–0.5 mg once daily PO for 7 days; 0.11–0.22 mg/kg IM, SC
Trichlorfon (Neguvon)	3% solution to whole body q3 days	None
Trifluomeprazine (Nortran)	0.55–2.2 mg/kg PO, sid to bid	Same
Triiodothyronine	4 μg/kg q8h (13 mg/kg/day) PO	Same
Trimethobenzamide (Tigan)	For dogs over 15 kg only. 10 mg IM or 100-mg suppository	None
Trimethoprim plus sulfadiazine (Tribrissen)	15 mg (combined)/kg q12h or 30 mg (combined)/kg q24h PO, SC	None
Tripelennamine	1.0 mg/kg q12h PO; 1 ml/20 kg IM	Same
Trisulfapyrimidine	50 mg/kg q12h PO	None
TSH (thyroid-stimulating hormone)	5 units IV (response test); post sample in 4 hours	5 units IM or SC
Tylosin	10 mg/kg q8h PO; 5 mg/kg q12h IV, IM	Same
Vermiplex	*Single-dose Method:* 1 #000 capsule/0.23 kg 1 #00 capsule/0.57 kg 1 #0 capsule/1.14 kg 1 #1 capsule/2.27 kg 1 #2 capsule/4.55 kg 1 #3 capsule/9.1 kg 1 #4 capsule/18.2 kg Can be repeated in 2–4 weeks.	Same
	Divided-dose Method: Divide body weight by 5 and administer appropriate size capsule once daily for 5 days. Can be repeated in 2–4 weeks.	Same
Vinblastine (Velban)	3.0 mg/M² weekly IV or 0.1–0.5 mg/kg weekly	Same
Vincristine (Oncovin)	0.025–0.05 mg/kg q 7–10 days; 0.5 mg/M² IV weekly or biweekly	Same
Viokase	Mix into food 20 minutes prior to feeding; 1–3 tsp/lb of food	Same
Vi-Sorbin	1–3 tsp/day PO	½ tsp/day PO
Vitamin A	400 units/kg/day PO for 10 days	Same
Vitamin B₁₂	100–200 μg/day	50–100 μg/day
Vitamin D	30 units/kg/day PO for 10 days	Same
Vitamin E	500 mg/day PO	100 mg/day PO
Vitamin K₁ (phytonadione)	5–20 mg IV, IM, or SC q12h	1–5 mg IV, IM, or SC q12h
Xylazine (Rompun)	1.1 mg/kg IV; 1.1–2.2 mg/kg IM, SC	Same
Yomesan	157 mg/kg PO. Overnight fast. Repeat in 2–3 weeks.	Same

A CATALOGUE OF CONGENITAL/HEREDITARY DISORDERS OF DOGS (BY BREED)

Breed	Mode*	Disorders
Aberdeen Terrier		Primary uterine inertia
Afghan Hound	R	Cataract (bilateral)
	R	Elbow joint malformation
		Necrotizing myelopathy
Airedale Terrier		Cerebellar hypoplasia
		Trembling of the hind quarters
		Umbilical hernia
Alaskan Malamute	R	Anemia with chondrodysplasia
	R	Dwarfism
	R	Factor VII deficiency
		Hemeralopia
		Renal cortical hypoplasia
American Foxhound		Deafness
		Microphthalmia
Antarctic Husky	D	Entropion
	SLR	Hemophilia A
Australian Shepherd	R	Microphthalmia/multiple colobomas
Basenji	R	Coliform enteritis
		Hemolytic anemia
		Inguinal hernia
	D	Persistent pupillary membrane
		Pyruvate kinase deficiency
		Umbilical hernia
Basset Hound	D	Achondroplasia
	SLR	Anomaly of third cervical vertebra
		Inguinal hernia
	ID	Platelet disorder
		Primary glaucoma
Beagle		Atopic dermatitis
		Bladder cancer
		Bundle branch block
		Cataract (unilateral)
	D	Cataract with microphthalmia
	P	Cleft lip and palate
		Distemper

Breed	Mode*	Disorders
	R, P	Epilepsy
	R	Factor VII deficiency
	SLR	Hemophilia A
		Hypercholesterolemia
		Intervertebral disc disease
		Lymphocytic thyroiditis
	R	Mononephrosis
		Multiple epiphyseal dysplasia
		Necrotizing panotitis
	P	Otocephalic syndrome
	R	Primary glaucoma
	P	Pulmonic stenosis
		Renal hypoplasia
	R	Retinal dysplasia
	R	Short tail
		Thyroiditis
		Unilateral kidney aplasia
Bedlington Terrier	R	Renal cortical hypoplasia
		Retinal dysplasia
Bernese Sennehund	P	Cleft lip and palate
Black and Tan Coonhound	SLR	Hemophilia B
Bloodhound		Distemper
Blue Tick Hound		Globoid cell leukodystrophy
Border Collie		Central progressive retinal atrophy
Border Terrier	R	Aortic and carotid body tumors
		Cataract (bilateral)
		Craniomandibular osteopathy
		Hemivertebra
		Mastocytoma
		Oligodendroglioma
		Patella luxation
		Pituitary tumor
Boxer		Abnormal dentition (extra incisor)
		Aortic and carotid body tumors
		Aortic stenosis
		Atrial septal defects

Breed	Mode*	Disorders
	SLR	Cystinuria
		Dermoid cysts
		Endocardial fibroelastosis
		Fibrosarcoma
		Gingival hyperplasia
		Histiocytoma
		Intervertebral disc disease
		Mastocytoma
		Melanoma
		Oligodendroglioma
		Persistence of right venous valve
		Pulmonic stenosis
	P	Subaortic stenosis
		Superficial corneal ulcer
Brussels Griffon		Short skull
Bull Mastiff		Abnormal dentition (extra incisor)
Bull Terrier	R	Deafness
		Inguinal hernia
		Umbilical hernia
Cairn Terrier		Craniomandibular osteopathy
	SLR	Cystinuria
	R	Globoid cell leukodystrophy
	SLR	Hemophilia A
	SLR	Hemophilia B
		Inguinal hernia
Ceylon		Hairlessness
Chihuahua		Collapsed trachea
		Dislocation of the shoulder
	SLR	Hemophilia A
	R	Hydrocephalus
		Hypoplasia of dens
		Mitral valve defects
		Patella luxation
		Pulmonic stenosis
Cocker Spaniel	P	Behavioral abnormalities
	R	Cataract (bilateral)
		Cataract with microphthalmia
	P	Cleft lip and palate
	R	Cranioschisis
		Distichiasis
	D	Factor X deficiency
		Hip dysplasia

Breed	Mode*	Disorders
English Bulldog		Abnormal dentition (extra incisor)
		Anasarca
		Arteriovenous fistula
	P	Cleft lip and palate
		Hemivertebra
	R	Hydrocephalus
		Hypoplasia of trachea
		Mitral valve defects
		Oligodendroglioma
		Predisposition to dystocia
		Pulmonic stenosis
		Short skull
	R	Short tail
		Spina bifida
English Cocker Spaniel	SLR	Hemophilia A
	R	Juvenile amaurotic idiocy
	R	Neuronal ceroidlipofuscinosis
English Springer Spaniel	D	Cutaneous asthenia
	ID	Factor XI deficiency
	R	Retinal dysplasia
Foxhound		Deafness
		Osteochondrosis of the spine
Fox Terrier	R	Ataxia
		Atopic dermatitis
		Deafness
		Dislocation of the shoulder
		Esophageal achalasia
		Glaucoma
		Goiter
		Lens luxation
		Oligodontia
		Pulmonic stenosis
French Bulldog		Hemivertebra
German Shepherd	P	Atopic dermatitis
		Behavioral abnormalities
	D	Cataract (bilateral)
	P	Cleft lip and palate
	SLR	Cystinuria
		Dermoid cyst
		Ectasia syndrome
		Enostosis
	R, P	Epilepsy
		Esophageal achalasia

Breed	Disorder	Inheritance
	Hydrocephalus	R
	Inguinal hernia	
	Intervertebral disc disease	
	Over- and undershot jaw	
	Patent ductus arteriosus	P
	Primary glaucoma	
	Primary peripheral retinal dystrophy	
	Renal cortical hypoplasia	
	Skin neoplasms	
	Tail abnormalities	R
	Umbilical hernia	
	Ununited anconeal process	P
Collie	Bladder cancer	R
	Collie eye anomaly	R
	Cyclic neutropenia	
	Deafness	
	Epilepsy	R, P
	Hemophilia A	SLR
	Inguinal hernia	
	Iris heterochromia	ID
	Microphthalmia	
	Nasal solar dermatitis	
	Optic nerve hypoplasia	
	Patent ductus arteriosus	P
	Umbilical hernia	
Dachshund	Achondroplasia	D
	Cleft lip and palate	P
	Cystinuria	SLR
	Deafness	
	Diabetes mellitus	
	Ectasia syndrome	
	Intervertebral disc disease	
	Iris heterochromia	ID
	Microphthalmia	
	Osteopetrosis	
	Over- and undershot jaw (Long-Haired Dachshund)	
	Renal hypoplasia	
Dalmatian	Atopic dermatitis	
	Deafness	R
	Excess uric acid excretion	
	Globoid cell leukodystrophy	
Doberman Pinscher	His bundle degeneration	
	Polyostotic fibrous dysplasia	
	Renal cortical hypoplasia	R
	Spondylolisthesis	
	Hemophilia A	SLR
	Hip dysplasia	P
	Pancreatic insufficiency	R
	Persistent right aortic arch	
	Pituitary dwarfism	P
	Renal cortical hypoplasia	
	Subaortic stenosis	P
	Ununited anconeal process	P
	Von Willebrand's disease	D
German Shorthaired Pointer	Amaurotic idiocy	R
	Eversion of nictitating membrane	R
	Fibrosarcoma	
	Lymphedema	D
	Melanoma	
	Subaortic stenosis	
Golden Retriever	Cataract (bilateral)	D
	Cataract with microphthalmia	
Gordon Setter	Generalized progressive retinal atrophy	
Great Dane	Cystinuria	SLR
	Deafness	
	Eversion of nictitating membrane	
	Iris heterochromia	ID
	Mitral valve defects	
	Spondylolisthesis	
	Stockard's paralysis	P
Great Dane × Bloodhound	Paralysis of the hind limbs	
Greyhound	Esophageal achalasia	SLR
	Hemophilia A	
	Predisposition to dystocia	
	Short spine	R
Griffon	Dislocation of the shoulder	
Griffon Bruxellois × Dachshund	Susceptibility to rickets	
Irish Setter	Carpal subluxation	SLR
	Generalized myopathy	
	Generalized progressive retinal atrophy	R
	Hemophilia A	SLR
	Persistent right aortic arch	R
	Quadriplegia with amblyopia	
Irish Terrier	Cystinuria	SLR

Breed	Mode*	Disorders
St. Bernard		Aphakia with multiple colobomas
		Dermoid cysts of cornea
		Eversion of nictitating membrane
	SLR	Hemophilia A
	SLR	Hemophilia B
	P	Stockard's paralysis
St. Bernard × Great Dane		Paralysis of the hind limbs
Samoyed		Atrial septal defects
		Diabetes mellitus
	SLR	Hemophilia A
		Pulmonic stenosis
Scottish Terrier		Bladder cancer
		Atopic dermatitis
		Achondroplasia
		Craniomandibular osteopathy
	SLR	Cystinuria
		Deafness
		Melanoma
		Primary uterine inertia
	R	Scottie cramp
	D	Von Willebrand's disease
Sealyham Terrier		Atopic dermatitis
		Lens luxation
	R	Retinal dysplasia
Shetland Sheepdog		Bladder cancer
	R	Collie eye anomoly
	SLR	Hemophilia A
	ID	Hip dysplasia
		Iris heterochromia
		Nasal solar dermatitis
	P	Patent ductus arteriosus
Shiba Ina	R	Short spine
Shih Tzu	P	Cleft lip and palate
		Renal cortical hypoplasia
Siberian Husky	ID	Iris heterochromia
Silver Grey Collie	ID	Cyclic neutropenia
		Iris heterochromia
Skye Terrier	R	Hypoplasia of the larynx

Breed	Mode*	Disorders
Jack Russell Terrier		Ataxia
		Lens luxation
Keeshond	P	Conus septal defects
	R, P	Epilepsy
		Mitral valve defects
	P	Tetralogy of Fallot
Kerry Blue		Hair follicle tumor
	P	Ununited anconeal process
King Charles Spaniel		Diabetes mellitus
Labrador Retriever	ID	Carpal subluxation
		Cataract (bilateral)
		Craniomandibular osteopathy
	SLR	Cystinuria
	SLR	Hemophilia A
	R	Retinal dysplasia
Labrador × American Foxhound	D	Diaphragmatic hernia
Labrador × Poodle	D	Lymphedema
Lhaso Apso		Inguinal hernia
		Renal cortical hypoplasia
Mexican, Turkish, and Chinese Breeds	D	Hairlessness
Miniature Pinscher	D	Dislocation of the shoulder
Miniature Poodle	R	Achondroplasia
		Cerebrospinal demyelination
	SLR	Cystinuria
		Dislocation of the shoulder
		Ectasia syndrome
		Ectodermal defect
	R	Generalized progressive retinal atrophy
		Globoid cell leukodystrophy
		Hypoplasia of dens
		Partial alopecia
		Patella luxation
	P	Patent ductus arteriosus
Miniature Schnauzer	R	Cataract (bilateral)
	R	Pulmonic stenosis
	D	Von Willebrand's disease

Breed	Inheritance	Disorder
Mongrel	SLR	Black hair follicular dysplasia
		Cystinuria
		Multiple cartilaginous exostoses
Newfoundland		Eversion of nictitating membrane
	P	Subaortic stenosis
Norwegian Dunkerhound		Deafness
		Microphthalmia
Norwegian Elkhound	R	Generalized progressive retinal atrophy
		Keratoacanthoma
		Renal cortical hypoplasia
Old English Sheepdog	R	Cataract, bilateral
Otterhound	ID	Platelet disorder
Pekingese		Distichiasis
		Hypoplasia of dens
		Inguinal hernia
		Intervertebral disc disease
		Short skull
		Trichiasis
		Umbilical hernia
Pointer	R	Bithoracic ectomelia
	R	Cataract (bilateral)
	R	Neuromuscular atrophy
		Neurotropic osteopathy
		Umbilical hernia
Pomeranian		Dislocation of the shoulder
		Hypoplasia of dens
	P	Patella luxation
		Tracheal collapse
Poodle (see also Miniature, Standard, and Toy Poodle)		Atopic dermatitis
	P	Behavioral abnormality
	SLR	Cystinuria
		Distichiasis
	R	Epilepsy
	P	Patent ductus arteriosus
Pug		Male pseudohermaphroditism
		Trichiasis
Rhodesian Ridgeback		Dermoid sinus
Rottweiler		Diabetes mellitus
Springer Spaniel	D	Ehlers-Danlos syndrome
	ID	Factor XI deficiency
	R	Retinal dysplasia
Staffordshire Bull Terrier	R	Cataract (bilateral)
	P	Cleft lip and palate
Standard Poodle	R	Cataract (bilateral)
Swedish Lapland	R	Neuronal abiotrophy
Swiss Dogs		Generalized progressive retinal atrophy
Swiss Sheepdog	P	Clefts of lip and palate
Tervueren Shepherd	R	Epilepsy
Toy Poodle		Ectasia syndrome
		Fibrosis of the plantaris muscle
	R	Generalized progressive retinal atrophy
		Patella luxation
	P	Patent ductus arteriosus
		Tracheal collapse
Vizsla	SLR	Hemophilia A
Weimaraner		Eversion of nictitating membrane
	R	Fibrosarcoma
	SLR	Hemophilia A
		Melanoma
		Spinal dysraphism
		Umbilical hernia
Welsh Corgi	SLR	Cystinuria
		Generalized progressive retinal atrophy
		Predisposition to dystocia
West Highland White Terrier		Atopic dermatitis
		Craniomandibular osteopathy
	R	Globoid cell leukodystrophy
		Inguinal hernia
Whippet		Partial alopecia
Yorkshire Terrier		Hypoplasia of dens
		Patella luxation
	R	Retinal dysplasia

Breed	Mode*	Disorders
All Breeds	D	Blood group incompatability
Brachycephalic breeds		Pituitary cysts
		Stenotic nares and elongated soft palate
Giant Breeds		Elbow dysplasia
		Hip dysplasia
		Osteogenic sarcoma
Many Breeds	P	Behavioral abnormalities
	SLR	Cryptorchidism
	D	Demodectic mange
		Dewclaws
		Ectropion
		Elbow dysplasia (especially large and giant breeds)
		Entropion
		Esophageal dilation
		Hip dysplasia (especially large and giant breeds)

Breed	Mode*	Disorders
Many Miniature Breeds		Collapsed trachea
		Glycogen storage disease
		Legg-Calve-Perthes syndrome
		Patellar luxation
		Predisposition to dystocia
		Tracheal collapse
Miscellaneous		White breed deafness

Modified from Patterson, D. F.: A catalogue of genetic disorders of the dog. *In* Kirk, R. W. (ed.): Current Veterinary Therapy VII. Philadelphia, W. B. Saunders Co., 1980.

*Mode of inheritance: R = recessive; D = dominant; ID = incomplete dominance; SLR = sex-linked recessive; and P = polygenic.

COMPENDIUM OF FELINE VACCINES, 1983*

Vaccine	Manufacturer	Type		Vaccine Components					Remarks
		MLV	Inact.	FPV	FVR	FCV	FP$_n$	Rabies	
Annumune	Fort Dodge		x					x	
Biorab-1	Burns-Biotec		x					x	
Biorab-3	Burns-Biotec		x					x	
Cytorab	Wellcome		x					x	
Dura-Rab 1	Wildlife		x					x	
Eclipse I	Fromm	x		x					
Eclipse I-KP	Fromm		x	x					
Eclipse III	Fromm	x		x	x	x			
Eclipse III-KP	Fromm	x	x	x(i)	x	x			
Eclipse III-KP-R	Fromm	x	x	x(i)	x	x		x(i)	
Eclipse IV	Fromm	x		x	x	x	x		
Eclipse IV-KP	Fromm	x	x	x(i)	x	x	x		
Eclipse IV-KP-R	Fromm	x	x	x(i)	x	x	x	x(i)	
Endurall-K	Norden		x					x	
Endurall-R	Norden	x						x	
Fel-o-Vax PCT	Fort Dodge		x	x	x	x			
Feline Panleukopenia	CEVA		x	x					
Felipan	Wellcome		x	x					
Felocell	Norden	x		x					
Felocell CVR	Norden	x		x	x	x			
Felocine	Norden		x	x					
Felomune CVR	Norden	x			x	x			IN
FVR-C-P	Pitman-Moore	x	x	x(i)	x	x			
FVR-C-P (MLV)	Pitman-Moore	x		x	x	x			
Leukogen-L	Bio-Ceutic	x		x					
Pan-Rab	Douglas		x	x				x	
Panacine	Beecham	x		x					
Panacine RC	Beecham	x		x	x	x			
Panagen	Pitman-Moore		x	x					
Panagen LL	Pitman-Moore	x		x					
Panavac	Beecham		x	x					
Panavac RC	Beecham	x	x	x(i)	x	x			
Panavac RCP	Beecham	x	x	x(i)	x	x	x		
Premune RC/KP	Wellcome	x	x	x(i)	x	x			
Premune RCN/KP	Wellcome	x	x	x(i)	x	x	x		
Premune RCPN	Wellcome	x		x	x	x	x		
Psittacoid	Fromm	x					x		
Rabcine	Beecham		x					x	
Rabguard-TC	Norden		x					x	Trien.
Rabmune	Schering		x					x	
Rabvac	Fromm		x					x	
Rhinoid-C	Fromm	x			x	x			
Rhinoid-C-Psittacoid	Fromm	x			x	x	x		
Rhinolin-CP	Bio-Ceutic	x		x	x	x			IN
Trimune	Fort Dodge		x					x	
Trirab	Wellcome		x					x	

*Modified from *Veterinary Pharmaceuticals and Biologicals 1982–1983*. Santa Barbara, CA: Veterinary Medicine Publishing Co., 1983; Compendium of Animal Rabies Vaccines, 1983 *In* Kirk, *Current Veterinary Therapy VIII*. Philadelphia: W. B. Saunders, 1983, p. 1137. Compiled by F. W. Scott, Cornell Feline Health Center, Ithaca, N.Y.

Notes: (i) = Inactivated component of mixed MLV/inactivated vaccine.
FCV = Feline calicivirus.
FP$_n$ = Feline pneumonitis (chlamydia).
FPV = Feline parvovirus (panleukopenia).
FVR = Feline viral rhinotracheitis.
IN = Intranasal administration.
Inact. = Inactivated (killed).
MLV = Modified live virus (attenuated).
Trien. = Triennial.

COMPENDIUM OF CANINE VACCINES, 1983*

Vaccine	Manufacturer	Type		Vaccine Components										Remarks
		MLV	Inact.	CDV	CAI	CA2	CPI	Lep.	Bor.	Rab.	MV	CPV	FPV	
Adenomune-5	Dellen	x		x	x	x(i)	x						x(i)	
Adenomune-7	Dellen	x		x	x	x(i)	x	x(i)					x(i)	
Annumune	Fort Dodge		x							x				
Biorab-1	Burns-Biotec		x							x				
Biorab-3	Burns-Biotec		x							x				
Bordegen C	Pitman-Moore		x						x					
Bronchicine	Dellen		x						x					
Canine Distemper-Hepatitis	Colorado Serum	x		x	x									
Canine Distemper-Hepatitis	CEVA	x		x	x									
Canine Distemper-Hepatitis-Leptospira	CEVA	x	x	x	x			x(i)						
Canine Distemper-Hepatitis-Leptospira	Colorado Serum	x		x	x			x(i)						
Cytogen d-h	Wellcome	x		x	x									
Cytogen d-h-1	Wellcome	x	x	x	x			x(i)						
Cytogen d-h-p	Wellcome	x	x	x	x		x	x(i)						
Cytogen d-h-p-1	Wellcome	x	x	x	x		x	x(i)						
Cytorab	Wellcome	x	x							x				
D-Vac-5	Bio-Ceutic	x	x	x	x		x	x(i)						
D-Vac-HL (L)	Bio-Ceutic	x	x	x	x			x(i)						
D-Vac-M	Bio-Ceutic	x		x							x			
DHP	CEVA	x		x	x		x							
DHPL	CEVA	x	x	x	x		x	x(i)						
Distemperoid	Fromm	x		x										
Dura-Rab 1	Wildlife		x							x				
Duramune DHLP + PV	Fort Dodge	x	x	x	x		x	x(i)				x		
Duramune-PV	Fort Dodge	x										x		
Endurall-K	Norden		x							x				
Endurall-R	Norden	x								x				
ERA Strain Rabies	Wellcome	x								x				
Fromm CP	Fromm	x					x						x(i)	
Fromm CP-DH	Fromm	x		x	x		x							
Fromm CP-DHL	Fromm	x	x	x	x		x	x(i)						
Fromm DH	Fromm	x		x	x									
Fromm DHL	Fromm	x	x	x	x			x(i)						
Galaxy IV	Fromm	x		x		x	x						x(i)	
Galaxy V	Fromm	x	x	x		x	x	x(i)				x		
Galaxy VI	Fromm	x	x	x		x	x	x(i)				x		
Galaxy VI MP	Fromm	x		x		x	x					x		
Galaxy VI MP-L	Fromm	x	x	x		x	x	x(i)				x		
Galaxy VI MHP	Fromm	x		x		x	x	x(i)				x		
Galaxy VI MHP-L	Fromm	x		x		x	x	x				x		
Intra-Trac-I	Burns-Biotec	x					x		x					IN
Intra-Trac-II	Burns-Biotec	x							x					IN

Product	Manufacturer	CDV	CA1	CA2	CPI	Lep	CPV	Rab	Bor	MV	FPV
Leptoferm C-I/Bordetella	Norden					x			x		
Leptoferm C-I	Norden					x					
Leukogen-L	Bio-Ceutic					x					
Naramune 2	Bio-Ceutic				x				x		
Neurogen-TC	Bio-Ceutic							x			
Parvac	Fromm						x				
Parvocine-MLV	Dellen						x				
Parvoid	Fromm						x				
Parvoid II	Fromm						x				
PV-Vax	Pitman-Moore						x				
Rabcine	Beecham							x			
Rabguard-TC	Norden							x			
Rabies Vacc	Guardian							x			
Rabmune	Schering							x			
Rabvac	Fromm							x			
Sentrypar	Beecham						x				
Sentryvac-DH	Beecham	x	x	x							
Sentryvac-DH/L	Beecham	x	x	x		x(i)					
Sentryvac-DHP	Beecham	x	x	x	x						
Sentryvac-DHP/L	Beecham	x	x	x	x	x(i)					
Tissuvax 5	Pitman-Moore	x	x	x	x	x(i)					
Tissuvax 6	Pitman-Moore	x	x	x	x	x(i)					
Tissuvax D-H-P	Pitman-Moore	x	x	x	x						
Tissuvax D-H-P/PV	Pitman-Moore	x	x	x	x		x				
Trimune	Fort Dodge							x			
Trirab	Wellcome							x			
Unirab	Bio-Ceutic							x			
Vanguard CPV (ML)	Norden						x				
Vanguard CPV (killed)	Norden						x(i)				
Vanguard D-M	Norden	x								x	
Vanguard DA₂	Norden	x		x							
Vanguard DA₂L	Norden	x		x		x(i)					
Vanguard DA₂P	Norden	x		x	x						
Vanguard DA₂P+CPV	Norden	x		x	x		x				
Vanguard DA₂PL	Norden	x		x	x	x(i)					
Vanguard DA₂PL + Bordetella	Norden	x		x	x	x(i)			x		
Vanguard DA₂PL + CPV	Norden	x		x	x	x(i)	x				
Vanguard DMP	Norden	x			x					x	

*Modified from *Veterinary Pharmaceuticals and Biologicals 1982–1983.* Santa Barbara, CA: Veterinary Medicine Publishing Co., 1983; Compendium of Animal Rabies Vaccines, 1983 *In* Kirk: *Current Veterinary Therapy VIII.* Philadelphia: W. B. Saunders, 1983, p. 1137. Compiled by F. W. Scott, Cornell Feline Health Center, Ithaca, N.Y.

Notes: (i) = Inactivated component of mixed MLV/inactivated vaccine.
  Bor. = *Bordetella bronchiseptica.*
  CA1 = Canine adenovirus-1 (infectious canine hepatitis).
  CA2 = Canine adenovirus-2.
  CDV = Canine distemper virus.
  CPI = Canine parainfluenza.
  CPV = Canine parvovirus.
  FPV = Feline parvovirus (feline panleukopenia).
  IN = Intranasal administration.
  Inact. = Inactivated (killed).
  Lep. = Leptospirosis (usually *L. canicola* plus *L. icterohaemorrhagiae*).
  MLV = Modified live virus (attenuated).
  MV = Measles virus.
  Rab. = Rabies virus.

INDEX

Note: Page numbers in *italics* refer to illustrations; page numbers followed by (t) refer to tables.
Additional pertinent information, still current, found in *Current Veterinary Therapy VII*, is designated within brackets by the edition and page number.

Luteinizing hormone(s) (*Continued*)
 feline pregnancy maintenance and, 935
 feline reproduction and, 933, *934*
 immunization against, as
  contraception, 905–906
Luteinization, preovulatory, 886
Lyell's disease, 473–474
Lymphadenopathy, 435–438
 hilar, and fungal pneumonia, 249
Lymphatics, peripheral, diseases of,
  [VII:337]
Lymphedema, [VII:337]
Lymphocyte(s), in pleural fluid, 268t,
  269
 pulmonary defense and, 196
Lymphokine(s), in immunotherapy, 451
Lymphoma, 435–438
Lymphopenia, in heartworm disease, 353
Lymphosarcoma(s), 593, 593t
 and primary hyperparathyroidism,
  880–881, 881t
 clinical staging of, 435, 436t
 immunotherapy for, 452
 transmissible, 413–415
 treatment of, 435–438
Lysis, vertebral, with diskospondylitis,
  719, *719*
Lysosomal storage disease(s), 744–746

MacConkey (MAC) agar, appearance of
  bacterial colonies on, 1155
Macdonaldius oschei, infection by, in
  reptiles, 605
Macropalpebral fissure(s), 537
Macrophage(s), alveolar, pulmonary
  defense and, 196, 216
 in pleural fluid, 268t, 269
Macula, 558
Magnesium, in total parenteral nutrition,
  659
Magnesium ammonium phosphate (MAP)
  calculus(i). See *Struvite urolith(s)*.
Malabsorption, osmotic diarrhea and,
  776, 776t, 777t
Malabsorptive diarrhea, 774–776, 775t
Malaria, avian, 645–646
Malassezia pachydermatitis, appearance
  of, on Levine EMB agar, 1155
Malassimilation syndrome, osmotic
  diarrhea and, 776, 776t, 777t, 779t
Maldevelopment, congenital, causes of,
  131–138. See also *Developmental
  toxicology, Genetic toxicology,
  Teratogenesis*, and *Mutagenesis*.
Maldigestion, osmotic diarrhea and, 776,
  776t, 777t
Malocclusion, in rabbits, 654
Mammal(s), gestation in, 130, 130t
 viral teratology of, 133–134, 134t
Mammary adenocarcinoma(s), feline,
  immunotherapy for, 452
Mammary gland(s), lactating, post-
  partum infection of, 960–961
 non-neoplastic disorders of, [VII:1224]
Mange, auricular, 672–674
 demodectic, canine, 484–487
  feline, 487–488
  in nondomestic carnivores, 662
 ear, 672–674
 head, 493–494

Mange (*Continued*)
 notoedric, 493–494
  in nondomestic carnivores, 662
 otodectic, 662, 672–674
  in nondomestic carnivores, 662
 psoroptic, in nondomestic carnivores,
  662
 sarcoptic, in nondomestic carnivores,
  661–662
Mannitol, in glaucoma, 570, 570t
Manx cat(s), corneal dystrophy in, 563
Mast cell neoplasia, and ulcerogenesis,
  768
Mastication, muscles of, inflammation of,
  in canine polymyositis, 681–682, 682t,
  683
Mastitis, in rabbits, 670
 post-partum, 960–961
Mastocytoma(s), canine, 415–418
Mastocytosis, systemic, and ulcerogenesis, 768
Masturbation, as indication for
  progestin therapy, 65
Maternal antibody(ies), definition of,
  1134
Maternal disease(s), puerperal,
  959–961
Maturation, social, of puppy, 57
Medroxyprogesterone acetate, as
  contraceptive, 905
 progestin therapy and, 69–70
Megaloblastic anemia, and folate
  deficiency, 753
Megalocornea, 558
Megaureter, in ureteral ectopia, 1045
Megestrol acetate, as oral contraceptive,
  903–904, 904t
 in estrus control in queens, 937
 in skin disorders, 459
 progestin therapy and, 69
Melanoma(s), epibulbar, 590
 uveal, 592, 593, 593t
Membrane(s), increased permeability of,
  pulmonary edema and, 254–255
 nictitating, diseases of, 548–549 See
  also *Nictitating membrane(s)*.
 pupillary, persistent, 558
 tympanic, diseases of, 51
  in otitis media–interna, 729–731
Membranous labyrinth, anatomy of,
  726–727, *726*
Meningioma(s), 731
Meningitis, 735–738
Meningoencephalitis, granulomatous,
  732–735
Mephentermine, in shock, 17, 20–21t,
  22
Mesothelial cell(s), in pleural fluid, 268t,
  269
Metabolic acidemia, and anuric uremia,
  991
Metabolic acidosis, 208–209, 209t
 alkalinizing agents in, 209, 210t
 and anion gap, 208, 209t
 and canine chronic polyuric renal
  failure, 1005
 and feline chronic polyuric renal
  failure, 1014–1015
 shock and, 8t
Metabolic alkalosis, 208–209, 211t
Metabolic disease(s), and episodic
  weakness, 698t, 700–701

Metabolic disease(s) (*Continued*)
 and ulcerogenesis, 767
Metabolic myocardial disease(s), 328
Metabolism, abdominal surgery and, 39,
  39
 and acid-base balance, 207–208, *207,
  208*, 212t
 and cataracts, 574
 burns and, 39, *39*
 effect of glucocorticoids on, 855–856
 effect of injury on, 6–7
 inborn errors of, 744–746
 infection and, 39, *39*
 in vitro, correction values for, 214t
 ovariohysterectomy and, 39, *39*
 skeletal trauma and, 39, *39*
 starvation and, 39, *39*
Metaldehyde poisoning(s), 106–107
Metal poisoning(s), incidence of, 78t, 79,
  80t
Metaphyseal sclerosis, in lead poisoning,
  109
Metestrus, 892–893
 cytology during, 937
 endoscopy during 919, *919, 920*
 vaginal smear during, 910
Methenamine, in urinary tract infections,
  1096
Methylphenidate, in narcolepsy, 758
Metoclopramide, in gastric stasis, 764
Metritis, 943
 acute, [VII:1214]
 post-partum, 960
Metronidazole, in diarrhea, 788
 in meningitis, 738
Mibolerone, as oral contraceptive,
  904–905, 905t
Microbiologic specimen(s), collection and
  handling of, 41–42
Microbiology, urinary, 1052–1053
Microcirculation, effect of shock on, 4–5.
  See also individual system (e.g.,
  Respiratory system).
Microcornea, 558
Microcytosis, in hepatic encephalopathy,
  832
Microfilaria(e), detection of, in heart-
  worm disease, 352–353, 353t
 infection by, in caged birds, 644, *644*
Microfilaricide therapy, for heartworm
  disease, 355t, 356–357
Microorganism(s), in garbage, 163–164
Micropalpebral fissure(s), 537
Microscopy, electron, as viral diagnostic
  technique, 1143–1144, 1144t
 collection of specimens for, 1145
Microsporum, infection by, in nondomestic carnivores, 663
Microwave(s), as cancer therapy, 425
Micturition, disorders of, 722–726
 nerve function in, 722–723
Midbrain, effect of progestin therapy on,
  69–70
Middle ear, diseases of, 51–52
Miliary dermatitis, progestin therapy
  and, 67
Mineral(s), and skin disorders, 461
 diets low in, in feline urologic syndrome, 1113
 imbalances of, in renal failure,
  1019–1021
 in feline uroliths, 1077, 1077t